# Pathophysiology

## Adaptations and Alterations in Function

### 3RD EDITION

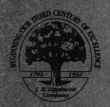

J. B. LIPPINCOTT COMPANY
Philadelphia

*Sponsoring Editor:* David P. Carroll
*Editorial Assistants:* Amy Stonehouse and Patty L. Shear
*Project Editor:* Dina Kamilatos
*Indexer:* Kathryn Pitcoff
*Designer:* Doug Smock
*Cover Designer:* Tom Jackson
*Production Manager:* Caren Erlichman
*Production Coordinator:* Nannette L. Winski
*Compositor:* G&S Typesetters, Inc.
*Printer/Binder:* Courier Book Company/Westford

3rd Edition

6  5  4  3

Library of Congress Cataloging-in-Publication Data

Bullock, Barbara L.
     Pathophysiology : adaptations and alterations in function /
Barbara L. Bullock, Pearl Philbrook Rosendahl ; with 18
contributors. — 3rd ed.
        p.      cm.
     Includes bibliographical references and index.
     ISBN 0-397-54861-3
     1. Physiology, Pathological.    I. Rosendahl, Pearl Philbrook.
II. Title.
     [DNLM:   1. Pathology.   2. Physiology.   QZ 4 B938p]
RB113.B85   1992
616.07—dc20
DNLM/DLC
for Library of Congress                                          91-46651
                                                                      CIP

Any procedure or practice described in this book should be applied by the health-care practitioner under appropriate supervision in accordance with professional standards of care used with regard to the unique circumstances that apply in each practice situation. Care has been taken to confirm the accuracy of information presented and to describe generally accepted practices. However, the authors, editors, and publisher cannot accept any responsibility for errors or omissions or for any consequences from application of the information in this book and make no warranty express or implied, with respect to the contents of the book.

Every effort has been made to ensure drug selections and dosages are in accordance with current recommendations and practice. Because of ongoing research, changes in government regulations and the constant flow of information on drug therapy, reactions and interactions, the reader is cautioned to check the package insert for each drug for indications, dosages, warnings and precautions, particularly if the drug is new or infrequently used.

# Contributing Authors to the Third Edition

**Roberta H. Anding,** M.S., R.D./L.D., C.D.E.
*Assistant Professor, University of Texas Health Sciences Center at Houston, School of Nursing, Houston, Texas*

**Carol Tull Bowdoin,** M.S.N., R.N., C.C.R.N.
*Critical Care Educator, Manatee Memorial Hospital, Bradenton, Florida*

**Barbara L. Bullock,** R.N., M.S.N.
*Education Instructor, Critical Care Division, Memorial Southwest Hospital, Houston, Texas*

**Martha Butterfield,** M.S.N., R.N.
*Associate Professor, Coordinator, Undergraduate Program, University of Tennessee at Chattanooga, School of Nursing, Chattanooga, Tennessee*

**Angela Smith Collins,** R.N., M.S.N., C.C.R.N.
*Critical Care Educator and Consultant in Nursing, Doctoral Candidate in Adult Health, University of Alabama at Birmingham, Birmingham, Alabama*

**Miguel F. da Cunha,** Ph.D.
*Professor, School of Nursing, University of Texas Health Sciences Center, Houston, Texas*

**Cherry Anderson Guinn,** Ed.D., R.N.
*Assistant Professor, School of Nursing, University of Tennessee at Chattanooga, Chattanooga, Tennessee*

**Doris J. Heaman,** D.S.N., R.N.
*Assistant Professor, School of Nursing, The University of Alabama in Huntsville, Huntsville, Alabama*

**Reet Henze,** B.S.N., M.S.N.
*Associate Professor, School of Nursing, The University of Alabama in Huntsville, Huntsville, Alabama*

**Pamela Holder,** D.S.N., R.N., O.C.N.
*Associate Professor of Nursing, Coordinator, Graduate Program, University of Tennessee at Chattanooga, Chattanooga, Tennessee*

**Bonnie M. Juneau,** Ph.D., R.N.
*Assistant Professor, Department of Acute and Continuing Care, University of Texas Health Sciences Center at Houston, School of Nursing, Houston, Texas*

**Gretchen Schaefer McDaniel,** R.N., D.S.N.
*Health Care Education and Research, Hoover, Alabama*

**Barbara R. Norwood,** M.S.N., R.N.
*Assistant Professor, School of Nursing, University of Tennessee, Chattanooga, Tennessee*

**Darlene H. Renfroe,** R.N., D.S.N.
*Clinical Researcher, Office of Clinical Practice Evaluation, University of Alabama Hospital, Birmingham, Alabama*

**Sharron Patton Schlosser,** D.S.N., R.N.
*Professor of Nursing, Ida V. Moffett School of Nursing, Samford University, Birmingham, Alabama*

**Camille P. Stern,** Ph.D., R.N.
*Associate Professor, Armstrong State College, Department of Nursing, Savannah, Georgia*

**Margaret L. Trimpey,** R.N.C., M.S.N.
*Associate Professor, School of Nursing, University of Tennessee at Chattanooga, Chattanooga, Tennessee*

**Joy H. Whatley,** R.N., D.S.N.
*Associate Professor, Ida V. Moffett School of Nursing, Samford University, Birmingham, Alabama*

To my husband, Pete, children, Sheila, Brian, and Doug,
and parents, Lois and Harry Radford,
with my love and appreciation.

# Contributing Authors to the Second Edition

**Gloria Anderson,** R.N., M.S.N.
*Associate Professor, University of Alabama School of Nursing in Huntsville, Huntsville, Alabama*

**Cheryl Bean,** R.N., D.S.N., C.S.
*Assistant Professor, University of Alabama School of Nursing at Birmingham, Birmingham, Alabama*

**Carol Bowdoin,** R.N., M.S.N.
*Formerly, Instructor, University of Alabama School of Nursing in Huntsville, Huntsville, Alabama*

**Barbara L. Bullock,** R.N., M.S.N.
*Cardiac Rehabilitation Program, St. Vincent's Hospital, Birmingham, Alabama*

**Ann Estes Edgil,** R.N., D.S.N.
*Associate Professor, University of Alabama School of Nursing at Birmingham, Birmingham, Alabama*

**Thomas Mark Fender,** R.N., M.S.N.
*Special Units Coordinator, Crestwood Hospital, Huntsville, Alabama*

**Dorothy Gauthier,** R.N., Ph.D.
*Associate Professor, University of Alabama School of Nursing; Birmingham, Birmingham, Alabama*

**Doris J. Heaman,** M.S.N.
*Assistant Professor, University of Alabama School of Nursing in Huntsville, Huntsville, Alabama*

**Reet Henze,** R.N., M.S.N.
*Associate Professor, University of Alabama School of Nursing in Huntsville, Huntsville, Alabama*

**Marcia Hill,** R.N., M.S.N.
*Manager, Dermatologic Therapeutics, The Methodist Hospital, Houston, Texas*

**Bonnie Juneau,** R.N., M.S.
*Assistant Professor, University of Texas Health Sciences Center, School of Nursing, Houston, Texas*

**Marianne T. Marcus,** R.N., M.Ed.
*Assistant Professor, University of Texas Health Sciences Center, School of Nursing, Houston, Texas*

**Gretchen McDaniel,** R.N., M.S.N.
*Formerly, Assistant Professor, Samford University School of Nursing, Birmingham, Alabama*

**Richard Pflanzer,** Ph.D.
*Associate Professor, Indiana University/Purdue University, Indianapolis, Indiana*

**Sharron P. Schlosser,** B.S.N., D.S.N.
*Associate Professor, Samford University School of Nursing, Birmingham, Alabama*

**Camille Stern,** Ph.D., R.N.
*Assistant Professor, Samford University School of Nursing, Birmingham, Alabama*

**Gloria Grissett Stuart,** R.N., M.S.N.
*Assistant Professor, University of Alabama School of Nursing in Huntsville, Huntsville, Alabama*

**Joan W. Williamson,** R.N., M.S.N.
*Associate Professor, University of Alabama School of Nursing in Huntsville, Huntsville, Alabama*

# Contributing Authors to the First Edition

**Gaylene Altman, R.N., M.S.**
*Assistant Professor, University of Washington School of Nursing, Seattle, Washington*

**Gloria Anderson, R.N., M.S.N.**
*Associate Professor of Nursing, University of Alabama School of Nursing in Huntsville, Huntsville, Alabama*

**Joseph L. Andrews, Jr., M.D.**
*Clinical Assistant Professor, Harvard Medical School, Boston, Massachusetts; Senior Staff, Respiratory Section, Lahey Clinic Medical Center, Burlington, Massachusetts*

**Pamela Appleton, R.N, M.N.**
*Assistant Professor of Nursing, University of Alabama School of Nursing in Huntsville, Huntsville, Alabama*

**Sue H. Baldwin, Ed.D.**
*Associate Professor of Nursing, University of North Alabama School of Nursing, Florence, Alabama*

**Anne Roome Bavier, M.N.**
*Associate Professor, Medical-Surgical Nursing Program, Yale University School of Nursing, New Haven, Connecticut*

**Joan P. Bufalino, R.N., M.S.N.**
*Clinical Nurse Specialist, Department of Surgery, Loyola University Medical Center, Maywood, Illinois*

**Barbara L. Bullock, R.N., M.S.N.**
*Assistant Professor, Ida V. Moffett School of Nursing, Samford University, Birmingham, Alabama*

**Concepcion Y. Castro, R.N., M.S.**
*Associate Professor, College of Nursing, University of Rhode Island; Project Director, Primary Health Care—Family Nurse Practitioner Program, College of Nursing, University of Rhode Island, Kingston, Rhode Island*

**Jules Constant, M.D.**
*Clinical Associate Professor of Medicine, Department of Medicine, State University of New York at Buffalo School of Medicine; Attending Physician, Buffalo General Hospital, Buffalo, New York*

**Virginia Earles, D.S.N.**
*Professor of Nursing, Russell Sage College, Troy, New York*

**Ann Estes Edgil, R.N., D.S.N.**
*Associate Professor, University of Alabama School of Nursing, Birmingham, Alabama*

**Thomas Mark Fender, B.S.N.**
*Orthopedic Specialist, Orthopedic Associates, Hunstville, Alabama*

**Shirley Freeburn, R.N., G.N.P., M.S.**
*Assistant Professor, School of Nursing, The University of Colorado Health Sciences Center, Denver, Colorado*

**Janet L. Gelein, R.N., M.S.N., G.N.P.**
*Doctoral Candidate, University of Rochester School of Nursing, Rochester, New York*

**Doris J. Heaman, M.S.N.**
*Assistant Professor, University of Alabama School of Nursing in Huntsville, Huntsville, Alabama*

**Reet Henze, R.N., M.S.N.**
*Associate Professor, University of Alabama School of Nursing in Huntsville, Huntsville, Alabama*

**Joan T. Hurlock, R.N.C., F.N.P., Ed.D.**
*Associate Professor of Nursing, University of Northern Colorado, Greeley, Colorado*

**Karen E. Jones, R.N., M.N.**
*Adjunct Assistant Professor, University of Alabama School of Nursing in Huntsville; Director of Nursing, Ambulatory Care Center of the School of Primary Medical Care, University of Alabama School of Nursing in Huntsville, Huntsville, Alabama*

**June H. Larrabee, R.N., M.S.**
*Assistant Professor of Nursing, University of Central Florida, Orlando, Florida*

**Carla A. Bouska Lee, R.N., Ed.S., F.A.A.N.**
*Assistant Professor and Chairperson, Nurse Clinician Department, College of Health Related Professions, Wichita State University, Wichita, Kansas*

**John A. R. Marino, M.D.**
*Chief, Division of Diabetes, Niagara Falls Memorial Medical Center, Niagara Falls, New York*

**Gretchen S. McDaniel, R.N., M.S.N.**
*Assistant Professor, Ida V. Moffett School of Nursing, Samford University, Birmingham, Alabama*

**M. S. Megahed, M.D., F.R.C.P.**
*Associate Clinical Professor, School of Nursing, State University of New York, Buffalo, New York*

**Frances Donovan Monahan, R.N., Ph.D.**
*Chair, Department of Nursing, Rockland Community College, Suffern, New York*

**Jennie L. Moore, R.N., M.P.H.**
*Formerly, Instructor in Nursing, University of Alabama School of Nursing in Huntsville, Huntsville, Alabama*

**Emilie Musci, R.N., M.S.N.**
*Assistant Professor, Department of Nursing, San Jose State University, San Jose, California*

**Betty Norris, R.N., M.S.N.**
*Cardiovascular Nurse Specialist, Baptist Medical Center, Birmingham, Alabama*

**Leah F. Oakley, R.N., M.S.N.**
*Clinical Nurse Specialist in Adult Health, Internal Medicine, Decatur, Alabama*

**Donna Rogers Packa, R.N., M.S.N.**
*Assistant Professor, School of Nursing, University of Alabama, Birmingham, Alabama*

**Marilyn Nelsen Pase, R.N., M.S.N.**
*Assistant Professor, University of Alabama School of Nursing in Huntsville, Huntsville, Alabama*

**Helen F. Ptak, R.N., Ph.D.**
*Associate Dean and Professor, School of Nursing, University of Texas Medical Branch; Director, Nursing Research and Evaluation, University of Texas Medical Branch Hospitals, Galveston, Texas*

**Cammie M. Quinn, R.N., M.S.N.**
*Department of Neurosurgery, University of Alabama Hospitals, Birmingham, Alabama*

**Pearl Philbrook Rosendahl, R.N., Ed.D.**
*Associate Professor, Boston University School of Nursing; University Hospital, Boston, Massachusetts*

**Sharron P. Schlosser, R.N., M.S.N.**
*Assistant Professor, Parent Child Health Nursing, Ida V. Moffett School of Nursing, Samford University; Staff Nurse, Department of Obstetrics and Gynecology, Baptist Medical Center, Birmingham, Alabama*

**Therese B. Shipps, R.N., M.S.**
*Adjunct Assistant Professor, Boston University, Boston, Massachusetts; Nursing Studies Coordinator, Mount Auburn Hospital, Cambridge, Massachusetts*

**Eileen Ledden Sjoberg, R.N., M.S.**
*Assistant Professor, Fitchburg State College, Fitchburg, Massachusetts*

**Carol A. Stephenson, R.N., Ed.D.**
*Assistant Professor, Harris College of Nursing, Texas Christian University, Fort Worth, Texas*

**Camille Stern, R.N., M.S.N.**
*Instructor, Ida V. Moffett School of Nursing, Samford University, Birmingham, Alabama*

**Metta Fay Street, M.S.**
*Assistant Professor and Community Health Coordinator, Ida V. Moffett School of Nursing, Samford University; Consultant, Bureau of Nursing, Jefferson County Department of Public Health, Birmingham, Alabama*

**Joan M. Vitello, R.N., M.S.N., C.C.R.N.**
*Graduate Student, University of Alabama, Birmingham, Alabama*

**Linda Hudson Williams, M.S.**
*Assistant Professor, University of Alabama School of Nursing in Huntsville, Huntsville, Alabama*

**Joan W. Williamson, R.N., M.S.N.**
*Associate Professor, University of Alabama School of Nursing in Huntsville, Huntsville, Alabama*

# Preface

Pathophysiology can be defined as the study of the physiologic and biologic manifestations of disease. The third edition of *Pathophysiology: Adaptations and Alterations in Function* provides a basis for this study by expanding the student's knowledge in the sciences and exploring how alterations in structure (anatomy) and function (physiology) disrupt the human body as a whole. Written for undergraduate and graduate students in nursing and other health-oriented disciplines, this text blends the conceptual and systems approaches. The overall mechanisms of disease are described first to set the stage for coverage of specific disease processes within each system.

Integral to the study of pathophysiology is an understanding of how the human body uses its adaptive powers to maintain the steady state. *Pathophysiology* begins its discussion of this adaptation at the cellular level. Because alterations cause a disruption in normal cellular processes, ultimately leading to tissue or organ alterations, the body's adaptive and compensatory mechanisms also occur at the cellular level. For this reason, cellular processes and alterations in these processes are discussed throughout the text. The concept of feedback and information sharing within the body is also explored in depth. In health the body functions in a negative feedback pattern that allows return to the normal or steady state. Some pathologic processes, however, establish a positive feedback pattern that, if unchecked, will result in death.

The understanding of disease processes is continually being updated and clarified by research. Continuing studies examine the fundamental nature of life and how it is altered by pathologic conditions. In this edition of *Pathophysiology*, every attempt has been made to provide the most current information available. Many new topics have been added and all of those carried over have been thoroughly edited and revised. A new unit on human development from reproduction through the aged adult has been added. It incorporates stress effects and sleep changes that affect adaptation. A new chapter incorporating normal and altered nutrition has been included to support the importance of this topic in health and disease. Other chapters have been completely rewritten or updated to reflect current concepts. The contributors have taken great care to provide currency, detail, and concept synthesis for every topic in the book.

This edition retains many features of the first and second edition, including the basic organization and presentation of topics. Physical and laboratory findings are emphasized in appropriate sections, but treatment regimens are included only to illustrate or clarify a process. Students are referred to the many current nursing and medical texts for information about treatment and nursing management.

This edition includes several features designed to make the text easy to use. A second color, used throughout, highlights both illustrations and text. The extensive artwork is expanded and refined so that it will be more useful in helping students to visualize complex subjects. Students are encouraged to use the Chapter Outlines and Learning Objectives as guides before reading each chapter and for review of content. For students and faculty who wish to pursue specific topics in greater depth, each chapter is thoroughly referenced and a bibliography is provided at the end of each unit.

*Pathophysiology: Adaptations and Alterations in Function*, Third Edition, is accompanied by a set of supplements to help students and instructors. The *Instructor's Manual* has been completely revised and contains key terms, chapter summaries, teaching strategies, and a bank of test questions. Study questions and answers are found in the *Instructor's Manual* and provide for synthesis of content. *Transparency Masters* of select illustrations in the text are also available.

Barbara L. Bullock, R.N., M.S.N

# Acknowledgments

Putting together a book of this magnitude requires contributions by many people. I gratefully acknowledge the contributors to previous editions. Their contributions provided the basis for the entire project. Contributors to each edition are acknowledged separately. The contributors to the third edition added new content and refined, updated, and expanded the second edition. Their diligence and attention to detail is greatly appreciated.

I also acknowledge the support and guidance provided by many talented persons at J. B. Lippincott Company, specifically, Dave Carroll, Senior Nursing Editor, and Dina Kamilatos, Project Editor. A special thank you goes to Ann West, who has helped me for years to make dreams become reality. Her enthusiasm and moral support made me believe that I really could accomplish the task. Marcia Williams, Medical Illustrator, has handled all of the major revisions of select pieces of art, making many suggestions for wonderful changes. The results are truly outstanding. Also, thanks go to Mary Murphy for her assistance in securing permissions.

I am also very grateful to Michelle McCarren, who again took on the typing and word processing of the entire manuscript and helped me to meet the deadlines. She produced virtually error-free copy and cheerfully endured my changes, revisions, and terrible handwriting.

My thanks also go to the third edition reviewers for their helpful comments and suggestions: Margaret M. Andrews, Ph.D., R.N.; Jeanne Cremeans, Ph.D., R.N.; Harriet R. Feldman, Ph.D., R.N.; Joan R. Hudiburg, M.S., R.D.; Laura R. Mahlmeister, R.N., Ph.D.; Nancy R. Mitchell, B.S.N., M.S.N.; Olive A. Santavenere, M.S., R.N., Doctoral Candidate; Martha O. Wood, R.N.C., M.S.N., C.R.N.P.; and Linda H. Youngstrom, A.B.D., M.S.N., R.N.

I could not have completed this project without the continuing support of my husband, Pete, my children, and my parents, to whom this book is dedicated. Pete and my parents, Lois and Harry Radford, spent weeks helping me put manuscript together. They checked figure numbers and cut and pasted all of the example figures in the text. Besides helping me to meet deadlines, they helped to make a tedious project fun.

# Contents

# Introduction to Pathophysiology: Adaptations and Alterations in Cellular Function

# CELLULAR DYNAMICS

**B**ecause the cell is the basis of life, it is appropriate to begin the study of pathophysiology with a review of normal cellular processes. Understanding of these processes is necessary for the understanding of concepts in every other unit of the text. The material can be found in many anatomy and physiology textbooks but is presented here as a convenient, accessible reference. Sources for the more detailed aspects of cellular function are listed in the bibliography at the end of Unit 1.

Chapter 1 describes normal cellular function, with special emphasis on the cellular organelles and on movement of materials across the cell membrane. Chapter 2 details the alterations in cells when they are exposed to a changing, hostile environment. Cellular adaptation, injury, and death are explored in terms of their effect on body function. Mechanisms by which the steady state can be maintained, even at the expense of altered intracellular metabolism, are explored. Altered cellular function ending in lethal change is described. Chapter 3 explains the principles of inheritance and relates them to the more common genetic disorders.

The reader is encouraged to use the learning objectives at the beginning of each chapter as a study guide outline for essential concepts. The bibliography at the end of the unit provides general and specific resources for further study.

# Cells: Structure, Function, Organization

## Chapter Outline

## Learning Objectives

1. Differentiate between intracellular and extracellular electrolyte composition.
2. Describe in detail the structure and function of the following organelles: cell membrane, mitochondria, ribosomes, endoplasmic reticulum, Golgi apparatus, lysosomes, microtubules, centrioles, nucleus, and nucleolus.
3. Explain the major ways by which adenosine triphosphate (ATP) is formed.
4. Describe the process of protein synthesis from DNA-RNA transcription to manufacture protein.
5. Compare the function of the smooth endoplasmic reticulum with the rough endoplasmic reticulum.
6. Explain briefly the negative feedback pattern seen with the reproduction of cells of the body.
7. Classify cells by their ability to regenerate.
8. Describe briefly the process of mitosis.
9. Explain the mechanisms of transport across the cell membrane.
10. Identify carrier-mediated transport, including the mechanism and what facilitates it.

11. Explain the purpose of the sodium-potassium pump.
12. Compare pinocytosis and phagocytosis.
13. Describe the purpose of exocytosis.
14. Draw a cell exhibiting ameboid motion.
15. Describe the process of muscle contraction.
16. Compare smooth, cardiac, and skeletal muscle contraction.
17. Explain briefly the electrical properties of cells, including depolarization and repolarization.
18. Define the *refractory periods*.
19. Describe the differences in structure among the four major types of cells in the human body.
20. Define the purposes of the three types of epithelial cells.
21. Differentiate among skeletal, cardiac, and smooth muscle on the basis of histologic appearance.
22. Describe briefly the components of the neuron.
23. List the major types of connective tissue cells.
24. Identify the structure and function of each type of connective tissue.

The cell is the basic structural and functional unit of the body; therefore, an understanding of the basic biology of the human cell is essential to the study of pathophysiology. All pathophysiologic processes reflect changes in normal cell function. This chapter reviews fundamental concepts of cell structure, function, and organization.

Cells are the units of tissues, organs, and finally, systems of the human body (Figure 1-1). The human body contains over 75 trillion cells, each of which performs specific functions. These functions are determined by genetic differentiation and are controlled by a highly specific information system that directs the activity of cellular organelles and inclusions.

Cells that have the major function of carrying out the activities of the organ are called *parenchymal cells*. This means that the parenchyma of an organ actually does its function. Some examples of parenchymal cells are hepatocytes, neurons, gastric parietal cells, osteocytes, and myocardial cells. Other cells make it possible for the parenchymal cells to perform their function by providing the supporting structure or architectural framework to hold the organ in place. Examples include neuroglia, gastric capillary endothelial cells, and cardiac connective tissue cells.

Although cells have different functions, they are alike in many ways. The similarities include how nutrients are used, what type of nutrients are needed, how oxygen is used, the disposition of excretory products, and the internal organization of protoplasm.

## CELLULAR ORGANELLES

The cell is composed of many different structures that carry out its complex functions. Within the cell are highly organized physical structures called *organelles*. These structures are suspended in the fluid medium called *protoplasm*. This substance includes the *cytoplasm,* which is outside the nucleus of a cell, and the *nucleoplasm,* which is inside the nucleus. The general structure of the cell and its organelles is schematically diagrammed in Figure 1-2.

Protoplasm is composed mostly of water but it contains specific amounts of electrolytes, proteins, lipids, and carbohydrates. The intracellular electrolyte balance is closely regulated and differs from that of extracellular fluid (Table 1-1). Proteins compose about 10% to 20% of the content of protoplasm and function to help the cellular inclusions maintain structural strength and form. Proteins also form the enzymes necessary for many intracellular reactions. Lipids make up a very small portion of the general cell and mainly join with proteins to keep the cell membranes insoluble in water. Lipids may be deposited in the cytoplasm of some cells when they are not needed for conversion to energy. Carbohydrates constitute a very small amount of the cytoplasm and are

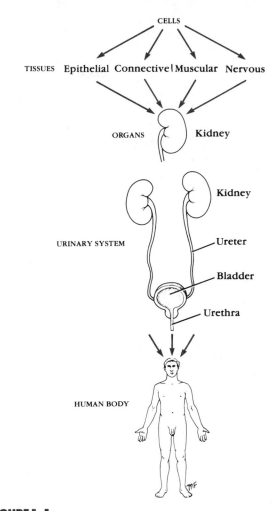

**FIGURE 1–1.**
Structural subunits of the body: cells, tissues, organs, and systems. (From R.S. Snell, *Clinical Histology for Medical Students.* Boston: Little, Brown, 1984.)

used mainly in forming adenosine triphosphate (ATP) for energy.

## The Plasma Membrane

All cells are surrounded by a limiting membrane, called the plasma membrane, that separates intracellular from extracellular fluids. Within the cell, some of the other organelles are bounded by a membrane that is similar in structure to the plasma membrane but named after the organelle (eg, mitochondrial membrane, lysosomal membrane, etc.).

The plasma membrane consists of a double layer of lipid molecules (the lipid bilayer) with proteins bound to each layer as well as within the layers (Figure 1-3). Lipids account for about half of the mass of the plasma membrane and consist of phospholipids (the most abundant), glycolipids, and others such as cholesterol.

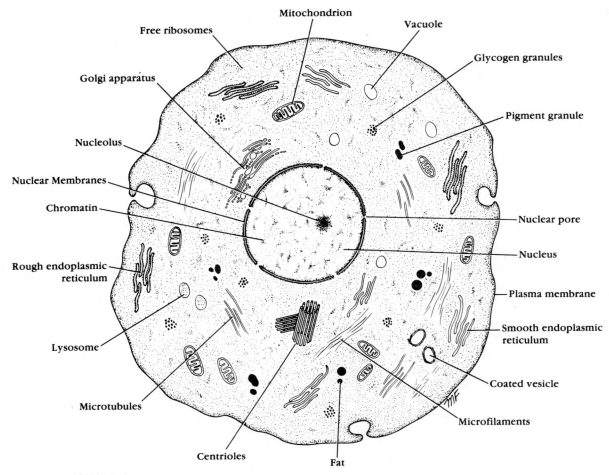

**FIGURE 1-2.**
The general structure of a cell and its organelles. (From R.S. Snell, *Clinical Histology for Medical Students.* Boston: Little, Brown, 1984.)

The phospholipid molecules are elongated; they have a polar end and a nonpolar end. Phospholipids in the bilayer are arranged so their polar (hydrophilic) region points toward the interior or exterior of the cell and their nonpolar (hydrophobic) regions are buried in the interior of the membrane. This arrangement allows the membrane to behave as a barrier, restricting the loss of intracellular material and governing material entry. The lipid bilayer gives the membrane the ability to conform to the changing shapes of cells and to fill in the gaps between the proteins in the membrane.[1]

Proteins are anchored in or on the lipid bilayer. Those bound to the inner or outer membrane surface are called *ectoproteins*. Those partially or completely embedded in the lipid bilayer are called *endoproteins*. Membrane proteins may have other types of molecules attached to them. Proteins on the outer membrane surface, for example, may have carbohydrates attached. These are called *glycoproteins*. Carbohydrates may also be attached to the polar region of the phospholipid molecules, forming *glycolipids*.

Membrane proteins not only form part of the molecular structure of the plasma membrane, but have many functional roles, such as transporting and exchanging materials between the cell and its environment. Other proteins are enzymes that help govern cell function or receptors that communicate chemically with the cell.

The plasma membrane exists in a fluid state at body temperature, and the protein and lipid components move; that is, the structure of the plasma membrane is dynamic, not static. Both proteins and lipids can move from one area of the membrane to another. Because the membrane is fluid and resembles a patchwork or mosaic of proteins and lipids, it is often called the *fluid mosaic membrane*.

## Mitochondria

Mitochondria are membranous, cigar-shaped organelles that synthesize ATP, a high-energy phosphate compound required by cells when they perform work (eg, contrac-

**TABLE 1-1.**
CHEMICAL COMPOSITIONS OF EXTRACELLULAR AND INTRACELLULAR FLUIDS

| | EXTRACELLULAR FLUID | INTRACELLULAR FLUID |
|---|---|---|
| $Na^+$ | 142 mEq/L | 10 mEq/L |
| $K^+$ | 4 mEq/L | 140 mEq/L |
| $Ca^{++}$ | 5 mEq/L | <1 mEq/L |
| $Mg^{++}$ | 3 mEq/L | 58 mEq/L |
| $Cl^-$ | 103 mEq/L | 4 mEq/L |
| $HCO_{3-}$ | 28 mEq/L | 10 mEq/L |
| Phosphates | 4 mEq/L | 75 mEq/L |
| $SO_{4--}$ | 1 mEq/L | 2 mEq/L |
| Glucose | 90 mg % | 0–20 mg % |
| Amino acids | 30 mg % | 200 mg % ? |
| Cholesterol Phospholipids Neutral fat | 0.5 g % | 2–95 g % |
| $P_{o_2}$ | 35 mm Hg | 20 mm Hg ? |
| $P_{co_2}$ | 46 mm Hg | 50 mm Hg ? |
| pH | 7.5 | 7.0 |
| Proteins | 2 g % (5 mEq/L) | 16 g % (40 mEq/L) |

Source: A.C. Guyton, *Human Physiology and Mechanisms of Disease* (4th ed.). Philadelphia: Saunders, 1987.

tion, secretion, conduction, transport, etc.). In a sense, mitochondria are like batteries in a cell, providing energy in a form that allows the cell to function normally (Figure 1-4).

Mitochondria are bounded by a double membrane, the inner one of which is thrown into a series of shelflike folds called *cristae* that project into the interior of the organelle. The folded inner membrane presents a large internal surface area on which chemical reactions that generate ATP take place.

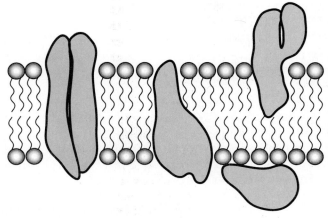

**FIGURE 1-3.**
The structure of the lipid bilayer.

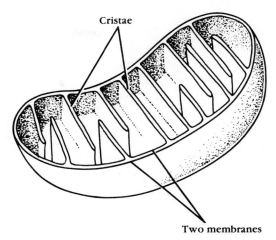

**FIGURE 1-4.**
Schematic representation of a mitochondrion. (From R.S. Snell, *Clinical Histology for Medical Students*. Boston: Little, Brown, 1984.)

Cells that are very active and have a high energy requirement, such as skeletal muscle cells, have many mitochondria, whereas less active cells, such as bone or cartilage cells, have fewer mitochondria. Usually, within a given cell, mitochondria tend to be most numerous in areas that are highly energy dependent, such as around the contractile elements of the muscle cell or at the terminus of a nerve cell where transmission occurs.

Mitochondria are able to regenerate themselves under conditions of increased energy need. They contain a special type of deoxyribonucleic acid (DNA) that resembles bacterial DNA rather than cellular DNA.

## Formation of ATP With Oxygen

The process used by mitochondria to form ATP is called *oxidative phosphorylation*. It requires simple forms of carbohydrates, proteins, and fats. These substances enter the mitochondria and, using oxidative enzymes, form ATP through the citric acid or Krebs cycle (Figure 1-5). High-energy phosphate radicals are formed that later release their energy when ATP is catabolized or reduced to adenosine diphosphate (ADP). By reentering the mitochondria, ADP can receive another phosphate radical and form ATP anew. The process of catabolizing ATP to ADP results in energy release. Adding the phosphate radical to the ADP is called *rephosphorylation*. This catabolizing and recombining of ATP to ADP and back to ATP has been called the *energy currency* of the cell, which is spent and remade over and over.[2]

The major source of *acetyl coenzyme A* (acetyl CoA), the common intermediary in carbohydrate, protein, and fat metabolism, is glucose. Fats and proteins can be metabolized to intermediates that can be fed into the Krebs cycle.

Approximately 95% of ATP is formed in the mito-

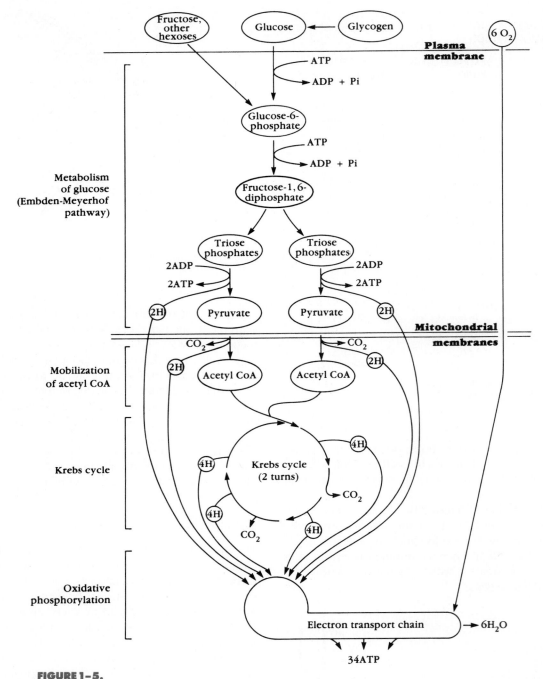

**FIGURE 1–5.**

Metabolism of glucose in the formation of ATP. (From C.P. Hickman, Jr., L.S. Roberts, and F.M. Hickman, *Integrated Principles of Zoology* [7th ed.]. St. Louis: Mosby/Times Mirror, 1984.)

chondria through a sequence of chemical reactions that require oxidative enzymes. The process involves glycolysis and then oxidation of the end product to form ATP. Many successive steps allow for the release of 38 moles of ATP for each mole of glucose. Actually, 40 moles of ATP are produced, with 2 moles being spent to initiate the process and 4 being produced outside the mitochondria. The efficiency in energy transformation is about 43%; the remaining 57% is given off as heat.[2]

## Formation of ATP Without Oxygen

A small amount of ATP can also be formed by glycolysis in the absence of oxygen. Figure 1-5 shows that glycolysis (Embden-Meyerhof pathway), itself, is an anaerobic process. Glycolysis proceeds to produce pyruvic acid (pyruvate). Important in the process is a coenzyme called *nicotinamide-adenine dinucleotide* (NAD), which functions to accept hydrogen ions. Normally, NAD picks up hydrogen and passes it to another acceptor to pick up more hydrogen. In the oxidative cycle, this acceptor is oxygen and the result is the formation of water. Without available oxygen, pyruvate is reduced to lactic acid. The system is inefficient but it can keep certain cells viable for short periods of time. In the normal, unstressed cell, anaerobic metabolism provides less than 5% of the ATP requirements of the cell. The lactic acid formed diffuses out of the cell into the tissues and plasma. This glycolytic process occurs during periods of intense muscular exertion in which oxygen consumption exceeds oxygen supply. Subsequently, the accumulation of lactic acid in the muscle causes pain. The process produces an *oxygen debt* of the muscle that requires deep breathing after exercise to restore the balance of ATP. The lactic acid remaining in the muscle cell can be reconverted to glucose or pyruvic acid in the presence of oxygen. Lactic acid that leaves the cell during exercise is carried to the liver, where it is converted to glycogen and carbon dioxide. The heart has been shown to be particularly capable of converting lactic acid to pyruvic acid until the lack of oxygen is severe enough that it produces more lactic acid than it can metabolize.

## Endoplasmic Reticulum

In some human cells, much of the cytoplasm is filled with an intricate, yet ordered, set of folded membranes that form small flattened sacs or tubes (Figure 1-6). All of the membranes are interconnected, giving rise to a netlike structure, the appearance of which is reflected by its name: endoplasmic reticulum (a net within the cytoplasm).

The outer membrane of the nuclear envelope is continuous with the membranes of the endoplasmic reticulum (ER). It is believed that the nuclear envelope develops from ER membranes after cell division.

Much of the surface of the ER may be covered with small particles or granules made up of ribonucleic acid (RNA) associated with protein. The particles, called *ribosomes*, give the outer membrane of the ER a rough or granular appearance; therefore, such endoplasmic reticulum is called *granular endoplasmic reticulum*. Other surfaces of the endoplasmic reticulum may be free of ribosomes; hence, they appear relatively smooth. This type of endoplasmic reticulum is called *agranular* or *smooth ER*.

The endoplasmic reticulum provides a large surface within the cell on which sequences of chemical reactions can occur. Enzymes and other substances are arranged in an assembly-line sequence to provide for efficient production of various types of proteins, carbohydrates, and lipids. In this way, the ER provides a large surface area for the production of substances responsible for the metabolic functions of the cell.[2]

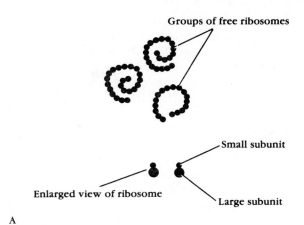

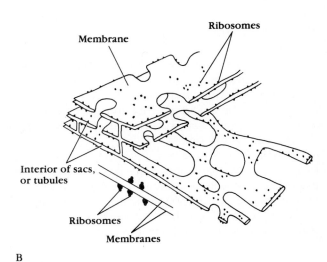

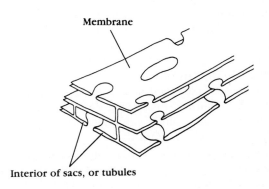

**FIGURE 1-6.**
Electron microscopic appearance of structures of **A.** Ribosomes, **B.** Rough endoplasmic reticulum, **C.** Smooth endoplasmic reticulum. (From R.S. Snell, *Clinical Histology for Medical Students.* Boston: Little, Brown, 1984.)

The granular ER is involved primarily with the production of proteins. Proteins such as hormones, for example, which are destined to be secreted, are put together on the ribosomes of this ER. Also, some of the proteins that form structural parts of the cell are produced here.

The smooth ER appears to be more involved with the formation of nonprotein substances, such as the fat-soluble triglycerides, fatty acids, steroids, and phospholipids. It is also involved in biotransformation of substances and in storing calcium in some cells.

The spaces between the folded membranes of the ER forming the fluid-filled interior of the saccules and tubules are called *cisternae*. These channels or canallike spaces allow molecules to be distributed from one area of the cell to another. In a sense, the endoplasmic reticulum also functions as an intracellular circulatory system.

## Polyribosomes

Some of the ribosomes within the cell are not bound to the endoplasmic reticulum. Instead, a number of ribosomes involved with the production of a specific protein molecule may be linked together, much like pearls on a string, forming a chain structure called a polyribosome (literally, many ribosomes).

Polyribosomes of several different lengths may be found in the cytoplasm and all are involved with the formation or synthesis of protein molecules. Most of the proteins made on the polyribosomes are for the cell's own use in building cell components (structural proteins) or in regulating cell activities (eg, enzymes).

## Golgi Complex

The Golgi complex, also called the Golgi apparatus or the Golgi body, is a series of concentric, flattened saccules with membranes resembling those of the smooth endoplasmic reticulum (Figure 1-7). In some cells, the Golgi membranes appear to be connected to the smooth ER and may be a specialized part of it. Membrane-bound vesicles are frequently observed near the Golgi membranes and represent packaged chemicals arriving at the Golgi complex for further processing or packaged substances leaving the Golgi complex destined for secretion by way of exocytosis (see p. 23).

The Golgi complex is predominant in various types of secretory cells, such as the pancreatic acinar cell, and plays several important roles in the process of secretion. Substances destined for secretion—a protein hormone, for example—may be produced on the granular ER and then transported through the cisternae of the ER to the Golgi apparatus. The Golgi apparatus may then prepare the hormone for release by packaging it within a mem-

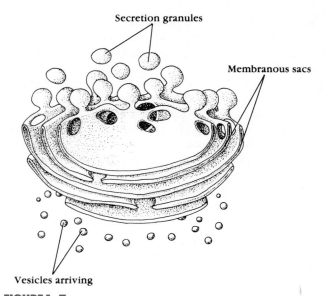

**FIGURE 1–7.**
Probable appearance of Golgi apparatus. (From R.S. Snell, *Clinical Histology for Medical Students*. Boston: Little, Brown, 1984.)

branous vacuole, which then moves toward the plasma membrane where the hormone is discharged into the extracellular environment.

Other functions of the Golgi apparatus include producing some substances such as polysaccharides, chemically modifying molecules produced by the ER (eg, activating enzymes), storing synthesized molecules, and producing digestive vacuoles called lysosomes.

## Lysosomes

Lysosomes (*lyse*—destroy, *some*—body), are membrane-bound organelles that are spherical and contain digestive enzymes. They originate from the Golgi complex and ER, and participate in intracellular digestive processes.

Lysosomes contain a variety of hydrolytic enzymes that break down protein, nucleic acids, carbohydrates, and lipids. When a cell ingests material by endocytosis, lysosomes fuse their membranes with those of the endocytotic vesicle, forming a common membrane-bound vesicle in which digestion can occur (Figure 1-8).

Lysosomes also digest "worn out" or damaged parts of the cell, thereby participating in the recycling of cell constituents. When a cell dies, the lysosomes it contains rupture, releasing enzymes that cause the cell to self-destruct (*autolysis*). It is not known why lysosomal enzymes are normally unable to digest their own lysosomal membrane.

Numerous lysosomes are present in cells that are very active in ingesting matter by phagocytosis. In some of the leukocytes, for example, lysosomes are so numerous they give the cytoplasm a granular appearance. Lyso-

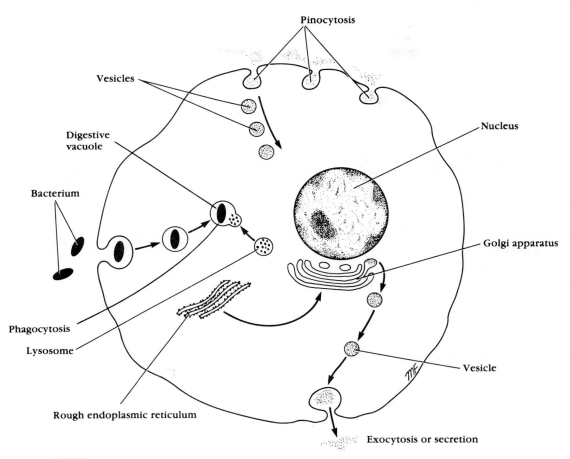

**Pinocytosis**

**Vesicles**

**Digestive vacuole**

**Bacterium**

**Phagocytosis**

**Lysosome**

**Rough endoplasmic reticulum**

**Nucleus**

**Golgi apparatus**

**Vesicle**

**Exocytosis or secretion**

**FIGURE 1–8.**
Schematic illustration of processes of endocytosis (pinocytosis and phagocytosis) and exocytosis. (From R.S. Snell, *Clinical Histology for Medical Students*. Boston: Little, Brown, 1984.)

somes are a critical part of the body's defensive phagocytic cells that are responsible for destroying foreign proteins.

## *Microtubules*

Microtubules are nonmembranous, cylindrical organelles, the walls of which are composed of 13 filaments of globular proteins called *tubulin* (Figure 1-9). They are hollow and have an internal diameter of approximately 250 angstroms (Å). An angstrom is a very small measurement equal to $10^7$ mm (one ten-millionth of a millimeter).

Microtubules may function in one or more of the following three ways: (1) to maintain the shape of a cell by providing structural support; (2) to act as an internal conduit for the movement of materials from one part of the cell to another; and (3) to provide for certain forms of cellular movement, such as ciliary motion.

Microtubules are commonly found in cells that possess long cellular extensions that require support; for

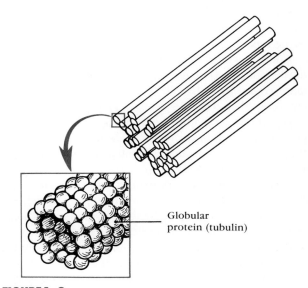

**Globular protein (tubulin)**

**FIGURE 1–9.**
Microtubules. (Adapted from R.S. Snell, *Clinical Histology for Medical Students*. Boston: Little, Brown, 1984.)

example, embedded in the cytoplasm of the long extensions of nerve cells (axons and dendrites) where they provide a certain amount of rigidity. If microtubules are destroyed, the cell processes lose their characteristic shape.

Because microtubules are usually oriented in the direction of material movement within the cytoplasm, they are believed to be involved with the intracellular transport of various substances. In certain nerve cells, for example, microtubules are numerous in the axon. Materials required for proper functioning of the terminals of the axon are synthesized in the cell body and transported down the axon to its terminals. If the axon is ligated (tied off), material will be observed damming up in the part of the axon nearest the cell body, and it will swell, much as a river does if its flow is restricted by a dam.

Studies have shown that the globular proteins making up the wall of the microtubule move along the length of the tubule in a sequential manner as one end of the tubule is being formed while the opposite end is being broken down. Some substances that are transported by the microtubules may attach to the protein subunits at the beginning of the tubule and move in association with the protein to the other end where they may be released.

In addition to intracellular transport, microtubules form parts of cilia and flagella, which are cellular structures specialized for movement.

## Cilia and Flagella

Cilia are short protoplasmic extensions on the free surface of some cells that line body cavities or hollow viscera. The lining of the upper respiratory tract, for example, contains ciliated cells, as does the lining of the uterine tubes.

Cilia (singular, cilium) are microtubule-containing cylinders enclosed by an extension of the plasma membrane (Figure 1-10). Usually, a single ciliated cell projects numerous cilia on its free surface, giving that portion of the cell surface a matlike appearance. One human cell type, the spermatozoon (sperm) or male reproductive cell, has a single elongated ciliumlike extension called a flagellum (plural, flagella).

Cilia and flagella are constructed from the same basic pattern and have three major parts: the stalk, which is a sheaf of tubules enveloped by the plasma membrane; a basal granule, from which the structure originates within the cytoplasm; and rootlet fibers, which extend from the basal granule into the cytoplasm.

In cross section, cilia and flagella are bounded by a sheath that encloses an array of 9 double microtubules arranged in a radial fashion, with two additional microtubules in the center. This arrangement is called the 9 + 2 pattern (see Figure 1-10). The compound tubular structure that is formed is called an *axoneme*. Ciliary motion

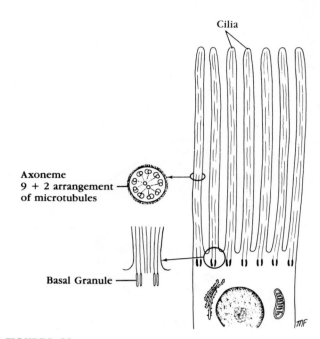

**FIGURE 1-10.**
A ciliated cell. (From R.S. Snell, *Clinical Histology for Medical Students.* Boston: Little, Brown, 1984.)

occurs when the microtubules, powered by ATP, slide past one another. Cilia move with a swift forward movement and a slow backward stroke (like a whip). Their movement is coordinated so stimulation is passed from one cilium to the next. On a sheet of ciliated cells, coordinated ciliary movement resembles the effect seen when wind ripples across a field of wheat.

Ciliary movement in the upper respiratory tract is an important part of the body's defense, helping to move inhaled particulate matter trapped in mucus toward the nasal and oral cavities where it may be discharged or swallowed. In the uterine tubes, ciliary motion helps move the ovum toward the uterine cavity.

Flagellar movement is undulating (wavelike), rather than whiplike. It is responsible for propelling sperm through body fluids at a rate of 1 to 4 mm per minute in a relatively straight line.

Microtubules, cilia, and flagella are nonmembranous organelles that are structurally related to the centriole. The centriole may be the source of microtubules, cilia, and flagella.

## Centrioles

Many human cells near the nucleus contain two hollow, cylindrical structures called centrioles which, like cilia, are composed of 9 sets of microtubules arranged in a radial fashion, but without the central pair of tubules (9 + 0 pattern). They are often found near the nuclear envelope lying at right angles to one another (Figure 1-11). The microtubules that make up the wall of the centriole are arranged in sets of three, lying in the same plane and embedded in a dense granular substance.

The function of the centrioles is to form and organize a complex array of microtubules, known as the spindle apparatus, which is needed to separate a single cell into two daughter cells when the cell divides (see pp. 16–18).

## Nucleus

The nucleus is a large membranous organelle frequently located near the center of a cell. The term *nucleus* is derived from a Latin word meaning "little nut," referring to the resemblance of a cell nucleus to a nut within a shell (the plasma membrane) or to a seed within a pod. It controls all of the cellular activities.

The nucleus is bound by a membranous envelope called the *nuclear envelope* (Figure 1-12). In contrast to the plasma membrane, it consists of two distinct membranes. The membranes are fused together periodically to form circular pores through which material can pass in and out of the nucleus. Protein molecules as large as 44,000 molecular weight can pass through these pores.[2] The inner membrane of the nuclear envelope represents the actual nuclear membrane, while the outer membrane of the envelope gives rise to and is continuous with membranes of the endoplasmic reticulum.

In some cells, the nucleoplasm appears homogeneous and undifferentiated. In others, distinct nuclear structures can be observed. Two commonly seen structures are the nucleolus and condensed strands of chromatin called *chromosomes*. These are readily identified during cellular mitosis.

The *nucleolus* (little nucleus) is a collection of dense fibers and granules forming a small spherical mass that is most visible when the cell is not in the process of reproducing itself (cell division) (see Figure 1-12). The nucleolus is composed primarily of RNA and protein, together with smaller amounts of DNA. These nucleic acids play key roles in the cellular synthesis of proteins. The granules of the nucleolus are precursors of ribosomes (particles of RNA and protein), which are the sites of protein synthesis in the cytoplasm.

Chromatin is composed of long molecules of DNA in association with protein. Chromatin fibers are too small to be seen with the light microscope. Prior to cell division, however, chromatin fibers coil and condense into compact structures that are visible when using the light microscope. These visible, x-shaped structures are called chromosomes (Figure 1-13). There are 46 chromosomes—23 pairs—in the human cell. The pairs of chromosomes differ from one another in size and shape (see Chap. 3).

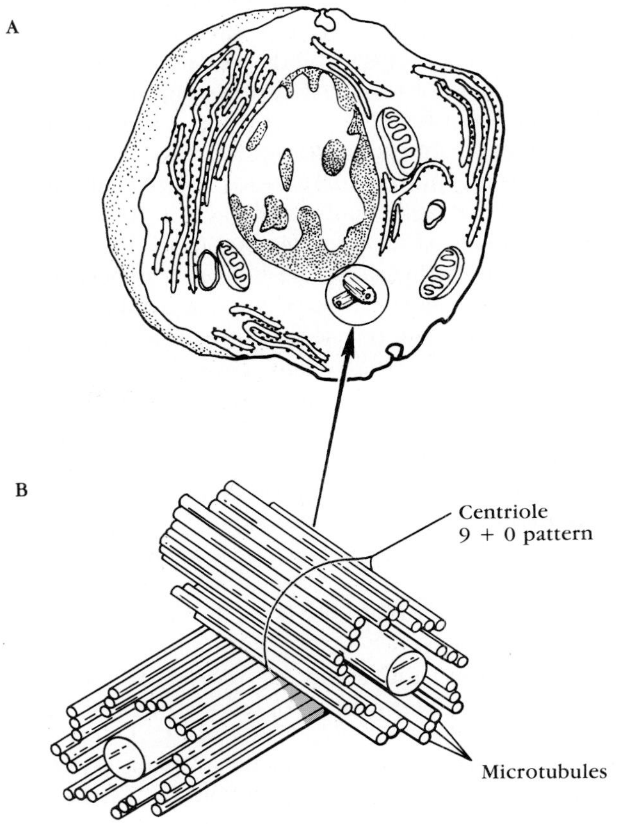

**A**

**B**

**Centriole 9 + 0 pattern**

**Microtubules**

**FIGURE 1-11.**
Centrioles. **A.** Placement in relationship to the nucleus. **B.** Appearance and composition of the centriole.

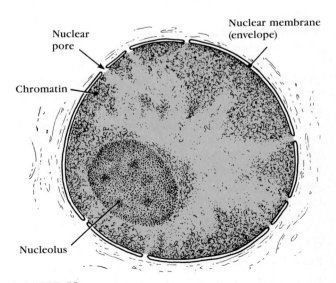

**Nuclear membrane (envelope)**

**Nuclear pore**

**Chromatin**

**Nucleolus**

**FIGURE 1-12.**
The nucleus.

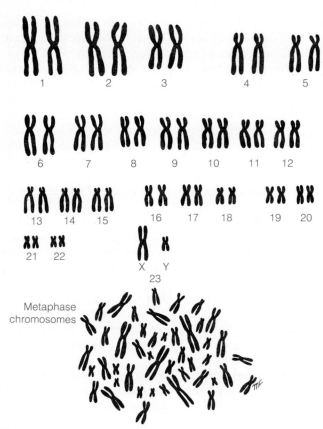

**FIGURE 1–13.**

Chromosomes. (Adapted from R.S. Snell, *Clinical Histology for Medical Students.* Boston: Little, Brown, 1984.)

## Genes

The nucleus directs and controls the activities of the entire cell through the genes. A gene is the linear sequence of nucleotides on DNA that code for the production of a single protein. The sequence is divided into units of three nucleotides, each called a *triplet.* The sequence of the nucleotide bases (*guanine, thymine, cytosine,* and *adenine*) determines the unique code and ultimately codes for a single amino acid. The genes determine the specific code that is transcribed as RNA. The gene is located on one of the two DNA strands called the *master strand,* which serves as the template (pattern) for *messenger RNA (mRNA)* transcription. Other parts of DNA serve as templates for *transfer RNA (tRNA)* or *ribosomal RNA (rRNA)* formation. The code, transmitted to the ribosomes, allows for the formation of several thousand types of proteins that are essential to the various functions of human cells.

## Protein Synthesis

Nearly all of the chemical reactions associated with normal cell function are enzyme dependent. All known enzymes are proteins, the synthesis of which is controlled by nuclear DNA. Therefore, the activity of the cytoplasmic organelles is regulated either directly or indirectly by the nucleus. In addition to enzymes, nuclear DNA contains the blueprints that specify construction of other types of proteins, such as hormones or structural proteins. The synthesis of proteins occurs in two major steps known as *transcription* and *translation* (Figure 1-14).

Transcription occurs in the nucleus and involves DNA and mRNA. During transcription, the DNA molecule partially unwinds into two separate strands. One strand acts as a template upon which mRNA is synthesized; the other strand acts as a cover. The genetic message carried by DNA in the form of a series of *triplets* is transcribed to mRNA by complementary base-pairing; thus, the formation of mRNA results in the synthesis of a molecule having a linear sequence of bases that are complementary to DNA. The mRNA molecule separates from the DNA template as fast as it forms.

After synthesis, the mRNA escapes the nucleus by way of pores in the nuclear envelope and enters the cytoplasm where it becomes associated with ribosomes, the organelle where amino acids are linked into the polypeptide chain of a protein. Within the ribosome, the genetic message carried by mRNA in the form of codons is deciphered, and correct amino acids are joined in the proper sequence to form a protein molecule. This process is translation, and it involves transfer RNA (tRNA). One or more specific tRNA molecules exist for each type of amino acid. Transfer RNA binds itself to a specific amino acid and carries it to the site of protein synthesis in the ribosome. Transfer RNA also contains a binding site (in the form of an anticodon) for mRNA; thus, as tRNA molecules bearing specific amino acids sequentially bind to mRNA in the ribosome, the amino acids are sequenced into a protein that is then released from the ribosome.

Once the mRNA template becomes associated with the ribosome, the process of peptide synthesis occurs rapidly, taking about one second for a new amino acid to be added to the peptide chain. Thus, the synthesis of a protein, such as the hormone insulin (51 amino acids), takes about 1 minute.

Also, several ribosomes may simultaneously translate a single strand of mRNA so protein synthesis may occur more rapidly.

## REPRODUCTIVE ABILITY OF CELLS

Most cells have the ability to reproduce themselves through the complex process of *mitosis.* In the adult, new cells take the place of old cells in a rigidly defined order that maintains cellular numbers, but allows for the replacement of only the needed cells. The turnover rate is billions of cells per day, but rigid controls inherently limit the number of cells to be reproduced.

Specific controls on the reproductive process pro-

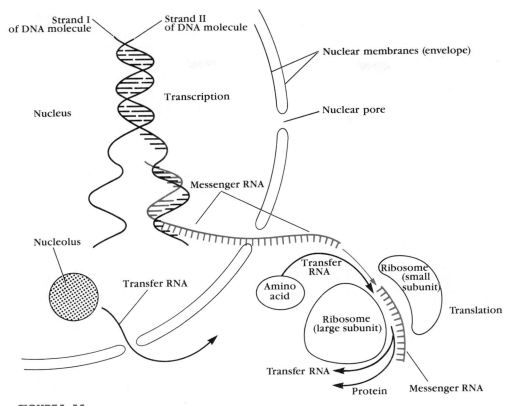

**FIGURE 1–14.**
Highly schematic picture of protein synthesis. (From R.S. Snell, *Clinical Histology for Medical Students.* Boston: Little, Brown, 1984.)

duce precisely the correct quantity of cells. For example, if the red blood cell (RBC) count decreases, specific stimulating factors cause the bone marrow to increase production of erythrocytes (RBCs), leading ultimately to increased numbers of circulating red blood cells (see Chap. 19). Another stage in the process of erythropoiesis (RBC production) occurs when the appropriate level of red blood cells is reached. Some factor, either diminished stimulation or an inhibitor, suppresses further production of RBCs.

## Regeneration of Cells

As stated earlier, almost all cells have the ability to reproduce themselves. This ability is called the regenerative capacity of cells.

*Labile cells* regenerate frequently and have a life span usually measured in hours or days. Some examples of labile cells are white blood cells and epithelial cells. Other cells retain the ability to regenerate or reproduce but do so only under special circumstances. These are called *stable cells,* and their life span is measured in years or, sometimes, the entire life span of an organism. Some examples of stable cells are osteocytes of bone, paren-

chymal cells of the liver, and cells of the glands of the body. In the normal liver cell, for example, mitotic figures are rare, but after injury, mitoses are abundant because the liver has a remarkable ability to repair itself.

The third type of cells, the *permanent cells,* live for the entire life of the organism. They include the nerve cell bodies and probably most of the muscle cells. The neuron does not divide after birth but has the ability, in certain circumstances, to regenerate its axon and dendrites (see Chap. 48). Myocardial muscle does not regenerate; when it dies, it is repaired by the formation of scar tissue.

## Reproduction of Cells

### The Cell Cycle

All human cells have a life cycle, called the cell cycle, that begins when the cell is produced by division of its parent and ends when the cell either divides to give rise to daughter cells or dies. A complete cell cycle consists of four stages labelled $G_1$, S, $G_2$, and M (Figure 1-15).

The $G_1$ stage is the time interval after the formation of the cell that precedes replication of DNA. The S stage is the time during which DNA replication occurs. The $G_2$

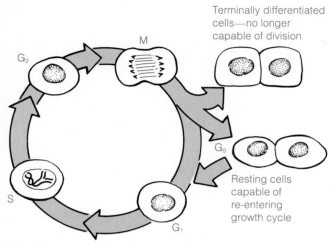

Terminally differentiated cells—no longer capable of division

Resting cells capable of re-entering growth cycle

**FIGURE 1–15.**
The cell cycle. The cycle consists of four stages: $G_1$, S, $G_2$, and M. Cell division occurs during the M phase. In the S phase, synthesis of DNA occurs. Daughter cells may undergo differentiation and no longer be capable of division, or they may enter $G_0$. Cells in $G_0$ are mitotically inactive but may be recalled to the growth fraction under appropriate conditions. (From D. O. Slauson and B. J. Cooper, *Mechanisms of Disease* [2nd ed.]. Baltimore: Williams & Wilkins, 1990.)

stage is the time interval after DNA replication and before the beginning of the M stage (mitosis), the stage during which cell division occurs. Cells not destined for an early repeat of the division cycle are commonly arrested at the $G_1$ stage or according to some systems of nomenclature, a $G_0$ stage (resting phase).[3] All of the stages between mitotic divisions are collectively called *interphase*.

The process by which a cell divides to form two identical daughter cells is mitosis. Before a cell can undergo mitosis, its chromosomes must duplicate themselves, a process called *replication*.

### Replication

Replication of DNA occurs during the S stage of interphase. During this time, the chromosomes appear to be spread out in a tangled mass known as chromatin. In replication, the two strands of the DNA molecule separate, and each serves as a template (pattern) for the formation of another strand (Figure 1-16). Each template and its complement then form a new DNA molecule. During mitosis, each daughter cell inherits a DNA molecule that consists of one new strand and one parental strand.

Each chromosome is furnished with a single centromere, an area that holds together the two daughter chromosomes produced when a chromosome replicates (see Chap. 3). After replication, the two identical, double-stranded molecules of DNA are called chromatids as long as they remain attached to each other by the centromere.

### Mitosis

Mitosis is described in terms of phases through which the cell passes as it divides (Figure 1-17). The phases are defined by the appearance of chromosomes under the light microscope and are designated (in sequence) as *prophase, metaphase, anaphase,* and *telophase.*

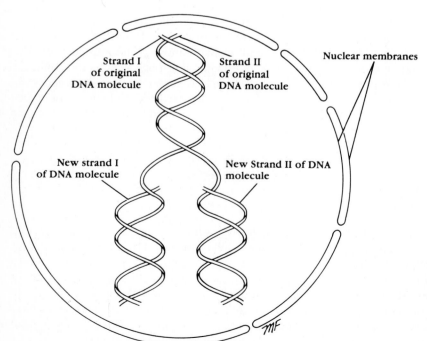

Strand I of original DNA molecule

Strand II of original DNA molecule

Nuclear membranes

New strand I of DNA molecule

New Strand II of DNA molecule

**FIGURE 1–16.**
Replication. The two strands of a DNA molecule first separate and a new strand is synthesized alongside each one. The result is that each newly formed, double-stranded molecule is identical to the original molecule whose strands became separated. (From R.S. Snell, *Clinical Histology for Medical Students.* Boston: Little, Brown, 1984.)

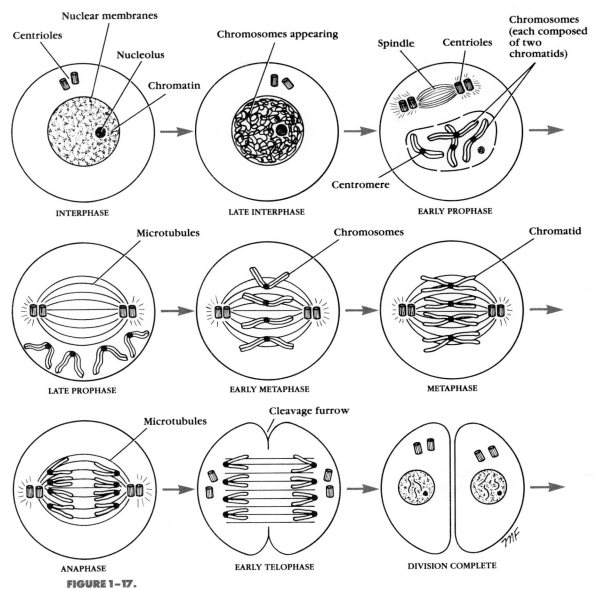

**FIGURE 1-17.**
Mitosis. (From R.S. Snell, *Clinical Histology for Medical Students.* Boston: Little, Brown, 1984.)

During prophase, the chromatin condenses into distinct chromosomes that are visible as pairs of *chromatids*, joined at their centers to form an X. The point of junction of the chromatin threads is called a *centromere*. In prophase, the nuclear membrane disappears, as does the nucleolus, and appears to be part of the cytoplasm. The centrioles migrate to opposite poles of the cell and a spindle of microtubules forms between the centrioles.

During metaphase, the assembly of the spindle is completed and the chromosomes align in a plane midway between the poles. This plane is called the *equatorial plane*. The chromosomes align at the equatorial plane because they experience an equal pull through the attached microtubules from the two poles of the spindle.

Anaphase starts with centromere division, which allows the newly divided chromosomes to move to opposite poles of the spindle. They assume a V shape as they are pulled through the cytoplasm by microtubules and filaments of the spindle apparatus.

At the beginning of telophase, two sets of daughter chromosomes are gathered at opposite poles. A new nuclear envelope is assembled from saccules of ER and surrounds each set of chromosomes. The chromosomes gradually unravel and disperse in the nucleoplasm, disappearing from view. The spindle disintegrates, but the duplicated centrioles remain and nucleoli reappear. As these events of telophase are occurring, a cleft forms in the plasma membrane and the cytoplasm is eventually divided equally between the two newly formed daughter cells by a process called *cytokinesis*.

# CELLULAR EXCHANGE

For the cell to produce its own protoplasm, synthesize chemicals for export, or derive energy from chemicals and convert the energy into useful work, the cell must acquire chemicals from the extracellular fluid (ECF). On the other hand, cell metabolism produces waste products which must be eliminated by the cell into the extracellular environment. Because the plasma membrane separates the intracellular fluid (ICF) from the ECF, all substances that either enter or leave the cell must pass through the plasma membrane.

In general, the mechanisms of cellular exchange can be divided into two categories: active and passive. *Active mechanisms* require the cell to expend energy (ATP) to effect solute movement across the plasma membrane, whereas *passive mechanisms* do not require energy expenditure by the cell. The mechanisms used in movement of substances across the cell membrane include diffusion, channel or pore diffusion, carrier-mediated, active or passive, and exocytosis or endocytosis (Figure 1-18).

## *Passive Movement Across the Cell Membrane*

### *Diffusion*

*Diffusion* is defined as the net movement of a substance from a region of higher concentration to a region of lower concentration. If the substance is equally distrib-uted between two regions, no concentration gradient exists and diffusion equilibrium is present.

The rate of net diffusion of a given substance, or the time that it takes for diffusion equilibrium to occur, is directly proportional to the concentration gradient, the cross-sectional or surface area of the diffusion pathway, and the temperature of the diffusing substance. The rate of net diffusion is determined by the amount of substance available, by kinetic motion, and by cell membrane openings through which the substance can move.[2] Additional factors include the atomic or molecular size and configuration, the ability of the diffusing solute to dissolve in lipids, and the presence or absence of an electrical charge on the diffusing solute particles.

The plasma membrane presents a barrier to the movement of materials in and out of the cell. Substances that diffuse through the membrane must either dissolve in the fluid structure of the plasma membrane and then diffuse from one side to the other, or they must pass through interruptions in the membrane called channels or "pores." Pores are fluid-filled channels formed by proteins within the membrane.

In general, substances with diameters greater than 8 Å are unable to, or else have difficulty in, passing through plasma membrane channels. Uncharged particles pass through the membrane more readily than charged particles (*ions*), and positively charged particles (*cations*) pass through less readily than do negatively charged particles (*anions*). Also, molecules that have a higher degree of lipid solubility tend to diffuse through plasma membranes more readily than molecules that are less soluble in lipids. How readily an ion or molecule

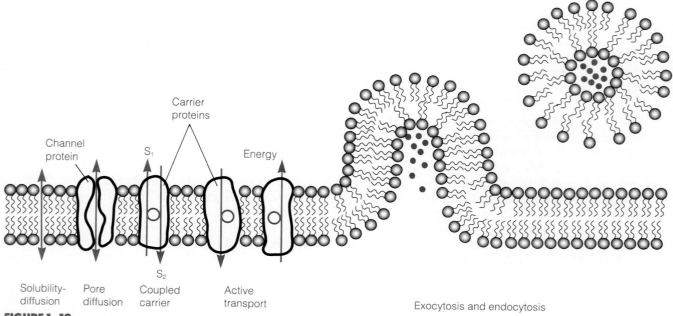

Carrier proteins

Channel protein    $S_1$    Energy

Solubility-diffusion    Pore diffusion    Coupled carrier    Active transport

$S_2$

Exocytosis and endocytosis

**FIGURE 1-18.**
Mechanisms for transport across the cell membrane.

diffuses in or out of a cell, therefore, depends upon both its physical and chemical properties, as well as the physical and chemical properties of the plasma membrane that the molecule or ion is attempting to cross.

The movement of oxygen molecules into cells and carbon dioxide molecules out of cells is an example of the process of diffusion. Oxygen molecules are being continually consumed by metabolic processes occurring within the cell, so that the concentration gradient favors diffusion of this gas into the cell. Carbon dioxide molecules are being continually produced during cellular metabolism, so the concentration gradient favors diffusion of this gas out of the cell.

## Osmosis

Osmosis is the net diffusion of water through a selectively permeable membrane that separates two aqueous solutions with different solute concentrations. The membrane is impermeable to one or more of the solutes.

When the concentration of nondiffusible solutes (substances dissolved in water that cannot diffuse through the membrane) is greater on one side of the membrane than the other, net diffusion of water (osmosis) occurs through the membrane toward the area of greater solute concentration until the solute:solvent ratio is equal on both sides of the membrane, or until a force of equal magnitude opposing the force created by the movement of water is applied. Water molecules will diffuse from an area of greater water concentration through a selectively permeable membrane to an area of lesser water concentration.

Consider a 500-ml beaker containing 280 ml of pure water divided into two equal compartments by a selectively permeable membrane (Figure 1-19). For purposes of discussion, consider the system to be unaffected by atmospheric pressure. Compartment A contains 140 ml of water, as does compartment B. If 8 gm of a nondiffusible solute, a solute to which the membrane was not permeable, were dissolved in the water in compartment A and 6 gm of nondiffusible solute were dissolved in the water in compartment B, net diffusion of water would occur from compartment B to compartment A until the solute:solvent ratios of each compartment became equal. At diffusion equilibrium, the solute:solvent ratio of compartment A would be 8 gm per 160 ml, and that of compartment B would be 6 gm per 120 ml, or 1 gm per 20 ml for the fluid in each compartment. A net diffusion of 20 ml water from compartment B to compartment A would have occurred.

During osmosis, pressure is created on the membrane as water moves from an area of higher concentration, through the membrane, to an area of lesser concentration. This pressure is called *osmotic pressure*. The magnitude of osmotic pressure depends upon the number of particles (solute particles) in the solution toward

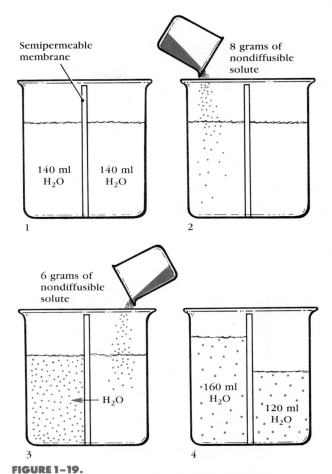

**FIGURE 1-19.**
Osmosis. **1.** A beaker of water with semipermeable membrane separating the sides. **2.** Add 8 gm of a nondiffusible substance to one side. **3.** Add 6 gm of a nondiffusible substance to the other side. **4.** The water will move toward the more concentrated side and make the concentrations equal, with more fluid on one side than the other.

which water is moving. The greater the number of nondiffusible particles in that solution, the greater its osmotic pressure.

Fluids that contain osmotically active particles in the same concentration as found in the plasma of blood are *isotonic*. If a human RBC is placed in an isotonic solution, it neither swells nor shrinks, because the net diffusion of water in or out of the cell is zero. An example of an isotonic solution is 0.9% sodium chloride in water (normal saline). Normally, the net volume of the cell remains constant. If a concentration difference for water occurs, the *water* will move, causing the cell to shrink or to swell.[2] Fluids that contain a higher concentration of osmotically active particles than blood plasma are termed *hypertonic fluids*. Red blood cells that are placed in a hypertonic solution shrink and shrivel (*crenation*) because net diffusion of water out of the cell occurs. *Hypotonic solutions* contain a lower concentration of osmotically active particles than does plasma; therefore, RBCs swell and

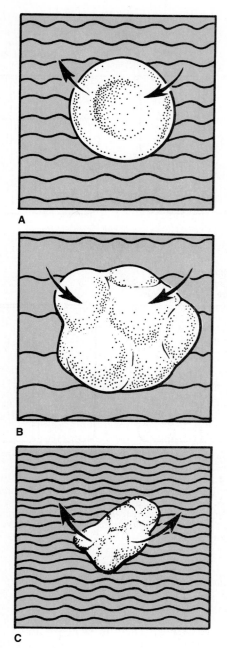

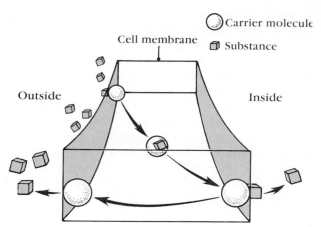

**FIGURE 1-21.**

Example of facilitated diffusion with a substance combining with a carrier molecule and moving it to the inside of the cell and down its concentration gradient, without the expenditure of energy. Each carrier molecule can only carry one specific substance.

**FIGURE 1-20.**

**A.** Isotonic solution (cell volume unchanged). **B.** Hypotonic solution (cell volume increased). **C.** Hypertonic solution (cell volume decreased).

hemolyze when placed in hypotonic solutions since the net diffusion of water is into the cell (Figure 1-20).

In the body, osmosis is important in maintaining plasma volume, interstitial and ICF volumes, and the volumes of other fluid compartments.

## Facilitated Diffusion

This process of assisted diffusion is especially important in moving glucose from the ECF to the ICF. Normally, there is a very small reserve of glucose for energy metabolism within the cell, so the cell is very dependent on the transport of glucose from the ECF. Glucose is not soluble in the lipid of the cell membrane and is too large to pass through the membrane pores. The mechanism of facilitated passive transport involves combining glucose with specific carrier molecules that are in the cell membrane. *Carrier systems* are composed of proteins that have receptors for specific solutes. After combining with the carrier molecule, glucose is carried into the cell by simple diffusion (Figure 1-21). This process requires no ATP but is assisted by the pancreatic hormone insulin, which has been shown to increase the rate of glucose transport sevenfold to tenfold. Substances move only from an area of high concentration to one of low concentration (down the concentration gradient). The process is enhanced when a greater differential exists between ICF and ECF. A maximum rate for movement of solutes exists and the mechanism can become saturated (see p. 22).

## Active Movement Across the Cell Membrane

### Active Transport

Many carrier systems transport solutes against a chemical or electrical gradient. These carrier-mediated transport systems always require the expenditure of energy and are often called "active transport" systems or simply "pumps." All of the body's cells are capable of active transport in one way or another. For example, when a meal low in carbohydrates is ingested, cells that line the intestinal tract transport glucose out of the intestine and toward the blood where the concentration of glucose may be much greater.

The *"sodium-potassium pump"* is an important example of active transport (Figure 1-22). As was noted earlier, the ICF normally contains a much higher concentration of potassium than the ECF. Conversely, the ECF contains a much higher concentration of sodium ($Na^+$) than potassium ($K^+$) (see Table 1-1). These balances must be rigidly maintained for proper cellular function. The $Na^+/K^+$ pump transports sodium ions out of the cell, thereby preventing their accumulation inside. It also returns potassium ions to the inside of the cell. This requires direct energy from ATP.

The sodium-potassium pump prevents accumulation of sodium within the cell; therefore, it also minimizes water influx and cellular swelling. Accumulation of sodium in ICF tends to cause osmosis of water toward the interior of the cell. The pumping of sodium ions out of the cell overcomes the continual tendency for water to enter the cell. When cellular metabolism ceases or decreases, adequate ATP to run the pump is not available and cellular swelling begins immediately.

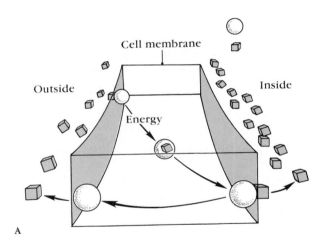

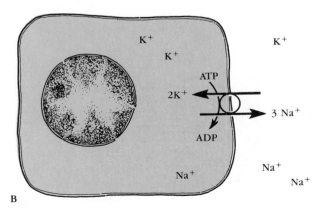

**FIGURE 1-22.**
**A.** Postulated carrier system for moving substances across the cell membrane; like facilitated diffusion, except movement is against a concentration gradient and requires energy. **B.** Postulated mechanism for moving sodium out of the cell and potassium to the interior of the cell.

## Carrier-Mediated Transport Systems

Although the phenomenon of carrier-mediated transport and the characteristics of transport processes have been studied for several years, the actual molecular mechanisms involved are not clear. Many carrier molecules are believed to be membrane-bound proteins (eg, glycoprotein) that become activated (capable of picking up and transporting) when the membrane becomes energized through the breakdown of ATP. On activation of the transport protein and its attachment to the substance to be transported, the protein changes its position in the membrane in a manner that effects the transfer of the substance from one side of the membrane to the other, as illustrated in Figure 1-21. Evidence also indicates that the binding of some substances to receptors on the membrane causes a pore or channel to form, thereby providing a less restrictive pathway for the passive movement of materials (eg, ions) across the membrane.[2]

Many types of solutes such as glucose, amino acids, and various inorganic ions (eg, $Na^+$, $Cl^-$, $K^+$) are transported across plasma membranes by carrier molecules. Some of these transport systems are active and others are passive. In general, carrier-mediated transport systems often display one or more of the following characteristics:

1. *Specificity*. Carrier systems are generally specific for a particular solute. For example, the system which transports glucose will not transport other organic solutes such as amino acids.
2. *Saturation*. Many systems have a maximum rate (called *transport maximum,* or *Tm*) at which a solute can be transported. If more solute is present than the system can handle, the system is said to be saturated and transporting solute at maximum rate. Below saturation level, the rate of transport varies directly with solute concentration (ie, the higher the solute concentration, the faster the rate of transport).
3. *Competition*. If the same carrier system transports two different solutes in the same direction, the rate of transport of each will be diminished by the presence of the other. In other words, the solutes compete for transport by the carrier, and some of each solute will be transported at the carrier's maximum rate.
4. *Energy dependency*. Many carrier systems require energy to function. Substances (metabolic inhibitors) that interfere with energy-producing reactions of the cell often stop transport processes.
5. *Gating of protein channels*. Gating refers to opening or closing of the channels formed by protein carriers. This opening or closing can be controlled by *voltage gating* or *ligand gating*. Voltage gating refers to a response to changes in the electrical potential of the cell membrane (see pp. 24–28). Ligand gating occurs with a physical change in the protein molecule, which results from binding of another molecule with the protein. This molecule is called a *ligand*. The ligand can be a chemical mediator, such as

acetylcholine, or a highly charged ion, such as sodium or potassium.[2]

## Endocytosis and Exocytosis

Endocytosis and exocytosis are methods for bringing particles into the cell and releasing secretions to the exterior of the cell. These processes are schematically illustrated in Figure 1-8. Both are essential in carrying out the functional capabilities of specific cells.

Endocytosis refers to the bringing in of protein and other substances through invagination of the outer cell membrane. This process occurs in the following two ways:

1. *Pinocytosis* involves movement of complex proteins and some strong electrolyte solutions into the cell. The protein is seen to adhere to the outer cell membrane, which stimulates invagination of the membrane. The material is encased or enclosed in a vesicle and floats into the cytoplasm. Lysosomes attach to the vesicle surface, release hydrolytic enzymes into the vesicle, and the enzymes break down the complex material for use within the cell. A residual body may be left within the vesicle or excreted through the cell membrane to the ECF. This process may be enhanced by cell membrane receptors which bind the ligands and internalize them rapidly. These coated vesicles allow for internalization of specific molecules without the ingestion of excess water. Once the coated vesicles are ingested, the lysosomes attach and process the material.[2]
2. *Phagocytosis* involves essentially the same process but the material brought into the cell is frequently a microorganism, especially a bacterium (see Chap. 20).

Exocytosis has been termed *reverse pinocytosis* and is an active release of soluble products to the ECF. Secretion granules are formed, as described earlier, by the Golgi complex. The formed secretion granules move to the inner cell membrane, adhere, and cause an outpouching of the membrane. The outpouched area ruptures and releases the contents of the secretion granules into the ECF. The secretory products are vital to maintenance of the steady state of the host and include secretions necessary for digestion, glandular secretion, neural transmission, and so on.

Both endocytosis and exocytosis require energy and are affected by cellular ability to synthesize ATP. Both processes require enzymatic activity to enhance the rate of the reactions.

## CELL MOVEMENT

Many cells exhibit the ability to move. Movement may involve locomotion from one place to another or it may involve movement of microtubules and microfilaments within the cell. Ciliary and flagellar movement are examples of microtubular and microfilament movement (see p. 12). Two additional forms of cell movement are ameboid locomotion and muscular contraction.

## Ameboid Locomotion

Ameboid locomotion refers to the ability of a cell to move from one location to another in a manner similar to the way a unicellar animal, called an amoeba, moves in its fluid environment. In the embryo, most of the cells exhibit ameboid motion by which they migrate to their appropriate location. This property of ameboid movement is retained by certain defensive cells of the body, especially the leukocytes, and allows them to move from the bloodstream to the tissue spaces to contact and destroy a foreign protein (see Chap. 12).

Using energy (ATP) and calcium ions, the process is accomplished by the forward projection of a portion of the cell called the *pseudopodium* (Figure 1-23). It probably depends on contraction of microfilaments in the outer portion of the cytoplasm to push out or project the pseudopodium. The remainder of the cell follows the projected area with a streaming motion. This process allows for the rapid movement of cells into an area.

## Muscular Contraction

Approximately 50% of the body mass is skeletal, smooth, and cardiac muscle. Contraction of these muscles make possible both involuntary and voluntary movements of the body. The details of muscular contraction are further described in Chapters 22, 40, and 44.

Both electrical and mechanical processes exist in muscle, with the initiation of most contractions through electrical stimulation from the nerve terminals. The electrical events are followed immediately by the mechanical

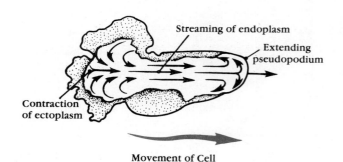

**FIGURE 1–23.**
Method of ameboid motion of a cell, showing contraction of ectoplasm, extended pseudopodium, and streaming of endoplasm toward the projected pseudopodium.

events in a sequential way. Electrical activation causes depolarization, which initiates the mechanical movement of contractile proteins between each other and causes a shortening of the muscle fiber. The muscle fiber is illustrated in Figure 1-24, which shows the subunits of the fiber and the form of two contractile proteins called *actin* and *myosin*.

Skeletal muscle has a striated appearance because of its regularly ordered proteins. These proteins make up the contractile portions of the muscle fiber. The process of skeletal muscle contraction basically follows a course: a nerve stimulation causes the release of acetylcholine at the neuromuscular junction. Acetylcholine, a chemical neurotransmitter, causes a change in muscle cell ion permeability, generating an *action potential* that is spread throughout the muscle cell membrane and to the T tu-

bules that carry the stimulus to the interior of the cell (see Figure 1-24). The transfer of stimulus by T tubules to the sarcoplasmic reticulum (SR) causes release of calcium from the SR. Calcium binds with the inhibitory protein *troponin*, causing troponin to interact with another protein, *tropomyosin*, resulting in the uncovering of the active sites on actin, which allows for free interaction with myosin. The actin filament is then pulled along the myosin filament, causing shortening of the entire sarcomere unit (Figure 1-25). Calcium is immediately taken back up into the SR, and troponin and tropomyosin regain their normal inhibitory function. Large quantities of ATP are necessary to provide energy to pump the calcium back into the SR. During this process, sodium also leaks into the cell. The sodium pump must be activated to prevent accumulation of water in the muscle cell.

Cardiac muscle is also striated and follows the same general pattern for contraction, but exhibits basic differences. Cardiac muscle is rapidly depolarized and contracts immediately after stimulation, but repolarizes much more slowly than skeletal muscle. This slow repolarization apparently protects cardiac muscle from tetany, a phenomenon that may occur in skeletal muscle. Also, impulses depolarize the entire muscle mass, either atrial or ventricular, rather than individual fibers, as seen with skeletal muscle. This characteristic occurs because the individual cells within cardiac muscle are connected to one another by low resistance electrical bridges (intercalated discs) that allow the electrical impulse to spread from cell to cell (Figure 1-26).

Smooth muscle cells are smaller than skeletal muscle cells. They form two major types of muscle units, *multiunit smooth muscle* and *visceral smooth muscle*. Multiunit smooth muscle is independently innervated by nerve signals and includes the piloerector muscles of hairs ("gooseflesh"), smooth muscle of larger blood vessels, and several muscles of the eye. Visceral smooth muscles are usually arranged in sheets, and the cell membranes contact each other so that ions can flow freely from one cell to the next. Contractions of visceral muscles are relatively slow and can be sustained for periods of up to 30 seconds. Rhythmic contractions or waves of contractions, such as intestinal peristalsis, result from the influence of nerve impulses, as well as from many chemical agents (see Chap. 40).

## ELECTRICAL PROPERTIES OF CELLS

Differences in electrical potential across the plasma membrane are characteristic of all living cells. The membrane potential exists because of unequal distribution of ions between the inner and outer surfaces of the membrane, the membrane's different permeability to various ions, and active transport systems that maintain ionic imbalance across the membrane.

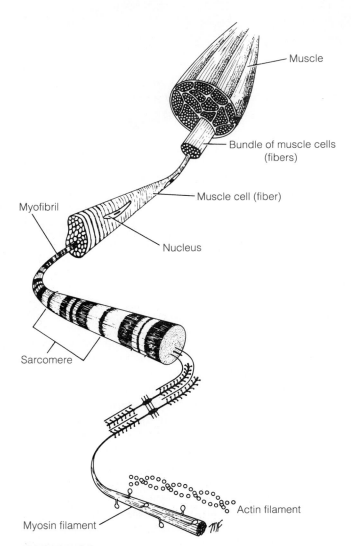

**FIGURE 1-24.**
Gross to microscopic components of a skeletal muscle fiber. (From R.S. Snell, *Clinical Histology for Medical Students.* Boston: Little, Brown, 1984.)

Muscle

Bundle of muscle cells (fibers)

Muscle cell (fiber)

Myofibril

Nucleus

Sarcomere

Actin filament

Myosin filament

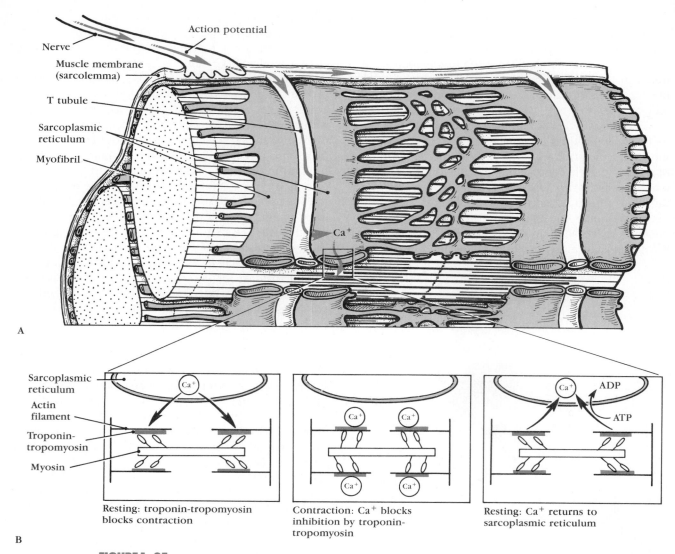

Nerve

Action potential

Muscle membrane
(sarcolemma)

T tubule

Sarcoplasmic
reticulum

Myofibril

Ca⁺

A

Sarcoplasmic
reticulum

Actin
filament

Troponin-
tropomyosin

Myosin

Ca⁺

Resting: troponin-tropomyosin
blocks contraction

Ca⁺    Ca⁺

Ca⁺    Ca⁺

Contraction: Ca⁺ blocks
inhibition by troponin-
tropomyosin

Ca⁺    ADP

ATP

Resting: Ca⁺ returns to
sarcoplasmic reticulum

B

**FIGURE 1–25.**
**A.** Schematic representation of depolarizing stimulus through a T tubule. **B.** Actin and myosin filament in the relaxed and contracted state.

The electrical charge for the inside of the cell is more negative than the outside. This *resting membrane potential* normally is about -70 to -85 millivolts from the inside to the outside of the cell when the cell is in the resting state. This equilibrium is attained and maintained through the sodium-potassium pump.

Some cells have the ability to respond to various types of stimuli, especially electrochemical stimuli. This response is called the cell's *excitability* and refers to the changing or altering of the electrical potential across the cell membrane. Two major types of cells, nerve and muscle, are considered to be excitable cells because they can change membrane potential, effect an action or response, and return to the resting state.

The excitable tissue or cell receives a stimulus, which rapidly changes its resting membrane potential. This action potential is followed by the action of the cell,

which may be a contraction, transmitting the action potential to the next cell, or other actions. The cell then returns to the normal resting state characterized by re-establishment of the resting membrane potential.

Many changes occur in the cell membranes when an *action potential* is elicited. The following discussion of the action potential is with reference to a neuron, but applies with minor variation to other excitable cells, such as skeletal and cardiac muscle.

When an adequate positive stimulus is applied to the neuron, a rapid and marked change occurs in the *membrane potential* at the point on the membrane of stimulus application. The positive stimulus increases the sodium permeability of the membrane, allowing sodium to begin entering the cell at a faster rate than it can be pumped out. As more sodium passes through the membrane, the membrane potential becomes less negative

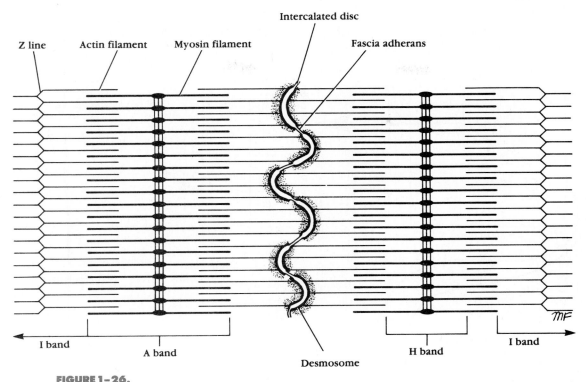

**FIGURE 1-26.**
Schematic microscopic representation of myocardial muscle cell. (From R.S. Snell, *Clinical Histology for Medical Students*. Boston: Little, Brown, 1984.)

(Figure 1-27). When the membrane potential has been reduced to a critical value called the *threshold*, additional sodium channels open, increasing the membrane's sodium permeability even more, resulting in a rapid influx of sodium. The membrane potential approaches zero and then actually becomes reversed, so the inside of the membrane is positive with respect to the outside. These changes characterize *depolarization* of the membrane.

Almost immediately after sodium influx begins to depolarize the membrane, an increase in potassium diffusion out of the cell begins and accelerates as the movement of sodium causes the inside of the membrane to become positive. Potassium leaves the cell for the same reasons that sodium entered—favorable electrical and chemical gradients coupled with an increase in membrane permeability. As potassium efflux accelerates, further diffusion of sodium into the cell is inhibited by a decrease in sodium permeability, and the net loss of positive charges ($K^+$) from the inside causes the membrane potential to return to zero and then become negative once again, reestablishing the resting potential. More potassium leaves the cell than is actually required to restore the resting potential. For a short time, the inside of the membrane is more negative than it normally is at rest. This increased internal negativity is termed *hyperpolarization*. The return of the membrane potential to resting level is completed by the $Na^+$-$K^+$ pump, which exchanges internal sodium for external potassium, thereby restoring the normal internal:external ratios of these ions.

The preceding activities that restore the resting membrane potential after depolarization of the membrane collectively characterize the phenomenon of *repolarization*.

The graphic representation (voltage versus time) of membrane depolarization and repolarization is called the action potential (see Figure 1-27). The duration of the action potential for a neuron is less than 0.5 msec. It must be remembered that the action potential represents the change in membrane potential only in the region of the membrane where an adequate positive stimulus has been applied. The entire plasma membrane does not simultaneously depolarize and then repolarize in response to an adequate stimulus. Once an action potential is generated, however, it spreads from one area of the membrane to another, resulting in the propagation of a nerve impulse.

A nerve impulse is a wave of depolarization followed by a wave of repolarization that travels along a nerve fiber away from the point of stimulation (Figure 1-28). When an adequate positive stimulus, one of sufficient strength or duration to reduce the membrane potential to *threshold* (sometimes called a threshold stimulus), is applied to the fiber, the membrane will depolarize, with the inside becoming positive with respect to the outside.

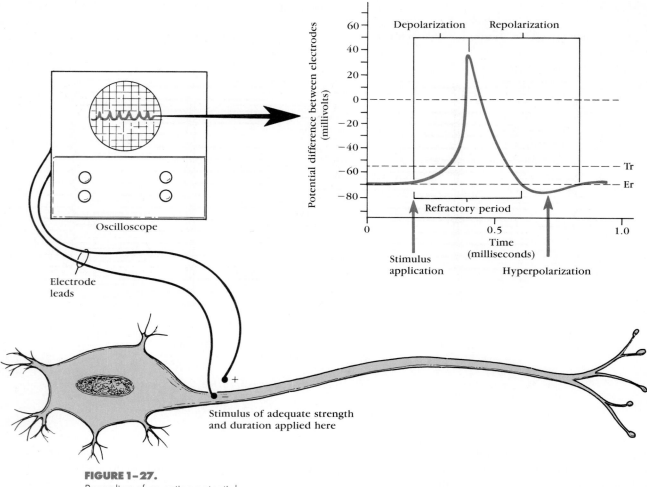

**FIGURE 1–27.**

Recording of an action potential.

Adjacent areas of the membrane remain polarized, inside negative, resulting in the flow of electrical current as positive charges are attracted to adjacent negative charges (see Figure 1-28). The flow of current reduces the membrane potential in adjacent areas of the membrane to threshold, allowing sodium to move in and depolarization to occur. The sequence of one area of depolarization inducing depolarization in an adjacent area results in a wave of depolarization that is propagated along the nerve fiber in a manner similar to the burning of a gunpowder fuse. As soon as the wave of depolarization passes a segment of the fiber, that segment is repolarized and its ability to respond to another stimulus is soon restored.

If an adequate (threshold) stimulus is applied to a nerve fiber, an action potential is generated at the site of stimulus and propagated away from the site. Once generated, each impulse is conducted in an identical manner without change in magnitude or velocity. Stimuli that fail individually or collectively to reduce the membrane potential to threshold fail to generate an action potential and therefore a nerve impulse. The response of a nerve

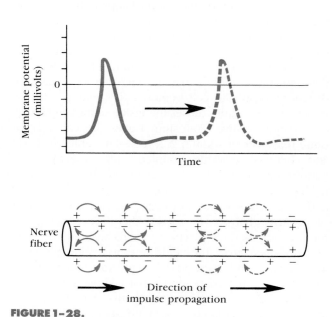

**FIGURE 1–28.**

Propagation of an action potential along nonmyelinated nerve fiber.

fiber to a stimulus is either maximal or zero. This property is the *all-or-none law*. In other words, weak stimuli do not generate weak impulses and strong stimuli, strong impulses.

After an action potential has been generated, a minimum amount of time is required before that area of the membrane becomes capable of responding in an identical manner to a second stimulus. This minimum period is called the *refractory period*. The length of the refractory period determines the maximum number of impulses that the fiber can conduct each second. Fibers with short refractory periods can conduct impulses at a higher frequency than fibers with long refractory periods.

## CELL ORGANIZATION

Although cells are the basic structural and functional units of the body, those that share a common function,

such as lining a body cavity or providing for movement of the skeleton, are organized into *tissues*. In turn, tissues are organized into more complex structures known as *organs*. Organs that share a common purpose, such as the formation and excretion of urine, are grouped into *systems,* which collectively make up the body.

The four basic types of tissues that compose the body are epithelial, muscular, nervous, and connective.

## Epithelial Tissues

Epithelial tissue provides a covering of most of the internal and external surfaces of the body. In this way, it may function as a protective barrier or it may be involved with absorption of materials, excretion of waste products, and secretion of specialized products into the cavities.

Epithelial tissue is classified according to its thick-

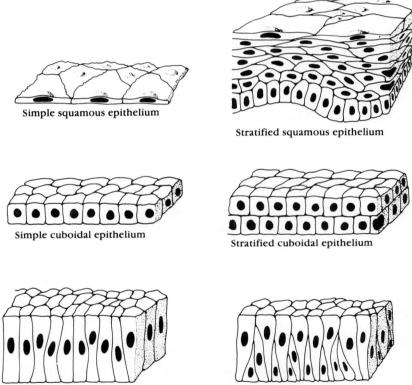

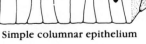

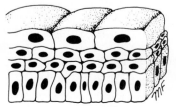

**FIGURE 1–29.**
Different types of epithelium. (From R.S. Snell, *Clinical Histology for Medical Students.* Boston: Little, Brown, 1984.)

Transitional epithelium

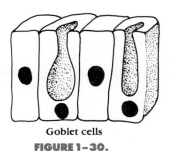
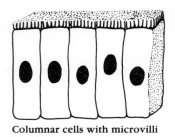
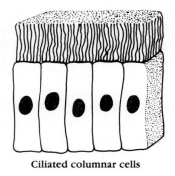

Goblet cells    Columnar cells with microvilli    Ciliated columnar cells

**FIGURE 1–30.**

Specialized columnar cells. (From R.S. Snell, *Clinical Histology for Medical Students.* Boston: Little, Brown, 1984.)

ness in number of layers. Simple squamous epithelium exists as single layers of flattened, pancakelike cells.

Simple cuboidal epithelial cells assume the appearance of cubes. Simple columnar epithelial cells have the appearance of columns (Figure 1-29).

Squamous epithelial cells may occur in single or multiple layers. Single layers allow for diffusion of material across the cell wall, while multiple layers provide for continuous replenishment or regeneration of cells. Simple squamous cells line the heart and blood vessels, form the alveoli, and exist in many other areas.

Cuboidal epithelial cells usually occur in single layers and frequently function in forming secretions. These

cells line the ducts and are the parenchymal cells of many glands.

Columnar epithelial cells, in various forms, line the walls of the gastrointestinal and respiratory systems and are involved with the secretion of mucus. They may exist as *goblet cells* or have projections called microvilli or cilia present on their surfaces (Figure 1-30).

Stratified squamous epithelium exists in multiple layers that replenish superficial layers as they are sloughed off. The skin is an excellent example of stratified squamous epithelium, but this tissue also lines the mouth, esophagus, vagina, and pharynx.

Transitional epithelial cells are usually considered to

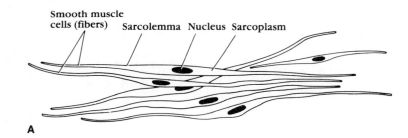

Smooth muscle cells (fibers)    Sarcolemma    Nucleus    Sarcoplasm

**A**

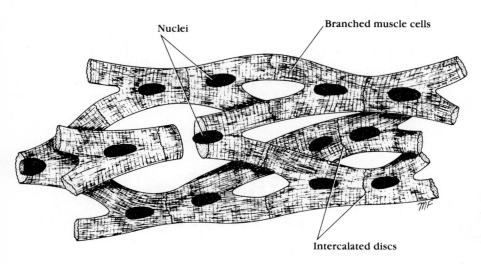

Nuclei    Branched muscle cells

Intercalated discs

**FIGURE 1–31.**

**A.** Group of smooth muscle cells (fibers). **B.** Group of branched cardiac muscle cells (fibers). (From R.S. Snell, *Clinical Histology for Medical Students.* Boston: Little, Brown, 1984.)

be cuboidal, except that their appearance varies depending on the stretch of the organ. Thus, at different times, they appear to be flattened or spheric. They are best exemplified by the epithelial cells in the bladder.

## Muscular Tissue

The microstructure and functions of the muscle cells that make up muscle tissues are discussed in depth in Chapter 43. In general, muscles are classified as skeletal, cardiac, or visceral according to their appearance and function (Figure 1-31; see also Figure 1-24).

Striated skeletal muscle provides for voluntary movement of the body. The characteristic striated appearance results from an ordered sequence of contractile proteins. These proteins form or constitute numerous myofibrils, the contractile units of the muscle cell. Skeletal muscle cells are multinucleate, with the nuclei located at the periphery of the cell under the cell membrane.

Cardiac muscle forms the walls of the heart, which are the working, or contractile, portions of this organ. Its appearance is similar to that of striated skeletal muscle, except that a nucleus is centrally located and the myocardial cells lie very closely approximated one to another. The importance of myocardial construction in relation to cardiac contraction is detailed in Chapter 22.

Visceral or smooth muscle does not exhibit the characteristic striations of skeletal or cardiac muscle, but smooth muscle cells have many fibrils that extend the length of the cell. A single nucleus lies near the center of each cell. Smooth muscle cells are located in the viscera, blood vessels, uterus, and many other areas.

## Nervous Tissue

Nervous tissue is made up of neurons, the cells that conduct nerve impulses, and glial cells that provide structural and functional support for the neurons. The typical nerve cell has a large central nucleus, multiple dendrites, and a single axon (Figure 1-32). The function of the neuron is described in Chapter 48.

## Connective Tissue

Connective tissue generally forms the framework for other cells and helps to bind together various tissues and organs. Many types of cells are included in the classification of connective tissue (Figure 1-33). Blood cells, described in detail in Unit 7, are specialized connective tissue cells.

Loose connective tissue (areolar tissue) contains numerous cells, especially fibroblasts and macrophages. It also attaches the skin to the body and helps to hold the

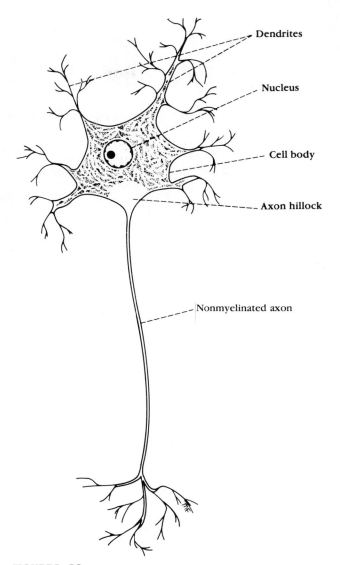

**FIGURE 1-32.**
A neuron. (From R.S. Snell, *Clinical Histology for Medical Students.* Boston: Little, Brown, 1984.)

organs and blood vessels in place. Spaces between cells allow for fluid storage and discharge of cellular products that are then returned to the bloodstream.

Dense irregular connective tissue is compact and forms the reticular layer of the dermis of the skin. Sheets of this tissue form sheaths of many types that can withstand stretching in the direction in which their fibers run. The layers of the dermis are composed of cells that constantly undergo synthesis and degradation. Collagen fibers interlace with each other to provide strength to the dermis. Collagen is a fibrous, insoluble protein that is an important part of connective tissue. Elastic fibers lie randomly dispersed throughout the dermis, which allows for flexibility.

Dense regular connective tissue is composed of

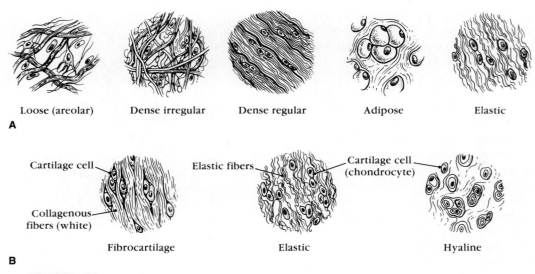

Loose (areolar)    Dense irregular    Dense regular    Adipose    Elastic

**A**

Cartilage cell

Collagenous
fibers (white)

Fibrocartilage

Elastic fibers

Elastic

Cartilage cell
(chondrocyte)

Hyaline

**B**

**FIGURE 1–33.**
**A.** Types of connective tissues. **B.** Types of cartilage.

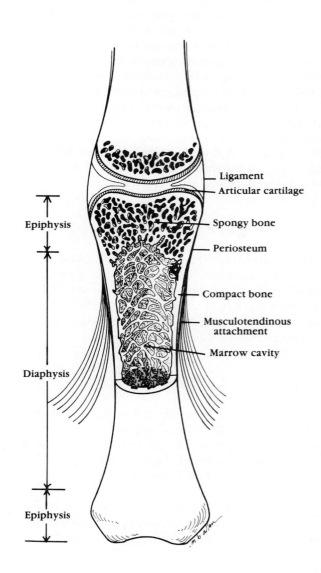

Ligament

Articular cartilage

Epiphysis

Spongy bone

Periosteum

Compact bone

Diaphysis

Musculotendinous
attachment

Marrow cavity

Epiphysis

**FIGURE 1–34.**
Vertical section through the proximal part of the femur shows the
arrangement of compact and spongy (cancellous) bone. (From
M. Borysenko et al., *Functional Histology* [2nd ed.]. Boston: Little,
Brown, 1984.)

white fibrous material. The cells are mainly fibrocytes, located in a regular or ordered plane. Rows of fibrocytes with large amounts of intracellular substance, especially collagen, form the tendons that attach muscle to bone. Ligaments that attach bone to bone and fascia that provide the coverings for muscles are included in this category of connective tissue. The aponeuroses, which are similar to tendons with a wider base, function to attach muscles to other structures.

Adipose tissue cells are those in which the cytoplasm is filled with lipid or fatty material. This storage area for lipids serves as a protective and insulating layer in the body. Layers of adipose tissue are normally present around the kidneys and intestines. In many areas of the body, substances not metabolized within the cell are converted to fat. This process is greatly influenced by insulin, a pancreatic hormone (see Chap. 39).

Elastic connective tissue allows for the properties of elasticity and extensibility, especially in the arteries and vocal cords. This is further discussed in Units 8 and 9.

Types of cartilage, a connective tissue that is made up of cells called chondrocytes, differ depending on the number of associated collagenous fibers. It provides structural strength with some degree of flexibility. It is present in the costal cartilage, trachea, intervertebral disks, external ear, and other areas. In children, the long bones have two ends, a diaphysis and an epiphysis, separated by epiphyseal cartilage, which allows for bone length to increase. Growth in length occurs as cartilage cells grow away from the shaft and are replaced by bone, resulting in an increased length of the shaft. When maturity is reached, this cartilage is entirely replaced by bone, a process called closure of the epiphysis (see Chap. 45).

Bone, the hardest of the connective tissues, provides the structural framework of the body, as well as a plentiful reservoir for the minerals calcium and phosphorus. It is composed of cells, fibers, and extracellular components, which are calcified and rigid. This material encloses the hematopoietic marrow, which supplies most of the blood cells of the body. Periosteum covers most bones and is lacking only in special areas. Bone tissue is organized in two ways: compact or cancellous (spongy) (Figure 1-34). *Compact bone* forms a solid mass and has few spaces in its continuity. *Cancellous bone* forms a network of intercommunicating projections called trabeculae. Compact bone generally is located on the outer shell, while spongy bone is usually in the internal framework. The principal cells of adult bone are osteocytes, which with the other bone cells—osteoblasts, osteoclasts, and osteoprogenitor cells—form and repair the bone tissue (see Chap. 45).

All of these distinct cells may be different functional states of the same cell type. Bone cells adjust their number in proportion to the amount of physical stress placed on them. For example, increased deposition of collagen fibers and inorganic salts occurs in response to prolonged increase in workload. Conversely, salts are pulled from bone when stress or weight bearing is decreased.

## REFERENCES

1. Hille, B. Membranes and Ions. In H.D. Patton et al., *Textbook of Physiology* (21st ed.). Philadelphia: W.B. Saunders, 1989.
2. Guyton, A.C. *Human Physiology and Mechanisms of Disease* (4th ed.). Philadelphia: W.B. Saunders, 1987.
3. Slauson, D.O., and Cooper, B.J. *Mechanisms of Disease* (2nd ed.). Baltimore: Williams & Wilkins, 1990.

# Alterations in Cellular Processes

## *Chapter Outline*

▶ **Stimuli That Can Cause Cellular Injury or Adaptation**
    **Physical Agents**
    **Chemical Agents**
    **Microorganisms**
    **Hypoxia**
    **Genetic Defects**
    **Nutritional Imbalances**
    **Immunologic Reactions**

▶ **Intracellular and Extracellular Changes Resulting from Cellular Adaptation or Injury**
    **Cellular Swelling**
    **Lipid Accumulation**
    **Free Radicals**
    **Glycogen Depositions**
    **Pigmentation**
    **Calcification**
    **Hyaline Infiltration**
▶ **Cellular Changes Due to Injurious Stimuli**
    **Atrophy**
    **Dysplasia**
    **Hypertrophy**
    **Hyperplasia**
    **Metaplasia**

▶ **Causes of Anoxic Cellular Injury and Death**
    **Ischemia**
    **Thrombosis**
    **Embolism**
    **Infarction**
    **Necrosis**
        **Coagulative Necrosis**
        **Colliquative Necrosis**
        **Special Types**
    **Somatic Death**

## *Learning Objectives*

1. Define *adaptation*.
2. Describe alterations in cells that can occur because of stimuli.
3. List the seven categories of stimuli that can cause cellular alterations.
4. Differentiate between endogenous and exogenous substances.
5. Describe the abnormal intracellular accumulations that result from noxious stimulation.
6. Discuss briefly extracellular changes resulting from cellular adaptation or injury.
7. Discuss the role of free radicals in the production of cell injury and death.

8. Define the common pigments that may accumulate in the cytoplasm.
9. Discriminate among the following pathologic cellular adaptations: atrophy, dysplasia, hypertrophy, hyperplasia, and metaplasia.
10. Define *autophagic vacuoles* and *residual bodies*.
11. Differentiate between ischemia and infarction.
12. Define and describe the factors that can produce thrombosis and embolism.
13. Describe the pathologic characteristic of infarcts.
14. Specify areas in which bacterial supergrowth may occur.
15. List and describe the major types of necrosis.
16. Explain the major changes that occur after somatic death.

The life cycle of a cell exists on a continuum that includes normal activities and adaptation, injury, or lethal changes. Adaptation may be the result of normal life cycle adjustments, such as growth during puberty or the changes of pregnancy. Stressful lifestyles produce physiologic changes that may lead to adaptation or disease. Other changes occur as the result of the aging process (see Unit 2). The pathologic changes exhibited may be obvious or very difficult to detect. The cell constantly makes adjustments to a changing, hostile environment to keep the organism functioning in a normal steady state. These adaptive adjustments are necessary to ensure the survival

**TABLE 2-1.**
STIMULI THAT CAN CAUSE CELLULAR INJURY

| STIMULI | INJURY |
| --- | --- |
| Physical agents | Trauma, thermal or electrical changes, irradiation |
| Chemical agents | Drugs, poisons, foods, toxic and irritating substances |
| Microorganisms | Viruses, bacteria, fungi, protozoa |
| Hypoxia | Shock, localized areas of inadequate blood supply, hypoxemia |
| Genetic defects | Inborn errors of metabolism, gross malformations |
| Nutritional imbalances | Protein-calorie malnutrition, excessive intake of fats, carbohydrates, and proteins |
| Immunologic reactions | Hypersensitivity reactions to foreign proteins |

of the organism. Adaptive changes may be temporary or permanent. The point at which an adapted cell becomes an injured cell is the point at which the cell cannot functionally keep up with the stressful environment affecting it. Injured cells exhibit alterations that may affect body function and be manifested as disease.[7]

Prevention of disease is dependent upon the capacity of the affected cells to undergo self-repair and regeneration. This process of repair prevents cellular injury and death, and may prevent the death of the host.

Specifically, adaptation is a return of the internal environment of the body to the steady state or normal balance after exposure to some alteration. The rigid electrolyte and water balance between the intracellular fluid (ICF) and extracellular fluid (ECF) must be maintained (see Chap. 8). The steady state may be attained at the expense of altered intracellular metabolism and may continue for a certain period of time, after which the cell, no longer able to adapt, may undergo injurious or lethal changes.

When cells are confronted with a stimulus that alters normal cellular metabolism, they may do any one or more of the following: (1) increase concentrations of normal cellular constituents; (2) accumulate abnormal substances; (3) change the cellular size or number; or (4) undergo a lethal change. These concepts are considered briefly in this chapter and delineated further in specific content areas. Categories of stimuli that can provoke changes and the types of changes that may occur are discussed in this chapter.

## STIMULI THAT CAN CAUSE CELLULAR INJURY OR ADAPTATION

Because the cell is constantly making adjustments to a changing, hostile environment, many agents potentially can cause cellular injury or adaptation. Cellular injury may lead to further injury and death of the cell, or the cell may respond to the noxious stimulation by undergoing a change that enables it to tolerate the invasion.

Stimuli that can alter the steady state are categorized as follows: (1) physical agents, (2) chemical agents, (3) microorganisms, (4) hypoxia, (5) genetic defects, (6) nutritional imbalances, and (7) immunologic reactions (Table 2-1).

### Physical Agents

Physical agents are factors such as mechanical trauma, temperature gradients, electrical stimulation, atmospheric pressure gradients, and irradiation. Physical stimuli directly damage cells, cause rupture or damage of the cell walls, and disrupt cellular reproduction. In addition to the direct damage from the physical agent, hypoxia may increase the extent of the injury.[7] Local swelling may decrease the microcirculation and produce hypoxia to the tissues.

### Chemical Agents

Chemical agents that can cause injury may include simple compounds, such as glucose, or complex agents, such as poisons. Therapeutic drugs often chemically disrupt the normal cellular balance. Chemicals produce a wide range of physiologic effects. Some chemicals directly damage the cells and cell membranes that they contact. Others may be taken into the cell and disrupt energy production or they may be changed within the cell to toxic metabolites.[7,9] The amount of disruption results in the ultimate outcome.

### Microorganisms

Microorganisms cause cellular injury in a variety of ways depending on the type of organism and the innate defense of the human body. Some bacteria secrete exotoxins, which are injurious to the host. Others liberate endotoxins when they are destroyed. Viruses interfere with the metabolism of the host cells and cause cellular injury by releasing viral proteins toxic to the cell (see Chap. 12).

## Hypoxia

Hypoxia is the most common cause of cellular injury and may be produced by inadequate oxygen in the blood or by decreased perfusion of blood to the tissues. The end results are disturbance of cellular metabolism and local or generalized release of lactic acid. Cellular and organ dysfunction result from lack of oxygen. This may lead to cellular, organ, and even somatic death. When cells try to adapt to the lack of oxygen, anaerobic cellular metabolism results in metabolic acidosis (see Chap. 9).

## Genetic Defects

Genetic defects can affect cellular metabolism through inborn errors of metabolism or gross malformations. The mechanisms for cellular disruption vary widely with the genetic defect but may result in intracellular accumulation of abnormal material (see Chap. 3).

## Nutritional Imbalances

Nutritional imbalances produce sickness and death in over one-half of the world's population. The imbalances include serious deficiencies of proteins and vitamins especially. Malnutrition may be primary or secondary, depending upon whether it is a socioeconomic problem in the underprivileged areas of the world or is self-induced or disease-induced. No matter what the cause, nutritional deficiency is a significant cause of cellular dysfunction and death. On the other hand, excessive food intake leads to nutritional imbalances and cell injury through the production of excessive lipids in the body. Excessive fat intake has been shown to be associated with cardiovascular diseases, and respiratory and gastrointestinal disorders.[2,6]

## Immunologic Reactions

Immunologic agents may cause cellular injury, especially when hypersensitivity reactions occur, causing the release of excess histamine and other substances. The cellular response to immunologic injury is inflammation, production of scar tissue, and even tissue death. Certain structures, such as the renal nephrons, are especially susceptible to immunologic damage. Immunologic injury is discussed in more detail in Chapter 16.

## INTRACELLULAR AND EXTRACELLULAR CHANGES RESULTING FROM CELLULAR ADAPTATION OR INJURY

Abnormal intracellular accumulations often result from an environmental change or an inability of the cell to process materials. Normal or abnormal substances that cannot be metabolized may accumulate in the cytoplasm. These substances may be endogenous (produced within the body) or exogenous (produced in the environment) and stored by an originally normal cell. Examples of abnormal exogenous substances include carbon particles, silica, and metals that are deposited and accumulate because the cell cannot degrade them or transport them to other sites.[1]

Common changes in and around cells include swelling, lipid accumulation in organs, glycogen depositions, pigments, calcification, and hyaline infiltration. These changes may be resolved or they may become permanent.

## Cellular Swelling

Cellular swelling is the initial response to disruption of cellular metabolism. It occurs most frequently with cellular hypoxia which impairs the cell's ability to synthesize adenosine triphosphate (ATP). It results in a shift of ECF to the intracellular compartment, causing cloudy intracellular swelling with enlargement of the cell.[3,5] Ultimately, organs are affected. Cellular swelling is frequently reversible when sufficient oxygen is delivered to the cell and normal ATP synthesis resumes. However, as the cell swells and injury progresses, damage to the cell membrane occurs, causing a true increase in its permeability.[7] When large molecules and enzymes leak out of (or into) the cell, severe injury or death results.[7] Continued accumulation of water in the cells often has the appearance of small or large vacuoles of water, which may represent portions of endoplasmic reticulum (ER) that have been sequestered.[4,5]

## Lipid Accumulation

Lipid accumulation refers to a fatty change process that occurs in the cytoplasm of parenchymal cells of certain organs. Fat droplets accumulate in the intracellular ER and Golgi complex as a result of improper metabolism.[9] The most common location for fatty change is the liver, but the heart and kidneys also can undergo fatty change when placed under abnormal stimulation.

Large, fatty intracellular accumulations have been shown to stimulate progressive necrosis, fibrosis, and scarring of organs. This leads to functional impairment of the involved organ.

Fatty change of the liver is very common. Pathologically, the liver is enlarged, yellow, greasy-looking, and infiltration may involve all or only a portion of the organ.[5] Microscopically, the cytoplasm may become filled with lipid, which pushes the nucleus and other cytoplasmic structures to one side (Figure 2-1). The pre-

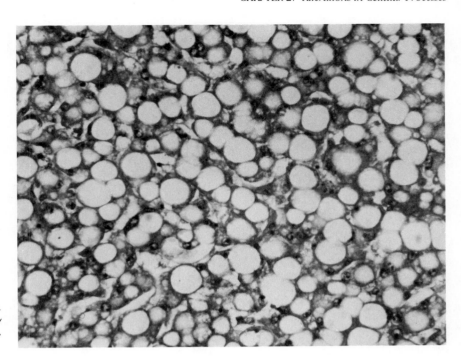

**FIGURE 2-1.**
Fatty change of the liver. (Magnification before reduction: ×400) (From F. Miller, *Peery and Miller's Pathology* [3rd ed.]. Boston: Little, Brown, 1978.)

dominant lipid involved in fatty change of the liver is triglyceride; its presence may be a result of increased synthesis or decreased secretion of this lipid from the cell.[2] This fatty change is the initial change seen in the alcoholic liver because alcohol increases free fatty acid mobilization, decreases triglyceride use, blocks lipoprotein excretion, and directly damages ER through the liberation of free radicals (see below). Protein-calorie malnutrition (PCM) causes a decrease in synthesis of cellular proteins necessary for attaching to and transporting the lipids from the cell, so that fatty change also occurs in PCM.[2,6] Other hepatotoxins such as carbon tetrachloride ($CCl_4$), may also cause this change.[5] The fibrous scarring of cirrhosis, discussed in Chapter 43, appears to result from a reaction to the lipid infiltration in the cytoplasm of hepatocytes.

The cells of the heart and kidneys also undergo fatty change under abnormal stimulation. It most commonly occurs in the heart after chronic hypoxia and may be patchy or diffuse. If diffuse, severe infections or toxic states are usually the causative factors. The kidneys show increased fatty change around the proximal convoluted tubules of the nephrons, often induced by exposure to certain nephrotoxins or poisons.[9]

Associated with intracellular lipid accumulation is *interstitial fatty infiltration*, a condition that occurs with obesity. Fat cells accumulate between the parenchymal cells of an organ, probably as a result of the transformation of interstitial connective tissue cells to fat cells.[5] This condition rarely seems to affect the function of the organ and localizes most frequently in the heart and pancreas of the extremely obese individual. Other effects of obesity involve fat cells laid down during gestation, during the first year of life, and immediately after puberty. The obese child develops an increased number of fat cells that remain for life but decrease in size after weight loss.[6] Adult-onset obesity, for the most part, occurs when caloric intake exceeds energy requirements and the excess is converted to fat. Areas of subcutaneous fat distribution are related to hereditary characteristics.

## Free Radicals

The generation of free radicals has been extensively studied as a mechanism of cell injury. Free radicals arise as a consequence of cellular oxidation-reduction reactions involving enzymatic and nonenzymatic reactions (Figure 2-2). The hydroxyl radical ($\cdot OH$) is particularly reactive, especially close to its site of formation.[7] Other free radicals can cause damage at some distance to the initial event.[7] Particularly dangerous is the *lipid peroxidation* process which, in several reactions, results in lipid peroxides which are unstable and break down to produce aldehydes and organic free radicals. This becomes a self-propagating interaction that can cause widespread membrane damage.[7] The membranes of intracellular organelles are very susceptible to lipid peroxidation. The end result is organelle dysfunction, especially for protein synthesis. Some of the free radicals are oxygen derived (superoxide anion, $O_2\text{-}$), and these may be released when ischemic tissue is reperfused, causing rapid cell death.[7]

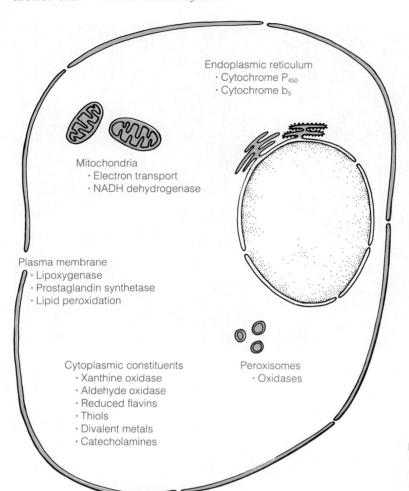

Endoplasmic reticulum
· Cytochrome $P_{450}$
· Cytochrome $b_5$

Mitochondria
· Electron transport
· NADH dehydrogenase

Plasma membrane
· Lipoxygenase
· Prostaglandin synthetase
· Lipid peroxidation

Cytoplasmic constituents
· Xanthine oxidase
· Aldehyde oxidase
· Reduced flavins
· Thiols
· Divalent metals
· Catecholamines

Peroxisomes
· Oxidases

**FIGURE 2–2.**
Cellular sources of free radicals. Free radicals can be derived via a number of cellular metabolic functions. (From D.O. Slauson and B.J. Cooper, *Mechanisms of Disease* [2nd ed.] Baltimore: Williams & Wilkins, 1990.)

Macrophages and neutrophils generate large amounts of superoxide anion during phagocytosis (see Chap. 20).

## Glycogen Depositions

Excess deposition of glycogen in organs and tissues occurs with different types of genetic disorders. One group, called *glycogen storage diseases* or *glycogenosis*, results from specific enzyme deficiencies. Different forms of glycogen accumulate in skeletal and cardiac muscle, as well as in the liver and kidneys. Glycogen disturbances also occur in diabetes mellitus with a greater than normal storage of glycogen in the proximal convoluted tubules and in the liver.[5] This disturbance is related to a deficiency in the pancreatic hormone, insulin.

## Pigmentation

Pigments are substances that have color and accumulate within the cells. Many types have been described, some

of which are normal components of cells and some abnormal ones that collect in cells under abnormal stimulation.[2] Pigments are often described as to source or origin: exogenous (outside the body) or endogenous (produced within the body).[5,8]

Lipofuscin pigmentation of the skin is common in the aging person. The pigment responsible is *lipofuscin* or *lipochrome*, which is the "wear and tear" pigment and is predominant in cells that have atrophied or are chronically injured.[2] It also may be present in the brain, liver, heart, and ovaries of an elderly individual. The pigments gradually accumulate with age and apparently do not cause cellular dysfunction.

*Melanin* is a pigment that is formed by the melanocytes of the skin. It is one of the pigments that imparts color to the skin. It also absorbs light and protects the skin from direct sun rays. Excessive deposition of melanin in the skin is common with Addison's disease (see Chap. 37), many skin conditions, and melanomas that arise from these cells. In the aged person, melanocyte activity is decreased and the skin becomes paler, with

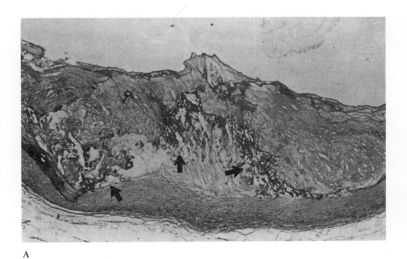

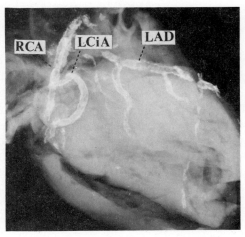

A                                                                    B

**FIGURE 2-3.**
Calcification. **A.** Photomicrograph of section of left anterior descending coronary artery. There is marked atheromatous thickening of the intima. Calcification of the wall (*arrows*) is prominent and is found microscopically at autopsy in the coronary arteries of a majority of patients over age 60 years. **B.** Radiograph of postmortem heart. Dense calcification is visible in virtually all branches of the coronary arteries, including the left anterior descending, left circumflex, and right coronary arteries. Note that the lumen in the presence of calcification may be quite adequate, but that in this patient, severe atherosclerosis has occluded the distal left anterior descending coronary artery and narrowed several branches. (From H.L. Abrams [ed.], *Coronary Arteriography.* Boston: Little, Brown, 1983.)

areas of hyperpigmentation called "liver spots" or lentigines.[5]

*Hemosiderin*, a derivative of hemoglobin, is a pigment that is formed from excess accumulation of stored iron. It is often a hemoglobin-derived substance, but may be formed due to excess intake of dietary iron or impaired use of iron. One example of localized hemosiderosis is the common *bruise*, which is an accumulation of hemosiderin after the erythrocytes in the injured area are broken down by macrophages. The excess hemoglobin thus released becomes hemosiderin. The colors occur as the hemoglobin is transformed first to biliverdin (green bile), then bilirubin (red bile), and the golden-yellow hemosiderin.[2] Deposits of hemosiderin in organs and tissues is called *hemosiderosis*, which may occur with excess of absorbed dietary iron, impaired use of iron, or the hemolytic anemias.[5] For the most part, accumulation of hemosiderin does not interfere with organ function unless it is extreme. In extreme hemosiderosis of the liver, fibrosis may result.

## Calcification

Pathologic calcification may occur in the skin, the soft tissues, blood vessels, heart, and kidneys. Normally, calcium is deposited only in the bones and teeth under the influence of various hormones. It may precipitate in areas of chronic inflammation or areas of dead or degenerating tissue.

Calcium that precipitates into areas of unresolved healing is called *dystrophic calcification* (Figure 2-3). It may be extracellular, intracellular, or both. It often localizes in the mitochondria and propagates from there. It is often a cause of organ dysfunction such as with atherosclerotic vessels or calcified cardiac valves.[2] Increased uptake of calcium into mitochondria is characteristic of injured cells.[7]

*Metastatic calcification* results from calcium-phosphorus imbalance associated with excess circulating calcium. Calcium precipitates into many areas, including kidneys, blood vessels, and connective tissue. These deposits rarely cause significant organ dysfunction.

## Hyaline Infiltration

*Hyaline* is a word that indicates a characteristic alteration within cells or in the extracellular space that appears as a homogeneous, glassy, pink inclusion on stained histologic section.[2,5] Because it does not represent a specific pattern of accumulation, different mechanisms are responsible for its formation. Intracellular hyaline changes may include excessive amounts of protein, aggregates of immunoglobulin, viral nucleoproteins, closely packed fibrils, or other substances.[1,5] Extracellular hyaline refers to the appearance of precipitated plasma proteins and other proteins across a membrane wall. This change is particularly well seen in and around the arterioles and the renal glomeruli. A variety of mechanisms causes the hyaline change, and the implications of this deposition differ depending on the underlying process.[2,9]

## CELLULAR CHANGES DUE TO INJURIOUS STIMULI

In some cases, the cell undergoes an actual change to adapt to an injurious agent. The changes often manifested are atrophy, dysplasia, hypertrophy, hyperplasia, and metaplasia. The adaptations are methods by which the cells stay alive and adjust workload to demand.

### Atrophy

Atrophy refers to a decrease in cell size resulting from decreased workload, loss of nerve supply, decreased blood supply, inadequate nutrition, or loss of hormonal stimulation.[5] The word implies previous normal development of the cell and cell loss of structural components and substance (Figure 2-4).

*Physiologic atrophy* occurs with aging in many areas and allows for survival of cells with decreased function. The cells tend to reproduce less readily. Physiologic atrophy begins in the thymus gland in early adulthood and in the uterus after menopause. Many cells in other glands and muscles also undergo atrophy with aging. These cells may develop an increase in the number of autophagic vacuoles in the cytoplasm that isolate and destroy injured organelles. The triggering mechanism for autophagia is unknown, but it may result in incompletely digested material called *residual* bodies.[2] An example of this is the lipofuscin or brownish pigment seen in the aging cell. Atrophy may progress to cellular injury and death, and the cells may be replaced with connective tissue, adipose tissue, or both.

*Disuse atrophy* is common after an extremity has been immobilized in a cast. The decreased workload placed on the affected muscles results in decreased size of the entire muscle. When the workload is again restored, the muscle often enlarges to its preinjury size.

Loss of nerve supply may also cause muscular atrophy. An example of this is the spinal cord injury that interrupts nervous stimulation to the muscles below the level of injury. The muscles gradually atrophy, and eventually musculature is replaced by fibrous tissue (see Chap. 44). Atrophy of muscles may also be seen with chronic ischemic disease of the lower extremities. The decreased blood supply impairs the metabolism within the cell, and atrophy occurs as a protective mechanism to keep the tissue viable.

### Dysplasia

Dysplasia refers to the appearance of cells that have undergone some atypical changes in response to chronic irritation. It is not a true adaptive process in that it serves

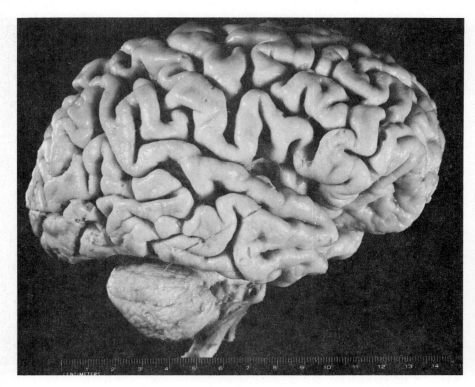

**FIGURE 2-4.**
Atrophy of the cerebral cortex. There has been pronounced shrinking of the rounded folds that normally constitute the brain's outer surface. Severe, generalized shrinkage of this sort is uncommon, and the cause is unknown. So-called senile changes in the brain of most elderly persons are much less severe than the degree of shrinkage shown here. (From F.K. Widmann, *Pathobiology: How Disease Happens.* Boston: Little, Brown, 1978.)

no specific function. Dysplasia is presumably controlled reproduction of cells, but it is closely related to malignancy in that it may transform into uncontrolled, rapid reproduction.[2] Epithelial cells are the most common types to exhibit dysplasia; changes include alterations in the size and shape of cells, causing loss of normal architectural orientation of one cell with the next. Dysplastic changes frequently occur in the bronchi of chronic smokers and in the cervical epithelium.[2]

## Hypertrophy

Hypertrophy is an increase in the size of individual cells, resulting in increased tissue mass without an increase in the number of cells. It usually represents the response of a specific organ to an increased demand for work. Hypertrophied cells increase their number of intracellular organelles, especially mitochondria. A good example of physiologic hypertrophy is the enlargement of muscles of athletes or weight lifters. The individual muscle cells enlarge but do not proliferate, and this provides increased strength. Limiting factors to hypertrophy exist, and these may have to do with limitation to the vascular supply or the capability of cells to produce energy. Hypertrophy may also be pathologic and frequently affects the myocardium (Figure 2-5).

## Hyperplasia

Hyperplasia is a common condition seen in cells that are under an increased physiologic workload or stimulation. It is defined as increase of tissue mass due to an increase in the number of cells. Cells that undergo hyperplasia are those that are capable of dividing and thus of increasing their number. Whether hyperplasia, rather than hypertrophy, occurs depends on the regenerative capacity of the specific cell.

*Physiologic hyperplasia* is a normal outcome of puberty and pregnancy. *Compensatory hyperplasia* occurs in organs that are capable of regenerating lost substance. An example is regeneration of the liver when part of its substance is destroyed. *Pathologic hyperplasia* is seen in conditions of abnormal stimulation of organs with cells that are capable of regeneration. Examples are enlargement of the thyroid gland secondary to stimulation by thyroid-stimulating hormone from the pituitary, and parathyroid hyperplasia due to renal failure (see Chap. 35).

Hyperplasia is induced by a known stimulus and almost always stops when the stimulus has been removed. This controlled reproduction is an important differentiating feature of hyperplasia from neoplasia. There is a close relationship between certain types of pathologic hyperplasia and malignancy (see Chap. 18).

## Metaplasia

Metaplasia is a reversible change in which one type of adult cell is replaced by another type. It is probably an adaptive substitution of one cell type more suited to the hostile environment for another.[3,8] Metaplasia is commonly seen in chronic bronchitis; the normal columnar, ciliated goblet cells are replaced by stratified squamous epithelial cells. The latter cells are better suited for survival in the face of chronic, irritating smoke inhalation or environmental pollution. Metaplasia increases the

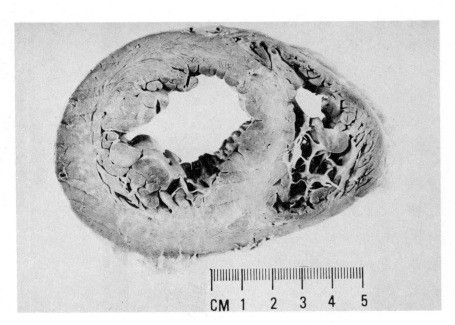

**FIGURE 2-5.**
Hypertrophy of the myocardium. (From F. Miller, *Peery and Miller's Pathology* [3rd ed.]. Boston: Little, Brown, 1978.)

CM  1    2    3    4    5

changes of cellular survival but decreases the protective aspect of mucus secretion. Certain types of metaplasia are closely related to malignancy, which probably indicates that chronic irritation causes the initial change.

## CAUSES OF ANOXIC CELLULAR INJURY AND DEATH

Lack of oxygen is the most common cause of cellular injury and death. The following conditions can produce this problem: ischemia, thrombosis, embolism, infarction, necrosis, and somatic death. In some instances, the injury is reversible or it may progress to a permanent, lethal change. Intracellular changes and their progression are detailed in Figure 2-6.

### Ischemia

Ischemia refers to a critical lack of blood supply to a localized area. It is reversible in that tissues are restored to normal function when oxygen is again supplied to them. Ischemia may precede infarction or death of the tissue,

or it may occur sporadically when the oxygen need outstrips the oxygen supply. It is important to differentiate between ischemia, a clinical change, and infarction, a pathologic change.

Ischemia usually occurs in the presence of atherosclerosis in the major arteries. Atherosclerosis, more fully described in Unit 8, is a lipid-depositing process with fibrofatty accumulations, or plaques, on the intimal layer of the artery. The medial layer of the artery may also become involved, predisposing it to atherosclerotic aneurysm formation. Atherosclerosis often gives rise to the formation of clots or thrombi on the plaque. These changes compromise blood flow through the artery, which then impairs oxygen supply to the tissues during increased need. In the later stages, the blood supply is impaired even at rest.

The classic conditions resulting from ischemia are *angina pectoris* and *intermittent claudication*. The former refers to pain from ischemia affecting the heart, and the latter refers to pain from ischemia of the extremities usually during activity. Ischemia is often relieved by rest and the tissues return to normal function. It may be progressive, however, and cause *ischemic infarction*, which involves cell death due to lack of blood supply or oxygen.

**Sequence of Events in Acute Ischemic Cell Injury**

| Lysosomes | Nucleus | Cytosol | Mitochondria | Cell Membrane | Endoplasmic Reticulum | Time |
|---|---|---|---|---|---|---|
| | | | ── Onset of Ischemia ── | | | O |
| | | | ▼ Mitochondrial Respiration | | | |
| | | | ▼ APT ; ▲ ADP : ATP | Inactivation of Sodium Pump | | |
| | | Glycolysis ▲ Pi | | Entry of Na;⁺ Loss of K⁺ | | |
| | | ▲ Lactate | Low Amplitude Swelling | | | |
| | | | | Entry of Water | | |
| | Clumping of Chromatin | ▼ pH | Loss of Matrix Granules | | Dilatation of ER | |
| | | | High Amplitude Swelling | | Detachment of Ribosomes ▼ Protein Synthesis | |
| | Pyknosis | | | | | Point of No Return |
| Swelling of Lysosomes | | | Loss of Matrical Enzymes + Cofactors | | | |
| ▲ Permeability of Lysosomal Membranes | | | Calcification and Flocculent Densities | ▲ Permeability to Large Molecules | | Necrosis |
| Release of Lysosomal Enzymes | | | | | | |
| | Digestion Karyorrhexis Karyolysis | Digestion | Digestion | Digestion | Digestion | |

**FIGURE 2-6.**

Progression of acute lethal anoxic cell injury. The cellular events that occur in injured cells are arranged here so that their temporal sequences and relationships to one another can be appreciated. (From D.L. Slauson and B.J. Cooper, *Mechanisms of Disease* [2nd ed.]. Baltimore: Williams & Wilkins, 1990.)

Lack of oxygen supply to the brain, heart, and kidneys can be tolerated for only a short time; damage is irreversible. The fibroblasts of connective tissue, however, have been shown to survive much longer periods of anoxia.

Ischemia occasionally occurs after vasospasm of coronary arteries or other vessels that are unaffected by atherosclerosis. Vasospasm may be induced by many factors including nicotine, exposure to cold, and, in some cases, stress. Vasospasm often occurs in association with atherosclerosis.

## Thrombosis

The word *thrombosis* refers to the formation of a clot on the intimal lining of the blood vessels or the heart. It may decrease blood flow or totally occlude the vessel.

The most common factor in thrombosis is disruption of the endothelial lining of the blood vessels and heart. This endothelial layer is continuous from the heart throughout the vascular circuit, including the capillaries and veins. When trauma, atherosclerosis, or other factors disrupt this layer, platelets may accumulate, and the intrinsic clotting mechanism is initiated (Figure 2-7). The body spontaneously initiates its fibrinolytic system to dissolve the clot and reopen the vessel. This may or may not be successful in reestablishing the flow of blood. Stasis of blood and increased blood viscosity also enhance coagulability of blood. Blood coagulation is described fully in Chapter 21.

Thrombosis most frequently occurs in the deep

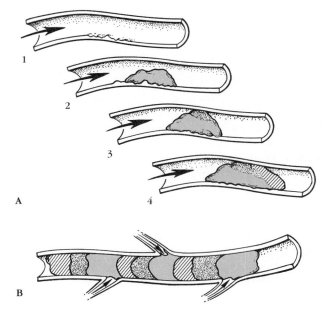

**FIGURE 2–7.**
**A.** Stages in the development of phlebothrombosis: (1) intimal damage, sluggish circulation; (2) platelet aggregation; (3) occlusion of the lumen of the vein; (4) blood clot propagates. **B.** Clot propagates clot at each point of entry of the small veins.

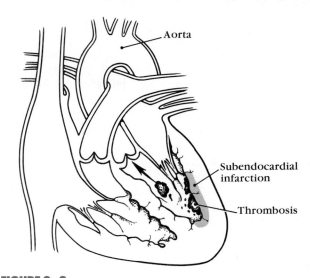

**FIGURE 2–8.**
Disruption of the endocardial surface, such as that after a subendocardial infarction, may lead to mural thrombosis that may become an arterial embolus.

veins of the legs, but *mural thrombosis* may occur on the endocardial lining of the heart. If this thrombosis occurs in the left ventricle, the risk for arterial embolization is quite high (Figure 2-8). Thrombosis in an artery can disrupt blood flow to the area supplied by the vessel and cause ischemia or infarction. Clots arising in the deep veins may detach, embolize, and lodge in the pulmonary arterial circuit (see Chap. 31).

## Embolism

A thrombus may break off and become a traveling mass in the blood. This process is called *thrombotic embolization*. The most common types of emboli are derived from thrombi, but other substances such as fat, vegetations from valves, or foreign particles also may embolize. The obstruction caused by an embolus is called an *embolism*.

If the embolus arises in the venous circuit, it is carried to and trapped in the vasculature of the pulmonary capillary bed. Depending on the size of the embolus, the clinical result may vary from being asymptomatic to death-producing (see Chap. 31).

If the embolus arises in the left side of the heart, it may travel to any of the arteries branching off the aorta. Arterial embolism may also occur from a larger artery, such as one affected by atherosclerosis, to a smaller artery. When it occludes the arterial tributary, it compromises blood flow to the area (see Chap. 27).

## Infarction

Occlusion of the blood supply from an artery causes *infarction*, which is a localized area of tissue death due to lack of blood supply. It is also termed *ischemic necrosis* and may occur in any organ or tissue.

Infarcts may have different pathologic characteristics. They are frequently classified as *pale infarcts, hemorrhagic infarcts*, and *infarcts with bacterial supergrowth*. Pale infarcts are seen in solid tissue deprived of its arterial circulation as a result of ischemia. Red or hemorrhagic infarcts are more frequent with venous occlusion or with congested tissues. The infarcted tissue has a red appearance, due to hemorrhage into the area, that may be poorly defined, causing difficulty in differentiating viable and nonviable tissue.[2,3] Bacterial supergrowth is common and may be present in the area or may be brought to the area.

The classification of *septic infarction* is added when there is evidence of bacterial infection in the area.[2] The lesion is converted to an abscess when it is septic and the inflammatory response is initiated. *Gangrene* is an example of infarction in which ischemic cell death is followed by bacterial overgrowth, leading to liquefaction of the tissues (Figure 2-9). This term is frequently used to describe conditions of the extremities and the bowel.[4]

## Necrosis

The term *necrosis* refers to cell or tissue death characterized by structural evidence of this death.[9] As cells die, the mitochondria swell, functions become disrupted, membranes rupture, and the lysosomal enzymes may be released into the tissues.[7,9] The nucleus undergoes specific changes that may include shrinking, fragmenting, or gradual fading.[9] Necrosis is commonly described in terms of coagulative, colliquative, and special types.[9]

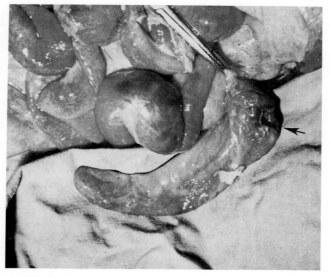

**FIGURE 2-9.**
Acute, gangrenous appendicitis with perforation. (From F. Miller, *Peery and Miller's Pathology* [3rd ed.]. Boston: Little, Brown, 1978.)

## Coagulative Necrosis

Coagulative necrosis usually results from lack of blood supply to an area. It is the most common pattern of necrosis and frequently occurs in organs such as the heart and kidneys, but it may result from chemical injury. The cell structure and its architectural outline may be preserved (structured necrosis), but the nucleus is lost. The outline may remain intact with the loss of intracellular organelles (structureless necrosis).

*Caseation* has long been described in relation to tuberculosis, but it may be present in a few other conditions. It is an example of structureless necrosis. The central area of necrosis is soft and friable and is surrounded by an area with a cheesy, crumbly appearance. The cellular architecture is destroyed. The area is walled off from the rest of the body and may become rimmed with calcium. Areas of caseous necrosis may localize in areas of tuberculous infestation.[5]

## Colliquative Necrosis

Colliquative necrosis most frequently occurs in brain tissue and results from fatal injury of the neuron. The breakdown of the neuron causes release of lysosomes and other constituents into the surrounding area. Lysosomes cause liquefaction of the cell and surrounding cells, leaving pockets of liquid, debris, and cystlike structures. Liquefactive necrosis is often described in brain infarction but may be seen with bacterial lesions because of the release of bacterial and leukocytic enzymes. Liquefaction may occur in an area of coagulative necrosis as a secondary change.[9]

## Special Types

*Fat necrosis* is a specific form of cellular death that occurs when lipases escape into fat storage areas. It particularly is seen in acute pancreatic necrosis and causes patchy necrosis of the pancreas and surrounding areas (see Chap. 39). Traumatic fat necrosis most commonly seen in the breast gives rise to a giant cell reaction that can resemble a carcinoma.[9]

*Gangrenous necrosis* is a combination of coagulative and liquefactive necroses. The term *gangrene* is applied to any black, foul-smelling area that is adjacent to living tissue.[9] The cause of tissue death is ischemia but bacteria and surrounding leukocytes cause liquefaction of the tissues. When the coagulative pattern is dominant, it is called *dry gangrene*. When the liquefactive process is more pronounced, it is called *wet gangrene*.[5]

Gas gangrene is a specific type of necrosis that can occur due to *clostridia* infections. Clostridia are gram-positive anaerobes that cause such conditions as tetanus, botulism, and food poisoning.[8] Gas gangrene usually occurs in large traumatic wounds in which the organisms cause destruction of the connective tissue framework. Gas bubbles are caused by a fermentative reaction causing a blue-black semifluid appearance of involved tissues.[8] If this material reaches the bloodstream, shock and disseminated intravascular coagulation (DIC) may be produced (see Chap. 21).

## Somatic Death

The body dies with the cessation of respiratory and cardiac function. The individual cells remain alive for different lengths of time, but irreversible changes occur and some of these make it difficult to determine exact premortem pathology. Postmortem changes include rigor mortis, livor mortis, algor mortis, intravascular clotting, autolysis, and putrefaction.

*Rigor mortis* develops because of depletion of ATP in the muscles, beginning in the involuntary muscles; in 2 to 4 hours it affects the voluntary muscles. The result is stiffening of the muscles, and the onset and disappearance varies among individuals. *Livor mortis* is the reddish blue discoloration of the body that results from the gravitational pooling of blood. *Algor mortis* is the term used for the cooling of the body that occurs after death. The rate of cooling depends on the premortem temperature and the postmortem environmental temperature. *Intravascular clotting* results in clots that are not adherent to the lining of the blood vessels and heart. They may be layered in appearance, with streaks or layers of yellowish, fatty material. *Autolysis* refers to the digestion of tissues from released substances, such as enzymes and lysosomes. Organs may be swollen and spongy in appearance. *Putrefaction* is caused by saprophytic organisms entering the dead body, usually from the intestines. This results in a greenish discoloration of the tissues and organs, and the organisms may produce gases, leading to foamy or spongy organs.[3,9]

## REFERENCES

1. Anderson, J.R. *Muir's Textbook of Pathology*. London: Edward Arnold, 1985.
2. Cotran, R., Kumar, V., and Robbins, S.L. *Robbin's Pathologic Basis of Disease* (4th ed.). Philadelphia: W.B. Saunders, 1989.
3. Golden, A. *Pathology: Understanding Human Diseases* (2nd ed.). Baltimore: Williams & Wilkins, 1985.
4. King, D.W., Fenoglio, C.M., and Lefkowitch, J.H. *General Pathology: Principles and Dynamics*. Philadelphia: Lea and Febiger, 1983.
5. Kissane, J.M. *Anderson's Pathology* (9th ed.). St. Louis: Mosby, 1990.
6. Lewis, C.M. *Nutrition and Nutritional Therapy in Nursing*. Norwalk, Conn.: Appleton-Century-Crofts, 1986.
7. Slauson, D.O., and Cooper, B.J. *Mechanisms of Disease* (2nd ed.). Baltimore: Williams & Wilkins, 1990.
8. Sodeman, W.A., and Sodeman, T.M. *Sodeman's Pathologic Physiology: Mechanisms of Disease* (7th ed.). Philadelphia: W.B. Saunders, 1985.
9. Walter, J.B. *Pathology of Human Disease*. Philadelphia: Lea & Febiger, 1989.

# chapter 3

## Miguel da Cunha

# Genetic Disorders

*Learning Objectives*

1. List the three broad types of genetic disorders.
2. Discuss briefly the chromosome set (karyotype) of human species.
3. Differentiate between the terms homozygous and heterozygous.
4. Define *allele, genotype,* and *phenotype.*
5. Draw a Punnett square to compute the progeny of specific genotypes.
6. Describe briefly autosomal dominant inheritance patterns.
7. Describe briefly autosomal recessive inheritance patterns.
8. Describe briefly X-linked dominant inheritance patterns.
9. Describe briefly X-linked recessive inheritance patterns.
10. Explain the three types of chromosomal aberrations.
11. Compare the inheritance pattern of multifactorial disorders with the inheritance pattern of single-gene disorders and chromosomal disorders.
12. Identify at least one disease or disorder that is determined by each type of inheritance pattern.
13. Identify the biochemical defect or structural alteration associated with phenylketonuria, albinism, sickle cell disease, and Marfan syndrome.
14. Differentiate between hemoglobinopathies and thalassemias.
15. Define *teratogen* and give examples of physical and chemical teratogenic agents.

Genes control the functions of a cell by determining what proteins are synthesized within the cell. Genes are also responsible for the transmission of characteristics from one generation to the next. This chapter describes the principles of inheritance, the classification of genetic disorders, and the mechanisms by which alterations in genetic material can produce structural or functional defects. Table 3-1 presents some essential terminology for the study of genetics. A large and diverse assortment of conditions has now been recognized as genetic diseases. It is likely that the expression of any disease is influenced by the genotype of the affected person.[6]

**TABLE 3–1.**
GENETIC TERMINOLOGY

| TERM | DEFINITION |
|---|---|
| Progeny | Offspring |
| Chromosome | Structure in the nucleus that contains deoxyribonucleic acid (DNA) that stores and transmits genetic information. Homologous chromosomes, respectively of paternal and maternal origin, are found in pairs in somatic cells |
| Gene | A segment of DNA that contains genetic information necessary to control a certain function, such as the synthesis of a polypeptide (protein); that segment is often referred to as a site, or locus, on a chromosome |
| Gamete | A mature male or female reproductive cell |
| Gametogenesis | Development of gametes |
| Alleles | Alternative forms of a gene at a given locus; for example, the alleles *H* and *h* of the gene HexA would determine synthesis (*H*), or no-synthesis (*h*) of the enzyme hexosaminidase A, whose absence causes Tay-Sachs Disease |
| Homozygous (homozygote) | An individual possessing a pair of identical alleles at a given locus on a pair of homologous chromosomes |
| Heterozygous (heterozygote) | An individual who has two different alleles at a given locus on a pair of homologous chromosomes |
| Homologous | Referring to chromosomes with matching genes, or to those genes individually |
| Karyotype | The chromosome constitution of an individual, usually represented by a laboratory-made display in which chromosomes are arranged by size and centromere position |
| Genotype | The basic combination of genes of an organism |
| Phenotype | The measurable expression of gene function in an individual (eg, eye color, hemoglobin type) |
| Pedigree chart | A schematic method for classifying genetic data |
| Dominant traits | Traits for which one of a pair of alleles is necessary for expression; eg, polydactyly |
| Recessive traits | Traits for which two alleles of a pair are necessary for expression; eg, cystic fibrosis |

## PRINCIPLES OF INHERITANCE

Gregor Mendel, an Austrian monk, is credited with discovering the basic principles of heredity. In 1865, Mendel presented the results of his experiments with garden peas, in which he crossed varieties with distinct characteristics and followed the progeny (offspring) of the crosses for at least two generations. Mendel proposed the idea of hereditary factors that are passed from one generation to the next, but his ideas were not accepted because the existence of chromosomes had not yet been recognized. In 1900, when chromosomes had been observed and their movements during cell division had been noted, Mendel's findings were rediscovered and accepted.

Mendel proposed two principles to describe the inheritance of characteristics in his garden peas. He concluded that the pea plant contains two inherited factors (now called alleles) for the determination of each characteristic. The principle of segregation describes the separation of these two alleles during gametogenesis, such that one half of the gametes receive one allele and the other half the other. The principle of independent assortment expresses the relationship between the alleles that determine different inherited characteristics. It states that pairs of alleles segregate independently of each other. Therefore, a gamete may contain either member of one allelic pair and either member of another pair. It is known that this principle is true, provided that the alleles are not linked, for example, located on different chromosomes. Mendel also recognized that some alleles are dominant and are expressed whenever one copy is present, whereas other alleles are recessive and require two copies for expression.

The distribution of genetic material, as proposed by Mendel, takes place during both divisions of meiosis. Mitosis, outlined in Chapter 1, is a type of cell division in which each of the two resulting daughter cells receives the same number of chromosomes as originally carried by the dividing mother cell. Therefore, mitosis is referred

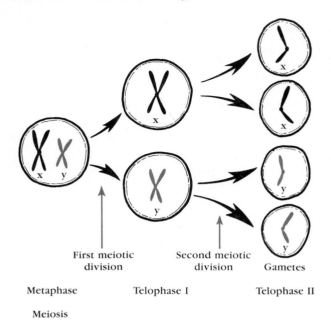

First meiotic
division

Second meiotic
division

Gametes

Metaphase            Telophase I                    Telophase II

Meiosis

**FIGURE 3–1.**
Selected stages in the process of meiosis. These are illustrated for the XY pair of chromosomes, the sex chromosomes in the male.

tional) division, by which each of the entering cells produces two daughter cells. In spermatogenesis, a process in which there is no cell loss, each original cell entering meiosis, therefore, results in four cells at the end of the completed process. The process of meiosis is outlined for one chromosome pair (the XY pair in a male) in Figure 3-1.

Studies in biochemical genetics reveal that the unit of heredity is the gene, which consists of a particular sequence of nucleotides in the deoxyribonucleic acid (DNA) of the chromosome. The sequence of nucleotides in a gene either determines the structure of a polypeptide chain or has a regulatory function in protein synthesis. Thus, the genes dictate which proteins are found in a cell and these proteins determine the form and function of the cell. Each chromosome is composed of thousands of genes arranged in linear order.

The karyotype (characteristic chromosome makeup) of each species defines the species chromosome number and morphology. In humans, the cell most commonly used for the study of chromosomes is the lymphocyte. To study the karyotype of an individual, cytogeneticists obtain lymphocytes from a blood sample and grow them in a nutrient medium. Colchicine is added to stop cell division in metaphase, allowing a large number of cells in the same stage of cell division to accumulate. Application of a hypotonic solution causes the cells to swell, separating the chromosomes from each other. They are then placed on a glass slide, stained, and photographed. The photographs are cut out, arranged into groups, and identified by number according to the length of the chromosome and position of its centromere (the constricted portion). A normal male karyotype is shown in Figure 3-2.

to as an equational process. This replenishment type of cell division is characteristic of somatic cells. Meiosis, one of the cell division types encountered during gametogenesis, consists of two division processes in tandem, referred to as meiosis I and II. During meiosis I, the number of chromosomes in the two initial daughter cells is reduced to one-half of the original mother cell chromosome number. This is the reductional portion of meiosis. Meiosis II, which rapidly follows, is a mitosis-like (equa-

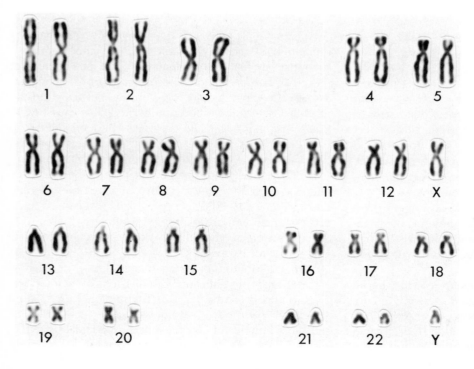

**FIGURE 3–2.**
Chromosomes from a normal human male are shown as they appear in metaphase and as they are displayed in a karyotype for study. The chromosomes have been individually cut out of the photomicrograph and arranged on the basis of size and position of centromere. (From K.A. May and L.R. Mahlmeister, *Comprehensive Maternity Nursing* [2nd ed.]. Philadelphia: J.B. Lippincott, 1990.)

Normal human somatic cells contain 23 pairs of chromosomes for a total of 46. Gametes contain only one member of each chromosome pair for a total of 23.

## CLASSIFICATION OF GENETIC DISORDERS

Generally, genetic disorders are classified into three broad groups: (1) single-gene, (2) chromosome, and (3) multifactorial. In these three groups, altered genetic material is passed from parent to offspring. Analysis of the genetics and pathophysiology of any genetic disorder first requires its categorization into one of these types. Table 3-2 shows examples of conditions that can be caused by genetic abnormalities.

Single-gene disorders result from mutation in a single gene. The mutated gene may be present on one or both chromosomes of a pair. In the former case, the matching gene on the partner chromosome is normal. Single-gene disorders may be recognized as hereditary by analysis of pedigree, the characteristic pattern of distribution of a specific trait in a family. Table 3-3 shows examples of some of the more common single-gene disorders and their frequency.

In chromosome disorders, the defect is due to an abnormality in chromosome number or structure. In contrast to single-gene disorders which involve mutated genes, the structure of the genes in chromosome disorders may be normal, but the genes may be present in multiple copies or may be situated on a different chromosome than is normally the case. For example, Down syndrome results from the presence of an extra chromosome 21 (trisomy 21). Chromosome disorders affect about seven infants per 1000 births and account for about one-half of all spontaneous first trimester abortions.[9]

Multifactorial disorders result from a combination of small variations in genes that, when combined with environmental factors, produce serious defects. Although they do not show the distinct pedigree patterns of single-gene disorders, multifactorial disorders tend to cluster in families. It has been estimated that as many as 10% of the population is affected by these conditions.[6]

Another group of disorders are alterations in fetal development caused by the environment. In this case, the conditions are not hereditary, but often involve a change in the expression of the cell's genetic material, which causes a defect in the structure and/or function of the cell. Environmental factors such as toxic chemicals, infectious agents, and irradiation are responsible for certain congenital abnormalities. Fetal development may also be affected by an unfavorable intrauterine environment due to maternal disease.

## SINGLE-GENE DISORDERS

### Terminology

Transmission patterns in hereditary disorders are described in specific terms that must be defined for precise understanding. The members of a pair of matching chromosomes (those carrying genes that influence the same traits) are termed homologous chromosomes. Each gene has a specific site or locus on a specific chromosome. Genes at the same locus on a pair of homologous chromosomes are called alleles. An individual in whom both members of a pair of alleles are the same is homozygous (a homozygote) with respect to that gene locus; when the members of a pair of alleles are different, the individual is heterozygous (a heterozygote) for that gene locus (Figure 3-3).

Genotype is the word used to describe the genetic constitution of an individual. The measurable expression of a gene in an individual is the phenotype.

An allele that is expressed when it is present on one (or both) chromosomes of a pair is dominant. An allele that is expressed only when it is present on both chromosomes of a pair (with the exception of the XY pair) is recessive. The terms *dominant gene* and *recessive gene* are commonly used. The trait (phenotype) which these genes determine can also be referred to as dominant or

**TABLE 3-2.**
COMMON EXAMPLES OF GENETIC DISORDERS

| DISORDER | CLASSIFICATION | GENETICS |
|---|---|---|
| Huntington disease | Single-gene disorder | Autosomal dominant |
| Cystic fibrosis | Single-gene disorder | Autosomal recessive |
| Hypophosphatemia (vitamin D-resistant rickets) | Single-gene disorder | X-linked dominant |
| Hemophilia | Single-gene disorder | X-linked recessive |
| Down syndrome | Chromosome disorder | Trisomy 21 |
| Turner syndrome | Chromosome disorder | 45,XO |
| Cleft lip/palate | Multifactorial | ? |

**TABLE 3-3.**
SELECTED EXAMPLES OF SINGLE-GENE DISORDERS

| DISORDER | OCCURRENCE | BRIEF DESCRIPTION |
|---|---|---|
| **Autosomal Dominant Inheritance** | | |
| Familial hypercholesterolemia (type II) | 1:200–1:500 | Deficiency in cell receptors for low density lipoproteins, hypercholesterolemia, xanthomas, coronary heart disease |
| Huntington disease | 1:18,000–1:25,000 (United States) | Progressive neurologic disease, involuntary muscle movements, mental deterioration with memory loss, personality changes |
| Neurofibromatosis | 1:3000–1:3300 | Disorder of neural crest-derived cells with skin and central and peripheral nervous system manifestations; café au lait spots, neurofibromas, and malignant progression are common; variable expression of manifestations |
| Tay-Sachs disease | 1:3600 (Ashkenazi Jews) | Lipid storage disease; progressive mental and motor retardation with onset at about age 6 months, deafness, blindness, convulsions, death by age 3–4 years |
| **X-Linked Dominant Inheritance** | | |
| Pseudohypoparathyroidism (Albright hereditary osteodystrophy) | Rare | Short stature, delayed dentition, hypocalcemia, hyperphosphatemia, mineralization of skeleton, round facies |
| Vitamin D-resistant rickets (familial hypophosphatemia) | 1:25,000 | Disorder of renal tubular phosphate transport; low serum phosphate, rickets, short stature |
| Polydactyly | 1:100–1:300 (blacks) 1:630–1:3300 (Caucasian) | Extra (supernumerary) digit on hands or feet |
| Polycystic renal disease (adult) | 1:250–1:1250 | Enlarged kidneys with cysts, hematuria, proteinuria, abdominal mass; may be associated with hypertension, hepatic cysts |
| **Autosomal Recessive Inheritance** | | |
| Albinism (tyrosinase negative) | 1:15,000–1:40,000 1:85–1:650 (American Indians) | Melanin lacking in skin, hair, and eyes; nystagmus; photophobia; increased susceptibility to neoplasia |
| Cystic fibrosis | 1:2000–1:2500 (Caucasians) 1:16,000 (American blacks) | Abnormal exocrine gland function with pancreatic insufficiency and malabsorption, chronic pulmonary disease, excessive salt in sweat |
| Cystinuria | 1:10,000 | Defect in transport of cystine, lysine, arginine, and ornithine in intestines and renal tubules, tendency toward renal calculi |
| Familial dysautonomia (Riley-Day syndrome) | 1:10,000–1:20,000 (Ashkenazi Jews) | Dysfunction of autonomic nervous system, sensory abnormalities, small stature, poor coordination, scoliosis, lack of tears leading to corneal ulcers |
| Hurler syndrome | 1–2:100,000 | Mucopolysaccharide disorder; mental retardation, coarse facies, skeletal and joint deformities, deafness, dwarfism, corneal clouding, onset age 6–12 months, fatal in childhood |
| Phenylketonuria (PKU) | 1:15,000 (United States) 1:5000 (Scotland) | Deficiency in phenylalanine by hydroxylase causing excess phenylalanine in blood and urine, mental retardation if untreated, normal development and life span with low phenylalanine diet |
| Sickle cell disease | 1:400–1:600 (American blacks) | Hemoglobinopathy with chronic hemolytic anemia, growth retardation, susceptibility to infection, painful crises, leg ulcers, dactylitis |

(continued)

## TABLE 3-3.
### SELECTED EXAMPLES OF SINGLE-GENE DISORDERS (continued)

| DISORDER | OCCURRENCE | BRIEF DESCRIPTION |
|---|---|---|
| **X-Linked Recessive Inheritance** | | |
| Color blindness (red green deutan) | 8:100 (Caucasian males)<br>4–5:100 (Caucasian females)<br>2–4:100 (black males) | Normal visual acuity, defective color vision with red-green confusion |
| Duchenne's muscular dystrophy | 1:3000–1:5000 males | Progressive muscle weakness, atrophy contractures, eventual respiratory insufficiency and death |
| G6PD (glucose-6-phosphate dehydrogenase) deficiency | 1:10 black American males<br>1:50 black American females | Enzyme abnormality with subtypes; manifestations involve RBC since it cannot replace unstable enzyme; usually asymptomatic unless person is under stress or exposed to certain drugs or infection, which increase need for chemical-reducing power generated by action of G6PD; decreased reducing power eventually results in denaturation of hemoglobin and hemolysis |
| Hemophilia A | 1:2500–1:4000 male births | Coagulation disorder due to deficiency of factor VIII |
| Hemophilia B | 1:4000–1:7000 male births | Coagulation disorder due to deficiency of factor IX |
| X-linked ichthyosis | 1:5000–1:6000 males | May be born with sheets of scales (collodion babies), dry scaling skin, corneal opacities, steroid sulfatase deficiency |

*Source:* Adapted from F. Cohen, *Clinical Genetics in Nursing Practice.* Philadelphia: Lippincott, 1984. Pp. 78, 81, 84, 87, 91. Additional material from J.M. Connor and M.A. Ferguson-Smith, *Essential Medical Genetics.* Oxford: Blackwell Scientific, 1984. Pp. 185, 186, 198.

recessive. In genetic disorders, a dominant disorder is one in which the person who carries the gene (in either a heterozygous or homozygous state) is clinically affected. To be clinically affected by a recessive disorder, the individual must be homozygous for the gene (with the exception of genes found on the X chromosome in a male). As gene loci found on the X chromosome in the male are not matched by corresponding loci on his Y chromosome, a recessive gene on the male's X chromosome will be expressed. A disorder carried on the X chromosome is an X-linked disorder. There are no known Y-linked genetic disorders of medical interest.

in a pedigree chart, which is a schematic method for classifying data. Some symbols used in constructing a pedigree chart are shown in Figure 3-4. Gene symbols are always expressed in italics. Usually a capital letter is used to signify a dominant allele and the lower case of the same letter is used to signify the corresponding recessive allele. By this method, a genotype may be shown as TT, Tt, or tt, as in Figure 3-5.

An example of a phenotype determined by a single pair of autosomal alleles is the ability to taste phenylthiocarbamide (PTC). The bitter taste of the drug is detected by persons with the dominant gene but not by persons

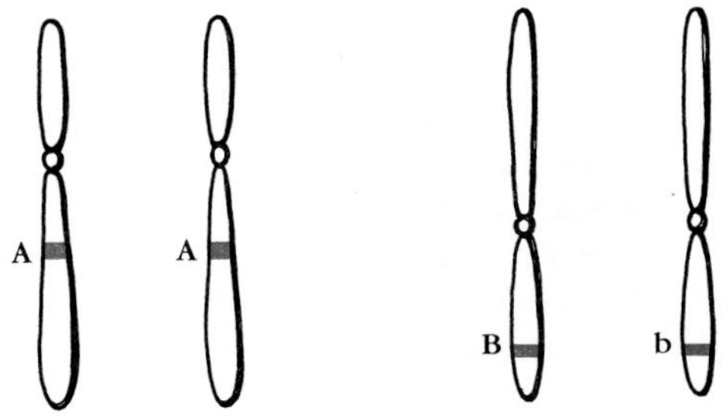

## *Principles of Transmission*

Phenotypes determined by single genes occur in fixed proportion in the progeny of a mating. The pedigree patterns of such traits are dependent on whether the gene is located on an autosomal chromosome (any chromosome other than a sex chromosome) or on the X chromosome, and whether the gene is dominant or recessive. These factors allow the following four basic patterns of inheritance for single-gene traits: (1) autosomal dominant, (2) autosomal recessive, (3) X-linked dominant, and (4) X-linked recessive.

Patterns of single-gene inheritance can be exhibited

### FIGURE 3-3.
Two pairs of homologous chromosomes. One pair has similar alleles at locus A. The other pair has dissimilar alleles at locus B. A person with these chromosomes would be homozygous for allele A and heterozygous for allele B.

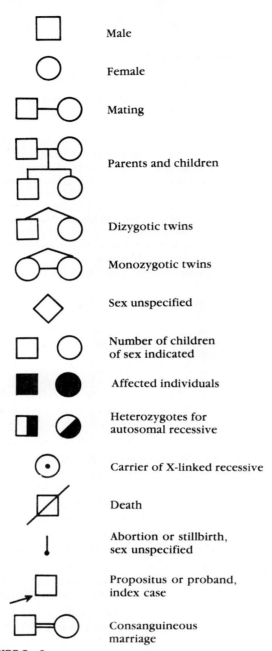

**FIGURE 3–4.**
Symbols used in pedigree charts.

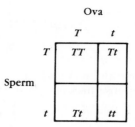

**FIGURE 3–5.**
Progeny of Tt and Tt mating.

spring, there is a 25% chance of being a dominant homozygote (TT) and a 50% chance of being a heterozygote (Tt). Both of these genotypes produce the phenotype, taster. There is a 25% chance of being a recessive homozygote (tt) and having the phenotype, nontaster.

Figure 3-6 illustrates all possible genotypes of offspring from matings involving a single pair of autosomal alleles. Using the same trait of PTC taster as an example, there are three possible genotypes for each male and female (TT, Tt, and tt) and six different combinations of genotypes that could be found in the offspring of each mating. With respect to autosomal dominant disorders, a common clinical situation is that of a couple in which one member is affected and the other is genetically normal (eg, Dd x dd). With autosomal recessive disorders, the typical situation is that of a couple of heterozygote carriers (Rr x Rr) who seek genetic advice after producing an affected child. The outcome of those matings and their implications are discussed in the following sections.

## Autosomal Dominant Inheritance

In autosomal dominant inheritance of a genetic defect, the abnormal allele is dominant and the normal allele is recessive. According to Mendelian laws, individuals with genotype DD and Dd would express an affected phenotype, whereas the genotype dd would result in a normal individual. Usually, the heterozygous person will display a more mild phenotype than the affected homozygote. For example, in achondroplastic dwarfism, the affected homozygous exhibits severe malformations, such as hydrocephalus, which usually result in severe mental retar-

homozygous for the recessive allele. Therefore, those with the genotype TT (homozygous dominant) or Tt (heterozygous) would be able to taste the drug and be classified as phenotype, taster. Persons with the genotype tt (homozygous recessive) would not be able to taste the drug and would be classified as phenotype, nontaster.

Figure 3-5 illustrates the use of a Punnett square to predict the genotypes and phenotypes of the progeny of a heterozygous (Tt) male and female. Mendel's law of segregation and the concept of dominance are used for this prediction. As shown in the genotypes of the off-

| | | Maternal genotype | | |
|---|---|---|---|---|
| | | **TT** | **Tt** | **tt** |
| **Paternal genotype** | **TT** | TT | TT, Tt | Tt |
| | **Tt** | TT, Tt | TT, Tt, tt | Tt, tt |
| | **tt** | Tt | Tt, tt | tt |

**FIGURE 3–6.**
Parental genotypes for autosomal alleles T and t and the genotypes that could be found in progeny of the various mating pairs.

dation in addition to the physical impairment. The heterozygous person, however, usually displays the typical physical manifestations and usually functions well in the societal structure. For this reason, it is usually safe to assume that the affected individual in a couple will be a heterozygote, whose disease did not impede him or her from developing the complex societal skills that led to courtship, marriage, mating, and reproduction. Therefore, in most cases, the typically observed mating is that of Dd x dd individuals. The stereotype pedigree of this pattern is shown in Figure 3-7. When either parent is heterozygous for the autosomal dominant allele (in this case the father) and the other parent is homozygous for the normal allele, each child has a 50% risk of receiving the dominant allele and thus being affected. Each child receives a normal allele from the normal parent. Although one-half of the children will theoretically receive the dominant allele, the chances are independent in each zygote formation, and in a small sample such as a family, the ratio of normal to affected children may be different than 1:1. Because the allele is autosomal and not X-linked, either sex may be affected. All affected children have an affected parent unless the disorder results from a fresh mutation.

Characteristics of autosomal dominant inheritance are summarized as follows: (1) affected persons usually have an affected parent; (2) affected persons mating with normal persons have equal chances of producing affected and unaffected offspring; (3) unaffected children born to affected parents will have unaffected children; and (4) males and females have equal chances of being affected.

## Autosomal Recessive Inheritance

In autosomal recessive disorders, the abnormal allele is recessive, the normal allele is dominant, and as a result, the genotypes RR and Rr will express a normal phenotype. Only an affected homozygote (rr) will express the disorder. The difference between the two unaffected individuals above is that the heterozygote has a certain risk of transmitting the defective allele (*r*); in fact, approximately 50% of their gametes will carry the defective allele. Because these persons are usually clinically normal but are able to transmit the disorder, they are referred to as heterozygous carriers. This accounts for the carrier state in autosomal recessive disorders. Because autosomal dominant disorders are expressed, no carrier state can exist for them. Because the dominant or normal allele masks the trait, most persons who are heterozygous for an autosomal recessive allele go undetected. When two heterozygous individuals mate (the most common pattern in autosomal recessive inheritance) and an offspring receives the recessive allele from each parent, the trait is expressed. *Consanguineous* marriage (marriage

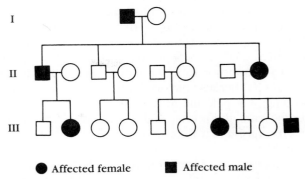

**● Affected female**  **■ Affected male**

**FIGURE 3-7.**
Stereotype pedigree of autosomal dominant inheritance.

of persons who are blood relatives) may increase this probability.

When a heterozygous person mates with a homozygous normal person, each offspring receives a normal allele from the normal parent and cannot express the trait. Figure 3-8 illustrates a stereotype pedigree of autosomal recessive inheritance. Note in generation I that when a homozygous normal male mates with a heterozygous female, each offspring receives a normal gene from the father. Fifty percent of the offspring receive the recessive allele from the heterozygous mother and are therefore carriers of the trait. Line II shows a heterozygous male mating with a heterozygous female. The progeny of this mating have a 1:4 risk of receiving a recessive allele from each parent and thus being affected with the trait.

Characteristics of autosomal recessive inheritance are summarized as follows: (1) the trait usually appears in siblings only, not in the parents; (2) males and females are equally likely to be affected; (3) for parents of one affected child, the recurrence risk is one in four for every subsequent birth; (4) both parents of an affected child carry the recessive allele; and (5) the parents of the affected child may be consanguineous.

## X-Linked Inheritance

Of the 23 pairs of chromosomes that determine the karyotype of the human, 22 pairs are autosomes and one

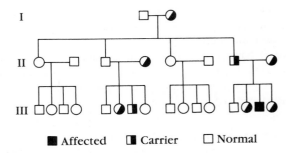

**■ Affected**  **◨ Carrier**  **□ Normal**

**FIGURE 3-8.**
Stereotype pedigree of autosomal recessive inheritance.

pair is sex chromosomes. Unlike the 44 autosomes that can be arranged in 22 homologous pairs, the two sex chromosomes are of unequal size and have different placement of their centromeres (see Figure 3-2). The two sex chromosomes in the female are XX and in the male are XY. Because the ovum must contain an X chromosome, if it is fertilized by a sperm containing an X chromosome, the product will be a female (XX). If the sperm contributes a Y chromosome, the product will be male (XY).

Transmission of genes on the sex chromosomes follows the same principles of inheritance as does transmission on the autosomes. The difference in the patterns of inheritance results from differences of morphology and gene complement in the two sex chromosomes. The X chromosome carries genes that are not matched on the Y chromosome. Because to date there are no known medically significant genes located on the Y chromosome, it seems that its major importance is sex determination and the organization of testes in the developing XY embryo. Therefore, for practical purposes, the genes located on the X chromosome are those involved in sex-linked inheritance.

Females inherit two X chromosomes, whereas males (XY) have only one. As the genes located on the male's one X chromosome have no counterparts on his Y chromosome (he is *hemizygous* for these genes), traits determined by either dominant or recessive X-linked genes are expressed in the male. The genes on the X chromosome cannot be transmitted from father to son, since fathers contribute a Y chromosome to sons, but are transmitted from father to all daughters through the one X chromosome. Recessive mutant genes on the X chromosome of a female may not be expressed because they are matched by normal genes inherited with the other X chromosome.

## X-Linked Dominant Inheritance

Genetic disorders caused by X-linked dominant genes are rare. The main characteristic of this inheritance pattern is that an affected male transmits the gene to all his daughters and to none of his sons. The affected female may transmit the gene to offspring of either sex (Figure 3-9).

Characteristics of X-linked dominant inheritance are summarized as follows: (1) affected males have normal sons and affected daughters; (2) affected females (heterozygous) have a 50% risk of transmitting the abnormal gene to each daughter or son; and (3) the disorder tends to be more severe in males (hemizygous) than in females (heterozygous).

## X-Linked Recessive Inheritance

Several genetic disorders associated with a recessive gene on the X chromosome have been identified. Again,

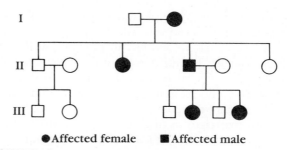

●Affected female    ■Affected male

**FIGURE 3–9.**

Stereotype pedigree of X-linked dominant inheritance.

the inheritance pattern of these disorders results from the morphologic difference in the X and Y chromosome. The recessive gene located on the one X chromosome of the male is not balanced by a dominant allele on the Y chromosome, and is thus expressed. The recessive gene should be expressed in the female only if she is homozygous. Therefore, X-linked recessive disorders are rare in females. Only matings between an affected male and a carrier or affected female should result in an affected female.

Occasionally, a carrier (heterozygous) female manifests some of the signs of a recessive disorder. This is due to the fact that during early embryogenesis, one or the other of the X chromosomes in each of the somatic cells (cells other than the gametes) of all females degenerate, leaving only one functioning X chromosome in each cell.[3] Thus, approximately one-half of the cells in a normal female express the genes on one of her X chromosomes, and the other half express the genes on her other X chromosome. If this "X-chromosome inactivation" is unequal, one of the X chromosomes may have a greater effect on the female's physiology than the other, resulting in the ability of a recessive gene on that chromosome to be expressed.[2]

Males affected with an X-linked recessive disorder cannot transmit the gene to sons, but transmit it to all daughters. An unaffected female who is heterozygous for the recessive gene transmits it to 50% of her sons and daughters. Figure 3-10 gives a stereotype pedigree of X-linked recessive inheritance.

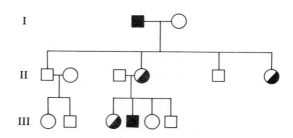

◗ Carrier female    ■ Affected male

**FIGURE 3–10.**

Stereotype pedigree of X-linked recessive inheritance.

Characteristics of X-linked recessive inheritance are summarized as follows: (1) males are predominantly affected; (2) affected males cannot transmit the gene to sons but transmit the gene to all daughters; (3) sons of female carriers have a 50% risk of being affected; and (4) daughters of female carriers have a 50% risk of being carriers.

## Pathophysiology of Single-Gene Disorders

Since the genes of a cell are primarily responsible for directing the synthesis of the cell's proteins, it is not surprising that the manifestations of single-gene disorders result from alterations in protein synthesis. In many cases, the affected protein is an enzyme, part of a synthetic or degradation pathway. In other instances, the altered protein is a constitutive protein, such as hemoglobin; is part of the cell membrane, such as a receptor of a transport protein; or is mainly supportive in function, namely collagen. Sometimes the disorder is classified by its pattern of transmission as a single-gene defect, but its basic pathology is not known.

### Altered Activity of an Enzyme in a Metabolic Pathway

Alterations in the activity of one enzyme in a metabolic pathway may have several results, including a deficiency in the end product of the pathway, or the accumulation of a toxic intermediate or a toxic byproduct. These possibilities are illustrated in Figure 3-11, which shows selected pathways for the metabolism of phenylalanine and tyrosine and metabolic blocks that are responsible for three genetic disorders—albinism, alkaptonuria, and phenylketonuria.

*ALTERATIONS IN AMINO ACID METABOLISM.* As indicated in Figure 3-11, both phenylalanine and tyrosine are normally available from the digestion of dietary protein. Phenylalanine is also converted to tyrosine, which has many uses in the cell, one of which is to produce melanin, the pigment in skin, hair, and eyes. In *classic albinism,* a deficiency in the enzyme tyrosinase results in decreased or absent melanin production. Manifestations of this condition are listed in Table 3-3. Another single-gene disorder, *alkaptonuria,* is due to the absence of homogentisic acid oxidase, which results in the accumulation of the pathway intermediate homogentisic acid (alkapton). Homogentisic acid is excreted in the urine and turns black in the presence of oxygen, which produces darkening of the urine. In later life, deposits of dark pigment may be noted in connective tissue and may lead to arthritis.

The most serious genetic disorder involving phenylalanine metabolism is *phenylketonuria* (PKU). In classic PKU, absence of phenylalanine hydroxylase from liver cells prevents the conversion of phenylalanine to tyrosine. Consequently, phenylalanine accumulates in the

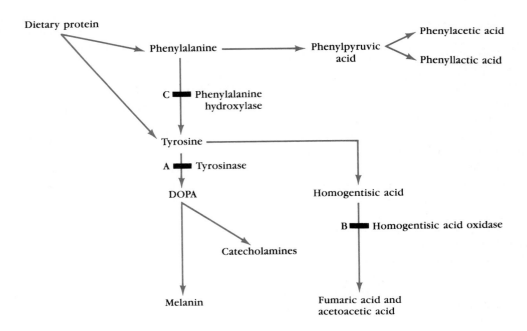

■■ = Blocked reaction

**FIGURE 3–11.**

Metabolism of phenylalanine and tyrosine. Arrows may represent one or more chemical reactions. The indicated enzyme defects result in (A) classic albinism, (B) alkaptonuria, and (C) classic phenylketonuria (PKU).

blood and some is converted to phenylpyruvic acid, phenyllactic acid, or phenylacetic acid. These compounds are excreted in the urine, giving it a characteristic musty odor. The excess of phenylalanine and its byproducts in the blood results in various metabolic disturbances, especially alterations in nervous system development, including delayed psychomotor development, seizures, hyperactivity, and mental retardation. In addition, excess phenylalanine in the blood inhibits the activity of tyrosinase. Since this enzyme is necessary for the synthesis of melanin and catecholamines, children with PKU tend to have lighter eyes and skin than their relatives and may show a decrease in circulating epinephrine. In the untreated infant, manifestations of PKU appear at approximately 3 to 6 months of age.

Fortunately, tests are available to detect phenylalanine or its metabolites in blood or urine. PKU screening is mandatory for newborns in most states.[12] The most commonly used test, the Guthrie bacterial-inhibition assay, which indicates phenylalanine level in the blood, is not positive until the infant has consumed enough protein to allow phenylalanine buildup. Therefore, if the test is performed during the first 3 days of life, as might occur with the current trend for early hospital discharge of mother and baby, it may have to be repeated, ideally before the infant is 3 weeks old.[11] In PKU-positive infants, neurologic damage can be prevented by restricting phenylalanine in the diet. The restrictive diet should be started as early as possible and followed until neurologic development is complete. Estimates regarding the age at which a normal diet may be allowed vary widely, from 3 years to never.[3] When a woman with PKU becomes pregnant, it is also necessary for her to resume her low-phenylalanine diet to protect the fetus.[3]

With the advent of widespread neonatal PKU screening, other causes of hyperphenylalaninemia have been identified, involving closely related aspects of phenylalanine metabolism. Classic PKU accounts for approximately 90% of all cases of hyperphenylalaninemia.[3] Other causes are deficiencies of related enzymes in the liver other than phenylalanine hydroxylase. Classic PKU exhibits autosomal recessive transmission; tests are available to detect heterozygous carriers.[12]

### ALTERATIONS IN CARBOHYDRATE METABOLISM.
Loss of activity of enzymes in the varied pathways for carbohydrate metabolism account for many single-gene disorders. These include alterations in the metabolism of glucose, galactose, or fructose, glycogen storage diseases, and disorders involving mucopolysaccharides. In *galactosemia,* deficiency of an enzyme needed for the conversion of galactose 1-phosphate to glucose 1-phosphate leads to the accumulation of galactose and galactose 1-phosphate in tissues. This interferes with normal liver and kidney function and produces other metabolic disturbances that may result in osmotic changes in the lens of the eye and cataract development.

*Glucose-6-phosphate dehydrogenase deficiency,* a relatively common disorder in American blacks, is described in Table 3-3. In *glycogen storage diseases,* various enzymes needed for the synthesis or breakdown of glycogen may be altered. The accumulation of glycogen in tissues, especially the liver, interferes with their functions. The most common glycogen storage disease is *von Gierke's disease,* in which developing liver pathology produces hepatomegaly, acidosis, increased glucose and lipids in the blood, and retarded growth.[12] *Mucopolysaccharides* are large complex carbohydrates that form part of the extracellular matrix of connective tissue. They are constantly being turned over in the tissues and are degraded by enzymes contained in the lysosomes of a cell. A deficiency in any of the necessary lysosomal enzymes leads to the accumulation of partially degraded mucopolysaccharides within the lysosome (one type of *lysosomal storage disease*). This interferes with various activities of the cell. Manifestations of one type of mucopolysaccharidosis, *Hurler syndrome,* are listed in Table 3-3.

### DISORDERS IN SPHINGOLIPID METABOLISM.
Accumulations of sphingolipids produce *lipid storage diseases* such as Gaucher and Tay-Sachs disease. Sphingolipids are lipids present in membranes, especially in the myelin of brain and other nervous tissue. The three classes of sphingolipids are sphingomyelins, cerebrosides, and gangliosides. Like many compounds in the body, sphingolipids are continually being turned over and a block in their metabolism can lead to their accumulation in various tissues. *Gaucher's disease* is the most common lipid storage disease, exhibiting a relatively high frequency in Ashkenazi Jews (Jews of European, as opposed to Mediterranean, origin). Glucocerebrosides accumulate in reticuloendothelial cells, producing Gaucher cells, which are found most often in the spleen, lymph nodes, liver, and bone marrow. Manifestations of this disease, which has several forms, include splenomegaly, hepatomegaly, osteoporosis, anemia, tendency to bleed, and, in some forms, neurologic damage and mental retardation. In *Tay-Sachs disease,* which is also most prevalent in Ashkenazi Jews, the accumulation of one type of ganglioside in the lysosomes of neurons results in the ballooning of neurons, the degeneration of axons, and demyelination, producing nervous system manifestations such as those indicated in Table 3-3. At present, there is no treatment for this disease. Fortunately, screening is available to detect heterozygous carriers of this autosomal recessive disorder.

### OTHER METABOLIC PATHWAY DEFECTS.
Other biochemical pathways that are known to be altered by single-gene mutations include ones that involve the metabolism of purines, pyrimidines, or heme, and those that are used for the biotransformation of certain drugs. The synthesis of heme occurs by way of several precursors called porphyrins. The *porphyrias* are disorders in which

an enzyme defect leads to the accumulation and excretion of porphyrins or porphyrin precursors. Some porphyrias are hereditary, whereas some are caused by the toxic effect of chemicals. Of the hereditary porphyrias, four types display autosomal dominant transmission and one is autosomal recessive.

General characteristics of porphyrias include the excretion of reddish urine, photosensitization of the skin and skin eruptions, excessive hair on the face and limbs, and neurologic and psychologic manifestations. This constellation of signs and symptoms may have led to afflicted persons being called the werewolves of European folklore. *Drug sensitivities* that are attributed to hereditary enzyme deficiencies include sensitivity to succinylcholine and isoniazid.[11]

## Loss or Alteration of Circulating Proteins

Other types of single-gene disorders can involve proteins that circulate in the bloodstream. Serum albumin is deficient in *analbuminemia,* producing oncotic pressure problems. Serum globulins that may be affected by single-gene mutations include complement components, alpha$_1$-antitrypsin, alpha$_2$-macroglobulin, transferrin, or various immunoglobulins (the immunoglobulins in *X-linked agammaglobulinemia* or *severe combined immunodeficiency*).[12] Clotting factor VIII, IX, or XI is absent from the blood in the *hemophilias.* Von Willebrand factor is a protein that interacts with and possibly stabilizes clotting factor VIII. It is also necessary for formation of a platelet plug. Lack of the factor occurs in *von Willebrand disease.*[10]

*HEMOGLOBIN ABNORMALITIES.* Disorders involving the synthesis of the protein component of hemoglobin include the *hemoglobinopathies* and the *thalassemia syndromes.* The hemoglobin molecule consists of the protein globin, plus four heme complexes. In adult hemoglobin, the globin component is made up of four polypeptide chains: two identical alpha chains and two identical beta chains. A single-gene mutation could change the structure of the alpha or the beta chains. Hundreds of variations in the globin chains have been identified.[11]

*Sickle cell anemia* results from a single-gene mutation that leads to the substitution of valine for glutamic acid at one location on the beta chains of adult hemoglobin (HbA), forming HbS. The hemoglobin of a person who is homozygous for the abnormal gene contains abnormal beta chains. Under low oxygen conditions, this hemoglobin tends to precipitate within erythrocytes and causes them to assume a characteristic sickle shape. These abnormal red blood cells tend to compromise blood flow to the tissues and also to lyse, resulting in anemia. A person who is homozygous for the gene is said to have *sickle cell disease.* A person who is heterozygous for the abnormal gene produces both HbS and HbA and

exhibits sickling of erythrocytes only under conditions of extremely low oxygen tension. This person may never exhibit signs of sickle cell anemia and is said to have the *sickle cell trait,* rather than the disease.

Manifestations of sickle cell anemia are discussed in more detail in Chapter 19.

Whereas hemoglobinopathies such as sickle cell disease involve an alteration in the structure of the globin component of hemoglobin, the thalassemias result from reduced synthesis of normal hemoglobin molecules. They are classed as alpha- and beta-thalassemias, depending upon which polypeptide chain is synthesized in reduced amounts (see Chap. 19).

*LIPOPROTEINS.* Hereditary alterations in the level and function of certain lipoproteins that are normally found in the blood occur in conditions such as *familial hypercholesterolemia, abetalipoproteinemia,* and *familial combined hyperlipidemia.*[7] Although these are thought to be single-gene disorders, they are influenced somewhat by the environment, and are therefore usually classed as multifactorial conditions.[1]

## Altered Cell Membrane Components

Familial hypercholesterolemia involves the lack of low-density lipoprotein receptors on liver cells and is thus an example of a *cell membrane defect* produced by a single-gene mutation. Other cell membrane defects may involve proteins that participate in the active transport of substances through the membrane. Conditions that are thought to result from defective membrane-transport proteins include *cystinuria* and *vitamin D-resistant rickets,* both of which are described in Table 3-3.

## Collagen Disorders

Several hereditary disorders are believed to result from abnormalities in the synthesis of collagen. This protein, which is the most abundant protein in the body, has a complex structure with several levels of organization. Eight different types of collagen are present in the various connective tissues in the body.[1] One example of a collagen disorder is *osteogenesis imperfecta,* which is discussed in Chapter 45.

Another is *Marfan syndrome,* which results from an autosomal dominant gene defect or, in 15% of the cases, a new mutation.[1] In this disorder, a defect in the structure of collagen or another connective tissue protein, elastin, is thought to be the basis for changes in skeletal, ocular, and cardiovascular tissues. Among the manifestations of Marfan syndrome are a tall, thin stature with arachnodactyly (excessively long fingers), lax ligaments allowing hyperextension of the limbs, dislocation of the optic lenses, and a tendency toward formation of dissecting aneurysms of the aorta. The stature of Abraham Lincoln and the violin virtuosity of Paganini have been attributed to Marfan syndrome.

### Single-Gene Disorders in Which the Basic Defect Is Unknown

Among the disorders that appear to be transmitted as single-gene defects are several for which the basic physiologic deficiencies are not known. These include cystic fibrosis, the muscular dystrophies, and Huntington's disease, all of which are mentioned briefly in Table 3-3 and discussed in greater detail in specifically related chapters.

Preliminary studies indicate that some manifestations of cystic fibrosis may be due to faulty control of channels for the diffusion of chloride through cell membranes.[5] Other possible basic defects in cystic fibrosis include hypersecretion of calcium by mucous glands, increased intracellular calcium, and the production of serum glycoproteins, which inhibit the activity of cilia.[11]

*Huntington disease* is an autosomal dominant disorder in which symptoms do not usually appear until 35 years of age or later. By the time of diagnosis, the affected person may have already reproduced, with a 50% chance of passing this lethal trait to each of his offspring. There is no treatment for the disease and progressive neurologic deterioration is inevitable. Until recently, there has been no way to identify persons carrying the gene for Huntington's disease before symptoms appear. Using modern techniques for analyzing DNA, researchers have noted a characteristic pattern of fragments produced when the DNA of chromosome 4 from cells of persons with the disease is cleaved by a particular enzyme, one of several called *restriction enzymes*.[3,8] Similar treatment of DNA from persons who do not carry the gene yields different fragments. Thus, a test is available for predicting which young persons will eventually develop the symptoms of Huntingdon's disease.[2] Use of the predictive test must be accompanied by consideration of the impact of a positive result on the person and the family.

## CHROMOSOME DISORDERS

*Chromosomal aberrations* (deviations from normal) may be either numeric or structural and may affect either autosomes or sex chromosomes. Rarely are both simultaneously affected. Chromosome aberrations resulting in two or more cell lines with different chromosome numbers produce *mosaics*. In these situations, one or more of the cell lines will be abnormal.

### Numerical Aberrations

Deviations or abnormalities in chromosome number are classified in terms of loss or gain of chromosome sets. As discussed earlier, the normal chromosome number in humans is 46 (23 pairs). To compare abnormalities with the normal karyotype, several terms must be defined.

Normal somatic cells, with two sets of 23 chromosomes, are said to be *diploid* (double) or 2N; gametes, with a single set of 23, are *haploid* (single) or N. A cell with an exact multiple of the haploid number is *euploid*. Euploid numbers may be 2N, 3N (*triploid*), or 4N (*tetraploid*). Chromosome numbers that are exact multiples of N but greater than 2N are called *polyploid*. *Aneuploid* refers to a chromosome complement that is abnormal in number but is not an exact multiple of N. An aneuploid cell may be *trisomic* (2N + 1 chromosomes) or *monosomic* (2N—1 chromosomes). Any cell with a chromosome number that deviates from the characteristic N and 2N is *heteroploid*.

*Disjunction* is the normal separation and migration of chromosomes during cell division. Failure of the process called *nondisjunction* in a meiotic division results in one daughter cell receiving both homologous chromosomes and the other receiving neither. It is the primary cause of aneuploidy. If this deviation in normal process occurs during the first meiotic division, one-half of the gametes will contain 22 chromosomes and one-half will contain 24. If joined with a normal gamete, a gamete produced in this manner will produce either a monosomic (2N—1) or trisomic (2N + 1) zygote. Normal disjunction and nondisjunction at the first and second meiotic divisions of the ovum are illustrated in Figure 3-12. The figure also shows the union of normal sperm with gametes of varying chromosome complement. A common example of a disorder that results from an abnormality of chromosome number is *trisomy 21*, or *Down syndrome*. This disorder can result when nondisjunction of chromosome 21 occurs at meiosis, producing one gamete with an extra chromosome 21 (N + 1 = 24) and one gamete with no chromosome 21 (N − 1 = 22). Union of the 24-chromosome gamete with a normal sperm produces a 47-chromosome zygote, trisomy 21.

The overall incidence of Down syndrome is one per 700 live births. The incidence increases with increasing maternal age. As it has been determined that in 20% to 30% of cases the extra chromosome is of paternal origin, the role of increased paternal age is being investigated. Presently, it is suggested that in couples in which the father is age 55 years or older, the mother's age-specific risk should be doubled to estimate the couple's risk of having an infant with trisomy 21.[3]

Clinical diagnosis of trisomy 21 is often based on facial appearance. The palpebral fissures are upslanting with speckling of the edge of the iris, the nose is small, and the facial profile flat. Figure 3-13 illustrates other manifestations of trisomy 21. The simian crease (a single midpalmar fold) is found in approximately 50% of persons with Down syndrome and in approximately 5% to 10% of nonafflicted persons.[3] The presence of mental re-

First meiotic division
Nondisjunction
Normal disjunction
Second meiotic division
Normal
Nondisjunction
Fertilization with normal sperm
Normal
Trisomes
Monosome

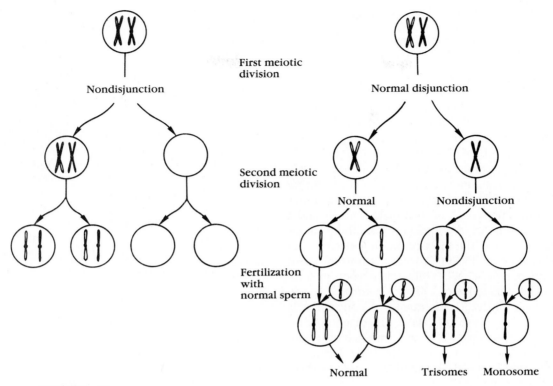

**FIGURE 3-12.**
Process of nondisjunction at the first and second meiotic divisions of the ovum and fertilization with normal sperm.

tardation is consistent in children with Down syndrome, but the degree may vary. The average IQ is approximately 50; infrequently, values may range up to 70 or 80.

## *Structural Aberrations*

Deviations in the normal structure of chromosomes result from the chromosome material and reassembling in an abnormal arrangement. These changes in structure may be either stable (persisting through future cell divisions) or unstable (incompatible with cell division). Stable types of structural abnormalities include the following:

1. *Deletion,* loss of a portion of a chromosome. The missing segment may be a terminal portion of the chromosome, resulting from a single break, or an internal section, resulting from two breaks.
2. *Duplication,* presence of a repeated gene or gene sequence. A deleted segment of one chromosome becomes incorporated into its homologous chromosome.
3. *Inversion,* reversal of gene order. The linear arrangement of genes on a chromosome is broken and the order of a portion of the gene complement is reversed in the process of reattachment.
4. *Translocation,* transfer of part of one chromosome to a nonhomologous chromosome. This occurs when two chromosomes break and the segments are rejoined in an abnormal arrangement.

Trisomy 21
• Mental retardation
• Epicanthic folds
• Small head
• Macroglossia
• High arched palate
• Spade hands
• Simian crease
• Hypermobile joints
• Hypotonia

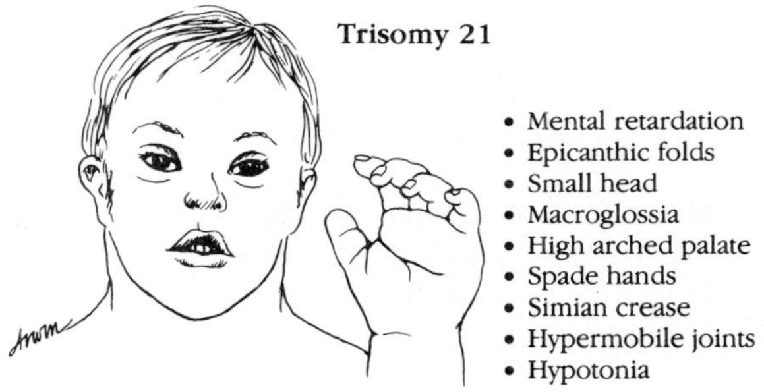

**FIGURE 3-13.**
Down's syndrome phenotype. (From R.D. Judge, G.D. Zuidema, and F.T. Fitzgerald, *Clinical Diagnosis, A Physiologic Approach* [4th ed.]. Boston: Little, Brown, 1982.)

## *Mosaics*

Nondisjunction occurring in cell division other than gametogenesis results in two or more cell lines with different chromosome numbers. Persons with at least two cell lines with different karyotypes are labeled mosaics. Although several different mosaics have been described,

most of the cases of different cell lines involve sex chromosome constitution.

## Sex Chromosome Aberrations

In comparison to other hereditary disorders, sex chromosome aberrations are fairly common. Of the types found in males, the incidence is about one in 400 births; of the types found in females, about one in 650 births.[6]

Most sex chromosome abnormalities are due to numeric aberration resulting from nondisjunction during meiosis. The disorders are described by the total number of chromosomes present. A normal male is 46,XY and a normal female is 46,XX. Any variation from these values constitutes a disorder. The most common genotype with female phenotype is 45,XO (Turner's syndrome) and with male phenotype, 47,XXY (Klinefelter syndrome).

The overall incidence of *Turner's syndrome* is one per 2500 female births. The frequency at conception is higher, but 99% spontaneously abort. The diagnosis may be suggested in the newborn by the presence of redundant neck skin and peripheral lymphedema. Diagnosis can also be made later during the investigation of short stature or primary amenorrhea.

The incidence of 47,XXY (*Klinefelter syndrome*) is one per 1000 males. The risk increases with increased maternal age.[3] Diagnosis is usually made during adult life as a result of the investigation of infertility. This syndrome is the most common cause of hypogonadism and infertility in men. Other manifestations include long lower extremities, sparse body hair with a female distribution, and, in approximately 50%, breast development.

## MULTIFACTORIAL DISORDERS

Multifactorial inheritance includes the disorders in which a genetic susceptibility combined with the appropriate environmental agents interact to produce a phenotype that is classified as disease.

Although the word *polygenetic* is sometimes used to describe multifactorial disorders, the former term more accurately describes disorders determined by a large number of genes, each with a small effect, acting additively.[6] To date, there is no method of establishing the exact effects of environmental factors or the additive effects of genes in determining the expression of a trait.[6] For this reason, multifactorial inheritance is more difficult to analyze than other types of inheritance. Multifactorial traits tend to cluster in families, but their genetic patterns are not clearly predictable, as they are with single-gene traits and chromosome disorders.

A characteristic of multifactorial inheritance is the unimodal distribution of a trait in the population (note the presence of only one peak in the curve in Figure 3-

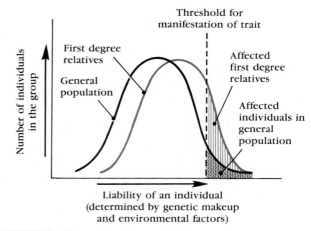

**FIGURE 3-14.**
Threshold model for multifactorial inheritance. First-degree relatives of the affected individual have more genetic and/or environmental factors, which increase their risk of manifesting the disorder.

14). Some normal characteristics are distributed unimodally and have family patterns that are characteristic of multifactorial inheritance, for example, stature and intelligence.[6] The correlation among relatives with such traits is proportional to their genes in common (inherited from a common ancestral source). The more distant the relationship, the fewer genes they have in common.[6] Abnormalities that are thought to be multifactorial include congenital heart disease, congenital dislocation of the hip, neural tube defects, cleft lip, cleft palate, and atherosclerotic heart disease.

The *threshold model* of multifactorial inheritance (see Figure 3-14) can be used to explain some of the features of the family distribution of multifactorial disorders. It is based on collecting information on the frequency of the disorders in the general population and in different categories of relatives (eg, first-degree relatives such as parents, siblings, and offspring, or second-degree relatives such as aunts, uncles, nieces, and nephews). Through this method of analysis, the empiric risk (recurrence risk based on experience) can be estimated. Knowledge of genetic and environmental factors in the pathogenesis of the disorder is not considered.

## ENVIRONMENTAL ALTERATIONS IN FETAL DEVELOPMENT

The effect of environmental influences on fetal development has been a subject of increasing concern. Reasons for this include the facts that more women have entered the workplace, the level of environmental chemical exposure is increasing for all people, and birth defects due to environmental exposure are preventable. Publicity generated by the thalidomide damage in the 1960s brought the problem to the attention of the general public.

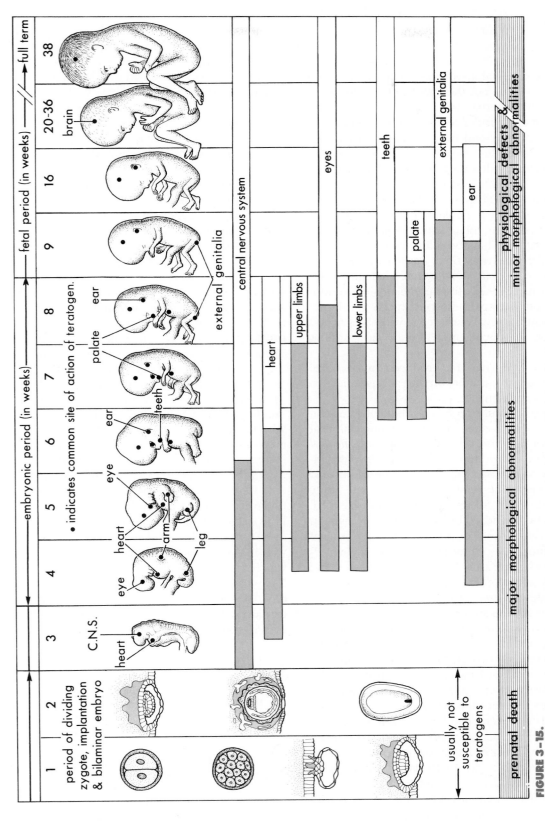

**FIGURE 3–15.**

Schematic illustration of the sensitive or critical periods in human development. Dark bar denotes highly sensitive periods; light bar indicates stages that are less sensitive to teratogens. (From K.L. Moore, *Before We Are Born* [2nd ed.]. Philadelphia: W.B. Saunders, 1983.)

A *teratogen* is an agent that acts on the embryo or fetus, causing abnormalities in form or function. Teratogenic agents can also be referred to as fetotoxic or developmentally toxic. Exposure to these agents results in a wide spectrum of consequences from no apparent effect to altered fetal growth, abnormal development in one or more systems, congenital anomalies, carcinogenesis, or fetal death. Whether or not the agent causes damage is the result of both maternal and fetal factors, including dose of the agent (and virulence if it is a microorganism), timing of the exposure, and host susceptibility (that of both mother and fetus).

Exposure of the mother during the first 2 weeks after fertilization may not affect the fetus since implantation has not yet occurred. Exposure of the fetus during this time may result in failure to implant or other lethal event. During the first trimester, teratogenic agents are likely to produce gross structural abnormalities because organogenesis is occurring at this time. Particularly sensitive periods for different organs are illustrated in Figure 3-15. After the first trimester, only the nervous system continues to differentiate. Fetotoxic effects in the last two-thirds of gestation mainly involve interference with the size and number of cells, producing more minor structural or functional defects.

Teratogenic effects may be produced by chemical agents, microorganisms, irradiation, and abnormalities in the maternal environment.

Although the harmful effects of alcohol consumption during pregnancy have been recognized since Biblical times, it was not until 1973 that the name *fetal alcohol syndrome* (FAS) was used to describe a specific constellation of abnormalities seen in the children of chronic alcoholic mothers.[13] The Fetal Alcohol Syndrome Study Group of the Research Society on Alcoholism has proposed that FAS be diagnosed by the presence of signs in each of three categories: (1) prenatal and/or postnatal growth retardation; (2) central nervous system involvement; and (3) characteristic facial dysmorphism.[13] The term *fetal alcohol effects* (FAE) is sometimes used to describe the manifestations of fetal alcohol exposure when all of the criteria for FAS are not present.

Abundant evidence links *maternal cigarette smoking* to fetal damage. Problems include an increased spontaneous abortion rate, an increased perinatal mortality rate, an increased incidence of maternal complications such as placenta abruptio and placenta previa, decreased birth weight and size in later childhood, an increased incidence of preterm delivery, and lower Apgar scores at 1 minute and 5 minutes after birth.[3] The mechanism by which cigarette smoking produces damage is not known, but may be related to a lack of available oxygen or to toxicity of certain products of the smoke.

*Microorganisms* that infect a pregnant woman may damage the fetus by direct infection or by altering the maternal environment. Consequences of maternal infection include increased reproductive loss, prematurity, congenital malformations, and growth retardation. Fetotoxic effects can be produced by certain viruses, bacteria, fungi, and protozoa, with the majority attributable to viruses. Among these are cytomegaloviruses, rubella, varicella zoster, herpes simplex 1 and 2, and Venezuelan equine encephalitis virus. In the United States, most fetal damage is produced by members of the STORCH group of infections, which are composed of syphilis (a bacterial infection), toxoplasmosis (a protozoan infection), rubella, cytomegalovirus, and herpes simplex.

Exposure to *radiation* at any time during gestation can produce detrimental effects and the question of what dose level may be considered safe is controversial. Diagnostic exposure of less than 5 rad to the fetus during the first trimester is generally considered safe with respect to teratogenic effects.[4] However, exposure to 1 to 2 rads has been reported to increase the possibility of leukemia 1.5-fold to 3-fold.[2] Fifty rad can produce microcephaly, mental retardation, cataracts, abnormalities in the genital and skeletal systems, and other defects. Mechanisms of radiation damage that have been noted include the killing of brain cells (which cannot be replaced), chromosome breakage, production of aneuploidy resulting in Down or Turner syndrome, and destruction of specific tissues (eg, the fetal thyroid by radioactive iodine).

Advances in the treatment of chronic diseases, such as diabetes mellitus, have resulted in an increase in the number of women with metabolic or genetic disorders who survive and become pregnant. These pregnancies are often at high risk due to the *altered maternal environment* in which the fetus must develop. Probably the hyperglycemia and ketoacidosis that accompany poorly controlled diabetes are the cause of the threefold to fourfold increase in congenital anomalies and the other problems encountered with offspring of diabetic women.

The possibility of damage to offspring of mothers with PKU was previously mentioned. Other conditions in which the maternal physiology has been known to affect the fetus include hyperthermia (from fever, sauna, or hot tub), Marfan syndrome (due to stress on the maternal cardiovascular system), homocystinuria, histidinemia, myotonic dystrophy, and acute intermittent porphyria.

## *REFERENCES*

1. Byers, P.H. Disorders of collagen biosynthesis and structure. In C.R. Scriver, A.L. Beaudet, W.S. Sly, and D. Valle (eds.), *The Metabolic Basis of Inherited Diseases* (6th ed.). New York: McGraw-Hill, 1989.
2. Caskey, C.T. Disease diagnosis by recombinant DNA methods. *Science* 236:1223, 1987.
3. Cotran, R., Kumar, V., and Robbins, S. *Robbin's Pathologic Basis of Disease* (4th ed.). Philadelphia: W.B. Saunders, 1989.
4. Creasy, R.K., and Resnick, R. *Maternal-Fetal Medicine*. Philadelphia: W.B. Saunders, 1984.

**5.** Frizzell, R.A., Rechkemmer, G., and Schoemaker, R.L. Altered regulation of airway epithelial cell chloride channels in cystic fibrosis. *Science* 233:558, 1986.

**6.** Gelehrt, T.D., and Collins, F.S. *Principles of Medical Genetics.* Baltimore: Williams & Wilkins, 1990.

**7.** Goldstein, J.L., and Brown, M.S. Familial hypercholesterolemia. In C.R. Scriver, A.L. Beaudet, W.S. Sly, and D. Valle (eds.), *The Metabolic Basis of Inherited Diseases* (6th ed.). New York: McGraw-Hill, 1989.

**8.** Gusella, J.F., Wexler, N.S., Conneally, P.M., Naylor, S.L., Anderson, M.A., Tanzi, R.E., Watkins, P.C., Ottina, K., Wallace, M.R., Sakaguchi, A.Y., Young, A.B., Shoulson, I., Bonilla, E., and Martin, J.B. A polymorphic DNA marker genetically linked to Huntington's disease. *Nature* 306:234, 1983.

**9.** Hassold, T.J. Chromosome abnormalities in human reproductive wastage. *Trends in Genetics* 2:105, 1986.

**10.** Hilgartner, M.W., and Pochedly, C. (eds.). *Hemophilia in the Child and Adult* (3rd ed.). New York: Raven Press, 1989.

**11.** King, R.A., Rotter, J.I., and Motulski, A.G. (eds.). *The Genetic Basis of Common Disease.* New York: Oxford University Press, 1990.

**12.** Muir, B.L. *Essentials of Genetics for Nurses.* New York: Wiley, 1983.

**13.** Rosett, H.L., and Weiner, L. *Alcohol and the Fetus: A Clinical Perspective.* New York: Oxford University Press, 1984.

## UNIT BIBLIOGRAPHY

Anderson, J.R. *Muir's Textbook of Pathology.* London: Edward Arnold, 1985.

Ayala, F.J., and Kiger, J.A. *Modern Genetics* (12th ed.). Menlo Park, Calif.: Benjamin-Cummings, 1984.

Dixon, K.C. *Cellular Defects in Disease.* Boston: Blackwell Scientific, 1982.

Elkeles, R.S., and Tavill, A.S. *Biochemical Aspects of Human Disease.* Oxford: Blackwell Scientific, 1983.

Ferguson, G.C. *Pathophysiology, Mechanisms and Expressions.* Philadelphia: W.B. Saunders, 1984.

Fisher, J.H., and Klinger, K.W. Closing in on the cystic fibrosis gene(s). *Am. Rev. Respir. Dis.* 132:1149, 1985.

Gelehrt, T.D., and Collins, F.S. *Principles of Medical Genetics.* Baltimore: Williams & Wilkins, 1990.

Golden, A. *Pathology, Understanding Human Disease* (2nd ed.). Baltimore: Williams & Wilkins, 1985.

Guyton, A.C. *Textbook of Medical Physiology* (8th ed.). Philadelphia: W.B. Saunders, 1990.

King, D.W., Fenoglio, C.M., and Lefkowitch, J.H. *General Pathology, Principles and Dynamics.* Philadelphia: Lea & Febiger, 1983.

King, K.A., Rotter, J.J., and Matulski, A.G. *The Genetic Basis of Common Disease.* New York: Oxford University Press, 1990.

Kolata, G. Closing in on the muscular dystrophy gene. *Science* 230:307, 1985.

MacLeod, A., and Sikora, K. *Molecular Biology and Human Disease.* St. Louis: Blackwell Scientific, 1984.

Moore, K.L. *Before We Are Born.* Philadelphia: Saunders, 1977.

Mottet, N.K. *Environmental Pathology.* New York: Oxford University Press, 1985.

Muir, B.L. *Essentials of Genetics for Nurses.* New York: Wiley, 1983.

Perez-Tamayo, R. *Mechanisms of Disease: An Introduction to Pathology* (2nd ed.). Chicago: Yearbook, 1985.

Rosett, H.L., and Weiner, L. *Alcohol and the Fetus: A Clinical Perspective.* New York: Oxford University Press, 1984.

Scriver, C.R., Beaudet, A.L., Sly, W.S., and Valle, D. *The Metabolic Basis of Inherited Diseases* (6th ed.). New York: McGraw-Hill, 1989.

Selkurt, E. *Basic Physiology for the Health Sciences* (2nd ed.). Boston: Little, Brown, 1982.

Sheldon, H. *Boyd's Introduction to the Study of Disease* (10th ed.). Philadelphia: Lea & Febiger, 1988.

Snell, R.S. *Clinical Anatomy for Medical Students* (2nd ed.). Boston: Little, Brown, 1981.

Snell, R.S. *Clinical Histology for Medical Students.* Boston: Little, Brown, 1984.

Sodeman, W.A., and Sodeman, T.M. *Sodeman's Pathologic Physiology: Mechanisms of Disease* (7th ed.). Philadelphia: W.B. Saunders, 1985.

Taussig, M.J. *Processes in Pathology and Microbiology* (2nd ed.). Boston: Blackwell Scientific, 1984.

Thompson, J.S., and Thompson, M.W. *Genetics in Medicine* (4th ed.). Philadelphia: W.B. Saunders, 1986.

Tortora, G., Evans, R., and Anagnostakos, N. *Principles of Human Physiology.* Philadelphia: Harper & Row, 1982.

Walter, J.B. *Pathology of Human Disease.* Philadelphia: Lea & Febiger, 1989.

Walter, J.B., and Israel, M.S. *General Pathology.* New York: Churchill Livingstone, 1987.

# DEVELOPMENT

Throughout life, developmental changes affect the ability of the human body to maintain the steady state. Periods of growth are common in certain stages while degenerative changes are dominant in others. A variety of factors affect the rate of these various changes. Because of the extensive nature of this topic, no attempt has been made to deal with all aspects of development but only to present normal developmental changes and the more common susceptibilities to disease at different developmental levels.

Chapter 4, Biophysical Development of Reproduction, discusses fetal development and factors affecting labor and delivery. Further information relating to the female reproductive system may be found in Chapter 56. Chapter 5, Biophysical Development of Children, describes physiologic changes occurring from the neonatal period through adolescence. While it is recognized that societal and cultural factors have a great impact on development, these have been briefly discussed or omitted due to the extensiveness of these topics.

Chapter 6, Biophysical Developmental Changes of Adults, presents a topic with a great deal of controversy and variability. Biophysically, adults do not age at the same rate. Some generalities are made and several sociocultural concepts are discussed due to their biophysical impact. The impact of nutrition, sleep cycle changes, physical fitness and stress are considered.

Chapter 7, Biophysical Changes of the Older Adult, deals with the theories of aging and the bodily systems affected. Older adults age at different rates and have different systemic problems but the changes seem to be an innate process. The societal and cultural impact of an aging society is only briefly alluded to due to the extensiveness of the topic.

The reader is encouraged to use the learning objectives at the beginning of each chapter as a study guide outline for essential concepts. The unit bibliography provides general and specific resources for further study.

# chapter 4

Sharron P. Schlosser
Joy H. Whatley

# Biophysical Development of Reproduction

## Chapter Outline

## Learning Objectives

1. Identify the stages of fetal development and discuss the biophysical development associated with each stage.
2. Discuss the process of placenta formation.
3. Trace the circulation of blood through the placenta and fetus.
4. Relate the effects of maternal illnesses on the biophysical development of pregnancy.
5. Discuss the effects of sexually transmitted diseases and infections on the biophysical development of the pregnancy and the fetus.

6. Identify and define fetal factors that affect biophysical development.
7. Identify demographic, obstetric, miscellaneous, and medical factors that place a fetus at risk for less than optimal outcome of pregnancy.
8. Compare the normal nutritional requirements for a woman in the childbearing years with the additional requirements needed during pregnancy and lactation.

(continued)

**9.** Discuss selected nutritional conditions that affect the biophysical development of pregnancy.

**10.** Discuss common agents that have a teratogenic effect on the pregnancy or fetus.

**11.** Differentiate currently used techniques and studies to assess fetal well-being.

**12.** Discuss the risks and benefits of currently used prenatal diagnostic screening procedures.

**13.** Identify and discuss the various theories regarding initiation of labor.

**14.** Identify and define the four stages of labor; discuss the processes occurring in each stage.

**15.** Examine the alterations associated with the four Ps: power, passage, passenger, and psyche; describe the adaptation problems associated with each.

---

The period of gestation begins with fertilization of the ovum and continues throughout development of the fetus. The duration of gestation is approximately 280 days or 10 lunar months from the last menstrual period. Typically, the period of gestation is divided into three 3-month periods termed *trimesters*. During this time, two processes account for the biophysical development of the fetus—*hyperplasia* and *hypertrophy*.[10] The early first trimester (first 12 weeks following conception) is characterized by hyperplasia where the mitotic cellular division accounts for an increase in the number of cells, while the size of cells remains relatively stable. The second trimester (weeks 13 to 24) is characterized by both hyperplasia and hypertrophy. The process of hypertrophy predominates the third trimester (weeks 25 to birth). During this trimester, the fetus experiences a very rapid period of growth whereby the number of cells does not change, but rather those cells present increase significantly in size. This chapter is concerned with prenatal development and the birth process. Factors affecting biophysical development, as well as prenatal diagnostic studies, are discussed. The genetics of reproduction is found in Chapter 3.

## FETAL DEVELOPMENT

### Stages

The biophysical development of the fetus is traditionally divided into three stages: the germinal period, the embryonic period, and the fetal period.

### Germinal Period

The germinal period is also referred to as the period of the ovum or the period of the zygote and extends from conception to approximately 2 weeks. Within hours of fertilization, generally in the outer third of the fallopian tube, the process of mitosis begins. Mitotic cellular division continues every 10 to 12 hours throughout the zygote's journey through the fallopian tube. At this time, the mass of cells is referred to as a *morula*. After approximately 4 days in the fallopian tube, the morula reaches the uterine cavity. At this point, the cells of the morula begin to differentiate and are known as the blastocyst (Figure 4-1). A fluid-filled cavity appears while the cells differentiate into two layers. The cells along the outer layer are termed trophoblast and will begin the implantation in the endometrium to form the placenta. The inner cluster of cells is termed the inner cell mass or embryoblast, and eventually develops into the embryo.

For an additional 3 to 4 days, the blastocyst remains free within the uterine cavity, edging toward the site of implantation. As the blastocyst comes into contact with the endometrium, proteolytic enzymes from the trophoblast allow the blastocyst to virtually digest its way into the endometrium (see Figure 4-1). This invasion of the soft and succulent endometrium erodes the maternal blood vessels in the endometrium, forming pools of maternal blood. It is here within the placenta that exchange of nutrients and waste products occurs throughout pregnancy. By approximately the 11th day, the implantation process is complete and the blastocyst appears as a slight bulge on the endometrium.

The implanting trophoblasts also secrete human chorionic gonadotropin (HCG). This hormone is responsible for positive pregnancy tests, as well as the continued functioning of the corpus luteum and resultant production of progesterone.

### Embryonic Period

The embryonic period begins with the complete implantation of the blastocyst (approximately the end of the sec-

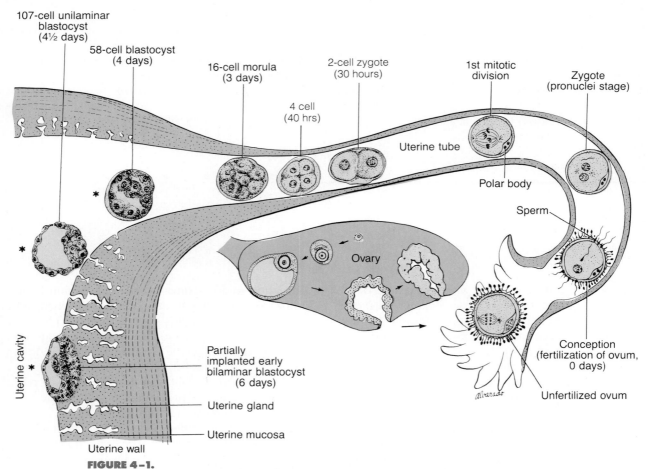

**FIGURE 4–1.**
Transport of the ovum into the fallopian tube, and fertilization within the tube followed by cleavage (cell division) to the 8- to 16-cell stage. The product, now referred to as a morula, is delivered into the uterus where it develops into a blastocyst and implants in the endometrium on the sixth to seventh postfertilization day. (Modified from R.F. Gasser, *Atlas of Human Embryos.* Hagerstown: Harper and Row, 1975 by S.J. Reeder and L.L. Martin, *Maternity Nursing* [16th ed.]. Philadelphia: J.B. Lippincott, 1987.)

ond week) and extends through the eighth week of prenatal development. Four major accomplishments are associated with this period of development: (1) rapid growth, (2) placenta formation and function, (3) early structural development of organs, and (4) development of a form which is recognizable as a human being.

The cells of the inner cell mass begin a rapid differentiation and are referred to as the embryonic disc. At this point, two germ layers have evolved. The primitive yolk emerges from the endoderm while the ectoderm gives rise to the amniotic sac. By about the 16th day, the cells of the embryonic disc have further differentiated into a third primary germ layer, the mesoderm (Figure 4-2). These three layers will eventually give rise to all major fetal organs. Table 4-1 lists the structures evolving from each of the three layers. Figure 4-3 shows the primary germ layers and the systems that develop from them.

Cephalocaudal and proximodistal principles of development become evident as one explores the developing embryo. By the 22nd day, the ectoderm has folded into the neural tube from which the brain, head, and spinal cord will develop. During this same time, two tubes form in the mesoderm; by the 22nd day, they have fused to form the fetal heart, which becomes the first functioning organ of the fetus (Figure 4-4). Eyes, ears, nose, and mouth begin to take shape by the 22nd day. By the 26th day, arm and leg buds appear. Development continues as the elbows and knees appear and fingers and toes lose their webbing. External genitalia are evident but not distinguishable. By the end of the embryonic period, the circulation is well-established. The embryo measures approximately 3 cm (1.2 inches) in a crown to rump measurement and weighs only about 1 to 2 grams.

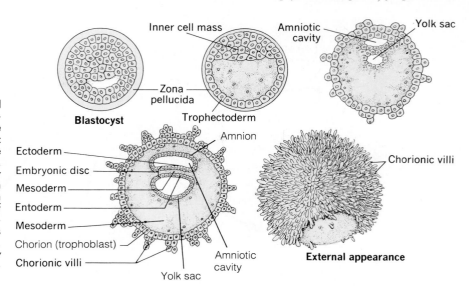

**FIGURE 4-2.**
Early stages of development. (Top, left and center): The cells are separated into a peripheral layer and an inner cell mass. The peripheral layer is called a blastodermic vesicle. (Top, right): The formation of the amniotic cavity and yolk sac is indicated. The former is lined with ectoderm, the latter with entoderm. (Bottom, left): The location of the embryonic disc and the three germ layers is shown, together with beginning of the chorionic villi. (Bottom, right): The external appearance of the developing mass is shown; the chorionic villi are abundant. (From S.J. Reeder and L.L. Martin, *Maternity Nursing* [16th ed.]. Philadelphia: J.B. Lippincott, 1987.)

## Fetal Period

The fetal period begins with the ninth week and terminates with the birth of the fetus. As the embryo enters this stage of biophysical development, the head accounts for about 50% of the overall body length and human characteristics are evident. Bones begin to harden, muscles develop, and sex is distinguishable by the fourth lunar month. The placenta is completely formed and fetal circulation established by the third lunar month. Reflexes appear and movement becomes evident to the mother by 20 weeks gestation. Lanugo (soft, downy hair) develops over the body by the fifth lunar month, while vernix caseosa (a cheese-like substance) appears on the skin in the sixth lunar month. Figure 4-5 illustrates the month-by-month development of the fetus.

## Support Structures

### Placenta

As noted earlier, the blastocyst is covered with a layer of cells known as trophoblast. Those trophoblasts in direct contact with the endometrium produce fingerlike projections called chorionic villi that invade and digest the endometrium (see Figure 4-2). This invasive process results in erosion of the maternal blood vessels in the endometrium and formation of maternal lakes filled with maternal blood. The placenta is formed from the fusion of the endometrium and enlarging chorionic villi. Tiny blood vessels also form in the chorionic villi. These vessels carry fetal blood that does not mix with the maternal blood. The processes of diffusion and active transport account for the exchange of nutrients, oxygen, and waste

products in the placenta following its complete development by the third month. The levels of estrogen and progesterone, originally produced by the corpus luteum, are now maintained by the placenta. The placenta functions as a barrier to infection, as an endocrine gland in the production of estrogen and progesterone, as well as the organ of metabolic and nutrient exchange. The fetal surface of the placenta is covered with the amnion. At term (38 to 42 weeks), the placenta is a rather large organ covering almost one-half of the internal uterine wall. At this time, it measures approximately 15 to 20 cm (5.9 to 7.9 inches) in diameter, 2.5 to 3.0 cm (1.0 to 1.2 inches) in thickness, and weighs about 400 to 600 grams (14 to 21 ounces).

The umbilical cord results from the elongation of the body stalk, which is responsible for connecting the embryo to the yolk sac. Tiny blood vessels develop and extend into the chorionic villi. As the body stalk elongates,

**TABLE 4-1.**
EVOLUTION OF BODY ORGANS FROM PRIMARY GERM LAYERS

| ENDODERM | MESODERM | ECTODERM |
|---|---|---|
| Gastrointestinal system | Skin | Epidermis |
| Liver, pancreas | Bones | Hair, nails |
| Trachea, lungs | Muscle | Urethra |
| Pharynx | Heart, blood | Teeth enamel |
| Thyroid | Spleen | Nervous system |
| Tonsils | Kidneys, ureters | Mammary glands |
| | Ovaries, uterus | |
| | Testes | |

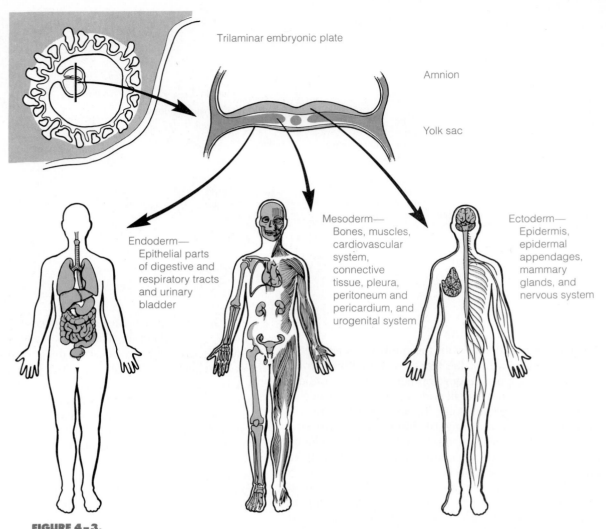

**FIGURE 4-3.**
The body systems and the primary germ layers from which they develop. (From K.M. Van De Graaff and S.I. Fox, *Concepts of Human Anatomy and Physiology.* Dubuque, Iowa: Wm. C. Brown, 1989.)

these tiny vessels merge into the umbilical vein and two umbilical arteries. These blood vessels are surrounded by a special connective tissue referred to as Wharton's jelly. At term, the umbilical cord measures approximately 2 cm (0.8 inch) in diameter and about 55 cm (22 inches) in length.

## Fetal Membranes

Fetal membranes consisting of both the chorion and amnion constitute the "bag of waters." The trophoblasts not directly involved with the implantation process soon begin to degenerate and form the chorion or outer lining. The amnion is a smooth membrane evolving from the ectoderm and forming the inner lining of the bag of waters (Figure 4-6). Amniotic fluid, ranging from 500 to 1500 cc, is secreted by the amnion. Amniotic fluid functions to regulate temperature, aid in fetal movement, and protect the developing fetus from injury.

## Yolk Sac

The yolk sac arises from the endoderm about the eighth or ninth day after conception. It is responsible for production of red blood cells for about 6 weeks until the fetal liver is capable of this function. However, it is not responsible for the developing embryo's nutrition.

## Fetal Circulation

Three unique structures function during fetal development to provide sufficient blood flow for metabolic and

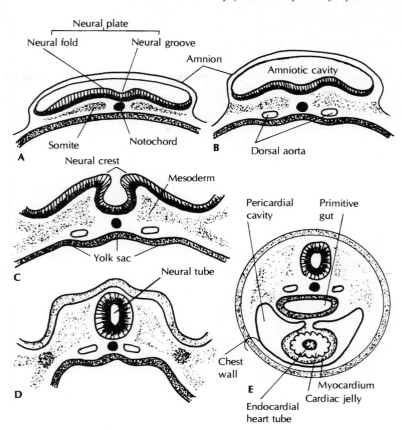

**FIGURE 4-4.**
Schematic representation of growth and folding of the germ layers. **A.** About 18 days; **B.** About 20 days; **C.** About 22 days; **D.** About 25 days; **E.** About 28 days. (From C.S. Schuster and S.S. Ashburn, *The Process of Human Development: A Holistic Approach.* Boston: Little, Brown, 1986.)

nutrient functions of the placenta. These structures include the ductus venosus, the foramen ovale, and the ductus arteriosus. Oxygenated and nourished blood from the placenta enters the fetus through the umbilical vein. Soon after entering the abdominal wall, the umbilical vein branches. The smaller branch enters the hepatic circulation and later empties into the inferior vena cava through the hepatic vein. The second, larger branch enters the inferior vena cava directly through the ductus venosus. Blood from the inferior vena cava empties directly into the right atrium where it mixes with blood from the superior vena cava. The majority of this blood passes through the foramen ovale and directly into the left atrium where it mixes with deoxygenated blood from the lungs. This blood is then pumped into the left ventricle and out to the fetal body through the aorta. The remaining blood in the right atrium is pumped through the tricuspid valve into the right ventricle and out the pulmonary artery. Only a small portion of this blood continues to the nonfunctioning lungs to nourish them, while the remainder passes through the ductus arteriosus and enters the body circulation directly. Deoxygenated blood returns to the placenta through the umbilical arteries where the process repeats itself (Figure 4-7).

## FACTORS AFFECTING BIOPHYSICAL DEVELOPMENT

### Maternal Factors

The event of conception activates a complex chain of events. Additional energy is needed for cell division, while hormones are helping to prepare body systems to accommodate the developing pregnancy and fetus. Alteration and adaptation to pregnancy involves all maternal body systems. Since the mother reacts as a total unit or system to the developing fetus, the intrauterine environment operates at an optimal level only to the degree that the maternal system is capable of adapting and adjusting to the developing fetus. Maternal illnesses and infections affect the intrauterine environment and the biophysical development of the pregnancy and fetus.

### Illnesses

*HYPERTENSIVE DISORDERS OF PREGNANCY.* Hypertension occurs in 5% to 7% of pregnancies. It is the third leading cause of maternal mortality and a major cause of infant morbidity in the United States. *Toxemia*

## Fetal Development

### 1st Lunar Month

The fetus is 0.75 cm to 1 cm in length.

Trophoblasts embed in decidua.

Chorionic villi form.

Foundations for nervous system, genitourinary system, skin, bones, and lungs are formed.

Buds of arms and legs begin to form.

Rudiments of eyes, ears, and nose appear.

4 weeks

### 2nd Lunar Month

The fetus is 2.5 cm in length and weighs 4 g.

Fetus is markedly bent.

Head is disproportionately large, owing to brain development.

Sex differentiation begins.

Centers of bone begin to ossify.

Heart begins to beat.

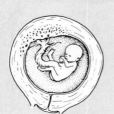

8 weeks

### 3rd Lunar Month

The fetus is 7 cm to 9 cm in length and weighs 28 g.

Fingers and toes are distinct.

Placenta is complete

Fetal circulation is complete.

Face develops human appearance.

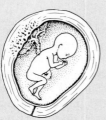

3 months

### 4th Lunar Month

The fetus is 10 cm to 17 cm in length and weighs 55 g to 120 g.

Sex is differentiated.

Rudimentary kidneys secrete urine.

Heartbeat is present.

Nasal septum and palate close.

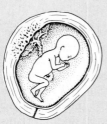

4 months

### 5th Lunar Month

The fetus is 25 cm in length and weighs 223 g.

Lanugo covers entire body.

Fetal movements are felt by mother.

Heart sounds are perceptible by auscultation.

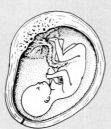

5 months

### 6th Lunar Month

The fetus is 28 cm to 36 cm in length and weighs 680 g.

Skin appears wrinkled.

Vernix caseosa appears.

Eyebrows and fingernails develop.

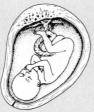

6 months

### 7th Lunar Month

The fetus is 35 cm to 38 cm in length and weighs 1200 g.

Skin is red.

Pupillary membrane disappears from eyes.

The fetus has an excellent chance of survival.

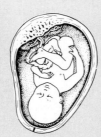

7 months

### 8th Lunar Month

The fetus is 38 cm to 43 cm in length and weighs 2.7 kg.

Fetus is viable.

Eyelids open.

Fingerprints are set.

Vigorous fetal movement occurs.

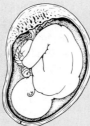

8 months

### 9th Lunar Month

The fetus is 42 cm to 49 cm in length and weighs 1900 g to 2700 g.

Face and body have a loose wrinkled appearance because of subcutaneous fat deposit.

Lanugo disappears

Amniotic fluid decreases.

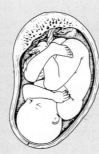

9 months

### 10th Lunar Month

The fetus is 48 cm to 52 cm in length and weighs 3000 g.

Skin is smooth.

Eyes are uniformly slate colored.

Bones of skull are ossified and nearly together at sutures.

**FIGURE 4–5.**
Fetal development. (Adapted from S.J. Reeder and L.L. Martin, *Maternity Nursing* [16th ed.]. Philadelphia: J.B. Lippincott, 1987.)

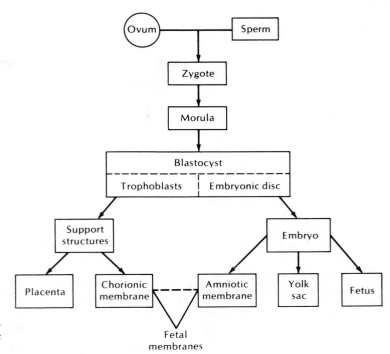

**FIGURE 4-6.**
Origin of embryo and support structures. (From C.S. Schuster and S.S. Ashburn, *The Process of Human Development: A Holistic Approach.* Boston: Little, Brown, 1986.)

was the term used in the past to categorize the several hypertensive states that occurred during pregnancy. In 1972, the Committee on Terminology of the American College of Obstetricians and Gynecologists developed a new classification system to replace the broad classification, toxemia. Toxemia included the major characteristics of hypertension, edema, and proteinuria. In the new classification, hypertension in pregnancy is defined as a diastolic blood pressure of at least 90 mm Hg, or a systolic blood pressure of at least 140 mm Hg, or a rise of 30 mm Hg over a baseline nonpregnant value.[3]

*Gestational hypertension* is the name given to hypertension that occurs only during pregnancy. It generally develops during the latter half of pregnancy with no associated symptoms and usually disappears within 10 days after delivery. Gestational hypertension should be differentiated from *chronic hypertension*, which occurs before the 20th week of gestation and continues more than 42 days after delivery.

Proteinuria, edema, or both, in the presence of hypertension, is defined as *pregnancy induced hypertension (PIH)*. PIH usually occurs after the 20th week of gestation. When proteinuria, edema, or both develop in the person who already displays hypertension before pregnancy, it is called *superimposed preeclampsia.* Progression of PIH can cause convulsions, which is termed *eclampsia*, in the absence of associated cerebral disorders such as epilepsy.

The cause of PIH is still unknown. In the later stage

of pregnancy, a sensitivity to the increased amount of angiotensin II, which is a vasoconstrictor, may occur. Only a small amount of angiotensin is required to elevate the blood pressure causing vasoconstriction and decreased peripheral blood flow to occur (Figure 4-8). Diminished placental blood flow also occurs and affects fetal perfusion. The glomerular filtration rate is decreased in response to the decreased blood flow to the kidneys. The glomerular capillaries become edematous and allow protein to be excreted in the urine. This produces a decrease in the serum albumin level.

Due to the decreased blood flow to the kidneys, serum levels of blood urea nitrogen (BUN), uric acid, and creatinine become elevated. Sodium is conserved and urine output is decreased. Sodium retention increases angiotensin II sensitivity.[4]

Although maternal mortality is low, hypertension during pregnancy, whatever the cause, places the mother at increased risk for eclampsia, cerebral vascular accidents, cardiopulmonary insufficiency, aspiration pneumonias, premature separation of the placenta which contributes to death from hypovolemic shock, and disseminated intravascular coagulation (DIC). The infant is often growth retarded or small for gestational age, and may be born prematurely due to placental insufficiency. The infant also may suffer hypoxia and acidosis if the mother experiences a seizure.

HELLP syndrome is a variant of PIH that can be fatal for both mother and fetus. It occurs in 2% to 12% of the

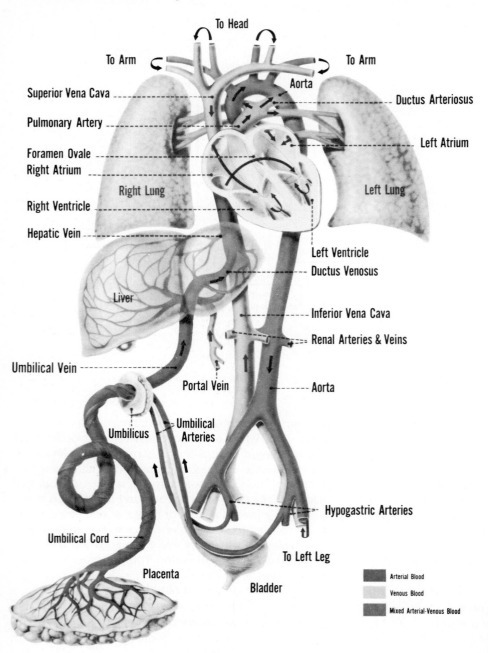

To Head

To Arm

To Arm

Aorta

Superior Vena Cava

Ductus Arteriosus

Pulmonary Artery

Left Atrium

Foramen Ovale

Right Atrium

Right Lung

Left Lung

Right Ventricle

Hepatic Vein

Left Ventricle

Ductus Venosus

Liver

Inferior Vena Cava

Renal Arteries & Veins

Umbilical Vein

Portal Vein

Aorta

Umbilicus

Umbilical Arteries

Hypogastric Arteries

Umbilical Cord

To Left Leg

Placenta

Bladder

Arterial Blood

Venous Blood

Mixed Arterial-Venous Blood

**FIGURE 4–7.**
Fetal circulation. (Ross Clinical Education Aid No. 1, Courtesy of Ross Laboratories.)

5% to 7% of persons who develop PIH. The characteristics of HELLP are hemolysis (H), elevated liver enzymes (EL), and a low platelet count (LP). HELLP always occurs in association with PIH. However, since HELLP syndrome symptoms may be present before the symptoms of PIH, it is often misdiagnosed as DIC, acute hepatitis, gallbladder disease, and other conditions.[10] Figure 4-9 outlines the pathophysiology that occurs in HELLP syndrome.

*DIABETES MELLITUS.*    Diabetes mellitus, the inability to properly metabolize glucose, is a challenging condition during pregnancy (see Chap. 39). White devel-

oped a classification system for the diabetic who is pregnant[15] (Box 4-1). Diabetes occurs in one of 100 to 500 pregnancies. Of these the maternal mortality is 0.5%, while perinatal mortality is approximately 10%. Perinatal mortality refers to fetal and infant death from 28 weeks gestation to 4 weeks after birth.

The maternal mortality rate for the pregnant diabetic has decreased in recent years. However, the pregnant diabetic is still at risk for higher mortality than the general obstetric population. The increase in maternal mortality may be influenced by the increased frequency of PIH, which progresses to eclampsia in approximately

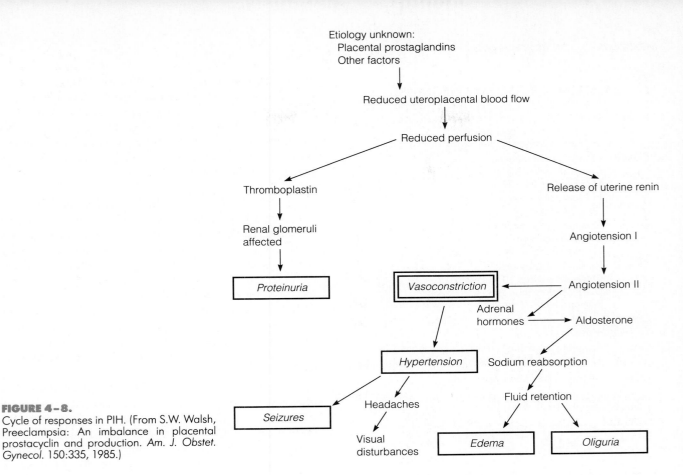

**FIGURE 4–8.**
Cycle of responses in PIH. (From S.W. Walsh, Preeclampsia: An imbalance in placental prostacyclin and production. *Am. J. Obstet. Gynecol.* 150:335, 1985.)

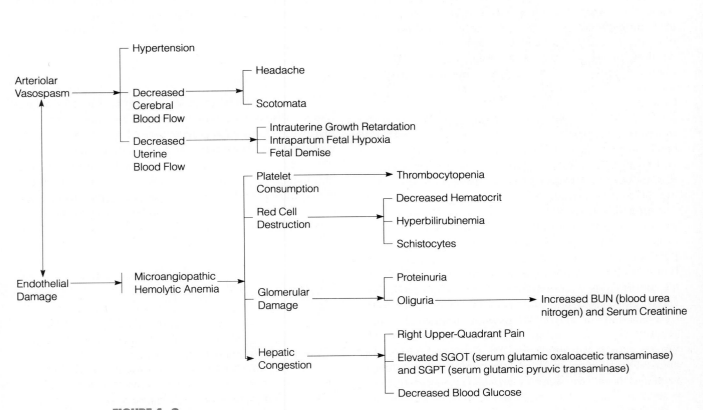

**FIGURE 4–9.**
Pathophysiology of HELLP syndrome. (From A.A. Whittaker, et al., Hemolysis, elevated liver enzymes, and low platelet count syndrome. Nursing care of the critically ill obstetric patient. *Heart Lung* 15:402–408, July 1986.)

**BOX 4-1.**
## CLASSIFICATION OF DIABETES IN PREGNANCY

| | |
|---|---|
| Class A | Patient with abnormal glucose tolerance test with normal fasting blood sugar<br>Controlled with diet alone |
| Class B | Insulin-treated diabetic<br>Onset after age 20<br>Duration less than 10 y<br>No vascular disease or retinopathy |
| Class C | Insulin-treated diabetic<br>Onset between ages 10 and 20 y<br>Duration between 10 and 20 y<br>No vascular disease or retinopathy |
| Class D | Insulin-treated diabetic<br>Onset before age 10 y<br>Duration more than 20 y<br>Retinopathy |
| Class E | Any pregnant diabetic with calcification of the pelvic vasculature |
| Class F | Any pregnant diabetic with diabetic nephropathy |
| Class R | Any pregnant diabetic with proliferative retinopathy |
| Class T | Pregnancy after renal transplant |

Source: Adapted from P. White, Classification of obstetrical diabetes. Am. J. Obstet. Gynecol. 130:228, 1978.

25% of pregnant diabetes, by infection and by hemorrhage. Spontaneous abortions occur more frequently due to compromised placental circulation associated with diabetic vascular complications. Polyhydramnios (excess amniotic fluid) occurs in about 10% to 25% of pregnant diabetics due to increased osmotic pressure, increased secretion of amniotic fluid, and diuresis from fetal hyperglycemia.

The fetal mortality rate is 10 times greater than the mortality rate for fetuses born to nondiabetic mothers. Fetal mortality may be attributed to fetal hyperglycemia and hyperinsulinemia. A previous history of stillbirth, PIH, or vascular involvement increases the frequency of intrauterine fetal death.

After delivery, there is also a 2% to 5% increase in the rate of infant mortality for the infant of a diabetic mother (IDM). Complications frequently occurring in IDMs include hypoglycemia, hypocalcemia, hyperbilirubinemia, and respiratory distress syndrome. Congenital abnormalities, particularly in the cardiac, renal, and central nervous systems, occur two to three times more frequently in the IDM. *Macrosomia* (abnormally large bodies) is present in infants whose mothers are in White's classes A through C and is associated with an increased frequency of traumatic complications during vaginal delivery. *Intrauterine growth retardation* (IUGR) is seen in infants whose mothers are in classes D through F due to the vascular complications occurring in these groups.

Gestational diabetes mellitus (GDM), also called class A diabetes, is defined as carbohydrate intolerance with onset during pregnancy. Approximately 2% to 3% of pregnant women develop GDM during pregnancy. Of this number, 20% to 50% will require insulin to maintain normal blood glucose levels. Many women with GDM will develop overt diabetes later in life.

*CARDIAC DISEASE.*    The increase in blood volume that occurs in pregnancy may begin as early as 6 weeks gestation. The blood volume rises slowly in the first trimester, reaching a peak about 30 to 34 weeks gestation. A woman who is healthy and without a cardiac disorder can withstand the additional stress from the increased blood volume. However, when there is cardiac pathology, the pregnancy may be complicated. The complications that can occur are related to the degree of disability as categorized in the New York Heart Association functional classification of heart disease defined in Box 4-2.[9]

The three major types of heart disease that affect pregnancy are rheumatic heart disease, congenital anomalies, and changes in the heart resulting from hypertension (see Chaps. 25 and 26). Maternal risks associated with cardiac disease are increases in the rates of spontaneous abortion and premature labor. Premature birth, respiratory acidosis, and growth retardation related to low oxygen levels in the mother are seen in infants born of mothers who suffer from cardiac disease.

## Sexually Transmitted Diseases and Infections

Sexually transmitted diseases (STDs) and infections are specific diseases or syndromes that are transmitted primarily through sexual contact (see Chap. 57). A pregnant woman, the unborn fetus, and the neonate suffer severe symptoms and complications as a result of a STD during pregnancy. More than 20 STDs have been identified which cause a wide variety of complications during pregnancy, such as spontaneous abortion, premature birth, IUGR, stillbirth, congenital anomalies, and neonatal

**BOX 4-2.**
## CLASSIFICATION OF HEART DISEASE

| | |
|---|---|
| Class I | No symptoms of cardiac insufficiency on exertion; no limitations of physical activity |
| Class II | Symptoms felt on ordinary exertion; a slight limitation in physical activity |
| Class III | Symptoms felt even during limited activity |
| Class IV | Symptoms occurring during any physical activity, even at rest |

**TABLE 4–2.**
EFFECTS OF INFECTIONS DURING PREGNANCY

| INFECTION | MATERNAL EFFECTS | FETAL EFFECTS |
|---|---|---|
| Condylomata acuminata | Vulvar warts; may require cesarean birth | None noted |
| Cytomegalovirus disease | Asymptomatic or mimics mononucleosis | Increase in perinatal mortality; fetal malformations |
| Gonorrhea | Asymptomatic or vaginal discharge; scarring of the fallopian tubes, which can affect ability to conceive | Fetal death, mental retardation, ophthalmia neonatorum |
| Herpes simplex Type II | Vulvovaginitis | Increased perinatal mortality; fetal malformations |
| Influenza | Can produce critical illness if pneumonia develops | Fetal death and congenital anomalies |
| Hepatitis Infectious (Type A) Serum (Type B) | Abortion or premature labor | Fetal death, fetal deformities, congenital hepatitis |
| Monilial vaginitis | Thick, irritating vaginal discharge | Thrush in newborn |
| Poliomyelitis | More susceptible during pregnancy | Increased perinatal mortality |
| Rubella (German measles) | Fever and typical rash, abortion | Increased perinatal mortality and congenital defects |
| Rubeola (3-day measles) | Fever and typical rash, abortion | Increased perinatal mortality; congenital or neonatal infection will produce rash |
| Syphilis | May be asymptomatic or produce primary and secondary lesions | Fetal death, congenital syphilis |
| Toxoplasmosis | Asymptomatic | Increased perinatal mortality, congenital anomalies, congenital toxoplasmosis |
| Chlamydia | Often asymptomatic | Increased incidence of preterm labor and postnatal eye and respiratory infection |
| Urinary tract infections | Asymptomatic or fever, chills, dysuria, urinary frequency, and pain; abortion and premature labor | No effects unless sulfonamides are used in late pregnancy; they may cause jaundice |
| Varicella | Typical lesions; may precipitate shingles | Fetal death, growth retardation, and fetal malformations |

Source: M. A. Auvenshine and M. G. Enriquez, Comprehensive Maternity Nursing: Prenatal and Women's Health. Boston: Jones and Bartlett, 1990.

death. Table 4-2 lists infections and their effects on the mother and fetus during pregnancy.

## Fetal Factors

The first 2 months of pregnancy represent an especially vulnerable time in the biophysical development of the embryo. Spontaneous abortion is most likely to occur, often before the woman is even aware that she is pregnant. Factors associated with spontaneous abortion include uterine anomalies, abnormal implantation, and genetic anomalies of the embryo. Genetic influences on biophysical development are discussed in Chapter 3. Fetal factors most associated with altered development include placental anomalies and multiple pregnancies.

## Placental Anomalies

As discussed earlier, the fertilized ovum begins its implantation process approximately 1 week after conception. Normally, this implantation occurs in the upper por-

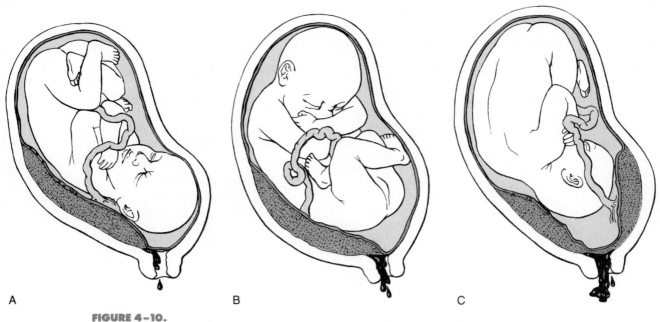

**FIGURE 4–10.**
Placenta previa. **A.** Low implantations, **B.** Partial placenta previa. **C.** Central (total) placenta previa.
(From S.J. Reeder and L.L. Martin, *Maternity Nursing* [16th ed.]. Philadelphia: J.B. Lippincott, 1987.)

tion of the body of the uterus. The formation of the placenta occurs in this position and is complete by the third lunar month.

*PLACENTA PREVIA.* Placenta previa involves an implantation in the lower portion of the uterus (Figure 4-10). This implantation may involve only the lower uterine segment or it may completely cover the cervix. The most frequent symptom associated with placenta previa is painless vaginal bleeding in the third trimester of pregnancy. The threat to the fetus depends upon the degree to which the birth canal is blocked or the development of hemorrhage. Conservative treatment and vaginal delivery may provide a healthy newborn when the placenta is implanted in the lower segment. However, the only way to insure the baby's survival when there is a complete previa is through cesarean delivery. Although the exact cause of placenta previa is unknown, several factors have been associated with it. These factors include advanced maternal age, increased parity, uterine scarring, multiple gestation, and enlarged placenta. Ultrasonography is especially helpful in identifying the exact location of the placenta. Risks for the fetus are also determined by the length of gestation and maturity of the fetus at the time of delivery.

*ABRUPTIO PLACENTA.* Another placental anomaly associated with high risk for poor fetal outcome is abruptio placenta (Figure 4-11). In this condition, the placenta

begins an abrupt premature separation from the uterine wall. The severity of the outcome depends upon the amount of hemorrhage and whether or not a clot forms. Generally, an immediate delivery is essential if the fetus is to survive and develop normally. The exact cause of abruptio placenta has not been determined but the condition is often associated with diabetes, pregnancy-induced hypertension, and chronic hypertension. There has also been an increased frequency associated with high parity, overdistention of the uterus, and physical injury, as well as cigarette smoking and the use of cocaine. Frequently, the woman presents with complaints of severe abdominal pain and a hard, boardlike abdomen. Fetal maturity at the time of emergency delivery will greatly influence fetal outcome.

*ECTOPIC PREGNANCY.* Ectopic pregnancy represents a third implantation anomaly. This condition involves the implantation of a fertilized ovum outside of the uterine cavity (Figure 4-12). The most common site is the fallopian tube where the fertilized ovum may get caught or become too large to proceed through the tube. The frequency of ectopic pregnancy has increased due to the increased number of women of childbearing age with a history of pelvic inflammatory disease or the use of intrauterine device for contraception, either of which can cause scarring and alterations within the tube. Ectopic pregnancy represents a life-threatening condition for the mother due to the hemorrhage and emergency surgery

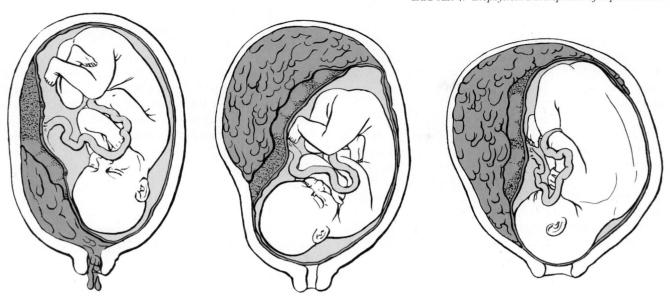

**FIGURE 4–11.**

Abruptio placentae at various separation sites. (Left) External hemorrhage. (Center) Internal or concealed hemorrhage. (Right) Complete separation. (From S.J. Reeder and L.L. Martin, *Maternity Nursing* [16th ed.]. Philadelphia: J.B. Lippincott, 1987.)

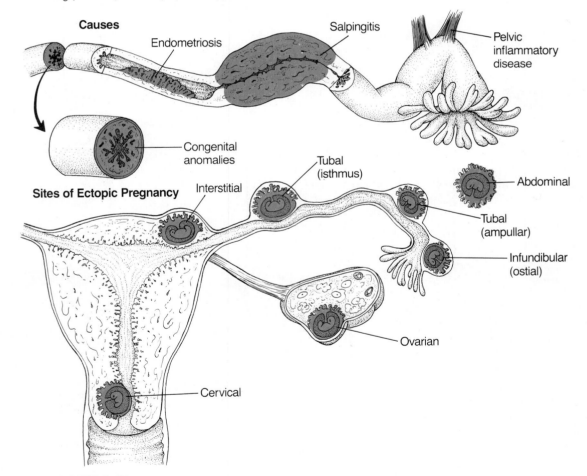

**FIGURE 4–12.**

Causes and sites of ectopic pregnancy. (From S.J. Reeder and L.L. Martin, *Maternity Nursing* [16th ed.]. Philadelphia: J.B. Lippincott, 1987.)

associated with a ruptured ectopic pregnancy. If this condition is diagnosed before tubal rupture, hemorrhage may be avoided and surgery scheduled for removal of the affected tube. Pregnancy tests and ultrasonography aid in the diagnosis of the presence of a fetal sac outside of the uterus.

*PLACENTAL INSUFFICIENCY.* Placental insufficiency is most often associated with fetal and uterine growth retardation and may produce dysfunction of maternal—placental or fetal—placental circulation which compromises fetal nutrition and oxygenation. Occasionally, the placenta may be too small or inadequately developed to support fetal growth and development. Causes of placental insufficiency include multiple pregnancy,

postmaturity, systemic diseases, hypertension, and abnormalities of the placental membranes.

Infarctions, usually found on the maternal side of the placenta, may develop when the blood supply is decreased and necrosis occurs. Infarctions appear as circular lesions ranging from dark red to yellowish white in color. Fetal risk is greatest when the infarctions occur in the central portion of the placenta and interfere with fetal circulation.

## Multiple Gestations

Multiple gestations constitute yet another risk factor to fetal growth and development and have increased greatly

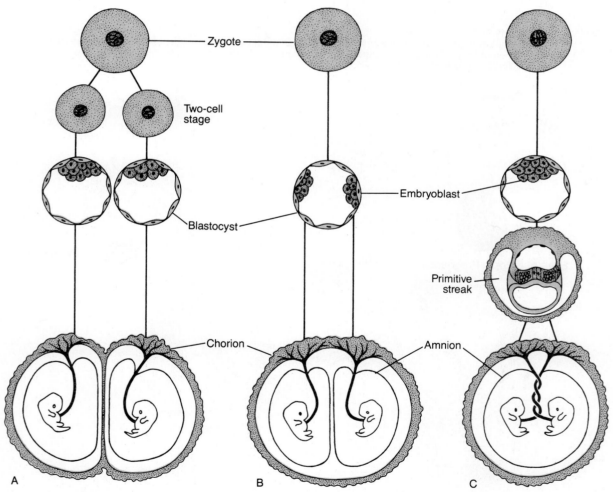

**FIGURE 4–13.**
Membranes and placenta in twin pregnancies. **A.** Two placentas, two amnions, two chorions (from eith dizygotic twins of monozygotic twins with early cleavage of the zygote. **B.** and **C.** Single ovum twins. **B.** One chorion and two amnions and one placenta **C.** One chorion and one amnion (note entanglement of cords, a danger when there is only one amnion) (From S.J. Reeder and L.L. Martin, *Maternity Nursing* [16th ed.]. Philadelphia: J.B. Lippincott, 1987.)

due to the use of fertility drugs in the treatment of infertility. The most common form of multiple gestation is twinning. There are two major types of twins. *Monozygotic* (identical) twins occur when one ovum, fertilized by one sperm, splits following conception (Figure 4-13). Genetically, monozygotic twins are identical. Depending upon the stage of development when cleavage occurs, the twins may share amnions, chorions, or both (see Figure 4-13).

*Dizygotic* (fraternal) twins occur when two individual ova are fertilized by two separate sperm. Two placenta, two chorions, and two amnions are present. The only similarities between dizygotic twins are those similarities associated with other siblings in the same family (Figure 4-14).

Due to the limited intrauterine space, prematurity is the most common problem associated with multiple gestation. Abnormal positioning is more frequent and may necessitate cesarean delivery. Monozygotic twins are especially at risk for transfusion syndrome where one infant is well nourished and developed while the other twin is pale, anemic, and displays evidence of intrauterine growth retardation (IUGR). In monozygotic twins, the umbilical cords may also become entangled, leading to fetal demise of one twin.

## Environmental Factors

### Maternal Nutrition

Pregnancy is a unique developmental time. At no other stage in the life cycle does the well-being of one individual, the fetus, depend so directly on the well-being of another individual, the mother. The nutritional status of the mother is a critical determinant of her own well-being, as well as that of the fetus. Proper nutrition during pregnancy reduces the risks for maternal complications such as PIH and anemia, ensures adequate tissue growth, and promotes optimal infant birth weights. Table 4-3 lists the recommended daily allowances for nonpregnant women as compared to Table 4-4, which includes the recommended daily allowances for pregnant and lactating women.

Inadequate maternal nutrition has a direct effect on fetal brain development. When maternal nutrition is insufficient, the fetal brain will not develop properly. Inadequate maternal nutrition also has a significant effect on infant birth weight. Infants with low birth weight are at risk for more frequent illness, hearing and vision disabilities, behavioral disorders, and learning problems than infants whose is the normal range.

Several maternal conditions or factors aid in identi-

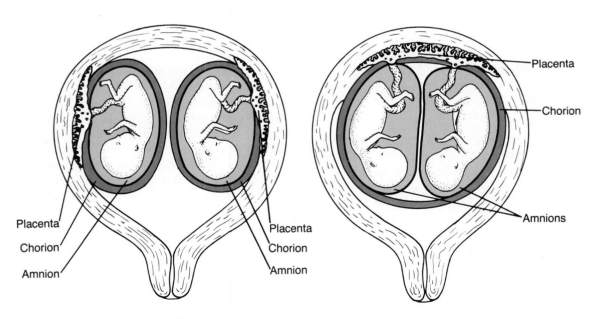

**A. Fraternal twins**          **B. Identical twins**

**FIGURE 4-14.**
Twin pregnancies. **A.** Fraternal twins with two placentas, two amnions, and two chorions. **B.** Identical twins with one placenta, one chorion, and two amnions. (From S.J. Reeder and L.L. Martin, *Maternity Nursing* [16th ed.]. Philadelphia: J.B. Lippincott, 1987.)

**TABLE 4–3.**

RECOMMENDED DAILY DIETARY ALLOWANCES
FOR WOMEN (NONPREGNANT)

| | AGES | | | |
|---|---|---|---|---|
| | 11–14 | 15–18 | 19–22 | 23–50 |
| Energy, kcal | 2200 | 2100 | 2100 | 2000 |
| Protein, g | 46 | 46 | 44 | 44 |
| Vitamin A, RE | 800 | 800 | 800 | 800 |
| IU | 4000 | 4000 | 4000 | 4000 |
| Vitamin D, $\mu$g | 10 | 10 | 7.5 | 5 |
| Vitamin E, Q-TE | 8 | 8 | 8 | 18 |
| Ascorbic acid, mg | 50 | 60 | 60 | 60 |
| Niacin, mg | 15 | 14 | 14 | 13 |
| Riboflavin, mg | 1.3 | 1.3 | 1.3 | 1.2 |
| Thiamin, mg | 1.1 | 1.1 | 1.1 | 1.0 |
| Vitamin $B_6$, mg | 1.8 | 2.0 | 2.0 | 2.0 |
| Folacin, $\mu$g | 400 | 400 | 400 | 400 |
| Vitamin $B_{12}$, $\mu$g | 3 | 3 | 3 | 3 |
| Calcium, mg | 1200 | 1200 | 800 | 800 |
| Phosphorus, mg | 1200 | 1200 | 800 | 800 |
| Iodine, $\mu$g | 150 | 150 | 150 | 150 |
| Iron, mg | 18 | 18 | 18 | 18 |
| Magnesium, mg | 300 | 300 | 300 | 300 |
| Zinc | 15 | 15 | 15 | 15 |

Source: *Food and Nutrition Board, Committee on Dietary Allowances, National Research Council. Recommended Dietary Allowances (9th ed.). Washington, D.C.: National Academy of Sciences, 1980.*

fying those women who are nutritionally at risk. Some of these conditions are: (1) adolescence, (2) overweight, (3) underweight, (4) inadequate weight gain, (5) excessive weight gain, (6) anemia, (7) smoking, alcohol, and drug use, (8) pica, (9) poor diet, and (10) medical problems such as diabetes. Several of these factors are discussed in the following section.

*ADOLESCENCE.* The pregnant adolescent has increased nutritional needs to provide for the developing musculoskeletal system. Musculoskeletal growth is not complete at puberty and growth may continue for 1 to 2 years after puberty. Additionally, the pregnant adolescent must meet her own nutritional needs, as well as those required by the developing fetus. The recommended daily allowances for the pregnant adolescent are reflected in Table 4-4.

*PICA.* Pica is the practice of eating nonfood substances such as laundry starch, dirt, or clay which may result in a less than optimal intake of essential nutrients. The nonfood items may contain lethal substances such as lead, which can seriously affect the fetus.

*IRON DEFICIENCY ANEMIA.* Iron deficiency anemia during pregnancy is defined as a hemoglobin of 10 gm or less during the second and third trimesters.[8]

Mild anemia, a hemoglobin of 11 gm, presents no real threat to the mother but it is evidence that the maternal nutritional status is less than optimal.

Iron deficiency anemia results from a decrease in hemoglobin production due to the expenditure of iron stores. Iron stores become depleted from insufficient intake of iron, blood loss, malabsorption, and hemolysis.[8] Ferrous sulfate, 320 mg three times a day, and vitamin C, 500 mg per day, are usually given for iron deficiency anemia.[8] However, these supplements should never be considered a replacement or substitute for proper nutrition. The influence of diabetes on nutritional status in pregnancy is discussed in Chapter 39. The effects of anorexia and bulimia on nutritional status is described in Chapter 10.

### Teratogens

A teratogen is a substance or agent that produces abnormalities in embryonic or fetal development. The most common teratogens that affect pregnancy and the fetus are tobacco, possibly caffeine, drugs including alcohol, infections, and radiation. Approximately 20% to 40% of women in the childbearing age in the United States smoke in spite of recent evidence supporting the negative effects of smoking during pregnancy.[1] Fetal tobacco syndrome is a phrase that has recently been introduced to refer to the specific conditions that result from prenatal exposure to tobacco smoke.[2] Clinical implications on caffeine use during pregnancy are not as clear as those for alcohol and tobacco. In one report, an increase in spontaneous abortions, stillbirths, and premature births was shown to be associated with maternal consumption of more than 600 mg of caffeine, or more than eight cups of coffee per day.[1] Approximately 20 million people in the United States have used cocaine on at least one occasion. There are no available national data on maternal cocaine use, but cocaine use during pregnancy produces serious physiologic effects on both mothers and fetuses (Figure 4-15).[1] The most serious effect of alcohol use during pregnancy occurs in fetal alcohol syndrome (FAS), which results from the consistent intake of more than 80 to 100 gm (2.8 to 3.5 ounces) of alcohol each day.[1]

## PRENATAL DIAGNOSTIC STUDIES

Prenatal diagnostic studies of fetal well-being and maturity provide much needed information regarding pregnancy status. Careful selection of tests can predict placental insufficiency, fetal anomalies, genetic abnormalities, and the ability of the fetus to survive in the existing intrauterine, as well as extrauterine, environment. Since maternal morbidity and mortality associated with childbearing are low, the focus of prenatal assessment of fetal well-being is to decrease fetal death and disease.

**TABLE 4–4.**

RECOMMENDED DIETARY ALLOWANCES FOR PREGNANT
AND LACTATING WOMEN

| | AGES | | | | Differences for Lactation |
|---|---|---|---|---|---|
| | 11–14 | 15–18 | 19–22 | 23–50 | |
| Energy, kcal | 2500 | 2400 | 2400 | 2300 | +200 |
| Protein, g | 76 | 76 | 74 | 74 | −10 |
| Vitamin A, RE | 1000 | 1000 | 1000 | 1000 | +200 |
| IU | 5000 | 5000 | 5000 | 5000 | +1000 |
| Vitamin D, $\mu$g | 15 | 15 | 12.5 | 10 | same |
| Vitamin E, Q-TE | 10 | 10 | 10 | 10 | +1 |
| Ascorbic acid, mg | 70 | 80 | 80 | 80 | +20 |
| Niacin, mg | 17 | 16 | 16 | 15 | +3 |
| Riboflavin, mg | 1.6 | 1.6 | 1.6 | 1.5 | +0.2 |
| Thiamin, mg | 1.5 | 1.5 | 1.5 | 1.4 | +0.1 |
| Vitamin $B_6$, mg | 2.4 | 2.6 | 2.6 | 2.6 | −0.1 |
| Folacin, $\mu$g | 800 | 800 | 800 | 800 | −300 |
| Vitamin $B_{12}$, $\mu$g | 4 | 4 | 4 | 4 | same |
| Calcium, mg | 1600 | 1600 | 1200 | 1200 | same |
| Phosphorus, mg | 1600 | 1600 | 1200 | 1200 | same |
| Iodine, $\mu$g | 175 | 175 | 175 | 175 | +25 |
| Iron, mg | 18+ | 18+ | 18+ | 18+ | +6 |
| Magnesium, mg | 450 | 450 | 450 | 450 | same |
| Zinc | 20 | 20 | 20 | 20 | +5 |

Source: *Food and Nutrition Board, Committee on Dietary Allowances, National Research Council. Recommended Dietary Allowances (9th ed.). Washington, D.C.: National Academy of Sciences, 1980.*

Assessment of fetal health and well-being ideally begins before conception. Those persons anticipating parenthood should prepare physically and psychologically by attaining and maintaining physical health, eating nutritiously, and avoiding substances such as drugs, alcohol, and cigarettes prior to conception. Women taking prescription medications for a preexisting medical condition should confer with their physician prior to conception.

## Risk Factors

Once conception has occurred, pregnancy presents a slightly greater risk of morbidity and mortality over the nonpregnant state. Factors that increase mortality and morbidity have been categorized into demographic, obstetric, medical, and miscellaneous conditions. Persons identified in any of these categories may require prenatal diagnostic studies to monitor the development of the pregnancy and fetus. Demographic factors that frequently place a woman at risk during pregnancy are maternal age of 15 years and under and 35 years or over, persons of a nonwhite race, single women, and those women who are dependent on welfare or public assistance. Obstetric risk factors are related to infertility, previous abortion, pre-

mature or low birth weight infant, postterm pregnancy, incompetent cervix, PIH, and multiple gestation. Miscellaneous factors that place a pregnancy at risk are related to maternal nutrition, smoking, and alcohol use. Medical factors that place a pregnancy at risk are anemia, heart disease, diabetes mellitus, sexually transmitted diseases (STDs), psychiatric disorders, and any other chronic medical condition.[8]

## Prenatal Diagnostic Techniques

Several antenatal diagnostic tests are currently available to assess fetal health and well-being. Selective use of the tests provides information concerning the development of the fetus and fetal adaptation to the intrauterine environment. Table 4-5 lists diagnostic tests and their most frequent use by trimesters.

### Ultrasonography

Ultrasound, or sonography, is a noninvasive procedure that uses high-frequency sound waves above 20,000 cycles per second to provide images of the fetus, placenta, and uterus as early as 4 to 5 weeks after the last menstrual

# EFFECTS OF MATERNAL COCAINE USE ON MOTHERS AND FETUSES/BABIES

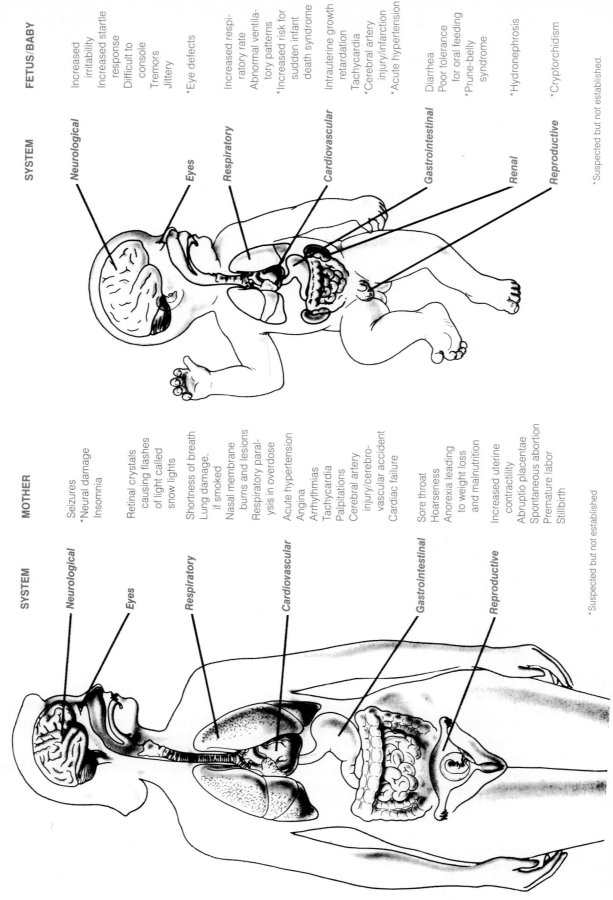

| SYSTEM | MOTHER |
|---|---|
| *Neurological* | Seizures<br>*Neural damage<br>Insomnia |
| *Eyes* | Retinal crystals causing flashes of light called snow lights |
| *Respiratory* | Shortness of breath<br>Lung damage, if smoked<br>Nasal membrane burns and lesions<br>Respiratory paralysis in overdose |
| *Cardiovascular* | Acute hypertension<br>Angina<br>Arrhythmias<br>Tachycardia<br>Palpitations<br>Cerebral artery injury/cerebrovascular accident<br>Cardiac failure |
| *Gastrointestinal* | Sore throat<br>Hoarseness<br>Anorexia leading to weight loss and malnutrition |
| *Reproductive* | Increased uterine contractility<br>Abruptio placentae<br>Spontaneous abortion<br>Premature labor<br>Stillbirth |

*Suspected but not established

| SYSTEM | FETUS/BABY |
|---|---|
| *Neurological* | Increased irritability<br>Increased startle response<br>Difficult to console<br>Tremors<br>Jittery |
| *Eyes* | *Eye defects |
| *Respiratory* | Increased respiratory rate<br>Abnormal ventilatory patterns<br>*Increased risk for sudden infant death syndrome |
| *Cardiovascular* | Intrauterine growth retardation<br>Tachycardia<br>*Cerebral artery injury/infarction<br>*Acute hypertension |
| *Gastrointestinal* | Diarrhea<br>Poor tolerance for oral feeding<br>*Prune-belly syndrome |
| *Renal* | *Hydronephrosis |
| *Reproductive* | *Cryptorchidism |

*Suspected but not established.

**FIGURE 4–15.**
The dangers of prenatal cocaine use. (MCN 13, 174–179, 1988.)

**TABLE 4–5.**
PRENATAL DIAGNOSTIC TESTS AND MOST FREQUENT USE BY TRIMESTERS

| FIRST TRIMESTER, WEEKS 1–13 | SECOND TRIMESTER, WEEKS 14–27 | THIRD TRIMESTER, WEEKS 28–40 |
|---|---|---|
| **Ultrasound (Crown-Rump Length/CRL)**<br>▶ Diagnose pregnancy<br>▶ Assess gestational age<br>▶ Identify congenital anomalies<br>▶ Evaluate vaginal bleeding<br>▶ Confirm multiple gestations<br>▶ Assess fetal growth<br>▶ Augment other prenatal tests<br>▶ Evaluate pelvic mass<br><br>**Doppler Ultrasound**<br><br>**Chorionic Villus Sampling** | **Ultrasound (Biparietal Diameter/BPD)**<br>▶ Assess gestational age<br>▶ Confirm multiple gestations<br>▶ Assess fetal growth<br>▶ Identify structural abnormalities of fetus such as hydrocephalus<br>▶ Guide amniocentesis and fetoscopy procedures<br>▶ Determine placenta location and condition<br><br>**Doppler Ultrasound**<br><br>**Duplex Scanning**<br><br>**Amniocentesis (Up to 20 weeks)**<br>▶ Determine genetic make-up<br>▶ Determine isoimmunization (20–22 weeks)<br><br>**Alpha-Fetoprotein**<br><br>**AchE**<br><br>**Placental Grading**<br><br>**Fetoscopy (16–20 weeks)**<br><br>**Percutaneous Umbilical Blood Sampling (PUBS)** | **Ultrasound**<br>▶ Determine fetal position<br>▶ Estimate fetal size<br><br>**Doppler Ultrasound**<br><br>**Duplex Scanning**<br><br>**Amniocentesis**<br>▶ Determine fetal lung maturity<br>▶ Determine blood grouping<br>▶ Detect amnionitis<br><br>**Phosphatylglycerol (PG)**<br><br>**Shake Test**<br><br>**Placental Grading**<br><br>**Percutaneous Umbilical Blood Sampling (PUBS)**<br><br>**Fetal Biophysical Profile** |

period (LMP). The first ultrasound scanning used a static B-scan method that provided two-dimensional images in cross section. The B-scan method also provided data on tissue density and consistency. Currently, real-time (B-scan) ultrasound is the newest and most sophisticated form of sonography. This method provides continuous cross section pictures of internal structures and the motion that occurs in these structures. With this method, an entire field can be scanned to show movement such as the fetal heart beating or the motion of an extremity.[3] Diagnosis of a pregnancy can be performed as early as 4 to 5 weeks after the LMP through the use of static scanning. At this time, the gestational sac that is implanted in the endometrial cavity can be pictured since it is filled with fluid, is echo-free, and is surrounded by solid uterine tissue. Early diagnosis of pregnancy expedites determination of the expected date of delivery (EDC), identifies persons with risk factors, and promotes planning and referral needed for persons identified as high risk.

The most frequent use of ultrasound during the first trimester is to determine gestational age. Due to the rapid growth that occurs during the first trimester, the most accurate time to determine the EDC is between weeks 7 and 13 after the LMP.[8] Through the use of real-time ultrasound, gestational age can be estimated to within 1 to 3 days exactness by measuring the fetal crown-rump length.

After 14 weeks gestation, the biparietal diameter (BPD), the widest transverse diameter of the fetal head, is measured to determine gestational age. The optimal time to assess gestational age using BPD measurement is between 16 and 20 weeks gestation. At this time, ultrasound is accurate to within plus or minus 1 week.

In addition to determination of gestational age, ultrasound is used to identify congenital anomalies, particularly in the large structures of the head and trunk. If fetal anomalies are identified, additional studies, such as amniocentesis or fetal blood sampling, are done to identify possible chromosomal disorders.

Assessment of placental condition and location is also possible since ultrasound, unlike radiography, detects soft tissue. Assessment of placental location is important, particularly in the presence of vaginal bleeding. Ectopic pregnancy can also be ruled out when an intrauterine pregnancy is identified. In cases where there is intraabdominal pathology, such as an ovarian cyst, and examination of the abdomen is difficult, ultrasound helps to determine the presence of a pregnancy.

Ultrasound can also be used to grade the placenta. Assessment of a mature placenta, in combination with adequate BPD measurements, indicates fetal lung maturity. Scores resulting from placental grading range from 0, immature, to 3, mature.

Since a large number of fetuses are aborted during the first trimester, serial ultrasounds done in weekly intervals help to authenticate fetal growth or deterioration. Serial sonograms are also used to assess fetal growth and well-being in high-risk situations, such as maternal diabetes and Rh sensitization.[3]

Ultrasound is also used to identify the presence of multiple gestation. Multiple gestation often produces associated risk factors such as prematurity and hypertension.

## Doppler Ultrasound

Doppler ultrasound is a diagnostic technique used to assess the movement of blood in blood vessels and body organs such as the uterus and the fetal heart. Doppler ultrasound differs from the ultrasound technique described above because images of body structures are not provided with this method. The doppler sends out sound waves at a particular frequency which are directed at moving red blood cells. The sound waves which locate and "bounce off" the RBCs return at a different frequency. The rate at which the RBCs move causes the change in frequency.[13]

Two types of doppler instruments may be used prenatally. One type is the continuous wave (CW) doppler. The other type is the pulsed-wave (PW) doppler. The CW doppler sends out continuous ultrasound waves. The velocity of the RBCs in the path of the wave can be recorded. The CW doppler is used in prenatal clinics and doctors' offices to assess fetal heart rate and blood flow through the fetal heart. Blood flow through the fetal heart can be detected as early as 8 weeks gestation with the CW doppler, while auscultation of the fetal heart with a manual fetoscope can only be accomplished at 16 to 20 weeks gestation.[13]

The PW doppler sends out pulses of ultrasound waves each second instead of a continuous sound wave. The sound wave pulses locate and "bounce off" different areas in the blood vessel. By sampling the sound waves as they return at different time intervals, velocity of blood flow in various areas of the blood vessel can be evaluated.[13]

PW ultrasound can also be combined with real-time ultrasound. This combination method of ultrasound is called duplex scanning. Specific blood vessels such as placental vessels, the umbilical vein, the fetal aorta and carotid arteries and the fetal heart can be located with real-time ultrasound. The PW doppler is then used to measure the velocity of blood flow in specific vessels. Duplex scanning is a useful assessment tool during the second and third trimesters when high-risk vascular conditions exist.[13]

## Chorionic Villus Sampling

Chorionic villus sampling (CVS) is a relatively new technique used during the first trimester of pregnancy to diagnose chromosomal abnormalities and biochemical disorders. It can be performed as early as nine weeks following the LMP. Chorionic villi are vascular extensions from the blastocyst that provide an attachment with the endometrium and result in the formation of the placenta. Chorionic villi sampling may be performed transvaginally or transabdominally. However, the success rate for the transvaginal method is more successful at 96%.[14] Viability and gestational age are determined by ultrasound prior to performing a CVS. A gonorrhea cervical culture is also collected and analyzed prior to performing a CVS. The woman must have a negative gonorrhea culture to prevent dissemination of neisseria gonorrhea into the bloodstream following the test.

Using ultrasound for direction, a plastic catheter is placed in the chorion frondosum and a specimen of chorionic villi is removed (Figure 4-16). The sample is placed in a sterile culture medium and studied in a cytogenetic laboratory. Women who are Rh negative and unsensitized to Rh positive blood should receive anti-D globulin RhoGam.[14]

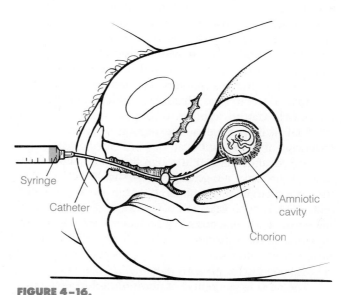

**FIGURE 4-16.**
Diagram of the uterus at 10 weeks gestation with biopsy catheter in position.

Syringe

Catheter

Amniotic cavity

Chorion

Because CVS is a relatively new procedure, data related to the risks associated with it are incomplete and in the process of being compiled by the International Registry of the World Health Organization. The risks associated with CVS are similar to those following amniocentesis and may include amniotic fluid leakage, infection, intrauterine fetal death, IUGR, Rh isoimmunization, spontaneous abortion, septic shock, and damage to the placental membranes.[6] There is less than 1% error in interpretation of the test results. Infection can occur since the catheter is passed transvaginally, and the risk increases with the number of catheters used. Higher infection rates are noted in primigravidas because of the opposition of the cervix to passage of the catheter. In addition, there is the potential for mistakes to occur if maternal tissue is analyzed or multiple gestation is present but unnoticed.

The greatest benefit of CVS is that the procedure can be performed during the first trimester, as opposed to amniocentesis, which cannot be done until approximately 14 to 16 weeks gestation when sufficient amniotic fluid is present. Because cell division occurs rapidly and the cells do not have to be grown in a laboratory, direct microscopic analysis can be done during the metaphase of mitosis. Preliminary results can then be obtained as early as 24 to 48 hours, and these results verified in 5 to 10 days. First-trimester termination of pregnancy then becomes an option when an abnormality is identified. Another benefit of CVS over amniocentesis is that CVS uses living tissue rather than dead, sloughed epithelial cells, permitting identification of more potential disorders.

## Amniocentesis

Amniocentesis is a procedure that involves the aspiration of amniotic fluid from the uterus by way of an abdominal puncture. The test can be performed in any trimester of pregnancy as long as sufficient fluid is present. When it is done in the first trimester, it is usually for genetic studies; in the second trimester, for Rh isoimmunization studies; and in the third trimester, for assessment of fetal lung maturity. Amniocentesis is preceded by ultrasound to confirm fetal viability and gestational age, locate the position of the placenta, and identify pockets of amniotic fluid. The site for needle insertion is chosen to avoid the placenta and fetus, but to also provide an adequate amount of fluid. Approximately 20 cc of amniotic fluid are aspirated for analysis. RhoGam is given to the Rh negative, unsensitized mother after the procedure.

*AMNIOCENTESIS FOR GENETIC STUDIES.* Of the 2300 identified genetic disorders that affect humans, over 70 can be diagnosed by amniocentesis.[3] The test is considered a conventional part of prenatal care especially in advanced maternal age. Most women who are age 35 years or older at the time of delivery will have amniocentesis performed. At age 35, the risk for cytogenetic abnormality, most frequently trisomy 21, is one in 80, and the risks increase with advanced maternal age.

In many cases, amniocentesis can identify missing enzymes that indicate a fetal biochemical abnormality. Biochemical disorders involve lipid, amino acid, and mucopolysaccharide abnormalities; neural tube defects (NTDs); trisomy 21; hemophilia; and muscular dystrophy.[3]

Amniocentesis is also appropriate when a previous pregnancy has involved a fetus or infant with a chromosomal abnormality, NTD, or in cases where parents have a genetic disorder or a known translocation carrier. One of every 500 people carry a balanced chromosomal translocation. This translocation in a parent who is phenotypically normal will produce genetic imbalance in the offspring.

Single gene x-linked (sex-linked) recessive disorders, such as hemophilia and muscular dystrophy, can be identified by amniocentesis through fetal sex determination. The recurrence risk for x-linked recessive transmission is 25% with each pregnancy for male fetuses. Females are carriers and are unaffected. Therefore, amniocentesis is indicated in pregnancies where the mother is a known carrier of an x-linked disorder.

Autosomal recessive single gene disorders, such as sickle cell anemia, can also be diagnosed by amniocentesis. Discussion of recurrence risks for autosomal recessive single gene disorders is found in Chapter 3.

*ALPHA-FETOPROTEIN.* The level of alpha-fetoprotein (AFP), which is increased in the presence of an NTD, can also be determined through amniocentesis. AFP, which is produced by the fetal yolk sac and liver, reaches its highest level at about 13 weeks gestation. AFP in maternal serum (MSAFP) reaches its highest serum peak around 30 weeks gestation. The protein enters the maternal serum through the placenta and the amniotic fluid through the fetal urine. The normal level of AFP at 18 weeks gestation is 18.5 mg per ml amniotic fluid. AFP levels may be increased in situations of fetal leakage, hemorrhage, or multiple pregnancy. The actual procedure of amniocentesis can also increase AFP levels so that an MSAFP should be done before the test to prevent errors in interpretation of AFP. In families with an increased risk for NTDs, MSAFP combined with ultrasound is recommended. If the MSAFP level is increased and the sonar is normal, an amniocentesis may be necessary to make the diagnosis of a possible NTD.

*ACETYLCHOLINESTERASE.* Acetylcholinesterase (AchE) is a new test that is more reliable than AFP or MSAFP to diagnose NTDs. AchE is produced in the fetal central nervous system and is more fetal-specific than

AFP or MSAFP. Increased levels of AchE indicate an NTD, while decreased levels indicate recent fetal demise.

*AMNIOCENTESIS FOR RH ISOIMMUNIZATION.*
An Rh negative mother with an antibody titer of 1:8 or 1:16 or higher should have the first amniocentesis at approximately 24 to 25 weeks gestation. Through amniocentesis, the quantitative amount of bilirubin is determined, indicating the degree of fetal red blood cell (RBC) hemolysis. Depending upon the severity of hemolysis, an intrauterine fetal blood transfusion of Rh negative blood may be indicated to decrease maternal antibody formation and to correct fetal anemia that results from hemolysis. In severe cases, fetal hydrops and fetal demise can result if intrauterine treatment is not performed.

*AMNIOCENTESIS FOR FETAL LUNG MATURITY.*
The most frequent use of amniocentesis in the third trimester is to assess fetal lung maturity. Fetal lung maturity is measured by two phospholipids produced by fetal lung tissue, lecithin, and sphingomyelin. Due to their detergent effect, lecithin and sphingomyelin mix with amniotic fluid in the lung to promote a decreased surface tension and protect the alveoli from collapse. If both lecithin and sphingomyelin, which are expressed as a ratio (L/S), are adequate, breathing of the neonate after delivery will prevent collapse of the alveoli. If the L/S ratio is inadequate, alveoli collapse and respiratory distress syndrome (RDS) may develop.

The L/S ratio of 2:1 indicates two times as much lecithin as sphingomyelin and is usually an acceptable indicator of fetal lung maturity. Prior to 30 to 32 weeks gestation, there is more sphingomyelin than lecithin. At about 32 weeks gestation, lecithin and sphingomyelin are equal in amount. At 35 weeks, lecithin increases rapidly and sphingomyelin remains constant.

*SHAKE TEST.*    In an emergency labor and delivery situation where there is no time to perform an L/S ratio, a shake test or foam test may be done at the bedside to determine fetal lung maturity. To determine the detergent action of lecithin and sphingomyelin, the specimen is rigorously shaken or agitated. After a 15-minute delay, mature fetal lungs are diagnosed if bubbles or foam remain on top of the amniotic fluid.

*PHOSPHATIDYLGLYCEROL.*    Phosphatidylglycerol (PG) and phosphatidylonisitol (PI) are two other phospholipids that are also associated with fetal lung maturity. PG is used in conjunction with L/S ratio. When the L/S ratio is low, a positive PG level may indicate fetal lung maturity.

## Fetoscopy

Fetoscopy is an experimental procedure used to diagnose and treat the fetus in utero. It is used in combination with ultrasound to locate the placenta and umbilical cord and to assess fetal growth. A needlescope, a flexible endoscope and needle, is inserted into the uterus to the fetus through the maternal abdomen. Fetal skin tissue and samples of blood can be collected for diagnosis of genetic disorders. Intrauterine blood transfusions can be performed in cases of severe fetal anemia that result from hemolysis where there is blood incompatibility.

There is a 5% risk for spontaneous abortion after fetoscopy. Bleeding, infection, injuries to the fetus, amniotic fluid leakage, and premature birth may also occur.

These risks along with its cost and the lack of availability of the procedure in prenatal centers, have limited its present use.

## Percutaneous Umbilical Blood Sampling

Percutaneous umbilical blood sampling (PUBS) is a new experimental procedure that allows direct entry to fetal circulation. The PUBS procedure produces a pure specimen of fetal blood that permits a speedy fetal karotype, blood typing, antibody testing, acid-base evaluation, assessment of isoimmune hemolytic anemia, and intrauterine fetal blood transfusion.[5,12]

Through the use of ultrasound, the placenta and cord are located before the procedure. Needle insertion and aspiration of the fetal blood sample take place near the insertion of the cord into the placenta because less movement of the cord occurs at this location. However, maternal intervillous blood lakes are situated near the insertion of the umbilical cord into the placenta, which result in an increased chance of contamination with maternal blood.

Potential complications following the PUBS procedure are chorioamnionitis, premature labor and rupture of the amniotic membranes, bleeding, and injury to the umbilical cord. Infection occurs in 1% of procedures.[5]

Through the PUBS procedure, direct assessment of fetal hemoglobin concentration is possible. Direct transfusion of RBCs to the fetus will immediately correct fetal anemia and is preferred over intraabdominal transfusion of packed RBCs, which take several weeks to be absorbed across the peritoneal membrane.[5]

## Fetal Biophysical Profile

A fetal biophysical profile involves evaluation of five variables that are assessed using real-time ultrasound. The five variables are: fetal movement (FM), fetal breathing movements (FBM), fetal tone (FT), amniotic fluid volume (AFV), and placental maturation. These variables are assessed and scored by the sonographer. Each variable receives a score of 2 if it is assessed as normal and a score of 0 if it is abnormal.[3] Table 4-6 includes a list of variables and the criteria for determining the score. High scores indicate fetal well-being and low scores indicate the need

**TABLE 4–6.**
BIOPHYSICAL PROFILE

| VARIABLES | NORMAL (SCORE = 2) | ABNORMAL (SCORE = 0) |
|---|---|---|
| Fetal breathing movements | One or more episodes in 30 min, each lasting >30 sec | Episodes absent or no episode of >30 sec in 30 min |
| Gross body movements | Three or more discrete body/limb movements in 30 min (episodes of active continuous movement considered as a single movement) | Less than three episodes of body/limb movements in 30 min |
| Fetal tone | One or more episodes of active extension with return to flexion of fetal limb(s) or trunk; opening and closing of hand considered normal tone | Slow extension with return to flexion; movement of limb in full extension, or fetal movement absent |
| Reactive fetal heart size | Two or more episodes of acceleration (>15 beats per min) in 20 min, each lasting >15 sec and associated with fetal movement | Less than two episodes of acceleration or acceleration of <15 beats per min in 20 min |
| Qualitative amniotic fluid volume | One or more pockets of fluid measuring >1 cm in two perpendicular planes | Pockets absent or pocket <1 cm in two perpendicular planes |

| SCORE | INTERPRETATION | RECOMMENDED MANAGEMENT |
|---|---|---|
| 10 | Normal infant, low risk for chronic asphyxia | Repeat testing at weekly intervals; repeat twice weekly in diabetic patients and patients >42 weeks |
| 8 | Normal infant, low risk for chronic asphyxia | Repeat testing at weekly intervals; repeat twice weekly in diabetic patients and patients >42 weeks; oligohydramnios is indication for delivery |
| 6 | Suspected chronic asphyxia | Repeat testing within 24 h; oligohydramnios or repeat score <6 is indication for delivery |
| 4 | Suspected chronic asphyxia | Indications for delivery are >36 weeks and favorable cervix; if <36 weeks and lecithin/sphingomyelin ratio <2.0, repeat test in 24 h; repeat score <6 or oligohydramnios is indication for delivery |
| 2 | Strong suspicion of chronic asphyxia | Extend testing time to 120 min; persistent score <4, regardless of gestational age, is indication for delivery |

Reprinted with permission from F. A. Manning, I. Morrison, I. R. Lange, et al.: Fetal assessment based on fetal biophysical profile scoring: Experience in 12,620 referred high risk pregnancies. Am. J. Obstet. Gynecol. 151:345, 1985.

for additional testing. Indications for assessment of the fetal biophysical profile are hypertension, diabetes, postmature pregnancy, and suspected IUGR.

## BIOPHYSICAL FACTORS AFFECTING LABOR AND DELIVERY

### Initiation of Labor

After approximately 266 days of being nourished and nurtured within the mother's womb, the fetus is ready for its transition to extrauterine life. The exact cause of the onset of labor has not been identified. However, various theories or a combination of theories are now being accepted as possible explanations for the initiation of labor.

### Theories of Onset

*HORMONAL STIMULATION.* Throughout pregnancy estrogen and progesterone play an important role in maintaining the gestation. Estrogen is believed to increase the oxytocin receptors in the uterus while progesterone exerts a relaxing effect. Although research findings continue to be inconsistent, estrogen may increase while progesterone may decrease at or near term.[7] Oxytocin, produced by both the fetus and mother, has a stimulating effect on the smooth muscle of the uterus, thus producing uterine contractions.

*UTERINE DISTENTION THEORY.*   This theory is based on the knowledge regarding the stretching of uterine muscle as it increases in size during pregnancy. During pregnancy, progesterone exerts a relaxing effect on the myometrium. As the pregnancy approaches term, the level of progesterone declines, thus allowing the overdistended uterus to begin contracting.

*PROSTAGLANDIN THEORY.*   Prostaglandin levels are known to increase just before the onset of labor. This action may be a response to estrogen stimulation.[7] Prostaglandin exerts a stimulating effect on the smooth muscle of the myometrium, possibly leading to the onset of the contractions of labor.

## Premonitory Signs

Some evidence of impending labor is noted by most women. These premonitory signs include lightening. Lightening heralds the entry of the presenting part into the pelvis. This process is accompanied by downward movement of the uterus and a release of pressure on the diaphragm. This movement, however, is often accompanied by leg cramps, pelvic pressure and urinary frequency, increased vaginal secretions, and venous stasis.

*BRAXTON-HICKS CONTRACTIONS.*   Braxton-Hicks contractions, present throughout pregnancy, become stronger, regular, and begin to produce cervical changes. These contractions sometimes become so uncomfortable that the woman goes to the hospital or physician's office for evaluation. Cervical dilatation is the most accurate way of differentiating between true and false labor.

*CERVICAL CHANGES.*   Cervical changes are another indication of the onset of labor. Softening (ripening) of the cervix occurs as a result of Braxton-Hicks contractions. Cervical dilatation and effacement may also occur prior to the onset of regular contractions.

*SHOW.*   Show is the pink-tinged secretion associated with the expulsion of the mucus plug from the cervix as it begins to dilate and efface. Labor usually begins within 24 to 48 hours of expulsion of the mucus plug. Show should be differentiated from the blood-tinged discharge associated with rupture of small vessels during vaginal examination.

*RUPTURE OF THE MEMBRANES.*   Rupture of the membranes may precede the onset of labor or occur during the process. There is increased risk of infection with prolonged rupture of the membranes. The color of the amniotic fluid should be noted when membranes rupture since meconium-stained fluid may be associated with fetal distress. There is also risk of prolapsed cord when the membranes rupture if the presenting part is not adequately engaged in the true pelvis or if there is abnormal fetal positioning, including breech position.

## Stages of Labor

The process of labor and delivery has been divided into four stages. *Stage one* begins with the first regular uterine contractions and ends with complete cervical dilatation (10 cm) (Figure 4-17). *Stage two* begins with complete dilatation and ends with expulsion of the fetus. The *third stage* of labor begins with delivery of the fetus and ends with delivery of the placenta. The *fourth stage* of labor encompasses the first hour or so after the delivery of the placenta.

### First Stage

The first stage of labor is divided into three phases: latent, active, and transition. Although both physical and emotional changes are associated with each stage, only the physical changes are discussed.

The *latent phase* begins with the first regular uterine contractions. Contractions are usually mild, lasting 15 to 20 seconds, and occurring every 5 to 7 minutes. The cervix effaces and dilates up to 3 to 4 cm. The average latent phase is 8.6 hours for nulliparas and 5.3 hours for multiparas.

The *active phase* ends when cervical dilatation reaches 8 cm. It is accompanied by cervical effacement and fetal descent in the birth canal. Uterine contractions become moderate in intensity and occur every 3 to 5 minutes, lasting 35 to 40 seconds.

*Transition* is associated with cervical dilatation between 8 and 10 cm. Contractions occur every 2 to 3 minutes, last 60 to 90 seconds, and are moderate to severe in intensity. Transition is also associated with nausea, vomiting, diaphoresis, periods of amnesia, and increased anal pressure.

### Second Stage

The second stage of labor is also referred to as the expulsion stage. In nulliparas, delivery usually occurs within 2 hours. The second stage of labor averages only 15 minutes in multiparas. As the fetus progresses through the birth canal, it undergoes a series of movements referred to as the mechanism or movements of labor. These movements include descent, flexion, internal rotation, extension, restitution, external rotation, and expulsion. These movements are illustrated in Figure 4-18.

The mother experiences an involuntary urge to

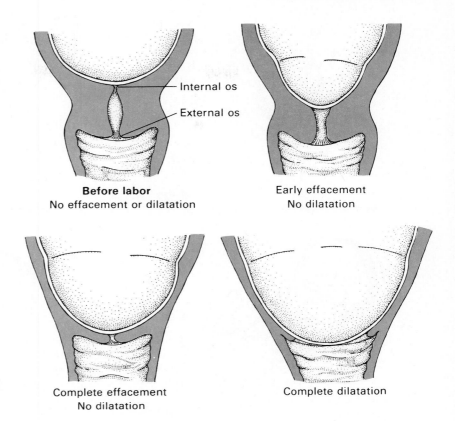

Internal os

External os

**Before labor**
No effacement or dilatation

Early effacement
No dilatation

Complete effacement
No dilatation

Complete dilatation

**FIGURE 4-17.**
Stages in cervical effacement and dilatation. (From S.J. Reeder and L.L. Martin, *Maternity Nursing* [16th ed.]. Philadelphia: J.B. Lippincott, 1987.)

push. Intraabdominal pressure works with the uterine contractions to expel the fetus. As the presenting part begins to emerge, the perineum bulges and flattens out. The anus dilates and the labia separate. Intense rectal pressure, pain, stretching, tearing, and burning of the perineum are common sensations as the woman delivers the fetal head. Upon delivery of the fetal head, the mother experiences a sense of relief and decrease of pain and pressure. A small perineal incision, called an episiotomy, may be performed to avoid laceration and aid in delivery of the fetus.

### Third Stage

The third stage of labor is referred to as the placental stage and involves separation and delivery of the placenta. After delivery of the infant, the uterus contracts, thus decreasing its size and surface area for placental attachment. Separation of the placenta results in bleeding and the formation of a hematoma. This hematoma further enhances placental separation. Membranes separate as the placenta descends the birth canal. Evidence that the placenta has separated include the following: (1) a firm, globular-shaped uterus that rises in the abdomen, (2) a sudden gush of blood, and (3) lengthening of the umbilical cord as it protrudes from the vagina. The length of

the third stage ranges from about 5 to 30 minutes. The risk for complications is increased after 30 minutes.

The most common mechanism for delivery of the placenta is Schultz's mechanism (Figure 4-19A). Placental separation occurs first in the center and results in delivery of the fetal side first. The second mechanism for placental delivery is referred to as the Duncan mechanism (Figure 4-19B). In this mechanism, separation occurs first along the outer edges, causing the placenta to roll and present the maternal side first. There is increased risk of retained placental parts when the Duncan mechanism occurs.

### Fourth Stage

Technically, the immediate postpartum period is not a true stage of labor. However, it is a critical period of adaptation. The uterus should remain firmly contracted, in the midline, and midway between the symphysis pubis and umbilicus. Relaxation of the uterus results in hemmorhage and even maternal death if not immediately treated by fundal massage and/or oxytocic drugs to control the bleeding. Although there may be a slight drop in blood pressure and slight increase in pulse immediately after delivery, vital signs should return to prelabor values very quickly. A shaking chill may be experienced in the

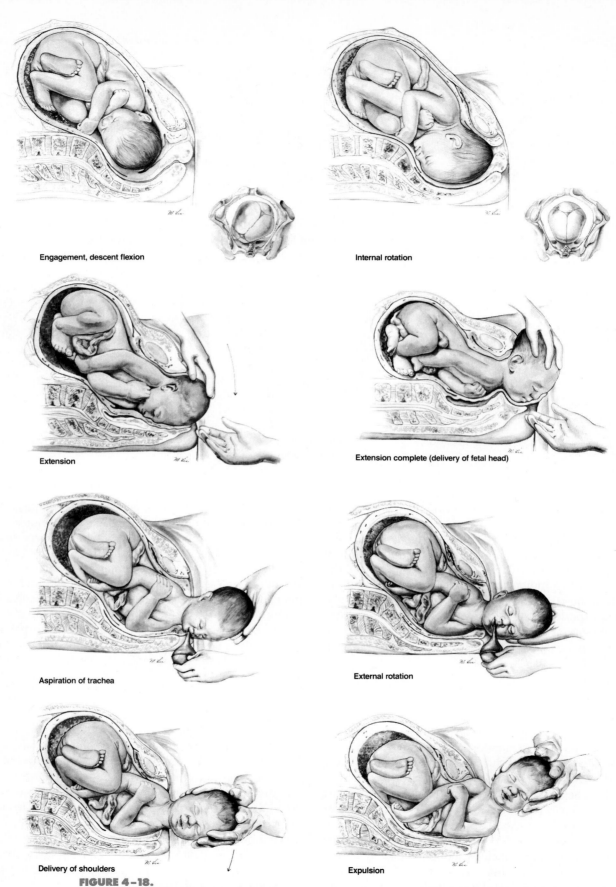

Engagement, descent flexion

Internal rotation

Extension

Extension complete (delivery of fetal head)

Aspiration of trachea

External rotation

Delivery of shoulders

Expulsion

**FIGURE 4-18.**
Mechanism of delivery for a vertex presentation. (From N. Whitley, *A Manual of Clinical Obstetrics.*
Philadelphia: J.B. Lippincott, 1985.)

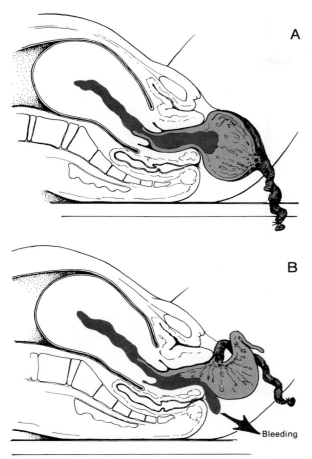

**FIGURE 4–19.**
Expulsion of the placenta by **A.** Schultze's mechanism, whereby the placenta is turned inside out within the vagina and is delivered with the glistening fetal surfaces to the outside, and by **B.** the Duncan mechanism, whereby the placenta is rolled up in the vagina and is delivered with the maternal surface to the outside. (From S.J. Reeder and L.L. Martin, *Maternity Nursing* [16th ed.]. Philadelphia: J.B. Lippincott, 1985.)

recovery room in response to the exertion of labor, anesthesia, and sudden release of intraabdominal pressure. The mother may also complain of thirst and hunger. A summary of the four stages of labor is found in Box 4-3.

## Alterations and Adaptations

The accomplishment of a spontaneous delivery requires the interaction of numerous factors. Problems in adaptation can occur as a result of alterations in any of the four Ps—*power, passage, passenger,* and *psyche.* Power represents the frequency, duration, and intensity of contractions, as well as the pushing effort of the woman. Passage refers to the size and type of pelvis, as well as ability of the cervix and vagina to respond and allow passage of

the fetus. Passenger is used to refer to the fetus, its head size, position, presentation, attitude, and umbilical cord. Psyche, critical in the birth process, includes the effects of anxiety, tension, and fear, which can lengthen the duration of labor and delivery. Specific problems associated with alterations in power, passage, and passenger are discussed in the following section.

### Power

The timing, strength, and efficiency of uterine contractions in producing cervical dilatation and effacement are major forces in the timely descent and delivery of the fetus. Uterine contractions must be rhythmical and of adequate force to facilitate delivery. There must also be adequate rest and relaxation between contractions to allow for sufficient uteroplacental exchange. Alterations in the contraction forces occur when contractions occur continuously, are prolonged, or are insufficient to produce dilatation and effacement. Any of these alterations may result in dysfunctional labor and may even predispose to additional alterations such as dehydration, exhaustion, infection, and fetal compromise.

*DYSFUNCTIONAL LABOR.* Four labor patterns are reflective of dysfunctional labor. These are *hypertonic labor, hypotonic labor, precipitous labor,* and *prolonged labor.* The characteristics, maternal implications, and fetal or neonatal implications of each pattern are reflected in Table 4-7.

*PRETERM LABOR.* Preterm labor refers to the onset of labor between 20 and 38 weeks gestation. Labor prior to 38 weeks gestation occurs in 5% to 10% of all pregnancies. As much as 75% of neonatal morbidity and mortality can be attributed to preterm delivery of the fetus. Even when the preterm neonate survives, long-term complications such as physical and mental handicaps are also attributed to complications of preterm delivery.

Although the exact cause of preterm labor is unknown, fetal, maternal, and placental factors have been known to contribute to the onset of preterm labor. Table 4-8 reflects low-, medium-, and high-risk factors associated with preterm labor. Table 4-9 reflects one system for determining risk of preterm labor and delivery.

Early diagnosis is essential if preterm labor is to be interrupted. Contractions occurring at less than 10-minute intervals for 30 to 60 minutes and resulting in cervical dilatation and effacement are strongly suggestive of preterm labor. Conservative management consisting of bedrest, increased fluids, and prenatal assessment is instituted prior to tocolytic therapy. Increased prenatal assessment includes more frequent office visits and possibly home fetal monitoring.

Two major *tocolytics* used in current practice are

## BOX 4-3.
### SUMMARY OF STAGES OF LABOR

**First Stage—Dilating Stage**
 Definition: period from first true labor contraction to complete dilatation of cervix
 What is accomplished: effacement and dilatation of cervix
 Forces involved: uterine contractions

**Second Stage—Expulsive Stage**
 Definition: period from complete dilatation of cervix to birth of baby
 What is accomplished: expulsion of baby from birth canal; facilitated by certain positional changes of fetus (descent, flexion, internal rotation, extension, external rotation, and expulsion)
 Forces involved: uterine contractions plus intraabdominal pressure

**Third Stage—Placental Stage**
 Definition: period from birth of baby through birth of placenta
 What is accomplished: separation of placenta; expulsion of placenta
 Forces involved: uterine contractions; intraabdominal pressure

**Fourth Stage—Recovery**
 Definition: period covering first hour after delivery
 What is accomplished: early adaptation to labor and delivery process
 Forces involved: uterine contractions; effects of any anesthesia

Adapted from S.T. Reeder and L.L. Martin. *Maternity Nursing: Family, Newborn, and Women's Health Care.* Philadelphia: J.B. Lippincott, 1987.

ritodrine hydrochloride (Yutopar) and terbutaline sulfate (Brethine). Both medications are beta-sympathomimetic agents that act on type II beta receptors in uterine muscle, bronchioles, and the diaphragm to produce uterine relaxation, bronchodilation, vasodilation, and muscle glycogenolysis. In addition to uterine relaxation, the mother may experience hypotension and a resultant increase in heart rate. Other new drugs used in the treatment of preterm labor include calcium channel blockers and prostaglandin inhibitors.

Magnesium sulfate, a central nervous system depressant, may be administered intravenously in an attempt to control preterm labor. This drug is believed to act by blocking the function of calcium and thus inhibiting uter-

## TABLE 4-7.
### COMPARISON OF DYSFUNCTIONAL LABOR PATTERNS

| PATTERN | CHARACTERISTICS | MATERNAL IMPLICATIONS | FETAL/NEONATAL IMPLICATIONS |
|---|---|---|---|
| Hypertonic | Occurs in early labor (latent phase) | Exhaustion | Fetal distress |
| Primary uterine inertia | Occurs most often in nullipara<br>Irregular, ineffective contractions<br>Lack of uterine relaxation between contractions<br>Little to no progress in dilatation of cervix<br>Failure of presenting part to descend | Dehydration<br>Uterine rupture<br>Infection of uterus<br>Vaginal lacerations if delivery is difficult | Sepsis<br>Birth injury |
| Hypotonic | Occurs in active labor | Exhaustion | Fetal distress |
| Secondary uterine inertia | Established contraction pattern converts to one in which contractions occur less often, decrease in intensity, and decrease in duration | Dehydration<br>Infection of uterus<br>Increased risk of postpartum hemorrhage | Birth injury |
| Precipitous labor | Labor less than 3 h in length | Ruptured uterus<br>Lacerations<br>No one in attendance for delivery | Increased risk for cerebral hemorrhage<br>Fetal hypoxia<br>No immediate care to clear airway, maintain body temperature |

**TABLE 4–8.**
LOW-, MEDIUM-, AND HIGH-RISK FACTORS FOR PRETERM LABOR

| LOW-RISK FACTORS | MEDIUM-RISK FACTORS | HIGH-RISK FACTORS |
|---|---|---|
| Any three of the following factors together equals a high-risk factor | Any two of the following factors together equals a high-risk factor | **Maternal Factors**<br>Abdominal surgery during pregnancy |
| **Maternal Factors** | **Maternal Factors** | Acute systemic bacterial infections |
| Age: under 16 or over 40 y | Age: under 16 y | Incompetent cervix |
| Anemia | Chemical abuse | Intrauterine infections |
| Bacteriuria | Cone biopsy | Maternal trauma |
| Cholestasis of pregnancy | Hyperthyroidism | Multiple gestation |
| Chronic renal disease | Narcotic addiction | Pregnancy-induced hypertension |
| Chronic cardiovascular disease | One second trimester abortion | Previous preterm labor |
| Fibroid tumors | Poorly controlled diabetes mellitus | Two or more second trimester abortions |
| Low socioeconomic factors | Pyelonephritis | Untreated Cushing's disease |
| Poor prenatal care | Unexplained vaginal bleeding after 16 wk gestation | **Fetal Factors** |
| Repeat first trimester abortions | Uterine anomalies | Congenital adrenal hyperplasia |
| Single parent status |  | Fetal infections |
| Smoking | **Placental Factors** | Multiple gestation |
| Stature: under 5 ft tall | Placenta previa | Oligohydramnios |
| Strenuous demanding work |  | Polyhydramnios |
| Weight: under 100 lbs prepregnancy weight |  |  |
| **Fetal Factors** |  |  |
| Breech presentations after 30 wk gestation |  |  |

Source: J. Holmes and L. Magiera, Maternity Nursing. *New York: Macmillan, 1987.*

ine contractions. Magnesium toxicity resulting in respiratory depression and depression of the patellar reflex is a common problem associated with its use.

Ethanol, a central nervous system depressant, acts to inhibit the release of oxytocin by the posterior pituitary. Due to side effects of nausea and vomiting and secondary aspiration in the mother this drug is rarely used in treatment of preterm labor.

*POSTTERM LABOR.* Postterm labor is a term used to refer to labor occurring after 42 weeks gestation. The cause is unknown but has been associated with anencephaly in the fetus, administration of prostaglandin synthetase inhibitors (aspirin and ibuprofen), and low serum and urine estriol levels.

The greatest risks in postterm pregnancy are related to placental aging and a decreased transfer of oxygen and nutrients to the fetus. Amniotic fluid volume may also decrease resulting in umbilical cord compression and fetal death. Most often postmature neonates are pale with dry, cracked, and peeling skin. The neonate may appear alert but distressed. Both lanugo and vernix tend to be absent. Hair and fingernails are long. Depending upon the degree of oxygen deprivation to which the fetus

was subjected, the amniotic fluid, umbilical cord, and skin may be meconium-stained with a green to yellow appearance. This neonate is at increased risk for meconium aspiration, asphyxia, hypoglycemia, cold stress, and polycythemia.

After 40 weeks gestation, it is essential that close surveillance of the fetus be instituted. This increased surveillance includes physician examinations, nonstress testing, and contraction stress testing when indicated.

*CERVICAL FACTORS.* One of the most common cervical conditions affecting biophysical development of reproduction is *incompetent cervix*. Incompetent cervix refers to the condition in which the cervix is unable to support the weight of the enlarging uterus during pregnancy. Factors predisposing to incompetent cervix include cervical conization or biopsy, prior second-trimester abortion, prior difficult delivery, and DES (diethylstilbestrol) exposure. During subsequent pregnancies, pressure from the enlarging uterus causes painless cervical dilatation. If detected early, McDonald's procedure can be performed and a suture placed around the cervical os (Figure 4-20). At or near term, the suture can be removed and the woman allowed to deliver vaginally.

**TABLE 4-9.**
SYSTEM FOR DETERMINING RISK OF SPONTANEOUS PRETERM DELIVERY[a]

| PTS | SOCIOECONOMIC FACTORS | PREVIOUS MEDICAL HISTORY | DAILY HABITS | ASPECTS OF CURRENT PREGNANCY |
|---|---|---|---|---|
| 1 | Two children at home<br>Low socioeconomic status | Abortion × 1<br>Less than 1 y since last birth | Works outside home | Unusual fatigue |
| 2 | Maternal age <20 y or >40 y<br>Single parent | Abortion × 2 | Smokes more than 10 cigarettes per d | Gain of less than 5 kg by 32 wk |
| 3 | Very low socioeconomic status<br>   Height <150 cm<br>   Weight <45 kg | Abortion × 3 | Heavy or stressful work<br>Long, tiring trip | Breech at 32 wk<br>Weight loss of 2 kg<br>Head engaged at 32 wk<br>Febrile illness |
| 4 | Maternal age <18 y | Pyelonephritis | | Bleeding after 12 wk<br>Effacement<br>Dilation<br>Uterine irritability |
| 5 | | Uterine anomaly<br>Second-trimester abortion<br>Diethylstilbestrol exposure<br>Cone biopsy | | Placenta previa<br>Hydramnios |
| 10 | | Preterm delivery<br>Repeated second-trimester abortion | | Twins<br>Abdominal surgery |

[a] Score is computed by adding the number of points given any item. The score is computed at the first visit and again at 22–26 wk gestation. A total score of 10 or more places client at high risk of spontaneous preterm delivery.
Source: S.J. Reeder and L.L. Martin, Maternity Nursing: Family Newborn and Women's Health Care. Philadelphia: J.B. Lippincott, 1987.

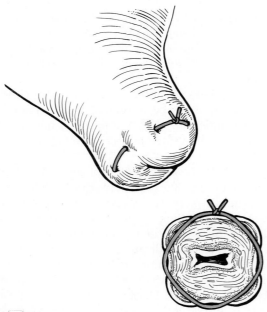

**FIGURE 4-20.**
A cross section of an incompetent cervix showing a cerclage suture in place. The suture is removed at term to allow cervical dilatation and delivery.

This procedure must be repeated with each subsequent pregnancy.

An alternative procedure is the Shirodkar procedure in which a purse-string suture is placed around the internal cervical os to maintain a closed cervix. This procedure may be performed prior to pregnancy and left in place. This procedure necessitates cesarean delivery in subsequent pregnancies.

### Passenger

The fetus, as a passenger, must be able to accommodate and descend through the woman's pelvis. The fetal head represents the most important part of the passenger and in most deliveries is the presenting part. When size or mobility of the fetal head prevents descent through or accommodation to the pelvis, vaginal delivery is difficult or impossible.

In addition to the size and mobility of the fetal head, the position, presentation, and attitude of the fetus affect accommodation to and descent through the pelvis. Position refers to the relationship of a particular fetal point to the front, sides, or back of the maternal pelvis.

*MALPOSITION.* Malposition refers to any position other than occiput anterior and can influence labor and birth (Figure 4-21). An occiput posterior presentation presents a larger diameter to the maternal pelvis. This position increases pressure on the sacral nerves, causing the woman to complain of low back pain and pelvic pressure during labor.

Presentation refers to the fetal part which enters, or presents to, the maternal pelvis. Attitude is the term used to refer to the relationship of fetal parts to each other. The most common presentation is cephalic and requires the least adaptation in the birth process. In the normal cephalic presentation, the occiput is the presenting part and the fetal head is completely flexed on the chest. This position allows the smallest diameter of the fetal head to present to the maternal pelvis.

*MALPRESENTATIONS.* Malpresentations include brow, face, breech, and shoulder presentations (see Figure 4-21). Any one of the malpresentations may result in the need for a cesarean delivery. In a brow presentation, the fetal head is partially extended. This causes the largest anteroposterior (occipitomental) diameter to present to the maternal pelvis. Difficult vaginal delivery may result in cerebral and neck compression, as well as trachea and larynx damage. The fetus is also at risk for increased infection if labor is prolonged.

In a face presentation, the fetal head is hyperextended and the occiput may even be in contact with the fetal back. The presenting part is the face. Edema and bruising are common if a face presentation is delivered vaginally. The neonate may also suffer physical injury to the neck if the delivery is difficult. With the utilization of ultrasound to document the breech position and tocolytic therapy to relax the uterine muscles and prevent contractions, an attempt is sometimes made to turn the fetus to a vertex position. An adequate amount of amniotic fluid and a complete or footling breech which is not engaged at the pelvic inlet are important prerequisites for successful version.[7]

Breech deliveries account for approximately 3% of term deliveries. Prolapsed cord is a common complication during labor. The fetus is also at risk for physical injury, including brachial plexus palsy, fractures, and spinal cord injury if vaginal delivery is attempted and difficult.

These presentations are classified according to the attitude of the hips and knees of the fetus. The most common classifications include complete breech, frank breech, and footling breech. In a complete breech presentation, both the fetal knees and hips are flexed. The buttocks and feet present to the maternal pelvis.

A frank breech represents the most common breech presentation and is characterized by flexions of the fetal thighs and extension of the knees. The presenting part to the maternal pelvis is the buttocks.

The footling breech is characterized by extension of knees and legs. Either one foot (single footling) or two feet (double footling) present to the maternal pelvis.

Shoulder presentation is also referred to as transverse lie. In this presentation, the fetal shoulder presents to the maternal pelvis. The acromion process of the scapula may be located either anterior or posterior and to either the woman's right or left side.

A summary of all fetal positions may be seen in Figure 4-21. Any malposition or malpresentation may necessitate a cesarean delivery, depending upon the size of the fetus, maternal pelvis, and progress of labor. Cesarean delivery is frequently indicated in shoulder, face, and some breech presentations. Prolapsed cord is most often associated with shoulder and breech presentations.

*PREMATURE RUPTURE OF THE MEMBRANES.* Premature rupture of the membranes (PROM) refers to the spontaneous rupture of the membranes or leakage of amniotic fluid prior to the onset of labor. Preterm rupture occurs prior to 37 weeks gestation. Predisposing factors include multiparity, incompetent cervix, maternal age >35 years, low weight gain during pregnancy, and cervical damage from surgical instrumentation. Diagnosis can usually be confirmed with Nitrazine Paper which turns dark blue in the presence of amniotic fluid and ferning.

Risk for the development of chorioamnionitis (infection of the chorion and amnion) is increased, especially if delivery does not occur within 24 hours of rupture. Signs of chorioamnionitis include maternal tachycardia and fever, fetal tachycardia, foul smelling amniotic fluid, and uterine tenderness. When the membranes rupture over 48 hours prior to delivery, the fetus is at increased risk for septicemia, pneumonia, and infection of the umbilical cord.

PROM early in pregnancy is more threatening due to prematurity of the fetus, possible malposition, risk of prolapsed cord, and infection. Occasionally corticosteroids are used to increase fetal lung maturity and lessen the chance of respiratory distress syndrome in the preterm neonate.

*PROLAPSED UMBILICAL CORD.* A prolapsed umbilical cord is one which descends into the birth canal prior to the presenting part (Figure 4-22). As a result, pressure is placed on the umbilical cord which can interfere with fetal circulation. The progress of labor is not affected nor is the woman's physical adaptation. However, this condition represents an obstetrical emergency for the fetus and requires immediate action.

Prolapsed umbilical cord is frequently associated

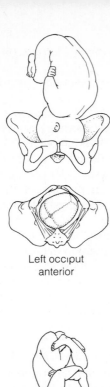
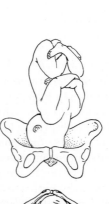
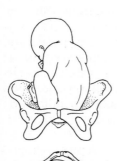
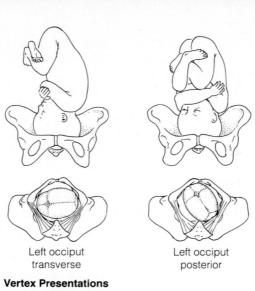
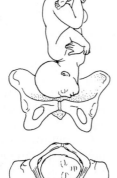
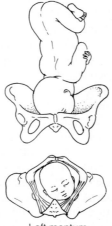
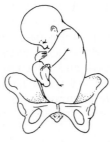
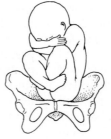

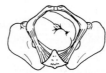

Left occiput
anterior

Left occiput
transverse

Left occiput
posterior

**Vertex Presentations**

Left mentum
anterior

Left mentum
transverse

Left mentum
posterior

**Face Presentations**

Left
sacrum
anterior

Left
sacrum
transverse

Left
sacrum
posterior

**Breech Presentations**

**FIGURE 4–21.**
Fetal presentations. (Redrawn from R.C. Benson, *Handbook of Obstetrics and Gynecology* [7th ed.]. Los Altos, Calif.: Lange, 1980 in Reeder and Martin.)

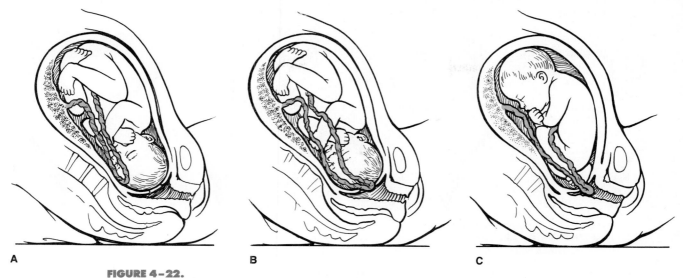

**FIGURE 4-22.**
Umbilical cord prolapse **A.** Occult prolapse and compression of cord by fetal head. **B.** Forelying cord palpable in cervical os. **C.** Complete cord prolapse with breech presentation. (From *Childbirth Graphics*, K.A. May and L.R. Mahlmeister, *Comprehensive Maternity Nursing*. Philadelphia: J.B. Lippincott, 1990.)

with rupture of the membranes when the presenting part is not fully engaged in the pelvis or in malpresentations. The umbilical cord may prolapse in varying degrees. It may protrude from the vagina, may prolapse into the vagina but not be visible to the naked eye, or may be compressed from pressure of the presenting part.

Evidence of cord compression can also be noted on fetal monitoring. Compression of the umbilical cord and reduction in blood flow between fetus and placenta result in variable decelerations on the monitor. Reduced blood flow leads to increased peripheral resistance and increased fetal blood pressure. This response stimulates the baroceptors in the aortic arch and carotid sinuses, which produces a slowing of the fetal heart rate.

Perinatal mortality depends upon the degree of cord compression and time between diagnosis and delivery. Knee-chest and Trendelenburg position can aid in circulation until delivery is possible. A gloved hand to provide pressure on the presenting part may also be used to relieve compression on the cord. The administration of oxygen to the mother increases the oxygen supply to the fetus.

*Passage*

The passage through which the fetus must pass includes not only the bony pelvis, but the cervix, vagina, and introitus as well. Size and shape of the pelvis are key factors in determining whether the woman can deliver the fetus vaginally. There are four classifications of pelves:

(1) gynecoid, (2) android, (3) anthropoid, and (4) platypelloid (Figure 4-23). The gynecoid pelvis is most often referred to as the typical female pelvis. Pelvic measurements for this type of pelvis are sufficient for the average full-term fetus.

The android pelvis is more characteristic of the male pelvis but is found in approximately 20% of women. Pelvic measurements of the android pelvis are generally not sufficient to allow vaginal delivery of the average full-term fetus.

The anthropoid pelvis is characterized by a narrowed side-to-side measurement with a widened measurement from front to back. Measurements are usually adequate for vaginal delivery of the average term fetus.

The pelvic measurements of the platypelloid pelvis are usually inadequate to allow vaginal delivery of the term fetus. This pelvis reflects a widened measurement from side to side and a narrowed measurement from front to back.

In determining the adequacy of the pelvis for vaginal delivery, it is important to examine the sacrum, the ischial spines, and the pubic arch. A concave sacrum provides optimal capacity, while a sacrum that is flat or convex decreases pelvic capacity. A fixed sacrum may also interfere with descent of the presenting part. Sharp ischial spines decrease the transverse pelvic measurement, while a pubic arch that is narrow with a decreased angle will prevent the fetal head from pivoting as it passes under the arch. Ideally, the pubic arch is wide with at least a 90 degree angle.

Gynecoid          Android          Anthropoid          Platypelloid

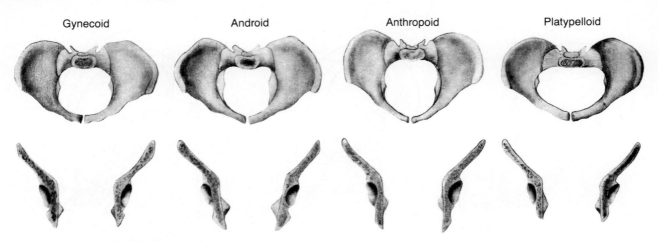

**FIGURE 4-23.**
Caldwell-Maloy classification of pelvic types. (Top) The typical shape of the inlet for each type is shown. A line has been drawn through the widest transverse diameter, dividing the inlet into an anterior and posterior segment. The longitudinal line illustrates the anteroposterior diameter of the inlet. (Bottom) The typical interspinous diameter of each type is depicted. (From S.J. Reeder and L.L. Martin, *Maternity Nursing* [16th ed.]. Philadelphia: J.B. Lippincott, 1987.)

In making a determination regarding the adequacy of the pelvis, the examiner must consider not only pelvic measurements but the position and size of the fetus as well. Radiographic pelvimetry and computed tomography (CT) pelvimetry are useful tools in determining pelvic adequacy relative to fetal size.

## REFERENCES

1. Aaronson, L.S., and Macnee, C.L. Tobacco, alcohol, and caffeine use during pregnancy. *J. Obstet. Gynecol. Neonatal Nurs.* 18:279, 1989.
2. Alexander, L.L. The pregnant smoker: Nursing implications. *J. Obstet. Gynecol. Neonatal Nurs.* 16:167, 1987.
3. Auvenshine, M.A., and Enriquez, M.G. *Comprehensive Maternity Nursing: Prenatal and Women's Health.* Boston: Jones and Bartlett, 1990.
4. Dickason, E.J., Schult, M.O., and Silverman, B.L. *Maternal-Infant Nursing Care.* St. Louis, Mo.: Mosby, 1990.
5. Dunn, P.A., Weiner, S., and Ludomirski, A. Percutaneous umbilical blood sampling. *J. Obstet. Gynecol. Neonatal Nurs.* 17:308, 1988.
6. Hogge, J.S., Hogge, A., and Golbus, M.S. Chorionic villus sampling. *J. Obstet. Gynecol. Neonatal Nurs.* 15(1):24, 1986.
7. Martin, L.L., and Reeder, S.J. *Maternity Nursing* (17th Ed.). Philadelphia: J.B. Lippincott, 1991.
8. May, K.A., and Mahlmeister, L.R. *Comprehensive Maternity Nursing: Nursing Process and Childbearing Family.* Philadelphia: J.B. Lippincott, 1990.
9. New York Heart Association. *New York Heart Association: Nomenclature and Criteria for Diagnosis and Diseases of the Heart and Blood Vessels* (Ed. 5). New York: Author, 1955.
10. Poole, J.H. Getting perspective on HELLP Syndrome. *MCN* 13:432, 1988.
11. Schuster, C.S. Intrauterine development. In C.S. Schuster and S.S. Ashburn (eds.). *The Process of Human Development: A Holistic Approach.* Boston: Little, Brown, 1986.
12. Seeds, J.W. PUBS: Important new aid for prenatal diagnosis. *Contemporary OB/GYN* 2:117, 1988.
13. Sherwen, L.N., Scoloveno, M.A., and Weingarter, C.T. *Nursing Care of the Childbearing Family.* Norwalk, Connecticut: Appleton and Lange, 1991.
14. Stringer, M.R. Chorionic villi sampling: A nursing perspective. *J. Obstet. Gynecol. Neonatal Nurs.* 17(1):19, 1988.
15. White, P. Classification of obstetric diabetes. *Am. J. Obstet. Gynecol.* 130:228, 1978.

# chapter 5

Joy H. Whatley
Sharron P. Schlosser

# Biophysical Development of Children

## Chapter Outline

## Learning Objectives

1. Discuss the respiratory, cardiovascular, thermoregulation, and hepatic adaptations of the neonate during transition from intrauterine to extrauterine life.

2. Describe the biophysical development occurring during the neonatal period.

3. Describe the physiologic changes occurring in each body system during the various stages of childhood.

4. Identify the basic nutritional needs of children and adolescents.

(continued)

## NEONATE

The neonatal period, the first 28 days of life, represents a time of dramatic anatomic and biochemical changes as the neonate adapts from intrauterine to extrauterine life. Prior to delivery, the fetus was dependent upon the mother for oxygen, elimination, nutrition, thermoregulation, and fluid balance. One minute following birth, the normal newborn changes from a dependent intrauterine existence to an independent being who is capable of oxygenating, perfusing, and heating his or her own body. The vital occurrence that must follow birth is the change of respiration from the placenta to respiration of the newborn lungs.[64]

### Intrauterine Pulmonary Adaptation

Fetal respiratory movements have been documented as early as the 13th week of gestation. The fetal respirations increase in frequency and strength as the pregnancy approaches term. About 3 days prior to birth, the frequency decreases dramatically. Since the intrauterine oxygen needs are met by the placenta, fetal breathing movements apparently contribute very little to the oxygen needs of the fetus. It is thought that the fetal breathing movements may stimulate the synthesis, release, and distribution of surfactant.[42]

In utero, in addition to the fetal breathing movements, the fetal lungs produce fluid that helps prevent their collapse. Surfactant, produced by type II alveolar cells beginning at approximately 20 to 24 weeks gestation and, continuing to term, increases and is part of the lung fluid as term approaches. Surfactant helps to stabilize the alveoli and decrease surface tension, preventing alveoli collapse. It also helps to establish a functioning residual capacity. Maternal health stressors, such as pregnancy induced hypertension (PIH) or heroin abuse, stimulate an increase in surfactant production. It is thought that the mother, who is stressed, produces more steroids. Prior to term, the mother may be given steroids to enhance fetal lung maturity when the fetus needs to be removed from the intrauterine environment prior to term.

Fetal lung fluid is significant in births that involve certain presentations and for cesarean births. During vaginal delivery, the infant's chest is squeezed and then re-expands rapidly. It is thought that the thoracic compression in a vaginal delivery plus the effect of gravity in the vertex presentation help to force out fetal lung fluid just before the first breath. The small amount of fetal lung fluid that remains in the lungs after birth is absorbed by the lymphatic system. The cesarean section delivery does not allow for the thoracic compression or for drainage of fluid by gravity. Therefore, the infant delivered by cesarean section or a presentation other than vertex is at a greater risk for respiratory problems.

### Extrauterine Pulmonary Adaptation

It is thought that several stimuli are responsible for the initiation of respiration. These stimuli are mechanical, sensory, chemical, and thermal in nature. Figure 5-1 outlines the interaction of stimuli in the initiation of respiration.

The mechanical forces are the thoracic compression that occurs with vaginal delivery and the change from intrauterine to extrauterine pressure subsequent to uterine contraction in labor. In addition to expelling fetal lung fluid, the thoracic compression creates a negative intrathoracic pressure that helps the lungs reexpand or "recoil," pulling in a small amount of air. When the uterus is relaxed, the intrauterine pressure is 15 cm $H_2O$. If the membranes are still intact, the 15 cm $H_2O$ pressure is evenly dispersed and cannot influence the amount of pressure in the lungs. Upon rupture of the membranes

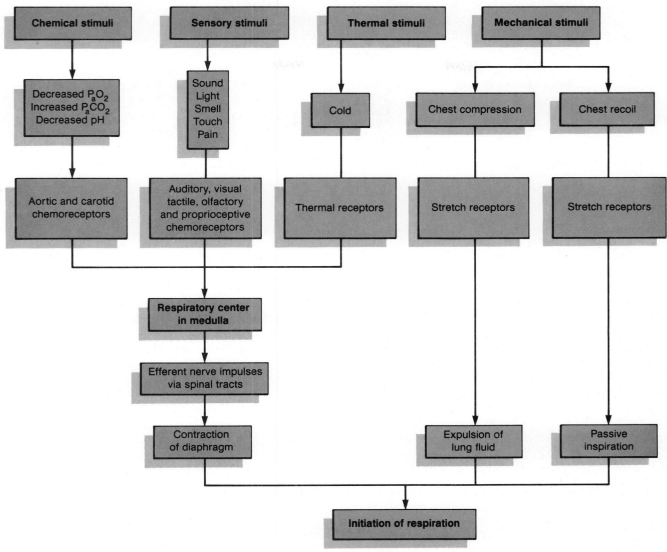

**FIGURE 5-1.**
Interaction of stimuli in the initiation of respiration. (From K.A. May and L.R. Mahlmeister, *Comprehensive Maternity Nursing*, Philadelphia: J.B. Lippincott, 1990.)

and descent of the fetus into the lower uterine segment, uterine contractions provide up to 75 cm $H_2O$ pressure that produces the thoracic compression and expels lung fluid.

The neonate is overstimulated during the birth process. Sensory stimuli which probably contributes to the initiation of respiration are bright lights, noise, and the sensation of weight with the addition of gravity.

Cold is a powerful thermal stimulus in the initiation of the first breath. The normal intrauterine temperature is 37°C. The delivery room may be as cold as 22°C. Extreme cooling of the infant will increase the oxygen needs and produce respiratory and metabolic acidosis.

Chemical changes in transition occur as a result of transient asphyxia. Mild asphyxia (hypercapnia, hypoxia,

and acidosis) normally occur at delivery. If chemical changes are prolonged, the respiratory center will become depressed. Drugs given to the mother near the time of delivery may also depress the respiratory center. The normal infant usually takes the first breath within 30 seconds following delivery, and a normal neonatal breathing pattern is established within 90 seconds.

After respirations are initiated, the range will be from 30 to 60 respirations per minute. It is not unusual for the respirations to be 80 per minute for the first few minutes following birth. Characteristics of newborn respirations are irregularity of rate, rhythm, and depth. As respirations continue, the partial pressure of oxygen ($PaO_2$) increases, the partial pressure of carbon dioxide ($PaCO_2$) decreases, and blood pH approaches adult values (Table 5-1). Pul-

**TABLE 5-1.**
ARTERIAL BLOOD GAS VALUES PRIOR TO THE INITIAL BREATH
COMPARED TO ADULT VALUES

|  | SUBSTANCE | VALUES |
|---|---|---|
| **Before Initial Breath** | *Oxygen* <br> *Saturation* | 10–20% |
|  | *Carbon dioxide* <br> *Partial pressure or tension* | 58 mm Hg |
|  | *Arterial pH* | 7.28 |
| **Adult** |  |  |
|  | *Oxygen* <br> *Saturation* | 96–100% |
|  | *Carbon dioxide* <br> *Tension* | 35–45 mm Hg |
|  | *Arterial pH* | 7.35–7.45 |

monary blood vessels that were constricted in utero dilate due to the increased oxygen levels, causing an increase in blood flow to the infant's lungs. The results of pulmonary transition are the following: (1) surfactant production is maintained; (2) residual volume is established; (3) physiologic acid-base balance continues; (4) blood flow to the lungs is increased; and (5) vital signs are within normal limits.[13]

## Extrauterine Circulatory Adaptation

The anatomic and biochemical changes that occur during conversion from fetal to adult circulation are closely related to the changes that occur in the respiratory system. These changes result from the alterations in systemic and pulmonary pressures after the initial breath, establishment of respirations, and from clamping the umbilical cord. Figure 5-2 outlines the alterations in pulmonary vascular resistance and neonatal circulation following the first breath. The major cardiovascular changes that occur in response to initiation of respiration and clamping the umbilical cord are closure of the foramen ovale, closure of the ductus arteriosus, and closure of the ductus venosus (see also Chap. 25).

### Closure of the Foramen Ovale

After the initial breath and after clamping the umbilical cord, a large amount of blood is returned to the heart and lungs. Pulmonary arteries dilate in response to the increased $PO_2$ and the pulmonary pressure is decreased. Pressure drops in the right side of the heart, while it increases in the left atrium. The increase in the left atrial pressure causes the functional closure of the foramen ovale within a few hours after birth. It may be several

months before permanent closure of the foramen ovale occurs. Right to left shunting of blood may continue until permanent closure occurs, which explains the nonpathologic murmurs heard in the neonate during this time.[33]

### Closure of the Ductus Arteriosus

The ductus arteriosus is sensitive to increases in oxygen concentration. As the $PaO_2$ levels increase after the first breath, the ductus arteriosus is stimulated to constrict. Functional closure occurs within 15 hours after delivery. Permanent closure is usually accomplished within 3 weeks.

### Closure of the Ductus Venosus

The mechanism that causes the ductus venosus to close is unknown. When the umbilical cord is clamped, the ductus venosus, which connected fetal portal circulation with the inferior vena cava, can no longer carry blood. Fibrosis of the ductus venosus occurs within 3 to 7 days after birth.[5]

## Extrauterine Thermoregulation Adaptation

Thermoregulation is the ability of the neonate to produce heat to maintain a normal body temperature. In the newborn, the balance between heat production and heat loss, or the maintenance of a stable body temperature, is possible with limited fluctuations in the environmental temperature.[5]

Newborns are prone to heat loss because of their unique anatomic characteristics in combination with exposure to environmental influences that occur at deliv-

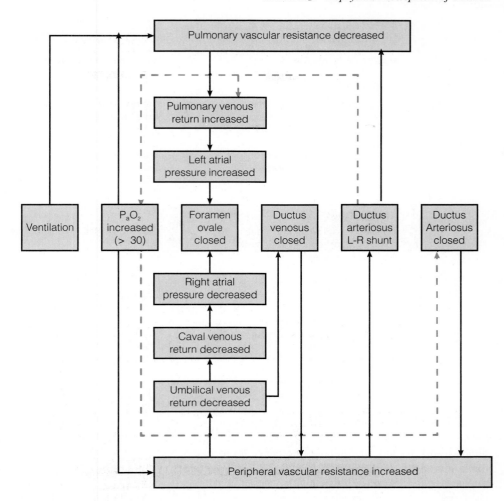

**FIGURE 5-2.**
Alterations in pulmonary vascular resistance and neonatal circulation following initiation of respiration. Broken lines indicate hypothesized mechanisms involved in alterations in pulmonary vascular resistance. (From C. Smith and N. Nelson, *The Physiology of the Newborn Infant* [4th ed.]. Springfield, Ill.: Charles C. Thomas, 1976.)

ery. Factors contributing to loss of heat are: (1) a large surface area in relation to body weight; (2) a limited metabolic capability; and (3) limited fat deposits. A decreased amount of adipose tissue results in decreased thermal regulation. The skin of the newborn is thin and blood vessels lie close to the skin surface, which result in transfer of heat to the environment. The newborn is wet at delivery, and the environmental temperature in the delivery room is much lower than the intrauterine temperature.

Four specific mechanisms cause heat loss in the neonate: (1) evaporation, which is the conversion of water on the wet newborn skin to vapor; (2) convection, or the transfer of heat in response to cool air; (3) conduction, which is the transfer of heat when the infant is placed on a cool surface; and (4) radiation, or the transfer of heat from the infant to the cool surface in contact with the infant's skin. Table 5-2 outlines the major environmental factors that contribute to neonatal heat loss.

The neonate responds to heat loss through vasomotor control, thermal insulation, limited shivering, muscular activity, and nonshivering thermogenesis.[5] Vasomotor control helps to control heat loss through vasocon-

striction of the blood vessels in the skin. The amount of thermal regulation in the newborn is directly related to his or her amount of white fat, which is a heat-retaining tissue. Fat accumulation begins about 32 weeks gestation so that premature and intrauterine growth retarded (IUGR) babies are at an increased risk for heat loss due to inadequate thermal regulation capability. Shivering, a major mechanism of heat production in adults, is limited in the newborn. Muscular activity contributes somewhat to heat production but is not a significant source of heat. Nonshivering thermogenesis is the primary mechanism for heat production in the neonate. In response to a decrease in skin temperature, thermal receptors transmit impulses to the central nervous system (CNS). Norepinephrine, in response to stimulation of the sympathetic nervous system, is released by the adrenal glands and nerve endings in a special type of adipose tissue, brown fat. Brown fat is remarkably vascular and is metabolized to produce heat. Brown fat makes up about 1.5% of total body weight and is found between the scapulae, behind the sternum, and around the neck, head, heart, great vessels, kidneys, and adrenal glands.[5]

Nonshivering thermogenesis and the increase in the

**TABLE 5-2.**
ENVIRONMENTAL FACTORS CONTRIBUTING TO NEONATAL HEAT

| MAJOR MECHANISMS | ENVIRONMENTAL FACTORS |
|---|---|
| **Evaporation** | |
| Loss of heat when water on the infant's skin is converted to a vapor | Wet blankets or diapers in contact with skin |
| | Water or urine on skin |
| **Convection** | |
| Transfer of heat when a flow of cool air passes over the infant's skin | Drafts from open windows |
| | Drafts from open portholes on isolette |
| | Drafts from air-conditioning ducts |
| | Flow of unheated oxygen over face |
| **Conduction** | |
| Transfer of heat when the infant comes in direct contact with cooler surfaces and objects | Cold mattresses, cold sidewalls in crib or isolette |
| | Cold blankets, shirts, diapers |
| | Cold hands of care-giver |
| | Cold weight scale |
| | Cold stethoscope |
| **Radiation** | |
| Transfer of heat from the infant to cooler surfaces and objects not in direct contact with the infant | Cold sidewalls of crib or isolette |
| | Cold outside building walls and windows |
| | Cold equipment in infant's environment |

metabolic rate are effective mechanisms for heat production. However, they also cause increased demands for glucose and oxygen. Normal term infants counterbalance these increased demands by increasing their respiratory rate and releasing glucose that is stored in the liver. If cold stress continues or the neonate is compromised, brown fat and glucose will become expended. This depletion of brown fat and glucose leads to a decrease in surfactant production and an increase in pulmonary vascular resistance. In this situation, an external heat source is essential to maintain a normal body temperature.[33]

## *Extrauterine Hepatic Adaptation*

Prior to birth, the placenta is responsible for the breakdown and excretion of bilirubin whereas after birth, the liver assumes this role. However, it is thought that the liver of the normal neonate may produce inadequate amounts of glucuronyl transferase, which is needed to change indirect or unconjugated bilirubin to direct bilirubin (see Chap. 42). Bilirubin is the end product of the breakdown of red blood cells (RBCs). The normal lifespan of the RBC in the neonate is only 80 to 120 days. As the RBCs become older, they become fragile and hemoglobin is split into two fragments, heme and globin. Heme is the unconjugated, indirect fraction which is fat soluble. Direct bilirubin is water soluble and can be excreted by the kidneys. The unbound or indirect form of bilirubin can exit the vascular system and infiltrate other extravascular tissues, such as the skin or sclera, which causes jaundice or icteric (yellow) skin color.

## *Physiologic Hyperbilirubinemia*

The most frequent factors thought to contribute to physiologic jaundice are the shorter life span of RBCs, decreased production of liver enzymes, and increased numbers of RBCs in the neonate.[5,6] Physiologic jaundice occurs in approximately 50% of newborns who are most frequently around 48 hours of age. Physiologic jaundice usually disappears by 1 week of age, and bilirubin levels generally do not exceed 12 mg per 100 ml. When jaundice occurs as early as 24 hours of age, it is considered pathologic, not physiologic.

Phototherapy, the process of exposing the newborn's skin to intense fluorescent light, is frequently used to treat physiologic jaundice. Phototherapy causes a structural alteration of bilirubin in the skin of the newborn by oxidizing the unconjugated, indirect bilirubin which is fat soluble into a water soluble form. The water soluble form, or direct, conjugated bilirubin is excreted in bile, urine, and feces without going through the usual conjugation process in the liver.[49]

## *Biophysical Development*

Normal values and variations of normal for weight, head circumference, chest circumference, temperature, pulse,

**TABLE 5-3.**
BIOPHYSICAL MEASUREMENTS OF NORMAL FULL-TERM NEONATE

| VALUE | AVERAGE FINDINGS | NORMAL VARIATIONS |
|---|---|---|
| Weight | 3400 gm (7 1/2 lbs); birth weight is regained within 2 wk | 2500–4000 gm (5 1/2–8 lbs, 13 oz); acceptable weight loss is 5–10% of birth weight |
| Head circumference | 33–33.5 cm (13–14 in) | 32–37 cm (12 1/2–14 1/2 in); molding of head can affect head circumference |
| Chest circumference | 30–33 cm (12–13 in) | 2 cm less than head circumference; breast engorgement can affect chest circumference |
| Length | 50 cm (20 in) | 44–55 cm (18–22 in) |
| Temperature | Rectal 36.5–37°C (97.7–98.6°F) Axillary 36.1–36.5°C (97–97.7°F) | Environmental temperature extremes, sepsis, and altered neurologic function can contribute to hypothermia or hyperthermia |
| Apical pulse | 120–160 beats per min (bpm) | 100 bpm while sleeping, 178 bpm while crying; at one month ranges from 138 bpm asleep to 165 bpm awake |
| Respirations | 30–60 breaths per min (bpm) | First hour following birth normal tachypnea, > 60 bpm, and grunting, flaring, and retracting may occur |
| Blood pressure | 74/42 mm Hg | Varies with activity level. Systolic: 60–82 mm Hg. Diastolic: 42–50 mm Hg. At 10 days of age: systolic 94–100 mm Hg; diastolic slightly increased |

Source: Adapted from D.R. Marlow and B.A. Redding, Textbook of Pediatric Nursing. *Philadelphia: W.B. Saunders, 1988.*

respirations, and blood pressure of the normal, full-term neonate are found in Table 5-3.

## *INFANT*

## *Biophysical Development*

### *Biologic Growth*

The period of infancy encompasses the first year following birth. The rapid, continuous growth that began at conception proceeds in a specific and orderly manner. Evidence of this rapid growth pattern can be seen in the month-by-month changes in the infant. Specific measures of height, weight, and chest and head circumference, as well as dentition, reflexes, and motor development provide evidence of these changes. A summary of average biologic growth on a month-by-month basis is found in Table 5-4. One must remember that these findings only represent the norm and that individual infants vary. Individual variation may be more evident when dealing with premature infants.

During the period of infancy, the baby grows an average of 2.5 cm (1 inch) per month during the first 6

months of life, and about 1.5 cm (0.5 inch) per month from 7 to 12 months. This rate of growth indicates a gain of approximately 50% of birth length during the first year of life. Although this growth occurs primarily in the trunk, the head continues to constitute a large proportion of the infant's body surface.

The normal weight gain provides for the doubling of the birth weight during the first 6 months of life and tripling of the birth weight by 12 months. By 1 year of age, the average weight is 9.75 kg (21.5 pounds).

Head circumference represents another area of rapid growth during infancy, indicative of brain maturation. From birth to 6 months, the head increases in size by approximately 1.5 cm (0.5 inch) per month, and 0.5 cm (0.25 inch) per month from 7 to 12 months. This accounts for approximately 33% increase during this first year of life. This growth is accompanied by closure of the posterior fontanel (soft spot at the sagittal and lambdoid sutures). The anterior fontanel (soft spot at the coronal, frontal and sagittal sutures) closes between 12 and 18 months.

Chest measurements can also indicate the overall growth of the individual infant. By the time the infant is 1 year of age, the head and chest should be about equal in size. The chest also changes in contour during this

**TABLE 5–4.**
BIOPHYSICAL MEASUREMENTS OF THE INFANT

| | 1 MONTH | 3 MONTHS | 5 MONTHS | 6 MONTHS | 7 MONTHS | 9 MONTHS | 12 MONTHS |
|---|---|---|---|---|---|---|---|
| **Weight** | 4.4 ± 0.8 kg (10 ± 1.5 lb); gains about 680 gm/mo (1.5 lb) for first 6 mo | 5.7 ± 0.8 kg (12.3 ± 2 lb) | At least 2 × birth weight; mean age for doubling 3.8 mo | 7.4 ± 1 kg (16.5 ± 2.5 lb); gains about 340 gm/mo (0.75 lb) | | | 10 ± 1.5 kg (22 ± 3 lb); 3 × birth weight |
| **Head Circumference** | Increases 1.5 cm (0.5 in) per mo for first 6 mo | | | 43 cm (17 in); increases 0.5 cm (0.25 in) permo6–12mo | 46 cm (18 in); increased by one-third since birth; head and chest measurement equal | | |
| **Length** | Approximately 53 ± 2.5 cm (21 ± 1 in); increases about 2.5 cm (1 in) per mo for first 6 mo | 60 ± 2 cm (23.5 ± 1 in) | | 65.5 ± 3 cm (26 ± 1 in); gains about 1.25 cm (0.5 in) permo6–12mo | 74.5 ± 3 cm (29 ± 1.5 in); length increased almost 50% | | |
| **Pulse** | 130 ± 20 | 130 ± 20 | | 120 ± 20 | 115 ± 20 | | |
| **Respirations** | 35 ± 10 | 35 ± 10 | | 31 ± 9 | 30 ± 10 | | |
| **Blood Pressure** | 80/50 ± 20/10 | 80/50 ± 20/10 | | 90/60 ± 28/10 | 96/66 ± 30/24 | | |
| **Dentition** | | | | two lower central incisors 6 ± 2 mo | upper central 7.5 ± 2 mo; lower lateral 7 ± 2 mo | upper laterals 9 ± 2 mo | 6–8 deciduous teeth |

Source: Adapted from D.R. Marlow and B.A. Redding, Textbook of Pediatric Nursing. Philadelphia: W.B. Saunders, 1988.

time, as the lateral diameter becomes larger than the anteroposterior diameter.

### Dentition

The eruption of the primary teeth represents a continuation of development begun in utero. The first of 20 deciduous (temporary) teeth erupts between 5 and 7 months of age. During the period of teething, the infant may drool, chew on hard objects, and become irritable. There is no physiologic basis for high temperature and diarrhea. If the infant refuses to eat, however, teething may be associated with low-grade fever due to some dehydration.

### Neuromuscular Development

Neuromuscular development follows the general principles of cephalocaudal and proximodistal as the infant refines both gross and fine motor skills. Gross motor skills include head control, sitting, standing, and walking. Fine motor skills make use of the hands and fingers.

Head lag, noted as the neonate is pulled from a lying to sitting position, becomes minimal by age 4 months. Increased head control becomes evident as the infant progresses to lifting the head and chest while supporting weight on the forearms. By age 6 months, the infant can lift the head, chest, and abdomen, and support weight on hands. This development facilitates rolling over. The infant can willfully roll from front to back at age 5 months and from back to front at age 6 months. As the back becomes straighter and stronger, the infant develops the ability to sit by leaning forward for support at age 7 months and unsupported at age 8 months.

Prior to about 7 months of age, the infant is unable to support weight on feet and legs. However, by age 9 months the infant has developed the ability to stand while holding onto furniture. The ability to crawl well occurs by age 10 months, taking steps while holding furniture or having hands held by age 11 months, and walking with one hand held by age 12 months. Walking unsupported occurs between age 12 and 15 months.

During the first 2 to 3 months of life, grasping occurs as a reflex. Gradually, the infant progresses from a visual grasp to palmar grasp, and finally to pincher grasp of smaller objects by age 9 to 10 months.

## Sensory Development

Sensory development involves the eyes, ears, tongue, nose, and skin. In addition to visual acuity, visual development is concerned with binocularity and stereopsis. In binocularity, the infant develops the ability to fuse two ocular images into one cerebral image. This ability should be well developed by age 4 months. Strabismus occurs when there is a lack of binocularity and may result in blindness if left untreated.

Stereopsis, or depth perception, is developed by age 7 to 9 months. Throughout infancy, children display a preference for the human face. By age 6 months, infants respond to facial expressions and recognize the face of strangers. This ability contributes to the stranger anxiety evident by age 7 or 8 months.

The parachute reflex develops by age 7 months and persists indefinitely. This reflex response produces forward extension of hands and fingers when the infant, suspended in a horizontal prone position, is suddenly thrust downward.

The ability to hear is evident from birth as the neonate responds to loud noise with a startle reflex. The quieting effect of low-pitched sounds, such as the human heartbeat or lullaby, is thought to originate from prenatal time. By age 3 months, the infant attempts to locate sound by turning the head in the direction of the sound. The infant begins to imitate sounds at about age 4 months and responds to his or her own name by age 4 to 6 months. By the time the infant is 1 year of age, he or she can recognize the sound of words such as "no" and the names of other family members.

Smell, touch, and taste continue to develop throughout infancy. The preference for various tastes is present at age 7 months and continues to develop throughout childhood.

## Factors Affecting Development and Health

### Sleep

The infant should begin to sleep through the night at 8-hour to 10-hour intervals by age 3 to 4 months. Total sleep needs, including naps, are variable, but average 13 to 15 hours per day. Persistent night feedings where the infant continues to awaken for a night feeding, night crying, and nightmares are the most common sleep problems during infancy.

### Nutrition

The primary food during infancy is milk. For breast-fed infants the only supplements needed are iron and fluoride, and vitamin D if the mother's diet is deficient. Fluoride is a dietary supplement needed by infants who are bottlefed.

There has long been a controversy over when solid food should be introduced into the infant's diet. Most authorities advocate the introduction of solid food at about age 5 to 6 months. Several developmental factors support this time frame: (1) the gastrointestinal tract should be sufficiently mature to allow digestion of the more complex solid foods, (2) there is disappearance of the tongue thrust or extrusion reflex, and (3) the infant has the ability to control the head and neck. Additionally, the eruption of the primary teeth facilitates biting and chewing.

When the decision is made to introduce solid foods, new foods should be introduced one at a time and in small amounts (approximately 1 teaspoon the first time). Cereal is the first food because of its high iron content. Fruit, vegetables, and meat are then added sequentially. Egg yolk is generally introduced before egg white because of the sensitivity associated with egg white. Crackers and Zwieback are finger foods recommended at about age 6 months.

By age 12 months, the infant generally has sufficient maturity to drink from a cup and indicates readiness for weaning. Weaning occurs gradually as the bottle is replaced one feeding at a time. Dental caries related to bottle feeding are a significant health problem associated with the milk or juice bottle at bedtime. From the time primary teeth erupt, care should be taken to clean the teeth with a damp cloth.

*Malnutrition, failure to thrive*, and *colic* are alterations associated with nutrition. Malnutrition reflects poor or inadequate nutrition, as well as overnutrition. Iron-deficiency anemia and vitamin deficiencies are the most common examples of inadequate nutrition. Overnutrition occurs frequently with the introduction of solid foods and no decrease in milk intake. Social, cultural, and economic factors contribute to malnutrition.

Failure to thrive (FTT) is a condition associated with a weight below the third percentile when charted on a growth chart. FTT can be further classified as organic or inorganic. Organic FTT is associated with such physical conditions as heart disease, cystic fibrosis, gastroesophageal reflux, and malabsorption, as well as endocrine and renal dysfunction. Inorganic FTT is a failure to grow in the absence of diagnosed disease. Psychosocial problems including inadequate parent-child bonding isolation, and caregiver inadequate coping, between the infant and primary caregiver are the basis for inorganic FTT. On occasion, a combination of physical and psychosocial problems may be present.

Colic is a common condition associated with early infancy. It occurs primarily in the first 3 to 4 months of life and is characterized by paroxysmal intestinal cramping associated with increased gas, abdominal distention, and pain. The infant exhibits loud crying accompanied by drawing of the legs on the abdomen. Tolerance for food continues to be good with the infant demonstrating a steady gain in weight.

## Immunity and Immunizations

The immune system of the infant does not respond to environmental antigens even though the cells of the system are present. Infants are not able to localize antigens at a site of infection. Early in life maternal antibodies provide some protection from infection both from maternal–placental transmission and through breast feeding. As these antibodies decline in numbers and effectiveness the infant must actively produce specific antibodies to combat a wide array of infectious organisms. Between the ages of 9 and 12 months the infant still does not react adequately. Both T and B lymphocyte function gradually increase and immunity to many antigens is attained through natural exposure and through immunizations (see Chap. 14).

The advent of immunizations has been instrumental in decreasing mortality and morbidity from communicable diseases in children. Immunizations should include diphtheria-tetanus-pertussis (DTP), trivalent oral poliovirus (OPV), measles-mumps-rubella (MMR), and Haemophilus influenzae B (Hib). The Committee on Infectious Diseases of the American Academy of Pediatrics and the Advisory Committee on Immunization Practices of the US Public Health Service recommend that immunizations commence at age 2 months with DTP and OPV and follow the recommended intervals. The MMR immunization is recommended at age 15 months and Hib at age 24 months, unless the infant is at increased risk for the disease.

## Alteration and Adaptation

### Sudden Infant Death Syndrome

Sudden infant death syndrome (SIDS) represents the major cause of death during the period between age 1 week and 1 year. It is especially devastating for the family since it involves the loss of an apparently normally developed, healthy infant. Even the postmortem examination sometimes fails to reveal the cause of death. Major characteristics associated with SIDS are summarized in Box 5-1.

Although the specific cause of SIDS remains unknown, chronic hypoxia, prolonged apnea, or both may contribute to the death. Figure 5-3 shows some factors that may be causative in some SIDS deaths. Pulmonary edema, inflammatory changes of the upper respiratory passage, and petechial hemorrhages in the lungs and pericardium are characteristic findings on postmortem examination.

### Accidents

Accidents represent another important cause of injury and death in infants, especially from age 6 to 12 months. During this period, the infant is growing and developing rapidly. Curiosity leads to an irresistible urge to explore. This exploration involves the use of hands, legs, and the mouth, and places the infant in a vulnerable position. Accidents during the first year of life commonly involve suffocation, aspiration, falls, burns, poison, and motor vehicles. Many of the accidents can be prevented by paying special attention to the environment and the use of child safety restraints when traveling.

### Otitis Media

Otitis media, the second most common disease of infants and young children, frequently occurs as a complication of nasopharyngitis.[32] Inflammation of the middle ear is especially common in infants and young children because they have a short, straight eustachian tube with undeveloped cartilage within it. Peak incidence for otitis media occurs between the ages of 6 months and 2 to 3 years. It is also more prevalent during winter months.

Eustachian tubes function to protect the middle ear from nasopharyngeal secretions, drain normal middle

**BOX 5–1.**
MAJOR CHARACTERISTICS ASSOCIATED WITH SUDDEN INFANT DEATH SYNDROME

| | |
|---|---|
| Family background | Highest in low birth weight, premature infants of adolescent mothers; underweight white males; black infants; and infants of multiple births |
| Siblings | No greater risk than general population when matched for maternal age and birth order |
| Previous health | Detailed history may show abnormalities |
| Age | Greatest in 1–6 mo old; peak incidence 2–4 mo |
| Sex | Males greater risk |
| Season of year | Fall and winter months |
| Time of day | Between midnight and 9 AM |

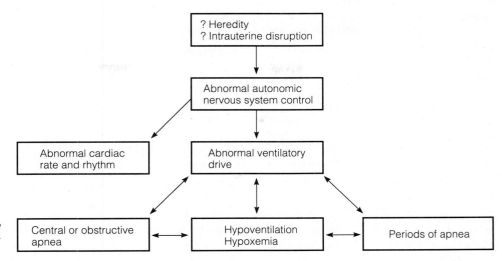

**FIGURE 5–3.**
Some physiologic factors that may be causative in deaths from sudden infant death syndrome.

ear secretions, and equalize pressure between the middle ear and the external ear. The eustachian tubes can become obstructed from allergy, infection, enlarged adenoids, or nasopharyngeal tumors. This obstruction prevents drainage of normal secretions from the middle ear (serous otitis media). Negative middle ear pressure occurs when air which normally escapes is absorbed. When the tube becomes fully or partially open, organisms then enter the middle ear where they multiply and produce infection. Organisms most frequently associated with otitis media are *Streptococcus pneumoniae, Haemophilus influenzae,* and *Staphylococcus aureus.* Continued or untreated otitis media can result in hearing loss from negative ear pressure, effusion in the middle ear, or damage to the tympanic membrane. Consequently, hearing loss may lead to speech and language problems.

Although acute otitis media may be asymptomatic, classic clinical manifestations include fever, severe pain, irritability, lethargy, anorexia, vomiting, and diarrhea. Sucking and chewing increase the pain. Findings from otoscopic examination include reddened and bulging tympanic membrane with absence of normal landmarks and light reflex.

Severe pain and fever are usually absent in serous otitis media. However, the child may experience a feeling of fullness and a popping sensation when swallowing. If air is present above the fluid, the child may experience a feeling of motion. Otoscopic examination reveals a dull, gray tympanic membrane which may be either bulging or depressed. Landmarks are obscured. A visible fluid level may be present if there is air above the fluid.

## EARLY CHILDHOOD

The years from 1 through 5 are referred to as early childhood. These years encompass what is also referred to as the toddler (age 1 to 3 years) and preschool (age 3 to 5

years) periods. During this time, biologic growth slows and the various systems mature.

## *Biophysical Development*

### *Biologic Growth*

During early childhood, biologic growth levels off. By age 2 1/2 years, the average toddler has quadrupled the birth weight and increased height by two-thirds. At age 2 years, the average toddler weighs 27 pounds and measures 34 inches. This height represents approximately one-half of the predicted adult height. Increase in leg length accounts for the major gain in height of about 4 to 5 inches per year for the toddler and 2 1/2 inches per year for the preschooler.

The toddler gains 4 to 6 pounds per year while the preschool child gains about 4 pounds per year. By age 6 years, the preschool child weighs about 48 pounds and stands about 46 inches tall. Table 5-5 summarizes early childhood growth by year.

### *Body Proportion*

During early childhood, the head continues to be relatively large in comparison to the body. By age 2 years, the chest is larger than the head. Between age 1 and 2 years, the head circumference increases about 1 inch. By age 5 years, this increase is only about 1/2 inch per year.

The toddler characteristically displays a long trunk with short extremities. Immature abdominal muscles contribute to the protruding or "pot-bellied" abdomen. The typical 2 year old also displays flat feet and slightly bowed legs.

The body of the preschool child begins to resemble that of an adult. The preschooler becomes taller and thinner as the lower extremities grow faster than the

**TABLE 5–5.**
BIOPHYSICAL MEASUREMENTS OF EARLY CHILDHOOD

|  | 2 YEARS | 3 YEARS | 4 YEARS | 5 YEARS |
|---|---|---|---|---|
| **Weight** | 11.8–12.7 kg (26–28 lb) | 12.5–16.5 kg (27.5–36.3 lb) | 13.5–19.5 kg (29.7–42.9 lb) | 15.4–21.4 kg (33.9–47 lb) |
| **Height** | 82.5–85.0 cm (32.5–34 in); about one-half adult height | 90.5–101.5 cm (35.5–40 in) | 95–109 cm (37.5–43.3 in) | 103–115 cm (40–45.3 in) |
| **Head Circumference** | 49–50 cm (19.6–20 in) | | | |
| **Pulse** | 110 ± 20; average 100/min | 105 ± 15; average 95/min | 100 ± 10; average 92/min | 95 ± 15; average 90/min |
| **Respirations** | 26–28/min | 25 ± 5/min | 24 ± 4/min | 22 ± 3/min |
| **Blood Pressure** | 99/64 ± 26/24 | 100/67 ± 24/25 | 100/66 ± 20 | 100/60 ± 14/10 |
| **Dentition** | 16 temporary teeth; 30 mo—full set temporary | | | |

Source: Adapted from D.R. Marlow and B.A. Redding, Textbook of Pediatric Nursing. Philadelphia: Saunders, 1988.

head, trunk, and arms. The protruding abdomen also disappears.

## Dentition

The 2-year-old toddler has about 16 primary teeth. By age 2 1/2 years, all 20 deciduous teeth have erupted. There is very little change in dentition during the preschool years.

## Physiologic Development

Physiologic development occurs as the individual systems mature. By the end of the toddler period, all systems are mature with the exception of the endocrine and reproductive systems.

## Genitourinary System

By age 2 years, the urinary tract of the toddler has matured sufficiently to concentrate urine. Completion of the myelinization process provides for increased sphincter control and increased bladder capacity. Once the genitourinary system has attained sufficient maturity, the child is physically ready for toilet training.

## Nervous System

The total number of brain cells is complete by 1 year of age. However, these cells continue to increase in size until the brain is 75% the adult size by age 3 years. Complete myelinization of the spinal cord provides the basis for control of urinary and intestinal elimination. Matura-

tion of the nervous system also accounts for the improved coordination evident during early childhood.

## Gastrointestinal System

Increased stomach capacity and delayed emptying of the stomach allows the child to eat three basic meals per day with between-meal snacks. Anal sphincter control is possible as the spinal cord achieves complete myelinization.

## Immune System

Continuing maturation of the immune system provides adult levels of immunoglobin G (IgG) during the toddler period. Adult levels of immunoglobin M (IgM) are reached toward the end of infancy. During the preschool years, the child achieves adult levels of immunoglobin A (IgA). Development of immunoglobins D and E continues during early childhood, but adult levels are not reached until later childhood (see Chap. 14).

## Motor Development

Large muscles, legs, and arms account for the most growth during early childhood, with muscles growing faster than bones. The individual in early childhood becomes a more coordinated person as hand/eye coordination and small muscle coordination improve, especially in the preschool years. The clumsy little toddler at age 2 years who learns to ride a tricycle continues to refine the ability to run, skip, jump, and climb. The preschool child develops an ability to catch and throw a ball, but throwing is not accurate at this age.

Fine motor development concentrates on the smaller muscles of the fingers. At age 2 years, the toddler has fat fingers and incomplete myelinization. As myelinization is completed, fine motor skills improve, allowing the child to use crayons, pencils, and scissors with increasing skill.

## Factors Affecting Development

### Nutrition

The toddler needs approximately 1300 calories and the preschooler needs about 1800 calories to maintain nutritional status and promote adequate growth.[4] Protein intake should be about 1.8 and 1.5 gm per kg of body weight, respectively, for the toddler and preschooler.[4] These recommendations represent an increase during this period due to the rapid growth in the muscles of the body (see Chap. 10). Calcium requirements are about 800 mg per day. The child eats at least five to seven times per day.

There continues to be a great deal of controversy over the need for dietary supplements. The best guide in determining whether a child should be placed on supplements is a review of the normal dietary intake. If a child's nutritional intake is consistently below the daily recommendations, then dietary supplements are definitely indicated.

Children in early childhood should also be observed for adverse reactions to various foods and food substances. Food substances known to produce adverse reactions include sugar, artificial coloring, and various preservatives. Allergic reactions to foods may be evidenced by urticaria, itching, headache, and changes in behavior, including hyperactivity.

### Accidents

Between ages 1 and 4 years, the leading cause of death is accidents. The number of deaths from accidents in this period is surpassed only by the rate of death from accidents among adolescents. The incidence of accidents is closely related to the development occurring in the child at this time. Children in this age group exhibit tremendous curiosity about the world that surrounds them. They explore this world with their hands and mouths and display increasing control of fine motor skills. Additionally, children of this age are walking, climbing, running, and learning to ride tricycles and other motion toys. Thus, major areas of injury include motor vehicles, drowning, burns, poisoning, falls, and aspiration and suffocation. Table 5-6 indicates the ranking of accidents by sex for children in early childhood.

**TABLE 5–6.**

### RANKINGS OF ACCIDENTAL DEATHS BY SEX IN EARLY CHILDHOOD

| RANKING | BOYS | GIRLS |
|---------|------|-------|
| 1 | Motor vehicle | Motor vehicle |
| 2 | Drowning | Burns |
| 3 | Burns | Drowning |
| 4 | Suffocation | Falls |
| 5 | Falls | Suffocation |

### Control of Bodily Functions

It is during the early childhood years that the individual gains control of bodily functions. Most children are physically mature enough to begin toilet training at about age 2 years. However, individual variation in development and cultural practices may prevent the child from gaining control of bodily functions until age 3 or 4 years. The absence of control of bodily function by age 4 to 5 years indicates the need for assessment and evaluation of the individual child for *enuresis* and *encopresis*. Both of these conditions represent alterations associated with bodily function.

Enuresis is defined as involuntary voiding after the age at which bladder control should have been achieved. This involuntary voiding occurs most often at night. Primary enuresis occurs when there is an absence of a long, dry, symptom free period. Secondary or acquired enuresis occurs after at least a year of dryness.[4,6] This condition occurs twice as often in boys as in girls and affects 5% to 17% of children age 3 to 15 years who are otherwise considered normal.[61]

No one cause of enuresis has been identified. One very common factor is urinary tract infection or obstruction.[19] An abnormal stream, including dribbling, is often indicative of a physiologic problem.[19] Enuresis has been associated with a history of bedwetting in parents, siblings, or other close relatives of affected children. Additionally, a higher frequency of enuresis has been found among children of lower socioeconomic groups and in black children.[62] Maturational lags characterized by frequent urination, small bladder capacity, and delayed inhibitory control, and dysfunction of the reticular activating system in rapid eye movement (REM) sleep have been shown to contribute to enuresis.[19] Diagnostic evaluation includes a complete family and child's history, as well as a urinary workup. Urine cultures should be ordered to rule out an infection, and bladder capacity should be determined.

Clinical management includes electronic conditioning devices to alert the child, and drug therapy. Tofranil is frequently used to inhibit urination. Bladder training may be used in an attempt to increase bladder capacity.

Withholding fluids before bedtime and interrupting sleep also help in achieving bladder control at night.

Encopresis is the repeated voluntary or involuntary passage of stool into clothing after the age when toilet training should have been achieved.[50] Primary, or continuous, encopresis occurs when the child has never achieved bowel control. Secondary, or discontinuous, encopresis occurs when the child has achieved bowel control prior to the onset of incontinence. This condition occurs more often in males than in females and affects 1.5% to 5.7% of children.[50] Encopresis is a physiologic, as well as behavioral, disorder, and is now referred to as idiopathic fecal incontinence (IFI), unless a psychiatric disorder is a direct contributing factor.[52] Emotional problems associated with encopresis include fear of parents, altered parent-child relationships and psychosocial stress associated with life changes such as sibling's birth or starting school.

Clinical manifestations of IFI include a history of chronic constipation, often beginning in infancy, painful defecation, complaints of poor appetite, abdominal pain, and distention. Passage of small, hard, formed stool with diarrhea is indicative of impaction. Frequently stools are extremely large and accompanied by blood.

Diagnosis is based upon a complete history and physical examination. Neurologic assessment, including deep tendon reflexes, sensory function, muscle strength, and tone of lower extremities are suggestive of spinal cord pathology.[52] Abdominal examination reveals tenderness, masses, and organ enlargement. A KUB flat plate of the abdomen will reveal any stool retained in the colon.

Therapeutic management of IFI includes a diet high in fiber, lubricants, cathartics, and behavior reinforcement.[52] The high fiber diet is directed toward the prevention of constipation. Mineral oil helps soften the stool and reduce its size. The administration of cathartics aids in establishment of regularity, but most children achieve bowel control without medication in 6 to 12 months.

### Hearing and Vision Problems

The most common long term handicapping disorder that affects children is hearing impairment.[32] Routine auditory screening during early childhood will aid in diagnosis and prevention of speech disorders associated with hearing loss. Normal hearing function and disorders of hearing are discussed in Chapter 49.

Hearing impairment in the child may be classified as: (1) conduction, (2) sensorineural, (3) mixed, and (4) central auditory dysfunction. Conduction hearing losses are the most common type and may be caused by congenital anomalies, such as ear malformation and atresia or acquired loss due to otitis media, trauma or blockage from a foreign body. Surgical correction may be possible.

Sensorineural hearing loss in children may be due to rubella, cytomegalovirus, meningitis, *Streptococcus pneumoniae,* hyperbilirubinemia, Down syndrome, exposure to excessive noise, and drugs, such as gentamycin and chemotherapeutic agents. Head injury may also lead to a sensorineural hearing loss. Central auditory dysfunction includes birth trauma and hypoxia at birth, as well as infantile autism and conversion hysteria.

Approximately 20 to 35 per 1000 children experience some visual impairment, even with glasses.[62] Visual impairment refers to visual loss that cannot be corrected with prescription glasses and, in childhood, can produce delays in the child's growth and development. Normal visual function and disorders of vision are found in Chapter 49.

The causes of visual impairment may be classified into four groups: (1) familial or genetic factors, (2) prenatal factors, (3) perinatal factors, and (4) postnatal factors. Familial or genetic factors include Tay-Sachs disease, Down syndrome, Crouzon disease, galactosemia, and retinoblastoma. Prenatal factors that may lead to visual impairment in the child include syphilis, rubella, and toxoplasmosis. Visual impairment may include blindness and cataracts. Prematurity, maternal infection, and high oxygen concentrations associated with respiratory distress syndrome are among perinatal factors producing visual impairment. Measles, mumps, rubella, chicken pox, poliomyelitis, leukemia, myasthenia gravis, and juvenile rheumatoid arthritis, as well as trauma, constitute postnatal factors responsible for visual impairment.

Visual disorders seen most often in children include errors of refraction, amblyopia, strabismus, cataracts, and glaucoma. Infections and trauma also constitute major visual alterations to which children must adapt. Specifically, errors of refraction are seen in farsightedness, nearsightedness, astigmatism, and anisometropia.

## MIDDLE CHILDHOOD

The years from age 6 to 12 are referred to as middle childhood. This period is one of quiescence in biophysical development when compared to the rapid growth and development noted in infancy and early childhood, as well as the growth spurts associated with youth and adolescence. This period of physical quiescence allows for control and mastery of skills which, up until now, were unrealistic.

### Biophysical Development

#### Biologic Growth

Biophysical growth and development proceed at a slower, but steadier, pace during the middle childhood years. The average gain in height during middle child-

**TABLE 5-7.**
BIOPHYSICAL MEASUREMENTS OF MIDDLE CHILDHOOD

| | 6–8 YEARS | 8–10 YEARS | 10–12 YEARS | 12 YEARS |
|---|---|---|---|---|
| **Weight** | 17.5–25.5 kg (39.5–55.5 lb) | 22–32 kg (48–70 lb) | 25.5–39.5 kg (57–85 lb) | Boys: 30–48 kg (73–97 lb) Girls: 30–50 kg (68–108 lb) |
| **Height** | 110–124 cm (43.5–48.5 in) | 121.5–136.5 cm (47.5–53.5 in) | 131.5–147.5 cm (52–58 in) | Boys: 142–158 cm (56–62 in) Girls: 144–160 cm (57–63 in) |
| **Pulse** | 90 ± 15/min | 85 ± 10/min | 90 ± 20/min | Boys: 90 ± 20/min Girls: 85 ± 20/min |
| **Respirations** | 21 ± 3/min | 20 ± 3/min | 19 ± 3/min | 19 ± 3/min |
| **Blood Pressure** | 100/60 ± 16/10 | 102/60 ± 16/10 | 109/58 ± 16/10 | 113/59 ± 18/10 |
| **Dentition** | Begins to lose temporary teeth; first permanent molars, medial and lateral incisor | | Acquires cuspids, first and secondary premolars | |

Source: *Adapted from D.R. Marlow and B.A. Redding,* Textbook of Pediatric Nursing. *Philadelphia: J.B. Saunders, 1988.*

hood is 2 to 3 inches per year. The school-age child gains an average of 5 to 7 pounds per year. By age 12 years, children are approximately 58 to 59 inches tall and weigh about 86 pounds, although boys tend to be slightly shorter than girls (Table 5-7). However, wide variations occur in height and weight indicative of the influence of genetics and nutrition on physical development. Periodic measurements of both height and weight are helpful in early diagnosis of significant deviations and are essential in determining appropriate medication dosage.

### Body Proportion

School-age children are significantly different from preschoolers and adolescents in body proportions. Arms and legs increase significantly in length. Both the brain and bones of the head remain relatively stable, while the facial structure shows the greatest growth. As a result, the head constitutes less of the body surface (Figure 5-4). The waist also decreases in relation to height.

### Dentition

By age 5 to 6 years, children begin to lose baby teeth, which are replaced by permanent teeth. This process tends to occur earlier in girls than in boys. At the same time, the facial structure changes, with the jaw lengthening and the face increasing in size. By age 12 to 13 years, permanent teeth should have erupted with the exception of the second and third molars.

### Physiologic Development

#### Musculoskeletal Changes

The steady weight gain during this period of development is due primarily to the increase in size of the skeleton and muscles. Skeletal growth continues until the epiphyseal disc closes and ossifies (see Chap. 45). Damage to the epiphyseal disc is especially important during the middle childhood years. Injury during this time can result in premature fusion of the ossification centers and a permanent shortening of the bone.

Adequate nutrition, including protein, vitamins, and minerals, is especially important to the growth of healthy bone. Kidney disease, endocrine problems, inadequate metabolism and food absorption, as well as interference with growth hormone production, can alter bone maturation.

Muscle tone improves and the "baby fat" of earlier years decreases as muscle mass and strength increase. Boys have more muscle cells than girls, thus contributing to their greater strength. Girls tend to have more fat than muscle tissue.

Increased muscle tone helps account for the improved posture during the middle years. However, increased muscle tissue and strength does not indicate muscle maturity. Therefore, school-age children are at increased risk for muscular injury from overuse.

Sheldon developed a classification schema for body build which still provides the basis for more current classification systems.[32] He proposed that there are three ba-

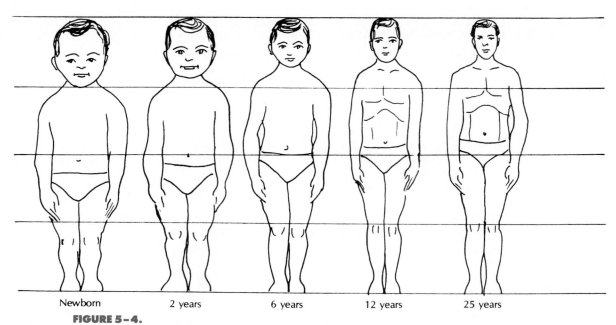

**FIGURE 5–4.**
Body proportions and form will change as individuals progress through the early years of the life cycle. (From C.S. Schuster and S.S. Ashburn, *The Process of Human Development: A Holistic Life Span Approach.* Boston: Little, Brown, 1986.)

sic body builds: endomorphic, mesomorphic, and ectomorphic. The endomorphic individual is one with a short, fat build who appears soft and round. The broad-shouldered individual with a strong muscular body is referred to as mesomorphic. The tall, thin person is the ectomorph. Although children are most often a combination of body builds, their self-concept may be influenced by the reaction of others to the predominant body build.

### Central Nervous System

Growth for the brain and head is minimal during middle childhood. Primary changes in the nervous system are evidenced in the myelinization process. The myelin sheath increases in thickness and results in improved conduction of nerve impulses. The effects of a maturing nervous system and improved nerve impulse conduction are seen as the clumsy child of age 6 years becomes a coordinated sports participant in later childhood.

### Other Systems

The maturation of the gastrointestinal system accounts for the decreased complaints of stomach aches and increased tolerance to food. Due to increased capacity and intake, the school-age child is also able to tolerate longer intervals between meals.

Middle childhood is also associated with maturation of the urinary system. Increased kidney size and function allow the child to better control elimination and adhere to a more controlled schedule.

The development of a mature immune system helps to account for the period of health associated with the school years. Tonsils and adenoids are enlarged and believed to contribute to the production of antibodies when the child is exposed to various antigens (see Chap. 14). Therefore, tonsillectomies and adenoidectomies should be considered only when there is a history of frequent severe infection of the tonsils, adenoids, or middle ears, or when breathing, or perhaps swallowing, is impaired.

The cardiovascular system continues to mature during middle childhood. The heart continues to grow, although at a slower rate. As the cardiovascular system matures, cardiac output increases, heart rate decreases, and blood pressure increases. This increased cardiac output increases oxygenation essential for the energy expenditures of the school-age child.

### Motor Development

The years of middle childhood are associated with smoother and more coordinated motor development. Perfection of gross motor development during these years allows the school-age child to learn to ride a bicycle, jump rope, swim, and skate. Running and climbing are mastered also. Motor development during these years allows children to participate in team and individual sports since they now have strength and skills to hit or kick a ball, throw, and catch.

Myelinization of the CNS accounts for the improvement in fine motor skills seen during the early school years. This fine motor development is evidenced as the child progresses from large printing with large pencils and crayons at age 6 years to smaller writing with a regular pencil by age 10 years. A preference for the right or left hand emerges early in the school years. Mastery of fine motor skills is also seen as school-age children learn to play musical instruments, sew, and work with models.

## Factors Affecting Development

### Physical Fitness

Exercise is especially important in biophysical development during the middle childhood years. Physical exercise allows the child to improve muscle tone and strength, as well as balance and coordination. School-age children generally display tremendous energy and thus need guidance in directing this energy. However, a survey of school fitness indicated that American children are not physically fit. The primary factor in the lack of fitness is the amount of time spent watching television. By the age of 18, the average child will spend more time watching television (15,000 hours) than in school (11,000 hours).[44]

Sports participation is common for children of this age group. However, parents must be certain that the child is truly interested in the sport and that adequate protective equipment is provided. Placement of children in a sport for which they are not physically prepared or interested in may lead to problems with self esteem or injury.

### Nutrition

Overall caloric needs decrease during this period of growth and development (see Chap. 10). However, it is important that a well-balanced diet be maintained to promote growth and to prepare for the increased needs of adolescence. Implementation of this well-balanced diet becomes increasingly more difficult, however, since the child is progressively more independent in determining what is actually eaten.

### Allergic Disorders

Allergic disorders in childhood include: (1) urticaria, (2) allergic rhinitis, and (3) asthma; they account for over 25% of school absence from chronic health problems.[48] Urticaria represents a skin reaction characterized by pruritus and pale wheals. Allergic rhinitis is the most common allergic disorder affecting children.[32] Hay fever and seasonal rhinitis are terms used to refer to allergic rhinitis, which occurs with the various seasons. The release of histamine in response to inhaled irritants causes the symptoms of nasal congestion, itching, sneezing, and watery discharge in predisposed children.

It is estimated that school-age children account for approximately 2% to 5% of all asthmatics and that the condition accounts for 25% of all school absences in children under age 17 years.[32] During middle childhood, asthma occurs more often in boys than in girls. However, during adolescence the incidence is about equal in boys and girls[32] (see Chap. 30).

### Learning Disabilities

The term "learning disabilities" is associated with children of normal intelligence who exhibit disorders in understanding or using written or spoken language. Manifestations of learning disabilities vary and may include problems with the ability to listen, speak, read, write, spell, or do math.[56]

Approximately 5% to 20% of school-age children have been shown to exhibit some type of learning disability.[8] The condition is more common in boys than in girls, which suggests some type of sex-linked predisposition.[1]

The diagnosis of learning disability has been subdivided to include attention deficit disorders, as well as specific learning disabilities.[27] Attention deficit disorders are those disorders in which the child is either overfocused or underfocused.[32] When the child is underfocused, he or she may be considered "hyperactive" and have difficulty maintaining attention long enough to learn. The overfocused child concentrates on only one area for too long a period of time. Specific learning disabilities generally involve a developmental delay.[27]

There is no single causative factor for learning disabilities. Problems associated with oxygen deprivation in the prenatal, perinatal, or postnatal periods, as well as complications of labor and delivery may be contributing factors. Encephalitis, meningitis, and lead poisoning in early childhood may also contribute to the disorder.[1]

Other contributing factors include diet and environment. Malnutrition, including vitamin B deficiencies, as well as caffeine and sugar, may contribute to attention problems. Attention deficit disorders occur more often in children from lower socioeconomic status, in families who move often, and in families who do not reward learning.[21]

## ADOLESCENCE

The period of adolescence is considered a transitional time from childhood to adulthood. During this time, rapid physical, intellectual, emotional, and social developmental changes occur. Although changes occur in all four domains and are interrelated, it is the purpose of this section to consider mainly the biophysical changes that occur during this stage of development. Alterations and adaptation specific to the adolescent are also discussed.

## Overview of Growth and Development Stages

Prepuberty or pubescence is considered to be a 2-year to 3-year period between childhood and adolescence. This stage of development is characterized by rapid physical growth and the appearance of secondary sex characteristics. Puberty begins in girls with the onset of menarche which is the onset of monthly flow of bloody fluid from the uterus, called the menses. On the average, menarche occurs in the United States at age 12.5 to 12.8 years. Puberty ends between ages 12 to 14 years in girls. In boys, puberty occurs with the ability to produce spermatozoa and the occurrence of nocturnal emissions and ends 1 to 2 years later than with girls. The onset of puberty occurs earlier in girls and is thought to be due to the more rapid maturation of the CNS.[48] The developmental stage of adolescence officially begins with the appearance of secondary sex characteristics and ends when somatic growth is complete. Adolescence is generally divided into three stages: early adolescence, ages 12 to 13 years; middle adolescence, ages 14 to 16 years; and late adolescence, ages 17 to 21 years. At the end of adolescence, the individual should be psychologically mature and capable of becoming a contributing, independent member of society.[32] Table 5-8 gives specific values and norms related to adolescent physical development.

## Physical Development

### Musculoskeletal System

Although all body systems undergo rapid maturation during the time of intense growth, the most noticeable change is observed in body height. The skeletal system, which doubles in mass during adolescence, grows at a faster rate than the supporting muscles. Because of this fact, the adolescent often appears clumsy and to be lacking in coordination.[32] Boys generally average an eight-inch gain in height during this growth spurt, girls usually average just over three inches each year. By age 18 years, most adolescents have attained 99% of the adult height.[16]

Lean body mass and nonlean body mass, which is primarily fat, double during puberty. The increase in skeletal mass, muscle mass, and nonlean muscle mass contributes significantly to the increased weight gain that occurs in adolescence. Muscles increase in both the number of individual cells and size in boys, while muscles in girls increase only in size.[16] Androgen is thought to be responsible for the increased muscle mass that occurs in boys. By age 17 years, boys possess two times greater muscle mass than girls, which contributes to the two to four times greater strength of boys.[48] When physically mature, girls average two times as much body fat as boys.[16]

After the appearance of secondary sex characteristics, the rate of growth declines. Ossification slows, the epiphyses of the long bones mature due to the influence of the sex hormones, and growth of the long bones ceases.[48]

Following menarche and nocturnal emissions, the adolescent may grow two to three more inches. How-

**TABLE 5-8.**
AVERAGE BIOPHYSICAL DEVELOPMENT OF THE YOUNG, MIDDLE, AND LATE ADOLESCENT

| | YOUNG ADOLESCENTS, 12–13 YEARS | | MIDDLE ADOLESCENTS, 14–16 YEARS | | LATE ADOLESCENTS, 17–21 YEARS | |
|---|---|---|---|---|---|---|
| | Males | Females | Males | Females | Males | Females |
| **Height** | 154–172 cm (60–68 in) | 153–167 cm (60–66 in) | 164–180 cm (65–71 in) | 155–169 cm (61–66.5 in) | 163–182 cm (64–72 in) | 156–170 cm (61–67 in) |
| **Weight** | 38–60 kg (84–132 lb) | 40–60 kg (88–132 lb) | 50–60 kg (110–132 lb) | 42–64 kg (92–141 lb) | 50–80 kg (110–176 lb) | 48–72 kg (106–158 lb) |
| **Heart Rate** | 65 beats/min ± 8 | 65 beats/min ± 8 | 63 beats/min ± 8 | 66 beats/min ± 8 | 70 beats/min ± 10 | 70 beats/min ± 10 |
| **Respirations** | 19/min ± 3 | 19/min ± 3 | 17/min ± 3 | 17/min ± 3 | 17/min ± 3 | 17/min ± 3 |
| **Blood Pressure** | 114/68 ± 10/14 | 112/66 ± 10/12 | 116/70 ± 12/14 | 114/70 ± 12/14 | 126/74 ± 26/16 | 126/74 ± 26/16 |
| **Dentition** | Second molars | Second molars | — | — | Third molars | Third molars |
| **Visual Acuity** | 20/20 | 20/20 | 20/20 | 20/20 | 20/20 | 20/20 |
| **Hearing** | Adult | Adult | Adult | Adult | Adult | Adult |

Adapted from: D.R. Marlow and B.A. Redding, Textbook of Pediatric Nursing. Philadelphia: W.B. Saunders, 1988.

ever, most of this growth is due to an increase in length of the trunk, not growth of long bones. Greater long bone growth usually occurs in boys due to the longer prepubertal stage.[48]

The relationship between growth in height and weight to maturation of the reproductive system is high, probably due to the activation of the hypothalamus, which is thought to have been suppressed during early childhood. The maturation of height and the reproductive system is genetically and environmentally determined, causing norms for this group to be variable. Some children may grow as much as six or seven inches in a year, while others may grow only one inch. Assessing growth in adolescents must be individualized, considering parental height, previous patterns of growth, sexual maturity, and environmental factors.[48]

## Central Nervous System

In comparison to all other body systems, the CNS does not undergo the rapid increase in growth during puberty. By age 10 years, growth of the cerebellum, cerebrum, and brain stem is basically complete. Myelinization of the greater cerebral commissures and reticular formation of the CNS continue until middle adulthood. At puberty, brain tissue is quantitatively and qualitatively mature.[48] During childhood, adult visual abilities and normal adult hearing were attained.[16]

## Respiratory System

The increase of vital capacity of the lungs corresponds with the height of the individual: the greater the height, the larger the vital capacity. As the vital capacity increases, the respiratory rate decreases in both boys and girls.[48] Since the lungs grow at a slower pace than other body systems, the supply of oxygen may not be adequate, causing the adolescent to feel constant fatigue.[32]

## Cardiovascular System

Like the lungs, the heart also grows at a slower pace than other body systems. However, during puberty the heart does experience rapid growth. Due to the increased growth, the heart pumps blood with greater strength.

This increased pumping strength causes an elevation in blood pressure. During the height of the growth period, the pulse rate may increase momentarily. However, the increased body size allows stabilization of the pulse at a slower rate. Blood volume is directly correlated with weight, therefore, it increases more rapidly in boys. By late adolescence, boys averages 5000 ml of blood while girls averages 4200 ml.[48] Pulse, respiration, and blood pressure values are within the adult range by age 15 or 16[16] (see Table 5-8).

## Gastrointestinal System

The digestive tract enlarges during adolescence. Because of the increased need for food required for growth, the size of the stomach enlarges in both length and width to accommodate the additional food. Gastric acidity also increases to aid in digestion of the additional food intake. The increased acidity combined with the stress of coping with the many other physiologic changes occurring during adolescence may lead to gastric ulcer symptoms.[48]

## Integumentary System

During adolescence, the sebaceous glands of the face, chest, and back become overactive and secrete increased amounts of sebum. Small pores trap the sebaceous material beneath the skin, producing a pimple or acne (see Chap. 47).[32]

## Basal Metabolic Rate

During puberty, the thyroid gland increases thyroxin secretion under the influence of the thyroid-stimulating hormone (TSH) from the anterior pituitary. The increased thyroxin levels cause an increase in total body metabolism. The basal metabolic rate (BMR) increases during periods of growth, reaching a peak at puberty. The increase in BMR also causes an increase in body temperature, often causing the teenager to complain of feeling too warm. As the growth rate slows, the BMR gradually declines. Because of the rapid rate of overall body growth and the slower rate of growth of the heart and lungs, the young adolescent may not have enough energy for strenuous physical activity, which contributes to the feeling of fatigue.[48]

## Nutritional Needs

The increased need for calories coincides with the increased rate of overall body growth and higher BMR. At the height of growth periods, girls may consume 2600 calories per day and boys 3600 or more.

Protein needs correspond closely to the rate of growth. The recommended food intake should consist of 15% protein, 30% fat, and 55% carbohydrate[37] (see Chap. 10). Higher proportions of proteins may be necessary in the earlier years in response to the rapid growth occurring at that time.

Adequate calcium intake is necessary for growth of bone and formation of teeth. Due to the periods of rapid skeletal growth, the adolescent may consume inadequate calcium, particularly boys. Girls on weight reduction diets may intake less than adequate calcium. Iron needs for girls vary depending upon the amount of blood lost during menstruation. For replacement and maintenance, an intake of 1.2 gm of iron daily is recommended.[38] Vitamin

C is another nutrient that is often inadequate since fruits and vegetables are often avoided by the adolescent.[48]

## Physiologic Development

The onset of puberty is a complex, poorly understood process beginning with differentiation of the gonads in the embryo. The function and maturation of the gonads remain unstimulated and dormant until puberty. It is generally thought that the events of puberty are influenced by the anterior pituitary in response to stimulation from the hypothalamus. The gonadotropin-releasing factor (GnRF) stimulates the anterior pituitary to produce gonadotropic hormones that, in turn, stimulate the gonads to begin functioning. The gonadotropic hormones are follicle-stimulating hormone (FSH), luteinizing hormone (LH), and luteotropic hormone (LTH) or prolactin. FSH stimulates the growth of ova in girls and Leydig cells in the testes. At the time, that estrogen and testosterone are produced by the ovaries and testes respectively, the adrenal cortex increases the production of androgen. The increased amounts of androgen that are produced at puberty are antagonistic to the pituitary growth hormone (GH) that is produced by the anterior pituitary (see Chap. 36). This antagonistic effect is partially responsible for the decline in rate of body growth.

Estrogen, testosterone, and androgen are the hormones responsible for the development of the secondary sex characteristics. The secondary sex characteristics that appear depend upon which hormone is produced in the greatest amount, since males and females produce both male and female hormones. The androgens produce the male characteristics while the estrogens produce the female characteristics. The appearance of secondary sex characteristics are orderly, yet widely variable. Since there is such a wide variation in sexual maturity and development of the adolescent in comparison to chronological age, Tanner developed a staging system to describe and label the different stages for use in comparing the adolescent's stage of sexual maturity.[54] Tables 5-9 and 5-10 and Figures 5-5, 5-6, and 5-7 help to identify the stage of development in both males and females to detect abnormalities and assist the adolescent in what to expect at succeeding stages. Table 5-11 delineates the specific somatic changes occurring in both boys and girls as a response to puberty.

## Alterations and Adaptations in Adolescence

The developmental stage of adolescence is described as identity versus role confusion.[15] It has been identified as a time of conflict, confusion, and intense emotions. Relationships with parents change and are replaced with peer relationships. At the same time that adolescents are searching for independence from parents and authority figures, they also still maintain an element of dependence. During this developmental stage, adolescents are formalizing behavioral decisions and practices for adult life. In an effort to explore all possible boundaries and options, adolescents often participate in risk-taking behaviors. Risk-taking may be demonstrated in a number of behaviors. Accidents, suicides, and homicides are the leading causes of death among adolescents in the United States. Teenage drivers contribute significantly to vehicular fatalities, both their own and those of others.[11] Drug and alcohol use are common among junior high school and high school students. Cigarette smoking, which is currently becoming more prevalent among female than male adolescents, is associated with respiratory symptoms during the teen years. Sexual activity is widespread and contributes significantly to pregnancy and sexually transmitted diseases (STDs).[31] Other alterations and adaptations that occur in response to the physiologic and psychosocial changes of adolescence are eating disorders and acne.

**TABLE 5-9.**
CLASSIFICATION OF SEXUAL MATURITY STAGES IN FEMALES

| STAGE | PUBIC HAIR | BREASTS |
|---|---|---|
| 1 | Preadolescent | Preadolescent |
| 2 | Sparse, light pigmentation, straight | Breast and papilla small mound; areola increases in diameter |
| 3 | Darker, begins to curl and increase in amount | Breast and areola enlarged |
| 4 | Coarse, curly, abundant in quantity but less than adult | Areola and papilla form secondary mound |
| 5 | Adult feminine triangle to medial surface of thighs | Mature, erect nipple, areola part of general breast contour |

Source: *Adapted from R.E. Behrman and V.C. Vaughn,* Nelson Textbook of Pediatrics. *Philadelphia: Saunders, 1987.*

**TABLE 5–10.**
CLASSIFICATION OF SEXUAL MATURITY IN MALES

| STAGE | PUBIC HAIR | PENIS | TESTES |
|---|---|---|---|
| 1 | None | Preadolescent | Preadolescent |
| 2 | Scanty, long, slightly pigmented | Slight enlargement | Enlarged scrotum, pink |
| 3 | Darker pigmentation, small in amount, begins to curl | Longer | Larger |
| 4 | Resembles adult type, coarse and curly, but less in amount than adult | Larger, glans and breadth increase in size | Larger, dark pigmentation |
| 5 | Adult distribution to medial surface of thighs | Adult | Adult |

Source: *Adapted from R.E. Behrman and V.C. Vaughn,* Nelson Textbook of Pediatrics. *Philadelphia: Saunders, 1987.*

## Eating Disorders

Obesity, anorexia nervosa (AN), and bulimia nervosa (BN) have increased significantly in the adolescent in the last decade. They are specific syndromes that represent a disturbance in eating behavior and psychological adjustment. Left untreated they can become life-threatening and seriously affect future development (see also Chap. 10).

*OBESITY.* Obesity is thought to be caused by an increase in the number of fat cells or adipocytes that accumulate in subcutaneous tissue. It is proposed that these

**STAGE 1**
Preadolescent—no pubic hair except for the fine body hair (vellus hair) similar to that on the abdomen

STAGE 2

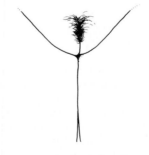

Sparse growth of long, slightly pigmented, downy hair, straight or only slightly curled, chiefly along the labia

STAGE 3

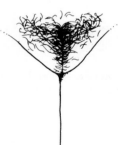

Darker, coarser, curlier hair, spreading sparsely over the pubic symphysis

STAGE 4

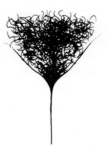

Coarse and curly hair as in adults; area covered greater than in stage 3 but not as great as in the adult and not yet including the thighs

STAGE 5

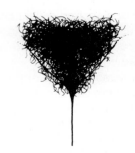

Hair adult in quantity and quality, spread on the medial surfaces of the thighs but not up over the abdomen

**FIGURE 5–5.**
Sex maturity rating in girls: Pubic hair. (From B. Bates, *Physical Examination.* Philadelphia: J.B. Lippincott, 1986.)

**STAGE 1**

Preadolescent. Elevation of nipple only

**STAGE 2**                                    **STAGE 3**

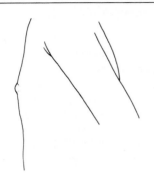                           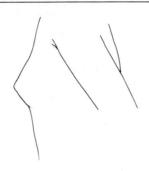

Breast bud stage. Elevation of breast and      Further enlargement and elevation of
nipple as a small mound; enlargement           breast and areola, with no separation
of areolar diameter                            of their contours

**STAGE 4**                                    **STAGE 5**

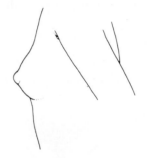                           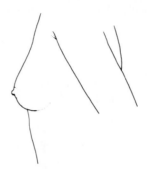

Projection of areola and nipple to form a      Mature stage; projection of nipple only.
secondary mound above the level of             Areola has receded to general contour
breast                                         of the breast (although in some normal
                                               individuals the areola continues to
                                               form a secondary mound).

**FIGURE 5-6.**
Sex maturity ratings in girls: Breasts
(From B. Bates, *Physical Examination*.
Philadelphia: J.B. Lippincott, 1986.)

adipocytes occur in infancy when the infant ingests increased calories. The potential then exists for the presence of increased weight later in life. The obese person may also have increased insulin levels, which result in a decrease in lipolysis and increased fat utilization and uptake.[32]

Diagnosis of obesity is made when the weight to height ratio and the skin fold thickness are greater than the 95th percentile. Obesity is present in 5% to 25% of children and adolescents.[14] The risk or potential for obesity is greater for the child who has obese parents. If both parents are obese, the risk for the child is 80%. If only one parent is obese, the risk for obesity in the child is still 40%.[62]

Many theories have been proposed as to the cause of obesity; however, there remains no definite answer. Increased caloric intake in infancy related to bottle-feeding and the early introduction of solid food has been proposed as a possible cause.[53] Another theory suggests that replication of fat cells occurs during a sensitive period and that obese children have increased numbers and larger fat cells, which are present for life.[29] Both these theories have been challenged. Another theory is the appestat or set-point theory.[16] This theory proposes that each person possesses an internal control system that keeps body weight stable. Through body metabolism, this set-point is maintained. If excess calories are consumed, the BMR increases to burn the additional calories. When calories are reduced, the BMR decreases.

Many causal and environmental factors have also

In assigning SMRs in boys, observe each of the three characteristics separately because they may develop at different rates. Record two separate ratings: pubic hair and genital. If the penis and testes differ in their stages, average the two into a single figure for the genital rating.

| | PUBIC HAIR | GENITAL | |
| --- | --- | --- | --- |
| | | PENIS | TESTES AND SCROTUM |
| **STAGE 1** | Preadolescent—no pubic hair except for the fine body hair (vellus hair) similar to that on the abdomen | Preadolescent—same size and proportions as in childhood | Preadolescent—same size and proportions as in childhood |
| **STAGE 2** 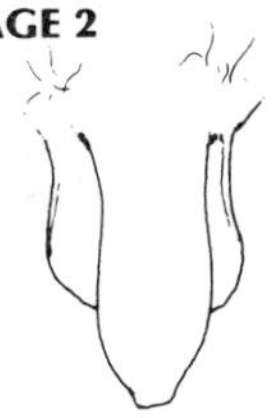 | Sparse growth of long, slightly pigmented, downy hair, straight or only slightly curled, chiefly at the base of the penis | Slight or no enlargement | Testes larger; scrotum larger, somewhat reddened, and altered in texture |
| **STAGE 3** 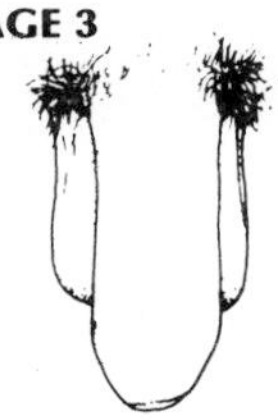 | Darker, coarser, curlier hair spreading sparsely over the pubic symphysis | Larger, especially in length | Further enlarged |
| **STAGE 4** 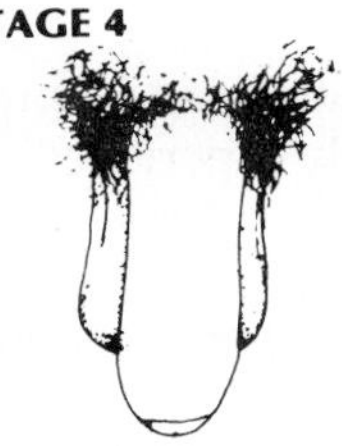 | Coarse and curly hair, as in the adult; area covered greater than in stage 3 but not as great as in the adult and not yet including the thighs | Further enlarged in length and breadth, with development of the glans | Further enlarged; scrotal skin darkened |
| **STAGE 5** 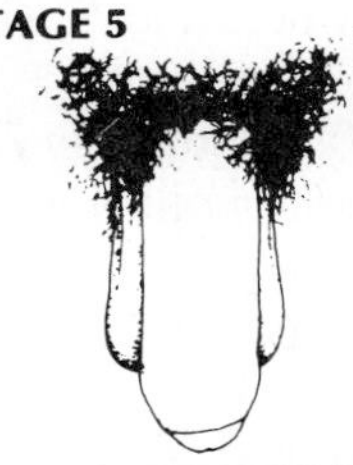 | Hair adult in quantity and quality, spread to the medial surfaces of the thighs but not up over the abdomen | Adult in size and shape | Adult in size and shape |

(Illustrations through the courtesy of W.A. Daniel, Jr, Division of Adolescent Medicine, University of Alabama, Birmingham)

**FIGURE 5–7.**
Sex maturity ratings in boys. (From B. Bates, *Physical Examination*. Philadelphia: J.B. Lippincott, 1986.)

been cited as contributing to childhood obesity. Examples of these are inactivity, possibly attributed to increased television and video games, tiredness during physical activity, and avoidance of activity leading to poor physical condition and further weight gain.[58]

*ANOREXIA NERVOSA.* Anorexia nervosa is a disorder of eating that involves self-induced starvation, an intense fear of fatness, dissatisfaction with body shape, and the belief that being thin and having control over body weight is essential for happiness.[17] Amenorrhea occurs in females, and males experience a decrease in sex drive. To achieve weight loss, the anorexic individual may restrict food, abuse laxatives and diuretics, cause self-induced vomiting, or engage in excessive exercise. Although the syndrome is labeled "anorexia," there is no loss of appetite.[36]

Anorexia nervosa affects about one in 200 white, ado-

**TABLE 5-11.**

SOMATIC CHANGES AS A RESPONSE TO PUBERTY

| STEP | MALES | FEMALES | BOTH SEXES |
|------|-------|---------|------------|
| 1 | | | Apocrine gland development |
| 2 | Bone structure thickens and strengthens | Internal pelvis increases in diameter | Pelvic changes |
| 3 | Growth of testes and scrotum | Growth of ovaries and uterus | Growth in size of gonads |
| 4 | | | Breast enlargement |
| 5 | | | Appearance of pubic hair |
| 6 | Growth of penis | Growth of labia and vagina | Growth of external genitalia |
| 7 | Nocturnal emissions | Menarche | External puberty |
| 8 | | | Axillary hair |
| 9 | Spermatogenesis, sperm in urine and semen | Oogenesis, ovulation | True puberty |
| 10 | Broadening of shoulders | Broadening of hips | Broadening of body frame |
| 11 | | | Vocal changes throughout |

Source: *Adapted from C.S. Schuster and S.S. Ashburn,* The Process of Human Development: A Holistic Life Span Approach. *Boston: Little, Brown, 1986.*

lescent females from middle to upper socioeconomic classes. The most common age for problems to begin is at 12 years, with peak years from ages 13 to 14 and 17 to 18. Although less common, AN may occur in females until the mid-30s and in young males.

The anorexic individual may present a variety of complaints. Amenorrhea may occur before weight loss, although it is more common after weight loss. Additionally, nonspecific gastrointestinal symptoms are present. Hypertrophy of the parotid gland occurs, causing a chipmunk-like face. Dry skin with the texture of sandpaper, yellow discoloration of the palms of the hands, and thin scalp hair associated with lanugolike hair over the face and body are common. Hypotension and hypothermia are late developing symptoms. If vomiting is used as a weight control measure, enamel erosion of the teeth occurs in response to frequent exposure to the high acidity of vomitus. Left untreated, AN has a 15% to 21% mortality rate from starvation.[2]

The physiologic manifestations that occur in AN are the result of starvation. Cognitive changes that occur are loss of concentration and of general interests, mood swings, irritability, depression, apathy, and sleep disturbances. Amenorrhea, an early symptom of AN, is caused by a reversal of gonadotropic secretion as seen in pubescence. Low levels of LH and FSH are associated with estrogen deficiency. The estrogen deficiency may contribute to the osteoporosis common in AN.

In addition, some anorexic individuals have problems concentrating urine due to water deprivation. This may be caused by defective osmoregulation or vasopressin secretion. Many anorexic individuals experience abnormal thermoregulatory responses when exposed to heat and cold.

In spite of the extreme low body weight, most anorexics experience hypothyroid symptoms of constipation, cold sensitivity, hypotension, bradycardia, dry skin and hair, and low levels of $T_4$ (thyroxine), and $T_3$ (triiodothyronine).[60]

Gastrointestinal symptoms are also common in AN. Gastric emptying is delayed and intestinal motility is decreased. This produces the complaints of bloating, constipation, and abdominal pain. Increased hepatic enzymes may indicate fatty infiltrates of the liver.

Other changes that occur in the individual with AN are left ventricle thinning and decreased cardiac chamber size, which cause hypotension and a decrease in cardiac output. When an electrolyte imbalance is associated with AN, cardiac dysrhythmias are common. Renal insufficiency usually contributes to dehydration.[22]

*BULIMIA NERVOSA.* Bulimia is a Greek term, "bous limos," which means "ox-hunger."[25] The term "ox-hunger" is used to explain the binge eating that occurs in this disorder. Binging is a secretive, rapid eating of large amounts of high caloric foods. The number of calories consumed in one binge can range from 500 to 10,000, with the mean being 3415.[34] Binges increase in frequency and eventually become the way of meeting nutritional needs since considerable food is absorbed in spite of the purging. After binging, the individual purges through self-induced vomiting, or laxative, or diuretic abuse.

The number of individuals affected with BN in the United States is not known. However, the frequency is increasing. One research study of college students found that 13% of the student population displayed major symptoms of BN.[20,40] Like AN, onset of BN most frequently occurs in adolescent females.

The physical changes associated with AN may also occur with BN. Although amenorrhea may occur, it does not occur as frequently in BN. The individual with BN has physical difficulties associated with repetitive purging. Swelling of the parotid glands and tooth enamel erosion may be present from the self-induced vomiting. Epigastric distress from chronic esophagitis and gastrointestinal bleeding also occur. Dilation and rupture of the esophagus can occur from binging. Some of the most serious complications of BN are hypokalemic alkalosis from persistent vomiting, cardiac dysrhythmia from hypokalemia, dehydration from laxative abuse, potassium depletion with cardiac arrest, and spastic colitis. Frequently, the adolescent with BN is also involved in drug and alcohol abuse, promiscuity, and stealing.[36]

Diagnosis of BN is made from the following American Psychiatric Association criteria:

1. There are reoccurring episodes of binging.
2. During binging, the individual has a feeling of lack of control over eating behavior.
3. The individual regularly engages in purging behaviors, strict dieting, fasting, or excessive exercise to prevent weight gain.
4. Binge eating occurs a minimum of twice per week for at least 3 months.
5. The individual is overly concerned with body shape and weight.[3]

## Acne Vulgaris

Acne vulgaris is the classic skin condition of adolescents. Between ages 9 and 20 years, approximately 80% of adolescents will experience varying degrees of acne.[51] It is caused primarily by increased androgen production, which stimulates hair follicles and sebaceous gland structures on the skin of the face, neck, shoulders, and upper chest. It occurs in nearly all boys and 80% of girls.

The pathophysiology of acne vulgaris involves three mechanisms: androgens, obstruction of follicles, and bacteria. During puberty, the secretion of androgen, in addition to its role in the appearance of secondary sex characteristics, leads to increased size of sebaceous glands and increased production of sebum. If sebum is secreted into open follicles, it flows on to the skin and evaporates. In acne vulgaris, the follicles become obstructed. The ducts leading from the glands to the skin may be small and unable to handle the large amount of material produced. This causes the sebum to occlude ducts and dilate glands. Normal skin bacteria colonize sebaceous follicles and free fatty acid is released which irritates surrounding tissue. The whitehead or closed comedo can continue to dilate until it becomes an open comedo (blackhead), or it can rupture below the skin and spread into surrounding tissue. The skin reacts like a localized foreign body responding to the comedo core and to acids from the ruptured comedos. When two or three comedos merge, cysts or nodules form. If bacteria is present, abscesses can form.[48]

Acne vulgaris generally subsides spontaneously by age 20. However, general management includes a balanced diet, good hygiene, adequate sleep and exercise, avoidance of known irritants, and the reduction of emotional tension. Diet restrictions have been found to have little effect on acne vulgaris.

## Accidents and Suicide

Accidents are the leading cause of death in adolescence. Motor vehicle accidents account for the greatest number of accidental deaths and most often are associated with alcohol intoxication. In addition to intoxication, peer pressure, high energy levels, and feelings of immortality contribute to the reckless, risk-taking behavior of adolescents.[16]

Adolescents are also prone to injuries from snowmobiles, minibikes, and motorcycles. Injuries may be sustained from falls, collisions, burns, or even hearing loss. Most deaths from motorcycles result from head injuries, most of which could be prevented by using a safety helmet.[32]

Suicide is the second leading cause of injury and death in adolescents. The frequency of suicide has increased in the past decade, with the greatest increase occurring in 15- to 24-year-olds.[39] Nationally, an average of 13 adolescents successfully commit suicide every day. For each fatality, it is estimated that between 50 and 200 adolescents attempt suicide and survive.[39] Suicidal behavior affects all educational levels and ethnic, socioeconomic, and religious groups.

Adolescent males are more successful with suicide, but more females admit to having difficulty with stress and depression.[41] Males choose more violent means of suicide, such as firearms, hanging, reckless behavior, and use of motor vehicles. Females choose more passive means like prescription and nonprescription drugs, poison ingestion, and cutting the wrists. Impulsive suicide occurs more frequently in this age group than in any other group.

Adolescents at risk for suicidal behavior have vegetative symptoms of depression such as sleep or appetite disturbances, somatic complaints, truancy, substance abuse, sexual promiscuity, or a proneness to accidents.[18] Possible precursors or crisis events have been identified that affect an adolescent's ability to cope with life. Some of the more common events are divorce or separation; death or an extreme change in health of a family member or close friend; break-up of a romantic relationship; pregnancy, abortion, adolescent birth, and the anniversary of these events; poor personal achievement; friendship squabbles; and overachievement expectations.[41]

Advanced warning and talk of suicide usually occur in adolescents contemplating suicide. These warnings should be responded to. However, adolescents frequently distance themselves from help by severing important relationships and not communicating with parents, family, and friends.[18]

## *Substance Use*

Statistics gathered from three National Institute on Drug Abuse surveys (the 1985 National Household Survey, the 1989 National High School Senior Survey, and the Drug Abuse Warning Network—DAWN) indicate a significant decrease in the use of many illicit substances among adolescents. The statistics are reflected in Figures 5-8 and 5-9 and show a tapering off from the peak levels seen in the 1970s and early 1980s. Table 5-12 indicates that a serious substance abuse problem still exists. Before graduation from high school more than 90% of high school seniors have tried alcohol, which is the most popular drug of adolescents. One-third of high school seniors report that most of their friends get drunk at least once a week; 55% have used marijuana; 62% have used other illicit drugs; and 30% use cigarettes.[63]

Substance use is a problem of adolescence, and the etiologic factors are related to the psychosocial development occurring at this age. Any combination of the following may be an incentive for adolescent substance abuse: (1) emotional influences: attempting to increase self-esteem and self-confidence, as an emotional escape, to decrease tension and anxiety, and to assert independence; (2) physical influences: to feel relaxed, block pain, increase sensation, and energy or endurance; (3) social influences: to be accepted in the peer group, overcome shyness or loneliness, or escape problems; (4) intellectual influences: attempting to decrease boredom and mental fatigue, and improving attention span; and (5) environmental influences: the popular acceptance of substance use, the changing role of the family, and the influence of negative role models.[26,28]

Adolescents use and abuse both licit and illicit chemical substances.[59] The used and abused licit and illicit substances found in Table 5-13 indicate types of substances used along with their actions and effects. In the 1989 National High School Senior Survey, a correlation was found between marijuana and cocaine use by seniors and the perceived harmfulness of the use of these drugs. Perceptions of harmfulness in the use of marijuana in-

creased from 1980 to 1989 while reported use of the drug decreased. When perceived harmfulness of cocaine use began to increase in 1987, reported use of cocaine by seniors declined. Although there may be several factors contributing to this phenomenon, efforts to educate children and adolescents to the dangers of drug use seem to be effective.

*ALCOHOL.*    Drunk driving is the leading cause of death among 15- to 24-year-olds. Other facts about alcohol are listed below:

1. Drunk driving accidents account for 25,000 deaths each year. Of these deaths, 5000 are adolescents.
2. Forty to 60% of fatal crashes to young people are alcohol related.
3. Drunk driving accidents cause 130,000 injuries per year to adolescents.
4. Thirty-one percent of high school students are alcohol misusers (drink a minimum of six times per year).
5. Daily use of alcohol occurs in 6% of high school students.
6. The average age to begin drinking is age 13 years.
7. Adolescent females drink almost as much as adolescent males.[32]

*NICOTINE.*    Nicotine is physically and psychologically addicting. Long-term use of this substance contributes to respiratory diseases, cancer, and cardiovascular diseases. The number of adolescents who smoke is increasing while the age at which adolescents begin to smoke is decreasing. The proportion of females who smoke regularly is the same or greater than the proportion of males who smoke regularly.[61]

Smokeless tobacco is a tobacco product that is placed in the mouth and not ignited. Examples of smokeless tobacco are snuff and chewing tobacco. Smokeless tobacco has been found to be carcinogenic. Regular use of these substances cause foul-smelling breath, periodontal disease, erosion, and loss of teeth.[61]

## *Adolescent Sexuality*

There are 21 million adolescents in the United States between the ages of 15 and 19. Eleven million of these are sexually active.[12] By age 17 years, 50% of adolescent females have become sexually active. More than 1.5 million adolescents admit to having four or more sex partners.[12] The average age of the first sexual experience for white males is 14.5 years.[12]

Many physical and psychosocial problems occur as the adolescent begins to physically mature and develop secondary sex characteristics. At this time, the adolescent is physically capable of procreation yet is still emotionally, socially, and intellectually too immature to handle the responsibilities and problems associated with sexual activity. The physical and psychosocial well-being of sexually active adolescents is at risk from two significant threats: STDs and unwanted pregnancy.

## Percentage of High School Seniors Reporting Drug Use in the Past 30 Days, 1975-1989

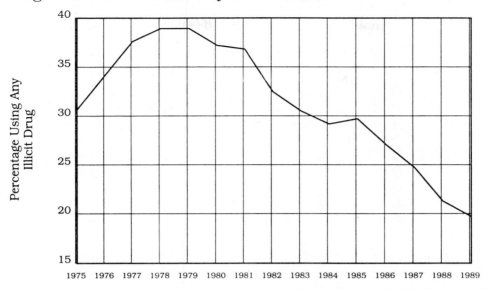

Source: NIDA - High School Student Survey, 1990

**FIGURE 5-8.**

Tapering off of drug use as reported by high school seniors. (Source: National Institute on Drug Abuse, Office of National Drug Control Policy. White Paper. Washington, DC: 1989.)

## Percentage of High School Seniors Reporting Lifetime Cocaine Use, 1975-1989

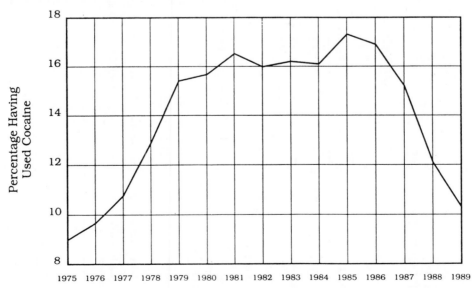

Source: NIDA High School Student Survey, 1990

**FIGURE 5-9.**

Sharp decline in cocaine use since 1987 by high school seniors. (Source: National Institute on Drug Abuse, Office of National Drug Control Policy. White Paper. Washington, DC: 1989.)

**TABLE 5-12.**
CURRENT DRUG USE: 1972–1985

| DRUG | YOUTH: AGE 12–17 | | | | | | | YOUNG ADULTS: AGE 18–25 | | | | | | |
| | '72 | '74 | '76 | '77 | '79 | '82 | '85 | '72 | '74 | '76 | '77 | '79 | '82 | '85 |
| | Percent | | | | | | | Percent | | | | | | |
|---|---|---|---|---|---|---|---|---|---|---|---|---|---|---|
| Marijuana & Hashish | 7.0 | 12.0 | 12.3 | 16.6 | 16.7 | 11.5 | 12.3 | 27.8 | 25.2 | 25.0 | 27.4 | 35.4 | 27.4 | 21.9 |
| Hallucinogens | 1.4 | 1.3 | 0.9 | 1.6 | 2.2 | 1.4 | 1.1 | — | 2.5 | 1.1 | 2.0 | 4.4 | 1.7 | 1.6 |
| Cocaine | 0.6 | 1.0 | 1.0 | 0.8 | 1.4 | 1.6 | 1.8 | — | 3.1 | 2.0 | 3.7 | 9.3 | 6.8 | 7.7 |
| Heroin | — | — | — | — | — | — | — | — | — | — | — | — | — | — |
| Nonmedical Use of: | | | | | | | | | | | | | | |
| Stimulants | — | 1.0 | 1.2 | 1.3 | 1.2 | 2.8 | 1.8 | — | 3.7 | 4.7 | 2.5 | 3.5 | 4.7 | 4.0 |
| Sedatives | — | 1.0 | — | 0.8 | 1.1 | 1.3 | 1.1 | — | 1.6 | 2.3 | 2.8 | 2.8 | 2.6 | 1.7 |
| Tranquilizers | — | 1.0 | 1.1 | 0.7 | 0.6 | 0.9 | 0.8 | — | 1.2 | 2.6 | 2.4 | 2.1 | 1.8 | 1.7 |
| Analgesics | — | — | — | — | 0.6 | 0.7 | 1.9 | — | — | — | — | 1.0 | 1.0 | 2.1 |
| Alcohol | — | 34.0 | 32.4 | 31.2 | 37.2 | 26.9 | 31.5 | — | 68.3 | 68.0 | 70.0 | 75.9 | 87.9 | 71.5 |
| Cigarettes | — | 25.0 | 23.4 | 22.3 | 12.1* | 14.7 | 15.6 | — | 48.8 | 49.4 | 47.3 | 42.6* | 36.5 | 37.2 |

—Not Available
*For 1979, includes only persons who ever smoked at least 5 packs.
**Less than one-half of 1 percent.
Source: National Household Survey on Drug Abuse, 1985, National Institute on Drug Abuse, Division of Epidemiology and Statistical Analysis.

**TABLE 5-13.**

MOST COMMON ADDICTIVE SUBSTANCES USED BY ADOLESCENTS

| CHEMICAL SUBSTANCE | ACTION, EFFECTS |
| --- | --- |
| **Narcotics** | |
| Opium, heroin, morphine, metha-done, Dilaudid, Demerol, codeine, Percodan, Darvon | Decreased blood pressure, dysrhythmias, nausea, vomiting, constipation, cramps, constricted pupils, convulsions, shallow slow breathing, urine retention, thrombosed veins, needle marks, swollen nasal mucosa |
| **Hallucinogens** | |
| LSD (d-Lysergic acid diethylamide), mescaline, psilocybin mushrooms phencyclidine (PCP), marijuana, nutmeg | Elevated blood pressure, flushing, tremors, distortions of perception, hallucinations, euphoria, ataxia, emotional lability, hunger, dry mouth, coughing, elation, relaxation |
| **Depressants** | |
| **Barbiturates** Amytal, Butisol, Luminal, Nembutal, Seconal, Tuinal | Decreased inhibitions, relaxation, slurred speech |
| **Barbiturate-like Substances** Doriden, Noludar, Placidyl, Quaalude, Sopor, alcohol | |
| **Stimulants** | |
| **Amphetamines** Benzedrine, Dexedrine, Diphentamine | Euphoria, anorexia, alertness, elevated blood pressure, increased motor activity |
| **Cocaine** Methylphenidate: Ritalin | |
| **Volatile Substances** | |
| Toluene, hydrocarbons or fluorocarbons, glue, gasoline, cleaning solvents, typing correction fluid, thinners, aerosol sprays | Mental confusion, giddiness, decreased inhibition |

Source: *United States Department of Health, Education and Welfare, National Institute on Drug Abuse, 1980.*

*SEXUALLY TRANSMITTED DISEASES.* Although they make up only 20% of the total United States population, adolescents experience much higher rates for STDs.[61] One in seven adolescents currently has an STD.[7] It is estimated that 25% of the 20 million persons with STDs are high school students.[30] The most common STDs affecting adolescents are *Chlamydia trachomatis, Neisseria gonorrhea,* human papillomavirus (wart virus), and acquired immune deficiency syndrome (AIDS) or HIV infection.

Unique biological, behavioral, and developmental phenomena cause these diseases to be a specific concern of adolescents. The immature cervix of the adolescent undergoes major physiologic changes in the endocervical transformation region. The infectious agents chlamydia, gonorrhea, and papillomavirus invade the columnar cells of the immature cervix. This invasion of the immature cervix contributes to the increased prevalence in adolescents. The immune system is basically untested at this time. Therefore, it does not provide the adolescent

with the localized antibody response from repeated exposure to infectious organisms. The role of cervical mucus in anovulatory menstruation and pelvic infection is poorly understood. The cervical mucus of adolescents is clear and watery due to the estrogen levels. This clear, watery mucus enhances the transport of pathogens to the upper genital tract.[7]

The major modes of HIV infection are unsafe sexual practices and substance abuse. Since both sexual activity and substance abuse are prominent behaviors in the adolescent, AIDS is an enormous risk to adolescents.[12]

In 1989, there were 98,255 diagnosed cases of AIDS in the United States. Of this number, 20,545 affected individuals were ages 20 to 29 years. In most cases, the time frame for developing AIDS is approximately 5 years. It is estimated that 21% of people who were diagnosed with AIDS in their 20s acquired the disease during adolescence.[24] Much public concern exists that future HIV rates in adolescents may far exceed present rates unless unsafe sex practices and drug behaviors are changed.[24] The contribution of homosexual behavior to HIV infection is covered in Chapter 15.

*ADOLESCENT PREGNANCY.* The United States has the highest adolescent pregnancy rate of any developed country in the world.[33] Every day in the United States more than 3200 girls become pregnant. Annually in the United States 11% of the total adolescent population become pregnant. Adolescent girls give birth to 1300 infants each day. Even with these figures, the nation's pregnancy rate stabilized in the 1980s except for those adolescents age 15 years and younger, a statistic which reflected an increase in sexual activity in this young group. Five hundred abortions are performed each day on adolescents. Forty to 50% of adolescents experience repeat pregnancies within 24 months of the initial pregnancy.[35] Fifteen percent of adolescents experience a repeat pregnancy within 12 months. Only one-third of adolescents use birth control consistently. Sixty-two percent of pregnancies result from total lack of use of birth control.[23]

Identification of the causes of adolescent pregnancy has met with limited success. Several interrelated factors contribute to the adolescent birth rates. Socioeconomic factors may play a major role. Adolescents from minority groups and lower socioeconomic groups have an increased risk for pregnancy, often begin sexual activity at an earlier age, and more frequently have illegitimate births than those from the majority and higher socioeconomic groups.[5] Girls from the lower socioeconomic groups usually have lower self-esteem and limited educational achievement.

Absence of family support, especially maternal support, appears to predispose adolescents to increased risk for pregnancy. Many times the adolescent lives in a single-parent home and competes with siblings for parental attention. Often adolescents view pregnancy as the means of providing a change of direction for the future. Negative as this change may be, the adolescent sees the change as a way of escaping a bad home environment, boring home town, or poor school experience, or a way of getting the boyfriend to marry her.

The extent of psychosocial risks to the pregnant adolescent depends on several factors: availability of care, family support, socioeconomic status, and developmental level of the adolescent. Adolescent childbearing results in more negative consequences than positive outcomes for the individual and society. It has been called the "syndrome of failure." Interruption or termination of education is a major contributing factor to the syndrome. Eight of 10 pregnant adolescents less than 17 years of age do not complete high school; four of 10 less than 15 years of age do not complete the eighth grade. Teen fathers are 40% less likely to graduate from high school than nonfathers. The limited education decreases job opportunities, which causes the adolescents to depend on a welfare system or have a marginal existence. The divorce rate is 72% for 14- to 17-year-olds and 46% for 18- to 19-year-olds. Children born to adolescent parents have a much higher incidence of poor school performance and impaired intellectual functioning. Adolescent pregnancy represents a cycle of repetition. Twenty-five percent of adolescent mothers and 50% of adolescent fathers were children of at least one adolescent parent.[55]

Parenting by adolescent mothers is less than optimal because of several maternal factors: insensitivity to infant behavior; harsh, impulsive physical punishment; tendency to spend less than the needed time for play and stimulation with the infant; and lack of knowledge of normal infant and child growth and development. Maternal behavior affects infant development and well-being so that these maternal characteristics are reason for concern. The extent to which the mother adapts to the infant may depend on the degree of maternal self-esteem, her knowledge of growth and development, and educational and developmental status.[45]

Adolescent lifestyle, vulnerability to complications, lack of adequate prenatal care, nutritional deficiencies, and noncompliance with health regimens predispose the pregnant adolescent and fetus to less than optimal pregnancy outcomes. Adolescents receiving adequate prenatal care do not have an increased incidence of physical and medical complications over those of older women. Problems usually arise from poverty and social conditions more than from age.

Adolescents most frequently have preterm labor and delivery and small for gestational age infants, partially due to the socioeconomic status, poor nutrition, lower prepregnancy weight, and delayed prenatal care. Adolescent pregnancy is also associated with PIH. In the general population, PIH occurs in 5% of pregnancies. In the adolescent population, it is estimated to occur in 7% to 34% of pregnancies. Spontaneous abortions occur more frequently in the pregnant adolescent who is age 15 years and younger.[33]

Sexually transmitted diseases, chlamydia, and trichomoniasis, which contribute to preterm birth and infant mortality, are more common in the adolescent. Adolescents who are in the 15- to 19-year group have the second highest rate for gonorrhea. Infections late in pregnancy contribute to chorioamnionitis, postpartum endometritis, and neonatal septicemia.

Pregnant adolescents are at increased risk for anemia. The fetal and adolescent stages of development are the two most rapid growth periods and are associated with the greatest iron requirements. Combining irregular eating habits with rapid growth presents an even greater risk for iron deficiency anemia.

*MENSTRUAL DISORDERS.* Several common problems or concerns associated with the menstrual cycle in adolescence are premenstrual syndrome, dysmenorrhea, and amenorrhea (see Chap. 56).

Premenstrual syndrome (PMS) occurs from 1 to 12

days before the menses. It is a treatable condition with symptoms of nervous tension, irritability, depression, feelings of a bloated abdomen, edema of the fingers and legs, and headaches. The actual cause of PMS is unknown because of its complex nature. PMS affects school performance, causes increased tension and problems in the home, and increases emotional upsets.[32]

Two types of dysmenorrhea occur in adolescents. The most common type is primary dysmenorrhea in which all pelvic organs are normal. In secondary dysmenorrhea, known pathology such as endometriosis or pelvic inflammatory disease exists.

Primary dysmenorrhea is thought to be due to increased prostaglandin production. The increased levels of prostaglandins produce uterine hyperactivity and contractions. In addition to the abdominal discomfort, the person may also experience nausea and vomiting, pallor, and syncope. The abdominal discomfort is usually mild to severe and generally lasts from a few hours up to 2 days.

Diagnosis of dysmenorrhea is based on a thorough history and physical examination. The physical examination should include pelvic exam, Pap smear, and gonorrhea culture.[32]

Two types of amenorrhea occur in the adolescent: primary and secondary. Primary amenorrhea occurs when menarche is delayed past age 17 years. Secondary amenorrhea occurs when one or more menstrual cycles have occurred followed by an absence of menses for 4 or more months.

Primary and secondary amenorrhea may be caused by chromosome or endocrine disorders, or structural abnormalities. Strenuous physical activity such as cross country running and marathon swimming frequently produce amenorrhea. Pregnancy is the most common cause of secondary amenorrhea.

*HOMOSEXUALITY.* Homosexual activity is a widely publicized risk factor for AIDS and the major mode for its transmission during adolescence. Partial responsibility for this transmission is the fact that many heterosexual males admit to engaging in some homosexual activity during adolescence. Approximately 17% to 37% of adolescent males engage in at least one homosexual activity to orgasm.[43] It is estimated that one of 10 individuals is homosexual. Self-recognition of homosexual activity occurs around age 17 years.[24]

It is not known what produces a homosexual orientation. However, there are many theories. Since homosexual activity occurs in most societies, many think there is a biologic basis for the behavior.[47] Other theories suggest a genetic connection and hormonal influences.[47] Review of literature indicates that homosexual males have normal testosterone levels and homosexual females also have testosterone levels consistent with healthy, nonlesbians.[47] Another theory, the psychoanalytic theory, refers to homosexuality as developmental and related to preoedipal and oedipal periods.[47] Social process theory explains homosexual behavior as a learned behavior occurring within an interpersonal setting involving family and peers.[47] Research involving 979 homosexual and 477 heterosexual males and females found that orientation to homosexuality was not statistically associated with ineffective parenting, seduction, or traumatic experiences with the opposite sex, labeling, or any other environmental theory.[46]

Development of homosexual behavior occurs in four stages: sensitization, identity confusion, identity assumption, and commitment.[57]

The stage of sensitization occurs before puberty. During this time, the children do not consider themselves as homosexual but realize that they are different from their peers. Girls stated that they felt different because they felt unfeminine, unattractive, and not interested in boys. Boys stated that they were interested in the arts, not sports, and were often called "sissies."[57]

During identity confusion, the adolescents begin to think that maybe they are homosexual because of their lack of heterosexual interests and their gender-atypical interests. Most homosexual (gay) males have self-realization around age 17 years, and homosexual (lesbian) females around age 18 years. Most adolescents deny their feelings during the stage of identity confusion hoping to "repair" themselves. They assume heterosexual relationships even to the point of pregnancy and try to escape through substance abuse.[57]

During the third stage, the adolescent assumes the homosexual identity and shares it with others. Gay males assume this identity around age 20 years and lesbians around age 21 years.[57]

In the fourth stage, commitment to the homosexual identity is made. Internally, the person has a valid self-identity as gay or lesbian and is satisfied with that identity. Externally this is the stage of "coming out" or disclosing the homosexual identity to society. The time that it takes for disclosure to occur varies because of the homophobia in our society. It is extremely frightening for gay or lesbian adolescents or adults to reveal their sexual identity.[46,57]

## SUMMARY

Adolescence is a time of rapid developmental change. These dramatic changes cause the individual to be physically mature enough to reproduce, but emotionally and socially immature and unable to handle the responsibilities of sexual activity. Unplanned pregnancy and STDs are two major threats to the sexually active adolescent's well-being. The threat of AIDS is particularly significant for this age group. Other alterations and adaptations affecting adolescent growth and development, such as accidents, suicide, acne, and eating disorders, have also been presented. Good hygiene, adequate nutritional requirements, and safe health practices, as well as meaningful education about sexuality are essential to attain and maintain high level physical and emotional well-being during and after the events of puberty.

# REFERENCES

1. Ack, M., et al. When the child is learning disabled. *Patient Care* 16:17, 1982.
2. Akridge, K. Anorexia nervosa. *J. Obstet. Gynecol. Neonatal Nurs.* 18:25, 1989.
3. American Psychiatric Association. *Diagnostic and Statistical Manual of Mental Disorders* (3rd ed.). Washington, D.C.: Author, 1987.
4. Ashburn, S.S. Biophysical development of the toddler and preschooler. In C.A. Schuster and S.S. Ashburn (eds.), *The Process of Human Development: A Holistic Life Span Approach*. Boston: Little, Brown, 1986.
5. Auvenshine, M.A., and Enriquez, M.G. *Comprehensive Maternity Nursing: Perinatal and Women's Health*. Boston: Jones & Bartlett, 1990.
6. Behrman, R.E., and Vaughn, V.C. (eds.). *Nelson Textbook of Pediatrics*. Philadelphia: W.B. Saunders, 1987.
7. Bell, T.A., and Hein, K. Adolescents and sexually transmitted diseases. In K.K. Holmes, P.A. Mardh, P.F. Sparling, and P. Weisner (eds.), *Sexually Transmitted Diseases*. New York: McGraw-Hill, 1984.
8. Binder, F.Z., and Butler, J.E. Children with learning disabilities. *Issues in Comprehensive Pediatric Nursing* 3, 1978.
9. Bloom, A. Acquired immune deficiency syndrome in childhood. *Public Health* 102(2):97, 1988.
10. Bobak, I.M., Jensen, M.D., and Zalar, M.K. *Maternity Nursing and Gynecologic Care: The Nurse and the Family*. St. Louis: Mosby, 1989.
11. Brown, R.C., Sanders, J.M., and Schonberg, S.K. Driving safety and adolescent behavior. *Pediatrics* 77:603, 1986.
12. Davidson, J., and Grant, C. Growing up is hard to do . . . in the AIDS era. *MCN* 13:352, 1988.
13. Dickason, E.J., Schultz, M.E., and Silverman, B.L. *Maternal Infant Nursing Care*. St. Louis: Mosby, 1990.
14. Dietz, W.H. Childhood obesity: Susceptibility, cause and management. *J. Pediatr.* 103:676, 1983.
15. Erikson, E. *Childhood and Society*. New York: W.W. Norton, 1963.
16. Foster, R.L., Hunsberger, M., and Anderson, J. *Family Centered Nursing Care of Children*. Philadelphia: W.B. Saunders, 1989.
17. Garner, D.M. Cognitive therapy for bulimia nervosa. *Adolescent Psychiatry* 13:358, 1986.
18. Gemma, P.B. Coping with suicidal behavior. *MCN* 14:101, 1989.
19. Gibson, L.Y. Bedwetting: A family's recurrent nightmare. *MCN* 14:270, 1989.
20. Halmi, K.A., Falk, J.R., and Schwartz, E. Binge eating and vomiting: A survey of the college population. *Psychol. Med.* 81(11):697, 1981.
21. Henker, B., and Whalen, C.K. Hyperactivity and attention deficits. *Am. Psychol.* 44:216, 1989.
22. Herzog, D.B., and Copeland, P.M. Eating disorders. *N. Engl. J. Med.* 313(5):295, 1985.
23. Holmes, J., and Magiera, L. *Maternity Nursing*. New York: Macmillan, 1987.
24. Janke, J. Dealing with AIDS and the adolescent population. *Nurse Pract.* 14(11):35, 1989.
25. Jones, S.L., Doheny, M.O., Jones, P.K., and Bradley, N. Binge eaters: A comparison of eating patterns of those who admit to binging and those who do not. *J. Adv. Nurs.* 11:545, 1986.
26. Kinney, J., and Leaton, G. *Understanding Alcohol*. St. Louis: Mosby, 1982.
27. Kinsbourne, M., and Caplan, P.J. *Children's Learning and Attention Problems*. Boston: Little, Brown, 1979.
28. Kleber, H.D. Cocaine abuse: Historical, epidemiological, and psychological perspectives. *J. Clin. Psychiatry* 49(2):3, 1988.
29. Knittle, J.L., et al. The growth of adipose tissue in children and adolescents: Cross-sectional studies of adipose cell numbers and size. *J. Clin. Invest.* 63:238, 1979.
30. Kroger, R., and Weisner, P.J. Sexually transmitted disease education: Challenge for the 80s. *J. School Health* 51(4):242, 1981.
31. Marks, A., and Fisher, M. Health assessment and screening during adolescence. *Pediatrics* 80:131, 1987.
32. Marlow, D.R., and Redding, B.A. *Textbook of Pediatric Nursing*. Philadelphia: W.B. Saunders, 1988.
33. May, K.A., and Mahlmeister, L.R. *Comprehensive Maternity Nursing*. New York: J.B. Lippincott, 1990.
34. Mitchell, J.E., Pyle, R.L., and Eckert, E.D. Frequency and duration of binge-eating episodes in patients with bulimia. *Am. J. Psychiatry* 141:835, 1981.
35. Moore, M.M. Recurrent teenage pregnancy: Making it less desirable. *MCN* 14:104, 1989.
36. Muscari, M.E. Effective nursing strategies for adolescents with anorexia nervosa and bulimia nervosa. *Pediatric Nurs.* 14(6):475, 1988.
37. Narins, D.M., Belkengren, R.P., and Sapala, S. Nutrition and the growing athlete. *Pediatric Nurs.* 9:163, 1983.
38. National Research Council. Committee on Dietary Allowances. *Recommended Dietary Allowances*. Washington, D.C.: National Academy of Sciences, 1980.
39. Pfeffer, C.R. *The Suicidal Child*. New York: Guilford Press, 1986.
40. Pyle, R.L., Mitchell, J.E., Echert, E.D., Halvorson, P.A., Newman, P.A., and Goff, G.M. The incidence of bulimia in freshmen college students. *International Journal of Eating Disorders* 2(3):75, 1983.
41. Rankin, W.W. Teenage suicide. *J. Pediatric Nurs.* 4(2):130, 1989.
42. Reeder, S.J., and Martin, L.L. *Maternity Nursing: Family, Newborn, and Women's Health Care*. Philadelphia: J.B. Lippincott, 1987.
43. Remafedi, G.J. Preventing the sexual transmission of AIDS during adolescence. *J. Adolescent Health Care* 9(2):139, 1988.
44. Rothenberg, M.B. In My Opinion . . . Role of Television in Shaping Attitudes of Children. *Child Health Care* 13:148, 1985.
45. Ruff, C. How well do adolescents mother? *MCN* 12:249, 1987.
46. Sanford, N.D. Providing sensitive health to gay and lesbian youth. *Nurse Pract.* 14(5):30, 1989.

47. Savin-Williams, R. Theoretical perspectives accounting for adolescent homosexuality. *J. Adolescent Health Care* 9:95, 1988.

48. Schuster, C.S. Biophysical development of the school-ager and the pubescent. In C.S. Schuster and S.S. Ashburn (eds.), *The Process of Human Development: A Holistic Life Span Approach*. Boston: Little, Brown, 1986.

49. Sherwen, L.N., Scoloveno, M.A., and Weingarten, C.T. *Nursing Care of the Childbearing Family*. Norwalk, Connecticut: Appleton and Lange, 1990.

50. Sprague-McRae, J.M. Encopresis: Developmental, behavioral and physiological considerations for treatment, 1990.

51. Stone, A.C. Facing up to acne. *Pediatric Nurs.* 8:229, 1982.

52. Stroh, S.E., Stern, H.P., and McCarthy, S.G. Fecal incontinence in children: A clinical update. *MCN* 14:252, 1989.

53. Taitz, L.S. Infantile overnutrition among artificially fed infants in the Sheffield region. *Br. Med. J.* 1:315, 1971.

54. Tanner, J.M. *Growth at Adolescence*. Oxford: Blackwell Scientific, 1962.

55. *Teenage Pregnancy: The Problem That Hasn't Gone Away*. New York: Alan Guttmacher Institute, 1980.

56. *The Law and Disabled People*. Washington, D.C.: U.S. Government Printing Office, 1980.

57. Troiden, R.R. Homosexual identity development. *J. Adolescent Health Care* 9:105, 1988.

58. Tucker, L.A. Television, teenagers, and health. *J. Youth Adolescence* 16:415, 1987.

59. United States Department of Health, Education and Welfare. National Institute on Drug Abuse, 1989.

60. Warren, M. Anorexia nervosa and related eating disorders. *Clin. Obstet. Gynecol.* 28(3):588, 1985.

61. Whaley, L.F., and Wong, D.L. Health promotion of the adolescent and family. In L.F. Whaley and D.L. Wong (eds.), *Nursing Care of Infants and Children*. St. Louis: Mosby, 1987.

62. Wilson, M.H. Obesity. In C.W. Hoekelman, *Primary Pediatric Care*. St. Louis: Mosby, 1987.

63. Zarek, D., Hawkins, J.D., and Rogers, P.D. Risk factors for adolescent substance abuse. *Pediatric Clin. N. Am.* 34:481, 1987.

64. Ziai, M., Clarke, T., and Merritt, T. *Assessment of the Newborn: A Guide for the Practitioner*. Boston: Little, Brown, 1984.

## chapter 6

Pam Holder   Barbara R. Norwood
Barbara L. Bullock   Cherry A. Guinn
Margaret L. Trimpey   Martha Butterfield

# Biophysical Developmental Changes of Adults

## Chapter Outline

## Learning Objectives

1. Identify the developmental tasks and conflicts characteristic of each stage of adulthood.
2. Specify physiologic changes that occur during adulthood.
3. Describe the significance of lifestyle patterns during each stage of adult development.
4. Discuss destructive lifestyles and disease processes that are commonly experienced by the adult.
5. Discuss the importance of sleep as a basic human need upon which the physical and emotional health of an individual depends.
6. Describe the physiology of sleep.
7. Explain the major characteristics of each stage of sleep.
8. Discuss the effects of aging on the sleep cycle.
9. Identify common sleep pattern disturbances.
10. Explain why adults are less physically fit today.
11. Discuss the concept of emotions and emotional response.

12. Describe the general adaptation syndrome according to Hans Selye's studies.
13. Explain the chemical and hormonal mediators important in the stress response.
14. Differentiate between the general and local adaptation syndromes.
15. Describe the three physiologic mechanisms that respond to stress stimulation.
16. Describe and give examples of how personalities and attitudes can contribute to the development of disease.
17. Relate diet and stressful living conditions to coronary artery disease.
18. Explain briefly the effects of catecholamines on lipids.
19. Describe the effect of stress on the immune system.
20. Relate stress to the development of stress, duodenal, and gastric ulcers.

*(continued)*

**21.** Identify some effects of stress on skin, musculoskeletal, and respiratory systems.

**22.** Describe the hazards of smoking tobacco.

**23.** Discuss the detrimental effects of substance abuse.

**24.** List signs and symptoms of the most common eating disorders.

**25.** Discuss the relationship of sedentary lifestyles and the development of disease.

Adulthood is usually defined as the years from the early 20s to the mid 60s, which is the largest portion of a person's life span. During this period, human beings are usually their most productive. It is a time of job achievement and recognition, childrearing, and the establishment of values and attitudes that will be transmitted to succeeding generations. Most adults are in relatively good health; however, the prevalence of both chronic disease and fatal illness increases with age. Accidental deaths and suicides/homicides cause a higher percentage of deaths during young adulthood, while illness and disability are more frequently seen in later adulthood.[58] Alterations to health may result from self-destructive lifestyle habits rather than nonpreventable biologic phenomena.[53] This chapter explores adult developmental changes, lifestyle patterns, destructive lifestyles, and some of the disease processes that are commonly experienced by the adult.

## ADULT DEVELOPMENT

The life cycle, or life span begins at birth and ends at death.[71] Chapters 4 and 5 have chronicled the developmental changes through adolescence. Chapter 7 describes changes characteristic of the older adult. Recently, attempts have been made to identify developmental characteristics of the adulthood years. Several theorists have figured prominently in our understanding of developmental changes in the adult. These are described briefly below.

### Developmental Theorists

Recognizing that physical and cognitive growth is mostly completed by adulthood, early developmental theorists described personality and psychosexual growth as if it ended at adolescence. Erikson was the first to suggest that development continued into adulthood. He conceptualized eight stages that encompassed the life span. During each stage, individuals successfully or unsuccessfully resolved specific emotional and social conflicts before moving to the next stage.[15] Figure 6-1 shows the usual developmental tasks, as defined by Erikson, and their approximate placement along the life cycle. The developmental tasks may be resolved in a healthy or unhealthy manner, and the method of resolution is important for later stages of development to proceed smoothly.[58]

Havighurst advanced the theory by organizing information about adult development into tasks each individual needs to accomplish during certain periods of life. Like Erikson, Havighurst related the successful achievement of developmental tasks of one stage to happiness and the potential for success in later stages.[24]

Research by Gould and Levinson has resulted in developmental stages that roughly approximate certain ages. Figure 6-2 shows Levinson's life cycle transitions, especially focusing on those of early and middle adulthood. Vaillant modified Erikson's adult stages, which allows for the agreement about the nature of adult stages that is shown in Figure 6-3.[58]

Each stage of the adult development process contains transitions or turning points that are commonly identified as maturational crises. While maturational crises can be anticipated and prepared for, the individual experiences stress as they occur. The impact of stress depends on the overall coping ability of the person, the intensity of the stressor, and the number of stressors that occur within a particular time frame.[60]

### Young Adulthood

Neurologic development is complete by age 20. The young adult continues to refine and develop intellectual and cognitive processes. The potential for improved judgment and problem solving is influenced by the types of life experiences the individual has. Reaction times to various stimuli usually peak during young adulthood until the late twenties.

For the most part, physical development is also complete. Men may experience some physical growth after adolescence as their bodies reach the peak in muscular strength and reproductive ability. Athletic ability may reach a peak due to muscular strength capability during the 20s.[53] Except for accidents and injury, this is normally the healthiest period of life.

## PHASES OF THE LIFE CYCLE

| | Infancy | Early childhood | Middle and late childhood | Adoles-cence | Young adulthood | Middle adulthood | Late adulthood |
|---|---|---|---|---|---|---|---|
| 1 | Basic trust vs. mistrust | | | | | | |
| 2 | | Autonomy vs. shame, doubt | | | | | |
| 3 | | | Initiative vs. guilt | | | | |
| 4 | | | | Industry vs. inferiority | | | |
| 5 | | | | | Identity vs. role confusion | | |
| 6 | | | | | | Intimacy vs. isolation | |
| 7 | | | | | | | Generativity vs. stagnation |
| 8 | | | | | | | Ego integrity vs. despair |

**FIGURE 6-1.**
Erikson's eight stages of development (From J.W. Santrock, *Adult Development and Aging*. Dubuque, Iowa: W.C. Brown, 1985.)

The early years of this developmental stage are a time of transition from adolescence into adulthood. Young people may seem caught in both worlds as they attempt to consolidate the sense of identity that was developed during adolescence with the independence that comes from completing an education, beginning an occupation, and moving away from parental decision making. This is the time when young people validate the perception they have of their identity as they move through new experiences. Ideally, the earlier years of adulthood are a time to try out differing lifestyles, jobs, and new relationships before settling down. In addition, the young person begins the process of developing a life plan that will help set the course of his or her life.

The early 20s, however, may be a period of prolonged struggle with adolescent identity issues, especially if the person must remain dependent on parents while in school, unemployed, or searching for a job. The transition may be even more difficult if the young person continues to live at home.

A major task of young adulthood is choosing and developing a career. The career decision is so important that most people feel pressure to begin the process in early adolescence and to complete it before the end of their formal education. A choice must be made, despite the fact that young people do not always have a true picture of their abilities or how well they are suited for a particular occupation. Men usually understand the role of work in their lives, while women may have conflict with the choices and responsibilities presented.

A second major task of young adulthood is developing the capacity for an intimate relationship. Intimacy implies a shared identity. For healthy relationships to develop, individuals must feel secure enough in their own identities to not fear losing themselves when they become intimate with another. The inability to form intimate relationships at this period may result in isolation and a diminished ability to deal with stress.

A major developmental task is developing a satisfying sexual pattern. Sexual activity occurs frequently in early

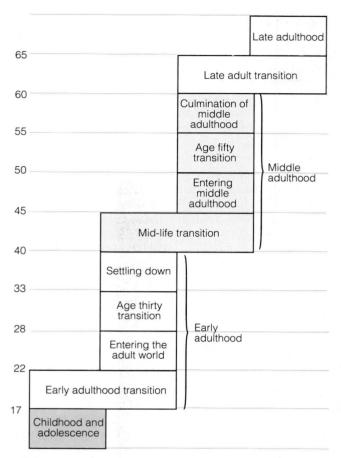

**FIGURE 6-2.**
Development periods in the eras of early and middle adulthood. (From J.W. Santrock, *Adult Development and Aging*, Dubuque, Iowa: W.C. Brown, 1985.)

tion or divorce can result in poor nutrition, inadequate or disturbed sleep, and high levels of stress. Nutrition alterations are described in Chapter 10. Alterations in sleep and the effects of stress are found later in this chapter.

Destructive lifestyles often have their beginning in late adolescence or early adulthood. The effect of these lifestyles may not be apparent until middle or late adulthood. Examples of destructive behaviors are cigarette smoking, excessive alcohol consumption, high fat or cholesterol dietary intake, illegal drug abuse, and risky sexual practices. These behaviors can lead to chronic lung and liver diseases, myocardial infarction, acquired immune deficiency syndrome (AIDS), neurologic dysfunction, and many other conditions. The use of illegal drugs also places individuals at high risk for accidental and homicidal death.

## Adulthood

The stage of adulthood is variously described as the years between age 30 and age 45. While there are no major

adulthood, and there are a variety of options available to young adults.[58] The choice of sexual patterns is individual for each person.

Marriage, childbearing and childrearing are often components during early adulthood. The demands on a couple to adequately perform the work role and successfully balance it with home responsibilities can limit the time and energy necessary to develop their own relationship. They may find themselves in conflict about money, responsibility, and decisionmaking, as well as over traditional or nontraditional values about male-female roles. Children add stress to the marital relationship and to career decisions for both men and women. Some couples postpone having children because of career factors.

The inability of a couple to develop and maintain the relationship itself or to cope effectively with external pressure can lead to separation and divorce. Regardless of the circumstances, divorce is an intensely stressful event. Divorce has been compared to death without either the comfort of formalized mourning or the social supports that accompany the death of a spouse.[19] Separa-

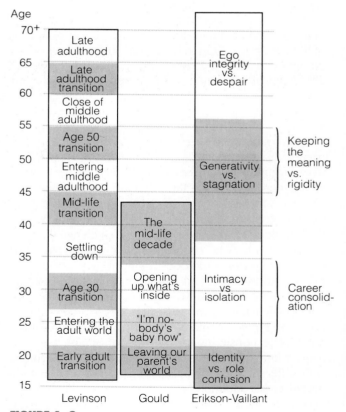

**FIGURE 6-3.**
A comparison of the adult stages of Levinson, Gould, and Erikson-Vaillant. (From J.W. Santrock, *Adult Development and Aging*, Dubuque, Iowa: W.C. Brown, 1985.)

physical changes in adulthood, gradual loss of skin elasticity and a few gray hairs remind the individual that aging is occurring. These changes are a source of stress that are compounded by career pressures and family problems. Good nutrition, proper rest, and physical activity can lessen the effects of aging, but the rate of onset of signs of aging is largely determined by genetic factors.

The adult developmental conflict involves increasing independence and self-reliance (see Figure 6-3). Individuals are expected to be productive, contributing members of society who participate in the maintenance and continuation of social values. The major tasks include career and parenting.

The transition to adulthood, at about age 30 years, may be marked by the conflict between stabilizing or modifying the structure of life. The individual must decide between "settling down" and strengthening relationships and career goals or making changes in the existing life plan before it is too late to do so.[30] Changes, especially in the area of work or relationships, may introduce considerable turmoil without providing guarantees of either success or happiness.

After the transition period, adult men focus on settling down and becoming their own persons.[30] They usually place primary importance on career advancement and productivity. Even though many men take more responsibility for childrearing than did their counterparts in previous generations, the career usually absorbs most of their energies. Women who combine work and family, on the other hand, find that they must divide their energies between the two. Career advancement often becomes more difficult for women than for men.

Whatever the occupation, there will be stress associated with it. Although studies have not found a specific correlation between stress-related disorders and specific occupations, there is definitely stress associated with work.[36] Some jobs are repetitive and monotonous, some are dangerous or physically demanding, and others may occur in a repressive or restrictive environment. Persons experience stress when their jobs make demands beyond their abilities or when work does not challenge them.

For couples who choose to have children, parenting is a major task of adulthood. For those who choose not to have children, other fulfillments must be found. Parenthood provides the couple with the opportunity to transmit personal, family, and societal values to a new generation. Some persons may feel that parenthood creates a sense of responsibility for the lives of others, while for some it limits their freedom to take risks and experiment with different roles or occupations. The traditional expectation that adulthood is the stage of life when women devote themselves exclusively to the task of mothering, raising children, and maintaining a household has been challenged by the events of the past 30 years. Yet neither remaining in the home and being a full time mother nor combining work and parenting is fully or comfortably accepted by all segments of American society. Role conflict invariably is generated for both men and women related to career and parenting responsibilities.

Couples who have divorced may find childrearing complicated by their relationship after the divorce. Both parents may find themselves taking on roles and responsibilities previously handled by the other.[74] Children live with one parent in most cases, with the noncustodial parent fulfilling his or her role intermittently. There may be struggles over money, discipline, privileges, time, and a variety of other concerns. Remarriage adds to the difficulty of raising children after divorce. When one or both of the couple bring children to a new marriage, the task of blending the two families can seem overwhelming.

A significant number of couples want to bear children and find themselves unable to conceive. A period of significant stress begins, and self-concepts change as the couple begins to search for causes of infertility. The infertility workup itself is frustrating, time consuming, and expensive, and in the end treatment is not always successful.

At around age 35 years for women and between ages 40 and 45 years for men, the mid-life crisis is viewed as another transition period. This period serves as a bridge between adulthood and middle age. It is a time when the individual determines if the dreams of early adulthood match the realities of life. The individual begins to recognize the limits to achievement and to the time available to accomplish the plans made in early adulthood. Men worry that the opportunities for advancement are decreasing as younger workers begin to challenge their positions. Women who chose a career as young adults are forced to make a decision about having children before their "biological clock" makes the decision for them. They must also contend with the fact that the risks of complications with pregnancy and childbirth increase with age.

Other issues emerge during the mid-life crisis. People begin to recognize the inevitability of aging and death.[19] Their parents are aging and may become dependent on their children. The "sandwich" generation may be caught between responsibilities for their children and responsibilities for their parents. Decisions must be made about whether to accept and value life as it is or to make changes before middle age.

## Middle Age

Intelligence, memory, and learning do not decrease in the period between ages 45 and 65 years unless there are problems associated with central nervous system (CNS) functioning. There is, nevertheless, a gradual slowing of the functional capacity of all organ systems. Of particular concern is the increase of disease processes, such as cardiovascular disease and cancer.

Sexual relationships change according to physiologic changes. Women experience menopause and men experience a plateau of sexual responsiveness (stable testosterone levels), which leads to slower response and recovery time. Adaptation to these changes maintains the capacity for satisfying sexual relationships.

When individuals effectively resolve the internal confrontation and the need for change generated by the midlife crisis, they are able to adapt to middle age. Middle age can be a period of giving something back to society, of economic productivity, and of preparation for retirement. Without successful resolution, middle-agers may feel a sense of impoverishment, dissatisfaction, and boredom.

As the last child leaves home, parents may feel free to emphasize other interests in life or they may develop feelings of loneliness and depression. How stressful this time is depends on how the couple engaged in childrearing. If childrearing has absorbed the emotional energy of the couple, they will have to restructure the marital relationship to again make it meaningful for them.

There is a tendency for people to become more introspective as they move through middle age. They begin to look at life in relation to the time left, not in terms of the time since birth. Individuals assess their place in time in terms of a "social clock" that tells them if their lives are in step with others of the same age.[43] They then sense if events are occurring too early or too late in life. Men have the chance to experience the feminine (nurturing, creative, expressive) side of their personality. Women may feel able to express the masculine (aggressive, task-oriented, rational) side to theirs. Care should be taken when making generalizations since men and women tend to use different criteria to evaluate middle age.

## PHYSIOLOGIC DEVELOPMENTAL CHANGES DURING ADULTHOOD

Physiologic changes are an ongoing process. Cell death begins even during embryonic development, as does cell renewal. Over the years, there is gradual decrease in cell function and the number of cells. Because of aging, the human passes through stages of immaturity, maturity, and deterioration.[53] Theories regarding the physiologic changes of aging are varied and focus on aging at the cellular level or the wearing out of biologic systems. Cells apparently gradually lose the capacity for self-repair.[53] An in-depth discussion of the theories of aging is found in Chapter 7.

### Biophysical Changes in Young Adulthood and Adulthood

Physical changes of aging have more variations among adults than children. Aging rarely progresses uniformly throughout the bodily systems. Persons of the same age appear to be of different ages.[10]

Gradual physical decline occurs in many systems of the body. The reserve in the systems accounts for continued optimal organ function.

Young adults begin to have a few physical signs of aging. The skin may develop a few wrinkles and loss of elasticity may produce some sagging. Hair changes may include graying or balding depending on the genetic heritage of the individual.

Muscle growth continues until about the age of 39 and muscle loss begins after that. Active muscles, especially those that are routinely exercised, atrophy more slowly than sedentary muscles.

The gradual changes in the sensory system do not interfere with functioning until late adulthood. Visual acuity often declines early in adulthood and minute perceptual changes for the colors of blues, greens, and violets occur.[10] Hearing also declines slowly and often becomes a significant problem late in life. Hearing loss may be accelerated by loud, high-pitched sounds such as those of loud rock music.[51]

Cardiopulmonary changes are insignificant in adulthood unless these systems are weakened by substance or nicotine abuse. There is normally a gradual functional loss especially in the lungs which is accelerated by cigarette smoking. Cocaine abuse has been shown to produce myocardial weakening and coronary artery spasm.[12,42]

The endocrine system is affected by decreased secretion and decreased tissue receptiveness to hormone. The endocrine system affects all bodily activities including metabolism and sexual functioning.

The reproductive system is at peak function in the young adult. This is often the period of reproduction and an active sexual life. The woman's reproductive function declines rapidly after age 30 and this is evidenced by changing menstrual function with cyclic changes.[42]

### Biophysical Changes in Middle Age

The physical changes in the 40s and 50s are also variable but all persons show signs of aging. These signs are expressed throughout all of the body systems.

The integumentary system shows wrinkling due to collagen fiber changes. Over the life cycle, the water content of the body decreases from about 61 to 53 percent while fat content increases from 14 to 30 percent.

The bony skeleton ceases its growth after full height has been reached. Bone mass rapidly declines after the age of 40 (see Chap. 45). Calcium loss becomes pronounced during the menopausal years in women but men also lose calcium at a later age and at a slower rate than do women. Osteoporosis is most common in whites and least common among blacks.[51] The use of calcium, Vitamin D and estrogen supplements may decrease the rate of demineralization of the bone. Studies are supporting estrogen replacement in early menopause to decrease the rate of bone loss. Loss of height is common during the aging process. It may be due to a change in the normal 130 degree angle of the hip-femur joint to an angle of 135 degrees or greater.[42]

Muscle strength and mass are directly related to muscle use. Muscle loss is caused by decreased muscle use. Changes in collagen fibers cause a sagging or drooping of muscles, especially those of the face, breast and abdomen.[10]

Some individuals experience a gradual decline in central nervous system function which may be seen as a decline in mental functioning and mood. Slower reflexes and decreased responsiveness to changes in the environment are common alterations.[42] CNS function is not often impaired (even though brain cell loss is continuous) due to the large reserve of CNS neurons. Middle aged CNS changes are offset by experience and problem solving ability.[51]

Visual changes may become marked after age 40. Presbyopia from loss of elasticity in the lens of the eye causes loss of near vision (see Chap. 49). Hearing and smell loss may become noticeable at around age 50.

Cardiopulmonary changes are very dependent upon lifestyle and genetic factors. Middle aged individuals with high blood pressure, high cholesterol levels and those who smoke are at much higher risk for cardiopulmonary problems than those without these risk factors (see Chap. 25). Maintaining an active lifestyle prevents loss of myocardial tone. Lung tissue becomes thicker, stiffer, and less elastic with age but this process is markedly accelerated by smoking.[42] Repeated respiratory illnesses such as pneumonia, asthma, and bronchitis alter the lung tissue.

Genitourinary problems include stress incontinence or urinary tract infections (UTIs) which are common problems especially with women. Stress incontinence is caused by a decrease in urethral muscle support and decreased sphincter control.[42] Some problems with incontinence can be improved by changing voiding patterns, treating UTIs, or even surgery.

The gastrointestinal tract exhibits a decline in gastric juice secretion so that total daily acid production decreases.[42] Ptyalin in the saliva decreases sharply after age 40.[42,51] Stress and lifestyle changes may affect gastric acid production. Pancreatic enzymes may also gradually decrease from the ages of 20 to 60 years.[51]

The endocrine system usually exhibits no marked changes but it is affected by stress and illness which markedly affect the regulation of blood sugar and electrolyte balance. Middle aged adults have an increased incidence of adult onset diabetes mellitus which is related to familial hereditary factors and obesity.

The reproductive system undergoes the most marked changes in middle life especially in women. During the climacteric period in women the ovaries cease to function and the menstrual cycle ceases either suddenly or erratically. The menopause usually occurs in women at approximately 51 years of age but may occur earlier or later.[10,42] The resultant estrogen deficiency and pituitary influences cause "hot flashes" and other symptoms (see Chap. 56). Symptoms are aggravated by stress and family changes that may be occurring at this time. The male climacteric is a much slower process and is related to decline in testosterone production (see Chap. 55). Male sexual performance declines in middle age and impotence in males over the age of 50 is a common problem.

## LIFESTYLE PATTERNS AFFECTING ADULTS

### Nutrition

A significant proportion of adults in the United States have chronic diseases that are caused by nutritional imbalance. Worldwide, nutritional inadequacies are major determinants of resistance to disease and increased mortality. Nutrition is a major environmental factor in the achievement of longevity, in resistance to disease, and in the tolerance and response to stress (see Chap. 10).

Dietary needs of adults vary according to the amount of energy expended in the course of everyday living. Decreased metabolic needs without decreased intake leads to the development of excess fat, the "middle-age spread." The kinds of foods consumed by many Americans also contribute to the development of excess fat. The most common dietary practice among Americans is the disproportionate intake of dietary fats and cholesterol at the expense of complex carbohydrates and fiber.[35]

Public education is producing an improvement in the American diet. Even fast food restaurants are beginning to provide foods with less fat and cholesterol. Further education is necessary, especially for persons in poverty-stricken circumstances, to prepare low-fat, nutritious meals. The rate of obesity in the United States is very high (see Chap. 10). Excess weight is often accompanied by elevated blood levels of cholesterol and triglycerides. These lipids are involved in producing the lesions of atherosclerosis, which may lead to coronary artery disease. Poor nutrition also can lead to hypertension, diabetes mellitus, gastrointestinal problems, renal dysfunction, and periodontal disease.

### Sleep

Sleep is an essential component in the quality of life for all people. The amount of sleep needed varies among different individuals. Sleep is a basic human need upon which the physical and emotional health of an individual depends.

## Functions of Sleep

The function of sleep is primarily to allow the body to restore itself and prepare for the next day. The heart and respiratory rate decrease during sleep, thus preserving respiratory and cardiac function. During sleep the body conserves energy by lowering the basal metabolic rate (BMR). Epithelial and specialized cells are also repaired and revitalized during sleep. Although the function of dreaming is unknown, some researchers believe that memory and problem solving relate to these nightly adventures.[57]

Several factors can alter the quantity and quality of an individual's sleep. These factors have been identified as physical illness, sleep schedule variations, stress (emotional), exercise and fatigue, weight loss/gain patterns, environmental factors, a person's lifestyle, and various drugs and substances.[57] These factors impact people's sleep patterns in various ways throughout their lifetime.

## Sleep Patterns

The pattern of an individual's sleep can be identified in a sleep lab. A sleep laboratory is set up (usually in a hospital or clinic) to resemble a bedroom with an "at home" atmosphere. The individual is attached to several leads. The electroencephalogram (EEG), which measures brain activity, the electrocardiogram (ECG), which measures electrical impulses of the heart, the electromyogram (EMG), which measures muscle tone, and the electrooculogram (EOG), which measures eye movement, are essential instruments to provide information and documentation on the physiology of sleep. In addition to this information, the individual's oxygen concentration and blood pressure are also monitored.

While the subject sleeps, the technician records sleep activity observed or heard through a microphone and video camera. A comprehensive graph of the subject's vital functions, brain waves, eye movements, and muscle activity are recorded during this sleep time. Typical measures obtained include total sleep and awake time, rapid eye movement (REM), and various sleep stages.

## Physiology of Sleep

Sleep and wakefulness physiology is a very complex phenomenon associated with many neurochemical transmitters and various areas of the brain. The coordinating mechanisms either activate or suppress the center in the brain that controls sleep. The reticular activating system (RAS) located in the upper brainstem area contains certain cells that maintain a person's state of being awake and alert. The catecholamine-releasing neurons that release dopamine may be the cause of wakefulness.[5,9] Other observations have suggested that cholinergic synapses (acetylcholine producing) facilitate wakefulness and REM sleep.[57] The spontaneous activity in the RAS excites the cerebral cortex and the peripheral nervous system. The feedback from these areas to the RAS tends to sustain the wakefulness state.[21] It is thought that the neurons in the RAS fatigue and are susceptible to inhibition by sleep-producing chemicals.[21]

Sleep may be the result of the release of serotonin or other mediators from special cells in the ralphe nuclei of the pons and medulla. Serotonin may play a role in synthesis of a hypnogenic factor that directly causes sleep. Serotonin levels are actually high in the waking state and become lower in slow-wave and REM sleep.[57]

Sleep is composed of a set of physiologic processes involving a sequence of states within the CNS.[25] Each sequence can be readily identified with an EEG, EMG, and EOG by the various levels of activity that are measured. Two distinct phases of sleep have been identified by these instruments. They are REM, active sleep, and non-REM, quiet sleep.

As the individual falls asleep, he or she enters non-REM sleep, which is characterized by four progressive stages. Non-REM sleep is recognized by snoring, slow regular respiration, absence of body movement, and slow regular brain activity. Each stage of non-REM sleep is progressively deeper. At the end of Stage IV, individuals enter Stage III, then Stage II, then finally they enter into REM sleep (Table 6-1).

REM, or active sleep, is characterized by irregular respirations, absence of snoring, rapid eye movement, and twitching of the face and fingers. It usually takes about 90 minutes for an individual to reach REM sleep. Each person is different, but a typical night's sleep consists of four to six sleep cycles beginning with Stage I and progressing through REM sleep (Figure 6-4).

## Effects of Aging on Sleep Cycle

The characteristics of sleep-waking cycles and the percentage of time spent in the various stages of sleep change over the life cycle.[57] Infants apparently have the highest amount of REM sleep, while young adults (20 to 40 years of age) spend 50% of their sleep time in Stage II, 25% in REM, 10% in Stage III, 10% in Stage IV, and 5% in Stage I.[39]

Total sleep time and the total nightly amounts of sleep are age-dependent, and generally sleep time is greatest in infancy and gradually decreases in childhood. The total sleep time stabilizes in adulthood until it starts

**TABLE 6–1.**
PHASES OF SLEEP

**NonREM Sleep**

| | |
|---|---|
| Stage 1 | Lightest level of sleep<br>Lasts a few minutes<br>Decreased physiologic activity begins with gradual fall in vital signs and metabolism<br>Person easily aroused by sensory stimuli, such as noise<br>If person awakens, feels as though daydreaming |
| Stage 2 | Period of sound sleep<br>Relaxation progresses<br>Arousal is still easy<br>Lasts 10–20 min<br>Body functions continue to slow down |
| Stage 3 | Initial stages of deep sleep<br>Sleeper is difficult to arouse and rarely moves<br>Muscles completely relaxed<br>Vital signs decline but remain regular<br>Lasts 15–30 min |
| Stage 4 | Deepest stage of sleep<br>Very difficult to arouse sleeper<br>If sleep loss has occurred, sleeper will spend considerable portion of night in this stage<br>Stage responsible for restoring and resting the body<br>Vital signs significantly lower than during waking hours<br>Lasts approximately 15–30 min<br>Sleepwalking and enuresis may occur |
| **REM Sleep** | Stage of vivid, full-color dreaming (less vivid dreaming may occur in other stages)<br>Usually begins every 50–90 min after sleep has begun<br>Typified by automatic response of rapidly moving eyes, fluctuating heart and respiratory rates, and blood pressure<br>Loss of skeletal muscle tone<br>Responsible for mental restoration<br>Sleeper most difficult to arouse<br>Duration of REM sleep increased with each cycle and averages 20 min |

Source: P. Potter and A. Perry, Fundamentals of Nursing Concepts, Process and Practice. *St. Louis: Mosby, 1989.*

to decrease with old age (Figure 6-5). In addition, the number of awakenings that occur during sleep tends to increase after age 40 years. Most of these awakenings occur during REM sleep.[39] Figure 6-6 illustrates a typical pattern of sleep in an elderly person.

*Sleep Pattern Disturbances*

Sleep pattern disturbances most often fall into four basic groups: (1) disorders of initiating and maintaining sleep; (2) disorders of excessive somnolence; (3) disorders of

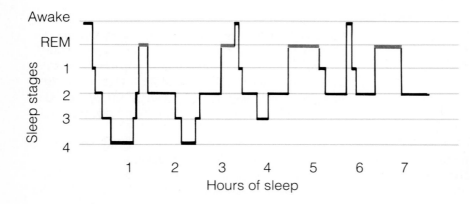

**FIGURE 6–4.**
The course of a typical night's sleep in a young adult. (From Kales and Kales, 1970.) (Source: M.R. Rosenzweig and A.L. Leiman, *Physiological Psychology* [2nd ed.] New York: Random House, 1989.)

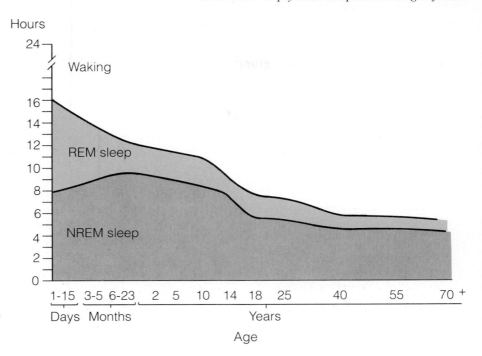

**FIGURE 6–5.**

Changes in sleep with age in humans. (From Roftwang, Muzio, and Dement, 1966.) (Source: M.R. Rosenzweig and A.L. Leiman, *Physiological Psychology* [2nd ed.]. New York: Random House, 1989.)

sleeping-waking schedule; and (4) dysfunctions associated with sleep, sleep stages, or partial arousals (Box 6–1). Individuals may suffer with one or more types of disturbances that can be either acute or chronic. Acute episodes are not usually a problem due to their short duration. However, chronic disturbances usually require intervention.

*DISORDERS OF INITIATING AND MAINTAINING SLEEP.* This problem can be caused by any number of factors, both internal and external. Several aspects of an individual's sleep environment can alter sleep patterns. Examples of these aspects are noise, uncomfortable beds, and sick children. Internal factors such as stress, pain, and ingested chemicals can alter sleep patterns.

Insomnia is a common term used to refer to sleep pattern disturbances. It is a subjective feeling in which individuals do not perceive themselves as getting enough sleep. Insomnia with chronic difficulty falling asleep or going back to sleep may indicate an underlying or psychologic disorder. The prevalence of insomnia ranges from about 15% of adults in Scotland to about 33% of adults in Los Angeles.[57]

*DISORDERS OF EXCESSIVE SOMNOLENCE.* Excessive daytime sleepiness may indicate either sleep apnea or narcolepsy. Sleep apnea may result from obstruction of the airway or changes in the pacemaker respiratory neurons in the brainstem.[57] Obstructive apnea occurs with progressive relaxation of the muscles of the chest, diaphragm, and throat, causing airway obstruction for as long as 30 seconds.[17,57] The individual still attempts to breathe as the chest and abdomen continue to move. Each breath gets stronger until the obstruction is relieved. Obstructive apnea most frequently occurs in the morbidly obese individual. Defects in the brain's respi-

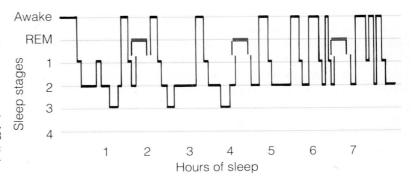

**FIGURE 6–6.**

The customary pattern of sleep in an elderly person. This record is characterized by frequent awakenings, absence of stage 4 sleep and a reduction of stage 3 sleep. (Adapted from Kales and Kales, 1974.) (Source: M.R. Rosenzweig and A.L. Leiman, *Physiological Psychology* [2nd ed.]. New York: Random House, 1989.)

## BOX 6-1.
## A CLASSIFICATION OF SLEEP DISORDERS

1. Disorders of initiating and maintaining sleep (insomnia)
   Ordinary, uncomplicated insomnia
     Transient
     Persistent
   Drug-related
     Use of stimulants
     Withdrawal of depressants
     Chronic alcoholism
   Associated with psychiatric disorders
   Associated with sleep-induced respiratory impairment
     Sleep apnea
2. Disorders of excessive somnolence
   Narcolepsy
   Associated with psychiatric problems
   Associated with psychiatric disorders
   Drug-related
   Associated with sleep-induced respiratory impairment
3. Disorders of sleep-waking schedule
   Transient
     Time zone change by airplane flight
     Work shift, especially night work
   Persistent
     Irregular rhythm
4. Dysfunctions associated with sleep, sleep stages, or partial arousals
   Sleepwalking (somnambulism)
   Sleep enuresis (bed-wetting)
   Sleep terror
   Nightmares
   Sleep-related seizures
   Teeth grinding
   Sleep-related activation of cardiac and gastrointestinal symptoms

Source: M.R. Rosenzweig and A.L. Leiman, Physiological Psychology (2nd ed.). New York: Random House, 1989.

ratory center that paces respiration are involved in central apnea. The impulse to breathe temporarily fails and air flow and chest wall movement cease. Central apnea may be the cause of crib death (SIDS) in infants due to immaturity of the respiratory neurons. It may be associated with head injury or brain tumors or lesions.

Narcolepsy is a condition in which the individual complains of excessive daytime sleepiness. There is also an abnormality in REM sleep.[57] During the day, the individual may suddenly fall asleep and REM sleep can occur within 15 minutes. Sleep attacks can occur at any time and may be due to brainstem dysfunction that involves failure of a waking mechanism to suppress the brainstem centers controlling REM sleep.

Depressive disorders cause a variety of sleep disorders, from difficulty falling asleep to extended sleep periods. Analysis of sleep character shows a marked decrease in Stage III and IV sleep, with increase in Stages I and II and frequent, vigorous REM sleep. A major avenue of study is the neurotransmitter imbalance seen in a high percentage of depressed persons. Measures of sleep are being used as a prognostic tool in the treatment of depression.[57]

*DISORDERS OF SLEEP-WAKING CYCLES.* When people work the evening or night shift or travel by air across numerous time zones, the sleep-waking cycles are disrupted. Irregular patterns characterize the sleep, and frequently their sleep cycles are shortened.

*DYSFUNCTIONS ASSOCIATED WITH SLEEP, SLEEP STAGES, OR PARTIAL AROUSALS.* Sleepwalking (somnambulism), night terrors, and bedwetting are common sleep disorders. These are occasional problems in adults and seem to occur mainly in Stage III and IV sleep. Certain illnesses such as peptic ulcer disease and cardiovascular disease seem to be aggravated during the normal intense REM sleep periods.[57] In one study, 32 of 39 episodes of chest pain in cardiovascular patients occurred during REM episodes.[27]

## Physical Fitness

Between the ages of 20 to 40 years, the adult begins to view life more seriously and advancement becomes a predominant task. Major life goals are established. A positive self-image, including body image, is very important. Body image goals for most Americans are for physical beauty and fitness. However, the minority of men and women are physically fit. The reasons for this disparity include inconvenience, discouragement, fear of death, and approach-avoidance behavior.[28] Approach-avoidance behavior is manifested when the person who initially takes part in a fitness program begins to see the program requiring more exertion and effort and then drops out of the program. He or she becomes torn between the need and desire for fitness and the tendency to avoid such behavior. Other reasons for not attaining physical fitness include social constraints and commitments, limited convenient access to facilities, loss of interest, declining physical ability, and breakdown of social contacts and networks.[46]

Primitive man's survival depended to a great extent on his physical prowess or efforts. Today, most persons survive through the use of intellect rather than physical abilities. In a highly technological society, there is little reason for many persons to move very much. Machines do much of the work that used to require great physical effort. Major modes of transportation have changed from walking or horseback riding, which requires much physical activity, to driving a car, which requires minimal hand and foot movements. Leisure time activities have changed from participation to observation. Thus, it has become virtually impossible to maintain fitness through activities of daily living.

Individuals in the adulthood age group tend to exercise sporadically. This can lead to detrimental effects of the exercise since the body is put under stress for which the cardiovascular system is not conditioned. Sporadic exercising can lead to angina or even to myocardial infarction. The ideal physical fitness program must be tailored to the individual, increased gradually, and performed regularly over time to prevent unwanted effects.

Recent efforts have been made to overcome one of the often cited reasons for lack of participation in a physical fitness program, that of inconvenience. Businesses have begun to provide facilities in the work place for physical fitness, some of which are extended to retirees. Other programs are being offered in neighborhood settings instead of in centrally located health care facilities.

Adults between ages 40 and 65 years begin to look at life in terms of the amount of time remaining rather than the amount of time lived since birth. Emphasis is focused on self-development, reexamination, and reevaluation. Physical changes become more dramatic, with the most common being weight gain. These changes may result in increasing stress and frustration. Selye reported research that supported regular exercise as a means to resist stress.[60] Successful aging, which can be defined as free of pathology and long-lived, occurs when a person is moderately physically active, a nonsmoker, has a positive outlook on life, and maintains a functional role in society.[47]

There are many advantages to remaining physically fit. The benefits of exercise include improved cardiovascular health, improved flexibility, improved skeletal and muscle strength, increased endurance, and increased respiratory capacity.[36] In addition, increased mobility, physical and psychological stimulation, and relaxation increase the benefits of physical activity. Many studies indicate that sedentary living habits and cigarette smoking are contributing factors to the development of atherosclerosis.[40] A positive relationship between exercise levels and lipoproteins has been identified, and it has been hypothesized that triglyceride levels can be reduced with regular, vigorous, physical activity. Medical research supports the therapeutic benefits of exercise, including its effect on rehabilitation of patients with coronary heart disease. Exercise reconditions heart and skeletal muscles, decreases heart rate and blood pressure, and thus decreases cardiac workload. There is evidence to suggest that exercise may retard age-related declines in neuromuscular efficiency and psychomotor speed.[65]

Lack of activity leads to increases in illness and costs society billions of dollars for health care services. Research suggests that atrophy secondary to inactivity may be responsible for approximately 50% of physical decline in the elderly.[63] Physical activity may not increase the quantity of life, but rather may increase the quality of life for the adult.[37] Even the ancient Greek physician Hippocrates realized the benefits of physical activity when he suggested that if one exercises one will become "healthy,

well-developed and age slowly"; and if one does not exercise, one will become "liable to disease, defective in growth, and age quickly."[46]

## Stress

As previously discussed, adults experience certain amounts of stress during each stage of the development process. *Stress* has been defined as the nonspecific response of the body to any demand placed upon it.[59] Stress-producing factors are called *stressors*; these may be physiological, psychological, or both. Reactions to stressors may be adaptive or maladaptive. The stressors may be pleasant or unpleasant, and may evoke many different emotional or psychologic responses while eliciting the similar physiologic reactions. Closely associated with stress is the concept of *emotions*. This concept includes a wide range of behaviors, expressed feelings, and changes in body states.[57] The literature is conflicting between the concepts of stress and emotions. Basically, stress can be viewed as the physiologic response aspects of emotion, while emotion, itself, can encompass the reported feelings and response to the stressor. Stressors may be the actual physical threats or perceived threats. They also may be the emotional side of joys or sorrows that elicit a physiologic response.

## Theories of Emotion

Several theories have attempted to explain the relationship between emotions and visceral activity. Three prominent theories are the James-Lange theory, the Cannon-Bard theory, and Schachter's cognitive theory. These are briefly described below, and the reader is referred to the bibliography for further reading.

The first theory of emotions, the James-Lange theory, suggests that strong emotions and skeletal muscle/autonomic nervous system activation are inseparable factors. An example of this is fear, which is a reaction to stimuli, and the results are noted as an emotion.[57] This theory emphasizes peripheral physiologic events in emotions.

The Cannon-Bard theory focuses on the brain and emotion with cerebral integration of emotional experience (stressor) and emotional response (stress). This theory emphasizes that some emotions are an emergency response of the sympathetic nervous system (SNS) to a sudden threatening condition.[57] These emotions provoke a nonspecific response of increased heart rate, glucose mobilization, and other SNS responses.[60]

Schachter's cognitive theory suggests that individuals interpret visceral activation in terms of the specific stimulus, the surrounding situation, and their cognitive states.[57] This allows for differences among individuals that are molded by experience. Therefore, an emotional state results from the interaction of physiologic stimulation, activation, and interpretation.[57]

As studies proceed in linking emotion to physiologic responses, it has been discovered that even when the physiologic receptors are blocked, the emotional response to a stimulus is not reduced. Other studies have demonstrated a specific pattern of autonomic arousal for each different emotion.[57] The study of emotional responses is in its infancy, but the relationship of stimulus to physiologic response is intriguing.

The ability to cope successfully with emotions directly affects the health status of the adult. Many health problems are related to inability to handle the stresses of everyday living. Because stress is the greatest threat to health during adulthood, it is important to understand the body's response to stress. A review of systems theory is presented as a basis for explaining the physiologic reaction.

### Systems Theory

Systems theory is a model for organizing and examining relationships among units. It describes closed systems as those that do not interact or exchange energy with their environments. The sciences of physics and physical chemistry are limited to the examination of closed systems. Conversely, open systems do exchange matter, energy, and information with their environments.[73] A relative state of balance, or dynamic equilibrium, called the steady state is achieved. Man, as an open, physiologic organism, uses relationships among his component parts to achieve a state of equilibrium, or *steady state*. The steady state exists when the composition of the system is constant despite continuous exchange of components of the system. The three fundamental qualities of open systems are structure, process, and function. *Structure* refers to the arrangement of all defined elements at a given time. *Process* is the transformation of matter, energy, and information between the system and the environment. *Function* relates to the unique manner that each open system uses to achieve its required end.[41]

A feedback scheme is used to describe the fundamental qualities of open systems. In the human, this means that if a factor becomes excessive or inadequate in the body, alterations in function will be initiated to decrease or increase that factor in an attempt to bring it into normal range. The processes used in this scheme include input, throughput, output, and feedback.

*Input* is the energy, matter, or information absorbed by the system. *Throughput* is the transformation of this energy into useful information, matter, or energy that is used by the system. The excess information, matter, or energy is discharged to the environment in a process called *output*.

*Feedback*, an essential component, is the process of self-regulation by which open systems determine and control the amount of input and output of the system. The two types of feedback are called *negative* and *positive feedback*. Negative feedback refers to a process of returning to the steady state, while positive feedback indicates movement away from the steady state.[41] In the human body, negative feedback indicates a return to the balanced steady state. Positive feedback, unchecked, will produce illness and finally, death. In the human organism, negative feedback can be readily illustrated by many functions. Figure 6-7 illustrates the feedback system used to maintain the balance of thyroid hormones. Loss of hormonal control, for example, causes disease states because the body's response becomes detrimental to the maintenance of the steady state.

In considering the open systems theory, one must enlarge the perspective beyond the physiologic and pathophysiologic bases. The individual, as a system, has physiologic, psychosocial, environmental, and other stressors (Figure 6-8). These stressors may unite to produce adaptive coping responses, or they may result in physical changes that are pathophysiologic.

### Effects of Stress

The study of the effects of stress on the human body was pioneered by Hans Selye.[60] He studied the nonspecific response of the body to a demand and noted differences in individual abilities to withstand the same demands. He defined *stress* as a specific syndrome that is nonspecifically induced. He also defined *stressors* as tension-producing stimuli that potentially could cause disequilibrium.[56] The perception of the significance of the stressor is important and varies among individuals. It is believed that psychologic stressors have as great an impact on dis-

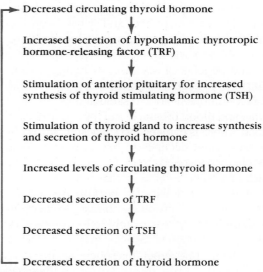

**FIGURE 6-7.**
Feedback system illustrating functions that keep the circulating thyroid hormone in balance.

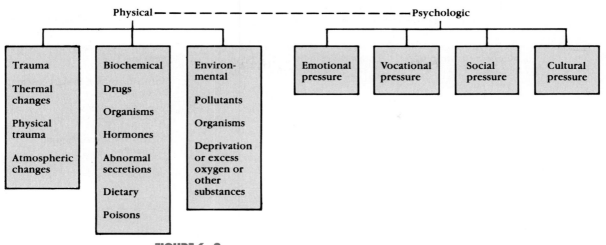

**FIGURE 6-8.**
Stressors, types of stimuli that can provoke the stress response.

ease states as physical stressors. Selye noted that laboratory animals reacted physiologically to different stressors by enlargement of the adrenal cortex, atrophy of the thymus gland, and development of gastric ulcers. Further study revealed a pattern including fatigue, loss of appetite, joint pains, gastric upset, and other similar nonspecific complaints.

Selye noted a similarity in sickness patterns, which initially he called "the syndrome of just being sick," then later described as the *general adaptation syndrome* (GAS).[60] The GAS may be elicited by a variety of stimuli or stressors and may be of a physiologic, psychogenic, sociocultural, or environmental nature. GAS is described in the following three stages: (1) alarm reaction, (2) stage of resistance, and (3) stage of exhaustion (Figure 6-9).

In the *alarm stage*, the defensive abilities of the body are mobilized. The hypothalamus is activated, releasing corticotropin-releasing factor (CRF). CRF stimulates the adenohypophysis to release adrenocorticotropic hormone (ACTH). Glucocorticoids are then released. The so-called *fight-or-flight* mechanism is activated mainly through the SNS, which releases two catecholamines, *norepinephrine* and *epinephrine*. The physiologic action of these hormones causes vasodilation in the heart and skeletal muscles. These hormones also cause vasoconstriction (in the skin, viscera, and kidneys), increased blood pressure, and increased rate and force of cardiac contractions. All of these physiologic actions prepare the body for an assault.

In the *stage of resistance*, levels of corticosteroids, thyroid hormones, glucagon, and aldosterone are increased (see Figure 6-9). The adrenal cortex enlarges and becomes hyperactive. A hypermetabolic state exists, increasing blood sugar for available energy and stabilizing the inflammatory response. The immune system becomes depressed. There is depression of T cells and B cells, and atrophy of the thymus gland, which leads to a

depression of primary antigen-antibody response, probably due to the effect of excess ACTH. The end result, immunologically, is suppression and atrophy of immune tissue (see Chap. 15). If infection is present, this suppression causes delayed clearing of the organisms and delayed healing.

If stage 3, *exhaustion*, occurs, resistance to the stressor is depleted and death ultimately occurs (see Figure 6-9). Exhaustion is frequently caused by the lack of immunologic defense and is considered to be an immunodeficiency secondary to stress. Selye proposed that exhaustion is a correct term for aging, a wearing down of the human body from lifelong stress.[60] This conclusion is not totally supported in much of the recent literature (see Chap. 7).

Individuals differ in what produces stress and in their reactions to stressors. The response to the same stressor can also vary from one day to the next. Localized reaction to stressors is called the *local adaptation syndrome* (LAS), which is well illustrated by the process of inflammation. The usual outcome of inflammation is localization and destruction of the foreign substance that triggered the process.[54] The LAS assumes the same general pattern as the GAS, with an acute phase followed by a resistance phase and exhaustion. Exhaustion of the LAS causes breakdown of the localizing mechanisms and spreading of the process, and ultimately leads to the generalized response and GAS.

## Adaptation

Adaptation is defined as adjustment of an organism to a changing environment. It refers to adjustments that are made as a result of stimulation or change, with the end result of modifying the original situation. An adaptive response is a type of negative feedback that maintains the organism in the steady state. Physiologic adaptation refers

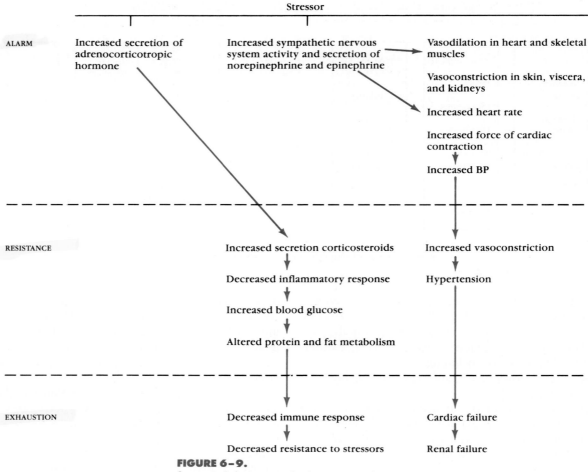

Stressor

ALARM

Increased secretion of adrenocorticotropic hormone

Increased sympathetic nervous system activity and secretion of norepinephrine and epinephrine

Vasodilation in heart and skeletal muscles

Vasoconstriction in skin, viscera, and kidneys

Increased heart rate

Increased force of cardiac contraction

Increased BP

RESISTANCE

Increased secretion corticosteroids

Decreased inflammatory response

Increased blood glucose

Altered protein and fat metabolism

Increased vasoconstriction

Hypertension

EXHAUSTION

Decreased immune response

Decreased resistance to stressors

Cardiac failure

Renal failure

**FIGURE 6-9.**

Stages in Selye's general adaptation syndrome.

to the adjustments made by the organs and systems to stress or physiologic disruption. This response is often called *compensation* for abnormal stimuli. *Maladaptation* is disruptive. It moves toward positive feedback, a disordering of the physiologic response. This positive feedback can be considered a vicious cycle—if not interrupted, it can become disruptive to the individual.

Physiologic responses to stress stimuli (stressors) fall into three separate and interactive mechanisms: neurologic, endocrine, and immunologic. These mechanisms may promote adaptation to the stressor. Long-term application of stressors ultimately causes end-organ dysfunction through these same mechanisms.[2]

*NEUROLOGIC MECHANISMS.* Both the voluntary and autonomic divisions of the nervous system are reactive to stress. The voluntary system is mediated through the cerebral cortex, which is responsive to the stress stimulus. The cerebral cortex directs the muscles to move to avoid danger and effects the flight response. The combination of vasodilation in the skeletal muscle and the voluntary flight response are sometimes termed the *musculoskeletal response* to a stressor.

The autonomic nervous system (ANS) is involuntary and is regulated through the hypothalamus. In the stress response, stimulation of the SNS occurs. Two hormones, epinephrine and norepinephrine, which are classified as *catecholamines*, are important factors in the stress response. Both are synthesized in the adrenal medulla and released when the SNS is activated. Norepinephrine is also synthesized and secreted at adrenergic (sympathetic) nerve terminals throughout the body, and is directly released when the SNS is stimulated. Epinephrine is excreted rapidly in the urine after being biotransformed in the liver. Norepinephrine, liberated at the axon ending, is actively taken up, restored, or biotransformed.

The primary action of epinephrine is to increase the rate and force of cardiac contraction. It is secreted as part of the stress response from the SNS stimulation of the adrenal medulla. It is interesting to note that epinephrine is a potent stimulus for glycogenolysis in the liver, which leads to an increased blood glucose level.[21] In addition to accelerating the degradation of glycogen, epinephrine diverts blood from the viscera to the skeletal muscles.

Norepinephrine is secreted in small quantities in the

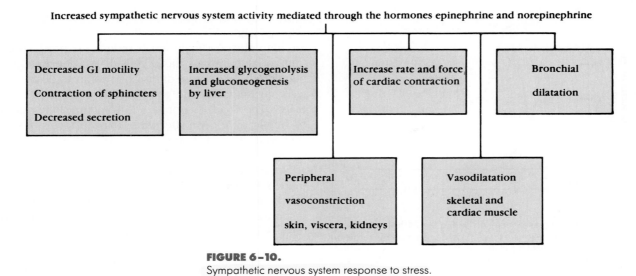

**FIGURE 6-10.**
Sympathetic nervous system response to stress.

flight-or-fight response and in acute physical or mental stress. Studies have shown a constant increase in norepinephrine levels in individuals under chronic, unremitting stress. Norepinephrine exerts its primary control over the arterioles, leading to intense vasoconstriction and increased peripheral vascular resistance (PVR), causing increased blood pressure and increased cardiac workload (Figure 6-10).[13] The vasoconstriction to the gut and reduced blood flow to the gastric mucosa is implicated in the development of stress ulcers.

Besides the above effects, epinephrine and norepinephrine are responsible for bronchial dilation, increased respiratory rate, inhibition of the gastrointestinal tract, and pupillary dilation. These hormones may be significant in the development of hyperlipidemia and of stress-induced cardiovascular disease.

*ENDOCRINE MECHANISMS.* The endocrine hormones are increased in the stress response through hypothalamic stimulation of the pituitary, leading to stimulation of target organ secretion. This relationship is illustrated in Figure 6-11. Stimulation of the pituitary can increase secretion of ACTH, antidiuretic hormone (ADH), thyroid-stimulating hormone (TSH), and others. Secretion of aldosterone is also increased from the adrenal cortex.

The target organs of ACTH are the adrenal glands. Stimulation from this hormone causes an increased synthesis of the glucocorticoids, especially cortisol, cortisone, and small amounts of hydrocortisone. These substances increase serum glucose and alter the metabolism of carbohydrates, fat, and protein. Gluconeogenesis, glycogenolysis, protein catabolism, and lipolysis are increased. The result is more available fuel for energy.

In individuals with a day-wake/night-sleep cycle, the glucocorticoids are thought to be synchronized by light.

Their concentration in blood and urine decreases during sleep and rises to its highest levels in the early morning.[21] This pattern of glucocorticoid secretion follows a particular rhythm called the *circadian rhythm* or *pattern.* The early morning high level drops about 10 AM, increases slightly again about 2 PM, and gradually declines until 10 PM (Figure 6-12). Changes in circadian rhythm may relate to illness in that phase relationships seem to be

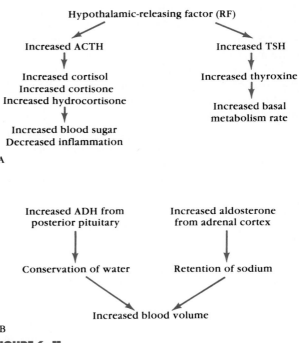

**FIGURE 6-11.**
**A.** Effects of stress on hypothalamic-pituitary-target organ axis.
**B.** Related hormonal effects of stress, possibly due to sympathetic stimulation.

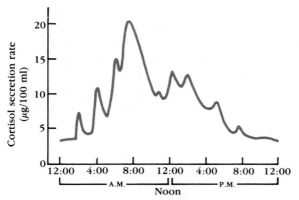

**FIGURE 6-12.**

A typical pattern of cortisol secretion during the 24-hour day. Note the oscillations in secretions as well as a daily secretory surge an hour or so after awakening in the morning. (From A.C. Guyton, *Textbook of Medical Physiology* [7th ed.]. Philadelphia: W.B. Saunders Co., 1986.)

consistent in particular maladies. For example, persons with peptic ulcer disease frequently have increased gastric acid secretion causing pain in the late night or early morning hours. Low blood levels of glucocorticoids increase the sensitivity to sounds, tastes, and smells. Continued high blood levels of the glucocorticoids produce suppression of the immune system.

The stress response increases the secretion of TSH from the anterior pituitary, which leads to increased synthesis and secretion of the thyroid hormones and an increased BMR. The effects of this increase are small and not well-coordinated with other effects of stress.[13] The thyroid hormone, thyroxine, apparently makes the body more responsive to the effects of epinephrine and may be the major effector of prolonged stress.

Numerous studies have shown an increase in ADH (vasopressin) secretion from the posterior pituitary in stressful situations. The general release of ADH in *any* stress reaction has not been shown consistently, but release during hypotensive episodes or in response to pain does seem to be consistent.[13] The release of ADH related to the stress of surgery would account for the decrease in urine output that can occur postoperatively. Vasopressin promotes water conservation and antidiuresis (see Chap. 36).

An increased level of aldosterone is present frequently in the stress response and may, like the elevated level of ADH, be a response to hemodynamic alterations or occur when there is associated renin release. Aldosterone functions in sodium and water retention (see Chap. 37).

*IMMUNOLOGIC MECHANISMS.* Stress, especially chronic, unremitting stress, apparently lowers the body's defense, a response at least partly due to increased production of corticosteroids (Figure 6-13). Corticosteroids

suppress the inflammatory response by affecting lymphocytes and granulocytes. The B cells are depressed, and the high glucocorticoid levels reduce the production of immunoglobulins by the B cells. Sleep deprivation has been reported to cause diminished ability to destroy bacteria, presumably due to suppression of granulocytic cells.[26] The T cell response, and sometimes the number of T cells, have been affected by various forms of stress, such as death of a spouse, excessive exercise, and taking exams.[26] Acceleration of normal thymic atrophy in the adult has been noted during periods of stress. The immune suppression after overwhelming insult to the body may be lifesaving in preventing a bodywide inflammatory response, but the end result of suppression may cause delayed healing and decreased resistance to infections.

## Stress and Disease

### Factors Related to Development of Disease

Many studies have been conducted to relate stress effects with actual disease development. Psychologic and physical stressors have been studied correlating personality traits, genetic predisposition, and environmental, emotional, occupational, and social factors with specific diseases.

A maladaptive response of the body to stressors increases the risk of disease development. It is commonly accepted that psychophysiologic arousal can cause specific end-organ pathology in certain individuals. The chronicity of the arousal state and hyperstimulation of the end organ are necessary factors in the production of pathology.[38] Other factors that increase the risk of disease include genetic predisposition and organ susceptibility. Each can be influenced by the amount of physical stress, emotional stress, or both placed on the individual at one time.

*GENETIC PREDISPOSITION.* Stressors of sufficient strength or intensity can cause an alteration in normal functioning of the body. If one has a genetic or hereditary susceptibility to the stressors, the alteration may be manifested as disease.

Genetic susceptibility refers to myriad conditions that "run in the family" and seem to make the individual react in a particular way to certain stressors. A common example is an exaggerated allergic response that predisposes members of families to specific pollens. When the pollen count is seasonally high, these persons suffer different types of allergic responses. In this example, the stressor is the pollen count, but the response is heightened by a hyperactive, hereditary, immune reaction (see Chap. 16).

Many other diseases seem to be familial and development of actual disease may or may not require addi-

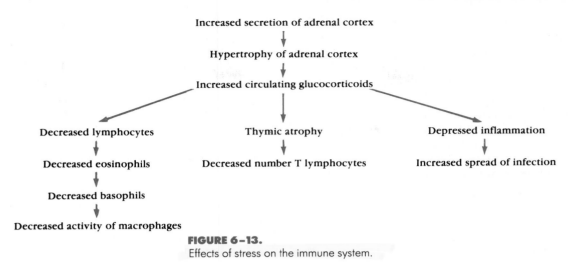

**FIGURE 6–13.**
Effects of stress on the immune system.

tional stressors to trigger the process. Coronary artery disease, for example, may develop in an individual with or without the associated risk factors of obesity, type A personality, hypertension, or others.

*ORGAN SUSCEPTIBILITY.* In different individuals, all organs are not equally resistant to stressors. Some persons under equal stress conditions develop cardiovascular disorders, while others develop peptic ulcers. Still others may suffer migraine headaches or other maladies. The weak-organ theory suggests that certain organs have increased susceptibility in certain individuals. Why the heart is the target organ in some persons and the stomach is targeted in others is not known.[76] It is known that numerous ailments are induced, or at least aggravated, by stressful living conditions.

## Stress-Induced Diseases

Stress has been described in terms of adaptive reaction patterns and systematically related to bodily manifestations.[75] Selye referred to the production of disease as maladaptation and categorized stress-induced diseases as indicated in Box 6-2.[60] In the subsequent material, the following are discussed in relation to their stress connection: (1) cardiovascular diseases, (2) immune deficiency diseases, (3) digestive diseases, (4) cancer, and (5) other conditions.

*CARDIOVASCULAR DISEASE.* For many years it has been recognized that stress is important in the etiology of coronary artery disease. It can be in the form of emotional, occupational, societal, cultural, hereditary, and physical stressors. The importance of occupation has received great attention in recent years.

Several theories of the pathogenesis of coronary artery disease resulted from studies of the relationship between high-fat, stressful living situations and develop-

ment of disease. Individuals who develop hypercholesterolemia have a greater risk of developing atherosclerotic heart disease than those with normal cholesterol levels. The mechanism for the production of hypercholesterolemia is unclear. In contrast, however, studies supported the protective nature of certain serum lipoproteins called high-density lipoproteins (HDLs), which may delay or prevent the development of atherosclerosis. The HDLs occur in greater serum concentrations in women than in men, which is consistent with studies showing that estrogen increases HDL levels while androgens tend to decrease them. During stressful periods, the serum cholesterol has been shown to rise, leading to the conclusion that lipid-regulating mechanisms are responsive to stress. According to some researchers, catecholamine release leads to an increased rate of lipolysis, increased serum free fatty acids, and a subsequent rise in serum cholesterol.[12,21]

**BOX 6-2.**
SELYE'S CLASSIFICATION
OF STRESS-INDUCED DISEASES

1. Hypertension
2. Heart and blood vessel disease
3. Kidney disease
4. Eclampsia
5. Arthritis
6. Skin and eye inflammation
7. Infections
8. Allergic and hypersensitivity diseases
9. Nervous and mental diseases
10. Sexual derangements
11. Digestive diseases
12. Metabolic diseases
13. Cancer
14. Diseases of resistance

Correlate studies also link serum lipid levels and personality patterns. Stress-induced lipemia is considered to be the principal mechanism for stress-induced atherosclerosis. Stress can also potentiate the sequence of blood coagulation. These two factors can lead to myocardial infarction.[14] Stress may also induce coronary artery vasospasm, myocardial hypoxia, and direct myocardial injury. This may alter postinfarction adaptation.[38] Emotional stress can precipitate anginal pain and aggravate heart failure.[2] Life stressors such as bereavement and loss of employment are significant risk factors for myocardial infarction. Depression significantly increases the risk of death after infarction.[14]

The catecholamines produce peripheral vasoconstriction and sclerosis of the smooth muscles of the blood vessels, both of which increase the blood pressure. This observation has led to the theory that chronic stress can produce high blood pressure.[50] The increased blood pressure leads to a weakening and tearing of the linings of the blood vessels, thus providing a focal point for the deposition of cholesterol plaques on the vessel lining. The end result is narrowing of the lumina of vessels, leading to increased peripheral vascular resistance and a further increase in blood pressure levels. To compensate for the elevated blood pressure, the left ventricle undergoes hypertrophy and requires a greater supply of blood and oxygen. A relationship between high blood pressure and coronary artery disease has not been found consistently, but the correlation is significant enough to consider hypertension as a major risk factor.[2]

The increase in frequency of coronary artery disease has prompted investigations into many facets of current lifestyles in the United States. One area of study is the commonly observed personality pattern in which the individual feels a loss of control over his or her occupational or social environment. One study identified a behavior pattern consistent with hypertension and heart attack. It includes competitiveness in work, fast work pace, time pressure, and inability to relax at work or play. Other risk factors also were studied, but the personality pattern apparently offered the greatest risk.[75]

IMMUNE DEFICIENCY.    The decreased immune response after stressful situations appears to be due to increased secretion of glucocorticoids from the adrenal cortex. The major effect is suppression of T lymphocytes, which, in turn, decreases the cell-mediated immune response. Both T and B lymphocytes are affected by glucocorticoid release, but the lymphopenia (decreased numbers of lymphocytes) is due to redistribution rather than actual loss of T cells. Physiologically or psychologically stressful events precipitate a decrease in lymphocytes and other leukocytes.[2]

The administration of glucocorticoids in conditions of hypersensitivity or exaggerated response has long been shown to be beneficial. This is especially true in such conditions as rheumatoid arthritis, acute asthmatic attacks, and specific types of malignancy, especially leukemia.

Conversely, the stress-induced response of decreased immunity can be very detrimental in conditions such as cancer. It is often seen that an individual who was declared "cured" of cancer may undergo relapse after an acute stressful situation, such as the death of a loved one. The stress-induced depression of the immune system may allow for an increased rate of malignant growth (see Unit 6).

DIGESTIVE DISEASES.    The relationship of stress and peptic ulcers has been studied for many years. Three types of stress-induced ulcer disease are described in this section and in further detail in Chapter 41.

Overwhelming stress frequently leads to the development of stress ulcers. These may be related to gastric mucosal ischemia and gastric acid secretion. The ischemia is a result of vasoconstriction by the circulating catecholamines. The mechanism for the related gastric acid secretion is not entirely understood, but may be due to cerebral stimulation of the dorsal motor nucleus of the vagus nerve.[26] Hypersecretion has only been demonstrated clearly in the development of Cushing's ulcers, which are associated with brain lesions. Stress ulcers are very frequent in individuals who experience overwhelming conditions such as shock due to trauma, surgery, burns, or infections.[2]

An increased rate of gastric secretions between meals has been demonstrated in persons who have duodenal ulcers, while those with gastric ulcers often have normal or decreased secretion of hydrochloric acid. It would appear that duodenal ulcers result from a chronic increase in gastric acid secretion and affect the duodenum before the alkalinizing secretions can buffer the acid. Gastric ulcers seem to be related to gastritis and to decreased resistance of the gastric mucosa.[20]

Stress has been indicated in many other digestive conditions, including such diverse ones as constipation, diarrhea, ulcerative colitis, and Crohn's disease. Personality and stress factors with ulcerative colitis and regional enteritis have been studied extensively, leading to much additional knowledge of the very complex pathogenesis of these disorders. Anger and anxiety may precipitate or exacerbate ulcerative colitis.[2]

CANCER.    Specific agents (stressors) are linked with cancer causation. These carcinogens are discussed in Unit 6. Numerous studies have linked psychosocial attitudes with development and progression of cancer. The findings vary, but depression, isolation, introverted personality, and feelings of hopelessness tend to support development of the disease. Individuals who suffer a major loss of chronic stressors also have increased risk of cancer development.[2]

The relationship of stress to cancer may be that depression of the immunologic response by the stress allows cancer to be initiated.[26] Local exposure to carcinogen stressors may result in tumorigenesis. Stress can be viewed as having a twofold influence on malignancy: (1) it increases the production of abnormal cells and (2) it decreases the capability of the body to destroy these cells.[59]

What is known is that all individuals are exposed daily to a host of potential carcinogens and resistance is multifactorial, including physiologic and behavioral responses and attitudes.[56]

*OTHER SYSTEM EFFECTS OF STRESS.* The skin is a target organ for stress reactivity, and when stress occurs, the vessels constrict and peripheral blood flow decreases. Some of the vasospastic conditions such as Raynaud's phenomenon are partly stress induced. Other stress-related disorders include eczema, urticaria, psoriasis, and acne.[2]

The musculoskeletal system exhibits stress effects by chronically tensed muscle, producing the common syndromes of backache, headache, and colon spasms.[2] Arthritis, especially rheumatoid arthritis, is aggravated by high degrees of stress, and symptoms may be exacerbated at these times.

The respiratory system participates in the acute stress reaction by hyperventilation. Stress may be exhibited also by heightened allergic sinusitis and episodes of bronchial asthma. Onset of acute asthmatic attacks may occur with sleeplessness, worry, and grief.[2]

## Destructive Lifestyles

Given proper diet, exercise, rest, and the ability to cope with the stresses of adult living, adulthood should be characterized by peak physical condition and performance. However, a number of destructive lifestyle patterns place adults at risk for the development of illnesses. Cigarette smoking, substance abuse, eating disorders, and sedentary lifestyles are examples of unhealthful behaviors that often originate in response to stress and contribute to destructive lifestyle patterns.

### Smoking

The controversy surrounding the use of tobacco has been evident for a long time. In 1859, Fairholt stated that "tobacco was a comfort to the poor, a luxury for the rich, and ... united all classes in a common pleasure."[16] The modern period of cigarette manufacture began after the Civil War; however, cigarettes did not begin to be mass manufactured until about 1890.[33] Prior to that time, snuff was the tobacco form of choice in both America and Europe.

The literature is replete with evidence regarding the hazardous effects of smoking. Cigarette smoking has been found to decrease or totally paralyze the mucociliary escalator system (see Chap. 28). It has also been clearly implicated as a major cause of emphysema and chronic bronchitis. The risk of lung cancer increases with the number of cigarettes smoked. The male smoker is 10 times as likely to develop lung cancer as is the male nonsmoker.[64] The American Cancer Society has estimated that 85% of lung cancer can be attributed to cigarette smoking.[6] The nicotine in cigarettes has been shown to increase the risk of heart disease.[44] Smoking has also been associated with the development of cancer of the bladder.[12] The newest development in research of cigarette smoking has shifted from the effects on the smoker to the effects on the nonsmoker exposed to what has been called environmental tobacco smoke or passive smoke.[66]

Many factors must be taken into account when one considers why people continue to smoke in the face of clear evidence that smoking cigarettes is a health hazard. Cigarettes are both accessible and relatively inexpensive. Smoking has been seen as an acceptable habit within society and is a form of gratification behavior for the smoker. One must learn to smoke. Learning this behavior requires practice. Once this behavior is learned, it has become a habitual behavior. There are several factors that affect whether or not a behavior becomes a habit, including social forces, interpersonal influence, and exposure through the media that depicts the behavior as desirable. There are five types of smoking: (1) habitual, which is done automatically; (2) pleasureful, which provides positive gratification; (3) anxiety-reducing, which alleviates tension; (4) addictive, which is done to relieve anguish produced by not smoking; and (5) contagion, in which other people's smoking causes distress if one is not also smoking.[67] Thus, smoking is seen as purposeful as well as pleasurable to the smoker, and as such, is a habit that is not readily changed. Adolescents view smoking as mature behavior while rationalizing that the health hazards could never happen to them. As a result, the behavior learned at this age is carried with them into adulthood.

### Substance Abuse

Many people cope with the stressors of life by the use of substances that alter their mood or perception. The majority use substances that fall into one of the following categories: sedatives, narcotics, or stimulants (Table 6-2). Although alcohol belongs in the sedative group, it is usually discussed separately because of its distinct properties. A major problem with psychoactive drug use is the potential for abuse and dependence.

Abuse occurs when a person continues using the substance despite the fact that it is creating problems in major areas of his or her life. Individuals are considered

**TABLE 6-2.**
PROBLEMS WITH PSYCHOACTIVE SUBSTANCE USE

| SUBSTANCE | POTENTIAL PROBLEMS |
| --- | --- |
| **CNS Depressants** | |
| Alcohol | Based on alcohol blood levels, CNS depressant effects increase from sedation and anxiety relief to incoordination, slurred speech, ataxia, stupor, unconsciousness, circulatory collapse, and death. Tolerance develops. Chronic use can lead to peripheral nerve injury; polyneuritis; dementia; myocardial lesions; pancreatitis; impaired liver function; nutritional deficiencies, especially B complex; fetal alcohol syndrome. Withdrawal without treatment can progress from nausea and vomiting, tremors, restlessness, tachycardia, and hypertension to hallucinations, seizures, profound confusion, delirium, and death. |
| Tranquilizers | Potentiates the effect of alcohol; cross-tolerance with alcohol and sedatives; physical dependence; may accumulate in body with slow excretion by kidneys; fetal deformities. Withdrawal is similar to alcohol. |
| Barbiturates | Decreases cortical function; ataxia; depresses respiratory centers in medulla; shortens REM sleep; accelerates function of hepatic microsomal enzymes (decreases effectiveness and speeds tolerance); when dependence develops, even temporary abstinence leads to withdrawal symptoms. Withdrawal is similar to alcohol. |
| **CNS Stimulants** | |
| Amphetamines | Potentiates endogenous catecholamine activity which elevates mood and increases alertness and concentration. Intoxication produces excitation, hyperactive reflexes, hostility, aggression, convulsions. Prolonged use can lead to dysrhythmias, cerebral vascular spasm, CVA, paranoidlike state, severe abdominal pain. Physical dependency occurs. Withdrawal leads to fatigue, lethargy, depression. |
| Cocaine | Immediate and short-lived CNS stimulation similar to amphetamines. Chronic use is associated with multisystem problems including dysrhythmias, CVA, pulmonary edema, perforation of the nasal septum, anorexia, CNS disturbances, and sexual dysfunction. Psychologic dependence can occur. |
| **Narcotics** | Relieves pain and anxiety and produces a temporary euphoria. CNS depression, pupillary constriction, depressed respirations occur. I.V. abuse can lead to malnutrition, infection, contaminant toxicity, hepatitis, thromboembolic complications, and AIDS. Tolerance develops with repeated use. Withdrawal includes yawning, tearing, chills and fever, tremors, muscle spasms, and tachycardia. Withdrawal, though uncomfortable, is not life-threatening. |

Adapted from *R.T. Malseed and G.S. Harrigan*, Textbook of Pharmacology and Nursing Care. *Philadelphia: J.B. Lippincott, 1989.*

dependent on psychoactive substances when they use larger quantities than they originally intended to and when they are unable to control or decrease its use. In addition, much of life revolves around securing or using the substance. When individuals need to increase the amount of the substance to achieve the desired effect, they have developed tolerance to it.[1,34]

## Eating Disorders

The most common eating disorders of early adulthood are *anorexia nervosa* (AN) and *bulimia nervosa* (BN) (see Chap. 10). Anorexia nervosa usually begins in adolescence but may continue into adulthood. Bulimia is thought to occur more often in early adulthood. Although treated as two separate disorders, many of the behaviors overlap.

Anorexia nervosa is a potentially life-threatening illness that is characterized by at least 15% loss of body weight, a voluntary refusal to eat, an obsessive concern about food and gaining weight, a distorted body image, and a tendency toward strenuous exercise.[8] The majority of cases (95%) are women. The anorexic person sees herself as fat, no matter what her weight. Often the only control she feels over her life is the control she is able to exert over food and its consumption. Therefore, it is common for the individual to deny the need for treatment and resist attempts to force her to gain weight.

Physical symptoms of AN include weight loss; an emaciated, malnourished appearance; slow pulse; and amenorrhea.[22] Other symptoms are lanugo, brownish discoloration of the skin, hypotension, "delayed gastric motility, and a hypothyroid-like state manifest by dry skin, listlessness, and dry falling hair."[8] In addition, there may be anemia, lymphocytosis, leukopenia, hypocholesterolemia, hypoglycemia, and hypoproteinemia. Changes occur in the gonadotropins and ovarian hormones. Death may result in 5% to 21% of cases from malnutrition, infection, or cardiac problems.[32]

Bulimia is characterized by "binge eating," consuming a large amount of food quickly, and "purging," the process of eliminating what is eaten by vomiting and the use of laxatives, enemas, or both. Diagnostic criteria require a minimum average of two episodes of binge eating a week within a 3 month period.[1] Bulimics tend to be somewhat overweight or of normal weight, but they too are concerned with the size and shape of their bodies. Unlike people with AN, those with BN are aware of the abnormality of their eating patterns but are unable to stop.

The dentist may be the first to identify bulimia from tooth enamel erosion resulting from the high acid content of the vomitus. Concentrated urine, abnormal electrolytes, fever, poor skin turgor, weakness, and lethargy may occur if body fluids are depleted.[8] One particular danger occurs with abuse of syrup of ipecac.[48] A cumulative systemic toxicity can result that affects the neuromuscular, gastrointestinal, and cardiovascular systems. Cardiotoxicity and death can result.

*Obesity* is the most common problem in the United States. The nation as a whole overconsumes calories and remains undernourished because of an imbalanced diet. Recent surveys show that the average energy intake has increased and that the US population is getting heavier.[61] Weight gain leading to obesity occurs when energy intake chronically exceeds energy expenditure.[55] Data from cross-sectional studies indicate that obesity increases with age throughout the adult years.[11] The weight loss industry is a multibillion dollar business as more and more people try to lose excess weight. Often unsupervised or fad diets are imbalanced and the end result is an obese person who is markedly malnourished (see Chap. 10).

Obesity is characterized by a number of metabolic changes related to lipid metabolism. Obese individuals often have elevated serum cholesterol and triglyceride levels and lower high-density lipoprotein concentrations. These changes increase the risk for coronary heart disease.

### Sedentary Lifestyles

In 1985, less than half of the US adult population reported exercising on a regular basis, and only a quarter had done so for 5 years or more.[70] The current best estimate is that only about 10% to 20% of adults participate in exercise required for cardiorespiratory benefit. In one community-based study of cardiovascular disease, physical inactivity was estimated to account for as much as 23% of cardiovascular risk.[45] Recent surveys indicate that fewer than 10% of Americans older than age 18 years meet the criteria for exercise proposed in the 1990 objectives for the nation, and the amount of physical activity at work and in the home has declined steadily with increasing automation and labor-saving aids.[7]

Television viewing is the most pervasive pasttime in the United States today.[65] Following sleep and work, it is the nation's third most time-consuming activity. The typical adult watches TV nearly four hours daily.[49] When the TV is on, activity ceases and time for exercise is reduced significantly. Due to decreased calorie expenditure, adults who view 3 hours of television or more each day have twice the risk of obesity and an even higher risk of super-obesity.[68]

An increase in physical activity together with a decrease in total energy intake and a decrease in dietary fat are needed to control obesity in sedentary affluent societies. Food intake is better regulated at higher levels of physical activity. Physically active people change to higher carbohydrate intake at the expense of dietary fat. There is increasing evidence that the carbohydrate-to-fat ratio in the diet relates to obesity.[62]

Physical exercise is characterized by an increase in lean body mass and by healthy changes in lipid and carbohydrate metabolism. There is a decrease in adipose tissue, an increase in high-density lipoprotein concentration, a decrease in cholesterol level, and lower blood pressure. Changes in carbohydrate metabolism include an increase in glucose uptake and an increase in insulin sensitivity in muscle; mobilization of free fatty acids from the adipose tissue; and a higher capacity to oxidize free fatty acids in the muscle cells. Exercise produces a metabolic status that maintains energy balance.[61]

Individuals in sedentary occupations are more prone to cancer of the colon.[72] Physical activity is associated with a reduced intestinal transit time, supporting the hypothesis that the bowel mucosa has reduced exposure to potential carcinogens. In addition, physical exercise and leanness are associated with less cancer of the reproductive system in female athletes, whereas obesity is associated with increased risk for cancer of the breast and endometrium in postmenopausal women.[18] Exercise may prevent bone loss in healthy postmenopausal women and possibly in women with osteoporosis.[18]

During the past several decades, numerous well-designed scientific studies have documented the beneficial effects of habitual exercise.[4,52] Emerging scientific evidence strongly supports the long-held notion that exercise is beneficial to health in a number of ways, including reducing the risk of cardiovascular disease, enhancing musculoskeletal integrity; improving weight control, hypertension control, and glucose tolerance; and enhancing mood and energy levels.[3] Furthermore, research has shown that even a modest improvement in fitness level among the most unfit confers a substantial health benefit.[3] A brisk half-hour walk once a day has been enough exercise to offer significant protection against death from a wide range of diseases.[29]

The adult years are an important time for education and medical care to preserve health and prevent or delay the onset of chronic disease. Despite the vast resources—scientific, economic, and human—devoted to health care, it is a disturbing fact that close to 60% of all deaths that occur annually in the United States are premature, and an equivalently high proportion of the disability and illness could be avoided.[69]

Cardiovascular disease, cancer, stroke, and injuries—the leading causes of adult death in this country, accounting for nearly 75% of deaths annually—are intimately linked to preventable risk factors.[70] Many of these factors, including smoking, improper nutrition, alcohol misuse, overweight, lack of exercise, and maladaptive responses to stressful experience, can be modified by changes in personal behavior or social choices.[23]

## REFERENCES

1. American Psychiatric Association. *Diagnostic and Statistical Manual of Mental Disorders* (3rd ed.). Washington, D.C.: Author, 1980.

2. Asterita, M. *The Physiology of Stress*. New York: Human Sciences Press, 1985.

3. Blair, S., Kohl, H., Paffenbarger, R., Clark, D., Cooper, K., and Gibbons, L. Physical fitness and all-cause mortality: A prospective study of healthy men and women. *JAMA* 262:2395, 1989.

4. Butler, R., and Goldberg, L. Exercise and prevention of coronary heart disease. *Primary Care* 16(1):99, 1989.

5. Canavan, T. The psychobiology of sleep. *Nursing 84* 2:682, 1984.

6. *Cancer Facts*. New York: American Cancer Society, 1987.

7. Centers for Disease Control. Progress toward achieving the 1990 national objectives for physical fitness and exercise. *Morbidity and Mortality Weekly Report* 38:449, 1989.

8. Chitty, K. Applying the nursing process for clients with eating disorders. In H.S. Wilson and C.R. Kneisl (eds.), *Psychiatric Nursing* (4th ed.). Menlo Park, Calif.: Addison-Wesley, 1991.

9. Chuman, W. The neurological basis of sleep. *Heart Lung* 12:177, 1983.

10. Clark-Stewart, A., Perlmutter, M., and Friedman, S. *Lifelong Human Development*. New York: Wiley, 1988.

11. Colditz, G., Willett, W., Stampfer, M., London, S., Segal, M., and Speizer, F. Patterns of weight change and their relation to diet in a cohort of healthy women. *Am. J. Clin. Nutr.* 51:1100, 1990.

12. Cotran, R.S., Kumar, V., and Robbins, S.L. *Robbins' Pathologic Basis of Disease* (4th ed.). Philadelphia: W.B. Saunders, 1989.

13. Dunn, A.J., and Kramaarcy, N.R. Neurochemical responses in stress: Relationships between the hypothalamic-pituitary-adrenal and catecholamine systems. In L.L. Iverson and S.D. Iverson, *Drugs, Neurotransmitters and Behavior*. New York: Plenum Press, 1984.

14. Elliott, G.R., and Eisdorfer, C. *Stress and Human Health: Analysis and Implications of Research. A Study by the Institute of Medicine National Academy of Sciences*. New York: Springer, 1982.

15. Erikson, E.H. *Childhood and Society* (2nd ed.). New York: Norton, 1963.

16. Fairholt, F. *Tobacco: Its History and Associations*. London: Chapman and Hall, 1859.

17. Feirman, J. Disordered sleep. *Emerg. Med.* 17:160, 1985.

18. Frisch, R., Wyshak, G., and Albright, N. Lower lifetime occurrence of breast cancer and cancers of the reproductive system among former college athletes. *Am. J. Clin. Nutr.* 45(suppl):328, 1987.

19. Gould, R.L. *Transformations: Growth and Change in Adult Life*. New York: Simon & Schuster, 1978.

20. Greenberger, N.J., and Winship, D.H. *Gastrointestinal Disorders: A Pathophysiologic Approach* (3rd ed.). Chicago: Yearbook, 1986.

21. Guyton, A.C. *Textbook of Medical Physiology* (8th ed.). Philadelphia: W.B. Saunders, 1991.

22. Halmi, R. Pragmatic information on eating disorders. *Psych. Clin. N. Am.* 5(2):371, 1982.

23. Hamburg, D., Elliott, G., Parron, D. (eds.). *Health and Behavior: Frontiers of Research in the Behavioral Sciences*. National Academy Press, August 27–29, 1984.

24. Havighurst, R.J. *Human Development and Education*. New York: Longman, 1972.

25. Hoch, C., and Reynolds, C. Sleep disturbances and what to do about them. *Geriatr. Nurs.* 7:24, 1986.

26. Irwin, J., and Anisman, H. Stress and pathology: Immunological and central nervous system interactions. In C.L. Cooper, *Psychosocial Stress and Cancer*. New York: Wiley, 1984.

27. Kales, A., and Kates, J. Evaluation, diagnosis, and treatment of clinical conditions related to sleep. *JAMA* 213:2229, 1970.

28. Kasch, F., and Boyer, J. *Adult Fitness Principles and Practice*. Palo Alto, CA: National Press, 1968.

29. Lemonick, M. Take a walk and live. *Time*. p. 90, November 13, 1989.

30. Levinson, D.J., et al. *The Seasons of a Man's Life*. New York: Ballantine, 1978.

31. Leviton, D., and Santoro, L. *Health, Physical Education, Recreation, and Dance for the Older Adult: A Modular Approach*. Reston, VA: American Alliance for Health, Physical Education, Recreation and Dance, 1980.

32. Lippi, B. Physiologic aspects of eating disorders. *J. Am. Acad. Child Psych.* 22(2):108, 1983.

33. Mackenzie, C. *Sublime Tobacco*. New York: Macmillan, 1958.

34. Malseed, R., and Harrigan, G. *Textbook of Pharmacology and Nursing Care*. Philadelphia: J.B. Lippincott, 1989.

35. McGinnis, J., and Hamburg, M. Opportunities for health promotion and disease prevention in the clinical setting. *West. J. Med.* 149:468, 1988.

36. McLean, A. Occupational psychiatry. In H. Kaplan, A. Freedman, and B. Sadock (eds.), *Comprehensive Textbook of Psychiatry* (3rd ed.). Baltimore: Williams & Wilkins, 1980.

37. McPherson, B. (ed.). *Sport and Aging.* Champaign, Ill.: Human Kinetics, 1986.

38. Meerson, F.Z. *Adaptation, Stress and Prophylaxis.* New York: Springer-Verlag, 1984.

39. Mendelson, W., Gillin, J., and Wyatt, R. *Human Sleep and Its Disorders.* New York: Plenum Press, 1977.

40. Miller, D., and Allen, T. *Fitness: A Lifetime Commitment.* Minneapolis, Minn.: Burgess, 1979.

41. Miller, J. Living systems: Basic concepts. In W. Gray et al., *General Systems Theory and Psychiatry.* Boston: Little, Brown, 1969.

42. Mourad, L.A., and Ashburn, S.S. Biophysical Development During Middlescence in C.S. Schuster and S.S. Ashburn, *The Process of Human Development* (2nd ed.). Boston: Little, Brown, 1986.

43. Neugarten, B. Adult personality: Toward a psychology of the life cycle. In W.C. Sze (ed.), *The Human Life Cycle.* New York: Jason Aronson, 1975.

44. The 1988 Report of the Joint National Committee on Detection, Evaluation, and Treatment of High Blood Pressure. *Arch. Intern. Med.* 148(5), 1988.

45. Oberman, A. Exercise and the primary prevention of cardiovascular disease. *Am. J. Cardiol.* 55:10D, 1985.

46. Ostrow, A. *Physical Activity and the Older Adult: Psychological Perspectives.* Princeton, New Jersey: Princeton Book Company, 1984.

47. Palmore, E. Predictors of successful aging. *The Gerontologist* 19(5):427, 1980.

48. Parks, B., and Fischer, R. Misuse of syrup of Ipecac. *Pediatr. Nurs.* 13(4):261, 1987.

49. Pearl, D., Bouthilet, L., and Lazer, J. (eds.). *Television and Behavior: Ten Years of Scientific Progress and Implications for the Eighties* (Vol. 2). Washington, D.C.: Government Printing Office, 1982.

50. Pelletier, K. *Mind as a Healer, Mind as a Slayer.* New York: Dell, 1977.

51. Perlmutter, M. and Hall, E. *Adult Development and Aging.* New York: Wiley, 1985.

52. Powell, K., Thompson, P., Caspersen, C., and Kendrick, J. Physical activity and the incidence of coronary heart disease. *Ann. Rev. Public Health* 1(8):253, 1987.

53. Rogers, D. *The Adult Years: An Introduction to Aging* (3rd ed.). Englewood Cliffs, New Jersey: Prentice Hall, 1986.

54. Roitt, I., Brostoff, J., and Male, D. *Immunology* (2nd ed.). Philadelphia: J.B. Lippincott, 1989.

55. Romieu, I., Willett, W., Stampfer, M., Colditz, G., Sampson, L., Rosner, B., Hennekens, C., and Speizer, F. Energy intake and other determinants of relative weight. *Am. J. Clin. Nutr.* 47:406, 1988.

56. Rosch, P.J. Stress and cancer. In C.L. Cooper, *Psychosocial Stress and Cancer.* New York: Wiley, 1984.

57. Rosenzweig, M.R., and Leiman, A.L. *Physiological Psychology* (2nd ed.). New York: Random House, 1989.

58. Santrock, J.W. *Adult Development and Aging.* Dubuque, Iowa: W.C. Brown, 1985.

59. Selye, H. Stress, cancer, and the mind. In S.B. Day, *Cancer, Stress and Death.* New York: Plenum Press, 1968.

60. Selye, H. *The Stress of Life.* New York: McGraw-Hill, 1956.

61. Simopoulos, A. Nutrition and fitness. *JAMA* 261(10):2862, 1989.

62. Sims, E., and Danforth, E. Expenditure and storage of energy in man. *J. Clin. Invest.* 79:1019, 1987.

63. Smith, E., and Serfass, R. (eds.). *Exercise and Aging.* Hillside, New Jersey: Enslow, 1981.

64. Smoking and cancer. *Morbidity and Mortality Weekly Report* 31(11):77, 1982.

65. Spirduso, W. Physical fitness, aging, and psychomotor speed: A Review. *J. Gerontol.* 35:850, 1980.

66. Tollison, R. (ed.). *Clearing the Air: Perspectives on Environmental Tobacco Smoke.* Lexington, Mass.: Lexington Books, 1988.

67. Tomkins, S. Psychological model for smoking behavior. *Am. J. Public Health* 56:17, 1966.

68. Tucker, L., and Friedman, G. Television viewing and obesity in adult males. *Am. J. Public Health* 79(4):516, 1989.

69. U.S. Department of Health, Education and Welfare (DHEW). *Healthy People: A Report of the Surgeon General.* Publication No. (PHS) 79–55071. Washington, D.C.: Government Printing Office, 1979.

70. U.S. Department of Health and Human Services (DHHS). *Health United States: 1986.* Publication No. (PHS) 87–1232. Hyattsville, Md.: National Center for Health Statistics, 1986.

71. Van Hoose, W.H., and Worth, M.R. *Adulthood in the Life Cycle.* Dubuque, Iowa: W.C. Brown, 1982.

72. Vena, J., Graham, S., Zielezny, M., Brasure, J., and Swanson, M. Occupational exercise and risk of cancer. *Am. J. Clin. Nutr.* 45(suppl):318, 1987.

73. von Bertalanffy, I. *General Systems Theory: Foundations, Development and Applications.* New York: Brazillier, 1986.

74. Weiss, R. *Going It Alone: The Family Life and Social Life of Single Parents.* New York: Basic Books, 1979.

75. Wheatley, D. *Stress and the Heart.* New York: Raven Press, 1977.

76. Wolff, H.G. *Stress and Disease* (2nd ed.). Springfield, Ill.: Charles C. Thomas, 1968.

# chapter 7

Gretchen McDaniel

# Biophysical Changes of the Older Adult

## Chapter Outline

▶ **Biologic Theories of Aging**
  **Early Theories of Aging**
  **Modern (or Recent) Theories of Aging**
    Free Radical Theory
    Waste Product Theory
    Immunologic Theory
    Cross-Link Theory
    Somatic Mutation Theory
    Genetic Aging Theory
▶ **Biophysical Effects of Aging and Susceptibility to Disease**
  **General Effects**
  **Nervous System**
  **Cardiovascular System**
    Anatomic Changes
    Physiologic Changes
    Conduction System Changes
    Arterial Changes
    Venular Changes
    Diseases Related to the Aging Cardiovascular System

**Respiratory System**
  Anatomic Changes
  Functional Changes
**Genitourinary System**
  Anatomic Changes in the Kidneys
  Physiologic Changes in the Kidneys
  Diseases and Problems with Aging Kidneys
  Bladder Changes
  Gynecologic Changes in the Elderly Woman
  Reproductive Changes in the Elderly Man
**Gastrointestinal System**
  Normal Anatomic Changes
  Esophageal Changes
  Stomach Changes
  Colon Changes
  Pancreatic Changes
  Liver Changes

**Musculoskeletal System**
  Characteristic Changes in Anatomic Structure and Function
  Joint Changes
  Problems Related to Skeletal Degeneration
  Fractures and Risk of Falling
**Skin and Dermal Appendages**
  Changes in the Skin, Nails, and Hair
  Diseases Associated with Aging Skin
**Sensory System**
  Vision Changes
  Hearing Changes
  Other Sensory Changes
**Aging and Cancer**
▶ **Drugs and the Elderly**

## Learning Objectives

1. Discuss important research on the aging process.
2. Describe the biologic cellular theories: free radical, waste product, immunologic, cross-link, somatic mutation, and genetic aging theories.
3. List the general effects of aging.
4. Describe the causes and effects of nervous system alterations.
5. Relate anatomic alterations in the cardiovascular system to the resultant physiologic changes.
6. Describe how the arterial changes in the elderly alter blood flow and pressure.
7. Discuss causes and effects of hypertension in the elderly.
8. Describe the physiologic result of respiratory changes due to aging.
9. Explain why elderly persons are at risk for the development of respiratory failure after stressful situations.
10. Compare renal function of the young adult with that of the elderly.

11. List common organisms that can cause bladder infection in the elderly.
12. Describe the effects of lack of estrogen in postmenopausal women.
13. Describe the effects of hormone changes in elderly men.
14. Discuss briefly the many factors that cause digestive disturbances in the elderly.
15. Characterize the alterations in body movement that occur as a consequence of aging.
16. Explain the factors that lead to increased risk of bone fractures in the elderly.
17. List the joint changes that are common in the elderly, at what age they begin, and when they become symptomatic.
18. Describe the characteristic changes in skin, nails, and hair associated with aging.
19. Explain how sensory alterations affect adjustment in the aging process.

*(continued)*

The phenomenon of aging is variable and complex in nature. It is very difficult to define what aging is or to establish the facts about the process. Much of the confusion arises from the difficulty of distinguishing between normal aging and changes secondary to disease. The causes of aging have been investigated for centuries, yet no researcher has been able specifically to identify any single causative factor. Science and medicine have concentrated on preventing and curing illness in the earlier stages of life, which has resulted in an increased life expectancy in the United States. Worldwide, however, the life span of human beings has not increased. The variability of life span for humans seems to be a function of several factors: heredity, culture, race, nutrition, and environment. Total life span seems to be limited to 90 to 105 years, which supports the belief that aging is an innate process.

## BIOLOGIC THEORIES OF AGING

A major problem encountered in aging theories is the fact that so many of them were developed with the biases of several disciplines, rather than with an objective, interdisciplinary approach. Biology, sociology, and psychology all arrived at different explanations for the changes that occur with the aging process. Some theories have been thoroughly researched, whereas others do not enjoy the support of clinical testing or the acceptance of the medical community.

### Early Theories of Aging

Until the nineteenth century, most of the interest in the aging process was concerned with ways to prevent it. The ancient Egyptians tried to find the fountain of youth. Hippocrates (C. 460 to 377 B.C.) perceived aging as stemming from a decrease in body heat, a natural, irreversible, and unavoidable phenomenon. Galen (C. 130 to 201 A.D.) had a similar theory postulating that the increased coldness and dryness of aging resulted from changes in body humor. Also, Galen viewed aging as a lifelong process as opposed to an event occurring late in the life span. Mai-

monides, a Jewish philosopher in the 12th century, believed the life span could be prolonged if suitable precautions were taken by an individual.[25] Leonardo da Vinci stimulated later development of theories of biologic aging through his descriptions and drawings.[9]

Theorists in the 18th and 19th centuries claimed that life was intrinsic energy which gradually decreased over time to the point of death. Darwin viewed aging as the body's inability to respond to stimuli as a result of decreased nervous and muscular tissue irritability. The predominant aging theories in the early 1990s included the "auto intoxication" theory and the "wear and tear" theory.[25]

### Modern (or Recent) Theories of Aging

To understand differences among theories of aging it is necessary to examine the processes that take place within the aging organism. Of importance to research is the number of times cells replicate themselves.[20] Research evidence has shown that the number of times normal diploid human fibroblasts can replicate themselves in vitro is limited. Hayflick reported, "The sum of population doublings undergone by normal fetal human fibroblasts both before and after preservation is always equal to 50 + 10."[20] Cells isolated from older persons show progressively fewer doublings before finally stopping.

Other researchers noted that the homeostatic mechanisms that govern immunity and cell replication decrease as a person grows older. Both cell division and ribonucleic acid (RNA) synthesis of protein slow down. There is also increasing heterogenicity of cells in terms of size, shape, and mitotic capabilities.

Common in metabolism of the older person is increased collagen cross-linking. Cross-linkages are stable molecules that prevent deoxyribonucleic acid (DNA) strands from dividing in the normal cell reproductive cycle. Cross-linkage molecules accumulate and affect proteins in elastin and collagen, resulting in cell death. The cell death results in decreased elasticity of blood vessels and skin.[12]

This section describes biologic cellular theories of aging. No one theory answers all the questions, but each provides a clue to the aging process and certain interrelationships that do appear to exist.

## Free Radical Theory

The free radical theory has been described as a unitary approach to the study of the phenomena of aging. It proposes that free radicals serve as central agents in the changes observed with aging at the tissue, cellular, and subcellular levels.[10] Free radicals are parts of molecules that have broken off or molecules that have had an electron stripped from their structure. Free radicals are a normal part of metabolic reactions that form part of a structural system and are not free to diffuse within the cells. Diffusible free radicals damage or alter the original structure or function of other molecules by attaching themselves to them.[10] The free radical theory has been linked to the idea of oxygen toxicity. Oxidation of protein, fat, carbohydrate, and other elements in the body results in the formation of these free radicals.[11] Lipofuscin, a pigmented material that accumulates in some organs with aging, is associated with oxidation of unsaturated lipids. Lipofuscin is thought to have a relationship to free radicals and the aging process because of this lipid oxidation.[25] Diffusible free radical end products and compounds can cause cellular disruption. In the aging process, the number of free radical compounds appears to increase faster than body cells can repair the damage. Some scientists consider the cell membrane as the key to survival and believe that the greatest damage could be perpetrated by free radicals at this membrane level.[12]

Vitamin E and coenzyme Q are thought to protect the mitochondria from the hazards of the free radical activity.

Vitamin E may function as an antioxidant and binding agent in the antioxidation process, which supports the use of antioxidants such as vitamin E in an attempt to delay cellular aging.

Free radical activity is also fostered in the body by such environmental factors as smog, byproducts of the plastics industry, gasoline, and atmospheric ozone. The human body appears to be bombarded from both external and internal sources of free radicals. If this theory is as fundamental to aging as proponents believe, careful monitoring of the environment and proper food selection should lead to better health in old age.

## Waste Product Theory

The waste product theory is derived as a result of observing increased pigment in aging cells. The pigment, called lipofuscin, is a dark, irregular, granular inclusion within cells.[11] There is some evidence that lipofuscin occurs in cells as a result of a variety of processes such as autophagocytosis, oxidation of lipids, and copolymerization of organic molecules. It has been suggested that lipofuscin forms as an end product of free radical-induced lipid peroxidation. This suggestion provides a connection between oxygen consumption, free radicals, lipofuscin, and aging.[27] The actual effect of lipofuscin on cell function is not known.

## Immunologic Theory

The immunologic theory asserts that aging is an autoimmune process. The body's immune system fails to recognize its own cells as the cells change with age.

Autoimmune responses damage or destroy cells, leading to cell death.[14] Tissue damage and increased susceptibility to infection may be caused by the presence of autoantibodies and decreased numbers of immunocompetent cells (see Unit 5). Whether or not the diminished capacity for immune responses is a cause of aging is not known, but it certainly is the source of many of the disease problems of the aged, such as increased frequency of autoimmune disease, cancer, and infections of all types.

Aging affects all parts of the immune system, but especially the T cells. A decline in T cell-dependent immune function begins at sexual maturity with the onset of involution of the thymus gland. This factor is associated with increased frequency of diseases such as cancer and autoimmune diseases. Macrophages that play a major role in protecting the body against infection do not seem to diminish in number as the body ages. The B cell number remains elevated, but responsiveness to stimulation by antigens decreases markedly, probably because of dependence on T cell stimulation.

## Cross-Link Theory

The cross-link theory, also called the collagen theory, suggests that strong chemical reactions create strong bonds between molecular structures that are normally separate. Cross-linking produces irreparable damage to DNA and leads to cell death. Cross-link agents are so numerous and varied in the diet and in the environment that they are impossible to avoid.[12] Connective tissue changes are an indicator that cross-linkage has occurred. Collagen, which makes up a large part of the proteins of the body, is the substance that maintains strength, support, and structural form. As a result of the chemical action of cross-linkage, aging collagens become more insoluble and rigid, resulting in inhibition of cell permeability. Passage of nutrients, metabolites, antibodies, and gases through the blood vessel walls is inhibited. The linings of the lungs and gastrointestinal tract are also affected.

Elastin, another of the fibrillar proteins present in connective tissue, is very prone to cross-linkage. It differs from collagen on the basis of its chemical composition and physical properties. Both elastin and collagen respond to cross-linkage in the same manner. Aging elastin becomes frayed, fragmented, and brittle, leading to many changes in connective tissue throughout the body. A good example of this is skin changes, such as loss of turgor, elasticity and tone, and dryness. Cross-linkage also affects cell division because its molecules prevent division of the strands of the DNA. If only one strand is affected, no damage results. If the cross-link molecule attaches itself to both sides of the DNA, the cell dies because division is prevented. Such cell death has a profound effect on the elasticity of blood vessels and skin. As a result of the changes in collagen and elastin, cross-linkage is thought to be a primary cause of aging.

### Somatic Mutation Theory

The somatic mutation theory asserts that spontaneous mutation occurs in DNA. This mutation occurs by hydrolysis, miscoding of enzymes, or irradiation. The mutation may be perpetuated during cell replication if not corrected by repair enzymes. Mutant cells decrease the efficiency of cellular function, and thus organ function declines.[14]

### Genetic Aging Theory

The genetic aging theory is based on the belief that the life span is programmed before birth into the genes in the DNA molecule. This means that a person fortunate enough to have long-lived parents or grandparents has a life expectancy longer than it would have been with short-lived parents. This theory is supported by genealogical studies that have indicated that children whose parents died before age 60 had an average life expectancy of almost 20 years less than children whose parents died at age 80.[25]

## BIOPHYSICAL EFFECTS OF AGING AND SUSCEPTIBILITY TO DISEASE

In 1980, over 15 million Americans were in the young aged (65 to 74 years) population. The older aged, or persons older than 75 years, numbered approximately 10 million.[14] Many physical and chemical changes that occur as a person ages have been identified through research, even though the exact causes of aging cannot be isolated. Specific age-related changes that occur from the young aged to older aged have not yet been defined through research. Some of the changes are harmful in that they interfere with the healthy function of cells and tissues. Others have not been found to be harmful.

Aging leads to a gradual diminution in the functional capacity of the organ systems. It must be realized, however, that the process is extremely variable among different individuals. Chronologic age, therefore, is a poor index of physiologic age or of performance, and advancing years are not necessarily equated with illness. If one problem is identified, however, others must be looked for because several diseases are characteristic of the elderly.[24]

### General Effects

The appearance of the aging person characteristically is altered. Stature is lost, body proportions are changed, skin is dry and wrinkled, hair is thinning and gray, and there are changes in body movement characterized by slowness, stiffness, and diminished coordination and balance. The intervertebral disks become thin, as do the vertebrae themselves, leading to reduction in height. The thoracic curve of the vertebral column increases, resulting in a kyphosis. This plus changes in lung elasticity result in increased anteroposterior diameter of the chest. The cervical curve increases to compensate for the thoracic curve, causing a tilting of the head. Height loss, therefore, is in the trunk. The length of the long bones is unchanged. Thus, the effect is a short trunk and long limbs, which is just the opposite of that of the child (Figure 7-1).

The total body composition is altered. Lean body mass is reduced, which includes fat-free body tissues such as nerves, organ parenchyma, and skeletal muscle. Increased amounts of fat are laid down in mesenteric or perinephritic areas rather than in subcutaneous fat. Decreased subcutaneous fat leads to increased skin folding. Amounts of total body potassium, water, and intracellular fluid decrease; however, there is no change in the amount of extracellular fluid. The bone mineral mass is reduced, with increased bone porosity (Figure 7-2). The total effect of these losses is reduced total body density.

Weight changes are characteristic. In men, the average maximum weight is 172 pounds at ages 35 to 54 years. This falls to 166 pounds at ages 55 to 64. In women, the average maximum weight is 152 pounds at 55 to 64 years, 146 pounds at ages 65 to 74, and 138 pounds at ages 75 to 89 (Table 7-1). The weight of women declines less proportionately than that of men.[26]

Visible changes in movement are primarily due to alterations in the nervous system, with diminished muscle

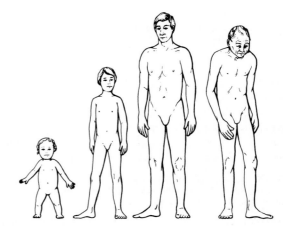

**FIGURE 7-1.**
Changes in body proportions throughout the life span.

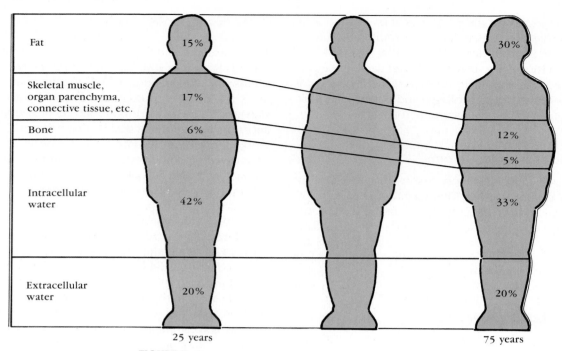

**FIGURE 7–2.**
Changes in major body components with the aging process.

strength and joint mobility contributing only minimally. Movement is an extremely complex activity requiring integration of many portions of the nervous system. Intact sensory information going to the brain must be coupled with integration of cortical, basal ganglionic, and cerebellar function. The extrapyramidal system is subject to early changes in function due to diminished presence of neurotransmitters. Vascular supply to all portions of the brain is critical to coordinated function for movement. Locomotion becomes increasingly precarious with aging.

Fasting blood sugar, blood volume, serum pH, red blood cell count, and osmotic pressure are unchanged with aging in the absence of disease. The ability to respond to severe stresses is altered, however. For example, normal pH may be well maintained under normal circumstances, but should ventilatory failure or metabolic acidosis occur, the elderly person takes much longer to restore normal pH. Responses to events such as infection may be diminished or slowed. An elderly person may have an infectious illness with subnormal or normal temperature and a normal heart rate.

## Nervous System

The general integrative effects of aging are strongly affected by alteration in the central nervous system (CNS). Because of its dependency on oxygen, the CNS responds to change in the circulatory system, such as arteriosclerosis, which can lead to decreased oxygen supply. A decreased oxygen supply to the brain leads to changes in mental acuity, sensory interpretation, and movement, and a generally reduced capacity to cope with numerous environmental events. The onset of such changes is extremely variable from one individual to another.

Nerve impulses decrease their rate of conduction by about 10%, which may lead to ischemia, generally lower basal metabolism, and temperature changes in nerve fi-

**TABLE 7–1.**
AVERAGE HEIGHTS AND WEIGHTS BY AGE AND SEX:
U.S. HEALTH EXAMINATION STUDY 1960–62

| Age (Yrs.) | MALES | | FEMALES | |
| --- | --- | --- | --- | --- |
| | Height (In.) | Weight (Lbs.) | Height (In.) | Weight (Lbs.) |
| 18–24 | 68.7 | 160 | 63.8 | 129 |
| 25–34 | 69.1 | 171 | 63.7 | 136 |
| 35–44 | 68.5 | 172 | 63.5 | 144 |
| 45–54 | 68.2 | 172 | 62.9 | 147 |
| 55–64 | 67.4 | 166 | 62.4 | 152 |
| 65–74 | 66.9 | 160 | 61.5 | 146 |
| 75–79 | 65.9 | 150 | 61.1 | 138 |

*Based on a nationwide probability sample of 7710 persons. Averages and fiftieth percentiles were quite equal. Both secular trends and aging changes are mirrored by such measures as the three-inch difference in height of younger and older males.*
Source: Public Health Service Publication 1000, Series 11, No. 8. Washington, D.C.: Government Printing Office, 1965.

bers.[6] The transmission strength of signals from the brain to the body parts decreases as a result of the dwindling number of neurons and the degenerating myelin sheath with age. The signals become slightly blurred and the threshold for arousal of an organ system may be altered. Adaptation to physiologic stressors does not occur as rapidly in the elderly as in younger persons. The increased recovery time within the autonomic system causes an organ to take longer to return to base level activity after stressful situations.

Physical changes also occur in the brain. The brain loses an average of 100 gm in weight between 25 and 70 years of age.[21] Diminished numbers of neurons result, with the loss being greater in some areas than others. In the older aged individual, there is a change in the cortex and white matter volume. White matter volume decreases by 11% between the ages of 70 and 90 years. During this period, there is a 2% to 3% decline in the cortex.[21] Little loss occurs in the brainstem. Atrophy of the convolutions of the brain is common, with widening of the sulci and gyri, especially in the frontal lobe. Dilatation of the ventricles also is common. Despite these anatomic changes, there is little loss of the total amount of DNA, nucleic acid, or protein.

The intracellular accumulation of lipofuscin pigment has been studied extensively. A major accumulation of this pigment is in storage vacuoles and is quantitatively correlated with age.

The amount per cell varies but there can be enough to fill the cytoplasm and force the nucleus into an abnormal position. Although little is known about the effect of lipofuscin on cell function, it is thought that its accumulation can hamper oxygen use.[4]

Neurofibrillary tangles frequently occur in the aging brain, but these are not exclusive to the older adult. This abnormal tissue appears to interrupt intraneuron communication. A large number of neurologic tangles has been found in people with neurologic disorders, such as Alzheimer's disease and senile dementia.[14] Because of physiologic and metabolic changes in the brain and the reduced oxygen consumption, less intracellular energy is produced; glucose use is diminished and cerebral blood flow is reduced. The electroencephalogram (EEG) of the older adult remains within the normal limits of other age groups except that it is about one cycle slower.

Substantial metabolic changes within the synaptic complexes are related to neurotransmitter production. Changes in neurotransmitter effects are known to be related to many brain functions related to neuroendocrine events such as sleep, temperature control, and especially mood. Depression is associated with reduced levels of norepinephrine in the brain, a common occurrence in older persons. Despite these changes, intellectual function in the older adult seems to be sustained.

The effects of general changes in the brain are associated with the common characteristics of aging. These include decreasing motor strength; lack of dexterity and agility; difficulties in association, retrieval, and recall; diminished memory and cognitive ability and change in affect; and often depression. The behavior resulting from these changes causes concern to the person and family.

## Cardiovascular System

Under normal circumstances, the aging heart adapts and allows the person to maintain an average level of activity. Anatomic and physiologic changes cause reduced stroke volume and cardiac output (Table 7-2). The heart begins to have difficulty adapting to the workload, especially when unusual demands are made on it. Also, if the workload is increased by such conditions as hypertension, valvular disease, or myocardial infarction, it can result in altered cardiac adaptation.

### Anatomic Changes

Anatomic changes in the heart lead to diminished contractility and filling capacity. Loss of muscle fiber in the heart with localized hypertrophy of individualized fibers

**TABLE 7-2.**
AGE CHANGES IN HEART RATE, CARDIAC OUTPUT, AND BLOOD VOLUME

| | AGE (YEARS) | | | | | | |
|---|---|---|---|---|---|---|---|
| | 20 | 30 | 40 | 50 | 60 | 70 | 80 |
| Maximum heart rate | | 190 | 182 | 174 | 164 | 155 | 146 |
| Resting heart rate | | 76 | 72 | 68 | 66 | 62 | 59 |
| Cardiac index (L/min/m²) | 3.5–3.7 | 3.5 | 3.0 | 2.8–3.1 | 2.6–3.7 | 2.4–3.6 | 2.4 |
| Blood volume (L/m²) | 2.7 | | | 2.6 | 2.6 | 2.5 | |

*Values include several studies and are means for groups.*
Source: M. A. Matteson, and E. S. McConnell, Gerontological Nursing: Concepts and Practice. *Philadelphia: Saunders, 1988. (From R. D. Kennedy, and F. I. Caird, Physiology of aging of the heart. Cardiovas. Clin. 12(1):3, 1981.)*

is due to an increased amount of collagenous material that surrounds every fiber. Thickening of the semilunar and atrioventricular valves causes increased resistance to blood flow. The end result is a heart encased in a more rigid collagen matrix, which leads to the diminished contraction and decreased filling capacity of the heart chambers.

## Physiologic Changes

The numerous physiologic changes that occur in the heart include alterations in the conduction system, loss of contractile efficiency, and decreased levels of circulating catecholamines. The evidence of changes in the heart differs at rest and with exercise. After age 60 years, peripheral vascular resistance increases 1% per year.[12] The change in peripheral resistance coupled with the anatomic and physiologic changes previously described produces numerous alterations in the capacity of cardiac performance. Cardiac output may be reduced and decreases approximately 1% per year.[12] The heart rate increase that occurs in response to stress is less effective, and the range of optimal heart rate narrows (Table 7-3). Mild tachycardia or bradycardia may lead to a significant deficit in blood flow in vital organs.

All these factors combined result in a heart that no longer has the capacity to meet all the demands that it met in earlier years. Excessive fluid load, excessive workload (as in shock or hemorrhage), and insult to the heart muscle, such as ischemia or infarction, are met by a heart muscle less able to compensate. Output may be inadequate relative to demands, which leads to many circulatory problems, such as cardiogenic shock and congestive heart failure. Even in situations of mild stress, all organs are less well perfused and therefore function inadequately.

## Conduction System Changes

The changes in the conduction system of the heart of the elderly are due to alterations in the conduction system per se and to ischemia due to interrupted blood supply through the coronary arteries. Disturbances of the autonomic nervous system and the local chemical (ionic) environment of the pacemaker cells may initiate dysrhythmias. The conduction impulses may be blocked as a result of increased fibrous tissue and fat in the myocardium, as well as loss of fibers in the bifurcating main bundle of His and the junction of the main bundle and its left fascicles.[5] Parts of the system may become irritable and susceptible to irregular discharge. Digitalis administration is a common cause of dysrhythmias in the elderly that can be potentiated by low serum potassium levels. A real danger exists when potassium-depleting diuretics are used in association with digitalis. Cardiac dysrhythmias contribute to poor cardiac output and may result in cardiac arrest.

## Arterial Changes

Blood vessels are markedly affected by degenerative changes in aging, particularly the arteries. Basic to the problems of all arteries is the progressive stiffness due to the cross-linkage effect on elastin and smooth muscle with an increase in the amount of collagen present. This generalized problem in the arteries leads to increased peripheral resistance. The major arteries demonstrate these changes as follows:[22]

1. The tunica intima becomes thickened and less smooth as arteriosclerotic streaks are accumulated.
2. In the tunica media, muscle fibers are replaced with collagen or connective tissue and calcium material.
3. The ability to expand or stretch decreases due to the changes of the intimal layers.
4. Higher blood pressures become common in the older adult, resulting from the decreased interior diameter of the arteries and diminished stretchability.
5. The aorta and its branches tend to dilate and become tortuous.

In addition, *atherosclerosis* develops. Fatty streaks in the intima have been found to be present in the first year

---

**TABLE 7-3.**
PHYSIOLOGIC CARDIOVASCULAR CHANGES WITH AGE

| AT REST | WITH EXERCISE |
|---|---|
| Heart rate unchanged | Maximal heart rate down |
| Left ventricular stroke volume down | Maximum $O_2$ consumption down |
| Cardiac output down | Atrioventricular $O_2$ up |
| Left ventricular end-diastolic pressure unchanged | Left ventricular end-diastolic pressure up |
| Ejection time up | Maximum cardiac output decreases |
| Systolic blood pressure up | Systolic blood pressure increases |
| Systemic vascular resistance up | Systemic vascular resistance up |

Source: Adapted from M. A. Matteson and E. S. McConnell, Gerontological Nursing: Concepts and Practice. Philadelphia: W.B. Saunders, 1988. (Data from: J. Lindenfeld and B. M. Groves, Cardiovascular function and disease in the aged. In R. W. Schrier, (ed.), Clinical Medicine in the Aged. Philadelphia: W.B. Saunders, 1982.)

of life. These may or may not be related to the subsequent development of atherosclerotic changes. As a person ages, the number of atheromatous plaques increases, resulting in raised areas with a central core of degenerative lipid on the tunica intima. These plaques are most numerous in the major arteries, particularly the aorta and iliac, coronary, and carotid arteries. They also occur frequently in the renal and femoral arteries. Pathologically they cause two problems: (1) thrombosis and occlusion in the lumen of the artery and (2) destruction of the tunica media leading to aneurysm. Aneurysms occur most typically in the abdominal or thoracic aorta. Arterial changes are widespread and result in diminished circulation to all organs and tissues. Of particular consequence is reduced circulation to the brain and to the kidneys. Renal plasma flow is reduced approximately 6 ml per year from 600 ml per minute per kidney in early adulthood to 300 ml per minute per kidney by age 80 years.[22]

### Venular Changes

The thin-walled veins have valves formed from the internal layer that assist the blood to flow toward the heart, but prevent a reversal of the flow. Veins constrict and enlarge, store large quantities of blood, and make it available when it is required by the circulation, and can actually propel blood forward.[19]

Because muscle contractions in the legs provide the upward propelling force for venous return, every time the legs are moved or the muscles are tensed, a certain amount of blood is propelled toward the heart. Varicose veins occur when the valves of the venous system are destroyed. They are quite common in older persons, and are usually caused by inactivity, constricting clothing, and crossing legs at the knees. The venous stasis that occurs with varicose veins further complicates the circulatory problems.

A major vascular problem of aging is that of venous thrombosis and pulmonary emboli. Immobilization from increased time spent sitting and in bed enhances the risk of thrombosis.

### Diseases Related to the Aging Cardiovascular System

Hypertension substantially increases in frequency with age, even though it is not an essential aspect of aging. Approximately 40% of Caucasians and greater than 50% of blacks over the age of 65 have hypertension.[25] The systolic pressure gradually increases with age due to decreased aortic elasticity. The increase in diastolic pressure is less marked and results from increased resistance in the peripheral blood vessels. The diastolic pressure tends to level off in later life. Cardiac output and blood volume are also factors in the regulation of blood pres-

sure. Blood pressure is elevated through increased resistance to blood flow due to arteriolar constriction. Blood pressure lowers when arteriolar relaxation reduces resistance to blood flow.

Benign essential hypertension is the most common type in persons over 70 years, with more than 90% of all cases in this category.[29] Elevated pressure usually develops slowly with little untoward effect in benign essential hypertension. Complications due to hypertension account for a significant number of the deaths in the United States.

Hypertension contributes considerably to diseases of the cardiovascular system. It is associated with increased frequency of coronary artery disease and myocardial infarction, and with hemorrhagic problems and infarcts in the brain. It is also associated with major hemorrhage from cerebral arteries and resultant strokes.

Transient cerebral ischemic attacks may occur prior to major strokes. These attacks are due to arterial occlusion or hypotension. The occlusive phenomena occur most frequently in the carotid artery. The signs are hemiparesis, hemianopsia, aphasia, and loss of vision in one eye. The vertebral artery is more often involved with hypotensive states, causing the person to fall forward on the knees without loss of consciousness, vertigo, vomiting, dysarthria, visual blurring, or diplopia.[8]

The baroreceptors in the aorta and carotid arteries become less sensitive to pressure changes, and sudden changes in position may cause dizziness or syncope. Pressure on the carotid sinus may cause serious slowing of the heart rate and may be elicited by twisting and turning of the head.

## Respiratory System

Alterations in the respiratory system in the aged impose many limitations that are not always obvious when the person is at rest but appear with exertion or stress. Under usual circumstances, older persons are capable of maintaining usual daily activities, but various changes make them more susceptible to pulmonary infections. Various consequences of the aging respiratory system are presented in Figure 7-3. Among aged individuals, influenza and pneumonia are the fourth leading causes of death, with bronchitis, emphysema, and asthma ranking eighth.[13]

### Anatomic Changes

Loss of elasticity affects the older person's pulmonary compliance and results from increased cross-linkage in collagen and elastin fibers around the alveolar sacs. Pressure builds up within the alveolar sacs during inspiration, some of which tends to be retained during expiration, and finally results in an increased residual air volume. In

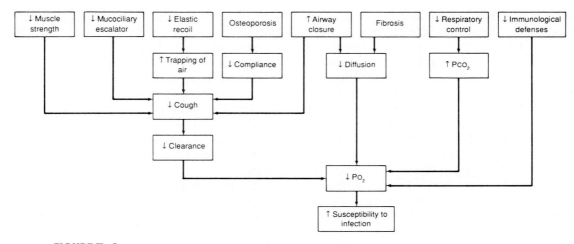

**FIGURE 7–3.**

Aging of the respiratory system and its consequences. (From K.K. Esberger and S.T. Hughes, *Nursing Care of the Aged.* Norwalk, Conn.: Appleton and Lange, 1989.)

addition, there is a decrease in the quantity of air that can be taken in during normal breathing.

Changes in the costal cartilage result in a diminution of chest wall compliance, which is further complicated by skeletal deformities of the thorax and postural changes such as stooped shoulders. In the older adult, the changes in the muscular system lead to a decline in the strength of muscles that assist respiration. Degeneration of the intervertebral disks of the thoracic spine results in increased anteroposterior diameter of the chest and a chest wall that is less compliant during respiration.

The end result of the loss of elasticity, the muscle weakness and changes in the structure of the chest, is difficulty in expiration of air. Results of pulmonary function studies are altered as a result of this reduced capacity to empty the lungs. Total lung capacity is changed little, but vital capacity is gradually and progressively reduced. The forced expiratory volume and maximum breathing capacity are both reduced, while the residual volume and functional residual capacity of the lungs are increased (Figure 7-4). The residual volume increases 50% between ages 30 and 90 years. The maximum breathing capacity is diminished by 60% between ages 20 and 80 years.[17] Actual air flow is reduced 20% to 50% throughout the adult years.

### Functional Changes

The main functional respiratory problems in the elderly person without pulmonary disease are reduced ventilation of all alveoli, especially at the bases of the lungs, and reduced oxygen partial pressure in the arterial blood. The partial pressure of arterial oxygen ($PaO_2$) declines with age, averaging 75 mm Hg in the seventh decade. The partial pressure of carbon dioxide ($PCO_2$), however, remains the same unless disease is superimposed on the

diminished ventilation; this is probably due to the higher rate of diffusion of carbon dioxide. With the structural and mechanical changes described above, the bases of the lungs are ventilated less and less. The part of the lungs that is well perfused is the part of the lungs not being ventilated. Blood must be shunted to the ventilated upper portions of the lungs. The redistribution of blood is usually insufficient to compensate and the arterial partial pressure of oxygen falls. The condition becomes

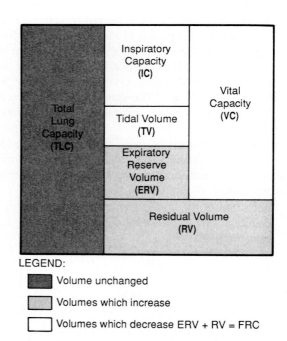

**FIGURE 7–4.**

Changes in lung volume with aging. TLC does not change with aging. As the amount of air trapped increases, the amount of air that is moved by breathing is decreased. (From K.K. Esberger and S.T. Hughes, *Nursing Care of the Aged.* Norwalk, Conn.: Appleton and Lange, 1989.)

worse when the elderly person lies down, and nocturnal hypoxemia may be a major cause of confusion.

Functional deficits may not impair function under baseline conditions with minimal physical exertion. Changes in the capacity to increase the work of breathing due to structural changes in the chest wall, and the structural changes that reduce the maximum breathing capacity, however, put the elderly person at risk for respiratory infections. The need to increase oxygen intake rapidly or to blow off carbon dioxide rapidly due to acidemia may cause decompensation and rapid respiratory failure in an elderly person with no respiratory disease per se. Sudden increases in physical activity or sudden psychologic stress may overwhelm a respiratory system that handles moderate stress well.

An elderly person with little previous difficulty may develop respiratory failure rather rapidly after stress such as surgery, excessive exercise, a sudden rise in environmental pollution (as in smog crises), or infection such as pneumonia. The assumption must be made that all elderly individuals are at risk for respiratory failure. Respiratory failure is evidenced by a diminishing $PaO_2$ and a rising $PaCO_2$ associated with a drop in arterial pH.

Potential causes of respiratory failure are surgery, the use of depressant drugs, lung infections, bedrest, pulmonary edema due to circulatory problems, and pulmonary embolism. Pulmonary embolism occurs frequently in elderly patients who are immobilized due to bone fractures or other conditions requiring bedrest. Any acute condition such as trauma, burns, or myocardial infarction in the elderly may be complicated by respiratory failure. The potential of unrecognized pulmonary changes, particularly those due to environmental effects, is present in all persons over age 40 years.

In addition to functional changes, which are normal alterations with aging, most persons in modern Western society have lung changes due to chronic environmental pollution. Inhalants such as smoke, various industrial end products, and the end products of combustion of petrochemicals have a profound effect on respiratory function. They cause decreased ciliary action, increased mucus production, and deposition of foreign materials in the functional alveoli and in intercellular spaces. These pollutants have two main effects: (1) they increase the obstructive component in lung function and (2) they decrease the compliance of the lung tissue through deposits of foreign material increasing its stiffness. The latter is common among miners and industrial workers who constantly inhale coal dust or asbestos.

## Genitourinary System

Genitourinary conditions in older adults are common problems that many of these individuals are reluctant to discuss. In addition to causing embarrassment, they are bothersome and frequently thought of as another sign of growing old. Renal dysfunctions are potentially life-threatening and become more so because of delay in detection and treatment.

### Anatomic Changes in the Kidneys

The urinary tract undergoes many changes with age. The kidneys are affected by involutional processes, and normal age-related changes occur in renal vascular anatomy and function independent of disease. The nephrons begin to degenerate and disappear by the seventh month in utero. The normal young adult has approximately 800,000 to 1 million nephrons in each kidney.[19] These gradually degenerate and their number is reduced by one-third to one-half by the seventh decade.[17] Changes in kidney size, volume, and filtering surface over the life span are shown in Table 7-4.[18]

In addition to the loss of nephrons, there is some degeneration of the remaining nephrons. The degeneration starts as a sclerosis or scarring of the glomeruli, followed by atrophy of the afferent arterioles. The glomeruli, deep in the cortex of the kidney, retain one capillary that enlarges and acts as a shunt between the afferent and efferent arterioles. The compensation that does occur results from enlargement of the remaining nephrons. Despite enlargement of the nephrons, the net weight of each kidney decreases by about 20% to 30% and occurs primarily in the cortex.[12]

### Physiologic Changes in the Kidneys

Due to the loss of nephrons or functional units of the kidneys, a decline in function is to be expected with age. The kidneys do not concentrate urine as well because of the loss of nephrons. Under normal circumstances, however, the kidneys are capable of maintaining acid-base balance.

The renal filtration rate decreases about 6% per decade. As general arteriosclerosis occurs throughout the body, the arterioles in the kidneys are also affected. The result is that some of the blood is diverted to other parts

**TABLE 7–4.**
CHANGE IN KIDNEY SIZE, VOLUME, AND FILTERING SURFACE ACROSS THE LIFE SPAN

|  | At Birth | Young Adult | Over 65 Years | Percentage Loss |
|---|---|---|---|---|
| Kidney mass (gm) | 50 | 270 | 185 | 31 |
| Kidney volume (mL) | 20 | 250 | 200 | 20 |
| Filtering surface area (m²) | 0.02 | 1.6 | 0.9 | 43 |

of the body and does not pass through the glomerular filtration system. Gradual decreases in renal blood flow and glomerular filtration rate are related to decreases in cardiac output, renal mass, and filtering surface of the kidneys.[25]

The physiologic alterations result in slower renal adaptation to excess acid or alkaline loads in the elderly. Even minor stress can cause disruption in kidney function, and aged kidneys have difficulty in restabilizing.

## Diseases and Problems with Aging Kidneys

Renal function in the elderly may be compromised by one or more of the following: (1) inadequate fluid intake, (2) fluid loss due to vomiting or diarrhea, (3) shock due to hemorrhage, (4) acute or chronic cardiac failure, (5) septicemia due to gram-negative bacteria, and (6) injudicious use of diuretics.[15] Any one of these may result in renal ischemia and acute renal shutdown if not promptly corrected.

The minimum urinary output should be 400 ml daily. Output of 20 ml per hour or less may herald acute renal failure. Acute renal failure (ARF) frequently arises in the elderly and carries a mortality in persons 70 years and over of 80%. The dangers of ARF include: (1) fluid overloading, leading to congestive heart failure and pulmonary edema, and (2) rising serum potassium level, which may cause cardiac arrest.

Diseases of the kidneys, regardless of the cause, create long-term problems. In addition to the various pathologic events associated with such diseases, the elderly also must adapt to the normal changes of aging. The most frequent chronic kidney disease in the elderly is pyelonephritis. Associated physiologic conditions are hypertension, sodium and water retention, marked sodium or water loss, retention of potassium, and loss of serum protein. The greatest concern is inability of the kidneys to handle changing concentrations of hydrogen ion. The responses to increased hydrogen ion concentration are slowed and diminished, leading to metabolic acidosis.

Several antibiotics often used in infections of the elderly are nephrotoxic, including tetracycline, cephaloridine, and gentamycin. Occasionally, penicillin also has this effect. It is not uncommon for an elderly person who has sepsis from an infection followed by treatment with one of these antibiotics to develop ARF. It is difficult to ascertain under such circumstances whether renal failure is caused by the antibiotic or by the shock associated with the infection.

## Bladder Changes

Two of the most common and bothersome problems the elderly encounter are nocturnal frequency of micturition and urinary incontinence. Among changes that contribute to these problems are loss of muscle tone that results in relaxation of the perineal muscles in the female, prostatic hypertrophy in the male, bladder diverticuli, sphincter relaxation, and altered bladder reflexes (Figure 7-5). Frequently, bladder capacity is reduced. Incomplete emptying of the bladder predisposes the elderly person to residual urine and infection.

*Escherichia coli* is the most frequent cause of bladder infection in women, while *Proteus* species are the most common in men.[11] Bladder infections can result from poor hygienic practices or from anything that impedes urinary flow, such as neoplasms, strictures, or a clogged indwelling catheter. Urine may become alkaline in the presence of an infection, leading to the formation of small inorganic salt calculi. Hematuria, gross or microscopic, may occur with urinary tract infections (see Chap. 33).

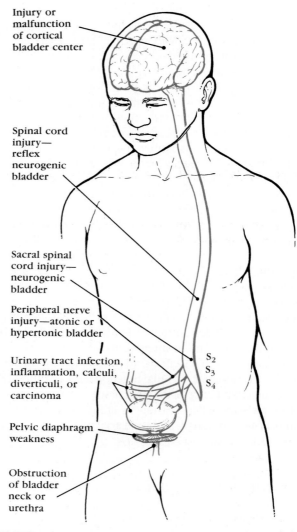

Injury or malfunction of cortical bladder center

Spinal cord injury— reflex neurogenic bladder

Sacral spinal cord injury— neurogenic bladder

Peripheral nerve injury—atonic or hypertonic bladder

Urinary tract infection, inflammation, calculi, diverticuli, or carcinoma

$S_2$
$S_3$
$S_4$

Pelvic diaphragm weakness

Obstruction of bladder neck or urethra

**FIGURE 7-5.**
Stresses that contribute to urinary incontinence.

## Gynecologic Changes in the Elderly Woman

In the elderly woman, objective gynecologic findings are directly related to the effects of estrogen deprivation. General atrophy occurs in the reproductive system, causing a reduction in the size of the uterus and cervix; thinning of the vaginal walls; changes in mucous secretions; and greater friability and susceptibility of vaginal tissue to irritation and infection. Due to diminished secretions, the vagina loses normal flora that create its protective acid environment. Atrophic changes result in a vulva that is pallid and has a loss of subcutaneous fat accompanied by a flattening and folding of the labia. Breast tissue thins and sags as a result of replacement of atrophying glandular tissue with fat.

## Reproductive Changes in the Elderly Man

Physiologic changes in the elderly man are also due to lowered hormone production and occur much more gradually than in the female. The testes undergo cellular change with no significant change in size. Fat content increases in testicular cells, accompanied by a decrease in the number of cells. The number of sperm ejaculated decreases by up to 50% by age 90 years. Sperm change in size and shape and lose their fertilization ability.[3] Androgen production begins to decline at age 30 and continues to decline until age 90 years.

Most elderly men have some benign prostatic hyperplasia, which is considered to be a normal aging change. The changes result in a prostate that is more fibrous and has irregular thickening. The frequency of prostatic cancer also increases with age (see Chaps. 34 and 55).

## Gastrointestinal System

### Normal Anatomic Changes

The gastrointestinal system is the source of many diseases in the elderly that range from simple dyspepsia to carcinomas. Contributing to the prevalence of these conditions are many normal features of aging (Table 7-5). The grinding surfaces of the molars have worn down, and many elderly persons have lost most or all of their teeth. With the loss of chewing ability, they may eat soft food, thereby developing gum and digestive problems. Altered taste sensation due to a decline in numbers of taste buds fosters a poor appetite, and this can result in malnutrition.

### Esophageal Changes

Changes in esophageal motility begin to occur with aging. Degenerative changes in smooth muscle that lines the lower two-thirds of the esophagus result in a delay in esophageal emptying, dilatation of the esophagus, and an increase in nonpropulsive contractions.[1,6] Obstructive phenomena can occur as a result of tumors, rings, or strictures.

**TABLE 7–5.**
GASTROINTESTINAL CHANGES OF AGING

| CHANGE | COMPLICATION OR ASSOCIATION |
|---|---|
| Loss of teeth | Poor intake, large bolus |
| Loss of tongue papilla, taste, and smell | Poor appetite, weight loss |
| Reduced salivary ptyalin | Slightly reduced carbohydrate digestion |
| Reduced esophageal peristal | Delayed emptying, presbyesophagus |
| Irregular nonperistalitic esophageal waves | Delayed emptying, presbyesophagus |
| Poor relaxation of esophageal sphincter | Delayed emptying, presbyesophagus |
| Hiatal hernia | Esophagitis, bleeding |
| Thinned gastric mucosa and muscularis; decreased gastrin, gastric acid, pepsin, intrinsic factor | Atrophic gastritis, iron deficiency anemia, pernicious anemia, ulcer, carcinoma |
| Decreased colonic muscle tone; decreased colonic motor function | Constipation |
| Diverticulosis | Diverticulitis |
| Reduced liver weight and blood flow | None |
| Decreased liver inducible enzymes | Altered drug metabolism |
| Reduced serum albumin | Weakness, weight loss |
| Increased globulin | None |
| Cholelithiasis | Cholecystitis |

Source: M. O'Hara-Devereaux, L. H. Andous, and C. D. Scott (eds.), Eldercare: A Practical Guide to Clinical Geriatrics. New York: Grune & Stratton, 1981, p. 100.

The risk of hiatal hernia in persons over 50 years of age may be as high as 40% to 60%. Small hiatal hernias are so common that they are frequently considered a normal finding on radiographs.[30] Difficulty in swallowing is one of the primary symptoms. Hiatal hernias can mimic pulmonary distress and angina; therefore, radiographs should be performed to verify the diagnosis.

### Stomach Changes

It is thought that the stomach mucosa becomes thinner; however, in some studies it has been indicated that gastric mucosa remains normal in individuals up to ages 80 and 90 years.[1] It is generally thought that gastric acid secretion is decreased with age. Pernicious anemia is common in the elderly because vitamin $B_{12}$ is dependent on the gastric intrinsic factor for its absorption (see Chap. 40). Gastric motility and gastric emptying appear to decrease with age.

### Colon Changes

Constipation is one of the most frequent complaints of the elderly. In a large percentage, constipation is due to cultural eating patterns, decreased exercise, decreased gastric motility, low fluid intake, and the ingestion of drugs such as antihypertensives and sedatives. Constipation in the elderly is compounded by the abuse of purgatives, laxatives, and enemas, which are employed to resolve constipation—a vicious cycle is created.

Diseases of the colon that are common in the elderly include diverticulosis, diverticulitis, polyposis, and cancer of the colon (see Chap. 41). Diverticulosis is considered to be a disease of aging, with the majority of diverticuli arising in the sigmoid colon. Most of the diseases are asymptomatic but occult blood in the stool is common, especially with colon cancer.

### Pancreatic Changes

The pancreas changes with age are associated with pancreatic ductal epithelial hyperplasia and intralobular fibrosis.[1] On rare occasions, this fibrosis may lead to atrophy. There is a decline in the volume of pancreatic secretions and a diminished enzyme output with advanced age. However, the importance of these changes in causing dysfunction or nutritional impairment has not been thoroughly researched.[1]

### Liver Changes

There is a decrease in liver size and hepatic blood flow with advancing age. Hepatocytes tend to be larger with an increased nuclear DNA. A brown atrophied appearance of the liver is seen in older persons as a result of deposited lipofuscin granules in hepatocytes. However, this trait has also been found in younger individuals who have cachexia or malnutrition.[1] Hepatic parenchymal fibrosis may be present but has no apparent functional significance.

## Musculoskeletal System

One of the most visible characteristics of aging is the change in posture and patterns of movement. Successful portrayal of an old person by an actor nearly always includes certain features of body movement, such as stooped posture, muscular rigidity, slow movement, and lack of coordination and stability. Alterations in neuromuscular function result from the combined effect of changes in the muscles, the peripheral motor neurons, the myoneural synapses, and the CNS. Diet, heredity, and hormonal balances also are influences on the musculoskeletal system.

### Characteristic Changes in Anatomic Structure and Function

General wasting of skeletal muscles occurs due to loss of muscle fibers. Muscle strength, endurance, and agility are affected by the decrease in muscle mass. All muscle activity in the elderly is affected by the degree of oxygen supply and its alterations, which are due to reduced circulatory and respiratory function. The peripheral motor neurons also have some decrease in protein synthesis, with thickening at the myoneural junction and decrease in acetylcholine levels.

The general decrease in movement, coupled with muscle stiffness and slowness, particularly in initiating movement, is attributable primarily to prolongation of contraction time, latency period, and relaxation period of motor units, as well as changes in the extrapyramidal system. A resting tremor may also be present. These changes are considered normal. If the extrapyramidal function becomes severely impaired, Parkinson's syndrome, chorea, or dystonia of various types may appear.

In addition to the wasting of skeletal muscles, loss of minerals causes the bones to become more brittle. The amount of trabecular bone begins to decrease in the mid 30s. By age 90 years, women lose 43% of trabecular bone, while men lose 27% by age 80 years. Cortical (compact) bone loss begins to occur in the mid 40s in women and 50s in men. This bone loss results in a change in cortical-trabecular bone ratio from 55:45 at age 15 years, to a ratio of 70:30 at age 85 years.[25] Reduction in height results from hip and knee flexion, kyphosis of the dorsal spine, and shortening of the vertebral column (see Chap. 45).

## Joint Changes

Joint changes in the elderly include the following: (1) erosion of the cartilagenous surface of the joints, (2) degenerative changes of the soft tissue in the joints, and (3) calcification and ossification of the ligaments, especially those around the vertebrae. The name given to the degenerative processes of the joints is *osteoarthritis*. Once again, it is difficult to determine how much of this process is normal aging because it is present in all persons to some degree. It may begin at age 20 years, and by age 50 years radiologic changes may be present.[17]

The cartilage of the joints loses elasticity, becomes dull and opaque, and then softens and frays, denuding the underlying bone. The underlying bone develops a proliferation of fibroblasts, and new bone is formed. At the joint margins, extensive proliferation produces bony outgrowths or spurs. When spurs project into the joint, they can cause considerable pain and limitation of motion. Pieces of cartilage and bone may break off to form loose bodies in the joint that require surgical removal.

Changes in joints are probably the result of long-term trauma. Alterations resulting from osteoarthritis are easily seen in the fingers with the development of Heberden's and Bouchard's nodes (Figure 7-6). When overgrowth of the bone margins occurs on the fingers, most often in women, it may be unsightly but is generally not painful. When bone overgrowth occurs about the hip, the femoral head may become trapped, painful, and immobile. Hip replacement surgery may be required. The cartilaginous disks that exist between the vertebrae undergo the same pathologic changes that take place in the other joints. The degenerative changes are contributed to by the predisposing factors of aging, extensive involvement in physical activities leading to injury, excessive use of the joint, and obesity. These pathologic changes are accompanied by pain and limitation of motion.

## Problems Related to Skeletal Degeneration

*Osteoporosis* is basically caused by an increase of bone absorption over bone formation. This primarily affects trabecular bone and also the cortices of long bones. The outer surfaces of long bones continue to grow slowly throughout life, but with osteoporosis, the inner surfaces are resorbed at a slightly faster rate. The end result is a long bone that is slightly longer in external diameter but with thinner walls and with markedly diminished trabecular bone in its ends. Vertebral bodies, which have a larger percentage of trabecular bone, are severely affected by this process.[2]

In osteoporosis, there is evidence of decreased calcium absorption from the gastrointestinal tract. Also, the disease has some relationship with gonad deficiency, as its frequency is greatly increased in postmenopausal women. Immobilization and lack of weight bearing on the skeletal system causes osteoporosis at any age. Also, elevated levels of cortisone, either exogenous or endogenous, cause the condition. Regardless of the underlying pathologic process, osteoporosis occurs to a degree in all elderly persons, but is much more marked in women.

Of primary concern in osteoporosis is the tendency for bone fracture, most frequently of the vertebrae and the femurs. Studies in the elderly show that 34% of fractures of the femur are due to accidents.[3] Twenty-five percent are due to a "drop attack," which is a sudden fall due to postural instability that results from changes in the hindbrain and cerebellum. The person suddenly falls to the ground without warning or with a momentary vertigo. In examining all the causes of falls for 384 persons evaluated in one study, the most frequent cause was tripping, the second most frequent was loss of balance, and the third most frequent was drop attack.[3] Forty-three percent of the total sample had neurologic disease.

Kyphosis, or curvature of the spine, in older persons frequently occurs as a result of osteoporosis of the vertebrae. Vertebral atrophy also occurs. Due to the progressive degeneration, the number of cells diminishes, the water content decreases, and the tissues lose turgor and become friable. The combined changes in the vertebrae and disks result in curvature of the spine. Kyphosis

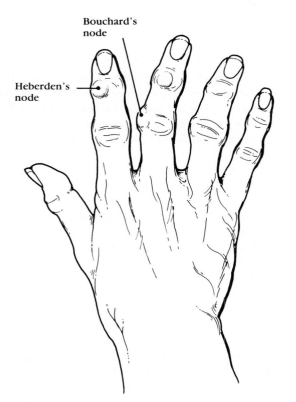

**FIGURE 7–6.**
Heberden's and Bouchard's nodes in an elderly individual. Note the lateral deviation of the third and ring fingers.

causes decreased respiratory capacity of the chest wall and conditions due to impingement on various spinal nerves from the narrowed disks and vertebral changes. These problems are most often related to the lumbar and cervical spine. Compression fractures of the spine are also common.

### Fractures and Risk of Falling

In the aged individual, there is an increased risk for falling and bone fractures. This may be due to cerebral vascular disease which often causes difficulty in locomotion of the elderly. Arteriosclerosis of the carotid and vertebral arteries resulting in ischemia may cause transient paralysis or lightheadedness, poor balance, and falling episodes. When such events occur, the person becomes anxious and tense about moving, and coordination is reduced even further. Older persons who fear falling tend to take fewer and fewer risks; the result is increased immobility. Individuals who have had cerebrovascular accidents tend to have hemiparesis or hemiplegia. Those who recover from such episodes tend to have some motor disability that creates difficulty in walking, postural changes both in sitting and standing, residual spasticity, and footdrop. These factors increase the risk for falling.

Injury from falling is a very real problem for the elderly. Fractures of the hip and wrist are frequent, as is head injury. The fractures are often the result of osteoporosis causing decreased bone strength. Hospitalization and surgical procedures for fractures carry a high risk.

## Skin and Dermal Appendages

### Changes in the Skin, Nails, and Hair

Next to alterations in the musculoskeletal system, changes in the integument are the most obvious with aging. With loss of elasticity, wrinkles, lines, and drooping eyelids occur. Exposed areas, such as the hands, develop age spots or excessive skin pigmentation. The skin becomes dry, thin, fragile, and prone to injury. Nails become dry and brittle. Toenails become susceptible to fungal infection and appear thickened; there is a lifting of the nail plates. The rate of change is very individual and is dependent on such factors as nutrition, genetics, emotions, and environment. Changes that occur in the various layers of the skin are depicted in Figure 7-7.

Numerous problems occur due to the changes in the skin. The loss of water, which is the basis for many problems in the elderly, results from atrophy of all skin layers, with diminished vascularity and decreased elasticity. Lack of water leads to pruritis and decubitus ulcers. Lesions such as tumors, warts, and keratoses may arise with no pain; however, lesions such as herpes zoster may be very painful. Sebaceous and sweat glands become less active and contribute to dry skin.

Another inevitable change is the loss of pigment, or graying; its onset and degree may vary greatly. There is also generalized thinning of the hair, contributed to by a decrease in the density of hair follicles. In older females, the hair appears finer and more sparse; some axillary and pubic hair is lost. Often, an increase in facial hair is noted due to decreased estrogen production after menopause. Older males frequently have hair growth in ears and nares, and the eyebrows grow more bushy. Men are more susceptible to alopecia than women, with genetics playing a part in the degree and rapidity of balding.

### Diseases Associated with Aging Skin

The skin often reflects other disease conditions such as liver or cardiac disease. Relatively minor skin problems, such as overgrowths of epidermal tissue, cause cosmetic problems but rarely need surgical excision. *Senile telangiectasias*, small scarlet growths scattered over the skin, increase in number after middle age. *Hyperkeratotic warts*, raised brown or black epidermal overgrowths, also develop in increased numbers with age. These two types of lesions, together with others that occur less frequently, have no clinical significance and do not require removal unless irritated by clothing or jewelry. Cancers of the skin are very common, especially in fair-skinned individuals or in sun-damaged skin (see Chap. 47).

## Sensory System

Few persons escape sensory deficits as they age. They become more vulnerable to injury, more isolated from society, and less able to care for their personal needs as these deficits occur. Deficits are greatest in sight, hearing, taste, smell, and touch, and interfere with the ability to communicate.

### Vision Changes

With age, changes take place in both the structural and functional aspects of the eyes. Eyelids become thinner and wrinkled, and skin folds result from loss of orbital fat, leading to proptosis. Inversion or eversion of the lids is common, and the conjunctivae are thinner and more fragile.

*Arcus senilis*, a bluish gray ring, may surround the corneal limbus and be visible against the darker pigments of the eye. Arcus senilis is a harmless change and does not affect visual acuity. Light brown patches may occur in the irides, changing their appearance but not their ability to regulate pupil size. The lenses may develop changes that cause vision problems such as loss of elasticity or presbyopia (see Chap. 49).

Cataracts may develop as a result of loss of soluble proteins and with loss of lens transparency. The cloudy,

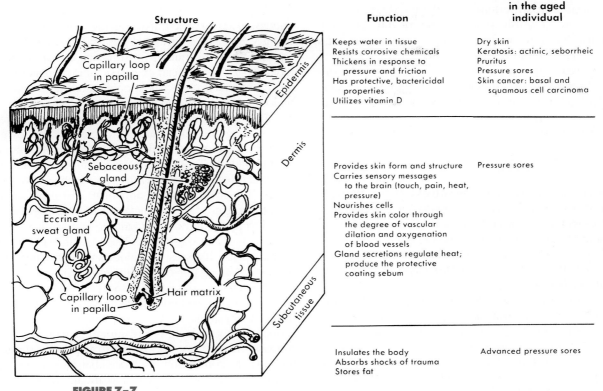

| Structure | Function | Skin condition in the aged individual |
|---|---|---|
| Epidermis | Keeps water in tissue<br>Resists corrosive chemicals<br>Thickens in response to pressure and friction<br>Has protective, bactericidal properties<br>Utilizes vitamin D | Dry skin<br>Keratosis: actinic, seborrheic<br>Pruritus<br>Pressure sores<br>Skin cancer: basal and squamous cell carcinoma |
| Dermis | Provides skin form and structure<br>Carries sensory messages to the brain (touch, pain, heat, pressure)<br>Nourishes cells<br>Provides skin color through the degree of vascular dilation and oxygenation of blood vessels<br>Gland secretions regulate heat; produce the protective coating sebum | Pressure sores |
| Subcutaneous tissue | Insulates the body<br>Absorbs shocks of trauma<br>Stores fat | Advanced pressure sores |

**FIGURE 7-7.**
How structure and function of the skin change with age. (From R. Ebersole and P. Hess, *Toward Healthy Aging* [2nd ed.]. St. Louis: Mosby, 1985.)

hazy lens results in visual loss. Reduced transmission of light causes distant objects to become hazy. Surgical excision may become necessary if the cataracts become too dense.

Glaucoma is another major eye problem that affects the aged. Glaucoma accounts for about 10% of all blindness in the United States.[13] Intraocular pressure rises rapidly in acute glaucoma and slowly in chronic glaucoma. Peripheral vision and night vision are both affected. The decline in peripheral vision may occur slowly and interferes with driving ability. Medications and surgery are now available to treat glaucoma. Early treatment is essential because the blindness that results is irreversible.

### Hearing Changes

With aging, changes may develop in the functional ability of the ears, as well as their external appearance. Population studies indicate that beginning in the third decade of life, hearing gradually deteriorates.[16]

The external ears undergo very little change other than some slight elongation of the lobes. Cerumen decreases in amount but contains a greater amount of keratin, which easily becomes impacted and difficult to remove. Impacted cerumen can block sound waves and cause temporary hearing loss until it is removed.

Sclerosis or atrophy of the tympanic membrane affects the middle ear usually by reducing the number of high frequency sound waves reaching the inner ear. Loss of cells at the base of the cochlea leads to retrocochlear loss of efficiency. The ability to hear high-frequency sounds is reduced first, and is followed by loss of ability to hear lower frequencies. The term used to describe progressive hearing loss in the aging is *presbycusis*. This bilaterally symmetric perceptive hearing loss starts at about the fourth decade, but the effects are usually not noticeable at their outset.

Exposure to excessive noise, recurrent otitis media in younger years, trauma to the ears, and certain drugs contribute to hearing loss. Persons living or working in highly industrialized areas experience more hearing loss than those in nonindustrial areas.

### Other Sensory Changes

The aging process does not have as dramatic an effect on taste, smell, and touch as it does on vision and hearing, but these senses are also reduced. There is an obvious decrease in ability to taste sweet and salty flavors due to a decrease in the number of taste buds. Diet becomes an important factor because the aging person tends to eat more sweets and to salt food more heavily. The sweets lead to obesity and increased dental problems, and the salt may aggravate hypertension when it exists. Olfactory function may diminish, resulting in inability to smell, which also interferes with appetite. It also can present a hazard in the case of fire or smoke.

A decrease in tactile sensation may be noted by difficulty discriminating temperature changes. Older persons tend to burn themselves because of this change. Minor injuries occur as a result of occasional unawareness of pain or pressure.

## Aging and Cancer

Cancer is a serious problem, regardless of age. Because cancers are multifaceted diseases whose prevalence often increases with age, a brief discussion of cancer and aging is presented here. Even though the prevalence of cancer is higher in older persons, certain types are diagnosed less frequently, including cervical cancer and sarcoma. Several factors are associated with cancer, although the exact etiology is unknown. Constant irritation from smoking a pipe can cause oral cancers, chewing tobacco can result in cancer of the mouth, and smoking cigarettes can lead to carcinoma of the lung. The percentage of lung cancer was once highest in men, but the disease is increasing in women due to the increase in number of women who smoke.

Environmental factors such as air pollution, food additives, asbestos, and certain chemicals are carcinogenic. According to the National Research Council, evidence indicates that most common cancers are influenced by diet, although there are no precise estimations of the impact of foods on cancer. Support exists for a viral cause of certain malignancies (see Chap. 18).

Chemical carcinogens produce different effects at different periods of life. Chemical carcinogenesis occurs most readily in the aged. The assumption is that there is either an accumulated effect on the DNA of the cell or an accumulated risk for a cell to become malignant.

The majority of persons with carcinoma of the colon are in the older age group. This cancer is usually very slow-growing and remains localized for a long time. Early surgical removal is beneficial.

Cancer of the prostate is the most common tumor of men over age 85 years.[17] The disease is known to metastasize to the pelvis, vertebrae, and other bony sites, as well as to the brain. Breast cancer is common in elderly women and is often discovered during examination for other conditions.

Chronic lymphocytic leukemia, lymphosarcoma, and myeloma are malignancies with a high frequency in the elderly population. Hodgkin's disease tends to run a rapid course in the aged, while malignancies of the lung, oral cavity, larynx, and gastrointestinal tract seem to have a similar prognosis in young and old.

## DRUGS AND THE ELDERLY

Aged persons use one-third of all prescribed drugs in this country. Most take several drugs and also use over-the-counter agents frequently.[28] All drugs can pose risks to elderly persons and can decrease their mental, physical, and functional status.[23] Nutritional status may be impaired by long-term use of certain drugs.

The elderly are the least able to tolerate injudicious use of drugs because many physiologic changes make them respond to medication in more variable ways than younger adults. These physiologic changes result in a system that is less able to distribute, metabolize, and excrete drugs. The liver, kidneys, and heart are most involved with drug excretion and metabolism. Because they may have lost some of their efficiency, compounds may accumulate and cause toxicity. The cumulative effects of trauma, prior illnesses, accidents, and disabilities further reduce the aging person's ability to handle drugs.

Pharmacokinetic (drug disposition in the body) factors have been studied in relationship to absorption in the gastrointestinal tract, which would theoretically be reduced in the elderly as a result of changes in intestinal mucosa, blood flow, and motility. At present, however, there is no convincing evidence that alterations in absorption actually occur.[7] With age, the total body composition changes, with a higher percentage of fat tissue and less lean tissue and water. The disposition of drugs that are selectively used in different tissues is affected. Also, body size decreases; thus, the concentration of the drug in the body is higher for standard dosages. Plasma binding by albumin in the elderly decreases 20%. Drugs that are normally plasma focused are therefore increased in concentration in the tissues.

Metabolism of drugs by the liver is diminished in the elderly by poor circulation to the liver, by a reduction in the hepatic mass, and by the possible decrease in hepatic enzymes. Any disease of the liver will aggravate this considerably. Some of the most common drugs metabolized by the liver that have increased half-life in the elderly are the antidepressants diazepam (Valium) and chlordiazepoxide (Librium).

Another problem is reduced excretion due to diminished renal function. Renal reserve is markedly reduced as people age, and the ability to excrete drugs is also markedly reduced. Drug action in the elderly is also altered by changes in tissue responses. There may be an increased threshold to the drug's actions. Also, there may be a decrease in the number of receptive sites for the drug, coupled with a decrease in the necessary enzymes. A summary of alterations in the pharmacokinetic variables in the elderly is presented in Table 7-6.

Listed high among drugs that can be dangerous to the elderly are antibiotics, such as tetracyclines and gentamycin. Antibiotics are excreted by the kidneys, and re-

**TABLE 7–6.**
ALTERATION OF PHARMACOKINETIC VALUES IN THE ELDERLY,
INCLUDING CLINICAL IMPORTANCE

| FACTOR | ALTERED PHYSIOLOGY | CLINICAL IMPORTANCE |
|---|---|---|
| Absorption | Elevated gastric pH<br>Reduced gastrointestinal blood flow<br>Possible changed number of absorbing cells<br>Possible altered gastrointestinal motility | Studies have not supported any loss of absorptive ability |
| Distribution | Decreased total body water<br>Decreased lean body tissue mass/ kg body weight<br>Increased body fat | Higher concentration of drugs distributed in body fluids<br><br>Possible longer duration of action of fat-soluble drugs |
| Protein binding | Decreased serum albumin concentrations | Increased unbound plasma concentrations of highly protein-bound drugs |
| Metabolism | Decreased hepatic blood flow; decreased hepatic mass; possible decreased enzyme activity | Decreased hepatic clearance, drugs will have decreased clearance |
| Elimination | Decreased glomerular filtration rate<br>Decreased renal plasma flow<br>Altered tubular function | Decreased renal clearance of drugs and metabolites |

duced kidney function can lead to toxic accumulation of the agents. Mental disturbances, gastrointestinal side effects, and rashes are some toxic effects.[7] When diuretics, which cause potassium loss, are given in combination with digoxin, the danger of dysrhythmias is greatly increased. The effect of digitalis on the conduction system is enhanced by low serum potassium levels. Many of the antihypertensive agents have diverse side effects, but they all possess the ability to cause hypotension. Orthostatic hypotension can lead to falls and fractures. Elderly persons should be warned of this possibility, and when taking antihypertensives they should be cautioned not to rise too rapidly from a supine or sitting position.

The elderly person does not display the toxic effects of digoxin, such as gastrointestinal and ocular symptoms, that usually arise in younger adults. This makes digoxin one of the drugs that places the older individual at grave risk. Digoxin blood levels are not always a good guide to toxicity because the elderly person reacts more commonly with electrocardiogram changes and confusion. Toxic blood levels may not be seen but the effects may be present.

Many elderly persons develop nutritional problems from long-term use of medications such as laxatives. Mineral oil can interfere with absorption of nutrients and vitamins in the intestinal tract, and its use should be discouraged.

## REFERENCES

1. Altman, D.F. Changes in gastrointestinal, pancreatic, biliary, and hepatic function with aging. *Gastroenterol. Clin. N. Am.* 19:227, 1990.
2. Barzel, U. Common metabolic disorders of the skeleton in aging. In W. Reichel (ed.), *Clinical Aspects of Aging* (3rd ed.). Baltimore: Williams & Wilkins, 1980.
3. Birren, J.E., and Schaie, K.W. (eds.). *Handbook of the Psychology of Aging* (3rd ed.). San Diego: Academic Press, 1990.
4. Burggraf, V., and Donlon, B. Assessing the elderly. *Am. J. Nurs.* 85:976, 1985.
5. Caird, F., Dall, J., and Williams, B. The cardiovascular system. In J.C. Brockehurst (ed.), *Textbook of Geriatric Medicine and Gerontology* (3rd ed.). New York: Churchill Livingstone, 1985.
6. Carnevali, D.L., and Patrick, M. *Nursing Management for the Elderly* (2nd ed.). Philadelphia: J.B. Lippincott, 1986.
7. Carruthers, S. Pharmacokinetics. In I. Rossman (ed.), *Clinical Geriatrics* (3rd ed.). Philadelphia: J.B. Lippincott, 1986.
8. Carter, A. The neurologic aspects of aging. In I. Rossman (ed.), *Clinical Geriatrics* (3rd ed.). Philadelphia: J.B. Lippincott, 1986.
9. Clark, K. *Leonardi da Vinci*. London: Cambridge University Press, 1939.
10. Cotran, R. Cell injury and Adaptation. In S.L. Robbins and V. Kumar (eds.), *Basic Pathology* (4th ed.). Philadelphia: W.B. Saunders, 1987.

11. Davies, I. Biology of aging—Theories of aging. In J.C. Brockehurst (ed.), *Textbook of Geriatric Medicine and Gerontology* (3rd ed.). New York: Churchill Livingstone, 1985.

12. Ebersole, P., and Hess, P. *Toward Healthy Aging: Human Needs and Nursing Response* (3rd ed.). St. Louis: Mosby, 1990.

13. Eliopoulos, C. *Gerontological Nursing* (2nd ed.). Philadelphia: J.B. Lippincott, 1987.

14. Esberger, K.K., and Hughes, S.T. *Nursing Care of the Aged.* Norwalk, Conn.: Appleton & Lange, 1989.

15. Faubert, P., Shapiro, W., Porush, J., and Kahn, A. Medical renal disease in the aged. In W. Reichel (ed.), *Clinical Aspects of Aging* (3rd ed.). Baltimore: Williams & Wilkins, 1989.

16. Fisch, L. Special senses—The aging auditory system. In J.C. Brockehurst (ed.), *Textbook of Geriatric Medicine and Gerontology* (3rd ed.). New York: Churchill Livingstone, 1985.

17. Gioiella, E., and Bevil, C. *Nursing Care of the Aging Client: Promoting Healthy Adaptation.* Norwalk, Conn.: Appleton-Century-Crofts, 1985.

18. Goldman, R. Aging of the excretory system. In C. Finch and E. Schneider (eds.), *Handbook of the Biology of Aging* (2nd ed.). New York: Van Nostrand Reinhold, 1985.

19. Guyton, A.C. *Textbook of Medical Physiology* (8th ed.). Philadelphia: W.B. Saunders, 1990.

20. Hayflick, L. Current theories of biological aging. *Fed. Proc.* 34:9, 1975.

21. Hubbard, B.M., and Squier, M. The physical aging of the neuromuscular system. In R. Tallis (ed.), *The Clinical Neurology of Old Age.* New York: John Wiley & Sons, 1989.

22. Kohn, R. Heart and cardiovascular system. In C. Finch and E. Schneider (eds.), *Handbook of the Biology of Aging* (2nd ed.). New York: Van Nostrand Reinhold, 1985.

23. Lamy, P.P. Drugs and the elderly: A new look. *Fam. Comm. Health* 5:34, 1982.

24. Malasanos, L., et al. *Health Assessment* (4th ed.). St. Louis: Mosby, 1990.

25. Matteson, M.A., and McConnell, E.S. *Gerontological Nursing: Concepts and Practice.* Philadelphia: W.B. Saunders, 1988.

26. Rossman, I. Anatomic and body composition changes with aging. In C. Finch and E. Schneider (eds.), *Handbook of the Biology of Aging* (2nd ed.). New York: Van Nostrand Reinhold, 1985.

27. Sohal, R., and Allen, R. Relationship between metabolic rate, free radicals, differentiation and aging: A unified theory. In A. Woodhead, A. Blachett, and A. Hollaender (eds.), *Molecular Biology of Aging.* New York: Plenum Press, 1985.

28. Vestal, R.D., and Cusack, B.J. Pharmacology of aging. In E.L. Schneider and J.W. Rowe (eds.), *Handbook of the Biology of Aging* (3rd ed.). San Diego: Academic Press, 1990.

29. Williams, G.H., and Braunwald, E. Hypertensive vascular disease. In E. Braunwald et al., *Harrison's Principles of Internal Medicine* (11th ed.). New York: McGraw-Hill, 1987.

30. Winsberg, F. Roentgenographic aspects of aging. In I. Rossman (ed.), *Clinical Geriatrics* (3rd ed.). Philadelphia: J.B. Lippincott, 1986.

## UNIT BIBLIOGRAPHY

Aaronson, L.S., and Macnee, C.L. Tobacco, alcohol, and caffeine use during pregnancy. *J. Obstet. Gynecol. Neonatal Nurs.* 18:279, 1989.

Ack, M. When the child is learning disabled. *Patient Care* 16:17, 1982.

Akridge, K. Anorexia nervosa. *J. Obstet. Gynecol. Neonatal Nurs.* 18:25, 1989.

Alexander, L.L. The pregnant smoker: Nursing implications. *J. Obstet. Gynecol. Neonatal Nurs.* 16:167, 1987.

American Psychiatric Association. *Diagnostic and Statistical Manual of Mental Disorders* (3rd ed.). Washington, D.C.: Author, 1987.

Asterita, M. *The Physiology of Stress.* New York: Human Sciences Press, 1985.

Avershine, M.A., and Enriquez, M.G. *Comprehensive Maternity Nursing: Perinatal and Women's Health.* Boston: Jones & Bartlett, 1990.

Bahlmann, J., and Liebau, H. *Stress and Hypertension.* New York: Karger, 1982.

Baker, D.A. Dangers of varicella-zoster virus infection. *Contemporary OB/GYN* 35(5):51, 1990.

Behrman, R.E., and Vaughn, V.C. (eds.). *Nelson Textbook of Pediatrics.* Philadelphia: Saunders, 1987.

Bell, T.A., and Hein, K. Adolescents and sexually transmitted diseases. In K.K. Holmes, P.A. Mardh, P.F. Sparling, and P. Weisner (eds.), *Sexually Transmitted Diseases.* New York: McGraw-Hill, 1984.

Belsky, J. *The Psychology of Aging.* Monterey, Calif.: Brooks/Cole, 1984.

Beregi, E. *Centenarians in Hungary: A Sociomedical and Demographic Study.* New York: Karger, 1990.

Binder, F.Z., and Butler, J.E. Children with learning disabilities. *Issues in Comprehensive Pediatric Nursing* 3, 1978.

Binstock, R.H., and George, L.K. *Handbook of Aging and the Social Sciences.* San Diego: Academic Press, 1990.

Birren, J.E., and Schaie, K.W. *Handbook of the Psychology of Aging* (3rd ed.). San Diego: Academic Press, 1990.

Bloom, A. Acquired immune deficiency syndrome in childhood. *Public Health* 102(2):97, 1988.

Bloom, B.L. *Stressful Life Event Theory and Research.* Rockville, Md.: U.S. Dept. of Health Service, 1985.

Bobak, I.M., Jensen, M.D., and Zalar, M.K. *Maternity Nursing and Gynecologic Care: The Nurse and the Family.* St. Louis: Mosby, 1989.

Brown, R.C., Sanders, J.M., and Schonberg, S.K. Driving safety and adolescent behavior. *Pediatrics* 77:603, 1986.

Burchfield, S.R. *Stress, Psychological and Physiological Interactions.* Washington, D.C.: Hemisphere, 1985.

Burke, D.S., Brundage, J.F., Goldenbaum, M., Gardner, L.I., Peterson, M., Visintine, R., Redfield, R.R., and The Walter Reed Retrovirus Research Group. Human immunodeficiency virus infections in teenagers: Seroprevalence among applicants for U.S. military service. *JAMA* 263(15):2074, 1990.

Crumley, F.E. Substance abuse and adolescent suicidal behavior. *JAMA* 263(22):3051, 1990.

Cumings, S. Stress, cigarettes and ulcers. *Gastroenterology* 85(5):1232, 1985.

Davidson, J., and Grant, C. Growing up is hard to do . . . in the AIDS era. *MCN* 13:352, 1988.

Dickason, E.J., Schultz, M.O., and Silverman, B.L. *Maternal Infant Nursing Care*. St. Louis: Mosby, 1990.

Dietz, W.H. Childhood obesity: Susceptibility, cause and management. *J. Pediatr.* 103:676, 1983.

Dinsmore, M.J. Group B streptococcus still poses a challenge. *Contemporary OB/GYN* 35(5):93, 1990.

Dotevall, G. *Stress and Common Gastrointestinal Disorders*. New York: Praeger, 1985.

Dunn, P.A., Bhutani, V., Weiner, S., and Ludomirski, A. Care of the neonate with erythroblastosis fetalis. *J. Obstet. Gynecol. Neonatal Nurs.* 17:283, 1988.

Dunn, P.A., Weiner, S., and Ludomirski, A. Percutaneous umbilical blood sampling. *J. Obstet. Gynecol. Neonatal Nurs.* 17:308, 1988.

Ebersole, P., and Hess, P. *Toward Healthy Aging* (2nd ed.). St. Louis: Mosby, 1986.

Erikson, E. *Childhood and Society*. New York: W.W. Norton, 1963.

Foster, R.L., Hunsberger, M., and Anderson, J. *Family Centered Nursing Care of Children*. Philadelphia: W.B. Saunders, 1989.

Gabbe, S.G. Latest methods of determining fetal lung maturity. *Contemporary OB/GYN* 35(2):89, 1990.

Garner, D.M. Cognitive therapy for bulimia nervosa. *Adolescent Psychiatry* 13:358, 1986.

Gemma, P.B. Coping with suicidal behavior. *MCN* 14:101, 1989.

Gibson, L.Y. Bedwetting: A family's recurrent nightmare. *MCN* 14:270, 1989.

Gormly, A.V., and Brodzinsky, D.M. *Lifespan Human Development* (4th ed.). New York: Holt, Rinehart and Winston, 1989.

Griffin, M.R., Ray, W.A., Mortimer, E.A., Fenichel, G.M., and Schaffner, W. Risk of seizures and encephalopathy after immunization with the diphtheria-tetanus-pertussis vaccine. *JAMA* 263:1641, 1990.

Halmi, K.A., Falk, J.R., and Schwartz, E. Binge eating and vomiting: A survey of the college population. *Psych. Med.* 81(11):697, 1981.

Hansen, B.D. Prader-Willi syndrome. *J. Obstet. Gynecol. Neonatal Nurs.* 18:392, 1989.

Hemenway, J.A. Sleep and the cardiac patient. *Heart Lung* 9:453, 1980.

Henker, B., and Whalen, C.K. Hyperactivity and attention deficits. *Am. Psychologist* 44:216, 1989.

Herzog, D.B., and Copeland, P.M. Eating disorders. *N. Engl. J. Med.* 313(5):295, 1985.

Hill, A.S., Cochran, C.K., and Dickerson, C. Nursing care of the infant with erythroblastosis fetalis. *J. Pediatr. Nurs.* 4:395, 1989.

Hodgen, G.W. Uses of GnRH analogs in IVF/GIFT. *Contemporary OB/GYN* 35(6):1012, 1990.

Hogge, J.S., Hogge, A., and Golbus, M.S. Chorionic villus sampling. J. Obstet. Gynecol. Neonatal Nurs. 15(1):24, 1986.

Holmes, J., and Magiera, L. *Maternity Nursing*. New York: Macmillan, 1987.

Homer, P., and Holstein, M. *A Good Old Age?* New York: Simon & Schuster, 1990.

Janke, J. Dealing with AIDS and the adolescent population. *Nurse Pract.* 14(11):35, 1989.

Jones, S.L., Doheny, M.O., Jones, P.K., and Bradley, N. Binge eaters: A comparison of eating patterns of those who admit to binging and those who do not. *J. Adv. Nurs.* 11:545, 1986.

Kaplan, H.L., and Sadock, B.J. *Pocket Handbook of Clinical Psychiatry*. London: William & Wilkins, 1990.

Kinney, J., and Leaton, G. *Understanding Alcohol*. St. Louis: Mosby, 1982.

Kinsbourne, M., and Caplan, P.J. *Children's Learning and Attention Problems*. Boston: Little, Brown, 1979.

Kleber, H.D. Cocaine abuse: Historical, epidemiological, and psychological perspectives. *J. Clin. Psych.* 49(2):3, 1988.

Knittle, J.L., et al. The growth of adipose tissue in children and adolescents: Cross-sectional studies of adipose cell numbers and size. *J. Clin. Invest.* 63:238, 1979.

Kroger, R., and Weisner, P.J. Sexually transmitted disease education: Challenge for the 80s. *J. School Health* 51(4):242, 1981.

Lagrew, D.C. Strategies for managing emboli in pregnancy. *Contemporary OB/GYN* 35(1):113, 1990.

*Law and Disabled People, The.* Washington, D.C.: U.S. Government Printing Office, 1980.

LeFrancois, G.R. *Of Children: An Introduction to Child Development* (6th ed.). Belmont, Calif.: Wadsworth, 1989.

Markides, K.S., and Cooper, C.L. Aging, Stress and Health. New York: Wiley, 1989.

Marks, A., and Fisher, M. Health assessment and screening during adolescence. Pediatrics 80:131, 1987.

Marlow, D.R., and Redding, B.A. (eds.). *Textbook of Pediatric Nursing* (6th ed.). Philadelphia: Saunders, 1988.

May, K.A., and Mahlmeister, L.R. *Comprehensive Maternity Nursing*. New York: Lippincott, 1990.

McKerns, K.W., and Pantic, V. *Neuroendocrine Correlates of Stress*. New York: Plenum Press, 1984.

Milsum, J.H. *Health, Stress and Illness: A Systems Approach*. New York: Praeger, 1984.

Mitchell, J.E., Pyle, R.L., and Eckert, E.D. Frequency and duration of binge-eating episodes in patients with bulimia. *Am. J. Psych.* 141:835, 1981.

Moore, M.M. Recurrent teenage pregnancy: Making it less desirable. *MCN* 14:104, 1989.

Munck, A., and Guyre, P. Glucocorticoid hormones in stress: Physiological and pharmacological actions. *News Physiol. Sci.* 1:69, 1986.

Muscari, M.E. Effective nursing strategies for adolescents with anorexia nervosa and bulimia nervosa. *Pediatr. Nurs.* 14(6):475, 1988.

Narins, D.M., Belkengren, R.P., and Sapala, S. Nutrition and the growing athlete. *Pediatr. Nurs.* 9:163, 1983.

National Research Council. Committee on Dietary Allowances. *Recommended Dietary Allowances*. Washington, D.C.: National Academy of Sciences, 1980.

New York Heart Association. New York Heart Association: *Nomenclature and Criteria for Diagnosis and Diseases of the Heart and Blood Vessels* (ed. 5). New York: Author, 1955.

Ott, M.J., and Jackson, P.L. Precocious puberty: Identifying early sexual development. *Nurse Pract.* 14(11):21, 1989.

Pace-Owens, S. Gamete intrafallopian transfer (GIFT). *J. Obstet. Gynecol. Neonatal Nurs.* 18:93, 1989.

Perlmutter, M. *Adult Development and Aging*. New York: Wiley, 1985.

Pfeffer, C.R. *The Suicidal Child*. New York: Guilford Press, 1986.

Poole, J.H. Getting perspective on HELLP syndrome. *MCN* 13:432, 1988.

Pyle, R.L., Mitchell, J.E., Echert, E.D., Halvorson, P.A., Newman, P.A., and Goff, G.M. The incidence of bulimia in freshmen college students. *Intl. J. Eating Disorders* 2(3):75, 1983.

Rankin, W.W. Teenage suicide. *J. Pediatr. Nurs.* 4(2):130, 1989.

Reber, A.M. *Nutrition and Aging* (2nd ed.). Denton, Tx.: Center for Studies in Aging, 1988.

Reeder, S.J., and Martin, L.L. *Maternity Nursing: Family, Newborn, and Women's Health Care*. Philadelphia: J.B. Lippincott, 1987.

Remafedi, G.J. Preventing the sexual transmission of AIDS during adolescence. *J. Adolesc. Health Care* 9(2):139, 1988.

Rhodes, A.M. Options and issues for pregnant adolescents. *MCN* 13:427, 1988.

Rogers, D. *The Adult Years: An Introduction to Aging* (3rd ed.). Englewood Cliffs, New Jersey: Prentice Hall, 1986.

Rosenzweig, M.R., and Leiman, A.L. *Physiological Psychology* (2nd ed.). New York: Random House, 1989.

Ruff, C. How well do adolescents mother? *MCN* 12:249, 1987.

Sanford, N.D. Providing sensitive health to gay and lesbian youth. *Nurse Pract.* 14(5):30, 1989.

Santrock, J.W. *Adult Development and Aging*. Dubuque, Iowa: W.C. Brown, 1985.

Santrock, J.W. *Children* (2nd ed.). Dubuque, Iowa: W.C. Brown, 1990.

Savin-Williams, R. Theoretical perspectives accounting for adolescent homosexuality. *J. Adolesc. Health Care* 9:95, 1988.

Schmidt, J., Boilanger, M., and Abbott, S. Peripartum cardiomyopathy. *J. Obstet. Gynecol. Neonatal Nurs.* 18:465, 1989.

Schrader, B.D., Heverly, M.A., and Rappaport, J. Temperament, behavior problems, and learning skills in very low birth weight preschoolers. *Res. Nurs. Health* 13:27, 1990.

Schuster, C.S., and Ashburn, S.S. (eds.). *The Process of Human Development: A Holistic Life Span Approach* (2nd ed.). Boston: Little, Brown, 1986.

Seeds, J.W. PUBS: Important new aid for prenatal diagnosis. *Contemporary OB/GYN* 31(2):117, 1988.

Selye, H. *The Physiology and Pathology of Exposure to Stress*. Montreal: Acta, 1950.

Selye, H. *Stress Without Distress*. Philadelphia: Lippincott, 1974.

Selye, H. *Selye's Guide to Stress Research*. New York: Van Nostrand Reinhold, 1983.

Shaffer, D.R. *Developmental Psychology: Childhood and Adolescence* (2nd ed.). Pacific Grove, Calif.: Brooks/Cole, 1989.

Shiffman, S., and Wills, T.A. *Coping and Substance Use*. Orlando, Fla.: Academic Press, 1985.

Smith, J. The dangers of prenatal cocaine use. *MCN* 13:174, 1988.

Sprague-McRae, J.M. Encopresis: Developmental, behavioral and physiological considerations for treatment. *Nurse Pract.* 15(6):8, 1990.

Stephens, M.A. *Stress and Coping in Later Life Families*. New York: Hemisphere, 1990.

Steptoe, A., Ruddel, H., and Neus, H. *Clinical and Methodological Issues in Cardiovascular Psychophysiology*. New York: Springer-Verlag, 1985.

Stone, A.C. Facing up to acne. *Pediatr. Nurs.* 8:229, 1982.

Stringer, M.R. Chorionic villi sampling: A nursing perspective. *J. Obstet. Gynecol. Neonatal Nurs.* 17(1):19, 1988.

Stroh, S.E., Stern, H.P., and McCarthy, S.G. Fecal incontinence in children: A clinical update. *MCN* 14:252, 1989.

Taitz, L.S. Infantile overnutrition among artificially fed infants in the Sheffield region. *Br. Med. J.* 1:315, 1971.

Tanner, J.M. *Growth at Adolescence*. Oxford: Blackwell Scientific, 1962.

*Teenage Pregnancy: The Problem That Hasn't Gone Away*. New York: Alan Guttmacher Institute, 1980.

Thomas, L.E. *Research on Adulthood and Aging*. Albany: State University of New York, 1989.

Troiden, R.R. Homosexual identity development. *J. Adolesc. Health Care* 9:105, 1988.

Tucker, L.A. Television, teenagers, and health. *J. Youth Adolesc.* 16:415, 1987.

U.S. Dept. of Health, Education, and Welfare. National Institute on Drug Abuse, 1980.

Vander Zanden, J.W. *Human Development* (4th ed.). New York: Alfred A. Knopf, 1989.

Warren, M. Anorexia nervosa and related eating disorders. *Clin. Obstet. Gynecol.* 28(3): 588, 1985.

Whaley, L.F., and Wong, D.L. (eds.). *Nursing Care of Infants and Children* (3rd ed.). St. Louis: Mosby, 1987.

White, P. Classification of obstetric diabetes. *Am. J. Obstet. Gynecol.* 130:228, 1978.

Wilson, D., and Molly-Martinez, T. Promoting driving safety for teens and adults. *Nurse Pract.* 14(10):28, 1989.

Wilson, M.H. Obesity. In C.W. Hoekelman, *Primary Pediatric Care*. St. Louis: Mosby, 1987.

Woolfolk, R.L., and Lehrer, P.M. *Principles and Practice of Stress*. New York: Guilford Press, 1984.

Zarek, D., Hawkins, J.D., and Rogers, P.D. Risk factors for adolescent substance abuse. *Ped. Clin. N. Am.* 34:481, 1987.

Ziai, M., Clarke, T., and Merritt, T. *Assessment of the Newborn: A Guide for the Practitioner*. Boston: Little, Brown, 1984.

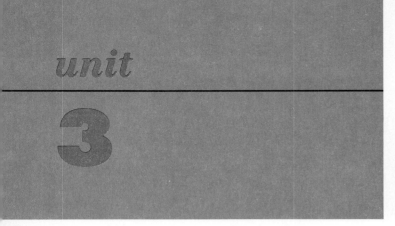

unit

3

# FLUID, ELECTROLYTE, ACID-BASE, NUTRITIONAL BALANCE, AND SHOCK

The maintenance of the steady state of fluid, electrolyte, and acid-base balance is achieved through the complex cooperation of various systems of the body. Continual movement and exchange of water results in a regulated balance between plasma and interstitial and intracellular fluid (ICF). Nutritional balance also participates in maintaining the steady state of the body. Because the subject encompasses many other systems, the intent of this unit is to provide the basis for further exploration in the specific systems of the body.

Chapter 8 summarizes water and electrolyte balance and explores the major alterations that can occur with disease states. Edema is presented in this chapter because it represents a shift of fluid volume between compartments. Specific reference to electrolyte and water regulation is found in many other areas of the text. Chapter 9 deals with the basic concepts of the regulation of acid-base balance and how alterations in the balance can result. Respiratory alterations are described in greater detail in Unit 9 and the metabolic alterations are specifically explored in Unit 10. Other systems that function in the regulation of hydrogen ion concentration are noted in Units 7, 11, 12, and 15. Chapter 10 is a newly incorporated chapter covering the principles of nutrition and alterations in nutritional balance. Chapter 11 explores the underlying mechanisms of shock. Alterations in cardiac output are also detailed in Unit 8.

The reader is encouraged to use the learning objectives as a study guide outline; the bibliography listed at the end of the unit can aid in further investigation of the topic.

# Normal and Altered Fluid and Electrolyte Balance

## Chapter Outline

▶ **Regulation of Fluid and Electrolyte Balance**

  **Water**
    Osmolality
  **Regulation of Water and Sodium Balance**
    Thirst
    Renal Regulation
    Antidiuretic Hormone (ADH)
    Aldosterone
    Prostaglandins
    Glucocorticoids
    Atrial Natriuretic Hormone (ANH)
  **Fluid Balance in Body Compartments**
  **Movement of Fluids at the Capillary Line**

**Water-Sodium Deficits and Excesses**
    Hypovolemia
    Hypervolemia
  **Sodium**
    Hyponatremia
    Hypernatremia
  **Potassium**
    Hypokalemia
    Hyperkalemia
  **Calcium**
    Relationship of Calcium to Phosphate
    Hypocalcemia
    Hypercalcemia

**Phosphate**
    Hypophosphatemia
    Hyperphosphatemia
  **Chloride**
  **Magnesium**
    Hypomagnesemia
    Hypermagnesemia
▶ **Edema**
  **Decreased COP**
  **Increased Capillary Hydrostatic Pressure**
  **Increased Capillary Permeability**
  **Obstruction of the Lymphatics**
  **Sodium and Body Water Excess**
  **Types of Edema**
  **Distribution of Edema**

## Learning Objectives

1. Describe the mechanisms by which water and sodium balance is normally regulated.
2. List the normal serum concentrations of the major electrolytes and plasma proteins.
3. Show the relationship of fluid and electrolyte composition between the intracellular and extracellular compartments.
4. Describe in detail the normal fluid dynamics at the capillary line.
5. Define the terms *hydrostatic pressure, oncotic pressure, colloid osmotic pressure,* and *outward and inward forces* as they relate to capillary fluid dynamics.
6. Describe briefly the role of the lymphatic system in controlling extravascular fluid volume.
7. Describe the role of sodium in controlling osmotic pressure in the extracellular fluid.
8. Explain the probable effects of atrial natriuretic hormone on fluid volume and sodium regulation.
9. Differentiate between volume imbalances and osmolar imbalances.
10. Differentiate the clinical effects of hypernatremia and hyponatremia.

11. Define *dilutional hyponatremia.*
12. Discuss how the syndrome of inappropriate antidiuretic hormone can cause hyponatremia.
13. Describe the function of potassium in the body.
14. Differentiate the pathophysiologic changes resulting from hypokalemia and hyperkalemia.
15. Discuss the numerous functions of calcium in the body.
16. List several causes of hypocalcemia.
17. Describe the physiologic effects of hypocalcemia and hypercalcemia.
18. List the functions of phosphate in the body.
19. Explain the relationship between calcium and phosphates in body functions.
20. Explain how hypochloremia is related to metabolic alkalosis.
21. Describe the effects of magnesium on the body.
22. Discuss the five pathologic mechanisms that can produce edema and their relationship to each other.

(continued)

**23.** Diagram the positive feedback mechanism associated with decreased colloid osmotic pressure.

**24.** Differentiate between pitting and nonpitting edema.

---

The volume and composition of body fluids must remain constant to support life. Continual movement and exchange of water and electrolytes occur and are regulated by the body to compensate for wide variations in intake and output that may result from environmental changes or disease states. The protein composition of plasma is also important in regulating fluid movement at the capillary line. This chapter presents a brief review of water and electrolyte balance and alterations that can occur with stress and disease.

## REGULATION OF FLUID AND ELECTROLYTE BALANCE

### Water

Water balance refers to an equilibrium maintained between intake and output. Water, a necessary solvent, is used in the many metabolic processes of the body and carries waste products for excretion through the urine, skin, lungs, and feces. Water cushions, protects, lubricates, insulates, and provides structure for and resilience to the skin.

Water accounts for approximately 60% of body weight in the adult. This amount normally decreases with age and is affected by other components of body composition. The lean individual has a greater percentage of body water than the obese person because fat cells contain less water than muscle cells. The amount of water necessary to maintain life in the adult is about 1500 ml per day. Water intake, although intermittent, is usually higher than necessary, with an average total of 2000 ml per day. Water is ingested in liquids and in foods, and is also produced by oxidation of foodstuffs. It is directly conserved by the antidiuretic hormone (ADH) and indirectly conserved by aldosterone.

The composition of the body fluids is regulated by the kidneys, gastrointestinal tract, nervous system, and lungs, with input from the heart and glands. Hormones, especially aldosterone and ADH, regulate the composition of plasma and other fluid compartments.

The intake of water must be balanced by output. The kidneys rid the body of excess water. Obligatory urinary output to eliminate waste and maintain minimal renal function is 300 to 500 ml per 24 hours. The volume of urinary excretion can be increased tremendously, and usually totals approximately 1500 ml per 24 hours. Water is also lost through the lungs (300 ml/24 hours), skin (500 ml/24 hours), and feces (200 ml/24 hours). This loss is termed insensible loss. In the adult, body water gains and losses are balanced at a total of 2500 ml per 24 hours.

Water imbalance can occur as a result of excess or depletion of body fluids. It often is closely associated with changes in sodium concentration. Body water loss is aggravated by elevated body temperature, diarrhea, vomiting, and other excessive depletion such as occurs through kidneys, skin, lungs, and gastrointestinal tract. Water excess is often due to sodium retention, but it may occur with excess ADH secretion or excessive ingestion of water.

### Osmolality

To determine the osmotic pressure of a solute, the osmolality of the solution must be determined. Osmolality is defined as the number of osmols of a substance contained within a liter of fluid. One osmole is the number of molecules in one gram molecular weight of undissociated solute.[7] A solution with one osmole in each kilogram of water has an osmolality of one osmole per kilogram. A solution with 1/1000 osmole per kilogram has an osmolality of 1 milliosmol per kilogram.[7] Normal serum osmolality is 290 milliosmols per kilogram. Electrolytes, primarily sodium, determine serum osmolality, and serum osmolality can easily be estimated by doubling the serum sodium value. An elevated osmolality is indicative of either excessive solutes, especially sodium, or inadequate fluid volume.[17]

### Regulation of Water and Sodium Balance

#### Thirst

Thirst, defined as the conscious desire for water, is the principal regulator of water intake. It is usually first expressed when the osmolality of plasma reaches about 295 mosm per kg.[14] Osmoreceptors located in the thirst center in the hypothalamus are sensitive to changes in the osmolality of extracellular fluids (ECFs).

When osmolality increases, the cells shrink and the sensation of thirst is experienced. The mechanism by which thirst occurs is twofold. First, in instances of volume depletion of hypovolemia, decreased renal perfusion stimulates the release of renin, which eventually leads to the production of angiotensin II (see also Chap. 26). Angiotensin II stimulates the hypothalamus to release neural substrates responsible for generating the sensation of thirst.[8] Secondly, osmoreceptors in the hypothalamus detect elevations in osmotic pressure and activate nervous pathways that result in the thirst sensation. Thirst may also result from depleted circulatory volume due to hemorrhage or from decreased cardiac output secondary to pump failure. Thirst may be induced by dryness of the mouth in true hyperosmolar states or may occur to relieve the unpleasant dry sensation that results from reduced salivation. The sensation may be diminished or unrecognized in elderly and confused individuals or in individuals with decreased levels of consciousness, resulting in inadequate fluid consumption.

Generally, the thirst sensation prompts the individual to consume water, thereby correcting the hypovolemia or state of increased osmolality. Once the thirst sensation has been satisfied, intake of fluid ceases. However, excessive intake of water that is unrelated to thirst has a psychogenic basis. Obsessive preoccupation with and indulgence in excessive water intake can lead to fluid volume overload, decreased serum osmolality, and decreased osmotic pressure.

## Renal Regulation

The kidneys regulate the volume and electrolyte concentration of body fluids. Extracellular fluid is filtered through the renal glomeruli. Selective reabsorption and excretion of water and solutes occur in the renal tubules. Glomerular filtration rate and renal perfusion, reflective of cardiac output, determine the rate of this process. Hy-

povolemic states result in reduced urinary output, which reflects the body's attempt to conserve or retain volume. The mechanism by which this occurs is related to decreased renal perfusion. Underperfused kidneys release renin, which converts first to angiotensin I and then to angiotensin II. The latter hormone stimulates the release of aldosterone from the adrenal cortex. The action of aldosterone is to facilitate renal reabsorption of sodium and water, thus increasing circulating fluid volume.

## Antidiuretic Hormone

Antidiuretic hormone is formed in the hypothalamus and stored in the neurohypophysis of the posterior pituitary. The area of ADH storage and release may overlap with the thirst center, which accounts for the integration of thirst and ADH release.[7] The major stimuli for ADH secretion are increased osmolality and decreased volume of ECF. Secretion may also occur with the stress of trauma, surgery, pain, and some anesthetics and drugs. The hormone increases reabsorption of water at the collecting ducts, thereby conserving water to correct the osmolality and restore the volume of ECF (Figure 8-1).

Also called vasopressin, ADH has a minor vasoconstrictive effect on the arterioles that can increase blood pressure. A significant decrease in ADH secretion secondary to lesions or trauma of the hypophyseal tract results in diabetes insipidus, which is characterized by a massive increase in urinary output. Blood volume depletion does not result in diabetes insipidus as long as the thirst mechanism remains intact. Increased secretion of ADH, stimulated by pituitary hypersecretion or by extrapituitary tumors, results in a marked decrease in serum osmolality, an increase in blood volume, and a decrease

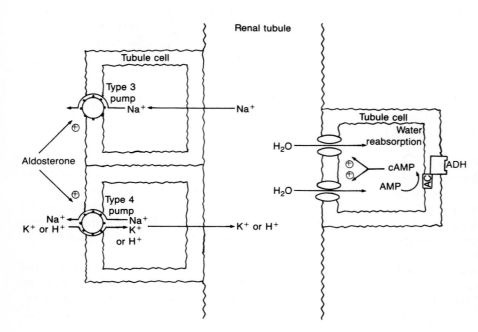

**FIGURE 8-1.**

Location and influence of aldosterone and ADH receptors. Aldosterone stimulates sodium pumps and exchange pumps in the serosal membranes of renal tubule cells, creating a gradient that draws sodium out of the renal tubule and pushes potassium and hydrogen into the tubule. ADH activates an adenylate cyclase-linked receptor on the serosal membrane of tubule cells that initiates formation of cyclic AMP, which promotes aggregation of proteins in the luminal membrane that serve as water channels. (From A.K. Swonger and M.P. Matejski, *Nursing Pharmacology.* Philadelphia: J.B. Lippincott, 1991.)

in urinary output. This is known as the syndrome of inappropriate ADH secretion (SIADH) (see Chap. 36).

### Aldosterone

Aldosterone, a hormone secreted by the adrenal gland, acts on the renal tubules to increase the sodium uptake. The increased sodium retention causes an increase in water retention. Aldosterone release is stimulated by changes in potassium concentration, by serum sodium concentrations, and by the renin-angiotensin system (see Chap. 26). Normally, the rate or amount of aldosterone secretion is closely regulated by the potassium concentration and is very effective in controlling hyperkalemia.

### Prostaglandins

The prostaglandins are naturally occurring fatty acids that are present in many of the tissues of the body and function in the inflammatory response, blood pressure control, uterine contractions, and gastrointestinal motility. In the kidneys, renal prostaglandins cause vasodilation and, in most cases, promote sodium excretion by inhibiting the response of the renal distal tubules to ADH. Prostaglandin-mediated renal vasodilation protects the kidneys from ischemia when levels of vasoconstrictors, such as angiotensin II and norepinephrine, increase.[1]

### Glucocorticoids

The glucocorticoids secreted by the adrenal cortex exert weak mineralocorticoid activity, thus promoting the resorption of sodium and water. This increases blood volume and sodium retention. Therefore, alterations in glucocorticoid levels cause alterations in the blood volume balance.

### Atrial Natriuretic Hormone

The atrial natriuretic hormone (ANH), first identified in 1981, is a 28-amino acid peptide, released from myocytes in the coronary sinuses of the atria in response to increased atrial stretch. Although ANH is released on a continual basis in healthy persons, its release is accelerated by any condition that results in increased atrial stretch, especially fluid volume excess (Box 8-1). Much research is being done to determine the physiologic function of this hormone in the body.[5,9,18] Figure 8-2 indicates some reputed systemic effects. It has been shown in laboratory studies to have the following effects: (1) increases the kidneys' ability to excrete both water and sodium; (2) improves glomerular filtration rate and hence increases sodium filtration by dilatation of the afferent and efferent arterioles;[4] (3) inhibits the reabsorption of sodium by the collecting ducts; (4) inhibits renin secretion

**BOX 8-1.**
CONDITIONS THAT MAY ENHANCE SECRETION OF ATRIAL NATRIURETIC HORMONE

Any condition resulting in fluid volume excess or vasoconstriction is a candidate
Conditions resulting in fluid volume excess
  Congestive heart failure
  Chronic renal failure
  Nephrosis
  Cirrhosis
  Cushing's disease
  Toxemia of pregnancy
  Premenstrual syndrome
Conditions resulting in vasoconstriction
  Hypertension: essential, secondary, portal
  Pain
  Stress
Cardiac conditions that result in atrial distension
  Congestive heart failure
  Cardiomyopathies
  Myocarditis
  Valvular heart disease: congenital heart defects, rheumatic heart disease
  Myocardial ischemia and infarction
  Restrictive disorders: pericarditis, cardiac tamponade
  Arrhythmias: paroxysmal atrial tachycardia, atrial fibrillation and flutter

Source: M.H. Birney, and D.G. Penney, Atrial natriuretic peptide: A hormone with implications. Heart Lung 19(2):174, 1990.

by the juxtaglomerular apparatus, thereby preventing release of aldosterone from the adrenal cortex; and (5) inhibits release of ADH.[3,20]

In clinical studies, especially in congestive heart failure, there has been a variable response to the hormone.[5] The foremost role appears to be regulation of plasma volume through renal, and perhaps interstitial, fluid escape.[4]

## Fluid Balance in Body Compartments

Fluids are maintained in strict volume and concentration in each of the three compartments: (1) extracellular, intravascular (plasma), (2) extracellular, extravascular (interstitial fluid), and (3) intracellular. Figure 8-3 shows the relationship of fluid balance and composition of these three compartments. In normal distribution, about 70% of body fluid is intracellular and the rest is extracellular in the form of interstitial, plasma, and secretion or excretion fluids. The relationship of cations, anions, and volumes must be maintained rigidly to preserve life. Interstitial fluid and plasma basically contain the same electrolyte composition, but plasma contains a large amount

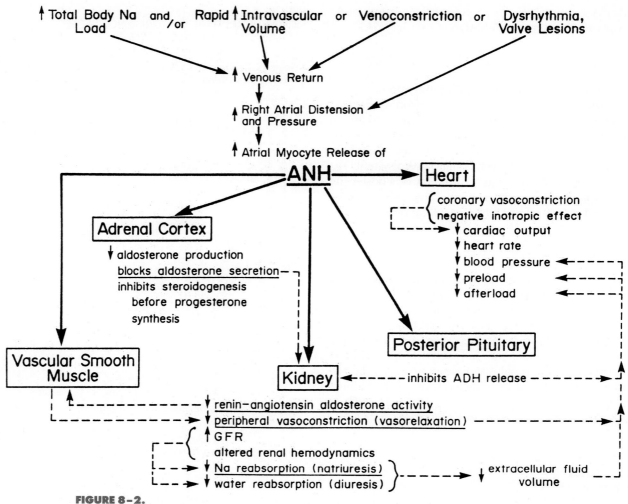

**FIGURE 8–2.**

Schema of major reputed effects of atrial natriuretic hormone (ANH) in control of vascular pressure and volume, and its likely antagonism to renin-angiotensin-aldosterone system. Rectangles enclose major sites of action; short vertical arrows indicate increase or decrease; heavy solid arrows and dashed arrows indicate interactions. (From M.H. Birney, D.G. Penney, Atrial natriuretic peptide: a hormone with implications. *Heart Lung* 19:2, 174–83, 1990.)

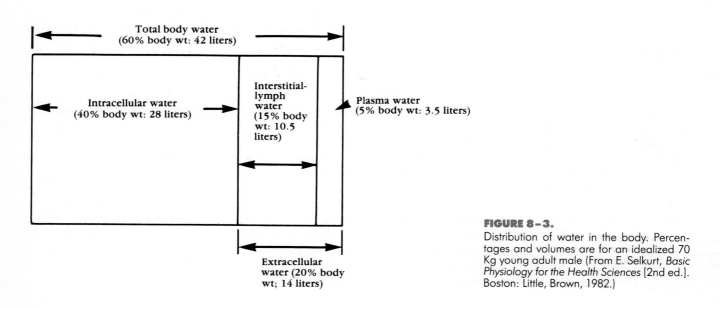

**FIGURE 8–3.**

Distribution of water in the body. Percentages and volumes are for an idealized 70 Kg young adult male (From E. Selkurt, *Basic Physiology for the Health Sciences* [2nd ed.]. Boston: Little, Brown, 1982.)

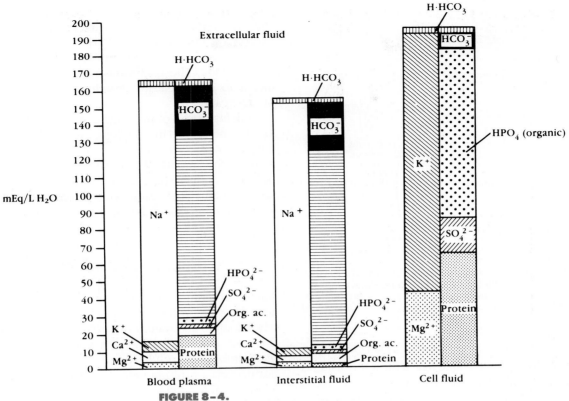

**FIGURE 8–4.**
Electrolyte composition of the body fluid compartments.

of protein. The composition of intracellular electrolytes is quite different from that of extracellular electrolytes, but the numbers of charges (cations and anions) are basically equal in the compartments (Figure 8-4). To maintain life, fluid containing oxygen and nutrients from the blood is filtered into the interstitial spaces and carried to the ICF, while excess carbon dioxide and other cellular waste products are returned to the bloodstream to be circulated and excreted by the lungs and kidneys. The process requires the constant movement and exchange of fluids and gases (see Chap. 1).

## Movement of Fluids at the Capillary Line

The capillaries are formed of endothelium, which is permeable to all of the solutes and water of the plasma. It is impermeable to the large molecules and cells in the plasma. Substances move through the gaps or spaces in the endothelial cells and some substances, such as carbon dioxide, oxygen, and small solutes, move through the endothelial membrane as well. The process occurs by diffusion, so that near equilibrium exists at the capillary line. The amount of fluid leaving the capillary nearly equals the amount reabsorbed. This equilibrium occurs mostly through a balance achieved between the hydro-

static pressure of the blood and the colloid osmotic pressure within the capillaries.

Blood entering the capillary comes in at a *hydrostatic pressure* that is generated by the heart. This hydrostatic pressure varies in the different systemic arterioles, but is always higher at the arteriolar end of the capillary than at the venular end (Figure 8-5). As fluid filters out of the capillary into the tissue spaces, the hydrostatic pressure decreases. The high pressure exerted at the arteriolar end of the capillary has been called a simple *outward force*, or pushing force, which moves fluid from the vessel to the interstitial spaces.[7] The average hydrostatic pressure at the arteriolar end is 32 mm Hg and drops to 15 mm Hg at the venous end.[7] This hydrostatic pressure provides the main outward force, but it is enhanced by a negative interstitial pressure and the interstitial fluid colloid osmotic pressure (ISCOP) as shown in Figure 8-5.

The ISCOP results from plasma proteins that are leaked into the interstitial spaces and that exert a colloid, or water-pulling, effect. The pressure exerted by the plasma proteins, the *colloid osmotic* or *oncotic pressure (COP)*, is an osmotic pulling or *inward force* that draws water toward it. Because the plasma proteins cannot move into the interstitial area, they exert their colloidal effect by drawing water back into the vessel. The average COP is 25 mm Hg, a pressure that remains constant across the capillary.

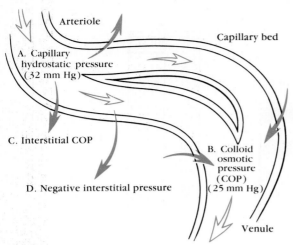

**FIGURE 8–5.**
Fluid dynamics at the capillary line. A. Capillary hydrostatic pressure is higher at the arteriolar end and tends to push fluid out. B. Colloid osmotic pressure (COP) generated by the plasma proteins maintains a constant inward pull or force. C. Interstitial COP is an outward force. D. Negative interstitial pressure is an outward force.

Referring to Figure 8-5, note that at the arteriolar end of a schematic capillary the hydrostatic pressure exceeds the colloid osmotic pressure by about 7 mm Hg, causing fluid movement to the interstitial area. At the venous end, the hydrostatic pressure has dropped to 15 mm Hg, and is now lower than the colloid osmotic pressure, which causes the movement of fluid into the capillary. The COP in the capillaries is mainly generated by albumin because it is the most abundant of the plasma proteins. Table 8-1 lists the relative concentrations of plasma proteins.

It has been noted that while the amount of fluid filtered out of the vessel nearly equals that reabsorbed, a larger amount is filtered into the tissue spaces than is reabsorbed. Also, small amounts of protein escape into

**TABLE 8–1.**
CONCENTRATION OF MAJOR PLASMA PROTEINS

| PROTEINS | CONCENTRATION |
|---|---|
| Total serum proteins | 6.0–8.0 gm/dl |
| albumin | 3.2–5.6 gm/dl |
| globulin | 2.3–3.5 gm/dl |
| fibrinogen | 150–400 mg/dl |
| Electrophoresis | |
| albumin | 52–65% of total |
| globulin | |
| Alpha$_1$ | 2.5–5% of total |
| Alpha$_2$ | 7–13% of total |
| Beta | 8–14% of total |
| Gamma | 12–22% of total |

Source: J. Wallach, *Interpretation of Diagnostic Tests* (4th ed.). Boston: Little, Brown, 1986.

the tissue spaces during the process of fluid movement and cannot be reabsorbed by the blood vessels. These excesses of fluid and protein are absorbed by the *lymphatic system* and returned through lymphatic channels to the blood. The lymphatic system provides the only means to return plasma proteins in the tissues to the bloodstream.[7]

Edema does not normally occur until there is a 17-mm Hg increase in the gradient favoring filtration, or the outward force.[7] This is because the lymph channels can increase the amount of fluid carried and thus can compensate for increased fluid escaping into the tissue spaces. Edema does result when there is significant alteration in the balance of the inward (COP) or outward (hydrostatic) forces.

## Water-Sodium Deficits and Excesses

Water and sodium imbalances are categorized as *volume* and *osmolar*. Volume, or isotonic, imbalances occur when sodium and water increase or decrease together in the same ratio that is normally found in the ECFs. Osmolar imbalances result when there is an alteration in the normal relationship of water to solutes in the ECFs. The serum sodium level is the best indicator of osmolality of blood because it is the most abundant solute in the vascular space.[11]

### Hypovolemia

Hypovolemia, or extracellular volume depletion, is an isotonic imbalance in which water and electrolytes are lost together in the same proportion as exists normally. The serum sodium level remains normal. Hypovolemia occurs when there is an abrupt decrease in intake of fluids or when the extracellular volume is decreased due to such conditions as hemorrhage, diarrhea, vomiting, burns, excessive diaphoresis, draining wounds, ascites, or severe uncontrolled diabetes mellitus. Hypovolemia results in a decrease in the size of the extracellular space and circulatory collapse that eventually depletes cellular fluid. Signs and symptoms of hypovolemia are related to the cause of the imbalance (Table 8-2). Regardless of the cause of the fluid volume loss, it is important to note that once symptoms are manifested, the volume depletion is quite advanced. This is due to the fact that interstitial fluid and, to a lesser extent, ICF move to the intravascular spaces to maintain circulation.

### Hypervolemia

Hypervolemia, or extracellular volume excess, is an isotonic imbalance in which water and electrolytes are gained together in the same proportion as exists normally in the ECF. The serum sodium level remains normal. Hypervolemia may result from excessive administra-

**TABLE 8-2.**
NORMAL FLUID AND ELECTROLYTE CONCENTRATIONS AND IMBALANCES

| FLUID AND ELECTROLYTE | VALUES | SOURCE AND CAUSE OF IMBALANCES | FUNCTIONS AND CLINICAL MANIFESTATIONS |
|---|---|---|---|
| **Water** | Average intake 2000 mL/d | Intake of fluids, water in foods, oxidation of foodstuffs | Removes waste products; cushions, protects, lubricates, insulates, and provides structure and resilience to skin |
| Hypervolemia | Extracellular fluid volume expansion; normal serum sodium | Excessive administration of isotonic solution; disease states that affect fluid and electrolyte homeostasis, renal, liver, congestive heart failure, malnutrition, and hyperaldosteronism; excessive administration of cortisone | Increase in extracellular fluid space; weight gain; dyspnea; cough, rales; distended abdomen; neck vein distention; bounding pulse; hypertension; hoarseness; normal skin turgor, sweating, edema |
| Hypovolemia | Extracellular fluid volume depletion; normal serum sodium | Decrease in fluid intake; loss of fluids through hemorrhage, draining wounds, diarrhea, vomiting, diaphoresis, renal disease, burns, fever, fluid shifts, decreased aldosterone secretion, uncontrolled diabetes mellitus | Decrease in extracellular fluid space; thirst, weakness, abdominal pain; nausea; diminished stools, anorexia; weight loss, decreased skin turgor; decreased sweating, tearing and salivation, decreased venous pressure; elevated pulse and respiratory rate; hypotension; oliguria, anuria, decreased body temperature (in the absence of infection) |
| **Sodium** | 136–145 mEq/L | Supplied by diet; excreted by kidney; balance normally regulated by aldosterone; dominant extracellular fluid cation | Regulates fluid volume by maintaining osmotic pressure between compartments; functions in acid-base balance; functions in neuromuscular and muscular excitability |
| Hypernatremia | >150 mEq/L | Excess loss of water over sodium through gastrointestinal system, lungs, or skin; excess administration of sodium through diet, hyperalimentation, renal insufficiency, dialysis, or hypothalamic lesions | Causes cellular shrinking due to hypertonic extracellular fluid, leads to central nervous system irritability, tachycardia, dry, flushed skin, hypotension; thirst excessive, elevated temperature, rapid pulse, weight loss, oliguria, anuria |
| Hyponatremia | <130 mEq/L | Dilutional hyponatremia from congestive heart failure, cirrhosis, nephrosis; sodium depletion, loss of body fluids, without replacement or replacement with hypotonic fluids; diuretic therapy | Causes cellular swelling, may lead to cerebral edema, headache, stupor progressing to coma; peripheral edema, polyuria, absence of thirst, decreased body temperature, rapid pulse, hypotension, nausea, vomiting |
| **Potassium** | 3.5–5.0 mEq/L | Balance maintained by dietary intake, excess excreted by kidneys; increased potassium in plasma excreted under influence of aldosterone by kidneys; dominant cation in intracellular fluid | Regulates osmolarity of intracellular fluid, functions in neuromuscular and muscular excitability; competition with $H^+$ and $Na^+$ in renal tubule helps maintain acid-base balance |
| Hyperkalemia | >5 mEq/L | Renal failure or renal insufficiency—acute or chronic; hemolysis of red blood cells; acute increase in potassium intake | Main effect is depression of conductivity in heart, peaked T waves, widened QRS on ECG; muscle cramping, paresthesias, nausea, diarrhea, associated with metabolic acidosis |
| Hypokalemia | <3.5 mEq/L | Lack of dietary intake; vomiting, gastric suction, potassium-depleting diuretics, aldosteronism, salt-wasting kidney diseases; major gastrointestinal surgery without replacement | Cardiac effect-increased irritability, onset of U wave on ECG, dysrhythmias, vomiting, paralytic ileus; thirst; associated with metabolic alkalosis; affects renal tubular function causing inability to concentrate urine |

(*continued*)

**TABLE 8–2.**
NORMAL FLUID AND ELECTROLYTE CONCENTRATIONS AND IMBALANCES (Continued)

| FLUID AND ELECTROLYTE | VALUES | SOURCE AND CAUSE OF IMBALANCES | FUNCTIONS AND CLINICAL MANIFESTATIONS |
|---|---|---|---|
| **Calcium** | 4.4–5.1 mEq/L 8.8–10.2 mg/dl | Regulated by parathyroid hormone (PTH) and calcitonin; supplied by diet, absorbed under influence of activated vitamin D; 99% stored in bones and teeth; excreted by kidney and gastrointestinal tract | Blocks sodium at cell membrane, decreased membrane excitability; enhances coagulation process; essential in complement cascade; makes up much of crystalline matrix of bone; reciprocal relationship with phosphate |
| Hypercalcemia | >5.5 mEq/L >10.5 mg/dl | Excessive vitamin D, immobility, renal insufficiency; hyperparathyroidism, malignancies of bone or blood | Decreased neuromuscular excitability, muscle weakness, central nervous system depression, stupor to coma; ECG may show shortened Q-T interval; if due to increased absorption from bones, increased risk of fracture; vomiting, constipation, kidney stones |
| Hypocalcemia | <4.0 mEq/L <8.5 mg/dl | Hypoparathyroidism, surgical or idiopathic; malabsorption of calcium; insufficient or inactivated vitamin D; dietary lack of calcium or vitamin D; hypoalbuminemia | Increased neuromuscular excitability; Trousseau's and Chvostek's signs positive; skeletal muscle cramps, tetany, laryngospasm, asphyxiation, death |
| **Phosphate** | 3.0–4.5 mg/100 mg | Supplied in diet; inverse relationship to calcium | Stored in bone; promotes acid-base balance; essential to metabolism at cellular level |
| Hyperphosphatemia | >4.5 mg/100 ml | Renal failure; decreased PTH | See hypocalcemia |
| Hypophosphatemia | <3.0 mg/100 ml | Increased excretion through gastrointestinal tract; antacid ingestion; vitamin D deficit; diabetic ketosis, hyperparathyroidism, malnutrition, alcoholism | Anorexia; weakness, bone pain; osteomalacia; muscle weakness; tremors; hyporeflexia; confusion seizures; coma; hemolytic anemia, bleeding disorders, leukocyte malfunction |
| **Chloride** | 100–106 mEq/L | Major anion of extracellular fluid; supplied by diet, excreted by kidney, gastrointestinal tract | Functions in acid-base balance; essential in gastric acid; follows sodium in loss and gain |
| Hypochloremia | <95 mEq/L | Diuretic therapy, hyponatremia, metabolic alkalosis due to chloride loss, bicarbonate gain | Signs of hyponatremia and metabolic alkalosis |
| **Magnesium** | 1.6–2.4 mEq/L 1.8–3.0 mg/dl | A major cation in extracellular fluid and bones; suplied in diet, excreted by kidneys; competes at renal tubule for reabsorption; PTH increases excretion | Promotes many intracellular enzyme reactions; depresses neuromuscular excitability, peripheral vasodilation |
| Hypomagnesemia | <1.5 mEq/L | Malabsorption related to gastrointestinal disease; excess loss of gastrointestinal fluids; acute alcoholism and cirrhosis of the liver; diuretic drug therapy; pancreatitis; sometimes hyper- or hypoparathyroidism | May cause hypocalcemia and hypokalemia; neuromuscular irritability increased, positive Chvostek's and Trousseau's signs, tetany, convulsions; tachycardia, hypertension |

Source: J. Wallach, Interpretation of Diagnostic Tests (4th ed.). Boston: Little, Brown, 1986; W.N. Kelley, Textbook of Internal Medicine. Philadelphia: J.B. Lippincott, 1989; and M.H. Maxwell, C.R. Kleeman, and R.G. Narins, Clinical Disorders of Fluid and Electrolyte Metabolism (4th ed.). New York: McGraw-Hill, 1987.

tion of isotonic solutions or of adrenal glucocorticoid hormones. This imbalance also may occur in disease states such as chronic renal failure, liver disease, congestive heart failure, malnutrition, and hyperaldosteronism when homeostatic mechanisms for fluid and electrolyte balance are impaired. Hypervolemia results in expansion of the extracellular space and circulatory overload. Signs and symptoms reflect the overload (see Table 8-2).

## Sodium

Sodium is the major cation of the ECF (see Table 8-2). It regulates the osmotic pressure of the ECF and markedly affects the osmotic pressure of ICF. Sodium intake comes from the diet; requirements for body needs vary according to age and size. Adolescents need between 900 and 2700 mg of sodium daily. Adults can maintain sodium balance with less than 500 mg per day. One teaspoon of salt contains approximately 2 gm of sodium.[10] The average daily intake in the United States is 2.3 to 6.9 gm.[10]

Sodium is also an essential component in neuromuscular excitability and is responsible for depolarization of the cell membranes of excitable cells. It participates in acid-base balance by combining with the bicarbonate radical. Sodium exists in combination with various anions, especially chloride and bicarbonate. Sodium concentration is directly regulated by aldosterone and indirectly by ADH, ANH, and the glucocorticoids.

### Hyponatremia

Deficits of serum sodium result from actual loss from body fluids or from excessive gains in extracellular water that dilute the sodium concentration. This imbalance may be caused by inadequate sodium intake, diuretic therapy, adrenal insufficiency, and administration of hypotonic solutions to replace fluid lost through diaphoresis, vomiting, or gastrointestinal suctioning. Conditions that may result in water gain include psychogenic polydipsia, inadequate excretion of water secondary to renal disease or brain lesions, or administration of hypotonic solutions after surgical procedures or trauma.[17] The cells become swollen as water moves from ECF to ICF to compensate for the solute deficit. The neuromuscular system is particularly sensitive to this imbalance (see Table 8-2).

### Hypernatremia

Serum sodium excess results from decreased intake or increased output of water. Overingestion of sodium may also cause this imbalance. Conditions that may lead to hypernatremia include impaired thirst sensation, dysphagia, profuse diaphoresis, watery diarrhea, polyuria due to diabetes insipidus, excessive water loss from the lungs, and excessive administration of hypertonic solu-

tions. Cells shrink and dehydration occurs as water moves from the ICF to the ECF to compensate for the solute excess. Brain cells are also sensitive to this imbalance (see Table 8-2).

## Potassium

Potassium is normally concentrated in the ICF. It directly affects the excitability of nerves and muscles, and contributes to the intracellular osmotic pressure (see Table 8-2). Secretions and excretions contain large amounts of potassium. The source of potassium is the diet, which normally provides much more than is needed by the body. Urine potassium concentrations vary, providing an efficient mechanism for the excretion of excess potassium to maintain a narrow range of normal serum concentrations.

Potassium moves into the cell during the formation of new tissues, the anabolic phase. During tissue breakdown, the catabolic phase, potassium leaves the cell. Potassium will not move into cells if there is a deficit of oxygen, glucose, or insulin.

The human body very effectively excretes potassium but has little mechanism for renal conservation. Potassium deficit occurs in 2 to 3 days if there is no intake. This deficit is enhanced by conditions such as surgery that increase anabolic needs. Anything that increases the excretion of potassium, such as diuretics, may also cause the depletion.

The major route for the loss of potassium is the kidneys, but some loss can occur through gastrointestinal secretions or the skin. In the kidneys, the final excretion of potassium is under the control of aldosterone at the distal tubules. At this point, hydrogen, potassium, and sodium tend to compete with each other for excretion. Sodium is usually preferred for absorption in the presence of aldosterone. If the plasma hydrogen ion concentration is elevated above normal, the tubules preferentially tend to excrete hydrogen and conserve potassium, which leads to the hyperkalemia often seen in association with acidosis. The reverse is true in alkalosis: when the hydrogen concentration is low, potassium is preferentially excreted and hydrogen is conserved, thus causing hypokalemia associated with alkalosis (see Chap. 9).

### Hypokalemia

A serum deficit of potassium may be caused by any of the following: (1) lack of intake; (2) diuretics (potassium-depleting); (3) major gastrointestinal surgical procedures, especially with nasogastric suctioning and incomplete replacement; (4) excessive gastrointestinal secretions; (5) hyperaldosteronism; (6) malnutrition; and (7) trauma or burns.

Hypokalemia affects every system. In the gastrointestinal system, anorexia, nausea, vomiting, and paralytic ileus may occur. In the muscles, flaccidity and weakness may be exhibited, and finally may lead to respiratory muscle weakness and arrest. Cardiac dysrhythmias are common and the electrocardiogram (ECG) may show the presence of a U wave when it was not previously present (Figure 8-6). Ventricular tachycardia and cardiac arrest may occur when the levels are very low. Central nervous system depression and decreased deep tendon reflexes also may be noted. Hypokalemia causes decreased ability of renal tubules to concentrate waste, leading to increased water loss.

Hypokalemia causes an increased sensitivity to digitalis and may precipitate the effects of digitalis toxicity in persons taking a preparation of the drug. Hypokalemia enhances automaticity and may precipitate ventricular fibrillation (see Chap. 23).

## Hyperkalemia

Excess potassium is usually secondary to temporary or permanent kidney dysfunction. It frequently occurs in association with renal failure. It also may be present transiently (with normal renal function) after major tissue trauma or after the rapid transfusion of stored bank blood. As blood is stored, the red blood cells begin to break down and release their potassium into the surrounding fluid. A unit of blood 1 day old has approximately 7 mEq per liter of potassium, while a unit that is 21 days old has 23 mEq per liter.[13]

Hyperkalemia mainly affects the cardiovascular system. A decreased membrane potential causes a decrease in the intensity of the action potential, resulting in a dilated, flaccid heart. Various kinds of conduction defects

may be noted together with ectopic dysrhythmias. The ECG shows tall peaked T waves, a short Q-T interval, and widening of the QRS complex (see Figure 8-6C). In the gastrointestinal system, nausea, vomiting, and diarrhea are common. Initial irritability of the skeletal muscles gives way to weakness and flaccid paralysis. Digital numbness and tingling may be described.

## Calcium

Calcium is present in the body in the form of calcium salts and as ionized and protein-bound calcium (see Table 8-2). Ninety-nine percent is in the bones and teeth in the crystalline form, which gives hardness to these structures. Of the 1% that is circulating, approximately 40% is bound to plasma proteins, especially albumin. The ionized form of calcium is the active portion and functions in membrane integrity, coagulation, muscle contraction, and in the electrophysiology of the excitable cells.

Calcium can be released from its bound form, especially in the presence of a decreased serum pH. The reaction simply stated is a reversible equation:

$$Ca^{++} (\text{protein bound} + H^+) \leftrightarrows$$
$$Ca^{++} (\text{ionized}) + H^+ (\text{protein complex})$$

The reaction is driven toward the right in acidosis, causing an increase in ionized serum calcium. In alkalosis, the reaction is driven more toward the left, which can cause hypocalcemia. This is the method used by the body plasma proteins to buffer hydrogen ion[19] (see Chap. 9).

Calcium concentration in the blood is under the influence of *parathyroid hormone* (PTH) and *calcitonin*. Parathyroid hormone is released by the parathyroid

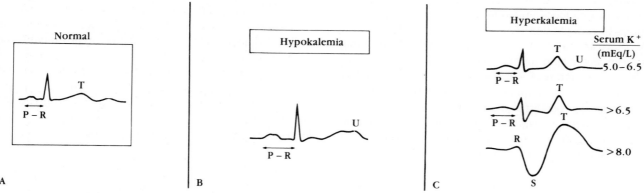

**FIGURE 8-6.**

Altered cardiac conduction in hypokalemia and hyperkalemia. A. Normal electrocardiogram in the adult. B. In hypokalemia, the T wave is flattened and the U wave is prominent. C. In hyperkalemia, the ECG changes do not always correspond to the serum potassium values given, but the progression from minor to severe changes correlates to some degree with the potassium level. With potassium concentration less than 6.5 mEq/L, the early ECG abnormality is peaking or tenting of the T waves. The next change shown with a level of potassium concentration greater than 6.5 includes flattening of the P wave, prolongation of the P-R interval, and widening of the QRS complex, with development of a deep S wave. With severe hyperkalemia (8.0 mEq/L) ventricular fibrillation or cardiac arrest is imminent (From R. Schrier, *Manual of Nephrology*, Boston: Little, Brown, 1981.)

glands when the extracellular ionized calcium level is decreased (see Chap. 38). Calcitonin enhances the deposition (uptake) of calcium into bone when increased calcium levels are present, and it inhibits bone reabsorption. Calcitonin is produced by C cells in the thyroid gland. It functions to reduce serum calcium and phosphate levels but may have more important roles in bone development in the fetus.[12]

Calcium stabilizes the cell membrane and blocks sodium transport into the cell. Because of this, decreased calcium levels increase the excitability of cells, while increased levels decrease excitability.

Vitamin D affects calcium absorption and bone deposition and reabsorption. Vitamin D is produced in the skin through the action of ultraviolet light and is present also in most American diets. It is changed by the liver to 25-hydroxycholecalciferol by hydroxylation and is further metabolized by the kidneys with the aid of PTH to form the most active type 1,25-dihydroxycholecalciferol (see Chap. 45). This substance is important in enhancing calcium uptake from the gastrointestinal tract and functioning with PTH in bone reabsorption.[7,12,19]

## Relationship of Calcium to Phosphate

Phosphate is an anion that is also regulated by PTH and activated vitamin D. Normally, the total concentration of calcium and phosphate is constant. If the calcium level increases, the phosphate level decreases. Calcium joins with phosphate to form calcium phosphate ($CaHPO_4$). When an excessive amount of $CaHPO_4$ is formed, it is not ionizable, and hypocalcemia results.

## Hypocalcemia

When calcium levels decrease, the blocking effect of calcium on sodium also decreases. As a result, depolarization of excitable cells occurs more readily as sodium moves in. Therefore, when the calcium levels are low, increased central nervous system (CNS) excitability and muscle spasms occur. Convulsions and tetany may be the result.

Hypocalcemia may be associated with decreased activation of vitamin D, which often results from renal or liver disease. Pancreatitis may cause decreased serum calcium due to the release of pancreatic lipase, which combines with fatty acids and calcium. Blood transfusions may cause hypocalcemia, as calcium binds with the citrate used in blood preparation, thus removing ionizable calcium from the blood.[15] Hyperphosphatemia, hypoalbuminemia, parathyroid disease, administration of agents such as adrenocorticotropic hormone (ACTH) or glucagon, surgical removal of the parathyroid glands, gastrointestinal tract disease, and neoplastic conditions may all be associated with hypocalcemia.

The results of hypocalcemia are spasms and tetany, increased gastrointestinal motility, cardiovascular problems, and osteoporosis. Muscle tetany is both common and dangerous, especially when it involves laryngeal spasm. Trousseau's sign of hypocalcemia is elicited when a blood pressure cuff is inflated on an extremity for 1 to 3 minutes and a contraction of the fingers occurs. Chvostek's sign is elicited when the facial nerve at the temple is tapped resulting in a twitch on that side of the face (Figure 8-7). Cardiac problems include decreased cardiac contractility and occasionally symptoms of heart failure. The cardiac action potential changes are seen on the ECG by prolongation of the S-T segment and resultant Q-T prolongation (Figure 8-8).[2,16]

## Hypercalcemia

Excessive levels of calcium increase the blocking effect on sodium in the skeletal muscles. This leads to decreased excitability of both muscles and nerves, eventually contributing to flaccidity. Hypercalcemia is associated with decreased phosphate levels. The major cause is hyperparathyroidism, which results in increased PTH, which increases calcium uptake from the bones into the circulating blood. Some malignant tumors secrete PTH-like substances that function similarly to true PTH. Excessive ingestion of vitamin D may cause the condition and occasionally, it occurs with prolonged immobilization.

Hypercalcemia causes skeletal muscle weakness, anorexia, nausea and vomiting, constipation, weight loss, and increased excretion of calcium in the urine. The increased circulating calcium may be deposited anywhere, but the kidneys are most vulnerable. Calcium deposition

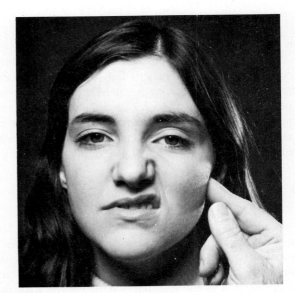

**FIGURE 8-7.**
Facial muscle contraction in Chvostek's sign. (From M. Beyers and S. Dudas, *The Clinical Practice of Medical Surgical Nursing* [2nd ed.]. Boston: Little, Brown, 1984.)

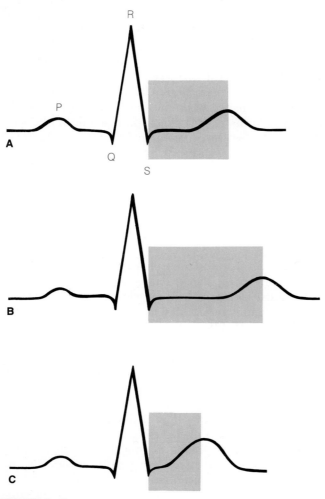

**FIGURE 8-8.**
**A.** Normal electrocardiogram tracing. **B.** Changes in the T wave and ST segment with hypocalcemia. **C.** Changes in the T wave and ST segment with hypercalcemia.

may result in kidney stones. Increased amounts may also be deposited in the arteries and cardiac valves. Central nervous system changes may include depression, bizarre behavior, and memory impairment. Acute hypercalcemia in persons on hemodialysis for renal failure can present symptoms suggestive of dementia.[2] Cardiac effects include shortening of the Q-T interval on the ECG with virtually no S-T segment (see Figure 8-8).[16]

## Phosphate

Phosphate functions with calcium to support bone formation. Phosphate is the primary intracellular anion. It assists with energy transfers within the cells.[13] Approximately 85% of body phosphate is in the bones, while the remaining 15% is intracellular.[19] It promotes acid-base balance of the body by acting as a buffer in the extracellular fluid. It also participates in the metabolism of glucose, fat, and protein.

## Hypophosphatemia

Hypophosphatemia occurs in alcoholism, malnutrition, diabetic ketoacidosis, and hyperthyroidism. A deficit may also result from antacid use because aluminum hydroxide, aluminum carbonate, and calcium carbonate combine with phosphate to promote loss of phosphate through the feces. This imbalance is characterized by hematologic malfunctions, encephalopathies, and musculoskeletal disorders (see Table 8-2).

## Hyperphosphatemia

Hyperphosphatemia can occur in renal failure or when parathyroid hormone levels are decreased. Because calcium is inversely related to phosphate, the clinical manifestations of hyperphosphatemia resemble those of hypocalcemia.

## Chloride

The chloride ion is the major anion of ECF (see Table 8-2). The amount of chloride in the fluid closely parallels the sodium content. Chloride is a component of hydrochloric acid in the stomach. It also serves an essential role in the transport of excess carbon dioxide by red blood cells (See Chap. 19). Chloride moves into the cells by passive transport.

Chloride depletion (hypochloremia) especially results from loss of gastrointestinal secretions, such as that occurring from vomiting, excessive diarrhea, and nasogastric suctioning. Diuretic therapy commonly causes hypochloremia together with hyponatremia, but urinary loss of chloride may be greater than loss of sodium. Metabolic alkalosis results as bicarbonate is conserved to maintain cation-anion balance. The clinical manifestations of hypochloremia are usually related to the associated metabolic alkalosis (see Chap. 9).

## Magnesium

Magnesium is found mostly within the cells and in the bones (see Table 8-2). This cation activates a number of intracellular enzyme systems and is required for protein and nucleic acid synthesis. Magnesium is particularly essential in promoting neuromuscular integrity.[13]

## Hypomagnesemia

The most common cause of decreased serum magnesium is excessive ingestion of alcohol. Other causes include malnutrition, diabetes mellitus, liver failure, and poor intestinal absorption. The clinical manifestations include increased neuromuscular irritability, paresthesia, tetany, and convulsions.

### Hypermagnesemia

This condition is rare but may occur in individuals with renal failure, especially if they ingest magnesium-containing antacids.[13] Clinical manifestations include lethargy, coma, cardiac dysrhythmias, respiratory failure, and death. Because dialysis in persons with chronic renal failure does not remove magnesium well, these individuals should be restricted from ingesting magnesium-containing medications.

## EDEMA

The word *edema* refers to the expansion or accumulation of interstitial fluid volume. It may be localized or generalized, pitting or nonpitting, depending on its etiology. Edema is usually thought of as accumulation of excess fluid in the skin; however, the mechanism causing skin edema also can cause fluid shifts in other vulnerable areas of the body. These fluid shifts are sometimes termed *third-space* shifts, and include ascites, pleural or pericardial effusions, and pulmonary edema.[13] Table 8-3 summarizes the etiologic mechanisms that may lead to the formation of edema and fluid shifts. Five interrelated mechanisms are commonly described: (1) decreased COP; (2) increased capillary hydrostatic pressure; (3) increased capillary permeability; (4) lymphatic obstruction;

and (5) sodium and body water excess.[7] Some forms of edema result from more than one mechanism.

## Decreased COP

When the plasma proteins are depleted in the blood, the inward forces are decreased, allowing the filtration effect to favor movement into the tissues. This leads to accumulation of fluid in the tissues with a decreased central volume of plasma. The kidneys respond to the decreased circulating volume by activating the renin-angiotensin-aldosterone system, resulting in additional reabsorption of sodium and water. Intravascular volume increases temporarily. However, because the plasma protein deficit has not been corrected, the colloid osmotic pressure (ie, the inward force) remains low in proportion to capillary hydrostatic pressure. Consequently, intravascular fluid moves into the tissues, worsening the edema and the circulatory status.

Hypoproteinemia causes decreased colloid osmotic pressure and may result from malnutrition, neoplastic wasting, liver failure, or protein loss from burns, kidneys, or the gastrointestinal tract. Albumin is the primary protein affected because it is the most abundant and also because its molecules are rather small and can pass through damaged capillary endothelium or glomeruli. Loss of protein into the tissues causes decreased reabsorption of tissue fluids and edema. This is a positive feedback response because as the central blood volume becomes depleted, the kidneys conserve more sodium and water,

---

**TABLE 8–3.**
EXAMPLES OF ETIOLOGIC MECHANISMS FOR THE FORMATION OF EDEMA

| ETIOLOGIC MECHANISMS | TYPES OF EDEMA |
| --- | --- |
| Increased capillary pressure | Congestive heart failure<br>Phlebothrombosis<br>Cirrhosis of the liver with portal hypertension |
| Vasodilatation | Inflammation<br>Allergic reactions<br>Burns (direct vascular injury) |
| Decreased colloid osmotic pressure | Liver failure<br>Protein malnutrition<br>Nephrosis<br>Burns |
| Lymphatic obstruction | Surgical removal of lymph structures<br>Inflammation or malignant involvement of lymph nodes<br>  and vessels<br>Filariasis |
| Sodium/body water excess | Congestive heart failure<br>Renal failure<br>Aldosteronism<br>Excess sodium intake |

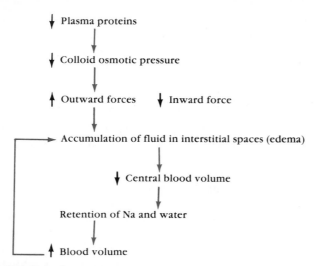

**FIGURE 8-9.**
Positive feedback of compensatory mechanisms for decreased colloid osmotic pressure.

and additional edema is formed (Figure 8-9). This response can be terminated by restoring intravascular protein levels, which increases the intravascular COP and subsequently its volume.

The accumulation of ascitic fluid in cirrhosis of the liver is partly related to hypoproteinemia from decreased hepatic production of albumin and partly to increased hydrostatic pressure created by portal hypertension (see Chap. 43).

## Increased Capillary Hydrostatic Pressure

The most common cause of increased capillary pressure is congestive heart failure in which increased systemic venous pressure is combined with increased blood volume. These manifestations are characteristic of failure of the right ventricle or right heart failure. Left heart failure may also lead to an increase in pulmonary capillary pressure (PCP). When the pressure exceeds 25 mm Hg, pulmonary edema can occur (see Chap. 24).

Other causes of increased hydrostatic pressure include renal failure with increased total blood volume, increased gravitational forces from standing for long periods of time, impaired venous circulation, and hepatic obstruction. Venous obstruction produces localized, rather than generalized, edema because only one vein or group of veins is usually affected.

## Increased Capillary Permeability

Direct damage to blood vessels, such as with trauma and burns, may cause increased permeability of the endothelial junctions. Localized edema may occur in response to an allergen, such as a bee sting. In certain individuals this allergen may precipitate an anaphylactic response with widespread edema initiated by the histamine type of reaction (see Chap. 16).

Inflammation causes hyperemia and vasodilation, which lead to accumulation of fluids, proteins, and cells in an affected area. This results in edematous swelling (exudation) of the affected localized area (see Chap. 13).

## Obstruction of the Lymphatics

The most common cause of lymphatic obstruction is the surgical removal of a group of lymph nodes and vessels to prevent the spread of malignancy. Radiation therapy, trauma, malignant metastasis, and inflammation may also lead to localized lymphatic obstruction. *Filariasis*, a rare parasitic infection of the lymph vessels, can cause widespread obstruction of the vessels.

Lymphatic obstruction leads to retention of excess fluid and plasma proteins in the interstitial fluid. As proteins accumulate in the interstitial spaces, more water moves into the area. The edema is usually localized.

## Sodium and Body Water Excess

With congestive heart failure, cardiac output is decreased as the force of contraction decreases. To compensate, increased amounts of aldosterone cause the retention of sodium and water. Plasma volume increases, as does venous intravascular capillary pressure. The failing heart is unable to pump this increased venous return, and fluid is forced into the interstitial space (see Chap. 24). Hypervolemia also can occur with renal insufficiency and renal failure. The kidneys cannot adequately excrete the solute load and hypervolemia results (see Chap. 35).

## Types of Edema

*Pitting* edema refers to the displacement of interstitial water by finger pressure on the skin, which leaves a pitted depression. After the pressure is removed, it often takes several minutes for the depression to be resolved. Pitting edema often appears in dependent sites, such as the sacrum of a bedridden individual. Similarly, gravitational hydrostatic pressure increases the accumulation of fluid in the legs and feet of an upright individual.

*Nonpitting* edema may be seen in areas of loose skin folds such as the periorbital spaces of the face. Nonpitting edema may occur after venous thrombosis, especially of the superficial veins. Persistent edema leads to trophic changes in the skin. These changes may progress to stasis dermatitis and ulcers that heal very slowly (see Chap. 27).

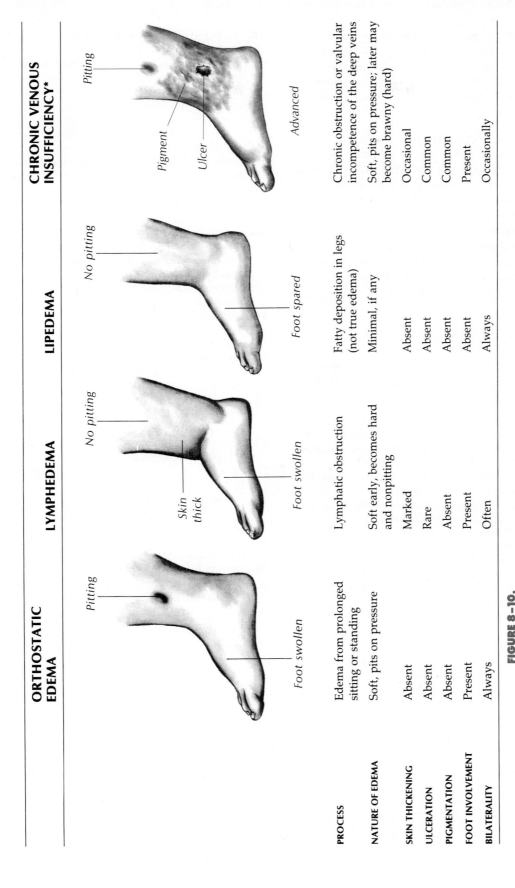

|  | ORTHOSTATIC EDEMA | LYMPHEDEMA | LIPEDEMA | CHRONIC VENOUS INSUFFICIENCY* |
|---|---|---|---|---|
| PROCESS | Edema from prolonged sitting or standing | Lymphatic obstruction | Fatty deposition in legs (not true edema) | Chronic obstruction or valvular incompetence of the deep veins |
| NATURE OF EDEMA | Soft, pits on pressure | Soft early, becomes hard and nonpitting | Minimal, if any | Soft, pits on pressure; later may become brawny (hard) |
| SKIN THICKENING | Absent | Marked | Absent | Occasional |
| ULCERATION | Absent | Rare | Absent | Common |
| PIGMENTATION | Absent | Absent | Absent | Common |
| FOOT INVOLVEMENT | Present | Present | Absent | Present |
| BILATERALITY | Always | Often | Always | Occasionally |

**FIGURE 8–10.**
Some peripheral causes of edema. (From B. Bates, A Guide to Physical Examination. Philadelphia: J.B. Lippincott, 1986.)

Nonpitting, brawny edema is also associated with thick, hardened skin and color changes. It occurs when serum proteins become trapped and coagulated in the tissue spaces. Figure 8-10 shows some different causes of edema and the mechanisms that may produce them.

## Distribution of Edema

The distribution of edema can give clues as to its cause. If it is localized in one extremity, it is probably due to venous or lymphatic obstruction. Edema resulting from hypoproteinemia is generalized but is especially pronounced in the eyelids and face in the morning, due to the recumbent position assumed at night and the aid of gravitational forces. Edema of heart failure is usually greatest in the legs of an ambulatory individual, and it tends to accumulate throughout the day.[6]

## REFERENCES

1. Andreoli, T.E. Disorders of fluid volume, electrolyte, and acid-base balance. In J.B. Wyngaarden and L.H. Smith (eds.), *Cecil's Textbook of Medicine* (17th ed.). New York: W.B. Saunders, 1985.

2. Benabe, J.E., and Martinez-Maldonado, M. Disorders of calcium metabolism. In M.H. Maxwell, C.R. Kleeman, and R.G. Narins (eds.), *Clinical Disorders of Fluid and Electrolyte Metabolism* (4th ed.). New York: McGraw-Hill, 1987.

3. Birney, M.H., and Penney, D.G. Atrial natriuretic peptide: A hormone with implications. *Heart Lung* 19(2):174, 1990.

4. Delaney, V.B., and Bourke, E. Diuretics. In J.W. Hurst et al., *The Heart* (7th ed.). New York: McGraw-Hill, 1990.

5. Delaney, V.B., and Bourke, E. The interrelationship of heart disease and kidney disease. In J.W. Hurst et al., *The Heart* (7th ed.). New York: McGraw-Hill, 1990.

6. Fishman, A.P. Heart failure. In J.B. Wyngaarden and L.H. Smith (eds.), *Cecil's Textbook of Medicine* (17th ed.). New York: W.B. Saunders, 1985.

7. Guyton, A.C. *Textbook of Medical Physiology* (8th ed.). Philadelphia: W.B. Saunders, 1990.

8. Hollenberg, N.K., and Dzau, V.J. The renin-angiotensin system. In M.H. Maxwell, C.R. Kleeman, and R.G. Narins (eds.), *Clinical Disorders of Fluid and Electrolyte Metabolism* (4th ed.). New York: McGraw-Hill, 1987.

9. Humes, H.D., and Cox, M. Principles of the renal regulation of fluid and electrolytes. In W.N. Kelley, *Textbook of Internal Medicine*. Philadelphia: J.B. Lippincott, 1989.

10. Lewis, C.M. *Nutrition and Nutritional Therapy in Nursing*. Norwalk, Conn.: Appleton-Century-Crofts, 1986.

11. Marcus, M.T. Fluid and electrolyte balance. In E.A. Mahoney and J.P. Flynn (eds.), *Handbook of Medical-Surgical Nursing*. New York: Wiley, 1983.

12. Marx, S.J., and Bourdeau, J.E. Calcium metabolism. In M.H. Maxwell, C.R. Kleeman, and R.G. Narins (eds.), *Clinical Disorders of Fluid and Electrolyte Metabolism* (4th ed.). New York: McGraw-Hill, 1987.

13. Metheny, N.M., and Snively, W.D. *Nurse's Handbook of Fluid Balance* (4th ed.). Philadelphia: J.B. Lippincott, 1983.

14. Morrison, G., and Singer, I. Hyperosmolal states. In M.H. Maxwell, C.R. Kleeman, and R.G. Narins (eds.), *Clinical Disorders of Fluid and Electrolyte Metabolism* (4th ed.). New York: McGraw-Hill, 1987.

15. Plumer, A.L. *Principles and Practice of Intravenous Therapy* (4th ed.). Boston: Little, Brown, 1987.

16. Rardon, D.R., and Fisch, C. Electrolytes and the heart. In J.W. Hurst et al., *The Heart* (7th ed.). New York: McGraw-Hill, 1990.

17. Reineck, H.J., and Stein, J.H. Sodium metabolism. In M.H. Maxwell, C.R. Kleeman, and R.G. Narins (eds.), *Clinical Disorders of Fluid and Electrolyte Metabolism* (4th ed.). New York: McGraw-Hill, 1987.

18. Schlant, R.C., and Sonnenblick, E.H. Normal physiology of the cardiovascular system. In J.W. Hurst et al., *The Heart* (7th ed.). New York: McGraw-Hill, 1990.

19. Schrier, R.W. *Renal and Electrolyte Disorders* (3rd ed.). Boston: Little, Brown, 1986.

20. Stanton, B.A., and Koeppen, B.M. Control of body fluid volume and osmolality. In R.M. Berne and M.N. Levy (eds.), *Principles of Physiology*. St. Louis: Mosby, 1990.

# chapter 9

## Barbara Bullock
## Bonnie Juneau

# Normal and Altered Acid-Base Balance

## Learning Objectives

1. Define *pH*.
2. List the normal values of the blood gases and pH of the different body fluids.
3. Differentiate between volatile and nonvolatile acids.
4. Diagram the dissociation of carbonic acid.
5. Describe the major buffer systems.
6. Describe specifically how the carbonic acid-bicarbonate system is affected by the respiratory and renal systems.
7. Explain how the kidneys maintain a constant hydrogen ion concentration in the plasma.
8. Describe the activity of hemoglobin as a protein buffer.
9. Differentiate between acidosis and alkalosis on the basis of physiologic disruption.
10. Describe the pathophysiology that underlies respiratory acidosis.
11. Compare respiratory acidosis and metabolic acidosis with respect to pathophysiology and compensatory mechanisms.
12. Define the term anion gap and relate it to an acid-base abnormality.
13. Differentiate the etiology of respiratory and metabolic alkalosis.
14. Describe the clinical manifestations of respiratory and metabolic alkalosis.

## NORMAL ACID-BASE BALANCE

All living cells of the human body are surrounded by a fluid environment called extracellular fluid (ECF). The chemical composition of the ECF is regulated within narrow limits that provide an optimal environment for maintaining normal cell function. The extracellular concentration of potassium ions, for example, is normally maintained within a range of 3.5 to 5.0 mEq per liter.

Deviation from normal serum potassium concentration can affect transmission of nerve impulses, electrical conduction in the heart, and the contraction of skeletal, cardiac, and smooth muscles.

The most precisely regulated ion concentration in extracellular fluid is that of the hydrogen ion, normally ranging from 37 to 43 nEq per liter. A nanoequivalent (nEq) is $10^{-9}$ equivalent, a very small measurement; the abbreviation saves writing a lot of zeros.[4] Deviation from normal hydrogen ion concentration can upset normal reactions of cellular metabolism by altering the effectiveness of enzymes, hormones, and other chemical regulators of cell function. It can also affect the normal distribution of other ions (such as sodium and potassium) between the intracellular and extracellular fluids, thereby disturbing a variety of cell and tissue ion-dependent functions, such as conduction, contraction, and secretion. Therefore, normal ECF hydrogen ion concentration is essential for normal body functions. The concentration is determined by the types and amounts of acids and bases present and its regulation is commonly called acid-base balance.

When hydrogen ions are formed, they rapidly react with water molecules to form the *hydronium ion* ($H^+ + H_2O \leftrightarrows H_3O^+$). It is the hydronium ion that gives a solution or body fluid its acidity. In usual practice, it is referred to as if it were a single hydrogen ion.[4]

## *Fundamental Concepts*

### *Electrolytes*

An electrolyte is a substance that *dissociates* and forms ions when mixed with water; the process is called *ionization*. It results in the formation of *cations* (positively charged electrolytes, such as sodium), and *anions* (negatively charged electrolytes, such as chloride). Ionic solutions readily conduct electric current, hence the term *electrolyte*.

An *acid* is any electrolyte that ionizes in water and forms hydrogen ions and anions. The anion formed is called the *conjugate base* of the acid. An acid is a *hydrogen ion donor* and thus elevates the hydrogen ion concentration of the solution to which it is added. The strength of an acid is determined by its degree of ionization in water. Strong acids completely ionize in water and readily liberate hydrogen ions. Hydrochloric acid (HCl) is a strong acid because 99.9% of the HCl molecules ionize in pure water. Weak acids partly ionize in water and therefore do not liberate hydrogen ions as readily as strong acids. The acidity of the solution depends on how much the acid dissociates.[4]

A *base* is any substance that can bind hydrogen ions. An *alkali* is a substance that contains a base. A strong base binds hydrogen ions readily. Hydroxides such as sodium hydroxide (NaOH) contain the hydroxyl (OH) ion, a strong base. A weak base binds hydrogen ions less readily. Sodium bicarbonate is a weak alkali containing the bicarbonate ion, a weak base. When *sodium bicarbonate* (NaHCO$_3$) is added to water, it completely dissociates. A small percentage of the resulting bicarbonate ions binds hydrogen ions and forms carbonic acid ($HCO_3^- + H^+ \leftrightarrows H_2CO_3$).

Since a base is a hydrogen ion acceptor, the addition of a base to a solution containing hydrogen ions lowers the hydrogen ion concentration; the opposite occurs when an acid is added.

## *pH and Hydrogen Ion*

The pH is simply a negative logarithm of hydrogen ions ($H^+$) in a solution. One liter of water contains 0.0000001 gm of hydrogen ions. This figure is equal to $1/10^7$ as shown by the following equation:

$$0.0000001 = 1/10,000,000$$
$$= 1/(10 \times 10 \times 10 \times 10 \times 10 \times 10 \times 10)$$
$$= 1/10^7 = 10^{-7}$$

This simplified formula denotes the negative notation of a pH of 7 for neutral water. For any given solution, the numeric value of pH decreases as the hydrogen ion concentration increases. Therefore, since water is neutral at a pH of 7, when hydrogen ions are added to it, the solution becomes more acidic. The greater the hydrogen ion concentration, the more acidic the solution and the more the pH number falls. Acidic solutions range in pH between 0 and 7. Alkalotic or basic solutions, on the other hand, have less hydrogen ion concentration and range in pH between 7 and 14. The smaller the hydrogen ion concentration, the more alkaline the solution. Table 9-1 shows the Sorensen pH scale as it relates to the approximate pH compositions of body fluids. Note that the relationship between the pH and the hydrogen ion figures is logarithmic rather than linear. This means that an increase or decrease of one pH unit represents a tenfold change in hydrogen ion concentration.[8]

In the fluids of the human body, the acceptable pH range is 7.35 to 7.45. Normal blood gas values are indicated in Table 9-2. Levels below 7.35 indicate a state of acidosis, while levels above 7.45 indicate alkalosis. When the hydrogen ion concentration is in the normal range of 40 nEq per liter, the pH is 7.40.

The broadest range of hydrogen ion concentration in extracellular fluids compatible with mammalian life is 16 to 125 nEq per liter, corresponding to a pH range of approximately 6.8 to 7.8. Cells of the human body usually function normally when the pH of extracellular fluid (interstitial fluids and plasma) remains constant at about 7.40.

Alterations in plasma $H^+$ concentration alter the functioning of many enzyme and hormone systems; for example, acidosis depresses the function of epinephrine. $H^+$ concentration also affects neurologic functioning and the distribution of other ions.

In the processes of cellular metabolism, acid is continually being formed. Excess hydrogen is produced daily and must be eliminated from the body to maintain a steady state. The acids formed are of two types: (1) *volatile* acids that are excretable by the lungs; and (2) *nonvolatile* acids that are excreted by the kidney.

**TABLE 9-1.**
pH SCALE SHOWING THE CONCENTRATION OF HYDROGEN IONS
FROM pH 0 TO pH 14

| H+ CONCENTRATION (gm/L) | SCIENTIFIC NOTATION | pH UNITS | | EXAMPLES |
|---|---|---|---|---|
| 1.0 | $10^0$ | $-\log 10^0$ | = 0 | |
| 0.1 | $10^{-1}$ | $-\log 10^{-1}$ | = 1 | |
| 0.01 | $10^{-2}$ | $-\log 10^{-2}$ | = 2 | Gastric juice |
| 0.001 | $10^{-3}$ | $-\log 10^{-3}$ | = 3 | Gastric juice |
| 0.0001 | $10^{-4}$ | $-\log 10^{-4}$ | = 4 | |
| 0.00001 | $10^{-5}$ | $-\log 10^{-5}$ | = 5 | Urine |
| 0.000001 | $10^{-6}$ | $-\log 10^{-6}$ | = 6 | Urine/saliva |
| 0.0000001 | $10^{-7}$ | $-\log 10^{-7}$ | = 7 | Pure water |
| | | | 7.4 | Arterial blood |
| 0.00000001 | $10^{-8}$ | $-\log 10^{-8}$ | = 8 | Pancreatic juice/bile |
| 0.000000001 | $10^{-9}$ | $-\log 10^{-9}$ | = 9 | |
| 0.0000000001 | $10^{-10}$ | $-\log 10^{-10}$ | = 10 | |
| 0.00000000001 | $10^{-11}$ | $-\log 10^{-11}$ | = 11 | |
| 0.000000000001 | $10^{-12}$ | $-\log 10^{-12}$ | = 12 | |
| 0.0000000000001 | $10^{-13}$ | $-\log 10^{-13}$ | = 13 | |
| 0.00000000000001 | $10^{-14}$ | $-\log 10^{-14}$ | = 14 | |

Note: The approximate pH of some of the body fluids is indicated.
Source: Adapted from M. Toporek, Basic Chemistry of Life. St. Louis: Mosby, 1981.

## Metabolism: Volatile and Nonvolatile Acids

### Volatile Acids

A volatile acid is defined as an acid that can be excreted from the body as a gas. Either the acid itself or a chemical product of the acid can be converted to a gas and excreted. Carbonic acid, produced by the hydration of carbon dioxide in body fluids, is a volatile acid. The formation can be expressed in the equation:

$$CO_2 + H_2O \leftrightarrows H_2CO_3$$
$$\text{(carbonic anhydrase)}$$

Note that the enzyme carbonic anhydrase is necessary to accelerate the reaction. A normal adult produces about 300 liters of carbon dioxide per day from metabolic reactions. This results in the production of a large amount of carbonic acid. Normally, the lungs excrete carbon dioxide as rapidly as cell metabolism produces it; therefore, carbonic acid is not allowed to accumulate in the body and alter ECF pH.

### Nonvolatile Acids

A nonvolatile acid, also called a fixed acid, cannot be eliminated by the lungs and must be excreted by the kidneys. All metabolic acids present in body fluids except carbonic acid are classified as nonvolatile, and include sulfuric acid, phosphoric acid, lactic acid, ketoacids (acetoacetic acid, beta-hydroxybutyric acid), and smaller amounts of other inorganic and organic acids.

To some extent, fixed acids are neutralized by fixed bases in our diet. Fruits and vegetables contain such alkaline substances as potassium citrate. In a typical American diet, however, metabolic breakdown of foodstuffs leads to an excess of fixed acids (about 50 to 100 mEq/day), and these acids (or their conjugate bases) must be eliminated by the kidneys in order to maintain normal ECF pH.

**TABLE 9-2.**
NORMAL VALUES FOR ARTERIAL BLOOD GASES

| ELEMENT MEASURED | NORMAL VALUE |
|---|---|
| pH | 7.35–7.45 |
| $PCO_2$ | 35–45 mm Hg |
| $HCO_3^-$ | 24–28 mEq/L |
| $PO_2$ | 80–100 mm Hg |
| Hemoglobin saturation | 95–100% |
| Base excess | +2 to -2 |

## Regulation of Body Fluid pH

As previously stated, ECF pH is normally maintained between 7.35 and 7.45. This occurs by four well-integrated mechanisms: (1) chemical buffers, (2) regulation of carbon dioxide concentration by the respiratory system, (3) regulation of plasma bicarbonate concentration by the kidneys, and (4) hydrogen ion migration.

## Chemical Buffers

Chemical buffers constitute the first line of defense against changes in body fluid pH. They act within a fraction of a second for immediate defense against either increases or decreases in hydrogen ion concentration.

A chemical buffer is a mixture of two or more chemicals that minimize changes in the pH of a solution when either acids or bases are added. Buffers minimize changes in pH by taking up hydrogen ions when acids are added to body fluids, or by releasing hydrogen ions when the pH of body fluids becomes too high. The function of buffers is to convert strong acids, which would strongly decrease overall pH, into weak acids, which have a minimal effect on pH. Buffers also convert strong bases, which strongly increase overall pH, into weak bases, which have a minimal effect on pH.

The most important chemical buffers in the body fluids consist of weak acids plus the salts of their conjugate bases, together referred to as acid-base buffer pairs. In ECF fluids, the salts are primarily sodium salts, and in the intracellular fluids (ICFs), they are primarily potassium salts. Important chemical buffer pairs of the body fluids include the *bicarbonate, phosphate,* and *protein-*

*ate buffer systems*. The carbonic acid-bicarbonate system buffers volatile and nonvolatile acids in the interstitial fluid and in plasma. The phosphate buffer system is a major buffer of metabolic acids in the ICF. Proteinate buffers are found in plasma proteins, hemoglobin, and in ICF proteins. These buffers can react with both volatile and nonvolatile acids.[4] Figure 9-1 indicates how hemoglobin functions in the pulmonary capillary to remove $CO_2$ from the body and how it picks up $CO_2$ from the systemic tissue cell. Other important chemical buffers are intracellular organic phosphate complexes, such as adenosine triphosphate, adenosine diphosphate, creatine phosphate, and the hydroxyapatite crystal complex of bone.

Buffering of metabolically produced acids occurs, both intracellularly and extracellularly, in interstitial fluids and in blood. The majority of chemical buffering reactions takes place inside of the body's cells.

When acid or base is added to ECF, approximately half of the added ions eventually diffuse into cells where they are buffered. These ions or others that affect acid-base balance are exchanged across the cell membrane for intracellular ions or are accompanied into cells by ions of opposite charge. For example, if an acid is added to ECF, some of the hydrogen ion is buffered chemically within the ECF. Some is also diffused across cell membranes into cells. Because the hydrogen ion is positively charged, it must either be exchanged across the cell membrane for another cation, such as $Na^+$ or $K^+$, or

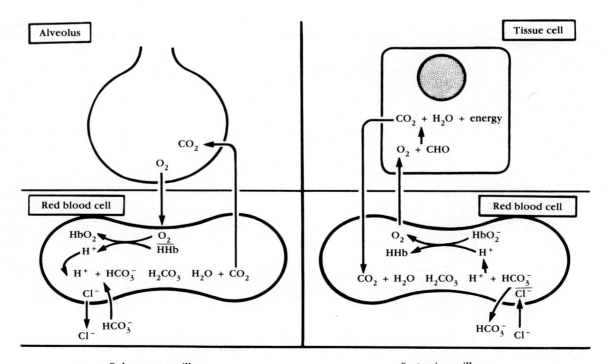

**FIGURE 9-1.**

Hemoglobin as an important blood buffer. (From: E. Selkurt, *Basic Physiology for the Health Sciences* [2nd ed.]. Boston: Little, Brown, 1982.)

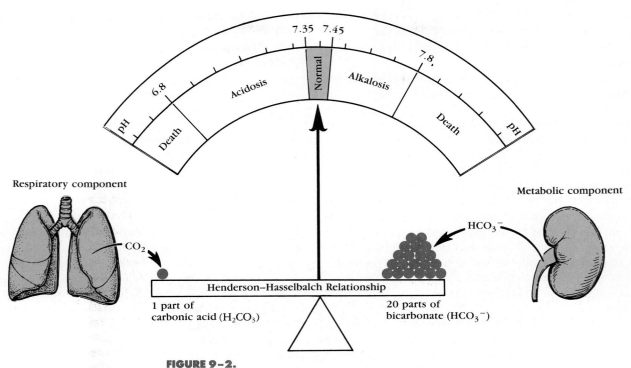

**FIGURE 9-2.**
Mechanisms for the defense against changes in body fluid pH.

be accompanied into the cell by an anion, such as $Cl^-$. Although both processes occur, the movement of cations out of the cell is quantitatively more important. In metabolic acidosis, for example, extracellular potassium levels, as measured in blood plasma, are frequently elevated, as intracellular stores are depleted to allow intracellular buffering of hydrogen ions (see p. 204). Often, in metabolic acidosis, plasma chloride is also reduced.

The carbonic acid-bicarbonate system is the most important extracellular buffer because it can be regulated by both the lungs and the kidneys. Normally, the carbonic acid ($H_2CO_3$)-bicarbonate ($HCO_3^-$) ratio is maintained at approximately 1:20 (Figure 9-2). This ratio keeps the pH at approximately 7.40. The actual content required to maintain this balance is 1.2 mmol per liter of $H_2CO_3$ to 24 mEq per liter of $HCO_3^-$. As long as the ratio of 1:20 is maintained, the pH will also be stabilized. If, for example, a retention of carbon dioxide and a reciprocal compensatory retention of bicarbonate occurs, the amounts might be 2.0 mmol per liter of $H_2CO_3$ and 40 mEq per liter of $HCO_3^-$, which would still maintain the ratio (2:40 instead of 1:20) and the pH would remain 7.40. The respiratory system works very rapidly in the excretion or retention of $CO_2$, while the renal system functions much more slowly to retain or excrete $HCO_3^-$, as is discussed in the subsequent sections.

### Respiratory Regulation of Plasma PCO₂

The respiratory system plays an important role in acid-base balance by controlling the partial pressure of carbon dioxide ($PCO_2$) in arterial blood. As excess carbon dioxide is formed during cellular processes, most of it is picked up by the red blood cells and carried to the lungs. Carbon dioxide reacts with body water to form carbonic acid, which then dissociates into hydrogen ion and bicarbonate ion, as the following reaction sequence indicates:

$$\underset{\text{Dehydration}}{\overset{\text{Hydration}}{CO_2 + H_2O \quad \leftrightarrows}} \quad \underset{\text{Association}}{\overset{\text{Dissociation}}{H_2CO_3 \quad \leftrightarrows}} \quad H^+ + HCO_3^-$$

These reactions are readily reversible. The hydration of dissolved carbon dioxide to form carbonic acid and the dehydration of carbonic acid to form carbon dioxide and water are slow reactions if uncatalyzed. The enzyme carbonic anhydrase, present in red blood cells, renal tubular cells, and other cells speeds up these reactions. The dissociation of carbonic acid to hydrogen ion and bicarbonate ion, or the reaction in the opposite direction, occurs virtually instantaneously. As long as the rate at which carbon dioxide is being eliminated from the body by the lungs equals the rate at which carbon dioxide is produced, no net change in the hydrogen ion concentration of that reaction will occur.

An increase in carbon dioxide tension results in the liberation of hydrogen ions; thus, the pH decreases. If alveolar ventilation is decreased, metabolically produced carbon dioxide accumulates in the blood, carbonic acid concentration rises, and blood pH falls.

A decrease in carbon dioxide tension results in less free hydrogen ions and consequently, a more alkaline pH. If ventilation is stimulated so that elimination of carbon dioxide temporarily exceeds its production, the blood $PCO_2$ moves to a lower level and alkaline blood pH results. Thus, changes in alveolar ventilation profoundly influence blood pH.

Alveolar ventilation is normally adjusted so that pH changes in the arterial blood are kept to a minimum. Increases of hydrogen ion concentration in body fluid (decreased pH), specifically in arterial blood and cerebrospinal fluid, result in a reflex increase in respiratory rate and depth. This respiratory response acts to blow off more carbon dioxide. The result is that the hydrogen ion concentration is decreased toward normal. Excess carbonic acid in the blood (due to failure to eliminate carbon dioxide adequately) is a powerful stimulus to ventilation. The increase in ventilation serves to diminish the retention of carbon dioxide and thereby minimizes the accumulation of carbonic acid in the blood. The ventilatory response also is reactive to acidosis from other acids. Fixed, nonvolatile acids cause a marked increase in ventilation rate and depth.

Decreases of body fluid hydrogen ion concentration (increased pH) depress respiratory activity. This allows carbon dioxide to build up in the blood. Consequently, more hydrogen ions are made available, minimizing the alkaline shift in pH. A decrease in respiration due to an alkaline pH is usually not very marked. This occurs because decreased ventilation produces *hypercapnia* (high serum carbon dioxide), which stimulates ventilation. In individuals with healthy lungs, increased levels of $PCO_2$ represent the greatest stimulus to breathe. Hypoxia stimulates respiration when the partial pressure of arterial oxygen ($PaO_2$) falls to 60 mm Hg or less (see Chap. 28).

The respiratory system normally changes its activity to minimize shifts in pH. Respiratory activity responds rapidly to acid-base stresses and shifts blood pH toward normal in minutes. A person who is hypoventilating begins to accumulate carbon dioxide rapidly and, as a reflex, increases the rate and depth of breathing to restore the blood pH. Conversely, respiratory rate is slowed when the pH elevates and the pH goes toward normal. An increase in alveolar ventilation of two times normal can increase the pH of blood 0.23 pH units. Conversely, depressing ventilation to one-fourth of normal decreases the pH by 0.4 pH units.[2]

## Renal Regulation of Plasma $HCO_3^-$

The major role of the kidneys in maintaining acid-base balance is to conserve circulating stores of bicarbonate and excrete hydrogen ions. The kidneys maintain ECF pH by: (1) increasing urinary excretion of hydrogen ions and conserving plasma bicarbonate when the blood is too acidic, and (2) increasing urinary excretion of bicarbonate and decreasing urinary excretion of hydrogen ions when the blood is too alkaline.

Renal mechanisms for hydrogen ion regulation are slower (taking hours or days) than are chemical buffer or respiratory mechanisms. Renal compensation for acid-base disturbances can be complete, however, because the kidneys actually excrete hydrogen ions and eliminate them from body fluids. Neither chemical buffering nor respiratory mechanisms can eliminate these metabolic hydrogen ions from the body.

Renal control of acid-base balance involves three processes that occur simultaneously along the length of the nephron: (1) reabsorption of filtered bicarbonate, (2) excretion of titratable acid, and (3) excretion of ammonia. All three mechanisms involve secretion of hydrogen ions into the urine and return of bicarbonate to the plasma.

Quantitatively, the *reabsorption of filtered bicarbonate* is the most important process in renal acid-base regulation. Approximately 4500 mEq of sodium bicarbonate are filtered each day. Normally, all but 1 or 2 mEq of sodium bicarbonate are resorbed into the plasma.

Figure 9-3 illustrates the cellular mechanisms involved in the resorption of filtered bicarbonate. Carbon dioxide in the tubular epithelial cell reacts with intracellular water to form carbonic acid. The reaction is catalyzed by the enzyme *carbonic anhydrase*. Carbonic acid dissociates to form hydrogen ions and bicarbonate ions. The hydrogen ions are actively secreted by the luminal cell membrane into the urine in exchange for sodium ions. The bicarbonate ion moves passively across the peritubular membrane into the blood, accompanying the actively reabsorbed sodium ion. In urine, hydrogen ions react with bicarbonate ions to form carbonic acid, which then dissociates into carbon dioxide and water. Water is either reabsorbed osmotically or eliminated in the urine, depending upon the body's water balance. Both blood

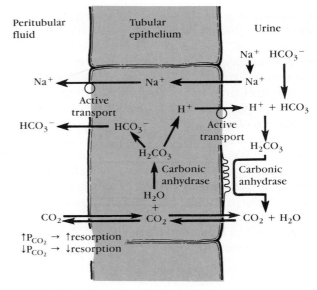

**FIGURE 9-3.**
Resorption of filtered bicarbonate.

and urine carbon dioxide are in equilibrium with carbon dioxide in tubular cells and provide the main impetus for cellular generation of bicarbonate.

The kidneys also excrete hydrogen ions in the form of *titratable acids*, which consist mostly of dihydrogen phosphate ($H_2PO_4^-$) formed when hydrogen in the tubular fluid combines with monohydrogen phosphate ($HPO_4^-$). For each hydrogen ion excreted in the form of titratable acid, an equivalent quantity of sodium bicarbonate is added to the blood (Figure 9-4). Approximately 10 to 20 mEq of titratable acid per day are excreted in the urine of an individual eating an average American diet.

Approximately 40 mEq of hydrogen ions are excreted per day, combined with *ammonia*. If a chronic acid load is imposed upon the body, the production and excretion of ammonia may increase more than tenfold over several days.

The cellular mechanisms of ammonia excretion are illustrated in Figure 9-5. Ammonia is produced in the tubular cells from amino acid metabolism. Ammonia, readily soluble in the luminal membrane, diffuses out of the tubular cell into the urine, where it combines with hydrogen ions to form ammonium ($NH_4$) ions. Ammonium ions penetrate cell membranes poorly, so they are effectively trapped in urine and excreted in combination with chloride.[3] For each hydrogen ion excreted with ammonia, an equivalent quantity of sodium bicarbonate is added to the blood. Normally, the kidneys produce up to 40 mEq of $HCO_3^-$ per day from $NH_4$ formation.[4]

### Hydrogen Ion Migration

A more obscure, but nonetheless effective, compensatory mechanism involved in acid-base derangements is hydro-

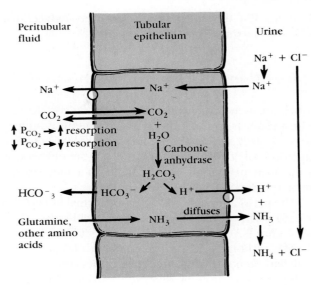

**FIGURE 9-5.**
Excretion of ammonia.

gen ion migration. In instances of increased hydrogen ion concentration, potassium passively diffuses from the intracellular to the extracellular environment. Along the same electrical gradient created by potassium migration, the hydrogen ion enters the cell. Thus, the extracellular environment becomes less acidic and more hyperkalemic. In alkalotic conditions, extracellular potassium enters the cell. Again, along the same electrical gradient created by the movement of potassium, hydrogen leaves the cell, thus making the extracellular environment less alkalotic and more hypokalemic (see p. 204).[7] Figure 9-6

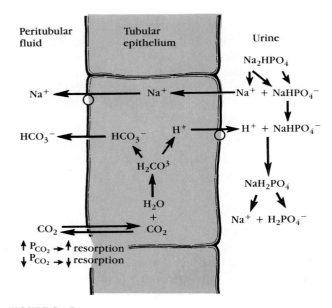

**FIGURE 9-4.**
Production of titratable acid.

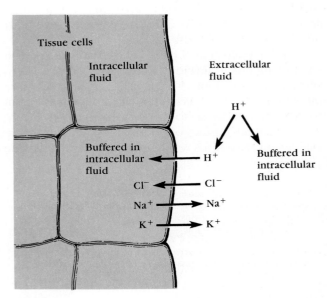

**FIGURE 9-6.**
Ion movements associated with intracellular buffering of H+.

illustrates ion movement associated with intracellular buffering of extracellular hydrogen ions.

## Integration of Defense Mechanisms

As previously noted, the body mechanisms for defense against changes in fluid pH consist of chemical buffers, the respiratory and renal mechanisms, and hydrogen ion migration. All of the mechanisms function simultaneously to maintain pH within normal limits, but they do not function independently of one another.

The pH of arterial blood is within normal limits (7.35 to 7.45) when the bicarbonate:carbonic acid ratio is 20:1 (see Figure 9-2).

The carbonic acid concentration in plasma is very small and cannot be measured directly. It is proportional to the concentration of dissolved carbon dioxide, so $PCO_2$ is often used to calculate $H_2CO_3$ levels. Note that it is the ratio of bicarbonate to $PCO_2$ that determines pH, rather than the absolute amounts of bicarbonate and carbon dioxide. Plasma bicarbonate is controlled by the kidneys, while arterial $PCO_2$ is controlled by the lungs. Thus, the effectiveness with which chemical buffers operate depends upon efficient respiratory and renal mechanisms to maintain proper buffer ratios. In this regard, the lungs and kidneys are sometimes referred to as physiological buffers. Integration of mechanisms for defense against changes in body fluid pH were described earlier.

## ALTERED ACID-BASE BALANCE

Since the hydrogen ion concentration of blood ultimately affects the hydrogen ion concentration of all body fluids, and because blood is readily accessible for chemical analysis, arterial blood is used as a representative body fluid in assessing acid-base balance.

Clinical evaluation of the acid-base status of a person involves the determination of arterial blood pH, $PCO_2$, and $HCO_3^-$ (see Table 9-2). Usually, pH and $PCO_2$ are measured and $HCO_3^-$ is determined from a nomogram based upon the Henderson-Hasselbach equation (Figure 9-7). Sometimes, instead of determining $HCO_3^-$ from the Henderson-Hasselbach relationship, total carbon dioxide

---

**Most laboratories measure pH and $PCO_2$ directly and calculate $HCO_3^-$ using the Henderson-Hasselbach equation:**

$$\text{Arterial pH} = 6.1 + \log \frac{(HCO_3^-)}{0.03 \times PCO_2}$$

**where 6.1 is the dissociation constant for $CO_2$ in aqueous solution and 0.03 is a constant for the solubility of $CO_2$ in plasma at 37°C.**

**FIGURE 9–7.**
Henderson-Hasselbach equation. (From J. Wallach, *Interpretation of Diagnostic Texts* [4th ed.]. Boston: Little, Brown, 1986.)

---

content of arterial plasma is measured.[9] This is the sum of plasma bicarbonate plus dissolved carbon dioxide plus carbonic acid. It is measured by acidifying the plasma sample to remove all the carbon dioxide. In a normal sample of plasma, 95% of the total carbon dioxide is bicarbonate.

In addition to arterial pH, $PCO_2$, and $HCO_3^-$, hemoglobin saturation, $PO_2$, and concentrations of selected electrolytes are determined.

## Acidosis and Alkalosis

Acidosis in the body fluids refers to an elevation of the $H^+$ concentration above normal or a decrease in the $HCO_3^-$ below normal, resulting in a decrease in the pH of the body fluids to below 7.35. The source of the excess hydrogen ion or altered $H_2CO_3:HCO_3^-$ ratio can be respiratory (volatile) or metabolic (nonrespiratory or nonvolatile). *Acidemia* is defined as an acidic condition of the blood signified by an arterial pH value less than 7.35. The physiologic processes causing the acidemia define the term *acidosis* (literally, "a condition of becoming acidic").

Alkalosis refers to a decrease in the $H^+$ concentration of the body fluids or an excess of the $HCO_3^-$, thus increasing pH of the body fluids to above 7.45. The source of the depletion of hydrogen ion is either elimination of carbon dioxide (hyperventilation), or a metabolic excess of primary base bicarbonate. *Alkalemia* is defined as an alkaline condition of the blood signified by arterial pH greater than 7.45. The physiologic processes causing the alkalemia define the term *alkalosis* (literally, "a condition of becoming alkalotic"). Table 9-3 summarizes some factors that tend to cause acidosis and alkalosis.

Disturbances of acid-base balance may arise from respiratory or metabolic causes. Metabolic causes are sometimes termed nonrespiratory because they are not necessarily related to abnormal metabolism. The four primary types of acid-base disturbances are: (1) respiratory acidosis, (2) respiratory alkalosis, (3) metabolic acidosis, and (4) metabolic alkalosis.

## Etiology and Clinical Manifestations of Acidosis and Alkalosis

### Respiratory Acidosis

Respiratory acidosis is caused by failure of the respiratory system to remove carbon dioxide from body fluids as fast as it is produced in the tissues. Essentially, any condition which impairs or interferes with breathing can result in respiratory acidosis. Impairment of breathing leads to an increase in arterial $PCO_2$ above 45 mm Hg, with a decrease in pH value to 7.35 or less.

**TABLE 9–3.**
DISTURBANCES OF ACID–BASE BALANCE

| ARTERIAL BLOOD pH | PRIMARY ABNORMALITY | INDICATOR OF PRIMARY ABNORMALITY | EXAMPLES OF CAUSATIVE FACTORS | COMPENSATORY MECHANISMS |
|---|---|---|---|---|
| Alkalemia pH > 7.45 | Respiratory alkalosis | Decreased $PCO_2$ < 35 mm Hg | Hypoxia, anxiety, pulmonary embolus, pregnancy, other causes of hyperventilation | Kidneys retain hydrogen ions and excrete bicarbonate |
| | Metabolic alkalosis | Increased $HCO_3^-$ > 26 mEq/L | Treatment with diuretics and hormones that augment renal excretion of $H^+$, $K^+$, and $Cl^-$; fluid loss from stomach by vomiting or nasogastric suction; Cushing's disease, aldosteronism, excessive ingestion of alkali | Alveolar ventilation decreases, more $CO_2$, is retained. Kidneys increase $H^+$ retention and excrete bicarbonate |
| Acidemia pH < 7.35 | Respiratory acidosis | Increased $PCO_2$ > 45 mm Hg | Obstructive lung disease, depression of respiratory center by drugs or disease, other causes of hypoventilation | Kidneys increase $H^+$ excretion and bicarbonate retention |
| | Metabolic acidosis | Decreased $HCO_3^-$ < 22 mEq/L | Diarrhea (loss of $HCO_3^-$), diabetic acidosis, lactic acidosis, renal failure, aspirin poisoning, treatment with ammonium chloride | Alveolar ventilation increases, more $CO_2$ is eliminated; kidneys increase $H^+$ excretion and bicarbonate retention |

Causes include obstructive lung disease, interference with movements of the thoracic cage (eg, poliomyelitis), decreased activity of the respiratory center (due to brain trauma, hemorrhage, narcotics, anesthetics, etc.), and neuromuscular disease (such as myasthenia gravis, Guillain-Barré syndrome). Individuals with severe respiratory acidosis usually show signs and symptoms of respiratory insufficiency such as cyanosis; rapid, shallow breathing; and disorientation. Acute respiratory acidosis can produce carbon dioxide narcosis with symptoms of headache, blurred vision, fatigue, and weakness. Prolonged acidosis may produce severe central nervous system (CNS) symptoms, including increased intracranial pressure and permanent damage.[6] When the pH falls below 7.10, dysrhythmias and peripheral vasodilatation may cause severe hypotension.[6]

## *Respiratory Alkalosis*

Respiratory alkalosis is caused by the loss of carbon dioxide from the lungs at a faster rate than it is produced in the tissues. This leads to a decrease in arterial $PCO_2$ below 35 mm Hg. Any condition resulting in excessive loss of carbon dioxide due to alveolar hyperventilation will cause respiratory alkalosis. Respiratory alkalosis is easily produced by voluntary overbreathing. Other causes include high altitude, anxiety, fever, meningitis, aspirin poisoning, pneumonia, pulmonary embolus, and other factors that increase respiratory center activity.

Symptoms of respiratory alkalosis are related to nervous system irritability and include lightheadedness, altered consciousness, various paresthesia, cramps, and carpopedal spasm from clinical hypocalcemia (see Chap. 8).[6]

## *Metabolic Acidosis*

Metabolic acidosis results from either an abnormal accumulation of fixed acids or loss of base. The arterial blood pH falls below 7.35, and the plasma bicarbonate is usually decreased below 22 mEq per liter.

Metabolic acidosis may result from the systemic accumulation of either hydrochloric or nonhydrochloric acids.[1] The determination of the cause is aided by determining the anion gap (see p. 205). It may be caused by kidney failure in which the kidneys are unable to replenish bicarbonate stores used for buffering strong acids produced by metabolism. In diabetes mellitus, ketoacid production due to incomplete oxidation of fats may lead to a severe metabolic acidosis. Anaerobic metabolism of glucose during strenuous exercise or circulatory shock may lead to lactic acidosis. Excessive administration of chloride can cause an excessive loss of $HCO_3^-$ and metabolic acidosis. Loss of pancreatic bicarbonate from the intestine during chronic diarrhea or bilious vomiting produces metabolic acidosis, often with serious consequences in children. Acid-producing overdoses include acetylsalicylic acid, ethylene glycol, methyl alcohol, and paraldehyde.

Symptoms of severe metabolic acidosis include deep, rapid respiration (Kussmaul's breathing), disorientation, and coma. Clinical manifestations of metabolic acidosis depend on the pH level. Arterial pH of less than 7.10 can produce severe ventricular dysrhythmias and reduction of cardiac contractility. Production of lactic acidosis may occur with associated hypotension.[5] Lethargy and coma can develop, but neurologic symptoms are less prominent in metabolic acidosis than in respiratory acidosis because the CNS is more sensitive to carbon dioxide changes than to pH shifts.[6] The chronic acidosis of renal failure retards bone growth and causes a variety of bone disturbances, probably due to buffering of acidosis by bone calcium.[6]

### Metabolic Alkalosis

Metabolic alkalosis results from either a loss of hydrogen ions or addition of base to body fluids. It is defined as a disorder that results in primary, not secondary, increase in plasma $HCO_3^-$.[1] The plasma bicarbonate increases to above 26 mEq per liter and the arterial blood pH increases above 7.45. Secondary increase in plasma $HCO_3^-$ occurs with chronic respiratory acidosis to keep the pH at or about normal levels (see Chap. 30).

One cause of metabolic alkalosis is ingestion of excessive amounts of base (eg, sodium bicarbonate, or baking soda) to treat stomach ulcers and indigestion. Administration of sodium bicarbonate in a cardiac arrest situation can produce a "post code" metabolic alkalosis. Another cause is vomiting of gastric contents in which hydrochloric acid is lost from the body. Endocrine disorders (eg, Cushing's disease) and treatment with certain types of drugs (eg, thiazide) may augment renal excretion of $H^+$, $K^+$, and $Cl^-$ and lead to metabolic alkalosis. Symptoms include apathy, mental confusion, shallow breathing, tetany, and spastic muscles. Clinical manifestations of metabolic alkalosis include weakness, muscle cramps, and dizziness, which may be due to hypokalemia or hypocalcemia. Neurologic symptoms include paresthesia and lightheadedness.[6]

### Effects of pH Changes on Potassium, Calcium, and Magnesium Balance

Integrated into the direct effects of acidosis and alkalosis on the physiologic process are the compounding effects on potassium and calcium balance. Other electrolytes, such as magnesium and phosphate, are also affected, but the systemic effects of potassium and calcium imbalances can be life-threatening.

Hydrogen is preferentially excreted or retained over other cations by the renal system to maintain the blood pH. When the arterial pH falls, the excessive $H^+$ is excreted through the kidneys. It cannot be excreted unless a cation is retained. Potassium is the cation usually retained, so hyperkalemia develops in acidosis. Potassium may also shift out of ICF because more than 50% of the excess $H^+$ is buffered intracellularly. The $K^+$ and small amounts of $Na^+$ leave the cell to maintain electroneutrality.[1] The reverse is true with alkalosis. The kidney retains $H^+$ to normalize the blood pH and $K^+$ is wasted. The intracellular hydrogen is donated to the ECF and $K^+$ is retained intracellularly.

Thus, hyperkalemia is associated with acidosis, and hypokalemia is associated with alkalosis (see Chap. 8). Severe symptoms such as cardiac dysrhythmias and coma can result.

Changes in the arterial pH affect the ionized calcium levels in blood. The calcium in an alkalotic serum binds with serum proteins, producing the clinical effect of hypocalcemia.[10] The result can be hypocalcemia, tetany, spasm, and dysrhythmias (see Chap. 8). In an acidic environment, more calcium may be released from the plasma proteins, and ionized calcium levels may rise transiently. The effect is not so pronounced as that seen with alkalemia.

Serum magnesium levels also may change in response to the pH levels. Hypomagnesemia is often seen in acidosis. The symptoms include weakness, mental depression, and tetany similar to that of hypocalcemia.

## COMPENSATION AND CORRECTION

There are two ways in which an abnormal pH of arterial plasma may be returned toward normal: (1) compensation and (2) correction. In correction, the primary cause of the acid-base disturbance is repaired. For example, if respiratory acidosis is caused by partial blockage of the respiratory tree, removing or reducing the obstruction improves ventilation and allows blood pH to return toward normal. Correction of an acid-base disturbance is the primary aim of persons concerned with the delivery of health care to affected individuals.

In compensation, the system or systems not responsible for causing the acid-base disturbance make physiologic adjustments to return blood pH toward normal. For example, in respiratory acidosis (high $PCO_2$), the kidneys compensate by increasing the return of bicarbonate to the blood to return the $HCO_3^-$:$H_2CO_3$ ratio to normal. All processes of compensation are directed at returning the bicarbonate:carbonic acid ratio to 20:1 and restoring the normal pH of arterial plasma.

The kidneys compensate for respiratory acidosis (high $PCO_2$) by elevating the plasma bicarbonate above 26 mEq per liter. The kidneys compensate for respiratory alkalosis (low $PCO_2$) by lowering the plasma bicarbonate below 22 mEq per liter. Similar compensations are made by the kidneys in nonrenal causes of metabolic acidosis and alkalosis.

The respiratory system attempts to compensate for metabolic acidosis (low $HCO_3^-$) by lowering the arterial $PCO_2$ below 35 mm Hg through hyperventilation. It attempts to compensate for metabolic alkalosis by elevating the arterial $PCO_2$ above 45 mm Hg through hypoventilation.

## INTERPRETATION OF BLOOD GAS DATA

Major disturbances of acid-base balance are rarely completely compensated. Arterial pH is returned toward normal during compensation, but rarely to normal. Therefore, the arterial pH indicates whether a process of acidosis or alkalosis is present. The arterial blood $PCO_2$ and the plasma bicarbonate concentration indicate which process, respiratory or metabolic, is responsible for the abnormal pH and which process is compensatory.

For example, the following blood gas data indicate an acid-base abnormality: pH = 7.22; $PCO_2$ = 30 mm Hg; $HCO_3^-$ = 12 mEq per liter. To interpret the data, one must look at the pH to see if there is acidemia or alkalemia. In this case, the arterial pH is below normal range (7.35 to 7.45) and indicates acidemia. The body does not overcompensate, so the pH is reflective of the cause. The plasma $PCO_2$ and bicarbonate are then examined for indications of acidosis and alkalosis. Here, the bicarbonate concentration is below normal range (22 to 28 mEq per liter) and indicates metabolic acidosis. The arterial $PCO_2$ is below normal range (35 to 45 mm Hg) and indicates respiratory alkalosis. Since there is acidemia, the primary disturbance is one of metabolic acidosis while the compensatory process is respiratory. Therefore, the data suggest partially compensated metabolic acidosis.

Sometimes two primary disturbances of acid-base balance may be present simultaneously in the same individual. For example, a person with severely impaired pulmonary function may have a combined respiratory acidosis due to retention of carbon dioxide, and metabolic acidosis due to lactic acid production caused by inadequate oxygenation of the blood. In this example, a severe acidemia will be seen. Examples of acid-base disturbances and blood values are shown in Table 9-3.

## THE ANION GAP

Preliminary assessment of arterial $PCO_2$, $HCO_3^-$, and pH is helpful in determining which, if any, of the four major types of acid-base disturbances is present. Other measurements, computations, and tests are performed to confirm the preliminary diagnosis and establish the exact cause of the disturbance. The anion gap is commonly used in the differential diagnosis of metabolic acidosis.

The number of milliequivalents per liter of cations in plasma is normally balanced by an equal number of milliequivalents per liter of anions: $Na^+ + K^+ + Mg^{++} + Ca^{++}$ + other cations = $Cl^- + HCO_3^- + HPO_4^{--} + SO_4^{--}$ + proteinate$^-$ + other anions. Only the concentrations of $Na^+$, $K^+$, $Cl^-$, and $HCO_3^-$ are measured routinely; $Mg^{++}$, $Ca^{++}$, and other cations are considered unmeasured cations (UC); and $HPO_4^{--}$, $SO_4^{--}$, proteinate$^-$, and other anions are considered unmeasured anions (UA).

According to the principle of electroneutrality, plasma ionic balance can be expressed in the form of an equation between cations and anions: $[Na^+] + [K^+] + [UC] = [Cl^-] + [HCO_3^-] + [UA]$.

If the equation is rearranged so that measured ions are on one side and unmeasured ions are on the other side, the result is $[Na^+] + [K^+] - [Cl^-] - [HCO_3^-] = 16 \pm 4$ mEq/L.

Notice that $K^+$ is included in determining the anion gap. Since plasma $K^+$ is small compared to $Na^+$, $Cl^-$, and $HCO_3^-$, it is sometimes excluded from anion gap computations, in which case the normal value for the anion gap becomes $12 \pm 4$ mEq per liter. In other words, it is normal for the measured $Na^+$ to exceed the sum of $Cl^-$ and $HCO_3$ by $12 \pm 4$ mEq per liter when the plasma K is not calculated.[1] In metabolic acidosis, the anion gap may be normal, increased, or decreased, depending on the etiology (Table 9-4).

A normal anion gap in metabolic acidosis occurs in such conditions as diarrhea, ammonium chloride inges-

**TABLE 9-4.**
DIFFERENTIAL DIAGNOSIS OF METABOLIC ACIDOSIS (AFTER KAEHNY)

| LOW OR NORNAL ANION GAP (HYPERCHLOREMIC) | INCREASED ANION GAP |
|---|---|
| Gastrointestinal loss of $HCO_3^-$<br>    Diarrhea<br>    Small bowel or pancreatic<br>    drainage or fistula<br>    Ureterosigmoidostomy, ileal<br>    loop conduit<br>    Anion-exchange resins | Increased acid production<br>    Diabetic ketoacidosis<br>    Lactic acidosis<br>    Alcoholic ketoacidosis<br>    Inborn errors of metabolism |
| Renal loss of $HCO_3^-$<br>    Renal tubular acidosis (RTA)<br>    Diamox | Ingestion of toxic substances<br>    Salicylate overdose<br>    Paraldehyde poisoning<br>    Methyl alcohol<br>    Ethylene glycol |
| Miscellaneous<br>    Dilutional acidosis<br>    Addition of HCl or its<br>    congeners<br>    Hyperalimentation acidosis | Failure of acid excretion<br>    Acute renal failure<br>    Chronic renal failure |

Source: R.W. Schrier, Renal and Electrolyte Disorders (3rd ed.). Boston: Little, Brown, 1986.

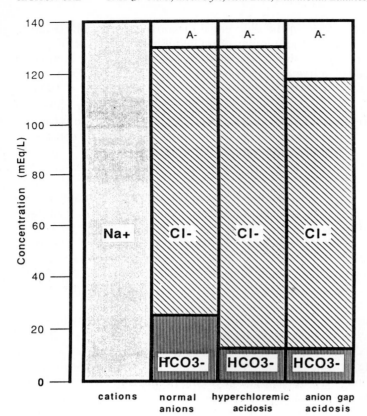

**FIGURE 9–8.**
The difference between the measured serum cation content (primarily $Na^+$) and the measured serum anion content (primarily $Cl^-$ and $HCO_3$) equals the "anion gap." In the normal state, these unmeasured anions ($A^-$) are usually sulfates, phosphates, and anionic serum proteins such as albumin. (From W.N. Kelley, *Textbook of Internal Medicine.* Philadelphia: J.B. Lippincott, 1989.)

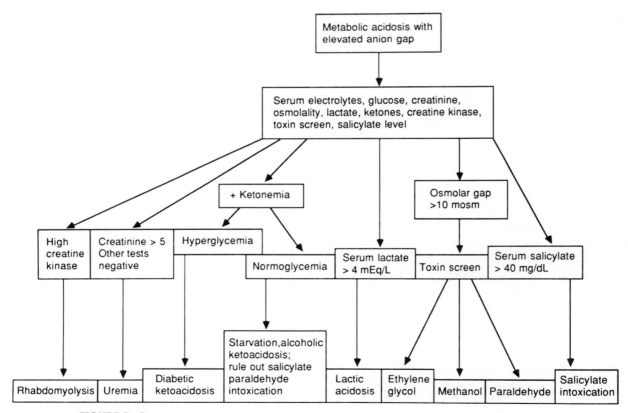

**FIGURE 9–9.**
Diagnostic approach to high-anion-gap acidosis. (From: W.N. Kelley, *Textbook of Internal Medicine.* Philadelphia: J.B. Lippincott, 1989.)

tion, and renal dysfunction. A high anion gap may be present with accumulation of organic acids, such as ketoacids and lactic acids, as well as certain drugs and poisons. A normal gap is maintained by increasing chloride ions so that the sum of the $HCO_3^-$ and $Cl^-$ remain constant. This situation is often called *hyperchloremic acidosis*. A high anion gap occurs when the sum of $HCO_{3-}$ and $Cl^-$ decrease due to the accumulation of other acids (Figure 9-8).

In clinical practice, the initial determination of high-anion-gap acidosis versus normal-anion-gap acidosis leads to distinct laboratory investigations.[1] Figure 9-9 shows the laboratory tests that can be used to differentiate causative factors in high-anion-gap acidosis. Normal-anion-gap acidosis is further delineated by history and physical examination, as well as by $HCO_3^-$ and $K^+$ studies. Diarrhea is the most common cause of normal-anion-gap acidosis and there is often associated hypokalemia. Persons receiving hyperalimentation intravenous fluids with hydrochloric acid or those with renal tubular acidosis may have a hyperkalemic/hyperchloremic metabolic acidosis[1] (see Table 9-4).

# REFERENCES

1. Breyer, M.D., and Jacobson, H.R. Approach to the patient with metabolic acidosis or alkalosis. In W.N. Kelley, *Textbook of Internal Medicine*. Philadelphia: J.B. Lippincott, 1989.
2. Guyton, A. *Textbook of Medical Physiology* (8th ed.). Philadelphia: W.B. Saunders, 1990.
3. Humes, H.D., and Cox, M. Principles of the renal regulation of fluid and electrolytes. In W.N. Kelley, *Textbook of Internal Medicine*. Philadelphia: J.B. Lippincott, 1989.
4. Keyes, J.L. *Fluid, Electrolyte and Acid-Base Regulation*. Monterey, Calif.: Wadsworth Health Sciences Division, 1985.
5. Rice, V. Acid-base derangements in the patient with cardiac arrest. *Focus on Critical Care* 14(6):53, 1987.
6. Rose, B.D. *Clinical Physiology of Acid-Base and Electrolyte Disorders* (2nd ed.). New York: McGraw-Hill, 1984.
7. Shoemaker, W.C. Fluids and electrolytes in the acutely ill adult. In W.C. Shoemaker, *Textbook of Critical Care* (2nd ed.). Philadelphia: W.B. Saunders, 1989.
8. Toporek, M. *Basic Chemistry of Life*. St. Louis: Mosby, 1981.
9. Wallach, J. *Interpretation of Diagnostic Tests* (4th ed.). Boston: Little, Brown, 1986.
10. Zaloga, G.P., and Chernow, B. Hypocalcemia in critical illness. *JAMA* 256:1924, 1986.

# chapter 10

Roberta H. Anding

# Normal and Altered Nutritional Balance

## Chapter Outline

## Learning Objectives

1. Discuss the nutritional terms *macronutrients* and *micronutrients*.
2. Discuss the mechanisms by which carbohydrates are used in the body for energy production.
3. Identify foods high in dietary fiber and their benefit in the diet.
4. List at least three alternate sources of sucrose.
5. Identify essential and nonessential amino acids.
6. Discuss the functions of protein in the body.
7. Describe the importance of nitrogen balance.
8. List the main functions of fat.
9. Compare saturated, monosaturated and polyunsaturated fats as to structure and function.
10. List the functions and sources of water-soluble and fat-soluble vitamins.
11. Compare deficiency and toxicity with water-soluble and fat-soluble vitamins.
12. Discuss the functions of the essential trace minerals.
13. Describe protein calorie malnutrition including its components marasmus and kwashiorkor.
14. Discuss insulin/glucagon changes in starvation.
15. Define *ketoadaptation* and the risks involved with its failure.
16. Compare hypertrophic and hyperplastic obesity.
17. Discuss the multifaceted process of weight control.
18. Explain the risks of android versus gynoid obesity.
19. Compare anorexia nervosa and bulimia in relation to etiology, manifestations and nutritional imbalances produced.

(continued)

***Learning Objectives*** (continued)

**20.** List the physiologic effects of vomiting, laxative and diuretic abuse.

**21.** Describe the diagnostic clues to the problems of anorexia nervosa and bulimia.

Nutritional balance is a major factor in promoting health and preventing disease. Balance can be altered by excessive or deficient quantities of essential nutrients. Vitamins, minerals, carbohydrates, proteins, and fats all provide these essential nutrients. This chapter presents an overview of the macronutrients, micronutrients, and the effects of an imbalance of each. Macronutrients include carbohydrates, proteins, and lipids. Micronutrients include the vitamins and particular trace minerals. Other minerals and water balance are discussed in Chapter 8. Water is essential for the absorption of nutrients and elimination of wastes from the body. Further discussion of nutrition is found in Unit 12, especially in relation to absorption and nutrient production. Alterations of nutritional balance affect all of the body processes and are discussed throughout the book.

# MACRONUTRIENTS

## Carbohydrates

Carbohydrates function to supply the body with energy. The simpler forms of carbohydrates, called simple sugars, are monosaccharides and disaccharides. Monosaccharides contain one sugar unit; disaccharides contain two (Figure 10-1). The more complex carbohydrates are classified as starches, or polysaccharides. They are also sources of dietary fiber. Polysaccharides contain 20 or more sugar units (monosaccharide molecules). Oligosaccharides are intermediate carbohydrates containing three to 10 sugar units. Glycogen, also referred to as animal starch, is the storage form of carbohydrate and is stored in liver and muscle (Figure 10-2).

In the United States, carbohydrates supply 45% of energy, with one-half coming from simple sugars and one-half from complex carbohydrates. Dietary goals for Americans include decreasing the amount of simple sugars and increasing the amount of complex carbohydrate intake. Table 10-1 lists forms of carbohydrate (CHO) and food sources.

### Functions

Dietary carbohydrate yields four calories (kcal) per gram (gm), whereas dextrose administered intravenously yields 3.4 kcal per gm. Certain tissues of the body, particularly the brain and red blood cells, rely on glucose as a preferred energy source. In the absence of adequate carbohydrate, *gluconeogenesis* ensues to synthesize glucose from noncarbohydrate sources, primarily protein. Most gluconeogenesis occurs in the liver (see Chap. 42). To spare protein, the daily consumption of 100 grams of carbohydrate is necessary. The provision of adequate carbohydrate will also prevent ketosis, which results from fat breakdown.

### Dietary Fiber

Complex carbohydrates are also sources of dietary fiber. Dietary fiber refers to the foodstuffs that remain undigested as they enter the large intestine.[78] Certain fibers, the water-soluble forms, are digested or fermented by the bacteria in the large intestine. Fiber, therefore, cannot always be defined as the undigested portion of CHO-containing foods. Current intake of fiber in the United States averages 10 to 13 gm per day.[80] Recommended goals for dietary fiber range from 20 to 35 gm per day to up to 40 gm per day.[136]

Adequate fiber intake has proposed benefits that include decreased risk of chronic diseases such as cancer

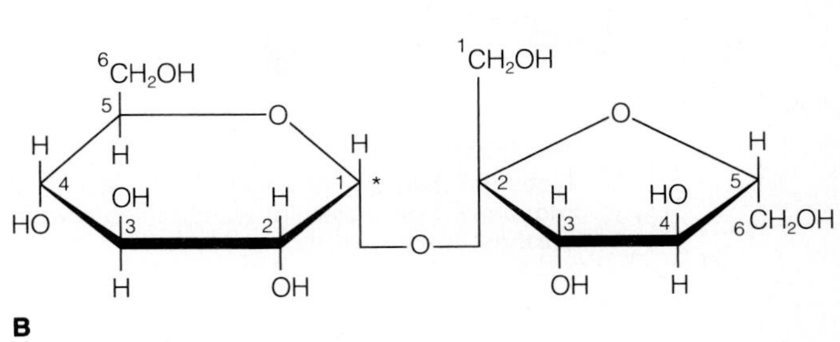


**FIGURE 10-1.**
**A.** Structure of monosaccharide glucose. **B.** Structure of disaccharide sucrose. (Redrawn from B. Luke, *Principles of Nutrition and Diet Therapy*. Boston: Little, Brown, 1984.)

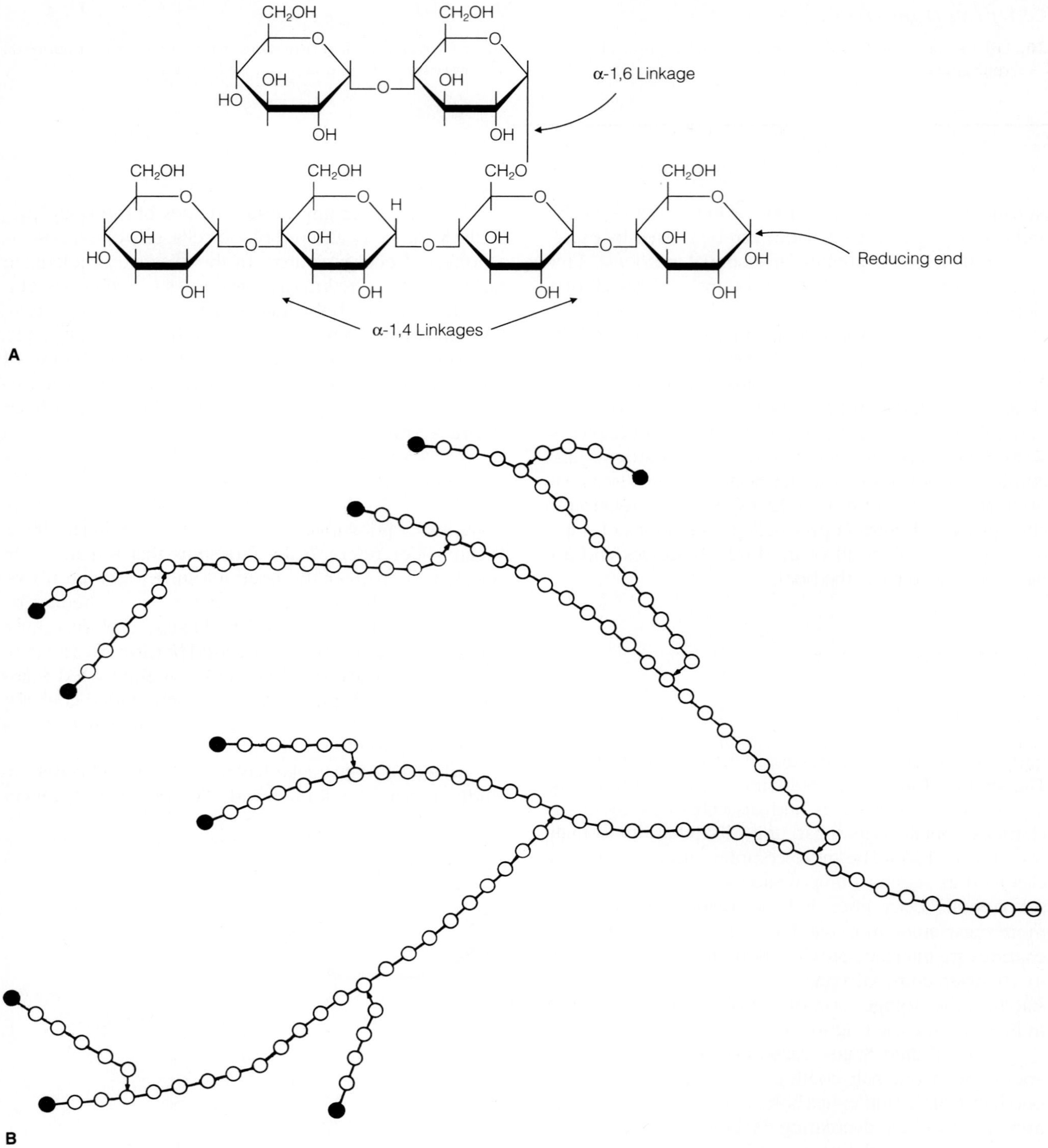

**FIGURE 10–2.**
Types of linkages in glycogen. Each chain is extended and branched, further producing a polysaccharide of high molecular weight. (Redrawn from I. Danishefsky, *Biochemistry for Medical Science.* Boston: Little, Brown, 1981.)

**TABLE 10–1.**

| TYPE OF CARBOHYDRATE | FOOD SOURCES |
|---|---|
| Monosaccharides | |
| Glucose | Breakdown of product (complex carbohydrates) |
| Fructose | Fruits, honey, corn syrup |
| Disaccharides | |
| Maltose | Grains |
| Lactose | Milk, milk products, filler in nondairy products |
| Sucrose | Sugar, honey, maple syrup |
| Oligosaccharides | Dried beans, peas (carbohydrate used in enteral medical nutrition products) |
| Polysaccharides | Breads, grains, starches |

**TABLE 10–3.**
ALTERNATE SWEETENERS

| CALORIC | NONCALORIC |
|---|---|
| Fructose 1.0–1.8 × | Aspartame[a] 180–200 × |
| Sugar Alcohols 0.5 × | Cyclamate |
| Sorbitol | Acesulfame 200 × |
| Mannitol | Saccharin 375 × |

[a]*Although aspartame is a dipeptide (protein), it is used as a carbohydrate alternative.*
*Source: Adapted from Diabetes Care 11(2):174–82, 1988.*

of the colon, diverticular disease, constipation, or hemorrhoids. Dietary fiber may also be used as an adjunct to the treatment of gastrointestinal (GI) disorders, diabetes, and coronary artery disease.[33,59,123,136] Classification of fiber is based on its solubility, which determines its physiologic function. Table 10-2 lists the type, function, and representative food sources of dietary fiber and amounts of water-soluble/insoluble fiber.[33]

Increasing dietary fiber should be done gradually to minimize GI discomfort. It requires a concomitant increase in fluid, especially water, to maintain GI motility. Increased dietary fiber in elderly individuals may create problems due to decreased ability to increase fluid intake and chronic ingestion of constipating medications. These factors may lead to fecal impactions, which are often difficult to recognize clinically. Intake of large amounts of fiber also is associated with the development of *bezoars*, an accumulation of fiber in the stomach, and may cause

a decreased absorption of minerals, particularly divalent calcium, zinc, and iron.[123]

### Alternate Sweeteners

To reduce simple sugar consumption and as an adjunct to weight control, Americans have increased consumption of alternatives to sucrose. Sweeteners can be classified as caloric and noncaloric. Table 10-3 lists sweeteners and their relative sweetening power as compared to sucrose.

*FRUCTOSE.* Fructose is a naturally occurring CHO found in fruit and honey. It has a slow postprandial rise in blood glucose when compared to sucrose. Excessive consumption of fructose is linked with hypertriglyceridemia (see Chap. 42).[94]

*SORBITOL AND MANNITOL.* Sorbitol and mannitol are sugar alcohols that contain 4 kcal per gm. Slow absorption from the GI tract causes intestinal gas and osmotic diarrhea. Children are particularly sensitive to the laxative effects of sorbitol.

**TABLE 10–2.**
CLASSIFICATION OF DIETARY FIBER

| TYPE | FUNCTIONS | GENERAL FOOD SOURCES | EXAMPLES: FOOD/ AMOUNT | TOTAL FIBER (g) | SOLUBLE (g) |
|---|---|---|---|---|---|
| Insoluble | Increases fecal bulk | Wheat bran, most vegetables | All Bran 1/3 c | 8.8 | 1.6 |
| | | | Whole wheat bread (1 slice) | 1.5 | 0.3 |
| | Decreases intestinal transit time | | Tomato 1/2 c | 1.0 | 0.2 |
| | | | Orange 1 | 2.0 | 0.5 |
| | | | Grapefruit 1/2 | 1.7 | 0.6 |
| Soluble | Delays gastric emptying time | Citrus fruit, oat bran, dried beans, and peas | Oat bran 1/2 c | 2.1 | 1.0 |
| | | | Blackeyed peas 1/3 c | 8.2 | 3.7 |
| | Decreases postprandial rise in blood glucose | | Kidney beans 1/3 c | 3.8 | 1.7 |
| | | | Lentils 1/3 c | 2.6 | 1.1 |
| | Hypocholesterolemic effect | | | | |

*Adapted from J.W. Anderson, Fiber and health: An overview. Nutr. Today Nov/Dec 1986.*

*ASPARTAME.* Aspartame is a dispeptide of phenylalanine and aspartic acid. Although technically noncaloric, it is extremely sweet and very small amounts are required to achieve desired sweetness. Safety issues concerning aspartame include the following:

1. There are nonspecific side effects including headache, nausea, and dizziness.[24]
2. Methanol production forms as a byproduct of aspartame metabolism. Methanol is formed when aspartame is improperly stored or through normal metabolism of the dispeptide.[64,90]
3. Aspartame has the potential to alter neurotransmitters in the brain. High levels of aspartame alter the level of phenylalanine and its metabolic product, tyrosine, in experimental animals. Phenylalanine and tyrosine are precursors of norepinephrine and dopamine. Consumption of a high carbohydrate meal exacerbates these effects while blocking the increase in tryptophan and serotonin normally seen after a high CHO meal.[149] Phenylalanine and tryptophan, both aromatic amino acids, may compete for transport across the blood barrier.
4. Aspartame use is contraindicated in individuals with phenylketonuria.

The Food and Drug Administration (FDA) has set an acceptable daily intake (ADI) for aspartame at 50 mg per kg. This is equivalent to approximately 14 soft drinks per day or 71 packets of the table top version, Equal.

*CYCLAMATES.* Cyclamates were banned by the FDA in 1970 after animal studies indicated a potential cancer risk, as well as testicular atrophy and chromosomal damage. Further review failed to establish cyclamates as carcinogenic.[39]

## Derangements of Carbohydrate Metabolism

Alterations of carbohydrate usage can be caused by defects in absorption, metabolism, or storage. Table 10-4 lists representative defects of carbohydrate metabolism and the cause.

## Protein

The recommended dietary allowance for protein is 8 gm per kg of ideal body weight for healthy individuals. Current average intake of protein in the United States is 75 to 110 gm, or approximately 1.5 times the needed amounts. Protein must be consumed daily because there is no storage or reserve of protein in the body. All protein in the body is functional. Any loss of body protein represents a loss of physiologic function.

Amino acids are the building blocks of protein. The key component of the molecule is the amine group, which is the nitrogen component. Twenty amino acids are required by the body, of which nine are essential, indicating dietary need. Eleven amino acids are synthesized by the liver (Table 10-5). Table 10-6 lists the essential and nonessential amino acids, as well as chemical classification.

Protein metabolism/catabolism is controlled by the liver, and excretion of the end products of protein metabolism (urea nitrogen and creatinine) is dependent on the kidneys.

Dietary protein can be classified as complete (high biologic value) or incomplete (low biologic value). Complete proteins contain all the essential amino acids in proper proportion, indicating the ability to perform physiologically the functions of protein. Incomplete proteins alone cannot function as proteins and are *deaminated*, the process of removing the amine group and converting the remaining carbon skeleton (keto analog) to glucose or ketones. Box 10-1 lists examples of complimentary proteins. Complimentary proteins, or mutual supplementation, is the process of combining two plant proteins that are deficient in one or more essential amino acids, thereby improving overall protein quality.

## Functions

The primary function of protein is to build and repair tissue in healthy individuals. Protein requirements are greatest during periods of rapid growth and develop-

**TABLE 10–4.**
DEFECTS OF CARBOHYDRATE METABOLISM

| DISEASE STATE | TYPE OF DEFECT | CLINICAL PRESENTATION |
|---|---|---|
| Diabetes mellitus | Metabolic defect in insulin secretion or utilization | Hyperglycemia |
| Lactose intolerance | Absorption deficiency of lactose | Diarrhea, gas cramps, bloating |
| Glycogen storage | Storage deficiency of glucose 6-phosphatase deficiency (von Gierke's disease) | Hepatomegaly, severe hypoglycemia, hyperlipidemia |

**TABLE 10–5.**
THE 20 COMMON AMINO ACIDS

| STRUCTURAL FORMULA | COMMON NAME | THREE-LETTER ABBREVIATION | STRUCTURAL FORMULA | COMMON NAME | THREE-LETTER ABBREVIATION |
|---|---|---|---|---|---|
| **Amino acids with nonpolar side chains** | | | $HO-\langle\bigcirc\rangle-CH_2-CHCO_2 \\ \quad\quad\quad\quad +NH_3$ | Tyrosine | Tyr |
| $H-CHCO_2 \\ \quad +NH_3$ | Glycine | Gly | | | |
| $CH_3-CHCO_2 \\ \quad\quad +NH_3$ | Alanine | Ala | $HSCH_2-CHCO_2 \\ \quad\quad\quad +NH_3$ | Cysteine | Cys |
| $(CH_3)_2CH-CHCO_2 \\ \quad\quad\quad\quad +NH_3$ | Valine* | Val | $CH_3SCH_2CH_2-CHCO_2 \\ \quad\quad\quad\quad\quad +NH_3$ | Methionine* | Met |
| $(CH_3)_2CHCH_2-CHCO_2 \\ \quad\quad\quad\quad\quad +NH_3$ | Leucine* | Leu | $\overset{O}{\underset{NH_2}{\parallel}}CCH_2-CHCO_2 \\ \quad\quad\quad +NH_3$ | Asparagine | Asn |
| $CH_3CH_2\overset{CH_3}{\underset{+NH_3}{\overset{\vert}{CH}}}-CHCO_2$ | Isoleucine* | Ile | $\overset{O}{\underset{NH_2}{\parallel}}CCH_2CH_2-CHCO_2 \\ \quad\quad\quad\quad +NH_3$ | Glutamine | Gln |
| $\langle\bigcirc\rangle-CH_2-CHCO_2 \\ \quad\quad\quad\quad +NH_3$ | Phenylalanine* | Phe | **Amino acids with acidic side chains** | | |
| | | | $HO_2CCH_2-CHCO_2^- \\ \quad\quad\quad\quad +NH_3$ | Aspartic acid | Asp |
| $\begin{matrix}CH_2 \\ CH_2 \\ CH_2\end{matrix}\begin{matrix}CHCO_2 \\ NH_2^+\end{matrix}$ | Proline | Pro | $HO_2CCH_2CH_2-CHCO_2 \\ \quad\quad\quad\quad\quad +NH_3$ | Glutamic acid | Glu |
| **Amino acids with polar but neutral side chains** | | | **Amino acids with basic side chains** | | |
| $\text{(indole)}-CH_2-CHCO_2^- \\ \quad\quad\quad\quad\quad +NH_3$ | Tryptophan* | Trp | $NH_2CH_2CH_2CH_2CH_2-CHCO_2 \\ \quad\quad\quad\quad\quad\quad\quad +NH_3$ | Lysine* | Lys |
| $HOCH_2-CHCO_2 \\ \quad\quad\quad +NH_3$ | Serine | Ser | $NH_2\overset{NH}{\overset{\parallel}{C}}NHCH_2CH_2CH_2-CHCO_2 \\ \quad\quad\quad\quad\quad\quad\quad +NH_3$ | Arginine* | Arg |
| $CH_3 \\ HOCH-CHCO_2 \\ \quad\quad +NH_3$ | Threonine* | Thr | $\text{(imidazole)}-CH_2-CHCO_2 \\ \quad\quad\quad\quad\quad +NH_3$ | Histidine* | His |

*These amino acids cannot be made by the body but must be obtained from the food we eat.*
*From G.H. Schmid, The Chemical Basis of Life: General, Organic, and Biological Chemistry for the Health Sciences. Boston: Little, Brown, 1982.*

---

ment. Table 10-7 compares protein requirements during stages of the life cycle.

Blood proteins, albumin and globulin, are hydrophilic molecules that contribute to blood oncotic pressure and thereby function in fluid balance and blood pressure (see Chap. 8). Deficiencies of protein can eventually cause leaking of fluid into the extracellular spaces with resulting edema. Proteins regulate acid-base balance through their buffering capabilities. Proteins function in the transport of nutrients and the enzymatic reactions of metabolism. Proteins also function in clotting, connective

tissue, and visual pigments. As an energy source, protein yields 4 kcal per gm.

## Alterations in Protein Requirements

Disease processes, through their impact on absorption, metabolism, or excretion, impact protein requirements. Decreased protein tolerance may also be observed. Table 10-8 lists various disease states and protein requirements or restrictions. Altering the amount and type of amino acids may compensate for the inability of the body to me-

**TABLE 10–6.**
CLASSIFICATION OF AMINO ACIDS

| CLASSIFICATION | ESSENTIAL AMINO ACIDS | NONESSENTIAL AMINO ACIDS |
|---|---|---|
| Neutral—one amine group ($^-NH_2$) and one carboxyl group $(-\overset{\overset{O}{\|}}{C}-OH)$ | | |
| Aliphatic (carbon-carbon chain) | Threonine<br>Valine[a]<br>Leucine[a]<br>Isoleucine[a] | Glycine<br>Alanine<br>Serine |
| Aromatic—contains benzene ring | Phenylalanine | Tyrosine[b] |
| Heterocyclic (multiringed) | Tryptophan<br>Histidine | Proline |
| Sulfur-containing | Methionine | Cysteine[b] (Cystine) |
| Basic—two amine groups and one carboxyl group | Lysine | Arginine |
| Acidic—one amine group and two carboxyl groups | | Aspartic acid<br>Asparagine[c]<br>Glutamic acid<br>Glutamine[c] |

[a] Branched-chain amino acids.
[b] These amino acids are classed as semi-essential.
[c] Asparagine and glutamine contain an amine group attached to the additional carboxyl group.
Source: G.M. Wardlaw and P.M. Insel, Perspect. Nutr. Boston: Times Mirror/ Mosby, 1990, p. 157.

tabolize the substrate. The branch chain amino acids, *valine*, *isoleucine*, and *leucine*, may be preferred amino acids in liver disease and trauma because they help to decrease muscle proteolysis.

*NITROGEN BALANCE.*   Nitrogen balance (NB), or equilibrium, is the amount of protein required to allow for normal physiologic functioning. Nitrogen balance studies are useful in determining the amount of protein required to remain in nitrogen homeostasis (achieve or maintain a positive NB). The NB can be calculated as follows: NB = (protein intake in grams x .16)—(24-hour urine urea nitrogen in grams + 3 gm). The extra 3 gm of urea nitrogen added to the equation is that amount normally lost in fecal material. Table 10-9 summarizes the interpretation and management of nitrogen balance studies.

## Lipids

Fats are the most concentrated source of energy, supplying 9 kcal per gm. Excessive saturated fat consumption

**BOX 10–1.**
EXAMPLES OF COMPLEMENTARY PROTEINS

Rice and beans
Croutons and split pea soup
Tortilla and beans
Corn bread and chili beans
Chick peas and tahini (sesame seed)
Tofu and sesame seeds

**TABLE 10–7.**
PROTEIN REQUIREMENTS DURING LIFE CYCLE

| | gm/kg |
|---|---|
| Infancy | |
| 0–6 mo | 2.2 |
| 7–12 mo | 1.6 |
| 1–3 y | 1.2 |
| 4–6 y | 1.1 |
| 7–10 y | 1.0 |
| 11–14 y | 1.0 |
| 15–18 y | .8–.9  (.9 for males; .8 for females) |
| Adults | .8 |
| Adults (50+) | .8 |

Source: Adapted from 1989 RDAs, Food and Nutrition Board, National Academy of Sciences.

**TABLE 10-8.**
ALTERATIONS IN PROTEIN REQUIREMENTS IN SELECT DISEASE STATES

| DISEASE | PROTEIN REQUIREMENTS |
|---|---|
| Renal disease | |
|   Early renal failure | |
|   (serum creatinine 2–6 mg/mL) | .6 gm/kg (75% HBV) (Human Biologic Value) |
|   Advanced renal failure | .3 gm/kg |
|   Dialysis—hemo | 1.0–1.2 |
|             peritoneal | 1.2–1.5 |
|   Nephrotic syndrome | .6 g plus urinary losses |
| Neoplastic disease | 1.5–2.5 g/kg |
| Liver disease | |
|   Hepatic encephalopathy | 50 g/d with increased amounts of BCAA (Branched Chain Amino Acids) |
|   Cirrhosis with encephalopathy | Decreased AAA (Aromatic Amino Acids) |
| | .8 gm–1.0 g/kg |
| Trauma | 1.0–105 gm/kg |
| Sepsis | 1.5–2.0 gm/kg |

is highly correlated with atherosclerosis and cancer incidence. A national dietary goal is to decrease saturated fat to about 10% of total dietary intake, balancing the total fat intake with polyunsaturated and monounsaturated fats.

## Functions

Current average fat intake in the United States is 38%; however, physiologic requirement for essential fatty acids is 4% of the total kcal. The main functions of fat include: (1) caloric source, (2) providing satiety, (3) insulation of the body, (4) transport of fat-soluble vitamins, and (5) prostaglandin (eicosanoid) formation by essential fatty acids, and (6) providing substrate for hormones, including cholecalciferol and estrogen.

## Families of Fatty Acids

Fatty acids are carbon chains of varying lengths with a carboxyl or acid group at one end and a methyl group at the other. Figure 10-3 illustrates the structure of a fatty acid.

A fatty acid is saturated if all the bonds between carbon atoms are single bonds. Saturated fats solidify at room temperature and can be of animal or plant origin.

**TABLE 10-9.**
INTERPRETATION AND MANAGEMENT OF NITROGEN BALANCE RESULTS

| NITROGEN BALANCE RESULT | INTERPRETATION OF NET BODY PROTEIN CHANGE | MANAGEMENT |
|---|---|---|
| Zero | Breakdown equals synthesis: normal state for healthy adults | Continue same protein intake unless anabolism/repletion is indicated (pregnancy, wound healing, etc.) |
| Negative (ie, less than zero) | Breakdown exceeds synthesis: undesirable state in all cases | Confirm that protein is of high quality and that calories are adequate, then increase protein intake by 6.25 g for each gram of $N_2$ under desired balance |
| Positive (ie, more than zero); anabolism goal: positive (4–6 g of $N_2$ per day) | Synthesis exceeds breakdown: desirable in growth, pregnancy, anabolic states, and repletion states of stress and disease | Continue current nutritional support; monitor tolerance of increased protein intake |

Source: A. Skipper, (ed.). Dietitian's Handbook of Enteral and Parenteral Nutrition. *Rockville, Md.: Aspen, 1989.*

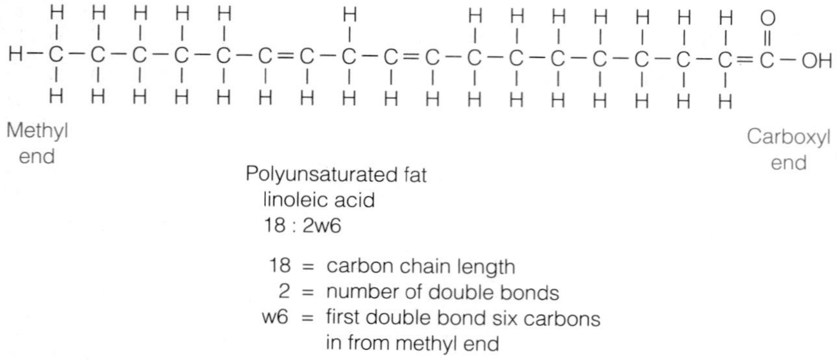

Methyl
end

Carboxyl
end

Polyunsaturated fat
linoleic acid
18 : 2w6

18 = carbon chain length
2 = number of double bonds
w6 = first double bond six carbons
in from methyl end

**FIGURE 10-3.**
Structure of a fatty acid.

Saturated fats are the most atherogenic (atherosclerosis-causing) family of fatty acids. Table 10-10 lists common food sources of saturated fat and cholesterol.

Monounsaturated fats are those containing a single double bond. Dietary sources include olive oil, peanut oil, or canola (rapeseed) oil. Monounsaturated fats lower serum cholesterol[50] (see Chap. 25).

Polyunsaturated fats are long chain fatty acids (greater than or equal to 18 c in the chain). Essential fatty acids, linoleic (omega 6), and alpha linolenic (omega 3) acids must be consumed in the diet. The physiologic function of these essential fatty acids is in the phospholipid layer in the cell wall and as precursors to the eicosanoids, prostaglandins, prostacyclins, thromboxanes, and leukotrienes. These compounds are integral to such vital body functions as regulation of blood pressure, blood clotting platelet aggregation, the immune response, inflammation, and the initiation of labor. Modification of

dietary lipids can impact physiologic function. Figure 10-4 illustrates the process of eicosanoid production from dietary precursors.

In polyunsaturated fats, the position of the first double bond determines the eicosanoids synthesized. If the first double bond is located at the third carbon atom from the methyl end, it is an omega 3 polyunsaturated fat. If the first double bond is located at the sixth carbon atom from the methyl end, it is an omega 6 fatty acid. A summary of the difference in physiologic effects is found in Table 10-11. Dietary sources of omega 6 fatty acids are corn, safflower, and sunflower oil. Dietary sources of omega 3 fatty acids are soybean oil, canola oil, and cold water fish. Polyunsaturated fats have been shown to have a hypocholesterolemic effect.[79]

Greenland Eskimos have approximately one-tenth the risk of heart attacks as compared with Danish people.[6] Although both populations consume high fat diets,

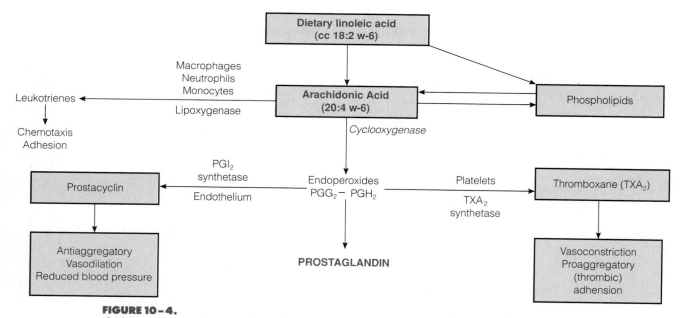

**FIGURE 10-4.**
Outline of pathway showing relationship between dietary linoleic acid and eicosanoid synthesis. The conversion of endoperoxide (PGH2) into proaggregatory thromboxane by platelets is normally counteracted by the production of antiaggregatory prostacyclin by the endothelial lining of blood vessels. The balanced production of these modulates platelet functions. (From J.E. Kinsella, *Nutrition Today.* Nov/Dec, 7–14, 1986.)

**TABLE 10-10.**

COMMON FOOD SOURCES OF CHOLESTEROL AND SATURATED FAT

| FOOD | CHOLESTEROL (mg) | SATURATED FAT (gm) |
|---|---|---|
| Ground beef (27% fat), 3 oz | 80 | 7.0 |
| Lean ground beef (15% fat), 3 oz | 50 | 5.0 |
| Chicken—white meat (no skin), 3 oz | 70 | 1.0 |
| Cheese, most varieties, 1 oz | 30 | 5.0 |
| Whole milk, 1 c | 33 | 5.0 |
| Skim milk, 1 c | trace | .3 |
| Butter, 1 T | 30 | 7.0 |
| Corn oil margarine, 1 T | 0 | 2.0 |
| Canola oil, 1 T | 0 | 1.0 |
| Corn oil, 1 T | 0 | 1.8 |
| Coconut oil, 1 T | 0 | 12.0 |

**TABLE 10-11.**

EFFECTS OF PRODUCTS MADE FROM OMEGA-3 (w-3) AND OMEGA-6 (w-6) FATTY ACIDS IN MAN

| SITE OF SYNTHESIS | w-6 (LINOLEIC ACID) | w-3 (EPA, DHA) |
|---|---|---|
| Cells lining blood vessels | Form prostaglandin $I_2$, which inhibits blood clotting | Form prostaglandin $I_3$, which inhibits blood clotting |
| Platelets[a] in the blood | Form thromboxane $A_2$, which is a strong promoter of blood clotting | Form thromboxane $A_3$, which is a very weak promoter of blood clotting |

*The net result is that omega-3 fatty acids reduce the tendency for blood to clot.*
*[a] Plate-like fragments in the bloodstream that contribute to blood clotting.*
Source: G.M. Wardlaw and P.M. Insel, St. Louis, Toronto, Boston: Times Mirror/Mosby, 1990.

Eskimos eat primarily cold water fish and Danes eat saturated fat. Fish oils decrease platelet aggregation and prolong bleeding times. The cholesterol lowering effect of fish oils is slight through the reduction of very low density lipoproteins (VLDL), a primary carrier of triglycerides.

When consuming a mixed diet, most individuals ingest a greater amount of omega 6 fatty acids. However, omega 6 and omega 3 fats compete for the enzymes responsible for desaturation and elongation to their respective metabolites. Affinity of the substrate for the enzyme increases with increasing number of double bonds, indicating omega 3 fatty acids can prevent the conversion of the omega 6 fatty acids to their metabolically active end products.

## Fatty Acid Metabolism

The metabolism of fatty acids is, in part, determined by the length in the carbon chain. Dietary fats are mostly made up of triglycerides: 3 fatty acid chains of varying length esterified to a glycerol backbone. Figure 10-5 illustrates the structure of a triglyceride. Long-chain triglycerides are hydrolyzed in the intestinal lumen by pancreatic lipase to monoglycerides and free fatty acids (FFA). Poorly soluble in water, bile salts enhance solubility through miceller formation (see Chap. 42). Micelles are transported passively across the intestinal cell wall where re-esterification occurs. Chylomicrons are the transport vehicle for re-esterified triglyceride. Chylomicrons are released into the lymphatic system, then to venous circulation. Lipoprotein lipase cleaves the triglyceride into FFA and monoglyceride. In the fed state,

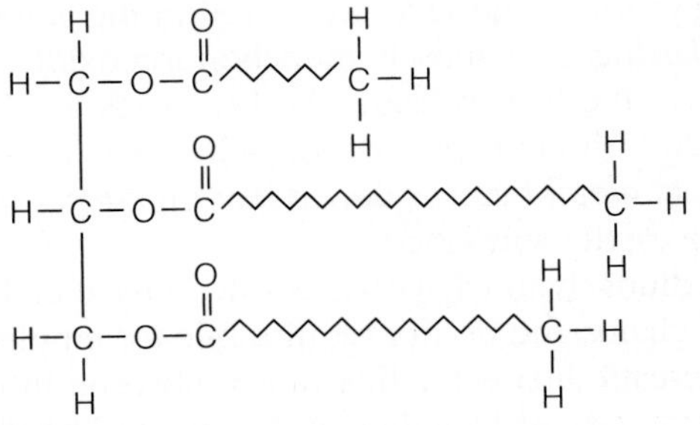

**FIGURE 10-5.**
The structure of a triglyceride. Three fatty acids attached to a glycerol backbone.

**TABLE 10–12.**

FOOD AND NUTRITION BOARD, NATIONAL ACADEMY OF SCIENCES—NATIONAL RESEARCH COUNCIL RECOMMENDED DIETARY ALLOWANCES (RDAs)[a]

| AGE (YEARS) AND SEX GROUP | WEIGHT[b] | | HEIGHT[b] | | PROTEIN | FAT-SOLUBLE VITAMINS | | | |
|---|---|---|---|---|---|---|---|---|---|
| | | | | | | vita-min A | vita-min D | vita-min E | vita-min K |
| | kg | lb | cm | in. | | | | | |
| | | | | | gm | $\mu$g RE[c] | $\mu$g[d] | mg $\alpha$-TE[e] | $\mu$g |
| **Infants** | | | | | | | | | |
| 0.0–0.5 | 6 | 13 | 60 | 24 | 13 | 375 | 7.5 | 3 | 5 |
| 0.5–1.0 | 9 | 20 | 71 | 28 | 14 | 375 | 10 | 4 | 10 |
| **Children** | | | | | | | | | |
| 1–3 | 13 | 29 | 90 | 35 | 16 | 400 | 10 | 6 | 15 |
| 4–6 | 20 | 44 | 112 | 44 | 24 | 500 | 10 | 7 | 20 |
| 7–10 | 28 | 62 | 132 | 52 | 28 | 700 | 10 | 7 | 30 |
| **Males** | | | | | | | | | |
| 11–14 | 45 | 99 | 157 | 62 | 45 | 1000 | 10 | 10 | 45 |
| 15–18 | 66 | 145 | 176 | 69 | 59 | 1000 | 10 | 10 | 65 |
| 19–24 | 72 | 160 | 177 | 70 | 58 | 1000 | 10 | 10 | 70 |
| 25–50 | 79 | 174 | 176 | 70 | 63 | 1000 | 5 | 10 | 80 |
| 51+ | 77 | 170 | 173 | 68 | 63 | 1000 | 5 | 10 | 80 |
| **Females** | | | | | | | | | |
| 11–14 | 46 | 101 | 157 | 62 | 46 | 800 | 10 | 8 | 45 |
| 15–18 | 55 | 120 | 163 | 64 | 44 | 800 | 10 | 8 | 55 |
| 19–24 | 58 | 128 | 164 | 65 | 46 | 800 | 10 | 8 | 60 |
| 25–50 | 63 | 138 | 163 | 64 | 50 | 800 | 5 | 8 | 65 |
| 51+ | 65 | 143 | 160 | 63 | 50 | 800 | 5 | 8 | 65 |
| pregnant | | | | | 60 | 800 | 10 | 10 | 65 |
| lactating | | | | | | | | | |
| 1st 6 months | | | | | 65 | 1300 | 10 | 12 | 65 |
| 2nd 6 months | | | | | 62 | 1200 | 10 | 11 | 65 |

[a]The allowances, expressed as average daily intakes over time, are intended to provide for individual variations among most normal persons as they live in the United States under usual environmental stresses. Diets should be based on a variety of common foods in order to provide other nutrients for which human requirements have been less well defined. Revised 1989. Designed for the maintenance of good nutrition of practically all healthy people in the United States.

[b]Weights and heights of Reference Adults are actual medians for the U.S. population of the designated age, as reported by NHANES II. The median weights and heights of those under 19 years of age were taken from P.V.V. Hamill, T.A. Drizd, C.L. Johnson, R.B. Reed, A.F. Roche, and W.M. Moore: Physical growth. National Center for Health

monoglycerides and FFAs are stored in the adipose cell. In the fasting state, muscle mitochondria oxidize FFA for energy or the liver releases the fatty acids as VLDL (see Chap. 26). The transport of long-chain fats across mitochondrial membranes is dependent on *carnitine*, which acts as a carrier substance.

Medium-chain triglycerides (MCT) have eight to ten carbon chains and do not require bile for emulsification or pancreatic lipase for hydrolysis. Absorption of these triglycerides is intact and degradation into FFAs acids occurs through intracellular lipase. Albumin carries FFA into portal circulation, then to the liver for oxidation. Rapid metabolism of MCT occurs as carnitine is not needed for transport into the cell. In diseases affecting fat digestion or absorption, MCT oil can be a valuable caloric source. MCT oil does not provide essential fatty acids.

Cholesterol is a sterol found only in animal products. There is no required intake for cholesterol as humans can synthesize cholesterol when dietary supply is inadequate. The richest dietary sources include liver, egg yolk, whole milk, whole milk cheese, beef, and pork. Physiologic functions of cholesterol include its role in forming many hormones, in keeping the cell membrane insoluble in water, and in forming bile salts. It is not necessary to

| vitamin C | thiamin | riboflavin | niacin | vitamin B$_6$ | folate | vitamin B$_{12}$ | calcium | phosphorus | magnesium | iron | zinc | iodine | selenium |
|---|---|---|---|---|---|---|---|---|---|---|---|---|---|
| | WATER-SOLUBLE VITAMINS | | | | | | MINERALS | | | | | | |
| ——— mg ——— | | | mg NE$^f$ mg | | ——— µg ——— | | ——————— mg ——————— | | | | | ——— µg ——— | |
| 30 | 0.3 | 0.4 | 5 | 0.3 | 25 | 0.3 | 400 | 300 | 40 | 6 | 5 | 40 | 10 |
| 35 | 0.4 | 0.5 | 6 | 0.6 | 35 | 0.5 | 600 | 500 | 60 | 10 | 5 | 50 | 15 |
| 40 | 0.7 | 0.8 | 9 | 1.0 | 50 | 0.7 | 800 | 800 | 80 | 10 | 10 | 70 | 20 |
| 45 | 0.9 | 1.1 | 12 | 1.1 | 75 | 1.0 | 800 | 800 | 120 | 10 | 10 | 90 | 20 |
| 45 | 1.0 | 1.2 | 13 | 1.4 | 100 | 1.4 | 800 | 800 | 170 | 10 | 10 | 120 | 30 |
| 50 | 1.3 | 1.5 | 17 | 1.7 | 150 | 2.0 | 1200 | 1200 | 270 | 12 | 15 | 150 | 40 |
| 60 | 1.5 | 1.8 | 20 | 2.0 | 200 | 2.0 | 1200 | 1200 | 400 | 12 | 15 | 150 | 50 |
| 60 | 1.5 | 1.7 | 19 | 2.0 | 200 | 2.0 | 1200 | 1200 | 350 | 10 | 15 | 150 | 70 |
| 60 | 1.5 | 1.7 | 19 | 2.0 | 200 | 2.0 | 800 | 800 | 350 | 10 | 15 | 150 | 70 |
| 60 | 1.2 | 1.4 | 15 | 2.0 | 200 | 2.0 | 800 | 800 | 350 | 10 | 15 | 150 | 70 |
| 50 | 1.1 | 1.3 | 15 | 1.4 | 150 | 2.0 | 1200 | 1200 | 280 | 15 | 12 | 150 | 45 |
| 60 | 1.1 | 1.3 | 15 | 1.5 | 180 | 2.0 | 1200 | 1200 | 300 | 15 | 12 | 150 | 50 |
| 60 | 1.1 | 1.3 | 15 | 1.6 | 180 | 2.0 | 1200 | 1200 | 280 | 15 | 12 | 150 | 55 |
| 60 | 1.1 | 1.3 | 15 | 1.6 | 180 | 2.0 | 800 | 800 | 280 | 15 | 12 | 150 | 55 |
| 60 | 1.0 | 1.2 | 13 | 1.6 | 180 | 2.0 | 800 | 800 | 280 | 10 | 12 | 150 | 55 |
| 70 | 1.5 | 1.6 | 17 | 2.2 | 400 | 2.2 | 1200 | 1200 | 320 | 30 | 15 | 175 | 65 |
| 95 | 1.6 | 1.8 | 20 | 2.1 | 280 | 2.6 | 1200 | 1200 | 355 | 15 | 19 | 200 | 75 |
| 90 | 1.6 | 1.7 | 20 | 2.1 | 260 | 2.6 | 1200 | 1200 | 340 | 15 | 16 | 200 | 75 |

*Statistics Percentiles. Am. J. Clin. Nutr. 32:607, 1979. The use of these figures does not imply that the height-to-weight ratios are ideal.*
$^c$*Retinol equivalents. 1 retinol equivalent = 1 µg retinol or 6 µg β-carotene. See text for calculation of vitamin A activity of diets as retinol equivalents.*
$^d$*As cholecalciferol. 10 µg cholecalciferol = 400 IU of vitamin D.*
$^e$*α-Tocopherol equivalents. 1 mg d-α tocopherol = 1 α-TE. See text for variation in allowances and calculation of vitamin E activity of the diet as α-tocopherol equivalents.*
$^f$*1 NE (niacin equivalent) is equal to 1 mg of niacin or 60 mg of dietary tryptophan.*

consume cholesterol per se, because the liver efficiently produces it from saturated fat in the diet (see Chap. 42).

## MICRONUTRIENTS

The micronutrients include the water-soluble and fat-soluble vitamins, as well as the minerals. Some of the minerals (electrolytes) are discussed in Chapter 8, and other necessary trace minerals are covered in this section. A basis for understanding the functions is presented in this chapter with application of materials throughout specific sections in the text. Table 10-12 lists the recommended daily allowances as determined by the National Research Council of the Food and Nutritional Board, National Academy of Sciences, for different age groups.

### Water-Soluble Vitamins

Vitamins are organic compounds needed for metabolism of foodstuffs. Vitamins provide no energy but facilitate energy-yielding chemical reactions. The B vitamins and vitamin C are water soluble and are not stored in appre-

**TABLE 10–13.**
FUNCTIONS AND ALTERATIONS IN WATER-SOLUBLE VITAMINS

| VITAMIN | FUNCTION | FOOD SOURCES | DEFICIENCY | FACTORS INFLUENCING REQUIREMENTS | SIGNS AND SYMPTOMS | TOXICITY |
|---|---|---|---|---|---|---|
| Thiamine | Metabolism through oxidative rxn | Pork, whole grains, organ meats | Beri beri, chronic alcoholism | Alcoholism,[135] fever, infection, hyperthyroidism, burns, trauma, chronic antacid use | Anorexia, fatigue, peripheral neuropathy, footdrop, cardiomegaly, depression | Nausea and vomiting |
| Riboflavin | Coenzyme flavin, mononucleotide, citric acid, beta-oxidation[109] | Milk, dairy products | Cheiclosis, ariboflavinosis | Thyroid dysfunction, burns, trauma, diabetes, alcoholism, oral contraceptives,[83] tricyclic antidepressants | Seborrheic dermatitis, scrotal dermatitis, growth failure, photophobia | None known |
| Niacin | Coenzyme NAD, NADP, formation of ATP, oxidation/reduction, reactions, immune competence | Mushrooms, enriched grain products, tuna, chicken, can be synthesized from dietary tryptophan | Pellegra | Alcohol, thyroid disorders, neoplasia,[8] isoniazid for TB, burns | Diarrhea, dermatitis, dementia, weakness, fatigue | In large amounts, nicotinic acid functions as a vasodilator; nausea, vomiting, hypocholesterolemic effect[118] |
| Pyridoxine (B₆) | Coenzyme form, pyridoxical phosphate, transamination of amino acids, synthesis of hemoglobin, neurotransmitter synthesis | Meat, fish, poultry, bananas, cantaloupe, broccoli | Irritability, depression | Uremia,[77] burns,[7] advancing age, neoplastic disease,[103] liver disease,[5] medication, uremia, isoniazid, hydralazine, high protein diets, asthma,[107] degenerative diseases[87] | Stomatitis, glossitis, cheilosis, anemia (after prolonged deficiency) | Irreversible nerve damage,[1] ataxia |
| Folic acid | One carbon transfer rxn, synthesis of RBC, nucleotides, RNA, DNA, proteins | Orange juice, liver, green leafy vegetables | Megaloblastic anemia/ macrocytic anemia | Fevers, burns, alcoholism,[57] ileal disease, inflammatory bowel disease, gluten-induced enteropathy, gastrectomies, periods of increased growth, medications, methotrexates, common deficiency in elderly, adolescent females[25] | Smooth, sore tongue; dementia; diarrhea; weight loss | May mask B₁₂ deficiency |

(continued)

**TABLE 10–13.**
FUNCTIONS AND ALTERATIONS IN WATER-SOLUBLE VITAMINS (Continued)

| VITAMIN | FUNCTION | FOOD SOURCES | DEFICIENCY | FACTORS INFLUENCING REQUIREMENTS | SIGNS AND SYMPTOMS | TOXICITY |
|---|---|---|---|---|---|---|
| $B_{12}$ | Coenzyme transfer of methyl ($CH_3$) groups, synthesis of nucleic acids and choline, RBC formation | Animal protein | Megaloblastic anemia, pernicious anemia | Vegetarian, gastrectomy patients, ileal resection, gastric bypass surgery,[16] intestinal parasites, medications such as neomycin, potassium chloride | Loss of appetite, weight loss, glossites, leukopenia, thrombocytopenia, tingling in extremities,[10] dementia[70] | None known |
| Ascorbic acid (vitamin C) | Collagen formation, cartilage formation, synthesis of bile, acts as a reducing agent, wound healing | Green peppers, citrus fruit, strawberries, broccoli, cabbage | Scurvy | Cigarette smoking,[69] alcoholic, oral contraceptive users, cancer, surgical patients, burns | Capillary fragility, hemorrhagic disorders, fatigue, anorexia, muscle pain, gingivitis | Diarrhea, nausea, excess converted to oxalate and form kidney stones, interfere with urine glucose tests, rebound scurvy[86] |

ciable amounts. Megadoses defined at 10 times recommended dietary allowance (RDA) are taken by some individuals, and toxicity may develop. The RDAs are summarized in Table 10-12.

Disease states can significantly increase the need for water-soluble vitamins. Table 10-13 summarizes function, food sources, deficiency disease, signs and symptoms of the deficiency, factors influencing or increasing requirements, and toxicity symptoms.

## Fat-Soluble Vitamins

The fat-soluble vitamins are A, D, E, and K, and are absorbed together with dietary fat. They are readily stored in fatty tissues and are more likely than water-soluble vitamins to cause a toxicity reaction. Toxicity symptoms may occur at levels as low as 10 times the RDA. Deficiency states may be encountered in individuals with steatorrhea, or fat malabsorption. However, because stores of these vitamins exist, the development of deficiency symptoms occur over a period of time. Table 10-14 lists the fat-soluble vitamins, chemical name, function, food sources, deficiency disease, clinical signs and symptoms of deficiency, conditions that influence requirements, and toxicity.

## Trace Minerals

Minerals are inorganic compounds that are vital in human nutrition and cell function (see also Chap. 8). Min-

erals function in a variety of metabolic roles, including enzyme cofactors, hormones, nerve conduction, and structural components. Bioavailability refers to the amount of mineral absorbed and used by the body. Various factors influence the bioavailability of a particular mineral, such as binding effect, fiber, and the physiologic need of the body.[26] Minerals are necessary in a variety of body functions including acid-base balance, osmotic pressure, cell membrane permeability, enzyme system activation, and nerve and muscle responsiveness. The activities of the minerals are discussed in the respective sections of the text. The important trace minerals are summarized in Table 10-15. The functions, food sources, disease states, and influencing requirements, as well as factors influencing bioavailability are presented in this table.

## MALNUTRITION

Malnutrition is defined as an inadequate intake of macronutrients, vitamins, or minerals that impairs the physiologic functioning of the body. It may be the result of inadequate intake or due to increased requirements. The incidence of malnutrition has been estimated to affect 50% of hospitalized patients.[13]

*Protein calorie malnutrition (PCM)* is a continuum with *marasmus* (starvation or semi-starvation) at one end and *kwashiorkor* (protein deficiency, also known as hypoalbuminemic malnutrition) at the other (Figure 10-6). Protein calorie malnutrition, as seen in the hospital, is generally classified into three categories:

**TABLE 10–14.**
FUNCTIONS AND ALTERATIONS IN FAT-SOLUBLE VITAMINS

| VITAMIN | FUNCTION | FOOD SOURCES | DEFICIENCY | FACTORS INFLUENCING REQUIREMENTS | SIGNS AND SYMPTOMS | TOXICITY |
|---|---|---|---|---|---|---|
| Vitamin A (retinoids) beta carotene (precursor) | Visual adaptation[4] adrenal hormone biosynthesis, mucopolysaccharide and glycoprotein synthesis, maintenance of epithelial structure, wound healing, immunocompetence | Whole milk, butter, carrots | Xerophthalmia | Preterm infants, gastrointestinal dysfunction,[48] respiratory ailments,[117] burns,[48] trauma | Night blindness, keratinization of epithelial cells, diarrhea | Nausea, vomiting, alopecia, hypercalcemia, long bone tenderness, pregnant women[128] and persons with chronic renal disease[46] may be more susceptible |
| Vitamin D cholecalciferol, synthesized via ultraviolet light | Absorption of calcium and phosphorus,[106] calcium reabsorption from kidney, removal of calcium and phosphorus from bone, immunoregulatory[89] | Milk, dairy products | Rickets, osteomalacia | Tropical sprue, regional enteritis, pancreatic insufficiency, gastric resection, jejunoileal bypass, chronic renal failure, hypoparathyroidism, medications (anticonvulsants, cimetidine, isoniazid),[11] total parenteral nutrition | Bone pain, increased serum alkaline phosphatase, decreased serum calcium levels, bone demineralization | Nausea, vomiting, anorexia, headache, diarrhea, confusion, calcification of soft tissue |
| Vitamin E (tocopherols) | Antioxidant, cell membrane integrity, immunoregulatory[112] | Vegetable oil | Hemolytic anemia | Increased intake of polyunsaturated fats, steatorrhea, protein calorie malnutrition, infancy, cystic fibrosis,[120] short bowel syndrome,[65] respiratory distress syndrome, retrolental fibroplasia,[100] bronchopulmonary dysplasia, smoking | Increased platelet aggregation, neurological abnormalities, decreased serum creatinine, excessive creatinuria | Nausea, headache, antagonist to vitamin K |
| Vitamin K (phylloquinone) diet (menaquinone) gut flora | Clotting factors | Greens, broccoli, cauliflower | Hemorrhagic disease | Stage of life cycle (newborn, elderly), renal failure, ulcerative colitis, chronic pancreatitis, biliary dysfunction, medications (antibiotics, coumadin,[95] cholestyramine[49]) | Prolonged bleeding times | With prescription menadione, jaundice, anemia |

**TABLE 10-15.**
FUNCTIONS AND ALTERATIONS IN TRACE MINERALS

| MINERAL | FUNCTION | FOOD SOURCES | DEFICIENCY | FACTORS INFLUENCING REQUIREMENTS | SIGNS AND SYMPTOMS | TOXICITY |
|---|---|---|---|---|---|---|
| Zinc | Ligand in albumin, nucleotides, thymus integrity, cellular immunity, sexual maturation | Oysters, wheat germ, crab, shrimp, red meat | Growth retardation, delayed secondary sex characteristics | Trauma,[92] burns, surgery, inflammatory bowel, short bowel syndrome, increased intake of fiber, recovery from malnutrition,[119] total parenteral nutrition[114] | Hair loss, inflammation of skin, poor wound healing, decreased taste | Decreased use of copper, iron[58]; decrease in HDL cholesterol; diarrhea; nausea and vomiting; immunosuppression |
| Copper | Component of enzymes of iron metabolism, crossbinding of collagen, myelination of nerves | Meat, liver, cocoa, legumes, nuts, affected by soil conditions | Rare, induced by copper; free total parenteral nutrition; microcytic hypochromic anemia; increased serum cholesterol levels[31] | Short bowel, chronic diarrhea, Crohn's disease, celiac disease, burns, antacids, high zinc intake[147] | Skeletal demineralization, impaired glucose tolerance, depigmentation of hair | Vomiting |
| Selenium | Antioxidant, glutathione, peroxidase | Fish, organ meats, eggs, shellfish | Muscle pain, muscle wasting, heart disease | AIDS,[35] cystic fibrosis,[140] cancer[122] | Growth retardation, muscle pain/weakness, cardiomyopathy | Narrow range of essentiality to toxicity; nausea, vomiting; death |
| Iron | Essential component of hemoglobin, respiratory oxidation, enzyme cofactor, hydroxylation of lysine and proline | Heme: liver, lean red meat, oysters; nonheme: green leafy vegetables | Hypochromic, microcytic anemia | Vegetarians, runners, periods of rapid growth, bioavailability decreased with tannins,[54] calcium carbonate, magnesium oxide,[3] zinc/copper,[55] oxalate | Shortness of breath, impaired motor development[137] spoon-shaped nails (koilonychia), increased susceptibility to infection[29] | Excess unbound iron, promotes bacterial/fungal growth,[141] hemochromatosis |

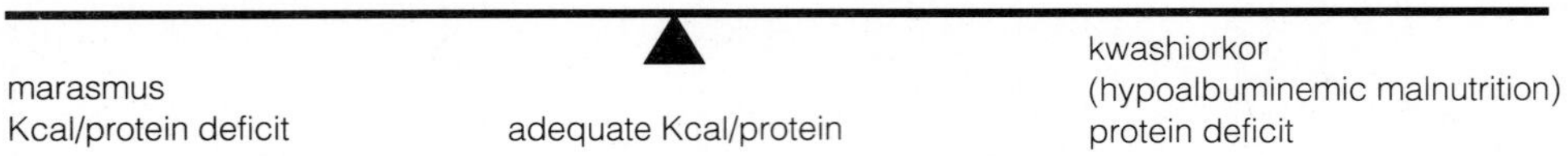

marasmus
Kcal/protein deficit                     adequate Kcal/protein

kwashiorkor
(hypoalbuminemic malnutrition)
protein deficit

**FIGURE 10–6.**
The continuum of marasmus and kwashiorkor. Balance requires adequate Kcal and protein. Alteration in either will tip the delicate balance.

1. *Marasmus:* This is semi-starvation caused by poor intake or poverty, where fat and muscle provide most of the calories required. It is characterized by a reduction of body weight but a preservation of serum proteins and immune competence unless it is very severe. The maintenance of serum proteins is at the expense of somatic (muscle) and visceral (organ) protein.

2. *Kwashiorkor:* Kwashiorkor means "the disease that the first child gets when the second one comes" and is typically seen in underdeveloped countries where children are weaned from the breast to a protein-poor gruel. The pathogenesis of kwashiorkor is evidenced by a low ratio of protein to calories as well as a "flaky paint" dermatitis and hair changes.[111] *Hypoalbuminemic malnutrition*, or hospital-based kwashiorkor, develops in persons who have the stress of injury or infection with poor intake or inappropriate nutrition support. There is a generalized protein loss with increasing impairment of visceral function, evidenced by a decrease in immunocompetence and hypoalbuminemia. This condition is also known as *stressed starvation.*

3. *Combined malnutrition:* This third and most serious form of macronutrient malnutrition is commonly seen in the elderly or individuals with chronic disease. The stress of illness or trauma is superimposed on a marasmic individual. This person needs early nutritional intervention to increase survival rate.

## Calorie Reserves in Starvation

During starvation, physiologic sources of calories include glycogen, somatic and visceral protein, and fat. In the early hours of a fast, glycogen serves as the primary energy source. Metabolism favors glucose homeostasis to support tissues dependent on glucose as a sole energy source, such as the brain, nerves, red blood cells, and renal medulla. During the initial stage of starvation, a fall in arterial blood glucose levels causes a decrease in *insulin*, which is a major anabolic hormone. As insulin levels fall, the levels of the counterregulatory or catabolic hormones increase. The major catabolic hormone involved in the process is *glucagon*. The decrease in the insulin:glucagon ratio stimulates glycogenolysis and the release of hepatic glucose. Glycogenolysis is the major source of glucose for approximately 24 hours. Gluconeogenesis from protein serves as the major source of glucose after the initial stage of starvation. Urinary excretion of nitrogen (from protein catabolism) increases as losses of 12 gm of nitrogen per day become common. As the fast continues, the decreased level of insulin allows li-

polysis and the release of FFAs, oxidation of fatty acids, and the synthesis of ketones. The brain cannot use FFAs because fatty acids do not cross the blood brain barrier. Ketones and ketoacids can cross the blood brain barrier and serve as an alternative energy source for the brain, a major consumer of glucose. This process is known as *ketoadaptation*. The rate of protein breakdown is slowed and urinary nitrogen losses become approximately 3 to 5 gm per day. Serum proteins (also known as the proteins of homeostasis) are preserved until the individual is close to death and fat reserves are exhausted. At this point, gluconeogenesis increases, nitrogen excretion increases, and death is likely.

Concomitantly, a decrease in metabolic rate reduces the caloric need of the body and slows the rate of deterioration. A decrease in voluntary work and loss of lean body mass from metabolically active organs such as the pancreas and gut may also contribute to a decrease in metabolic activity. Cardiac workload decreases and bradycardia lowers the basal metabolic rate.

## Nutritional/Metabolic Consequences of Stress

Hypoalbuminemic malnutrition, or stressed starvation, has a profound and significantly different effect on body composition, protein utilization, and organ function when compared to marasmus. Neuroendocrine control mechanisms are altered and mediate changes in nutritional status. Increases in catecholamines, as well as increased levels of glucagon, increase the blood glucose level. This is often referred to as "stress diabetes." The hyperglycemia does stimulate insulin release, but insulin resistance, coupled with increases in glucagon levels, allows hyperglycemia to persist. Gluconeogenesis is accentuated and losses of protein continue at a greater rate than with simple starvation alone. In this hypermetabolic state, there is an increase in lipolysis, but there is a marked decline in ketone production, possibly due to adequate levels of circulating insulin. This failure to ketoadapt has the greatest clinical implications for the individual who is obese. Often viewed as having ample calorie reserves, the major calorie source in stressed starvation is protein and not fat. Therefore, an obese individual may not be perceived at nutritional risk based on physical size rather than the degree of stress. In clinical nutrition, the provision of intravenous dextrose prevents ketoadaptation. When dextrose is given, nutritional support, including adequate protein, should begin as soon as possible.

Skeletal muscle is catabolized to gain access to the branched chain amino acids (BCAA), which serve as energy substrates through gluconeogenesis. Hepatic protein synthesis shifts from the production of the proteins of homeostasis (albumin, transferrin, prealbumin, and retinol binding protein) to the production of acute phase reactants such as interleukin I, ceruloplasmin, and clotting factors, thereby contributing to hypoalbuminemia. Alterations in the serum levels of the proteins of homeostasis can be used to assess the degree of nutritional depletion (Table 10-16). Hypoalbuminemia has deleterious effects on wound healing and makes nutritional repletion difficult. Box 10-2 summarizes the effects of hypoproteinemia.

Hypermetabolism is a hallmark feature of stress and this causes calorie and protein requirements to increase. Factors influencing calorie and protein requirements include the type of stress such as infection, fractures, trauma, fever, and respiratory support. Figure 10-7 illustrates the percent change in metabolic activity and increased caloric need in various forms of stress. To promote anabolism, 150 kcal should be provided for each gram of nitrogen given. Alterations in plasma levels of BCAA, glutamine, and arginine may indicate unique roles for these amino acids in the critically ill.[30,121]

## DISORDERS OF WEIGHT MANAGEMENT

### Obesity

#### Incidence

Obesity is the most common nutritional disorder in the United States. Although weight reduction promotions are a multimillion dollar industry, Americans are becoming

## BOX 10-2.
### EFFECTS OF HYPOPROTEINEMIA

1. Decreased wound tensile strength
2. Poor wound healing
3. Decreased blood volume
4. Decreased bone marrow activity—anemia, leukopenia
5. Decreased coagulation mechanisms
6. Increased atrophy of spleen, lymph tissue
7. Decreased antibody production
8. Decreased cell-mediated immunity—resistance to infection
9. Decreased resistance of liver to toxic agents
10. Decreased urine output and water retention
11. Decreased pulmonary function and ventilation
    atrophy of respiratory muscles
    retained secretions
    decreased albumin—interstitial edema
    decreased serum buffering capacity
12. Increased tendency to develop decubitus ulcers
13. Diarrhea

Source: Adapted from A. Barrocas, G.L. Webb, W.R. Webb, and C.M. St. Romain, Hypoproteinemia in Nutritional Considerations in the Critically Ill 75(7): 849, 1982.

more obese than ever. Despite the fact that calorie intake has decreased by 10% in the last century, the frequency of obesity has doubled during that time span.[101] Since 1975, obesity in children ages six to 11 years has increased by 54%, and by 39% in the 12- to 17-year-old group. It has been estimated that 40% of children who are obese at age seven years will also be obese adults.[91] At present, 34 million Americans are obese and 13 million more are severely obese.[132]

#### Definition

Obesity is generally defined as being 20% above ideal body weight (IBW) and severely obese as 40% above IBW. A quick estimation of the IBC can be performed as

## TABLE 10-16.
### RELATIONSHIP BETWEEN NUTRITIONAL DEPLETION AND SERUM PROTEINS

| INDICATOR | NORMAL | DEGREE OF DEPLETION | | |
|---|---|---|---|---|
| | | Mild | Moderate | Severe |
| Albumin (g/dl) | 3.5–5.5 | 2.8–3.4 | 2.1–2.7 | < 2.1 |
| Transferrin (mg/dl) | 180–260 | 150–200 | 100–149 | < 100 |
| Prealbumin (mcg/dl) | 200–300 | 10–15 | 5–9 | < 5 |
| Retinol-binding protein[a] (mcg/dl) | 40–50 | — | — | — |

Note: To convert albumin (g/100 ml) to international standard units (nmol/L), multiply by 37.06. To convert transferrin (mg/100 ml) to standard international units (g/L), multiply by 0.01.
[a] Levels of < 3 mg/100 ml suggest compromised protein status. The actual degree of depletion (mild, moderate, and severe) has not been defined.
Adapted from: E.N. Whitney, C.B. Cataldo, and S.R. Rolfes. Understanding Normal and Clinical Nutrition (3rd ed.) St Paul: West 1991.

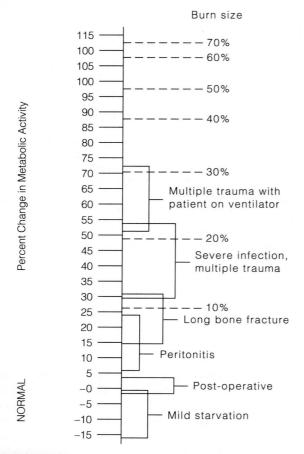

**FIGURE 10–7.**
Estimate of increased energy needs with stress. (Redrawn from D.W. Willmore, *The Metabolic Management of the Critically Ill.* New York: Plenum, 1977.)

shown in Box 10-3. Resting metabolic expenditure (REE) is defined as the amount of calories the body uses at rest for involuntary metabolic activities in the nonfasting state. It is influenced by a variety of factors. Resting energy expenditure decreases with age, starvation, inactivity and loss of lean body mass. Lean body mass is lost during dieting. It is increased by fever, physiological stress and physical activity. In most individuals, the REE accounts for about 75% of the total daily energy expenditure. Voluntary physical activity accounts for the remaining 25%. Although many formulas and techniques exist for the calculation of REE, it may be estimated by using the individual's IBW × 10. Additionally, Table 10-17 provides the REE and total calorie allowance per day throughout the life cycle for normal weight individuals. Body mass index, also known as the Quetelet index, can also be used in defining obesity.[42] A body mass index of 30 kg per m² can be categorized as obese. Table 10-18 illustrates the Body Mass Index.

### *Types of Cellular Obesity*

Hypertrophic obesity is characterized by an increase in the size of the existing adipocyte, or fat cell. Hypertrophy is present in all obesity and 80% to 90% of adult onset obesity is hypertrophic. Hyperplastic obesity is defined as an increase in the number of fat cells available to fill. Hyperplasia occurs primarily during periods of rapid growth, such as infancy and adolescence, and is often called "juvenile-onset" obesity. Weight loss and weight maintenance are more difficult to achieve in hyperplastic obesity.[19]

---

**BOX 10–3.**
## QUICK ESTIMATION OF IDEAL BODY WEIGHT

**Men:**

For 5 feet, consider 106 pounds a reasonable weight.

For each inch over 5 feet, add 6 pounds.

Subtract 6 pounds for each inch under 5 feet.

Add 10 percent for a large-framed individual; subtract 10 percent for a small-framed individual.

*Example:* A man 5 feet 8 inches tall (medium frame) would start at 106 pounds, add 48, and arrive at a reasonable weight of 154 pounds.

**Women:**

For 5 feet, consider 100 pounds a reasonable weight.

For each inch over 5 feet, add 5 pounds.

Subtract 5 pounds for each inch under 5 feet.

Add 10 percent for a large-framed individual; subtract 10 percent for a small-framed individual.

*Example:* A woman 5 feet 6 inches tall (medium frame) would start at 100 pounds, add 30, and arrive at a reasonable weight of 130 pounds.

Source: E.N. Whitney, C.B. Cataldo, and S.R. Rolfes. *Understanding Normal and Clinical Nutrition* (3rd Ed.) St. Paul: West, 1991.

**TABLE 10–17.**
MEDIAN HEIGHTS AND WEIGHTS AND RECOMMENDED ENERGY INTAKES
(UNITED STATES)

| AGE | WEIGHT | | HEIGHT | | AVERAGE ENERGY ALLOWANCE | | |
|---|---|---|---|---|---|---|---|
| (Years) | (kg) | (lb) | (cm) | (inches) | REE[a] (kcal/day) | kcal per kg | kcal per day[c] |
| **Infants** | | | | | | | |
| 0.0–0.5 | 6 | 13 | 60 | 24 | 320 | 108 | 650 |
| 0.5–1.0 | 9 | 20 | 71 | 28 | 500 | 98 | 850 |
| **Children** | | | | | | | |
| 1–3 | 13 | 29 | 90 | 35 | 740 | 102 | 1300 |
| 4–6 | 20 | 44 | 112 | 44 | 950 | 90 | 1800 |
| 7–10 | 28 | 62 | 132 | 52 | 1130 | 70 | 2000 |
| **Males** | | | | | | | |
| 11–14 | 45 | 99 | 157 | 62 | 1440 | 55 | 2500 |
| 15–18 | 66 | 145 | 176 | 69 | 1760 | 45 | 3000 |
| 19–24 | 72 | 160 | 177 | 70 | 1780 | 40 | 2900 |
| 25–50 | 79 | 174 | 176 | 70 | 1800 | 37 | 2900 |
| 51+ | 77 | 170 | 173 | 68 | 1530 | 30 | 2300 |
| **Females** | | | | | | | |
| 11–14 | 46 | 101 | 157 | 62 | 1310 | 47 | 2200 |
| 15–18 | 55 | 120 | 163 | 64 | 1370 | 40 | 2200 |
| 19–24 | 58 | 128 | 164 | 65 | 1350 | 38 | 2200 |
| 25–50 | 63 | 138 | 163 | 64 | 1380 | 36 | 2200 |
| 51+ | 65 | 143 | 160 | 63 | 1280 | 30 | 1900 |
| **Pregnant** (2nd and 3rd trimesters) | | | | | | | +300 |
| **Lactating** | | | | | | | +500 |

[a] REE (resting energy expenditure) represents the energy expended by a person at rest under normal conditions.
[b] Recommended energy allowances assume light to moderate activity and were calculated by multiplying the REE by an activity factor.
[c] Average energy allowances have been rounded.
Source: Recommended Dietary Allowances. © 1989 by the National Academy of Sciences, National Academy Press, Washington, D.C.

## Regulation of Body Weight

In most individuals, body weight is maintained within a narrow range over time by short- and long-term regulation. Short-term regulation refers to the onset of eating on a meal-to-meal basis and is largely dependent on appetite. Long-term regulation refers to the modulation of intake and output so that body weight is maintained within a range.[133,134] It is a multifaceted process influenced by genetics, thermogenesis, hormones, enzymatic activity, and activity level.

*APPETITE CONTROL.* Appetite is regulated internally by the hypothalamus. The lateral hypothalamus, or *hunger center*, initiates food consumption after receiving clues, such as hypoglycemia, indicating macronutrient depletion. The ventromedial hypothalamus, or *satiety center*, monitors rising nutrient levels and signals the termination of hunger.[73] Many physiologic clues are directed to the hypothalamus. The gut releases brain-gut peptides, including cholecystokinin and bombesin, throughout the process of eating, signaling satiety.[45] Increasing nutrient levels in the blood, rising blood glucose levels, and tryptophan also cue satiety.[18] Tryptophan, an amino acid precursor to serotonin, is a powerful regulator of carbohydrate intake.[43,146] Norepinephrine release by the sympathetic nervous system (SNS) stimulates feeding, and epinephrine and dopamine inhibit feeding.[62] Obesity may, in part, be due to a defect in the stimulation and inhibition of the SNS.[17,99]

External factors such as the type, appearance, and smell of food; the social impetus to eat; and environmental stressors also increase or decrease food intake. Control of appetite through internal and external manipulations is essential in controlling obesity.[14]

*GENETIC INFLUENCES.* Obesity is highly familial. Adoption studies have demonstrated positive correlations between parents and their biological children, and

**TABLE 10–18.**

BODY WEIGHTS IN KILOGRAMS ACCORDING TO HEIGHT AND
BODY MASS INDEX[a,b]

| HEIGHT, cm | BODY MASS INDEX, kg/m² | | | | | | | | | | | | | |
|---|---|---|---|---|---|---|---|---|---|---|---|---|---|---|
| | 19.0 | 20.0 | 21.0 | 22.0 | 23.0 | 24.0 | 25.0 | 26.0 | 27.0 | 28.0 | 29.0 | 30.0 | 35.0 | 40.0 |
| | BODY WEIGHT, kg | | | | | | | | | | | | | |
| 140.0 | 37.2 | 39.2 | 41.2 | 43.1 | 45.1 | 47.0 | 49.0 | 51.0 | 52.9 | 54.9 | 56.8 | 58.8 | 68.6 | 78.4 |
| 142.0 | 38.3 | 40.3 | 42.3 | 44.4 | 46.4 | 48.4 | 50.4 | 52.4 | 54.4 | 56.5 | 58.5 | 60.5 | 70.6 | 80.7 |
| 144.0 | 39.4 | 41.5 | 43.5 | 45.6 | 47.7 | 49.8 | 51.8 | 53.9 | 56.0 | 58.1 | 60.1 | 62.2 | 72.6 | 82.9 |
| 146.0 | 40.5 | 42.6 | 44.8 | 46.9 | 49.0 | 51.2 | 53.3 | 55.4 | 57.6 | 59.7 | 61.8 | 63.9 | 74.6 | 85.3 |
| 148.0 | 41.6 | 43.8 | 46.0 | 48.2 | 50.4 | 52.6 | 54.8 | 57.0 | 59.1 | 61.3 | 63.5 | 65.7 | 76.7 | 87.6 |
| 150.0 | 42.8 | 45.0 | 47.3 | 49.5 | 51.8 | 54.0 | 56.3 | 58.5 | 60.8 | 63.0 | 65.3 | 67.5 | 78.8 | 90.0 |
| 152.0 | 43.9 | 46.2 | 48.5 | 50.8 | 53.1 | 55.4 | 57.8 | 60.1 | 62.4 | 64.7 | 67.0 | 69.3 | 80.9 | 92.4 |
| 154.0 | 45.1 | 47.4 | 49.8 | 52.2 | 54.5 | 56.9 | 59.3 | 61.7 | 64.0 | 66.4 | 68.8 | 71.1 | 83.0 | 94.9 |
| 156.0 | 46.2 | 48.7 | 51.1 | 53.5 | 56.0 | 58.4 | 60.8 | 63.3 | 65.7 | 68.1 | 70.6 | 73.0 | 85.2 | 97.3 |
| 158.0 | 47.4 | 49.9 | 52.4 | 54.9 | 57.4 | 59.9 | 62.4 | 64.9 | 67.4 | 69.9 | 72.4 | 74.9 | 87.4 | 99.9 |
| 160.0 | 48.6 | 51.2 | 53.8 | 56.3 | 58.9 | 61.4 | 64.0 | 66.6 | 69.1 | 71.7 | 74.2 | 76.8 | 89.6 | 102.4 |
| 162.0 | 49.9 | 52.5 | 55.1 | 57.7 | 60.4 | 63.0 | 65.6 | 68.2 | 70.9 | 73.5 | 76.1 | 78.7 | 91.9 | 105.0 |
| 164.0 | 51.1 | 53.8 | 56.5 | 59.2 | 61.9 | 64.6 | 67.2 | 69.9 | 72.6 | 75.3 | 78.0 | 80.7 | 94.1 | 107.6 |
| 166.0 | 52.4 | 55.1 | 57.9 | 60.6 | 63.4 | 66.1 | 68.9 | 71.6 | 74.4 | 77.2 | 79.9 | 82.7 | 96.4 | 110.2 |
| 168.0 | 53.6 | 56.4 | 59.3 | 62.1 | 64.9 | 67.7 | 70.6 | 73.4 | 76.2 | 79.0 | 81.8 | 84.7 | 98.8 | 112.9 |
| 170.0 | 54.9 | 57.8 | 60.7 | 63.6 | 66.5 | 69.4 | 72.3 | 75.1 | 78.0 | 80.9 | 83.8 | 86.7 | 101.2 | 115.6 |
| 172.0 | 56.2 | 59.2 | 62.1 | 65.1 | 68.0 | 71.0 | 74.0 | 76.9 | 79.9 | 82.8 | 85.8 | 88.8 | 103.5 | 118.3 |
| 174.0 | 57.5 | 60.6 | 63.6 | 66.6 | 69.6 | 72.7 | 75.7 | 78.7 | 81.7 | 84.8 | 87.8 | 90.8 | 106.0 | 121.1 |
| 176.0 | 58.9 | 62.0 | 65.0 | 68.1 | 71.2 | 74.3 | 77.4 | 80.5 | 83.6 | 86.7 | 89.8 | 92.9 | 108.4 | 123.9 |
| 178.0 | 60.2 | 63.4 | 66.5 | 69.7 | 72.9 | 76.0 | 79.2 | 82.4 | 85.5 | 88.7 | 91.9 | 95.1 | 110.9 | 126.7 |
| 180.0 | 61.6 | 64.8 | 68.0 | 71.3 | 74.5 | 77.8 | 81.0 | 84.2 | 87.5 | 90.7 | 94.0 | 97.2 | 113.4 | 129.6 |
| 182.0 | 62.9 | 66.2 | 69.6 | 72.9 | 76.2 | 79.5 | 82.8 | 86.1 | 89.4 | 92.7 | 96.1 | 99.4 | 115.9 | 132.5 |
| 184.0 | 64.3 | 67.7 | 71.1 | 74.5 | 77.9 | 81.3 | 84.6 | 88.0 | 91.4 | 94.8 | 98.2 | 101.6 | 118.5 | 135.4 |
| 186.0 | 65.7 | 69.2 | 72.7 | 76.1 | 79.6 | 83.0 | 86.5 | 89.9 | 93.4 | 96.9 | 100.3 | 103.8 | 121.1 | 138.4 |
| 188.0 | 67.2 | 70.7 | 74.2 | 77.8 | 81.3 | 84.8 | 88.4 | 91.9 | 95.4 | 99.0 | 102.5 | 106.0 | 123.7 | 141.4 |
| 190.0 | 68.6 | 72.2 | 75.8 | 79.4 | 83.0 | 86.6 | 90.3 | 93.9 | 97.5 | 101.1 | 104.7 | 108.3 | 126.4 | 144.4 |
| 192.0 | 70.0 | 73.7 | 77.4 | 81.1 | 84.8 | 88.5 | 92.2 | 95.8 | 99.5 | 103.2 | 106.9 | 110.6 | 129.0 | 147.5 |
| 194.0 | 71.5 | 75.3 | 79.0 | 82.8 | 86.6 | 90.3 | 94.1 | 97.9 | 101.6 | 105.4 | 109.1 | 112.9 | 131.7 | 150.5 |
| 196.0 | 73.0 | 76.8 | 80.7 | 84.5 | 88.4 | 92.2 | 96.0 | 99.9 | 103.7 | 107.6 | 111.4 | 115.2 | 134.5 | 153.7 |
| 198.0 | 74.5 | 78.4 | 82.3 | 86.2 | 90.2 | 94.1 | 98.0 | 101.9 | 105.9 | 109.8 | 113.7 | 117.6 | 137.2 | 156.8 |
| 200.0 | 76.0 | 80.0 | 84.0 | 88.0 | 92.0 | 96.0 | 100.0 | 104.0 | 108.0 | 112.0 | 116.0 | 120.0 | 140.0 | 160.0 |

[a] Each entry gives the body weight in kilograms (kg) for a person of a given height and body mass index.
[b] Desirable body mass index range in relation to age (from Bray[7]).

| Age Group, y | Body Mass Index, kg/m² | Age Group, y | Body Mass Index, kg/m² |
|---|---|---|---|
| 19–24 | 19–24 | 45–54 | 22–27 |
| 25–34 | 20–25 | 55–64 | 23–28 |
| 35–34 | 21–26 | 65+ | 24–29 |

Source: G.A. Bray, D.S. Gray, Obesity, Part 1. Pathogenesis. West Med J 149:429, 1988.

little or no correlation in body weight between adoptees and their adoptive parents.[104,126] It is estimated that 25% of all obesity is linked to genetic factors.[20]

A "thrifty gene" theory has been proposed as one possible expression of obesity. A thrifty metabolism is described as having high metabolic efficiency, meaning that a higher proportion of excess kcal is stored as fat, better equipping the individual to withstand starvation, or diet-ing.[40] When overfed, lean individuals gain a higher proportion of lean body mass. The amount of lean body mass is a major determinant of the human basal metabolic rate.[41]

*BROWN ADIPOSE TISSUE.* Brown adipose tissue (BAT) is a richly innervated, highly vascular tissue possessing metabolic activity through its mitochondria. BAT has a high capacity for heat production and is involved in thermogenesis. Most fat in the human body does not possess metabolic activity but functions as a storage depot. During periods of overconsumption, often called "luxus consumption," BAT may be involved in the increased rate of heat production seen in lean individuals.[61] BAT is under the control of the SNS. Under conditions of overconsumption, failure to stimulate BAT results in the storage of excess calories as fat rather than being released as heat.[61] It has been estimated that 50 gm of BAT could increase energy turnover by 10% to 15%.[124] Current research is focusing on pharmacologic agents that can activate brown fat.[61]

Another facet of thermogenesis is the thermic effect of food or diet-induced thermogenesis. When food is eaten, the basal metabolic rate rises and kcal expenditure can be 10% to 15% of the meal. The thermic effect of food is blunted in reduced, formerly obese individuals and may contribute to the regain of lost weight.[61]

*SET POINT THEORY.* The set point theory of obesity implies that body weight, like body temperature, is regulated at a physiologically, possibly genetically, predetermined level. Obesity can be defined in this context as a regulation at an elevated set point.[74] In normal starvation, a decrease in metabolic rate accompanies restricted intake. Obese individuals decrease metabolic rate accordingly but exhibit minimum weight loss, indicating a physiologic process that appears to be defending the present weight.[72] Interventions in individuals with regulated body weight at a higher level may prove disappointing to client and practitioner alike.[145] At present, methods to alter set point are not proven to work.

*ENZYME ACTIVITY: CONTROL OF LIPOLYSIS.* Lipoprotein lipase (LPL) is the enzyme that facilitates the removal of lipid from the blood. Lipoprotein lipase hydrolyzes triglyceride into FFAs and glycerol. The FFAs enter the fat cell and are re-esterified. LPL activity increases during periods of weight gain in all individuals. However, after weight reduction in the obese, LPL activity remains elevated and may contribute to rapid regain of weight often seen after dieting attempts.[37]

Adenyl cyclase also stimulates lipolysis but within the cell. It increases FFA concentration. This, in turn, decreases hepatic clearance of insulin.[98] The activity of adenyl cyclase is greater in abdominal depots than in gluteal fat and may contribute to the health risks associated with obesity by hyperinsulinemia.

## Endocrine Aspects of Obesity

*UNIQUE ROLE OF INSULIN.* The major health risks of obesity, such as cardiovascular disease, hypertension, noninsulin dependent diabetes mellitus, and cancer, are generally ascribed to obesity in general. Excess body weight, or increasing body mass index, heretofore has been the major determinant of risk. However, upper body obesity, known as *android obesity*, is now considered a better predictor of risk, especially cardiovascular risk, than body weight alone.[68] Lower body obesity, or *gynoid* obesity, is an overall health risk but is not seen as a risk factor. Figure 10-8 provides a nomogram for calculating the waist-to-hip ratio used in determining upper body versus lower body obesity. Table 10-19 compares the general features of android versus gynoid obesity.

Obesity is often accompanied by an increase in beta cell secretion, peripheral resistance to insulin, and resultant hyperinsulinemia. Indeed, hyperinsulinemia may precede the development of obesity and be a cause rather than a consequence. Hyperinsulinemia is responsible for the "deadly quartet": upper body obesity, glu-

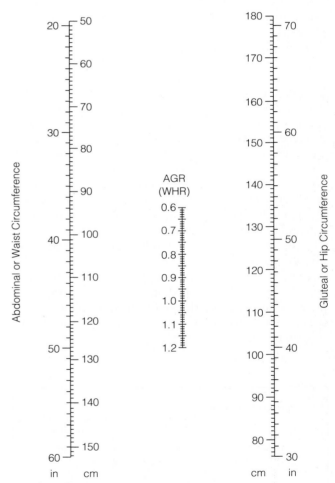

**FIGURE 10-8.**
The abdominal (waist) and gluteal (hips) ratio (AGR) can be determined by placing a straight edge between the column for waist circumference and reading the ratio from the point where this straight edge crosses the AGR or waist–hips ratio (WHR) line. The waist or abdominal circumference is the smallest circumference below the rib cage and above the umbilicus, and the hips or gluteal circumference is the largest circumference at the posterior extension of the buttocks. (From G.A. Bray and D.S. Gray, Obesity. Part I: Pathogenesis. *West. J. Med.* 149:429, 1988.)

**TABLE 10–19.**
TERMS FOR THE TWO DIFFERENT DISTRIBUTIONS
OF BODY FAT

| ANDROID | GYNOID |
| --- | --- |
| Upper body | Lower body |
| Apple | Pear |
| Abdominal | Visceral, gluteal, femoral |
| Central | Peripheral |
| Subscapular skinfold thickness > 25 | Subscapular skinfold thickness < 25 |
| Waist-to-hip girth ratio > 0.85 | Waist-to-hip girth ratio < 0.85 |

cose intolerance, hypertriglyceridemia, and hypertension.[71] Research over the last decade has focused on the link between android obesity and hyperinsulinemia and the increased risk of diabetes, hypertriglyceridemia, and lowered high density lipoprotein (HDL) levels, hypertension, and coronary artery disease.[9,38,81,85,105,113,125,131] The proposed mechanism is dependent on the evidence suggesting that abdominal fat is more metabolically active than peripheral or gluteal fat. Increases in adenyl cyclase in the cell and lipoprotein lipase in the blood allow an increase in FFA concentration which decreases hepatic clearance of insulin. This, coupled with a positive energy balance and increasing levels of plasma free testosterone (android),[98] yields a cascade effect with hyperinsulinemia as the end result [103,116] (Figure 10-9). Therefore, many of the generalized overall health risks of obesity may be attributed to hyperinsulinemia.[76]

The management of the individual with upper body obesity may differ from conventional treatment of obesity. Diet therapy for obese individuals usually consists of a traditional high carbohydrate, low fat diet. However, persons with upper body obesity, hyperinsulinemia, and hypertension may require lower carbohydrate, higher unsaturated fat diets as high carbohydrate may exacer-

bate hyperinsulinemia.[98] Hypertensive, hyperinsulinemic persons should be treated cautiously with diuretics and beta blockers because these medications can worsen glucose tolerance.[36]

Other endocrine disorders associated with obesity are summarized in Box 10-4.

## Inactivity

Inactivity, or lack of exercise, contributes to the development and maintenance of obesity. Television watching has been positively correlated with the development of obesity in children. The prevalence of obesity increases 2% per each hour of daily television viewing.[34] Although obese individuals use more calories per any given activity, most obese individuals choose to be less active when compared to their lean counterparts.

Benefits of exercise for obese individuals include an increase in metabolically active lean body mass, decrease in hunger, increase in basal metabolic rate, and decrease in insulin levels. Cardiovascular endurance improves and HDL cholesterol levels may rise with exercise (see Chap. 26). Exercise should be strongly encouraged as an adjunct to weight control.

In addition to exercise, traditional management of

**BOX 10–4.**
MAJOR ENDOCRINE ABNORMALITIES IN OBESITY

Pancreas
    Hyperinsulinemia
Pituitary—growth hormone
    Decreased basal levels and response to stimulation
Pituitary—prolactin
    Decreased response to stimulation
Pituitary—testis
    Increased free testosterone
    Low total serum testosterone and sex-hormone-binding globulin
    Total testosterone = bound-biologically inactive free-mediator of androgen effects
    High serum estrogens
Pituitary—ovary
    High serum estrogens and androgens
Pituitary—adrenal
    Increased cortisol turnover with normal serum levels
Pituitary—thyroid
    Increased serum $T_3$
Parathyroid
    Increased serum parathyroid hormone
    Decreased serum 25-OH-vitamin D
Miscellaneous
    Abnormal vasopressin regulation
    Increased serum endorphins
    Increased serum norepinephrine
    Increased serum lipids

Source: Modified from A.R. Glass, Endocrine aspects of obesity. Med. Clin. N. Am. 73:139, 1989.

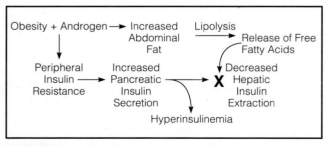

**FIGURE 10–9.**
A possible scheme for the development of hyperinsulinemia with upper-body obesity. (From N.M. Kaplan, The deadly quartet: Upper body obesity, glucose intolerance, hypertriglyceridemia, and hypertension. *Arch. Intern. Med.* 149:1514, 1989.)

obesity includes weight loss diets and behavior modification. Other options include surgery for severe obesity and pharmacologic interventions.

## Anorexia Nervosa

### Definition and Incidence

Anorexia nervosa (AN) is an eating disorder considered to be a psychologic disorder with physiologic manifestations. It is characterized by the following: (1) a relentless pursuit of thinness that does not diminish as weight loss progresses; (2) disturbed body image; and (3) amenorrhea. The eating pattern and weight loss are not viewed as abnormal. Although AN has been recognized since the middle ages, the psychogenesis of the disorder has changed in modern times. In present day culture, weight control is seen as a form of self-control. The disorder affects primarily women, and the frequency of AN is approximately 1% to 3% in the United States.[60] The diagnostic criteria are presented in Box 10-5.

### Etiology

The etiology of AN is multifactorial. Societal pressures toward thinness and increased expectations of women are possible explanations. The young women are usually from enmeshed, or overly close, families.[75] Family conflicts go unresolved and feelings are repressed. Mothers are often viewed as overbearing and fathers as underinvolved. Hence, anorectics can be viewed as the symptom bearer for a dysfunctional family. Persons with AN are usually overachievers and thought of as the "perfect little girl." Although many women in this culture are preoccupied with weight, anorectics can be differentiated on the basis of their sense of ineffectiveness, lack of personal fulfillment, interpersonal distress, and fear of maturity.[60]

Behavioral disturbances seen in anorectics mimic those exhibited in individuals undergoing simple starvation. Landmark research by Keys described a "starvation syndrome" where normal young male volunteers were put on restrictive diets for several months. Subjects in this study developed a preoccupation with food and food preparation, as well as elaborate food rituals. Cognitively, the men experienced difficulty with decisionmaking and a decrease in alertness. Socially, the subjects withdrew from group activities and became isolated, depressed, and experienced a decrease in sex drive.[75] These biologic effects of starvation are also seen in anorectics. This underscores the importance of weight loss in the development of symptoms seen in AN.

### Medical Complications

The medical complications of AN are dependent on the variant of the disease manifested. Clinically, two major variants exist: "restrictors," who control weight through caloric restriction alone, and "bulimic anorectics," who alternate kcal restriction with binging and purging.[88] It is estimated that 30% to 50% of anorectics use various purging behaviors.[129] Medical complications are most severe in bulimic anorectics.[52] The mortality rate for both variants of the disorder are as high as 15% to 20%.[56] The physical signs and symptoms associated with AN are summarized in Box 10-6.

RESTRICTORS: COMPLICATIONS OF SEMI-STARVATION. Cardiac abnormalities account for the majority of deaths associated with AN.[116] Reductions in cardiac muscle mass, decrease in cardiac chamber size, and alterations in myocardial contractility have been documented.[47] Clinical presentation includes hypotension, sinus bradycardia, and abnormal exercise tolerance.[115] Overzealous nutritional repletion may precipitate congestive heart failure. Refeeding edema is associated with an increase in intracellular and extracellular volume and heart failure.[129] Decreased basal metabolic rate and subnormal body temperature are associated features of star-

---

**BOX 10-5.**
DIAGNOSTIC CRITERIA FOR ANOREXIA NERVOSA

▸ Refusal to maintain body weight over a minimal normal weight for age and height, eg, weight loss leading to maintenance of body weight 15% below that expected; or failure to make expected weight gain during period of growth, leading to body weight 15% below that expected

▸ Intense fear of gaining weight or becoming fat, even though underweight

▸ Disturbance in the way in which one's body weight, size, or shape is experienced, eg, the person claims to "feel fat" even when emaciated, believes that one area of the body is "too fat" even when obviously underweight

▸ In females, absence of at least three consecutive menstrual cycles when otherwise expected to occur (primary or secondary amenorrhea) (A woman is considered to have amenorrhea if her periods occur only following hormone, eg, estrogen, administration)

*Source: American Psychiatric Association. Diagnostic and Statistical Manual of Mental Disorders III-R. Washington, D.C.: American Psychiatric Association, 1987.*

## BOX 10-6.
### PHYSICAL SYMPTOMS AND SIGNS IN ANOREXIA NERVOSA

Presenting Physical Symptoms
  Weight loss
  Amenorrhea, no cyclic symptoms or physical changes or menstruation (anovulatory)
  Hyperactivity (mental and motor)
  Aberrant behavior, irritability, isolation or withdrawal, sleep disturbances
  Hyperacusis or optic hyperesthesia
Physical Signs
  Cachexia, emaciation, debilitation or dehydration, possible signs of shock or impending shock
  Covert infectious processes (pneumonia or sepsis; immunologic problems [late], anergy-negative skin tests)
  Skin changes (dryness, yellowish palms and soles, desquamation, and "dirty" appearance to skin)
  Scalp and pubic hair loss or lanugo hair or increased pigmented body hair
  Hypothermia (rectal temperature below 96.6°F)
  Bradypnea (respiratory compensation for alkalosis)
  Bradycardia, "quiet" heart (decreased basal metabolic rate); pulse below 60 bpm usual
  Hypotension often below 80/50 mm Hg
  Heart murmur (infrequent)
  Edema of lower extremities
  Signs of estrogen deficiency (skin dryness; osteoporosis; small uterus and cervix; vaginal mucosa is pink, dry; and gross and microscopic evidence of deficient estrogen)
  Signs of decreased androgen (no acne, no oily skin)

Source: G.D. Comerci, Medical complications of anorexia nervosa and bulimia nervosa. Med. Clin. N. Am. 74(5):1293, 1990.

vation. Consequently, resting caloric expenditure can decrease to approximately half normal.[130] This is a compensatory mechanism to preserve physiologic functioning, although at a lowered rate. Therefore, refeeding chronically starved individuals requires a conservative intake of kcal at approximately 75% of basal requirements.[27] Clinicians faced with a cachectic client often begin parenteral dextrose solutions either alone or as part of a total parenteral nutrition program. These solutions cause an increase in insulin production by the beta cell. Increasing levels of insulin force phosphate into the cell, resulting in hypophosphatemia. Phosphate participates in many enzymatic reactions as either adenosine triphosphate (ATP) or 2,3-diphosphoglycerate. Profound muscular weakness and progressive encephalopathy, coma, and death may develop. Hematologic disturbances associated with hypophosphatemia include hemolytic anemia and impaired leukocyte and thrombocyte function. Although the ideal form of nutritional repletion needs to be delineated for anorectics, care should be given to not increase feeding too rapidly and to monitor electrolyte disturbances. Recommended weight gain per day should not exceed one-quarter to one-half pound per day.[27]

*METABOLIC DISTURBANCES.* Metabolic findings in anorexia are similar to those seen in starvation, and a summary is found in Table 10-20. Restrictors normally experience a "fixed hypoglycemia" secondary to ketoadaptation and adequate glucogenic substrates. As weight loss progresses to a critical point, fat reserves are exhausted and gluconeogenic precursors are diminished.

Profound hypoglycemia and hypoglycemic coma may develop. Hence, severe hypoglycemia represents a grave prognosis and prompt medical treatment is warranted.[108] Elevation in uric acid may be present and also can serve as an index of severity. Strenuous exercise, starvation alcohol consumption, and thiazide diuretics contribute to hyperuricemia.[51]

*ENDOCRINE ABNORMALITIES.* Hypogonadism is a characteristic feature of AN, and loss of needed body fat contributes to amenorrhea. Lack of estrogen, cortisol excess, and malnutrition are central to the pathogenesis of the bone disease exhibited in women with the disorder. In most women, the onset of the disorder occurs before peak bone mass is achieved (approximately age 24 years). Therefore, the prolonged duration of amenorrhea increases the severity of osteopenia.[12] Increased exercise may increase the risk of pathologic fractures. Osteonecrosis and femoral head collapse have also been reported.[139]

*GASTROINTESTINAL DISORDERS.* Gastrointestinal disorders are often presented as a reason to eliminate certain foods from the diet. Nausea, epigastric pain, bloating, flatus, and early satiety are common complaints in AN. Gastric emptying time is often delayed but is secondary to decrease in food intake and subsequent malnutrition. As gradual refeeding commences, emptying time improves and normalization occurs while body mass index is still subnormal.[127]

## TABLE 10-20.
### LABORATORY FINDINGS IN ANOREXIA NERVOSA

**Chemical/Metabolic**

Normal results on most laboratory tests early in process

Elevated BUN levels, secondary to dehydration; decreased glomerular filtration rate

Hypercarotenemia

Elevated serum cholesterol levels (early; may decrease later)

Decreased transferrin, associated anemia (usually normal protein and albumin-globulin ratio); low complement, fibrinogen, and prealbumin

Elevated serum lactic dehydrogenase and alkaline phosphatase (possibly related to growth)

Depressed phosphorus level (a late and ominous sign); depressed magnesium and calcium levels (calcium may be elevated)

Possible depression of plasma-zinc, urinary zinc, and urinary copper levels

Fixed hypoglycemia, possible hypoglycemic coma

Negative nitrogen balance

Elevated uric acid

**Endocrine**

Low leutinizing hormone (LH); low or pseudo-normal follicle-stimulating hormone (FSH); deficiency of gonadotropin-releasing hormone (GnRH); normal prolactin; low testosterone in men and low estradiol in women

Elevated circulating cortisol (normal production; does not suppress with dexamethasone)

Low normal fasting glucose (increased insulin binding by red blood cells and growth hormone deficiency reported)

Low normal thyroxine ($T_4$); reduced triiodothyronine ($T_3$); elevated reverse $T_3$; normal TSH

Possible elevation of parathyroid hormone (PTH) secondary to hypomagnesemia with resultant hypercalcemia

Elevated resting growth hormone levels

**Hematologic**

Leukopenia with relative lymphocytoses (bone marrow hypoplasia), absolute lymphopenia

Thrombocytopenia

Very low erythrocyte sedimentation rate, almost always

Anemia late (especially with rehydration)

Source: Adapted from G.D. Comerci, Medical complications of anorexia nervosa and bulimia nervosa. Med. Clin. N. Am. 74(5):1293, 1990.

*NEUROPATHY.* Chronic malnutrition contributes to the development of peripheral neuropathy. Compression neuropathies may also develop due to excessive loss of supportive subcutaneous tissue.[84]

## Bulimia

### Definition and Incidence

Bulimia, meaning "ox hunger," is a disorder of weight maintenance characterized by a preoccupation with weight, an increased interest in dieting, and ultimate control of weight through caloric restriction alternating with binge eating and purging. Purging is generally accomplished through use of vomiting, laxative abuse, and/or diuretic abuse. Actual incidence of bulimia is controversial, but estimates are that 4% to 10% of adolescent and young women are affected.[150] It is a disorder almost exclusively confined to women. Affected males are gener-

ally those who pursue interests or careers where body image and weight are of paramount importance, such as wrestlers, jockeys, and dancers. Most of the women are from upper socioeconomic classes. The age of onset is generally in the late teens. A bulimic episode is considered an "out of control" experience and the food consumed is deemed excessive. The average calories consumed during a binge are 500 to 10,000. Foods chosen are high in calories, nondiet, and easily consumed. As opposed to AN, affected persons are aware that the eating habits are abnormal but are unable to stop voluntarily.[102] Shame and secrecy accompany this disorder and prevent appropriate diagnosis and treatment. Box 10-7 lists the diagnostic criteria for bulimia.

### Etiology

The psychogenesis of bulimia is complex. Bulimia is considered a "disorder of maturation" and usually occurs at

**BOX 10–7.**
DIAGNOSTIC CRITERIA FOR BULIMIA NERVOSA

- ▸ Recurrent episodes of binge eating (rapid consumption of a large amount of food in a discrete period of time)
- ▸ A feeling of lack of control over eating behavior during the eating binges
- ▸ The person regularly engages in either self-induced vomiting, use of laxatives or diuretics, strict dieting or fasting, or vigorous exercise to prevent weight gain
- ▸ A minimum average of two binge eating episodes a week for at least 3 mo
- ▸ Persistent overconcern with body shape and weight

Source: *American Psychiatric Association. Diagnostic and Statistical Manual of Mental Disorders III-R. Washington, D.C.: American Psychiatric Association, 1987.*

a time of separation from home or loved ones. It signals difficulty in making the transition from adolescence into young adulthood.[144] As with anorexia, increased societal expectations of women, difficulty in defining the female role, and a desire for thinness are central to the development of the disorder. Family or individual history are often significant for affective disorders such as depression.[82] In addition, childhood sexual abuse is more common in bulimic women than in the general population.[21] As opposed to the anorectic's family, families of bulimic women often exhibit overt conflict and less cohesion. Bulimic women sense greater neglect and rejection. Mothers are disengaged or distant from their daughters. Daughters, in turn, feel anxious and disorganized.[148]

Dieting initiates the disorder; however, the maintenance of the disorder is attributed to the new role binging and purging takes on. The rapid consumption of large amounts of food followed by a purgative behavior functions in the reduction of anxiety. Therefore, anxiety reduction contributes to the continuance of the bulimic behavior.[148]

## Medical Complications

*ELECTROLYTE ABNORMALITIES: EFFECTS OF LAXATIVES, DIURETICS, AND VOMITING.* Electrolyte disturbances are a common manifestation in bulimic anorectics and bulimics, and are dependent on the purgative method used.

Hypokalemia is a common and dangerous electrolyte disturbance. Continual vomiting and laxative and diuretic abuse precipitate hypokalemia as 80% of body potassium is excreted in the urine and 20% in the feces.[32]

Other causative factors in the development of hypokalemia include decreased plasma volume, metabolic alkalosis, and coexisting magnesium deficiency.[53] Chronic laxative abuse may produce nephropathy and a urine concentration deficit. The resultant polyuria and hypovolemia result in hyperaldosteronism and the development of edema.[143]

Chronic laxative abuse affects GI and renal functioning and, therefore, impacts the development of electrolyte abnormalities. Gastrointestinal effects include atrophy of smooth muscle, progressive loss of innervation, and decrease in colonic mysenteric neurons.[28] Cathartic colon, a permanent alteration in bowel function, may result in severe constipation, as well as GI bleeding. Anemia, steatorrhea, and protein-losing enteropathy may be present. Effects on the renal system include dehydration and sodium loss. Hyponatremia stimulates the renin aldosterone system, resulting in sodium and fluid retention and hypokalemia. Abrupt cessation of laxatives promotes secondary hyperaldosteronism and peripheral edema results. Weaning from laxatives prevents the rapid weight gain, reduces anxiety, and decreases the likelihood of returning to laxatives.[142] Diarrhea from laxative abuse causes electrolyte abnormalities but does not cause a significant malabsorption of calories. Ingestion of 50 laxative tablets results in a calorie loss of only 12%, indicating that 88% of the calories from the binge have been absorbed. Therefore, laxative abuse is an ineffective method of weight control.[15,96]

Acid-base disturbances occur in bulimia secondary to the purgative method employed. Metabolic alkalosis is the most common.[138] Loss of hydrogen ion in vomiting and in diuretic abuse leads to an increase in plasma bicarbonate, contributing to alkalosis.

Metabolic acidosis can occur during the starvation or restricting phase when ketoacids are being used as a primary energy source. Additionally, laxative abuse causes a profound bicarbonate loss and leads to metabolic acidosis. Figure 10-10 illustrates the electrolyte/acid base abnormalities seen in eating disorders. The physical signs and symptoms associated with bulimia are summarized in Table 10-21.

*ENDOCRINE ABNORMALITIES.* The endocrine disturbances in bulimia are not clearly defined or understood. Endocrine dysfunction exists and may be related to poor nutritional intake, starvation during the restrict-

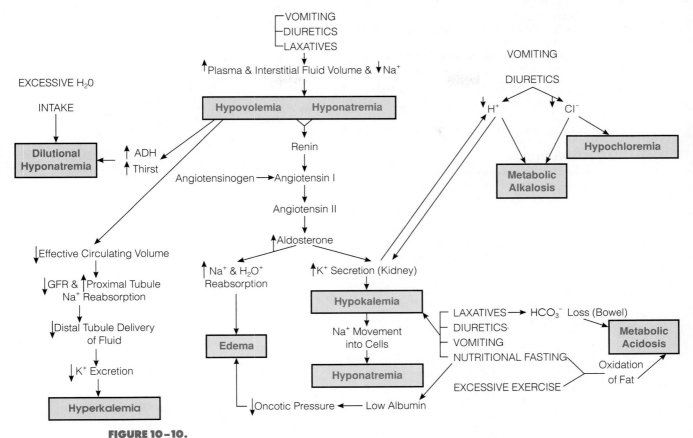

**FIGURE 10–10.**
Pathophysiology explanation of selected fluid electrolyte and acid-base manifestations of AN and bulimia according to methods of weight control. (From P.O. Dardis and S.L. Hopland, Anorexia Nervosa. Fluid, Electrolyte, and Acid-Base Manifestations. *JCPN* 3:3, 1990.)

ing phase, and secondary to an affective disorder.[93] Menstrual and ovulatory disturbances occur in normal weight bulimics and the etiology is unknown.[22]

*UPPER GASTROINTESTINAL DISORDERS.* Dysphagia may develop in bulimics secondary to a poor or absent pharyngeal gag reflex and increased duration of dry swallow. The defect in swallowing may be attributed to desensitization from prolonged vomiting, as well as being a learned response.[110] Bulimics often have increased stomach capacity due to repeated binging, but gastric emptying time may be increased or normal.[44,67] Gastric rupture and esophageal tears are the most severe form of upper GI disorders.

*ORAL PATHOLOGIES.* In bulimic anorectics and bulimics who vomit, enamel erosion is the most common oral pathology. Other oral abnormalities include dentin hypersensitivity, caries, xerostomia, parotid gland enlargement, and periodontal disease. The low pH of vomitus is the major cause. Post vomiting rinsing with tap water may contribute to the pathology of oral disease as it

reduces the buffering capacity of saliva.[2] Due to the secretive nature of bulimia, it may be the oral pathologies that provide the first diagnostic clue to health professionals, particularly the dental hygienist and dentist.

*DERMATOLOGIC COMPLAINTS.* Bulimics often exhibit a fine, dry rash on the hands secondary to dehydration. Calluses on the knuckles may be present when the fingers are used for vomiting.

## Nutritional Deficiencies of Anorexia Nervosa and Bulimia

The nutritional deficiencies exhibited in individuals with eating disorders are many and varied. Chronic protein deficiency, hypoalbuminemia, and negative nitrogen balance are seen in both anorectics and bulimics.[63] Vitamin deficiencies, especially water-soluble vitamins, can be evidenced by angular stomatitis, mucosal ulcers, and hair loss.[52] Zinc deficiency is commonly seen in restrictors and bulimics, and may impair appetite regulation. Defi-

**TABLE 10-21.**
PHYSICAL SYMPTOMS AND SIGNS IN BULIMIA NERVOSA

**Presenting Physical Symptoms**

Weight may be normal, overweight, or underweight

Complaints of bloating, diarrhea, swelling

Hyperactivity (mental and motor); exceptions common

Constant or extreme thirst and increased urination (hypokalemic nephropathy-hypovolemia)

May present with depression, anxiety, despair, and suicidal ideation

**Physical Signs**

Usually well-groomed and good hygiene; definite exceptions, especially patients with a severe character disorder or chronic addictive conditions

Usually normal weight or mild to moderate obesity (exception: food restrictors or anorexia nervosa patients with associated bulimia, vomiting, purging)

Generalized or localized edema at lower extremities (compensatory renal retention of sodium and water, ie, hypovolemia with secondary hyperaldosteronism or pseudo-Bartter's syndrome)

Physical findings of extreme weight loss (self-starvation) if bulimia, vomiting, and purging are complications of anorexia nervosa or food restriction

Loss of scalp hair, skin changes of anorexia nervosa

Amenorrhea, effects of estrogen deficiency

Hypothermia

Swelling of parotid and other salivary glands

Dental enamel dysplasia and discoloration due to gastric juices (vomiting)

Bruises and lacerations of palate and posterior pharynx; lesions of fingernails, fingers, and dorsum of hand(s) (due to self-induced vomiting)

Pyorrhea and other gum disorders

Diminished reflexes, muscle weakness, paralysis, and, infrequently, peripheral neuropathy with muscle weakness and paralysis

Muscle cramping (with induced hypoxia or positive Trousseau's sign)

Signs of hypokalemia (cardiac dysrhythmias, hypotension, decreased cardiac output, weak pulse, poor-quality heart sounds, abdominal distention, ileus, acute gastric dilatation, myopathy, shortness of breath, depression, and mental clouding)

Source: *G.D. Comerci, Medical complications of anorexia nervosa and bulimia nervosa. Med. Clin. N. Am. 74(5): 1293, 1990.*

ciency of zinc results in altered taste acuity, altered taste sensitivity, and impairment in the sense of smell.

The deficiency of zinc may contribute to the chronicity of eating disorders. It develops secondary to poor intake, impaired absorption, and the consumption of low zinc foods during a binge.[66]

# *REFERENCES*

1.  Albin, R.L., et al. Acute sensory neuropathy-neuronopathy from pyridoxine overdose. *Neurology* 37:17, 1987.
2.  Altshuler, B.D., Dechow, P.C., Waller, P.A., and Hardy, B.W. An investigation of the oral pathologies occurring in bulimia nervosa. *Intl. J. Eating Disorders* 9:191, 1990.
3.  Babior, B.M., Peters, W.A., Briden, P.M., and Cetrulo, C.L. Pregnant women's absorption of iron from prenatal supplements. *J. Reprod. Med.* 30:355, 1985.
4.  Bauernfiend, J.C. Vitamin A deficiency, a staggering problem of health and sight. *Nutr. Today* pp. 34–46, March/April 1988.
5.  Baker, H., et al. Inability of chronic alcoholics with liver disease to use food as a source of folates, thiamin and vitamin B6. *Am. J. Clin. Nutr.* 28:1377, 1975.
6.  Bang, H.O., et al. The composition of the Eskimo food in northwestern Greenland. *Am. J. Clin. Nutr.* 33:2657, 1980.
7.  Barlow, G.B., and Wilkinson, A.W. Plasma pyridoxal phosphate levels and tryptophan metabolism in children with burns and scalds. *Clin. Chim. Acta.* 64:79, 1975.
8.  Basu, T.K., et al. Excretion of 5-hydroxyindoleacetic acid and N'-methylnicotinamide in advanced cancer patients. *Eur. J. Cancer* 9:527, 1973.
9.  Baumgartner, R.M., Roche, A.F., Chumlea, W.C., Survogel, R.M., and Gevech, C.J. Fatness and fat patterns: Associations with plasma lipids and blood pressures in adults, 18 to 57 years of age. *Am. J. Epidemiol.* 126:614, 1987.
10. Beck, W.S. Cobalamin and the nervous system. *N. Engl. J. Med.* 318:752, 1988.
11. Bengoa, J.M., Bolt, M.J., and Rosenberg, I.H. Hepatic vitamin D 25-hydroxylase inhibition by cimetidine and isoniazid. *J. Lab. Clin. Med.* 104:546, 1984.
12. Biller, B.M.K. Mechanism of osteoporosis in adult and

adolescent women with anorexia nervosa. *J. Clin. Endocrinol. Metab.* 68:548, 1989.

13. Bistrain, B.R., et al. Prevalence of malnutrition in general medical patients. *JAMA* 235:1567, 1976.

14. Blundell, J.E. Appetite disturbance and the problems of overweight. *Drugs* (39 Suppl.) 3:1–29, 190.

15. Bo-Linn, G.W., et al. Purging and caloric absorption in bulimic patients and normal women. *Ann. Intern. Med.* 99:14, 1983.

16. Boylan, L.M., Sugerman, H.J., and Driskell, J.A. Vitamin E, vitamin B6, vitamin B12 and folate status of gastric bypass surgery patients. *J. Amer. Diet. Assoc.* 88:579, 1988.

17. Bray, G.A., York, D.A., and Fisher, J.S. Experimental obesity: A homeostatic failure due to defective nutrient stimulation of the sympathetic nervous system. *Vitamins and Hormones* 45:1, 1989.

18. Bray, G.E. Nutrient balance and obesity: Classification and evaluation of the obesities. *Med. Clin. N. Am.* 73:29, 1989.

19. Bray, G.E. Obesity. In M.L. Brown (ed.), *Present Knowledge in Nutrition* (6th ed.). Washington, D.C.: Internal Life Sciences Institute, Nutrition Foundation, 1990.

20. Bray, G.A., and Gray, D.S. Obesity Part I—Pathogenesis. *West. J. Med.* 149:429, 1988.

21. Bulik, C.M., Sullivan, P.F., and Rorty, M. Childhood sexual abuse in women with bulimia. *J. Clin. Psychol.* 50(12): 460, 1989.

22. Cantopher, T., Evans, C., Lacey, J.H., and Pearce, J.M. Menstrual and ovulatory disturbances in bulimia. *Br. Med. J.* 297:836, 1988.

23. Casper, R.C., Elke, E.D., and Halmi, K. Bulimia: Its incidence and clinical importance in patients with anorexia nervosa. *Arch. Gen. Psychol.* 37:1030, 1980.

24. Centers for Disease Control, Division of Nutrition, Center for Health Promotion and Education. Evaluation of consumer complaints related to aspartame use. *Morbid. Mortal. Weekly Rep.* 33:605-607, 1990.

25. Clark, A.J., et al. Folacin status in adolescent females. *Am. J. Clin. Nutr.* 46:302, 1987.

26. Clydesdale, F.M. The relevance of mineral chemistry to bioavailability. *Nutr. Today* pp. 23–27, March/April 1989.

27. Comerci, G.D. Medical complications of anorexia nervosa and bulimia. *Med. Clin. N. Am.* 74(5):1293, 1990.

28. Cummings, J.H., Sladin, G.E., James, O.F.W., Sarner, M., and Misiewicz, J.J. Laxative induced diarrhea. A continuing clinical problem. *Br. Med. J.* 1:531, 1974.

29. Dallman, P.R. Iron deficiency and the immune response. *Am. J. Clin. Nutr.* 46:329, 1987.

30. Daly, J.M., et al. Immune and metabolic effects of arginine in the surgical patient. *Ann. Surg.* 208:512, 1988.

31. Danks, D.M. Copper deficiency in humans. *Ann. Rev. Nutr.* 6:13, 1988.

32. Dardis, P.O., Hofland, S.L. Anorexia nervosa. Fluid and electrolyte and acid base manifestations. *J. Child Adolesc. Psychol. Mental Health Nurs.* 3(3):85, 1990.

33. Demark-Wahnefried, W., Bowering, J., and Cohen, P.S. Reduced serum cholesterol with dietary change using fat modified and oat bran supplemented diets. *J. Am. Diet. Assoc.* 90:223, 1990.

34. Dietz, L., and Gortmaker, S.L. Do we fatten our children at the television set? Obesity and television in children and adolescents. *Pediatrics* 75:807, 1985.

35. Divorhin, B.M., Rosenthal, W.S., Worniser, G.P., and Werss, L. Selenium deficiency in the acquired immunodeficiency syndrome. *JPEN* 10:405, 1986.

36. Dornhorst, A., Powell, S.H., and Pensky, J. Aggravation by propranolol of hyperglycemic effect of hydrochlorothiazide in type II diabetics without alteration of insulin secretion. *Hypertension* 11:244, 1985.

37. Elliot, D.L., et al. Obesity: Pathophysiology and practical management. *J. Gen. Int. Med.* 2:188, 1987.

38. Ferrarinini, E., et al. Insulin resistance in essential hypertension. *N. Engl. J. Med.* 317:350, 1987.

39. Food and Drug Administration. *Cancer Assessment Committee Report.* Washington, D.C.: U.S. Government Printing Office, FDA Docket No. 82F-0320, 1984.

40. Forbes, G.B. Do obese individuals gain weight more easily than nonobese individuals? *Am. J. Clin. Nutr.* 52:224, 1990.

41. Forbes, G.B. Lean body mass—Body fat interrelationships in humans. *Nutr. Rev.* 45:225, 1987.

42. Ganrow, J.S., and Webster, J. Quetelet's index (W/H²) as a measure of fatness. *Int. J. Obesity* 9:147, 1985.

43. Garattini, S., et al. Progress in assessing the role of serotonin in the control of food intake. *Clin. Neuropharmacol. II* (Suppl. 1) 8–32, 1988.

44. Geliebter, A., Melton, P.M., Roberts, D., McCray, R.S., Gage, D., and Haskim, S.A. The stomach's role in appetite regulation in bulimia. *Ann. N. Y. Acad. Sci.* 575:512, 1989.

45. Gibbs, J., and Smith, G.P. Satiety: The role of peptides from the stomach and the intestine. *Fed. Proc.* 45:1391, 1986.

46. Gotloib, L., Sklan, D., and Mines, M. Hemodialysis: Effect of plasma levels of vitamin A and carotenoid. *JAMA* 239:239, 1978.

47. Gottdiener, J.S., Gross, H.A., Henry, W.L., Borer, J.S., and Ebert, M.H. Effects of self induced starvation on cardiac size and function in anorexia nervosa. *Circulation* 58:425, 1978.

48. Gottschilich, N.M., Warden, G.D., and Michel, M. Diarrhea in tube fed burn patients: Incidence, etiology, nutritional impact and intervention. *JPEN* 12:338, 1988.

49. Gross, L., and Brotman, M. Hypoprothrombinemia and hemorrhage associated with cholestyramine therapy. *Ann. Intern. Med.* 72:95, 1970.

50. Grundy, S. Monounsaturated fatty acids, plasma cholesterol and coronary heart disease. *Am. J. Clin. Nutr.* 45:1168, 1987.

51. Gupta, M.A., and Kavanaugh-Danelon, D. Elevated serum uric acid in eating disorders: A possible index of strenuous physical activity and starvation. *Int. J. Eating Disorders* 8:463, 1989.

52. Hall, R.C.W., and Beresford, T.P. Medical complications of anorexia and bulimia. *Psychol. Med.* 7:165, 1989.

53. Hall, R.C., et al. Refractory hypokalemia secondary to hypomagnesemia in eating disorders patients. *Psychosomatics* 29(4):435, 1988.

54. Hallberg, L. Bioavailability of dietary iron in man. *Ann. Rev. Nutr.* 1:123, 1981.

55. Hallberg, L., Brune, M., and Rossander, L. Iron absorption in man: Ascorbic acid and dose-dependent inhibition by phytate. *Am. J. Clin. Nutr.* 49:140, 1989.

**56.** Halmi, K. Anorexia nervosa: Demographic and clinical features in 94 cases. *Psychol. Med.* 36:18, 1974.

**57.** Halsted, C.H., Robles, E.A., and Mezey, E. Intestinal malabsorption in folate deficient alcoholics. *Gastroenterol.* 64:526, 1973.

**58.** Hambidge, K.M., Krebs, N.F., Sibley, L., and English, J. Acute effects of iron therapy on zinc status during pregnancy. *Obstet. Gynecol.* 4:593, 1987.

**59.** Harju, E., Heikkila, J., and Larmi, T.K. Effect of guar gum on gastric emptying after gastric resection. *JPEN* 8:18, 1984.

**60.** Herzog, D.B., and Copeland, P.M. Eating disorders. *N. Engl. J. Med.* 315:295, 1985.

**61.** Himms-Hajen, J. Brown adipose tissue thermogenesis and obesity. *Prog. Lipid Res.* 28:67, 1989.

**62.** Hoebel, B.G. Neurotransmitters in the control of feeding and its rewards: Monoamines, apiates and brain gut peptides. In A.J. Stunkard and E. Stellar (eds.), *Eating and Its Disorders.* New York: Raven Press, 1984.

**63.** Hooker, C., and Hall, R.C.W. Nutritional assessment of patients with anorexia and bulimia: Clinical and laboratory findings. *Psychol. Med.* 7(3):27, 1989.

**64.** Horwitz, D.L., and Bauer-Nehrling, J.K. Can aspartame meet our expectations? *J. Am. Diet. Assoc.* 83:142, 1983.

**65.** Howard, L., Ovesen, L., Satya-Murti, L.O., and Chu, R.C. Reversible neurological symptoms caused by vitamin E deficiency in patients with short bowel syndrome. *Am. J. Clin. Nutr.* 36:1243, 1982.

**66.** Humphries, L., Vivian, B., Stuart, M., and McClain, C.J. Zinc deficiency and eating disorders. *J. Clin. Psychol.* 50:456, 1989.

**67.** Hutson, W.R., and Wald, A. Gastric emptying time in patients with bulimia nervosa. *Am. J. Gastroenterol.* 85:41, 1990.

**68.** Jointhorp, B. Obesity and adipose distribution as risk factors for the development of disease. A review. *Infusionstherapie* 17:24, 1990.

**69.** Kallner, A.B., et al. On the requirements of ascorbic acid in man: Steady state of turnover and body pool in smokers. *Am. J. Clin. Nutr.* 34:1347, 1981.

**70.** Kanax, D.S., and Carmel, R. Low serum cobalamin levels in primary degenerative dementia. *Arch. Intern. Med.* 147:429, 1987.

**71.** Kaplan, N.M. The deadly quartet: Upper body obesity, glucose intolerance, hypertriglyceridemia and hypertension. *Arch. Intern. Med.* 149:1514, 1989.

**72.** Keesey, R.E. The body weight set point: What can you tell your patients? *Postgrad. Med.* 83:114, 1988.

**73.** Keesey, R.E. A set point analysis of the regulation of body weight. In A.J. Stunkard (ed.), *Obesity.* Philadelphia: W.B. Saunders, 1980.

**74.** Keesey, R.E. A set point theory of obesity. In K.D. Brownell and J.P. Foreyt (eds.), *Handbook of Eating Disorders: Physiology, Psychology and Treatment of Obesity, Anorexia and Bulimia.* New York: Basic Books, 1986.

**75.** Keys, A., et al. *The Biology of Human Starvation.* Minneapolis, Minn: University of Minnesota Press, 1950.

**76.** Kissebah, A.H., Freedman, D.S., and Peiris, A.N. Health risk of obesity. *Med. Clin. N. Am.* 73:111, 1989.

**77.** Kopple, J.D., and Swendseid, M.E. Vitamin nutrition in patients undergoing maintenance hemodialysis. *Kid. Int.* (Suppl.) 7:79, 1975.

**78.** Kritchevsky, D. Dietary fiber. *Ann. Rev. Nutr.* 8:301, 1988.

**79.** Lands, W.E.M. Renewed questions about polyunsaturated fats. *Nutr. Rev.* 44:189, 1986.

**80.** Lanza, E., et al. Dietary fiber intake in the U.S. population. *Am. J. Clin. Nutr.* 46:790, 1987.

**81.** Lavaroni, I., et al. Risk factors for coronary artery disease in healthy persons with hyperinsulinemia and normal glucose tolerance. *N. Engl. J. Med.* 320:702, 1989.

**82.** Levy, A.B., Dixon, K.N., and Stern, S. How are depression and bulimia related? *Am. J. Psychol.* 146:162, 1989.

**83.** Lewis, C.M., and King, J.C. Effect of oral contraceptive agents on thiamin, riboflavin, and pantothenic acid status in young women. *Am. J. Clin. Nutr.* 33:832, 1980.

**84.** MacKenzie, J.R., La Ban, N.M., and Sacheyfio, A.H. The prevalence of peripheral neuropathy in patients with anorexia nervosa. *Arch. Phys. Med. Rehabil.* 70(12):827, 1989.

**85.** Maicardi, V., Camellini, L., Bellodi, G., Coscelli, C., and Ferramini, E. Evidence for an association of high blood pressure and hyperinsulinemia in obese man. *J. Clin. Endocrin. Metab.* 62:1302, 1986.

**86.** Maye, S.T., et al. Rebound effect with ascorbic acid in adult males. *Am. J. Clin. Nutr.* 48:379, 1988.

**87.** Merrill, A.H., and Henderson, J.M. Diseases associated with defects in vitamin B6 metabolism or utilization. *Ann. Rev. Nutr.* 7:137, 1987.

**88.** Mitchell, J.E. Medical complications of anorexia and bulimia. *Psychol. Med.* 1(3):229, 1984.

**89.** Monolagas, S.C., Provedini, D.M., and Tsoukas, C.D. Interactions of 1-25,dihydroxy vitamin D3 and the immune system. *Mol. Cell. Endocrinol.* 4(3):113, 1985.

**90.** Monte, W.C. Aspartame: Methanol and the public health. *J. Appl. Nutr.* 36:42, 1984.

**91.** Morgan, B.L.G. Obesity. *Nutr. Health* 8:1, 1988.

**92.** Moser, P.B., Borel, J., Mauerus, T., and Anderson, R.A. Serum zinc and urinary zinc excretion of trauma patients. *Nutr. Rev.* 5:253, 1985.

**93.** Newman, M.M., and Halmi, K.A. The endocrinology of anorexia nervosa and bulimia nervosa. *Endocrinol. Metab. Clin. N. Am.* 17(1):195, 1988.

**94.** Nikkila, E.A., and Kekki, M. Effects of dietary fructose and sucrose on plasma triglyceride metabolism in patients with endogenous hypertriglyceridemia. *Acta. Med. Scand. Suppl.* 542:221, 1972.

**95.** O'Reeley, R.A., and Rytand, D.A. Resistance to warfarin due to unrecognized vitamin K supplementation. *N. Engl. J. Med.* 303:160, 1980.

**96.** Oster, J.R., Materson, B.J., and Rogers, A.I. Laxative abuse syndrome. *Am. J. Gastroenterol.* 74:451, 1980.

**97.** Parillo, M., Coulston, A., Hollenbeck, C., and Reaven, G. Effect of a low fat diet on carbohydrate metabolism in patients with hypertension. *Hypertension* 11:244, 1988.

**98.** Peiris, A.N., Mueller, R.A., Smith, G.A., Struve, M.F., and Kissebah, A.H. Relationship of androgenic activity to splanchic insulin metabolism and peripheral glucose utilization in premenopausal women. *J. Clin. Endocrinol. Metab.* 64:162, 1986.

**99.** Peterson, H.R., et al. Body fat and the activity of the autonomic nervous system. *N. Engl. J. Med.* 318:1077, 1988.

**100.** Phelps, D.C., Rosenbaum, A.L., Isenberg, S.J., Leake, R.D., and Dorey, F.J. Tocopherol efficacy and safety for preventing retinopathy of prematurity: A randomized, controlled, double masked trial. *Pediatrics* 79:489, 1987.

**101.** Pi-Sunyer, F.X. Exercise in the treatment of obesity. In F.T. Frankle and M.U. Yang (eds.), *Obesity and Weight Control.* Rockville, Md.: Aspen, 1988.

**102.** Pope, H.G., et al. Anorexia and bulimia among 300 female suburban shoppers. *Am. J. Psychol.* 141:292, 1984.

**103.** Potera, C., Rose, D.P., and Brown, R.S. Vitamin B6 deficiency in cancer patients. *Am. J. Clin. Nutr.* 30:1677, 1977.

**104.** Price, R.A., and Stunkard, A.J. Commingling analysis of obesity in twins. *Hum. Hered.* 39:121, 1989.

**105.** Reaven, G.M., Hollenbeck, C., Jen, C-Y, Wu, M.D., and Chen, Y-DI. Measurement of plasma glucose, free fatty acid, lactate and insulin for 24h in patients with NIDDM. *Diabetes* 37:1020, 1988.

**106.** Reichel, H., et al. The role of the vitamin D endocrine system in health and disease. *N. Engl. J. Med.* 320:980, 1989.

**107.** Reynolds, R.D., and Nalta, C.L. Depressed plasma pyridoxal phosphate concentrations in adult asthmatics. *Am. J. Clin. Nutr.* 41:684, 1985.

**108.** Rich, L.M., Caine, M.R., Findling, J.W., and Shaker, J.L. Hypoglycemic coma in anorexia nervosa. Case report and review of the literature. *Arch. Intern. Med.* 150(4):894, 1990.

**109.** Rivlin, R.S. Riboflavin metabolism. *N. Engl. J. Med.* 283:463, 1970.

**110.** Roberts, M.W., et al. Dysphagia in bulimia nervosa. *Dysphagia* 4(2):106, 1989.

**111.** Rossow, J.E. Kwashiorkor in North America. *Am. J. Nutr.* 49:58, 1989.

**112.** Rundos, C., Peterson, V.M., et al. Vitamin E improves cell-mediated immunity in the burned mouse: A preliminary study. *Burns* 11:11, 1984.

**113.** Saad, M.F., Knowler, W.C., Pettitt, D.J., Nelson, R.G., Mott, D.M., and Bennett, P.H. Sequential changes in serum insulin concentration during development of non insulin dependent diabetes. *Lancet* 1:1356, 1989.

**114.** Sanstead, H.H. Discovery of zinc deficiency in patients receiving total parenteral alimentations: Clinical correlations. *Nutrition* 5:21, 1989.

**115.** Schochen, D.D., Holloway, J.D., and Powers, P. Weight loss and the heart: Effects of anorexia nervosa and starvation. *Arch. Intern. Med.* 149:877, 1989.

**116.** Schwartz, D., and Thompson, M. Do anorectics get well? Current research and future needs. *Am. J. Psychol.* 138:319, 1981.

**117.** Shenai, J.P., Kennedy, K.A., Chytil, F., and Stahlman, M.T. Clinical trial of vitamin A supplementation in infants susceptible to bronchopulmonary dysplasia. *J. Pediatr.* 111:269, 1987.

**118.** Shepherd, J. Effects of nicotinic acid therapy on plasma high density lipoprotein subfraction distribution and composition on apolipoprotein A metabolism. *J. Clin. Invest.* 63:858, 1979.

**119.** Simmer, K., et al. Nutritional rehabilitation in Bangladesh—The importance of zinc. *Am. J. Clin. Nutr.* 47:1036, 1988.

**120.** Sitrin, M.D., et al. Vitamin E deficiency and neurologic disease in adults with cystic fibrosis. *Ann. Intern. Med.* 107:51, 1987.

**121.** Souba, W.W., Smith, R.J., and Wilmore, D.W. Glutamine metabolism by the intestinal tract. *JPEN* 9:608, 1985.

**122.** Stead, R.J. Selenium deficiency and possible increased risk of carcinoma in adults with cystic fibrosis. *Lancet* 2:862, 1985.

**123.** Stevens, J., et al. Comparison of the effects of psyllium and wheat bran on gastrointestinal transit time and stool characteristics. *J. Am. Diet. Assoc.* 88:323, 1988.

**124.** Stock, M.J. Thermogenesis and brown fat: Relevance to human obesity. *Infusionstherapie* 16:282, 1989.

**125.** Stout, R.W. Insulin and atheroma: 20 year perspective. *Diabetes Care* 13:631, 1990.

**126.** Stunkard, A.J., Foch, T.T., and Hrubec, Z. A twin study of human obesity. *JAMA* 256:51, 1986.

**127.** Szmukler, G.I., Young, G.P., Lichtenstein, M., and Andrew, J.T. A serial study of gastric emptying time in anorexia nervosa and bulimia. *Aust. N. Z. J. Med.* 20(3):220, 1990.

**128.** Teratology Society. Teratology Society position paper: Recommendations for vitamin A use during pregnancy. *Teratology* 35:267, 1987.

**129.** Vaisman, N., Corey, M., Rossie, M.F., et al. Changes in body composition during refeeding in patients with anorexia nervosa. *J. Pediatr.* 113(5):925, 1988.

**130.** Vaisman, N., et al. Energy expenditure and body composition in patients with anorexia nervosa. *J. Pediatr.* 113(5):919, 1988.

**131.** Van Gaal, L.F., Vansant, G.A., and De Leeuw, I.H. Upper body obesity and the risk for atherosclerosis. *J. Am. Coll. Nutr.* 8:504, 1989.

**132.** Van Itallie, T.B. Health implications of overweight and obesity in the United States. *Ann. Intern. Med.* 103:983, 1985.

**133.** Van Itallie, T.B., Smith, N.S., and Quartermain, D. Short term and long term components in the regulation of food intake: Evidence for a modulatory role of carbohydrate status. *Am. J. Clin. Nutr.* 30:742, 1977.

**134.** Vaselli, J.R., and Maggio, C.A. Mechanism of appetite and body-weight regulation. In F.T. Frankle and M.U. Yang (eds.), *Obesity and Weight Control.* Rockville, Md.: Aspen, 1988.

**135.** Victor, M., and Adams, R.D. On the etiology of the alcoholic neurologic diseases, with special reference to the role of nutrition. *Am. J. Clin. Nutr.* 9:379, 1961.

**136.** Vinik, A.I., and Jenkins, D.J.A. Dietary fiber in the management of diabetes. *Diabetes Care* 11:160, 1988.

**137.** Walter, T., et al. Iron deficiency anemia: Adverse effects on infant psychomotor development. *J. Pediatrics* 84(1):7, 1989.

**138.** Warren, S.E. Acid base and electrolyte disturbances in anorexia nervosa. *Am. J. Psychol.* 136(4A):415, 1979.

**139.** Warren, M.P., et al. Femoral head collapse associated with anorexia nervosa in a 20 year old ballet dancer. *Clin. Orthop.* 251:171, 1990.

**140.** Watson, R.D., Cannon, R.A., Kurland, G.S., Cox, K.L., and Frates, R.C. Selenium responsive myositis during prolonged home parenteral nutrition in cystic fibrosis. *JPEN* 9:58, 1985.

**141.** Weinberg, E.D. Infection and iron metabolism. *Am. J. Clin. Nutr.* 30:1485, 1977.

**142.** Willard, S.G., Winstead, D.K., Anding, R., and Dudley, P. Laxative detoxification in bulimia nervosa. In W.G. Johnson (ed.), *Advances in Eating Disorders* (Vol. 2). Greenwich, Connecticut: JAI Press, 1989.

**143.** Wolff, H.P., Vecsei, P., and Kruch, R., et al. Psychiatric disturbance leading to potassium depletion, sodium depletion, raised plasma renin concentration and secondary hyperaldosteronism. *Lancet* 1:257, 1968.

**144.** Wooley, S.C., and Kearney-Cooke, A. Intensive treatment of bulimia and body image disturbance. In K.D. Brownell and J. Foreyt (eds.), *Handbook of Eating Disorders.* New York: Basic Books, 1986.

**145.** Wooley, S.C., and Wooley, O.W. Should obesity be treated at all? In A.J. Stunkard and E. Stellar (eds.), *Eating and Its Disorders.* New York: Raven Press, 1984.

**146.** Wurtman, J.J. Carbohydrate craving, mood changes and obesity. 49 Suppl:37, 1988.

**147.** Yadrick, M.K., Kenney, M.A., and Winterfelt, E.A. Iron, copper, and zinc status: Response to supplementation with zinc or zinc and iron in adult females. *Am. J. Clin. Nutr.* 49:145, 1989.

**148.** Yates, A. Current perspectives on eating disorders: I. History, psychological and biological aspects. *J. Am. Acad. Child Adolesc. Psychol.* 28:813, 1989.

**149.** Yokogoshi, H., Roberts, C.H., Caballero, B., and Wurtman, R.J. Effects of aspartame and glucose administration on brain and plasma levels of large neutral amino acids and brain 5-hydroxyindoles. *Am. J. Clin. Nutr.* 40:1, 1984.

**150.** Zuckerman, D., et al. Prevalence of bulimia among college students. *Am. J. Pub. Health* 76:1135, 1986.

# chapter 11

Barbara L. Bullock<br>Bonnie Juneau

# Shock

## Chapter Outline

▶ **Maintenance of Tissue Perfusion**
    **Cardiac Output**
    **Total Peripheral Resistance**
    **Autonomic Response**
    **Intravascular Fluid Volume**
    **Hormones**
      Catecholamines
      Renin-Angiotensin-
        Aldosterone System (RAA)
      Antidiuretic Hormone (ADH)
▶ **Shock—An Overview**

▶ **Stages of Shock**
    **Nonprogressive Shock**
    **Progressive Shock**
    **Irreversible Shock**
▶ **Classifications of Shock**
    **Hypovolemic Shock**
      Hemorrhage
      Dehydration
      Burns
      Trauma
    **Cardiogenic Shock**
      Pump Failure
      Decreased Venous Return
      Progression of Cardiogenic
      Shock

**Vasogenic Shock**
    Neurogenic Shock
    Septic Shock
    Anaphylactic Shock
▶ **Complications of Shock**
    **Lactic Acidosis**
    **Adult Respiratory Distress**
      **Syndrome**
    **Disseminated Intravascular**
      **Coagulation**
    **Organ Ischemia and Necrosis**

## Learning Objectives

1. Discuss the physiologic mechanisms responsible for maintaining normal tissue perfusion.
2. Discuss compensatory responses to the shock state.
3. Describe the stages of shock.
4. List causes, indicators, and consequences of irreversible shock.
5. Identify the etiologies of shock relative to their designated classification.
6. Differentiate among the pathologic processes associated with each classification of shock.
7. List and explain the basis for symptoms associated with each classification of shock.
8. Define *toxic shock syndrome*.
9. Explain the basis for the development of the complications of shock.

The occurrence of the shock state is a most dreaded and yet predictable development in innumerable pathologic conditions ranging from hemorrhage to spinal cord injury. It is a complex problem that causes multiorgan effects, and the etiology does not begin and end with a single pathophysiologic alteration.[21] The interactions, including compensatory mechanisms, cause changes in volume, flow, and oxygen transport no matter what the initiating event is. These changes are the main factors that lead to survival or circulatory failure and death.[21] Therapy can alter the interactions; however, it should address not only the primary insult but the systemic effects of the insult. The physiology of tissue perfusion that underlies normal metabolism is reviewed in the first part of this chapter as a basis for understanding the alterations that occur when that balance is disturbed.

## MAINTENANCE OF TISSUE PERFUSION

Any discussion of the state of shock must be preceded by an overview of the physiologic mechanisms that maintain and regulate normal blood pressure (BP). Basically, BP is the product of cardiac output (CO) times total peripheral resistance (TPR) and can be expressed by the equation BP = CO x TPR. Any condition or derangement that increases or decreases either CO or TPR may potentially raise or lower BP accordingly. Alterations in BP due to an increase or decrease either in CO or in TPR are transient and momentary in healthy individuals who have intact and functional autonomic nervous systems (see Chap. 22). Because there is an inverse relationship between CO and TPR, an increase or decrease in one component prompts an opposite response in the other so that BP remains constant. For example, if CO decreases, TPR automatically increases and BP returns toward normal. The physiologic mechanisms responsible for activating this inverse relationship and maintaining BP are generated by autonomic nervous system response.

## Cardiac Output

Cardiac output is defined as the volume or load of blood ejected by the left ventricle each minute. In the average-sized adult, this volume equals 5 liters. It is usually slightly less in females due primarily to lower body weight, size, or both. Cardiac output volume, although relatively consistent in most individuals, is not an absolute or constant value because it may be influenced directly or indirectly by many factors. Cardiac output is the product of stroke volume (SV) times heart rate (HR) (the equation: CO = SV x HR). Stroke volume is that quantity of blood ejected by each ventricle with each cardiac contraction. It is determined or influenced by factors such as the volume (preload) and compliance, contractility, and afterload of the ventricles.[5] The relationship between these functional factors and SV as they pertain to CO is represented in Figure 11-1.

Circulating blood volume with an adequate venous return plays a very significant role in determining SV. Conditions that alter either atrial pressure, ventricular function, or venous return affect SV and consequently, CO. If SV increases or decreases, an automatic opposite response in HR serves to maintain constant CO. For example, a decrease in venous return results in a decreased

SV. Cardiac output remains constant, however, because the decreased SV indirectly prompts an increase in HR.

The second determinant of CO is HR. Heart rate is mediated by autonomic nervous system (parasympathetic and sympathetic) influence on the sinoatrial (pacemaker) node. Parasympathetic innervation decreases HR through vagal stimulation, whereas sympathetic innervation increases HR.

## Total Peripheral Resistance

Total peripheral resistance (TPR) is determined primarily by the diameter of the arteries and, to a lesser extent, that of the veins. Resistance is high in vessels with small diameter (vasoconstriction) and low in vessels with larger diameter (vasodilation). Therefore, systemic BP is increased when vessels are constricted and decreased when vessels are dilated. Like HR, blood vessel diameter, and hence resistance, is under the influence of the autonomic nervous system. Sympathetic stimulation results in vasoconstriction, whereas parasympathetic stimulation results in vasodilation.

## Autonomic Response

The influence of the autonomic nervous system on peripheral resistance and HR has a critical role in regulating BP. The effects of autonomic nervous system innervation focus on two areas in the medulla of the brainstem: the cardiac center and the vasomotor center. Both centers respond promptly to autonomic innervation through stimulation by the sympathetic branch or inhibition by the parasympathetic branch.

Sympathetic stimulation of the cardiac center results in acceleration of HR, while parasympathetic stimulation results in deceleration of HR. Similarly, sympathetic stimulation of the vasomotor center produces vasoconstriction and an increase in TPR. Parasympathetic stimulation of the vasomotor center produces vasodilation and a decrease in TPR (see Chap. 48).

The structures responsible for instigating autonomic activity are the baroreceptors located in the aortic arch and carotid sinuses. The baroreceptors are sensitive to changes in the degree of stretch or tension in the walls of these major arteries. Decreased stretch or tension is indicative of low CO and/or decreased peripheral vascular resistance consistent with low BP. Conversely, increased stretch or tension indicates elevated CO and/or increased peripheral vascular resistance consistent with high BP. Marked decrease in stretch in the arterial wall prompts a reflex at the baroreceptors, resulting in sympathetic stimulation of the cardiac center, which then causes acceleration of HR, increased CO, and a simultaneous stimulation of the vasomotor center, which, in

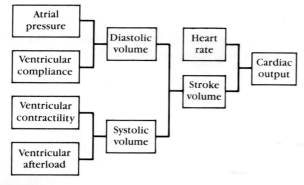

**FIGURE 11-1.**
Physiologic determinants of cardiac output. (From R.I. Vick, *Contemporary Medical Physiology*, Menlo Park, Calif: Addison-Wesley, 1984.)

turn, increases peripheral resistance. The net effect is an elevation in BP.[8,11] In the case of increased stretch in the arterial wall, the baroreceptors respond by stimulating parasympathetic activity. Increased parasympathetic activity elicits a decelerating effect from the cardiac center, resulting in a decreased HR and hence, CO, and a concomitant decrease in TPR through inhibition of vasomotor center activity. The overall effect is a reduction in BP.

Autonomic nervous system innervation stabilizes BP by modifying HR and thus, CO, and/or by changing TPR. It performs a critically significant physiologic function in BP regulation. Absence of autonomic nervous system influence in BP control can lead to irreversible shock and death.

## Intravascular Fluid Volume

Fluid volume ranks equally in significance with autonomic nervous system influence in BP regulation. Without sufficient quantities of circulating intravascular volume, autonomic nervous system innervation would be ineffective and virtually useless in executing normal, as well as compensatory/adaptive, physiologic functions related to BP control.

Normally, fluid volume contributes to BP control in a maintenance-type fashion. Physiologically, adequate circulating fluid volume ensures adequate venous return, which, consequently, with other factors such as ventricular function and HR being normal, ensures adequate CO. This provides a major contribution to BP maintenance. Increases or decreases in circulating fluid volume can either raise or lower BP accordingly.

An additional component in the fluid volume influence over BP is the process of autoregulation. Autoregulation is the mechanism whereby blood vessels either constrict or dilate in response to respective increases or decreases in the amount of intravascular fluid volume circulating to the tissues.[5] This constriction or dilatation is called a myogenic response.[5] In the case of increased volume and pressure, autoregulation results in vasoconstriction to normalize or equilibrate acceptable blood flow to tissues and organs. Vasoconstriction in peripheral vessels increases TPR and systemic BP (Figure 11-2).

Low or inadequate fluid volume and pressure induce autoregulative vasodilation to increase the amount of blood flow to tissues and organs. Vasodilation reduces TPR, thereby lowering BP. Another explanation for autoregulation is that as volume and pressure decrease, there may be an accumulation of vasodilator metabolites in the area that cause vasodilation, and restore flow to the tissues.[5]

Intravascular fluid volume is determined in large measure by the body's sodium content through the following mechanisms. Increased sodium content activates

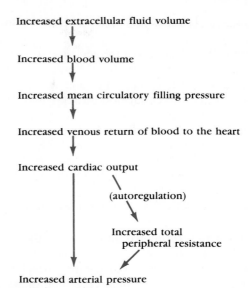

**FIGURE 11-2.**
Effects of increased volume on blood pressure. (From A.C. Guyton, *Textbook of Medical Physiology* [7th ed.]. Philadelphia: W.B. Saunders, 1986.)

the thirst response through hypothalamic stimulation.[4] Thirst induces voluntary water intake, thereby diluting sodium levels and offsetting sodium excess. A second and probably concurrent mechanism instigated because of excessive extracellular sodium is the increased release of antidiuretic hormone (ADH or vasopressin) from the posterior pituitary. Antidiuretic hormone is released in response to either increased serum osmolarity, as would be the case in sodium excess, or to conditions of water deficit. Activity of ADH, like increased oral intake, increases water volume and raises BP by increasing venous return and CO. Increased intravascular volume also raises BP (see Chap. 26).

## Hormones

Hormones that are responsible for BP regulation are the catecholamines (epinephrine and norepinephrine), renin-angiotensin-aldosterone (RAA), and ADH. Each regulates BP through different, but equally effective, mechanisms.

### Catecholamines

The catecholamines, released by the adrenal medulla, as well as by various adrenergic terminals located throughout the body, are categorized basically as short-term, immediate determinants of BP and operate in the following ways. Epinephrine increases both the rate of cardiac contractions and TPR. Both effects raise BP. In instances of hypotension, epinephrine is quite effective in instituting compensatory measures to elevate BP by increasing both CO and TPR. The role of norepinephrine in restoring and maintaining BP is related to improving and strengthening myocardial contractility, thereby increasing SV and consequently, CO. Both epinephrine and norepinephrine are released into the circulation through stimulation of autonomic adrenergic sympathetic nervous system influence on the adrenal medulla and various other sympathetic terminals located throughout the body.

### Renin-Angiotensin-Aldosterone System

The role of the RAA system in BP restoration is shown in Figure 11-3.

This system is prompted into action by the effects of hypotensive episodes on renal perfusion. Low or decreased renal perfusion stimulates the juxtaglomerular apparatus to release renin. Renin has little or no direct effect on BP, but it acts on angiotensin, a plasma protein, to produce angiotensin I, which then is converted in the lungs to angiotensin II. Angiotensin II has two profound effects on BP restoration. First, it is a very potent vasoconstrictor and as such, produces a generalized increase in TPR, thereby elevating BP. Second, angiotensin II stimulates the hypothalamus to induce thirst and prompts the release of aldosterone from the adrenal cortex. Aldosterone increases the resorption of sodium from the distal tubules and collecting ducts. Increased sodium resorption obliges a concomitant resorption of water. These mechanisms increase BP by elevating intravascular fluid volume.

### Antidiuretic Hormone

Antidiuretic hormone, also called *vasopressin,* is secreted by the posterior pituitary in response to hyperosmolarity,

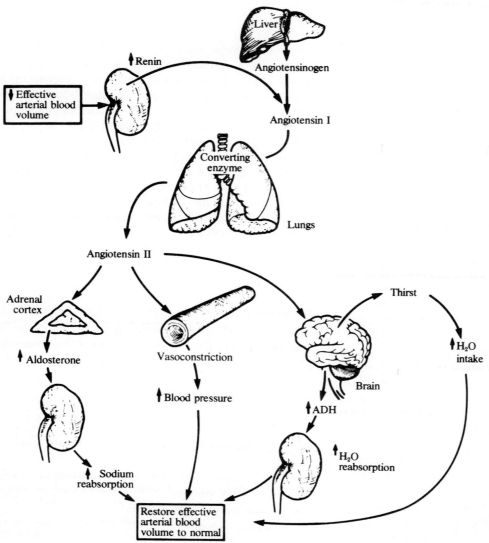

**FIGURE 11-3.**

Influence of the renin-angiotensin-aldosterone system on blood pressure. (From E. Selkurt, *Basic Physiology for the Health Sciences* [2nd ed.]. Boston: Little, Brown 1982.)

water deficit, or low blood volume. The mechanisms by which these states prompt ADH secretion vary, but result in quite effective compensation for each state.

Hyperosmolarity (especially due to hypernatremia) and water deficit conditions are detected by osmoreceptors located in the supraoptic nuclei of the hypothalamus. These structures, in turn, stimulate pituitary release of ADH. The action of the hormone is that of water conservation. It is accomplished by a poorly understood mechanism that results in increased resorption of water, mainly in the collecting ducts of nephrons. Increased resorption of water dilutes or offsets the hyperosmolar condition and corrects the water deficit. In addition, increased resorption of water raises intravascular volume, augments venous return, improves CO, and thereby raises BP. Increased vascular volume also raises BP through autoregulation.

The second condition that stimulates secretion of ADH is low blood volume. This results in decreased stretch on the pressure sensors in the atria and in the baroreceptors in the carotid sinus and aortic arch, which, in turn, stimulate the secretion of ADH. In addition to its water conservation action, ADH also produces a vasoconstrictive effect on arterioles, ultimately raising BP.[11]

## SHOCK—AN OVERVIEW

Shock is defined as a condition in which there is an overall or generalized reduction of adequate blood flow and oxygen delivery to the capillaries and tissues of the body.[11,21,24] It is typically manifested by hypotension; tachycardia; oliguria; cool, moist skin; restlessness; and altered levels of consciousness. It usually is induced by such conditions as hemorrhage, heart failure, sepsis, and neurologic damage.

Regardless of its etiology or pathologic basis, every form or classification of shock is characterized by compromised or inadequate tissue and organ perfusion. In effect, a discrepancy exists between tissue need for oxygen and various nutrients and actual supply of those elements. The ultimate result of this discrepancy is multisystem deterioration and related loss of function. Table 11-1 presents the general etiologic classification of circulatory shock.

Compromised tissue and organ perfusion characteristic of shock is caused by *low cardiac output*, or *reduced tissue perfusion pressure*, or both. Every type of shock can easily be grouped with or related to one or sometimes both of these categories. The various forms of shock are presented separately in this chapter.

## STAGES OF SHOCK

There are essentially three stages of the shock state. Various authors refer to them by different names: initial, pro-

gressive, and final;[8] nonprogressive, progressive, and irreversible;[11] early, tissue hypoperfusion, and cell and organ injury;[4] and compensated, decompensated, and irreversible shock.[5] Despite the variation in nomenclature, the basic fact remains that individuals experiencing shock progress through fairly distinguishable phases ranging from compensation to various states or degrees of decompensation. The terms *nonprogressive, progressive,* and *irreversible shock* are used in this discussion.

Table 11-2 indicates differences in the clinical picture according to the degree of shock.

## Nonprogressive Shock

Nonprogressive shock represents the initial or early phase during which, in response to the initial insult, several physiologic compensatory mechanisms are activated. Frequently, when these mechanisms are fully operational they may compensate for the shock state, depending on the extent of the insult.

During this early phase, CO, TPR, or both are decreased as a consequence of the initial insult, regardless of its origin or nature. These decreases result in decreased stretch or tension in the walls of major arteries. Baroreceptors situated in these arterial walls, specifically in the aortic arch and carotid sinuses, detect the reduced stretch and activate the autonomic nervous system response.

The sympathetic branch of the autonomic nervous system (SNS) responds to baroreceptor innervation by instigating two processes. First, sympathetic activity stimulates the cardiac center to increase HR by inhibiting vagal tone, thereby increasing CO. Second, and simultaneously, sympathetic activity stimulates the vasomotor center to increase TPR through vasoconstriction. Both of these responses represent an effort to raise BP compensatorily and thus improve or restore adequate tissue and organ perfusion. They are usually operational within several seconds to minutes.

Another compensatory mechanism set into motion in this early stage of shock is activation of the RAA system. Renin, released in response to low renal perfusion, triggers the eventual production of angiotensin II. Angiotensin II exerts its effects on BP by vasoconstriction and by both stimulation of the thirst mechanism and release of aldosterone from the adrenal cortex. The vasoconstrictive effect raises BP by increasing TPR, and the other effects do so by increasing circulating intravascular fluid volume. The RAA system is fully activated about 20 minutes after the initial stimulus, so its action follows that of the SNS.

Still another compensatory activity is increased secretion of ADH. Vasopressin is released in response to low pressure in the atria, aortic arch, and carotid sinuses. Its action is directed primarily toward water conservation

**TABLE 11–1.**
GENERAL ETIOLOGIC CLASSIFICATION OF CIRCULATORY SHOCK

**Reduction of Intravascular Volume
(Hypovolemic Shock)**
**Loss of Blood Volume—Hemorrhage**
External loss
  Trauma
  Gastrointestinal bleeding
  Severe hemoptysis
Internal or sequestered blood loss
  Hemothorax
  Hemoperitoneum
  Retroperitoneal hemorrhage
  Ruptured aortic aneurysm
  Fractures
**Loss of Plasma Volume**
**Loss of protein-rich body fluids**
  Burns
  Desquamated-exudative lesions
Dehydration
  Gastrointestinal loss
    Vomiting
    Diarrhea
  Renal loss
    Diabetic ketoacidosis
    Hyperosmolar nonketotic diabetes
    Diabetes insipidus
    Adrenal insufficiency
    High-urine-output renal failure
    Overly aggressive diuretic therapy
  Cutaneous loss
    Nonreplaced perspiration or insensible loss
  Internal or sequestered loss
    Peritonitis
    Pancreatitis
    Budd-Chiari syndrome
    Bowel ischemia and infarction

**Increased Vascular Capacitance (Vasogenic,
Veno-Vasodilatory Shock, Distributive Shock)**
**Neurogenic**
Spinal cord injury
Cerebral damage
Severe dysautonomia
**Toxic, Humoral**
Septicemia
Endotoxemia
Anaphylaxis
**Drugs**
Anesthesia
Sympatholytics
Adrenergic blockers
Veno-vasodilators
Barbiturates
Narcotics

**Failure of the Heart as a Pump (Cardiogenic Shock)**
**Impaired Systolic Performance**
Myocardial injury or depression
  Myocardial ischemia-infarction
  Myocarditis
  Cardiomyopathy
  Drugs (eg, doxorubicin, cocaine)
  Septic shock
  Acidosis
Misdirected systolic ejection
  Papillary muscle or chordal rupture
  Ruptured ventricular septum or free wall
Cardiac dysrhythmias
  Marked bradycardia or tachycardia
  Ventricular fibrillation
**Inadequate Ventricular Diastolic Filling**
Extracardiac or extravascular compression
  Pericardial tamponade
  Tension pneumothorax
  Positive-pressure ventilation
Obstruction to blood flow
  Pulmonary embolization
  Cardiac tumors (eg, myxoma)
**Valvular Incompetence or Malfunction**
Acute severe aortic or mitral valvular regurgitation
Obstruction or incompetency of prosthetic heart valve

**Miscellaneous Causative Factors**
**Microcirculatory Injury and/or Obstruction**
Thrombotic thrombocytopenic purpura
Disseminated intravascular coagulation
Anaphylaxis
Septic shock
Trauma
**Tissue and Cell Membrane Injury**
Septic shock
Pancreatitis
Prolonged hypoxia or shock

Source: *W. N. Kelley et al.,* Textbook of Internal Medicine. *Philadelphia: J.B. Lippincott, 1989.*

**TABLE 11-2.**
CLINICAL PICTURE EXHIBITED ACCORDING TO DEGREE OF SHOCK

| | NONPROGRESSIVE | PROGRESSIVE | IRREVERSIBLE |
|---|---|---|---|
| Sensorium | Oriented to time, place, person | Remains oriented; words slurred | Disoriented |
| Pulse | Rate increased Quality, full to decreased | Rate, very high Quality, decreased and variable | Rate, over 150 Quality, weak, thready, difficult to feel |
| Blood pressure | Normal to low (10–20% decrease but may be slightly increased as compensatory mechanism) | Decreased 40–50 mm Hg below normal (20–40% decrease) | Systolic less than 80 Diastolic may not be heard |
| Urinary output | 35–50 mL/h | 20–35 mL/h | Less than 20 mL/h |
| Color | Pale | Pale | Mottled |
| Capillary refill | Circulation return slightly slowed | Circulation return slowed | Circulation return very slow; skin pale both before and after Large differences between rectal and big toe temperature |
| Blood gases | pH normal | pH below 7.35 | pH very low; 7.0–7.2 |

and arteriolar vasoconstriction. Both of these actions tend to elevate BP.

Symptoms that predominate in this initial stage are directly related to compensatory activity. The individual is usually awake and alert but somewhat anxious. Heart rate is elevated but BP is normal, indicating the presence of SNS activity. Without the influence of the SNS, the BP would be decreased. The skin is usually pale, moist, and cool owing to sympathetic activity. Pupillary dilatation may be evident. Over time, the hematocrit becomes depressed when the condition is due to hemorrhage, because interstitial fluid is absorbed into the blood vessel and dilutes the blood. Respirations may be shallow, and the rate is increased in response to inadequate tissue oxygen delivery. Urinary output is slightly reduced because of impaired renal perfusion and ADH and aldosterone activity. The individual usually complains of thirst. Bowel sounds may be hypoactive, related to compensatory vasoconstriction and reduced blood delivery to nonessential organs such as the intestines. Muscle weakness and hyporeactive reflexes may be present for the same reason.

The shock state usually resolves within a matter of several hours, as long as the initiating event is not overwhelming and compensatory mechanisms are intact and functional. Otherwise, shock progresses to a more advanced stage in which compensatory mechanisms become virtually incapable of restoring BP.

## Progressive Shock

Progressive shock, commonly referred to as uncompensated shock, represents a condition in which compensatory responses fail to restore BP and tissue perfusion. In addition, the deleterious effects of prolonged tissue and organ hypoperfusion with resultant ischemic deterioration begin to compound the worsening clinical picture. It is, in fact, during this stage that the potentially devastating complications of shock usually begin to develop (see p. 258).

In the progressive stage, the effects of ischemia to, as well as exhaustion of, organs generating compensatory responses become evident. The medullary vasomotor center reacts to decreased perfusion and oxygen deprivation by completely ceasing its activity. Similarly, the myocardium, subjected to inadequate coronary artery perfusion and increased work in efforts to sustain CO, begins to deteriorate and is unable to generate adequate CO. Figure 11-4 shows the effect of shock on contractility. Despite the underlying mechanism causing the alteration, myocardial depression results.[2] Additional factors responsible for myocardial ineffectiveness are related to the influence of lactic acid and the myocardial depressant factor. Lactic acid is produced both in the myocardium, itself, and in tissues throughout the body as a byproduct of anaerobic glycogenesis consistent with stages of oxygen deprivation. It has a very potent ability to suppress

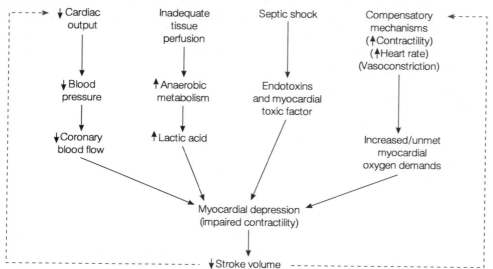

**FIGURE 11-4.**
Effect of shock on contractility. (From K.M. Burns, Vasoactive drug therapy in shock, *Crit. Care Nurs. Clin. N. Am. 2:2, 167–178, 1990.)*

myocardial contractility. The myocardial suppressant factor is thought to exert a potent negative inotropic effect (see Chap. 22). It is released by the pancreas, which suffers from compromised splanchnic organ circulation consistent with shock states.[5] Eventually, myocardial contractility is impaired and heart failure with pulmonary edema ensues.

Renal integrity is compromised relatively early in this stage of shock. The kidneys are quite sensitive to low perfusion pressure and respond rather quickly to reduced glomerular filtration by activating the RAA system. The kidneys, like the gastrointestinal system, skin, and splanchnic organs, are targeted as nonessential organs and are further compromised by selective vasoconstriction induced by sympathetic activity. The more essential organs, the heart and brain, are not affected by sympathetic vasoconstriction. Renal effects of the shock state and preferential vasoconstriction are seen in the form of acute tubular necrosis secondary to ischemia, and rather prompt acute renal failure (see Chap. 35).

The kidneys are not the only organs affected by hypoperfusion, ischemia, and selective vasoconstriction. Lung tissue also undergoes ischemic deterioration, resulting in adult respiratory distress syndrome, or shock lung (see Chap. 29). The ischemic gastrointestinal tract undergoes necrotic changes and releases endotoxins, vasodilating substances that further compound shock. Liver function deteriorates and this organ becomes incapable of performing metabolic or biotransformation functions.[3]

Symptoms associated with the progressive stage of shock are related to organ failure and the development of complications. Levels of consciousness and orientation decrease. Bradycardia and hypotension progress, urine output ceases, pulmonary and peripheral edema develop, and tachypnea with dyspnea becomes prominent. Abdominal distention and paralytic ileus are common.[3] The person appears critically ill, with cold, diaphoretic,

and ashen skin. The arterial pH becomes acidotic due to lactic acid accumulation. Recovery at this point depends on the underlying condition and rapid, effective, therapeutic management.

## Irreversible Shock

Irreversible shock denotes the final progression and is basically the point at which the individual becomes refractory or unresponsive to all forms of therapeutic management. There is progressive decrease in the CO and BP, together with increased severity of the metabolic acidosis. Ischemic cell death occurs and is manifest by renal, heart, pulmonary, and brain dysfunction.[4] Progressive renal and heart failure, manifestations of respiratory difficulties, and coma mark the ultimate outcome of the condition. Survival is virtually impossible. Figure 11-5 summarizes the different types of feedback that can lead to the progression of shock.

## CLASSIFICATIONS OF SHOCK

It is convenient to classify shock according to either etiology or associated physiologic impairment. For example, hypovolemic shock is caused by loss of intravascular volume, cardiogenic shock is the result of cardiac decompensation, and vasogenic shock denotes widespread vasodilation. In addition, various shock states, or at least shock-promoting status, can be categorized under one of those three broad classifications or headings: hypovolemic, cardiogenic, or vasogenic. Subsumed under the heading of hypovolemic shock are conditions such as hemorrhage, burns, dehydration, and trauma. Cardiogenic shock includes pump failure and decreased venous return referring to insufficient quantity of blood entering

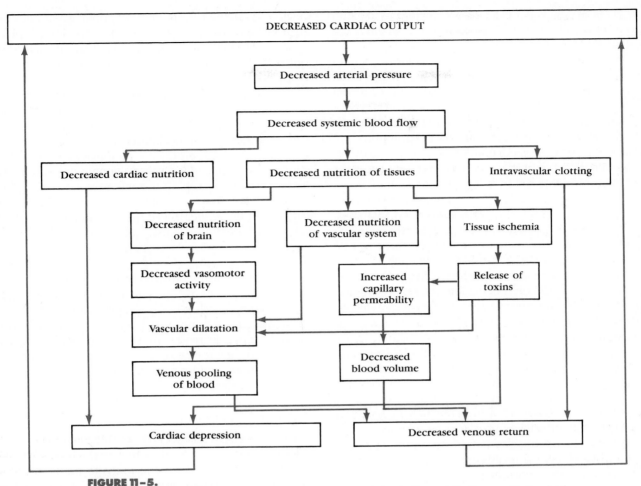

**FIGURE 11–5.**
Different types of feedback that can lead to progression of shock. (From A.C. Guyton, *Textbook of Medical Physiology* [7th ed.]. Philadelphia: W.B. Saunders, 1986.)

the heart. Vasogenic or distributive shock is the broad heading under which nervous system failure, septicemia, and anaphylaxis are grouped.

## Hypovolemic Shock

Hypovolemic shock, or that shock state resulting from loss of circulating fluid volume, may be caused by or result from any condition that significantly depletes normal volumes of whole blood, plasma, or water. The underlying pathology, regardless of the exact type of fluid loss, is related to actual circulatory fluid pressure/volume deficits. Decreased circulating fluid volume decreases venous return, which reduces CO and, therefore, lowers BP. As a consequence, lowered BP impedes tissue and organ perfusion and oxygen delivery. These consequences of lowered BP are potential first steps leading eventually to ischemia, necrosis, organ malfunction, and shock. Compensatory mechanisms are activated to adjust for the reduced tissue and organ perfusion. These mech-

anisms, discussed previously, include SNS stimulation to increase cardiac rate and TPR, activation of the RAA system, and increased secretion of ADH.

These mechanisms, working together, effectuate an increase in BP. If treatment to correct or remove the underlying cause of fluid volume loss is initiated, the shock remains in the nonprogressive stage and crisis is averted or resolved. If the fluid volume loss is overwhelming or therapeutic measures are not effective, this initial stage of shock may progress to the irreversible stage.

## Hemorrhage

Hemorrhagic shock occurs as a result of massive loss of whole blood. Some conditions that produce drastic loss of blood include gastrointestinal bleeding, postoperative hemorrhage, hemophilia, uterine lesions, childbirth, and trauma. For the shock state to ensue, blood loss must be extensive. Minimal loss of blood, up to 10% of the total volume, does not produce noticeable changes in BP or CO. Blood losses of up to 45% of the total blood volume reduce both CO and BP to zero.[11] Symptoms depend upon the actual volume of blood lost and whether the loss was sudden and abrupt or gradual.

In addition to the compensatory mechanisms, certain humoral substances are released in hemorrhage in an attempt to restore the steady state. In shock due to abrupt hemorrhage, adrenocorticotropic hormone (ACTH) is increased, which, in turn, increases glucocorticoid levels. The *glucocorticoids* maintain capillary integrity and combat the effects of the mediators of the inflammatory response. Erythropoietin levels increase and stimulate bone marrow to produce red blood cells. Circulating volume of *2-3,diphosphoglycerate*, a substance that interacts with hemoglobin to promote the release of oxygen, increases. This increases the liberation of oxygen, thereby reducing the effects of the tissue and organ hypoxia characteristic of shock.[19] The *prostaglandins*—$PGE_2$, $PG_{12}$, $PGF_2$-alpha, and $PGA_2$—play a mixed role in hemorrhagic shock, exerting beneficial and detrimental effects. Both $PGE_2$ and $PG_{12}$ dilate liver and renal vessels, thereby improving, to some extent, perfusion to these organs; $PGF_2$-alpha and $PGA_2$ constrict blood vessels. While $PG_{12}$ retards aggregation of platelets, $PGA_2$ exerts the opposite effect and actually promotes platelet aggregation. This latter action has been implicated in the development of disseminated intravascular coagulation in hemorrhagic shock (see Chap. 21). Activation of the *complement system* is beneficial in hemorrhagic shock because of its role in cell lysis but detrimental because it promotes leukocyte dysfunction, which potentiates the development of adult respiratory distress syndrome[18] (see Chap. 29).

In addition to these humoral agents released in hemorrhagic shock, other substances released in response to cellular deterioration actually have the potential for perpetuating the shock state. For example, lysosomal enzymes extend cellular damage, depress myocardial contractility, and constrict coronary vessels. The kinins depress myocardial contractility, promote vasodilation, and together with histamine, make capillaries more permeable, contributing to fluid volume loss. Serotonin causes potent arteriolar constriction and thus impedes microcirculation. Lactic acid, generated by anaerobic metabolism, depresses myocardial contractility. Endotoxins are released in response to gastrointestinal ischemia and result in vasodilation and myocardial depression.[18] All of these substances—lysosomal enzymes, kinins, histamine, serotonin, lactic acid, and endotoxins—are released in response to cellular damage and as such, are normal byproducts of injured cells. Their overall effect in hemorrhagic shock, however, is to perpetuate the vicious cycle of decreased perfusion and hypoxia.

## Dehydration

Dehydration results from extensive and profound loss of body fluid. Conditions that classically cause dehydration are profuse sweating; extensive gastrointestinal fluid loss related to diarrhea, vomiting, or upper gastrointestinal suctioning; diabetes insipidus; ascites; the diuretic phase of acute renal failure; Addison's disease; hypoaldosteronism; lack of adequate fluid volume intake; osmotic diuresis; and injudicious use of diuretics.

For dehydration to produce a shock state, it must be quite severe because fluid shifts from the interstitial spaces and even the intracellular compartments to maintain intravascular volume. Simple and even moderate dehydration does not produce symptomatology consistent with shock because fluid moves along a pressure gradient from tissue spaces to the intravascular space. Fluid volume in the vascular compartment is maintained at the expense of the tissues. Once fluid volume loss becomes severe, however, the transfer of water is not sufficient to maintain intravascular volume, and the shock state ensues.

The mechanisms involved in producing shock from dehydration are much the same as those that produce shock with hemorrhage. Fluid lost from the body diminishes vascular volume, which reduces venous return. Cardiac output decreases, BP falls, and tissue and organ perfusion declines. Physiologic adaptive mechanisms are activated in an attempt to restore BP, fluid volume, and ultimately, perfusion.

## Burns

Burns, especially third-degree burns, can cause hypovolemic shock. The mechanism by which this type of shock occurs is related not so much to fluid loss, as to loss of plasma proteins through the burn surface. Loss of plasma proteins significantly decreases colloidal osmotic pressure. In an effort to restore colloidal and hydrostatic pressure equilibrium, water leaves the vascular space and enters the interstitium (see Chap. 8). As a consequence, intravascular volume decreases, venous return is also decreased, CO is inadequate, and BP falls.

Shock secondary to burns also may be caused by hemorrhage and sepsis. Burn surfaces promote platelet aggregation and activation of factor XII, which leads to localized intravascular clot formation. These localized clots can impair microcirculation, resulting in tissue ischemia and necrosis, and can consume factors of coagulation, causing disseminated intravascular coagulation (DIC). Sepsis can result from extensive burns because of loss or destruction of the body's natural barrier—that is, the skin—to bacterial invasion. In addition, burned surfaces apparently release toxins into systemic circulation that can injure intestinal capillaries, thereby permitting the release of intestinal bacteria and endotoxins into systemic circulation. The mechanisms of septic shock are discussed on pages 253–255.

## Trauma

Trauma, in the forms of crushing injuries to muscles and bones, gunshot wounds, and penetration of blood vessels, the viscera, or other vital organs by knives or sharp instruments, produces the shock state primarily through extensive and sudden blood loss. An astounding amount of blood lost internally due to trauma can be concealed in tissue, organs, and third spaces for variable lengths of time before symptoms of shock are manifested. For example, the thigh muscle can hold up to 1000 ml of blood resulting from a fractured femur or a tear in a femoral vessel without a noticeable increase in thigh diameter.[8] Loss of 1 liter of whole blood represents a significant hemorrhage, especially if it goes undetected and uncorrected. It consequently perpetuates and compounds the shock state. Because of the massive blood loss usually associated with extensive trauma, traumatic shock is practically identical to hemorrhagic shock in terms of pathologic mechanisms and adaptive responses.

Another aspect of trauma is that loss of plasma, even without overt blood loss, often occurs.[10,11] Loss of plasma alone from capillary damage can lead to hypovolemia extensive enough to produce shock. Similarly, release of endotoxin and intestinal bacteria due to injury or ischemia to the gastrointestinal tract results in septic shock, which compounds the trauma-induced shock.

## Cardiogenic Shock

That shock state that is directly attributable to impaired or compromised CO is referred to as cardiogenic shock. There are essentially only two categories of conditions that can induce shock of cardiac origin: *pump failure*, actual inability of the heart to contract effectively, and *decreased venous return*, inability of sufficient quantities of blood to enter the heart.

### Pump Failure

Pump failure shock is always directly attributable to heart failure, which most frequently results from massive myocardial infarction. Other conditions causing cardiogenic shock from pump failure include the myocardiopathies, drug toxicity, dysrhythmias, etc. (see Table 11-1). The mechanism by which myocardial infarction causes pump failure is related to extensive myocardial damage that results in greatly diminished CO. The predominant and prevailing defect accounting for low CO is impaired myocardial contractility with loss of functional myocardium (see Chap. 24). Pump failure results when nearly half of myocardial tissue is nonfunctional.

### Decreased Venous Return

Decreased venous return is a category of cardiogenic shock that is not caused by inadequate circulating volume but by actual impedance of blood flow into the heart. It is the consequence of conditions such as cardiac tamponade, acute pericardial effusion, and mediastinal shifts that essentially squeeze or compress the heart to such an extent that venous inflow is impaired.[14] Decreased venous return always results in decreased CO and, hence, lowered BP with impaired tissue and organ perfusion.

## Progression of Cardiogenic Shock

In response to low CO, regardless of the cause, compensatory mechanisms are activated for the purpose of improving or restoring tissue perfusion by increasing BP through acceleration of HR and elevation of TPR. The decreases in SV, CO, and perfusion brought about by impaired myocardial contractility are compounded and worsened by the autonomic sympathetic responses intended to improve them. The autonomic response increases HR, thus increasing oxygen demand and decreasing diastolic filling time, both of which further compromise an ischemic myocardium. In addition, autonomically mediated vasoconstriction increases afterload, forcing the failing myocardium to work even harder in its attempt to sustain adequate CO. Selective vasoconstriction shunts blood away from organs such as the kidneys, skin, and splanchnic organs and toward the heart and brain, resulting in additional reduction of tissue and organ perfusion. Eventually, these selectively deprived organs experience and demonstrate the effects of inadequate perfusion. A schema depicting the sequential and intricate pattern of cardiogenic shock development is shown in Figure 11-6.

Left ventricular filling pressure and cardiac index obtained through use of a flow-directed, balloon-tipped pulmonary artery (Swan-Ganz) catheter are universal values for determining not only the extent of cardiac decompensation, but also the prognosis for survival in cardiogenic shock. Generally, those with high left ventricular end-diastolic pressure or pulmonary artery end-diastolic pressure (greater than 12 to 15 mm Hg) and/or low cardiac index (less than 2 L/min/m²) have statistically higher rates of mortality (see Chap. 24). The higher the left ventricular or pulmonary artery end-diastolic pressure and the lower the cardiac index, the greater is the likelihood of death from cardiogenic shock.[5]

In addition to pressure values recorded from the Swan-Ganz cather, other signs indicative of cardiogenic shock include varying degrees of pulmonary edema, hypotension, decompensation such as oliguria/anuria, ascites, cold and diaphoretic skin with pallor, decreased or altered sensorium, and abdominal distension with hypoactive or absent bowel sounds. Bradycardia and hypotension denote advanced stages of shock and usually are indications that sympathetic compensatory activity has failed and that survival is not likely.

Early recognition and prompt treatment of conditions that result in cardiogenic shock may actually preclude its development. This is true especially in cardiogenic shock secondary to venous inflow impedance. If the shock state is related to acute myocardial infarction, however, prompt treatment may or may not alter the

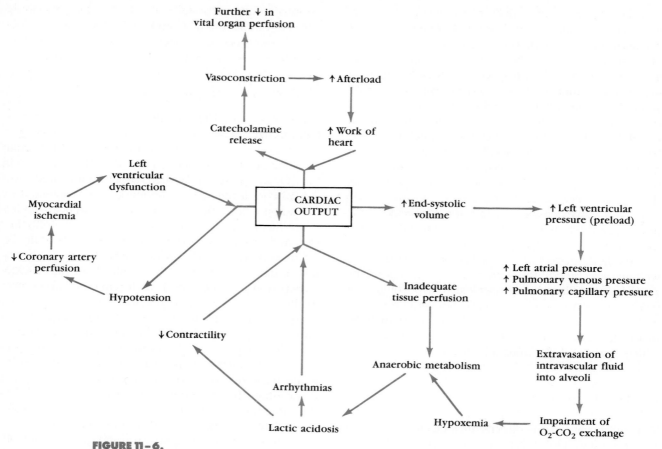

**FIGURE 11–6.**
Pathologic development of cardiogenic shock. (From B. Hammon, Cardiogenic shock: A review. *J. Emerg. Nurs.* 9:4, 1984.)

eventual outcome depending on the extensiveness of the infarct.

## Vasogenic Shock

The shock state that develops as a consequence of profound and massive vasodilatation as opposed to hypovolemia or cardiac dysfunction is referred to as low-resistance or distributive, that is, vasogenic, shock.[14] The term "distributive" shock is used because central blood volume is redistributed to peripheral vascular beds, especially venous beds.[14] The primary defect is a marked increase in vascular capacity or vasodilatation relative to the amount of circulating blood volume. Blood volume per se is not reduced, but rather the circulatory capacity to accommodate that volume is increased. Categories of conditions that result in extensive vasodilatation or increased vascular capacity include *vasomotor center depression, sepsis,* and *anaphylaxis.*

Regardless of the initiating event or insult, the sequence of pathologic events that culminates in vasogenic shock is uniform and consistent. Profound arteriolar dilatation and vasodilatation related to the vasomotor center depression, sepsis, or anaphylaxis lead to a relaxation or reduction of TPR. Reduced TPR results in a decrease in the volume of blood returning to the heart. This is related to blood vessel size or diameter and velocity or force of blood flow. The smaller the vessel, the more brisk is the blood flow through it. Similarly, the larger the vessel diameter, the less forceful, more sluggish, and slower is the blood flow through it. Dilated vessels are unable to generate sufficient force or pressure to propel blood adequately. Hence, in vasodilatation, venous return to the heart is reduced. The consequence of diminished venous return is decreased filling pressures in the chambers of the heart, with subsequent diminution of heart muscle fiber stretch or tension, such as decreased preload, which lowers SV. The consequence of reduced SV is impaired perfusion of tissues and organs, which deprives them of needed oxygen and nutrients. This sets the stage for the vicious cycle of positive-feedback, shock-related pathology. The sequence of events in vasogenic shock is displayed in Figure 11-7.

The vasodilatation that promotes or leads to the shock state interferes with or impairs tissue and organ

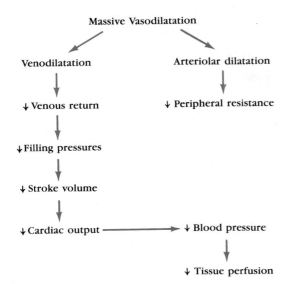

**FIGURE 11–7.**
Sequence of events leading to vasogenic shock. (From V. Rice, Shock: A clinical syndrome. *Crit. Care Nurse,* March-April: 46, 1981.)

perfusion for a variable time prior to the actual development of shock. Thus, the onset of shock actually compounds and worsens the already existing perfusion deficit. In addition, compensatory mechanisms instituted to restore BP and hence, tissue perfusion, are hampered and even offset by the underlying disease process, namely, vasomotor failure or potent vasodilator substances.

One of the major compensatory mechanisms activated in the shock state, the sympathetic vasomotor stimulation, may be futile and ineffective in vasogenic shock, owing to the nature of the primary defect. As long as the initiating vasodilatatory event prevails, vasomotor response is unable to contribute to the restoration of BP and tissue perfusion. Activation of the RAA system and secretion of ADH are also altered.

Pure symptoms of vasogenic shock are very difficult to distinguish from those of the primary condition due to the predominant feature of vasodilatation. Therefore, some overlap or dual causation of symptoms is unavoidable. Symptoms include hypotension; tachycardia; cool, moist to diaphoretic skin; fever; oliguria; hypoactive bowel sounds; increased hematocrit; anxiety; and tachypnea.

## Neurogenic Shock (Vasomotor Center Depression)

Neurogenic shock, also known as spinal shock, is the result of loss of vasomotor tone that induces generalized arteriolar and venous dilatation. This leads to hypotension, with pooling of blood in storage or capacitance vessels and splanchnic organ capillaries. Vasomotor tone is controlled and mediated by the vasomotor center in the medulla and the sympathetic fibers extending down the

spinal cord to peripheral blood vessels, respectively. Thus, any conditions that depress medullary function or spinal cord integrity and innervation can potentially precipitate neurogenic shock. One example of such a condition is head injury that directly or indirectly adversely affects the medullary area of the brainstem. Indirect injury results from cerebral edema, with increased intracranial pressure that accompanies head trauma or ischemia of the brain. Other instances that may promote neurogenic shock from medullary brainstem depression are deep general anesthesia and drug overdose, especially barbiturates, opiates, and tranquilizers.[11] Spinal cord injury and high spinal anesthesia may also induce neurogenic shock or profound vasomotor failure because of interference with or interruption of sympathetic pathways to blood vessels, which blocks vasoconstrictive responses and promotes vasodilatation. Syncopal episodes, or fainting, are considered to be a mild form of neurogenic shock that is relatively transient and inconsequential.

## Septic Shock

Septic shock is defined as a severe and profound condition of generalized vascular collapse, secondary to a systemic infection commonly caused by a gram-negative organism. The development of the shock state due to infection is believed to be related to the release of endotoxin from the bacterial cell wall. For this reason, septic shock is commonly referred to as *endotoxin shock* or simply *toxic shock.* Toxic shock is usually caused by gram-negative organisms but may be caused by viruses, fungi, or gram-positive bacilli. Gram-positive bacteria produce toxins on the surface of their cell wells, called exotoxins. Shock produced by these organisms is called *exotoxic shock.*[13] Table 11-3 summarizes the most frequently occurring gram-negative bacteremias and their sites of origin.

Endotoxin, a lipopolysaccharide made up of the layers of the bacterial cell wall, is capable of interacting with and influencing the activity of other cells and plasma proteins throughout the body. The net symptomatic effects of endotoxin activity include fever, abnormal clotting, hypotension, and elevated complement levels.[10] In addition to being released by bacteria in systemic circulation, endotoxin is released from necrotic bowel.[4,15]

The release of endotoxin by the bacterial cell wall initiates the process by which septic shock develops. Endotoxin is liberated from gram-negative bacteria through phagocytic activity of the macrophage system. If the bacterial infection is relatively minor, endotoxin is eventually neutralized and rendered harmless by the cells of the mononuclear phagocyte system.[23] In more extreme infections, the release of greater quantities of endotoxin virtually overwhelms the defensive system, thereby allowing endotoxin activity to prevail and the shock state to de-

**TABLE 11-3.**
GRAM-NEGATIVE ORGANISMS AND THEIR SITES OF ORIGIN

| ORGANISM | SITES OF HOSPITAL-ACQUIRED BACTEREMIA |
|---|---|
| *Escherichia coli* | Urinary tract, abdominal abscesses, peritonitis |
| *Klebsiella* sp. | Lungs, abdominal wound, intravenous lines, urinary tract |
| *Serratia* sp. | Peritoneal catheter, intravenous lines, urinary tract, lungs, intravascular pressure-monitoring equipment |
| *Pseudomonas aeruginosa* | Lungs, urinary tract, cutaneous wounds, intravenous lines |
| *Bacteroides* sp. | Subphrenic abscesses, abdominal wounds, decubiti |
| *Erwinia* sp. | Intravenous infusion sets |
| *Acinetobacter* sp. | Intravenous lines |
| *Citrobacter* sp. | Urinary tract |

Source: *Reprinted by permission from R. Gleckman and A. Esposito, Gram-negative bacteremic shock: Pathophysiology, clinical features, and treatment. South. Med. J. 74(3):336, 1981.*

velop. Endotoxin liberated into systemic circulation triggers and promotes the activation of several noxious substances, such as histamine, lysosomal enzymes, bradykinin, and serotonin, that significantly compromise capillary wall integrity. As a result of capillary damage, leakage of plasma occurs that produces marked fluid volume loss. The inevitable consequence of this plasma loss is a circulating fluid volume deficit with resultant hypotension. This capillary insult is also the basis for the development of adult respiratory distress syndrome in septic shock (Figure 11-8).[20]

Recent research has identified another role of the macrophage system in producing septic shock. The macrophage system apparently activates substances known to mediate shock. These substances include acid hydrolases, complement, coagulation factors, prostaglandins, and the monokines. Monokines are initially beneficial in shock as they mobilize body nutrient stores for energy. If the shock state is protracted, however, these substances actually lead to metabolic deterioration in the form of muscle tissue catabolism, depletion of carbohydrate stores, hypoglycemia, ineffective use of fat, and retarded to absent production of ketone bodies.[6]

The overall systemic effects of septic shock are shown in Figure 11-9. The process is initiated by some form of infectious agent that enters the body and overwhelms normal defenses to foreign invasion. As a consequence of host defense activity, mediators of shock such as histamine, bradykinin, complement, prostaglandins, and serotonin are liberated. The collective effects of these and other mediators are vasodilatation, capillary endothelial cell damage, platelet aggregation with microemboli formation, myocardial depression, and impaired myocardial contractility. The alterations in peripheral venules and arterioles, as well as those of myocardial function impair tissue and organ perfusion, leading to hypoxia-induced lactic acid glycogenesis. Lactic acidemia

further depresses myocardial contractility, TPR, and the vital organ functions. Death ensues predictably unless this chain of events is interrupted.[15,21]

Essentially three identifiable patterns of response or states are associated with septic shock. The initial one, referred to as the *hyperdynamic state*, presents the familiar picture of acute infection with chills, fever, and warm, dry, flushed skin (hence, the synonymous term "pink shock"). Tachycardia, tachypnea with respiratory alkalosis, and little alteration of BP occur in the early stage. Blood pressure is relatively normal because CO remains quite high, despite early widespread vasodilatation and the beginning stage of increased capillary permeability induced by endotoxin-stimulated release of vasoactive substances. In fact, the predominant physiologic feature of the hyperdynamic state is high CO, which is attributable to an intact and functional compensatory sympathetic response to decreased peripheral resistance.[11]The second or intermediate state in septic shock is called *normodynamic* and basically represents a transitional period between the first and third states. It is that pattern or state during which the effects of endotoxin liberation begin to become manifested by signs and symptoms such as hypotension, oliguria, cool skin, and thirst.[17] Tachycardia persists in an attempt to restore BP and tissue perfusion.

The final state is called *hypodynamic* and can be equated with the irreversible stage of hemorrhagic shock. The affected person is obviously acutely ill and moribund, with cold, clammy, diaphoretic skin, anuria, severe hypotension, tachycardia, and tachypnea. Metabolic acidosis from increased tissue catabolism and lactic glycogenolysis is usual. Effects of myocardial depression are evidenced by pulmonary edema and low CO. Once septic shock has progressed to this state, survival is doubtful and therapeutic measures are usually futile.

A special condition called *toxic shock syndrome (TSS)*

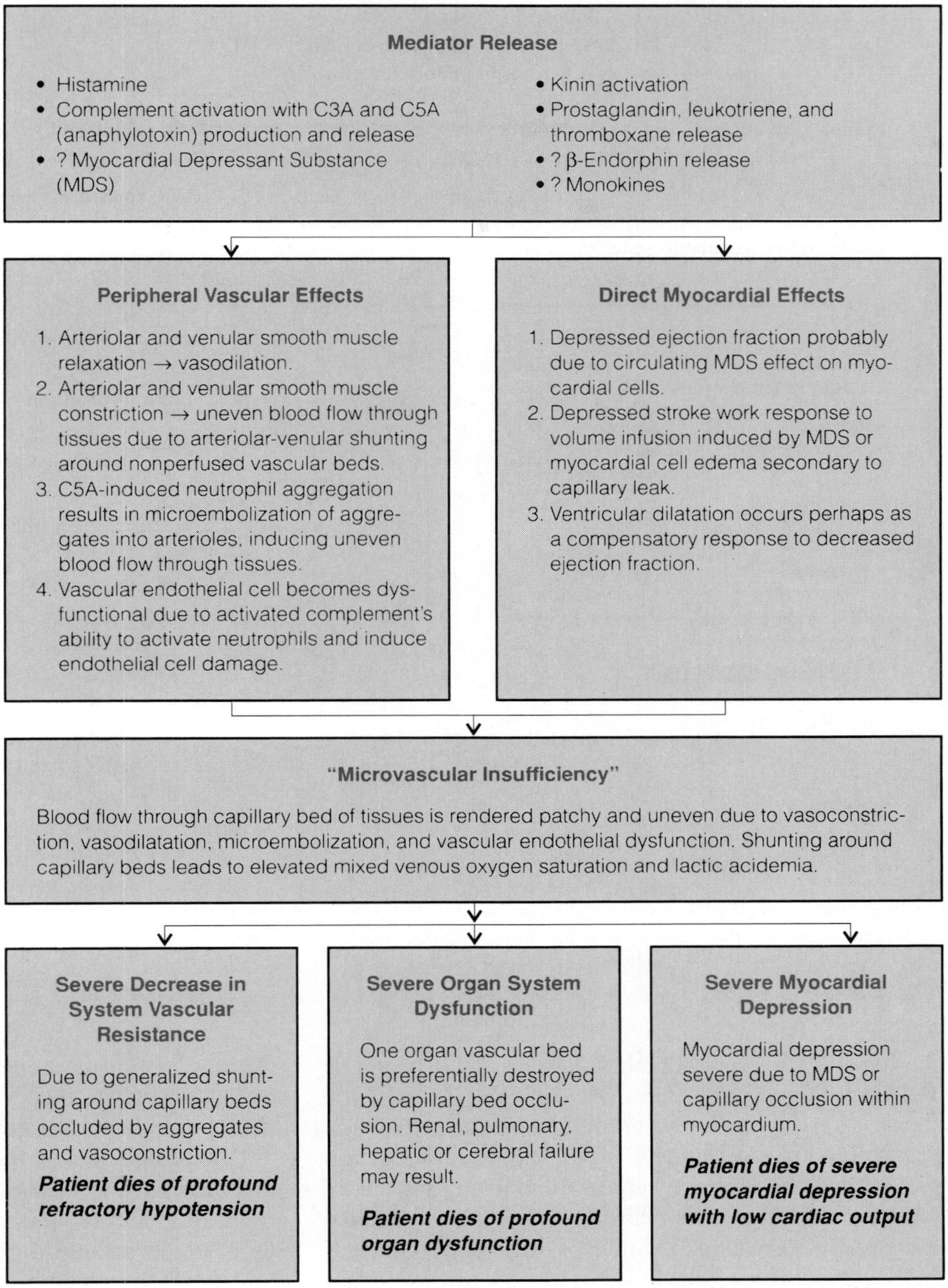

**Mediator Release**

- Histamine
- Complement activation with C3A and C5A (anaphylotoxin) production and release
- ? Myocardial Depressant Substance (MDS)

- Kinin activation
- Prostaglandin, leukotriene, and thromboxane release
- ? β-Endorphin release
- ? Monokines

**Peripheral Vascular Effects**

1. Arteriolar and venular smooth muscle relaxation → vasodilation.
2. Arteriolar and venular smooth muscle constriction → uneven blood flow through tissues due to arteriolar-venular shunting around nonperfused vascular beds.
3. C5A-induced neutrophil aggregation results in microembolization of aggregates into arterioles, inducing uneven blood flow through tissues.
4. Vascular endothelial cell becomes dysfunctional due to activated complement's ability to activate neutrophils and induce endothelial cell damage.

**Direct Myocardial Effects**

1. Depressed ejection fraction probably due to circulating MDS effect on myocardial cells.
2. Depressed stroke work response to volume infusion induced by MDS or myocardial cell edema secondary to capillary leak.
3. Ventricular dilatation occurs perhaps as a compensatory response to decreased ejection fraction.

**"Microvascular Insufficiency"**

Blood flow through capillary bed of tissues is rendered patchy and uneven due to vasoconstriction, vasodilatation, microembolization, and vascular endothelial dysfunction. Shunting around capillary beds leads to elevated mixed venous oxygen saturation and lactic acidemia.

**Severe Decrease in System Vascular Resistance**

Due to generalized shunting around capillary beds occluded by aggregates and vasoconstriction.

***Patient dies of profound refractory hypotension***

**Severe Organ System Dysfunction**

One organ vascular bed is preferentially destroyed by capillary bed occlusion. Renal, pulmonary, hepatic or cerebral failure may result.

***Patient dies of profound organ dysfunction***

**Severe Myocardial Depression**

Myocardial depression severe due to MDS or capillary occlusion within myocardium.

***Patient dies of severe myocardial depression with low cardiac output***

**FIGURE 11–8.**
Sequential steps in the pathogenesis of septic shock in patients who die. Surviving patients would have the sequential steps interrupted at some stage prior to the last three mechanisms of patient death (bottom three boxes). (Modified from J.E. Parrillo, S.M. Ayres, *Major Issues in Critical Care Medicine.* Baltimore: Williams and Wilkins, 1984.)

may produce septic shock. It also may be a relatively mild condition that resolves on treatment. Toxic shock syndrome is highly correlated to the use of tampons in menstruating women (85% of cases).[7] The causative organism, *Staphylococcus aureus*, is absorbed and releases a large amount of pyogenic exotoxin called TSS toxin 1.[7] Signs and symptoms of infections include fever, nausea and vomiting, diarrhea, peritoneal irritation, conjunctivitis, hypotension, renal dysfunction, headache, hypocalcemia, diffuse erythroderma, and desquamation of the palms and soles of the feet.[7] Circulatory collapse and death are rare.

### Anaphylactic Shock

Anaphylactic shock, or anaphylaxis, is the most drastic, acutely developing, and rapidly progressing of all forms of shock. Onset often occurs within a matter of seconds, and profound peripheral vascular collapse may become well-established in only a few minutes. Without immedi-

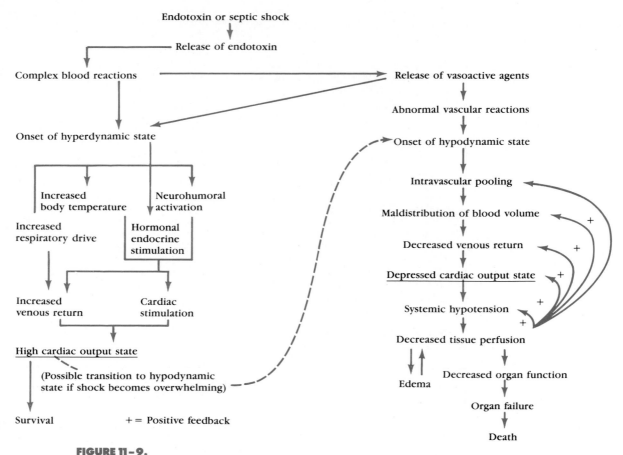

**FIGURE 11-9.**

Septic shock may develop after either of two major pathways through a hyperdynamic (high cardiac output) or a hypodynamic (low cardiac output) state. (From I. Hinshaw, Overview of endotoxin shock, in R.A. Cowley and B.F. Trump, *Pathophysiology of Shock, Anoxia, and Ischemia.* Baltimore: Williams and Wilkins, 1982.)

ate treatment, irreversible shock develops quite promptly and death occurs in an hour or so.[22] This form of the shock state is induced by an antigen-antibody reaction that occurs when an antigen to which the individual had previously been sensitized enters the body by any one of a variety of routes. Anaphylaxis rarely occurs on initial exposure to an antigen. Antigens that are commonly known to precipitate anaphylaxis are therapeutic drugs (ie, antibiotics, anesthetics, and contrast media, particularly those containing iodine) and foreign protein such as that found in blood products and snake and insect venom[12] (Table 11-4).

Anaphylaxis, or type I hypersensitivity reaction, is brought about or initiated by the action of immunoglobulin E (IgE) (see Chap. 16). An antibody present in serum, IgE binds to mast cells and basophils when stimulated by exposure to a specific antigen. Upon a second or repeat exposure, the antigen adheres to the mast cell or the basophil, resulting in the release of substances that mediate shock.[4,12] These substances, which essentially include histamine, bradykinin, leukotrienes, and prosta-

glandins, mediate shock by different mechanisms and produce most of the overt symptomatology associated with anaphylactic shock (Figure 11-10).

Histamine dilates blood vessels, constricts respiratory smooth muscle, and increases vascular permeability. Bradykinin also causes vasodilatation and makes capillaries more permeable, but apparently has little or no effect on respiratory smooth muscle. The leukotrienes $C_4$, $D_4$, and $E_4$ (formerly called SRS-A, or slow-reacting substances of anaphylaxis) constrict bronchial smooth muscle and increase venule permeability.[9] The prostaglandins exert a variety of effects depending on their type. They increase, decrease, or do not influence vascular permeability, blood vessel size, or respiratory smooth muscle.

The mechanism by which antigen-antibody reactions induce shock is directly related to the effects of the substances liberated at the outset of the reaction. Specifically, the shock state develops as a consequence of hypotension from profound vasodilatation and low CO secondary to central fluid volume deficits due to increased capillary permeability and peripheral pooling of blood.[16] Compen-

**TABLE 11-4.**
AGENTS COMMONLY IMPLICATED IN ANAPHYLACTIC AND
ANAPHYLACTOID REACTIONS

| | |
|---|---|
| Antibiotics | Penicillin and penicillin analogs, cephalosporins, tetracyclines, erythromycin, streptomycin |
| Nonsteroidal antiinflammatory agents | Salicylates, aminopyrine |
| Narcotic analgesics | Morphine, codeine, meprobamate |
| Other drugs | Protamine, chlorpropamide, parenteral iron, iodides, thiazide diuretics |
| Local anesthetics | Procaine, lidocaine, cocaine |
| General anesthetics | Thiopental |
| Anesthetic adjuncts | Succinylcholine, tubocurarine |
| Blood products and antisera | Red cell, white cell, and platelet transfusions, gamma globulin, rabies, tetanus, diphtheria antitoxin, snake and spider antivenom |
| Diagnostic agents | Iodinated radiocontrast agents |
| Foods | Eggs, milk, nuts, legumes (peanuts, soybeans, kidney beans), fish, shellfish |
| Venoms | Bees, wasps, hornets, snakes, spiders, jellyfish |
| Hormones | Insulin, ACTH, pituitary extract |
| Enzymes and other biologicals | Acetylcysteine, pancreatic enzyme supplements |
| Extracts of potential allergens used in desensitization | Pollen, food, venoms |

Source: W.C. Shoemaker, et al. Textbook of Critical Care (2nd ed.). Philadelphia: W.B. Saunders, 1989.

satory mechanisms are not capable of reversing or retarding the progression of this form of shock because the initial shock-producing insult develops rapidly and acutely.

In addition to overwhelming hypotension and tissue and organ ischemia, anaphylactic shock is often characterized by severe laryngeal spasm, edema, and bronchoconstriction. These pathologic developments compound the shock state by adding further hypoxemia to the overall pattern of response. Hypoxemia perpetuates the cycle of anaerobic metabolism and lactic acid production.

Signs and symptoms of anaphylaxis include profound hypotension, tachycardia, urticaria, pruritis, fever, dyspnea with hoarseness or stridor with wheezing, oli-

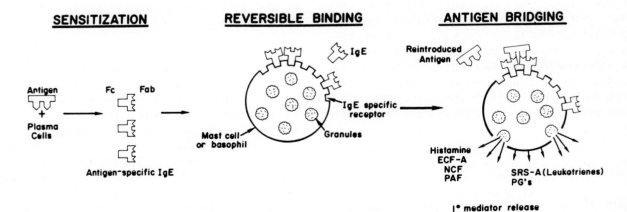

**FIGURE 11-10.**
The sequence of events leading to mediator release. During the initial exposure to antigen (sensitization) antigen-specific IgE is synthesized by plasma cells. The Fc portion of the IgE molecules then reversibly binds to receptors on mast cells or basophils. When antigen is subsequently reintroduced, two cell-bound IgE molecules are linked by a divalent antigen molecule (antigen bridging). This initiates a series of biochemical events leading to primary mediator release. (From W.C. Shoemaker, *Textbook of Critical Care* [2nd ed.]. Philadelphia: W.B. Saunders, 1989.)

guria, cool and moist skin with pallor, cyanosis, and anxiety. The individual has a recent history of contact with a known allergen or an antigen capable of inducing the anaphylactic reaction. Respiratory complications, such as stridor and inspiratory wheezing, may precede respiratory arrest.

## COMPLICATIONS OF SHOCK

Complications that are directly caused by the shock state are devastating and often fatal. These complications stem from and are actually produced by the pathologic processes inherent in shock. The three most common processes that induce severe complications are: vasodilatation with inadequate tissue and organ perfusion, damage to the capillary endothelial lining, and activation of clotting factors. Complications of these processes include lactic acidosis, adult respiratory distress syndrome (ARDS), disseminated intravascular coagulation, and organ necrosis.

### Lactic Acidosis

The basis for lactic acidosis in shock is the relentless production of lactic acid related to continual hypoxia of tissues from impaired perfusion. Impaired perfusion is secondary to vasodilatation and, to some extent, compensatory selective vasoconstriction. Hypoperfusion to tissues deprives them of oxygen. Cells are not able to metabolize nutrients appropriately without oxygen. In the absence of sufficient oxygen, cells are forced to metabolize nutrients anaerobically, which invariably results in the production of lactic acid.

Lactic acid exerts two major effects on the body. First, and probably of primary importance, it depresses myocardial contractility. Depressed contractility interferes with CO, which further reduces the already compromised perfusion and oxygenation of tissue. A vicious cycle of positive feedback is thereby established. The second untoward effect of lactic acid production is that it contributes acid to the body, leading to metabolic acidosis and further impairment of cellular metabolic function (see Chap. 9).

### Adult Respiratory Distress Syndrome

Adult respiratory distress syndrome develops secondary to shock because of at least two processes associated with the shock state. Apparently, pulmonary ischemia from hypoperfusion and aggregation of platelets in pulmonary capillaries significantly damage the endothelial lining of the pulmonary capillaries, causing them to lose selective permeability. As a consequence, water, electrolytes, red blood cells, and plasma proteins are extravasated into the interstitium of the lungs. This greatly impedes pulmonary compliance. Later, these fluids and blood components penetrate the alveoli, leading to frank pulmonary edema, further reduction in compliance, bronchospasm, atelectasis, and ultimately, significant hypoxemia.[4] A schema of the pathologic events leading to ARDS is depicted in Figure 11-11 (see also Chap. 29).

### Disseminated Intravascular Coagulation

Disseminated intravascular coagulation is a complex coagulopathy that occurs rather frequently among individuals who are acutely ill, especially those who have experienced some form of shock. The bases for the development of DIC are abnormal platelet aggregation and activation of factors of clotting, both of which are prominent features of shock. In response to the platelets and clotting factors, generalized coagulation occurs in the microcirculation and impedes capillary flow. In addition, the clotting process consumes fibrin, platelets, and other factors of clotting, and initiates fibrinolysis. Active fibrinolysis produces and releases fibrin degradation products, which are the end products of fibrin, fibrinogen, and plasmin lysis. The presence of these fibrin degradation products plus the consumption of platelets and other clotting factors interrupts subsequent coagulation and leads to widespread bleeding.[4]

Symptoms of microcirculation (capillary) coagulation are present, including cool skin with mottling and cyanotic nail beds and concomitant signs of profuse bleeding, especially from puncture sites, incisions, and the gastrointestinal tract. The overall picture of DIC is one of a vicious cycle of coagulation and anticoagulation (see Chap. 21).

### Organ Ischemia and Necrosis

Organ ischemia with resultant necrosis and loss of function are the inevitable consequences of shock, particularly if the condition is protracted or progresses to the irreversible stage. Organ ischemia occurs secondary to shock as a consequence of hypotension, selective vasoconstriction of sympathetic activity, platelet aggregation with microcirculation clotting, and capillary endothelial damage. Organ systems that undergo the most pronounced damage are the heart, brain, kidneys, liver, and lungs. Necrotic lesions secondary to the shock state have been identified in liver, myocardial, renal, and lung tissue with resultant dysfunction or complete loss of function.[4,21]

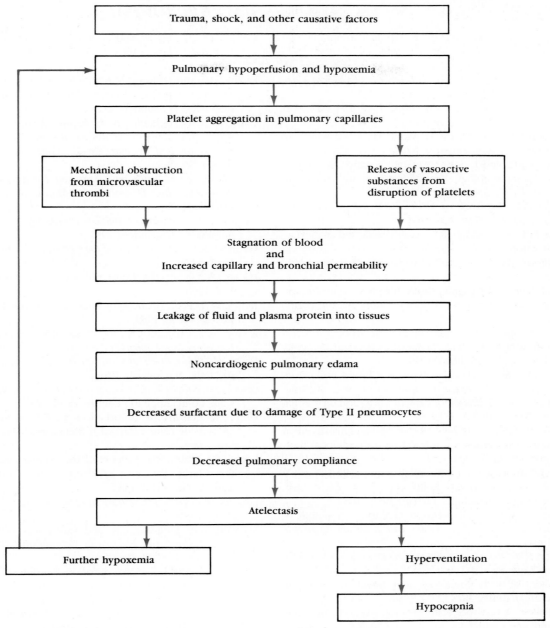

**FIGURE 11–11.**
Sequential development of adult respiratory distress syndrome. (Reprinted with permission from the February issue of *Nursing 82*, Copyright © 1982, Springhouse Corp., 111 Bethlehem Pike, Spring-house, PA 19477. All rights reserved.)

## *REFERENCES*

1. Baumgartner, J.D., Vaney, C., and Perret, C. An extreme form of the hyperdynamic syndrome in septic shock. *Intensive Care Med.* 10:245, 1984.

2. Burns, K.M. Vasoactive Drug Therapy in Shock. *Critical Care Nurs. Clin. N. Am.* 2: June, 1990.

3. Collins, A. Gastrointestinal Complications in Shock. *Crit. Care Nurs. Clin. N. Am.* 2: June, 1990.

4. Cotran, R., Kumar, V., and Robbins, S.L. *Robbins' Pathologic Basis of Disease* (4th ed.). Philadelphia: W.B. Saunders, 1989.

5. Ferguson, D.W., and Abboud, F.M. The pathophysiology, recognition, and management of shock. In J.W. Hurst et

al. (eds.), *The Heart* (7th ed.). New York: McGraw-Hill, 1990.

6.  Filkins, J.P. Monokines and the metabolic pathophysiology of septic shock. *Fed. Proc.* 44:300, 1985.

7.  Fisher, C.J., and Panacheck, E.A. Toxic shock syndrome. In W.A. Shoemaker et al. (eds.), *Textbook of Critical Care* (2nd ed.). Philadelphia: W.B. Saunders, 1989.

8.  Ganong, W.F. *Review of Medical Physiology* (15th ed.). Norwalk, Conn.: Appleton Lange, 1991.

9.  Gaunder, B.N., and Winkle, D. Anaphylaxis: Managing and preventing a true emergency. *Nurse Pract.* May:17, 1984.

10. Gleckman, R., and Esposito, A. Gram-negative bacteremic shock: Pathophysiology, clinical features, and treatment. *South Med. J.* 74:335, 1981.

11. Guyton, A.C. *Textbook of Medical Physiology* (8th ed.). Philadelphia: W.B. Saunders, 1991.

12. Haupt, M.T., and Carlson, R.W. Anaphylactic and anaphylactoid reactions. In W.C. Shoemaker et al. (eds.), *Textbook of Critical Care* (2nd ed.). Philadelphia: W.B. Saunders, 1989.

13. Hoyt, N.J. Preventing septic shock: Infection control in the intensive care unit. *Crit. Care Nurs. Clin. N. Am.* 2:287, 1990.

14. Leier, C.V. Approach to the patient with hypotension and shock. In W.N. Kelley et al., *Textbook of Internal Medicine*. Philadelphia: J.B. Lippincott, 1989.

15. Parrillo, J.E. Septic shock in humans: Clinical evaluation, pathogenesis, and therapeutic approach. In W.C. Shoemaker et al. (eds.), *Textbook of Critical Care* (2nd ed.). Philadelphia: W.B. Saunders, 1989.

16. Perkins, R.M., and Anas, N.G. Mechanisms and management of anaphylactic shock not responding to traditional therapy. *Ann. Allergy* 54:202, 1985.

17. Phair, J.P. Approach to bacteremia (gram positive/negative and septic shock). In W.N. Kelley et al., *Textbook of Internal Medicine*. Philadelphia: J.B. Lippincott, 1989.

18. Runciman, W.B., and Skowronski, G.A. Pathophysiology of hemorrhagic shock. *Anesthesia and Intensive Care* 12: 193, 1984.

19. Schrier, R.W. *Renal and Electrolyte Disorders* (3rd ed.). Boston: Little, Brown, 1986.

20. Schumer, W. Pathophysiology and treatment of septic shock. *Am. J. Emerg. Med.* 2:74, 1984.

21. Shoemaker, W.C. Shock states: Pathophysiology, monitoring, outcome prediction, and therapy. In W.C. Shoemaker et al. (eds.), *Textbook of Critical Care* (2nd ed.). Philadelphia: W.B. Saunders, 1989.

22. Silverman, H.J., VanHook, C., and Haponik, E. Hemodynamic changes in human anaphylaxis. *Am. J. Med.* 77: 341, 1984.

23. Stroud, M., Swindell, B., and Bernard, G.R. Cellular and humoral mediators of sepsis syndrome. *Crit. Care Nurs. Clin. N. Am.* 2:151, 1990.

24. Summers, G. The clinical and hemodynamic presentation of the shock patient. *Crit. Care Nurs. Clin. N. Am.* 2: 287, 1990.

## UNIT BIBLIOGRAPHY

Cotran, R.S., Kumar, V., and Robbins, S.L. *Robbins' Pathologic Basis of Disease* (4th ed.). Philadelphia: W.B. Saunders, 1989.

Falkner, B., and Gazdick, M.A. Fluids and electrolytes. In S.S. Zimmerman and J.H. Gildea, *Critical Care Pediatrics*. Philadelphia: W.B. Saunders, 1985.

Gann, D.S., and Amaral, J.R. Pathophysiology of trauma and shock. In G. Zuidema, R. Rutherford, and W. Ballinger, *The Management of Trauma* (4th ed.). Philadelphia: W.B. Saunders, 1985.

Gonick, H.C., and Buckalew, V.M. *Renal Tubular Disorders: Pathophysiology, Diagnosis and Management*. New York: Dekker, 1985.

Guyton, A.C. *Textbook of Medical Physiology* (8th ed.). Philadelphia: W.B. Saunders, 1991.

Hazinski, M.F. *Nursing Care of the Critically Ill Child*. St. Louis: Mosby, 1984.

Hurst, J.W., et al. *The Heart* (7th ed.). New York: McGraw-Hill, 1990.

Kelley, W.N., et al. *Textbook of Internal Medicine*. Philadelphia: J.B. Lippincott, 1989.

Kenner, C.V., Guzzetta, C.E., and Possey, B.M. *Critical Care Nursing: Body, Mind, Spirit* (2nd ed.). Boston: Little, Brown, 1985.

Keyes, J.L. *Fluid, Electrolyte and Acid-Base Regulation*. Monterey, Calif.: Wadsworth, 1985.

Lewis, C.M. *Nutrition and Nutritional Therapy in Nursing*. Norwalk, Conn.: Appleton-Century-Crofts, 1986.

Linton, A.L. Electrolyte disturbances. In W.J. Sibbald, *Synopsis of Critical Care* (2nd ed.). Baltimore: Williams & Wilkins, 1984.

Lowry, S.F. Nutritional support of the traumatized patient. In G.T. Shires, *Principles of Trauma Care* (3rd ed.). New York: McGraw-Hill, 1985.

Luke, B. *Principles of Nutrition and Diet Therapy*. Boston: Little, Brown, 1984.

Maxwell, M.H., Kleeman, C.R., and Narins, R.G. *Clinical Disorders of Fluid and Electrolyte Metabolism* (4th ed.). New York: McGraw-Hill, 1987.

Moore, G.L. Metabolic and nutritional problems in trauma. Unpublished presentation at First Annual Symposium on Trauma. Vanderbilt University, Nashville, 1985.

Plumer, A.L. *Principles and Practice of Intravenous Therapy* (4th ed.). Boston: Little, Brown, 1987.

Rice, V. (ed.). Shock. *Crit. Care Nurs. Clin. N. Am.* 2(2):143–343, 1990.

Robinson, C.H., and Weigley, E.S. *Basic Nutrition and Diet Therapy* (5th ed.). New York: Macmillan, 1984.

Shoemaker, W.C., et al. *Textbook of Critical Care* (2nd ed.). Philadelphia: W.B. Saunders, 1989.

Vander, A.J. *Renal Physiology* (4th ed.). New York: McGraw-Hill, 1991.

Whitney, E.N., Cataldo, C.B., and Rolfes, SR. *Understanding Normal and Clinical Nutrition* (3rd ed.). St. Paul: West Publishing Co., 1991.

# Bodily Defense Mechanisms

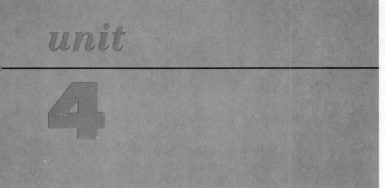

Infectious Agents

Inflammation and Resolution of Inflammation

# INFLAMMATION AND REPAIR

The inflammatory response is the body's reaction to tissue injury. It usually is initiated by an injurious substance and results in removal of the foreign material. It is a beneficial response that must be present for the maintenance of life. The most common causes of inflammation are infectious agents. Chapter 12 presents a condensed review of the classifications of organisms that can cause inflammation. It also describes the normal mechanisms used by the body to prevent or inhibit an organism's entrance. The student may want to expand the study of microbiology as it relates to pathophysiology; a reference list is included. Chapter 13 details acute and chronic inflammation and their resolution. Both normal and aberrant resolutions are presented. The effects of the inflammatory process as they alter specific organs and systems are studied in other sections of this textbook.

The reader is encouraged to study Units 4 and 5 together to maximize understanding of inflammation and immunity. Use of the learning objectives will facilitate understanding by providing an organized approach to the topic. The bibliography at the end of the unit provides additional sources for investigation.

# Infectious Agents

## Learning Objectives

1. Describe the major defense mechanisms of the host.
2. Define *organotropism, opportunistic infections,* and *pathogenic and nonpathogenic organisms.*
3. List the major characteristics of each type of infectious agent.
4. Explain how infectious agents are classified.
5. Describe the mode of viral infection and how viruses multiply.
6. List the events that occur as a cell is infected by a virus.
7. Describe at least six viral infections, differentiating DNA and RNA viruses, incubation periods, mode of transmission, and clinical effects.
8. Describe the pathologic effects of the rickettsial organism in spotted and typhus fevers.
9. Discuss the role of toxins produced by bacterial organisms.
10. Describe at least six gram-positive and gram-negative bacterial infections in terms of pathogenesis and clinical effects.
11. List three major classifications of fungi that are infectious to humans and describe the relationships among them.
12. List the protozoa that may be pathologic to humans.
13. Explain how protozoa move and reproduce.
14. Briefly describe three infections that may result from protozoa.
15. Categorize the types of helminths and describe how each can cause pathology in humans.

Infectious diseases are produced by living organisms: viruses, rickettsia, bacteria, fungi, protozoa, and nematodes. These diseases have been present in enormous numbers and have caused epidemics by their contagiousness. Although developments in nutrition, insect control, immunization, sanitation, and drug therapy have decreased the mortality and morbidity of infectious diseases, microbial infections have not been eliminated.[9] Microbes have developed mutant strains that are resistant to once-effective antimicrobial therapy. Infectious diseases still occur in great numbers and often are fatal to very young or debilitated victims. People in less developed countries have a much greater risk of contracting and dying from infectious diseases than do those in industrialized countries.[9]

## HOST-PARASITE RELATIONSHIPS

The occurrence of infectious diseases depends on many factors, including the virulence of the organism, the number of invading organisms, the defense mechanisms of the body, and the pathogenesis of the infection. *Virulence* is the ability of the infecting organism to cause disease, requiring a receptive host in which it can settle and multiply. The mechanisms by which an organism can cause disease require epithelial attachment, penetration into tissues, production of toxins, and the ability to cause alterations in the genome of the new host.[1] The number of invading organisms must be sufficient to overwhelm the host's defenses. *Organotropism* is the term used for the high selectivity of infectious organisms for specific tissues.[1] Some organisms are *opportunistic,* that is, normally *nonpathogenic* but *pathogenic* when the immune defense of the host is compromised.[1] The importance of opportunistic infections has been underscored by the emergence of many unusual infections in people infected with the human immunodeficiency virus that causes acquired immune deficiency syndrome (see Chap. 15).

The defense mechanisms of the human body reside on the external and internal surfaces and include physical, chemical, and immune barriers. Whether or not the organism can cause disease largely depends on the success or failure of these mechanisms and barriers to provide adequate defense. The main physical external barrier to infection is the skin, an intact epidermis being almost impervious to infection. The mucous membranes lining various organs also remove organisms by secreting mucus, which provides a washing effect and prevents organisms from adhering to membranes. Chemical secretions, such as hydrochloric acid in the stomach and the normally acid-pH urine, contribute to the sterile environment in the organs. The immune system targets pathogens for destruction. When organisms gain access to the body, lymphocytes recognize and destroy them, often without producing disease manifestations. The competence of the immune system, therefore, plays a major role in the outcome of infectious disease (see Chap. 14).

The defense mechanisms can be grouped into physical or chemical characteristics, immune factors, and nature of the host (Table 12-1). Clinically apparent infections occur when the defense mechanisms have not been sufficient to hold the growth of the organism in check.

The pathogenesis of infection depends on the capability of the specific organism and its ability to bypass or inactivate the defense mechanisms of the body. Manifestations of infections can be ascribed to injury, dysfunction, destruction of host cells, and alterations in the steady state.[7] Once actual infection is established, it often causes nonspecific signs and symptoms that characteristically include fever, chills, muscle pain, lymph node enlargement, and variable elevation in the white cell count. Each microorganism is distinct and has its own means of invasion and reproduction. The major classifications of living organisms are described in this chapter. The effects of the resultant diseases also are described in the chapters relating to specific organs and systems.

Infections may produce illness, as described earlier, or they may be inapparent or *subclinical,* in which state they are so mild that signs and symptoms are not seen. A particular form of subclinical infection is the *carrier state,* in which the person remains a reservoir of infection and

**TABLE 12-1.**
DEFENSE MECHANISMS OF THE BODY

| MECHANISM | CHARACTERISTICS OF DEFENSE |
|---|---|
| Physical | Intact epidermis<br>Mucus-secreting membranes<br>Mucus blanket movement in respiratory tract<br>Connective tissue |
| Chemical | Hydrochloric acid in stomach<br>Acid pH of urine<br>Lysozyme enzyme present in many secretions<br>Resident flora in mouth, on skin, in large intestine |
| Immune | Specific antigen–antibody reactions<br>Immunoglobin A<br>Inflammatory response |
| Host factors | Age<br>Sex<br>Genetic susceptibilities<br>Nutritional balance<br>Stress—physiologic or emotional<br>Presence of other diseases |

retains the ability to infect others.[1] Another important form of infection is *latent infection,* in which bouts of disease occur, interrupted by periods of no disease manifestation or infectivity. Herpes viral infections are common latent infections that can be reactivated by stress, other infection, or other factors.[1]

All infectious organisms are communicable (transmissible) from one member of the same species to another. The modes of transmission vary, and depend on the source, quantity of organisms, transit survival, and a susceptible new host.[1]

The human organism has the ability to contact and combat a multitude of potential pathogens in the environment. This is evidenced by the state of relative disease freedom in most people. This active defense is maintained through the complex immune system, which demonstrates a high degree of selectivity for organisms. The defensive ability of this system is affected by age, genetic factors, psychologic factors, and environmental and nutritional factors.

## VIRUSES

Viruses are the smallest infectious agents known. They are not complete cells in themselves and essentially exist as parasites on living cells. These organisms use the biochemical products of other living cells to replicate.

## Structure, Reproduction, and Pathogenesis

Viruses vary in size, appearance, and behavior. They are classified as either DNA or RNA viruses, according to their genetic material. Many contain nucleic acid, which is protected by a closed protein shell called the *capsid.* Some are surrounded by a lipid envelope.

Mature virus particles are called *virions* and contain a core of nucleic acid of either DNA or RNA.[4] Viruses appear to be species- and organ-specific and apparently can replicate only in permissive or receptive cells. Some viruses enter a receptive cell by pinocytosis, after which the process of multiplication can begin.

The structure of the virus has been studied with the electron microscope and is described according to its appearance. The complete infective particle is called a *virion.* The *capsid* is the protein coat, which is made up of protein subunits called *capsomeres.* The viral nucleic acid and the capsid are called the *nucleocapsid.*[4] Complex virions may contain additional layers, or envelopes.

The protein covering of the virus is type-specific. The surface structure is responsible for attachment to particular cell receptors. Infection depends on the compatibility of the viral surface with the host cell receptors and the ability of viral nucleic acid to use the host cell to manufacture viral products. All viruses are similar in their method of attachment to the specific receptors on the host cell membrane, the so-called lock-and-key attachment. Some have amino acids that are similar to the actively transported substances in the cell membrane of the host. Viruses can fool the cell, attach themselves to receptor sites on the host cell, and block the movement of normally transported materials.

Viruses affect and infect specific cells. Some B lymphocytes, for example, carry receptors for the Epstein–Barr virus, whereas cells in the tracheal lining have receptors for the influenza virus. Viruses produce specific diseases that involve specific tissues, but their modes of transmission and diseases produced are numerous. Cells respond to viral infection in different ways. There may be no apparent cellular change because viral DNA may adopt a symbiotic relationship with the host cell. Cellular pathologic effects, such as death or virus-induced hyperplasia, may occur. Cytopathic effects are common and include aggregation of host cells into clusters with shrinkage, lysis, and fusion of the cells. The effects differ and are influenced by the effects of the virus on cellular synthesis of macromolecules, alteration in cellular organelles such as the lysosomes, and changes in the host cell membrane (Figure 12-1).

Although no one virus is typical, the replication and transmission of this organism have been assessed extensively by studying the bacteriophage (virus that attacks bacteria). The genetic material of the bacteriophage is enclosed in an angular head or protein-containing capsid. The hollow head contains the viral genetic material and connects with a hollow cylinder of protein surrounded by protein contractile fibers. The contractile fibers coil around the cylinder like a spring. At the end of

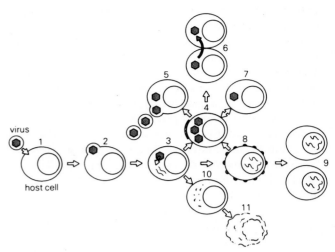

**FIGURE 12–1.**

A generalized viral life cycle. The virion becomes absorbed by its receptors to a host cell (**1**). The virus then penetrates the cell and becomes uncoated (**2** and **3**). Infection may take several courses, depending on the viral species. Some viruses replicate their components, which then assemble in the host cell (**4**) and are released by budding from the cell membrane (**5**). Alternatively, the virus can spread by cell-to-cell contact (**6**), without being released. Viruses also remain dormant within cells, to be reactivated at a later date (**7**). Some viruses are capable of inserting their genetic material into the host cell genome, where they remain latent (**8**). The cell subsequently may become productive (**4**) or, in certain circumstances, can undergo neoplastic transformation (**9**). Some virus infections may be abortive (**10**), either because the host cell is nonpermissive for infection or because the virus is defective. Both abortive infections and productive infections can lead to cell death (**11**). (From I. Roitt, J. Brostoff, and D. Male, *Immunology* [2nd ed.]. Philadelphia: J.B. Lippincott, 1989.)

the tail, the fibers and an enzyme are important in attaching the virion to the host cell (Figure 12-2).

Viral multiplication usually occurs in several steps. The first step is recognition and attachment of the virus to the host cell. The mechanism varies with the type of virus. The accumulation of viral particles in the cell ultimately results in lysis of the cell and viremia.[9] The tail of the virus may adsorb to specific receptor sites on the host

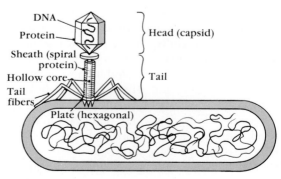

**FIGURE 12–2.**
A bacteriophage.

Labels: DNA, Protein, Sheath (spiral protein), Hollow core, Tail fibers, Head (capsid), Tail, Plate (hexagonal)

cell and then digest part of the host cell wall through lysosomal-like enzymes. The hole produced by the virus allows viral genome to be injected into the recipient cell. The viral shell (capsid and tail) remains attached to the host cell (as a "ghost" on the outside of the cell wall) after the genetic material has been injected. Within the host cell, the viral particles may alter protein synthesis, cause chromosomal changes, or alter the genes of the host.[8] Synthesis of new viral DNA, proteins, and shells occurs, and new DNA is assembled into the hollow protein shells, a process that continues until the host cell rup-

tures and releases swarms of new infective viruses (Figure 12-3). The formed particles can survive outside the host cell for variable periods of time, often until a new susceptible host cell can be found.

Each type of virus infects the host cell in a unique manner. The resulting signs and symptoms of the viral disease reflect the manner in which the virus has affected the host.[8] Some viruses are *endogenous,* and can remain latent within the host for years, only to be later reactivated. Examples of this type are herpes zoster and genital herpes. In most cases, the disease results from exposure

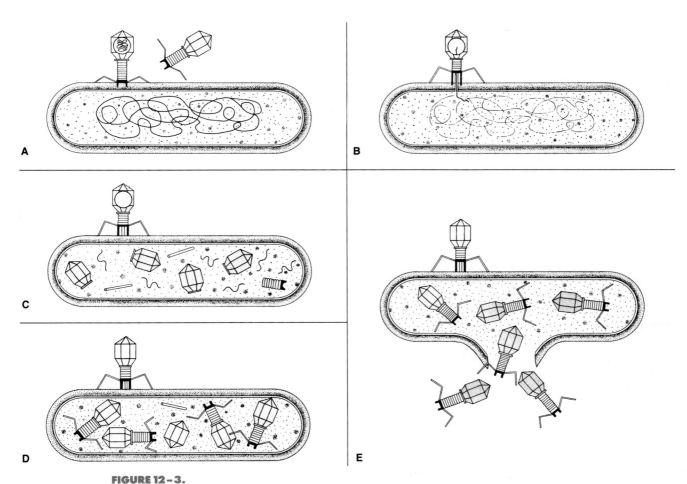

**FIGURE 12-3.**

Development of a virulent phage in a susceptible bacterium. (**A**) The polyhedral head of the phage is attached to the outer surface of the bacterium by its tail and tail fibers. (**B**) Within a few seconds or minutes, the bacterial cell wall and membrane have been perforated by the lytic enzymes in the tail, and the DNA of the phage has entered the bacillus through the phage tail. Note the retraction of the tail sheath. The opening through the cell wall is resealed. The inert protein coat of the phage remains on the outside of the cell. Disintegration of cell DNA begins at once. The phage, as such, is no longer demonstrable. (**C**) During the next 12 minutes, phage protein heads, tails, and DNA replicons are being synthesized. (**D**) About 12 minutes later, after a brief period of maturation during which some of the heads, tails, and DNA molecules have been assembled, infective phage virions are first demonstrable by artificial rupture of the cell. (**E**) About 12 minutes later, the assembly of parts into phage virions is complete, and the now eviscerated cell, an inert sac, ruptures by enzymatic lysis of the cell wall, liberating many new phage particles. Their number is characteristic of the burst size of the phage involved—in this case six. The whole process (**A**–**E**) occupies about 30 to 40 minutes in this particular virus–cell system. In this diagram, the phage virions have been drawn about three times larger proportionately to show more clearly certain structural details. (From M. Frobisher, *Fundamentals of Microbiology* [9th ed.]. Philadelphia: W.B. Saunders, 1974.)

to an *exogenous virus,* either through direct contact with another infected host or through indirect transmission, such as by means of contaminated water or shellfish.[4]

Viral infections stimulate the immune system's antibody production. Neutralizing antibodies are formed during viremia, but the main host defense is through cell-mediated immunity (see Chap. 14).[9] The initial response to viral infestation usually is by the mononuclear cells, such as monocytes and lymphocytes. At the site of entry of viruses into the body, the immunocompetent (antigen-specific) cells accumulate and initiate the inflammatory process. Macrophages often attach to the virus and enhance T- and B-cell interaction (see Chap. 14). Exposure to viral agents initially causes the synthesis of specific IgM antibodies, which is followed after about 10 days by the synthesis of IgG antibodies. When the virion is sufficiently coated with antibody, it is rendered noninfectious. The specific T lymphocytes provide for long-term immunity. Viruses and other substances stimulate the production of *interferon,* an antiviral protein that inhibits viral spread from cell to cell.[5]

After attachment, an *eclipse* stage may be entered, during which viral DNA becomes part of the host chromosome and remains *latent.* The greater the capability to initiate a rapid reproductive cycle, the more virulent the virus.

Activation or induction causes the latent viruses to become active and reprograms the cell for viral reproduction. It has been suggested that activation may be initiated by cold temperatures, carcinogens, or materials in food, air, or water.

Each virus responds to a specific induction mechanism. Sometimes a few cells with viruses within them escape induction, so that not all affected cells are lysed. In this way the host cell carries viral DNA as part of its own DNA, and the virus can remain latent in the host tissues throughout the life of the cell.

Viral infections produce many diseases, including hepatitis, meningoencephalitis, pneumonia, rhinitis, skin diseases, and numerous other disorders that affect almost every body system. Research is being conducted in many other disease conditions, such as multiple sclerosis, diabetes mellitus, and cancer, in the hopes of finding a viral connection.[9] Although there are multitudes of types of viruses, most of them can be classified into DNA or RNA structural viruses. Table 12-2 presents this classification, listing the common disease-producing groups, their modes of transmission, and the resulting symptomatology.

## RICKETTSIA

Rickettsia, once thought to be related to viruses because of their small size, are obligate, parasitic organisms. They possess all of the features of bacteria except that they can multiply only within certain cells of susceptible hosts.[9] Their normal reservoir most often is the arthropods, especially ticks, mites, lice, and fleas, in which they multiply without causing disease. Most rickettsial diseases are transmitted to humans through the bite or feces of the infected arthropod. An exception to this is Q fever, which probably is spread from person to person by respiratory droplet. The classification of rickettsia is based on the clinical features and epidemiologic aspects of the diseases they cause. The organisms are classified into the (1) spotted fever group, (2) typhus group, and (3) others, including Q fever.

All rickettsial diseases cause fever, and most cause a rash that is the result of rickettsial multiplication in the endothelial cells of the small blood vessels. The cells become swollen and necrotic, leading to the vascular lesions noted on or through the skin. Aggregations of lymphocytes, granulocytes, and macrophages accumulate in the small vessels of the brain, heart, and other organs.

Laboratory tests demonstrate the presence of rickettsial antigen and antibodies. Broad-spectrum antibiotics, such as tetracycline, suppress the growth of rickettsia, but full recovery requires an intact immune system that can develop antibodies against the organism.[11]

The most common diseases resulting from rickettsial infection include Rocky Mountain spotted fever and the typhus fevers (Table 12-3).

## BACTERIA

Unlike viruses, bacteria do not require living cells for growth. They are free-living organisms that use the nutrients of the body as a food source and a favorable environment for growth.

Bacteria can attach to epithelial tissue and, like viruses, prefer to infect specific sites. Pathogenic effects of bacterial infection usually result from substances such as enzymes or toxins produced by the bacteria or from injury caused by the inflammatory response of the body to the bacteria.

Bacteria are classified in many ways. They may be gram-positive or gram-negative, depending on the chemical composition of their cell walls and their absorption of staining dye. *Gram-positive bacteria* stain purple because their cell walls resist decolorization by acetone-alcohol. *Gram-negative bacteria* are first decolorized and then stained with a red dye to make them stand out.

Bacteria also are classified by their morphology. Spherical bacteria are *cocci;* rod-shaped are *bacilli;* and spiral bacteria are *spirochetes.* They can be pyogenic (pus-producing), granulomatous, aerobic, or anaerobic. Organisms such as *Mycobacterium tuberculosis* elicit a granulomatous inflammatory response that involves a chronic inflammatory process with a nodule of granula-

*(text continues on page 272)*

**TABLE 12-2.**
COMMON VIRUSES THAT CAUSE PATHOLOGIC EFFECTS IN HUMANS

| TYPE | NUCLEIC ACID PRESENT | INCUBATION PERIOD | EPIDEMIOLOGY | CLINICAL MANIFESTATIONS |
|---|---|---|---|---|
| Herpesviruses<br>Varicella (chicken pox) | DNA | 10–21 days | Highly contagious through respiratory droplets | Fever, disseminated vesicular eruption profuse on trunk and on oral mucosa; increased risk in immunosuppressed people |
| Zoster (shingles) | DNA | Variable | | Follows chicken pox—may occur years after a primary attack; spreads down peripheral nerves of skin; active ganglionitis causes burning or dull pain; vesicles follow nerve fibers |
| Herpes simplex<br>Type 1 | DNA | 2–12 days | Skin contact (oral) | Fever, vesicular eruption of mucous membranes, conjunctivitis, oral lesions (fever blisters); encephalitis occasionally results when virus ascends to central nervous system; manifestations more severe in immunosuppressed people |
| Type 2 | DNA | 2–5 days | Skin contact (genital); attack rate with sexual contact 1:3 | Genital vesicles, fever, burning, urinary urgency in males; dysuria, vulvar burning, dyspareunia in females |
| Epstein-Barr | DNA | 30–50 days | Respiratory droplet, transfusion | Sore throat, lymphadenopathy, splenomegaly, supraorbital edema; causative agent of infectious mononucleosis; virus has been isolated from Burkitt's lymphoma |
| Cytomegalovirus | DNA | ?20–50 days | Saliva, urine, feces, semen, transplacental, transfusion | Vary with age of onset: *Congenital:* failure to thrive, jaundice, respiratory distress; may be fatal *Postnatal:* infection may cause anemia, hepatomegaly, lymphocytosis *Adult form:* fever, lymphocytosis, Guillain-Barré syndrome *Immunosuppressed people:* interstitial pneumonia, hepatitis, increased frequency of rejection of transplanted organs |
| Pox viruses<br>Variola (smallpox) | DNA | 7–17 days | Respiratory droplets | Global eradication declared in 1979 because of worldwide immunization; still a potential concern because of laboratory research; high fever, vesicles on mucous membranes, papules on face and trunk, bone marrow depression |

*(continued)*

| TYPE | NUCLEIC ACID PRESENT | INCUBATION PERIOD | EPIDEMIOLOGY | CLINICAL MANIFESTATIONS |
|---|---|---|---|---|
| Vaccinia | DNA | About 2 wk after vaccination | Inoculation for smallpox | Probably hybrid of variola or cowpox virus; may cause widespread eczematous reaction or encephalomyelitis that causes death in 30%–40% of patients |
| Adenovirus (many strains identified) | DNA | 5–10 days | High frequency in children and military recruits; respiratory aerosol or droplet | Febrile pharyngitis; headache, regional lymphadenopathy, nasal obstruction and discharge, conjunctivitis, *pneumonia* |
| Papovavirus (warts—many types) | DNA | 1–20 months | Skin contact, contact with contaminated secretions; sexually transmitted | Solid, rounded tumors with horny projections 1–2 cm in size; often asymptomatic unless located on area of irritation; often found on hands, neck, shins, forearms, genital area |
| Picornavirus—coxsackie viruses A & B (many strains) | RNA | 2–5 days | Fecal-oral contact; insects may be passive vectors | Depend on type; acute myocarditis, fever, muscle and pleuritic pain, vesicular lesions on soft palate and tonsils, pharyngitis; associated with many systemic problems |
| Coronavirus | RNA | 3 days | Respiratory droplet | Common cold, rhinitis, pneumonia, bronchitis |
| Rhinovirus (many strains) | RNA | 1–2 days | Respiratory droplet | Common cold; fever, cough, croup, and pneumonia may develop in children; sore throat, nasal congestion, and nasal discharge without fever common in adults |
| Poliovirus | RNA | 2–5 days | Fecal-oral contact | Undifferentiated febrile illness may spread to involve anterior horn cells of spinal cord and motor nuclei of cranial nerves; causes various muscle paralyses, hemiplegia, paraplegia; bladder and respiratory muscle dysfunction; poliovaccines can prevent disease |
| Orthomyxovirus—influenza A, B, and C | RNA | 18–36 hours, up to 7 days | Epidemic, new strains evolve frequently; transmitted by infected respiratory secretions | Respiratory symptoms, cough, headache, muscle pain, fever, chills, sneezing, nasal discharge, prostration common; symptoms among strains similar |
| Mumps | RNA | 15–21 days | Very communicable in crowded conditions; transmitted by upper respiratory tract secretions | Painful enlargement of salivary glands; orchitis occurs in 20%–35% postpubertal males; small percentage develop meningitis or may affect other glands |
| Arenavirus—rubella | RNA | 14–21 days | Very communicable; disease confers immunity; nasopharyngeal transmission | Rash begins on face, spreads to trunk and extremities; lasts 1–5 days; enlarged lymph nodes common; joint pains and encephalomyelitis rare complications |

(*continued*)

| TYPE | NUCLEIC ACID PRESENT | INCUBATION PERIOD | EPIDEMIOLOGY | CLINICAL MANIFESTATIONS |
|---|---|---|---|---|
| Rhabdovirus—rabies | RNA | Variable; average 2–6 wk in humans | Animal bite of nonimmunized domestic dogs or cats, or of wild animals such as skunks, foxes, raccoons, bats, wolves | Virus introduced through mucous membranes or epidermis; replicates in striated muscle and then spreads up peripheral nerve bundles to central nervous system; passes to all organs but major effects on CNS; acute encephalitis, brain stem dysfunction and death; rapidly fatal if not treated; hydrophobia (excessive salivation) characteristic |
| Arbovirus—four groups cause CNS disease | RNA | 4–14 days | Mosquito bite transmits to humans; can multiply in horses, birds, bats, snakes, insects | Age-related; younger people often have high fever and convulsions; headache, fever, drowsiness, confusion, disorientation; some manifest mainly by lethargy, "sleeping sickness"; muscle weakness; residual effects range from none to convulsions; speech difficulties |
| Unclassified hepatitis A | RNA similar to picorna-viruses | 15–45 days | Fecal-oral enhanced by poor hygiene, overcrowding, contaminated food, water; sexual; percutaneous | Onset acute, most frequent in young people; causes anorexia, malaise, and other symptoms followed by jaundice; dark urine, clay-colored stools; recovery usually complete |
| Hepatitis, non-A, non-B (epidemic and parenteral types) | RNA | 15–160 days | Not known; possible fecal-oral or percutaneous | Clinical course variable; debilitation and liver dysfunction not infrequent |
| Hepatitis B | DNA-type | 45–160 days | Percutaneous, sexual, fecal-oral | Chronic active hepatitis may occur; jaundice, liver dysfunction may progress to liver failure; recovery slow |
| Hepatitis D | RNA | ?2–10 weeks | Blood, homosexual contact | People susceptible to hepatitis B or HBV carriers can be infected; clinical picture like HBV; may progress to chronic hepatitis |
| Human immunodeficiency virus | RNA retrovirus | Not known | Homosexual or heterosexual contact; parenteral transmission; perinatal transmission | May be dormant; may cause AIDS-related complex (ARC) or clinical AIDS; immunodeficiency affects resistance to cytomegalovirus and Epstein-Barr virus with high percentage affected; pneumonia caused by *Pneumocystis carinii*; series of opportunistic infections; Kaposi's sarcoma; with ARC, swollen lymph glands, fatigue, weight loss occur; clinical AIDS usually results in death |

**TABLE 12–3.**
COMMON RICKETTSIA THAT CAUSE PATHOLOGIC EFFECTS IN HUMANS

| RICKETTSIA | MORPHOLOGY | EPIDEMIOLOGY | CLINICAL EFFECTS |
|---|---|---|---|
| Spotted fevers (*R. rickettsii*; Rocky Mountain spotted fever) | Small organism, stains purple; usually gram-negative cell wall antigen; elaborates endotoxinlike substance | Multiply in nucleus and cytoplasm of infected cells of ticks and mammals; commonly occurs in Western hemisphere; transmitted by bite of infected tick or through skin abrasions contacting tick feces or tissue juices; incubation 3–12 days | Swelling and degeneration of endothelial cells, vascular damage, myocarditis, pneumonitis; peripheral vascular collapse may cause death; impairment of hepatic function and consumption coagulopathy may occur; severe headache, muscle pain, fever for 15–20 days; characteristic rash begins as small discrete, non-fixed pink lesions on wrists, ankles, forearms, etc., becomes petechial; mortality 7%–10% |
| Typhus fevers (*R. prowazekii*; epidemic typhus) | Small, gram-negative organism; always multiplies within cytoplasm of cells | Inhalation of dried louse feces; louse feces often rubbed into broken skin as with scratching of bite; incubation approximately 1 wk | Intense headache; continuous pyrexia for 2 wk; macular rash in axilla spreads to extremities, becomes petechial; peripheral vascular collapse as with Rocky Mountain spotted fever |
| *R. typhi* (endemic typhus) | Similar to *R. prowazekii* | Transmitted by fleas, widespread in U.S., especially southeastern and Gulf Coast states | Headache, fever, chills; fever up to 12 days; rash generalized, dull red macular, over thorax and abdomen; prognosis good with or without treatment |
| Q fever (*R. burnetti*) | Appearance similar to other rickettsiae | Inhalation of infected dust, of ticks on body and lice feces; sheep, goats, cows often affected; incubation 2–4 wk; present throughout the world | Fever, headache, weakness, interstitial pneumonitis, dry cough, chest pain; hepatitis and endocarditis may follow; rash not characteristic |
| Trench fever (*R. quintana*) | Appearance like other rickettsiae | Transmitted by body louse feces into broken skin; found in Europe, Africa, North America; incubation usually 1–4 wk | Headache, fever, malaise, pain, tenderness, splenomegaly, macular rash common; recovery usually rapid |

tion tissue and actively growing fibroblasts and capillary buds (see Chap. 29).

A unique group of organisms, the *chlamydiae,* sometimes are grouped separately from bacteria because they do not synthesize their own adenosine triphosphate, but they do possess DNA and RNA and form their own cell walls.[9] These organisms are obligate, intracellular pathogens that respond well to broad-spectrum antibiotics.

## Pathogenesis

All bacteria are capable of localizing in specific organs and often produce acute inflammatory reactions. The degree of tissue damage depends on the number of bacteria present, the virulence of the organisms, the site of infestation, and the resistance of the host to the organism. The bacteria must resist engulfment by the defensive neutrophil cell. Some elaborate toxins kill or depress the phagocytic cell; others develop resistant strains to escape recognition. Some of these organisms are *facultative intracellular bacteria* that counteract the defensive phago-

cyte after being interiorized. In this way latent foci can be reactivated years after the initial infection.[9] The most common example of this is tuberculosis. Table 12-4 presents a classification of some of the more common bacteria that affect humans. The list is necessarily incomplete because there are thousands of bacterial organisms.

The virulence of bacteria is enhanced by the elaboration of endotoxins and exotoxins. *Endotoxins* are produced by many gram-negative organisms and, when released, are pyrogenic and confer antigenic specificity to the toxin.[9] These enhance chemotaxis, and some activate complement by the alternate pathway (see Chap. 13). *Exotoxins* usually are produced by gram-positive bacteria. These toxins have specific effects on target organs; for example, elaboration of diphtherial toxin causes the formation of a thick membrane on the respiratory structures and toxic effects on the heart and nervous system.

*Coagulase,* an enzyme produced by many staphylococcal organisms, can initiate the coagulation sequence and produce coagulation in various areas. Coagulase also may cause the deposition of fibrin on the surface of staphylococci that may inhibit the ability of defensive

(text continues on page 276)

**TABLE 12–4.**
BACTERIA THAT CAUSE PATHOLOGIC EFFECTS IN HUMANS

| BACTERIA | GRAM STAIN | MORPHOLOGY | EPIDEMIOLOGY | CLINICAL EFFECTS |
|---|---|---|---|---|
| *Pseudomonas aeruginosa* | Gram-negative | Motile rod; greenish yellow pigment formed; saprophytic but can establish infection and invade when host resistance is decreased | Commonly present on skin and mucous membranes; often attacks debilitated, immunosuppressed, burned, premature, or elderly people; transmitted by contact, especially to urinary tract, lungs, or damaged skin | Purulent drainage from wounds; characteristic greenish mucous from site of infection; bacteremia carries a 75% mortality; high fever, confusion, chills followed by circulatory collapse and sometimes leukopenia |
| *Proteus* | Gram-negative | Active motile rod; hydrolyzes urea; actively decomposes protein | Commonly present in decaying matter, soil, water, and human intestine; affects skin, urinary tract, ears, and other areas secondarily in susceptible people | Localized purulent infections may spread and cause bacteremia, symptoms of bacteremia; usually sensitive to penicillin therapy |
| *Enterobacter, Klebsiella* | Gram-negative | Short, plump, nonmotile rods; type-specific capsular antigens | Urinary tract and respiratory infections, especially pneumonia; often found in immunosuppressed, alcoholics, or people with diabetes mellitus | Symptoms of pneumonitis; productive cough, weakness, anemia; may resemble TB; responds well to aminoglycoside therapy |
| *Shigella* | Gram-negative | Nonmotile rods; aerobic or nearly anaerobic | GI tract resident; transmitted through fecal-oral route, or through contaminated food, water, swimming pools; common in countries where sanitation is poor; incubation usually less than 48 h | Fever, colicky abdominal pain, diarrhea; liquid, greenish stools may contain various amounts of blood; dehydration may result |
| *Escherichia coli* | Gram-negative | Non–spore-forming rods; different strains characterized by their antigens | Normal inhabitant of colon; may spread to urinary tract directly or through bloodstream; opportunistic organism in debilitated people | Accounts for more than 75% of urinary tract infections; abscesses may form on any area; bacteremia characterized by fever, chills, dyspnea; may develop endotoxic shock |
| *Salmonella* *S. typhi* (typhoid fever) | Gram-negative | Motile; type identified by specific antigens | Ingestion of contaminated foods, water, or milk; transmitted through fecal contamination of foodstuffs; totally transmitted by human carriers; incubation period about 10 days | Rare in U.S.; onset of fever, chills, abdominal pain, and distention; rash of small macules on upper abdomen and thorax; without treatment often causes intestinal bleeding and perforation |
| Other *Salmonella* organisms | Gram-negative | Varies with type | Food contamination; disease onset within hours of food ingestion | Enteritis, massive vomiting, diarrhea, dehydration, fever; antibiotic treatment normally not helpful |
| *Haemophilus* *H. influenzae* | Gram-negative | Small, pleomorphic nonmotile, aerobic non–spore-forming | Respiratory transmission, especially to very young and aged | Nasopharyngitis may be epidemic, especially in impoverished and rural populations; often outbreaks during winter months may develop into pneumonia, ear infections, rarely meningitis |
| *H. pertussis* (*Bordetella pertussis*) | Gram-negative | Small, aerobic, slow-growing | Respiratory droplets; very contagious; incubation about 1 wk | "Whooping cough"; characterized by catarrhal stage followed by paroxysmal cough and laryngeal stridor; without immunization, epidemics occur; immunization or disease does not provide lifelong immunity |

(*continued*)

| BACTERIA | GRAM STAIN | MORPHOLOGY | EPIDEMIOLOGY | CLINICAL EFFECTS |
|---|---|---|---|---|
| *Chlamydia* (*C. trachomatis*) | Gram-negative | Obligate, intracellular parasite, unique reproductive cycle; sometimes classified as separate species | Mainly sexually transmitted; incubation 5–10 days | Urethritis, less severe than gonococcal; commonly causes epididymitis in males, macupurulent cervicitis in females; no immunity has been demonstrated |
| *Staphylococcus* | Gram-positive | Spherical, grapelike clusters of organisms on solid media | | |
| *S. aureus* | Gram-positive | Coagulase positive; remains viable on surfaces of furniture or clothing | Commonly resides on skin and mucosal surfaces; invades skin through hair follicles, thence to bloodstream; occasionally through urinary or respiratory tract | Most common cause of *skin infections*, furuncles, boils, and carbuncles; may have localized lymphadenopathy; impetigo results from exfoliative toxin from a form of *S. aureus*; *pneumonia* more common in hospitalized patients; causes fever, tachycardia with localized areas of pneumonia; also may cause empyema; *bacteremia* may produce fever, tachycardia with abscess throughout the body; often fatal, nearly 50% mortality; *acute osteomyelitis* commonly caused by this organism; may result from skin or blood-borne infection or from open or closed trauma of affected bone; high fever and bone pain; may cause much osseous destruction; usually responds well to antimicrobials; urinary tract infections most frequently result from contamination of indwelling catheter, ascends to kidneys from bladder |
| *Streptococci* | Gram-positive | Spherical, anaerobe nonmotile, non–spore-forming | | |
| Group A, *S. pyogenes* (at least 60 subtypes), B hemolytic | Gram-positive | | Respiratory droplet | Streptococcal *pharyngitis* very common in crowded living situations, greatest frequency ages 5–15 yr; fever, extremely painful and inflamed pharynx, tonsils, uvula; *scarlet fever* may result when a specific strain of *Streptococcus* A produces a toxin causing rash, diffuse erythema, with petechiae on soft palate, scarlet "strawberry" tongue in early stages; later, tongue becomes beefy in appearance, called "raspberry" tongue; desquamation of skin occurs up to 3–4 wk after the disease; may occur before rheumatic fever; *rheumatic fever* may follow acute streptococcal infection and apparently is immune reaction to organism; *acute glomerulonephritis* also may follow streptococcal infection; *erysipelas,* an acute infec- |

(*continued*)

| BACTERIA | GRAM STAIN | MORPHOLOGY | EPIDEMIOLOGY | CLINICAL EFFECTS |
|---|---|---|---|---|
| | | | | tion of the skin and subcutaneous tissue from *S. pyogenes*, causes malaise, itching, erythema that spreads rapidly with edema and encrustation; localized skin lesions, cellulitis, and pneumonia may also result |
| Group B, *S. agalactiae* | Gram-positive | | Frequently colonize in the female genital tract, throat, and rectum; may be transmitted to susceptible person directly or by respiratory contact | May occur in puerperium to cause septicemia, pulmonary involvement, and meningitis in newborns |
| *S. pneumoniae* (pneumococcus) | Gram-positive | Diplococcal form, lancet-shaped | Transmitted by respiratory tract droplet; rapidly progressive once established | Preceded by "cold" or "sinus" complaints; fever, chills, pleuritic pain, cough productive of rusty sputum; hypoxia occurs with infiltration of lung tissue; progresses to atelectasis in one or more lobes; responds well to antibiotic therapy |
| *Neisseria* *N. meningitides* | Gram-negative | Single cocci, grows well in media with small amount of oxygen | Resides in nasopharynx of carriers, spreads through respiratory droplets; transmitted by bloodstream to meninges | *Meningococcemia* begins with cough, headache, sore throat followed by high fever and sometimes manifestations of endotoxic shock; *meningitis* evidenced by presence of meningococcus in cerebrospinal fluid and neurologic symptoms |
| *N. gonorrhoeae* (gonorrhea) | Gram-negative | Diplococcus | Humans only natural hosts; transmitted almost solely through sexual intercourse; incubation period usually less than 1 wk | Men develop dysuria, urethral discharge; because of penicillin treatment, complications are rare; women have dysuria, vaginal discharge, abnormal menstrual bleeding, Bartholin's gland may be involved; pelvic inflammatory disease may result |
| *Corynebacterium diphtheriae* (diphtheria) | Gram-positive | Nonmotile rod, club-shaped; elaborates exotoxin | Most frequently transmitted through respiratory tract but may be transmitted by skin, genitalia; incubation 1 day to 1 wk | Respiratory effect on pharynx, larynx, and trachea; formation of thick, leathery membrane on these structures, causing respiratory obstruction; exotoxin effects: heart, causing myocarditis; nervous system, causing peripheral neuritis, motor denervation; peripheral vascular collapse occurs in late stages; without antitoxin protection, mortality about 35% with 90% of those having laryngeal involvement |
| *Clostridium tetani* (tetanus) | Gram-positive | Anaerobic, motile rod, spore-bearing; exotoxin production | Found in soil and intestinal tract of humans and some animals; puncture or laceration of skin usual mode of entry; incubation variable, usually about 14 days | Exotoxin attacks CNS, causing muscle rigidity and spasms; pain and stiffness of jaw early symptoms; *lockjaw* refers to inability to open jaw; laryngospasm may lead to hypoxia; overall mortality 40%–60% |

*(continued)*

**TABLE 12–4.**
BACTERIA THAT CAUSE PATHOLOGIC EFFECTS IN HUMANS (*Continued*)

| BACTERIA | GRAM STAIN | MORPHOLOGY | EPIDEMIOLOGY | CLINICAL EFFECTS |
|---|---|---|---|---|
| *Mycobacterium*<br>M. tuberculosis<br>(tuberculosis) | | Aerobic, acid-fast; resists de-colorization with acid or acid alcohol; curved, spindle-shaped | Respiratory droplet; reinfection or activation of dormant infec-tion; incubation 4–8 wk if not walled off | *Primary TB:* usually lung involve-ment, macrophages wall off vi-able organisms; these may be seen on radiograph as rims of calcification; *clinical TB:* fever, pleurisy, night sweats, cough, weight loss; can spread to bone or cause liquefaction and cavi-tation of lung |
| M. leprae | | Hansen's bacillus; acid-fast rod | Prolonged exposure, especially familial; skin or nasal mucosa may be portal of entrance; in-cubation about 3–5 yr; little immunity has been demon-strated; endemic regions: tropical countries and few states in U.S. | Destructive lesions of skin, pe-ripheral nerves, upper respira-tory passages, testes, hands, and feet; treatment may be curative |
| *Treponema palli-dum* (syphilis) | | Spiraled organism, with fi-brile, 3 at each end, contrac-tile elements for motility | Almost always transmitted by sexual contact; incubation av-erages 3 wk | Organism can penetrate any mucous membrane, enters blood and lymphatics; primary lesion at site of infection heals; secondary effects are lymph-adenopathy, rash, arterial in-flammation; tertiary syphilis in-volves CNS changes, dementia, inflammatory changes of aorta, etc. |

phagocytes to destroy the bacteria. Laboratory tests often note whether or not a bacterium is coagulase-positive.[2]

## FUNGI

Fungal or mycotic diseases are caused by yeasts and molds. They are divided into three groups, according to the part of the body they infect. *Systemic* or *deep mycoses* affect the internal organs or viscera. The pathogens in-volved can attack major systems and organs and may cause death. *Subcutaneous mycoses* infect the skin, sub-cutaneous tissue, fascia, and bone. Infection usually oc-curs from direct contamination with fungal spores or my-celia (mycelia are filamentous parts of fungi) fragments into wounds or broken areas of the skin. *Superficial my-coses* involve only the epidermis, hair, and nails. The principal habitat of the organisms is mammalian skin.[9]

Unlike bacteria, most pathogenic fungi produce no extracellular toxic substances. They usually stimulate hy-persensitivity to their antigenic components or metabo-lites that is thought to cause their pathogenicity. Of the many thousands of species of fungi, only about 50 cause pathology in humans. The structure of pathogenic fungi is similar to that of other fungi. Long, branching filaments

called *hyphae* are produced, which may divide into a chain of cells by forming walls or septa. As hyphae grow and branch, they form a mesh of growth called a *myce-lium*. Fungi reproduce sexually by spores when there is fusion or asexually by nuclei when there is no fusion.[8]

Saprophytic fungi that grow in the soil usually cause a systemic mycosis. The infection is transmitted from the soil or the droppings of fowl to humans through the in-halation of spores. Most deep mycoses are caused by free-living organisms and are limited to certain geo-graphic locations.[3] The severity of the disease depends on the degree of hypersensitivity of the host. The usual pathologic lesion is a chronic inflammatory granuloma that can produce abscess and necrosis.

Saprophytic fungi in the soil or on vegetation also can cause subcutaneous mycotic infection. This infection is opportunistic, in that it occurs by direct implantation through a crack or sore on the skin. As with the systemic mycoses, necrotic granulomatous lesions of any area may occur.

The superficial mycoses may represent allergic reac-tions to fungi. These organisms do not invade deeper tis-sues or become disseminated.

Table 12-5 summarizes some of the common human fungal infections. The reaction to these organisms often

**TABLE 12-5.**
COMMON FUNGI THAT CAUSE PATHOLOGIC EFFECTS IN HUMANS

| FUNGUS | MORPHOLOGY | EPIDEMIOLOGY | CLINICAL EFFECTS |
|---|---|---|---|
| Superficial dermato-phytoses: tinea pedis (athlete's foot), tinea capitis (scalp ringworm), tinea corporis (body ringworm) | Branching hyphae on microscopic examination; found on keratinized portion of skin, nail plate, and hair | Contact with fungus through skin; maceration or poor hygiene favor acquisition | Fissuring of toe webs, itching, irritation, areas of alopecia, and scaling; circumscribed lesion with round borders of inflammation leads to designation of *ringworm*; treatment curative |
| Systemic candidiasis (*C. albicans*) | Small, yeastlike cells; blastospores with budding; forms clusters of round growths on cornmeal agar | Contact with normal flora of mouth, stool, vagina; may be superficial or systemic in susceptible immunosuppressed people | *Oral* lesions: white plaques on mouth and tongue, may cause fissures and open sores; *urinary tract infection* after broad-spectrum antibiotic therapy or in person with diabetes mellitus; *vaginal* discharge may be profuse and irritating; *Candida* in serum may cause disseminated abscesses |
| Coccidioidomycoses (*C. immitis*) | Yeastlike cells; no budding is formed; divided into multiple small cells | Soil saprophyte in southern U.S., Mexico, South America; infection occurs with inhalation of arthrospores; symptoms begin 10–14 days after inhalation | *Primary form:* respiratory infection causes flulike symptoms, sometimes pneumonia; pleural effusion may occur; *progressive form:* dissemination to regional lymph nodes, skin, meninges, etc. may occur, especially with immunosuppressed, other than Caucasian; fever, cough, chest pain, pulmonary coin lesion |
| Histoplasmosis (*H. capsulatum*) | Dimorphic fungus; forms cottony white growth on glucose agar | Grows as mold, prefers moist soil; airborne exposure by cleaning chicken coops, working with soil | Cough, fever, weight loss, hilar adenopathy; progressive fibrosis of mediastinal structures; difficult to diagnose; treatment with amphotericin B may or may not be helpful; ultimate prognosis poor for disseminated type |
| Blastomyosis (*B. dermatitidis*) | Dimorphic fungus; budding, round, yeastlike cells | Majority of cases in southeast, central and mid-Atlantic U.S.; infection acquired by inhalation of fungus, reservoir unknown; incubation may be about 4 wk | Fever, cough, weight loss, chest pain, pneumonia, large skin lesions; responds well to treatment with amphotericin B |
| Cryptococcosis (*C. neoformans*) | Yeastlike, budding | Infection through inhalation in lungs, often opportunistic with immunosuppressed people (AIDS, lymphoma, etc.); fungus excreted in pigeon droppings | More common in males; pulmonary infection causes chest pain, cough, infiltrates; meningoencephalitis causes headache, dementia, confusion, cranial nerve palsies, cerebral edema, and death 2 wk to several years after diagnosis |

depends on host resistance and nutritional balance. Systemic fungal infections are more commonly seen in people who have a depressed immune resistance.

## PROTOZOA

Protozoa are complex, unicellular organisms that may be spherical, spindle-shaped, spiral, or cup-shaped.[8] Many absorb fluids through the cell membrane, and all possess the ability to move from place to place. Pathogenesis caused by protozoa often occurs in the gastrointestinal tract, genitourinary tract, and circulatory system. Table 12-6 summarizes several common protozoal diseases in humans.

The protozoa may be divided into four groups, or *subphyla.* The *flagellates* (Mastigophora) have flagella, or undulating membranes. They are considered to be some of the more primitive protozoa. This group includes members of *Giardia, Trichomonas,* and *Enteromonas* genera, which infect the intestinal or genitourinary tract.[2] Other flagellates, such as *Leishmania,* tend to be localized to skin, tissue, or mucous membranes. *Trypanosoma* organisms cause a systemic disease that frequently is fatal.[9] *Trichomonas vaginalis,* a common protozoal infection in women, is discussed in Chapter 57.

**TABLE 12–6.**
COMMON PROTOZOA THAT CAUSE PATHOLOGIC EFFECTS IN HUMANS

| PROTOZOA | MORPHOLOGY | EPIDEMIOLOGY | CLINICAL EFFECTS |
|---|---|---|---|
| Amebiasis (*Entamoeba histolytica*) | Motile trophozoite usually seen in active disease; cysts form usual means of disease transmission; anaerobic | Cysts transmitted from human feces; contaminated food, poor personal hygiene | Chronic, mild diarrhea to fulminant dysentery; stools may contain mucus and blood, may persist for months or years; numerous trophozoites found in stools; fever, abdominal cramps, and hepatomegaly common |
| Malaria (*Plasmodium vivax, Plasmodium ovale, Plasmodium malariae, Plasmodium falciparum*) | Asexual phase passed in human body; multiple in liver, called *exoerythrocytic* cycle; then enter RBCs and multiply, *trophozoite* stage; as RBCs hemolyze, segments called *merozoites* released into blood | Transmitted by bite of infected female *Anopheles* mosquito; incubation period varies with type of organism from 10 days–7 wk | Anemia due to loss of RBCs; hemolyzing process with release of parasites causes chills and fever; immunologic mechanisms cause normal as well as infected RBC hemolysis; debilitation progressive; hepatic complications may cause permanent damage |
| Toxoplasmosis (*Toxoplasma gondii*) | Intracellular protozoa exist in trophozoites; cysts and oocysts form; trophozoites invade all cells; cysts often take the form of transmission; oocysts transmitted through cycle by cat; form not seen in humans | Transplacental transfusion or fecal-oral cysts; may be in lamb or pork | Focal areas of necrosis, especially of eyes, but may cause CNS or disseminated effects; lymphadenopathy common in immunosuppressed people; CNS involvement leads to high mortality; may infect fetus of affected mother |
| *Pneumocystis carinii* | Pleomorphic forms, sporozoites, trophozoites, and cyst; primitive organelles; apparently does not have intracellular phase | Worldwide distribution; opportunistic protozoan; transmitted by airborne route, usually does not cause disease unless host is debilitated; especially seen in AIDS; incubation thought to be about 4–8 wk | Dyspnea, fever, nonproductive cough; progresses to pneumonia, bilateral diffuse infiltrates; cyanosis and arterial deoxygenation characteristic; frequently fatal in AIDS cases |

Typical ameboid characteristics are seen in the subphylum Sarcodina. Species of the genera *Entamoeba, Endolimax,* and *Iodamoeba* are representative of this group.

Organisms in the Sporozoa subphylum have a definite life cycle that usually involves two different hosts, one of which often is the arthropod and the other a vertebrate. *Plasmodium,* genus of the malaria parasites, is representative of this group.

Together with the Sporozoa, organisms in the subphylum Ciliata are the most complex of the protozoa. These organisms have cilia distributed in rows or patches and two kinds of nuclei in each individual. *Balantidium coli* is the only representative that is pathogenic to humans. It is a rare cause of infection, with only a few cases being recorded.

The *Pneumocystis carinii* is a protozoan organism that has received considerable attention since it has been identified as an opportunistic pathogen in people suffering from acquired immunodeficiency syndrome. The clinical features include dyspnea, fever, and cough. The progression of pulmonary symptoms and pneumonia often is chronic, occurring over several months. Pneumonia with diffuse pulmonary infiltrates often is the cause of death in these immunocompromised people.[10]

The motility of the protozoa is accomplished by pseudopod or by the action of flagella or cilia. In *pseudopod* movement, characteristic of many ameboid cells, the projection is actively pressed forward and rapidly followed by the rest of the organism. The movement usually is directional, toward a specific focus. *Flagella* are whiplike projections that cause rapid movement of the organism from place to place. *Cilia* are shorter and more delicate, and cover the entire outer surface of the organism. The synchronous action of these structures allows the organism to move rapidly.[6]

Reproduction may be sexual or asexual, depending on the species. The sexual cycle, when it occurs, takes place in the definitive host, whereas the asexual cycle takes place in the intermediate host.[8] Protozoa capable of sexual reproduction are called *gametes,* and those of asexual reproduction are called *zygotes.* Protozoa also have the ability to form cysts, which means that they can surround themselves with a resistant membrane. This prevents destruction and allows them to live for a long time.

**TABLE 12–7.**
COMMON HELMINTHS THAT CAUSE PATHOLOGIC EFFECTS IN HUMANS

| HELMINTHS | MORPHOLOGY | EPIDEMIOLOGY | CLINICAL EFFECTS |
|---|---|---|---|
| Trematodes (flukes; schistosomiasis, S. mansoni, S. haematobium, S. japonicum) | Blood flukes grow and mature in portal venous system; may attain 1–2 cm in length; life span 4–30 yr | Eggs of worm pair excreted in feces or urine of humans hatch miracidia that penetrate a specific snail host and transform into infective larvae; these penetrate human skin and are carried to rest finally in portal venous circulation; worldwide distribution | Usually asymptomatic; may cause dermatitis at focus of entry; cause mild fever and malaise; acute fever begins 1–2 mo after exposure, often associated with lymphadenopathy and hepatomegaly, eosinophil levels markedly elevated; mucosa of bowel may become ulcerative and ova may be recovered from stool specimens. S. haematobium causes hematuria with involvement of kidneys, ureters, bladder, and seminal vesicles |
| Cestodes (tapeworms; Taenia saginata [beef], Taenia solium [pork], Hymenolepis nana [dwarf], Dipylidium caninum [dog]) | Segmented ribbon-shaped hermaphroditic worms; absorb food through their surface; attach to host intestinal mucosa by sucking cups; length varies with species from 1 cm–10 m | Transmitted when raw or poorly cooked beef or pork eaten; other types may be transmitted by fecal-oral route, man to man or dog to man; usually matures in adult intestines | Weight loss, hunger, epigastric discomfort; in T. solium, encysted larvae may deposit in muscles, eyes, and brain; leads to eosinophilia, weakness, muscle pain; anemia may result from tapeworm competition for nutrition |
| Nematodes | Elongated, cylindric, unsegmented organisms from a few millimeters to a meter in length; life span 1–2 mo–10 yr | | |
| Trichinosis (Trichinella spiralis) | | Encysted larvae of T. spiralis ingested in poorly cooked pork or bear meat; larvae released in intestinal mucosa, multiply, and new larvae migrate into vascular channels throughout body; lodge in skeletal muscle, become encysted and grow for 5–10 yr | Severe inflammation of muscles in major infestation of muscle; may begin with diarrhea and fever; muscle pain, conjunctivitis, and rash may develop; eosinophilia common; neurotoxic symptoms and myocarditis may be seen |
| Enterobiasis (pinworm, threadworm; Enterobius vermicularis) | Female 10 mm, male 3 mm; live attached to mucosa of bowel; female deposits eggs on perianal skin at night, then dies | Fecal-oral transmission, transfer of eggs from anus to mouth; contamination of bed linens, remains viable 2–3 wk; common infection in humans | Pruritus of anal and genital region common, especially at night; bladder infection or other foci relatively rare; simultaneous treatment of entire families and group essential |
| Hookworm (Ancylostoma duodenale, Necator americanus) | Four prominent hooklike teeth attach worm to upper part of small intestine; adults about 1 cm in length | Affects about 700 million persons worldwide; greatest incidence in Africa, Asia, tropical Americas; transmitted by invasion of exposed skin by larvae, migrates through lungs and resides in GI tract; excretion of larvae in fecal material perpetuates cycle | Iron deficiency anemia and hypoalbuminemia result from chronic intestinal blood loss; most infections asymptomatic but may have GI distress or ulcerlike pain; eosinophilia common |

## *HELMINTHS*

The word *helminth* means worm, and usually refers to pathogenic worms, many of which are parasitic. The common intestinal helminths are divided into three general groups: (1) *nematodes,* or roundworms; (2) *trematodes,* or flukes; and (3) *cestodes,* or tapeworms. Helminths are complex organisms in both their structure and their life cycle. Many spend part of their developmental life in several locations and in various hosts such as fish, hogs, rats, snails, and humans. Their eggs, or larvae, often are eliminated in the feces or urine of humans and may be found in the feces on microscopic examination. The mode of infection for intestinal helminths often is through fecal-oral transmission or through broken skin.

Table 12-7 summarizes some common diseases caused by helminths. These conditions, although not often fatal, are an important source of disability worldwide.

# REFERENCES

1.  Bellanti, J.A. Host-parasite relationships. In J.A. Bellanti, *Immunology III*. Philadelphia: W.B. Saunders, 1985.
2.  Benenson, A.S. *Control of Communicable Diseases in Man* (14th ed.). Washington, D.C.: American Public Health Association, 1985.
3.  Bennett, J.E. Fungal infections. In J. Wilson et al., *Harrison's Principles of Internal Medicine* (12th ed.). New York: McGraw-Hill, 1991.
4.  Fields, B.N. The biology of viruses. In J. Wilson et al., *Harrison's Principles of Internal Medicine* (12th ed.). New York: McGraw-Hill, 1991.
5.  Jawetz, E., and Grossman, M. Introduction to infectious diseases. In M.A. Krupp, M.J. Chatton, and L.M. Tierney, *Current Medical Diagnosis and Treatment 1986*. Los Altos, Calif.: Lange, 1986.
6.  Plorde, J.J. Trichomonas and other protozoan infections. In J. Wilson et al., *Harrison's Principles of Internal Medicine* (12th ed.). New York: McGraw-Hill, 1991.
7.  Root, R.K. Infectious diseases: Pathogenic mechanisms and host responses. In L.H. Smith and S.O. Thier, *Pathophysiology: The Biological Principles of Disease* (2nd ed.). Philadelphia: W.B. Saunders, 1985.
8.  Smith, A.L. *Principles of Microbiology* (10th ed.). St. Louis: C.V. Mosby, 1985.
9.  von Lichtenberg, F. Infectious disease. In R.S. Cotran, V. Kumar, and S.L. Robbins, *Robbins Pathologic Basis of Disease* (4th ed.). Philadelphia: Saunders, 1989.
10. Walzer, P.D. *Pneumocystis carinii* pneumonia. In J. Wilson et al., *Harrison's Principles of Internal Medicine* (12th ed.). New York: McGraw-Hill, 1991.
11. Woodward, T.E. Rickettsial diseases. In J. Wilson et al., *Harrison's Principles of Internal Medicine* (12th ed.). New York: McGraw-Hill, 1991.

# Inflammation and Resolution of Inflammation

## Chapter Outline

▶ **Acute Inflammation**
  **Vascular Phase**
  **Cellular Phase**
    Margination and Pavementing
    Emigration
    Recognition and Phagocytosis
  **Mediators of Inflammation**
    Complement
    Autocoids (Arachidonic Acid
      Metabolites)
    Kinins
    Coagulation System
    Histamine and Serotonin
    Lymphokines
    Neutrophils

  **Exudates**
  **Summary of the Acute**
    **Inflammatory Response**
▶ **Chronic Inflammation**
▶ **Local and Systemic Effects of**
  **Inflammation**
  **Lymphadenopathy**
  **Fever**
  **Erythrocytic Sedimentation**
    **Rate**
  **Leukocytosis**
▶ **Resolution of Inflammation**
  **Simple Resolution**
  **Regeneration**

**Repair by Scar**
  Healing by First Intention
  Healing by Second Intention
**Factors That Delay Wound**
  **Healing**
**Aberrant Healing**
  Exuberant Granulation and
    Keloids
  Contracture
  Dehiscence and Evisceration
  Stenosis and Constriction
  Adhesions

## Learning Objectives

1. Define and describe different types of mechanical and physical wounds.
2. List factors that can cause inflammation.
3. Describe the vascular and cellular phases of acute inflammation.
4. Define *chemotaxis* and *chemotactic gradient*.
5. Explain leukocyte response in inflammation.
6. Describe directional emigration.
7. Draw or describe phagocytosis.
8. Briefly explain how organisms are killed.
9. Describe the functions of the major mediators of the inflammatory system.
10. Draw the classic and alternate pathways for complement activation.
11. Define the types of exudates and show familiarity with how they are named.
12. Differentiate chronic inflammation from acute inflammation.

13. Describe the reasons for the effects of inflammation, including fever, leukocytosis, lymphadenopathy, lymphangitis, lymphadenitis, and neutropenia.
14. Briefly explain the process of simple resolution in inflammation.
15. Explain why regeneration occurs in some tissues and not in others.
16. Describe the process of repair by scar tissue.
17. Define *cicatrization*.
18. Differentiate between healing by first intention and healing by second intention.
19. Define *epithelialization* in wound healing.
20. Describe exuberant granuloma and keloid scar formation.
21. Define *contracture* as a normal and abnormal part of wound healing.
22. Define *stenosis, constriction, adhesion, dehiscence*, and *evisceration*.

In the process of living, injury to the body tissues and organs inevitably occurs. Healing and repair of these tissues and organs must proceed for life to be maintained. Wound healing and inflammation are part of many disease processes and are modified or altered by many environmental and individual factors. Healing normally is preceded by inflammation, which provides a cellular environment conducive to healing.

Injury normally is prevented by the body's host defense system, which includes both physical and chemical barriers (Box 13-1). The inflammatory response, which includes white blood cells and their chemical mediators, provides a mechanism for ridding the body of microorganisms and decreasing their injury potential.[7]

A *wound* is a break or interruption of the continuity of a tissue caused by *mechanical* or *physical* means (Table 13-1). A mechanical wound is caused by some kind of trauma that damages the tissues. Physical wounds may result from organisms, chemical or thermal agents, or death of tissues or organs. Each type of wound results in inflammation, which is the reaction of the body to tissue injury.

Inflammation usually is a beneficial response to invasion by microbial agents or to tissue injury. It normally proceeds on a continuum from the inflammatory phase to the healing phase. Inflammation can be defined as a tissue reaction to injury that characteristically involves vascular and cellular responses working together in a coordinated manner to destroy substances recognized as being foreign to the body. The tissue is then restored to its previous state or repaired in such a way that the tissue or organ can retain viability. The process of inflammation is closely related to the process of immunity (see Chap. 14).

## BOX 13-1.
### MECHANISMS OF HOST DEFENSE

Physical and chemical barriers
  Morphologic integrity of skin, mucous membranes
  Sphincters
  Epiglottis
  Normal secretory and excretory flow
  Endogenous microbial flora
  Gastric acidity
Inflammatory response
  Circulating phagocytes
  Complement
  Other humoral mediators (bradykinins, fibrinolytic systems, acid cascade)
Reticuloendothelial system
  Tissue phagocytes
Immune response
  T lymphocytes and their soluble products
  B lymphocytes and immunoglobulins

*Wilson, J.D., et al. Harrison's Principles of Internal Medicine (12th ed.). New York: McGraw-Hill, 1991.*

Healing ideally involves the return of tissue to its previous state. Tissue regeneration also participates in the healing process. If the amount of tissue damaged is excessive, scar tissue may result.

Inflammatory states may be classified as *acute* or *chronic*. Acute inflammation involves the vascular and cellular changes that characterize the process. Chronic inflammation follows a persistent, self-perpetuating course, with the source of the inflammation being unresolved. The most common causes of inflammation include (1) infection from microorganisms in the tissues; (2) physical trauma, often causing free blood in the tissues; (3) chemical, irradiation, mechanical, or thermal injury, causing direct irritation to the tissues; and (4) immune reactions, causing hypersensitivity responses in the tissues.

## ACUTE INFLAMMATION

### Vascular Phase

When injury occurs large amounts of strong chemical substances are released in the tissue. These substances create a "chemical wall" called a *chemotactic gradient*, which provides a source toward which fluids and cells begin to move. The first reaction to injury is a neural reflex that causes vasoconstriction, which initially decreases the blood flow. It is rapidly followed by arteriolar and venular dilatation, the hyperemic response, which allows fluids to cross from the capillaries into the tissue spaces. The increased permeability allows protein-rich fluid high in fibrinogen to move into the area of high chemical concentration. This fluid may dilute the injurious chemicals and bring complement, antibodies, and other chemotactic substances to the area. The plasma proteins leaked into the tissues provide an osmotic gradient, or pull, that brings more water in from the plasma (Figure 13-1A).

### Cellular Phase

The components of the fluid exudation cause a characteristic response by the leukocytes commonly described as margination and pavementing, directional emigration, aggregation, recognition, and phagocytosis. The properties of the leukocytes allow for the destruction of the foreign material and the removal of cellular debris (see Chap. 20).

### Margination and Pavementing

Margination refers to the movement of granulocytes and monocytes toward the endothelial lining of the vessel. Because of the increased capillary permeability that results from the initial injury, the movement of blood

**TABLE 13-1.**
TYPES OF MECHANICAL AND PHYSICAL WOUNDS

| WOUND | DEFINITION |
|---|---|
| **Mechanical** | |
| Incision | Caused by cutting instrument; wound edges are in close proximity, aligned |
| Contusion | Caused by blunt instrument, usually disrupting skin or organ surface; causes hemorrhage or ecchymosis of affected tissue |
| Abrasion | Caused by rubbing or scraping of epidermal layers of skin or mucous membranes |
| Laceration | Caused by tissue tearing, with blunt or irregular instrument; tissue non-aligned with loose flaps of tissue |
| Puncture | Caused by piercing of tissue or organ with a pointed instrument accidentally, such as with a nail, or intentionally, such as a venipuncture |
| Projectile or penetrating | Caused by foreign body entering tissues at high velocity; fragments of foreign missile may scatter to various tissues and organs |
| Avulsion | Caused by tearing of a structure from its normal anatomic position; damage to vessels, nerves, and other structures may be associated |
| **Physical** | |
| Microbial agents | Living organisms may affect skin, mucous membranes, organs, and bloodstream; secrete exotoxins; or release endotoxins or affect other cells |
| Chemical agents | Agents toxic to specific cells include pharmaceutic agents, substances released from cellular necrosis, acids, alcohols, metals, and others |
| Thermal agents | High or low temperatures can produce wounds of various thicknesses; these in turn may lead to cellular necrosis |
| Irradiation | Ultraviolet light or radiation exposure affects epithelial or mucous membranes; large doses of whole-body radiation cause changes in CNS, blood-forming system, and GI system |

is slowed. The polymorphonuclear leukocytes (PMNs), mostly neutrophils, drop to the side of the capillary to form a layer closely approximated to the endothelial lining. This layer assumes a particular appearance called *pavementing* (Figure 13-1B). The platelets and a few red blood cells may join the PMNs on the endothelial lining. The endothelial cells normally are charged so that blood cells are repelled, but the changes that occur during inflammation appear to inhibit this property.

## Emigration

White blood cells move to the area of injury by emigration. Neutrophils move by ameboid motion toward the chemotactic signal (chemical gradient) by projecting a pseudopodium into the gap between two endothelial cells. This active process is followed by the cytoplasm streaming toward the projected extension (Figure 13-1C).[2] The entire leukocyte then arrives in the tissue spaces. The first leukocytes on the scene are neutrophils. Monocytes (macrophages) and lymphocytes arrive later. Red blood cells may passively leak into the tissues after the PMNs or after hydrostatic pressure changes.

Directional orientation for the movement of the PMNs is through chemotaxis. *Chemotaxis* is the directional movement of ameboid cells along a concentration gradient composed of substances such as bacterial toxins, products of tissue breakdown, activated complement factors, and other factors. The gradient provides a directional force that draws phagocytic cells to the area (Figure 13-1D).

## Recognition and Phagocytosis

Phagocytosis is a highly specific process that requires recognition of the foreign particle by the phagocyte before actual attack and engulfment can take place. The major phagocytes are neutrophils and macrophages. Neutrophils usually require the foreign material to be coated with a substance called *opsonin*. Opsonins include immunoglobulins, especially IgG, and the opsonic fragment of C3 (see Chap. 14).[2] Once the foreign particles are recognized, their receptors are attached by the leukocyte, and phagocytosis occurs. Macrophages also may respond to opsonized or other foreign material.

Phagocytosis involves the engulfment of foreign material. The cytoplasm of the phagocyte flows around the foreign particle and ingests it. Cytoplasmic lysosomes attach to the ingested particle and release hydrolytic enzymes into it, which often kill the microorganisms or dissolve foreign proteins (Figure 13-1E). In the process, the phagocyte often dies and releases its proteolytic enzymes

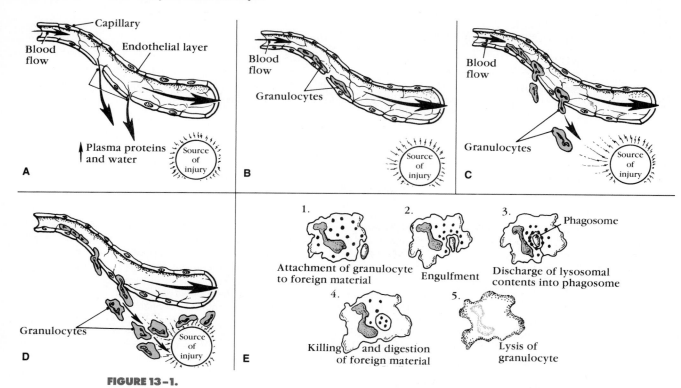

**FIGURE 13–1.**

Acute inflammation. (**A**) Vascular phase. Increased permeability of endothelial junctions allows the movement of plasma proteins into interstitial spaces, pulling water into the area and leading to edema. This increased permeability is induced by chemical mediators given off by the foreign agent or by cells' reaction. It occurs immediately after the injury, and primarily affects the venulae. (**B**) Cellular phase. Granulocytes marginate to the wall of the blood vessel. This also is probably a response to the chemical messengers. As groups stick to the endothelium, a pavementing pattern is seen. The leukocyte then begins to move by ameboid action toward the endothelial junctions. (**C**) Emigration. Granulocytes move by ameboid action through the endothelial gaps toward the chemotactic source. (**D**) Chemotaxis. Large numbers of granulocytes accumulate in the area of injury. (**E**) Phagocytosis engulfs and destroys foreign material. Many granulocytes also are destroyed and may release their lytic enzymes into surrounding tissues.

into the surrounding tissue, causing injury to surrounding cells and resulting in the digestion of the cell membrane of the phagocyte.

Accumulations of large numbers of phagocytes lead to pus accumulations and, eventually, the destruction and removal of foreign material. Phagocytosis localizes or walls off foreign material, preventing the spread of the process to other areas.

Phagocytosis is an energy-dependent process and stimulates the production of hydrogen peroxide within the lysosomes of the phagocyte. The pH of the lysosome drops to about 4.0, which enhances the action of the hydrolytic enzymes.[2] The quantities of hydrogen peroxide produced are apparently not sufficient to induce a bactericidal effect, but they increase in the presence of myeloperoxidase and a halide ion. Myeloperoxidase is present in the granules of the neutrophils.[9] Superoxide, formed during oxidative metabolism, has been studied in bacterial killing during phagocytosis.[9] These, and other tissue-injuring by-products, have been called free radicals, which function in bacterial killing and in tissue-damaging reactions.

Some organisms are virulent and quite resistant to destruction by the phagocytes. Others, such as the tuberculosis bacillus, are engulfed, but not destroyed, by macrophages and live within the cell for years.[2]

## Mediators of Inflammation

Many mediators of the inflammatory system are responsible for the effectiveness of the response and limitations on tissue damage. General factors that promote a beneficial inflammatory reaction include adequate blood supply, nutrition, age, and general health. This section deals with some of the major chemical mediators known to play an important role in promoting inflammation. Research has disclosed complicated interplay among the various mediators and a cooperative system with enhancers and depressors to the response.

### Complement

The complement system has been identified as a major mediator of the inflammatory response. It is essential in promoting the acute inflammatory reaction elicited by bacteria, some viruses, and immune complex disease.[6] The system contains at least 18 distinct proteins and their cleavage products. Complement components normally are present in the blood in the form of inactive proteins called *zymogens*.[6] These are sequentially activated, with each component activating the next in the series (Figure 13-2). The complement system enhances chemotaxis, increases vascular permeability, and, in the final conversion, causes cell lysis. Fixation or activation of complement at the C1 level is by antigen–antibody interaction. This *classic pathway* continues a reaction pattern until the C8 and C9 enzymes are activated (see Chap. 14).

The *alternate pathway* is initiated by cleavage or activation of the C3 portion by plasmin, trypsin, bacterial proteases, and other enzymes found in the tissues. The C5 fragment also can be activated by many of these same substances. These pathways may be important mediators of the inflammatory process to clear agents that have little immunologic specificity, such as some bacterial products and proteases present in normal tissue.[6]

The inflammatory process is greatly diminished in the absence of complement enzymes. Deficiency of C3 especially causes a depression of the response and poor clearing of infection (see Chap. 15).[4]

### Autocoids (Arachidonic Acid Metabolites)

*Prostaglandins* and related substances belong to a group of so-called autocoids or local, short-range hormones that exert their effects locally and are rapidly broken down.[2] These substances can be synthesized by most connective tissue, blood, and parenchymal cells. Through a complex conversion process, another group of active substances, called *leukotrienes*, is formed. Some of these substances (previously called slow-reacting substances of anaphylaxis, or SRS-A) are potent mediators of smooth-muscle contraction and increased chemotaxis (Figure 13-3).[9] During cell injury, phospholipids become available for conversion to prostaglandins. Other mediators of inflammation, such as bradykinin, also have been shown to stimulate prostaglandin synthesis. Some of the prostaglandins function as vasodilators by enhancing vascular permeability. This leads to edema, with increased concentrations of these substances in the fluids and exudates of inflammatory reactions. The mechanism by which prostaglandins increase fever is not known, but local production is thought to affect the hypothalamus, which then transmits the information to the vasomotor system, resulting in stimulation of the sympathetic nervous system.

### Kinins

Substances called kinins can cause vasodilation. *Bradykinin*, a small polypeptide, is activated by the enzyme *kallikrein*. Kallikrein, present in the body fluids in an inactive form, can be activated by a decreased pH of body fluids, changes in temperature, contact with abnormal surfaces, and activation of the Hageman factor (XII) of the clotting system.

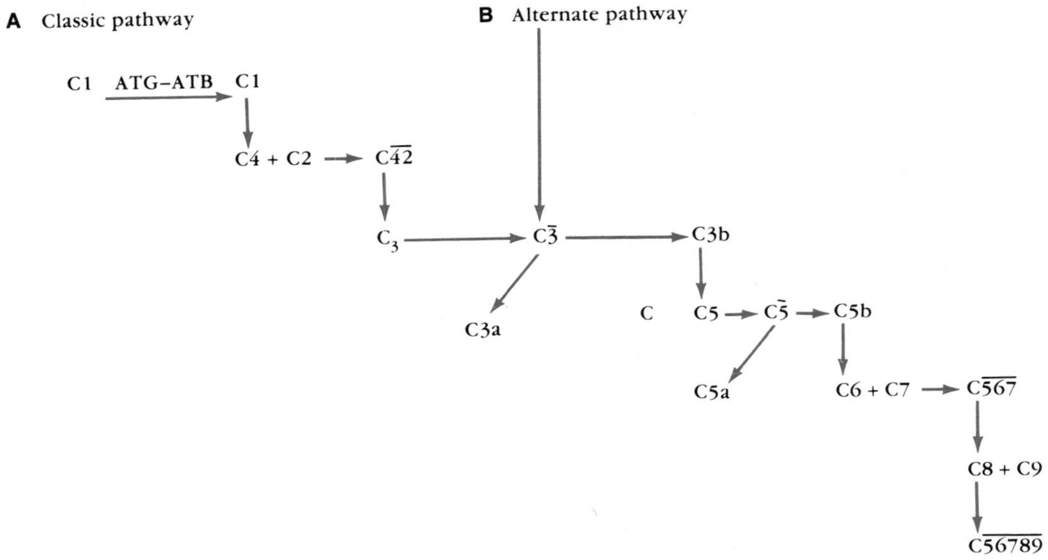

**FIGURE 13–2.**
Complement activation. (**A**) Classic pathway activated by ATG–ATB reaction. (**B**) Alternate pathway at C3 activated by endotoxins, trypsin, plasmin, and tissue proteases. (**C**) Alternate pathway at C5 activated by trypsin, bacterial proteases, and macrophages. C3a increases vascular permeability; anaphylotoxin causes liberation of histamine from mast cells and platelets; C3b is an opsonic factor; C5a increases chemotaxis and vascular permeability; C567 complex is chemotactic; C89 causes breakdown of cell membrane (cell lysis).

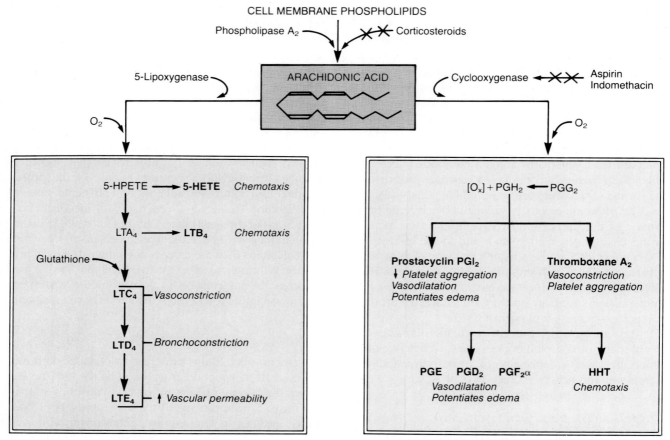

**FIGURE 13–3.**
Arachidonic acid metabolites in inflammation. The principal mediators are the leukotrienes (LTA4, LTB4, LTC4, LTD4, and LTE4), the prostaglandins (PGG$_2$, PGH$_2$, PGI$_2$, PGE, PGD$_{2a}$, PGF$_2$), and thromboxane A$_2$. Arachidonic acid may be converted to HPETE, which is a hydroperoxy derivative (hydroperoxy eicosatetranoic acid). It then may undergo peroxidation to HETE, which is a chemotactic stimulus for neutrophils. (From R. Cotran, V. Kumar, and S.L. Robbins, *Pathologic Basis of Disease* [4th ed.]. Philadelphia: W.B. Saunders, 1989. Reprinted by permission.)

The Hageman factor may be activated by endotoxins, cartilage contact, and contact with basement membrane tissue. Bradykinin is a powerful vasodilator; kallikrein, which can be converted to bradykinin, has been shown to have chemotactic properties.[9]

## Coagulation System

Factor XII, the Hageman factor, activated by surface-active agents, causes the activation of the coagulation proteins as well as conversion of prekallikrein to kallikrein. Kallikrein then causes further activation of the Hageman factor (Figure 13-4).[2] Complement also works in the coagulation system through activation of the Hageman factor. The process is not fully understood but may be an underlying factor in disseminated intravascular coagulation (see Chap. 21).[6] Plasminogen may be activated to plasmin in the process that lyses fibrin clots and also activates the alternate pathway of complement. Several factors in this system lead to increased vascular permeability.

## Histamine and Serotonin

In the immediate postinjury phase, histamine and serotonins are the major mediators of increased vascular permeability. Histamine is present mostly in mast cells, basophils, and platelets. Many agents promote its release from tissue, including mast cell and IgE reactions, C3 and C5a fragments, trauma, heat, and lysosomes of neutrophils.[3] The release is due to increased vascular permeability and histamine-releasing factors.

Some serotonin is present in the platelets, but the major source of this amine is the mucosal layer of the gastrointestinal tract. It is not present in mast cells of humans. Release from platelets occurs when platelet aggregation is stimulated.

## Lymphokines

Lymphokines are released from T lymphocytes during immunologic reactions (see Chap. 14). This group of va-

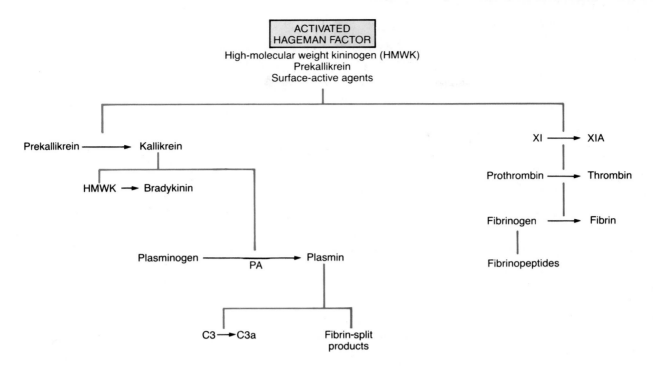

**FIGURE 13-4.**

Plasma mediator systems triggered by activation of Hageman factor. PA = plasminogen activator. (Adapted from R. Cotran, V. Kumar, and S.L. Robbins, *Pathologic Basis of Disease* [4th ed.]. Philadelphia: W.B. Saunders, 1989.)

soactive substances has a major role in immunologic reactions and also induces chemotaxis for neutrophils (PMNs) and macrophages.

## Neutrophils

The lysosomes of neutrophils contain potent proteins and proteases that can activate the alternate pathway for complement, release kininlike substance, and release cationic proteins, all of which increase vascular permeability.[2] As the neutrophils die and release their products into the surrounding tissue, chemotaxis and vasodilation are enhanced. Box 13-2 summarizes the most common chemical mediators of inflammation.

## Exudates

In the process of inflammation, different types of exudates are formed, the analysis of which may offer clues to the nature of the process. An exudate is fluid or matter collecting in a cavity or tissue space. The simplest exudate, the *serous* exudate, is the protein-rich fluid that escapes into the tissues in the early stages of inflammation. Because of its high protein content, it draws water, and thus is responsible for the edema at the site of an inflammatory reaction. Depending on the source of the inflammation, other types of exudates may be seen. These are

**BOX 13-2.**
MOST LIKELY MEDIATORS IN INFLAMMATION

Vasodilation
  Prostaglandins
  Histamine
  Serotonin
Increased vascular permeability
  Vasoactive amines
  C3a and C5a (through liberating amines)
  Bradykinin
  Leukotrienes C, D, E
Chemotaxis
  C5a
  Leukotriene B$_4$
  Other chemotactic lipids
  Bacterial products
Fever
  Endogenous pyrogen
  Prostaglandins
Pain
  Prostaglandins
  Bradykinin
Tissue damage
  Neutrophil and macrophage lysosomal enzymes
  Oxygen-derived free radicals
  Growth factors
  Platelet-activating factors (PAF)
  C8-C9

*Adapted from Cotran, R., Kumar, V., and Robbins, S.L. Robbins Pathologic Basis of Disease (4th ed.). Philadelphia: W. B. Saunders, 1989. Reprinted by permission.*

**TABLE 13-2.**
TYPES OF EXUDATES

| TYPE | DESCRIPTION |
| --- | --- |
| Serous | Exudate fluid high in proteins; without cells |
| Fibrinous | Exudate has high content of fibrin; may lead to development of adhesions |
| Hemorrhagic | Usually suppurative exudation also containing red blood cells |
| Purulent | Exudate that contains pus |
| Suppurative | Exudate with pus and tissue damage from breakdown of neutrophils and macrophages; polymorphonuclear leukocytes major cells in early suppurations; macrophages in old exudates |
| Abscess | Area of pus, usually located in an organ |
| Furuncle | Abscess of skin |
| Carbuncle | Extensive abscess of skin that tends to spread |
| Serofibrinous | Serous exudate with high fibrin content |
| Fibrinopurulent | Purulent exudate with high fibrin content |

described in Table 13-2, which shows that the nomenclature depends on the constituents of the exudates.

## Summary of the Acute Inflammatory Response

Acute inflammation begins with the invasion of the body by an agent recognized as being foreign. The initial response often is vasoconstriction, followed closely by vasodilatation. Vasodilatation, or hyperemic response, causes increased vascular permeability, which leads to the exudation of serous, protein-rich fluid into the area. This fluid, together with histamines and other substances, sets up a chemotactic gradient toward which leukocytes are attracted. These ameboid cells marginate and emigrate along the chemotactic gradient. The first cells to be delivered to the area are PMNs, which attack and phagocytize the foreign material once it is recognized as foreign. Recognition occurs through opsonization, which is the coating of the foreign material by antibody, or through fragments of the complement factors. Complement enhances hyperemia, chemotaxis, and opsonization, and causes cell lysis. When the foreign agent is destroyed, the cellular debris is removed by macrophages and neutrophils and the inflammation resolves (see pp. 289–291).

## CHRONIC INFLAMMATION

When an inflammatory process persists in the tissues and is not cleared by the body, certain patterns of response occur. The chronically inflamed area usually is infiltrated by mononuclear leukocytes, mostly macrophages and lymphocytes, whereas the acute process mostly contains PMNs. Certain types of chronic inflammation, such as

osteomyelitis, contain neutrophils for months, whereas some types of acute inflammation have increased numbers of lymphocytes in the early phase. When macrophages are the predominant cells, they divide and multiply, and release chemotactic substances that attract more macrophages. The inflammatory process may begin as a low-grade, poorly cleared inflammation, or as an acute inflammation that is not totally resolved by the body.

Chronic inflammation results in infiltration of the site with fibroblasts, increased amounts of collagen deposits, and varying amounts of scar tissue formation. The scar tissue and smoldering inflammation often cause organ dysfunction.

A distinctive pattern of chronic inflammation is the *granulomatous* inflammation, which is characterized by the accumulation of large *macrophages* or *histiocytes*. The offending foreign material is walled off from the rest of the body but not removed. In tuberculosis, the resulting granuloma is called a *tubercle*, which is characterized by caseous necrosis and calcium infiltration at the rim of the granuloma.[2] Calcium infiltration in injured tissue is usual in a chronic inflammatory process.

## LOCAL AND SYSTEMIC EFFECTS OF INFLAMMATION

All types of inflammation have in common the following five cardinal signs, which were described many centuries ago: calor (heat), dolor (pain), rubor (redness), tumor (swelling), and loss of normal function. These result from vasodilatation, exudation, and irritation of nerve endings. The vasodilatation is associated with the release of chemical mediators, as described earlier. Exudation results from fluid and white blood cell movement into the affected area. Nerve endings are irritated by chemical mediators, causing pain and sometimes loss of functioning.

## Lymphadenopathy

Lymphadenopathy is a sign of a severe, localized infection. It results when the local lymph nodes and vessels drain the infected material, which becomes enmeshed in the follicular tissue of the nodes.

Increased lymphatic flow is characteristic of localized inflammation. If an inflammation of the lymphatic vessel occurs, it is termed *lymphangitis*. If it affects the lymph nodes, it is termed *lymphadenitis*. The lymph system helps to keep infections localized and away from the bloodstream.

## Fever

Fever is an almost universal phenomenon of illness, particularly of inflammation. It is thought to be caused by the release of *endogenous pyrogens* from macrophages and possibly from eosinophils, which are activated by phagocytosis, endotoxins, immune complexes, and other products. These pyrogens (fever-producing substances) act on the temperature-regulating centers in the hypothalamus to elevate the thermostat set-point. In response to the pyrogens, the body generates an arachidonic acid and the prostaglandin $PGE_1$, which actively mediate the central responses and may further increase the hypothalamic set-point (see Table 13-1 and Figure 13-3).[8] The body then initiates heat conservation measures, including vasoconstriction, piloerection (gooseflesh), and shivering, to drive the body temperature up to a new level. These mechanisms, along with conscious heat conservation measures, such as covering the person with blankets, aid the body in attaining the new set-point. Therefore, the new set-point may be 38° to 40°C. Above 40°C the temperature control regulation can become seriously impaired, causing central nervous system damage.

When the set-point is reached or the stimulus is removed, the body initiates cooling measures, including vasodilation (flush) and sweating, to maintain the set-point. If the set-point returns to normal, the fever rapidly dissipates. This rapid resolution has been termed "breaking of the fever," and may signify that the causative agent has been destroyed. Effective antibiotic therapy can rapidly destroy a pyrogen that produces bacteria and cause a rapid recovery of the temperature control mechanism. Also, antipyretic agents, such as aspirin and acetaminophen, can interfere with prostaglandin synthesis and reduce fever.

The purpose of fever is unknown, but in the presence of elevated body temperature, the phagocytes act more quickly to accomplish their purpose. The metabolism of the body is increased, which may promote phagocytosis by increased blood flow. Fever in viral infections may stimulate interferon production, and thus may limit the course of the viral infection.[10]

## Erythrocyte Sedimentation Rate

The erythrocyte sedimentation rate is the rate at which red blood cells settle in a test tube. In inflammation, the rate is elevated, probably because of alterations in plasma components that occur during the inflammatory process.

## Leukocytosis

Leukocytosis refers to an elevation in the white blood cell count. The rise in the number of cells is selective, according to the causative agent. For example, pyogenic bacteria often cause an increase in the neutrophil count, whereas helminthic infections may cause eosinophilia (see Chap. 20).

In advanced or overwhelming infections, neutropenia may occur. This depletion of neutrophils indicates that the system is unable to mount an adequate defense.

## RESOLUTION OF INFLAMMATION

For the body to maintain a steady state, foreign material must be removed or isolated to prevent deleterious effects on the body. This is accomplished through (1) simple resolution, (2) regeneration, or (3) replacement by a connective tissue scar.

## Simple Resolution

Simple resolution involves no destruction of normal tissue and probably goes on continuously in the human body. The offending agent is neutralized and destroyed. The vessels return to their normal permeability, and excess fluid exudation is reabsorbed. Any defensive cells in the area are either reabsorbed or cleared by tissue macrophages.

## Regeneration

Regeneration refers to the replacement of lost or necrotic tissue by tissue of the same type. It is part of the reparative process to heal and reconstitute damaged tissue.[2] Intact, healthy neighbor cells surrounding the dead cells undergo mitosis and proliferate to replace the cells lost in the tissue. This process usually occurs to the greatest degree in epithelial tissue. Certain glands and organs can regenerate functional parenchymal cells if the architectural structure remains intact.

In the healthy human body, how cell growth and reproduction occur is still essentially unknown. Certain cells, such as hematopoietic and epithelial cells, reproduce continuously. Many others, such as bone and fibrous tissue, do not reproduce for years unless stimulated to do so. Still others, such as neurons, do not reproduce at all. If a person develops a deficiency of some cell types, these reproduce rapidly until a precisely adequate number is available. Other cells do not reproduce even when their numbers are depressed.

Little is known about mechanisms and controls that keep adequate numbers of cells in the human body. Control substances are probably secreted by cells that act as a feedback mechanism to stop or slow growth when an adequate number of cells is produced.[4] Cells removed from the body can be grown in a laboratory culture if the medium is suitable. These cells stop growing when small amounts of their own secretions are allowed to collect in the culture medium. Thus the secretions are probably the control substances that limit cell growth and reproduction.

Cells may be classified according to reproductive capability. Differences in reproductive ability cause these cells to react differently during wound healing. All of the *labile* cells undergo complete regeneration by the proliferation of reserve cells. *Stable* cells regenerate if they are stimulated to do so. For example, bone injury causes fibroblasts to differentiate into osteoblasts and osteocytes. Studies of muscle regeneration have shown that smooth muscle shows little regenerative ability, whereas voluntary muscle may partially regenerate if conditions are optimal.[5] Synovial cells in the tendons may be reformed under optimal healing conditions. *Permanent* cells do not regenerate, so their death requires replacement by scar tissue.

If tissue cells are to regenerate, they must preserve (1) part of the original structure and (2) the architectural framework of the injured tissue.

## Repair by Scar

Repair by scar occurs when dead tissue cells are replaced by viable cells that are of a different type than the original cells. The new cells form granulation tissue, which later matures to fibrous scar tissue.

Wound healing begins with inflammation. There is no distinct line between the time when inflammation ends and healing begins. Healing follows several typical steps or stages. The first stage requires a cleanup of cellular debris, organisms, or clot, which is carried out mostly by macrophages and a few neutrophils. Replacement of necrotic material, clot, or exudate by granulation tissue is called *organization*. *Granulation tissue* is proliferative connective tissue that is highly vascularized. The gradual laying down of *collagen* by these connective tissue cells eventually causes a dense fibrous scar to form.[5] Collagen is the main component that provides strength to healing wounds.[2,4] The scar begins as collagen bridges

the defect and provides the initial strength to a wound. Epithelialization also occurs from the wound margins across the surface of the wound (Figure 13-5).

As granulation tissue forms, it is very vascular and bleeds readily. As the scar forms, it tends to mold to the shape of the surrounding tissue, and increases in tensile strength by compressing the collagen. In the early weeks, the scar is red because of the many blood vessels infiltrating it. The new vessels originate by a budding or sprouting process called *angiogenesis*, or *neovascularization*. The new vessels are leaky and allow fluid and protein to pass through them into the extravascular spaces. This leakiness accounts for long-term edema after the acute inflammation has subsided. The red scar color fades as vessels become smaller, until the scar assumes a white, fibrous appearance. Wound remodeling occurs throughout healing. Contraction, or shortening, is effective in pulling the wound edges closer together in the early stages of scar formation.

*Cicatrization* denotes formation of mature scar tissue. It has been described as less vascular, pale, and

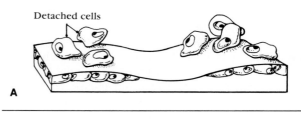

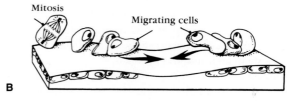

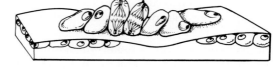

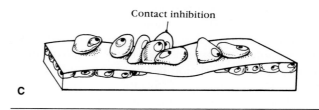

**FIGURE 13-5.**
Epithelialization of a wound. (**A**) With injury, epidermal cells detach from basement membrane and enlarge. (**B**) Undifferentiated basal cells migrate toward center of wound defect. (**C**) Contact inhibition occurs when migrating cells meet in the center and touch. (**D**) Basal cells proliferate to restore epidermis.

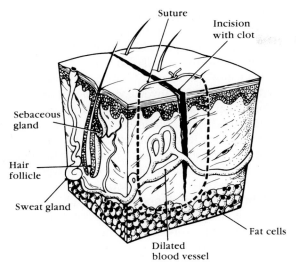

**FIGURE 13-6.**
Initial stage of healing by first intention.

contracting scar tissue. The *cicatrix* denotes the scar, which has less elasticity than most normal tissue.

### Healing by First Intention

First-intention healing refers to scar tissue that is laid down across a clean wound whose edges are in close apposition. The edges are sealed together by a blood clot, which dries to protect and seal the wound. The best example is a clean surgical wound closed by sutures (Figure 13-6).

An acute inflammatory reaction occurs within the first 24 hours, with neutrophilic infiltration of the area. By the third day, macrophages have moved in to clear up cellular debris, and fibroblasts begin to synthesize collagen on the margins of the incision.[1] By the 5th day, the collagen fibrils begin to bridge the defect. Maximum vascularization occurs at this time. Collagen continues to accumulate to form a firm, tough scar, progressively increasing in strength until about the 21st day.[1] Epithelialization across the superficial layers restores a smooth contour. The scar initially is bright red from the extensive vascularization, but it fades to a thin white line as vascularity decreases. Wound contraction occurs in all major scars, and this pulls the margins closer together.[1]

### Healing by Second Intention

Second-intention healing parallels first-intention healing, except that it occurs in larger wounds in which large sections of tissue have been lost or in wounds complicated by infection. Much more time is necessary to remove the necrotic debris and infection from this type of wound. The inflammatory reaction is more extensive with the larger wound surface, and occurs over a longer period.

Large amounts of granulation tissue must be formed. The wound must granulate from its margins and base, with collagen gradually filling the defect. Epithelialization across the granulation tissue occurs to provide a smooth surface. Wound contraction results, mostly caused by fibroblast contraction that tends to pull the wound edges into closer proximity (Figure 13-7).

Healing by second intention is similar to healing by first intention, except that more cellular debris must be cleared, much more granulation tissue is formed, and a large, often deforming scar results. This type of healing is required in third-degree burns, deep skin ulcerations, and infected and other large wounds. Structures normally found in the scarred area cannot be replaced, so hair follicles, sweat glands, and melanin-producing cells are lost.

## Factors That Delay Wound Healing

Many factors affect the body's ability to heal a wound. Oxygen deficiencies, malnutrition, and electrolyte imbal-

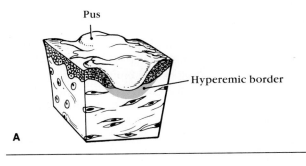

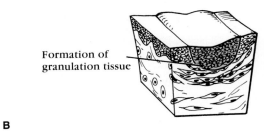

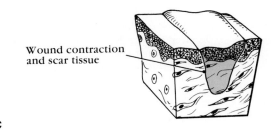

**FIGURE 13-7.**
Healing by second intention. (**A**) Hyperemic border around infected area. (**B**) Formation of granulation tissue. (**C**) Wound contraction and scar tissue.

ances are examples of conditions that can markedly affect the efficiency of the normal defense mechanisms. Immune suppression and clotting deficiencies also can disturb the primary closure of a wound surface. The effects of systemic bodily stress from injury or illness produce immune suppression, resulting in delayed healing (see Chap. 15). Table 13-3 lists local and general factors that can delay wound healing.

## Aberrant Healing

Aberrant means deviating from the normal, typical, or usual. In healing wounds, deviations from the normal may cause complications, deformity, and decreased function of the injured tissue. The results of aberrant healing depend on where the wound is located, the degree of deviation, and the modifying factors present in the patient. Aberrant healing results from an abnormality in healing mechanisms that leads to formation of excess scar tissue, contracture, constrictions, or adhesions.

## Exuberant Granulations and Keloids

Exuberant granulations, or "proud flesh," occur when there is an excessive accumulation of scar tissue. They may vary in size from small to very large protrusions of granulation tissue that block the epithelialization of the wound. Once removed, they do not return. Keloids are excessive, bulging, tumorous scars that extend beyond the confines of the original wound and seldom regress.[3]

They can result with any wound but occur most often around the face, neck, and shoulders.

Keloid formation probably results from abnormalities in collagen synthesis and degradation. Inadequate lysis of collagen by *collagenase* may be the main defect, or elevated levels of propylhydroxylase, necessary for collagen formation, may contribute to the excess scar formation. Research has demonstrated that in contrast to normal fibroblasts, keloid fibroblasts synthesize collagen at a rapid rate, possibly because of excessive histamine in the area. Keloid formation also may be a type of autoimmunity in people with elevated levels of serum immunoglobulins.[3] Dark-skinned people develop keloids more frequently than light-skinned people. Those under age 30 also have a propensity for development of these abnormalities. Keloids tend to recur after removal.

## Contracture

Wound contraction is a normal part of healing and involves migration of wound margins toward the center. Some wounds continue to contract after closure, and a disfiguring scar or disability results. The ability of a wound to close depends in part on the flexibility of the surrounding skin. The ability of skin to stretch on the scalp and tibial area is limited, especially if little subcutaneous tissue is present. Contractures may interfere with joint mobility or with other body movements such as breathing and head movement. They can occur in any area, skin, and subcutaneous tissue, as well as after bone fractures and tendon, muscle, or nerve injuries.

**TABLE 13-3.**
FACTORS THAT DELAY WOUND HEALING

| GENERAL FACTORS | LOCAL FACTORS |
| --- | --- |
| Age | Devitalized tissue |
| Nutrition status | Tissue damage at time of injury |
|   Vitamin deficiencies—particularly of A, D, C, K, thiamine, riboflavin, and pantothenic acid | Tissue destruction by dessication before closure |
|   Protein depletion | Cellular injury from use of excessively strong antiseptics |
| Fluid-electrolyte balance | Compromised tissue converted to an avascular state, such as by excessively restrictive dressings or an underlying expanding hematoma |
|   Dehydration, edematous conditions, or both | |
| Medication, such as immunosuppresives, glucocorticoids, and anticoagulants | Seroma or hematoma, which provide excellent conditions for bacterial growth |
| Diseases, such as diabetes mellitus, hemophilia, and other disease states in which nutrition, fluid-electrolyte imbalance, or methods of treatment compromise the normal progression of would healing | Bacterial infection |
| | Retained foreign body, including buried suture material |
| | Failure to close a dead space |
| | Closure under tension |
| | Improper approximation of wound edges |

Source: *Barnes, H. V. Clinical Medicine. Chicago: Yearbook, 1988. Page 103.*

## Dehiscence and Evisceration

Dehiscence is the surface disruption that results in the bursting open of a previously closed wound. This can occur as a result of interruption of primary or secondary healing. Dehiscence occurs when the strength of the collagen framework is not adequate to hold against the forces imposed on the wound. Poor collagen synthesis often is related to poor circulation.

Evisceration refers to the internal organs moving through a dehiscence. This most frequently occurs with the abdominal organs, but others also may eviscerate.

## Stenosis and Constriction

If scar tissue forms in and around tubular areas, such as the ureter or esophagus, a stricture may develop, leading to narrowing or obstruction of an opening. Scarring may occur around an incision line or as a consequence of inflammation.

## Adhesions

When serous or mucous membrane surfaces are inflamed, the exudate may cause scar tissue to bind or adhere to adjacent surfaces. Adhesions commonly occur in the peritoneal cavity between loops of bowel or abdominal viscera, especially after abdominal surgical procedures. Partial or complete intestinal obstruction can result from the fibrinous bands extending from organ to organ or from organ to peritoneal wall. Adhesions also frequently develop after pleuritis, causing dense fibrous pleural adhesions that obliterate the pleural space and restrict respiratory excursion.

## REFERENCES

1. Barnes, H.V., et al. *Clinical Medicine.* Chicago: Yearbook, 1988.
2. Cohen, I.K., and Diegelmann, R.F. The biology of keloid and hypertrophic scar and influence of corticosteroids. *Clin. Plast. Surg.* 4:2, 1977.
3. Cotran, R., Kumar, V., and Robbins, S.L. *Robbin's Pathologic Basis of Disease* (4th ed.). Philadelphia: W.B. Saunders, 1989.
4. Guyton, A. *Textbook of Medical Physiology* (8th ed.). Philadelphia: W.B. Saunders, 1991.
5. Kissane, J.M. *Anderson's Pathology* (9th ed.). St. Louis: C.V. Mosby, 1990.
6. Laurell, A.B. The complement system. In L.A. Hanson and H. Wigzell, *Immunology.* London: Butterworth, 1985.
7. Masur, H., and Fauci, A.S. Infections in the compromised host. In J.D. Wilson, J.D., et al., *Harrison's Principles of Internal Medicine* (12th ed.). New York: McGraw-Hill, 1991.
8. Root, R.K. Infectious diseases: Pathogenetic mechanisms and host responses. In L.H. Smith and S.O. Thier, *Pathophysiology: The Biological Principles of Disease.* Philadelphia: W.B. Saunders, 1985.
9. Slauson, D.O., and Cooper, B.J. *Mechanisms of Disease* (2nd ed.). Baltimore: Williams & Wilkins, 1990.
10. Walter, J.B. *Pathology of Human Disease.* Philadelphia: Lea & Febiger, 1989.

## UNIT BIBLIOGRAPHY

Balk, R.A., and Bone, R.C. The septic syndrome: Definition and clinical implications. *Crit. Care Clin.* 5:1, 1989.

Benenson, A.S. *Control of Communicable Diseases in Man* (14th ed.). Washington, D.C.: American Public Health Association, 1985.

Bettoli, E.J. Herpes: Facts and fallacies. *Am. J. Nurs.* 82:924, 1982.

Cormack, D.H. *Ham's Histology* (9th ed.). Philadelphia: J.B. Lippincott, 1987.

Cotran, R.S., Kumar, V., and Robbins, S.L. *Robbins' Pathologic Basis of Disease* (4th ed.). Philadelphia: W.B. Saunders, 1989

Dineen, P., and Hildick-Smith, G. *The Surgical Wound.* Philadelphia: Lea & Febiger, 1981.

DuPont, H.L. Infectious diseases. In W.N. Kelley, *Textbook of Internal Medicine.* Philadelphia: J.B. Lippincott, 1989.

Flynn, M.E. Influencing repair and recovery. *Am. J. Nurs.* 82: 1550, 1982.

Flynn, M.E., and Rovee, D.T. Promoting wound healing. *Am. J. Nurs.* 82:1543, 1982.

Fox, R.A. *Immunology and Infection in the Elderly.* Edinburgh: Churchill Livingston, 1984.

Gantz, N.M., et al. *Manual of Clinical Problems in Infectious Disease* (2nd ed.). Boston: Little, Brown, 1986.

Guyton, A. *Textbook of Medical Physiology* (8th ed.). Philadelphia: W.B. Saunders, 1991.

Kissane, J.M. *Anderson's Pathology* (9th ed.). St. Louis: C.V. Mosby, 1990.

LiVolsi, V.A., et al. *Pathology* (2nd ed.). Media, Pa.: Harwal, 1989.

Lynch, J.M. Helping patients through the recurring nightmare of herpes. *Nursing82* 12:52, 1982.

Morello, J.A., Mizer, H.E., and Wilson, M.E. *Microbiology in Patient Care.* New York: Macmillan, 1984.

Segreti, J. Nosocomial infections and secondary infections in sepsis. *Crit. Care Clin.* 5:172, 1989.

Smith, A.M. *Principles of Microbiology* (10th ed.). St. Louis: C.V. Mosby, 1985.

Stroud, M., Swindell, B., and Bernard, G.R. Cellular and humoral mediators of sepsis syndrome. *Crit. Care Nurs. Clin. North Am.* 2:2, 1990.

Taylor, D.L. Wound healing: Physiology, signs, and symptoms. *Nursing83* 13:44, 1983.

Walter, J.B. *Pathology.* Philadelphia: W.B. Saunders, 1990.

Wilson, G., Miles, A., and Parker, M.T. *Topley and Wilson's Principles of Bacteriology, Virology, and Immunity.* Baltimore: Williams & Wilkins, 1983-4.

Wilson, J.D., et al. *Harrison's Principles of Internal Medicine* (12th ed.) New York: McGraw-Hill, 1991.

# IMMUNITY

An intact, functioning immune system is essential to protect the human body from invasion by microorganisms and damage by foreign substances. The cells of the immune system, called immunocompetent cells, are developed during fetal life, during which time they develop self-tolerance, thus distinguishing self from nonself. Chapter 14 covers the basic immunologic response, including components of the immune system and the development of immunity. Chapter 15 describes the alterations in defense that can occur with primary or secondary immunologic deficiency. Acquired immune deficiency syndrome (human immunodeficiency virus disease) is covered in some depth because of its increased incidence in recent years. Chapter 16 describes the hypersensitivity or exaggerated immune responses. Autoimmune disease is considered a hypersensitive response, and the mechanisms are discussed in this chapter.

The topic of immunity is vast, and knowledge of the system's functioning is constantly expanding. It requires readers to be familiar with a new terminology. In studying immunity, the reader is encouraged to review or study the inflammatory process. The learning objectives are helpful as a study guide outline for learning. The bibliography at the end of the unit gives some direction for further research.

# chapter 14

Barbara L. Bullock

# Normal Immunologic Response

## Chapter Outline

## Learning Objectives

1. Identify the functions of the organs and cells of the immune system.
2. Differentiate between T and B lymphocytes on the basis of function.
3. Trace the development of immunocompetent T and B cells.
4. Compare antibody-mediated immunity with cell-mediated immunity.
5. Define *self* and *nonself* as they are used in immunology.
6. Differentiate between primary and secondary immune responses.
7. Compare the functions of the different classes of immunoglobulins.
8. Briefly describe the role of macrophages and polymorphonuclear leukocytes in the immune response.
9. Explain one theory of specificity in the immune reaction.
10. Define the process of *immunosurveillance*.
11. Discuss the process of developing active immunity.

---

The immune system consists of cells and organs that defend the body against invasion by microorganisms and damage by foreign substances. The inherent capacity to distinguish what is foreign from what belongs to the body is effected by particular cells called *immunocompetent* cells. These cells distinguish *self* from *nonself*. The development of *self-tolerance* involves the recognition of self proteins and is gained during fetal development. All other proteins to which the body is exposed are treated as foreign agents and are targeted for destruction by the immunocompetent cells.

This chapter describes the processes for the development of immunity and for the recognition of foreign-

ness. Table 14-1 lists some of the essential terminology used in describing this system. Knowledge in the area of immunology is rapidly expanding through both research and many applications to clinical situations. Chapters 15 and 16 detail the major abnormalities of the immune system.

## ORGANS OF THE IMMUNE SYSTEM

### Lymphoid Organs and Tissues

The lymphoid organs include the lymph nodes, thymus, spleen, and tonsils. The lymphoid tissues are composed

**TABLE 14–1.**
TERMS FREQUENTLY USED TO EXPLAIN IMMUNE RESPONSES

| TERM | DEFINITION |
|---|---|
| Antibody | Protein produced as the result of introduction of an antigen; also called immunoglobulins; secreted from plasma cells |
| Antigenic determinants | Specific areas or combining sites on the surface of the cell membrane of an antigen; determine specificity |
| Antigens | Foreign substances, usually proteins, capable of stimulating an immune response |
| Autoimmunity | Immunity to self-antigens; loss of self-tolerance |
| Complement | Series of enzymes, normally inactive, circulating in the bloodstream that, when activated by an antigen–antibody reaction, participate in the inflammatory response |
| Immunity | Development of protection of the body against agents that are foreign to it |
| Immunocompetent cells | Those cells that can recognize and react with antigen; T and B lymphocytes |
| Memory | Ability to respond to an antigenic challenge because of previous exposure to the antigen and development of a bank of specific immunocompetent cells to that antigen |
| Specificity | Property of reacting with one antigen only; both the antigen and the T or B lymphocyte have surface receptors that allow them to recognize each other specifically |
| Tolerance | State of unresponsiveness developed to a specific, known antigen |

of lymphocytes and plasma cells, which are present throughout the body, especially in the gastrointestinal tract and bone marrow. Lymphoid tissue often is described in terms of *primary* and *secondary lymphoid organs* (Figure 14-1). Lymphocytes travel throughout the lymphoid tissues and organs, entering and leaving the tissue spaces with ease. The two major classes of lymphocytes are the T and B lymphocytes. Their function is discussed on page 300–304. A network of lymphatic vessels conducts the lymph fluid to the vascular circulation and drains areas throughout the entire body.

## Lymph Nodes

Lymph nodes are distributed throughout the body and receive the lymph circulation. Human lymph nodes are from 1 to 25 mm in diameter and are round or kidney-shaped. These encapsulated secondary lymphoid organs often are seen at branches of the lymphatic vessels and are found in clusters at strategic locations, such as the neck and axillae.[15] A lymph node consists of an outer portion, called the *cortex,* and an inner portion, called the *medulla* (Figure 14-2). Some lymphocytes are formed in or reproduce in the thymus, especially in the cortical areas. They are then seeded into the bloodstream. In the paracortex is an area called the *thymus-dependent zone,* which is believed to contain chiefly T lymphocytes. The *germinal centers* contain mostly B lymphocytes but may contain a few T lymphocytes and macrophages.

The node consists of a stroma in which different types of free cells are held in place by reticular and collagen fibers. The lymph sinusoid is a thin-walled vessel through which lymph flows. The lymph sinus in the sub-

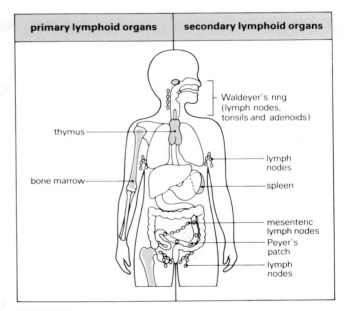

**FIGURE 14–1.**
Major lymphoid organs and tissues. The thymus produces T cells and the bone marrow, B cells. The secondary lymphoid organs and tissues contain mature T and B cells and accessory cells. In the mammalian fetus, the B cells initially are generated in the liver. In humans, the adult bone marrow also is a secondary lymphoid organ. Lymph nodes are present throughout the body (only a few are depicted here) and usually are found at the junctions of lymphatic vessels. The group of lymph nodes, including the tonsillar and adenoidal lymphoid tissue in the area of the neck and throat, is called the Waldeyer's ring of lymphoid tissue. Lymph nodes drain the tissue spaces and the lymph-borne antigens while lymphoid cells in the spleen respond to blood-borne antigens. Peyer's patches are unencapsulated masses of lymphoid tissue in the small intestine. (From I. Roitt, J. Brostoff, and D. Male, *Immunology* [2nd ed.]. Philadelphia: J.B. Lippincott, 1989.)

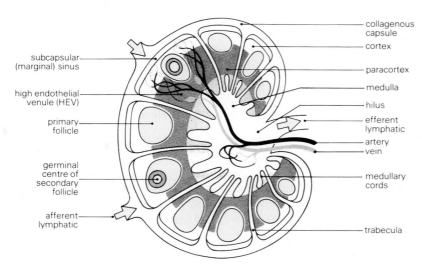

**FIGURE 14-2.**

Structure of a lymph node. Beneath the collagenous capsule is the subcapsular sinus, which is lined by phagocytic cells. Lymphocytes and antigens, if present, pass into the sinus by way of the afferent lymphatics from surrounding tissue spaces or adjacent nodes. The cortex contains aggregates of B cells (primary follicles), most of which (secondary follicles) have a site of active proliferation (germinal center). The paracortex mainly contains T cells, many of which are found in close apposition to the interdigitating cells (antigen-presenting cells). Each node has its own arterial and venous supply. Lymphocytes enter the node from the circulation through the specialized high endothelial venules in the paracortex. The medulla contains both T and B cells and most of the lymph node plasma cells organized into cords of lymphoid tissue. Lymphocytes can leave the node only through the efferent lymphatics. (From I. Roitt, J. Brostoff, and D. Male, *Immunology* [2nd ed.]. Philadelphia: J.B. Lippincott, 1989.)

capsular space is like a hollow space that conducts the lymphatic flow.[5] Basically, lymph nodes serve as a series of in-line filters, so that all lymph in the lymph vessels is filtered by at least one node. Lymph nodes receive lymph from an afferent lymphatic vessel, and the lymph then passes through the cortical, paracortical, and medullary regions (see Figure 14-2). Many lymphocytes and macrophages reside in these areas.

## Thymus

The thymus gland, a primary lymphoid organ, is located in the mediastinal area. It processes lymphocytes, and rapid production of lymphocytes occurs in this region from the early years of life until puberty. In the medullary area, lymphocytes appear to become more differentiated,

after which they enter the circulation (Figure 14-3). Many of the cells that are produced by the thymus die in the gland.[12] The thymus and other lymphatic tissues undergo marked changes in size in relation to age (Figure 14-4). The thymus grows rapidly in children, reaching maximum size at puberty, after which it gradually begins the process of involution, beginning in the cortical zone and progressing to the medullary area.[1] The gland never completely disappears, but in elderly people, it is a collection of reticular fibers, some lymphocytes, and connective tissue. During stress reactions, the cortical cells rapidly involute in size because of the effect of corticosteroids.[1]

Lymphocyte maturation is regulated by transformation of lymphocyte precursor cells into antigen-specific lymphocytes. This process occurs in the cortical and medullary areas under the influence of the *thymic hor-*

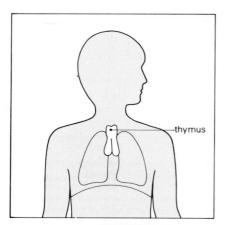

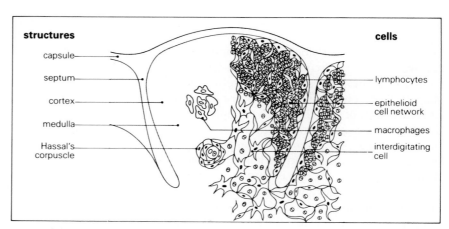

**FIGURE 14-3.**

Structure of the thymus. The bilobed thymus is an encapsulated organ divided into lobules by septa. The cortex contains densely packed dividing lymphocytes in a network of epithelial cells that extends into the medulla. The medulla contains fewer lymphocytes, but there are more bone marrow—derived interdigitating cells. Note the close association of the developing lymphocytes with epithelial and interdigitating cells. The function, if any, of the whorled epithelial structures termed Hassal's corpuscles is unknown. (From I. Roitt, J. Brostoff, and D. Male, *Immunology* [2nd ed.]. Philadelphia: J.B. Lippincott, 1989.)

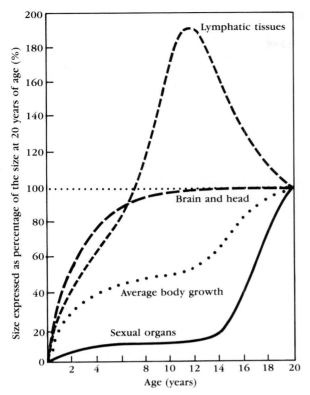

**FIGURE 14-4.**
Comparison of the growth curves for various tissues. Note that the lymphatic tissues achieve maximum growth and function in the early adolescent years (From L.A. Hanson and H. Wigzell, *Immunology*. London: Butterworth, 1985.)

*mones.* A group of hormones that affect cell activities has been identified, but not all of their effects are known.[1] These hormones are necessary to cause the differentiation of the stem cell precursor received from the bone marrow into mature T cells.[12] *Thymopoietin* secreted by the thymus and circulating in body fluids enhances T-cell immunity.[11]

## Spleen

The spleen is the largest lymphatic organ. It can function as a reservoir for blood in two areas, the venous sinuses and the pulp (Figure 14-5). As the spleen enlarges, the quantity of red blood cells within its *red pulp* (so called because of its dark red tissue that is rich in blood) also can increase. One of the main functions of the spleen is to process the red blood cells that squeeze through its pores. Red cells that are nearing the end of their life span often break down here (see Chap. 19). The macrophages in the splenic tissue clear the cellular debris and process hemoglobin.

Many phagocyte cells, especially macrophages, line the pulp and sinuses of the spleen. Groups of lymphocytes and plasma cells that can be seen with the naked eye throughout the parenchyma of the spleen are called

the *white pulp.* These cells function in the process of immunity.

### Mucosa-Associated Lymphoid Tissue

Aggregates of lymphoid tissue are found in many organs, especially those of the gastrointestinal, respiratory, and urogenital tracts. These systems normally are the main portals of entry for microorganisms.[15] Therefore, the presence of lymphoid tissue can, through secretory IgA and other immune factors, prevent entry of these microorganisms into the body.[15] The tonsils are aggregations of lymphoid tissue and are named according to their location (Figure 14-6). Those of the mouth and pharynx are called *palantine, lingual,* and *pharyngeal.* They are composed of lymphoid tissue and many lymphocytes. In the intestinal area, *Peyer's patches* are accumulations of lymphoid tissue, as is the vermiform appendix.

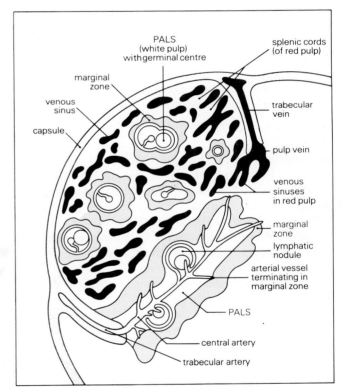

**FIGURE 14-5.**
Organization of lymphoid tissue in the spleen. The white pulp is composed of the periarteriolar lymphatic sheaths (PALS), frequently containing germinal centers with mantle zones. The white pulp is surrounded by the marginal zone. (Marginal zones contain specialized antigen-presenting cells, macrophages, and slowly recirculating B cells.) The red pulp contains venous sinuses separated by splenic cords. Blood enters the tissues by way of the trabecular artery and becomes the central artery, which gives rise to many branches; some end in the white pulp, supplying the germinal centers and mantle zones, but most empty into or near the marginal zones. Some arterial branches run directly into the red pulp, mainly terminating in the cords. The venous sinuses drain blood into pulp veins and then trabecular veins. (From I. Roitt, J. Brostoff, and D. Male, *Immunology* [2nd ed.]. Philadelphia: J.B. Lippincott, 1989.)

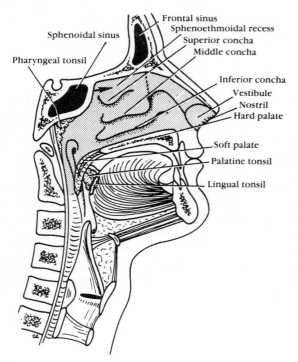

**FIGURE 14-6.**
Tonsils of the mouth and pharynx. (From R. Snell, *Clinical Anatomy for Medical Students* [2nd ed.]. Boston: Little, Brown, 1981.)

## CELLS OF THE IMMUNE SYSTEM

Mononuclear and polymorphonuclear leukocytes are involved in the immune response. Mononuclear T and B lymphocytes are considered to be the only *immunocompetent cells.* They provide for specificity, or recognition, of specific antigens by specific lymphocytes. An *antigen* is a substance recognized by the immunocompetent cells as being foreign, against which an immune reaction is initiated.

Polymorphonuclear leukocytes are *nonspecific cells* that interact with the lymphocytes and antigen to produce an inflammatory reaction (see Chap. 13). Phagocytic macrophages also play an important role in the immune response, in that macrophages can be used to process antigen. This role is further described on pages 305 and 306.

The interaction among B cells, T cells, and macrophages with antigen provides the basis for the development of immunity. The cell- or tissue-specific antigens provoke specialized cells (immunocytes) that protect the human organism from microorganisms, from foreign tissue, and from diseases caused by altered cells. This protective function is known as *immune surveillance.*[12] Through immune surveillance, the *immune response* may be triggered. The immune response is a complex sequence of events set off by the introduction of a foreign agent (antigen) and usually ends with the elimination of it.[10] This response requires recognition of the antigen

with the appropriate cellular and humoral mechanism to effect its elimination. The later introduction of the antigen to the body will not produce disease because of the large number of specific cells that recognize it and ultimately destroy it. This is *immunity.* The remainder of this chapter elucidates the process.

## B Lymphocytes

The B lymphocytes are responsible for *humoral-* or *immunoglobulin*-mediated–immunity. These cells originate in the bone marrow, and mature either there or in some other portion of the system. They are capable of proliferating and differentiating into *plasma cells* and *memory cells* when exposed to antigen. Plasma cells secrete large quantities of specific immunoglobulin.

Immunoglobulin secreted by plasma cells is called *antibody.* Antibody has exquisite specificity for antigen, so that within the many classes of antibody are molecules that recognize only their specific antigen.[20] The specificity resides in a portion of the molecule that has binding affinity for antigen.[4] Some lymphoblasts are formed by activation of a clone of specific B lymphocytes. These form numbers of new B lymphocytes that are similar to the original clone. The net effect is to increase the population of specific B cells for a specific antigen. These B cells circulate throughout the lymphoid tissue and are available to combat antigen whenever it is encountered. An expanded clone causes a rapid response when new contact occurs.[11] These are the methods for fighting infection through the primary and secondary immune response described on page 306–307.

The basic unit of every immunoglobulin molecule is a symmetric arrangement of four polypeptide chains. Two of the polypeptide chains, called *heavy chains (H),* are identical and have a greater molecular weight than the two *light chains (L).* These heavy and light chains are kept together as a symmetric four-chain molecule $(H_2L_2)$.[4] The chains are held together by disulfide bonds. Figure 14-7 shows a representative model of an immunoglobulin. The Fab (fragment, antigen-binding) portion is the *variable* portion, and the Fc (fragment, crystallizable) portion is the *constant* portion of the immunoglobulin class. The constant portion, or heavy chain, almost certainly directs the biologic activity of the antibody and perhaps the distribution or location of the immunoglobulin within the body.[20] The variable portion, or light chain, provides individual specificity for binding antigen and varies among immunoglobulin molecules.

Five major classes of immunoglobulins have been identified: IgG, IgM, IgA, IgE, and IgD. The classification depends on the structure of the heavy-chain portion of the molecule.[20] Table 14-2 lists the main properties of each major classification. The ability of the antibody to combine with a specific antigen resides in the Fab por-

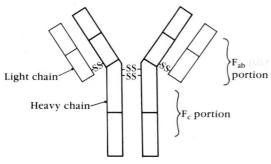

**FIGURE 14–7.**
Schematic appearance of an immunoglobulin showing two light and two heavy polypeptide chains. The constant portion, or Fc, accounts for the biologic activity, and the variable portion, of Fab, provides for the binding of specific antigen. SS, disulfide bonds.

tion of the molecule, whereas the biologic properties that determine how the antigen is destroyed or rendered harmless are found in the Fc portion of the molecule.[20]

## IgM

Often called the macroglobulin (because it is the largest), IgM is the first immunoglobulin produced during an immune response. It is made up of five units held together by a short peptide chain called the J chain. It makes up about 10% of normal immunoglobulins.[9] IgM is efficient in agglutinating antigen as well as in lysing cell walls. It is present in high concentrations in the bloodstream and

also early in the course of an infection. It can react efficiently with bacteria and viruses. The level of IgM normally decreases in about a week as the IgG response increases.[4,20] IgM activates (fixes) complement and has five binding sites for antigen.

## IgG

IgG makes up about 80% of the antibodies in plasma. During the secondary response, it is the major immunoglobulin to be synthesized. This antibody freely diffuses into the extravascular spaces to interact with antigen. The amount of IgG synthesized is closely related to the amount of *antigenic* stimulation presented to the host. In prenatal life, it diffuses across the placental barrier to provide the fetus with passive immune protection until the infant can produce an adequate immune defense. Various subtypes of IgG exist, each with slightly different biologic characteristics.[9] It has been shown to carry the major burden in neutralizing bacterial toxins partly through its ability to fix complement. This property functions in accelerating phagocytosis.

## IgA

Most IgA is in the form of *secretory* IgA in the external body secretions, such as saliva, sweat, tears, mucus, bile, and colostrum. It provides a defense against pathogens on exposed surfaces, especially those entering the respi-

**TABLE 14–2.**
IMMUNOGLOBULIN CLASSIFICATION

|  | IgG | IgA | IgM | IgD | IgE |
|---|---|---|---|---|---|
| Serum concentration (mg/dL) | 1000 | 200 | 120 | 3 | 0.05 |
| Molecular weight | 150,000 | 160,000 (serum) 400,000 (secretory) | 900,000 | 180,000 | 190,000 |
| Serum half-life (days) | 23 | 6 | 5 | 3 | 2 |
| Binds to mast cells | − | − | − | − | + |
| Fixes complement | + + | − | + + + | − | − |
| Antiviral activity | + | + + + | + | ? | ? |
| Antibacterial lysis | + | + | + + + | ? | ? |
| Total (%) | 75–80 | 10–15 | 6 | 1 | 0.002 |
| Crosses placenta | + | − | − | − | − |
| Function | Major antibody formed in secondary response; most common antibody in response to infection; long-lived | External secretions and surfaces, saliva, tears, mucus, bile, colostrum; protective function in preventing entry of microorganisms through portals of entry | First antibody formed in primary response; mediates cytotoxic responses; can produce antigen–antibody complexes that precipitate | Not known; found with IgM on surface of B cells | Reaginic antibody binds to mast cells and basophils; causes allergic symptoms through attaching to mast cells and release of histamine and other substances |

Key: −, negative; +, positive; + +, active; + + +, highly active.
Summarized from Cormack, D. Ham's Histology (9th ed.). Philadelphia: J.B. Lippincott, 1987; Roitt, I., Brostoff, J., and Male, D. Immunology. Philadelphia: J.B. Lippincott, 1989; Stites, D.P., and Terr, A.I. Basic Human Immunology. (7th ed.). Norwalk, Conn.: Appleton & Lange, 1990.

ratory and gastrointestinal tracts. More than 85% of plasma cells in the intestinal area produce IgA. Secretory IgA is derived from specific plasma cells. A *secretory component* is synthesized by exposed epithelial cells. These two factors interact to form specific defense against bacterial and viral antigens. The first exposure causes increased amounts of secretory IgA and secretory component to be formed, so that on second exposure, the body surfaces are defended by specific antibody when exposed to specific antigen.[7,8] Antibodies to IgA may inhibit the adherence of pathogens to mucosal cells. The structure of the IgA molecule appears to facilitate its transport into the external secretions.

### IgD

IgD is present in plasma and readily broken down (half-life in plasma, 2–8 days). Its exact function is not known, but its presence on lymphocyte surfaces together with IgM suggests that it may be the receptor that binds antigens to the cell surface. Its levels are elevated in chronic infections, but it has no apparent affinity for particular antigens.[4]

### IgE

IgE is called the reaginic antibody because it is involved in immediate hypersensitivity reactions. Concentrations normally are low in the serum, and the antibody apparently remains firmly fixed on the tissue surfaces, probably bound to mast cells. Contact with an antigen triggers the release of the mast cell granules. The released vasoactive amines cause the signs and symptoms of allergy and anaphylaxis (see Chap. 16). High serum levels of IgE occur in allergy-prone people and in those infected with certain parasites, especially helminths.

## Formation of Specific Antibodies

To be specific, an antigen and an antibody must fit together precisely, the way the right key fits into a lock (Figure 14-8). The antigen-binding, or variable, region of the antibody binds others of similar structure. A person is confronted every day with many different antigens, both environmental and synthetic, against which the body must provide defense. Figure 14-9 shows how this might work when the antibody is confronted with two microbes and responds to one.

Each immunoglobulin molecule has a *constant region* and a *variable region*. The constant region is similar in molecules of each class of immunoglobulin. The variable region must be able to bind many different antigens and provides for specificity. Several theories have been proposed to try to explain immunoglobulin specificity.

One of these, the *clonal-selection theory*, proposes

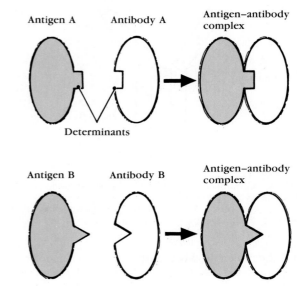

**FIGURE 14–8.**

Highly schematic appearance of specificity of antibody for antigen, the so-called lock-and-key response. The determinants on the surface of the antigen and antibody provide for recognition of antigen by antibody (ATG–ATB interaction).

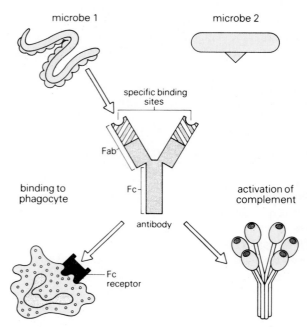

**FIGURE 14-9.**

Antibody—a flexible adaptor. When a microorganism lacks the inherent ability to activate complement or bind to phagocytes, the body provides a class of flexible adaptor molecules with a series of different shapes that can attach to the surface of different microbes. These flexible adaptor molecules are antibodies, and the body can make several million antibodies that are able to recognize a wide variety of infectious agents. Thus the antibody shown binds microbe 1, but not microbe 2, by its "antigen-binding portion" (Fab), while the Fc portion (which may activate complement) binds to Fc receptors on host tissue cells, particularly phagocytes. (From I. Roitt, J. Brostoff, and D. Male, *Immunology* [2nd ed.]. Philadelphia: J.B. Lippincott, 1989.)

that each lymphocyte contains all the genetic information necessary to produce all possible antibodies. Thus the gene for specific antibody is activated by contact with the antigen, and large amounts of the antibody are formed.[19] The binding of antigen stimulates the small number of B cells that recognize it to proliferate, producing sufficient cells to mount an immune response.[19] The clonal-selection model assumes that large amounts of antigenic stimulation trigger the immunocompetent lymphocyte to divide and make large amounts of specific antibody.[13]

When the B cell first encounters its specific antigen, it may become a *memory cell* or a *plasma cell*. Memory cells are a method of stockpiling a specific clone of B cells, so that immediate production of large quantities of the specific immunoglobulins results when the cells are exposed to a particular antigen.

## T Lymphocytes

The long-lived T lymphocytes account for about 70% to 80% of the blood lymphocytes. Their life span ranges from a few months to the duration of a person's life, and they account for long-term immunity. The T lymphocytes are thought to originate from stem cells in the bone marrow but are matured under the influence of the thymus gland. Sometimes they are called *thymocytes* because they mature in the thymus gland. The process proceeds from stem cell to prothymocyte to immature thymocyte to the mature, immunocompetent T lymphocyte.[20] These cells develop distinctive receptors on their cell surfaces, which makes their functions different from those of B cells. The T lymphocytes proliferate rapidly in the thymus and produce large numbers of antigen-specific cells.

The T lymphocytes leave the thymus to enter special regions called thymus-dependent zones, mainly in the paracortical region of the lymph nodes and part of the white pulp of the spleen. They may remain in the lymphoid tissue, enter the blood circulation, or enter the extravascular spaces to encounter antigens that correspond to the membrane receptors on their surfaces. If a T cell encounters its specific antigen, it divides and proliferates to form a clone of T cells that can destroy the antigen. The T lymphocyte can be functionally divided into three subgroups: killer, helper, and suppressor cells.

### Major Histocompatibility Complex

The maturation of T cells requires the influence of thymic hormones. The mature T lymphocyte has the ability to recognize products of genes in the *major histocompatibility complex (MHC)*.[8] A low reaction to *self*-MHC proteins is acquired, while a high reaction to *nonself* or foreign proteins is developed. The T cell becomes a major defender against infected host cells or nonself cells such as transplanted tissue.[16]

All nucleated cells contain histocompatibility antigens that are genetically determined and expressed on their membranes. The MHC genes are critical in initiating and regulating immunity. The MHC is found in the HLA (human leukocyte antigen) on chromosome 6. These HLA antigens are so named because they were first seen on the leukocyte population. The products of the MHC are expressed on the cell surface of nucleated cells, which are part of the genetic makeup of the individual.[8,16,20]

### Killer Cells

Killer T lymphocytes (cytotoxic T cells) bind to the surface of the invading cell, disrupt its membrane, and kill it by altering its intracellular environment. Killer T cells secrete *lymphokines*, which include such substances as chemotactic factor, migratory inhibition factor, macrophage activation factor, blastogenic factor, transfer factor, lymphotoxin, and interferon.[20] These substances may be *chemotactic*, establishing a chemical gradient that helps to bring leukocytes and other substances into the area.

Cytolytic T lymphocytes (CTLs) directly kill cells and are essential in killing virally infected cells. This is accomplished by binding to virally infected host cells and secreting cytotoxic substances into the host cytoplasm. This kills the cells and stops the spread of viral particles.[2] The recognition mechanism of the T cells must be tightly controlled to discriminate between self and nonself because they recognize the membrane proteins of the host cell rather than free antigen. Therefore, CTLs are the chief mechanisms to react to and reject foreign tissue.[16] The lymphokines secreted draw macrophages to the area and stimulate the production of interferon, which may function to suppress the spread of viruses from cell to cell (Figure 14-10).

### Helper T Cells

Helper T cells stimulate B lymphocytes to differentiate into antibody producers. A message from antigen-sensitized T lymphocytes also induces sensitized B cells to divide and mature into plasma cells, which begin to synthesize and secrete immunoglobulins. The synthesis of IgM seems to be the least dependent on T cell activity, whereas the IgA response is the most dependent.

### Suppressor T Cells

Suppressor T cells reduce the humoral response. The production of immunoglobulins against a particular antigen can be reduced or abolished in the presence of these cells. The mechanism of action may be to control the production of immunoglobulins either by regulating the proliferation of B cells or by inhibiting the activity of helper T cells.

Figure 14-11 summarizes the comparative formation and differentiation of T and B lymphocytes.

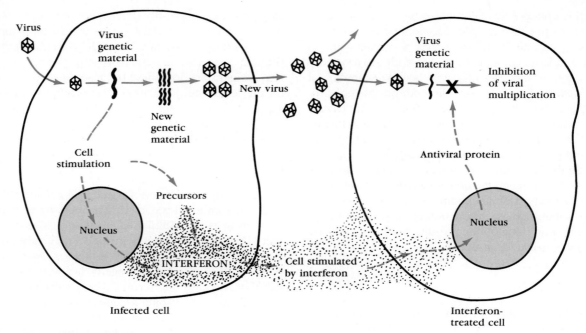

**FIGURE 14–10.**
Schematic representation of interferon activity. (From J.A. Bellanti, *Immunology III*. Philadelphia: W.B. Saunders, 1985.)

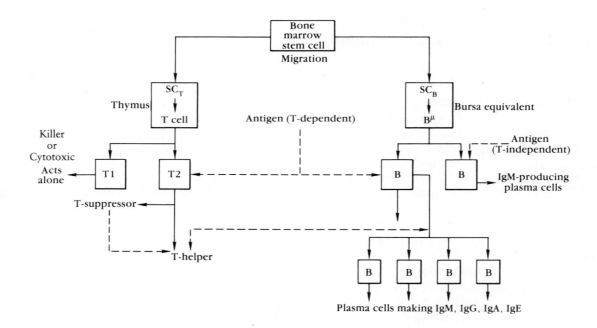

**FIGURE 14–11.**
Both T and B lymphocytes arise from the bone marrow stem cell (SC) and migrate to the thymus gland (T cell) or to an unknown bursa equivalent area (B cell), where they mature to immunocompetent cells. The T cells may act in cooperation with B cells or alone. Some antigens can stimulate B cells.

## Third-Population Cells

Some cells cannot be classified as T or B cells or macrophages because they lack the surface markers that are characteristic of these cells and are not phagocytic. Morphologically, these cells are mainly large granular lymphocytes, and account for up to 20% of blood lymphocytes. Third-population cells (TPCs) are functionally identified through their abilities to kill virus-infected cells, tumor cells, and IgG antibody–coated target cells. The ability to kill (lyse) target cells is called *natural killer activity or antibody-dependent cellular cytotoxicity,* depending on the specific activity of the cell.[14] TPCs also may release interferon or other cytokines and may be the cells involved with graft rejection or recognition of some foreign material.[14] As can be readily seen, the functions of TPCs overlap with those of T cells. TPCs seem to be more bone marrow–dependent and differ morphologically from T cells.

## Macrophages

Macrophages are the mature cells of the *mononuclear phagocyte system* that function in phagocytosis of antigen and in processing and presenting antigen to specific lymphocytes.[3,14] They are mature forms of blood monocytes, and migrate into the different tissues of the body and function as phagocytes. Tissue macrophages make up a network of phagocytic cells throughout the body. These have special names in different areas: Kupffer cells in the liver, alveolar macrophages in the lungs, peritoneal macrophages in the peritoneal cavity, histiocytes in the connective tissue, and others. In the central nervous system, the special cells of the neuroglia classification called *microglia* have the ability to undergo changes and develop the property of phagocytosis during pathologic states.[14] Figure 14-12 shows these different monocytes and macrophages.

Macrophages serve an essential function in removing

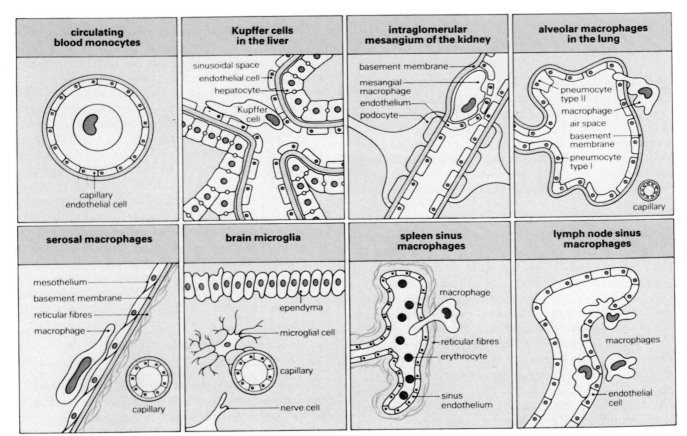

**FIGURE 14–12.**
Mononuclear phagocyte system. The cells of this system include circulating blood monocytes, and dispersed phagocytes in connective tissue or fixed to the endothelial layer of the blood capillaries that in the liver are known as Kupffer cells. Endothelium-fixed phagocytes include the intraglomerular mesangial cells in the kidney. Alveolar and serosal macrophages are examples of "wandering" macrophages, whereas brain microglia are cells that enter the brain around the time of birth and differentiate into fixed tissue cells. (From I. Roitt, J. Brostoff, and D. Male, *Immunology* [2nd ed.]. Philadelphia: J.B. Lippincott, 1989.)

foreign and devitalized material from the body. They are active at a site of injury during wound healing and in removing microorganisms, cellular debris, and necrotic material.

Macrophages also have an important cooperative role in the immune response, but how they function is not entirely understood. These cells trap and process antigens to present them to lymphocytes. They may play a secondary or accessory role in promoting lymphocyte activity and may function as an intermediary between specific T cells and specific B cells.[20]

The macrophage moves by ameboid motion toward a chemical concentration of soluble substances released into its environment by antigens or by lymphocytes. This is called movement toward a *chemotactic gradient*, or signal, that is elicited by soluble substances such as lymphokines (see Chap. 13). The macrophage migration inhibition factor and the macrophage-activating factor, which, respectively, tend to retain the macrophage in an area and increase its phagocytic activity, are especially important lymphokines.[20]

## Antigen, Immunogen, or Hapten Recognition

An *antigen* is a molecule that is capable of inducing a detectable immune response when introduced into the body. When an antigen stimulates an immune response, it is said to have *immunogenicity*.[3] It then stimulates the immune response, denoting an active production of antibodies or sensitized cells. Most antigens and immunogens are proteins, but other large molecules, such as polysaccharides and nucleoproteins, also may function in this way.

Several characteristics appear to determine whether a molecule can stimulate an immune response, and these include such aspects as size, foreignness, shape, and solubility. Some molecules become antigenic only when they are combined with a carrier. Called *haptens*, these substances fail to elicit an immune response because they are small. These molecules cannot serve as complete antigens until they are combined with protein carriers (Figure 14-13). An example is the contact allergens, which probably attach to proteins of the skin and stimulate the proliferation of a T-cell population sensitized to the substance. Later exposure to the allergen leads to a more rapid reaction.[17] Other examples include drugs, dust particles, dandruff, industrial chemicals, and poisons.[11]

## TYPES OF IMMUNITY

### Humoral Immunity

Humoral immunity refers to immunity effected by antibody synthesis or the production of specific immuno-

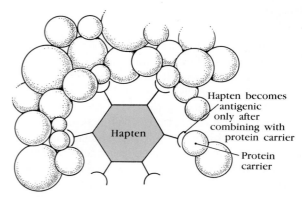

**FIGURE 14–13.**
Some molecules become antigenic only after they have combined with a carrier, usually a protein. These molecules, called hapten, when combined with a carrier, are fully antigenic.

globulin that coats the antigen and targets it for destruction by polymorphonuclear neutrophils. The interaction of antigen with antibody activates the classic pathway of the complement system (see Chap. 13).

Most antigens are recognized by T helper cells, which promote the activation of specific B cells. These B cells are "turned on" by either direct T-cell interaction or T-cell secretions. In some cases, a macrophage serves as an intermediary between the T and B cells. The B cell then divides and differentiates into a plasma cell that secretes specific immunoglobulin to target the antigen for destruction. Antigen recognition by T or B cell often is enhanced by macrophage interaction, which processes the antigen and presents it to the appropriate cell (Figure 14-14).

Certain antigens, designated as *thymus-independent antigens*, elicit strong B-cell responses without T-cell interaction. Examples include *Escherichia coli*, pneumococcal polysaccharide, dextrans, and other large polymers.[20]

Humoral immunity often is described in terms of the *primary* and *secondary* immune responses. This terminology refers to the time lapse between the introduction of antigen and the humoral or immunoglobulin response.

### Primary Response

The first time a particular antigen enters the body a characteristic pattern of antibody production is induced. As the antigen binds to specific B cells, activation occurs and causes the cells to proliferate and differentiate into specialized antibody-producing plasma cells. After about 6 days, antibodies specific to the antigen can be measured in the blood. This *lag* or *latent* phase is the time during which activation of T and B lymphocytes is taking place.[10] The first antibodies or immunoglobulins to be produced in measurable quantities usually are IgM. These are produced in large quantities, with levels in-

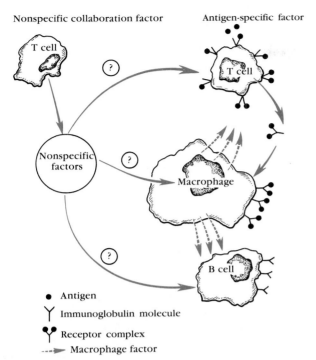

● Antigen

Y Immunoglobulin molecule

YP Receptor complex

--->▶ Macrophage factor

**FIGURE 14-14.**
The macrophage often enhances antigen recognition and probably serves as an intermediary between T and B cells.

creasing up to 14 days and then gradually declining in production to little IgM production after a few weeks.[5]

After the initial IgM elevation, IgG immunoglobulins appear at about day 10, peak at several weeks, and maintain high levels much longer. During the course of the primary immune response, the immunoglobulins improve in their ability to bind the inducing antigen. The mechanisms responsible for this change are not known, but probably firmer binding occurs because of greater precision in matching surface receptors. IgG is considered the highest-affinity antibody that binds antigenic groupings firmly.[6,11] After a time, a *steady-state phase* is reached, during which antibody synthesis and degradation are about equal. Then a *declining phase* occurs, when the synthesis of new antibody decreases.[10] Figure 14-15 shows primary and secondary immune responses to the same antigen.

## Secondary Response

The secondary response differs from the primary response in that the production of specific antibodies for the antigen begins almost immediately. More antibody is produced, and specific immunoglobulin is produced early and in large amounts.

The secondary response is called the memory response because the immune system responds much faster to a second exposure to a particular antigen. Both T and B memory cells are involved because in the pri-

mary response, lymphocytes proliferate and differentiate into T and B memory cells. If the antigen is introduced into the host a second time, these cells begin immediate production of antibodies of a higher binding capacity than in the primary response. Small amounts of antigen stimulate a highly specific response with the specific antibody.[19]

## Complement Activation

Complement is a system of at least 18 proteins and their fragments that circulate as functionally inactive molecules. They are capable of interacting with one another in a sequential activation cascade. They are designated by numbers, with nine numbers indicating the major molecules, and symbols or names indicating the components (see Chap. 13).

The *classic pathway* for the activation of complement involves binding the first component, C1, with a portion of the immunoglobulin molecule. This begins the cascade of complement activation, which is essential in promoting the inflammatory process. Figure 14-16 shows the major pathway of activation and the end results of the process. The system promotes inflammation by increasing vascular permeability, chemotaxis, and phagocytosis, and, finally, causes lysis of the foreign cell.[13] Activation of complement also promotes opsonization of target material (see Figure 14-16). Opsonization occurs with the fixation of complement proteins to antigen particles.[19] This sets the stage for phagocytosis by neutrophils or macrophages. Complement activation (fixation) is the result of complement-fixing antibody, especially IgG. The results

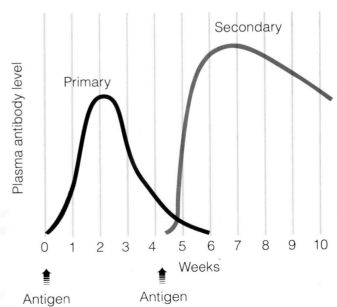

**FIGURE 14-15.**
Primary and secondary immune response by antibody to the same antigen.

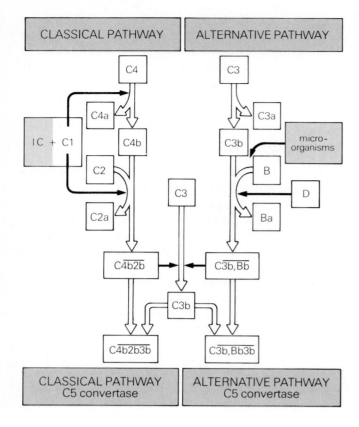

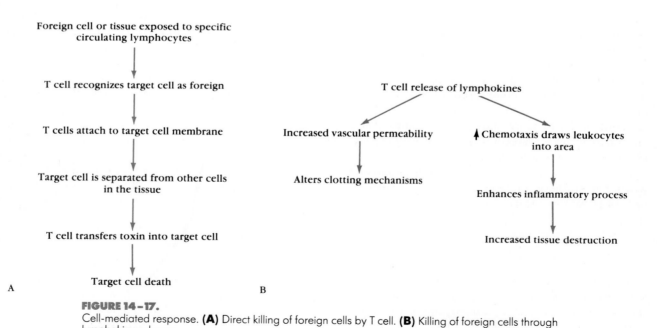

**FIGURE 14–16.**

Analogous action of the classic and alternative pathways. Both pathways generate a C3 convertase: C4b2b (classic pathway) and C3bBb (alternative pathway). In the classic sequence, C1 activated by complexed antibody splits C4 and C2 with the loss of the small fragments C4a and C2a; the major components form C4b2b. In the alternative route, preexisting C3b binds Factor B, which is split, releasing a small fragment Ba. The major fragment, Bb, remains bound to form C3bBb. This converts more C3, continuing the feedback cycle. Activator surfaces on microorganisms, for example, facilitate the combination of Factor B and C3b, and promote alternative pathway activation. The C3 convertases of both pathways may bind further C3b to yield the enzymes that activate the next component of the complement system, C5: classic pathway C5 convertase C4b2b3b, and alternative pathway C5 convertase, C3bBb3b. IC immune complexes. (From I. Roitt, J. Brostoff, and D. Male, *Immunology* [2nd ed.]. Philadelphia: J.B. Lippincott, 1989.)

**FIGURE 14–17.**

Cell-mediated response. **(A)** Direct killing of foreign cells by T cell. **(B)** Killing of foreign cells through lymphokine release.

of the components of the cascade cause some damage to normal tissue around the foreign tissue, and in some cases, this process can be damaging to the host. In most cases, an antigen–antibody (ATG–ATB) reaction is required for the activation of complement. The *alternate complement activation* described in Chapter 13 results in no immunologic memory, because there is no ATG–ATB reaction. The complement factors then can participate in inflammation with the result of destroying foreign material.

## Cell–Mediated Immunity

Cell-mediated immunity, caused by T-lymphocyte activity, is mediated through contact between T cells and antigen, with subsequent destruction of the antigen.[3] The T lymphocyte recognizes antigen by receptors on the surface of the T cell.[8] Destruction may occur through the release of soluble chemical compounds directly into the target cell membrane or through the secretion of lymphokines (Figure 14-17). Direct contact with an antigen frequently is called *killer activity*.

Killer activity is mediated through a group of cytotoxic T cells that function in the destruction of cells with identified surface antigens. The specific recognition is through the lock-and-key approach described earlier. The killer T lymphocyte may directly destroy the antigen by binding to the cell and producing a break in its membrane. This results in disruption of the intracellular osmotic environment and the death of the cell. The activated killer cell also may release cytotoxic substances directly into the target cell.[16]

The activated T lymphocytes release lymphokines, which affect other lymphocytes by enhancing or suppressing their activity. These cells also may create a chemotactic gradient that causes macrophages to accumulate in the area. The activation of a very few antigen-specific T cells leads to a reaction that involves a large number of mononuclear cells that destroy the antigen.[3] The specific antigen involved may be foreign tissue (transplant reactions), intracellular parasites (such as viruses or mycobacteria), soluble protein, or penetrating chemicals.[3] The chemotactic gradient also attracts eosinophils, basophils, and neutrophils to the area.

Cell-mediated immunity, often termed *delayed hypersensitivity* because the response usually takes days, involves the direct intervention of T cells in a response without a corresponding humoral immunity. It results in the accumulation of macrophages around the small blood vessels, resulting in destruction of vessels. This may lead to minor vascular lesions—for example, the wheal-and-flare response—or it may result in major destruction and massive necrosis. The antigen initially may react with a few specific T cells in the area and produce the chemotactic response as well as macrophage-inhibiting factor, which tends to keep macrophages in the area. The response seems to be dose-related, in that the greater the amount of antigen present, the greater the development of sensitized T lymphocytes. The end result is cytolysis of the antigenic cell. This mechanism, which involves the T cells and associated macrophages, is responsible for rejecting transplanted organs and, in this process, is called *cell-mediated lymphocytolysis*.[16] The *tuberculin reaction* is a good clinical example, in that people infected with *Mycobacterium tuberculosis* develop a wheal-and-flare response when injected intradermally with a lysate of tuberculin material.[3]

The T cells function in *immunosurveillance* to detect cells in the host that have foreign antigens on their surface. They can be thought of as defensive cells that patrol the blood and tissue spaces. This self-protective function prevents the transplantation of tissue from one person to another unless the antigens on the surface of the cells in the tissue are similar enough for the host tissue to accept the transplanted tissue as self.

## SUMMARY OF THE PROCESS OF IMMUNITY

As previously described, the term *immunity* refers to all of the mechanisms used by the body to prevent foreign material from causing harm to the body.[3] The agents may be microorganisms or other environmental factors. *Innate immunity* refers to those factors a person is born with to prevent disease. These factors, broadly speaking, can be physical barriers, such as skin, cough, or mucous membranes.[3] Chemical barriers also work cooperatively to decrease microorganism invasion. The internal factors include the cells of the mononuclear phagocyte system and leukocyte secretions.

*Acquired immunity* refers to passive and active immune processes. In early neonatal life, some of the mother's immunity, passed through the placenta prenatally, continues to protect the infant from disease. This *passive immunity* protects only for the first months of life. *Active acquired immunity* involves the response mounted by the person's own immune system. It requires all of the factors described earlier. Scientists have discovered the process of inducing acquired immunity through *vaccination*. The resultant individual response can be induced against microorganisms and their products as well as against thousands of natural and synthetic compounds.

The vaccine prepared uses the least amount of antigenic material to provide the maximum human response and, thus, protection from disease. People are vaccinated against antigens that are threatening to them in the environment in which they live. Table 14-3 lists the main immunizing preparations that are useful in humans.

**TABLE 14–3.**

IMMUNIZING PREPARATIONS (VACCINES AND ANTISERA) USEFUL IN HUMANS

| VACCINES | TYPE OF VACCINE |
|---|---|
| **Bacterial** | |
| Anthrax | Alum-precipitated antigen from culture filtrate |
| Cholera | Killed *Vibrio cholerae* |
| *Haemophilus influenzae* | Type b polysaccharide |
| Meningococcal meningitis | Polysaccharide, group A, C, Y, W135 of *Neisseria meningitidis* |
| Pertussis | Killed *Bordetella pertussis* |
| Plague | Killed *Yersinia pestis* (attenuated strain in some parts of the world) |
| Pneumococcal infection | Polysaccharide (capsule) of 23 serotypes of *Streptococcus pneumoniae* |
| Tetanus | Toxoid |
| Tuberculosis | Attenuated live bacille Calmette-Guérin (BCG) |
| Typhoid | Killed *Salmonella typhi* (attenuated) |
| Botulism | Toxoid, limited use in research workers |
| Brucellosis | Attenuated live *Brucella abortus* strain 19 (limited use in humans outside the United States) |
| **Rickettsial** | |
| Typhus fever | Formalin-inactivated *Rickettsia prowazekii* (attenuated, live; shows promise) |
| Rocky Mountain spotted fever | Inactivated *Rickettsia rickettsii* |
| **Viral** | |
| Hepatitis B | Inactivated HB surface antigen |
| Influenza | Inactivated; whole or "split" virus |
| Measles | Attenuated |
| Mumps | Attenuated |
| Polio | Attenuated or inactivated |
| Rabies | Inactivated |
| Rubella | Attenuated |
| Varicella | Attenuated |
| **Antisera** | |
| Botulism | Human immune globulin; equine immune globulin |
| Diphtheria | Equine immune serum |
| Hepatitis A | Pooled human serum globulin (ISG) |
| Hepatitis B | Specific anti-HB (HBIB) or ISG |
| Hypogammaglobulinemia | Pooled human ISG |
| Measles | Pooled human ISG |
| Rabies | Human immune globulin, RIG, equine immune serum |
| $Rh_{0(D)}$ | Immune (human) globulin vs. $Rh_{0(D)}$ factor |
| Tetanus | Human immune globulin (TIG) |
| Vaccinia | Vaccinia immune globulin |
| Varicella zoster | Zoster immune globulin (VZIG) |
| Antilymphocyte serum | Equine |
| Black widow spider | Equine antivénin |
| Coral snake bite | Equine antivenin |
| Crotalid snake bite | Polyvalent equine antiserum |

*Benjamin, E. and Leskowitz, S. Immunology: A Short Course. New York: Alan R. Liss, 1988.*

## REFERENCES

**1.** Alm, G., and Wigzell, H. Anatomy of the immune system. In L.A. Hanson and H. Wigzell, *Immunology*. London: Butterworth, 1985.

**2.** Bellanti, J.A. *Immunology III*. Philadelphia: W.B. Saunders, 1985.

**3.** Benjamini, E., and Leskowitz, S. *Immunology: A Short Course*. New York: Alan R. Liss, 1988.

**4.** Bennich, H. Immunoglobulins. In L.A. Hanson and H. Wigzell, *Immunology*. London: Butterworth, 1985.

**5.** Cormack, V.H., and Ham, A.W. *Ham's Histology* (9th ed.). Philadelphia: J.B. Lippincott, 1987.

**6.** Cotran, R.S., Kumar, V., and Robbins, S.L. *Robbins' Pathologic Basis of Disease* (4th ed.). Philadelphia: W.B. Saunders, 1989.

**7.** Ganong, W.F. *Review of Medical Physiology* (15th ed.). Los Altos, Calif.: Lange, 1991.

8. Goetzl, E.J., and Stobo, J.D. Immunology. In L.H. Smith and S.O. Thier, *Pathophysiology: The Biological Principles of Disease* (2nd ed.). Philadelphia: W.B. Saunders, 1985.

9. Goodman, J.W. Immunoglobulin structure and function. In D.P. Stites and A.I. Terr, *Basic Human Immunology*. (7th ed.). Norwalk, Conn.: Appleton & Lange, 1990.

10. Goodman, J.W. The immune response. In D.P. Stites and A.I. Terr, *Basic Human Immunology*. (7th ed.). Norwalk, Conn.: Appleton & Lange, 1990.

11. Guyton, A.C. *Textbook of Medical Physiology* (8th ed.). Philadelphia: W.B. Saunders, 1991.

12. Kamani, N.R., and Douglas, S.D. Structure and development of the immune system. In D.P. Stites and A.I. Terr, *Basic Human Immunology*. (7th ed.). Norwalk, Conn.: Appleton & Lange, 1990.

13. Laurell, A.B. The complement system. In L.A. Hanson and H. Wigzell, *Immunology*. London: Butterworth, 1985.

14. Lydard, P., and Grossi, C. Cells involved in the immune response. In I.M. Roitt, J. Brostoff, and D.K. Male, *Immunology* (2nd ed.). Philadelphia: J.B. Lippincott, 1989.

15. Lydard, P., and Grossi, C. The lymphoid system. In I.M. Roitt, J. Brostoff, and D.K. Male, *Immunology* (2nd ed.). Philadelphia: J.B. Lippincott, 1989.

16. Marrack, P., and Kapplar, J. The T cell and its receptor. *Sci. Am.* 254:32, 1986.

17. Perlmann, P., and Hammarstrom, S. Antigen-antibody reactions. In L.A. Hanson and H. Wigzell, *Immunology*. London: Butterworth, 1985.

18. Roitt, I.M. *Essential Immunology* (5th ed.). Oxford: Blackwell, 1985.

19. Roitt, I.M., Brostoff, J., and Male, D.K. *Immunology* (2nd ed.). Philadelphia: J.B. Lippincott, 1989.

20. Unanue, E.R., and Benacerraf, B. *Textbook of Immunology* (2nd ed.). Baltimore: Williams & Wilkins, 1984.

# chapter 15

Barbara L. Bullock
Miguel da Cunha

# Immune Deficiency

## Chapter Outline

## Learning Objectives

1. Differentiate between primary and secondary immune deficiency.
2. Differentiate between cell-mediated and humoral immune deficiency.
3. Describe severe combined immunodeficiency.
4. Briefly identify the genetic basis for immune deficiency.
5. Characterize the age of onset of signs and symptoms in the major described primary immune deficiencies.
6. Explain the different symptoms that can occur according to the types of cells affected.
7. Briefly describe complement abnormalities and how these affect the immune response.
8. List at least six disorders that can cause secondary immune deficiency.
9. Describe why secondary immune deficiency increases the risk for the host.
10. Specifically describe how stress alters the immune response.
11. Explain the effect of aging on T- and B-cell response.
12. List several immunosuppressive agents, giving benefits and drawbacks of their use.
13. Describe how cancer can disrupt the immune mechanism.
14. List three causes of malnutrition or protein depletion and explain how these can disrupt the immune response.
15. Describe the acquired immune deficiency syndrome.
16. Explain the changes in outlook for people with human immunodeficiency virus infection.
17. Discuss how opportunistic diseases become a real threat in immune deficiency.

The development of an immunocompetent system is essential to protect the human organism from foreign invasion. Therefore, any deficiency in any of the components of the immune system can alter the activity of the body's entire defense system. The effects of phagocytic dysfunction are described in Chapter 20. The major classifications of immune deficiency are *primary* and *secondary*. Primary immunologic deficiency is a developmental abnormality that results in failure of humoral immunity, the cell-mediated response, or both. Complement abnormalities are briefly described as one category of immune deficiency. Secondary immunologic deficiencies are acquired conditions that may be associated with disease states or result from medical treatment.

## PRIMARY IMMUNE DEFICIENCY

A primary defect in the immunologic system results from the failure of an essential part of the immune system to develop. The defect can occur at any point during the development of the immune system and may involve organ or cellular defects. Many types of primary immune deficiency states have been described according to the cell type affected and the developmental stage of the cellular system (Box 15-1). The more common disorders are described in the next section.

## *Stem Cell Deficiency (Severe Combined Immunodeficiency Disease)*

Severe combined immunodeficiency disease (SCID) is thought to arise from a deficiency of the stem cell population that forms the lymphocytes. It is manifested by T- and B-cell deficiency associated with a hypoplastic thymus. A tremendous decrease in the number and maturity of lymphocytes provides for little, if any, immune response to antigen. The loss of T cells usually is greater than that of B cells, and T-cell immaturity may be manifested by failure to differentiate to a mature form on antigen stimulation.[17] There are evidently two mechanisms for the development of SCID: (1) a defect in stem cell population and (2) abnormal differentiation of T cells because of abnormalities in the thymus gland.[7] The result is deficiency of both humoral and cell-mediated responses.

Stem cell deficiency severely depresses a person's ability to mount any type of immune response. The thy-

**BOX 15–1.**
CLASSIFICATION OF IMMUNE DEFICIENCY DISORDERS

**Antibody (B cell) immune deficiency diseases**
X-linked (congenital) hypogammaglobulinemia
Transient hypogammaglobulinemia of infancy
Common, variable, unclassifiable immune deficiency (acquired hypogammaglobulinemia)
Immune deficiency with hyper-IgM
Selective IgA deficiency
Selective IgM deficiency
Selective deficiency of IgG subclasses

**Cellular (T cell) immune deficiency diseases**
Congenital thymic aplasia (DiGeorge syndrome)
Chronic mucocutaneous candidiasis (with or without endocrinopathy)

**Combined antibody-mediated (B cell) and cell-mediated (T cell) immune deficiency diseases**
Severe combined immunodeficiency disease (autosomal recessive, X-linked, sporadic)
Cellular immune deficiency with abnormal immunoglobulin synthesis (Nezelof syndrome)
Immune deficiency with ataxia-telangiectasia
Immune deficiency with eczema and thrombocytopenia (Wiskott-Aldrich syndrome)
Immune deficiency with thymoma
Immune deficiency with short-limbed dwarfism
Immune deficiency with enzyme deficiency
Episodic lymphopenia with lymphotoxin
Graft-vs-host disease

**Phagocytic dysfunction**
Chronic granulomatous disease
Glucose-6-phosphate dehydrogenase deficiency
Myeloperoxidase deficiency
Chédiak-Higashi syndrome
Job syndrome
Tuftsin deficiency
Lazy leukocyte syndrome
Elevated IgE, defective chemotaxis, eczema, and recurrent infections

**Complement abnormalities and immune deficiency diseases**
C1q, C1r, and C1s deficiency
C2 deficiency
C3 deficiency (type I, type II)
C4 deficiency
C5 dysfunction, C5 deficiency
C6 deficiency
C7 deficiency
C8 deficiency

*Stites, D. P., et al. Basic and Clinical Immunology (7th ed.). Los Altos, Calif.: Lange Medical Publishers, 1990. Reprinted by permission.*

mus remains small and embryonic, resembling that of a 6- to 8-week-old fetus.[7] The few lymphocytes present are not activated by antigen. Few B cells are present, so all classes of immunoglobulins are depressed, resulting in lack of production of specific antibodies.

An infant with this condition is affected from birth and is unable to cope with a germ-laden environment. Such children are vulnerable to all forms of infections, and many die within the first year of life. The initial problem in early infancy is failure to thrive, which is followed in the first few weeks of life by serious infections, such as pneumonia and infectious diarrhea. Any type of infection may develop, and none responds well to treatment. If SCID is suspected within hours of birth, the child may be placed in a germ-free environment with a later attempt to perform bone marrow transplantation.

In some cases, full immunologic ability can be attained if *graft-versus-host disease* (GVHD) does not limit the success. This disorder occurs when immunocompetent cells are transplanted to recipients who lack the usual immune defense. The normal cells react against those of the recipient. Involvement of the skin, liver, and intestinal mucosa is most common (Figure 15-1). GVHD can be ameliorated by close matching of bone marrow for transplantation and, in some cases, pretreating bone marrow cells (Figure 15-2).[13]

## Deficiencies of Antibody Production

Several pathophysiologic defects in the immune system result in abnormal immunoglobulin synthesis or a deficiency of immunoglobulins. These can affect production of all of the immunoglobulins or of only specific classes.

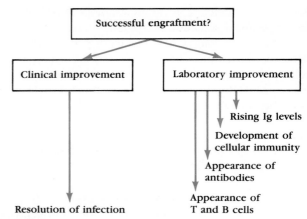

**FIGURE 15-2.**
Indirect evidence that bone marrow grafting is successful. (From M. Haeney, *Introduction to Clinical Immunology*. Boston: Butterworth, 1985.)

Antibody deficiency is suspected in people with persistent, recurrent, severe, or unusual infections. Different types of deficiencies can arise at any age (Figure 15-3). Examples include transient hypogammaglobulinemia of infancy, sex-linked hypogammaglobulinemia, IgA deficiency, and selective IgM or subclass IgG deficiency.

## X-Linked Agammaglobulinemia

A defect in the maturation of stem cells into B cells occurs in X-linked hypogammaglobulinemia (Bruton-type agammaglobulinemia). This congenital disease first appears in male infants at about age 5 to 6 months, when the maternally transmitted level of antibodies has decreased. The

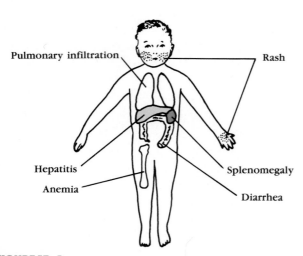

**FIGURE 15-1.**
Major clinical features of graft-versus-host in humans. (From M. Haeney, *Introduction to Clinical Immunology*. Boston: Butterworth, 1985.)

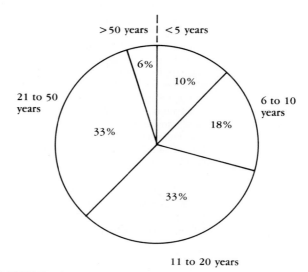

**FIGURE 15-3.**
Age at diagnosis of patients with primary defects of antibody synthesis. (From M. Haeney, *Introduction to Clinical Immunology*. Boston: Butterworth, 1985.)

B cells are virtually absent from the blood, and the basic defect seems to be failure of B cells to mature.[7]

Levels of immunoglobulins IgM, IgG, and IgA are low. Antigens are not cleared well from the body, causing infants with this condition to be extremely susceptible to bacterial infections, especially those caused by *Staphylococcus aureus, Streptococcus pyogenes, Haemophilus influenzae,* and pneumococci. The result is a high frequency of respiratory, sinus, and throat infections.[7]

The cellular immune system remains competent. Allograft rejection and the ability to resist viral, fungal, and parasitic infections are apparently normal. Autoimmune disease frequently occurs, especially rheumatoid arthritis and systemic lupus erythematosus.[13]

## Variable Immune Deficiency

Variable immune deficiency may be seen in various forms, with the common feature being hypogammaglobulinemia, usually of all antibody classes but sometimes of only IgG. These conditions may be congenital or acquired; in the latter case, they may be seen along with malnutrition or immune suppressant chemotherapy. Variable immune deficiency can manifest as a B-cell defect in which antigen is recognized and B cells proliferate but do not differentiate into plasma cells. In some cases, autoantibodies are directed at the T and B cells, which cause a general immune deficiency disorder. It may be associated with T-helper cell suppression or the presence of activated T-suppressor cells.[7] Autoimmune diseases and cancer occur with high frequency, but the main problem is the inability to clear infectious diseases from the body.[7,8]

## IgA Deficiency

Selective IgA deficiency, which occurs in apparently healthy people who may have normal serum levels of the other immunoglobulins, is the most common immune deficiency disorder (1 of every 600 persons). These people lack IgA in serum and external secretions. The disease has a hereditary basis.[7]

The presence of normal numbers of B cells with IgA expressed on their surface suggests failure in the synthesis and release of IgA rather than absence of IgA B lymphocytes. The defect appears to be in differentiation of IgA B lymphocytes, perhaps because of hyperactivity of IgA suppressor cells that prevents the differentiation. A defect in the helper cells specific for IgA synthesis also may be present. Acquired IgA deficiency may occur in persons treated with phenytoin and penicillamine.

The most common symptoms relate to those surfaces that normally are covered with mucosal secretions. Infections of the sinuses and respiratory tract are common. Related gastrointestinal problems include ulcerative colitis, pernicious anemia, and malabsorption states. About

50% of people with IgA deficiency also have some atopic disease.[8] The prevalence of autoimmune diseases, such as systemic lupus erythematosus and rheumatoid arthritis, is markedly increased, and the diagnosis can be supported by the presence of anti-IgA antibodies.[7] A high frequency of cancer in the respiratory and gastrointestinal tracts and lymphoid system has been reported.

The reason for this increased susceptibility to atopic disease, autoimmune disease, and cancer is not known, but one theory is that IgA normally interacts with many antigens on the mucosal surfaces and prevents their entry into the body.[8] A deficiency of IgA would allow the body to be exposed to more antigens than it can successfully combat. Because of increased antigenic stimulation, more antigen can react with IgE and produce allergic manifestations. Increased risk of production of antibody that will cross react with a self-antigen increases the risk of autoimmune disease. Chronic irritation and inflammation caused by the large amount of antigen could predispose the exposed tissue to malignant transformation.

## Deficiency of Cell-Mediated Immunity (DiGeorge Syndrome)

Selective immune deficiency affecting T cells but not B cells is rare. The complete DiGeorge syndrome consists of (1) low-set ears and slanted eyes; (2) hypoparathyroidism; (3) congenital heart defects, such as septal defects and truncus arteriosus; and (4) cellular immune deficiency.[13] It is associated with failure of the embryonic third and fourth pharyngeal pouches to develop, which results in hypoplasia or aplasia of the thymus gland. No familial history is found, so it is thought that the defect is due to an environmental agent or drug exposure before the 8th week of gestation. If the defect is not complete, T-cell function may become adequate by age 5 years.[13]

Among other causes of deficiency of cell-mediated immunity, the most common is an enzyme defect (purine nucleoside phosphorylase) that results in accumulation of by-products within T lymphocytes, causing a blockage of DNA synthesis. The congenital thymic hypoplasia causes a decrease or absence of T cells, and the neonate is extremely susceptible to fungal and viral infections. This defect has been successfully treated by transplantation of the thymus gland. If the disease is untreated, death resulting from overwhelming infection occurs in infancy.[7]

The immune defect is due to the developmental failure of the thymus and parathyroid glands. Lack of the thymus gland, and thus lack of the thymic hormone, results in failure of T cells to mature.

Persons with this condition are unable to reject allografts or react to skin test antigens. They have little or no resistance to intracellular infections by viruses, fungi, and some gram-negative bacteria. A decrease of T-cell helper function may depress the humoral response. In com-

**TABLE 15-1.**
CLINICAL PROBLEMS ASSOCIATED WITH
COMPLEMENT DEFICIENCIES

| COMPLEMENT PROTEIN | CLINICAL PROBLEMS |
| --- | --- |
| C1q | High frequency of immune complex disease |
| C1r | High frequency of immune complex disease |
| C2 | High frequency of immune complex disease |
| C3 | Recurrent pyogenic infection |
| C4 | High frequency of immune complex disease |
| C5 | Recurrent neisserial infection, high frequency of systemic lupus erythematosus |
| C6 | Recurrent neisserial infection |
| C7 | Recurrent neisserial infection |
| C8 | Recurrent neisserial infection |
| C9 | Asymptomatic |
| C11NH | Angioneurotic edema |
| Factor (C3bINA) | Recurrent pyogenic infection |
| Factor H | Recurrent pyogenic infection |
| Properdin (P) | Recurrent neisserial infection |

*Unanue, E.R. and Benacerraf, B. Textbook of Immunology (2nd ed.). Table 15.1, p. 306. Baltimore: Williams & Wilkins, 1984. Copyright © 1984 The Williams & Wilkins Co., Baltimore. Reproduced with permission from the publisher.*

plete DiGeorge syndrome, the corresponding failure of parathyroid development may lead to tetany caused by hypocalcemia.

## Complement Abnormalities

Complement factors are necessary to promote the inflammatory process. Complement deficiency has been detected in an increased number of persons with autoimmune disease (Table 15-1). Various symptoms occur, depending on the complement factor that is deficient.

Deficiency of complement inhibitors also can result in allergic reactions; the most frequent is hereditary angioedema, caused by a genetic deficiency of C1 esterase inhibitor. This produces uncontrolled activation of the complement system, causing angioedema in the skin, larynx, and gastrointestinal and genitourinary tracts.[7]

Deficiencies of complement 2 and 3 (C2 and C3) are fairly common. Deficiency of C2 is transmitted as an autosomal dominant trait, and people with this condition have a high frequency of systemic lupus erythematosus and other connective tissue disorders.[13,26]

Deficiency of C3 results in impairment of the inflammatory response and difficulty in clearing pyogenic and gram-negative infection. The deficiency can be inherited or acquired. The substance is used faster than it can be made in major systemic infections or in a nutritionally depleted host.[7]

# SECONDARY IMMUNE DEFICIENCY

## Multifactorial Secondary Immune Deficiency

Secondary immune deficiency states result from the loss of a previously effective immune system. They include any disorder that exhibits loss of immunocompetence as a result of another condition. A broad classification includes immune deficiency secondary to stress, malnutrition, systemic infection, cancer, renal diseases, radiation therapy, immunosuppressive drugs, or aging (Box 15-2). These conditions may lead to a loss of immunoglobulins, inadequate synthesis of immunoglobulins, loss of specific lymphocytes responsible for cell-mediated immunity, loss of phagocytic inflammatory cells, or a combination of these.

Even though decreased effectiveness of the immune system frequently is not life-threatening, it often results in decreased ability of the organisms to mount an inflammatory or immune response. Therefore, susceptibility to infection by bacteria, viruses, fungi, or all three is increased. In some cases, the loss of immunocompetence causes enough alteration in host resistance to increase morbidity and mortality.

Stress response has been the target of a great deal of research with respect to how it disrupts the physiologic functioning of the body. Stress appears to alter the immune response by neural interruption from the hypothalamus, which ultimately decreases the functioning of the thymus through secretion of glucocorticoids. Glucocorticoid hormones mainly diminish the inflammatory

**BOX 15-2**
CONDITIONS THAT CAUSE SECONDARY
IMMUNOSUPPRESSION

Immunosuppressive therapy
  Antimetabolites
  Corticosteroids
  Antibiotics
Radiation therapy
Cancer
  B-cell lymphoproliferative disorders
  T-cell deficiency
Acquired immune deficiency syndrome
Stress
Aging
Systemic infections
Renal disease
Malnutrition
  Cirrhosis
  Tumor cachexia
  Dietary deficiency
Burns
Trauma
Surgery

response by suppressing macrophages, decreasing the number of white blood cells, and causing regression of lymphatic tissue. This can enhance the spread of infection (see Chap. 6).

Immune system changes with aging have been studied extensively. Some studies have related aging changes to immune system deterioration. Most studies of immune system cell numbers show little change over the life span.[5,26] The activities of T cells may change because of an increased number of immature T cells in the blood. As a person ages, there is a decrease in thymic hormone, which may cause a decline in cell-mediated immunity.[5] When the T cells are less functional, there is a decrease in B-cell activation to mount specific antibody responses. In an older person, there is an increase in the production of autoantibodies and apparently nonfunctional monoclonal immunoglobulin proteins.[5] The results of immune system dysfunction include (1) a decrease in the ability to control infections; (2) possibly a decrease in immune surveillance, which leads to an increase in cancer; and (3) possibly an increase in autoimmune diseases related to increased autoantibody production.[5,7,26]

*Immunosuppression* usually refers to the pharmacologic suppression of the immune system. Drugs have been used extensively to decrease the rejection phenomenon in transplanted tissue, the rate of growth of malignant tumors, and the inflammation involved with autoimmune disorders. Agents used to achieve these effects are cytotoxic drugs, such as methotrexate, and corticosteroids, such as hydrocortisone. The cytotoxic drugs are toxic to cells that divide rapidly, including T and B lymphocytes as well as polymorphonuclear leukocytes. Corticosteroids suppress the inflammatory response. The result of immunosuppression is increased sensitivity to the environmental antigens. Superimposed infections may develop and spread readily. Many pharmacologic agents cause depression of the bone marrow formation of leukocytes, and thus affect all types of white blood cells.[27]

Systemic infection can deplete the host defense to the point at which further antigen stimulation may result in decreased resistance. Thus host resistance is decreased and opportunistic organisms may cause serious problems.

Cancer usually causes malnutrition as a result of protein wasting. Decreased synthesis of lymphocytes results. Immune deficiency caused by B lymphoproliferative disorders such as chronic lymphocytic leukemia and multiple myeloma results in impairment of the antibody responses, causing secondary infections with pyogenic bacteria.

Radiation therapy, usually instituted against cancer, affects rapidly proliferating cells and results in a decrease in all of the cells of the inflammatory response, including the T and B lymphocytes. Opportunistic infections, especially those caused by gram-negative bacteria, viruses, and fungi, occur with increased frequency.[25]

Renal disease probably causes most of its immuno-suppressive effects from proteinuria leading to hypoproteinemia or from acid–base disruptions that can affect the formation of lymphocytes, especially T cells. Many pathologic processes of the kidneys are treated with corticosteroids, and immunosuppression may result from drug therapy.

## *Acquired Immune Deficiency Syndrome (HIV Disease)*

Opportunistic diseases associated with acquired immune deficiency syndrome (AIDS) were first reported in the United States in mid-1981. Small clusters of *Pneumocystis carinii* pneumonia (PCP) and Kaposi's sarcoma (KS) were reported among young, otherwise healthy male homosexuals. Although they were not previously unknown diseases, PCP and KS had not affected that target population before 1981 and had remained fairly restricted to young malnourished children (PCP), elderly men of Mediterranean ancestry (KS), and immunosuppressed people (both PCP and KS). With subsequent reports of horizontal transmission of these diseases and of their occurrence among recipients of blood products (eg, factor VIII cryoprecipitate for hemophilia), the possibility of an infectious agent was raised. The virus that causes AIDS, a retrovirus (ie, RNA-containing), now termed human immunodeficiency virus type 1 (HIV-1), was discovered by French and American researchers in 1983-84. In addition to HIV transmission through sexual activity and through contaminated blood, reports of vertical perinatal transmission from infected women to their offspring established the third method of viral spread. The awareness that HIV was a blood-borne virus prompted the development of tests to screen donated blood for the presence of HIV antibodies that would reveal a previously infected donor. One such screening antibody test, the ELISA (enzyme-linked immunosorbent assay), was approved for general clinical use in 1985.

### *Modes of HIV Transmission*

Three modes of transmission of HIV have been identified since the beginnings of the epidemic: (1) through sexual activity, (2) through blood-to-blood contamination, and (3) through perinatal events.

Most of the cases reported in the United States occurred through *sexual activity* (man-to-man transmission), reflecting a high virus load in seminal fluid. Bidirectional heterosexual transmission, in which 75% of all cases are transmitted from man-to-woman and 25% from woman-to-man, confirms the high risk of seminal fluid. Although it is easy to conceptualize how the virus may be acquired by the recipient of infected semen, the portal of HIV entry into the circulation in man-to-woman transmission has not been clearly determined.[1] Woman-to-man spread may be achieved through contaminated vaginal fluids, cervical mucus, or menstrual blood, but the portal of entry in the male, likewise, has not yet been conclusively identified. Recent data on transmission of hepatitis B virus and HIV among homosexual males suggest that transurethral exposure is an important transmission method.[16] The recipient of unprotected anal or vaginal intercourse carries the highest risk of HIV infection, followed by the inserter in these two activities, respectively.[11] It is the sexual activity practiced, and not the gender or sexual orientation of the participants, that determines the risk factors in sexual transmission of HIV. For this reason, there is an increasing tendency, when reporting HIV statistics, to replace the term "groups at risk" by the concept of "activities at risk."

Blood-to-blood contamination accounts for the transmission of HIV among intravenous (recreational) drug users (IVDUs) through the sharing of hypodermic needles and devices; the recipients of blood products, including clotting factors; and, in rare instances, occupational infection of health care workers from HIV-positive patients. The frequency of HIV infection in IVDUs and in their sex partners and offspring has increased significantly in recent years, with a disproportionate number of cases among blacks and Hispanics. A recent study of 452 persons enrolled in a methadone treatment program revealed an overall HIV seroprevalence of 40%, with 49% in blacks (who account for 12% of the general U.S. population), 42% in Hispanics (who account for 7%), and 17% in non-Hispanic whites.[24] The rate of HIV infection among *hemophiliacs* averages 55% and is a function of frequency of clotting factors infusion (people with severe hemophilia being at increased risk) and the time when most infusions took place (new infections were virtually eliminated since 1985, with the development of viral-inactivation measures and donor antibody testing).[12] Likewise, HIV infection through blood transfusions has declined since 1985 because all units of donated blood are antibody-tested. However, because there is a window of time between infection and seroconversion, blood units can test antibody-negative but actually be virus-positive. The current risk of HIV transmission from screened blood is in the range of 1 in 38,000 to 1 in 153,000 units of donated blood.[2] This risk increases in areas of high HIV prevalence. The frequency of HIV infection following occupational exposure among *health care workers* is small, given their extensive contact with persons who are HIV-infected or their body fluids.[20]

*Perinatal transmission* from an HIV-positive woman may occur during gestation, during labor and delivery, or postpartum through breast-feeding.[23] Reported rates of transmission of HIV from pregnant women to their offspring range from 20% to 65%.[15] Because the virus can cross the placenta, variation in transmission rates appears to be related to maternal virus load; women who become pregnant soon after infection have a lower transmission risk than those who conceive many months or years after infection, or those who have previously given birth to HIV-positive children. Rates of HIV infection through vaginal versus cesarean delivery are not significantly different, which indicates that most infections occur during gestation. Transmission through breast milk has been challenged, since nipple fissures during lactation are a common occurrence and transmission through blood cannot be ruled out.

## Epidemiologic Trends

An estimated 1 to 1.5 million Americans are infected with HIV-1. As of September 30, 1991, the Centers for Disease Control (CDC) reports 126,159 deaths.[29]

The United States is witnessing the emergence of a new wave of people with HIV infection—the offspring of women who were infected through intravenous drug use or through sexual activity with an IVDU. The first wave was represented by homosexual and bisexual men infected through sexual activity, the second by IVDUs who acquired the virus through needle-sharing.

The frequency of new cases of HIV infection among homosexual men has decreased in recent years. This trend is probably due to intensive educational efforts directed at that community, resulting in stricter adherence to safer sex practices and a reduction in the number of sex partners. The majority of reported cases of AIDS in the United States (67%), however, continues to occur among homosexual and bisexual men, and projections for the decade of the 1990s indicate that this pattern will persist.

Educational outreach toward the IVDU community has not succeeded in reducing the number of new cases. This population currently accounts for 17% of all reported cases, a significant increase from the 5% reported in 1985. Impairment of mental ability and judgment caused by drug use precludes IVDUs from implementing risk-reduction activities, such as needle-cleaning with sterilizing solutions, avoidance of needle-sharing behavior, and the consistent use of condoms during sexual activity. Projections for the new decade suggest a further increase in the frequency of HIV infection among IVDUs. Because the virus often is transmitted from infected IVDUs to their (mostly heterosexual) sex partners, educational efforts are now being directed at these women in an attempt to empower them to take responsibility for implementing their own protective measures.[14] In the early 1980s, sexual activity was the most common source of HIV infection in women; in 1990, 51% of infections in women can be attributed to drug use.[29] HIV infection was the eighth leading cause of death among women in the reproductive age category, a rate that was increased by 40% in 1988. Projections for 1991 indicate that HIV infection will be among the five leading causes of death among women of child-bearing age.[4] Because 80% of infected children acquired the virus from their infected mothers, educational approaches aimed at women should, if successful, reduce infection rates among these mothers and their children.

## Natural History and Immunologic Aspects of HIV Infection

Once introduced into the blood circulation, HIV initiates the infective process by binding to a specific receptor glycoprotein (CD4) present on the surface of target host cells. Such CD4-positive cells include helper T cells; various antigen-presenting cells, including monocytes or macrophages in the central nervous system, peripheral blood, and lungs; dendritic cells in lymph nodes and peripheral blood; microglial cells and neurons; and others.[18] After binding, HIV enters the cell, loses its coat, and releases its two RNA molecules into the cytoplasm of the host cell. By a process called *reverse transcription*, the incoming viral RNA controls the synthesis of viral DNA and viral proteins, resulting in (1) the integration of viral DNA into the genome of the host cell in the form of a latent provirion, and (2) the production of new viral particles. Also, as a consequence of viral infection, large numbers of host cells are killed by mechanisms yet unknown.[3] The cumulative effects of increased numbers of viruses with the loss of helper T lymphocytes result in progressive, severe impairment of immune function, which renders the host vulnerable to the opportunistic diseases that are the hallmark of HIV infection. The production of host cells with an integrated provirion ensures the availability of viruses for future infection, as these provirions are activated into infective particles by yet undetermined factors.

In the intact immune system, the regulatory effects of helper T cells (T4 cells) are modulated by the action of suppressor T cells (T8 cells). For instance, T4 cells stimulate blast proliferation of antigen-activated B cells, and thus they indirectly stimulate the production of antibodies by the formed plasma cells. Conversely, T8 cells inhibit B-cell blast proliferation and therefore suppress antibody production. The balance between the two effects is achieved through a T4-T8 ratio of about 2:1, which means that in an intact immune system, the tendency is toward stimulation, not inhibition, of antibody production. The T4-T8 ratio is an important predictor of disease progression in HIV disease. When the ideal ratio of 2:1 falls to about 1:1, it reflects a reduction in T4 numbers and is indicative of significant immune suppression. Ratios below 0.5:1 signal impending opportunistic diseases. Reduction in total T4 cell count also is prognostic of immune dysfunction. When the normal count (650–1200 cells per cubic millimeter) drops to 500/mm³, significant impairment of immune function is expected; a reduction to 200/mm³ or less indicates impending opportunistic disease.[21] Although T4 cell count is the most reliable indicator of disease progress, the clinician should not be surprised to encounter people with markedly reduced counts (sometimes in the range of 10–100/mm³) who exhibit no signs or symptoms of immune dysfunction for long periods.

Impairment of T- and B-cell function creates a severe loss of cell-mediated and humoral immunity and results in (1) production of nonspecific immunoglobulins (including IgM hyperimmunoglobulinemia common in pediatric cases) and (2) impaired natural killer cell function, resulting in decreased cancer immunosurveillance ability.

## Clinical Course for HIV Infection

According to the current classification by the Centers for Disease Control (CDC), the spectrum of HIV disease encompasses the four groups shown in Box 15-3.[28]

The initial phase of HIV disease, or *group I disease*, is termed acute HIV infection, or *acute retroviral syndrome*.[30] This phase is represented by a transient mononucleosis-like symptomatology, which occurs about 10 to 14 days after infection. The symptoms usually include fever, myalgia, arthralgia, malaise, lymphadenopathy, gastrointestinal symptoms, sore throat, headache, and photophobia. In many cases, this flulike illness may be accompanied by a rash, a roseola-like eruption that occurs mainly on the trunk and limbs. This illness usually subsides within a few days, with the rash remaining for as long as 1 week, and the infected person returns to an asymptomatic status.[30] Virus multiplication continues during this period, and seroconversion usually occurs within 2 to 12 weeks (seroconversion time) after infection; thus most HIV-infected asymptomatic people (group II) will yield positive results on antibody tests such as the ELISA and the Western blot. From this point on, most people will continue to test HIV antibody-positive. Delayed seroconversion, up to 18 months, has been reported.[22]

*Group II disease* in CDC classification is represented by an asymptomatic phase whose duration, as of this writing, may be as long as 11 years (incubation period). In the absence of any symptomatology, infected people can be identified only by a positive HIV-antibody test. Antibodies produced against the HIV do not neutralize the virus, which means that anyone who tests HIV antibody-positive also must be considered virus-positive and a potential transmitter of HIV through sexual activity or blood-sharing. Despite the inaccuracy of the terminology that has been developed, people in this phase are commonly termed HIV-positive (virus) carriers.

Conversion to *group III disease* is signaled by the development of various nonspecific clinical manifestations, including persistent generalized lymphadenopathy, night fever and night sweats, rash, muscle pain, malaise, fatigue, persistent cough, and diarrhea. These early signs and symptoms of disease process are traditionally associated with a phase formerly termed *AIDS-related complex (ARC)*.

*Group IV disease*, commonly referred to as AIDS, or

## BOX 15–3.
### CENTERS FOR DISEASE CONTROL CLASSIFICATION FOR HIV INFECTION

Group I.   Acute HIV infection

Group II.  Asymptomatic HIV infection

Group III. Persistent generalized lymphadenopathy (PGL)
Lymphadenopathy (>1 cm diameter) at 2 or more extrainguinal sites lasting more than 3 months without another condition to explain the findings

Group IV.  Other HIV disease

Subgroup A:  Constitutional disease. One or more of the following: fever for >1 month, 10% weight loss, diarrhea lasting <1 month, and no other condition to explain the findings

Subgroup B:  Neurologic disease. One or more of the following: dementia, myelopathy, or peripheral neuropathy, and no other condition to explain the findings

Subgroup C:  Secondary infectious diseases

C-1:        One of the 12 specified symptomatic or invasive diseases that define AIDS: *Pneumocystis carinii* pneumonia, chronic cryptosporidiosis, toxoplasmosis, extraintestinal strongyloidiasis, isoporiasis, candidiasis (esophageal, bronchial, or pulmonary), cryptococcosis, histoplasmosis, *Mycobacterium avium* complex or *M. kansasii*, cytomegalovirus, chronic mucocutaneous or disseminated herpes simplex infection, or progressive multifocal leukoencephalopathy

C-2:        Symptomatic or invasive disease with one of the following: oral hairy leukoplakia, multidermatomal herpes zoster, recurrent *Salmonella* bacteremia, nocardiosis, tuberculosis, or oral candidiasis

Subgroup D:  Secondary cancers. Diagnosis of one of the following known to be associated with HIV infection: Kaposi's sarcoma, non-Hodgkin's lymphoma (small, noncleaved lymphoma or immunoblastic sarcoma), or primary lymphoma of the brain

Subgroup E:  Other conditions in HIV infection. Includes a variety of clinical findings that may be attributable to HIV disease, including chronic lymphoid interstitial pneumonitis, constitutional symptoms not meeting subgroup IV-A, patients with infectious diseases not meeting subgroup IV-C, and patients with neoplasms not meeting subgroup IV-D

*U.S. Centers for Disease Control. Classification system for human T-lymphotrophic virus type III/lymphadenopathy-associated virus infection. M.M.W.R. 35:334, 1986.*

fully developed AIDS, is characterized by the appearance of specific disease processes, and is further divided into five subgroups that identify the presenting condition. *Subgroup A* represents disease diagnosed by constitutional manifestations (fever, weight loss); *subgroup B*, by neurologic disease (AIDS dementia complex); *subgroup C*, by opportunistic infections (eg, PCP); *subgroup D*, by secondary cancers (eg, KS); and *subgroup E*, by other HIV-related conditions, such as lymphoid interstitial pneumonitis, a common condition among HIV-infected children. Recovery from Group IV disease has not been reported.

Although this classification system currently is adopted in most civilian clinical settings, the trend in describing the clinical progression of HIV infection has been moving toward a two-point classification: (1) asymptomatic HIV disease (formerly asymptomatic HIV-positive, or carrier) and (2) symptomatic HIV disease, to include early, nonspecific disease (formerly ARC) and late, specific disease (AIDS). This disease interpretation is based on the knowledge that HIV disease represents a continuum that begins with infection and, in the absence of successful therapeutic intervention, leads to AIDS.

## Treatment Approaches

Because the major clinical manifestations of HIV infection result from opportunistic diseases secondary to immunosuppression, palliative treatment is indicated for each individual disorder. For instance, fungal infections such as those caused by *Cryptococcus neoformans* can be successfully controlled by antifungal agents such as ketoconazole or amphotericin. PCP is the presenting disease in about 60% of all cases of HIV infection, and until recently, it accounted for 75% to 80% of all deaths. Intravenous and, more recently, aerosolized administration of pentamidine has achieved remarkable results in the prophylaxis and treatment of PCP. The management of KS is still not greatly successful in controlling tumor growth or metastasis. Treatment approaches for KS include chemotherapy with vinblastine, immunotherapy with interferon, and palliative radiation therapy.

In the future, total management of HIV infection will need to be approached on a three-prong basis: prophylactic vaccination of uninfected people coupled with antiviral agents and immune modulators ("immune boosters").

The development of an effective vaccine has been hindered by various obstacles: (1) variability of the viral genome because of the high mutation rate of the HIV; (2) anti-HIV antibodies are produced by infected people (the general aim of active immunization methods), but they are not efficient in neutralizing the virus; (3) lack of adequate animal models (with the exception of the chimpanzee and a recently developed mouse strain, other laboratory animals could not be infected with the virus); (4) definitive evidence of vaccine safety (genetically engineered vaccines must not contain any traces of infectious fragments of the virus); and (5) demonstration of efficacy (difficult to establish when progressing from animal models to clinical trials).

In the management of infected people, treatment approaches vary according to disease progression. In the early stages, when the immune system is not so severely compromised and opportunistic diseases are absent, treatment can be restricted to antiviral agents to prevent viral replication and disease progression. In the later stages, the presence of severe immune suppression and opportunistic diseases requires the combination of antiviral agents with immune modulators.

Immune modulators studied, so far unsuccessfully, include replacement methods (eg, lymphocyte transfer, bone marrow transplant, immunoglobulin replacement) and the use of biologic response modifiers, such as interleukin 2 and other cytokines, and interferons. New clinical trials that combine antiviral agents with immune modulators (interferon) are in progress.

The most promising approach is the development of antiviral agents that block reverse transcription and arrest intracellular viral replication. Such agents are active only against intracellular virus particles and not free-circulating viruses. As such, these drugs need to be taken for life, and therefore, they should have manageable side effects. The most successful of these agents is zidovudine (AZT), followed by some related compounds such as 2pr,3pr-dideoxyinosine (ddI). The use of zidovudine has significantly reduced the signs and symptoms of infection and extended the life span of symptomatic people. It is now being used by HIV-positive asymptomatic people in an attempt to delay disease development.[10] The most significant side effect of zidovudine is bone marrow suppression, with about 50% of the people developing anemia and becoming transfusion-dependent. A recent study has concluded that administration of erythropoietin in conjunction with zidovudine significantly increases red blood cell production.[9]

Initial results from studies on the effects of ddI have concluded that this drug is effective in increasing T4 count while decreasing viral titer.[6,19] Another encouraging finding is that, although not toxicity-free, the side effects of ddI (mostly pancreatitis and painful peripheral neuropathy) differed from those of zidovudine, which will permit the use of these two agents in combination.

Although antiviral therapy appears to be the most effective approach to the treatment of HIV disease, clinicians are beginning to realize that the control of this disease will require long-term administration of multiple-drug regimens not unlike the current approach to cancer chemotherapy. It also is apparent that the management of HIV disease in the future will be that of a chronic disease, by which a drug protocol will prevent asymptomatic HIV-positive people from developing disease process. In this sense, HIV disease in the future may be managed like controlled diabetes mellitus.

## REFERENCES

1. Alexander, N.J. Sexual transmission of human immunodeficiency virus: Virus entry into the male and female genital tract. *Fertil. Steril.* 54:1, 1990.

2. Alter, H.J., Epstein, J.S., Swenson, S.G., et al. Prevalence of human immunodeficiency virus type 1 p24 antigen in U.S. blood donors—an assessment of the efficacy of testing in donor screening. *N. Engl. J. Med.* 323:1312, 1990.

3. Broder, S. The life cycle of human immunodeficiency virus as a guide to the design of new therapies for AIDS. In V.T. DeVita, S. Hellman, and S.A. Rosenberg (eds.), *AIDS: Etiology, Diagnosis, Treatment, and Prevention* (2nd ed.). Philadelphia: J.B. Lippincott, 1988.

4. Chu, S.Y., Buehler, J.W., and Berkelman, R.S. Impact of the human immunodeficiency virus epidemic on mortality in women of reproductive age, United States. *J.A.M.A.* 264:225, 1990.

5. Cohen, H.J. Immune regulation. In W.N. Kelley, *Textbook of Internal Medicine.* Philadelphia: J.B. Lippincott, 1989.

6. Cooley, T.P., Kunches, L.M., Saunders, C.A., et al. Once-daily administration of 2pr,3pr-dideoxyinosine (ddI) in patients with the acquired immunodeficiency syndrome or AIDS-related complex. *N. Engl. J. Med.* 322:1340, 1990.

7. Cotran, R.S., Kumar, V., and Robbins, S.L. *Robbins' Pathologic Basis of Disease* (4th ed.). Philadelphia: W.B. Saunders, 1989.

8. Elson, C.O. Gastrointestinal disease with an immune basis. In W.N. Kelley, *Textbook of Internal Medicine.* Philadelphia: J.B. Lippincott, 1989.

9. Fischl, M.A., Galpin, J.E., Levine, J.D., et al. Recombinant human erythropoietin for patients with AIDS treated with zidovudine. *N. Engl. J. Med.* 322:1488, 1990.

10. Fischl, M.A., Richman, D.D., Frieco, M.H., et al. The efficacy of azidothymidine (AZT) in the treatment of patients with AIDS and AIDS-related complex: A double-blind, placebo-controlled trial. *N. Engl. J. Med.* 317:185, 1987.

11. Glasel, M. High-risk sexual practices in the transmission of AIDS. In V.T. DeVita, S. Hellman, and S.A. Rosenberg (eds.), *AIDS: Etiology, Diagnosis, Treatment, and Prevention* (2nd ed.). Philadelphia: J.B. Lippincott, 1988.

12. Goedert, J.J., Kessler, C.M., Aledort, L.M., et al. A prospective study of human immunodeficiency virus type 1 infection and the development of AIDS in subjects with hemophilia. *N. Engl. J. Med.* 321:1141, 1989.

13. Haeney, M. *Introduction to Clinical Immunology.* Boston: Butterworth, 1985.

14. Haile, B. *Drug Use Practices and Sexual Behavior Among IV Drug Users and Their Sexual Partners in Houston: Risk Factors for AIDS,* thesis. University of Texas Health Science Center, School of Public Health, Houston, 1990.

15. Halsey, N.A., Boulos, R., Holt, E., et al. Transmission of HIV-1infections from mothers to infants in Haiti. *J.A.M.A.* 264:2088, 1990.

16. Kingsley, L.A., Rinaldo, C.R., Lyter, D.W., et al. Sexual transmission efficiency of hepatitis B virus and human immunodeficiency virus among homosexual men. *J.A.M.A.* 264: 230, 1990.

17. Kissane, J.M., and Scotti, J. *Anderson's Synopsis of Pathology* (12th ed.). St. Louis: C.V. Mosby, 1991.

18. Koenig, S., and Faucci, A.S. AIDS: Immunopathogenesis and immune response to the human immunodeficiency virus. In V.T. DeVita, S. Hellman, and S.A. Rosenberg (eds.), *AIDS: Etiology, Diagnosis, Treatment, and Prevention* (2nd ed.). Philadelphia: J.B. Lippincott, 1988.

19. Lambert, J.S., Seidlin, M., Reichman, R.C., et al. 2pr,3pr-dideoxyinosine (ddI) in patients with the acquired immunodeficiency syndrome or AIDS-related complex: A phase I trial. *N. Engl. J. Med.* 322:1333, 1990.

20. Marcus, R., and the CDC Cooperative Needlestick Surveillance Group. Surveillance of health care workers exposed to blood from patients infected with the human immunodeficiency virus. *N. Engl. J. Med.* 319:1118, 1988.

21. Polk, B.F., Fox, R., Bookmeyer, R., et al. Predictors of the acquired immunodeficiency syndrome developing in a cohort of seropositive homosexual men. *N. Engl. J. Med.* 316:61, 1987.

22. Ranki, A., Valle, K.L., Krohn, M., et al. Long latency precedes overt seroconversion in sexually transmitted human immunodeficiency virus infection. *Lancet* 2:589, 1987.

23. Rogers, M.F., Ou, C-Y., Rayfield, M., et al. Use of polymerase chain reaction for early detection of the proviral sequences of human immunodeficiency virus in infants born to seropositive mothers. *N. Engl. J. Med.* 320:1649, 1989.

24. Shoenbaum, E.E., Hartel, D., Selwyn, P.A., et al. Risk factors for human immunodeficiency virus infection in intravenous drug users. *N. Engl. J. Med.* 321:874, 1989.

25. Stites, D.P., et al. *Basic and Clinical Immunology* (5th ed.). Los Altos, Calif.: Lange, 1984.

26. Stites, D.P., and Terr, A.I. *Basic Human Immunology* (7th ed.). Norwalk, Conn.: Appleton & Lange, 1990.

27. Unanue, E.R., and Benacerraf, B. *Textbook of Immunology* (2nd ed.). Baltimore: Williams & Wilkins, 1984.

28. U.S. Centers for Disease Control. Classification system for human T-lymphotrophic virus type III-lymphadenopathy-associated virus infections. *M.M.W.R.* 35:334, 1986.

29. U.S. Centers for Disease Control. *IV/AIDS Surveillance Report, September*. Atlanta: CDC, 1991.

30. Yarchoan, R., and Pluda, J.M. Clinical aspects of infection with AIDS retrovirus: Acute HIV infection, persistent generalized lymphadenopathy, and AIDS-related complex. In V.T. DeVita, S. Hellman, and S.A. Rosenberg (eds.), *AIDS: Etiology, Diagnosis, Treatment, and Prevention* (2nd ed.). Philadelphia: J.B. Lippincott, 1988.

# chapter 16

Barbara L. Bullock

# Hypersensitivity and Autoimmune Reactions

## Learning Objectives

1. Define *hypersensitivity reactions.*
2. Discuss the types of agents that can elicit hypersensitivity reactions.
3. Describe the types of hypersensitivity reactions according to underlying pathophysiologic mechanisms and how they are manifested as disease.
4. Differentiate between anaphylaxis and atopy.
5. Identify the mechanisms of red cell destruction seen with cytotoxic hypersensitivity reactions.
6. Describe the results of hemolysis with respect to transfusion reactions, erythroblastosis fetalis, and warm and cold antibody diseases.
7. Describe the development of Goodpasture's syndrome as a result of cytotoxic hypersensitivity.
8. Explain the underlying pathophysiology of immune complex disease.
9. Describe the mechanisms that occur in serum sickness.
10. Identify the pathophysiologic mechanism of Arthus reaction.
11. Describe the relation of hypersensitivity reactions and autoimmune disorders.
12. Describe the pathophysiologic mechanisms by which delayed hypersensitivity can result.
13. Identify the histology of contact dermatitis.
14. Describe transplant graft rejection using the transplanted kidney as an example.
15. Describe the classification of immune disruptions according to homologous, exogenous, and autologous source of antigen.
16. List at least six conditions that are probably the result of autoimmunity.
17. Name the main clinical finding that supports diagnosis of the autoimmune phenomena.
18. Describe systemic lupus erythematosus (SLE) in terms of pathology and resultant clinical effects.
19. List 10 of the 14 criteria issued by the American Rheumatism Association for the diagnosis of SLE.
20. Describe the basis for classifying rheumatoid arthritis as an autoimmune disease.
21. Explain the pathophysiologic results of rheumatoid arthritis on the joints and the other systems of the body.
22. Describe the syndrome of rheumatoid arthritis.

Tissue-damaging immune disorders have been classified in various ways to clarify their pathophysiologic basis. Four mechanisms of immunologically mediated disorders have been described according to the manner in which tissue injury occurs.[11] Some of these conditions also may be classified as autoimmune reactions. These are both discussed in this chapter.

The classic term for immunologic, tissue-damaging reactions is *hypersensitivity reactions,* which refers to an exaggerated response of the immune system to an antigen. The antigen that elicits the response is called an *allergen.* Allergens produce different responses, depending on a person's genetic predisposition for an exaggerated response. In some cases, the antigen that produces the response is unknown.

## CLASSIFICATIONS OF TISSUE INJURY CAUSED BY HYPERSENSITIVITY

The types of hypersensitivity reactions are described in this section according to the underlying pathophysiologic mechanisms and how they manifest themselves in different diseases (Table 16-1). Figure 16-1 shows a summary diagram of the four types of hypersensitivity reactions.

## Type I: Immediate Hypersensitivity: Anaphylaxis or Atopy

Anaphylaxis refers to an acute reaction usually associated with a wheal-and-flare type of skin reaction and vasodilation that may precipitate circulatory shock. Atopy, which results from the same mechanism, chronically recurs in responses that depend on the antigen, frequency of contact, route of contact, and sensitivity of the organ system to the antigen.

Atopy, or anaphylactic disease, is the most common of the immediate hypersensitivity reactions. These diseases, commonly called *allergies,* occur in organs that are exposed to environmental antigens.[2] The skin, respiratory tract, and gastrointestinal system are especially affected. Many types of antigens or allergens can initiate the hypersensitivity state in susceptible people. The most common of these are the environmental allergens, such as pollens, dander, foods, insect bites, and certain household cleaning agents. Drug sensitivity reactions can effect the same response. Other disease states that are classified in this group include hay fever, urticaria (hives), asthma, and atopic eczema. Susceptibility to allergy is inherited and may result from excessive IgE production.[13]

Pathophysiologically, the immune response is acti-

**TABLE 16-1.**
Classification of Hypersensitivity States

| TYPE | CAUSE | RESPONSIBLE CELL OR ANTIBODY | IMMUNE MECHANISM | EXAMPLES OF DISEASE STATES |
|---|---|---|---|---|
| I—Immediate hypersensitivity (Anaphylaxis, atopy) | Foreign protein (antigen) | IgE | IgE attaches to surface of mast cell and specific antigen, triggers release of intracellular granules from mast cells | Hay fever, allergies, hives, anaphylactic shock |
| II—Cytotoxic hypersensitivity | Foreign protein (antigen) | IgG or IgM | Antibody reacts with antigen, activates complement, causes cytolysis or phagocytosis | Transfusion, hemolytic drug reactions, erythroblastosis fetalis, hemolytic anemia, vascular purpura, Goodpasture's syndrome |
| III—Immune complex disease | Foreign protein (antigen) | IgG | Antigen–antibody complexes precipitate in tissue, activate complement, cause inflammatory reaction | Rheumatoid arthritis, systemic lupus erythematosus, serum sickness |
| IV—Delayed/Cell-mediated | Foreign protein, cell, or tissue | T lymphocytes | Sensitized T cell reacts with specific antigen to induce inflammatory process by direct cell action or by activity of lymphokines | Contact dermatitis, transplant graft reaction |

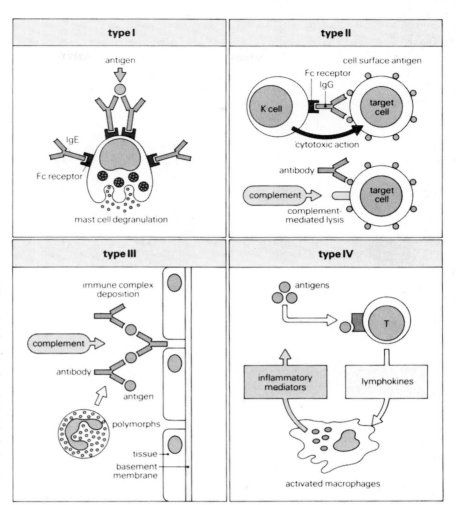

**FIGURE 16-1.**

Summary diagram of the four types of hypersensitivity reaction. *Type I.* Mast cells bind IgE by way of their Fc receptors. On encountering antigen, the IgE becomes cross-linked, inducing degranulation and release of mediators. *Type II.* Antibody is directed against antigens on a person's own cells (target cell). This may lead to cytotoxic action by K-cell or complement-mediated lysis. *Type III.* Immune complexes are deposited in the tissue. Complement is activated, and polymorphs are attracted to the site of deposition, causing local damage. *Type IV.* Antigen-sensitized T cells release lymphokines after a secondary contact with the same antigen. Lymphokines induce inflammatory reactions, and activate and attract macrophages, which release mediators. (From I. Roitt, J. Brostoff, and D. Male, *Immunology* [2nd ed.]. Philadelphia: J.B. Lippincott, 1989.)

vated when antigen binds to IgE antibodies attached to the surface of mast cells. Mast cells are present in profusion in connective tissue, skin, and mucous membranes. The reaction proceeds when the IgE molecule specific for a particular antigen becomes cross-linked on the surface of the mast cell and triggers the release of intracellular granules. These granules contain large quantities of histamine and other chemotactic substances. Histamine causes peripheral vasodilation and an increase in vascular permeability, resulting in local vascular congestion and edema. It also causes constriction of smooth muscle in the bronchioles, which accounts for the bronchiolar constriction often associated with the allergic reaction (Figure 16-2).

Testing for a reaction to a particular allergen is done with a needle prick to the skin. Sensitivity to the allergen on the needle is exhibited by a rapid wheal-and-flare reaction. A provocation test also may be performed in which the allergen is dropped on the mucous membrane of the eyes or nose.[7]

## Anaphylaxis and Anaphylactic Shock

Anaphylaxis is defined as an allergic hypersensitivity reaction of the body to a foreign protein or a drug. Anaphylactic shock occurs when the reaction becomes systemic, and thus a life-threatening event. In either case, the subject has been previously sensitized to the antigen. The antigen–antibody reaction occurs on the mast cells in the connective tissue and around small blood vessels. It causes the mast cells to release histamine and other mediators, which results in contraction of smooth muscle and increased vascular permeability. This causes bronchospasm and the loss of intravascular fluid into the tissue spaces in some cases. Edema follows and is particularly noticeable around the eyes. This edema, called *angioneurotic edema* or *angioedema,* may appear in the skin or mucous membranes. Laryngeal edema associated with bronchospasm often causes acute dyspnea and air hunger.[16]

Hives, or urticaria, may appear on any skin surface as

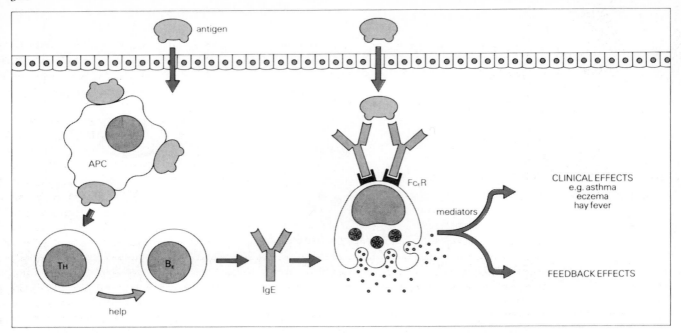

**FIGURE 16–2.**
Overall scheme for type I hypersensitivity. Antigen stimulates Be cells to produce specific IgE with T-cell help. This antigen-specific IgE binds to mast cells by way of Fce receptors (FceR), thus sensitizing them. When antigen subsequently reaches the sensitized mast cells, it cross-links surface-bound IgE and the cell degranulates, releasing mediators, which cause the symptoms associated with type I hypersensitivity. (From I. Roitt, J. Brostoff, and D. Male, *Immunology* [2nd ed.]. Philadelphia: J.B. Lippincott, 1989.)

cutaneous localized swellings. These are sudden, generalized eruptions of papules or wheals, and intense itching is exhibited.

Fluid shift from increased vascular permeability may be significant enough to result in decreased blood pressure and shock. Signs and symptoms of anaphylactic shock include urticaria, angioedema, dyspnea, hypoxia, and hypotension.[3] Some people experience vascular collapse without signs of respiratory distress. Other signs that are associated with anaphylaxis include leukopenia, decreased body temperature, and bradycardia.

### Bronchial Asthma

Atopic allergy may cause bronchial asthma, frequently induced by the inhalation of environmental antigens (see Chap. 30). The mechanism for bronchial asthma, like atopy, may result from interaction of antigen with specific IgE antibodies. The inflammation produces mucosal edema, increased secretion of mucus, and bronchospasm, all of which cause narrowing of the airways and increased airway resistance. The early signs and symptoms of asthma are dyspnea and wheezing. Repeated attacks result in hypertrophy of the smooth muscle, which can exaggerate bronchoconstriction and increase the severity of each subsequent attack. Bacterial or viral infections may precipitate asthmatic attacks.

### Atopic Eczema

An acute or chronic, noncontagious inflammatory condition, atopic eczema may occur after contact with irritants to which a person has a specific sensitivity.[6] In some cases, it results from a cell-mediated reaction (see Chap. 14), and in others, it is mediated by IgE, with liberation of chemotactic mediators into dermal areas.

Atopic eczema causes urticaria and angioedema. Urticaria involves the superficial capillaries, and angioedema involves the capillaries of the deeper skin layers. The wheals of urticaria have well-defined margins, erythema, and vesicles filled with clear fluid. Pruritus frequently is severe. Angioedema causes nonpitting swelling of localized areas of the skin.[4] This skin reaction to an allergen frequently is associated with respiratory hypersensitivity, especially hay fever or other type of allergy. Drug reactions may result in the same dermatologic manifestations, probably caused by the same mechanisms.[16]

## Type II: Cytotoxic Hypersensitivity

In type II hypersensitivity response, a circulating antibody, usually an IgG, reacts with an antigen on the surface of a cell. Because people normally have antibodies to antigen of the ABO blood group not present on their own membranes, the antigen may be a normal component of the membrane.[11] It also may be a foreign antigen, such as a pharmacologic agent, that adheres to the surface of the host's own cells. Antibodies produced to self red blood cells may produce an autoimmune hemolytic anemia. The cell is destroyed by the reaction on its surface either by phagocytosis or lysis. The effect on the host depends on the numbers and types of cells destroyed.

Examples of this hypersensitivity response include autoimmune hemolytic anemia, erythroblastosis fetalis, and Goodpasture's syndrome. These are briefly discussed after a review of some of the general pathophysiologic features.

The pathophysiology of type II hypersensitivity usually involves the activation of complement and resultant destruction of red blood cells or specific target cells. Coating of target cells with IgG antibody sets the stage for phagocytosis by the mononuclear phagocyte system. Another mechanism involves specific IgG or IgM activation of complement, with cytolysis resulting from complement activation through C89 (Figure 16-3). Red cell destruction may be triggered by IgG opsonization and the attachment of lymphocytes or macrophages to the cell surface.[4]

## Hemolytic Reactions

Examples of reactions that destroy red blood cells are transfusion reactions, erythroblastosis fetalis, autoimmune hemolytic anemia, and drug-induced hemolysis. The reaction of host antibody with the surface antigens on the red blood cells of an incompatible donor results in hemolysis. The surface antigens that make up the ABO and Rh systems are common sources of incompatibility (see Chap. 19).

Transfusion reactions result in hemolysis of donor red blood cells with the liberation of large quantities of hemoglobin into the plasma. Some of the hemoglobin is broken down into unconjugated bilirubin. If the amount of free hemoglobin is greater than 100 mg/dL of plasma, the excess diffuses into the tissue or through the renal glomeruli into the renal tubules.[7] Precipitation of large amounts of hemoglobin in the renal tubular fluid forms sharp needles in the acid urine, which can cause tubular damage and obstruction. Precipitation in the tubules of the shells of red blood cells also frequently contributes to tubular damage and renal failure. Transfusion reactions may increase the risk of renal failure by causing circulatory shock, renal vasoconstriction, and decreased renal blood flow.

The antigenic nature of mismatched blood transfusions depends on the type and Rh factor of the donor blood. For example, people with type A blood possess anti-B antibodies. Therefore, the incompatible blood is coated with antibodies, usually of the IgM class. This causes agglutination of the donor cells, and lysis rapidly follows.[2]

Signs and symptoms of a transfusion reaction include chills, fever, low back pain, hypotension, tachycardia, anxiety, hyperkalemia, nausea and vomiting, red or port wine–colored urine, and, occasionally, urticaria. These may progress to shock and irreversible renal failure.

*Erythroblastosis fetalis* may result if a mother without Rh antigens carries a child with Rh antigens, or if mother and fetus have ABO incompatibility. A mother who *lacks Rh antigens* on her red blood cells (Rh-negative) can be sensitized to the Rh antigen carried on the cells of the fetus by mixing her red blood cells with fetal red blood cells. If the woman again becomes pregnant with a fetus that has Rh antigens, her anti-Rh antibodies may cross the placenta and enter the fetal circulation. The result is destruction of fetal red blood cells through a hemolytic reaction. More commonly, *ABO blood group incompatibility* causes the free passage of antibodies from the mother through the placenta to the fetus.[4] Blood types interact in different ways, but the result is attachment and hemolysis of fetal red blood cells by maternal antibodies.[2,11]

Hemolysis of fetal red blood cells results in severe *anemia,* which may lead to heart failure. Also, the release of high concentrations of bilirubin from hemoglobin may result in brain damage, called *kernicterus,* as unconjugated bilirubin passes across the still permeable blood–brain barrier, causing edematous swelling of brain parenchyma. The mechanism by which unconjugated bilirubin crosses the blood–brain barrier is not clearly understood. The barrier apparently is more permeable in neonates and premature infants.[4] *Hyperbilirubinemia* is common in an affected infant who survives for more than several days. This increased bilirubin level usually is manifested as jaundice and is termed *icterus gravis.* The red cell activity in bone marrow increases, and extramedullary hematopoiesis begins in the liver,

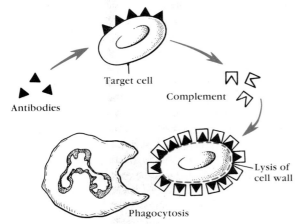

**FIGURE 16–3.**
Type II hypersensitivity response. The target cell is covered with antibody that activates complement and sets the stage for phagocytosis.

spleen, and perhaps other organs to compensate for lost red blood cells.

The risk of erythroblastosis fetalis in subsequent pregnancies can be reduced by administering anti-Rh antibodies to the mother within 72 hours after the birth of the first Rh-positive infant. More difficult to predict is ABO erythroblastosis, but the condition can be monitored if both parents are aware of their blood incompatibility.

Two types of hemolytic anemias with a probable autoimmune basis are *warm antibody disease* and *cold antibody disease*. Warm antibody disease is called *autoimmune hemolytic anemia* and usually is due to IgG antibody that attacks the host's own red blood cells. The disease can be life-threatening, depending on the amount of hemolysis. The red blood cells develop a limited life span, and the resulting anemia can be severe. Autoimmune hemolytic disease may develop for no known reason, or it may be associated with other autoimmune diseases, cancer, or systemic infection.[4] Cold antibody disease results when an autoantibody, usually IgM, binds to erythrocytes at temperatures below 31°C. These temperatures may be reached in the fingers or toes during very cold weather. The red blood cells thus coated with cold antibodies reenter the general circulation, activate complement, and hemolyze the red blood cells. These hemolytic attacks occur only after exposure to cold and tend to be self-limiting.[4] The major diagnostic criterion for hemolytic anemia is the Coombs' antiglobulin test. In this test, agglutination of red blood cells occurs when immunoglobulins are attached to the red blood cell membranes.[4]

*Drug-induced hemolysis* may result from drug–antibody complexes that bind passively to red blood cells and initiate the complement reaction. Other drugs may act as haptens and bind to a red blood cell carrier. Antibody is formed and induces hemolysis of the red blood cells. Some drugs produce changes in the surface antigens of the red blood cells, resulting in antibody production against the host's own erythrocytes. Most drug-induced hemolytic reactions stop once use of the drug is discontinued.

### Specific Target Cell Destruction

The best illustration of specific target cell hypersensitivity reaction is *Goodpasture's syndrome*, which is a rapidly occurring condition characterized by the development of *antiglomerular basement membrane antibodies (anti-GBM)*. These antibodies are directed at the glomerular basement membrane of the kidneys as well as the basement membrane of the pulmonary alveoli. The initiator is unknown, but the condition may rapidly progress to death because of the destruction of the basement membranes, which frequently leads to hemoptysis or uremia. Improvement in prognosis has been reported with use of plasma exchange to remove anti-GBM antibodies. Both pulmonary and glomerular improvement have been seen.[4] Bilateral nephrectomy also has arrested the pulmonary course of the disease.[4]

## Type III: Immune Complex Disease

Immune complex disease results in the formation of antigen–antibody complexes that activate a variety of serum factors, especially complement.[4] This results in precipitation of complexes in vulnerable areas, leading to inflammation as a consequence of complement activation. The end result is an intravascular, synovial, endocardial, and other membrane inflammatory process that affects the vulnerable organs (Figure 16-4). Each person apparently has some unique vulnerability in target organs.

Antigen–antibody complexes may be present in the plasma but may not cause disease manifestations. If the complexes are not removed by the mononuclear phagocyte system, they may lodge in the tissue, where they initiate an inflammatory reaction that leads to tissue destruction. The complexes frequently are small, and their size seems to determine whether they will be cleared and whether they can lodge at a place where significant damage can occur. The antigen–antibody complexes that remain in solution cause reactions when they circulate through the body and lodge in the tissue and small vessels.[14] Increased vascular permeability allows the complexes to be deposited in the extravascular spaces. Deposition also appears to be greater at points of high pressure, high flow, and turbulence.[6] Once precipitated, the immune complexes initiate the inflammatory process by activating complement and releasing vasoactive substances from the defense cells (Figure 16-5). Complement activation can be initiated through either the classic or the alternative pathway, depending on which immunoglobulin class is involved.[14] Box 16-1 summarizes the pathogenesis of inflammatory lesions in type III reactions.

### Serum Sickness

Serum sickness results from injection of large doses of foreign material and can cause various types of arthritis, glomerulonephritis, and vasculitis. First reported after passive immunization with horse serum (equine tetanus antitoxin), which contains at least 30 antigens, serum sickness can cause an acute reaction or a chronic condition. Antigen–antibody complexes form in the bloodstream and precipitate into vulnerable areas. It also occurs as an allergic reaction to penicillin and in some viral infections, especially viral hepatitis.[14]

If the antigen concentration is greater than the antibody concentrations, the resulting antigen–antibody complexes tend to be small and remain in solution for as

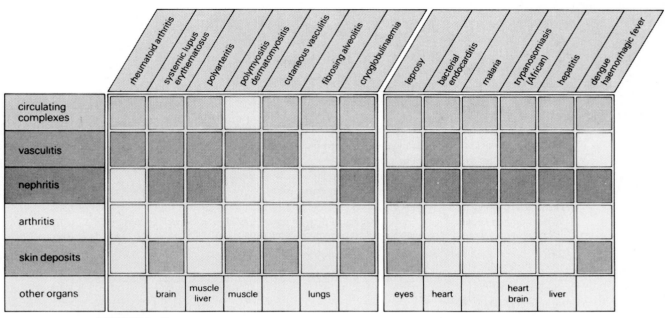

**FIGURE 16-4.**
Some of the main diseases in which immune complexes are implicated, indicating sites of deposition. Diseases on the left of the figure are primarily autoimmune; those on the right are caused by microbial antigens. (From I. Roitt, J. Brostoff, and D. Male, *Immunology* [2nd ed.]. Philadelphia: J.B. Lippincott, 1989.)

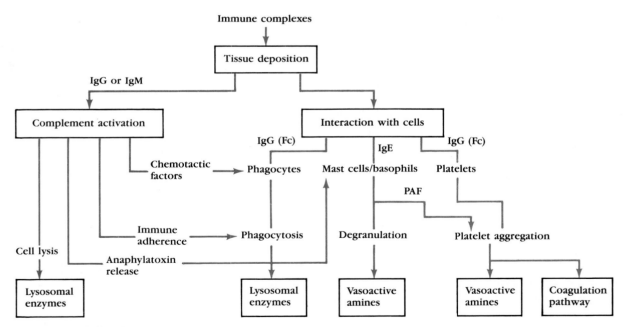

**FIGURE 16-5.**
Simplified view of the major pathways by which immune complex deposition may produce tissue damage. PAF, platelet aggregating factor. (From M. Haeney, *Introduction to Clinical Immunology.* Boston: Butterworth, 1985.)

**BOX 16–1.**
PATHOGENESIS OF INFLAMMATORY LESIONS IN TYPE III REACTIONS

Formation of antigen–antibody complexes (usually in antigen excess)

Fixation of complement by complexes

Release of complement components chemotactic for leukocytes

Damage to platelets, causing release of vasoactive amines

Increased vascular permeability

Localization of antigen–antibody complexes in vessel walls

Further fixation of complement and release of chemotactic factors

Infiltration with polymorphonuclear leukocytes

Ingestion of immune complexes by neutrophils and release of lysosomal enzymes

Damage to adjacent cells and tissues by lysosomal enzymes

Deposition of fibrin

Regression and healing if lesion is due to a single dose of antigen, or chronic deposition and inflammation if there is continuing formation of immune complexes

Stites, D. P., et al. *Basic and Clinical Immunology* (7th ed.). Norwalk, Conn.: Appleton & Lange, 1990. Reprinted by permission.

long as 8 to 15 days after initial injection. Immune complexes are deposited throughout the vasculature of the body; complement is activated, and neutrophils and macrophages move into the area in response to chemotactic signals. Phagocytosis of the immune complexes begins with the release of lysosomal enzymes into the area, which causes acute vasculitis with destruction of the elastic lamina of the arteries. Once phagocytosis of the immune complexes is complete, the inflammatory process decreases, leaving some scarring of the blood vessel walls.[4]

Renal glomerular deposits of complexes occur even when the immune complex concentrations are not high, probably because of the efficient filtering action of the kidneys. The complexes form characteristic deposits in the glomerular walls that activate complement and lead to destruction of glomerular tissue. Increased permeability of the glomerular basement membrane often produces hematuria and proteinuria.

### Arthus Reaction

Another type III disorder, the Arthus reaction, involves inflammation and cellular death at the site of injection of antigen into a previously sensitized person. Pathologically, it causes acute, localized edema with tissue inflammation and little vasculitis.[14] Antibody precipitation and complement activation cause all of the effects of inflammation, with activation of the complement fragments through C89, which destroys antigen and surrounding tissue.

Hypersensitive pneumonitis probably is an Arthus reaction from the inhalation of organic dusts.[16] This reaction is closely involved with the anaphylactic type I re-

sponse, except that IgG immunoglobulin seems to be necessary for Arthus reaction and IgE is involved with the type I reaction. It has been postulated that some relation exists between the reactions.[4]

### Other Type III Conditions

Many of the common autoimmune conditions are classified as immune complex disorders. The mechanism for inflammation and damage is the precipitation of immune complexes into vulnerable areas. Immune complex disorders are dynamic, constantly changing processes that are manifested in the tissues in which they become lodged. Systemic lupus erythematosus (SLE), rheumatoid arthritis, and some types of glomerulonephritis are examples. SLE and rheumatoid arthritis are discussed more fully on page 334 to 338. Glomerulonephritis is described in detail in Chapter 33.

### Type IV: Cell-Mediated Hypersensitivity

Type IV response is the result of specifically sensitized T lymphocytes. Activation causes a delayed-type response.

### Delayed Hypersensitivity

Delayed hypersensitivity responses are due to the specific interaction of T cells with antigen. The T cells react with the antigen and release lymphokines that draw macrophages into the area. The lymphokines include the macrophage migration inhibitory factor, the macrophage-activating factor, chemotactic factors, lymphotoxin,

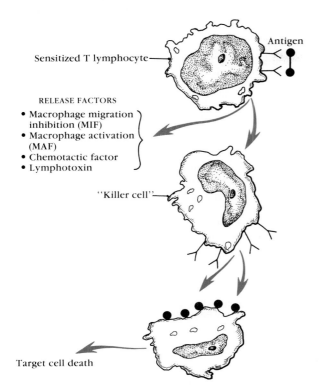

**FIGURE 16-6.**
Type IV cell-mediated hypersensitivity. The T lymphocyte contacts the foreign material, and through direct intervention or secretion of substances toxic to the foreign material, it destroys the foreign protein.

transfer factor, and other factors.[8] These substances enhance the inflammatory response that destroys the foreign material (Figure 16-6).

The tuberculin response is the best example of the delayed hypersensitivity response and is used to determine whether a person has been sensitized to the disease. Reddening and induration of the site begin within 12 hours of injection of tuberculin and reach a peak in 24 to 72 hours.[7] It is mainly a dermal reaction. The positive response occurs because of the persistent presence of mycobacterium organisms that the macrophages are unable to destroy.

Delayed hypersensitivity responses usually are caused by infectious agents, such as mycobacteria, protozoa, and fungi.[11] These organisms present a chronic antigenic stimulus, and the T lymphocytes and macrophages react, sometimes conferring protective immunity against later exposure.

## Granulomatous Hypersensitivity Response

Granulomatous hypersensitivity response is the most important form of delayed hypersensitivity because it results in the formation of granulomas in different areas of the body. The epithelioid cell is the characteristic morphologic feature and appears as a large, flattened cell that may be derived from activated macrophages. Sometimes the formation of multinucleate giant cells may occur.[11] Figure 16-7 shows a proposed scheme for the formation of giant cells from the monocyte/macrophage system. The granuloma may be surrounded by fibrosis, and necrotic material may be contained within it.[11]

Precise classification of diseases that manifest delayed hypersensitivity with or without granuloma formation is difficult. A wide variety of chronic diseases are included, most of which are related to infectious agents. Table 16-2 describes the common chronic diseases together with etiology, pathology, and clinical manifestations.

## Contact Dermatitis

A common allergic skin reaction, contact dermatitis seems to be a T-cell response with a delayed reaction. It occurs on contact with certain common household chemicals, cosmetics, and plant toxins. These may alter the normal skin protein so that it becomes antigenic, or they may act as haptens that combine with proteins in the skin.[11]

The area of contact becomes red and indurated, and vesicles begin to appear. This type of dermatitis is mainly confined to the epidermis. Lymphocytes and macrophages infiltrate the area and react against the epidermal

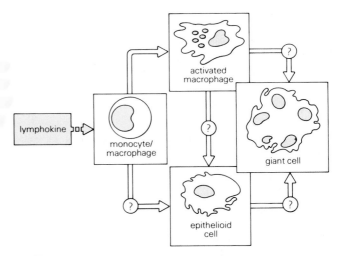

**FIGURE 16-7.**
Proposed scheme for the terminal differentiation of cells of the monocyte/macrophage system. The pathologic changes result from the inability of the macrophage to deal effectively with the pathogen. Lymphokines from active T cells induce monocytes and macrophages to become activated macrophages. Where prolonged antigenic stimulation exists, activated macrophages may differentiate into epithelioid cells and then into giant cells in vivo, in granulomatous tissue. The multinucleate giant cell may be derived from fusion of several epithelioid cells. (From I. Riott, J. Brostoff, and D. Male, *Immunology* [2nd ed.]. Philadelphia: J.B. Lippincott, 1989.)

**TABLE 16–2.**
Examples of Granulomatous Inflammations

| DISEASE | CAUSE | TISSUE REACTION |
|---|---|---|
| **Bacterial** | | |
| Tuberculosis | *Mycobacterium tuberculosis* | *Noncaseating tubercle (granuloma prototype)*: a focus of epithelioid cells, rimmed by fibroblasts, lymphocytes, histiocytes, occasional Langhans' giant cell; *caseating tubercle*: central amorphous granular debris, loss of all cellular detail; acid-fast bacilli |
| Leprosy | *Mycobacterium leprae* | Acid-fast bacilli in macrophages; granulomas and epithelioid types |
| Syphilis | *Treponema pallidum* | *Gumma*: Microscopic to grossly visible lesion, enclosing wall of histiocytes; plasma cell infiltrate; center cells are necrotic without loss of cellular outline |
| Cat-scratch disease | *Gram-negative bacillus* | Rounded or stellate granuloma containing central granular debris and recognizable neutrophils; giant cells uncommon |
| **Parasitic** | | |
| Schistosomiasis | *Schistosoma mansoni, S. haematobium, S. japonicum* | Egg emboli; eosinophils |
| **Fungal** | | |
| | *Cryptococcus neoformans* | Organism is yeast-like, sometimes budding; 5 to 10 $\mu$m; large, clear capsule |
| | *Coccidioides immitis* | Organism appears as spherical (30–80 $\mu$m) cyst containing endospores of 3 to 5 $\mu$m each |
| **Inorganic Metals and Dust** | | |
| Silicosis, berylliosis | | Lung involvement; fibrosis |
| **Unknown** | | |
| Sarcoidosis | | *Noncaseating granuloma*: giant cells (Langhans' and foreign-body types); asteroids in giant cells; occasional Schaumann's body (concentric calcific concretion); no organisms |

*Source: Cotran, R., Kumar, V., and Robbins, S. L. Robbins Pathologic Basis of Disease (4th Ed.) Philadelphia: Saunders, 1989.*

cells. Sterile, protein-rich fluid fills the blebs. If the blebs are opened, the antigen may be spread to a new area. The affected cells are destroyed, slough off, and are replaced by regenerating new cells.

## Transplant or Graft Rejection

Rejection of tissue and transplanted organs involves several of the hypersensitivity responses. Targeting of transplanted organs depends on whether the *histocompatibility antigens* are similar enough between the donor and the recipient to prevent activation of the rejection phenomenon. These surface antigens on cells distinguish them from other people and from other organs. These are the self-proteins to which a person develops tolerance. Identical twins have identical histocompatibility antigens, so that organs or tissue can be transplanted from one to the other with ease. Donor and recipient tissues are matched; the closer the match, the more likely the transplantation will be successful.[5] Table 16-3 indicates some principles of donor–recipient matching.

**TABLE 16 – 3.**

Principles of Donor-Recipient Matching

| PRINCIPLE | TESTING METHOD |
| --- | --- |
| No transplantation across ABO incompatibility | Hemagglutination |
| No transplantation in presence of positive T-cell crossmatch, i.e., anti–T-cell antibodies; avoid transplantation in presence of warm anti–B-cell bodies | Lymphocytotoxicity, leukagglutination |
| Attempt to obtain best HLA match from ABO-compatible potential donors (not critical in liver or heart transplantation) | Lymphocytotoxicity |
| Attempt to obtain transplant from donor inducing mixed lymphocyte response from ABO-compatible, satisfactorily matched, potential donors | Mixed lymphocyte culture reactivity |

*Bellanti, J.A. Immunology III. Philadelphia: W. B. Saunders, 1985. Figure 20–19. Reprinted by permission.*

Rejection is a complex reaction that involves both cell-mediated and humoral responses. It is defined as the process by which the immune system of the host recognizes, develops sensitivity to, and attempts to eliminate the antigenic differences of the donor organ.[5] Cytolytic T lymphocytes may either attack grafted tissue directly or secrete chemotactic lymphokines that enhance the activity of macrophages in tissue destruction. Humoral responses may be due to circulating antibodies that were formed during previous exposure to the antigen. After transplantation, the lymphocytes become sensitized as they pass through the donor site. When antibody is involved, it appears to target the vasculature of the graft, especially the graft site.[4,5]

The rejection phenomenon of a transplanted kidney has been studied extensively. It appears to involve both humoral and cell-mediated hypersensitivity. The sensitized lymphocytes interact with the graft proteins and release mediators that attract macrophages and polymorphonuclear leukocytes to the area. The lysosomal enzymes released by these cells cause endothelial destruction, especially of the blood vessels, that leads to decreased glomerular filtration rate and renal failure.

The T lymphocytes are directly cytotoxic to the donor cells. They also may activate B lymphocytes to form antibodies and immune complexes that activate complement and further damage the vascular endothelium.

The process may be acute or chronic. The more adequately matched the donor and recipient, the less acute the reaction. Also, recipients are given immunosuppressive drugs that delay the rejection. Chronic changes usually affect the vasculature and lead to organ ischemia and eventual failure.

Graft rejection is common, and most cadaver grafts are rejected within 5 years. Long-term survival of grafts has not been achieved except in twin or closely matched HLA transplants. Adequate immunosuppression has been helpful in prolonging graft survival.[4]

## AUTOIMMUNITY

The study of autoimmunity has been spurred by the discovery of antibodies directed toward specific cells in certain people. Many people demonstrate serum autoantibodies but show no evidence of disease. This is especially true in the elderly, and much research related to the loss of self-tolerance with aging is being conducted. Even people who have suffered myocardial infarction may exhibit myocardial autoantibodies but experience no further myocardial disruption. In diabetes mellitus, autoantibodies to the islet cells of the pancreas often are demonstrated, which leads to the theory that some forms of diabetes mellitus may be a result of an autoimmune attack on these cells.[13]

A wide spectrum of autoimmune responses has been divided clinically into systemic, non-organ–specific, and organ-specific diseases.[15] Figure 16-8 indicates common organ-specific and non-organ–specific diseases. The diseases are classified according to where they lie in a spectrum between organ-specific and non-organ–specific (Figure 16-9). Many of these are described in other sections of the book. The relations of destructive autoimmune reactions are most clearly demonstrated in myasthenia gravis, Graves' disease, rheumatoid arthritis, SLE, and others (Table 16-4). SLE, rheumatoid arthritis, and scleroderma are considered in further detail in the section below as well as in Chapter 45. The possibility of

**organ specific diseases**     **non-organ specific diseases**

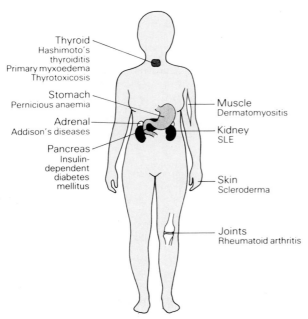

**FIGURE 16–8.**

Two types of autoimmune diseases—organ-specific and non–organ-specific. Although the non–organ-specific diseases produce symptoms in different organs, particular organs are more markedly affected by particular diseases, for example the kidney in systemic lupus erythematosus (SLE) and the joint in rheumatoid arthritis. (From I. Roitt, J. Brostoff, and D. Male, *Immunology* [2nd ed.]. Philadelphia: J.B. Lippincott, 1989.)

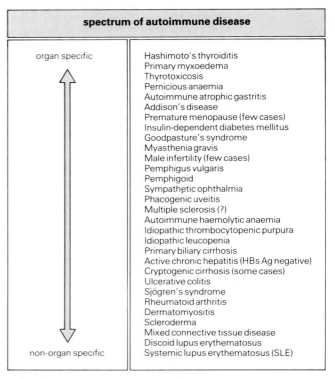

**FIGURE 16–9.**

Spectrum of autoimmune diseases. Autoimmune diseases may be classified as organ-specific or non–organ-specific, depending on whether the response is primarily against either antigens localized to particular organs or widespread antigens. (From I. Roitt, J. Brostoff, and D. Male, *Immunology* [2nd ed.]. Philadelphia: J.B. Lippincott, 1989.)

autoimmunity as a causative factor has been speculated in conditions as diverse as multiple sclerosis, hepatitis, and cancer. Autoantibodies, however, have not been consistently demonstrated in cancer. The appearance of *autoantibodies* and the symptomatology of a disease lend support for an autoimmune classification. Table 16-5 lists some of the pathologic lesions that may occur with autoantibodies.[11]

Observations of autoimmune phenomena have resulted in the following generalizations:

1. Specific autoimmune phenomena occur with greater frequency in certain families, which suggests a genetic disorder related to a fundamental disorder of thymic immune control.
2. Autoimmune diseases are more common in females than in males, which indicates a relation between the sex hormones and the immune response.
3. Elderly people have a greater prevalence of autoantibodies, which may be the result of genetic errors because of the immune system's wearing out through the aging process.
4. Viruses may play a role in the occurrence of autoimmunity because of their ability to disrupt the immune system at any one of several levels.
5. Sequestered tissue (tissue and protein not normally in contact with T and B cells) may be exposed to these cells through disease or disruption.
6. Tissue self-antigen is altered by disease or injury so that the host no longer recognizes it as self.[4,15]

## Systemic Lupus Erythematosus

SLE is a multisystem, chronic, rheumatic disease that may assume several forms. It frequently is fatal in people who develop significant involvement of the glomerular capillaries. The greatest frequency of the disease is found in women 20 to 40 years of age.

Pathologically, widespread degeneration of connective tissue occurs, especially in the heart, glomeruli, blood vessels, skin, spleen, and retroperitoneal tissue. Skin changes include atrophy, dermal edema, and fibrinoid infiltration. The renal glomeruli characteristically demonstrate fibrinoid changes, necrosis with scarring, and deposits of immunoglobulin and complement in the basement membrane.[10] Antinuclear antibody (ANA) is demonstrated in the serum of 80% to 100% of persons with SLE. The ANA may represent antibodies to DNA, to nucleoproteins, or to other nuclear components. The LE (lupus erythematosus) cell is present in about 76% of

**TABLE 16–4.**
Autoimmune Diseases

| CONDITION | AUTOANTIBODY | METHOD OF DETECTION |
|---|---|---|
| **Organ-specific diseases** | | |
| Myasthenia gravis | Antiacetylcholine | Immunoprecipitation of $^{125}$I-alpha-bungarotoxin-conjugated acetylcholine receptors |
| Graves' disease (diffuse toxic goiter) | Thyroid-stimulating immunoglobulin or anti-TSH receptor auto-antibody | Bioassay; measurement of adenylate cyclase activity after incubation of thyroid tissue with immunoglobulin from patient's serum, radio-receptor assay for antibodies competing with TSH for the receptor on thyroid membranes |
| Hashimoto's thyroiditis | Antibodies to thyroglobulin and to microsomal antigens | Radioimmunoassay, tanned erythrocyte agglutination, complement fixation, immunofluorescence assay |
| Insulin-resistant diabetes associated with acanthosis nigricans | Antiinsulin receptor | Inhibition of $^{125}$I-insulin binding to receptors on monocytes or adipocytes, activation of lipogenesis in adipocytes |
| Insulin-resistant diabetes associated with ataxia-telangiectasia | Antiinsulin receptor | |
| Allergic rhinitis, asthma, functional autonomic abnormalities | Antibodies to beta$_2$-adrenergic receptors | Binding of $^{125}$I-protein A to lung membranes preincubated with sera; ability of plasma to inhibit binding of $^{125}$I-iodohydroxybenzylpindolol (HYP) to calf lung membranes; immunoprecipitation of soluble receptors complexed with $^{125}$I-HYP in the presence of propranolol |
| Juvenile insulin-dependent diabetes | Antibodies to islet cells; antiinsulin antibodies | Immunofluorescence assay; competitive inhibition of insulin binding, stimulation of adipocytes |
| Pernicious anemia | Antibody to gastric parietal cells and to vitamin B$_{12}$-binding site of intrinsic factor | Immunofluorescence assay; radioimmunoassay |
| Addison's disease | Antibodies to adrenal cells | Immunofluorescence assay |
| Idiopathic hypoparathyroidism | Antibodies to antigens of parathyroid cells | Immunofluorescence assay |
| Spontaneous infertility | Antibodies to sperm | Agglutination and immobilization of spermatozoa |
| Premature ovarian failure | Antibodies to interstitial cells and corpus luteum cells | Immunofluorescence assay |
| Pemphigus | Antibodies to intercellular substance of skin and mucosa | Immunofluorescence assay |
| Bullous pemphigoid | Antibodies against basement membrane zone of skin and mucosa | Immunofluorescence assay |
| Primary biliary cirrhosis | Antibodies to mitochondrial antigens | Immunofluorescence assay |
| Autoimmune hemolytic anemia | Anti–red blood cell antibodies | Direct and indirect Coombs' tests |
| Idiopathic thrombocytopenic purpura | Antiplatelet antibodies | Immunofluorescence assay |
| Idiopathic neutropenia | Antineutrophil antibodies | Agglutination, immunofluorescence assay |
| Vitiligo | Antimelanocyte antibodies | Immunoprecipitation, immunofluorescence assay |
| Osteosclerosis and Meniere's disease | Anti–collagen type II antibodies | Radioimmunoassay |
| Chronic active hepatitis | Antinuclear antibodies; antihepatocyte antibodies | Immunofluorescence assay |
| Goodpasture's syndrome | Anti–basement membrane antibodies | Immunofluorescence assay, radioimmunoassay |
| **Systemic diseases (non–organ-specific)** | | |
| Rheumatoid arthritis and Sjögren's syndrome | Antigammaglobulin antibodies; antibodies to EBV-related antigens | Sensitized-SRBC agglutination, latex-immunoglobulin agglutination, radioimmunoassay, immunofluorescence assay, immunodiffussion |

(continued)

**TABLE 16–4.**
Autoimmune Diseases (continued)

| CONDITION | AUTOANTIBODY | METHOD OF DETECTION |
| --- | --- | --- |
| **Systemic diseases (non–organ-specific), continued** | | |
| Systemic lupus erythematosus | Antinuclear antibodies | Immunofluorescence assay |
| | Anti-dsDNA and anti-ssDNA | Farr assay, solid phase enzyme and radioimmunoassay, hemagglutination, counterelectrophoresis |
| | Anti-Sm antibodies | Hemagglutination, immunodiffussion, radioimmunoassay |
| | Antiribonucleoprotein antibodies | Hemagglutination, radioimmunoassay |
| | Antilymphocyte antibodies | Immunofluorescence assay, cytotoxicity |
| | Anti–red blood cell antibodies | Coombs' test |
| | Antiplatelet antibodies | Immunofluorescence assay |
| | Antineuronal cell antibodies | Immunofluorescence assay |
| | Antigammaglobulins | Radioimmunoassay |
| Scleroderma (systemic sclerosis) | Antinuclear antibody | Immunofluorescence assay |

Adapted from Stites, D. P., et al. Basic and Clinical Immunology (7th ed.). Norwalk, Conn.: Appleton & Lange, 1990. Reprinted by permission.

affected people. It is basically a mature polymorphonuclear leukocyte that has engulfed nuclear material. These cells may be clustered around masses of nuclear material and are then called LE rosettes.[4] The LE cell is the result of targeting by antinuclear antibodies.

The American Rheumatism Association issued a list of 14 criteria indicative of SLE.[9] If the person exhibits four or more of these, the diagnosis is probable (Table 16-6).

Stiffness and pain in the hands, feet, or large joints are common complaints. The joints appear red, warm, and tender but do not exhibit the deformities of rheumatoid arthritis. The exposed skin shows signs of a patchy atrophy. An erythematous rash frequently occurs in a butterfly pattern over the nose and cheeks. The dermis becomes edematous and infiltrated by lymphocytes, plasma cells, and histiocytes.

Renal involvement, a serious complication, results from the precipitation of immune complexes in the renal glomeruli. The complexes on the endothelial side of the basement membrane cause inflammatory lesions, thickened basement membrane, tubular atrophy, and interstitial spaces filled with lymphocytes and plasma cells. The course of renal involvement is characterized by remissions and exacerbations ranging in severity from mild

**TABLE 16–5.**
Direct Pathogenic Effects of Humoral Antibodies

| DISEASE | AUTOANTIGEN | LESION |
| --- | --- | --- |
| Autoimmune hemolytic anemia | Red cell | Erythrocyte destruction |
| Lymphopenia (some cases) | Lymphocyte | Lymphocyte destruction |
| Idiopathic thrombocytopenic purpura | Platelet | Platelet destruction |
| Male infertility (some cases) | Sperm | Agglutination of spermatozoa |
| Pernicious anemia | Intrinsic factor | Neutralization of ability to mediate $B_{12}$ absorption |
| Hashimoto's disease | Thyroid surface antigen | Cytotoxic effect on thyroid cells in culture |
| Thyrotoxicosis | TSH receptors | Stimulation of thyroid cells |
| Goodpasture's syndrome | Glomerular basement membrane | Complement-mediated damage to basement membrane |
| Myasthenia gravis | Acetylcholine receptor | Blocking and destruction of receptors |
| Acanthosis nigricans (type B) and ataxia-telangiectasia with insulin resistance | Insulin receptor | Blocking of receptors |

Roitt, I. Essential Immunology (5th ed.). Oxford: Blackwell Scientific Publications, Ltd., 1984. Table 10-4. Reprinted by permission.

**TABLE 16–6.**
Clinical Features of Systemic Lupus Erythematosus

| ORGAN SYSTEM | ARA CRITERIA FOR CLASSIFICATION OF SLE* | OTHER FEATURES |
|---|---|---|
| Constitutional | | Fever, malaise, anorexia, weight loss |
| Cutaneous | 1. Malar rash<br>2. Discoid rash<br>3. Photosensitivity<br>4. Oral/nasopharyngeal ulcers | Alopecia<br>Raynaud's phenomenon<br>Other rashes: subacute cutaneous LE, urticaria, bullous lesions<br>Vasculitis<br>Panniculitis (lupus profundus) |
| Musculoskeletal | 5. Nonerosive arthritis | Arthralgia/myalgia<br>Myositis<br>Ligamentous laxity<br>Avascular necrosis of bone |
| Cardiopulmonary | 6. { Pleuritis<br>Pericarditis | Pleural effusions<br>Myocarditis<br>Pneumonitis<br>Verrucous endocarditis (Libman-Sacks syndrome)<br>Interstitial fibrosis<br>Pulmonary hypertension |
| Renal | 7. { Proteinuria (>500 mg/24 h)<br>Cylindruria | Nephrotic syndrome<br>Celluria<br>Renal insufficiency<br>Renal failure |
| Neurologic | 8. { Psychosis<br>Seizure | Organic brain syndrome<br>Cranial nerve abnormalities<br>Peripheral neuropathies<br>Cerebellar signs |
| Gastrointestinal | | Serositis<br>Ascites<br>Vasculitis (bleeding/perforation)<br>Pancreatitis<br>Elevated levels of liver enzymes |
| Hematologic | 9. { Hemolytic anemia<br>Leukopenia (<4,000/mL)<br>Lymphopenia (<1,500/mL)<br>Thrombocytopenia (<100,000/mL) | Anemia of chronic disease<br>Lupus anticoagulant<br>Thrombosis<br>Splenomegaly<br>Lymphadenopathy |
| Other systems | | Sicca complex<br>Conjunctivitis/episcleritis |
| Laboratory | 10. ANA<br>11. { Anti-dsDNA<br>Anti-Sm<br>False-positive VDRL<br>LE preparation | |

*Any combination of four manifestations listed as American Rheumatism Association criteria meets the 1982 revised ARA guidelines for classifying patients with SLE; one or more features from within each bracket are considered as one manifestation.*
*Kelley, W. N. Textbook of Internal Medicine. Philadelphia: J.B. Lippincott, 1989.*

proteinuria to massive hematuria and proteinuria, finally resulting in total renal failure.[9]

Systemic problems, including fever, fatigue, anorexia, and weight loss, are common. Cardiopulmonary and neurologic manifestations also are seen. Besides antibody demonstration, hematologic abnormalities include anemia and leukopenia.

## Rheumatoid Arthritis

Rheumatoid arthritis is a chronic, systemic, inflammatory disease that specifically affects the small joints of the hands and feet in its early stages and involves the larger joints in later stages. It is nonsuppurative but finally results in the destruction of cartilage and joints. It also may produce lesions of the heart valves, pericardium, myocardium, and pleura.[10]

The pathophysiologic manifestations of rheumatoid arthritis appear to result from the development of antibody against IgG. These antibodies, called *rheumatoid factor (RF)*, belong to the IgM, IgG, and IgA classes.[4] The RF is present in 85% to 90% of persons with rheumatoid arthritis and may be stimulated by a self-antigen, an antigen in the synovial cavity, or an infectious antigen. The RF continues to interact with IgG even in the absence of any specific antigen.[1] Chronic antigenic stimulation, such as occurs in chronic respiratory infections, causes the production and destruction of large amounts of antibody. The RF–IgG complexes are present in the rheumatoid lesions and apparently activate complement or prostaglandins or other substances that promote the inflammatory response (Figure 16-10).

Acute attacks of rheumatoid arthritis occur as the RF–IgG complexes precipitate in the synovial fluid. Complement is activated and attracts polymorphonuclear leukocytes, whose main function appears to be phagocytosis of the complexes. The lysosomal enzymes released by these cells intensify the inflammatory reaction and increase destruction of the articular cartilage. Granulation tissue and inflammatory cells form a mass of tissue called *pannus* that erodes the articular cartilage. The joint space is destroyed, and the resultant scarring may completely immobilize the joint or cause bleeding and thrombosis in the area.

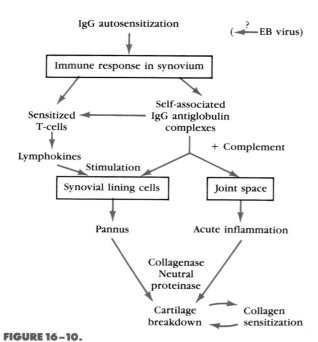

**FIGURE 16–10.**
Hypothetical scheme showing how initial autosensitization to IgG can lead to the pathogenetic changes characteristic of rheumatoid arthritis. (From I. Roitt, *Essential Immunology* [5th ed.]. Oxford: Blackwell Scientific, 1984.)

Rheumatoid subcutaneous nodules often are seen and are described as firm, nontender, oval masses, up to 2 cm in diameter. These are present on the forearms and sometimes the Achilles tendons, or attached to underlying periosteum or tendons.

Other systems also are affected. A necrotizing arteritis may lead to thrombosis of small arteries. Fibrinous pericarditis, cardiomyopathy, and valvular lesions may affect the heart. Pleuritis and interstitial fibrosis may affect the lungs. The rheumatoid nodules may occur on bone, and other effects are seen in the nervous system and the eyes.[1]

The signs and symptoms of rheumatoid arthritis are due to both systemic and local inflammatory lesions. Fatigue, weakness, joint stiffness, and vague arthralgias are early symptoms. The individual complains of morning stiffness, which gradually improves after rising. Joints in the hands or feet may be inflamed and swollen; these symptoms tend to spread symmetrically, so that the corresponding joints on the contralateral extremity become involved.

Laboratory values, besides the positive RF, include mild leukocytosis with eosinophilia and elevated erythrocyte sedimentation rate.

The course of rheumatoid arthritis is variable, with remissions and exacerbations. Some people have a relatively benign disease, whereas in others it progresses to severe deformity and total disability. Table 16-7 summarizes the criteria for classification of rheumatoid arthritis.

## Scleroderma

Scleroderma, also called systemic sclerosis, is a relatively uncommon condition that involves thickening and fibrosis of the skin together with vascular, organ, and immunologic derangements. It affects about four times as many women as men, with the highest onset between ages 25 and 50 years. Different forms of the disease exist, but the initial onset usually is marked by Raynaud's phenomenon. The condition may be more prevalent than is thought because of missed diagnosis.

The initial skin changes of edema may be accompanied by arthralgia or morning stiffness. This is followed by skin thickening that results from accumulation of collagen in the dermis.[12] The skin changes are continuous, causing taut restrictions over joints, thoracic cavity, and even the face. The serum ANA is positive in 90% of persons with systemic sclerosis, and other antibodies may be demonstrated. As the disease progresses, organ changes occur. Patchy fibrosis of the myocardium may be the result of intermittent myocardial ischemia. Pulmonary changes are varied and may include interstitial inflammatory fibrosis and vascular injury.[12] Progressive renal insufficiency and marked hypertension result from renovascular changes. The gastrointestinal changes are varied

**TABLE 16–7.**
1987 Revised Criteria for Classification of Rheumatoid Arthritis*

| CRITERION | DEFINITION |
| --- | --- |
| 1. Morning stiffness | Morning stiffness in and around the joints lasting at least 1 h before maximal improvement |
| 2. Arthritis of three or more joint areas | At least three joint areas have simultaneously had soft-tissue swelling or fluid (not bony overgrowth alone) observed by a physician. The 14 possible joint areas are right or left PIP, MCP, wrist, elbow, knee, ankle, and MTP joints. |
| 3. Arthritis of hand joints | At least one joint area swollen as above in a wrist, MCP, or PIP |
| 4. Symmetrical arthritis | Simultaneous involvement of the same joint areas (as in 2) on both sides of the body (bilateral involvement of PIPs, MCPs, or MTPs is acceptable without absolute symmetry) |
| 5. Rheumatoid nodules | Subcutaneous nodules, over bony prominences, or extensor surfaces, or in juxta-articular regions, observed by a physician |
| 6. Serum RF | Demonstration of abnormal amounts of serum RF by any method that has been positive in less than 5% of normal control subjects. |
| 7. Radiographic changes | Radiographic changes typical of RA on posteroanterior hand and wrist x-rays that must include erosions or unequivocal bony decalcification localized to or most marked adjacent to the involved joints (osteoarthritis changes alone do not qualify) |

*For classification purposes a patient shall be said to have RA if he has satisfied at least four of the seven criteria. Criteria 1 to 4 must have been present for at least 6 wk. Patients with two clinical diagnoses are not excluded. Designation as "classic," "definite," or "probable" is not to be made. Reprinted from Arthritis and Rheumatism Journal, copyright 1988. Used by permission of the American Rheumatism Association.
Kelley, W. N. Textbook of Internal Medicine. Philadelphia: J.B. Lippincott, 1989.

and include esophageal reflux, malabsorption, intussusception, and volvulus. Endocrine changes include hypothyroidism and reproductive disorders.[12]

Morbidity and mortality depend on the degree of organ involvement, and a 60% overall 5-year survival rate is reported in systemic sclerosis.[12]

# REFERENCES

1. Ball, G.V., and Koopman, W.J. Rheumatoid arthritis. In W.N. Kelley, *Textbook of Internal Medicine*. Philadelphia: J.B. Lippincott, 1989.
2. Bellanti, J.A. *Immunology III*. Philadelphia: W.B. Saunders, 1985.
3. Chatton, M.J. General symptoms. In M.A. Krupp et al., *Current Medical Diagnosis and Treatment 1986*. Los Altos, Calif.: Lange, 1986.
4. Cotran, R.S., Kumar, V., and Robbins, S.L. *Robbins' Pathologic Basis of Disease* (4th ed.). Philadelphia: W.B. Saunders, 1989.
5. Gelfand, M.C. Organ transplantation. In J.A. Bellanti, *Immunology III*. Philadelphia: W.B. Saunders, 1985.
6. Haeney, M. *Introduction to Clinical Immunology*. Boston: Butterworth, 1985.
7. Hanson, L.A., and Wigzell, H. *Immunology*. London: Butterworth, 1985.
8. Henney, C.S. T cell-mediated cytotoxicity. In D.P. Stites et al., *Basic and Clinical Immunology* (5th ed.). Los Altos, Calif.: Lange, 1984.
9. Kimberly, R. Lupus erythematosus—systemic and local forms. In W.N. Kelley, *Textbook of Internal Medicine*. Philadelphia: J.B. Lippincott, 1989.
10. Kissane, J.M. *Anderson's Pathology* (9th ed.). St. Louis: C.V. Mosby, 1990.
11. Roitt, I., Brostoff, J., and Male, D. *Immunology* (2nd ed.). Philadelphia: J.B. Lippincott, 1989.
12. Seibold, J.R. Scleroderma. In W.N. Kelley, *Textbook of Internal Medicine*. Philadelphia: J.B. Lippincott, 1989.
13. Steinberg, A.D. Mechanisms of disorder and immune regulation. In D.P. Stites and A.I. Terr, *Basic and Clinical Immunology* (7th ed.). Norwalk, Conn.: Appleton & Lange, 1991.
14. Strober, S., Grumet, C., and Stites, D.P. Immunologic disorders. In M.A. Krupp et al., *Current Medical Diagnosis and Treatment 1986*. Los Altos, Calif.: Lange, 1986.
15. Terr, A.I. Mechanisms of inflammation. In D.P. Stites and A.I. Terr, *Basic Immunology* (7th ed.). Norwalk, Conn.: Appleton & Lange, 1991.
16. Wells, J.V. Immune mechanisms in tissue. In D.P. Stites et al., *Basic and Clinical Immunology* (5th ed.). Los Altos, Calif.: Lange, 1984.

# UNIT BIBLIOGRAPHY

Albert, E.D., Bauer, M.P., and Mayr, W.R. *Histocompatibility Testing*. New York: Springer-Verlag, 1984.

Bellanti, J.A. *Immunology III*. Philadelphia: W.B. Saunders, 1985.

Benacerraf, B., and Unanue, R.E. *Textbook of Immunology* (2nd ed.). Baltimore: Williams & Wilkins, 1984.

Benjamin, E., and Leskowitz, S. *Immunology: A Short Course*. New York: Alan R. Liss, 1988.

Bowry, T.R. *Immunology Simplified* (2nd ed.). Oxford: Oxford University Press, 1984.

Cotran, R.S., Kumar, V., and Robbins, S.L. *Robbins' Pathologic Basis of Disease* (4th ed.). Philadelphia: W.B. Saunders, 1989.

Dean, J.H., et al. *Immunotoxicology and Immunopharmacology*. New York: Raven Press, 1985.

Ganong, W.F. *Review of Medical Physiology* (15th ed.). Norwalk, Conn.: Appleton & Lange, 1991.

Gershwin, M.E., Beach, R.S., and Hurley, L.S. *Nutrition and Immunity*. Orlando, Fla.: Academic Press, 1985.

Guyton, A.C. *Textbook of Medical Physiology* (8th ed.). Philadelphia: W.B. Saunders, 1991.

Haeney, M. *Introduction to Clinical Immunology*. Boston: Butterworth, 1985.

Hanson, L.A., and Wigzell, H. *Immunology*. London: Butterworth, 1985.

Helm, B., et al. The mast cell binding site on human immunoglobulin E. *Nature* 331:180, 1988.

Herberman, R.B., and Callewaert, D.M. *Mechanisms of Cytotoxicity by NK Cells*. Orlando, Fla.: Academic Press, 1985.

Hood, L.E., et al. *Immunology* (2nd ed.). Menlo Park, Calif.: Benjamin-Cummings, 1984.

Kelley, W.N. (ed.). *Textbook of Medicine*. Philadelphia: J.B. Lippincott, 1989.

Kissane, J.M. *Anderson's Pathology* (9th ed.). St. Louis: C.V. Mosby, 1990.

Mitchell, M.S. *The Modulation of Immunity*. Oxford: Pergamon Press, 1985.

Niemtzow, R.C. *Transmembrane Potentials and Characteristics of Immune and Tumor Cells*. Boca Raton, Fla.: CRC Press, 1985.

Paul, W.E. *Fundamental Immunology* (2nd ed.). New York: Raven Press, 1989.

Roitt, I. *Essential Immunology* (5th ed.). Oxford: Blackwell, 1985.

Roitt, I., Brostoff, J., and Male, D. *Immunology*. Philadelphia: J.B. Lippincott, 1989.

Samter, M. *Immunological Diseases*. Boston: Little, Brown, 1988.

Sodeman, W.A., Jr., and Sodeman, W.A. *Sodeman's Pathological Physiology: Mechanisms of Disease* (7th ed.). Philadelphia: W.B. Saunders, 1985.

Stites, D.P., and Terr, A.I. *Basic and Clinical Human Immunology* (7th ed.). Norwalk, Conn.: Appleton & Lange, 1991.

Waldmann, T.A., and Broder, S. Suppressor cells in the regulation of the immune response. *Prog. Clin. Immunol.* 3:155, 1977.

Wallach, J. *Interpretation of Diagnostic Tests* (4th ed.). Boston: Little, Brown, 1986.

Watkins, J. *Trauma, Stress, and Immunity in Anesthesia and Surgery*. Boston: Butterworth, 1982.

Watson, J.D., and Marbrook, J. *Recognition and Regulation in Cell-Mediated Immunity*. New York: Dekker, 1985.

Watson, R.R. *Nutrition, Disease Resistance and Immune Function*. New York: Dekker, 1984.

Williams, W.J. *Hematology* (4th ed.). New York: McGraw-Hill, 1989.

Wilson, J.D. *Harrison's Principles of Internal Medicine* (12th ed.). New York: McGraw-Hill, 1991.

Concepts of Altered Cellular Function

Benign and Malignant Neoplasia

# NEOPLASIA

The response of cells to the daily barrage of stimuli they receive may be growth or degeneration, alteration of normal metabolism, or even death. Cellular growth and proliferation often occur on a continuum from near-normal to grossly abnormal. Neoplasia refers to an alteration in cellular growth and development. This unit examines some of the factors related to neoplasia. Chapter 17 describes cell membrane changes in neoplasia and some related alterations in cellular characteristics. Chapter 18 describes the process of carcinogenesis and mechanisms for growth and spread of cancer.

The topic of neoplasia is inclusive, and investigative studies are revealing much new, important data. The extensive bibliography at the end of this unit is an attempt to provide current and important historical documentation for this vast subject.

Chapter 17 serves as an introduction to Chapter 18, and should be reviewed first to facilitate understanding. The reader is encouraged to study the unit by using the learning objectives at the beginning of each chapter. The unit bibliography provides sources for further investigation.

# Concepts of Altered Cellular Function

## Chapter Outline

▶ The Cell Life Cycle
▶ Outer Cell Membrane Changes as an Explanation for Neoplasia
   **Appropriate Cell Recognition**
   **Cellular Adhesion**
   **Intercellular Communication**
▶ Inner Cell Changes in Neoplasia
   **Changes in Nucleoplasm**
   **Changes in the Cytoplasm**
▶ Differentiation and Anaplasia

## Learning Objectives

1. Explain the physiology of each step in the cell's life cycle.
2. Relate the cell's life cycle to neoplasia.
3. Explain how doubling time is estimated.
4. Explain the difference between neoplastic and normal cells in relation to contact inhibition.
5. Discuss the role of each intercellular connection in cellular adhesion.
6. Discuss alterations in intercellular connections of neoplastic tissues.
7. Explain the role of contact inhibition in intercellular communication.

8. Discuss the role of the gap junction in intercellular communication.
9. Relate second messengers in the cytoplasm to growth and neoplasia.
10. Discuss the nucleus as the site of all hereditary information in relation to neoplasia.
11. Describe the concept of clonal evolution of cancer.
12. Relate cellular differentiation to neoplasia.
13. Discuss the histologic features of an anaplastic cell.
14. Explain the significance of poorly differentiated, highly anaplastic tumors.

The cell is constantly confronted by factors in its environment that stimulate or inhibit its activity. It responds to these factors by growth and proliferation or regression and degeneration. These two responses may occur simultaneously in a given cell population, or one may follow the other.[12] When cells are confronted with a stimulus that alters their normal metabolism, they may increase concentrations of normal cellular constituents, accumulate abnormal substances, change cellular size and number, or undergo lethal change. The stimuli that cause these alterations are grouped as follows: (1) physical agents, (2) chemical agents, (3) microorganisms,

(4) hypoxia, (5) genetic factors, and (6) immunologic factors.

Alterations in cellular growth and proliferation may be viewed as occurring on a continuum from near-normal changes to grossly abnormal alterations. Hypertrophy, hyperplasia, metaplasia, and dysplasia usually are classified as controlled adaptive cellular responses (see Chap. 2). They make the cell vulnerable to injurious agents that cause alterations in its normal controls of growth and development.

*Neoplasia* is defined as the development of an abnormal type of growth that is unresponsive to normal growth control mechanisms.[11] A *neoplasm* is a group or clump of neoplastic cells. *Benign neoplasia* refers to neoplastic cells that do not invade the surrounding tissue and do not metastasize. *Metastasis* refers to the ability of the cancer cell to disseminate and establish growth in another part of the body than where it originated.[8] *Malignant neoplasia* refers to neoplastic (cancer) cells that grow by invading surrounding tissue and metastasize to receptive tissue. All malignant neoplasms are classified as cancers and then further delineated as to their origin (see Chap. 18).

## THE CELL LIFE CYCLE

The cell life cycle is composed of all the steps in the process of reproduction or that period extending from one mitosis to the next.[1] In a normal cell population, inhibitory controls slow or stop reproduction, whereas stimulating factors cause the process to proceed more rapidly. Therefore, the actual length of a cell life cycle varies. The four "gap" phases are designated $G_1$, S, $G_2$, and M, with a fifth phase, $G_0$, being composed of cells leaving the normal cell cycle, which can be induced to reenter the cycle by specific stimuli (Figure 17-1).[9] The letter G is an abbreviation for "gap," and refers to the time between mitosis and synthesis ($G_1$) and synthesis and mitosis ($G_2$).

The symbol $G_0$ is used to describe the cell that performs all metabolic activities except for reproduction (mitosis). The cell remains at this level until some stimulus, such as the death of other cells of the same cell population, triggers the beginning of $G_1$. A cell may remain in the $G_1$ phase for long periods until some key process occurs to signal its entrance into the S phase of deoxyribonucleic acid (DNA) synthesis.[8]

Ribonucleic acid (RNA) and protein are synthesized in the G1 interval. The length of the G1 interval varies with each cell type, being shorter in cell populations with great activity. At a certain point in G1 the decision is made between proliferation and resting; this is called a *restriction point*.[4] The cell, stimulated to begin the synthesis of DNA, enters the S step. Synthesis of DNA occurs in the S step with replication of the chromosomes. The length of the S step varies and is followed by a period of inactivity called $G_2$. Little is known about this phase except that some RNA is synthesized in preparation for mitosis. Mitosis (M) occurs next, with cellular division creating two daughter cells that have identical genetic information (see Chap. 1). These daughter cells can mature and repeat the process, or they can enter a $G_1$ or $G_0$ interval until they are stimulated to reproduce.

The concept of the cell life cycle has helped in the basic understanding of the causes and effects of neoplasia. Neoplastic cell populations ignore normal growth limitations and enter the cell cycle repeatedly at different rates. The terms growth fraction, cell cycle time, cell loss, and doubling time are used in describing neoplastic tumors. *Growth fraction* refers to the proportion of cells in a given cell population undergoing cell cycle activity at any given time. Rapidly growing neoplasms have a larger number of cells in active reproduction at any given time than do slow-growing neoplasms. *Cell cycle time* usually is shorter in rapidly growing neoplasms than in normal cells. *Cell loss* refers to the number of cells lost in the process because of death or some other event. These three factors, when taken together, account for the *doubling time,* which is the rate at which a neoplasm doubles its cell population.

Cell replication depends on the degree and specialization of the particular cell. In general, the greater the degree of specialization, the less the tendency of the cell to reproduce. Neurons and cardiac muscle cells have lost the ability to reproduce entirely. Cells such as the skin, gastrointestinal mucosal cells, and blood cells continually reproduce to replace lost cells throughout life.

## OUTER CELL MEMBRANE CHANGES AS AN EXPLANATION FOR NEOPLASIA

All cells are surrounded by a limiting membrane that constantly exists in a dynamic state (see Chap. 1). The parts of the membrane have the capacity to redistribute and change the cell surface properties, which may have an effect on the cell's growth, metabolism, and behavior.[12]

The outer cell membrane is the point of contact between cells (Figure 17-2). Interactions that involve the outer cell membrane have been shown to function in the control of normal cellular growth.[1] Changes in the membrane are apparent in neoplastic cells and have been implicated in the failure of the neoplastic cells to respond

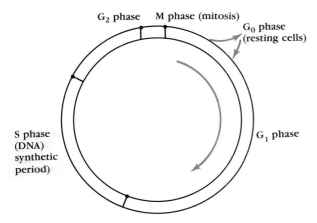

**FIGURE 17-1.**
The cell cycle. Interphase (GI), DNA synthesis (S), intermediate phase (G2), and mitosis (M) interval are shown. The G0 period may be entered from G1, and reentry from G0 to G1 may occur.

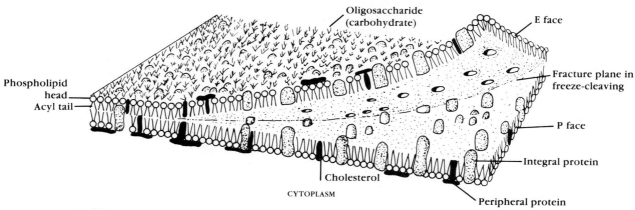

**FIGURE 17-2.**
Outer cell membrane demonstrating integrated structures that are associated with various surface properties of the cell. (From M. Borysenko et al, *Functional Histology* [2nd ed.]. Boston: Little, Brown, 1984.)

to normal growth-control mechanisms. They involve alterations in appropriate cell recognition, cellular adhesion, and intercellular communication. Escape from growth control could involve breakdown at any of these points.[10]

## Appropriate Cell Recognition

The mechanisms used by specific cells to recognize one another are not well defined. That recognition exists can be demonstrated by mixing cells of different types in culture media; specific cells eventually segregate themselves. Membrane enzymes and surface sugar residues are thought to contribute to recognition. One hypothesis is that sugar-binding enzymes, glycosyltransferases, in the outer cell membrane recognize sugar residues on glycoproteins in the membrane of neighboring cells.[11] In the neoplastic cells, glycolipids are altered. Glycoproteins or glycolipids, or both, may be missing from the membrane or have abnormal structure.[1,5]

## Cellular Adhesion

Cellular adhesion is a complex process that involves the development of connections between cells.[2] Three types of connections have been described.

1.  The *desmosome* is a mechanical way of holding cells together. Because it is composed of fibrous protein, it can be destroyed by a proteolytic enzyme, such as trypsin. Once the desmosome is gone, the cells separate (see Chap. 18).
2.  The *tight junction* involves the actual fusion of two cell membranes, forming barriers to the movement of ions and solutes from one side of the membrane to the

other.[6,11] Thus it is present where sharp physical separation is needed, such as in the endothelial lining of the cerebral blood vessels that form the blood–brain barrier.
3.  The *gap junction,* a pore passing through the outer cell membrane, permits the movement of low-molecular-weight substances from one adjoining cell to the next.[2]

A decrease in the number of desmosomal, tight, and gap junctions often occurs in the neoplastic cell population. This causes a decrease in cellular adhesion. The communication of cells evidently is dependent on the junctions described. When cells cannot communicate in this way, the loss of contact inhibition can lead to neoplastic change.[10] This reduction in tight cell connections disrupts the extracellular environment.

Junctional changes may not be involved in the early disruption of cellular adhesion. It is thought that glycosyltransferase, serum factors, cell surface proteins, cytoskeletal elements, and membrane glycoproteins all play a role in early cellular membrane changes.[1,10]

Cellular adhesion properties also include the electrical charge of the outer cell membrane. Under physiologic conditions, all mammalian cell surfaces have a negative charge, but this charge becomes more negative in neoplasia. The more aggressive the behavior of the neoplasm, the more negative the cell surface charge. This tends to push the cells away from one another.[10]

## Intercellular Communication

Contact inhibition, or density-dependent growth control, is observed when normal cells are grown in culture media. The cells move around freely in the culture media until they touch one another. On contact, they adhere to one another and form parallel lines. They then grow on

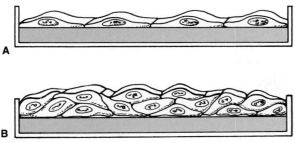

**FIGURE 17-3.**
(**A**) Normal cells are inhibited by a crowded environment. (**B**) Neoplastic cells continue to grow despite cell contact.

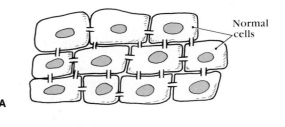

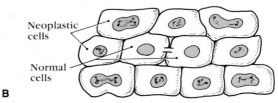

**FIGURE 17-4.**
(**A**) Demonstration of normal growth control information by the gap junction. (**B**) Isolation of normal cells from neighboring cells.

a single layer until they reach the edge of the culture dish. Growth then stops. The cells of a neoplasm, however, respond by continuing to divide and migrate until they are several layers deep. Clearly, normal cells respond to a crowded environment, but neoplastic cells do not, as they have lost their ability either to receive or to send the necessary information to stop growth (Figure 17–3).[10] Cancer cells have been described as antisocial, fairly autonomous units that do not respond to the constraints and regulatory signals imposed on normal cells.[3]

In addition to contact inhibition, agglutination by lectins has been used by researchers to study both the outer cell membrane and cell growth. Using lectins (sugar-binding proteins) as molecular markers during normal and neoplastic cell growth in culture media, investigators have observed that when the outer layer of protein is removed from their outer membrane, normal cells begin to reproduce and are agglutinated by lectin. Neoplastic cells, however, when subjected to a nonagglutinating lectin, grow to a single layer.[3]

Lectins have been used to study the cell cycle and growth signals. On entering mitosis, normally growing cells appear to experience a change on the outer cell membrane that leads to the next round of cell division by a messenger, or *go* signal. Sometime after that, but before the outer cell membrane returns to the nonagglutinable state, another messenger, or *stop* signal, is received that causes the cell to enter $G_0$, the resting phase. If the stop signal is not received, the cell is committed to another round of division. Therefore, normal growth apparently involves signals to stop cell division; these signals may be blocked in the neoplastic cell.

It is thought that normal cellular growth is controlled by growth stimulators and growth inhibitors. Many growth factors have been described, especially polypeptide growth factors, that stimulate a variety of cell-type proliferations.[3,7] Current research has focused on imbalances in the growth factors as a possible cause or contributor to neoplasia. The lack of response to growth inhibitor influences accounts for the *uncontrolled proliferation* characteristic of neoplastic cells. This factor has been described as that of *autonomy*.[8] In other words, the

cells reproduce through the cell cycle again and again as long as nutrients and oxygen are available.

Messengers carrying information on growth control move into the cell through the gap junction. With loss of gap junction, as occurs with neoplasia, the cell may become isolated from the growth-control messengers of its normal neighboring cells as well as its own (Figure 17-4).

## INNER CELL CHANGES IN NEOPLASIA

Just as changes occur in the outer cell membrane in neoplasia, changes occur within the cell. It is difficult to ascertain whether they are a function of the neoplasia or of the increased growth rate. The changes involve both the nucleoplasm and the cytoplasm.

### Changes in the Nucleoplasm

The nucleus is the location of the genes, the locus of all hereditary information. All cells of the body carry identical genetic information. Gene expression is modulated by poorly understood molecular interactions that allow the cells to carry out their intended functions.[9] Cells then expand clonally to function with varying degrees of autonomy, and as they differentiate, they can move from one part of the body to another.[7] The concept of *clonality* or *clonal evolution of cancer* is supported by the karyotype abnormalities in malignant cells that are inherited by all of the tumor cells.[8] A particular karyotype change is seen in most people with a particular form of cancer.[8] The most well-known example is the Philadelphia chromosome, observed in 85% of persons with chronic myelogenous leukemia (see Chap. 20). Karyotypic abnor-

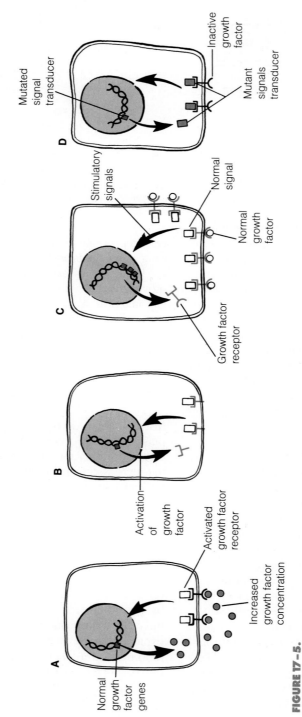

**FIGURE 17–5.**

Mechanisms of growth promotion by an oncogene. (**A**) The oncogene codes for a growth factor and stimulates tumor cells. (**B**) Growth factor receptor may be defective and constantly activated. (**C**) An increased number of growth receptors may cause amplification of oncogene. (**D**) Defective signal transducers may promote growth without an external trigger.

malities can be induced by certain substances, called *oncogenes*. This supports the concept that cancer is a disease of genetic disruption that alters the controls on cellular reproduction and function. Chapter 18 discusses this concept in much more depth.

## Changes in the Cytoplasm

The cytoplasm is a medium through which growth stimulators or inhibitors must move to reach the nucleus of the cell, where they interact with DNA. The exact nature of the messengers remains unclear.

The cytoplasm also contains many enzymes active in normal cellular anabolism and catabolism. Enzymatic changes are common in rapidly growing neoplastic cells.[3] Tumor cells do not reproduce more rapidly than normal cells, but the *growth fraction* places more cells in the *cell growth* than in the *cell loss* phase with loss of normal growth controls (see below). Figure 17-5 describes the mechanisms by which an oncogene may promote cell growth. Oncogenes, described in detail in Chapter 18, are substances that can give rise to malignant tumors.

## DIFFERENTIATION AND ANAPLASIA

During fetal development, cells undergo changes in their physical and structural properties as they form the different tissues of the body. This is cellular differentiation. Differentiated cells become specialized and differ from one another physically and functionally. Nerve cells, for example, are like other nerve cells, but they look and act differently from other types of cells. The more specialized and differentiated a cell is, the less likely it is to divide, and therefore, it is less susceptible to neoplastic change.

The controlling factors of cell differentiation are not well understood but probably involve selective repression of genetic information. Repressor substances in the cytoplasm are apparently responsible for differentiation, with the repressor substance in one cell acting to repress one genetic characteristic, and that of another cell acting to repress a different genetic characteristic. The full set of genetic information is always present, but parts of it are repressed.[6] Cells that look and act like the cell of origin (parent cells) are called *well-differentiated cells*. All benign tumors are well differentiated, often being impossible to differentiate from the normal. The cells of a malignant neoplasm are not as well differentiated as the cells of normal tissue. Neoplasms composed of cells that resemble the mature cells of the tissue of origin are called well-differentiated tumors.[3] Neoplasms composed of cells that bear little or no resemblance to the tissue of

origin are called *poorly differentiated* or *undifferentiated tumors*. The lack of differentiation is called *anaplasia* and is considered a hallmark in recognizing malignant tumors.[3]

Anaplasia describes the regression of a cell population from being well differentiated to being less differentiated. Anaplastic cells vary in morphology and may resemble the tissue of origin or may bear little resemblance to it.[3] Less differentiated (more anaplastic) tumor cells lose orientation to one another, and tumor cells can break off from the primary tumor and metastasize to other areas. The functional efficiency of anaplastic cells correlates with the level of morphologic differentiation.[3]

Well-differentiated cancer cells may elaborate relatively normal products of the tissue of origin, whereas poorly differentiated cancer cells may lose all specialized functional characteristics.[3] Very anaplastic tumors may elaborate a product that is completely foreign to the tissue of origin. An example is the elaboration of antidiuretic hormone from the small cell (oat cell) carcinoma of the lung (see Chap. 31).

The anaplastic cell usually is pleomorphic, which means that it has many shapes and sizes. Large hyperchromatic nuclei with irregular membranes are exhibited, having larger and more numerous nucleoli.[3]

The cytoplasmic organelles of the anaplastic cell are less numerous than those of a normal cell and are abnormal in form. Pseudopodia, microfilaments and clumps of membraneous sacs, and tubules usually are present. Less endoplasmic reticulum and fewer mitochondria are present, so that less cell work occurs. The nuclear membrane appears convoluted, irregular, and doubled on itself.[4]

Mitoses of anaplastic cells frequently are abnormal, and various chromosomal defects result. Most cells exhibit atypical and bizarre mitotic figures.[3] Few mitoses faithfully reproduce the abnormality, and new aberrations with chromosome deletions or translocations occur.

## REFERENCES

1. Cheville, N.F. *Cell Pathology* (2nd ed.). Ames: Iowa University Press, 1983.
2. Cormack, D.H. *Ham's Histology* (11th ed.). Philadelphia: J.B. Lippincott, 1987.
3. Cotran, R.S., Kumar, V., and Robbins, S.L. *Pathologic Basis of Disease* (4th ed.). Philadelphia: W.B. Saunders, 1989.
4. DeVita, V.T., Hellman, S., and Rosenberg, S.A. *Cancer, Principles and Practice of Oncology* (3rd ed.). Philadelphia: J.B. Lippincott, 1989.
5. Ganong, W.F. *Review of Medical Physiology* (12th ed.). Norwalk, Conn.: Appleton & Lange, 1991.
6. Guyton, A. *Textbook of Medical Physiology* (8th ed.). Philadelphia: W.B. Saunders, 1986.

7. LiVolsi, V.A. Neoplasia. In V.A. LiVolsi et al. (eds.), *Pathology* (2nd ed.). Media, Pa.: Harwal Publ., 1989.

8. Neiman, P. Oncogenes and neoplastic disease. In J.D. Wilson, et al. *Harrison's Principles of Internal Medicine* (12th ed.). New York: McGraw-Hill, 1991.

9. Pitot, H.C. *Fundamentals of Oncology* (3rd ed.). New York: Dekker, 1986.

10. Taussig, M.J. *Processes in Pathology and Microbiology* (2nd ed.). Boston: Blackwell, 1984.

11. Walter, J.B. *Pathology of Human Disease.* Philadelphia: Lea & Febiger, 1990.

12. Weiss, L. *Histology, Cell and Tissue Biology* (5th ed.). New York: Elsevier, 1983.

# chapter 18

Barbara L. Bullock

# Benign and Malignant Neoplasia

## Chapter Outline

## Learning Objectives

1. Define *neoplasm, tumor, aberrant cellular growth, benign, malignant, cancer, carcinoma, sarcoma,* and *metastasis.*
2. Define cancer at the clinical, cellular, and molecular levels.
3. Explain the morphologic differences in the subgroups of cancer.
4. Explain staging of cancers.
5. Compare the characteristics of benign and malignant neoplasms.
6. Discuss the concept of genetic instability in cancer development.
7. Describe the role of DNA and RNA viruses in altering the genetic code.
8. Classify chemical carcinogens, and identify the neoplasms with which they are associated.
9. Discuss irradiation as a cause of malignant neoplasms.
10. Relate dietary factors, sexuality, habits, hormones, and pre-

disposing lesions to the development of malignant neoplasms.
11. Explain important factors in primary tumor growth.
12. Describe the TMN classification for staging neoplasms.
13. Explain metastasis from invasion of the basement membrane to proliferation at a new site.
14. List characteristics of a receptive host environment for metastasis.
15. Describe the value of tumor markers in diagnosis and treatment of specific types of cancer.
16. Discuss the role of the immune system in the destruction of malignant cells.
17. Explain the mechanisms responsible for the development of local symptoms of neoplasms.
18. Briefly discuss paraneoplastic syndromes of the endocrine, nervous, hematologic, renal, and gastrointestinal systems.
19. Explain the anorexia-cachexia syndrome.

The capacity to undergo mitosis is inherent in all cells. Mitosis is repressed or controlled until a specific stimulation for growth occurs. Every time a normal cell passes through a cycle of division, the opportunity exists for it to become neoplastic. Cancer cells lack repression and, therefore, lose control of mitosis. The wonder, then, is

not that we have so many neoplasms, but that we have so few. Neoplastic disease affects one person in four and causes worldwide problems of morbidity and mortality (Figure 18-1).

Malignant neoplasms constitute more than 100 distinct disease entities. Cancer can strike at any age. It kills

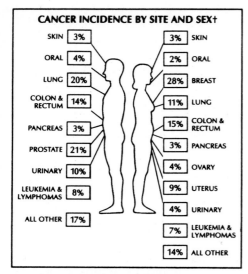

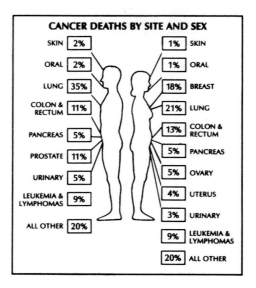

**FIGURE 18–1.**
1989 estimate of cancer deaths by site and sex. (From Cancer Facts and Figures 1989. New York, American Cancer Society, 1989.)

†Excluding non-melanoma skin cancer and carcinoma in situ.

more children aged 3 to 14 than any other disease.[2] The three leading death-producing cancers in men are cancer of the lung, colon and rectum, and prostate gland. For women, the most common cancers are those of the breast, lung, and colon and rectum. Even though breast cancer is much more frequently diagnosed in women than lung cancer, lung cancer became the leading cause of cancer deaths in women by 1989.[5] Advancing age increases the risk of developing cancer. The frequency rises sharply as age increases, with the death rate from cancer of the large intestine, for example, increasing 1000–fold between ages 20 and 80. Cancer follows heart disease as the second leading cause of death in the United States.[2]

This chapter compares benign and malignant neoplasms. Various causative factors are discussed, and metastasis is explored. The local and systemic effects of neoplasms are explained, using benign and malignant tumors as examples. Neoplasms of specific organs are described in the chapters that relate to each system.

## DEFINITIONS

Terms commonly used in discussions about abnormal cellular growth include neoplasm, tumor, aberrant cellular growth, benign, malignant, cancer, carcinoma, sarcoma, and metastasis (Table 18-1). A *neoplasm* refers to a new growth that is abnormal, and the word usually is used synonomously with *tumor*. *Aberrant cellular growth* refers to an alteration in normal cell growth. The transformation of a normal cell into one that escapes the host's usual controls on growth and differentiation is involved in all aspects of neoplasia.

*Malignant* and *benign* describe the ability or inability of abnormally dividing cells to invade normal tis-

sues and spread to distant sites in the host. Table 18-2 indicates the commonly accepted differences between benign and malignant growths.

Benign neoplasms are described on the basis of their cells of origin, microscopic architecture, or macroscopic patterns.[5] Adenomas, for example, refer to epithelial neoplasms with glandular patterns. Polyps and cystadenomas also are descriptions of types of benign neoplasm. Table 18-3 lists some common benign neoplasms.

Cancer always refers to a malignant growth and is characterized by the following features: (1) abnormal cell division, (2) invasion of surrounding normal tissues, and (3) spread to distant sites in the host. In humans, cancer consists of a large group of diseases with a variety of local and systemic signs and symptoms. Untreated, widespread systemic effects can cause the death of the host.

At the cellular level, cancer consists of diseases caused by abnormal cellular growth resulting from defective controls on cell reproduction. Cells lose their differentiation characteristics and become less like the normal parent cell. The loss of differentiation is called anaplasia, which is a characteristic feature of cancer (see Chap. 17). At the molecular level, cancer is caused by abnormal nucleic acid metabolism.[3]

Cancers may be divided into three broad subgroups: carcinomas, sarcomas, and leukemias and lymphomas. *Carcinoma* is a term often used interchangeably with cancer, but it actually refers to a group of abnormally dividing cells of epithelial origin that invade surrounding tissues and spread to distant sites in the host. *Sarcomas* arise in connective tissues, such as the fibrous tissues and blood vessels. These also invade surrounding tissues and spread to distant sites in the host. The *leukemias* and *lymphomas* arise in the blood-forming cells of the bone marrow and lymph nodes, and then invade the mononuclear phagocytic system and remaining body structures.

**TABLE 18-1.**
TERMS USED IN DISCUSSIONS OF NEOPLASIA

| TERM | DEFINITION |
|------|------------|
| Neoplasm | New growth, abnormal cellular reproduction |
| Aberrant cellular growth | Alteration in normal cellular growth |
| Tumor | A growth of neoplastic cells clustered together; may be benign or malignant |
| Benign | Characterized by abnormal cell division but does not metastasize or invade surrounding tissue |
| Malignant | Abnormal cell division with ability to invade, metastasize, and recur |
| Cancer | Malignant growth accompanied by abnormal cell division, invasion of surrounding tissues, and metastasis to distant sites |
| Carcinogenesis | Production or origination of a cancer |
| Carcinoma | Malignant growth originating in epithelial tissue |
| Sarcoma | Malignant growth originating in mesodermal tissues that form connective tissue, blood vessels, lymphatic organs |
| Metastasis | Ability to establish secondary tumor growth at a new location away from the primary tumor |

## CLASSIFICATION OF NEOPLASMS

Neoplasms are customarily classified according to their cell of origin and whether their behavior is benign or malignant. The terminology places the cell or type of tissue of origin as the first part of the name, and "oma" forms the last portion (see Table 18-3).

Epithelial benign tumors of squamous and basal cell origin are called *papillomas.* Glandular epithelial benign tumors are called *adenomas.* Papillomas or adenomas that grow at the end of a stem or pedicle are referred to as *polyps,* and they may or may not be neoplastic. As stated earlier, malignant neoplasms of epithelial origin are carcinomas. Those of glandular epithelial origin are called *adenocarcinomas,* such as adenocarcinoma of the breast.

Neoplasms of muscle cell origin are named accord-

ing to muscle type—for example *leiomyoma,* which means "smooth-muscle tumor." Malignant neoplasms of muscle cell origin are *sarcomas,* an example of which is *leiomyosarcoma.* Neoplasms of nerve cells and connective tissue cells are named in a similar manner. Neoplasms of the blood-forming cells and lymph nodes are named according to the type of blood cell affected.

Pigmented and embryonic cells also are indicated in the nomenclature of neoplasms. In normal embryologic development, three layers of cells become apparent. The outer layer is the *ectoderm,* which forms the skin and other structures in the adult human. The middle layer, or *mesoderm,* forms the supporting structures of bone, muscle, fat, blood, and connective tissue. Malignant tumors of these mesodermal or mesenchymal structures are called sarcomas. The inner layer is the *endoderm,* which ultimately forms the gastrointestinal tract and

**TABLE 18-2.**
A COMPARISON OF BENIGN AND MALIGNANT NEOPLASMS

| BENIGN | MALIGNANT |
|--------|-----------|
| Similar to cell of origin | Dissimilar from cell of origin |
| Edges move outward smoothly (encapsulated) | Edges move outward irregularly |
| Compresses | Invades |
| Slow growth rate | Rapid to very rapid growth rate |
| Slight vascularity | Moderate to marked vascularity |
| Seldom recur after removal | Frequently recur after removal |
| Necrosis and ulceration unusual | Necrosis and ulceration common |
| Systemic effects unusual unless it is a secreting endocrine neoplasm | Systemic effects common |

**TABLE 18–3.**

CLASSIFICATION OF COMMON BENIGN AND MALIGNANT NEOPLASMS

| CELL | BENIGN | MALIGNANT |
|------|--------|-----------|
| **Epithelial** | | |
| Squamous | Squamous cell papilloma | Squamous cell carcinoma |
| Basal cell | Basal cell papilloma | Basal cell carcinoma |
| Glandular | Adenoma | Adenocarcinoma |
| Pigmented | Benign melanoma | Malignant melanoma |
| **Muscle** | | |
| Smooth muscle | Leiomyoma | Leiomyosarcoma |
| Striated muscle | Rhabdomyoma | Rhabdomyosarcoma |
| **Nerve** | | |
| Nerve sheath | Neurilemmoma | Neurofibrosarcoma |
| Glial cells | Glioma | Glioblastoma |
| Ganglion cells | Ganglioneuroma | Neuroblastoma |
| Meninges | Meningioma | Malignant meningioma |
| **Connective tissue** | | |
| Fibrous | Fibroma | Fibrosarcoma |
| Fatty | Lipoma | Liposarcoma |
| Bone | Osteoma | Osteosarcoma |
| Cartilage | Chondroma | Chondrosarcoma |
| Blood vessels | Hemangioma | Angiosarcoma |
| Lymph vessels | Lymphangioma | Lymphangiosarcoma |
| Bone marrow | | Multiple myeloma |
| | | Leukemia |
| | | Ewing's sarcoma |
| **Lymphoid** | | Malignant lymphoma |
| | | Lymphosarcoma |
| | | Reticulum cell sarcoma |
| | | Lymphatic leukemia |
| | | Hodgkin's disease |
| **Other blood cells** | | |
| Erythrocytes | | Polycythemia vera (?) |
| Granulocytes | | Myelogenous leukemia |
| Monocytes | Mononucleosis (?) | Monocytic leukemia |
| Plasma cells | | Multiple myeloma |
| T or B lymphocytes | | Lymphocytic leukemia |

other structures.[20] Sometimes *blastoma* is used to denote that the tissue has a primitive or embryonic appearance. A *teratoma* is another embryonic-appearing tumor that comes from all three germ layers but appears as a highly disorganized array of cells. The teratoma is considered to be benign, whereas the *teratocarcinoma* is malignant. The teratocarcinoma also contains embryonal carcinoma cells that are a population of stem cells whose proliferation is responsible for the malignancy of these tumors.[16] Neoplasms of pigmented cells are named for their cell of origin, the melanocyte. Neoplasms of embryonic cell origin also may contain bits of the germinal layers, such as hair or teeth.

## BENIGN NEOPLASMS

Benign neoplasms consist of cells that are similar in structure to the cells from which they are derived. The cells of benign neoplasms are more cohesive than those of malignant neoplasms. Growth occurs evenly from the center of the benign mass, usually resulting in a well-defined border. The edges move outward, smoothly pushing adjacent cells out of the way (Figure 18-2). As this occurs, many of these tumors become encapsulated. The capsule, composed of connective tissue, separates the tumor from surrounding tissues. A benign neoplasm usually grows slowly and is limited to one area. Its blood

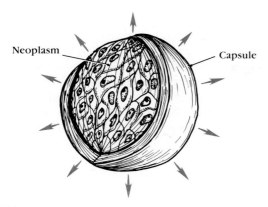

**FIGURE 18-2.**
Encapsulated benign neoplasm. Arrows indicate equal expansion from the center.

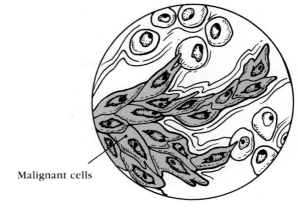

**Malignant neoplasm**

**FIGURE 18-3.**
Malignant neoplasm with irregular borders, indistinct from surrounding tissues.

supply is less profuse than that of a malignant neoplasm. A benign neoplasm seldom recurs after surgical removal, and seldom ulcerates, undergoes necrosis, or causes systemic problems. An exception is a secreting endocrine neoplasm, which causes symptoms resulting from excess hormone secretion. Benign tumors produce their effects from obstruction, pressure, and secretion. A benign tumor in an enclosed space such as the skull can produce serious disruption that may lead to death.[23] Intestinal obstruction may result from a benign tumor growing in that location. When benign endocrine tumors produce excess quantities of hormones, the effects can cause major physiologic problems.[23]

## MALIGNANT NEOPLASMS

Malignant neoplasms have atypical cell structure, with abnormal nuclear divisions and chromosomes. The malignant cell loses its differentiation or resemblance to the cell of origin. The tumor cells are not cohesive, and consequently, the pattern of growth is irregular; no capsule is formed, and distinct separation from surround-

ing tissues is difficult (Figure 18-3). Malignant cells invade adjacent cells rather than pushing them aside. Tumors have varying growth rates and develop a greater blood supply than normal tissues or benign neoplasms. The hallmark of a malignant neoplasm is its ability to metastasize or spread to distant sites. Box 18-1 summarizes the biologic characteristics of the tumor. It frequently recurs after surgical removal and can cause systemic problems.

## MECHANISMS OF CARCINOGENESIS

Most research related to the etiology of neoplasia concerns malignant tumors. Because cancer is not 1 disease, but more than 100 entities, it probably has a phenomenal number of causes. None of the theories that attempt to explain the peculiarities of the cancer cell has been completely successful. Cancer is revealing itself as a highly logical, coordinated process by which cells turn the usual benign life purposes to the most dangerous of ends.[2]

**BOX 18-1.**
BIOLOGIC CHARACTERISTICS OF THE MALIGNANT NEOPLASTIC CELL

Metastatic—transferring to other tissues by blood and lymph

Invasive—cells not contained by barriers of connective tissue and basement membrane

Anaplastic—large nuclei and nucleoli; fewer mitochondria and other organelles; concerned with replication and not with normal cell metabolism

Mitotic—greater mitotic activity

Nondifferentiated—haphazard growth pattern; does not resemble normal tissue

Nonencapsulated

*Reprinted by permission from Cell Pathology (2nd ed.), by N.F. Cheville. © 1983 by Iowa State University Press, 2121 South State Avenue, Ames, Iowa 50010.*

Many areas of study have evolved to explain the nature of the different diseases processes.

## Genetic Instability

The theory of somatic cell mutation was formulated by Bauer in 1928. It supports the concept that genetic abnormalities can be induced by mutational carcinogenic agents and heredity susceptibility. There is strong evidence that this mutational process is progressive and involves many steps.[5,14] Some cancers can develop as a result of more than one carcinogenic influence.

The clonal evolution of cancer cells results in changes in the nature of the original cancerous phenotype. These changes may be manifest as differences in morphology, special product elaboration, and antigenicity.[14] As morphology changes, tumors may begin to grow and metastasize more readily. Some tumors secrete hormonelike substances that produce physiologic results and account for some of the symptoms of the tumor. The antigenicity of tumors is becoming a vast area for research, with specific tumor markers helping to make diagnoses and prognostic estimates (see p. 363).

## Carcinogens

Since 1775, when Sir Percival Pott linked the occurrence of scrotal cancer in chimney sweeps and their exposure to soot, certain substances have been known to be capable of inducing neoplastic growth. These substances are *carcinogens* or *oncogenes*. Carcinogens are known to increase the likelihood that exposed people will develop a neoplasm. *Cocarcinogens* increase the activity of carcinogens. Some substances in higher doses and exposure rates are carcinogenic, whereas at lower doses and exposure rates, they may be cocarcinogenic. *Procarcinogens* are carcinogens that must be activated or modified in the cell.[14,20] Many procarcinogens in their original form cannot induce cellular changes but require metabolic activation in the body. Three types of carcinogens are examined in the subsequent pages: (1) chemical, (2) physical, and (3) viral.

Numerous substances have been identified as having cancer-causing abilities. These include chemical and physical agents as well as oncogenic viruses. It is thought that a number of steps are necessary for the expression of the fully malignant cell.[14] The change in the first cell is a random mutation. Whether that cell will reproduce or die depends on a number of interrelated factors. Carcinogenesis is now being described on the basis of these interrelated mechanisms (Figure 18-4). The substances must undergo molecular modification inside the cell to cause the cancer. Foreign substances normally are modified and detoxified by different enzymes, but certain people have enzymes that modify the carcinogens in such a way as to bind to the nuclear deoxyribonucleic acid (DNA). This modification is called *activation,* and it becomes the first step in cancer-causing mutations.[21] The individuality of enzyme systems may be one factor that accounts for susceptibility to different forms of cancers. In many cases, the DNA disruption can be repaired, and the process does not progress. The mutation that is produced also must affect particular genes to initiate the cancerous process.[21]

In the 1940s, Berenblum described a two-step mutational model that involved *initiation* and *promotion.* The initial mutation, called *initiation,* increases the sensitivity of the cell to surrounding promoters, and a larger population of initiated cells is formed. An *initiator* causes DNA structure alterations and is mutagenic.[14] A *promoter* stimulates replication of mutant cells but does not promote their mutation.[14] Initiation and promotion probably must go on for several cycles with subsequent mutations of initiated cells before a tumorous mass is formed.

## Chemical Carcinogenesis

Many agents are capable of causing neoplasms in either humans or animals. Chemical carcinogens can be grouped as polycyclic aromatic hydrocarbons, aromatic amines, alkylating agents, nitrosamines and other nitrosocompounds, naturally occurring products, drugs, metals, and industrial carcinogens (Table 18-4).

*Polycyclic aromatic hydrocarbons* are some of the most powerful carcinogens. They are present in the condensates of tobacco smoke, automobile exhaust, and other products of combustion. They also are produced from animal fats in broiling meats and in smoked meat and fish.[5] Cancers of the lips, tongue, oral cavity, head, neck, larynx, lungs, pancreas, and bladder are associated with exposure to polycyclic aromatic hydrocarbons.

*Aromatic amines* and *azo dyes* are another significant group of carcinogens. These include certain foods, naphthalene (a coal tar used in moth repellents and insecticides), and 2-acetylaminofluorene, an insecticide. The aromatic amines have been linked with cancer of the bladder. Some azo dyes were used to color foods, such as margarine and maraschino cherries, and are now federally regulated.[5]

*Alkylating agents* in controlled circumstances are used for therapeutic purposes but can be carcinogenic. Some agents are powerfully immunosuppressive, which may decrease the natural host resistance to cancer. Two common alkylating agents are nitrogen mustard (cyclophosphamide) and mustard gas. Both are implicated in the causation of leukemia and lymphoid neoplasms.[5]

*Nitrosamines* and other nitrosocompounds develop under physiologic conditions from chemical interactions between nitrites and other secondary amines. Numerous drugs and nicotine may supply the amines for the process

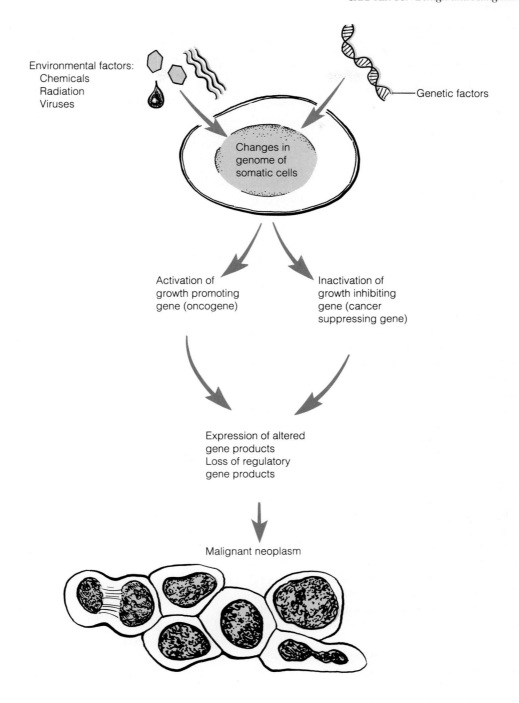

Environmental factors:
  Chemicals
  Radiation
  Viruses

Genetic factors

Changes in genome of somatic cells

Activation of growth promoting gene (oncogene)

Inactivation of growth inhibiting gene (cancer suppressing gene)

Expression of altered gene products
Loss of regulatory gene products

Malignant neoplasm

**FIGURE 18–4.**
Flow chart showing simplified scheme of cancer pathogenesis.

of converting nitrites to nitrosamines in the gastrointestinal tract. Nitrites are present in foods as additives. A number of drugs and nicotine may supply the amines for the process. These agents require activation and may be contributors to gastric carcinomas.[15]

*Naturally occurring products* implicated in the causation of malignant neoplasm include aflatoxin and the betel nut. Aflatoxin B is a mold, *Aspergillus flavus,* found on corn, barley, peas, rice, soybeans, fruit, some nuts, milk, and cheddar cheese. It has been linked to liver cancer in humans. Infection with hepatitis B virus has been correlated with liver cancer, raising the possibility that the virus and mold work together in carcinogenesis.[5] In animals, aflatoxin B has been shown to cause liver, stom-

## TABLE 18-4.
### SUMMARY OF CHEMICAL CARCINOGENS AND THEIR SITES OF ACTION

| CARCINOGENS | SOURCE | SITES OF ACTION |
| --- | --- | --- |
| Polycyclic aromatic amines | Soots, tars, cigarette smoke, benzpyrene | Lips, tongue, oral cavity, head, neck, larynx, lungs, bladder |
| Aromatic amines | Dyes, naphthalene, 2-acetylaminofluorene | Bladder |
| Alkylating agents | Nitrogen mustard and mustard gas, drugs (cyclophosphamide, melphalan) | Lungs, larynx, bladder, hemopoietic system |
| Nitrosamines and nitrosocompounds | 4-Nitrobiphenyl | |
| Naturally occurring products | Aflatoxin B, betel nut | Liver, oral cavity |
| Drugs | Griseofulvin, hycanthone, metronidazole, diethylstilbestrol | Cancers in rats, vagina, bladder, hemopoietic system |

ach, colon, and kidney cancer. Chewing the betel nut has been implicated in cancer of the oral cavity.

Several *drugs* besides the alkylating agents are known to have carcinogenic effects. Griseofulvin, an antifungal agent used to treat mycotic disease of the skin; hycanthone, an antihelminthic agent; and metronidazole, an antiprotozoal used to treat *Trichomonas vaginalis* and *Entamoeba histolytica,* cause cancer in rats. Diethylstilbestrol, used during the 1950s to prevent spontaneous abortion, increased the frequency of cancer of the vagina in the daughters of women who received this treatment. Studies also have shown increased prevalence of cancer in male offspring of treated mothers (see Chap. 55).

Alcohol deserves special mention as a cancer-causing drug. Heavy consumption is associated with cancer of the mouth, pharynx, esophagus, larynx, and liver.[12] Alcohol apparently enhances the effects of procarcinogens and carcinogens such as nicotine by increasing their solubility, altering liver metabolism, altering the intracellular metabolism of epithelial cells, and causing nutritional deficiencies.[12]

Asbestos, cadmium, chromium, and nickel are some of the *metals* involved in carcinogenesis. All are associated with cancer of the lung. Chromium and nickel also may cause nasal cavity tumors. Cadmium may be associated with cancer of the prostate gland. Asbestos may cause cancer of the pleural cavity and gastrointestinal tract.

Industrial compounds have been implicated in carcinogenesis. One example of these is polyvinyl chloride, which is used in the manufacture of plastics and may cause angiosarcomas of the liver.[11]

*Asbestos fibers* are associated with bronchogenic and gastrointestinal carcinomas in humans continuously exposed to the substances. The fibers are thought to function as promoters for other carcinogens such as cigarette smoke.[5] Chronic pulmonary tuberculosis also is associated with an increased frequency of lung carcinoma. Chronic injury of the mucosa of the lips and gums from dentures or pipe smoking leads to an increased occurrence of oral cancer.

*STEPS INVOLVED IN CHEMICAL CARCINOGENESIS.* Induction of cancer involves the sequential activation of substances and is roughly divided into two phases: *initiation* and *promotion* (see Figure 18-4). Initiating carcinogens induce permanent DNA changes in target cells.[7,15] Promoters are of many types and often are only effective for one type of cancer. These substances induce clonal proliferation of initiated cells by activating enzymatic pathways. Promoters are not tumorigenic by themselves.[15]

## Radiation Carcinogenesis

*Ionizing radiation* is a recognized cause of cellular mutations. Damage to DNA may be direct or indirect. Direct damage results from interaction of the electron itself with the DNA of the cell. Indirect damage occurs when a secondary electron interacts with a water molecule, giving rise to a free radical, which then damages DNA.[20] A long latent period often exists between exposure and the development of clinical disease. Firm evidence links exposure to large doses of irradiation to leukemia.

Overexposure to radiation from atomic bomb detonation has been extensively studied in survivors of Hiroshima and Nagasaki, Japan. The high prevalence of leukemia in these people supports the relation between leukemia and irradiation. Miners of radioactive elements have suffered a tenfold increase in lung cancer incidence.[5] Skin cancers were common in pioneers in x-ray technology because of excessive exposure to electromagnetic radiation.[5]

Even low doses of irradiation may cause cancer in susceptible people. The frequency of breast cancer increases with small, widely spread doses of irradiation, and that of thyroid cancer increases with head and neck radiography during childhood. Radiography of the fetus in utero increase its chances of developing childhood cancer.

*Ultraviolet radiation* from the sun is a major cause of skin cancers. Fair-complexioned people are more likely to develop skin cancers than their darker-complexioned counterparts because of the lack of melanin, which protects the latter from injurious effects of the sun (see Chap. 46).[17]

*MECHANISMS OF RADIATION CARCINOGENESIS.*
Ionizing radiation causes injury to DNA. The mutagenic property depends on radiation quality, dose, dose rate, DNA repair, and host factors.[5] The susceptibility of certain people is variable. The more rapidly reproducing cells, such as skin, mucosa, and blood, are more vulnerable.

## Oncogenic Viruses

Viruses are thought to cause some human malignant neoplasms and have been directly associated with tumor induction in animals. Viruses implicated in human cancers are called oncogenic viruses. Current evidence favors the view that viruses alter the genome of the infected cell, which then alters the progeny (offspring) of the host cell.[5]

The two types of oncogenic viruses are DNA and ribonucleic acid (RNA). The DNA viruses are incorporated into the genes of the host and then transmitted to subsequent generations. The genes are then expressed without the usual symptoms that accompany infections. Cells in which viral reproduction can take place are called *permissive cells*, but these cannot be transformed to neoplastic cells because they die with release of the virus. The *nonpermissive cells* that do not allow the virus to multiply can be transformed into neoplastic cells.[5] The viral DNA integrates into the chromosomes of the cell. The RNA viruses, or *retroviruses*, also contribute genetic information to the host cell. The mechanism for this viral transmission appears to involve a reversal of the normal processes. Thus the transcription and synthesis of DNA results from an RNA template using an enzyme called reverse transcriptase.[5] This explanation clarifies the process by which genes are expanded and new DNA sequences are developed without the parent structures being altered (Figure 18-5). As part of the genome of the host cell, the virus is not attacked and destroyed by the immune system. Present evidence favors the view that *reverse transcriptase* acts to accomplish *reverse transcription*, to degrade RNA

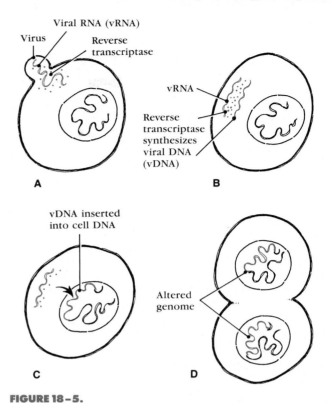

**FIGURE 18–5.**
Schematic showing how RNA viruses change the genome of the cell and cause replication of new cells with altered genome. (**A**) Virus infects the cell. (**B**) Alteration of cell RNA by virus (vRNA). (**C**) Alteration of cell DNA. (**D**) Duplication of the cell, with altered DNA going to the progeny.

in the new DNA–RNA complex, and to form the new DNA double strand.[5]

Some viruses associated with human malignant neoplasms are the C-type and B-type RNA viruses and certain DNA viruses. Although the mechanism is not clearly established, the C-type RNA viruses are implicated as causative agents in the development of certain types of leukemias; the B-type RNA viruses may be factors in causing breast cancer, and herpesviruses may be associated with cervical cancer. The Epstein-Barr virus, a DNA virus of the herpes type, has been closely associated with Burkitt's lymphoma and nasopharyngeal carcinoma. The human papillomavirus has many distinct types, and directly causes human warts (papilloma of the skin). The connection with skin cancers, anogenital malignancy, and carcinoma of the cervix is being studied.[5,15] Table 18-5 summarizes the viruses most closely implicated in the development of malignant neoplasia.

## Other Factors in Carcinogenesis

Epidemiologic studies have revealed other factors in the occurrence of neoplasms besides chemical and physical

**TABLE 18–5.**
VIRUSES IMPLICATED IN MALIGNANT NEOPLASIA

| VIRUS | ASSOCIATED CANCER |
| --- | --- |
| C-type RNA | Leukemia |
| B-type RNA | Breast cancer |
| Herpes II | Cancer of cervix |
| Epstein-Barr | Burkitt's lymphoma, nasopharyngeal cancers |
| Human papilloma virus | Cancer of cervix, anogenital cancers |

carcinogens. These factors are primarily related to habits of daily living and religious or cultural traditions. Some predispose people to the development of neoplasms, whereas others serve a protective function. For example, cancer of the stomach is more common in Japan than in the United States, whereas cancers of the intestine, breast, and prostate are less common. These differences are lost within a generation or two after the Japanese take residence in the United States.

## *Diet*

Dietary customs have been the subject of a great deal of research. Diets high in fat and low in fiber content have been implicated in cancers of the colon and breast. The mechanisms postulated for these connections include the estrogen hormone for breast cancer and the slowing of transit time in colon cancer. Food preservation seems to play a role in carcinogenesis. The nitrates used in some food preservatives can be activated, and nitrates in water and soil can be reduced to nitrites by the body. Foods preserved by salting, drying, or charring increase the consumer's risk of cancer of the stomach.[5,15]

## *Sexuality*

Customs and religious beliefs that involve sexuality seem to have a role in carcinogenesis. Cancer of the cervix is more likely to occur in women who begin having sexual intercourse at a young age and who have many sexual partners. The frequency of cervical cancer is lowest in nuns, virgins, and Jewish women. This finding is thought to be due to hygiene practices and circumcision. Cancer of the penis also is lowest among Jewish men who are circumcised shortly after birth. Cancer of the breast is more prevalent in women who have no children, who begin menses early, or who enter menopause late.[10] Kaposi's sarcoma, a virus-associated tumor, occurs mainly in victims of acquired immune deficiency syndrome (see Chap. 15).

## *Habits*

A person who consumes 6 oz of 80-proof alcohol a day over a period of time increases the risk of developing cancer of the esophagus two to three times. The risk is even greater for those who also smoke cigarettes. A person who smokes cigarettes increases the risk of lung cancer fourfold by smoking 9 to 10 cigarettes a day, or 10 or more times by smoking a pack or more a day. There also seems to be a relation between polluted air and cigarette smoking and the development of cancer.[2]

## *Hormones*

Alterations in hormonal balance resulting in increased hormonal levels over a prolonged time may promote the growth of neoplasms in the target cells. Cancer of the breast, endometrium, vagina, prostate, thyroid, and adrenal cortex are thought to be affected by altered hormonal influences.

## *Predisposing Lesions*

Many neoplastic changes in tissues are known to be precancerous. For example, chronic cystic disease of the breast predisposes a woman to cancer of the breast. Bronchial dysplasia seen with cigarette smokers often precedes bronchogenic carcinoma, and most hepatocellular carcinomas arise in cirrhotic livers.[5] Adenomatous polyps of the colon and rectum remain questionably precancerous.

## GROWTH OF THE PRIMARY MALIGNANT TUMOR

The growth rate of malignant tumors does tend to correlate with their level of differentiation. Therefore, the more undifferentiated or anaplastic a tumor, the greater is its potential for aggressive growth and dissemination.

The primary tumor usually grows for years before producing a clinically overt mass.[5] It depends on the cellular reproduction of tumor cells. Each time a cell reproduces, it doubles the tumor mass, from 1 to 2 to 4 to 8, and so on. It is estimated that a typical tumor has doubled 30 times before it becomes clinically observed. A 40-time doubling often proves to be fatal to the host. The *growth fraction* is the ratio of proliferating to nonproliferating cells. As the total volume of the tumor increases, the growth fraction usually decreases. Another factor that accounts for this is that many cells of the primary tumor are lost through death or shedding into a hostile environment.[19]

The rate of tumor growth is affected by many factors, including blood supply, nutrition, immune responsiveness, and, in some tumors, endocrine support. Studies have shown that many tumors elaborate a *tumor angiogenesis factor* that promotes directional blood vessel growth into the tumor mass.[8] The increased vascularity of a malignant tumor is critical to providing nutrients and oxygen to sustain its continued growth.[7,15] If a tumor outgrows its blood supply, central ischemic necrosis may occur. In a nutritionally depleted host, the tumor growth may slow because of a decrease in the supply of adequate nutrients.[5]

## STAGING OF NEOPLASMS

Staging is an effort to describe the extent of a neoplasm in terms that are commonly understood. The purposes of staging are to (1) determine treatment, (2) evaluate survival rates, (3) establish the relative merits of different methods of treatment, and (4) facilitate the exchange of information among treatment centers. The staging of cancers is based on the size of the primary tumor and the spread of tumor to regional lymph nodes or other distant areas.[5] The TMN classification varies slightly with different types of cancer but provides some general principles of staging. Box 18-2 shows a scheme for staging breast cancer.

The three capital letters are used to denote the following: T, the tumor or primary lesion and its extent; N, lymph nodes of the region and their condition; and M, distant metastasis.[20] Tumor in situ, or localized tumor, is abbreviated TIS. $T_x$ is used when the extent of tumor cannot be adequately assessed. Using the letter *T* and adding ascending numbers indicates increasing tumor size. The spread of cancer to regional lymph nodes is indicated by $N_1$, referring to "few," with $N_2$ referring to many nodal metastases. The presence or absence of distant metastasis is designated by an $M_0$ or $M_1$. When the amount or extent of metastasis cannot be assessed, $M_x$ is used.

## METASTASIS

The ability of a malignant neoplasm to spread to distant sites is *metastasis*. A clump of malignant cells, no longer attached to the original neoplasm, travels to and becomes established at a new site. The original cancer is the primary neoplasm, tumor, or site. Metastasis involves the release of many malignant cells, only some of which are able to survive the defense mechanisms and hostile environment.[24] Five phases are involved in metastasis: (1) invasion, (2) cell detachment, (3) dissemination, (4) arrest and establishment, and (5) proliferation (Figure 18-6).[19]

### Invasion

To invade normal adjacent cells, the malignant cells grow out from their original location into the neighboring location. To infiltrate a body cavity or blood vessel, the malignant cells must break through the basement cell membrane. They may escape into the bloodstream through gaps between endothelial cells as rapidly growing capillary tubes penetrate the basement membrane of the capillaries.

A major structural component of the basement cell membrane is type IV collagen. It has been suggested that an enzymatic action causes dissolution of the basement membrane so that tumor cells can penetrate it. This enzyme, *collagenase type IV*, actively attaches to and dissolves type IV collagen. Greatly damaged endothelium has high levels of collagenase IV, which may be significant for malignant cells to select invasion sites.[13]

---

**BOX 18-2.**
ABBREVIATED CLINICOPATHOLOGIC STAGING SCHEME FOR BREAST CANCER

| | |
|---|---|
| T0 | No palpable tumor |
| T1 | <2 cm |
| T2 | 2–5 cm |
| T3 | >5 cm |
| T4 | Grave local signs: chest wall fixation, edema, inflammation, ulceration |
| N0 | No palpable ipsilateral axillary nodes |
| N1 | Positive ipsilateral axillary lymph nodes |
| N2 | Ipsilateral matted or fixed axillary lymph nodes |
| N3 | Infra- or supraclavicular lymph node |
| M0 | No evidence of disease metastasis |
| M1 | Metastases present |
| Stage I | T1, N0, M0 |
| State II | T2, N0, M0 or T1–2, N1, M0 |
| Stage III | T3 or T4, any N, M0 or any T, N2–3, M0 |
| Stage IV | Any T, any N, M1 |

*Kelley, W. N. Textbook of Internal Medicine. Philadelphia: J.B. Lippincott 1989.*

**A.** Primary tumor grows and invades the surrounding tissues. Cells are easily shed and can invade the basement membrane of the highly vascular tumor bed. The increased vascularity is caused by the elaboration of tumor angiogenesis factor (TAF) or by procoagulant factors.

**B.** The tumor cells move between the endothelial capillar junctions or penetrate the basement membrane of the capillary.

**C.** The shed tumor cells become arrested in a capillary bed, often liver, lungs, or brain. At this point they can penetrate the capillary wall and establish in the new environment.

**D.** Proliferation at the new site requires a receptive environment, with blood supply and nutrition to encourage tumor growth. Most tumor cells are killed in the process of metastasis.

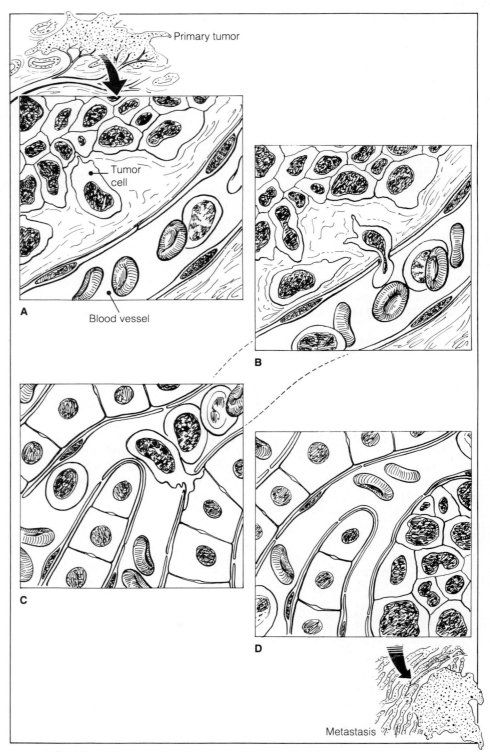

**FIGURE 18–6.**
Metastasis of tumor cells to nonadjacent tissues.

## Cell Detachment

After invading the neighboring tissues, body cavities, and blood vessels, malignant cells separate from the primary neoplasm and penetrate lymphatic or blood vessels. Tumor cells lack the normal property of adhesion and are easily shed into the surrounding tissues, blood, and lymph.

## Dissemination

The most common route that malignant cells take to distant sites from the primary neoplasm is through the lymphatic and blood vessels. Malignant cells move from lymphatic to blood vessels and vice versa. A malignant neoplasm of just a few grams may shed several million cells into the circulation each day. A large proportion of these cells die, and few possess the factors necessary for survival in the hostile, turbulent circulatory system.[18] To survive in the circulatory system and to effect arrest in the endothelium, malignant cells undergo a variety of cellular interactions that involve immunity and adherence.

### Lymphatic Dissemination

As the tumor invades surrounding tissue, it penetrates the small lymphatic vessels. Tumor cell emboli are shed into the vessels and trapped in the first lymph node encountered.[6] The lymph nodes of a group may become involved with disease or some may be skipped.[8] The lymph node often enlarges, which may be due to a localized reaction to the tumor cells or growth of the tumor within the node. Stimulation of the immune defense system may contain the material within the node or filter the tumor cells from the circulation. This may decrease the net spread of tumor.[9]

There are numerous venous-lymphatic communications by which tumor cells can pass between the blood vessels and lymph systems. The main communication lies at the thoracic duct, where lymphatic fluid empties directly into the venous circulation. Tumor cells brought to the lungs by the thoracic duct may be trapped in the pulmonary capillary bed or break into the pulmonary veins and reach the systemic circulation.[6]

### Bloodstream Dissemination

Just as the tumor spreads into and sheds its cells into the lymphatic system, it also can spread into the microcirculation. The spreading is facilitated when collagenase IV is present because this enzyme dissolves the capillary basement membrane and enhances dissemination. Tumor then may grow at the site of vascular spread, or it may embolize to other parts of the body. Most tumor cells do not survive the turbulence of circulating blood. The chances for survival improve if the tumor cells aggregate with one another or with host cells, such as platelets or leukocytes.

Metastasis requires entrapment in the capillary bed of distant organs.[9] Fibrin deposits often form around the new tumor and may protect it from destruction by immune defensive cells. After the tumor is carried to the lungs, it may invade branches of the pulmonary veins and be released into the systemic circulation to travel to the brain or viscera.[6] If the tumor is shed into the portal venous system, it often ends in liver metastasis.

The *vertebral vein plexus* provides some answers regarding the odd distributions of metastases of certain tumors. This plexus of veins has no valves, and communicates with all major vein systems.[6] It carries neoplastic cells from the prostate gland to the vertebra, pelvis, and femur in the absence of evidence of other metastatic disease. Cancer of the breast may metastasize specifically to the dorsal vertebra, as do lung cancers. Even some of the cerebral metastases may be a result of cells passing through the vertebral venous plexus.[6]

Adherence also is involved in the survival of malignant cells in the circulatory system, as well as their arrest in the endothelium of the capillary. Malignant cells form clumps that enter the capillary bed and adhere to endothelial cells lining the capillary, where they become entrapped or arrested. There the clump surrounds itself with fibrin, which protects it during growth.

## Arrest, Establishment, and Proliferation

After becoming trapped in the small vessels of the arteries or veins, the aberrant clump of malignant cells must break through the vessel into the interstitial spaces to continue to grow. Cell-free spaces in the endothelial lining of the capillary appear to be induced by the malignant cells, a process that involves alterations in cellular adhesion and consequent retraction of the endothelial cells. A new environment conducive to cellular growth must be established once the malignant cells are in the interstitial spaces.

Once the clump has grown to exceed about 2 cm in diameter, it can no longer supply its nutritional needs by diffusion. Its own blood supply becomes essential for further development. The establishment of a blood supply is the factor that changes a self-contained clump of malignant cells into a rapidly growing metastatic tumor. As in primary tumor growth, the clump of malignant cells secretes tumor-angiogenesis factor, which causes the blood vessels to send out new capillaries. These new capillaries grow toward and eventually penetrate the malignant cells, creating a blood supply through which the malignant cells receive nourishment and have their waste

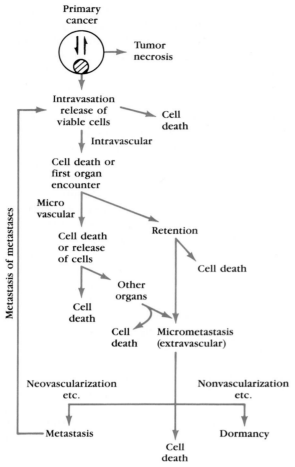

**FIGURE 18-7.**
Metastatic process showing cell loss and gain. Diagram shows intravascular metastasis to organ involvement. Note that more cells die in the process than survive and grow. (From I. Weiss and H.A. Gilbert, *Liver Metastasis*. Boston: G.K. Hall, 1982.)

products removed. Establishment and proliferation of these cells also depends on the immunologic and outer cell membrane properties discussed earlier. Thus the malignant cell adjusts its environment to further its own growth. Figure 18-7 shows the possible outcomes of metastasis from the primary tumor.

## Sites of Metastasis

Primary tumors have a great tendency to metastasize to and grow in specific organs. Because a small tumor can release several million tumor cells a day into the bloodstream, some eventually will arrest and survive at a receptive site.[9] Patterns of metastasis apparently are determined by individual cellular characteristics and by environmental factors.[18]

Certain primary malignant neoplasms metastasize more readily to specific sites. For example, cancer of the breast metastasizes to the lungs and brain, whereas cancer of the prostate or adrenals metastasizes to the bone. The site of the metastatic neoplasm is not randomly chosen but may be based on mechanical considerations involving cell size, pressure, vessel size, and other physical features. Also, the site of metastasis may be similar to the site that fostered the primary growth. Vascularity of the secondary site is a well-established need. The lungs may well be a popular site simply because malignant cells entering the venous system enter their first capillary network there.

## HOST DEFENSE MECHANISMS IN THE CONTROL OF NEOPLASIA

### Tumor-Associated Antigens

Investigations have shown that some human tumors have tumor-specific antigens on their cell surfaces. Various nonmalignant tissues also elaborate a number of different antigens. Among these are the oncofetal antigens, viral antigens, and histocompatibility determinants.[5] In a malignant neoplasm, the antigen-bearing cells are expanding, so that as the tumor grows, the total tumor-associated antigen (TAA) also increases. If treatment decreases the pool of TAA, measuring the amount of TAA can be helpful in plotting the course of certain cancers. These TAAs often are considered among the broad category of *tumor markers* (see below). The use of TAA as a target for clinical treatment is limited because its expression varies among cells within a tumor.

Oncofetal antigens are those normally present during embryonic development and reexpressed in some neoplastic tissue. Useful markers of this classification include the carcinoembryonic antigen (CEA), alphafetoprotein (aFP), and gross cystic disease protein. The CEA has been found in persons who have colon and pancreatic cancers, but about 5% of the normal population have positive CEA titers. The aFP levels elevate in persons with liver and pancreatic carcinomas. It also is elevated in conditions such as viral hepatitis.[22]

Histocompatibility antigens are being studied in neoplastic tissue, with the goal being to use a host-versus-tumor reaction to destroy the tumor or metastasis. If the immune system can recognize the tumor as foreign, the immunization prepared from host tumor or tumor cell membranes of a donor may cause the host to reject the tumor. In animal studies, these processes have been quite successful, but in humans, the response has been variable.[4]

The immune system has natural defenses of tumor destruction (see Chap. 14). When the tumor cell antigen is recognized by the immune system as being foreign, it may be destroyed by T-cell cytotoxic response, by natural killer (NK) cells, by macrophage intervention, or by B cells and complement activation. T cells and NK cells apparently contact the foreign material directly and destroy its membrane. Activated macrophages bind to and destroy neoplastic cells more readily than normal cells. In antibody reactions, the antibody apparently serves as a bridge between the effector (eg, NK cells, macrophages, and polymorphonuclear leukocytes) and target cells. When complement is involved, the final activated complement can cause the destruction of tumor cells.[1]

If the immune system is capable of destroying neoplastic tissue, how do tumor cells escape destruction? Many human tumors lack tumor-specific antigens, or the antigen is not expressed at the cell surface to be recognized as foreign. Some tumors can modulate the expression of antigen after exposure to the immune system. Immune suppression in individuals debilitated by systemic disease or irradiation or chemotherapy predisposes them to a higher than normal frequency of later cancers, especially leukemia and lymphoma. People with cancers may have specific and nonspecific suppressor factors, particularly active against T cells.[1]

## Tumor Markers

Tissue-specific markers are antigens that are found only in certain tissues. They can be used to diagnose the source of a neoplasm. A tumor marker is an abnormality that is specific for a particular type of cancer. Assays of the particular markers can be used to (1) screen high-risk people for the presence of cancer, (2) diagnose the exact nature of a cancer, (3) monitor the effectiveness of therapy, (4) detect recurrences of cancer, and (5) detect metastases using radioactive-labeled antibodies.[15] Because a particular substance is consistently found in the serum of people with a certain type of cancer, a measurement of that substance can be used to screen for cancer and to monitor for recurrences.[14] Table 18-6 lists some examples of tumor markers that can include tumor antigens, hormones, enzymes, and elevated amounts of normal electrolytes. Chromosomal abnormalities also have been identified in certain cancers, the most consistent of which is the Philadelphia chromosome in chronic myelogenous leukemia (see Chap. 20). The hormone, human chorionic gonadotrophin (HCG), has been used as a marker for trophoblastic tumors and testicular and ovarian germ cell tumors. The serum levels of HCG can be used to make decisions on discontinuing and reinstituting therapy.[15] Unit 16 presents more information on gonadotrophin-releasing tumors.

## CLINICAL MANIFESTATIONS OF NEOPLASMS

In their earliest stages of development, benign and malignant neoplasms are asymptomatic. The mass of cells simply is not large enough to interfere with any bodily

**TABLE 18–6.**
EXAMPLES OF TUMOR MARKERS

| MARKER | TYPE OF TISSUE OR CANCER |
|---|---|
| **General Markers** | |
| Leukocyte common antigen | Lyphomas |
| S-100 protein | Melanomas, schwannomas, chondromas |
| Carcinoembryonic antigen | Carcinomas especially of intestine or pancreas |
| Alpha-fetoprotein | Germ cell tumors, intestine or pancreatic tumors |
| **Specific Tissue Markers** | |
| Prostate-specific antigen | Prostate cancer |
| Thyroglobulin | Thyroid cancers |
| Calcitonin | Medullary thyroid carcinoma |
| Coagulation factor VIII–related antigen | Angiosarcoma |
| Myoglobin | Rhabdomyosarcoma |
| Parathyroid hormone | Parathyroid tumors, multiple myeloma, breast and lung cancer |
| Adenocorticotropic hormone | Adrenal tumors, oat cell carcinoma of lung |
| Antidiuretic hormone | Oat cell carcinoma of lung, renal cell carcinoma |
| Immunoglobulins | Plasma cell (multiple) myeloma |
| Human chorionic gonadotropin | Germ cell neoplasms of testes and ovaries |

Adapted from LiVolsi, V. A., et al., Pathology (2nd ed.), Media, Pa.: Harwal Publishing, 1989, and Mendelsohn, J. Principles of neoplasia, in J. D. Wilson et al., Harrison's Principles of Internal Medicine (12th ed.), New York: McGraw-Hill, 1991.

function. As it increases in size, local alterations in function occur.

As malignant neoplasms metastasize, they interfere with function at distant sites and disrupt the biochemical balance of the body.

## Local Manifestations

The nature and development of local symptomatology depends on the location of the neoplasm and on the size and distensibility of the space it occupies. A neoplasm located in the abdomen, which is large and distensible, may grow to considerable size without producing symptoms. A neoplasm the size of a pea located in the cranial vault, a rigid space containing vital sensory and motor functions, may cause major symptoms.

The mass of cells that makes up a primary or a metastatic neoplasm compresses surrounding tissues and organs and their blood supply. The resulting symptomatology is related to interference with blood supply, interference with function, and mobilization of compensatory mechanisms and immune responses.

Compression by the neoplasm interferes with the blood supply to the tissues and organs and decreases their oxygen and nutrient supply, resulting in ischemia and necrosis. In addition, waste products are not removed, and lactic acid accumulates. As lactic acid accumulates and blood vessels are eroded, the individual experiences pain and bleeding. Ischemic necrotic tissues may form sites of secondary infections.

The symptoms produced by interference with the function of the organ vary with the organ involved and the degree of interference. A carcinoma of the lung that obstructs a bronchus may cause atelectasis, abscess formation, bronchiectasis, or pneumonitis distal to the site. The obstruction inhibits removal of secretions and bacteria from the area distal to it. The person experiences coughing, which may or may not be productive, together with signs and symptoms of infection. Infection is common in structures obstructed by a neoplasm. Neoplasms of the colon obstruct the bowel. If the obstruction is incomplete, the person experiences pencil-thin stools, constipation, and cramping. Activated function, rather than an altered function, may occur. For example, compression of nerves or stretching of a nerve-rich membrane by a tumor stimulates the nerve and produces pain.

Compensatory mechanisms also vary with the organ involved. The cramping associated with obstruction of the bowel is the result of increased peristalsis in an attempt to force a fecal mass past the obstruction. Mobilization of the immune system awakens the inflammatory response. As a result, the person experiences increased pulse rate, elevated temperature, and elevated white blood cell count.

## Systemic Manifestations

Neoplasms have systemic as well as local effects. Systemic symptoms may be the first indication that a person has a neoplasm, or they may accompany more advanced metastatic disease. They include anorexia, nausea, weight loss, and malaise, as well as signs and symptoms of anemia and infection. These signs and symptoms occur away from the primary tumor or metastasis and are not a direct effect of either one. The term used to describe them is *paraneoplastic syndromes*.[5] Up to 75% of all persons with a malignant neoplasm experience a paraneoplastic syndrome sometime during their illness. Significant paraneoplastic syndromes involve the endocrine, nervous, hematologic, renal, and gastrointestinal systems.

Only those hormones produced by nonendocrine neoplastic tissues are considered to be paraneoplastic. Symptoms that occur as a result of endocrine paraneoplastic syndromes vary with the hormone produced. For example, all types of lung cancer can produce adrenocorticotropic hormone, causing the person to experience symptoms of Cushing's syndrome—moon face, salt retention, water retention, and so on. Another example is the hypercalcemia or hypocalcemia that can be caused either by the production of a parathyroid hormone-like or calcitonin-like agent by ectopic neoplastic tissues. This type commonly is found in multiple myeloma and breast and lung cancer.[8]

Persons with malignant tumors may experience neurologic difficulties that are due to direct effects of the neoplasm, its metastasis, or fluid, and electrolyte alterations. A few neurologic symptoms are paraneoplastic, however, and may be the primary signs of cancer. The possible neurologic symptoms can be grouped according to the area involved: cerebral, spinal cord, or peripheral nerve. Examples of cerebral symptoms are ataxia, dysarthria, hypotonia, abnormal reflexes, and dementia. Examples of spinal cord symptoms are muscle weakness, atrophy, spasticity, hyperreflexia, extensor-plantar responses, and paralysis. The syndromes associated with the spinal cord may resemble amyotrophic lateral sclerosis. Examples of peripheral nerve symptoms are sensory loss, weakness, wasting, and areflexia.

Hematologic alterations also most frequently result from the direct effects of the malignant neoplasm, its metastasis, or therapy. Some of these alterations may be paraneoplastic and include an increase in red blood cells (associated with an erythropoietin-secreting tumor), anemia, an increase or a decrease in granulocytes, and an increase or a decrease in thrombocytes.[8] Symptoms are related to the specific alteration. For example, in the case of anemia, the person may experience fatigue, cold feet, increased respirations, and palpitations. Coagulation alterations also occur frequently, resulting in either hemorrhage or thrombosis. Disseminated intravascular coagulation (DIC) is often initiated by tumor secretions (see Chap. 21). Nonbacterial thrombotic endocarditis, in either the presence or absence of DIC, is another cause of thrombosis or hemorrhage.

Renal paraneoplastic syndromes result from lesions of the glomeruli and obstructions that are caused by neoplastic products. The nephrotic syndrome with proteinuria may be experienced. Hodgkin's disease is the most common neoplastic cause of the nephrotic syndrome. Tumor antigens and other products of the immune response also have been identified in the glomeruli.

Gastrointestinal paraneoplastic syndromes include loss of protein into the gut, malabsorption, liver dysfunction, and anorexia-cachexia. More than 90% of those persons with advanced disease have a low serum albumin level. Loss of albumin into the gastrointestinal tract occurs as a result of (1) inflammation and ulceration of the mucosa, (2) intestinal lymph channel abnormalities (usually neoplastic obstruction), (3) congestive heart failure, and (4) causes of unknown origin. Hypoalbuminemia causes edema. The liver may enlarge in the absence of metastatic involvement. Other abnormalities, such as elevated levels of alkaline phosphatase, hyperglobulinemia, and hypocholesterolemia, and prolonged prothrombin time may occur. Anorexia, cachexia, weight loss, and taste changes are experienced by most persons with advanced malignant neoplasia.

The *anorexia-cachexia syndrome* may occur either early or late in the course of the disease. This condition may be the manifestation of an undiagnosed cancer. A wide range of other events may cause anorexia-cachexia, such as chemotherapy, radiation therapy, obstruction of the gastrointestinal tract, and toxicity. About one-third of persons with malignant neoplasms experience negative nitrogen balance because of excessive protein wasting. The person who experiences the anorexia-cachexia syndrome has anorexia; loss of strength (asthenia); loss of body fat, protein, and other nutrients; anemia; water and electrolyte imbalance; and increased metabolic rate and energy use. The end result is tumor-induced starvation of the body. There is marked protein and muscle loss as well as adipose tissue (Chapter 10 contains a complete discussion of malnutrition).

Taste plays an important role in appetite. Persons with malignant neoplasms may have altered taste perception. A dislike for meats and other protein foods correlates with a lower threshold for bitter taste, whereas satisfaction with sweets indicates an elevated threshold for sugars. Besides taste, hunger and satiety are controlled by other complex mechanisms, such as the satiety and feeding centers of the hypothalamus, and insulin, glucagon, and amino acid levels. The cause of the anorexia-cachexia syndrome is likely to involve alterations in these mechanisms as a result of the neoplasm.

Some paraneoplastic phenomena cause generalized effects from metabolic alterations. These include lactic acidosis, hyperlipidemia, amylase elevation, and various muscle and joint pains.[5] Fever frequently occurs; paraneoplastic fever refers to an unexplained temperature elevation that subsides with destruction of the cancer but recurs with its reappearance. It occurs with a variety of neoplasms—for example Hodgkin's disease, myxomas, hypernephroma, and osteogenic sarcoma.

## REFERENCES

1. Bast, R.C. Principles of cancer biology: Tumor immunology. In V.T. Devita, S. Hellman, and S.A. Rosenberg, *Cancer: Principles and Practice of Oncology* (3rd ed.). Philadelphia: J.B. Lippincott, 1991.
2. *Cancer Facts and Figures 1990.* Rochester, N.Y.: American Cancer Society, 1989.
3. Cheville, N.F. *Cell Pathology* (2nd ed.). Ames: Iowa State University Press, 1983.
4. Coombes, R.C., and Neville, A.M. Methods of tumor detection. In A.J.S. Davies and P.S. Rudland, *Medical Perspectives in Cancer Research.* Chichester, Engl.: Ellis Horwood, 1985.
5. Cotran, R.S., Kumar, V., and Robbins, S.L. *Robbins' Pathologic Basis of Disease* (4th ed.). Philadelphia: W.B. Saunders, 1989.
6. del Regato, J.A., Spjut, H.J., and Cox, J.D. *Ackerman and del Regato's Cancer Diagnosis, Treatment and Prognosis* (6th ed.). St. Louis: C.V. Mosby, 1985.
7. DeVita, V.T., Hellman, S., and Rosenberg, S.A. *Cancer: Principles and Practice of Oncology* (3rd ed.). Philadelphia: J.B. Lippincott, 1991.
8. Fidler, I.J., and Hart, I.R. Principles of cancer biology: Cancer metastasis. In V.T. DeVita, S. Hellman, and S.A. Rosenberg, *Cancer: Principles and Practice of Oncology* (3rd ed.). Philadelphia: J.B. Lippincott, 1991.
9. Fidler, I.J., and Hart, I.R. Biological diversity in metastatic neoplasms: Origin and implications. *Science* 217:998, 1982.
10. Hogan, R. *Human Sexuality: A Nursing Perspective* (2nd ed.). Norwalk, Conn.: Appleton-Century-Crofts, 1985.
11. Jakobovits, A., Banda, M.J., and Martin, G.R. Embryonal carcinoma-derived growth factors: Specific growth-promoting and differentiation-inhibiting activities. In J. Feramisco, B. Ozanne, and C. Stiles, *Cancer Cells.* New York: Cold Spring Harbor Laboratory, 1985.
12. Lewis, C.M. *Nutrition and Nutritional Therapy in Nursing.* East Norwalk, Conn.: Appleton-Century-Crofts, 1986.
13. Liotta, L.A. Biochemical mechanisms of tumor cell invasion and metastases. *Prog. Clin. Bio. Res.* 256:3, 1988.
14. LiVolsi, V.A., Merino, M.J., Brooks, J.S., et al. *Pathology* (2nd ed.). Media, Pa.: Harwal Publ., 1989.
15. Mendelsohn, J. Principles of neoplasia. In E. Braunwald et al., *Harrison's Principles of Internal Medicine* (11th ed.). New York: McGraw-Hill, 1987.
16. Merino, M.J. Special diagnostic tests. In V.A. LiVolsi et al., *Pathology* (2nd ed.). Media, Pa.: Harwal Publ., 1989.
17. Miller, E.C., and Miller, J.A. Mechanisms of chemical carcinogenesis. *Cancer* 47:5, 1055, 1981.

18. Nicholson, G.L. Tumor metastasis. In A.J.S. Davies and P.S. Rudland, *Medical Perspectives in Cancer Research*. Chichester, Engl.: Ellis Horwood, 1985.

19. Pardee, A.B. Principles of cancer biology: Biochemistry and cell biology. In V.T. DeVita, S. Hellman, and S.A. Rosenberg, *Cancer: Principles and Practice of Oncology* (2nd ed.). Philadelphia: J.B. Lippincott, 1985.

20. Pitot, H.C. *Fundamentals of Oncology* (3rd ed.). New York: Dekker, 1986.

21. Rensberger, B. Cancer: The new synthesis: Cause. *Science 84* 5(7):28, 1984.

22. Wallach, J. *Interpretation of Diagnostic Tests* (4th ed.). Boston: Little, Brown, 1986.

23. Walter, J.B. *Pathology of Human Disease*. Philadelphia: Lea & Febiger, 1990.

24. Weiss, L. *Principles of Metastasis*. Orlando, Fla: Academic Press, 1985.

## UNIT BIBLIOGRAPHY

Anderson, W.A.D., and Scotti, T.M. *Anderson's Pathology* (9th ed.). St. Louis: C.V. Mosby, 1990.

*Cancer Facts and Figures 1990*. New York: American Cancer Society, 1989.

Carter, R.L. *Precancerous States*. New York: Oxford University Press, 1984.

Chevilie, N.F. *Cell Pathology* (2nd ed.). Ames: Iowa State University Press, 1983.

Cotran, R.S., Kumar, V., and Robbins, S.L. *Robbins' Pathologic Basis of Disease* (4th ed.). Philadelphia: W.B. Saunders, 1989.

Creasey, W.A. *Diet and Cancer*. Philadelphia: Lea & Febiger, 1985.

Davies, A.J.S., and Rudland, P.S. *Medical Perspectives in Cancer Research*. Chichester, Engl.: Ellis Horwood, 1985.

del Regato, J.A., Spjut, H.J., and Cox, J.D. *Ackerman and del Regato's Cancer: Diagnosis, Treatment and Prognosis* (6th ed.). St. Louis: C.V. Mosby, 1985.

DeVita, V.F., Hellman, S., and Rosenberg, S.A. *Cancer: Principles and Practice of Oncology* (2nd ed.). Philadelphia: J.B. Lippincott, 1985.

Fidler, I.J., and Hart, I.R. Biological diversity in metastatic neoplasms: Origin and implications. *Science* 217:998, 1982.

Fraumeni, J.F. *Radiation, Carcinogenesis, Epidemiology, and Biological Significance*. New York: Raven Press, 1984.

Fraumeni, J.F. *Cancer Epidemiology and Prevention*. Philadelphia: W.B. Saunders, 1982.

Garfinkel, L., et al. Cancer in black Americans. *CA* 30:39, 1980.

Gropp, C., Havermann, K., and Scheuer, A. Ectopic hormones in lung cancer patients at diagnosis and during treatment. *Cancer* 46:347, 1980.

Haddox, M.K., Magun, B.E., and Russell, D.H. Differential expression of type I-type II cyclic AMP-dependent protein kinases during cell cycle and cyclic AMP-induced growth arrest. *Proc. Natl. Acad. Sci. USA* 77:3445, 1980.

Jakobivits, A., Banda, M.J., and Martin, G.R. Embryonal carcinoma-derived growth factors: Specific growth-promoting and differentiation-inhibiting activities. In J. Feramisco, B. Ozanne, and C. Stiles, *Cancer Cells*. New York: Cold Spring Harbor Laboratory, 1985.

Kerbel, R.S. Implications of immunological heterogeneity of tumors. *Nature* 280:358, 1979.

LiVolsi, V.A., Merino, M.J., Brooks, J.S., et al. *Pathology* (2nd ed.). Media, Pa.: Harwal Publ., 1989.

Moossa, A.R., Schimpff, S.C., Robson, M.C. *Comprehensive Textbook of Oncology* (2nd ed.). Baltimore: Williams & Wilkins, 1991.

Nicolson, G.L. Cancer metastasis. *Sci. Am.* 240:66, 1979.

Pilot, H.C. *Fundamentals of Oncology* (3rd ed.). New York: Dekker, 1986.

Rodgers, J.E. Catching the cancer strays. *Science 83* 4:42, 1983.

Saunders, G.F. *Symposium on Fundamental Cancer Research*. Houston: M.D. Anderson Hospital and Tumor Institute, 1982.

Slauson, D.O., and Cooper, B.J. *Mechanisms of Disease* (2nd ed.). Baltimore: Williams & Wilkins, 1990.

Wallach, J. *Interpretation of Diagnostic Tests* (4th ed.). Boston: Little, Brown, 1986.

Walter, J.B. *Pathology of Human Disease*. Philadelphia: Lea & Febiger, 1990.

Weiss, L. *Principles of Metastasis*. Orlando, Fla.: Academic Press, 1985.

# Organ and System Mechanisms: Adaptations and Alterations

*unit*

**7**

**Normal and Altered Erythrocyte Function**

**Normal and Altered Leukocyte Function**

**Normal and Altered Coagulation**

# HEMATOLOGY

This unit consists of three chapters that deal with the major functions of blood cells. Activities of some of the white blood cells (WBCs) are also discussed in Units 4 and 5.

Chapter 19 details erythrocytic activities, with special emphasis on the pathologic processes of erythrocytosis and anemia. Chapter 20 expands on leukocyte function and emphasizes nonmalignant and malignant disorders of the WBCs. Blood coagulation is explained in Chapter 21, providing a basis for understanding the normal clotting process and disorders of coagulation. Descriptions of crucial hematologic studies are included in all three chapters. The detailed contents of this unit provide for increased understanding of processes that involve blood cell disorders.

The reader is encouraged to use the learning objectives as an outline for study. The unit bibliography presents resources for additional study.

# Normal and Altered Erythrocyte Function

*Learning Objectives*

1. Describe the composition of whole blood.
2. Discuss the primary functions of blood.
3. Explain the stem cell theory.
4. Diagram the process for the development of erythrocytes.
5. Explain the structure and function of hemoglobin.
6. List five substances needed for erythropoiesis.
7. Review energy production in the erythrocyte.
8. Explain the factors that influence erythropoiesis.
9. Explain blood typing and transfusion reactions.
10. Describe the process of red blood cell destruction.
11. Differentiate between physiologic erythrocytosis and polycythemia.
12. Discuss the neoplastic process involved in polycythemia vera.
13. List and differentiate the morphologic characteristics of five types of anemia.
14. Explain how aplastic anemia can develop.
15. List and describe the cause and result of the hemolytic anemias.
16. Describe the precipitating cause of and environment that produces sickle cell anemia.
17. Explain why iron deficiency anemia is common in children and young women.
18. Explain the relation of intrinsic factor deficiency to the development of pernicious anemia.
19. Differentiate the causes of pernicious anemia and folic acid anemia.
20. Briefly explain why posthemorrhagic anemia may not occur immediately after an acute hemorrhage.
21. Briefly describe the laboratory findings and diagnostic tests that are helpful in diagnosing disorders of red blood cells.

All living cells require materials to survive and to perform functions that are necessary to maintain life. Blood and interstitial fluid provide the means by which essential substances are delivered to the cells and materials not needed are removed from the cells. Transportation of cellular and humoral messages by the blood helps to integrate physiologic processes, thus enabling the body to function as a unified whole.

Since ancient times there has been much interest in and curiosity about blood and its relation to life. Blood was known to be essential to human existence; loss of large amounts became associated with loss of life. The first description of red blood cells (RBCs) came with the discovery of the microscope by Leeuwenhoek (1632–1723). He examined the blood and described the red corpuscles.[16] Sophisticated and advanced technology now makes it possible to examine and describe blood components and their functions in minute detail.

## GENERAL PHYSICAL CHARACTERISTICS OF BLOOD

The primary roles of blood in general are to integrate body functions and to meet the needs of specific tissues. Two functions basic to meeting these goals are transportation and distribution of (1) respiratory gases to and from the tissues, (2) hormones to body tissues or organs, and (3) nutrients to the cells. In addition, blood is involved in regulating acid–base balance, thermoregulation, and electrolyte distribution. As detailed in Chapter 20, the leukocytes provide a defense mechanism for the body against invading microorganisms. Platelets aid in the coagulation process by affecting clot formation (see Chap. 21).

Blood consists of a clear yellow fluid called *plasma,* in which cells and many other substances are suspended. Proteins are the major solutes in plasma, and consist primarily of albumins, globulins, and fibrinogen. The composition of plasma is similar to that of interstitial fluid, except that it has a much higher protein concentration. This higher concentration of proteins in the blood maintains the intravascular volume by the exertion of colloid osmotic pressure. In addition to holding water in the intravascular spaces, plasma proteins bind substances such as lipids and metals such as iron, contribute to viscosity of blood, and participate in the coagulation of blood. They also are important in regulating acid–base balance.

Blood accounts for about 8% of total body weight.[9] The total blood volume is divided into two main categories, plasma and cells. Ninety-nine percent of the cells are RBCs. Table 19-1 summarizes the main substances present in blood.

The blood volume is the sum of volumes of plasma and formed elements of blood in the vascular system. It can be calculated from either plasma volume or cell volume, which, in the healthy man, average 45 mL/kg and 30 mL/kg body weight, respectively.[10] If the average man weighs 75 kg, the total blood volume (including plasma and cell volume) will be about 5500 to 6000 mL.

A wide variation in normal blood volumes exists because of the following factors:

1. *Weight.* Because fatty tissue contains little water, the total blood volume correlates more closely with lean body mass than with total body weight.
2. *Sex.* Because women usually have a higher ratio of fat tissue to lean tissue, the blood volume per kilogram for them usually is lower than that for men.
3. *Pregnancy.* Total blood volume gradually rises as a pregnancy progresses, with the greatest increase occurring primarily in plasma volume.
4. *Posture* or *position.* Volume tends to increase when a person is in bed for a period of time and decreases when he or she assumes the erect position. The variation in blood volume may result from alterations in capillary pressure that lead to changes in glomerular filtration.
5. *Age.* Percentage of blood volume is higher in the newborn and decreases with increasing age.
6. *Nutrition.* Lack of nutrients may cause a decrease in RBCs or plasma formation, thus decreasing the total blood volume.
7. *Environmental temperature.* The volume of blood increases when the environmental temperature is increased.
8. *Altitude.* At high altitudes, the environmental oxygen pressure is greatly decreased, and a greater number of RBCs are produced for oxygen transport.

Although numerous factors affect blood volume, it remains relatively stable in the healthy person. Several compensatory mechanisms contribute to this stability; for example, decreased RBC volume is followed by increased plasma volume, thus returning total blood volume to its normal level. In this situation, the total blood volume may be normal, but the ratio of plasma to cells is altered. Capillary dynamics and renal mechanisms play major roles in maintaining plasma volume.

General physical characteristics of the blood are summarized in Table 19-2. Oxygenated arterial blood is bright red, changing to dark red or crimson when oxygen is lost and carbon dioxide is added. The pH is regulated within the narrow limits of 7.35 to 7.45 (see Chap. 9). The relatively high viscosity of blood is primarily due to the suspension of cells and plasma components, which causes it to flow more slowly than water.

The circulation of blood provides for maintenance of a steady state in individual body cells. The constituency of blood rapidly and continuously changes, but the overall concentration of substances remains relatively constant. This constancy in the environment of individual body cells is essential for life.

**TABLE 19–1.**
COMPOUNDS PRESENT IN HUMAN BLOOD

| COMPOUND | CONCENTRATION AND FRACTION |
|---|---|
| Acetone | 0.3–2.0 mg/dL |
| Ammonia | 80—110 $\mu$g/dL |
| Bicarbonate | 24 mM/L |
| Bilirubin | Direct: 0.1–0.3 mg/dL; indirect: 0.2–1.2 mg/dL |
| Calcium | 8.5–10.5 mg/dL; 4.3–5.3 mEq/L |
| Carbon dioxide | 24–30 mEq/L |
| Chloride | 100–106 mEq/L |
| Cholesterol | 150–200 mg/dL |
| Copper | 70–150 $\mu$g/dL |
| Creatinine | 0.7–1.3 mg/dL |
| Glucose (fasting) | 60–100 mg/dL |
| Iron | 50–150 $\mu$g/dL |
| Lactic acid | 5–20 mg/dL |
| Lead | 0–10 $\mu$g/dL |
| Lipase | Below 2 U/mL |
| Lipids, total | 450–1000 mg/dL |
| Magnesium | 7.3–2.1 mEq/L; 1–2 mg/dL |
| Phosphatase, acid, total | Male, 0.5–11 U/L; female, 0.2–9.5 U/L |
| Phosphatase, alkaline | 25–100 U/L |
| Phosphorus, inorganic | 2.3–4.5 mg/dL |
| Potassium | 3.5–5.0 mEq/L |
| Protein | |
| Total | 6.0–8.0 g/dL |
| Albumin | 3.5–5.5 g/dL |
| Globulin | 2.0–3.0 g/dL |
| Sodium | 136–145 mEq/L |
| Transaminase | |
| SGOT (AST) | 7–45 U/L |
| SGPT (ALT) | 4–45 U/L |
| Triglycerides | 10–150 mg/dL |
| Urea nitrogen (blood urea nitrogen) | 4.0–8.5 mg/dL |
| Uric acid | Males, 4.0–8.5 mg/dL; females, 3.0–7.5 mg/dL |

Wallach, J. Interpretation of Diagnostic Tests (4th ed.). Boston: Little, Brown, 1986.

**TABLE 19–2.**
PHYSICAL CHARACTERISTICS OF BLOOD

| CHARACTERISTIC | NORMAL | EXAMPLE OF ALTERATIONS |
|---|---|---|
| Color | Arterial: bright red<br>Venous: dark red or crimson | Anemia |
| pH | Arterial: 7.35–7.45<br>Venous: 7.31–7.41 | Decreases in acidosis; increases in alkalosis |
| Specific gravity | Plasma: 1.026<br>RBC: 1.093 | |
| Viscosity | 3.5–4.5 times that of water | Increases in polycythemia; decreases in anemia |
| Volume | 5000 mL (70=kg male)<br>About 3 L in plasma<br>2 L blood cells | Decreases in dehydration<br><br>Increases in pregnancy |

## HEMATOPOIESIS

### Bone Marrow

In the adult, the bone marrow produces all of the blood cells and platelets. At birth, *red marrow* is present in all bone marrow cavities, and blood cells are formed there as well as in the liver and spleen.[4] In children, blood cells are produced in the marrow of all bones. By age 20 to 25 years, red marrow is present in the cranial bones, vertebrae, sternum, ribs, clavicles, scapulae, pelvis, and proximal ends of the femora and humeri. The other marrow areas become inactive and infiltrated with fat and are called *yellow marrow*. In the aged person, red marrow begins to leave the cranial bones and lower vertebrae.[9]

The blood supply to the marrow comes from large-lumina, thin-walled arteries that branch into a network of capillaries to become a bed of sinusoids. Between the sinuses lies the hematopoietic tissue in which blood cells are formed. The new cells enter the sinuses through small openings in the walls. Blood cells gain access to the sinusoids at a critical moment in their maturation phase, and maturation is completed in the circulatory system and tissues. Loss of integrity of the sinus walls or increased need may allow the release of immature cells into the circulation.

Hematopoiesis is a dynamic, constant process, with rapid turnover of blood cells and a constant need for new cells. Bone marrow can meet the body's changing needs for various types and numbers of cells. It maintains a reserve supply of cells for stressful and unexpected situations that create an increased demand. Normally, 75% of cells in the marrow are precursors to WBCs, and 25% are maturing red blood cells.[15]

### Stem Cell Theory

Most of the formed elements of the blood have a limited life span. Erythrocytes live an average of 120 days. Granulocytes circulate in the blood for an average of 6 hours and then move into the tissues, where they may live for several days.[8,15] Other cells, such as macrophages and lymphocytes, may live months or years. When cells are lost through use or age, they must be continually replaced through a rigidly controlled process.

The origin of cells that develop into mature erythrocytes, leukocytes, and platelets has been investigated for many years. The *stem cell theory* helps to explain the various stages of cell differentiation in the bone marrow.[15] The cellular elements finally present in blood are the more differentiated and mature cells. The pluripotential stem cells transform to committed precursors and finally differentiate (mature) into recognizable precursors of mature cells (Figure 19-1). Stem cells can be *pluripotent*, from which any type of blood cell can form, or *unipotent*,

from which only one type of cell develops.[15] The appearance of these cells cannot be distinguished by ordinary microscopic techniques.

Stem cells may be described based on their morphology, kinesis, or operation (function).

1.  *Morphologically,* they are small mononuclear cells that resemble lymphocytes. Occasional stem cells normally are present in the circulating blood.
2.  The *kinetic* definition recognizes the stem cell pool (compartment) as able to maintain itself and to produce cells that can become committed to a certain line of blood cells.
3.  The *operational* definition regards committed stem cells as colony-forming units (CFUs).

Complex feedback loops of humoral regulation of hematopoiesis are beginning to be recognized. Colony-stimulating and -inhibiting factors are important in regulating the proliferation and differentiation of blood cells.[6,15] As noted in Figure 19-1, the stem cell becomes committed to the lymphoid or trilineage myeloid stem cell lines. From that point, further changes determine the ultimate cell formed. The stem cell maintains the property of self-renewal. Pools of pluripotent or uncommitted cells must be present because once the cell line becomes differentiated (eg, proerythroblast), the cells are in active cell division and cannot self-replicate.[6] The pool apparently can recover if injured but not lethally damaged.[5] RBC formation is the most well understood of hematopoietic cell formation and differentiation (see p. 376). The reader is referred to Chapters 14, 20, and 21 for discussions of the other blood cells.

### Spleen

The spleen is a large, highly vascular organ with elements of the lymphoid and mononuclear phagocyte systems. It is located in the left upper abdominal cavity, directly beneath the diaphragm, above the left kidney, and behind the fundus of the stomach (Figure 19-2). The spleen is covered by peritoneum, and held in position by the peritoneal folds. It has a connective tissue capsule from which trabeculae (supporting strands) extend inside the organ and form a framework. Splenic pulp is present in the small spaces of this framework (Figure 19-3).

The major areas of the spleen are the *red pulp*, the *white pulp*, and the *venous sinuses*. As can be seen in Figure 19-3, a small splenic artery penetrates into the splenic pulp and terminates in highly porous capillaries. Cells move from these capillaries into the red pulp and then gradually squeeze through the trabecular network, eventually ending up in the venous sinuses.[6,10] This exposure of cells to phagocytic cells gives a large surface area to get rid of unwanted debris in the blood. Old RBCs, bacteria, platelets, or parasites, for example, can be

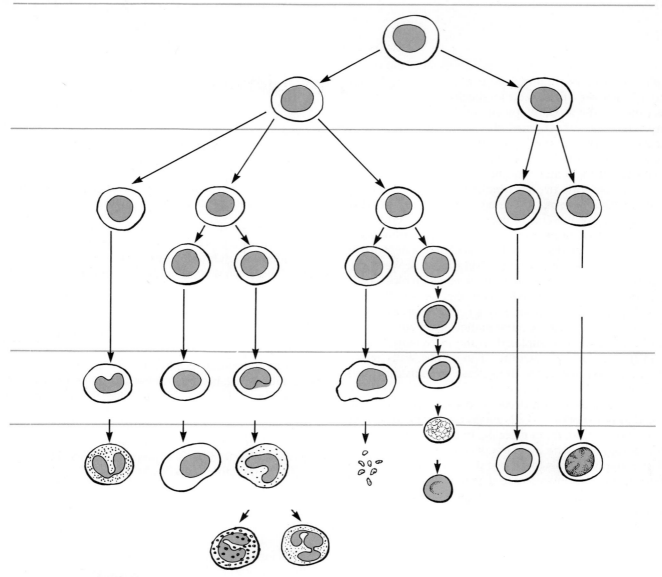

**FIGURE 19–1.**

Differentiation of Hematopoietic cells. (Modified from J.B. Wyngaarden and L.H. Smith, *Cecil Textbook of Medicine* [18th ed.]. Philadelphia: W.B. Saunders, 1988.)

removed from the circulation and destroyed. The destruction of old and imperfect RBCs sometimes is referred to as "culling." Reticulocytes and many platelets are stored in the spleen. Much of the spleen contains white pulp, which consists of a large number of phagocytic and immunocompetent cells. The cells also line the venous sinuses to cleanse the blood.[10] Splenic enlargement is seen in some infectious conditions in the same manner as is seen with lymph node enlargement.

Blood is brought to the spleen by the splenic artery, which divides into several branches before entering the

concave side of the spleen. The small arteries divide into smaller vessels and finally to arterioles and capillaries. After passing through the substance of the spleen just described, the capillaries empty into thin-walled veins that finally terminate in the splenic vein, which itself terminates in the portal vein.

The spleen is not a muscular organ, but dilatation of vessels within it can cause it to store several hundred milliliters of blood and release this blood into the circulation with vascular constriction.[10]

Although the spleen is not necessary for survival, it

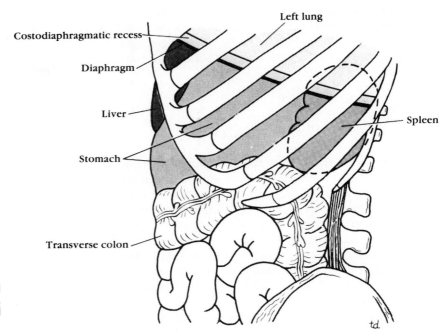

**FIGURE 19-2.**
Spleen, showing notched anterior border and relation to adjacent structures. (From R. Snell, *Clinical Anatomy for Medical Students* [2nd ed.]. Boston: Little, Brown, 1981.)

is involved in four general functions: (1) production of lymphocytes in the white pulp; (2) destruction of erythrocytes in the red pulp; (3) filtration and trapping of foreign particles in both areas, destroying bacteria and viruses; and (4) storage of blood.[6] In fetal life, the spleen is active in hematopoiesis, a function that mostly ends at or before birth. The normal adult spleen holds about 150 to 200 mL of blood, but because of its structure, the spleen often enlarges with increased volume when the systemic venous pressure becomes elevated, such as with right-sided heart failure.[10]

## ERYTHROPOIESIS

### Description of Erythrocytes

Erythrocytes are nonnucleated, biconcave disks. This shape provides a large surface-volume ratio that permits distortion of the cells without stretching their membrane. RBCs can traverse very small capillaries, and normal RBCs adapt to the sinusoids of the spleen, escaping without being trapped and destroyed. The unique shape of erythrocytes also is conducive to gas exchange. The red

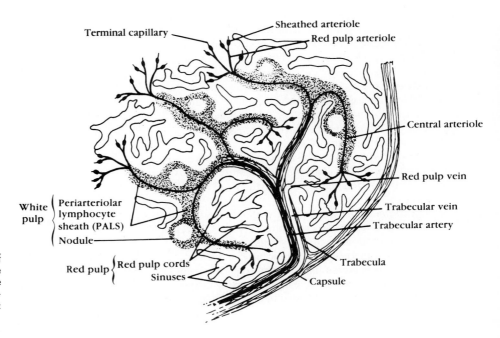

**FIGURE 19-3.**
Schematic representation of part of the spleen showing the relation of the vasculature to the red and white pulp. (From M. Borysenko, *Functional Histology* [2nd ed.]. Boston: Little, Brown, 1984.)

cell membrane is made of lipids and proteins, making it resilient, flexible, and water-insoluble. Erythrocytes contain hemoglobin, which binds loosely with oxygen and carbon dioxide to carry essential gases to and away from the tissues (see below).

## Development of Erythrocytes

Erythrocytes are formed in the blood islands of the yolk sacs during the first several weeks of gestation. During the second trimester of pregnancy, fetal RBCs are produced in the liver, spleen, and lymph nodes. After birth, the bone marrow becomes the principal site of RBC production. After adolescence, the red marrow of the membranous bones, especially the pelvic bone, sternum, ribs, and vertebrae, take over the major erythropoietic function. This marrow cell pool provides a constant supply of peripheral RBCs.

The mature RBC is the end result of several divisions and differentiations before reaching the final stage of maturity (Figure 19-4). During maturation, the nucleus decreases in size until it disappears, the total size of the cell shrinks, the amount of ribonucleic acid lessens, and hemoglobin synthesis increases.

The maturational process of the RBC appears to adhere to the following established sequence:

1. *Erythroid burst-forming unit.* This is the most primitive progenitor of RBCs. It is responsive to *erythropoietin,* an RBC-promoting hormone, and other lymphocyte- and monocyte-produced growth factors.[2]
2. *Erythroid colony-forming unit.* This produces a smaller clone of immature RBCs that also are influenced by other hormones, such as the catecholamines and thyroid and growth hormone.[2]
3. *Proerythroblast.* This immature cell formed from the erythroid colony-forming unit has a nucleus, which is large and centrally located, and contains from one to five nucleoli that are not clearly separated from the rest of the nucleus.
4. *Basophilic erythroblast.* The nucleus becomes smaller and hemoglobin synthesis begins. The cell contains small pinocytic vesicles that are thought to be involved in the uptake of ferritin (storage iron), which is necessary in the formation of hemoglobin.
5. *Polychromatic erythroblast.* The nucleus becomes even smaller and denser. This cell contains a mixture of basophilic material and red hemoglobin, giving it the name polychromatic.
6. *Late orthochromatic normoblast.* Hemoglobin synthesis is almost complete, reaching a concentration of 34% of cell volume. The nucleus continues to shrink and often assumes an odd shape before disappearing. The nucleus migrates into a pseudopod-like protrusion of cytoplasm. It is surrounded by a cytoplasmic membrane, which degenerates; the freed nucleus is ingested by surrounding macrophages.

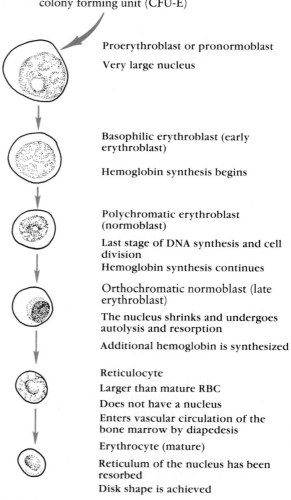

Uncommitted stem cell becomes committed as erythroid burst—forming unit and this erythroid colony forming unit (CFU-E)

Proerythroblast or pronormoblast
Very large nucleus

Basophilic erythroblast (early erythroblast)
Hemoglobin synthesis begins

Polychromatic erythroblast (normoblast)
Last stage of DNA synthesis and cell division
Hemoglobin synthesis continues

Orthochromatic normoblast (late erythroblast)
The nucleus shrinks and undergoes autolysis and resorption
Additional hemoglobin is synthesized

Reticulocyte
Larger than mature RBC
Does not have a nucleus
Enters vascular circulation of the bone marrow by diapedesis

Erythrocyte (mature)
Reticulum of the nucleus has been resorbed
Disk shape is achieved

**FIGURE 19–4.**
Development of red blood cells.

7. *Reticulocyte.* This large, nonnucleated, immature cell contains remnants of the Golgi apparatus, mitochondria, and other cytoplasmic organelles.[10] It normally remains in the marrow about 1 day and then in the bloodstream 1 day before becoming a mature erythrocyte.
8. *Mature erythrocyte.* This cell develops after resorption of the reticulum in the reticulocyte. It is a biconcave disk that is capable of altering its shape without damaging its membrane.

## Hemoglobin

The protein hemoglobin is a conjugated, oxygen-carrying red pigment with a molecular weight of about 64,500. The synthesis of hemoglobin begins in the erythroblast and continues through the normoblast stage. Small amounts of hemoglobin are formed for a day or so by the

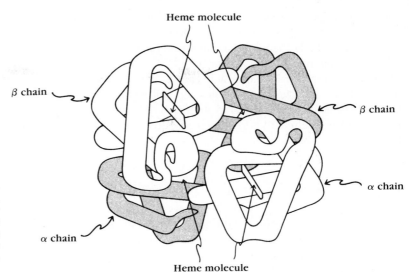

Heme molecule

β chain

β chain

α chain

α chain

Heme molecule

**FIGURE 19–5.**
Structure of the hemoglobin molecule. The hemoglobin molecule is made up of four polypeptide chains. Two identical chains are called α chains, and the other two identical chains are called β chains. Each chain encloses a heme molecule. (From G. Schmid, *The Chemical Basis of Life, General, Organic, and Biological Chemistry for the Health Sciences.* Boston: Little, Brown, 1982.)

reticulocytes. Two parallel processes are involved in hemoglobin synthesis: the formation of the porphyrin structure (heme) that contains iron and the formation of the polypeptide chains that make up globin (Figure 19-5). *Heme* is a large disk that contains iron and porphyrin, a nitrogen-containing organic compound.[11] The adult hemoglobin molecule (HbA) is composed of a globin (made of two alpha and two beta large polypeptide chains) with four heme (iron porphyrin) complexes. The structure of hemoglobin changes in the last 3 months of gestation from primarily fetal hemoglobin (HbF) to HbA. In certain congenital hemolytic anemias, the HbF persists, which, along with globin chain synthesis imbalance, provides the basis for the pathophysiology of these disorders (see pp. 383–385).[1] One iron atom is present for each heme molecule. Each of the four iron atoms of the molecule combines reversibly with an atom of oxygen, forming oxyhemoglobin. When oxygen concentration is high, as in the lungs, oxygen combines with hemoglobin; but when the concentration is lower, as in the tissues, oxygen is released. In the lungs, about 95% of hemoglobin becomes saturated with oxygen. The high density of hemoglobin in each RBC allows a large amount of oxygen to be transported. The disk shape of the erythrocytes provides a large surface area per unit mass of hemoglobin, enhancing gas exchange in the capillary system.

## Substances Needed for Erythropoiesis

Several substances are essential for the proper formation of RBCs and hemoglobin. Among these are amino acids, iron, copper, pyridoxine, cobalt, vitamin $B_{12}$, and folic acid. Iron is essential for the production of heme, and about 65% of body iron is present in hemoglobin. The total amount of iron in the body equals about 4 g, with 15% to 30% of this amount being stored as *ferritin*, primarily in the liver. Ferritin (storage iron) is formed from a combination of iron with a protein called *apoferritin*.[10] It is readily available for hemoglobin synthesis when needed through the aid of a beta-globulin called *transferrin*. Transferrin has specific binding capabilities that facilitate the transfer of iron across the membranes of immature erythrocytes. Transferrin also carries the iron released from worn-out erythrocytes to the bone marrow, where it is reused for hemoglobin synthesis. The presence of reduced ferrous iron allows the formation of hemoglobin, which is capable of binding and releasing oxygen normally. Oxidized ferric iron, however, results in the formation of *methemoglobin,* which cannot carry oxygen. Certain drugs, such as nitrates, phenacetin, sulfonamides, and lidocaine, may cause the production of excess ferric iron.[1]

Daily losses of iron are replaced by dietary intake or transferred to apoferritin to make ferritin. Iron is absorbed mostly in the duodenum by an active process that apparently continues until all of the transferrin is saturated. When transferrin can accept no more iron, absorption of iron almost entirely ceases in the duodenum. Conversely, if the stores are depleted, larger amounts of iron are absorbed. The result is a feedback mechanism that keeps a stable level of iron for hemoglobin synthesis.[9] Lack in the diet or poor absorption of iron leads to iron deficiency anemia (see p. 388).

Vitamin $B_{12}$ (cyanocobalamin) is essential for the synthesis of deoxyribonucleic acid (DNA) molecules in the forming RBCs. This large molecule does not easily penetrate the mucosa of the gastrointestinal tract, but must be bound to a glycoprotein known as the *intrinsic factor (IF)* for its absorption. The IF is secreted by the parietal cells of the gastric mucosa and binds to vitamin $B_{12}$ to protect it from the digestive enzymes. After absorption from the gastrointestinal tract, vitamin $B_{12}$ is stored in the liver and is available for the production of new erythrocytes. Long-standing lack of $B_{12}$ leads to maturation-failure anemia (pernicious anemia) (see p. 388).

Folic acid (pteroylglutamic acid) also is necessary for the synthesis of DNA, and promotes red cell maturation. Lack of folic acid causes folic acid anemia, a type of maturation-failure anemia that readily responds to dietary replacement.

## Energy Production in Erythrocytes

Mature erythrocytes cannot synthesize nucleic acids, complex carbohydrates, lipids, or proteins because they do not have a nucleus or other intracellular organelles. Because there are no mitochondria for oxidative metabolism, the energy of mature RBCs is generated from the metabolism of glucose by the Embden-Meyerhof (anaerobic) pathway and at least three other pathways that use oxygen in different ways (Figure 19-6). Even without a nucleus, the RBC is metabolically active and requires energy to provide for the following functions: (1) maintenance of osmotic stability through intact membrane pumps and active transport of sodium and potassium; (2) maintenance of iron in the reduced ferrous state; and (3) modulation of hemoglobin function by generating 2,3-diphosphoglycerate (2,3-DPG) in the process of generating energy.[11]

## Function of Red Blood Cells in Oxygen and Carbon Dioxide Transport

Most of the oxygen that crosses the alveolocapillary membrane to the blood combines with the heme portion of hemoglobin. This combination is in a loose bond called *oxyhemoglobin*. Hemoglobin saturation with oxygen usually is 95% in arterial blood, and oxygen is rapidly released when it reaches the tissues, which have an oxygen pressure ($PO_2$) of about 40 mm Hg. In normal venous blood, the $PO_2$ is about 40 mm Hg, with a hemoglobin saturation of about 70% (see Chap. 28).[10]

As stated before, hemoglobin becomes nearly saturated with oxygen as it passes through the lungs. This oxygen is unloaded at the tissue level to meet cellular needs. The affinity of hemoglobin for oxygen is affected by hydrogen ion concentration, carbon dioxide levels, and the amount of 2,3-DPG.[1] Increased levels of any of these causes a decreased affinity for oxygen and more effective oxygen unloading to the tissues. This could be viewed as a compensatory mechanism for tissue oxygenation (see Chap. 9). Elevated levels of 2,3-DPG have been seen with some chronic hypoxic states. Conversely,

if the 2,3-DPG levels are decreased or hydrogen and carbon dioxide levels are lowered, there may be a defect in oxygen unloading.[1]

Transport of carbon dioxide from the tissues of RBCs occurs in two major ways: (1) in combination with hemoglobin as carbaminohemoglobin (20%–25%) and (2) in the dissolved form of bicarbonate (70%). When carbon dioxide is released from the tissue cell, it diffuses into the RBC and combines with water, with carbonic anhydrase as the catalyst, to form carbonic acid. Carbonic acid ($H_2CO_3$) almost immediately dissociates into free hydrogen and bicarbonate ions. Free hydrogen attaches to hemoglobin because it is a powerful acid–base buffer, and bicarbonate is free to diffuse into the plasma or attach to a positive ion within the RBC. When bicarbonate diffuses into the plasma, it usually is replaced by chloride in the *chloride shift*. This is made possible by a bicarbonate–chloride carrier protein that rapidly moves these ions in opposite directions. The end result is a greater amount of chloride in venous RBCs than in arterial cells.[10]

## Factors That Influence Erythropoiesis

The normal life span of adult red blood cells is 120 days. Old RBCs are continuously destroyed, and new ones are regenerated daily for replacement. There normally is little variation in the rate of destruction and production, so that the total RBC mass in the body remains relatively constant. Erythropoiesis is controlled by the number of circulating RBCs; decreased numbers stimulate the activity of the bone marrow to increase production of RBCs. Erythropoiesis also is stimulated by a decrease in the $PO_2$ of arterial blood. Chronic hypoxemia, such as with chronic lung disease, produces an increase in the number of circulating RBCs.

*Erythropoietin* hormone stimulates the bone marrow to produce increased numbers of RBCs through conversion of certain stem cells to proerythroblasts. These stem cells are derived from pluripotent stem cells but are more sensitive to erythropoietin than are other stem cells. These cells are referred to as erythropoietin-responsive cells, which are part of a fast cycling system for RBC production. These cells also mature faster than other precursor cells.[8,15] Erythropoietin principally comes from renal glomerular epithelial cells, but some may be released from liver epithelium. The usual stimulus for erythropoietin secretion is hypoxia, but androgens and possibly other hormones have an effect on its secretion. The androgen connection accounts for the higher RBC count in men than in women.[8] A negative feedback system is established, with hypoxemia being a stimulus for erythropoietin and resulting in increased production of RBCs (Figure 19-7). The hypoxic stimulus is relieved, so that both the stimulus for erythropoietin synthesis and

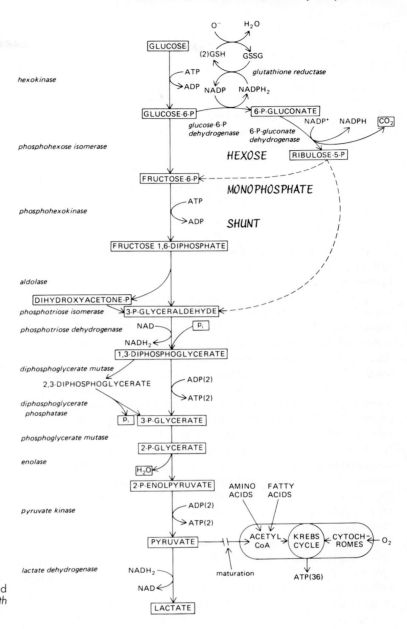

**FIGURE 19-6.**
Metabolism of glucose by red cells. (From J.H. Jandl and R.A. Cooper, *The Metabolic Basis of Inherited Disease* [*4th ed.*]. *New York: McGraw-Hill, 1978.*)

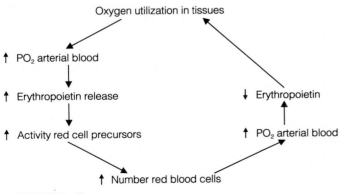

**FIGURE 19-7.**
Feedback mechanism for maintaining red blood cell population.

the rate of erythropoiesis decrease. Conversely, if the volume of circulating RBCs is increased, erythropoiesis is delayed.

## Antigenic Properties of Erythrocytes

More than 300 RBC antigens have been identified, the molecular structure of which is determined by genes at various chromosomal loci.[9] Because distinct RBC antigenic properties are genetically determined, the antigens and antibodies are almost never precisely the same among individuals.[9] The antigens in the blood of one person may react with plasma or cells of another, especially

**TABLE 19–3.**
BLOOD GROUPS

| PERCENTAGE OF POPULATION | TYPE | |
|---|---|---|
| 47 | O: | neither antigen A nor B |
| 41 | A: | antigen A on RBC; no anti-A antibodies; contains anti-B antibodies |
| 9 | B: | antigen B on RBC; no anti-B antibodies; contains anti-A antibodies |
| 3 | AB: | both antigen A and antigen B on RBC; no anti-A; no anti-B antibodies in plasma |

during or after a blood transfusion. The antibody to the RBC antigen attaches to the antigenic sites and may cause hemolysis or agglutination of the RBCs.

Blood is classified into different groups and typed according to the antigens present on the red cell membrane. The term *blood group* refers to any well-defined system of RBC antigens; 21 systems currently are recognized.[9] The term *blood type* refers to identification of the antigens to determine a person's blood group. The antigens most commonly present on RBC membranes are antigens A, B, and Rh. These make up the OAB system of antigens and the Rh system (Table 19-3). A person may inherit neither of these antigens (type O), or one (A or B) or both (A and B). Type O blood is referred to as the universal donor because it lacks A or B antigens. Type AB blood, referred to as the universal recipient, contains neither anti-A nor anti-B antibodies. Either may contain other antigens that can account for a blood transfusion reaction.

The Rh type is determined by the presence or absence of particular antigens on the RBC. Type Rh negative refers to the absence of these antigens, and Rh positive refers to the presence of the antigens. There are six types of Rh factors: C, D, E, c, d, and e. The most common is D, which, when present, accounts for the Rh+ (positive) designation. Blood that does not have the D antigen is called Rh− (negative). The other factors are considered in blood transfusion reactions. Eighty-five percent of whites and 95% of blacks in the United States are Rh+ .[7,10]

Types A and B surface antigens are called *agglutinogens*, and plasma antibodies that can cause agglutination are called *agglutinins*.[14,15] Antibodies to the agglutinogens are almost always present if the agglutinogen is not present on a person's RBCs.[8,10] For example, anti-A agglutinins are present in the plasma of someone who does not have a type A agglutinogen.

## Destruction of Erythrocytes

When RBCs are released into the circulation from bone marrow, they have a limited life span of about 120 days.[10]

The metabolism of glucose begins to fail in the aging erythrocytes, causing a gradual decrease in the amount of available adenosine triphosphate (ATP). Without an adequate supply of ATP, the cells are no longer able to maintain functions that are essential for life. The fragile cell membrane may rupture when passing through a tight spot in the circulation, such as the spleen, or it may be phagocytosed by macrophages in the spleen, liver, or bone marrow. After lysis of the RBC, hemoglobin is reduced, releasing iron, which is then recycled. After the iron is removed, the remainder of the components in the heme molecule are converted to bilirubin. Bilirubin is taken to the liver to be conjugated with glucuronide (see Chap. 42).

A few RBCs undergo intravascular destruction. When the RBC membrane is damaged, hemoglobin moves out of the cells and quickly becomes bound with a plasma globulin called *haptoglobin*. The resulting complex prevents renal excretion of hemoglobin. The complex is then taken up by phagocytic cells in the liver and processed. When the amount of hemoglobin presented for uptake exceeds renal absorptive capacity, free hemoglobin and methemoglobin appear in the urine.[7] The membranous remains of RBCs are called "ghosts" when they are present in blood samples.

## POLYCYTHEMIA

No general agreement has been reached regarding the use of the term *erythrocytosis* versus the term *polycythemia*. The term polycythemia is the more commonly used term for an increase above normal of circulating RBCs.[3] Erythrocytosis and *erythremia* are terms used more frequently now for conditions of *absolute polycythemia* in which there is an actual increase in total RBC mass. Erythrocytosis denotes an increase in RBCs secondary to a known stimulus, whereas erythremia refers to a primary, myeloproliferative disorder called polycythemia vera.

*Relative polycythemia* occurs when, through plasma loss, the concentration of RBCs becomes greater than normal in the circulating blood.[3] The term *myeloproliferative disorders* includes a large group of syndromes whose common denominator is the ability to proliferate hematopoietic elements. Table 19-4 lists the classifications and causes of polycythemia.

## Erythrocytosis

The most commonly recognized causes of erythrocytosis are as follows:

1. *Hypoxemia.* A decrease in oxygen availability to the tissue cells causes an increase in blood levels of erythropoietin, stimulating the marrow to produce more RBCs and caus-

**TABLE 19–4.**
CLASSIFICATIONS AND CAUSES OF POLYCYTHEMIA

| DISEASE TYPE | CHARACTERISTICS |
|---|---|
| Primary (erythremia) | |
| Polycythemia vera | Myeloproliferative disease of RBCs and often other blood cells |
| Secondary (erythrocytosis) | |
| Physiologic increase in erythropoietin (hypoxia) | Low arterial $O_2$ saturation |
| Respiratory failure | Hypoxia resulting from decreased pulmonary reserve because of obstructive, restrictive, or respiratory center disease |
| Cardiovascular | Hypoxia resulting from right-to-left shunting or chronic low-output cardiac failure |
|   Congenital heart disease | |
|   Congestive heart failure | |
| High altitude | Low $PO_2$ in inspired air |
| High-affinity hemoglobins | Increased affinity for oxygen by abnormal hemoglobins, eg, Chesapeake, Rainier, Little Rock |
| Chronic methemoglobinemia | Methemoglobinemia and carboxyhemoglobinemia decrease hemoglobin ability to transport oxygen |
|   Heavy smoking | |
| Inappropriate erythropoietin elaboration | |
| Renal disease (cysts, hypernephroma, renal carcinoma) | Tumors and cysts contain and release erythropoietin |
| Adrenal tumors | Increased secretion of androgens may stimulate increased RBC formation |
| Hepatocellular carcinoma/oat cell carcinoma | May secrete excessive amounts of erythropoietin-like hormone |
| Cerebellar hemangioblastoma/sub-tentorial tumors | Usually benign, cystic, hereditary with increased erythropoietin in cystic fluid |
| Uterine fibromyomas | Thought to impinge on kidney because of position and size and interfere with erythropoietin release |
| Relative polycythemia | Water deprivation, loss of plasma, electrolytes, gastrointestinal losses |
| Stress | |
| Burns | |
| Renal disease/diuretics | |
| Enteropathy | |
| Dehydration | |

*Adapted from Barnard, D.L. Clinical Haematology. Oxford: Heineman Med., 1989; and Beck, W.S. Hematology (4th ed.). Cambridge, Mass.: MIT Press, 1985.*

ing release of increased numbers of reticulocytes. In the process of acclimatization to high altitudes, plasma volume reduces, red cell volume slowly rises, and total hemoglobin increases, resulting in an increase in total blood volume. Hypoxemia frequently is noted in patients with pulmonic disease, and many of these affected patients have an associated erythrocytosis. Heavy smokers often have an increased hematocrit level, which is probably due to either an increase in red cell mass or a decrease in plasma volume, or both. This probably results from the high carbon monoxide levels in cigarette smoke that displace oxygen from the hemoglobin and reduce oxygen content.

2. *Overproduction of erythropoietin.* Inappropriate production of erythropoietin has been associated with renal disease, tumors, or conditions in which there is a disturbance of renal blood flow.

## Polycythemia Vera

Polycythemia vera is a myeloproliferative disorder in which there is increased production of all the formed elements (RBCs, granulocytes, and platelets) of blood. The cause of this condition is unknown. Polycythemia vera must be differentiated from polycythemia secondary to excessive erythropoietin secretion. It is associated with lower than normal levels of serum and excreted erythropoietin.[7] The condition is relatively rare, occurring most frequently in men between ages 40 and 60.

The abnormal proliferation often initially involves both white and red elements of the marrow. Thrombocytosis and erythrocytosis may be much greater than normal values. Current evidence supports the belief that the disease is a neoplastic disorder that stimulates abnormal erythropoietin-hypersensitive stem cells while supressing normal stem cells.[6]

The results of the proliferating cellular elements are increases in RBC count, blood viscosity, and blood volume. The liver and spleen become congested and packed with RBCs. The thick blood causes stasis and thrombosis in many areas, which may lead to infarction in any area. Vascular thrombosis mainly results from associated elevated platelet levels.[5] The course of the disease may change, resulting in aplastic, fibrotic, or even leukemic bone marrow.[7] The polycythemia may be gradually replaced by an anemia. The cause of anemia or leukemic change may be related to the effects of the chemotherapy used to treat the disease. A terminal acute myeloblastic leukemia is seen to result in patients treated with chlorambucil or marrow irradiation.[7]

The clinical onset of polycythemia vera is insidious. Most symptoms appear to be related to the increased blood volume, increased blood viscosity, and changes in cerebral blood flow. Light-headedness, visual disturbances, headaches, and vertigo may be described. Ruddy cyanosis of the face usually is apparent. Pruritus is a common complaint, possibly caused by histamine release from the basophils. Increased cardiac work may be manifested by eventual congestive heart failure. Thrombophlebitis and thrombosis of digital arteries, accompanied by gangrene, may occur. Associated laboratory values are increased hematocrit, hemoglobin, red cell mass, basophils, eosinophils, neutrophils, thrombocytes, leukocyte alkaline phosphatase, serum $B_{12}$ and $B_{12}$-binding protein, and uric acid. The RBC count may be 7 to 9 million/$\mu$L or higher, and the total blood volume is elevated.

## ANEMIAS

The term anemia refers to a condition in which there is a decrease in hemoglobin concentration, the number of circulating RBCs, or the volume of packed cells (hematocrit) compared with normal values. Anemias usually are categorized according to cause or morphology (Table 19-5). To diagnose the type of anemia present, one must determine the underlying mechanism of the disease. Almost all anemias can be divided into two kinds: (1) those caused by impaired RBC formation and (2) those caused by excessive loss or destruction of RBCs.[11] The reticulocyte count is of primary importance in diagnosis, as are the size, shape, color, and hemoglobin content of RBCs as determined on blood smear. Morphologic characteristics of RBCs usually are used in the classification of anemias. The terms used include the following:

**TABLE 19-5.**
CLASSIFICATION OF ANEMIAS

| TYPE | MORPHOLOGIC CHARACTERISTICS | CAUSES |
| --- | --- | --- |
| Aplastic | Normocytic, normochromic RBCs, depletion of leukocytes and platelets | Drug toxicity<br>Genetic failure<br>Radiation<br>Chemicals<br>Infections |
| Hemolytic | Normocytic, normochromic, increased number of reticulocytes | Mechanical injury<br>RBC antigen–antibody reaction<br>Complement binding<br>Chemical reactions<br>Hereditary membrane defects |
| Macrocytic or megaloblastic; pernicious or folic acid | Macrocytic with variation in size (anisocytosis), shape (poikilocytosis) of RBCs | Inadequate diet<br>Lack of intrinsic factor for pernicious anemia<br>Impaired absorption |
| Microcytic; iron deficiency; chronic blood loss | Microcytic, hypochromic | Inadequate diet<br>Blood loss, chronic<br>Increased need |
| Posthemorrhagic; acute hemorrhage | Normocytic, normochromic, increased number of reticulocytes within 48–72 h | Loss of blood leading to hemodilution from interstitial fluid within 48–72 h<br>Internal or external hemorrhage, leading to blood volume depletion |

1. *Normocytic/normochromic.* Normal size and color of RBCs imparted from hemoglobin concentration
2. *Microcytic/hypochromic.* Decreased size and color of RBCs caused by inadequate hemoglobin concentrations
3. *Macrocytic.* Large size of RBCs
4. *Anisocytosis.* Variations in RBC size
5. *Poikilocytosis.* Variations in RBC shape

Alterations in RBC size or hemoglobin content are common in anemias related to deficiencies of iron, folate, or vitamin $B_{12}$. The shape of the cells gives valuable clues in diagnosis of inherited membrane abnormalities, hemolytic anemias, and hemoglobinopathies. In addition, the blood smear provides information regarding red cell inclusions. Increased stimulus for erythrocyte production is indicated by an increased number of reticulocytes (polychromomatophilia) or normoblasts in the peripheral blood.

## Aplastic Anemia

Aplastic anemia occurs as a result of reduced bone marrow function and causes a decline in levels of all blood elements. The blood-forming cells do not mature. A severe anemia results, with the formed RBCs sometimes appearing morphologically as slightly macrocytic. The cells also may be normocytic and normochromic.

The cause of aplastic anemia is poorly understood, and in more than one-half of cases, it is not known.[15] Genetic failure of bone marrow development or injury to stem cells may prohibit the cells' reproduction and differentiation. Physical agents such as whole-body irradiation have been implicated. Chemical agents that may cause aplastic anemia include cytotoxic drugs used for treatment of malignant disease, antimicrobial agents such as chloramphenicol, anticonvulsants, and antiinflammatory drugs (Table 19-6). Aplastic anemia also may occur as a sequelae to systemic infections.

A routine blood examination and marrow aspiration and biopsy provide essential information regarding bone marrow function. The marrow is hypocellular or, in rare cases, hypercellular. Marrow biopsy reveals large areas of fat with clusters of lymphocytes, reticular cells, and plasma cells. Uptake of iron by the marrow is decreased and serum iron is increased. Smears usually show normocytic, normochromic RBCs that are profoundly decreased in number.[7,14]

The onset of symptoms is variable and usually gradual. Symptoms often are associated with the progressive anemia and concomitant decrease in oxygen transport. Weakness, dyspnea, headaches, and syncope are common. Symptoms resulting from associated leukopenia (decreased WBCs) include decreased immunologic defense and recurrent infections. The associated thrombocytopenia (decreased platelets) is variable, with bleeding

**TABLE 19-6.**
DRUGS LISTED BY THE COUNCIL ON DRUGS OF A.M.A. AS HAVING CAUSED APLASTIC ANEMIA IN 5 OR MORE INSTANCES

| | |
|---|---|
| Acetazolamide | Oxyphenbutazone |
| Acetophenetidin | Phenylbutazone |
| Acetylsalicylic acid | Phenytoin |
| Chloramphenicol | Potassium perchlorate |
| Chlordiazepoxide HCl | Primidone |
| Chlorothiazide | Prochlorperazine |
| Chlorpheniramine | Pyrimethamine |
| Chloropromazine | Quinacrine HCl |
| Chlorpropamide | Salicylamide |
| Colchicine | Streptomycin |
| Diphenylhydantoin sodium | Sulfadimethoxine |
| Epinephrine | Sulfamethoxypyridazine |
| Gold salts | Sulfisoxazole |
| Mepazine | Sulfonamides |
| Meprobamate | Tolbutamide |
| Methazolamide | Trimethadione |

*A.M.A. Registry on Adverse Reactions; The National Registry of Drug-Induced Ocular Side Effects; key case report.*
*In Jandl, J.A. Blood: Textbook of Hematology. Boston: Little, Brown, 1987.*

tendencies ranging from formation of small petechiae to severe bleeding.

Bone marrow transplantation may be a treatment option for the younger person if a compatible family donor is available. Blood components may be replaced by blood transfusions to allow time for bone marrow to recover in cases of transient marrow failure. Therapy with drugs and other chemical agents should be discontinued until recovery of the bone marrow begins. Splenectomy may be indicated if active hemolysis is associated.

The prognosis of aplastic anemia varies, depending on the causative agent. Gradual recovery of hematopoiesis can occur once the agent is discontinued. Severe, progressive anemia is a poor prognostic sign, with infection and hemorrhage being the most frequent causes of death.

### Red Blood Cell Aplasia

Pure RBC aplasia is much less common than aplastic anemia. It is characterized by severe normocytic, normochromic anemia. It may be immunologically mediated, drug-induced, or preleukemic, or it can occur after a viral infection. RBC aplasia frequently is secondary to end-stage renal failure[7,15] (see Chap. 35).

### Hemolytic Anemia

The life span of the RBC may be shortened by intrinsic or extrinsic factors that adversely affect the cell; the short-

**BOX 19-1.**
PATHOGENETIC CLASSIFICATION OF HEMOLYTIC ANEMIAS

**Primary defects of the red cell membrane**
Hereditary spherocytosis
Hereditary elliptocytosis
Acanthocytosis; spur cell anemia
Stomatocytosis
Paroxysmal nocturnal hemoglobinuria
Other membrane disorders

**Secondary defects of the red cell membrane**
Macroangiopathic hemolytic anemias
Microangiopathic hemolytic anemias
Thrombotic thrombocytopenic purpura
Burns
Other forms of mechanical hemolysis
Hemolysis caused by membrane lysins
  Clostridial sepsis; phospholipases
  Venoms; mixed lipases and lysins
  Chemical lysins
Immunohemolytic anemias
  Isoimmune hemolysis: transfusion reactions and erythroblastosis fetalis
  Idiopathic and secondary immunohemolytic anemias
    Warm-active antibodies
    Cold-active antibodies

**Hemolytic anemias caused by infection of red cells**
Malaria
Babesiosis
Other protozoan infections of red cells
Bartonellosis
Other bacterial infections of red cells

**Heinz Body hemolytic anemias**
Oxidative hemolysis in normal people
Oxidative hemolysis in genetically hypersusceptible people
  G6PD deficiency
  Other defects of the hexose monophosphate shunt
  Unstable hemoglobin diseases: congenital Heinz body hemolytic anemia
Favism

**Hemolytic anemias caused by genetic aberrations of glycolysis**
Pyruvate kinase deficiency
Other derangements of the Embden–Meyerhof pathway
G6PD deficiency
Other enzyme deficiencies that affect the hexose monophosphate shunt and glutathione
  metabolism

**Hemoglobinopathies**
Sickle cell syndromes, sickle cell anemia, and sickle cell trait
Thalassemias, alpha chain, and beta chain
Other hemoglobinopathies

**Hemolytic anemias secondary to generalized disorders**
Anemia of chronic liver disease
Anemia of acute or subacute infection
Anemia of metabolic disorders
Anemia of starvation; anorexia nervosa

**Spenomegaly syndrome (hypersplenism)**

Adapted from J. A. Jandl, Blood: *Textbook of Hematology. Boston: Little, Brown, 1987.*

ening may be compensated for by an increase in erythrocyte production. When erythrocyte survival is shortened to 20 days or less, increased erythropoiesis becomes unable to compensate for the rapid RBC destruction.[12]

There are a number of ways to classify hemolytic anemias. Categories often overlap, and no classification seems to be completely satisfactory. A pathogenetic classification of hemolytic anemias is found in Box 19-1, which indicates the wide diversity of causative conditions. The more common diseases are discussed in more detail in the next section.

## Abnormalities of the Red Cell Membrane

These inherited and acquired disorders of the red cell membrane include such conditions as hereditary spherocytosis, acquired immune hemolytic anemia, and glucose-6-phosphate dehydrogenase deficiency.

*Hereditary spherocytosis* is an inherited autosomal dominant condition that results in a red cell membrane defect. The red cells are spheric, and are prematurely destroyed in the spleen. The cells rapidly hemolyze in a hypotonic solution.[11]

Clinical signs depend on the amount of hemolysis present, and can include jaundice, splenomegaly, and signs of anemia. The splenic enlargement is characteristic and is a key determinant in clinical expression.[11] Crises in hereditary spherocytosis are related to associated problems, such as infections and gallstones.

*Acquired immune hemolytic anemia* results from destruction of the RBCs by the immune system. It is diagnosed by the Coombs' test. A *positive direct Coombs' test* means that a plasma protein, usually IgG or complement, has become fixed to the surface of an RBC. The type involving IgG is associated with lymphoma, systemic lupus erythematosis, and drug reactions, or it may be id-

iopathic. Some people with this type of disease have an antibody against a specific antigen on their own RBCs.

The IgG-related Coombs' test agglutination of RBCs sometimes is called *warm antibody disease* because antibody-coated cells adhere to macrophages in the spleen and precipitate RBC destruction at 37°C.[15] *Cold antibody disease* is mediated through the IgM antibodies, which, at temperatures below 30°C, trigger the complement sequence that destroys RBC membranes, leading to loss of hemoglobin. Most cold antibody disease is idiopathic, but it has been described with some of the myeloproliferative disorders. Hemolysis is localized to those body parts exposed to cold temperatures.[6,15]

The *indirect Coombs' test* uses normal RBCs exposed first to the suspected serum and then crossed with the Coombs' serum, which induces agglutination of RBCs if anti–red cell antibodies are present in the suspected serum. It often is used as a screening test to detect the presence of antibodies, especially in crossmatching blood for transfusions. Both direct and indirect Coombs' tests may be positive, especially in relation to drugs such as penicillin, quinidine, quinine, and methyldopa.[14] The signs and symptoms of anemia, hemolysis, and fever often are temporal, and remit after the drug is withdrawn.

*Blood transfusion reactions* are a good example of secondary defects of the red cell membrane. These reactions are immunologically mediated and directed at the antigens in the transfused blood that are deemed foreign. Figure 19-8 shows the process and the results of the immune attack. Major hemolysis usually results from incompatibilities of the ABO system or, occasionally, the Rh factor.[9] Other hemolytic reactions may be directed toward any of the other RBC antigens. Hemolysis usually occurs intravascularly, but it also may occur in extravascular spaces. Symptoms of the reaction usually involve the sudden onset of restlessness, anxiety, fever, chills, flushing,

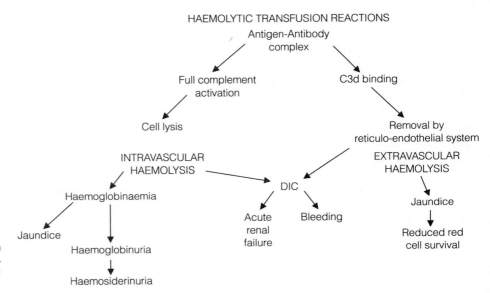

**FIGURE 19-8.**
Mechanisms of hemolytic transfusion reaction. (From A.S.J. Baughan, *Manual of Hemaetology.* Edinburgh: Churchill-Livingstone, 1985.)

chest or back pain, nausea, vomiting, and then early onset of disseminated intravascular coagulation, renal failure, and shock. Laboratory tests show hemoglobinemia, elevated bilirubin, and often a positive direct Coombs' test.[9] Early identification of the reaction and stopping further blood transfusion may be lifesaving.

*Glucose-6-phosphate dehydrogenase deficiency* is a deficiency of this X-linked red cell enzyme. It occurs in 13% of American black males, and 25% of black females are carriers. Levels of the enzyme reflect the susceptibility of the carrier to hemolysis. One in four carriers is subject to hemolysis. Oxidant drugs such as sulfonamides and primaquin may precipitate the development of hemolysis in susceptible people. Conditions that may precipitate an acute hemolytic episode include viral or bacterial infections and diabetic ketoacidosis. Two main variants of the disease have been described, with profound hemolytic anemia occurring in affected African blacks and people of Mediterranean descent. Once the infection is controlled or the triggering drug discontinued, recovery usually occurs.[11]

## Hemoglobinopathies

Two related genetic disorders are described as *sickle syndromes: sickle cell trait* and *sickle cell anemia*. These syndromes occur almost exclusively in blacks, and are demonstrated by the curved shape of the RBCs when they are exposed to decreased oxygen tension. About 10% of American blacks carry HbS on the hemoglobin molecule and about 0.2% exhibit the actual disease.[7] The designation HbS is given when there is substitution of an amino acid (valine) for the normal glutamic acid.[4] The sickle cell trait is carried by heterozygous individuals; sickle cell anemia occurs when an individual is homozygous.

The altered amino acid sequence alters the solubility of hemoglobin. At low blood pH and with decreased oxygen tension, the HbS precipitates out of solution and the cells become sickle-shaped and then become stuck in the small vessels.[4] After vascular obstruction, there is hemolysis of the RBCs. Symptoms depend on the number of hemolyzed and sickled RBCs.

Most people with the sickle cell trait have no symptoms unless they suffer a hypoxic episode, during which some hemolysis and anemia may be noted. Because sickle cell trait is heterozygous, RBCs require very low oxygen tension to precipitate the characteristic sickling effect, and overall RBC life span usually is not affected.

Sickle cell anemia causes symptoms beginning at about 6 months of age. The hemoglobin, HbS, when deoxygenated, distorts the RBC into a sickle or holly-leaf shape. Small blood vessels become blocked by aggregates of these sickle cells, and the blood supply to all parts of the body may be compromised. The damaged RBCs are trapped in the spleen, and the entire organ eventually may become infarcted.

Infections or hypertonic plasma greatly increase the chances of sickling. As the RBCs obstruct blood flow to the tissues, further deoxygenation and more sickling occurs. The characteristic shape usually returns to normal when oxygen again becomes available.

Hemolysis occurs when RBCs assume the sickle form, and average RBC survival time becomes 10 to 15 days. Bilirubin is released from the hemoglobin during hemolysis, and jaundice may become evident when increased conjugated and unconjugated bilirubin accumulates in the plasma.

The bone marrow often becomes hyperplastic, with evidence of increased erythropoiesis. Reticulocytes and even normoblasts may be released into the circulating blood.

Signs and symptoms of sickle cell anemia vary in severity from sickle crisis in acute hemolysis to impairment of growth and maturity. Because of increased susceptibility to infections, especially those caused by pneumococci, repeated episodes of painful crisis occur. These result from microinfarcts from the vasoocclusive phenomenon.[4,7] Anemia usually is severe, with most of the hemolysis occurring in the extravascular spaces. Chronic leg ulcers, attacks of abdominal pain, and neurologic complications of sudden onset are common. Joint pains may mimic osteomyelitis, and joint effusions are frequent.[4] Any organ may be permanently impaired. Severe renal impairment may lead to frank renal failure (see Chap. 35). The prognosis for sickle cell anemia is improving, and with proper oxygenation and hydration, more persons are surviving to adulthood.

*Thalassemias* are intrinsic, congenital disorders that result from defects in the synthesis of hemoglobin and cause a hypochromic, microcytic anemia. They are classified as *major* and *minor*, according to the features of the disease. Defects of both beta and alpha chains are known, and many forms have been diagnosed according to the number of these defects. Disease involving defects of beta chain synthesis occurs most frequently in inhabitants of the Mediterranean areas, Central Africa, Asia, the South Pacific, and parts of India.[1] Defects in alpha chain synthesis are most frequent among southern Orientals. The effects vary markedly, depending on whether the disorders are heterozygous or homozygous.[1]

Thalassemia major is homozygous, and exhibits ineffective erythropoiesis and peripheral hemolysis, which stimulates enlargement of the red marrow to increase RBC formation. Sometimes the liver also becomes involved in erythropoiesis, resulting in hepatomegaly. Clinical manifestations include profound anemia, wasting, jaundice, hepatomegaly, and characteristic "chipmunk" facies. Typical expansion of the bone marrow leads to thin cortical bone, causing enlargement of the bones of the face and jaws. The long bones become vulnerable to fracture. Growth retardation is common, as are marked splenomegaly and hepatomegaly. Death may occur early in fetal life, and the condition is diagnosed with severe hemolytic anemia along with hypochromic, microcytic RBCs.[1,4] A less severe form of the disease may permit the homozygote to survive to adulthood.[1]

Thalassemia minor is a heterozygous disorder that may be diagnosed in studies of persons having chronic, asymptomatic, mild anemia. It is diagnosed by blood smear, and must be differentiated from iron deficiency anemia.[14]

### Direct Physical Trauma

Direct physical trauma to red cells can induce hemolytic anemias. External trauma from blows, as may be inflicted in the martial arts, usually is self-limiting. Turbulent blood flow also can cause trauma to the RBCs. Trauma to circulating RBCs has been reported from prolonged exercise, artificial cardiac valves, extracorporeal circulation devices, and conditions in which fibrin deposited in the microvasculature causes fragmentation of RBCs. The results include mild to severe hemolysis and bilirubinemia. The degree of hemolysis is related to the severity of the symptomatology; for example, artificial cardiac valves may be replaced if significant hemolysis is noted.

## Maturation-Failure Anemia

Megaloblastic anemias refer to those that demonstrate large, immature, poorly functional erythrocytes. The two most common causes are vitamin $B_{12}$ deficiency and folate deficiency. Other conditions also may produce this type of anemia (Box 19-2).

---

**BOX 19–2.**
PATHOGENETIC CLASSIFICATION OF MEGALOBLASTIC ANEMIAS

I. Vitamin $B_{12}$ deficiency
   A. Dietary deficiency
   B. Deficiency of gastric intrinsic factor
      1. Pernicious anemia
      2. Gastrectomy
   C. Intestinal malabsorption
      1. Ileal resection or ileitis
      2. Familial selective vitamin $B_{12}$ malabsorption
      3. Competitive parasites or infections
         a. Fish tapeworm
         b. Bacterial overgrowth in malformed small bowel
   D. Increased requirement
II. Folate deficiency
   A. Dietary deficiency
   B. Impaired absorption
      1. Sprue
      2. Extensive small-bowel disease or resection
      3. Intestinal short circuits
      4. Anticonvulsants, oral contraceptives
   C. Increased requirement
      1. Pregnancy
      2. Hemolytic anemia
      3. Myeloproliferative and other hyperproliferative disorders
      4. Other causes
III. Drug-induced suppression of DNA synthesis
   A. Folate antagonists
   B. Metabolic inhibitors
      1. Of purine synthesis
      2. Of pyrimidine synthesis
      3. Of thymidylate synthesis
      4. Other inhibitors
   C. Alkylating agents
   D. Nitrous oxide
IV. Inborn errors
   A. Hereditary orotic aciduria
   B. Defective folate metabolism
   C. Lesch–Nyhan syndrome
   D. Defective transport of vitamin $B_{12}$
V. Erythroleukemia

Jandl, J. A. Blood: Textbook of Hematology. *Boston: Little, Brown, 1987.*

## Pernicious Anemia

Vitamin B$_{12}$ deficiency usually results from malabsorption of the vitamin because of a deficiency of the intrinsic factor that protects the vitamin so that it can be absorbed in the ileum (see Chap. 40). Pernicious anemia, which results from this deficiency, occurs most frequently in people over age 60 who have fair complexions and a family history of the disease.

Vitamin B$_{12}$ normally binds chemically with the intrinsic factor that promotes its absorption. In certain conditions, such as atrophy of the gastric mucosal cells, lack of secretion of the intrinsic factor leads to malabsorption of vitamin B$_{12}$. Normal erythrocyte maturation is dependent on adequate amounts of vitamin B$_{12}$ for the synthesis of DNA molecules. Without B$_{12}$, a *macrocytic* or *megaloblastic anemia* results, with marked anisocytosis and poikilocytosis. Ineffective erythropoiesis and increased erythroblast destruction result in hyperbilirubinemia. Although the most pronounced changes arise in the RBCs, mild neutropenia and thrombocytopenia also may occur.

The onset of symptoms usually is insidious, but may be hastened by conditions such as infection. Persons with pernicious anemia do not secrete hydrochloric acid (on gastric analysis) even after parenteral stimulation with histamine. Many of the signs and symptoms of pernicious anemia are common to any of the anemic states. Anorexia, fatigue, shortness of breath, and irritability are common. Soreness of the tongue characteristically occurs early in the illness and progressively worsens. The soreness is quickly relieved after adequate vitamin B$_{12}$ treatment. Symmetric numbness and tingling of the toes and fingers occur in 10% of these people and this may indicate early neurologic disease. Ataxia and loss of vibration sense also may be noted. Neurologic symptoms may not entirely remit after treatment.

### Folic Acid Anemia

A deficiency of folic acid produces anemia with characteristics similar to those of pernicious anemia. The two conditions cannot be distinguished morphologically. The RBCs are large (megaloblastic) with fragile membranes. A definite dietary deficiency can be demonstrated, and the anemia develops 1 to 2 months after a continued dietary deficiency. Folic acid anemia is common in alcoholism and chronic malnutrition. Increased frequency during pregnancy relates also to poor nutrition.[15] It usually responds well to oral dietary replacement unless malabsorption is a problem.

## Microcytic, Hypochromic Anemia

### Iron Deficiency Anemia

Iron deficiency anemia is characterized by deficient hemoglobin synthesis caused by a lack of iron. With severe deficiency, the RBCs become *microcytic* and *hypochromic* because of low concentrations of hemoglobin. This is the most common type of anemia, and it occurs in all geographic locations and in all age-groups.[11] The main causes of iron deficiency are increased loss, as in chronic or acute bleeding, and decreased dietary intake. The blood lost during menstruation accounts for a high frequency of iron deficiency in women. Iron deficiency is common among preschool children, presumably because of increased dietary need and poor dietary supply.[2]

Because iron is absorbed mostly in the duodenum and its ionization and absorption are enhanced by gastric hydrochloric acid, iron deficiency anemia may accompany pernicious anemia or gastrectomy. Also, malabsorption syndromes impair absorption of iron along with other nutrients.

Laboratory values reflect decreased levels of serum iron and apoferritin (iron-binding protein produced by the liver) in the early stages. Normal serum iron levels range from 12 to 300 $\mu$g/mL, but 20% of affected adults have normal iron indices.[13] Anemia, characterized by microcytic and variably sized hypochromic RBCs, is a relatively late manifestation.[13]

Clinical manifestations are nonspecific, and their onset is insidious. Fatigue, tachycardia, irritability, and pallor with epithelial abnormalities such as sore tongue or stomatitis may occur. Thinning or spooning of the nails (koilonychia) occasionally is encountered. Pica may be striking, with affected people craving dirt, starch, or ice.[2] Late manifestations may include cardiac murmurs, congestive heart failure, loss of hair, and pearly sclera.

## Posthemorrhagic Anemia

Posthemorrhagic anemia may occur after acute or chronic blood loss, although chronic blood loss usually results in iron deficiency anemia. Plasma and RBCs are both lost during a hemorrhage, so laboratory values may reveal a normal hemoglobin level and RBC count immediately after a hemorrhage. The dominant clinical picture is that of hypovolemia and shock.[4]

Blood volume is restored by the movement of fluid from the interstitial spaces into the capillaries, causing dilution of the remaining RBCs (dilutional anemia) with a maximum effect in 48 to 72 hours. This dilute blood carries too few RBCs to efficiently oxygenate the tissues. Anemia of a normocytic and normochromic type becomes apparent.[4] The bone marrow is stimulated to produce increased numbers of RBCs, but this process requires a period of time that varies according to the amount of blood lost. Within 7 days the reticulocyte count can be elevated to 10% to 15%.[15] In acute massive bleeding, this compensatory effect may not occur in time to be lifesaving without transfusions of whole blood.

## LABORATORY AND DIAGNOSTIC TESTS

### Hematologic Studies

Examination of the blood provides valuable information in the diagnosis and treatment of blood disorders. Normal hematologic values, summarized in Box 19-3, are based on the examination of statistically significant numbers of healthy people. They vary with age, environment, sex, genetics, and physiologic state. The most important erythrocyte studies are discussed in this section.

### Hemoglobin

The primary function of hemoglobin is to carry oxygen in the form of oxyhemoglobin; therefore, the oxygen-combining capacity of blood is directly proportional to the hemoglobin concentration. The hemoglobin level varies significantly with sex and age (see Box 19-3). Levels may be decreased in anemia or circulatory overload and are increased in polycythemia.

### Red Blood Cells

Erythrocytes are the mature circulating RBCs whose primary function is to transport oxygen and carbon dioxide. Increases and decreases in red cell counts usually vary in the same direction as the hemoglobin, as previously mentioned.

### Packed Cell Volume or Hematocrit

The packed cell volume is the ratio of packed cells to total volume in a sample that has been centrifuged. The

---

**BOX 19-3.**
NORMAL HEMATOLOGIC VALUES

| | |
|---|---|
| **Red blood cells** | |
| Infant, first day | $5.1 \pm 1$ million/$\mu$L |
| Child, 1 year | $4.5 \pm 1$ million/$\mu$L |
| Child, 6–10 yr | $4.7 \pm 1$ million/$\mu$L |
| Adult | |
|   Female | $4.8 \pm 0.6$ million/$\mu$L |
|   Male | $5.4 \pm 0.8$ million/$\mu$L |
| **Hemoglobin** | |
| Infant, first day | $19.5 \pm 5.0$ g/dL |
| Child, 1 year | $11.2 \pm 2.3$ g/dL |
| Child, 6–10 yr | $12.9 \pm 2.3$ g/dL |
| Adult | |
|   Female | $14.0 \pm 2.0$ g/dL |
|   Male | $16.0 \pm 2.0$ g/dL |
| **Volume packed RBC (hematocrit)** | |
| Infant, first day | $54 \pm 10$ mL/dL |
| Child, 1 year | $35 \pm 5$ mL/dL |
| Child, 6–10 yr | $37.5 \pm 5$ mL/dL |
| Adult | |
|   Female | $42 \pm 5$ mL/dL |
|   Male | $47 \pm 5$ mL/dL |
| **Erythrocyte sedimentation rate (Westergren method)** | |
| Female | 0–20 mm/h |
| Male | 0–13 mm/h |
| **Mean corpuscular volume** | |
| Female and male | $87 \pm 5$ $\mu$m$^3$ |
| **Mean corpuscular hemoglobin** | |
| Female and male | $29 \pm 2$ $\mu$g |
| **Mean corpuscular hemoglobin concentration** | |
| Female and male | $34\% \pm 2\%$ |
| **Reticulocyte count** | 0.5%–1.5% of erythrocytes |

Wallach, J. Interpretation of Diagnostic Tests (4th ed.). Boston: Little, Brown, 1986.

packed cell volume is used to determine RBC indices, calculate blood volume and total RBC mass, and roughly measure the concentration of RBCs.[16] Levels increase in conditions associated with hemoconcentration (burns, shock, and trauma), hypovolemia, and polycythemia. The hematocrit decreases in hypervolemic states (cardiac failure, overhydration with intravenous fluid), hemorrhage, and hemolysis.

### Erythrocyte Sedimentation Rate

Blood is a suspension of formed elements in plasma; therefore, when it is mixed with an anticoagulant and stands, the heavier RBCs sink to the bottom. The rate at which the RBCs settle is a function of fibrinogen and globulin. These proteins enhance clumping of erythrocytes, thus increasing the rate at which the cells fall. Other factors that affect the rate are alterations in the positive charge of plasma, the ratio of plasma protein fractions to each other, and changes in the erythrocyte surface.

The erythrocyte sedimentation rate (ESR) is a nonspecific test, but because the sedimentation rate is increased in many inflammatory conditions, it can serve in the differential diagnosis in such conditions as acute myocardial infarction, angina pectoris, rheumatoid arthritis, and osteoarthritis. A moderately increased ESR often is noted in patients over age 60.

### Mean Corpuscular Volume

The mean corpuscular volume (MCV) measures the volume and size of each RBC. The MCV increases in megaloblastic anemias (large cells) and decreases in iron deficiency (small cells).[13]

### Mean Corpuscular Hemoglobin

The mean corpuscular hemoglobin (MCH) gives the amount of hemoglobin by weight in the average RBC. Macrocytic cells with a large volume of hemoglobin show increased levels, as in macrocytic anemia. Levels of MCH are decreased in conditions related to hemoglobin deficiency, as in iron deficiency anemia.

### Mean Cell Hemoglobin Concentration

The mean cell hemoglobin concentration gives the average percentage of hemoglobin saturation or concentration of hemoglobin in the average red cell. Decreased levels occur in hemoglobin deficiency.

### Reticulocyte Count

The reticulocyte is a young, nonnucleated cell of the erythrocyte line. An elevated reticulocyte count is indicative of increased bone marrow activity, with early release of increased numbers of reticulocytes, as in hemolytic anemias.

### Bone Marrow Studies

Bone marrow may be obtained for examination by aspiration or biopsy. Data obtained from bone marrow examination are useful in the diagnosis, progression, and prognosis of blood disorders.

## Diagnostic Test

### Schilling Test

This test measures the absorption of vitamin $B_{12}$. Radioactive $B_{12}$ is administered orally and a 24-hour urine collection is begun. The presence of radioactivity in the urine indicates gastrointestinal absorption of vitamin $B_{12}$. Above 8% excretion of the radioactive dose is normal. This test is used in the diagnosis of pernicious anemia.

## REFERENCES

1. Bunn, H.F. Disorders of hemoglobin. In E. Braunwald et al., *Harrison's Principles of Internal Medicine* (11th ed.). New York: McGraw-Hill, 1987.
2. Bunn, H.F. Pathophysiology of the anemias. In J. Wilson et al., *Harrison's Principles of Internal Medicine* (12th ed.). New York: McGraw-Hill, 1991.
3. Braunwald, E. *Hypoxia, polycythemia and cyanosis.* In J. Wilson et al., *Harrison's Principles of Internal Medicine* (12th ed.). New York: McGraw-Hill, 1991.
4. Brooks, J.S. Hematopoietic and lymphatic systems. In V.A. LiVolsi et al., *Pathology* (2nd ed.). Media, Pa.: Harwal, 1989.
5. Castle, W.B. The polycythemias. In W.S. Beck, *Hematology* (4th ed.). Cambridge, Mass.: MIT Press, 1985.
6. Cormack, D.H. *Ham's Histology* (9th ed.). Philadelphia: J.B. Lippincott, 1987.
7. Cotran, R.S., Kumar, V., and Robbins, S.L. *Robbins' Pathologic Basis of Disease* (4th ed.). Philadelphia: W.B. Saunders, 1989.
8. Ganong, W.F. *Review of Medical Physiology* (15th ed.). Los Altos, Calif.: Lange, 1991.
9. Giblett, E.R. Blood groups and blood transfusion. In J. Wilson et al., *Harrison's Principles of Internal Medicine* (12th ed.). New York: McGraw-Hill, 1991.
10. Guyton, A. *Textbook of Medical Physiology* (8th ed.). Philadelphia: W.B. Saunders, 1991.
11. Jandle, J.A. *Blood: Textbook of Hematology.* Boston: Little, Brown, 1987.
12. Reich, P.R. *Hematology: Physiopathologic Basis for Clinical Practice* (2nd ed.). Boston: Little, Brown, 1984.
13. Wallach, J. *Interpretation of Diagnostic Tests* (4th ed.). Boston: Little, Brown, 1986.

14. Wallerstein, R.O. Blood. In M.A. Krupp, M.J. Chatton, and L.M. Tierney, *Current Medical Diagnosis and Treatment.* Los Altos, Calif.: Lange, 1986.

15. Weatherall, D.J., and Bunch, C. The blood and blood-forming organs. In L.H. Smith and S.O. Thier, *Pathophysiology:* *The Biological Principles of Disease.* Philadelphia: W.B. Saunders, 1985.

16. Wintrobe, M.M. *Blood, Pure and Eloquent.* New York: McGraw-Hill, 1980.

# Normal and Altered Leukocyte Function

## *Learning Objectives*

1. List and describe the five types of leukocytes.
2. Differentiate leukocytes on the basis of morphology and function.
3. Define the normal white cell count per microliter of blood and explain its significance.
4. Describe the differential white count and list the relative proportion of each cell type.
5. Describe phagocytosis and discuss its significance with respect to the destruction of microorganisms and immunologic integrity.
6. Compare the average life span of the five types of leukocytes.
7. Explain locomotion, diapedesis, degranulation, killing, chemotaxis, and opsonization with respect to phagocytosis and immunologic integrity.
8. Explain the function of the mononuclear phagocyte system.
9. Describe the characteristics of a myeloproliferative disorder.

10. Differentiate between malignant and nonmalignant disorders in leukocytes.
11. Explain the basis of classification of leukemias.
12. Differentiate between acute and chronic leukemia.
13. Differentiate generally between reactive lymphadenopathies and malignant lymphomas.
14. Differentiate Hodgkin's disease and other lymphomas on the basis of laboratory findings.
15. Describe the qualitative and quantitative alterations of leukocytes found in infectious mononucleosis.
16. Discuss the causative agent of infectious mononucleosis and its significance.
17. Explain the significance of Sternberg-Reed cells with respect to Hodgkin's disease.
18. Discuss the clinical features and pathologic alterations in multiple myeloma.

Leukocytes, larger and less numerous than erythrocytes, play a key role in the defense mechanisms of the body. As the name implies, leukocytes are almost white (the Greek *leukos* means "white"). Examination of a centrifuged tube of whole blood reveals a fuzzy gray-white layer between the packed red cells and the clear yellow plasma. This white layer, called the *buffy coat,* contains leukocytes and platelets.

The most important function of the leukocytes is to defend the body against invasion by foreign organisms and to produce, transport, and distribute defensive elements such as antibodies or other factors that are necessary for the immune response. The various types of leukocytes work together in an integrated system. Each type performs different functions in the defense mechanisms, and all functions are necessary for a total integrated and effective defense.

## NORMAL LEUKOCYTE FUNCTION

### Characteristics of Leukocytes

There normally are about 5000 to 10,000 leukocytes per microliter of adult human blood.[13] Of these, *granulocytes* (polymorphonuclear leukocytes, or polys) make up the largest portion of the total number, about 65%. The *agranulocytes* compose the remaining 35%. Granulocytes have large granules and horseshoe-shaped nuclei that differentiate and become multilobed, with two to five distinct lobes connected by thin strands. The background cytoplasm stains blue to pink with Wright's stain, which enhances their morphologic identification (Table 20-1).

Granulocytes are subdivided into three cell types: neutrophils, eosinophils, and basophils. The *neutrophils* are the most numerous, making up 50% to 70% of the total white cell count. They have small, fine, light pink or lilac acidophilic granules when stained, and a segmented, irregularly lobed, purple nucleus.

*Eosinophils* constitute about 1% to 5% of the normal white cell count. They have large, round granules that contain red-staining basic mucopolysaccharides and multilobed purple-blue nuclei.[3]

Like eosinophils, *basophils* constitute a small percentage of the white cells, ranging from 0% to 1% of the total count. The coarse, basophilic blue granules often conceal the segmented nucleus. The content of these granules includes histamine, heparin, and acid mucopolysaccharides.[3]

Lymphocytes and monocytes are the remaining white blood cell (WBC) types normally present in peripheral blood. They were termed *agranulocytes* because they were originally thought to have no granules. Their granules are very small, and stain quite differently than the large granules of granulocytes. Lymphocytes and monocytes also are called mononuclear leukocytes because they do not have the multilobed nucleus as the granulocytes do.

*Lymphocytes,* also called *immunocytes,* are cells with large, round, deep-staining nuclei and very little cytoplasm. The cytoplasm is slightly basophilic, and stains pale blue. They make up about 20% to 40% of the total white cell count.

The *monocyte* is a large mononuclear leukocyte with a prominent, multishaped nucleus that sometimes is kidney-shaped. The chromatin in the nucleus looks like lace, with small particles linked together by fine strands. Chromatin is less clumped than in the mature granulocyte or lymphocyte. The gray-blue cytoplasm is filled with many fine lysosomes that stain pink with Wright's stain. Monocytes constitute about 1% to 6% of the total white cell count. Figure 20-1 shows the different types of WBCs.

### White Cell Count

The white cell count is determined by counting cells in a diluted blood sample. The procedure can be done manually, but an electronic enumerator usually is used to count the leukocytes suspended in a dilute fluid that lyses the erythrocytes to prevent interference. Normal values range between 5000 and 10,000 white cells per microliter. The count is important as a diagnostic tool in cases of infection, cancer, and other disorders that cause alterations of these cells. Significant increases or decreases of the count are known as *quantitative alterations.*

**TABLE 20-1.**
STAINING CHARACTERISTICS OF LEUKOCYTES

| LEUKOCYTE | CYTOPLASM | CYTOPLASMIC GRANULES | NUCLEUS |
|-----------|-----------|----------------------|---------|
| Neutrophil | Blue to pink | Lilac | Purple-blue |
| Eosinophil | Blue to pink | Red | Purple-blue |
| Basophil | Blue to pink | Blue-black | Purple-blue |
| Lymphocyte | Pale blue | | Dark blue |
| Monocyte | Gray-blue | Pink | Blue lighter than lymphocytes |

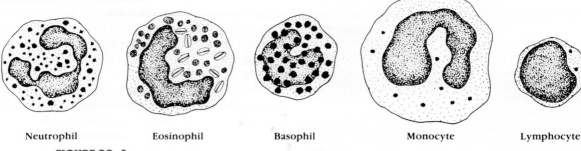

Neutrophil          Eosinophil          Basophil          Monocyte          Lymphocyte

**FIGURE 20–1.**
Characteristics of different types of leukocytes. (From M. Borysenko, *Functional Histology* [2nd ed.].
Boston: Little, Brown, 1984.)

## Differential White Cell Count

Each of the leukocytes has a specific function in the body's defense system. An attack by a foreign agent often elicits a response by a certain type of leukocyte. For example, a pyogenic bacterial infection may elicit an increase in neutrophils, or a parasitic infection might elicit an increase in eosinophils. Therefore, an increase or decrease in the normal percentage of leukocytes may have significant diagnostic value. The relative proportion of leukocyte cell types is called the *differential count*.

The differential count is determined on a smear of blood one cell layer thick. This layer is stained with a polychrome solution that contains both basic and acidic dyes, usually Wright's stain. The leukocyte cellular structure absorbs the dye differentially and permits evaluation not only of the relative proportions of the white cells, but also of cellular elements and platelets. Differentials may be counted manually or electronically (Table 20-2).

Normal differential white cell proportions vary with age. The neutrophils, for example, are significantly increased at birth, but fall below the normal adult level by 2 weeks of age. Lymphocytes, higher at birth and in early childhood, decrease in numbers until adult levels are reached (Table 20-3).[11]

An *absolute count* of a particular leukocyte often is necessary for diagnosis. This can be obtained by using a

**TABLE 20–2.**
NORMAL DIFFERENTIAL COUNT OF LEUKOCYTES

| LEUKOCYTES | COUNT (%) |
|---|---|
| Neutrophils, segmented | 50–70 |
| Neutrophils, bands or stabs | 0–5 |
| Eosinophils | 1–4 |
| Basophils | 0–1 |
| Lymphocytes | 20–40 |
| Monocytes | 1–6 |

**TABLE 20–3.**
NORMAL AGE-RELATED LEUKOCYTE DIFFERENTIAL COUNT IN PERIPHERAL BLOOD

| CELL TYPE | PERCENTAGE | NUMBER |
|---|---|---|
| **Segmental neutrophils** | | |
| Infant, first day | 47 ± 15 | 8870 |
| Child, 1 yr | 23 ± 10 | 2600 |
| Child, 10 yr | 46 ± 15 | 3700 |
| Adult, over 21 | 51 ± 15 | 3800 |
| **Band neutrophils** | | |
| Infant, first day | 14.2 ± 4 | 2580 |
| Child, 1 yr | 8.1 ± 3 | 990 |
| Child, 10 yr | 8.0 ± 3 | 645 |
| Adult, over 21 | 8.0 ± 3 | 620 |
| **Eosinophils** | | |
| Infant, first day | 2.4 | 450 |
| Child, 1 yr | 2.6 | 300 |
| Child, 10 yr | 2.4 | 200 |
| Adult, over 21 | 2.7 | 200 |
| **Basophils** | | |
| Infant, first day | 0.5 | 100 |
| Child, 1 yr | 0.4 | 50 |
| Child, 10 yr | 0.5 | 40 |
| Adult, over 21 | 0.5 | 40 |
| **Lymphocytes** | | |
| Infant, first day | 31 ± 5 | 5800 |
| Child, 1 yr | 61 ± 15 | 7000 |
| Child, 10 yr | 38 ± 10 | 3100 |
| Adult, over 21 | 34 ± 10 | 2500 |
| **Monocytes** | | |
| Infant, first day | 5.8 | 1100 |
| Child, 1 yr | 4.8 | 550 |
| Child, 10 yr | 4.3 | 350 |
| Adult, over 21 | 4.0 | 300 |

*J. Wallach, Interpretation of Diagnostic Tests (4th ed.). Boston: Little, Brown, 1986.*

special diluting fluid that lyses the erythrocytes and either lyses or does not stain the other white cells present. The specific leukocyte can then be counted without including the other cells.

## Genesis of Leukocytes

The multipotential or uncommitted stem cells in bone marrow are essentially responsible for blood cell and platelet formation. They differentiate into unipotential, or committed, stem cells that ultimately become WBCs, platelets, and erythrocytes (see Figure 19-1).

Neutrophils, basophils, and eosinophils are formed in the bone marrow, and can be stored there until needed. If the need is greater than the supply, immature forms may be released into the bloodstream.

Granulocytes and monocytes are thought to be derived from a common committed stem cell. The promonocyte also is formed and differentiated in bone marrow, and is released into the circulation as a mature monocyte. The monocyte can leave the blood for the tissues, where it enlarges and is transformed or matured into a lysosome-filled *macrophage*. The macrophage is much larger than the monocyte, which is important for the phagocytosis of large particles and debris.[6] Both granulocytes and monocytes have phagocytic properties.

Lymphocytes are thought to be formed from a separate committed stem cell in the bone marrow. In the fetus, proliferating stem cells migrate from the yolk sac to the liver, which is a major blood-forming organ during gestation.[7]

Unlike granulocytes and monocytes, most lymphocytes are differentiated not in the bone marrow, but in the lymphoid tissue, thymus, or spleen. Only large and small lymphocytes and plasma cells can be identified by morphology. Identification of B and T lymphocytes involves such laboratory techniques as cell marker studies and cytochemistry. Differentiation of the B and T lymphocytes in the lymphoid tissue is an important aspect of the immunologic response (see Chap. 14).

## Life Span of White Blood Cells

The life span of WBCs in the circulating blood usually is short. The average half-life of a neutrophil is about 6 hours.[8] During a serious infection, neutrophils often live 2 hours or less, until they are used or destroyed.

Granulocytes mature in the bone marrow. After myelocytes (precursors of granulocytes) stop dividing, maturing granulocytes accumulate as a reserve in the bone marrow. Under normal conditions, there is about a 5-day supply of granulocytes in this reserve. Once the granulocytes leave the marrow, they spend an average of 12 hours in the circulation and about 2 to 3 days in the tissues before they are destroyed.

Monocytes spend less time in the bone marrow pool than granulocytes. The life span of the monocyte in the circulation is about 36 hours, or about three times as long as that of granulocytes.[3] After the monocyte has been transformed into a mobile or fixed macrophage in the tissues, its life is long, ranging from months to years.

The life span of the lymphocytes varies tremendously. A small population of extremely long-lived cells may survive for many years. These cells are necessary for maintaining immunologic memory, and have the special ability to reenter cell division through specific stimulation by an antigen.

Most T lymphocytes of the peripheral lymphatic tissue recirculate about every 10 hours.[6] They follow a path from the blood to the lymphatic tissue, through the lymphatic channels, and back to the blood through the thoracic duct. The survival rate of T lymphocytes ranges from a few days to months and years. In general, most T lymphocytes have slow replacement rates and a long survival time.

The B lymphocytes are largely noncirculating. They remain mainly in the lymphoid tissue, and can differentiate under appropriate stimulation into plasma cells. Mature plasma cells, which have the ability to secrete specific antibodies, have a survival rate of about 2 to 3 days (see Chap. 14). Table 20-4 summarizes the life span of the various WBCs.

## Properties of Leukocytes

### Functional Classification

The properties of leukocytes can be best understood by separating them into two major functional groups: *phagocytes* and *immunocytes*. As discussed in the previous section, immunocytes and phagocytes are thought to be derived from a common stem cell in the bone marrow. The immunocytes, or lymphocytes, probably undergo a differentiation phase outside the bone marrow. Phagocytes mature in the bone marrow, and are released as mature granulocytes and monocytes into the circulation. Granulocytes and monocytes are classified as phagocytes. Monocytes must enter the tissues and differentiate into macrophages to exhibit the property of phagocytosis.

### Phagocytosis

The most important property of the phagocytes (granulocytes and macrophages) is phagocytosis. Phagocytosis is a process similar to that by which an ameba ingests and digests its nourishment. The phagocyte can change its shape by sending out processes from its protoplasm. Mi-

**TABLE 20–4.**
LIFE SPAN OF WHITE BLOOD CELLS

| CELL TYPE | IN CIRCULATING BLOOD | TISSUE LIFE |
|---|---|---|
| Granulocytes | 6–8 h; time shortened in acute infection | 2–3 days |
| Monocytes | Short transit time, often less than 36 h | Months or years as tissue macrophages |
| T lymphocytes | Remain in the blood a few hours but recirculate about every 10 h | Varies from a few days to years |
| B lymphocytes | Few circulate | Most remain in lymphoid tissue; when they become secreting plasma cells, they survive 2–3 days |
| Platelets | Most circulate; are totally replaced every 10 days | |

croorganisms, old cells, or foreign particles can then be enveloped or engulfed in a vacuole, or *phagosome,* formed by the fusing of the processes of protoplasm. Associated with ingestion of the foreign or devitalized material are rapid increase in cellular energy and the generation of hydrogen peroxide (Figure 20-2).

### Degranulation

Phagocytosis involves not only ingestion of a microorganism or particle, but also digestion or destruction of this foreign body. After the material has become engulfed in the phagosome, degranulation occurs. This process involves lysosomes (granules) fusing with the internal membrane of the phagosome and emptying their contents into its vacuole. The biochemical events of this morphologic phenomenon are incompletely understood.

The granules contain hydrolytic enzymes that cause the dissolution of the phagosome contents and, eventually, lysis of the phagocyte itself.

### Killing

Killing is the process by which the phagocytosed microorganism contained within the membrane-bound phagosome dies. Most of the hydrolytic enzymes contained in the granules serve a digestive function and are not directly involved in killing.[8] What actually kills the microorganism is peroxidation of hydrogen peroxide, which, in the presence of iodide, destroys the microbial membrane. Most bacteria can be killed by this process. Some organisms, such as acid-fast bacilli that cause tuberculosis and leprosy, are able to survive inside the phagocyte.

Dissolution is complex, and involves integrated ac-

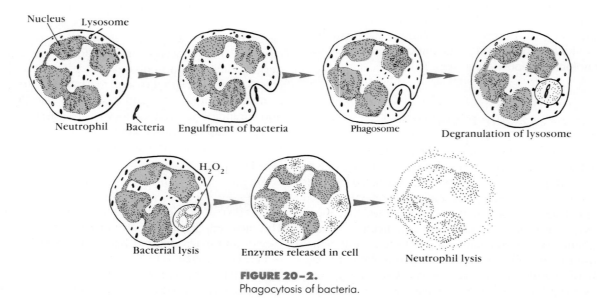

**FIGURE 20–2.**
Phagocytosis of bacteria.

tion of many hydrolytic enzymes. The phagocyte, as well as the foreign invader, often is lysed by its own enzymes and becomes part of the degradation products (see Figure 20-2).

The degradation products that remain after phagocytosis usually intensify the inflammatory process to varying degrees. The released lysosomal enzymes of degranulation or toxins released by the bacteria may damage the surrounding tissues. Degradation products include thromboplastic products that lead to vascular clotting (see Chap. 21).

Phagocytosis is promoted by other factors, such as temperature and electrical charge. Elevated body temperatures or increased heat at the site of infection enhances phagocytosis. Fever during an infection may serve as a protective mechanism within limits. The electrical charge on antigen surfaces also may enhance phagocytosis, as the charge on dead or foreign particles is different from that on living tissues and is considered to be a dominant factor in specificity.[6]

Increased glucose metabolism and cellular oxygen consumption are needed for phagocytosis because increased energy is necessary for the production of large amounts of hydrogen peroxide used to kill bacteria. Energy in the form of adenosine triphosphate is supplied by glycolysis in the WBC itself.

## Diapedesis

Phagocytes have the ability to accumulate at the site of invasion or injury. Like the ameba, they form pseudopod-like processes that allow them to move through avenues of the body. Granulocytes and monocytes can leave the circulation and enter tissue by a process called diapedesis. Diapedesis refers to the ability of the phagocyte to slip through the walls of the capillary vessel by ameboid motion. A small portion of the phagocyte slides through at a time until the entire cells leaves the circulation. Diapedesis allows phagocytes to accumulate at the invasion site (see Chap. 13).

## Chemotaxis

The phagocytes must be able to find the site of a bacterial invasion or recognize that infection has taken place. Specific phagocytes break down and digest necrotic material. Chemical substances, called chemotactic agents or mediators, are released from the infected or necrotic tissues and provide a signal for the leukocytes to move toward the source of the chemotactic agent. This process, called chemotaxis, is dependent on a concentration gradient. A greater concentration of the chemical causes more leukocytes to move toward the source. Other chemotactic agents include the complement system, plasminogen, the fibrinolytic system, kallikrien (the kinin system), and substances released from the phagocytes.

## Pinocytosis

Pinocytosis is the cellular engulfment by the phagocyte of tiny particles included in a droplet of fluid. It differs from phagocytosis in that in phagocytosis the membrane sends out processes to grasp a relatively large particle using a biochemical mechanism similar to muscle action. In pinocytosis, macrophages ingest and break down macromolecules. The role of pinocytosis in many macrophage activities is not totally understood.[6]

## Recognition of the Particle

Before a phagocyte can ingest a bacterium or particle, it must recognize the particle. Recognition of the foreign invader is achieved through mediation in one of two ways: opsonization and surface properties.[4]

*Opsonization* of the antigenic surface is necessary for the phagocyte to attach to the antigen. Opsonization is mediated by activation of the complement protein system or by specific antibodies. Activation of complement results in attachment of C3b to the surface of the particle, which, with specific antibody, allows it to be recognized and phagocytosed by the leukocyte.[4]

Some particles have special *surface properties* that cause them to adhere to the phagocyte and subsequently undergo phagocytosis. These physiochemical properties allow the particle to adhere to the cell membrane of the phagocyte while pseudopodia surround and engulf the particle. This type of phagocytosis is seen in the early phases of an illness and is most effective with tightly packed leukocytes. The exact mechanism of attachment of the phagocyte to the antigen before antibody formation, complement activation, or cell devitalization is not known.

## Function of Phagocytes

The functions of granulocytes and monocyte-macrophages overlap, but in general, granulocytes are the first line of defense against microbe invasion; neutrophils are adept at recognizing, ingesting, and killing pyogenic bacteria; and monocyte-macrophages are important in the final removal or cellular cleanup of debris after phagocytosis and cell lysis.

Monocyte-macrophages can ingest bigger particles and larger amounts of debris because of their larger size. Inert materials as large as wood or steel fragments can be engulfed by macrophages and removed from the site of inflammation. If a particle is very large, multinucleated foreign-body *giant cells* may be produced. The characteristic foreign-body giant cell may represent fusion of several macrophages.

Macrophages not only provide the final removal of microorganisms, but also clear the body of its own aged and damaged cells. Some macrophages possess the ability to break down and recycle old red blood cells (RBCs). Certain tissue macrophages break down hemoglobin, leaving products that can be recycled into new hemoglobin. Macrophages of the liver, spleen, and bone marrow can return the released iron to transferrin to be transported to the erythroid marrow for RBC synthesis.

Phagocytes contain antibacterial substances, peroxidase, and lysosomal enzymes necessary for phagocytosis and other activities. Macrophages are thought to participate in killing tumor cells that have been processed by the lymphocytes. Monocytes and granulocytes also interact with other biologically active substances, such as complement.

For the phagocytes to accomplish their defensive purpose, the following must occur: (1) they must accumulate in sufficient numbers at the right place; (2) they must attach to the foreign material or agent; (3) they must envelop or engulf the agent; and (4) they must dispose of the debris.[4,8] Alterations in any of these functions results in defective phagocytosis, which then results in a defective defensive response.

## Function of Basophils and Eosinophils

The precise function of basophils and eosinophils is not well understood, but it is known that these cells participate in inflammatory and allergic reactions.

### Basophils

Basophils contain histamine, heparin, and small quantities of bradykinin and serotonin. They are present in small numbers in the blood and in larger numbers in the connective tissue and pericapillary areas. Their function seems to be largely to prevent clotting in the microcirculation and to cause some of the signs and symptoms of allergic reactions.[7] People with allergies often have elevated levels of immunoglobulin E (IgE). Receptor sites for IgE have been found on the basophils. When these receptor sites are attacked, histamine and other substances are released that increase chemotaxis and also enhance the allergic response (see Chap. 16). The number of basophils increases in some of the myeloproliferative diseases, such as polycythemia vera.

### Eosinophils

Eosinophils weakly exhibit phagocytosis and chemotaxis.[7] They are present in large numbers in the mucosa of the intestinal tract and of the lungs. Because of this, they probably help to detoxify foreign proteins. The circulating level of eosinophils is increased in people with allergies, perhaps as a result of the cells removing and digesting the antigen–antibody complex. Eosinophilia is associated with worm infestation or parasitic infections. In trichinosis, the numbers of eosinophils can increase 25% to 50%.

## Mononuclear Phagocyte System

The mononuclear phagocyte system is the large system of stationary and mobile macrophages. It was formerly called the reticuloendothelial system, but the term mononuclear phagocyte system is a more clearly descriptive term for the functional capabilities of this system. Important in the body's defense, it is considered to be more a functional than an anatomic system. It includes all the fixed and mobile phagocytic cells in the liver, spleen, lymph nodes, and gastrointestinal tract. Fixed macrophages in these organs seem to exist in dynamic equilibrium with mobile macrophages. All tissue macrophages, including the Kupffer cells of the liver and alveolar macrophages in the lungs, originate from the mobile circulating macrophages. This system is important in preventing the spread of infection and removing cellular debris and products of metabolic degradation. Many of the metabolic products are conserved and recycled.

## Function of Immunocytes

Unlike monocytes and granulocytes, lymphocytes do not possess phagocytic capabilities, but protect the body against specific antigens. This specific immunity, discussed in Chapter 14, is integrated with other general immune responses. The lymphocytes move freely from the blood to the lymphoid tissues. They seem to patrol the tissue spaces for foreign material.

## NONMALIGNANT WHITE BLOOD CELL DISORDERS

## Quantitative Alterations of Granulocytes

Quantitative alterations of granulocytes result from several conditions that cause a significant increase or decrease in the number of leukocytes. This usually is measured by calculating the number of leukocytes in blood. Each cell type often is considered and counted individually to identify the causative condition.

### Neutrophils

A normal physiologic shift in the number of neutrophils can be influenced by several conditions. Physiologic leukocytosis (increase in number of leukocytes above

10,000/$\mu$L) can be caused by exercise, emotional stress, menstruation, sunlight, cold, and anesthesia. During pregnancy, the number of polymorphonuclear leukocytes consistently increases. This increase is even more exaggerated during labor and the first postpartum week. The newborn infant also has increased neutrophil levels.

*Neutrophilic leukocytosis (neutrophilia)* is defined as an absolute neutrophil count greater than 7500/$\mu$L blood. The *leukemoid reaction* refers to persistent neutrophilia of 30,000 to 50,000/$\mu$L, but the cells of this reaction usually are mature.[6] The total white count in this condition usually is greater than 10,000/$\mu$L blood.[13] A *shift to the left* occurs with increases in the number of leukocytes of nonsegmented neutrophils in circulating blood. When increased numbers of neutrophils are released in an inflammatory process, some may be in immature forms called *bands* or *stabs*, which have a short life span. An increased number of these cells in the peripheral blood often is a good indicator of an inflammatory process, especially an acute bacterial infection.[16] A leftward shift usually indicates an acute infectious process. When it returns to normal mature cells, the infection often is seen to be subsiding.[4] Neutrophilic leukocytosis occurs in such pathologic conditions as acute pyogenic infections, cancer, hemorrhage, hemolysis, tissue necrosis, and metabolic chemical toxic poisonings.

*Neutrophilic leukopenia (neutropenia)* occurs when the absolute neutrophil count is less than 2500/$\mu$L of blood.[13] Irradiation, anaphylactic shock, and systemic lupus erythematosus are specific causes of this decrease. Chemical agents that affect the hematopoietic system cause a decrease in the neutrophils. Antithyroid drugs, phenothiazines, and chemotherapeutic agents are only a few of the many drugs that can cause neutropenia (Box 20-1).

Nonpyogenic bacterial, viral, and rickettsial infections can cause a decrease in the neutrophil count. Any overwhelming bacterial infection may lead to a neutrophilic leukopenia because the vast numbers of cells used to fight the infections is much greater than the reserve supply.[16] The body's reserve ability to form neutrophils is exhausted, and the neutrophil count falls.

### Eosinophils

*Eosinophilic leukocytosis (eosinophilia)* is defined as an absolute eosinophil count that exceeds 500/$\mu$L of blood, and often is associated with allergy.[13] It is believed that this increase with allergic conditions is due to the tissue reactions associated with allergy-released products that specifically increase the production of eosinophils in the bone marrow.

Eosinophilic leukocytosis also occurs in response to parasitic infection. This is probably the most common cause of extremely large numbers of eosinophils. The mechanism by which the parasitic infections cause the increased count is not known. Eosinophilic leukocytosis also can be caused by pulmonary disorders, skin diseases, and cancer.[5,15]

*Eosinophilic leukopenia (eosinopenia)* occurs when the absolute eosinophil count is less than 50/$\mu$L of blood.[13] The decrease may be due to severe infection,

**BOX 20-1.**
CAUSES OF NEUTROPENIA

**Decreased production**
Hematologic diseases—idiopathic, cyclic neutropenia, Chediak–Higashi syndrome, aplastic anemia, infantile genetic disorders
Drug-induced—alkylating agents (nitrogen mustard, busulfan, chlorambucil, cyclophosphamide), antimetabolites (methotrexate, 6-mercaptopurine, 5-fluorocytosine), noncytotoxic agents (antibiotics [chloramphenicol, penicillins, sulfonamides], phenothiazines, tranquilizers [meprobamate], certain diuretics, antiinflammatory agents, antithyroid drugs, many others)
Tumor invasion, myelofibrosis
Nutritional deficiency—vitamin B$_{12}$, folate (especially alcoholics)
Infection—tuberculosis, typhoid fever, brucellosis, tularemia, measles, infectious mononucleosis, malaria, viral hepatitis, leishmaniasis

**Peripheral destruction**
Antineutrophil antibodies and/or splenic trapping
  Autoimmune disorders—Felty's syndrome
  Drugs—aminopyrine, methyldopa, phenylbutazone, mecurial diuretics, some phenothiazines

**Peripheral pooling**
Overwhelming bacterial infection
Hemodialysis
Cardiopulmonary bypass

*Braunwald, E., et al., Harrison's Principles of Internal Medicine (11th ed.). New York: McGraw-Hill, 1987.*

shock, or adrenocortical stimulation. Peripheral blood eosinophils are sensitive to adrenocortical hormones, and may be reduced or absent in stress, with Cushing's disease, or in patients being treated with corticosteroids.[15] There is no reported adverse effect of eosinopenia.[5]

### Basophils

*Basophilic leukocytosis (basophilia)* is defined as an absolute basophil count exceeding 50 to 100/$\mu$L of blood.[13] This usually is greater than 2% of the white cell differential, and is associated with myeloproliferative disorders, chronic granulocytic leukemia, and, occasionally, ulcerative colitis and certain skin diseases.[15]

*Basophilic leukopenia (basopenia)* occurs when the absolute basophil count is less than 20/$\mu$L of blood.[13] It often is associated with suppression of other granulocytes in drug-induced suppression, as well as severe infection, shock, and adrenocortical stimulation.

## Qualitative Alterations of Granulocytes

When granulocytes display defective physical and chemical functions, they are said to have qualitative abnormalities. Most of these defective functions are related to phagocytosis. The defects may be in phagocyte locomotion or in the phagocyte itself, such as that in the lazy leukocyte syndrome. There may be deficient chemotaxis generation and complement abnormalities. The latter are associated with collagen vascular disorders and, occasionally, bacterial infections. Some drugs, such as aspirin, corticosteroids, colchicine, and phenylbutazone, can cause dysfunction of the phagocyte.[5]

Normal human serum contains a low concentration of heat-stable globulin that impairs both chemotaxis and phagocytosis in vitro. This inhibitor is elevated in the sera of most people with leukemia.[5]

Ethanol causes a significant decrease in leukocyte migration and chemotaxis during acute intoxication. Chemotaxis also can be decreased by the use of some antibiotics, such as gentamicin, in therapeutic doses.[6,15]

*Granulomatous diseases* are rare qualitative defects of the granulocytes, especially neutrophils, that result in defective bactericidal activity. In chronic granulomatous disease (CGD), there is an inherited absence of neutrophil and monocyte oxidative metabolism. The enzymes are necessary for the actual killing of bacteria, without which leukocytes are unable to oxidize or destroy certain bacteria. Diagnosis can be made by the nitroblue tetrazolium (NBT) reduction test. NBT normally is reduced to a blue-black material called blue formazan, but in CGD, this reduction is not seen. The disease results in severe recurrent infections of the skin, lymph nodes, lungs, liver, and bones with catalase-positive microorganisms (those that destroy their own hydrogen peroxide).[5]

Several qualitative abnormalities of the granulocytes are inherited. Altered nuclear structure and appearance, excessive granulation of the cytoplasm, and hypersegmentation of neutrophils may occur. These alterations may affect phagocytosis or may have no clinical implications.

## Monocyte Abnormalities

*Monocytosis* infers an absolute monocyte count greater than 750/$\mu$L in children and 500 to 600/$\mu$L in adults.[13] This disorder arises in nonpyogenic bacterial infections such as active tuberculosis, subacute bacterial endocarditis, syphilis, and brucellosis. It is associated with recovery from such disorders as agranulocytosis, hematologic disorders, cancer, and collagen disease.[5]

*Monocytopenia* refers to a decrease in the blood monocyte counts, and it often is associated with other causes of leukopenia. It frequently is secondary to acute stress reactions or glucocorticoid administration. Overwhelming infections and immunosuppressive agents will decrease the monocyte count.

## Lymphocytic Disorders

*Lymphocytosis* must be defined according to a person's developmental stage. The absolute lymphocyte count from birth to age 3 years is 9000/$\mu$L of blood. From 4 to 12 years, it is 7000/$\mu$L, and in adults, it is 4000/$\mu$L.[13] Viral disorders that produce lymphocytosis include mumps, rubella, rubeola, hepatitis, and varicella. Lymphocytosis also occurs in pertussis and chronic lymphocytic leukemia. Numbers of atypical lymphocytes are increased in infectious mononucleosis, cytomegalic inclusion disease, and toxoplasmosis.

*Lymphopenia* is defined as an absolute lymphocyte count of less than 1400/$\mu$L in the child and less than 1000/$\mu$L in the adult.[13] This condition may be caused by such factors as stress, adrenocortical stimulation, alkylating agents, and irradiation. It is associated with Hodgkin's disease, lymphosarcoma, terminal uremia, and acute tuberculosis.

### Infectious Mononucleosis

A disease that often strikes young adults, infectious mononucleosis is characterized by cervical lymphadenopathy, fever, sore throat, and splenomegaly. Exudative tonsillitis is common.

The designation mononucleosis is misleading because the proliferating cells present in the lymph nodes, spleen, tonsils, and other organs are atypical lympho-cytes, not monocytes. Serology shows an increase in lym-phocytes, with 10% to 20% of these being abnormal.

Mononucleosis is caused by the Epstein-Barr virus (EBV). The EBV is transmitted primarily through oral se-cretions. Blood and sexual transmission are rare.[1] This is the same herpesvirus that causes the malignant Burkitt's lymphoma that occurs in some areas in Africa. If cultured infectious mononucleosis lymphocytes are transplanted into immunosuppressed animals, a malignant lympho-proliferative disorder results. Genetically determined de-fects in the immune response may be the key to this cancer.[4]

EBV subclinically infects from 50% to 80% of the world's population.[6] Large epidemiologic studies have shown that only people without antibodies against EBV are at risk for developing infectious mononucleosis. The active disease is associated with the brief appearance of IgM antibodies against EBV. The IgM antibody increase represents a primary response, and indicates recent ex-posure to the virus.

Infectious mononucleosis particularly affects the adolescent and young adult age-groups. By adulthood, 95% of the population have EBV antibodies.

Hematologic changes are characteristic of mono-nucleosis. At first, there may be a mild leukopenia, but by the second week, the white cell count reaches 15,000 to 30,000/$\mu$L of blood. Atypical lymphocytes make up 15% to 60% of the white cells in the 2nd through the 4th weeks. The atypical lymphocytes may take one of several forms, but the most common picture includes nuclear chromatin that is finely divided or clumped. The nucleo-lus usually is absent, and vacuoles often are present in the cytoplasm. If atypical lymphocytes are present in large numbers, the disease may hematologically re-semble acute leukemia or Hodgkin's disease; but the combination of fever, pharyngitis, lymphadenopathy, and antibody tests usually make the differential.[12]

EBV induces an increase in antibody formation by the B lymphocytes. The presence of this antibody forms the basis for laboratory diagnostic testing. The heterophil antibody titer and MonoSpot tests are used for differen-tial diagnosis. No correlation has been noted between the levels of EBV or antibody titer and severity of the disease.[7]

Symptoms of infectious mononucleosis disappear before the abnormal hematologic findings do. Clinical characteristics include fever, malaise, sore throat, and weakness. Splenomegaly and hepatic dysfunction may be present. Complications are infrequent but include he-molytic anemia, splenic rupture, encephalitis, hepatitis, and pulmonary complications.[12] Avoidance of contact sports and increased rest usually are prescribed for 6 to 8 weeks after diagnosis. Gradual recovery is the rule, and usually occurs in 2 to 4 weeks with no residual effects.

## Lymphadenopathy

Lymphadenopathies are characterized by enlarged lymph nodes. The nodes may be tender or nontender and mov-able or fixed. Nodes involved by lymphomas or leuke-mias tend to be large, firm, and movable, whereas those of metastatic spread of cancer tend to be adherent to sur-rounding structures. In acute infections, the nodes usu-ally are asymmetric with associated redness and edema.

Localized lymphadenopathy usually indicates drain-age of an inflammation that may be due to infection, neoplasm, or early lymphoma. Generalized lymphade-nopathy infrequently is caused by infection in the adult, more often being caused by a malignant or nonmalignant process.

Lymphadenopathies show individual pathologic fea-tures, depending on the causative agent. Suppurative lymphadenitis is characterized by neutrophils in the si-nusoids of the lymph nodes.

These nodes serve as filtration units for the regions infected by pyogenic bacteria. Lymph node enlargement may be due to reactive follicular hyperplasia of nonspe-cific origin. There usually is hyperplasia of follicular cen-ter cells, which may be due to stimulation of B cells in viral diseases, syphilis, or autoimmune diseases such as rheumatoid arthritis or systemic lupus erythematosus.

# MALIGNANT WHITE BLOOD CELL DISORDERS

## Leukemia

Leukemia is the name of a group of malignant diseases characterized by both qualitative and quantitative altera-tions in circulating leukocytes. It is associated with diffuse abnormal growth of leukocyte precursors in the bone marrow. The word *leukemia* is derived from the Greek *leukos* and *aima,* meaning "white" and "blood," refer-ring to the abnormal increase in leukocytes. This uncon-trolled increase eventually leads to anemia, infection, thrombocytopenia, and, in some cases, death. The fre-quency of all leukemias is about 13 per 100,000 per-sons per year, with both acute and chronic forms being slightly higher in males.[2]

## Classification

Classification of leukemia usually is based on (1) *the course and duration of the illness* and (2) *the abnormal type of cells and tissue involved.* The course of the illness has been subclassified into acute and chronic.

*Acute leukemia* is associated with rapid onset, a mas-sive number of immature leukocytes, rapidly progressive anemia, severe thrombocytopenia, high fever, infective lesions of the mouth and throat, bleeding into vital areas, accumulation of leukocytes in vital organs, and severe infection. Laboratory studies usually show some degree of anemia and thrombocytopenia. Most advanced laboratory methods can now identify the cell type that causes acute leukemia, but a small percentage of cases cannot be classified, except that the predominant cell is an undifferentiated stem cell (Table 20-5). Demonstration of leukemic cells in the peripheral blood cannot always be relied on. Open surgical biopsy of the bone marrow usually demonstrates the abnormal cells.

*Chronic leukemia* is characterized by gradual onset and leukocytes that are more mature. This disease mostly strikes older people. The clinical course progresses more slowly than, but can end with the onset of, acute leukemia. Laboratory analysis usually reveals a well-differentiated leukemic cell that can be classified as lymphocytic or granulocytic (Table 20-6).

Leukemia is further classified by the type of tissue and abnormal cell involved. Three broad categories based on tissue origin are (1) *myeloid,* which includes the granulocytes (neutrophils, eosinophils, or basophils); (2) *monocytic;* and (3) *lymphocytic.* If abnormal proliferation of granular leukocytes or their precursors is found in the blood or bone marrow, the leukemia may be called granulocytic, myelocytic, or myelogenous.

With abnormal proliferation of lymphocytes or monocytes, the disease is called lymphocytic or monocytic, respectively.

If the majority of cells are immature, the suffix "blastic" is used instead of "cytic." For example, lymphoblastic, myeloblastic, or monoblastic indicates immaturity of leukocytes.

Classification of the chronic leukemias has not been a diagnostic problem because sufficient abnormal mature cells often are present from which to make a diagnosis. Diagnosis and classification of acute leukemia present a greater challenge. Because of cellular immaturity, sometimes it is difficult to identify the cell type. Research and technologic advances have led to a more sophisticated

**TABLE 20-5.**

FRENCH-AMERICAN-BRITISH (FAB) CLASSIFICATION OF ACUTE LEUKEMIAS

| FAB CLASS | MORPHOLOGY |
| --- | --- |
| **Acute Lymphoblastic Leukemias** | |
| L1 | Small cells predominate but may vary, with some cells up to twice the diameter of small lymphocytes. Nuclei normally are round and regular with occasional clefts. Nucleoli often are not visible. Cytoplasm is scanty. Cell population is homogeneous. |
| L2 | Cells are heterogeneous in size, and share in features of both L1 and L3. Nuclei often show clefts. Nucleoli often are present. |
| L3 | There is a homogeneous population of large cells (3 to 4 times the diameter of small lymphocytes). Nuclei are round to oval with prominent nucleoli. Cytoplasm is abundant and deeply basophilic. |
| **Acute Myeloblastic (Myelocytic) Leukemias** | |
| M1 Acute myelocytic leukemia without differentiation | Myeloblasts predominate; distinct nucleoli; few granules or Auer rods |
| M2 Acute myelocytic leukemia with differentiation | Myeloblasts and promyelocytes predominate; Auer rods may be present |
| M3 Acute promyelocytic leukemia | Hypergranular promyelocytes, often with many Auer rods per cell; may have reniform or bilobed nuclei |
| M4 Acute myelomonocytic leukemia | Myelocytic and monocytic differentiation evident; myeloid elements resemble M2; peripheral monocytosis |
| M5 Acute monocytic leukemia | Promonocytes or undifferentiated blasts |
| M6 Acute erythroleukemia | Bizarre, multinucleated, megaloblastoid erythroblasts predominate; myeloblasts also present |
| M7 Acute megakaryocytic leukemia | Pleomorphic undifferentiated blasts; react with antiplatelet antibodies; myelofibrosis, or increased bone marrow reticulin |

Cotran, R.S., Kumar, V., and Robbins, S.L., Robbins' Pathologic Basis of Disease (4th ed.). Philadelphia: W.B. Saunders, 1989.

**TABLE 20–6.**
CHRONIC LEUKEMIAS

| TYPE | DESCRIPTION |
| --- | --- |
| Chronic myeloid leukemia | Chromosome marker, Ph$_1$ (Philadelphia) characteristic in 90% of cases. Granulocyte precursors dominate cell line. Marked elevation of leukocyte count usually >100,000 cells/mm$^3$. Thrombocytosis common. Marked lack of alkaline phosphatase in granulocytes. Accelerated phase may terminate in "blast" crisis, which appears like acute leukemia |
| Chronic lymphocytic leukemia | Various chromosomal abnormalities common. Similar to lymphatic lymphoma. B-cell neoplasm with long-lived nonfunctional B lymphocytes that infiltrate the bone marrow. Total leukocyte count may be 200,000 cells/mm$^3$. Hypogammaglobulinemia common with increased susceptibility to bacterial infections. Course variable with median survival of 4–6 years. |
| Hairy cell leukemia | Cell origin obscure, surface markers of T and B cells as well as monocytes. Genetic structure resembles B cells. Cells have fine, hairlike projections. Splenic and liver infiltration common; leukocytosis uncommon. Course is variable with median survival of 4 years. |

Cotran, R., Kumar, V., and Robbins, S.L., Robbins' Pathologic Basis of Disease (4th ed.). Philadelphia: W.B. Saunders, 1989.

identification and classification system that includes the use of cell marker studies, cell secretory activity, and cytochemistry, as well as morphology and response to therapy.

Many factors are thought to influence the development of leukemia. These can be divided into three groups: (1) genetic factors, (2) acquired diseases, and (3) chemical and physical agents.

Genetic factors present in an identical twin pose a great risk if the other twin has leukemia or Bloom syndrome. Bloom syndrome is caused by an autosomal recessive trait characterized by dwarfism, photosensitivity, and butterfly telangiectatic erythema of the face with numerous defects of the skin pigment and keratin development. Siblings of a person with leukemia and people with Down syndrome also are at significant risk for developing leukemia. Several chromosomal abnormalities have been associated with the onset of leukemia. The Philadelphia chromosome, now thought to be chromosome 22 rather than 21, as previously reported, is associated with chronic granulocytic leukemia. Acute leukemias often show abnormalities of chromosomes 8 and 21.[15]

Acquired diseases with some increased risk for leukemia include myelofibrosis, polycythemia vera, and sideroblastic refractory anemia. Multiple myeloma and Hodgkin's disease also represent increased risk for development of the disease.

Physical and chemical agents that pose significant risk include irradiation and long-term exposure to benzene. Some risk also is associated with the chemothera-peutic agent chloramphenicol and alkylating agents. Viral causation of leukemia in humans has been studied extensively, particularly because it has been noted in lower animals. Induction of leukemic changes in tissue cultures of human cells by ribonucleic acid viruses supports the possibility of viral transmission of certain forms of leukemia.[9] The human T-cell leukemia virus has been isolated from cells of persons with adult T-cell leukemia, an aggressive cancer composed of mature T-lymphoid cells.[2] The disease is found particularly in southwestern Japan, parts of the Caribbean, and central Africa.[2]

## Clinical Manifestations

Pathologic alterations caused by the disease process create characteristic signs and symptoms. *Acute lymphocytic leukemia (ALL)* usually occurs abruptly, with fever, fatigue, bleeding, signs of bone marrow dysfunction, and bone pain. Anemia is present in 90% of persons with ALL.[10] The WBC count is variable, sometimes normal to low. The bone marrow is crowded with lymphoblasts that may be morphologically indistinguishable from myeloblasts.[9] Infiltration of the lymph nodes, spleen, and liver is characteristic.[4]

*Acute myeloblastic* or *myelocytic leukemia (AML)* also arises abruptly with symptoms similar to those of ALL. Laboratory studies differentiate various forms of AML. The organ infiltration with AML is not as prominent as with ALL. Hemorrhages, small vascular occlusions, and disseminated intravascular coagulation (DIC) commonly occur. Anemia is characteristic, but elevated WBC above 100,000/$\mu$L occurs in only about 20% of cases.[4]

*Chronic myelocytic leukemia (CML)* accounts for 15% to 20% of cases, and may be discovered on routine physical examination, especially with evidence of an enlarged spleen. In about 90% of cases, the Ph₁ (Philadelphia) chromosome can be demonstrated. This chromosome represents the translocation from the long arm to chromosome 22 to another chromosome.[4] This aberration also is occasionally seen in ALL. Early signs are fatigability, weakness, weight loss, and anorexia. Bleeding, anemia, and infection are late manifestations. The WBC count is very high, from 50,000 to 500,000/$\mu$L. After about 3 years, about 50% of people affected enter an accelerated phase and finally a picture like acute leukemia.[2]

*Chronic lymphocytic leukemia* is a long-term disease, usually of elderly people and especially among Western peoples.[6,12] It is characterized by generalized lymphadenopathy and often is otherwise asymptomatic. Anemia, fatigue, and night sweats may be described. The WBC count may range from 20,000 to 150,000/$\mu$L. The leukemia cells are small and mature-looking but nonfunctional. The course and progression of the disease are variable, with median survival of 4 to 6 years.[4]

*Hairy cell leukemia* is a rare form that produces distinctive cells with hairlike projections. The origins of the cells are not known, but they are thought to be of B-lymphocyte lineage.[4] The disease occurs mainly in elderly men, with splenomegaly, hepatomegaly, and bone marrow failure resulting in *pancytopenia*. At least 50% of affected people survive for more than 8 years with appropriate chemotherapy.[2]

Infection caused by marrow failure and granulocytopenia is the most common cause of fatality in all types of leukemia. It may appear in any organ or area, and may be manifested by fever, chills, inflammation, and weakness. Bleeding of the skin, gingivae, or viscera often occurs because of thrombocytopenia. DIC caused by reduced platelets and coagulation factors may cause significant hemorrhage (see Chap. 21). Probably DIC is triggered by proteolytic enzymes or factors released by the leukemic cells that activate the clotting process.

Reduced appetite and hypermetabolism result in weight loss, weakness, fatigue, and pallor associated with anemia. The progression varies with the specific disease process. Calcium and magnesium abnormalities can be seen in serologic laboratory tests.

Leukemic infiltration of the meninges, central nervous system, and cranial nerves results in such clinical manifestations as headache, visual disturbances, nausea, and vomiting. Bone infiltration leads to bone tenderness and pain. Hepatosplenomegaly and infiltration of other viscera are manifested by abdominal tenderness and anorexia. Lymphadenopathy and neoplastic masses are due to local infiltration.

## Progression of the Disease

Chemotherapy has markedly increased the survival rates for acute leukemias. Untreated ALL usually is fatal within 3 months. Studies show that more than 60% of children who receive chemotherapy are alive after 5 years.[3] AML has a poorer record, even with treatment, with average survival of 1 to 2 years.

The chronic leukemias have a variable course that can be controlled by oral alkylating agents or irradiation. Progressive anemia and susceptibility to infection are hazards, and CML may terminate by transforming into AML.

## Malignant Lymphomas

Malignant lymphomas are solid neoplasms that contain cells of lymphoreticular origin. These tumors should be considered tumors of the immune system.[10] *Lymphoreticular organs* include the lymph nodes, spleen, bone marrow, thymus, liver, and the submucosa of the gastrointestinal and respiratory tracts.

Pathologically, lymphadenopathy is characteristic, with eventual involvement of the liver, spleen, and viscera. Diffusely diseased nodes are gray, with capsular infiltration occurring later in the process. The enlarged nodes may become adherent to one another and to surrounding organs and tissues.[4]

### Classification

The classification of malignant lymphomas usually is based on the predominant cell type and its degree of differentiation. The disease may be further divided into nodular and diffuse types, depending on the predominant pattern of cell arrangement. Table 20-7 shows the cellular origins of malignant lymphomas. With more specific antiserums, the lymphocyte origin of B cells, T cells, and monocytes can be delineated.

The diffuse lymphomas are more invasive than the nodular lymphomas. The more undifferentiated the cell, the more aggressive the tumor becomes. As with leukemia, most persons with lymphomas develop immune deficiencies that are followed by infection. A common staging classification for lymphomas is used; the later the stage, the greater the involvement, and the worse the prognosis (Table 20-8).

### Hodgkin's Disease

Hodgkin's disease is a malignant lymphoma that occurs in various distinct forms. It is characterized by proliferation of a tumor with normal tissue, reactive lymphocytes, plasma cells, and a scattering of the characteristic malig-

**TABLE 20–7.**
## THE MALIGNANT LYMPHOMAS

| | NON-HODGKIN'S | HODGKIN'S |
|---|---|---|
| Cellular derivation | 90% B Cell<br>10% T Cell<br>Rare monocytic | Unresolved |
| Sites of disease | | |
| Localized | Uncommon | Common |
| Nodal spread | Discontiguous | Contiguous |
| Extranodal | Common | Uncommon |
| Mediastinal | Uncommon | Common |
| Abdominal | Common | Uncommon |
| Bone marrow | Common | Uncommon |
| B systemic symptoms* | Uncommon | Common |
| Chromosomal translocation | Common | Yet to be described |
| Curability | <25% | >75% |

*Fever, night sweats, weight loss of greater than 10% of body weight.*
*From Wilson, J.D., Harrison's Principles of Internal Medicine (12th ed.). New York: McGraw-Hill, 1991.*

nant cells, called Sternberg-Reed cells. Infiltration of the nodes with eosinophils and plasma cells occurs, and this is associated with necrosis and fibrosis.

The histologic criteria in cancer of Hodgkin's disease are similar to those in non-Hodgkin's lymphomas. The Sternberg-Reed cell, which is a multinucleated, odd-looking giant cell with a prominent nucleolus, must be present to confirm the diagnosis. Hodgkin's disease appears to involve a defect in the T cells, and the total lymphocyte count is depressed. Infection often causes major complications.

Hodgkin's disease has been classified into four types: (1) lymphocyte predominant, in which there is diffuse replacement by lymphocytes; (2) mixed type, which includes several distinct cell patterns, both lymphocytic and histiocytic; (3) lymphocyte depletion, with a predominant pattern of large malignant cells; and (4) nodular sclerosing, which has extensive scarring.[4]

Staging of Hodgkin's disease uses the same classification as other lymphomas (see Table 20-8). Bone marrow examination and examination of the spleen for pathology after splenectomy often are the bases for staging.

**TABLE 20–8.**
## STAGING CLASSIFICATION FOR LYMPHOMAS

| STAGE | DEFINITION |
|---|---|
| I | Involvement of a single lymph node region (I) or of a single extralymphatic organ or site ($I_E$) |
| II | Involvement of two or more lymph node regions on the same side of the diaphragm (II) or localized involvement of an extralymphatic organ or site and of one or more lymph node regions on the same side of the diaphragm ($II_E$) |
| III | Involvement of lymph node regions on both sides of the diaphragm (III), which also may be accompanied by involvement of the spleen ($III_S$) or by localized involvement of an extralymphatic organ or site ($III_E$) or both ($III_{SE}$) |
| $III_1$ | Involvement limited to the lymphatic structures in the upper abdomen, that is, spleen, or splenic, celiac, or hepatic portal nodes, or any combination of these |
| $III_2$ | Involvement of lower abdominal nodes, that is, paraaortic, iliac, or mesenteric nodes, with or without involvement of the splenic, celiac, or hepatic portal nodes |
| IV | Diffuse or disseminated involvement of one or more extralymphatic organs or tissues, with or without associated lymph node involvement |

*E, extralymphatic site; S, splenic involvement. The presence of fever, night sweats, or unexplained loss of 10% of body weight in the 6 months preceding admission is denoted by the suffix letter B. The letter A indicates the absence of these symptoms. Biopsy-documented involvement of stage IV sites also is denoted by letter suffixes; marrow, M+; lung, L+; liver, H+; pleura, P+; bone, O+; skin and subcutaneous tissue, D+.*
*Adapted with permission from Wilson, J., et al., Harrison's Principles of Internal Medicine (12th ed.). © 1991 McGraw-Hill. Reprinted with permission of McGraw-Hill Publishers.*

As with other lymphomas, the later the stage, the poorer the prognosis.[11]

Common clinical manifestations of Hodgkin's disease are enlarged, palpable lymph nodes, fever, weight loss, and loss of energy. Node enlargement may cause compression on the spinal cord or other organs. The tumor may invade the vasculature or the lung parenchyma.

Anemia and immune deficiency with lymphocytopenia occur in the later stages. Biopsy may be needed to demonstrate Sternberg-Reed cells.[4] Immune deficiency, exacerbated by chemotherapy, leads to ineffective control of microbial invasion, especially fungal and protozoal. Infection is a common complication of both the disease and the tumor.

Treatment with chemotherapy and radiation therapy has markedly improved the prognosis for Hodgkin's disease, with 90% to 100% remission being reported.

## Multiple Myeloma

Multiple myeloma, or *plasma cell myeloma*, is a malignant neoplasm of plasma cells that damages the bone marrow and skeletal structure. The aberrant myeloma cells arise from a single clone of plasma cells that are B cell–derived and secrete anomalous circulating immunoglobulins, also called *paraproteins*. The immunoglobulins most often are of the IgG class, but may be IgA, IgM, or, rarely, IgD or IgE (see Chap. 14).[4]

Laboratory examination of the bone marrow shows proliferation of both mature and immature plasma cells, with about 20% or more having multinucleated forms. These cells often completely replace the bone marrow. Serum protein electrophoresis and immunoelectrophoresis are abnormal. Bence Jones proteinemia and proteinuria, which are proliferations of light chains of immunoglobulin molecules, are present in about 50% of affected people. A higher frequency of renal failure correlates with the amount of protein found in the urine, since the excreted light chains are thought to be toxic to the renal tubules.[3] About 1% of the affected plasma cells do not secrete antibodies.

The malignant neoplasm that arises in bone usually does not metastasize outside bone. The destructive lesions erode the bone and cause punched-out lytic lesions observable radiographically. These lesions can be visualized in any bone but are most frequent in the vertebral column, ribs, skull, pelvis, femurs, clavicles, and scapulae.[3] The bones can become so fragile that simple movements can cause fractures. Pathologic fractures usually occur because of the lesions, especially of the weight-bearing regions.

Calcium metabolism often is abnormal, causing some persons to have elevated serum calcium levels. There often is a normocytic, normochromic anemia, with variable depression of WBC and platelet counts.

Bone or back pain is the most common symptom.

Pallor and weakness caused by secondary anemia may occur.

In some cases, myeloma nephrosis occurs because of the infiltration and precipitation of the light chains (Bence Jones protein) in the distal tubules as the urine is concentrated. The laminated, crystalline casts in the distal tubules damage the kidney cells and obstruct the tubules. Pathologic interstitial inflammation and fibrosis further impair kidney function, leading to uremia.

Anemia, thrombocytopenia that leads to bleeding, and neutropenia resulting in infection are common results of the disorder. Vascular insufficiency may occur in the peripheral areas, and apparently is related to increased blood viscosity caused by high levels of circulating immunoglobulins. Survival statistics remain poor, and largely depend on the person's response to the chemotherapeutic regimen, with 2 to 3 years as the norm.[4] In about 10% of cases, the disease progresses very slowly, taking many years to run its course.

## REFERENCES

1. Benenson, A.S. *Control of Communicable Disease in Man* (14th ed.). Washington, D.C.: American Public Health Assoc., 1985.
2. Champlin, R., and Golde, D.W. The leukemias. In J. Wilson et al., *Harrison's Principles of Internal Medicine* (12th ed.). New York: McGraw-Hill, 1991.
3. Cormach, D.H. *Ham's Histology* (9th ed.). Philadelphia: J.B. Lippincott, 1987.
4. Cotran, R.S., Kumar, V., and Robbins, S.L. *Robbins' Pathologic Basis of Disease* (4th ed.). Philadelphia: W.B. Saunders, 1989.
5. Gallin, J. Disorders of phagocytic cells. In J. Wilson et al., *Harrison's Principles of Internal Medicine* (12th ed.). New York: McGraw-Hill, 1991.
6. Goetzl, E.J., and Stobo, J.D. Immunology. In L.H. Smith and S.O. Thier, *Pathophysiology: The Biological Principles of Disease* (2nd ed.). Philadelphia: W.B. Saunders, 1985.
7. Grossman, M., and Jawetz, E. Infectious diseases: Viral and rickettsial. In M.A. Krupp, M.J. Chatton, and L.M. Tierney, *Current Medical Diagnosis and Treatment 1986.* Los Altos, Calif.: Lange, 1986.
8. Guyton, A.C. *Textbook of Medical Physiology* (8th ed.). Philadelphia: W.B. Saunders, 1990.
9. Harmon, D.C. The leukemias. In W.S. Beck, *Hematology* (4th ed.). Cambridge, Mass.: MIT Press, 1985.
10. Nadler, L.M. The malignant lymphomas. In J. Wilson et al., *Harrison's Principles of Internal Medicine* (12th ed.). New York: McGraw-Hill, 1991.
11. Rosenthal, D.S. The malignant lymphomas. In W.S. Beck, *Hematology* (4th ed.). Cambridge, Mass.: MIT Press, 1985.
12. Schooley, R.T. Epstein-Barr virus infections including infectious mononucleosis. In J. Wilson et al., *Harrison's Principles of Internal Medicine* (12th ed.). New York: McGraw-Hill, 1991.
13. Wallach, I. *Interpretation of Diagnostic Tests* (4th ed.). Boston: Little, Brown, 1986.

14. Wallerstein, R.O. Blood. In M.A. Krupp, M.J. Chatton, and L.M. Tierney, *Current Medical Diagnosis and Treatment 1986*. Los Altos, Calif.: Lange, 1986.

15. Weatherall, D.J., and Bunch, C. The blood and blood-forming organs. In L.H. Smith and S.O. Thier, *Pathophysiology:* *The Biological Principles of Disease* (2nd ed.). Philadelphia: W.B. Saunders, 1985.

16. Wilkerson, E. Inflammation, infection and wound healing. In E. Howell, L. Widra, and G. Hill, *Trauma Nursing*. Glenview, Ill.: Scott, Foresman, 1988.

*chapter* **21**　　　Barbara L. Bullock

# Normal and Altered Coagulation

## *Chapter Outline*

▶ Hemostasis
　**Vasoconstriction**
　**Hemostatic Platelet Plug**
　　**Formation**
　**Characteristics and**
　　**Physiology of Platelets**
▶ General Mechanism of Blood
　Coagulation
　**Clotting Factors**
　**Formation of the**
　　**Prothrombin Activator**
　**Intrinsic Pathway**
　**Extrinsic Pathway**
　**Enzymatic Complexes**
　**Final Common Pathway to**
　　**Clot Formation**

**Clot Formation**
　Blood Clot Composition
　Clot Retraction
▶ Lysis of Blood Clots
▶ Anticoagulation Factors in
　Normal Blood
▶ Laboratory Tests for Coagulation
　Problems
　**Clotting or Coagulation Time**
　**Prothrombin Time**
　**Partial Thromboplastin Time**
　**Tests for Specific Deficiencies**
　**Platelet Count**
　**Bleeding Time**
　**Clot Retraction**

▶ Deficiencies in Blood
　Coagulation
　**Single Coagulation Factor**
　　**Deficiencies**
　　Hemophilia
　**Vitamin K Deficiencies**
　**Liver Disease**
　**Massive Transfusion**
　　**Syndrome**
　**Disseminated Intravascular**
　　**Coagulation**
　**Primary Fibrinolysis**
　**Antibody Anticoagulants**
　**Platelet Disorders**
　　Thrombocytopenia
　　Qualitative Platelet Disorders
　　Thrombocytosis
　　Hypercoagulation

## *Learning Objectives*

1. Define *hemostasis* and list the four major events included in this process.
2. Explain the role of vasoconstriction in hemostasis and the mechanism of stimulation.
3. Describe the function of the platelets and explain their role in the hemostatic process.
4. Describe the sequence of events in the coagulation process.
5. Describe briefly the essential clotting factors, where they are formed, and how they act.
6. Explain the common pathway of blood coagulation.
7. Differentiate between the intrinsic pathway and the extrinsic pathway in prothrombin activation.
8. Diagram the interrelationships of the major components involved in hemostasis.
9. Describe the composition of the blood clot.
10. Explain the action of the fibrinolytic system.

11. List several factors normally present in the blood that inhibit clotting.
12. Differentiate factors that enhance coagulation and those that inhibit coagulation in normal blood.
13. Explain the basis of common laboratory tests used to determine coagulation problems.
14. Explain briefly the role of liver function with respect to normal coagulation.
15. Differentiate the factor deficiencies that cause the various types of hemophilia.
16. Explain how uncontrolled bleeding occurs in disseminated intravascular coagulation.
17. Differentiate between thrombocytosis and thrombocytopenia, and list some causative conditions for each.
18. Describe some platelet disorders that are associated with hypercoagulability.

Coagulation is an essential, protective part of hemostasis that prevents blood loss when a vessel is damaged. Hemostasis refers to the arrest of bleeding. Coagulation is the ability of blood to change from a fluid to a semisolid mass. It involves the conversion of fibrinogen, a soluble macromolecule composed of three polypeptide chains, to fibrin monomers by action of the proteolytic enzyme thrombin. Polymerization of the monomers follows and spontaneously bonds fibrin monomers together. A fibrin-stabilizing factor acts on fibrin to cause cross-linkage bonding, which forms an insoluble, threadlike mesh on which a clot forms. This mechanism for clot initiation and formation involves a series of sequential cascadelike reactions that employ several factors in the blood and injured tissues.

## HEMOSTASIS

Hemostasis, the arrest of bleeding or circulation of the blood, is often divided into four main events: (1) vasoconstriction, (2) formation of a hemostatic platelet plug, (3) blood coagulation, and (4) clot formation. The interaction of all four events is essential for normal hemostasis. The general dynamic interaction of these events is illustrated in Figure 21-1.

## *Vasoconstriction*

Vasoconstriction is the result of many events that occur during an injury. Immediately after the wall of a vessel is injured, contraction of the vessel decreases the flow of blood in and out of the vessel. This contraction is due mainly to two factors: nervous reflexes and local myogenic spasms.[4] Nervous reflexes are probably initiated by pain impulses created by the tissue or vascular trauma. Local myogenic spasm is initiated by direct damage to the vascular wall and by the release of serotonin from platelets.

The greater the portion of vessel traumatized, the greater the degree of spasm. A sharply cut vessel bleeds longer than a crushed one.[4] A clean cut by a sharp razor blade, for example, bleeds longer than a scrape or jagged cut.

## *Hemostatic Platelet Plug Formation*

When a blood vessel is damaged, the endothelial lining is disrupted, exposing the underlying collagen. When platelets are exposed to collagen or other foreign surfaces such as antigen–antibody complexes, thrombin, proteolytic enzymes, endotoxins, or viruses, they undergo a dynamic change called viscous metamorphosis.

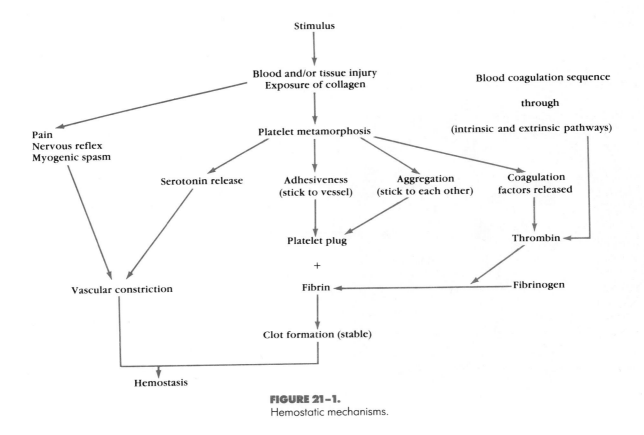

**FIGURE 21–1.**
Hemostatic mechanisms.

They begin to swell and form irregular shapes with processes protruding from their surfaces. They become sticky and adhere to the collagen and basement membrane of the vessel. The platelets release adenosine diphosphate, which attracts other platelets and aids in platelet adhesion and aggregation. Adenosine diphosphate also is released from disrupted red blood cells and damaged tissue. Enzymes released from the platelets cause the formation of thromboxane A (a type of prostaglandin) in the plasma.[4] Both adenosine diphosphate and thromboxane A activate nearby platelets that stick to the original platelets, thus, creating a cycle of platelet activation. The platelet plug results, causing the damaged endothelial vessel wall to adhere to the collagen fibers.[5] This plug is loose and arrests circulation only if the tear in the vessel is small. Later, a tight plug is formed by fibrin threads that result from the process of coagulation.

Hundreds of minute ruptures occur in the capillaries each day. The platelet plug is important because it can stop bleeding completely if the damage is small. A significant decrease in the number of platelets can lead to small hemorrhagic areas under the skin and in the internal tissue.[5] Usually, the plugging mechanism seals the tear in the vessel rather than occluding the lumen.

## Characteristics and Physiology of Platelets

Platelets are fragments of megakaryocytes formed in the bone marrow and released into the circulation. The normal platelet concentration in the blood is about 140,000 to 340,000 per $\mu$L.[10] Adequate numbers must be present for normal hemostasis and clotting.

Each platelet has four major functional regions: the peripheral, sol-gel, organelle, and membrane systems zones (Figure 21-2).[11] The peripheral zone includes the cell membrane and closely associated structures, in which are found the receptors for the various stimuli that trigger platelet activation, the substrate for adhesion and aggregation reactions, and a surface for coagulant protein interaction. Adhesion involves the platelet-collagen interaction that results in platelets sticking to the site of injury on the blood vessel. Aggregation is a calcium-requiring process of platelet-to-platelet association. The peripheral zone translates the signals of stimuli into chemical messages and initiates the physical alterations required for platelet activation.[3]

The sol-gel zone is composed of the platelet cytoplasm matrix. Here are the fiber systems that support the disklike shape of the unstimulated platelets and provide the contractile systems that allow the platelets to change shape, form pseudopods, and perform contraction and secretion functions. The organelle zone contains the cellular organelles, which are embedded in the sol-gel matrix and serve metabolic purposes. This zone is an important storage area for enzymes, serotonin, calcium, and protein constituents. The membrane systems region is comprised of canalicular systems or tiny surface-connected canallike structures that have access to the interior. In this region, plasma substances are able to enter and cellular products may be released or secreted. Prod-

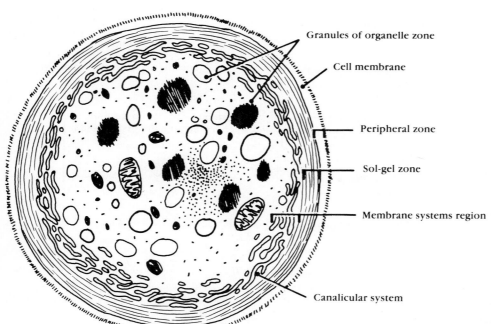

Granules of organelle zone

Cell membrane

Peripheral zone

Sol-gel zone

Membrane systems region

Canalicular system

**FIGURE 21–2.**
Major functional regions of the platelet.

ucts stored in secretory organelles are extruded to the outside through an energy-dependent process.[11]

Contractile physiology dominates the platelet response and is critical to the development of the hemostatic plug. The contractile ability allows shape changes and internal transformation. It facilitates the process of secretion and converts loosely clumped platelets into tightly packed masses that can seal a vascular rent. Contraction of the platelets provides the force for contraction of the platelet-fibrin meshwork and allows for retraction of a clot.

## GENERAL MECHANISM OF BLOOD COAGULATION

Three basic reactions constitute the sequential pathway for blood coagulation: (1) a prothrombin activator is formed by the intrinsic or extrinsic pathway in response to tissue or endothelial damage; (2) prothrombin activator catalyzes the conversion of prothrombin to thrombin; and (3) thrombin catalyzes the conversion of soluble fibrinogen to solid fibrin polymer threads. These fibrin threads form the meshwork on which plasma, blood cells, and platelets aggregate to make the clot (Figure 21-3). Before these three reactions can occur, other responses must take place. A group of reactants called clotting factors begin the process that terminates in the formation of the blood clot.

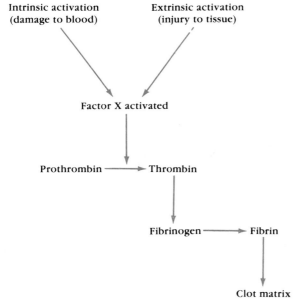

**FIGURE 21-3.**
Common pathyway of blood coagulation.

## Clotting Factors

The clotting factors are a series of plasma proteins that are generally inactive forms of proteolytic enzymes. Table 21-1 summarizes these factors and indicates the international nomenclature used for each. The enzymatic proteolytic actions cause successive reactions of the clotting process in a cascadelike sequence. One activated factor is important for the activation of the next factor. The inactive precursor enzyme is activated by peptide-bond cleavage. A low level or lack of even one of these inactive proteolytic enzymes can lead to abnormal bleeding and hemorrhage.[4]

Fibrinogen, prothrombin, and factors VII, IX, and X are essential procoagulation factors. Fibrinogen (factor I) is synthesized in the liver at a rate that usually corresponds to the rate of use or need. The levels of fibrinogen may be increased by adrenocorticotropic hormone, growth hormone, endotoxin, pregnancy, and occlusive arterial disease. Prothrombin (factor II) and factors VII, IX, and X are also synthesized exclusively in the liver by a process that requires vitamin K. These factors are affected by many conditions including pregnancy, oral contraceptives, and diethylstilbestrol.[9]

## Formation of the Prothrombin Activator

The coagulation process begins with the formation of the prothrombin activator, a substance or complex of substances. The mechanism is initiated by trauma to the tissues or blood, or contact of the blood with damaged endothelial cells, collagen, or other substances outside the blood vessel endothelium. This injury or contact leads to the formation of the prothrombin activator, which then leads to the conversion of prothrombin to thrombin.

The prothrombin activator is formed in one of two ways: (1) through the extrinsic pathway, initiated by trauma to the vessel wall or tissues outside the vessel; or (2) through the intrinsic pathway, which begins with trauma to blood components, and thus alters the platelets and factor XII (Figure 21-4).

Interplay of both the intrinsic and extrinsic systems is needed for normal clotting. Deficiency of a single protein in one of these pathways may lead to a clotting disorder. The intrinsic and extrinsic pathways converge on a final common pathway, leading to the formation of a fibrin clot (see Figure 21-3). Each precursor protein is important in the clotting process because it is necessary for the activation of the next.

The clotting process occurs by a cascade of zymogen activations. A zymogen is an inactive precursor that is converted to an active enzyme by the action of another enzyme.[9] The activated form of one factor sequentially catalyzes the activation of the next in cascade fashion, leading to clot formation.

**TABLE 21–1.**
BLOOD COAGULATION FACTORS

| FACTOR (INTERNATIONAL NOMENCLATURE) | COMMON SYNONYMS | REMARKS |
|---|---|---|
| I | Fibrinogen | Soluble macromolecule, synthesized in liver, fibrin precursor |
| II | Prothrombin | Synthesized in liver, vitamin K required for formation |
| III | Tissue thromboplastin; thrombokinase | Phospholipid; involved in activation of extrinsic pathway |
| IV | Calcium | Involved in several complexes of coagulation process |
| V | Proaccelerin; labile factor; Ac-globulin; Ac-G | Synthesized in liver; modifier protein, not enzyme; required in prothrombin activator complex |
| (VI) | Obsolete term | Same as factor V |
| VII | Proconvertin; stable factor; serum prothrombin conversion accelerator | Part of enzyme complex in extrinsic pathway; synthesized in the liver; vitamin K required for formation |
| VIII | Antihemophilic globulin (AHG); antihemophilic factor (AHF); anti-hemophilic factor A | Required for intrinsic pathway function; possibly synthesized in liver, spleen, RES, or kidneys |
| IX | Plasma thromboplastin component (PTC); Christmas factor; antihemophilic factor B | Synthesized in liver; requires vitamin K; needed for intrinsic pathway function |
| X | Stuart-Prower factor; Stuart factor | Synthesized in the liver; requires vitamin K, needed for both intrinsic and extrinsic pathways |
| XI | Plasma thromboplastin antecedent (PTA); antihemophilic factor C | Substrate in intrinsic activator enzymatic complex; needed for intrinsic system activation, area of synthesis unknown |
| XII | Hageman factor; contact factor; antihemophilic factor D | Involved in first step of activation of intrinsic system; area of synthesis unknown |
| XIII | Fibrin stabilizing factor (FSF); plasma transglutaminase | Causes amide cross-linkage fibrin; stabilizes clot formation, synthesized by platelets and possibly other proteins, may be activated by liver |

## Intrinsic Pathway

The intrinsic pathway for the initiation of coagulation is through activation of components already present in the blood. This mechanism for initiating clotting begins within the vessel. When the blood comes into contact with collagen or damaged endothelium, an intrinsic activator-enzymatic complex is formed. An important part of this complex is the Hageman factor (activated factor XII), a proteolytic enzyme. This complex enzymatically activates factor XI. Sequential events continue in cascade fashion. Activated factor XI enzymatically activates factor IX. Factor IX forms factor X activation complex, which consists of activated factor IX, factor VIII, calcium, and phospholipids. Activated factor X then combines with factor V, calcium, and phospholipids to form the prothrombin activator. Within seconds, the prothrombin activator initiates the proteolytic cleavage of prothrombin bonds to form thrombin. The amount of thrombin formed is closely related to the amount of prothrombin activator present. Once thrombin is formed, the final clotting process is set in motion (see Figure 21-4).

If factor VIII or the platelets are not at an adequate level, activation of factor X is impaired. Decreased factor VIII is the major problem in classic hemophilia, and decreased platelets result in bleeding disorders such as thrombocytopenia (see p. 420). All of the clotting factors are essential to the normal coagulation sequence.

## Extrinsic Pathway

The extrinsic pathway for coagulation is triggered by factors not normally present in the blood, such as sub-

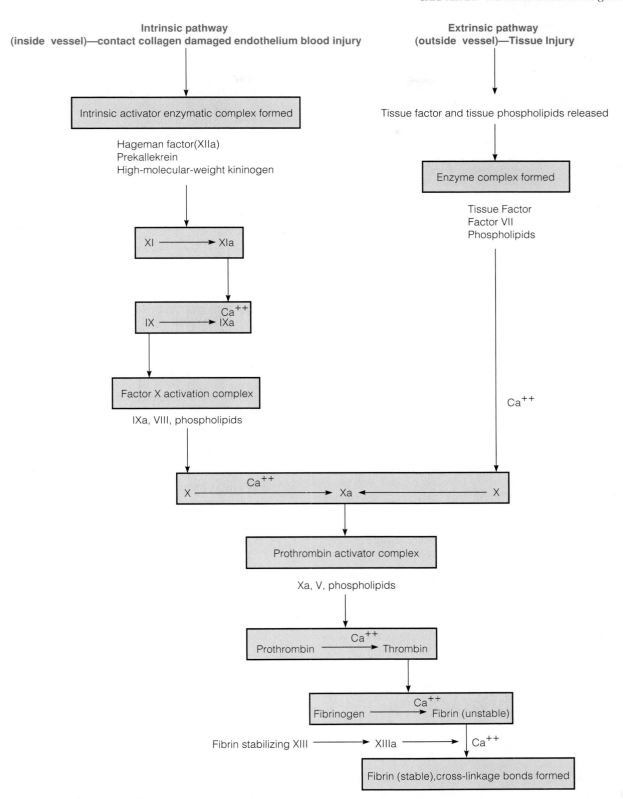

**FIGURE 21–4.**
Blood coagulation sequence. Key: a = activated enzyme; Ca++ = calcium is necessary in several reactions.

stances released from damaged tissues or other foreign materials. When the blood comes in contact with a traumatized vascular wall or extravascular tissue, substances called tissue factor and tissue phospholipids are released. Tissue factor is a proteolytic enzyme with cleavage ability, and tissue phospholipids are mainly those of the cell membrane.

The tissue factor plus factor VII, calcium, and phospholipids form a complex. This complex acts enzymatically on factor X to form activated factor X. Activated factor X then becomes part of the prothrombin activator complex, which enzymatically converts prothrombin to thrombin. Thrombin, in turn, enzymatically converts fibrinogen to fibrin (see Figure 21-4).

## Enzymatic Complexes

The cascade hypothesis used to describe the relationships among the protein constituents associated with blood coagulation has been the object of much study over the years. Most of the enzymes involved in the process and their precursors have been isolated and identified. The specificity of the proteolytic cleavages and activation processes in the coagulation transformations is quite well understood. Nonenzyme cofactor proteins are also essential for blood coagulation. Four principal enzymatic complexes involving these cofactors have been isolated:[4]

1. The *intrinsic* activator, which includes the Hageman factor (factor XII), prekallikrein, high-molecular-weight kininogen, and the substrate for the reaction factor XI
2. Factor VII, tissue factor, calcium, and phospholipids
3. Factor X activation, which is composed of activated factor IX, cofactor, factor VIII, calcium, and phospholipids
4. The *prothrombinase* complex, which includes activated factor X, activated factor V, calcium, and phospholipids

The significance of the cofactors and complex formation may be illustrated by the prothrombinase complex. The cofactors in this complex at physiologic concentrations lead to amplification of the reaction rate by 300,000 times.[9] It is obvious that without these cofactors and the interactions of the components in the complex, conversion of prothrombin to thrombin would be slowed tremendously.

## Final Common Pathway to Clot Formation

With the activation of factor X and formation of the prothrombin activator complex, the final common pathway for clot formation begins. Prothrombin activator complex causes the conversion of prothrombin to thrombin. Thrombin, in turn, enzymatically converts fibrinogen to fibrin. These reactions constitute the final coagulation pathway for both the intrinsic and extrinsic systems. The rate of the blood coagulation reaction is generally related to the amount of prothrombin activator formed and the degree of activation of factor X. If either is inhibited or stopped because of the absence of a clotting factor or other reasons, the coagulation process becomes altered and excess bleeding results.

## Clot Formation

Blood coagulation occurs faster with severe trauma to the vascular wall than with minor trauma. The general sequence of physical events takes place in a comparatively short time. After the vessel is severed, the platelets agglutinate and fibrin appears. A fibrin clot can form in as little as 15 seconds up to 6 minutes. Clot retraction follows and may take 30 to 60 minutes. After the clot is formed, it either dissolves or organizes into a fibrous mass.

### Blood Clot Composition

The blood clot is composed of a meshwork of polymerized fibrin threads that have become attached to blood cells, platelets, and plasma products. The fibrin threads adhere to the damaged vessel surface, holding the clot in place and preventing blood loss. The meshwork is produced by spontaneous aggregation of fibrin monomer to form polymer threads. Transglutaminase (factor XIII) acts on the fibrin to form covalent cross-links. This stabilizes the clot and makes it resistant to dissolution.[9,11]

### Clot Retraction

The contractile physiology of the platelet response is critical in clot retraction. Failure of a clot to retract often indicates a decrease in the number of platelets. The platelets entrapped in the clot continue to release fibrin-stabilizing factor. Stronger bonding of the fibrin threads occurs and causes the threads to contract. Clot retraction pulls the edges of a broken vessel closer together, which allows the vascular wall to mend. After contraction is completed, blood serum, which includes plasma and the clotting factors, is expressed from the clot.

## LYSIS OF BLOOD CLOTS

*Plasmin* or *fibrinolysin*, a proteolytic enzyme that resembles trypsin, is formed from inactive circulating plasminogen by the action of thrombin, which stimulates the production of *tissue-type plasminogen activator*.[11] It digests fibrin threads and causes lysis of the clot, along with destruction of blood clotting factors. Large amounts of the inactive enzyme plasminogen are incorporated into

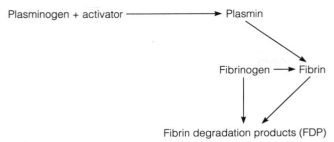

**FIGURE 21-5.**

Fibrinolysis. (Source: D.L. Barnard, *Clinical Haematology.* Oxford: Heinemann Med, 1989.)

the clot and activated by vascular endothelial factors, such as thrombin, activated factor XII, and lysosomal enzymes in damaged tissue (Figure 21-5).[5] Urokinase, a definite activator, is synthesized by renal cells and is present in the urine.[11] Bacterial organisms, especially streptococci, produce activators. In the case of the streptococcus organism, the activator is *streptokinase*, which has been used therapeutically to dissolve clots. Plasmin largely mediates the fibrinolytic system. This built-in, self-destructing system for clots breaks down and limits excessive clot formation. Plasmin is self-limiting and localizes the fibrinolytic activity to the region of the resolving clot. Inhibitors of plasmin prevent excessive proteolytic action.

Specific substances such as alpha$_2$-antiplasmin and alpha$_2$-macroglobulin inhibit plasmin action. Alpha$_2$-antiplasmin binds to fibrin by factor XIII during clot formation, so that the rate of fibrinolysis depends upon a balance of amounts of plasminogen, plasminogen activators, and antiplasmins within the clot.[11] The fibrinolytic system breaks down the clot so that healing can occur. Intravascularly, it assures patency of the vascular system.

The degradation products produced from fibrinolysis are called fibrinogen degradation products. They inhibit the formation of thrombin and limit the formation of the clot. A balance between the formation of thrombin and plasmin must be present for normal coagulation and clotting to occur.

## ANTICOAGULATION FACTORS IN NORMAL BLOOD

Anticoagulants inhibit coagulation and are important in keeping the blood fluid. An anticoagulant can be considered as any factor that prevents blood clotting. Factors that aid in the prevention of clotting include the smooth endothelial lining of the vessel, rapid blood flow through an area, negatively charged proteins on the endothelial surface, and anticoagulant substances in the blood.

A smooth endothelium and a monomolecular layer of negatively charged proteins adsorbed on the endothelium are essential for maintaining the fluidity of blood.[5]

Rapid blood flow dilutes the factors that promote coagulation, thus preventing initiation of the clotting process. An intact, smooth endothelium prevents contact activation of the intrinsic pathway, and the layer of negatively charged proteins repels clotting factors and platelets that might stick to the vessel wall.

Several plasma proteins can dampen the activity of proteolytic enzymes generated in the coagulation and fibrinolytic systems. These include antiplasmin, activated protein C inhibitor, antithrombin III, and alpha$_2$-macroglobulin.[5] These plasma proteins localize coagulation action at the site of injury and prevent propagation of the coagulation effect throughout the vascular system.

The most powerful anticoagulants in the blood are those that remove the excess thrombin formed during coagulation. These are *fibrin threads* and *antithrombin III*. During clot formation, 85% to 90% of thrombin becomes adsorbed to fibrin threads.[5] This adsorption effectively stops the action of thrombin on fibrinogen. Excess thrombin not adsorbed combines with the plasma protein antithrombin III, which blocks the effect of thrombin on fibrinogen and inactivates the thrombin.

Heparin, a potent anticoagulant, is present in the granules of the circulating basophils and the tissue mast cells. Its concentration in blood is very slight. Heparin acts as an anticoagulant mainly by inhibiting factor IX, factor X, and thrombin. It reacts with factors in both the intrinsic and extrinsic pathways.

## LABORATORY TESTS FOR COAGULATION PROBLEMS

### Clotting or Coagulation Time

One of the oldest tests for normal coagulation is based on the amount of time drawn blood takes to clot. This can be done simply by observing the clotting time in a test tube. Increased clotting time indicates that a problem exists, but normal clotting time does not rule out a hemostatic abnormality. The normal coagulation time (Lee-White) is 6 to 17 minutes in a glass tube or 19 to 60 minutes in a siliconized tube.[10]

Causes of prolonged clotting time include deficiencies of any factor in the intrinsic clotting system or in the common pathway, fibrinogen deficiency, or excessively rapid fibrinolysis. This test has long been used for persons receiving heparin therapy but is now being replaced by the partial thromboplastin time (PTT), which is a more sensitive measurement of the coagulation factors. Table 21-2 lists the laboratory tests for coagulation problems.

### Prothrombin Time

To perform the test for prothrombin time (PT), animal tissue extract and calcium are added to freshly drawn and

**TABLE 21-2.**

## NORMAL BLOOD COAGULATION VALUES

| TEST | NORMAL VALUES | SIGNIFICANCE OF ALTERED VALUES |
|------|---------------|--------------------------------|
| Clotting or coagulation time | 6–17 min (glass tube)<br>19–60 min (siliconized tube) | Prolonged in deficiency of all clotting factors except VIII and VII; used for heparin therapy control |
| Prothrombin time | 11–16 sec | Prolonged in deficiency of factors I, II, V, VII, and X; inadequate vitamin K in diet; extrinsic pathway |
| Partial thromboplastin time (PTT) | 60–90 sec | Prolonged by deficiency in factors I, II, V, VIII, IX, X, XI, and XII; intrinsic pathway; best single screening test; APTT most commonly used |
| Activated partial thromboplastin time (APTT) | 25–37 sec | |
| Platelet count | 140,000–340,000/$\mu$L (Rees-Ecker)<br>200,000–350,000/$\mu$L (Coulter Counter model B) | Increased in malignancy, myeloproliferative disease, iron deficiency anemia, collagen disorders, cirrhosis of the liver, thrombocytosis; decreased in thrombocytopenia, laboratory artifact, red blood cell count above 6.5 mil/mm$^3$ |
| Bleeding time | 4 min (Ivy method)<br>1–4 min (Duke method) | Prolonged in thrombocytopenia, drug-induced with aspirin, indomethacin, phenylbutazone, myeloproliferative diseases; normal in hemophilia A and B, hypoprothrombinemia, hypofibrinogenemia |
| Clot retraction | Begins: 30–60 min<br>Complete: 12–24 h | Prolonged in thrombocytopenia, thrombasthenia (oxygen release deficit) |

Source: J. Wallach, *Interpretation of Diagnostic Tests* (4th ed.). Boston: Little, Brown, 1986.

separated citrated plasma. The time the mixture takes to clot is given in seconds. The tissue extract bypasses the intrinsic clotting system so only factors VII, X, and V, prothrombin, and fibrinogen affect the test. Normal PT (11 to 16 seconds) is increased if any of the above factors is deficient.[10] The PT is often reported as a percentage of normal activity, which is a way of expressing the activity of factors in comparison to a normal control. Normal is always considered to be 100%. If the individual measures at 20%, only about one fifth of normal clotting activity exists. A person having faster clotting activity than the control can have greater than 100% activity. An *increased* PT refers to a longer time for clotting to occur, with clotting ability being less than normal. A *decreased* PT refers to the reverse. Deficiencies of factors XII, XI, IX, and VIII do not affect the PT.

The PT is often used to monitor the effects of the coumarin anticoagulants. Coumarin depresses the synthesis of factors VII, IX, X, and prothrombin.

## *Partial Thromboplastin Time*

Partial thromboplastin time is a relatively simple test for mild to moderate deficiencies of intrinsic clotting factors. It is useful for detecting many types of bleeding disorders due to decreased amounts of factors composing the intrinsic system. It is a general test that is used to monitor heparin therapy. Chemicals are often added to achieve an activated PTT (APTT). The resulting clotting time is accelerated.

The PTT increases (becomes longer) both in hereditary factor deficiencies and in acquired conditions such as disseminated intravascular coagulation (DIC) (see pp. 418–419). Therapeutic heparin is used to keep the PTT at 1.5 to 2.5 times the normal level. Deficiencies of all the factors prolong the PTT with the exception of factor VII. A person with a factor VII deficiency has a normal PTT and a prolonged PT. Partial thromboplastin time can be used to demonstrate circulating anticoagulants in plasma. If test plasma mixed with normal plasma has a longer PTT than normal plasma alone, it indicates that something in the test plasma has inhibited coagulation.

## Tests for Specific Deficiencies

Special tests can determine the absence of specific clotting factors. These are specific coagulation factor assays. Any of the other specific factors can be tested. Small amounts of blood are added to samples of plasma known to be deficient in a particular factor. If, for example, the added plasma corrects the PTT to normal for plasma known to be deficient in a particular factor, that factor is not deficient in the sample. The process is repeated until the tested plasma does not correct the PTT. This identifies the missing factor in the plasma of the individual being tested. Several special tests for coagulation factors are based on this laboratory method.

## Platelet Count

One of the most common laboratory tests, the complete blood count, usually includes the platelet count. Platelets normally range from about 140,000 to 340,000 per $\mu$L (Rees-Ecker) or 200,000 to 350,000 per $\mu$L (Coulter Counter Model B).[10] Platelets are difficult to count because of their inherent tendency to clump, adhere to the vessel, and aggregate. Electronic means of counting them offer the greatest accuracy.

Thrombocytosis, elevated platelet count, may occur in association with certain malignancies and with polycythemia vera.[3] Thrombocytopenia, decreased platelet count, may be secondary to many conditions or it may be idiopathic (see p. 422).

## Bleeding Time

To measure *bleeding time* an incision is made either on the earlobe (Duke method) or on the inner surface of the forearm (Ivy method). The time needed for active bleeding from the clean, superficial wound to stop is called the bleeding time. Normal bleeding time is less than 4 minutes by the Ivy method and 1 to 4 minutes by the Duke method.[10] The variables involved are vascular contractility and platelet aggregation.

*Secondary bleeding time* can be measured by noting

how long it takes for bleeding to cease after a scab is removed. Secondary bleeding time is prolonged in persons with deficiencies of factors in the intrinsic pathway or factor XIII, the fibrin-stabilizing factor.

## Clot Retraction

Measuring the clot retraction time consists of observing the time in which a clot retracts and expresses serum, and the degree of retraction. Whole blood is left in a test tube at 37°C. Clot retraction normally begins in about 30 minutes; by 4 hours, a well-defined clot is surrounded by clear serum. Complete retraction requires about 12 to 24 hours if measured at room temperature. The norm is 50% to 100% in 2 hours.[10] If platelet function or number is decreased, clot retraction is impaired.

# DEFICIENCIES IN BLOOD COAGULATION

Deficiency of any of the clotting factors can result in a defect or impairment of blood coagulation. This impairment may result from genetic deficiencies of clotting factors, or suppression or consumption of the major clotting components. Coagulation does not occur as an isolated, independent event but continually interacts with other mechanisms of the body, such as the inflammatory process. Alterations in the process can result in injury, hemorrhage, or death.

## Single Coagulation Factor Deficiencies

Single coagulation factor deficiencies are usually hereditary. The most common deficiencies are of factor VIII, IX, and XI. All cause bleeding that may involve any of the soft tissues or the joints.

### Hemophilia

Hemophilia loosely defines several different hereditary deficiencies of coagulation factors of the intrinsic pathway. The most common cause of this coagulation disorder is a deficiency in factor VIII, accounting for about 83% to 85% of cases of hemophilia.[4] Usually factor VIII is produced, but it is abnormal and does not promote coagulation.

The classic factor VIII deficiency is genetically transmitted through a sex-linked recessive gene. It affects men almost exclusively. Women are usually asymptomatic carriers but in rare cases may manifest the disease.[1] This type of hemophilia is called *classic hemophilia* or *hemo-*

*philia A.* It is characterized by spontaneous or traumatic subcutaneous and intramuscular hemorrhages. Hematuria and bleeding from the mouth, gums, lips, and tongue are common manifestations. Repeated joint hemorrhages cause extreme pain and deformity. The severity of the bleeding depends upon the coagulation factor levels with borderline factor VIII (0.05 $\mu$ per mL with a normal range of 0.5 to 2.0 $\mu$ per mL, causing problems only with post-traumatic or postsurgical bleeding). Levels less than 0.02 $\mu$ per mL result in spontaneous bleeding episodes.[1] Transfusion of normal factor VIII or fresh plasma relieves the bleeding tendency for a short time.

*von Willebrand's disease* is characterized by a quantitative and qualitative deficiency of factor VIII. Because of this deficiency, adhesion of platelets to the injury-exposed collagen is impaired. This condition produces a prolonged bleeding time with a mild to moderate bleeding disorder. Epistaxis, gastrointestinal bleeding, and menorrhagia are common.[1] von Willebrand factor is one of the products of factor VIII (VIII R).[11] This condition, usually of autosomal dominant basis, has been shown to be associated with some of the autoimmune or lymphoproliferative conditions.

Factor IX deficiency, called *hemophilia B* or *Christmas disease*, is sex-linked, recessive, and accounts for about 10% to 15% of cases of hemophilia. Clinically, it is indistinguishable from factor VIII hemophilia and requires laboratory differentiation.[1] Bleeding tends to be severe with crippling joint deformities. This condition is sometimes seen in association with severe protein-wasting glomerulopathies.[4]

Factor XI deficiency, called *hemophilia C* or *Rosenthal's disease*, is a mild bleeding disorder manifested by bruising, epistaxis, and menorrhagia. It is transmitted as an autosomal recessive trait and accounts for about 2% of hemophiliacs. The mildness of this disease is thought to be due to activation of factor XI through other mechanisms.[11]

## Vitamin K Deficiency

Many disorders can lead to deficiencies of several coagulation factors. One example is fat-soluble vitamin K, which is required for the synthesis of factors II, VII, IX, and X. These vitamin K-dependent factors can be monitored by PT. Deficiencies of vitamin K may result from several conditions. A newborn is normally deficient in vitamin K due to an immature liver and lack of intestinal bacteria that are important for the synthesis of the vitamin. The newborn is often given injections of vitamin K to help prevent any possible bleeding disorder that might occur.

Obstructive liver disease and malabsorption disorders can also cause a deficiency in vitamin K. Obstructive liver disease blocks the flow of bile necessary for the ab-

sorption of fat-soluble vitamins, and malabsorption disorders to not allow enough vitamin K to be absorbed into the circulation.

Coumarin anticoagulants are competitive inhibitors of vitamin K. Vitamin K can be injected as an antidote in case of excessive bleeding or possible hemorrhage due to overdose of these drugs.

## Liver Disease

Both coagulation disorders and platelet dysfunction are present in persons with significant liver disease. The liver is essential for the synthesis of the coagulation proteins and for the removal of activated coagulation products from the circulation.[1] Liver disease may produce platelet dysfunction and thrombocytopenia. Any form of severe liver dysfunction, such as that produced from hepatitis, shock state, poisoning, or acute alcohol-induced dysfunction, can produce abnormal coagulation. The abnormal coagulation results from the following: (1) reduced coagulation factor synthesis; (2) failure to remove activated products; (3) impaired clearance of the fibrinolytic enzymes; and (4) accompanying DIC.[1]

Replacement therapy, such as fresh frozen plasma, may be needed to stop bleeding, but it is only a temporary measure due to the short half-life of factor VII, which is only 5 hours.[1]

## Massive Transfusion Syndrome

If a large volume of blood is administered over a short time, there will be a decrease in circulating coagulation factors and platelets. Bank blood is usually deficient in factors V and VIII, and platelets.[1] It also is collected into bags that contain citric acid, which prevents clotting. If the amounts of blood administered are massive, a generalized bleeding disorder may occur.[1]

## Disseminated Intravascular Coagulation/Consumptive Coagulopathy

Disseminated intravascular coagulation involves both bleeding and clotting. It occurs as a complication of several clinical conditions that trigger senseless activation of the clotting factors within the circulating blood.[8] It can be caused by a wide range of factors and can be manifested as a life-threatening hemorrhage or a subclinical disorder noted only on laboratory examination.[1] The process begins with activation of the sequence causing coagulation. This hypercoagulable state produces thrombosis, especially in the small vessels.[7] Widespread coagulation acti-

**TABLE 21–3.**
ETIOLOGY OF DISSEMINATED INTRAVASCULAR COAGULATION

| CAUSATIVE AGENT OR CONDITION | PROBABLE MASSIVE COAGULATION STIMULUS |
|---|---|
| Infection | |
| Gram-negative bacteria | Endotoxemia; endothelial damage |
| Gram-positive bacteria | Fulminating sepsis; endothelial damage |
| *Rickettsia rickettsii;* (Rocky Mountain spotted fever) | Parasitization of endothelial cells; rupture walls of small vessels |
| *Plasmodium falciparum;* (falciparum malaria) | Injury to red cells and platelets; possible antigen-antibody reaction |
| Complications of pregnancy | |
| Amniotic fluid embolism | Circulating thromboplastins absorbed |
| Saline abortion | |
| Hydatidiform mole | |
| Puerperal sepsis | Vascular damage |
| Toxemia | |
| Large hemangiomas | Turbulence of blood, stasis Endothelial damage |
| Disseminated carcinoma | Circulating tissue thromboplastins from malignant tissue |
| Hemolytic transfusion RX anaphylaxis, hemolytic-uremic syndrome | Antigen–antibody reactions |
| Tissue damage | |
| Massive trauma | Thromboplastins released |
| Heat stroke | |
| Extensive burns | |
| Snake bites | |
| Extracorporeal circulation | Blood injury |

vation leads to consumption of clotting factors, such as platelets and fibrin. Secondary activation of the fibrinolytic system then occurs. Table 21-3 indicates some of the diverse factors that can initiate the coagulation sequence.

Persons who develop DIC are often critically ill as a result of the underlying pathology. The DIC often develops insidiously and widespread bleeding becomes the initial sign.

The clotting sequence is triggered either by endothelial damage that activates the intrinsic coagulation cascade or by release of thromboplastic substances. The resultant clotting causes occlusion of a large proportion of the small peripheral blood vessels. The clotting sequence activates the fibrinolytic system and thus causes diffuse fibrinolysis. The conversion of plasminogen to plasmin in the fibrinolytic system inhibits the proteolysis of fibrinogen by thrombin and may inhibit platelet aggregation. Fibrin degradation (split) products are formed by the lysis of plasmin, fibrinogen, and fibrin. These end products form a complex with the fibrin monomer, which prevents the laying down of the fibrin thread and platelet aggregation. Therefore, despite widespread clotting, the major problem is bleeding (Figure 21-6).

Uncontrolled bleeding occurs because of consumption of the clotting factors. Normal hemostasis is prevented so varying degrees of ecchymoses, petechiae, and bleeding from any opening may occur. The onset may be acute, such as that after acute obstetric emergencies, or it may gradually develop, as with disseminated cancers. Bleeding problems usually predominate, and venipuncture sites or incisions may bleed profusely.

Acrocyanosis often occurs in the digits and is manifest as cold, mottled fingers and toes. Hypoxemia may cause dyspnea, cyanosis, and air hunger. Neurologic or renal symptoms may result from microthrombi that occlude the small vessels.

Laboratory tests that are helpful include the PT, PTT, fibrinogen level, and platelet count. Both the PT and PTT are prolonged, while fibrinogen and platelet levels are depressed. Levels of fibrin split or degradation products are elevated.[1]

## Primary Fibrinolysis

Primary fibrinolysis results when massive amounts of plasminogen activator are released into the system. The activator, such as streptokinase, may be administered therapeutically to dissolve pulmonary emboli. Plasminogen activators can also be released by activator-rich neoplastic tissue, such as prostatic carcinoma. Severe anoxia, shock, or surgical procedures may also precipitate their release.

Disseminated intravascular coagulation and primary

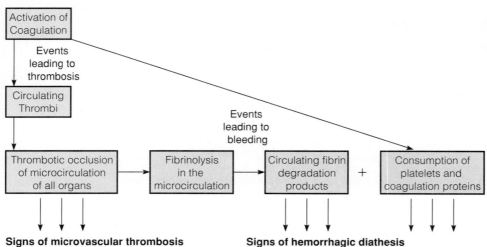

**FIGURE 21-6.**
Sequential events during DIC that
lead to both thrombotic and hemorrhagic manifestations. (Source:
V.J. Mander, *Microvascular Thrombosis in Hematology and Oncology,*
M.A. Lichtman, New York: Grune
and Stratton, 1980.)

**Signs of microvascular thrombosis**

- Neurologic : Multifocal, delirium, coma.
- Skin : focal ischemia, superficial gangrene.
- Renal : oliguria, azotemia, cortical necrosis.
- Pulmonary : acute respiratory distress syndrome.
- Gastrointestinal : acute ulceration.

**Signs of hemorrhagic diathesis**

- Neurologic : intracerebral bleeding.
- Skin : petechiae, ecchymoses, venipuncture oozing.
- Renal : hematuria.
- Mucous membranes : epistaxis, gingival oozing.
- Gastrointestinal

fibrinolysis reactions are similar. Both are associated with increased fibrinolytic activity, but primary fibrinolysis results in increased amounts of plasminogen activator in the plasma. In DIC, it is a secondary response to a hypercoagulable state.

### Antibody Anticoagulants

Antibodies to various coagulation factors have been observed in many disease states. About 10% of persons treated for hemophilia A develop an antifactor antibody to factor VIII.[1] Antibodies to paraproteins in those with multiple myelomas and antibodies to multiple coagulation factors in persons with systemic lupus erythematosus are other examples of antibodies that act as circulating anticoagulants. The development of antibodies to coagulation factors results in an increased risk of hemorrhage.

### Platelet Disorders

#### Thrombocytopenia

This quantitative platelet disorder involves the presence of a very low number of platelets in the circulatory system. If the platelet number falls below 50,000, there is a potential for hemorrhage associated with trauma, such as surgery or accidents. A platelet count of about 20,000 is associated with petechiae, ecchymoses, and sometimes bleeding from mucous membranes. With a count below 5000, a great risk exists for fatal hemorrhage through the intestinal tract or central nervous system.[2]

An abnormal decrease in the number of platelets may occur in several disorders, such as defective platelet production, increased platelet destruction, sequestration of platelets, and loss of platelets from the system. The two major types of thrombocytopenia are: idiopathic thrombocytopenic purpura (ITP) and secondary thrombocytopenia. Table 21-4 classifies causes of thrombocytopenia by mechanism. Figure 21-7 illustrates the evaluation of thrombocytopenia to determine the cause.

Idiopathic thrombocytopenia purpura is apparently an autoimmune condition that causes an increased rate of destruction of platelets. The result is either acute destruction of platelets, which often follows a viral infection, or chronic ITP, which may be associated with another autoimmune disease, such as autoimmune hemolytic anemia.[6] The pathogenesis appears to involve the production of autoantibodies directed against the platelets. Clinical manifestations include diffuse petechiae, ecchymosis, epistaxis, hemorrhages into the soft tissues, melena, or hematuria.

Secondary thrombocytopenia commonly occurs in association with drug hypersensitivity, viral infections, and some of the autoimmune conditions. The platelet count is depressed as a result of a superimposed hemorrhagic problem caused by the underlying condition. Some of the drugs that may induce secondary thrombocytopenia are chlorothiazide derivatives, gold thiomalate, diphenylhydantoin, acetaminophen, quinidine, sulfonamides, chloramphenicol, antimetabolites, and antihistamines. The drug usually acts as a hapten; the antibody–drug complex binds to platelets, fixes complement, and causes intravascular damage.[6]

### Qualitative Platelet Disorders

Qualitative platelet disorders include alterations that have a prolonged bleeding time with a normal platelet

**TABLE 21–4.**

CLASSIFICATION OF THE THROMBOCYTOPENIAS

| TYPE OF DISORDER | ETIOLOGY |
|---|---|
| **Decreased Production** | |
| Hypoproliferation | Toxic agents, especially drug toxicity; radiation, infection; constitutional factors (Fanconi's anemia, etc.); idiopathic aplastic anemia; paroxysmal nocturnal hemoglobinuria; myelophthisis (tumor, fibrosis, etc) |
| Infective thrombopoiesis | Megaloblastic anemia; Di Guglielmo's syndrome; familial thrombocytopenia |
| **Abnormal Distribution** | Congestive splenomegaly; myeloid metaplasia, lymphoma; Gaucher's disease |
| **Dilutional Loss** | Massive blood transfusion |
| **Dysfunction** | |
| Drug-induced | Drugs that cause platelet dysfunction include: aspirin, nonsteroidal antiinflammatory drugs, alcohol, antihistamines, tricyclic antidepressants, phenothiazines, sulphapyrazone |
| Systemic disease | Renal disease; liver disease; myeloproliferative diseases; hereditary protein disorders; leukemia and myelodysplasia |
| **Abnormal Destruction** | |
| Consumption | Disseminated intravascular coagulation, vasculitis; thrombotic thrombocytopenia (TTP) |
| Immune mechanism | Idiopathic thrombocytopenic purpura (ITP); drug-induced thrombocytopenia; chronic lymphocytic leukemia, lymphoma, LE; neonatal thrombocytopenia; posttransfusion purpura |

Source: *Adapted from W.S. Beck,* Hematology *(4th ed.). Cambridge, MA.: MIT Press, 1985; and D.L. Barnard,* Clinical Haematology. *Oxford: Heinemann Med., 1989.*

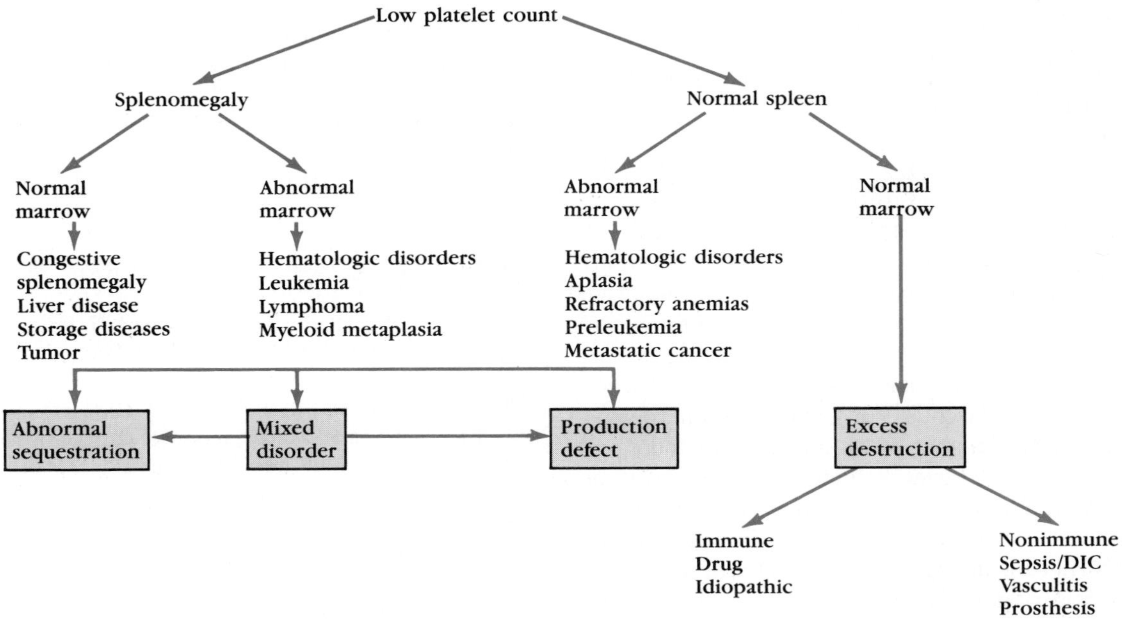

**FIGURE 21–7.**

A schematic approach to the clinical evaluation of thrombocytopenia. (Source: W.S. Beck, *Hematology* (4th ed.). Cambridge, Mass.: MIT Press, 1985.)

count in most instances. The disorders are due to a variety of defects of platelet function, such as in platelet adhesion in von Willebrand's disease, or in platelet aggregation as in thrombasthenia, a congenital disorder.

Qualitative platelet disorders can also be acquired. Drugs such as aspirin may impair the aggregation of platelets. In uremia, a dialyzable factor is formed that inhibits platelet aggregation.

## Thrombocytosis

Thrombocytosis (thrombocythemia) is an increased number of platelets in the peripheral blood. Counts of 400,000 to 1,000,000 per $\mu$L are usually asymptomatic, but counts greater than 1,000,000 per $\mu$L may result in thrombosis or bleeding when the excessive numbers of platelets are dysfunctional.[2] Physiologic thrombocytosis occurs in response to infection, trauma, and other conditions. It almost always occurs after splenectomy when all of the platelets are circulated in the blood because they can no longer pool in the spleen. Idiopathic thrombocythemia refers to a sustained platelet count of greater than 800,000 per $\mu$L. The condition is generally regarded as one of the myeloproliferative disorders due to its responsiveness to chemotherapy. It occurs with splenic enlargement and may be associated with other myeloproliferative disorders, such as chronic myelogenous leukemia and polycythemia vera. Affected individuals often exhibit peripheral thrombosis and episodes of spontaneous bleeding.

## Hypercoagulation

Hypercoagulation may involve accelerated rates of coagulation, hyperviscosity, and increased platelet activity or antithrombin III deficiency. The term refers to an increased propensity of the blood to clot. The condition has been seen in association with atherosclerosis, blood stasis, hemangiomas, and certain myeloproliferative diseases.

*Thrombotic thrombocytopenic purpura,* a rare disorder, is characterized by thrombocytopenia, anemia, neurologic deficits, and renal failure. Endothelial cell damage may be the activator in the disorder, with an immune vasculitis affecting the endothelial cells. Platelet adhesion and aggregation lead to obstruction of the vessel and ischemia of the surrounding tissues.[4]

Blood stasis in the small vessels is enhanced when the blood is more viscous. Polycythemia increases viscosity and affects the rate of blood flow. An increased number of any of the formed elements may increase the viscosity of blood. Giant hemangiomas may precipitate massive blood turbulence with stasis in the affected vascular bed. There is an increased platelet and fibrinogen turnover, and coagulation in and around the hemangioma is common.

Hyperfunction of platelets in the absence of thrombocytosis has been postulated as a mechanism for various pathologies. It is theorized that strokes and transient ischemic attacks in younger persons who have no evidence of arterial abnormalities or degenerative changes could be the result of hyperfunction of the platelets. Platelet clumping in small vessels may result in alterations of blood supply.[11]

Platelet activation and release of thromboxane $A_2$ may lead to coronary artery spasm, ischemia, and infarction. Platelet function in these cases can be examined by laboratory means for increased sensitivity to aggregating agents and increased release of thromboxane $A_2$ and other platelet factors.

Antithrombin III deficiency is an inherited familial disorder that results in thrombosis. The antithrombin III inactivates most of the active proteases involved in thrombin formation. A modest decrease in this inhibitor allows the proteases to remain active for a longer period, which results in the rapid formation of thrombi. Antithrombin III deficiency can also occur as an acquired disorder and is associated with liver disease or DIC. Oral contraceptives and heparin also reduce antithrombin III levels.

Myeloproliferative diseases of many sorts may elaborate factors, which initiate the coagulation sequence. Usually the coagulation pattern results in activation of the fibrinolytic system and DIC.

## REFERENCES

1. Barnard, D.L. *Clinical Haematology.* Oxford: Heinemann Med., 1989.
2. Chanarin, I. *Laboratory Haematology: An Account of Laboratory Techniques.* Edinburgh: Churchill-Livingstone, 1989.
3. Cormack, D.H. *Ham's Histology* (9th ed.). Philadelphia: J.B. Lippincott, 1987.
4. Cotran, R.S., Kumar, V., and Robbins, S.L. *Robbins' Pathologic Basis of Disease* (4th ed.). Philadelphia: W.B. Saunders, 1989.
5. Guyton, A.C. *Textbook of Medical Physiology* (8th ed.). Philadelphia: W.B. Saunders, 1990.
6. Handin, R.J. Hemorrhagic disorders II: Platelets and purpura. In W.S. Beck, *Hematology* (4th ed.). Cambridge, Mass.: MIT Press, 1985.
7. Handin, R.J., and Rosenberg, R.D. Hemorrhagic disorders III: Disorders of primary and secondary hemostasis. In W.S. Beck, *Hematology* (4th ed.). Cambridge, Mass.: MIT Press, 1985.
8. Jandl, J.A. *Blood Textbook of Hematology.* Boston: Little, Brown, 1987.
9. Rosenberg, R.D. Hemorrhagic disorders I: Protein interactions in the clotting mechanisms. In W.S. Beck, *Hematology* (4th ed.). Cambridge, Mass.: MIT Press, 1985.

**10.** Wallach, J. *Interpretation of Diagnostic Tests* (4th ed.). Boston: Little, Brown, 1986.

**11.** Weatherall, D.J., and Bunch, C. The blood and blood-forming organs. In L.H. Smith and S.O. Thier, *Pathophysiology: The Biological Principles of Disease* (2nd ed.). Philadelphia: W.B. Saunders, 1985.

## UNIT BIBLIOGRAPHY

Anderson, J.R. *Muir's Textbook of Pathology* (12th ed.). London: Arnold, 1985.

Back, R.R. Initiation of coagulation by tissue factor. *CRC: Critical Reviews in Biochemistry* 23(4):339, 1988.

Baker, W.F. Clinical aspects of disseminated intravascular coagulation: A clinician's point of view. *Seminars in Thrombosis and Hemostasis* 15(1):1, 1989.

Barnard, D.L. *Clinical Haematology*. Oxford: Heineman Med., 1989.

Baughan, A., Hughes, A., Patterson, K., and Stirling, L. *Manual of Haematology*. Edinburgh: Churchill-Livingstone, 1985.

Beck, W.S. *Hematology* (4th ed.). Cambridge, Mass.: MIT Press, 1985.

Begeman, H., and Rastetter, J. *Atlas of Clinical Hematology* (4th ed.). Berlin: Springer-Verlag, 1989.

Brown, B. *Hematology: Principles and Procedures* (5th ed.). Philadelphia: Lea & Febiger, 1988.

Carr, M.E. Disseminated intravascular coagulation: Pathogenesis, diagnosis, and therapy. *J. Emerg. Med.* 5(4):311, 1987.

Chanarin, I. *Laboratory Haematology: An Account of Laboratory Techniques*. Edinburgh: Churchill-Livingstone, 1989.

Cotran, R.S., Kumar, V., and Robbins, S.L. *Robbins' Pathologic Basis of Disease* (4th ed.). Philadelphia: W.B. Saunders, 1989.

Cozzolino, F., Torcia, M., and Miliani, A. Potential role of interleukin 1 as the trigger for diffuse intravascular coagulation in acute nonlymphoblastic leukemia. *Am. J. Med.* 84(2):240, 1988.

Donovan, E.V. *Essentials of Pathophysiology*. New York: Macmillan, 1985.

Ferguson, G.C. *Pathophysiology, Mechanisms and Expressions*. Philadelphia: W.B. Saunders, 1984.

Ganong, W.F. *Review of Medical Physiology* (15th ed.). Los Altos, Calif.: Lange, 1991.

Golden, A., Powell, D., and Jennings, C.D. *Pathology, Understanding Human Disease* (2nd ed.). Baltimore: Williams & Wilkins, 1985.

Guyton, A. *Textbook of Medical Physiology* (8th ed.). Philadelphia: W.B. Saunders, 1990.

Hardisty, R.M., and Weatherall, D.J. *Blood and Its Disorders* (2nd ed.). Boston: Blackwell, 1982.

Hauptman, J.G., Hassouda, H.I., Bell, T.G., Penner, J.A., and Amerson, T.E. Efficacy of antithrombin III in endotoxin-induced disseminated intravascular coagulation. *Circulatory Shock* 25(2):111, 1988.

Hocking, W.G. *Practical Hematology*. New York: Wiley, 1983.

Hughes-Jones, N.C. *Lecture Notes on Haematology* (4th ed.). Oxford: Blackwell, 1984.

Jandl, J.A. *Blood: Textbook of Hematology*. Boston: Little, Brown, 1987.

Kelley, W., et al. *Textbook of Internal Medicine*. Philadelphia: J.B. Lippincott, 1989.

Kissane, J.M. *Anderson's Pathology* (9th ed.). St. Louis: Mosby, 1990.

Krupp, M.A., Chatton, M.J., and Tierney, L.M. *Current Medical Diagnosis and Treatment 1986*. Los Altos, Calif.: Lange, 1986.

Mazza, J. *Manual of Clinical Hematology*. Boston: Little, Brown, 1988.

McDonald, G.A., Paul, J., and Cruickshank, B. *Atlas of Haematology* (5th ed.). Edinburgh: Churchill-Livingstone, 1988.

Miale, J.B. *Laboratory Medicine: Hematology* (6th ed.). St. Louis: Mosby, 1982.

Muller-Berghaus, G. Pathophysiologic and biochemical events in disseminated intravascular coagulation: Dysregulation of procoagulant and anticoagulant pathways. *Semin. Thromb. Hemost.* 15(1):58, 1989.

Rifkind, R.A., et al. *Fundamentals of Hematology* (3rd ed.). Chicago: Yearbook, 1986.

Sheldon, H. *Boyd's Introduction to the Study of Disease* (9th ed.). Philadelphia: Lea & Febiger, 1984.

Smith, L.H., and Thier, S.O. *Pathophysiology: The Biological Principles of Disease* (2nd ed.). Philadelphia: W.B. Saunders, 1985.

Sodeman, W.A., and Sodeman, T.M. *Sodeman's Pathologic Physiology* (7th ed.). Philadelphia: W.B. Saunders, 1985.

Spivak, J.L. *Fundamentals of Clinical Hematology* (2nd ed.). Philadelphia: Harper & Row, 1984.

Thompson, R.B. *A Concise Textbook of Hematology* (6th ed.). Baltimore: Urban & Schwarzenberg, 1984.

Turgeon, M.L. *Clinical Hematology: Theory and Procedures*. Boston: Little, Brown, 1988.

Williams, J.W., et al. *Hematology* (4th ed.). New York: McGraw-Hill, 1990.

Wilson, J., et al. *Harrison's Principles of Internal Medicine* (12th ed.). New York: McGraw-Hill, 1991.

Wintrobe, M.M., et al. *Clinical Hematology* (8th ed.). Philadelphia: Lea & Febiger, 1981.

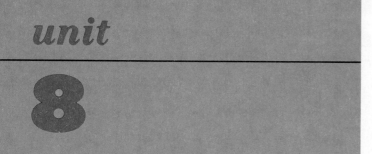

# CIRCULATION

The study of circulation requires an understanding of both normal dynamics and alterations of related structures that lead to the effects of compromised tissue perfusion.

Chapter 22 examines the anatomy of the heart and vessels. The physiology of the system is reviewed in sufficient depth to support the contents of subsequent chapters. An attempt has been made to relate the electrophysiology of the heart to electrocardiography. The major cardiac dysrhythmias are described in Chapter 23. The material presented in these two chapters provides a physiologic basis for much of the information in subsequent chapters.

Chapter 24 details heart failure, which commonly results from other heart conditions and may be the end result of other system dysfunctions. Chapter 25 details specific diseases of the heart and pericardium. Chapter 26 classifies and clarifies hypertension. Chapter 27 discusses arterial and venous peripheral vascular disease.

It is suggested that the reader use the learning objectives in each chapter and the bibliography at the end of the unit to enhance learning.

# chapter 22

Barbara L. Bullock

# Normal Circulatory Dynamics

*Chapter Outline*

*Learning Objectives*

1. Locate the major structures of the heart, including the chambers, valves, and vessels.
2. Compare the three layers that compose the atrial and ventricular walls.
3. Show the positions of the trabeculae carneae, the papillary muscles, and the chordae tendineae.
4. Differentiate the structures of the atrioventricular valves and the semilunar valves.
5. Locate the origin and the branches of both the right and left coronary arteries.
6. Trace the conduction system of the heart.
7. Structurally differentiate a myocardial muscle cell and a skeletal muscle cell.
8. Define *intercalated disk* and *syncytium.*
9. Review the general mechanism for skeletal muscle contraction.
10. Compare skeletal and cardiac muscle contraction.
11. Define *absolute and relative refractory periods in cardiac muscle.*
12. Describe cardiac metabolism and cardiac work.
13. Describe clearly the properties of the heart: automaticity, rhythmicity, excitability, and conductivity.
14. Define *diastolic depolarization* in the sinoatrial node and indicate why it is considered to be the pacemaker of the heart.
15. Relate the events of the cardiac cycle to the wave forms seen on an electrocardiogram tracing.
16. Describe the four interrelated factors of cardiac contraction: preload, afterload, contractility, and heart rate.
17. Define ventricular compliance.
18. Define *inotropic and chronotropic effects.*
19. Describe the events of the cardiac cycle.
20. Differentiate isovolumic contraction, ejection, and isovolumic relaxation as phases in ventricular systole.
21. Explain how a different stroke volume between the ventricles is compensated for or equalized.
22. List the normal pressures and oxygen saturations in the chambers of the heart and in the vessels.
23. Describe the factors responsible for generating heart sounds.

*(continued)*

Understanding the dynamics of normal cardiac contraction provides the basis for understanding the effects of alterations to structures within the heart, myocardial muscle, and vessels. The first part of this chapter is devoted to normal cardiac anatomy and physiology; the second part deals with the dynamics of circulation.

## ANATOMY OF THE HEART

The heart is a double pump that pumps its blood to the lungs and to the systemic arteries. It provides for oxygenation and nutrition of all of the tissues of the body.

The heart is composed of four pumping chambers: the right and left atria and the right and left ventricles. The right atrium and ventricle receive blood from the systemic veins and pump it to the lungs through the pulmonary artery. The left atrium and ventricle pump blood received from the pulmonary veins to the systemic arteries through the aorta. Figure 22-1 shows the general anatomy of the heart and blood vessels along with direction of blood flow.

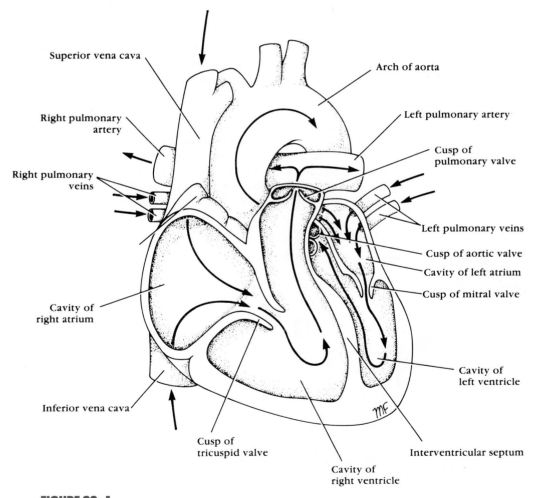

**FIGURE 22-1.**
Anatomy of the heart and great vessels. Arrows show the flow of blood through the heart. (From R.S. Snell, *Clinical Histology for Medical Students*, Boston: Little, Brown, 1984.)

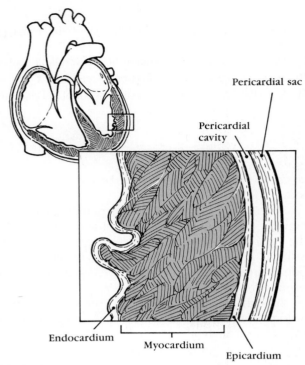

**FIGURE 22-2.**
Cross-section showing the layers of the ventricles. Note the thin endocardial layer in relation to the thick myocardium.

## Atria

The *right atrium* is a low pressure, thin-walled chamber that receives blood from the superior and inferior vena cava and from the veins draining the heart. The *left atrium* is slightly smaller than the right and receives blood from the four pulmonary veins that carry oxygenated blood from the lungs back to the heart.

The atrial walls are composed of three layers: (1) epicardium, a thin outer layer that is continuous with the outer layer of the ventricles; (2) myocardium, the middle or muscular layer of the atria, discontinuous with that of the ventricles; and (3) endocardium, a thin, continuous, inner layer that covers the inner surface of the atria, the valves, ventricles, and vessels entering and leaving the heart. The muscular layer of the atria is much thinner than that in the ventricles and accounts for the lower pressures maintained in these chambers. The atria serve mostly as storage reservoirs and as conductive passageways for the movement of blood to the ventricles.

Dividing the right atrium from the left atrium is the membranous atrial septum, a separation that prevents the communication of blood between the atria. This septum houses the fossa ovalis, which originated as a fetal communication, the foramen ovale (see Chap. 25).

## Ventricles

The ventricular walls are also composed of three layers: epicardium, myocardium, and endocardium (Figure 22-2). The right ventricle has been described as looking like a bellows, with a myocardial layer that is thicker than that in the atrial walls but thinner than that of the left ventricle. The left ventricle is more circular than the right. Its myocardial muscle layer is much thicker than that in the right ventricle, which allows it to achieve the high pressures required for systemic arterial circulation.

Separating the ventricles is the ventricular septum, a thick muscular structure that becomes membranous as it nears the atrioventricular valves (Figure 22-3). This septum contains the branches of the conduction tissue and provides an important fulcrum during contraction of the ventricles.

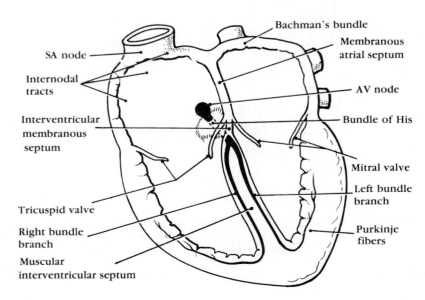

**FIGURE 22-3.**
Interventricular septum and branches of the conduction system.

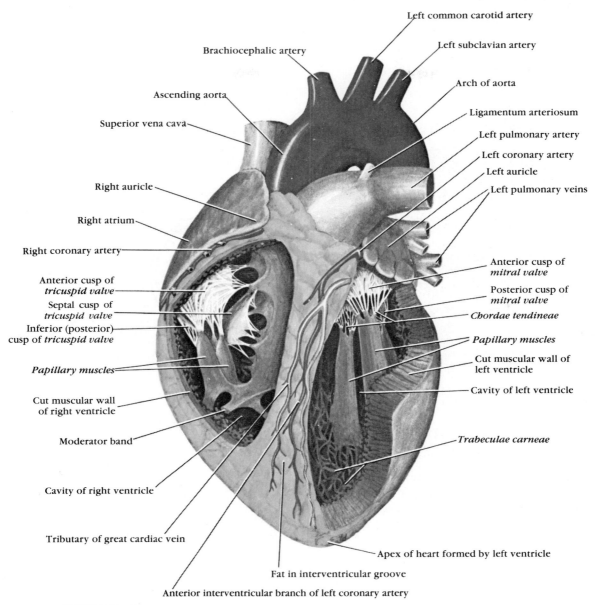

**FIGURE 22-4.**
The heart viewed from the left side. The anterior wall of the right ventricle and posterior wall of the left ventricle have been removed. Note the trabeculae carneae, or raised muscle bundle are more prominent in the left ventricle than the right (Source: R.S. Snell, *Atlas of Clinical Anatomy*. Boston: Little, Brown, 1978.)

The inner surface of the ventricles contains areas of raised muscle bundles that are undercut by open spaces. These muscle bundles are called the *trabeculae carneae*. The papillary muscles project from the trabeculated surface, giving rise to two groups of papillary muscles in the left ventricle and three groups in the right. These muscles give off strong fibrous strands called *chordae tendineae*, which attach to the margins of the atrioventricular valves (Figure 22-4).

## Atrioventricular Valves

The mitral or bicuspid valve and the tricuspid valve are called the atrioventricular (AV) valves. They separate the atria from the ventricles.

The mitral (bicuspid) valve lies between the left atrium and the left ventricle (see Figure 22-4). It is composed of two leaflets of fibroelastic tissue that slightly overlap each other when the valve is in the closed posi-

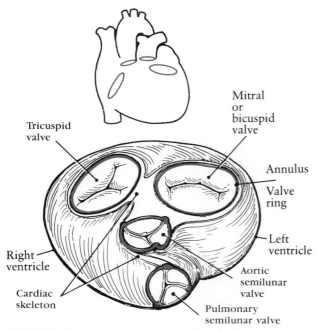

**FIGURE 22-5**
Fibrous rings of cardiac skeleton surround the heart valves as viewed from above. Valves are in the closed position.

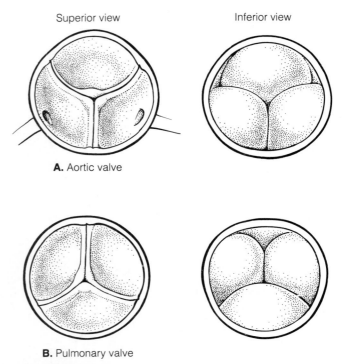

**A.** Aortic valve

**B.** Pulmonary valve

**FIGURE 22-6.**
**A.** Aortic valve in closed position viewed from above and below.
**B.** Pulmonic valve in closed position viewed from above and below.

tion (Figure 22-5). The margins of the valve are attached to the fibrous chordae tendineae.

The tricuspid valve is composed of three leaflets and lies between the right atrium and the right ventricle. The leaflets, also composed of fibrous tissue, are thinner than those of the mitral valve. These are also attached to chordae tendineae that project from the right ventricular papillary muscles (see Figure 22-4). The anulus (valve ring) that surrounds each valve is quite compliant and distorts its shape during ventricular contraction.[7,10]

## Semilunar Valves

The aortic and pulmonary valves are called semilunar valves because their cusps are cuplike in appearance (Figure 22-6). Each of the valves contains three cusps whose margins meet when the valves are in the closed position. The valve cusps meet when they are filled with blood during the diastolic or resting phase of the cardiac cycle (see pp. 443–445). Two coronary arteries arise from the aortic sinuses of Valsalva, which are pouchlike dilatations of the cusps. The coronary ostia (openings) are located in the upper one third of the aortic coronary cusps (Figure 22-7). In a small percentage of hearts, a third coronary artery arises from the right coronary sinus.

The aortic and pulmonic valves are similar in structure except that the aortic valve is composed of slightly thicker fibrous cusps than the pulmonary valve. Both valves are supported by strong fibrous tissue or valve rings.

## Veins

The superior and inferior venae cavae bring the systemic venous blood back to the heart. After passing through the systemic vascular (capillary) bed, the blood passes through venules, small veins, larger veins, and finally to the inferior and superior vena cava (see Figure 22-1).

The pulmonary veins, usually four in number, carry oxygenated blood from the lungs back to the left atrium. These bring the entire output of the right ventricle back to the left side of the heart to be circulated. Veins are distensible, thin-walled structures that can hold large volumes of blood. For this reason, veins are often called *capacitance vessels*.[14]

## Arteries

The two major arteries leading from the heart are the pulmonary artery and the aorta. The pulmonary artery leads from the right ventricle to the lungs. It branches into smaller and smaller vessels that finally become the pulmonary capillary bed where oxygen and carbon dioxide exchange occurs. The pulmonary capillaries then become venules and finally the four pulmonary veins described above.

The aorta is the main systemic artery and carries oxygenated blood to all of the tissues of the body. It gives off

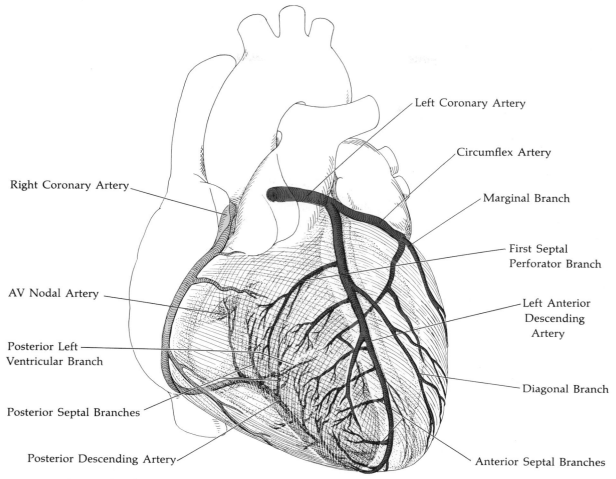

**FIGURE 22-7.**

Coronary arteries. The right and left coronary arteries arise from the aorta immediately above the aortic valve. The right coronary artery runs in the AV groove toward the posterior surface of the heart. In its course, it gives off branches that supply the right atrium and ventricle. At the posterior border of the interventricular septum, the right coronary artery gives off the AV nodal artery which supplies the atrioventricular node and then divides into a posterior descending artery and a posterior left ventricular branch. Septal branches arising from the posterior descending artery supply blood to the posterior one-third of the interventricular septum. Soon after its emergence from the aortic sinus, the left main coronary artery divides into the left anterior descending artery, which runs downward to the cardiac apex, and the circumflex artery, which winds around the left side of the heart in the AV groove. The left anterior descending artery, in turn, gives rise to a first septal perforator branch, which is a major supplier of nutrient blood to the right bundle branch and the anterior fascicle of the left bundle branch; a diagonal branch which courses laterally to nourish the anteriolateral aspects of the left ventricle, and anterior septal branches, which supply the anterior two-thirds of the interventricular septum. The circumflex artery gives off a marginal branch that nourishes the lateral aspect of the left ventricle. (Copyright 1987, Scientific American, Inc. All rights reserved. From Scientific American Medicine, Figure 1, Section 1, Subsection IX.)

branches that become smaller and smaller, terminating finally in systemic arterioles and capillaries where exchange for oxygen and nutrition takes place.

The aorta and pulmonary arteries are composed of three layers: tunica intima (endothelial layer or coat); tunica media (muscular layer); and tunica externa (outer, adventitial coat). These provide the structure necessary for the higher pressures generated in the arteries (see Chap. 27).

## Coronary Arteries

Two main coronary arteries arise from the sinuses of Valsalva of the aortic valve. The *right coronary artery* (RCA) arises from the right coronary sinus and the *left coronary artery* (LCA) arises from the left coronary sinus (see Figure 22-7). The RCA usually arises as a singular vessel from the right coronary ostium but two vessels may arise from this position. This second vessel, if present, is called the *conus artery*. When a single coronary artery arises on the right side, the conus artery is the first branch off the right main coronary artery.[9] The RCA travels in the AV groove (sulcus) and turns downward in the posterior surface to the posterior interventricular sulcus. Smaller arterial vessels branch off the main artery. In about 55% of human hearts, the RCA supplies blood to the sinoatrial node (SA) and in about 90% it supplies the AV node. In some hearts, the RCA supplies the posterior surface of the right and left ventricles and the posterior interventricular septum. It may extend to supply part of the lateral and apical surfaces of the heart. A variation in the amount of myocardial tissue supplied by the RCA accounts for the difference in myocardial pathology when the RCA is diseased.

The left main coronary artery arises from a single ostium in the left coronary sinus. It travels in the AV sulcus to the left for a few millimeters to a few centimeters, and then divides or bifurcates into the left anterior descending coronary artery and the left circumflex. At the point of the bifurcation, other branches called *diagonal arteries* may branch off. The diagonal arteries, one to four in number, supply the anterior surface of the left ventricle. The left anterior descending coronary artery descends in the anterior interventricular sulcus and supplies blood to the anterior left ventricle, the anterior interventricular septum, and the apex of the heart. The circumflex artery comes off the main LCA at a sharp angle and travels in the left AV sulcus to the posterolateral surface of the left ventricle. Its branches supply blood to the lateral left ventricle and various amounts of posterior wall. In a small percentage of persons the circumflex is dominant and supplies the entire left ventricle and interventricular septum.[9] The circumflex also supplies the SA node in approximately 45% of persons and usually supplies blood to the left atrium. Table 22-1 summarizes the normal blood supply to the myocardium and variations that may occur.

The coronary arteries divide into smaller and smaller branches that penetrate deep into the myocardial muscle. These form a network of capillaries that supply the myocardial cells. Numerous functional and nonfunctional anastomoses exist between the coronary vessels. These have been shown to enlarge when the flow in one arterial branch is decreased. Enlargement of anastomoses can improve blood flow to myocardial segments.[9] The endocardial layer is the only portion of the heart that receives oxygen and nutrients from the blood that circulates within the chambers. The rest of the heart receives its oxygen and nutrients from branches of the coronary arteries.

## Coronary Veins

The coronary veins provide for drainage of the myocardium and empty into the right atrium. They consist of the coronary sinus and its branches, the anterior right ventricular veins, and the thebesian veins (Figure 22-8). The majority of drainage from the left ventricle is received by the coronary sinus and its branches. The coronary sinus is basically an extension of the great coronary vein. The anterior cardiac veins drain the right ventricle and usually empty directly into the right atrium. The remaining venous blood empties into the heart through the small Thebesian veins. These are tiny venous outlets draining directly into the right atrium and ventricles.[9]

## Conduction System

Normal contraction of the heart is initiated by specialized conductive tissues, which are actually myocardial muscle

**TABLE 22–1.**
NORMAL BLOOD SUPPLY TO MYOCARDIUM

| CORONARY ARTERY | AREA SUPPLIED | VARIATIONS |
|---|---|---|
| Right coronary artery | SA node in 55% of hearts; AV node in 90% of hearts; posterior surface of right and left ventricles; posterior interventricular system | Dominant when supplies lateral and apical left ventricle |
| Left main coronary artery | | |
| Left anterior descending | Anterior left ventricle; apex of heart; anterior interventricular septum | In 5–10% of hearts supplies AV node; anterolateral left ventricle |
| Circumflex | SA node in 45% of hearts; left atrium; posterior lateral surface left ventricle | In 5–10% of hearts supplies AV node; dominant where supplies entire left ventricle; interventricular septum |

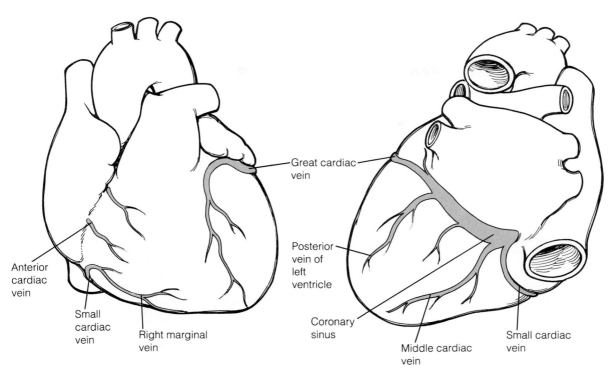

**FIGURE 22–8.**
Coronary sinus and its branches, anterior, middle, and posterior veins and great cardiac vein.

cells with fewer myofibrils than the other myocardial cells. Figure 22-9 shows the location of the conductive structures within the heart: the SA node, atrial internodal tracts, AV node, bundle of His, right and left bundle branches, and terminal or Purkinje network.

The sinus (SA) node is a small mass of cells located near the entrance of the superior vena cava into the right atrium. It normally serves as the pacemaker of the heart because of its ability to generate an impulse through automatic diastolic depolarization (see pp. 437–440).

The atrial internodal tracts extend from the SA node and are difficult to distinguish from the surrounding cardiac muscle. The pathways are designated as the *anterior, middle,* and *posterior internodal tracts.*[9] The electrical impulse generated by the SA node travels rapidly along these tracts to merge at the AV node. Bachman's bundle (the anterior internodal tract) conducts the impulse to the left atrium. The two remaining tracts travel through the right atrium.

The AV node and bundle of His form an interconnecting structure between the atria and ventricles that functionally joins the two units. The AV node lies in the right atrium at the juncture of the atrial septum. It is composed of dense fibrous tissue that continues into the bundle of His. The AV node along with the bundle of His pathway is the only muscular and functional connection between the atrial and ventricular muscles.[7] The slow

conduction in the AV node may be partly due to the unspecialized structure of its cells. The bundle of His directly connects with the AV node and crosses into the membranous portion of the ventricular septum. It is composed of fibrous tissue with a few myofibrils and terminates in the bifurcation of the common bundle into the right and left bundle branches.

The right and left bundle branches travel down the interventricular septum to terminate in the Purkinje network. The right bundle branch descends superficially in the endocardium of the right ventricular septum. It divides into numerous branches that penetrate the walls of the right ventricle. The left bundle divides into three *fascicles—posterior, anterior,* and *septal*—which travel in the left interventricular septum for varying distances. The posterior fascicle sends its branches to the lateral and posterior wall and papillary muscle. The anterior fascicle primarily goes to the anterior and lateral wall of the left ventricle. The septal fascicle travels to the interventricular septum and the apex of the left ventricle.[9] The fascicular branches subdivide into smaller and smaller subbranches and terminate in the Purkinje network.

The Purkinje network is composed primarily of Purkinje cells that have few myofibrils and are joined end-to-end by intercalated disks that aid in the property of accelerated conduction of the impulse[9] (see myocardial cellular structure below). A Purkinje fiber is composed

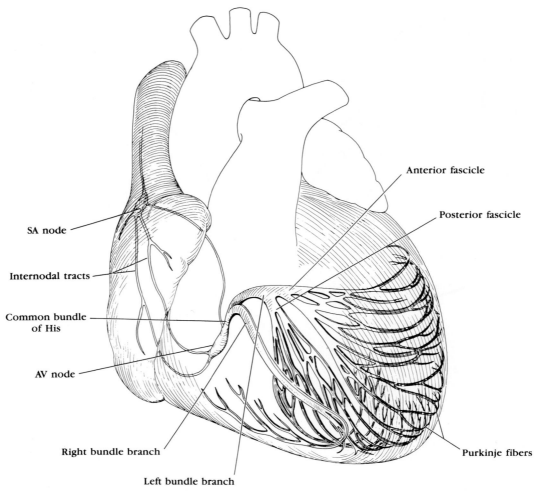

SA node

Internodal tracts

Common bundle
of His

AV node

Right bundle branch

Left bundle branch

Anterior fascicle

Posterior fascicle

Purkinje fibers

**FIGURE 22–9.**
Cardiac conduction system. The cardiac impulse originates in the sinus node and is conducted to the ventricles by way of the internodal tracts, the AV node, the bundle of His, and the right and left bundle branches, which terminate in the network of Purkinje fibers. The left bundle branch subdivides into an anterior and a posterior fascicle. (Copyright 1987, Scientific American, Inc. All rights reserved. From Scientific American Medicine, Figure 6, Section 1, Subsection VI.)

of many Purkinje cells in a series. These fibers lie in the deepest layer of the myocardium and supply the papillary muscles and apical parts of the ventricles. Thus, the apical portion of the ventricles contracts before the basal parts, facilitating the excitation of the right and left ventricles.[1]

## Myocardial Cellular Structure

Cardiac muscle cells are similar to skeletal muscle cells in many ways but have some fundamental differences. Cardiac muscle cells have a single central nucleus, while skeletal cells have peripheral nuclei. The muscle cells are closely approximated so that impulses generated in one myocardial cell can be passed easily to the next.

The myofibril is the contractile unit of the myocardial muscle cell. Its action occurs through the movement of actin on myosin in the sarcomere unit. The thin actin filament also contains two inhibitory proteins, *tropomyosin* and *troponin*. The activity of these proteins in muscle contraction is described in detail in Chapter 44.

The myocardial muscle cell has a poorly developed sarcoplasmic reticulum (SR) but a highly developed transverse tubular system. This tubular system probably contributes to the intracellular release of calcium.[6] The cardiac cell also contains a large number of mitochondria that have been shown to store calcium. Glycogen and lipid are also stored in the cells.

Cardiac muscle cells are close to one another. The end of one cell very closely approximates the next. The junctions of the cells consist of intercalated disks, which form a tight connection and allow impulses to pass rapidly from one cell to the next (Figure 22-10). The myocardial cellular structure allows the entire myocardial unit to contract when one cell is stimulated to threshold

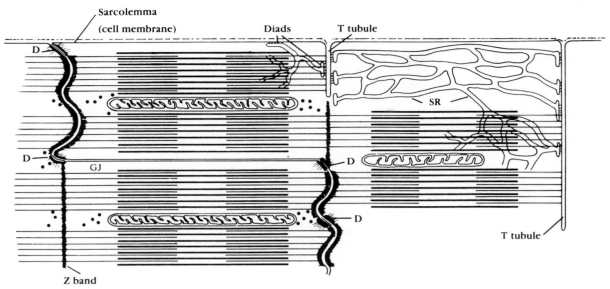

**FIGURE 22-10.**
A thin section through cardiac muscle as it might appear on electron microscopy. Positions of two cardiac muscle fibers are depicted in the area where their plasmalemmas associate to form the intercalated disk. Desmosomes (D) provide structural integrity to the disk. The gap junctions (GJ) are located in the horizontal part of the disk. The disk occurs where a Z band would have been. The T tubules occur at the Z lines. The sarcoplasmic reticulum (SR) forms a sleeve around the myofibrils, but here it is depicted along to show its pattern more clearly (Source: M. Borysenko, et al., *Functional Histology* (2nd ed.). Boston: Little, Brown, 1984.)

level. The heart behaves as a *syncytium*; that is, if one cell is stimulated, the entire unit contracts (see below).

## PHYSIOLOGY OF THE HEART

The physiology of the heart is considered in terms of the electrical and mechanical activities of the myocardial muscle. The cellular aspects are briefly outlined to provide greater understanding of the process. Table 22-2 provides definitions to understand the process.

### Contraction of Cardiac Muscle

Cardiac contraction occurs in much the same way as skeletal muscle contraction except that the muscle functions as a syncytium. This means that if one cardiac muscle cell is stimulated to threshold and contracts, the impulse spreads to all of the muscle cells and the entire unit contracts. The two separate syncytial units in the myocardium, atrial and ventricular, are functionally joined by the AV node and the bundle of His.

The mechanism for contraction is similar to that described in Chapter 44. The action potential generated causes the release of calcium from the SR into the sarcoplasm. Calcium binds with the inhibitory proteins troponin and tropomyosin, allowing actin to slide on myosin. Actin and myosin are the contractile proteins that make up the sarcomere units of the myocardial muscle cell. The calcium ion apparently has two major roles in excitation-contraction: as the trigger substance or initiator and as the regulator of contraction.[10] When the action potential is initiated, there is a rapid influx of sodium. As the action potential travels down the extensive T tubular system, it comes close to the terminal cisternae of the SR. The SR releases large amounts of free calcium that bind with troponin and, thus, inhibit both troponin and tropomyosin. Energy for the contraction is obtained from adenosinetriphosphate (ATP), which is split by an adenosinetriphosphatase (ATPase) site on the myosin filament when it interacts with actin (Figure 22-11).[10]

The amount of calcium available to inhibit troponin is directly related to the rate and amount of myocardial tension developed.[12] The T tubules possess a large number of voltage-dependent calcium channels. The more calcium that flows across the sarcolemma through these channels largely determines the amount of calcium released by the SR.[6] It is also possible that competition between sodium and calcium for binding sites affects myocardial contractility. Calcium must be returned to the SR through a continually active calcium pump that decreases the free calcium. A decreased level of calcium in the sarcoplasmic fluid restores the inhibition of actin and myosin by the troponin-tropomyosin complex.[5] The sarcomere unit then returns to the resting position.

Over recent years, *calcium channel* blockers have been developed to close or partially close the calcium

## TABLE 22-2.
DEFINITIONS OF CARDIAC PHYSIOLOGY TERMS

| TERM | DEFINITION |
| --- | --- |
| Cardiac action potential | A rapid sequence of changes in the electrical potential across the cell membrane resulting in systole and diastole |
| Syncytium | A cardiac property; if one cardiac muscle fiber is stimulated to threshold, the entire myocardial unit will contract |
| Inotropic state | Referring to contractility; (+) inotropic refers to increased contractility; (−) inotropic refers to decreased contractility |
| Chronotropic state | Refers to heart rate; (+) chronotropic refers to tachycardia; (−) chronotropic refers to bradycardia |
| Absolute refractory period | The period in the cardiac cycle during which the cell will not respond to a second stimulus regardless of the strength of the stimulus |
| Relative refractory period | The period in the cardiac cycle during which the cell will respond to a strong stimulus; main cause of ectopic beats |
| Automaticity | The spontaneous property of depolarizing and generating an action potential; enhanced automaticity increases irritability of conduction outside SA node |
| Rhythmicity | Regular, rhythmic generation of an action potential |
| Excitability | Ability of a cell to respond to stimulation from an adjacent cardiac muscle cell |
| Conductivity | Ability of muscle cell to transmit action potential from one cell to adjacent cell |
| Preload | Volume related; degree of myocardial muscle length, prior to contraction |
| Afterload | Pressure related; resistance against which the ventricles must pump |
| Contractility | Force of contraction generated by myocardial muscle |
| His-Purkinje system | Portion of conduction system including AV node, bundle of His, bundle branches, and Purkinje network |
| Cardiac work | The amount of oxygen consumption required for cardiac contractions, includes intramyocardial tension |

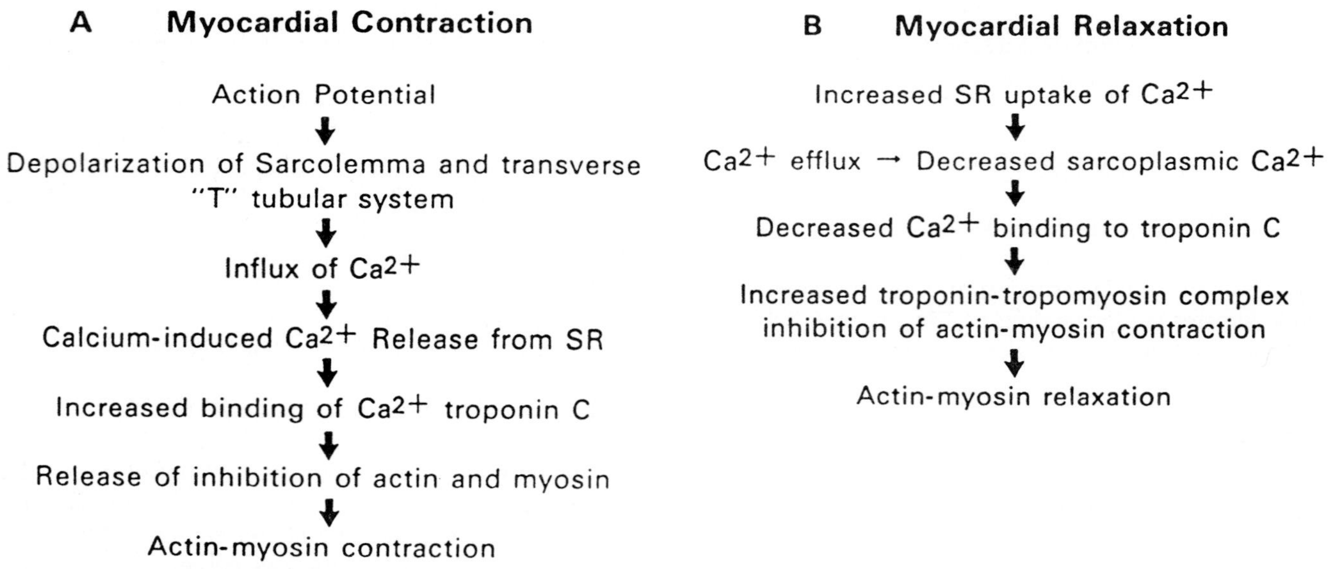

**A    Myocardial Contraction**

Action Potential
↓
Depolarization of Sarcolemma and transverse "T" tubular system
↓
Influx of $Ca^{2+}$
↓
Calcium-induced $Ca^{2+}$ Release from SR
↓
Increased binding of $Ca^{2+}$ troponin C
↓
Release of inhibition of actin and myosin
↓
Actin-myosin contraction

**B    Myocardial Relaxation**

Increased SR uptake of $Ca^{2+}$
↓
$Ca^{2+}$ efflux → Decreased sarcoplasmic $Ca^{2+}$
↓
Decreased $Ca^{2+}$ binding to troponin C
↓
Increased troponin-tropomyosin complex inhibition of actin-myosin contraction
↓
Actin-myosin relaxation

**FIGURE 22-11.**

Schematic diagram of the events that produce (A) myocardial excitation-contraction coupling, and (B) myocardial relaxation. With depolarization of the cardiac cell membranes (sarcolemma and transverse T system), the $Na^+$ channels open, followed by the $Ca^{++}$ channels. The initial transsarcolemmal influx of $Ca^{++}$ triggers the release of $Ca^{++}$ from the sarcoplasmic reticulum (SR) $Ca^{++}$ in higher concentration then binds to troponin C. This produces conformational changes in whole troponin (troponin 1-troponin C-troponin T complex) that relieves a troponin 1 interaction with actin, thereby allowing tropomysin to roll back into the grooves of the F-actin superhelix and allowing the interaction of actin and myosin to produce a contraction. The transsarcolemmal $Ca^{++}$ current has both a faster and a slower component. It is possible that the former may act to trigger the release of $Ca^{++}$ current from the SR, whereas the slow component may cause the SR to accumulate calcium. $Ca^{++}$ influx may also occur by the $Na^+$ $Ca^{++}$ exchanger. Relaxation is initiated by an unknown stimulus that produces the active uptake of $Ca^{++}$ by the SR $Ca^{++}$ binding to troponin C and relaxation. During relaxation, $Ca^{++}$ efflux may occur both by $Ca^{++}$ ATPase and by a $Na^+$ $Ca^{++}$ exchanger. (Source: J.W. Hurst, et al., *The Heart* (7th ed.). New York: McGraw-Hill, 1990.)

channels and, thus, decrease the myocardial tension. As described on page 443, the contractility or force of cardiac contraction is called its *inotropic state*. An increased (+) inotropism refers to increased force of contraction and energy use within the muscle fibers. In ischemic heart disease or hypertrophic cardiomyopathy, the result of decreased available calcium is a decrease in cardiac work or causing a negative (−) inotropic state. The end result is a decreasing blood pressure and cardiac ischemia. Obviously, the results of these pharmacologic agents could be detrimental if the inotropic state were not sustained to adequately maintain the blood pressure. The explanation of how some of the antidysrhythmic agents work is thought to relate to the blocking of *sodium channels*. This has led to classification of antidysrhythmic drugs according to their membrane/channel action.[8]

### Action Potential

When the myocardial muscle cell is at rest, the resting membrane potential is approximately −85 to −95 mV. When an action potential occurs, it changes the membrane potential from the negative to a slightly positive value. The action potential in cardiac muscle remains in plateau longer than in other excitable cells, which allows for a longer contraction in cardiac muscle. After the action potential, contraction occurs, and is followed by repolarization and a return to the resting state. As noted in Figure 22-12, these changes in potential and state of cardiac muscle can be described in terms of discrete phases:

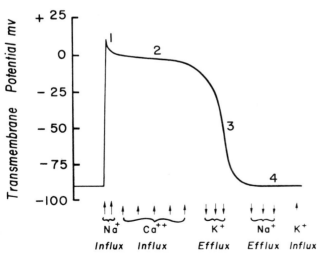

**FIGURE 22-12.**
Schematic action potential of human ventricular myocardium together with probable electrolyte movements. The initial phase O spike and overshoot is related to a sudden influx of Na+. This is followed by a slower, maintained influx of Ca++ during the plateau phase 2. The phase of Ca++ efflux is not well-defined for human ventricular myocardium, but presumably it occurs during phase 4. (Source: J.W. Hurst, *The Heart* (7th ed.). New York: McGraw-Hill, 1990.)

phase 0 denotes depolarization; phase 1 indicates complete depolarization and contraction; phase 2 is a plateau phase of maximum cardiac contraction; phase 3 is the period of repolarization; and phase 4 indicates the myocardium at rest.[12]

Restimulation during phases 1 and 2 does not cause the muscle to contract again. This is called the refractory period and occurs in both atrial and ventricular muscle. The *absolute refractory period* is the time during which the membrane is completely depolarized and/or contracting, when no stimulus can cause it to respond or contract again. The *relative refractory period* (phase 3) occurs when the muscle membrane is repolarizing and a strong stimulus will cause it to contract.

### Metabolism of Cardiac Muscle

Cardiac muscle requires constant production of ATP. Little is stored in cardiac muscle so oxygen and nutrients for energy production must be constantly supplied. Most ATP is produced in the numerous myocardial mitochondria using fatty acids and other nutrients, especially lactate and glucose. If one substance is not available, cardiac muscle can efficiently use the other.

The amount of ATP normally produced is equivalent to the work needed to pump incoming blood into the arteries with sufficient pressure to maintain vital body functions. *Myocardial work* is generated by the ventricular wall tension during systole and diastole. The wall tension generated during systole creates the pressure to eject blood into the arteries. Cardiac work is often expressed in terms of *myocardial oxygen consumption*. The amount of oxygen consumed is closely related to the amount of stress developed in the ventricular wall. The major factors that affect oxygen consumption include the amount of myocardial muscle mass, the contractile or inotropic state, heart rate, and intramyocardial tension generated.[10] The oxygen supply for this work is totally delivered from the coronary arteries. Increased oxygen is needed in stress situations because of enhanced contractility and tachycardia that is induced by the catecholamines.

The myocardial muscle takes up a large amount of the oxygen delivered to it from the coronary arteries. Oxygen extraction of up to 70% leaves little oxygen reserve. Increased systemic energy needs can be met only by increasing the heart rate and respiratory rate to increase oxygen delivery (Figure 22-13).

### Automaticity

The spontaneous property of generating an action potential by the conduction tissue is called *automaticity*. This occurs through a slow, sliding depolarization that creeps

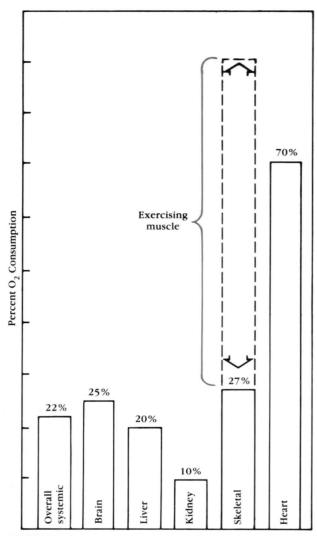

**FIGURE 22-13.**
Oxygen extraction by the heart and other organs. (Source: M. Jackle and M. Halligan, *Cardiovascular Problems.* Bowie, MD: Brady, 1980.)

toward threshold. When the threshold level is reached, spontaneous depolarization occurs. The action potential usually arises in the SA node where an inward leakage phenomenon allows sodium to drift into the cell. Self-initiation of the action potential (diastolic depolarization) then occurs. All parts of the conduction system retain the property of automaticity but do so at inherently different rates. Figure 22-14 shows that this phenomenon normally occurs because of an unstable membrane potential, with gradual, slow depolarization at the end of the cycle (phase 4). The rate of depolarization in phase 4 is more rapid in the SA node. Thus, it fires more frequently. These SA node impulses dominate other automatic regions simply because they are formed with greater frequency. The term *enhanced automaticity* usually refers

to increased irritability of cells of the conduction tissue outside the SA node.

Pharmaceutical agents, hypoxemia, and injury are examples of factors that can alter the threshold for myocardial response. Some drugs, for example, raise the threshold for generation of the action potential and thus decrease the rate of diastolic depolarization. This is especially effective if ectopic impulses are causing ventricular dysrhythmias (see Chap. 23).

Parasympathetic influences through the vagus nerve slow the rate of diastolic depolarization and decrease the rate of SA node automaticity. Sympathetic influences increase the automaticity and the rate of diastolic depolarization.

### Rhythmicity

Rhythmicity is an important property of the conduction tissue that is characteristic of all of the potential pacemakers of the heart. It refers to the rhythmic or regular generation of an action potential. The leakage phenomenon described above remains regular, allowing for the same amount of time from one depolarization to the next. Therefore, the action potential discharges regularly. Rhythmicity also may be affected by the sympathetic nervous system (SNS) and the parasympathetic system. A cyclic increase and decrease in cardiac rate due to respiratory influences on the vagus nerve result in an increased cardiac rate on inspiration and a decreased rate on expiration in certain persons. Rhythmicity may be interrupted by enhanced automaticity of influences such as nervous system stimulation, electrolyte imbalances, and pharmaceutical agents.

### Excitability

Excitability refers to the ability of the cell to respond to stimulation. In the heart, there are fast and slow conductors. The fast conductors include atrial and ventricular muscle cells and the Purkinje fibers, while the slow responses are those in the SA and the AV nodes. Different cardiac muscle fibers have been shown to have both fast and slow channels. The word *excitability* denotes the ability of the muscle cell to respond to an impulse in an adjacent muscle cell.[12]

### Conductivity

Impulse transmission in cardiac muscle is affected mostly by the structure of the intramyocardial cells, which allows the current to flow easily from one cell to the next. Therefore, threshold current from one cell rapidly passes

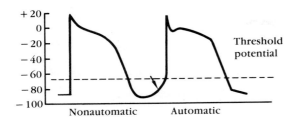

**A**

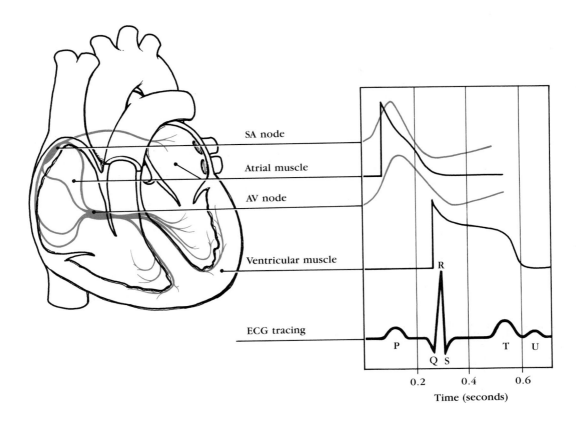

**B**

**FIGURE 22-14.**

**A.** Action of automatic and nonautomatic cells. The automatic cell slides toward threshold potential at regular intervals. **B.** Automatic and nonautomatic areas of the conduction system related to the ECG. (Source: M. Sokolow and M. McIlroy, *Clinical Cardiology* (4th ed.). Los Altos, CA: Lange, 1986.)

to and depolarizes the adjacent cell. Conductivity is effected through the intercalated disks, or the tight junctions between the myocardial muscle cells. It may be slowed or altered with intracellular damage, such as ischemia or infarction.

## Electrical Events of the Cardiac Cycle

As stated above, the cardiac cycle is initiated through specialized conduction tissue. These pacemaker cells spon-

taneously depolarize in a rhythmic fashion. The critical threshold is gradually reached; spontaneous depolarization occurs and is followed by repolarization.

The pacemaker of the heart is the sinus node because spontaneous depolarization occurs more frequently here than in the other potential pacers. This depolarization supersedes the discharge of the other potential pacers. During normal pacemaking activity, the sinus node impulse suppresses the His-Purkinje system that could be potential pacemakers.[1]

The cells of the His-Purkinje system (which includes

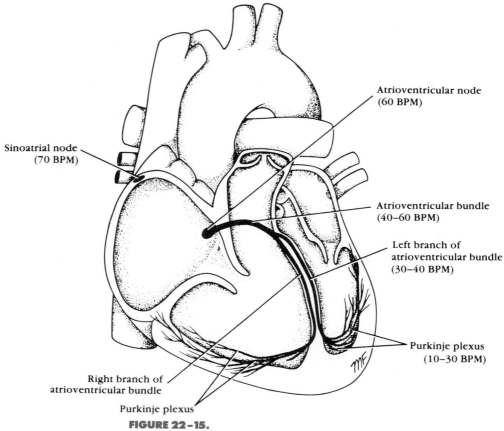

**Sinoatrial node**
**(70 BPM)**

**Atrioventricular node**
**(60 BPM)**

**Atrioventricular bundle**
**(40–60 BPM)**

**Left branch of**
**atrioventricular bundle**
**(30–40 BPM)**

**Purkinje plexus**
**(10–30 BPM)**

**Right branch of**
**atrioventricular bundle**

**Purkinje plexus**

**FIGURE 22–15.**
Approximate rates of inherent cardiac pacemakers.

AV node, bundle of His, and branches) are depolarized by the sinus impulse before their diastolic depolarization reaches threshold.[1] The conduction tissue has been referred to as a cascade of potential pacers that fire at different rates and can take over pacemaker function if the more rapid pacemaker is not operational.[7] Figure 22-15 shows the approximate potential rates of the inherent cardiac pacemakers.

Excitation of cardiac muscle normally follows a strict sequential pattern. The sinus node begins the excitation. This is due to the less negative resting membrane potential ($-55$ to $-60$ mV) in the sinus node than in the other cardiac muscle fibers and to increased membrane permeability to sodium. The impulse or action potential occurs and sends the excitation wave through the internodal pathways, causing depolarization of the atrial muscle and excitation of the AV node. At the AV node, the impulse is slowed as it passes through the dense fibrous tissue. This allows time for the atria to complete contraction before the depolarization wave is sent to the ventricles. The impulse is then sent down the bundle of His and the bundle branches to the Purkinje network, which causes rapid depolarization and contraction of the ventricles.

The electrocardiogram (ECG) graphically depicts these electrical events. Figure 22-16 shows the appearance of the ECG in relation to electrical activities. This activity creates an electrical field that is distributed to the body surfaces. For example, SA node depolarization is inscribed as the P wave. The PR interval is the time it takes for the impulse to traverse the AV node. As the impulse travels down each bundle, the QRS is formed. Finally, the T wave represents repolarization (see Chap. 23). Because the myocardium is depolarized from endocardium to epicardium, an electrode placed on the epicardial surface normally shows a positive inscription. If a large amount of muscle mass is depolarized, a large inscription is formed (Figure 22-17). Smaller muscle masses inscribe smaller R waves.

## Mechanical Events of the Cardiac Cycle

The mechanical events of cardiac contraction are regulated by the following interrelated factors: (1) preload, (2) afterload, (3) contractility, and (4) heart rate.[10]

### Preload

This term refers to the degree of stretch (myocardial muscle length) prior to contraction. A commonly used

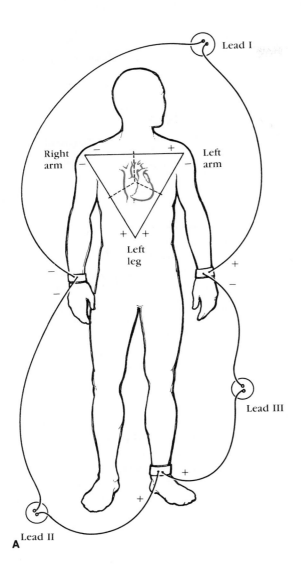

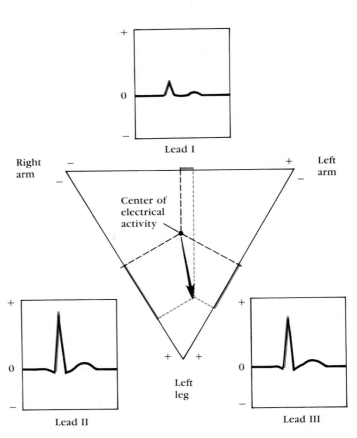

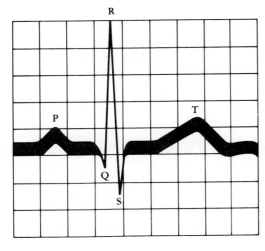

**FIGURE 22–16.**

**A.** The standard electrocardiographic leads with their attachments to the body. **B.** Electrocardiograms recorded with leads I, II, and III. **C.** The normal electrocardiogram from lead II. Each small square represents 0.04 seconds on the horizontal plane. Measurements are made of time required for impulses to pass through different portions of the conduction system. The P wave indicates SA node initiation of the impulse. The QRS indicates ventricular depolarization and the T wave reflects ventricular repolarization.

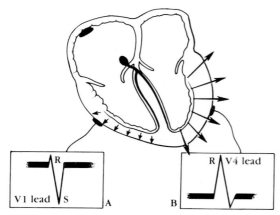

**FIGURE 22-17.**

**A.** As the depolarization wave spreads from endocardium to epicardium in the right ventricle, the small muscle mass produces a small positive wave in V1 or right ventricular lead of the 12 lead ECG. The deep S wave reflects left ventricular depolarization which is seen as moving away from the V1 lead. **B.** Endocardial to epicardial depolarization produces a tall R wave in V4 because of the thick muscle mass of the left ventricle.

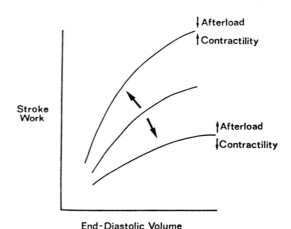

**FIGURE 22-18.**

Ventricular function curves with stroke work plotted as a function of the left ventricular end-diastolic volume. Each of these curves represents the effect of preload (end-diastolic volume on cardiac performance (stroke work) at a given afterload and contractile state. An increase in contractility or a decrease in afterload shifts the curve upward and to the left, such that the stroke work is greater for a given preload. A decrease in contractility or an increase in afterload shifts the curve downward and to the right such that the stroke work is less for a given preload (Source: W.N. Kelley, *Textbook of Internal Medicine*, Philadelphia: J.B. Lippincott, 1989.)

word for this property is *compliance*, the ratio of volume change to pressure change. Decreased compliance means increased stiffness; a compliant chamber can accept volume without an elevation in pressure.[12] Ischemia of cardiac muscle causes a decrease in compliance, while a normally functioning ventricle can increase volume without a significant increase of pressure, such as during exercise stress.

The inherent property of cardiac muscle that allows for an increased force of contraction due to increased initial fiber length is called *Starling's law of the heart*. It is now termed the *Frank-Straub-Wiggers-Starling Principle*.[10] The increased fiber length is related to increased volume of blood, which causes the initial stretch. When the fiber is stretched, it responds with an increased force of contraction. This has been related to the all-or-nothing law of the heart, which means that despite the strength of stimulus applied, cardiac muscle responds either to its fullest or not at all.[10]

In the normal, compliant ventricle, changes of volume can be accommodated quite readily. Ventricular compliance refers to the ability of the ventricle to accept more diastolic volume. Normally, right ventricular output equals that of the left, even though the stroke volumes between the chambers may vary slightly. Respiratory excursion, for example, may cause a temporary increase in right ventricular output. However, when the ventricle receives this increased volume, it increases its output to balance the minute cardiac output. Ischemia, pericardial restriction, and hypertrophy are examples of factors that can affect this compliance by limiting venous inflow or limiting the contractility that normally would occur. Increased ventricular distensibility without effective contraction may be present in heart failure (Figure 22-18).

End-diastolic volume and preload can be determined by a variety of factors. Intravascular blood volume depletion decreases preload, while overload of intravascular volume increases. Decreased efficiency or cardiac contractility, such as with heart failure, increases preload. Body position can greatly influence it because blood tends to pool in dependent parts of the body. Loss of effective negative intrapleural pressure can cause a significant decrease in preload.[13]

The concept of *wall stress* is important in cardiac physiology. Systolic wall stress is generated by the contraction event, and determines the extent of fiber shortening and oxygen consumption within the cardiac muscle. Wall stress during diastole determines intraventricular diastolic pressure and sarcomere length at the onset of the next contraction.[14]

## Afterload

This factor refers to the resistance that is normally maintained by the aortic and pulmonary valves, the condition and tone of the aorta, and the resistance offered by the systemic and pulmonary arterioles. Afterload is the net force per unit cross-sectional area across the myocardial wall during ejection. It is estimated by using LaPlace's law which is figured as follows: Wall stress $= PR/2h$, where $P = $ intracavitary pressure, $R = $ radius of curvature, and $h = $ wall thickness.[13] It is determined primarily by aortic impedance, which is mainly determined by systemic vascular resistance.[13] Because wall stress is difficult to measure, the mean arterial pressure or left ventricular systolic pressure is used to approximate afterload.[13] Increased blood viscosity and added preload also contribute to afterload. Pathologic states, such as hypertension and aortic stenosis, significantly increase afterload. As afterload increases, so does cardiac work and oxygen consumption.

Greater muscle mass is required to maintain cardiac output against chronic increased resistance. Over time, the ventricular muscle mass increases, leading to cardiac hypertrophy.

### Contractility

Contractility refers to the force of contraction generated by the myocardial muscle. This may be expressed in terms of the *inotropic state*, which is referred to as positive ( + ) if the force of contraction is increased and negative ( − ) if the force of contraction is decreased. This factor is influenced by both preload and afterload but it may occur independently of these influences. The SNS, through the influence of catecholamines, causes an increase in cardiac rate and force of contraction. Also, by increasing the recoil of ventricular muscle on diastole, diastolic ventricular pressure is decreased. This allows for greater filling, greater fiber stretch, and, therefore, a stronger contraction.[9] Contractility is difficult to measure independent of preload or afterload changes.[10,13]

### Heart Rate

Stress in any form stimulates the SNS, which leads to an increased cardiac rate. This increased rate leads to increases in cardiac output and ventricular contractility. Rate changes are often called the *chronotropic effect*, with a positive effect referring to an increased rate and a negative effect referring to the decreased rate.

## Phases of the Cardiac Cycle

The two major phases of cardiac activity are called *systole* and *diastole*. Systole refers to contraction, generally ventricular events. Diastole refers to relaxation, usually of the ventricles.[5] The events of the cardiac cycle from the atria through the ventricles relating systole and diastole are discussed in this section. Table 22-3 summarizes the commonly used terms in the cardiac cycle.

### Atrial Filling and Contraction

As the atria receive blood from the incoming veins, blood accumulates in these structures until ventricular pressures fall below atrial pressures. As the atrial pressure rises, the flow of blood passively opens the AV valves and blood flows into the ventricles. Approximately 70% of blood flow from the atria to the ventricles occurs passively. Atrial contraction, which follows atrial depolarization from the SA pathways, provides the "atrial kick" to move the remaining atrial blood into the ventricles.

### Ventricular Filling and Contraction

Rapid ventricular filling occurs after the AV valves open. Blood moves into the ventricles passively and then actively in response to the atrial kick. Ventricular depolar-

**TABLE 22–3.**
TERMS USED TO DEFINE THE CARDIAC CYCLE

| TERM | DEFINITION |
| --- | --- |
| Cardiac output | Amount of blood pumped from heart/minute; cardiac output = stroke volume × heart rate |
| Stroke volume | Amount of blood ejected from each ventricle/beat; this is not all of the blood in each ventricle, but about 60–75% of the volume, and is called the *ejection fraction* |
| End-diastolic volume | Amount of blood in the ventricle just before systole |
| Isovolumic contraction | Period of ventricular pressure rise prior to opening of semilunar valves |
| Ejection | Period when ventricular pressure exceeds arterial pressure, and blood is ejected from heart |
| Incisura | Inscription of a pressure recording that occurs when aortic valve closes; caused by a momentary reversal of pressures between aorta and left ventricle |
| Isovolumic relaxation | Rapid drop of pressure in ventricles toward diastolic pressure. Occurs prior to opening of atrioventricular valves and ventricular filling |
| Systole | Contraction of the heart |
| Diastole | Relaxation of the heart |

ization and contraction occur from the conduction pathways and Purkinje activation of the muscle. Ventricular systole occurs in discrete phases:

1. Ventricular pressure begins to rise, causing increased tension around the AV valve structures and closure of the mitral and tricuspid valves. This is called the *isovolumic contraction* period and occupies the time between onset of ventricular contraction and opening of the semilunar valves.
2. Blood is ejected from the ventricles when the pressure in the ventricles exceeds the diastolic pressures maintained in the aorta and the pulmonary artery. This increased pressure opens the semilunar valves and blood flows into the arteries.

3. After ejection of the stroke volume, the pressure in the ventricles begins to fall. At a certain point, the pressure falls below the arterial diastolic pressure and the semilunar valves close. On a pressure tracing, closure of the aortic valve is indicated by the *incisura* or *aortic dicrotic notch*. The *isovolumic relaxation phase* occurs as pressure continues to descend in the ventricles toward the low diastolic pressure. This lasts until the pressure in the ventricles falls below the atrial pressure, when rapid ventricular filling begins again. Figure 22-19 summarizes the events of the cardiac cycle.

The mechanical events occur at the same time in both the right and left sides of the heart. Figure 22-20 shows some significant differences between the cham-

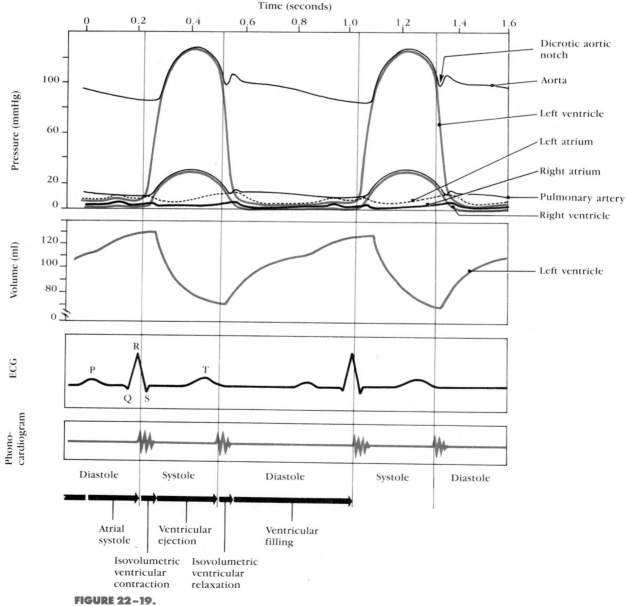

**FIGURE 22–19.**
Events of the cardiac cycle indicating changes in volume and pressure related to the ECG and heart sounds.

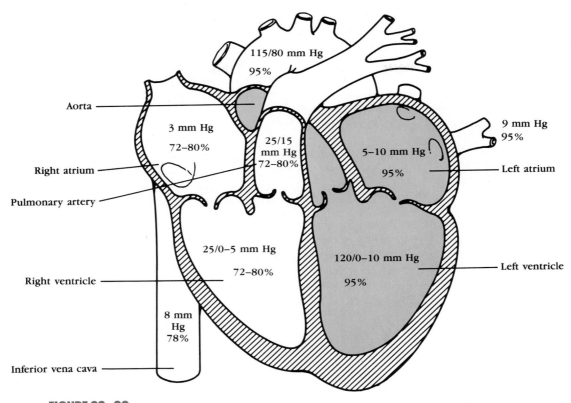

**FIGURE 22–20.**
Normal oxygen pressures and saturations in the great vessels and cardiac chambers.

bers in terms of pressure and oxygen saturation. It can be readily seen that left-sided pressures exceed the right. While both arteries maintain a diastolic pressure, the aortic pressure is much higher than the pulmonary. The diastolic pressure in both ventricles is normally very low, nearing zero.

## Heart Sounds

Two major distinct sounds are produced in the normal heart: S1, often called the mitral sound, and S2, which occurs with the closure of the semilunar valves. The S1 occurs when the ventricles begin contraction or during cardiac systole. It has always been attributed to closure of the AV valves but that may or may not be a component of the sound. The S1 is probably produced by the acceleration and deceleration of blood with tensing of the valve structures and cardiac vibrations.[11] Normally, this sound is best heard in the fifth intercostal space in the midclavicular line.

The second heart sound is mainly due to closure of the semilunar valves. It has two components: the aortic and pulmonary closure sounds. During the inspiratory phase of respiration, there is an increase in venous return to the right side of the heart, which increases the volume in the right ventricle, thereby increasing ejection time. The pulmonary valve closes slightly after the aortic valve, producing a physiologic splitting sound. This split

is more obvious in young persons and during hyperventilation. This sound is best heard in the aortic and pulmonary areas at the second intercostal spaces (Figure 22-21).

The third heart sound, S3 (ventricular gallop), may be normally heard in young children but is usually pathologic in adults. When heard, it occurs after the S2. It results from tensing of the chordae and AV ring during the end of the rapid filling phase.[11] It is most frequently heard when there is a dilated ventricle or volume overload, especially with heart failure.

The fourth heart sound, S4 (atrial gallop), occurs

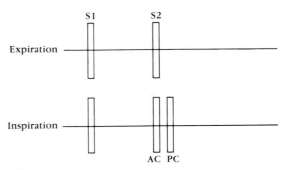

**FIGURE 22–21.**
Illustration of splitting of the second heart sound on inspiration. Note that aortic closure (AC) occurs first; pulmonic closure (PC) follows. On inspiration, two separate sounds may be heard.

with increased ventricular pressure during atrial contraction. It is heard immediately before S1 and may be associated with hypertension or decreased ventricular compliance. Both S3 and S4 are heard best at the apex with the bell portion of the stethoscope.

Figure 22-19 summarizes the relationship of S1 (systole) and S2 (diastole) to cardiac events. Also shown are the periods of the cardiac cycle as related to the ECG.

## Autonomic Influences on Cardiac Activity

The autonomic nervous system (ANS) provides an external influence on myocardial contractility and rate. This involves adjusting the heart rate and contractility to the demands of the body. The ANS has an enhancing or restraining effect on the inherent pacemaker system and can alter the automaticity of abnormal pacemaker systems.

### Sympathetic Nervous System

Fibers from the SNS are present in the atrial wall, ventricles, and SA and AV nodes.

When stimulated, these fibers release norepinephrine, which stimulates the rate of depolarization and the rate at which impulses are transmitted through the conduction tissue. Therefore, increased sympathetic tone increases cardiac rate and the contractility of myocardial muscle. The predominant effect is usually on the sinus node and causes a sinus tachycardia as occurs in response to exercise or fear. Stimulation of the SNS also can increase the irritability of myocardial muscle cells, causing abnormal or early depolarization, such as with premature atrial or ventricular contractions (see Chap. 23). These are usually referred to as *ectopic foci* because they are outside the SA node.

The effects of the SNS on the coronary arteries are somewhat more complex. Norepinephrine has been shown to cause coronary artery vasoconstriction and causes increased oxygen extraction by the myocardial cell. Some individuals have a hyperactive response to norepinephrine and exhibit coronary artery vasospasms during stressful situations. Ischemia results and causes the liberation of metabolites that, in turn, can cause vasodilation. Epinephrine, most of which is released from the adrenal glands, has a secondary dilating action on the coronary arteries. Prostaglandins, a group of chemically related substances, may be stimulated secondarily in the stress response. They are synthesized by the myocardial cells and arteries and usually dilate the coronary arteries.[5]

Normally, autoregulation of coronary blood flow appears to counteract the effects of neural stimulation. When ANS stimulation induces coronary vasoconstriction, coronary autoregulation usually overrides the mechanism and ischemia is prevented.[3] As long as the obstruction affects the larger coronary vessels, there is a progressive decrease in the distal coronary arteriolar bed.[3]

### Parasympathetic Nervous System

The parasympathetic nervous system (PSNS) is mediated through the chemical transmitter acetylcholine, which is released from vagal fibers (see Chap. 48). The major effect of vagal stimulation is on the SA node, atrial muscle, and the AV node. The result of stimulation is a restraining influence on the conduction tissue, with only a slight decrease in ventricular contractility. Vagal stimulation slows the heart rate by restraining the rate of diastolic depolarization in the conduction tissue.

### Baroreceptors

Baroreceptors are pressure-sensitive structures present mostly in the carotid sinus and the aortic arch. Decreased systolic blood pressure causes a reflex sympathetic response with increased pulse, increased contractility, and vasoconstriction. Increased pressure stimulates stretch receptors and causes a reflex vagal response, which results in decreased heart rate and passive vasodilation in the systemic arterioles.

### Chemoreceptors

The major chemoreceptor of the body is the medulla oblongata, but special receptors are also located in the carotid and aortic bodies. Chemical changes in the blood, especially of pH and carbon dioxide and oxygen levels, alter cardiac activity. A decreased pH or $PO_2$ causes a reflex sympathetic discharge that results in tachycardia, vasoconstriction, and increased myocardial contractility. A decreased $PCO_2$ and increased pH serve to reduce the vasoconstrictor effect, leading to passive vasodilatation.[7]

## ANATOMY OF THE ARTERIES, CAPILLARIES, VEINS, AND LYMPHATICS

### Arteries

The arteries are composed of three layers: tunica intima, tunica media, and tunica externa or adventitia (Figure 22-22). The layers contain variable amounts of collagen and muscle fibers according to the type of artery. Basically,

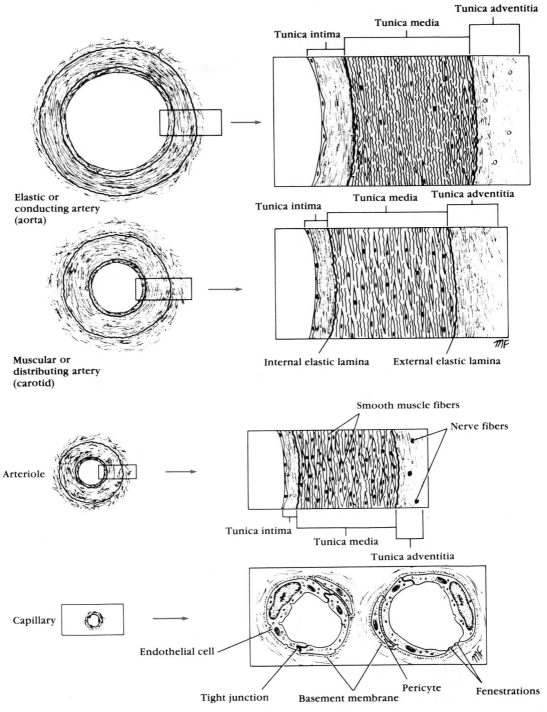

**FIGURE 22–22.**
Layers of the aorta, artery, arterioles, and capillary.

however, the outer coat supports or gives shape to the vessel, the middle or muscular coat regulates the diameter of the vessels, and the inner coat provides a smooth passageway for blood flow. The large arteries are called *elastic vessels* because they can stretch or increase their diameter to receive the stroke volume of the heart and then contract or resume their original shape, which pushes the blood forward. The *nutrient arteries* are branches of the elastic vessels; they supply oxygen and nutrients to the organs and tissues. The smallest branch of an artery is the *arteriole*, which leads into the capillary bed. The arteriole offers varying degrees of resistance to circulating blood by constricting or dilating its diameter. This mechanism regulates the volume and pressure in the artery and the capillary bed.

Blood pressure changes as blood courses down the arteries, being highest in the aorta and lowest in the capillary system (Figure 22-23). Vasoconstriction causes increased diastolic pressure (increased peripheral vascular resistance; PVR) and decreased capillary pressure. Vasodilatation causes decreased diastolic pressure (decreased PVR) and increased capillary pressure. The terminal portion of the arteriole contains precapillary sphincters that constrict and relax with autonomic stimulation or with local changes in temperature, pH, and oxygen levels.

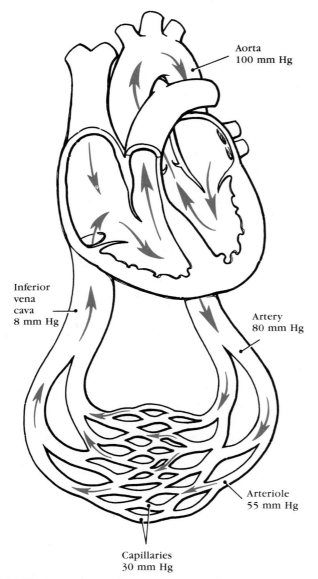

**Aorta**
**100 mm Hg**

**Inferior vena cava**
**8 mm Hg**

**Artery**
**80 mm Hg**

**Arteriole**
**55 mm Hg**

**Capillaries**
**30 mm Hg**

**FIGURE 22–23.**
Changes in pressure of blood from the aorta to the capillary bed to the great veins.

## Capillary Network

A network of tiny blood vessels provides the microcirculation through which materials enter or leave the circulating blood. A capillary consists of a single layer of endothelial cells. These cells are lined up in such a way to allow for the exchange of fluids, dissolved gases, and small molecules.[7] Large molecules, such as the plasma proteins, are held back in the capillaries and provide osmotic pressure. Capillary pressures differ in different organs and systems.

## Veins

The smallest veins are the venules, which receive their blood from the capillaries. These vessels have very thin walls through which some nutrients and oxygen may leave and waste products may enter. Capillaries and venules are often called *exchange vessels*.[7] Venules join together to form the veins. Many more veins than arteries are formed. These vessels contain approximately 75% of circulating blood volume at any one time. Because they have the capability to stretch and hold blood, they are called *capacitance vessels*. The larger veins have valves that are endothelial flaps or folds interspersed along the inner surface of the veins. These prevent the backflow of blood and are numerous in the lower extremities, especially in skeletal muscle areas.

## Lymph Vessels

Lymph vessels begin as blind-ended capillaries. They connect the lymph nodes and provide a secondary circulatory system. Approximately 2 liters of fluid are left in the interstitial spaces every day. This diffuses into the lymph capillaries. The lymph vessels effectively remove any excess plasma proteins that have leaked into the interstitial area.

The movement of lymph through the large lymphatic vessels occurs because of arterial pulsations and muscle movement. Backflow is prevented by the lymphatic vessel valves. Lymph flow in the thoracic duct is approximately 1.3 mL per kg of body weight per hour.[4] If the lymphatic circulation is decreased or blocked, *lymphedema* (edema of high protein content) occurs.

## FACTORS CONTROLLING ARTERIAL PRESSURE AND CIRCULATION

### Arterial Blood Pressure

Arterial blood pressure is determined by cardiac output and resistance to blood flow. The highest pressure is the *systolic pressure*, which is achieved by the contracting left ventricle in the ejection of its stroke volume. The *diastolic pressure*, maintained or stored as potential energy in the aorta during diastole, permits a continuous forward flow of blood. The difference between the systolic and diastolic pressures is the *pulse pressure*.

The sounds described in auscultating blood pressure are called *Korotkoff sounds* (Figure 22-24). They are generated after a cuff is placed around an extremity and pressure sufficient to occlude the blood flow is applied. As the cuff pressure is released, the beating sounds begin when the pressure falls below the systolic blood pressure. As the cuff pressure is continually released, the sounds become muffled and disappear at the point of diastolic pressure. It is generally appreciated that an error of 8 to 10 mm Hg (systolic pressure underestimated by 4 to 5 mm Hg and diastolic pressure overestimated by the same amount) occurs with this indirect measurement.[4] The sounds are basically produced by turbulence

of blood flow through the constricted segment. Flow of blood in an unconstricted artery is silent.[4]

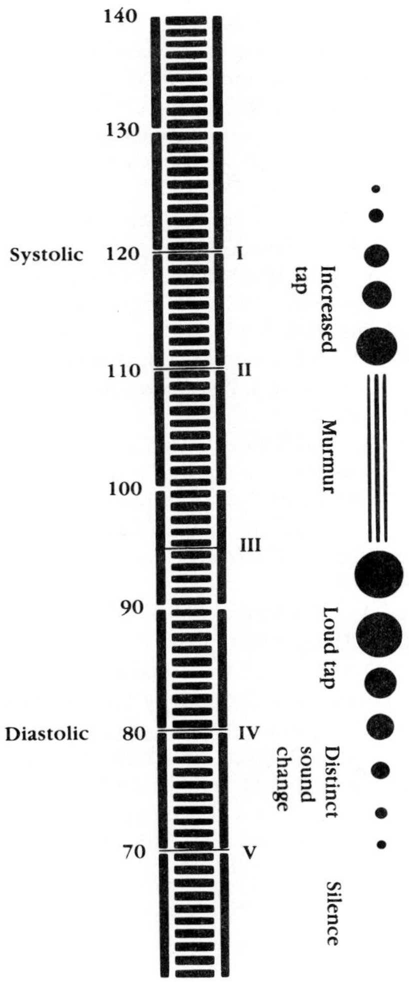

## Pulse Pressure

The pulse pressure is the difference between the systolic and diastolic pressures and normally is about 50 mm Hg.[4] Changes are affected by changes in the systolic or diastolic level. High systolic and low diastolic pressures increase or widen the pulse pressure. Low systolic and high diastolic pressures decrease or narrow the pulse pressure. Either component can be altered with a net effect of pulse pressure alteration.

Increased pulse pressure is usually the result of increased stroke volume, decreased peripheral volume, or decreased PVR. These factors might occur during exercise, fever, with aortic insufficiency, or sometimes with atherosclerosis. A narrowed pulse pressure can occur with increased PVR, decreased cardiac output, hypovolemia, or other conditions.[14]

## Direct and Indirect Determinants of Blood Pressure

Contraction of the left ventricle moves its stroke volume into the aorta. The left ventricle pumps against the elastic resistance of the aortic wall, the resistance offered by the arterioles, and the residual volume in the aorta. Therefore, direct determinants of arterial blood pressure include cardiac output, vascular resistance, aortic impedance (resistance to flow), and diastolic arterial volume.[2] Indirect determinants of blood pressure include the activity of the ANS and the renin-angiotensin-aldosterone system.

### Cardiac Output

The amount of blood ejected from the heart is partly determined by the length of end-diastolic fibers. Changes in stroke volume vary in healthy persons and increased ventricular volume at the end of diastole will, of itself, produce a stronger ventricular contraction. If an individual is hypovolemic, the decreased end-diastolic fiber length leads to a decrease in the force of ventricular contraction and, subsequently, a decrease in cardiac output and blood pressure.[14]

### Vascular Resistance

Vascular resistance is often called *peripheral vascular resistance* and refers to the impedance offered to blood flow by the arterioles. The major factor that determines resistance to blood flow from a major artery is the caliber

**FIGURE 22-24.**
Korotkoff sounds (Source: B. Dossey, C. Guzzetta, C. Kenner, *Critical Care Nursing: Body, Mind, Spirit* (3rd ed.). Philadelphia: J.B. Lippincott, 1992.)

or radius of the arteriole.[14] Constriction of the arterioles increases the resistance against which the heart has to pump and raises the blood pressure. Dilatation of the arterioles decreases the impedance offered and decreases blood pressure. Stimulation of the sympathetic nerves causes vasoconstriction, a mechanism that is important in blood pressure elevations with exercise or fear. Humoral mechanisms can cause an increased or decreased PVR. Prostaglandins, renin, kinins, and many other substances are under study in relation to their regulation of PVR.

The control of blood flow by the tissues is called *autoregulation* and probably occurs with selective opening and closing of capillary sphincters. Hyperemia occurs when the channels are open and cause increased amounts of blood flow to an area.

### Aortic Impedance

Aortic impedance is offered by the elastic aortic wall and the aortic valve. The aortic valve normally remains closed until the pressure in the left ventricle exceeds the pressure maintained in the aorta. After this occurs, the valve opens and the ventricle must pump against the resistance offered by the elastic aortic wall. When elasticity increases, such as with aging, more aortic impedance is offered to the left ventricle. Also, with narrowing of the aortic valve, impedance requires an increased ventricular force to eject its contents.

### Diastolic Arterial Volume

The amount of blood remaining in the aorta on diastole is related to all of the factors mentioned in the previous paragraph. If cardiac output is increased and PVR is also elevated, increased amounts of blood remain in the arterial circuit during diastole. This usually increases the diastolic pressure and the resistance against which the ventricle has to pump. If cardiac output is increased and PVR is decreased, the "run-off" decreases the diastolic volume and volume resistance against which the heart is pumping.

## FACTORS AFFECTING THE VENOUS CIRCULATION

Blood in the veins does not normally pulsate as it does in arteries. Movement of blood through the systemic veins is due to pressure differences; skeletal, thoracic, and visceral muscle pressures; and valves that prevent the backflow of blood. Pulsations may be seen in the jugular veins; these reflect the activity of the right atrium and right ventricle. Abnormalities in venous circulation can result from many conditions, such as fluid overloading, venous insufficiency, and constrictive pericarditis.

## REFERENCES

1. Biggers, J.T. The electrical activity of the heart. In J.W. Hurst et al. (eds.), *The Heart* (7th ed.). New York: McGraw-Hill, 1990.
2. Dustan, H.P. Pathophysiology of hypertension. In J.W. Hurst et al. (eds.), *The Heart* (7th ed.). New York: McGraw-Hill, 1990.
3. Factor, S.M. Pathophysiology of myocardial ischemia. In J.W. Hurst et al. (eds.), *The Heart* (7th ed.). New York: McGraw-Hill, 1990.
4. Ganong, W.F. *Review of Medical Physiology* (15th ed.). Norwalk, Conn.: Appleton & Lange, 1991.
5. Guyton, A.C. *Textbook of Medical Physiology* (8th ed.). Philadelphia: W.B. Saunders, 1990.
6. Hathaway, D.R., and Watanabe, A.M. Biochemical basis for cardiac and vascular smooth muscle contraction. In W.N. Kelley (ed.), *Textbook of Internal Medicine*. Philadelphia: J.B. Lippincott, 1989.
7. Little, R.C. *Physiology of the Heart and Circulation* (3rd ed.). Chicago: Yearbook, 1985.
8. Mason, J.W., and Hordeghem, L.C. Principles of cardiac electrophysiology. In W.N. Kelley (ed.), *Textbook of Internal Medicine*. Philadelphia: J.B. Lippincott, 1989.
9. Schlant, R.C., and Silverman, M.E. Anatomy of the heart. In J.W. Hurst et al. (eds.), *The Heart* (7th ed.). New York: McGraw-Hill, 1990.
10. Schlant, R.C., and Sonnenblick, E.H. Normal physiology of the cardiovascular system. In J.W. Hurst et al. (eds.), *The Heart* (7th ed.). New York: McGraw-Hill, 1990.
11. Shaver, J.A., and Salerni, R. Auscultation of the heart. In J.W. Hurst et al. (eds.), *The Heart* (7th ed.). New York: McGraw-Hill, 1990.
12. Sokolow, M., and McIlroy, M.B. *Clinical Cardiology*. Los Altos, Calif.: Lange, 1986.
13. Vatner, S.F., and Cox, D.A. Circulatory function and control. In W.N. Kelley (ed.), *Textbook of Internal Medicine*. Philadelphia: J.B. Lippincott, 1989.
14. Wallace, A.G., and Waugh, R.A. Pathophysiology of cardiovascular disease. In L.H. Smith and S.O. Thier (eds.), *Pathophysiology: The Biological Principles of Disease* (2nd ed.). Philadelphia: W.B. Saunders, 1985.

# Alterations in Cardiac Rhythms

## Chapter Outline

## Learning Objectives

1. Identify the limb and precordial leads of the electrocardiogram.
2. Identify the leads for examining electrocardiographic changes indicative of anterior myocardial infarction and inferior myocardial infarction.
3. Discuss the effects of digitalis toxicity and hyperkalemia on conduction of electrical impulses in the heart.
4. Trace the path of a normal sinus impulse from the sinoatrial node to the ventricles.
5. Define *dysrhythmia* and *escape rhythms*.
6. Discuss the factors that will alter hemodynamic stability during dysrhythmias.
7. List etiologic factors commonly associated with dysrhythmia development.
8. Discuss the two major mechanisms responsible for altered cardiac rhythms.
9. Identify and state the electrocardiographic characteristics for the following dysrhythmias: sinus bradycardia, atrial fibrillation, junctional rhythm.

10. List the three classifications of dysrhythmias and give an example of each.
11. Discuss the pathophysiology for each of the following dysrhythmias: atrial tachycardia, Wolff-Parkinson-White syndrome, and ventricular tachycardia.
12. Discuss the role of electrophysiologic mapping in the detection and treatment of dysrhythmias.
13. List the dysrhythmias classified as disturbances in impulse formation.
14. Discuss "R on T" phenomena.
15. Define hemiblock.
16. Discuss the relationship between dysrhythmias and coronary artery supply in the setting of acute myocardial infarction.
17. Compare and contrast the clinical significance of Mobitz type I and Mobitz type II atrioventricular block.
18. Identify the characteristic waveforms associated with atrial flutter.
19. Discuss the clinical significance of complete heart block.

(continued)

An alteration in the normal cardiac rhythm can be an unwelcome symptom to the individual or a life-threatening event. Cardiac rhythm abnormalities may be symptomatic of developing or chronic disease processes or may occur in otherwise healthy individuals. This chapter presents common alterations in cardiac rhythms, known as cardiac dysrhythmias, the pathophysiology of these events, and their hemodynamic consequences. Table 23-1 defines some important terms relating to normal electrophysiology and cardiac dysrhythmias.

## THE ELECTROCARDIOGRAM

Any discussion regarding alterations in cardiac rhythms must be prefaced with an overview of the basic concepts,

**TABLE 23-1.**
TERMS RELATING TO NORMAL ELECTROPHYSIOLOGY
AND CARDIAC DYSRHYTHMIAS

| TERM | DEFINITION |
|---|---|
| Absolute refractory period | Period where cardiac cell cannot accept any stimulus, regardless of intensity, to initiate an impulse |
| Accessory pathway | An extra or analogous pathway bypassing the AV node |
| Action potential | A change in electrical activity along the cell membrane initiating an impulse; each cardiac cell has five phases: 0, 1, 2, 3, and 4 |
| Automaticity | Electrical property of cardiac cells that permits spontaneous depolarization generating an electrical impulse; groups of these automatic cells make up the heart's primary pacemakers: SA node, AV node, and ventricles |
| Circus movement | Continuous stimulation of the myocardium through conduction pathways within the myocardium |
| Conduction | Flow of electrical impulses through the cardiac conduction system. Normal conduction occurs in this way from the SA node to the ventricles |
| Aberrant conduction | Impulses that are abnormally conducted through the ventricles due to a delay in the refractory period in the bundle branches; seen on the ECG as a change in QRS morphology |
| Antegrade conduction | Impulses flow forward through the conduction system |
| Retrograde conduction | Impulses flow backward through the conduction system |
| Compensatory pause | A pause that occurs after a premature complex; a premature beat that does not interrupt the cardiac cycle is a full compensatory pause and is equal to twice the R to R interval between two normal beats |
| Reentry | Phenomenon where an impulse returns to reexcite a previously stimulated region of the myocardium through a pathway; usually the impulse is sinus or ectopic in origin and occurs in an area of slowed conduction with unequal response time in the myocardium |
| Rhythm | |
| Active rhythm | A rhythm stimulated by a premature ectopic focus that maintains a rate faster than a normal pacemaker and assumes control of cardiac rhythm regardless of the underlying rhythm |
| Ectopic rhythm | Impulses that originate outside of the SA node due to the inability of the SA node to generate an impulse |
| Normal sinus rhythm | A series of impulses generated by the SA node and conducted through the conduction system in a normal fashion |
| Passive rhythm | Impulses generated by a lower pacemaker when the primary pacemakers slow or fail; also termed as escape rhythm |

purpose, and use of the electrocardiogram (ECG). Electrocardiographic tracings are indispensable to differentiate between normal and abnormal cardiac rhythms. The rhythm identified can provide evidence not detected through the usual diagnostic techniques. It should be noted that ECGs are not to be depended on solely to diagnose pathologic conditions. A comprehensive evaluation of the individual's history, physical examination, and other diagnostic tests are necessary to make differential diagnoses.

The ECG is a graphic recording of the heart's electrical activity. The waveforms produced are of: (1) the electrical activity (action potential) generated as electrical impulses spread through the conduction system, and (2) the recovery of myocardial cells following depolarization (Figure 23-1). These waveforms, labeled as the P, Q, R, S, and T waves, are recorded on graph paper with horizontal time and vertical voltage scales (Figure 23-2). Positive waveforms are those occurring above the line, while negative waveforms occur below the O or isoelectric line. The technology used to transmit and record this data consists of electrodes, monitoring cables, amplifier, and oscilloscope (monitor). These range in sophistication from simple ECG machines to complex computerized monitoring systems.

The electrical impulses are sensed by positive and negative electrodes placed in various locations on the body surface. One positive and one negative electrode make a lead. Leads record the magnitude, direction, and surface potential of impulses generated by cardiac cells. Electrical impulses moving toward a positive electrode produce a predominantly positive deflection of the QRS complex (R wave), while impulses traveling away from a positive produce predominantly negatively deflected QRS (QS) complexes (Figure 23-3).

The two types of leads are bipolar and unipolar. Bipolar leads were first identified by Einthoven as a triangular lead system composed of a positive and a negative electrode placed at equal distances from the heart.[10] The electrodes are placed on the left arm, right arm, and left leg and are termed limb leads (Figure 23-4). In lead I, the positive electrode is on the left arm with the negative on the right. In lead II, the negative electrode is on the right arm with the positive on the left leg. In lead III, the positive electrode is on the left leg with the negative on the left arm. The bipolar leads view the heart from the frontal plane gathering data from the superior, inferior, right, and left surfaces. The basic electrodes necessary for monitoring in the limb leads are the positive, negative, and ground electrodes.[19] In ECG machines and some

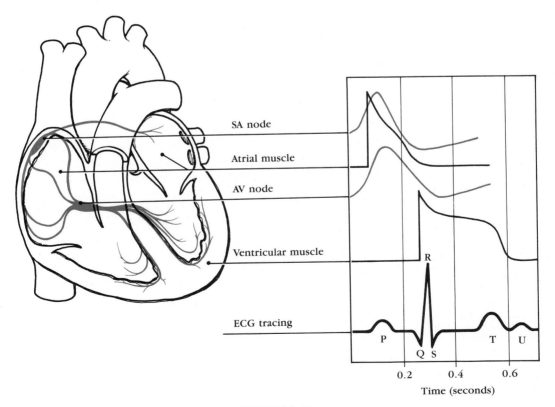

**FIGURE 23–1.**
Action potentials.

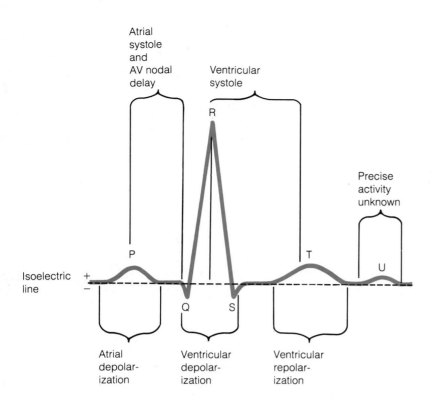

Atrial
systole
and
AV nodal
delay

Ventricular
systole

Precise
activity
unknown

R

P

T

U

Isoelectric
line    +
       −

Q    S

Atrial
depolar-
ization

Ventricular
depolar-
ization

Ventricular
repolar-
ization

**FIGURE 23–2.**
Correlation of mechanical and electrical activity within the heart.

monitoring systems, a fourth electrode is placed on the right leg to serve as an electrical ground.

The unipolar leads consist of the augmented limb leads and the precordial chest (V) leads. The augmented limb leads are so called because the electrical vol-

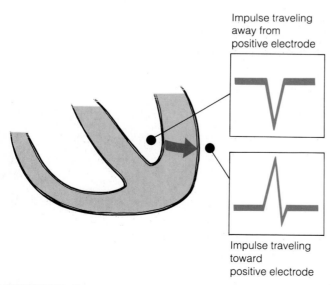

Impulse traveling
away from
positive electrode

Impulse traveling
toward
positive electrode

**FIGURE 23–3.**
Appearance of QRS complex relative to cardiac placement of a positive electrode.

tage is so small that it must be amplified to be seen. These leads also look at the frontal plane of the heart. A positive electrode is placed on either the left arm (AVL), right arm (AVR), or left leg (AVF) with a common reference point at the heart (see Figure 23-4).[10] All four electrodes are required to monitor or record the augmented leads.

Precordial leads provide six views (V1 through V6) of electrical activity of the heart on the horizontal plane (Figure 23-5). Due to the position of the electrodes in the precordial area, these leads are particularly useful in detecting ventricular activity and chamber hypertrophy, and also in providing a mirror image of posterior heart activity. The positive electrodes are placed in specific locations on the anterior chest wall and each gives specific important information that can be supportive of a diagnosis of myocardial ischemia or infarction (See Chap. 25). The majority of the electrical impulses move away from the electrode in V1, producing a small, positive R wave and deep, negative S wave. Due to the placement of the V2 through V6 electrodes and the flow of the forces, the R wave appears to grow, becoming more positive, biphasic in V3, and reaching maximum height in V4. This is known as *R wave progression* and is characteristic of normal ECGs. The R waves in V5 and V6 then become smaller (see Figure 23-5).

The 12 lead ECG is composed of the six limb and six precordial leads, giving a comprehensive view of the

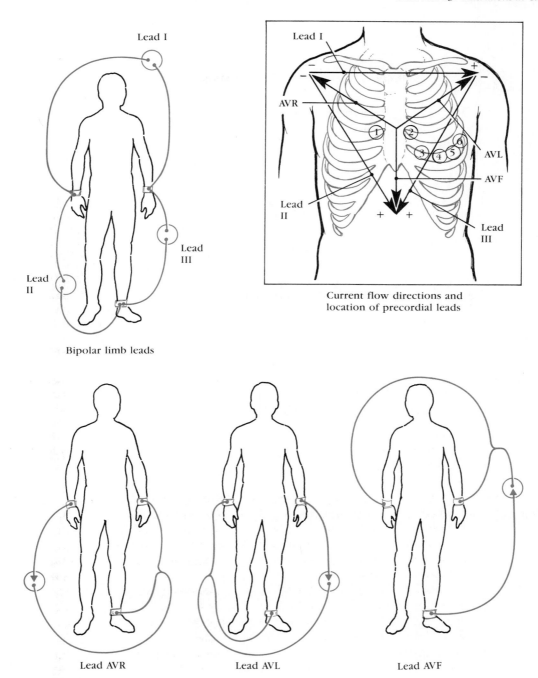

Current flow directions and
location of precordial leads

Bipolar limb leads

Augmented limb leads

**FIGURE 23-4.**
The ECG leads and 12 lead placement.

heart in two dimensions. Figure 23-6 illustrates a normal 12 lead ECG. It is useful in diagnosing acute myocardial infarction (MI), atrial and ventricular hypertrophy, and congenital defects; it can detect the dysrhythmias associated with acute or chronic heart disease. Suspect cardiac rhythms must be evaluated in all 12 leads. An ectopic rhythm is not identified from a single monitoring lead unless the rhythm requires immediate intervention.[16] Figure 23-7 exemplifies the need to view a dysrhythmia in all 12 leads to identify it. In a single lead, this rhythm appears to be a bradycardia. However, upon examination of all the leads, the undulating waves of atrial fibrillation (AF) can be seen (see p. 468).

In the diagnosis of acute MI, the 12 lead ECG assesses

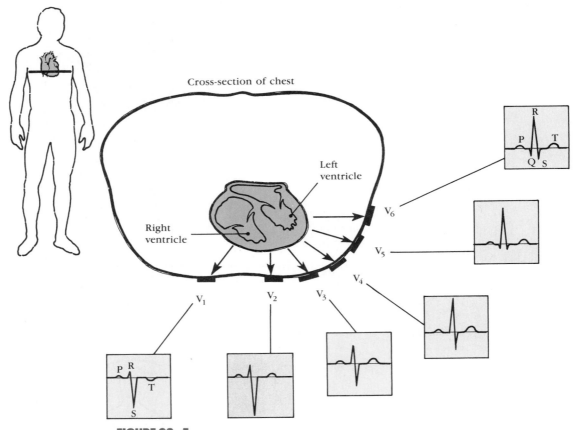

**FIGURE 23–5.**
Appearance of QRS complexes in precordial leads of a 12 lead ECG.

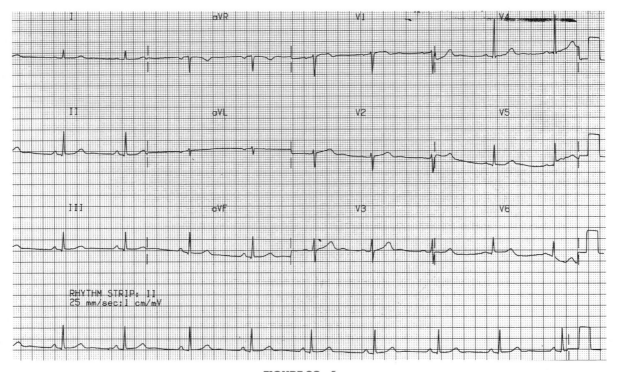

**FIGURE 23–6.**
Normal 12 lead ECG.

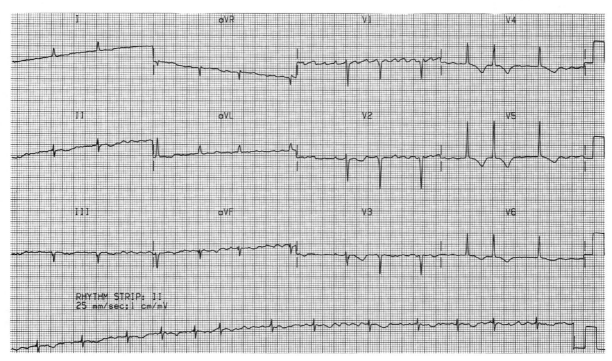

**FIGURE 23-7.**
The 12 lead ECG used to detect dysrhythmias: atrial fibrillation.

anatomic areas or surfaces of the heart perfused by the right and left coronary arteries. Patterns reflecting ischemia, injury, and necrosis can be detected by examining these areas (Figure 23-8). Leads I, II, and AVF view the inferior and posterior portions of the myocardium normally perfused by the right coronary artery. Leads I and AVL view the lateral portion of the left ventricle while leads V1 through V6 view the anteroseptal areas. Loss of R wave progression is characteristic of infarction in these areas. In addition, the precordial leads may indicate posterior infarction by their ability to mirror electrical activity from the posterior surface of the left ventricle. In this mirror image, R waves are positively deflected with inverted ST segments. Figure 23-9 illustrates ECG changes indicative of inferior MI with a complicating third degree block.

The movement of electrical forces (a wave of impulses) through the myocardium is called a *vector*. It is a mathematical value of magnitude, sense, and direction that is expressed as an arrow.[1] The electrical axis is defined as a vector that originates in the center of Einthoven's triangle.[1] A line drawn between two connections of a lead is called a lead axis.[5] The vector that represents the electrical axis gives the direction of the activation process as it is projected in the limb leads. A simple method of calculating the quadrant in which the electrical axis is located consists of using the maximal QRS deflection on two of the three bipolar leads on a hexax-

ial reference system (Figure 23-10). A brief description of the significance of axis deviation is in the following discussion.

Axis deviation is estimated by plotting the peak values of either the R wave or the S wave on two of the three bipolar leads of a hexaxial reference system. From that point, lines perpendicular to the lead axis are drawn. The QRS axis is obtained by connecting the center of the hexaxial lead system and the point where the two perpendicular lines cross.

An axis in the range of −30° to +90° is normal. An axis in the range of −30° to −90° is left axis. A left axis greater than −30° is abnormal, not due to cardiac anatomical position but most likely to a conduction defect. Left axis deviation of −30° is easily identified by an equiphasic QRS complex in lead II. An axis in the range of +90° to +180° is right axis deviation. Right axis deviation of +90° is recognized by an equiphasic QRS complex in lead I. An axis in the range of −90° to +180° is an indeterminate axis.[5]

Figure 23-11 shows the ECG appearance of the normal axis and deviations from them using leads I, II, and AVF. Abnormal left axis deviation may be due to left anterior hemiblock, inferior wall MI, Wolff-Parkinson-White syndrome, hyperkalemia, and a right ventricular pacemaker. Right axis deviation may be seen in normal individuals with a vertical heart position, right ventricular hypertrophy, left posterior hemiblock, extensive antero-

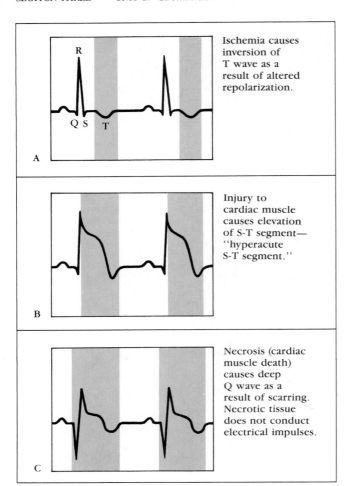

Ischemia causes inversion of T wave as a result of altered repolarization.

Injury to cardiac muscle causes elevation of S-T segment—"hyperacute S-T segment."

Necrosis (cardiac muscle death) causes deep Q wave as a result of scarring. Necrotic tissue does not conduct electrical impulses.

**FIGURE 23–8.**
These ECG patterns reflect (A) ischemia, (B) injury, and (C) necrosis.

lateral MI, left ventricular pacemaker, or dextrocardia (heart in right hemithorax).[1]

## NORMAL CONDUCTION

Chapter 22 details the normal cardiac anatomy, physiology, and electromechanical events. Normal cardiac rhythm is comprised of many single cardiac events, each the result of an electrical impulse originating in the sinoatrial (SA) node. Figure 23-12 shows normal cardiac conduction and correlates these electrical events occurring in the myocardium to the graphic representation on the ECG.

From the SA node, the impulse then spreads to the atria and AV node through the internodal pathways. The three pathways are designated the anterior, middle, and posterior internodal tracts. The anterior internodal tract, called *Bachman's bundle*, travels anteriorly around the superior vena cava down the atrial septum to the AV node and fibers also branch off to the left atrium.[18] The sinus impulses conducted by these specialized cells cause atrial depolarization and contraction. The electrical event is reflected on the ECG as the P wave. At the AV node, the impulse slows as it passes through the nodal fibers, thereby allowing the atria time to completely contract. This event constitutes the PR interval of the ECG complex. The impulse then flows through the bundle of His to the left and right bundle branches to reach the Purkinje fibers embedded in the ventricular muscle. Stimulation of the ventricles results in ventricular depolarization and contraction. The QRS complex represents this electrical event. Repolarization of the ventricles is reflected by the T wave.

These electromechanical events comprise one cardiac cycle or one heart beat. Sixty to 100 cardiac cycles per minute constitute a normal cardiac rhythm (Figure 23-13). A series of normal cardiac electrical events is known as normal sinus rhythm.

## NORMAL HEMODYNAMICS

The electrical events of the heart precede the mechanical events. The mechanical events of the cardiac cycle, systole and diastole, are responsible for adequate perfusion and oxygenation of systemic organs and tissues. Normal cardiac output (4 to 8 liters/min) is dependent upon stroke volume and heart rate (see Chap. 22). Any condition that alters these two components alters perfusion and oxygenation. Most of the dysrhythmias discussed in this chapter directly or indirectly alter cardiac output or tissue perfusion.

## CARDIAC DYSRHYTHMIAS

An alteration in the normal rhythm of the cardiac cycle is often labeled as dysrhythmia, arrhythmia, or ectopic rhythm. The term most widely accepted is dysrhythmia. A *dysrhythmia* is defined as an abnormality of the formation or conduction of an electrical impulse that causes an alteration in heart rate or regularity.[15] A dysrhythmia occurs when some factor alters the normal action potential of the heart. The two primary mechanisms that initiate alterations in normal cardiac rhythm are *abnormal automaticity* and *reentry phenomena*.[13,27]

Automaticity may be enhanced or depressed. In *enhanced automaticity*, the rate of pacemaker discharge is increased secondary to an accelerated rise of phase 4 (see Chap. 22). Conversely, *depressed automaticity* re-

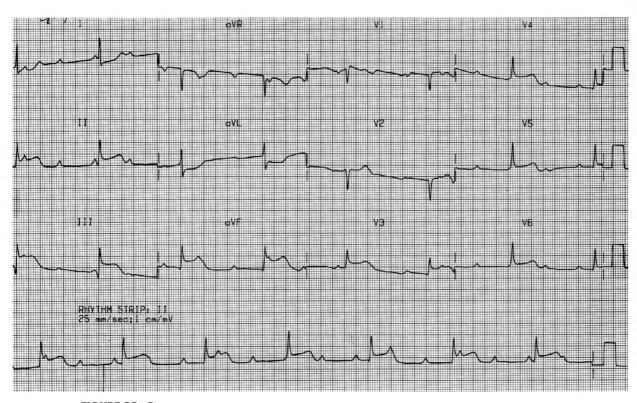

**FIGURE 23-9.**
Inferior MI with third-degree AV block. Note elevated ST segments in Leads II, III, and aVF. Some elevation of ST segments in V leads suggests possible septal injury.

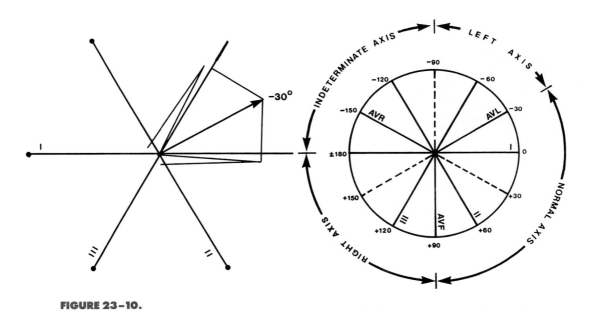

**FIGURE 23-10.**
Plot of QRS axis on hexaxial system (left) and range of axis (right) (Source: W.N. Kelley, *Textbook of Internal Medicine*. Philadelphia: J.B. Lippincott Co., 1989.)

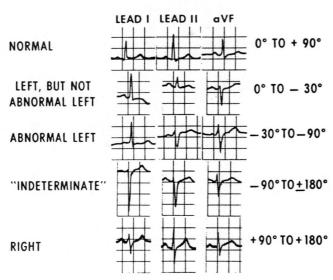

**FIGURE 23–11.**

Determination of the quadrant, or parts of the left superior quadrant, in which the electrical axis can be located according to maximal ventricular deflections. The "indeterminate" quadrant is also called "right superior" and "northwest." (Source: J.W. Hurst, *The Heart* (7th ed.). New York: McGraw-Hill, 1990.)

sults from a slowing of the rise of phase 4. Factors influencing automaticity are listed in Table 23-2.

During conditions that enhance automaticity, a second action potential may be generated at the end of phase 2 or early in phase 3. Should this after-potential be conducted, a premature beat ensues. The enhanced automaticity and secondary action potentials may trigger repetitive firing, producing tachydysrhythmias.[26]

Reentry develops when an impulse has the ability to reexcite tissue previously depolarized through anatomic or functional circuits.[13,27] The rate of impulse conduction and the length of the refractory period influence the presence of reentry phenomena. As illustrated in Figure 23-14, when all criteria are present, single or multiple impulses may enter the circuit generating ectopic beats or recurrent dysrhythmias. Continuous excitement of the myocardium by normal or anomalous paths is described as *circus movement*.[28] Sustained tachydysrhythmias are associated with the combination of reentry and circus movement.[26] Electrophysiologic mapping techniques have provided much new insight into the mechanisms responsible for dysrhythmias seen clinically. The techniques remain imprecise, however, and the findings are controversial.[8,11]

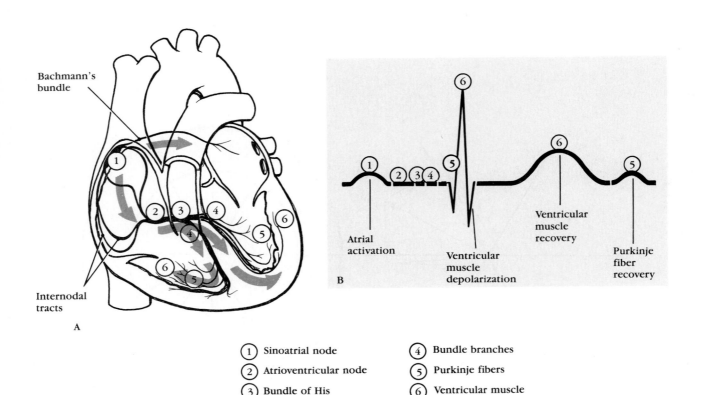

| | | | |
|---|---|---|---|
| ① Sinoatrial node | | ④ Bundle branches | |
| ② Atrioventricular node | | ⑤ Purkinje fibers | |
| ③ Bundle of His | | ⑥ Ventricular muscle | |

**FIGURE 23–12.**

**A.** Normal cardiac conduction. **B.** Correlation of electrical events of the heart and ECG tracing.

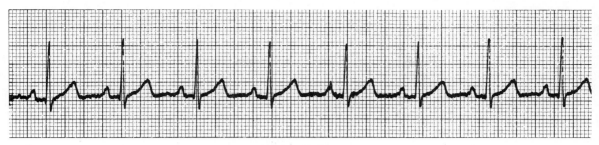

**FIGURE 23-13.**
Normal sinus rhythm.

Alterations in cardiac rhythms can result from many etiologies (Table 23-3). The most common include disease or injury to the cardiac muscle, structures, or conduction system; systemic diseases; drug intoxication; electrolyte imbalances; and exercise.[10] Figure 23-15 exemplifies the effect of drugs and electrolytes on the ECG.

Dysrhythmias are clinically significant as indicators of underlying heart disease or they may produce life-threatening electrical events with catastrophic hemodynamic results. Dysrhythmias may be present with or without clinical signs or symptoms and in individuals with and without advanced cardiac disease. Clinical symptoms in the individual with a normal heart are usually not noted unless the heart rate exceeds 180 beats per minute (BPM) or slows to below 40 BPM.[14] Due to the inability

of normal compensatory mechanisms to equilibrate, these extremely fast or slow rhythms can significantly reduce both cardiac output and systemic blood pressure, thus reducing perfusion to the brain, heart, kidneys, mesentery, and other vital centers.

The hemodynamic effects of dysrhythmias vary based on the heart rate; heart rhythm; synchronization of atrial and ventricular events; presence, stage, and etiology of underlying cardiac disease; existence of drug toxicity; and state of the vasomotor compensatory mechanisms.[2]

Dysrhythmias in the pediatric population, while similar in appearance to adult dysrhythmias, differ in subcellular mechanisms, rates, and prognosis.[6] Due to the scope of the topic, discussion in this chapter will be limited to adults.

**TABLE 23-2.**
FACTORS THAT ENHANCE AND DEPRESS AUTOMATICITY

| ENHANCING FACTORS | DEPRESSING FACTORS |
|---|---|
| Sympathetic nervous system stimulation<br>  fever<br>  pain<br>  anxiety | Parasympathetic nervous system stimulation<br>  vagotonia<br>  hyperkalemia<br>  drugs |
| High-output states<br>  hyperthyroidism<br>  anemia<br>  AV fistula | |
| Congestive heart failure | |
| Hypoxia | |
| High metabolic rates | |
| Toxic states | |
| Exercise | |
| Drugs<br>  vagolytics (atropine)<br>  sympathomimetics (epinephrine,<br>  norepinephrine) | |
| Catecholamines | |
| Hypokalemia | |
| Acid-base imbalance | |
| Trauma | |

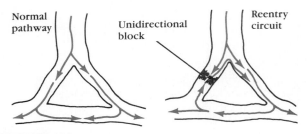

**FIGURE 23–14.**
Mechanism of reentry. In the reentry circuit, a unidirectional block permits the impulse to reenter the tissue and set up a circus movement. (Source: B.H. Yee, and S.I. Zorb, *Cardiac Critical Care Nursing.* Boston: Little, Brown, 1986.)

## CLASSIFICATION OF COMMON CARDIAC DYSRHYTHMIAS

Dysrhythmias are classified into three major groups according to the mechanisms and etiologies: disturbance in impulse formation, disturbances in impulse conduction, and combinations of the two.[8,14]

### Disturbance in Impulse Formation

The primary rhythms to be explored are SA, ectopic, and ventricular rhythms.

#### Sinoatrial Rhythms

Sinus bradycardia and sinus tachycardia (ST) are dysrythmias associated with *abnormal rates*. The PR and QRS intervals are normal.

*SINUS BRADYCARDIA.*    In sinus bradycardia, the heart rate is less than 60 BPM and is a regular sinus rhythm (Figure 23-16). Sinus bradycardia is usually not associated with pathologic findings unless it occurs as a sequela of sick sinus syndrome. Usually it occurs as a normal compensatory mechanism to reduce cardiac output secondary to increased vagal stimulation. With automaticity in the SA node decreased, the heart rate slows. This rhythm is expected in athletes, during sleep, and following MI.[19] If sinus bradycardia occurs after acute MI, junctional or escape rhythms may be precipitated. Bradycardia is thought to be due to a vagal reflex, a chemoreflex triggered by chemical stimuli from the left ventricular wall.[21]

*SINUS TACHYCARDIA.*    *Sinus tachycardia* occurs when the heart rate is in the range of 100 to 150 BPM. There is no change in QRS waveform or PR intervals (Figure 23-17). With the increased rate, there may be a slight variation in the R to R intervals. This feature is beneficial in distinguishing between atrial and STs at fast rates. Sinus tachycardia is a normal response to increased stress on the body. Such conditions as fever, exercise, and fear stimulate the normal sinus mechanism and increase heart rate. Sinus tachycardia is commonly seen as a normal compensatory response in hypotensive states requiring increased tissue perfusion. It may also develop in normal individuals after drinking caffeinated beverages or using tobacco products. Sinus tachycardia as the primary problem is mainly associated with sick sinus syndrome (see p. 464). Because the accelerated firing of the SA node is due to enhanced automaticity secondary to stimulation from the sympathetic nervous system, it may be an early symptom of congestive heart failure (CHF), MI, or pulmonary infarct.[22]

Clinical significance of ST is dependent upon the underlying disease process. Elevated heart rates can increase myocardial oxygen demand, thus increasing existing myocardial ischemia. Increased heart rate in the presence of myocardial ischemia may also lead to in-

**TABLE 23–3.**
ETIOLOGIES OF DYSRHYTHMIAS

| ETIOLOGY | EXAMPLES |
| --- | --- |
| Underlying cardiac disease | Coronary artery disease; cardiomyopathies; valvular lesions; congenital defects; rheumatic heart disease |
| Acute myocardial infarction | |
| Systemic/metabolic diseases | Diabetes; hypertension; pulmonary disorders; hyperthyroidism; anemia |
| Electrolyte imbalance | |
| Anesthesia | |
| Drug intoxication | Digitalis<br>Other prescription and illegal drugs |
| Central nervous system disorders | |
| Psychoneurogenic disorders | |
| Exercise | |

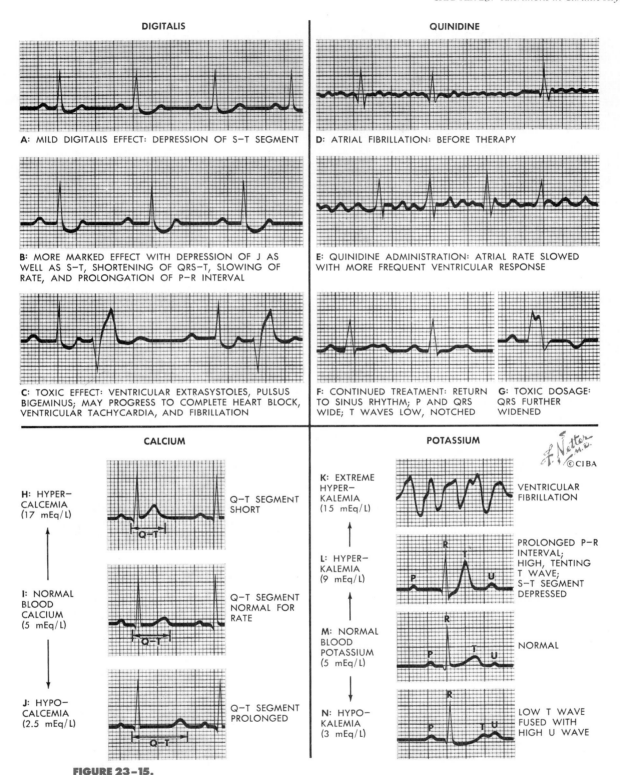

**FIGURE 23–15.**

Effects of drugs and electrolytes on the electrocardiogram. (Source: Copyright 1969, CIBA Pharmaceutical Company, division of CIBA-GEIGY Corporation; Reprinted with permission from the CIBA Collection of Medical Illustrations, illustrated by Frank H. Netter, MD. All rights reserved.)

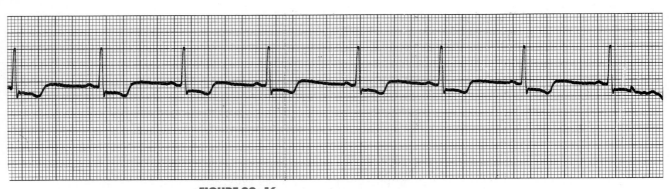

**FIGURE 23-16.**
Sinus bradycardia with associated ST segment depression.

creased ventricular irritability and trigger ventricular tachycardia (VT) (see p. 471).

*SINUS DYSRHYTHMIA. Sinus dysrhythmia* is an irregular rhythm arising from the SA node. Commonly called the respiratory rhythm, the cycles vary with respiratory rate, increasing with inhalation and decreasing with exhalation (Figure 23-18).[2,22] The PQRS complexes and intervals remain normal unless altered by other mechanisms. The irregularity can be attributed to factors that enhance vagal tone. Sinus dysrhythmia becomes clinically significant when the pauses between the RR intervals are long enough to allow atrial, junctional, or ventricular ectopic beats to escape.

*SICK SINUS SYNDROME. Sick sinus syndrome* (SSS) is a syndrome of alternating tachycardic and bradycardic rhythms associated with cerebral hypoperfusion and syncopal episodes.[22] It is a common cause of hypoperfusion and is usually treated with pacemaker insertion.

Although SSS is usually idiopathic and found in elderly individuals, it may be linked to: (1) dysfunction of the SA node secondary to inflammatory, collagen, or metastatic diseases; (2) influence of the autonomic nervous system, such as abnormal vagotonia; (3) effect of drugs, such as beta-blockers and antihypertensives; or (4) surgical injury.[13,23]

The tachycardia associated with this syndrome is a supraventricular (SVT) escape mechanism rather than one arising from the SA node.[13] The escape mechanism is triggered by the bradycardic rate as a compensatory mechanism. Without this escape mechanism, profound bradycardia and cerebral hypoperfusion will occur. The fast and slow rhythms may alternate with other rhythms, especially atrial tachycardia and AF. When the abnormal rhythm terminates, a long period of asystole or bradycardia may result in syncope.[13]

*SINUS ARREST. Sinus arrest* is a rhythm produced by a marked depression of sinus node activity secondary to coronary artery disease, acute infectious processes, enhanced carotid sinus and vagal tone, and the toxic effects of digitalis, quinidine, and salicylates.[23] Sinus arrest is notable for long pauses in cardiac rhythm and absent P waves (Figure 23-19). The rate and PQRST complexes of the underlying rhythm are normal unless altered by other mechanisms. The pauses generated by the failure of the SA node to fire produces an irregularity to the underlying rhythm. This dysrhythmia is clinically insignificant unless SA node depression is prolonged and atrial standstill results. The AV node may assume the pacemaker function or an escape rhythm may surface to maintain ventricular rate.

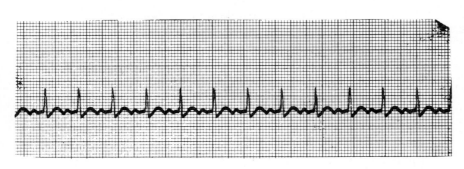

**FIGURE 23-17.**
Sinus tachycardia. (Source: B.H. Yee and S.I. Zorb, *Cardiac Critical Care Nursing.* Boston: Little, Brown, 1986.)

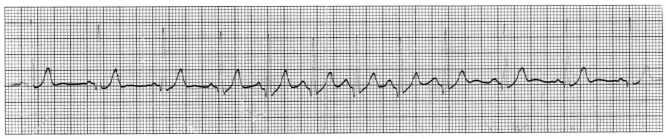

**FIGURE 23-18.**
Sinus dysrhythmia.

## Ectopic Atrial Rhythms

Ectopic atrial rhythms are those that originate outside the SA node. Usually these arise due to the inability of the primary pacemaker (SA node) to generate an electrical impulse. Thus, automatic cells within the atria or one of the latent pacemakers (the AV node or ventricles) initiate impulses to stimulate the myocardium to sustain the ventricular rate.[23] The dysrhythmias in this category are atrial rhythms, junctional escape rhythms, and ventricular rhythms.

### *PREMATURE ATRIAL CONTRACTIONS.* The primary ectopic beats that originate from the atria are *premature atrial contractions* (PACs). These impulses result from the enhanced automaticity secondary to emotional distress, use of tobacco and caffeine, electrolyte imbalance, atrial hypertrophy, hypoxia, digitalis toxicity, and chronic lung disease.[2]

The PACs appear on the ECG as premature beats that interrupt the underlying cardiac rhythm (Figure 23-20). They may appear alone or alternate with the intrinsic rhythm. The shape of the P wave of the PAC appears different from the sinus P and varies depending upon the origin of the ectopic focus in the atria. The PR interval and QRS complex of the PAC is usually normal unless affected by other mechanisms that alter conduction through the AV junction and the ventricles. A pause follows the PAC due to the early depolarization of the atria and the resetting of the SA node.[10] Occasionally, the PAC arises so soon after the sinus beat that it is nonconducted, producing a blocked PAC.

An individual who has a normal myocardium may experience PACs. Frequent PACs may produce palpitations and discomfort but they are otherwise clinically insignificant. In the presence of a diseased myocardium, PACs may precipitate AF, atrial flutter, and atrial tachycardias. Both PACs and subsequent atrial dysrhythmias are dangerous to the person who has suffered an acute MI. A decrease in cardiac output may further decrease myocardial perfusion and increase ventricular irritability, initiating VT. In the acute MI period, PACs may also indicate impending CHF or electrolyte imbalance.

Premature atrial contractions can occur at a critical time, the *critical coupling interval*, and can establish a reentry circuit, thus producing atrial tachycardia.[21]

Reentry from the premature atrial beat through the AV node back to the atria has been projected as the most common cause of PACs. Other reentry circuits may include the SA node, the atria, or accessory bypass tracts. The wave of depolarization proceeds through the fiber with slowed conduction; then it returns to a nearby fiber, causing reexcitation.[21] Increased rapidity of the firing through the reentry circuit can produce atrial flutter and even AF.[20]

### *ATRIAL TACHYCARDIA.* *Atrial tachycardia* is defined as three or more successive ectopic atrial beats in a

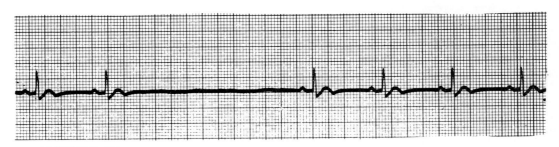

**FIGURE 23-19.**
Sinus arrest. (Source: B.H. Yee and S.I. Zorb, *Cardiac Critical Care Nursing*. Boston: Little, Brown, 1986.)

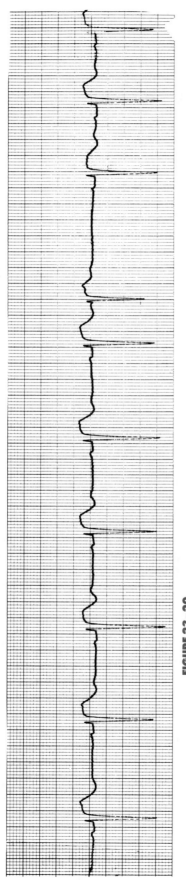

**FIGURE 23–20.**

Premature atrial complex with sinus bradycardia. Note varying sizes of QRS complexes, a phenomenon often seen in heart failure.

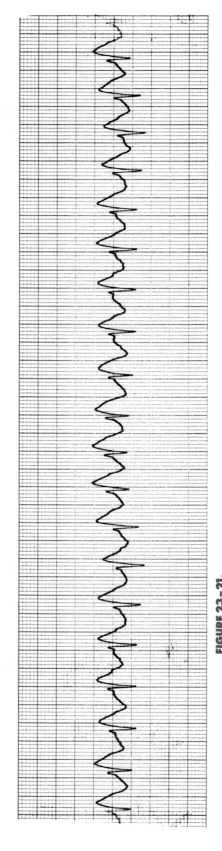

**FIGURE 23–21.**

Atrial tachycardia at rate of approximately 150. Rhythm is usually initiated by a premature atrial complex.

row at a rate of 160 to 250 BPM. This dysrhythmia is usually initiated by a PAC. Mechanisms responsible for sustaining the atrial tachycardia include reentry phenomena and abnormal impulses generated by digitalis excess.[8,20] Repeated stimulation of this reentry path results in atrial tachydysrhythmia.

Onset of tachydysrhythmia may be abrupt, thus, the term *paroxysmal atrial tachycardia* (PAT). The condition may be transient or chronic. Termination is often spontaneous or in response to vagal stimulation (Valsalva maneuver, carotid sinus stimulation, gag reflex, and so on).

Factors contributing to development of atrial tachycardias include hypoxia, alkalosis, increased catecholamine levels, hypokalemia, recent MI cardiomyopathy, atrial-septal defects, hypertension, conditions that increase atrial stretch (such as chronic obstructive pulmonary disease), and acute alcohol ingestion.[22] Paroxysmal atrial tachycardia often occurs in individuals with no known cardiac disease or in those under emotional duress. Rheumatic heart disease, mitral valve disease, pericarditis, coronary artery disease, and thyrotoxicosis are less common causes. Wolff-Parkinson-White (W-P-W) syndrome often manifests episodes of PAT.

Atrial tachycardia appears on the ECG as a continuous run of PACs (Figure 23-21). The P wave configuration differs from the sinus P due to its ectopic atrial origin. PR intervals may vary depending upon atrial rate and degree of AV block. When the atrial rate exceeds 200, the AV node often blocks every other beat producing a 2:1 AV block. The QRS and T waves remain normal. Persistently rapid ventricular rates may cause the QRS complex to take on an aberrant configuration (see p. 476).[9,13] These rhythms are often misdiagnosed as VT and treated inappropriately.

At rapid atrial rates, it is often difficult to distinguish between PAT and junctional tachycardia due to the merging of the P wave with the T wave of the previous beat. Junctional rhythms arise from the AV node or bundle of His. In the circumstances where the source of the rhythm is uncertain, it may be identified as *supraventricular tachycardia* (SVT or PSVT, if paroxysmal).

Atrial tachycardias have clinical significance for both diseased and healthy hearts. Symptoms associated with these dysrhythmias (weakness, palpitations, diaphoresis, shortness of breath, and hypotension) are related to the fall in cardiac output secondary to rapid ventricular rates. Therefore, the major factors to consider are the duration of the dysrhythmia and the existence of cardiac disease. Atrial tachycardia in the presence of a diseased myocardium often precipitates CHF and coronary insufficiency. It has been noted that CHF can also develop in nondiseased myocardiums with long-term, rapid atrial tachycardia.

*ATRIAL FLUTTER.*    The focus or foci for *atrial flutter* may originate anywhere in the atria. It occurs most commonly in individuals over the age of 40 with underlying cardiac disease, especially in infective endocarditis, coronary artery disease, and mitral stenosis. It also may occur after cardiac surgery and with digitalis toxicity.

The mechanisms most often attributed to atrial flutter are: (1) enhanced automaticity of an ectopic focus and (2) circus movement through the atria.[3,19,20] These mechanisms activate rapid depolarization of the atria. This is noted on the ECG as a characteristic sawtooth pattern (Figure 23-22). Atrial rate ranges from 250 to 350 BPM with ventricular rates 125 to 150, depending upon the rate of conduction through the AV node. The ratio of conduction is usually 2:1 to 4:1.[8] PR intervals cannot be distinguished. QRS intervals are normal but the QRS complexes may become aberrant with a wide and bizarre appearance when the rates are very rapid. Atrial flutter may progress to AF or it may respond to drugs, vagal stimulation, or electric countershock.

The clinical significance of atrial flutter is dependent upon the cardiac rate and degree of underlying heart dis-

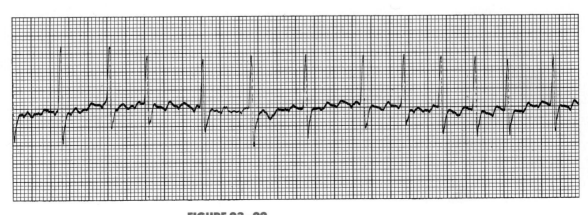

**FIGURE 23–22.**
Atrial flutter with 1:1, 1:2, and 1:3 conduction.

ease. Ventricular rates of 100 or less are usually asymptomatic. Higher rates may reduce coronary perfusion in individuals with ischemic heart disease.

*ATRIAL FIBRILLATION.    Atrial fibrillation* is commonly associated with numerous disease processes that enhance automaticity or increase atrial size such as rheumatic heart disease, pericarditis, hyperthyroidism, coronary artery disease, hypertension, chronic obstructive pulmonary disease, and digitalis toxicity.[15,22] It is the most common atrial dysrhythmia in the elderly population.

Atrial fibrillation is an irregular rhythm that can be established or paroxysmal. In the latter case, attacks of AF may spontaneously convert to sinus rhythm or may do so with electric cardioversion. The acute attack may continue and become established as chronic AF. The degree of hemodynamic disruption depends upon the underlying heart disease, the cardiac rate, and whether or not CHF ensues.

Atrial fibrillation can be identified on the ECG monitor as an irregular ventricular rhythm with chaotic atrial fibrillatory waves (Figure 23-23). Atrial rate will usually exceed 350 BPM, with ventricular rates between 50 and 200 BPM, depending on the rate of AV conduction. Elevated ventricular rates almost invariably occur unless the rhythm is treated with a digitalis preparation. The pulse manifests as an irregular rhythm with the apical rate being faster than the radial pulse. This *pulse deficit* is produced because the more rapid beats may not lead to a stroke volume sufficient to cause a perceptible pulse.[21] With very rapid rates, the apical pulse may be much higher than the radial rate. Because of the irregularity of the beat, it may become difficult to distinguish the S1 and S2 heart sounds, therefore, ascertaining the atrial beat is difficult.

Atrial contraction is responsible for 25% of the cardiac output. Thus, loss of AV synchronization may result in inefficient emptying of the atria and a decrease in left ventricular volume.[14] Chronic fibrillation can lead to cardiac dilatation and hypertrophy, predisposing these individuals to CHF or pulmonary edema.

Pulmonary or arterial embolization is an increased risk for persons with chronic AF. Emboli result from thrombus formation in the atria that loosen and travel the arterial circuit. The atrial appendages often contain thrombus formation or the entire atrial chambers may be filled with thrombi, a condition occurring especially in severe rheumatic mitral stenosis (see Chap. 25).

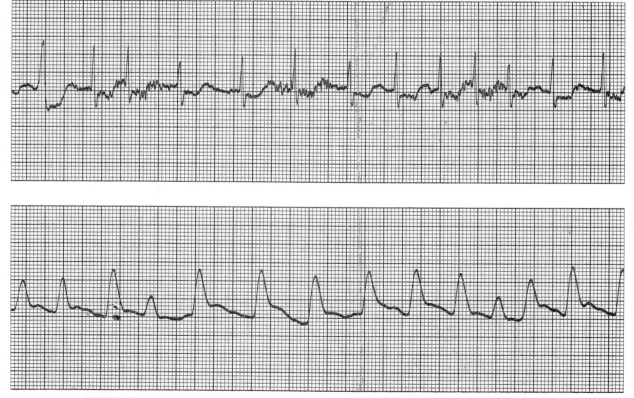

**FIGURE 23–23.**

Atrial fibrillation with simultaneous blood pressure monitoring. Note the changes in blood pressure (cardiac output) with each irregular beat.

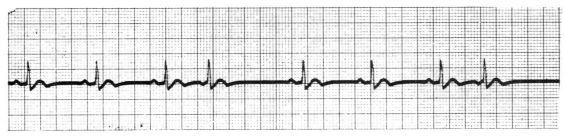

**FIGURE 23–24.**
Premature junctional contractions. (Source: B.H. Yee and S.I. Zorb, *Cardiac Critical Care Nursing.*
Boston: Little, Brown, 1986.)

## Escape Rhythms

Escape rhythms arise from the AV junction and act as secondary pacemakers when the SA node fails. They include premature junctional contractions (PJCs), junctional (nodal) rhythm, junctional tachycardia, and SVT tachycardia.

*PREMATURE JUNCTIONAL CONTRACTIONS. Premature junctional contractions* occur less commonly than their atrial and ventricular cousins. They originate as either premature or escape beats emitting from the bundle of His. The mechanisms involved include enhanced automaticity of the junctional sites and an AV nodal reentry phenomena as a result of digitalis toxicity, acute inferior MI, rheumatic fever, or profound slowing of the cardiac cycle.[13]

As with PACs, PJCs occur earlier in the cardiac cycle than the sinus beat. The atrial impulse is conducted in a retrograde fashion producing an inverted P wave in lead II that may precede, follow, or be buried in a normal QRS complex (Figure 23-24). The PR interval may vary, depending on the location of the focus and the rate of conduction. A PJC may be followed by a partial or full compensatory pause.

*JUNCTIONAL ESCAPE RHYTHM. Junctional escape rhythm* is considered to be a physiologically passive rhythm occurring when a sinus impulse fails to be generated or conducted. The impulse arises in the atrial-nodal junction or the nodal-His bundle junction.[21] By definition, an escape beat is late in the cycle and occurs when a higher pacemaker defaults.[14] When several junctional escape beats occur in a row, it is termed *junctional escape rhythm.* The rhythm then may become the pacemaker of the heart and control ventricular activity.

Junctional rhythm may be attributed to the presence of SA node disease or trauma, enhanced vagotonia, digitalis toxicity, hyperkalemia, acute MI, or the presence of sinus block, sinus arrest, sinus bradycardia, and second and third degree heart block.[14]

The ECG characteristics include a rate of 40 to 60 BPM, abnormal or absent P waves, and variable PR intervals with normal QRS complexes (Figure 23-25). Hemodynamic effect will be dependent on the underlying cause and duration of this rhythm, the ventricular rate, and the presence of cardiac disease. Junctional rhythm predisposes those with diseased myocardium to myocardial ischemia, intractable CHF, and syncopal attacks.[17]

*JUNCTIONAL TACHYCARDIA. Junctional tachycardia* may begin in any site within the AV junctional tissue and is stimulated by an ectopic focus. Thus, it is an active rhythm. It appears on the ECG as a series of PJCs. Junctional tachycardia may be paroxysmal and nonparoxysmal depending on onset, rate, and clinical significance.[28]

*Paroxysmal junctional tachycardia* usually occurs in the individual with nondiseased myocardium. It is initiated by a premature junctional ectopic focus. The rate ranges between 160 and 250 BPM. In the otherwise healthy individual, there is little hemodynamic effect. However, at very fast rates, individuals may describe palpitations, dizziness, or weakness.

*Nonparoxysmal junctional tachycardia* causes rates of 60 to 130 BPM. Junctional tachycardia of less than 100 BPM is often termed *accelerated junctional* or *idionodal rhythm.* Most of these tachycardias result from increased automaticity of the junctional tissues, which may result from released metabolites from ischemic and hypoxic cells.[21] This dysrhythmia is therefore closely associated

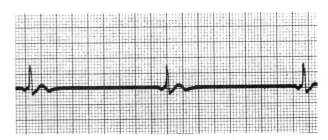

**FIGURE 23–25.**
Junctional rhythm. (Source: B.H. Yee and S.I. Zorb, *Cardiac Critical Care Nursing.* Boston: Little, Brown, 1986.)

with myocardial disease such as MI, myocarditis, or post open-heart surgery.[28]

*PAROXYSMAL SUPRAVENTRICULAR TACHYCARDIA.* *Paroxysmal supraventricular tachycardia* (PSVT) can be caused by an AV nodal reentry mechanism.[28] Here, reentry is through the slow and fast pathways within the AV node. The impulse is conducted first down the slow paths to the ventricles and returns up the fast paths to the atria. The impulse reactivates the ectopic focus and the process repeats until interrupted or spontaneous cessation occurs.[28] As discussed on page 467, it is difficult to differentiate between atrial tachycardia and SVT tachycardia due to the distortion caused by rapid rates. Usually PSVT ranges between 170 and 250 BPM, the P waves are indistinguishable, and the QRS normal unless altered by conduction defects in the bundle branches. Paroxysmal supraventricular tachycardia can be initiated by any of the ectopic foci. Symptoms include palpitation, nervousness, angina, syncope, or shock.[28] In the presence of acute MI, the resultant decrease in cardiac output and increased myocardial energy consumption will exacerbate further ischemic episodes.

## Ectopic Ventricular Rhythms

Ventricular dysrhythmias are impulse formations arising from ectopic foci in the ventricles. The main dysrhythmias are premature ventricular contractions, idioventricular rhythms, VT, and ventricular fibrillation.

*PREMATURE VENTRICULAR CONTRACTIONS. Premature ventricular contractions* (PVCs) originate from single or multiple foci below the level of the bundle of His.[28] These premature depolarizations interrupt the underlying cardiac rhythm. The hallmark of the PVC is a wide (greater than 0.12 seconds), irregular QRS complex with no associated P wave. The T wave is directed in the opposite direction to the T wave of the sinus beat, with a full compensatory pause afterward (Figure 23-26). The PVCs may occur singly, in multiples, or in regularly occurring combination with the underlying rhythm, such as *ventricular bigeminy* (occurring every other beat), or *ventricular trigeminy* (occurring every third beat). The proximity of the ectopic complex to the T wave is an indicator of electrical instability in the ventricle. When it falls at the T wave, it is called an *R on T phenomenon* and the condition is often predisposed to ventricular fibrillation. All PVCs 6 or more per minute, paired (coupled), or multifocal, must be treated as if there is underlying cardiac disease. This dysrhythmia is frequently a precursor of the life-threatening dysrhythmias of VT, or the lethal ventricular fibrillation.

The two mechanisms responsible for the appearance of PVCs are *enhanced automaticity* of ventricular tissue and *reentry*. The reentry phenomena involves microcircuits in the His-Purkinje tissue or macrocircuits in the bundle of His and bundle branch fibers.[12,28]

Premature ventricular contractions are detected in both healthy and diseased hearts. Premature ventricular ectopy is seldom seen in a young person and occurrence does increase with age. In healthy persons, ventricular ectopy is attributed to excessive use of caffeine and/or tobacco, emotional excitement, and exercise. The effects of catecholamine drugs (eg, isoproteronol, epinephrine), digoxin toxicity, electrolyte imbalances (hypokalemia and hypomagnesemia), hypoxia, myocardial ischemia, mitral valve prolapse, advanced anemia, and myocardial hypertrophy or aneurysm can produce PVCs in the diseased heart.[19,22] In myocardial ischemia, the ventricular myocardium is irritable due to the hypoxia and acidosis associated with decreased coronary artery perfusion. Thus, PVCs are the most common dysrhythmia associated with acute MI.

The hemodynamic effects of PVCs are usually transient and clinically insignificant. Premature ventricular contractions are associated with shortened left ventricular filling time, decreased stroke volume, and decreased

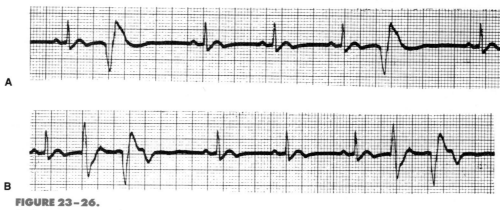

**FIGURE 23-26.**

**A.** Premature ventricular contractions, unifocal. **B.** Two multifocal couplets are noted. (Source: B.H. Yee and S.I. Zorb, *Cardiac Critical Care Nursing.* Boston: Little, Brown, 1986.)

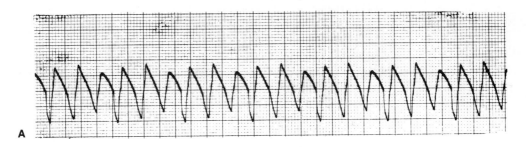

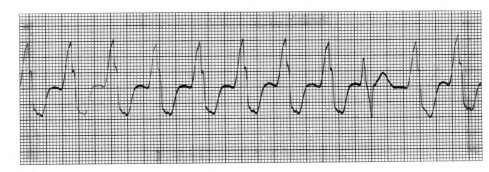

**FIGURE 23-27.**
**A.** Ventricular tachycardia. **B.** Slow ventricular tachycardia. (Source: B.H. Yee and S.I. Zorb, *Cardiac Critical Care Nursing*. Boston: Little, Brown, 1986.)

contractility thereby reducing the cardiac output with each abnormal beat. Thus, the frequency and the presence of cardiac disease are important factors in determining the significance of the dysrhythmia.

*VENTRICULAR TACHYCARDIA.* Six or more consecutive premature ventricular beats constitute the ventricular dysrhythmia termed *ventricular tachycardia.* Ventricular tachycardia appears on the ECG as a series of slightly irregular, wide, undulating waves. The only identifiable waves are the wide, distorted QRS greater than 0.12 second, the ST segment, and T wave (Figure 23-27). The ventricular rate ranges between 100 and 250 BPM. Ventricular tachycardia may be transient or may continue until the underlying cause is treated.

Ventricular tachycardia is often triggered by a PVC falling during the vulnerable period of ventricular diastole (R on T phenomena).[8] This ectopic rhythm is often a product of enhanced automaticity of the ventricular myocardium caused by acidosis, hypoxia, hypotension, or hypokalemia. Heart disease in the forms of coronary vasospasm, cardiomyopathy, mitral valve prolapse, and CHF are also commonly associated with the occurrence of VT. A special form of VT is called *torsades de pointes.* It is characterized by wide QRS complexes of changing amplitude occurring at a rate of 200 to 250 BPM.[28] The person affected invariably has a long QT interval, and the condition is associated with severe bradycardia, hypokalemia, and certain antidysrhythmic drugs.[28] It is a very dangerous dysrhythmia that often degenerates to ventricular fibrillation.[14]

Ventricular tachycardia is clinically significant and requires immediate intervention. Loss of consciousness and hypotension are indicators of the substantial reduction of cardiac output associated with this dysrhythmia. Immediate cardioversion is indicated. Untreated VT usually progresses to ventricular fibrillation.[7]

Often VT is mistaken for *supraventricular tachycardia (SVT) with aberration* (distortion of the QRS complex) (see p. 476). This is clinically significant because intervention with an inappropriate antidysrhythmic (such as verapamil versus procainamide or lidocaine) can result in profound hypotension, ventricular fibrillation, and death.[3] The use of age or hemodynamic stability as clinical parameters to distinguish these dysrhythmias is inadequate. Ventricular tachycardia has been found to occur in all ages and to be well tolerated hemodynamically in some individuals.[25] Box 23-1 lists commonly used criteria

**BOX 23-1.**
CRITERIA TO DIFFERENTIATE VENTRICULAR TACHYCARDIA FROM SUPRAVENTRICULAR TACHYCARDIA

1. Monophasic QRS with taller left peak in V1
2. RS pattern in V6
3. QRS wider than 0.14 favors VT; QRS equal to or less than 0.14 second favors SVT
4. AV disassociation or lack of 1:1 conduction indicates VT
5. Left axis deviation above −30° or right axis deviation greater than +120 favors VT

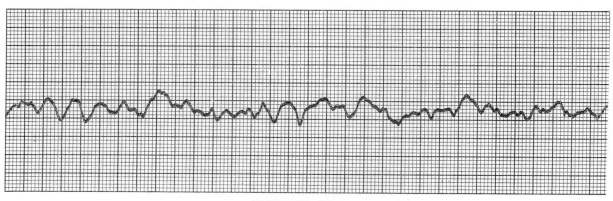

**FIGURE 23–28.**
Ventricular fibrillation.

for distinguishing VT from SVT.[3,4,13] While a 12 lead ECG is preferred, monitoring in V1 or MCL1 will provide adequate information when time is of the essence.[13]

*VENTRICULAR FIBRILLATION.*    The most serious of the cardiac dysrhythmias is *ventricular fibrillation.* It is the most common cause of sudden death and is often the terminal rhythm in advanced cardiac disease. Single or multiple ectopic foci fire in a chaotic manner producing an unsynchronous quivering of the myocardium.[7]

The ECG reveals indistinguishable waveforms undulating about the isoelectric line with varying degrees of amplitude (Figure 23-28). Ventricular fibrillation can range from 150 to 500 oscillations per minute.[28] It often profoundly disintegrates into slow idioventricular or agonal (dying heart) rhythm just prior to death (see below).

The etiologies for ventricular fibrillation are primarily the same as for PVCs and VT. In addition, cardiac pacing, cardiac catheterization, electrical shock, and hypothermia are known to stimulate this rhythm.

Because of its lethal potential, this dysrhythmia must be detected and treated immediately. Due to the quivering of the ventricles, no pump action takes place. Therefore, no cardiac output is produced. Electrical defibrillation is essential to prevent death. Brain damage occurs within 4 to 6 minutes without oxygenated perfusion to its tissues.

*IDIOVENTRICULAR RHYTHM.*    An escape rhythm, *idioventricular rhythm,* plays an important role in maintaining control of the ventricles when other SVT pacemakers and escape mechanisms have failed. This rhythm is readily identified on the ECG (Figure 23-29) by the wide, irregular QRS complexes and a slow rate between 30 and 40 BPM. Idioventricular rhythms are most commonly found in the presence of a high degree of AV block, usually complete. Idioventricular rhythm may also follow SA block, sinus arrest, ectopic atrial rhythms with AV block, or bilateral bundle branch block.[13] This rhythm is often a terminal rhythm in advanced stages of cardiac disease.

*Accelerated idioventricular rhythm* is a common result of reperfusion of the myocardium following thrombolytic therapy or balloon angioplasty. It is usually a transient dysrhythmia which occurs at a rate of 60 to 110

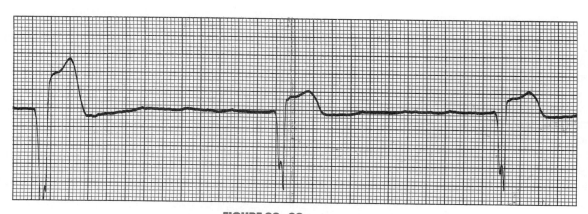

**FIGURE 23–29.**
Idioventricular (agonal) rhythm.

beats per minute.[17] It has the appearance of VT; if it is prolonged, hypotension and clinical signs of shock may develop. Accelerated idioventricular rhythm has been used as a criterion to indicate that reperfusion has been accomplished.[28]

## Disturbances in Conduction of Cardiac Impulses

Disturbances in conduction of cardiac impulses are described as various types of heart block. There are three major categories of conduction disorders: (1) SA block, (2) atrioventricular (AV) block, and (3) intraventricular block.

### Sinoatrial Block

Sinoatrial block is thought to be produced by the blockage of sinus impulses leaving the SA node. This mechanism occurs at the SA junction and is called an *exit block*.[13] Exit blocks are usually transient and produce pauses in the cardiac rhythm where the sinus impulse normally would have fallen. The PQRST waveforms are normal unless altered by other conditions. Ventricular rate and rhythm will vary due to the pauses. Normally, these pauses are an exact multiple of the sinus cycle.

An SA block can be caused by a variety of etiologies including excessive vagal stimulation, acute myocardial infectious processes, digitalis or quinidine intoxication, hyperkalemia, thyroid disorders, metastatic cancer, and degenerative diseases of the SA node.[8] The block occurs frequently after an acute inferior MI because the right coronary artery supplies the blood supply to the SA node in 60% of individuals.

An SA block can occur in healthy or diseased hearts. The duration of the pause, during which no cardiac output is produced, as well as the presence and degree of underlying cardiac disease, determines the clinical significance of this dysrhythmia. Prolonged pauses or episodes in which escape mechanisms fail may produce symptoms associated with a fall in cardiac output. Prolonged episodes of SA block may lead to ventricular standstill and death.

### Atrioventricular Block

Atrioventricular block can occur as either a physiologic mechanism or pathologic mechanism. The physiologic function protects the ventricular rate of the heart by blocking multiple impulses during states such as AF. The pathologic mechanism blocks impulses from reaching the ventricles by varying degrees of block based on the area of the AV junction involved.[14] The AV blocks derived from pathology in the AV node are sometimes transient and ischemic. Infranodal blocks involving bundle of His and bundle branches are permanent and require intensive management. The AV block is classified in degrees, reflecting the extent of the conduction disturbance.

FIRST DEGREE AV BLOCK. *First degree AV block* is a result of delayed conduction at the AV node between the SA node and the ventricles (Figure 23-30). The ECG reveals a sinus rhythm with a prolonged PR interval greater than 20 seconds.

First degree AV block is often seen in healthy elderly adults, secondary to degenerative changes in the AV node, and is generally clinically insignificant. It becomes significant for persons taking digoxin or beta-blockers because it may signal toxic levels. First degree AV block in clients with inferior wall MI is usually transient but may progress to Wenckebach's phenomenon. The occurrence of this dysrhythmia in persons with anterior wall MI is dangerous because the degree of block may progress rapidly to third degree heart block and trifascicular bundle branch block.[14] This dysrhythmia is also commonly associated with acute myocarditis, uremia, hyperkalemia, and rheumatic fever.

SECOND DEGREE AV BLOCK. In *second degree AV block*, the degree of block increases so that not every sinus impulse reaches the ventricle. The two major types

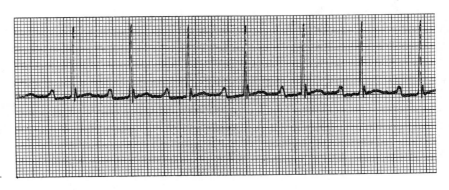

**FIGURE 23–30.**
First degree AV block.

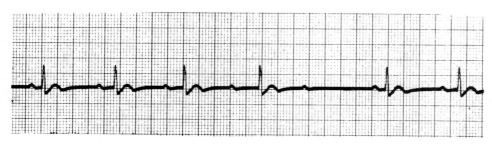

**FIGURE 23-31.**
Second degree AV block, Mobitz type I. (Source: B.H. Yee and S.I. Zorb, *Cardiac Critical Care Nursing.* Boston: Little, Brown, 1986.)

of second degree AV block are Mobitz type I (Wenckebach) and Mobitz type II.

Mobitz type I block produces a progressive delay in conduction at the AV node until a sinus impulse is completely blocked. This is seen on the ECG as a gradual lengthening of the PR interval until a QRS complex is dropped (Figure 23-31). The underlying rate is normal, the rhythm irregular, and the QRS complex of the sinus beats normal. Mobitz type I is usually a temporary dysrhythmia associated with ischemic heart disease, digoxin toxicity, and right coronary artery pathology.[2] In persons with acute inferior MI, it may progress to third degree AV block.

Mobitz type II block is usually caused by an infranodal conduction delay. Some sinus impulses are blocked within or distal to the bundle of His and do not reach the ventricles. The degree of block occurs at variable intervals. Thus, the ECG monitor shows constant PR intervals of the conducted beats with varying ratios of P waves to QRS complexes (Figure 23-32). Due to the level of conduction defect, the QRS complexes may be widened. Overall ventricular rhythm is regular with a normal or bradycardic rate.

The causes of Mobitz type II block include degenerative collagen diseases, Lev's disease (fibrocalcific changes in the conduction system), myxedema, and progressive conduction system disease.[19] By far, the most clinically significant condition is left coronary artery pathology associated with acute anterior MI. The degree of block is irreversible and will progress to complete heart block, which requires pacemaker insertion.

*THIRD DEGREE AV BLOCK.   Third degree* or *complete AV block* occurs when no sinus impulses reach the ventricles. The most prominent characteristic is the independent activity of the atria and ventricles (Figure 23-33). A slower idioventricular rhythm established in the bundle branches or lower system is responsible for ventricular contraction.

The most common cause of third degree AV block is acute inferior MI. It also may be caused by antidysrhythmic drugs, infections, anterior MI, rheumatic fever, open heart surgery, degenerative fibrosclerosis of the cardiac skeleton, fibrosis of the conduction system, cardiomyopathies, scleroderma, and severe coronary artery disease in the absence of infarction.[13,14]

Persons with third degree AV block may or may not be symptomatic depending on onset, etiology, and ventricular rate. Acute onset with a slow ventricular rate and symptomatic fall in cardiac output requires immediate pacemaker insertion. Syncopal episodes and ventricular fibrillation can occur. Stokes-Adams syndrome occurs when the established idioventricular pacemaker fails to initiate a ventricular beat, resulting in variable periods of ventricular asystole. Cerebral symptoms resulting from this include transient giddiness, loss of consciousness, convulsions, and sudden death, depending upon the duration of the asystole.[21]

## *Intraventricular Block*

Intraventricular blocks are conduction defects occurring in the bundle branch network. These give rise to several types of block: left bundle branch block (LBBB), right bundle branch block (RBBB), bifascicular block, and trifascicular block. Intraventricular blocks may be chronic and relatively benign or acute with serious implications in the setting of MI.

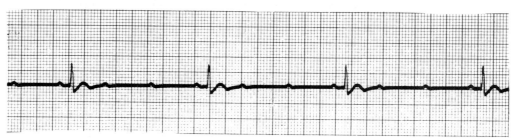

**FIGURE 23-32.**
Second-degree AV block, Mobitz type II. (Source: B.H. Yee and S.I. Zorb, *Cardiac Critical Care Nursing.* Boston: Little, Brown, 1986.)

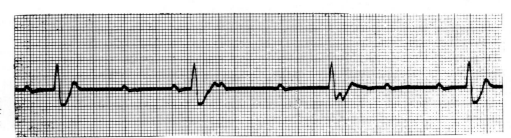

**FIGURE 23–33.**
Third-degree AV block. (Source: B.H. Yee and S.I. Zorb, *Cardiac Critical Care Nursing.* Boston: Little, Brown, 1986.)

*LEFT BUNDLE BRANCH BLOCK. Left bundle branch block* occurs when a lesion blocks the common left bundle. Due to its dual blood supply from the left and right coronary arteries and size, this block represents advanced cardiac disease.[1] Impulses are conducted normally from the atria until the area of block is reached. The impulse is then conducted down the right bundle normally, but the impulse is delayed at the left bundle and may be passed from muscle fiber to muscle fiber rather than through the normal channels to effect left ventricular depolarization. The block may be intermittent and take years to develop.[21]

A characteristic wide (greater than 0.12 seconds), notched QRS complex is produced. This is best seen as a negative QS complex in lead V1 and a positive RR complex in V6. The most common cause of this defect is atherosclerosis of the left main coronary artery, but it may be associated with Lenegre's disease (idiopathic fibrosis of the His-Purkinje system), Lev's disease (idiopathic fibrosis of the bundle branches), coronary artery disease, syphilis, trauma, tumors, congenital lesions, aortic stenosis, and acute infections.[20,21]

Left bundle branch block may be chronic and clinically insignificant. Sudden onset in the presence of anterior MI, however, may lead to a further progression of block. Figure 23-34 illustrates the bundle branch block configuration seen in leads I, V1, and V6.

*HEMIBLOCK.* A *hemiblock* represents a blockage of one of the divisions (or fascicles) of the left bundle branch. These blocks are identified on the ECG by examining the frontal leads and QRS axis.

A block in the anterosuperior division produces left anterior hemiblock. This fascicle is particularly vulnerable due to its location, size, and single blood supply from the left coronary artery.

Left posterior hemiblock develops from a block in the posteroinferior branch of the left bundle. Its development is significant in that it may indicate compromise of both the right and left coronary arteries. Due to the greater density of its fascicle, location, and dual blood supply, it is relatively rare. In addition to the etiologies previously listed, pulmonary disorders are also responsible for this block.

*RIGHT BUNDLE BRANCH BLOCK. Right bundle branch block* may occur in both healthy and diseased hearts. Due to the small size of the right fascicle, it can be affected by small insults such as altered blood flow from the left anterior descending artery. In RBBB, conduction proceeds from the atria to the septum and left bundle in the normal fashion. Conduction occurs from left to right producing an RSR pattern in V1 and QRS pattern in V6 characteristic of this conduction defect.

Etiologies for this bundle branch block include acute MI and any of the conditions that cause LBBB. It can also be produced after surgery to repair atrial-septal defects and tetralogy of Fallot. In the event of anterior MI, RBBB should be observed closely for the development of bifascicular block.

*BIFASCICULAR BLOCK. Bifascicular block* is a combination of RBBB and either type of hemiblock. The most common combination is with left anterior hemiblock because they share a common blood supply. This combination in the presence of anterior MI may be a precursor to trifascicular block.[14]

*TRIFASCICULAR BLOCK. Trifascicular block* results from the blocking of all fascicles of the bundle branch system, suggesting profound interruption to blood flow from the coronary arteries. If incomplete, a SVT escape rhythm with first or type II second degree block emerges. If block is complete, an escape rhythm

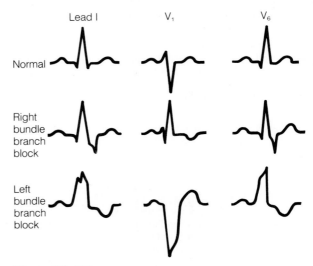

**Figure 23–34.**
Bundle branch block configurations seen in selected ECG leads.

below the block develops with a ventricular rate incompatible with life.

## Aberrant Conduction

Aberrant conduction is the movement of sinus or atrial impulses through either abnormal pathways or through normal pathways altered by enhanced automaticity or injury. Aberrant intraventricular conduction of atrial dysrhythmias was first described in the 1900s. Wide, notched, irregular QRS complexes occurring during atrial or AV junctional rhythms often simulate a ventricular ectopic rhythm. The irregular QRS is thought to occur due to a preexisting bundle branch block or ventricular preexcitation.[9] *Functional* or *phase 3* (RBBB) *aberration* is the most common form. The impulse is premature, reaching the intraventricular fibers during the electrical systole of the preceding beat. Functional aberrancy is pathological when the refractory period is abnormally prolonged, stimulating the involved fascicle at a rapid rate. *Rate dependent BBB aberrancy* develops when the sinus rate accelerates (due to exercise, stress, hypoxemia), making the normal cycle shorter than the bundle branch cycle. With the shortened cycle, the impulse is unable to be conducted normally and follows the longer bundle path. Thus, aberrant conduction will persist until the rate slows, restoring normal cycle length.[13] *Phase 4 (LBBB) aberration* occurs late in diastole and occurs in the setting of bradycardia or enhanced normal automaticity. It is always pathological and associated with organic heart disease.[14] It is important to differentiate aberrant conduction from other wide complex dysrhythmias for appropriate treatment. Box 23-2 lists criteria for identifying aberrant rhythms.[9,13]

Aberrancy during atrial dysrhythmias is of concern due to the potential for further hemodynamic compromise. The treatment for aberrantly conducted SVT occurring during AF is digitalis, propranolol, verapamil, or cardioversion to restore a more normal ventricular rate and improve cardiac output.

Determining aberrancy is especially important during atrial tachycardia where aberrantly conducted beats may be mistaken for VT and be inappropriately treated. This is clinically significant when AV conduction is 1:1 at a rapid rate, resulting in decreased cardiac output and hypotension.

Aberrancy in atrial flutter with varying degrees of block may look like ventricular bigeminy. Application of the aforementioned criteria would reveal the aberrantly conducted beats leading to appropriate treatment.

Alternating RBBB and LBBB aberrancy is not uncommon. The mechanism for this phenomenon is not known. However, it is useful to distinguish dual aberrancy from bifocal ectopy.[13]

Aberrancy should not be considered a primary disorder. It usually occurs secondary to other pathology within the heart. Alone, aberrancy is not treated. However, as previously discussed, identification and treatment of underlying mechanisms are extremely important to the clinical management of the person with dysrhythmias.

## Disturbances in Both Conduction and Impulse Formation

Dysrhythmias classified as disturbances in both conduction and impulse formation are frequently complicated, involving mechanisms not fully understood. The more common disorders are AV disassociation, preexcitation syndromes, and ventricular standstill.

*AV disassociation* may result from various mechanisms. Usually two separate pacemakers, one sinus and the other junctional, coexist and produce independent rhythms. It is thought to be produced by a slowing or failure of the SA node, accelerated impulse formation in the AV junction or ventricles, or complete SA or AV block. This condition usually occurs as a symptom of rhythm disturbance rather than a separate entity.

*Preexcitation syndrome* arises secondary to the existence of accessory pathways between the atria and ventricles (Figure 23-35). *Wolff-Parkinson-White (WPW)* and *Lown-Ganong-Levine (LGL)* syndromes are the most common forms. In these syndromes, the accessory pathways bypass the AV node producing accelerated conduction to the ventricles. Excitation of the involved accessory path permits ectopic atrial impulses to enter and establish a reentry circuit.[20,24] Atrial fibrillation, atrial flutter, and paroxysmal SVT tachycardia commonly develop in these syn-

---

**BOX 23-2.**
CLUES TO IDENTIFYING ABERRANT CONDUCTION

- ▸ Classic RBBB and LBBB patterns in V1, V2, V6
- ▸ Normal axis
- ▸ QRS of less than 0.14 sec
- ▸ Atrial ectopic beat precedes broad complex beat
- ▸ Aberrant beat is second in a row of nonaberrant SVT
- ▸ In RBBB pattern, initial deflection in V1 is identical to deflection of conducted beat

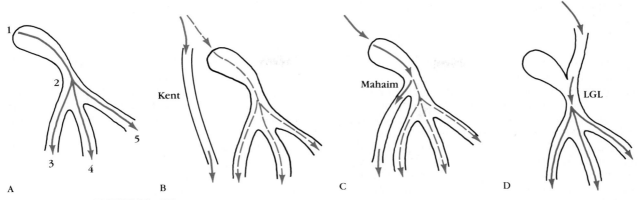

**FIGURE 23-35.**

Diagrammatic illustrations of accessory pathways. **A.** Normal conduction from atrium to (1) AV node, (2) bundle of His, (3) right bundle branch, (4) left anterior fascicle, and (5) left posterior fascicle. **B.** Lateral accessory pathway. This bypasses the AV node and enters a site in the ventricular myocardium (typical WPW). **C.** Mahaim fibers connected the distal AV node or His bundle with a portion of the ventricular myocardium. **D.** Accessory pathway connecting the atrium with the distal AV node or His bundle (LGL) (Source: M.J. Goldman, *Principles of Clinical Electrocardiography* (10th ed.). Los Altos, CA: Lange, 1979.)

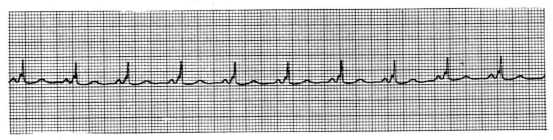

**FIGURE 23-36.**

Preexcitation. (Source: B.H. Yee and S.I. Zorb, *Cardiac Critical Care Nursing.* Boston: Little, Brown, 1986.)

dromes. The accelerated conduction of these dysrhythmias can cause severe hemodynamic compromise. When they exist alone, the preexcitation syndromes are clinically insignificant.

The ECG characteristics for both WPW and LGL are similar. Both exhibit a shortened PR interval (less than 0.10; Figure 23-36). The QRS complex differs in that in WPW there exists a delta wave (a slurring of the R wave) and a widened QRS complex (greater than 0.10). The QRS complex in LGL is normal. The underlying rate and rhythm are normal.

Preexcitation syndromes have been observed in persons with psychoneurotic disorders, hyperthyroidism, mitral valve prolapse, rheumatic heart disease, congenital defects, atrial-septal defects, and idiopathic subaortic stenosis.[14]

*Ventricular standstill* occurs when lower level pacemakers fail to produce escape rhythms. This often terminal dysrhythmia of a dying heart may also occur after numerous conditions, especially acute MI, advanced digitalis toxicity, carotid sinus stimulation, and after cardioversion of atrial, junctional, or VTs.[14] At the onset, the ventricles cease to contract. The P waves will continue for a short period before also ceasing (asystole). Intervention must be immediate because no cardiac output is produced and death will quickly ensue. Occasionally, erratic bizarre idioventricular complexes will surface after clinical death is established. These are probably idioventricular escape complexes which arise in the terminal portion of the Purkinje network. These terminal events are referred to as agonal or dying heart rhythm.

Clinical management of dysrhythmias depends on the preexistence of cardiac disease, the hemodynamic effects, and the timely identification of altered cardiac rhythms. Selection of appropriate treatment modalities necessitates a thorough understanding of the mechanism and etiologies of cardiac dysrhythmias.

## REFERENCES

1. Castellanos, A., and Myerburg, R.J. The resting electrocardiogram. In J.W. Hurst et al. (eds.), *The Heart* (7th ed.). New York: McGraw-Hill, 1990.

2. Conover, M.B. *Pocket Nurse Guide to Electrocardiography*. St. Louis: Mosby, 1986.

3. Conover, M.B. VT or SVT? *Critical Care Nurse* 9(2):16, 1989.

4. Cooper, J., and Marriott, J.L. Why are so many critical care nurses unable to recognize ventricular tachycardias in the 12 lead electrocardiogram? *Heart Lung* 18(3):243, 1989.

5. Fisch, C. Electrocardiography, exercise stress testing, and ambulatory monitoring. In W.N. Kelley, (ed.). *Textbook of Internal Medicine*. Philadelphia: J.B. Lippincott, 1989.

6. Garson, A. Arrhythmias in pediatric patients. *Med. Clin. N. Amer.* 68:1171, 1984.

7. German, L.D., and Ideker, R.E. Ventricular tachycardia: Mechanisms, diagnosis, and management. *Med. Clin. N. Am.* 68:970, 1984.

8. Gilmour, R.F., and Zipes, D.P. Basic electrophysiologic mechanism for the development of the arrhythmias. *Med. Clin. N. Am.* 68:795, 1984.

9. Goldschlager, N., and Goldman, M.J. Aberrancy of intraventricular conduction in association with supraventricular arrhythmias. *Electrocardiology: Essentials of Interpretation*. Los Altos, Calif.: Lange, 1984.

10. Kelley, S. *ECG Interpretation and Identifying Arrhythmias*. Philadelphia: J.B. Lippincott, 1984.

11. Kruthcher, K.L. Cardiac electrophysiologic mapping techniques. *Focus on Critical Care* 12:26, 1985.

12. Loeb, J.M. Cardiac electrophysiology. *Critical Care Quarterly* 7:9, 1984.

13. Marriott, H.J., and Conover, M.B. *Advanced Concepts in Arrhythmias*. St. Louis: Mosby, 1989.

14. Marriott, H.J., and Myerberg, R.J. Recognition of cardiac arrhythmias and conduction disturbances. In J.W. Hurst et al. (eds.), *The Heart* (7th ed.). New York: McGraw-Hill, 1990.

15. Mead, R.H., and Harrison, D.C. Clinical management of common cardiac abnormalities. In D.A. Zschoche (ed.), *Mosby's Comprehensive Review of Critical Care* (3rd ed.). St. Louis: Mosby, 1986.

16. Myerburg, R.J., and Kessler, K.M. Clinical assessment and management of arrhythmias and conduction disturbances. In J.W. Hurst et al. (eds.), *The Heart* (7th ed.). New York: McGraw-Hill, 1990.

17. Rakita, L., and Vrobel, T.R. Electrocardiography in critical care medicine. In W. Shoemaker et al., (eds.) *Textbook of Critical Care* (2nd ed.). Philadelphia: W.B. Saunders, 1989.

18. Schlant, R.C., Silverman, M.E., and Roberts, W.C. Anatomy of the heart. In J.W. Hurst et al. (eds.), *The Heart* (7th ed.). New York: McGraw-Hill, 1990.

19. Sidel, J.C. *Basic Electrocardiography*. St. Louis: Mosby, 1986.

20. Smith, W.M. Cardiac arrhythmias and conduction disturbances. In J.W. Hurst et al. (eds.), *The Heart* (7th ed.). New York: McGraw-Hill, 1990.

21. Sokolow, M., and McIlroy, M.B. *Clinical Cardiology* (14th ed.). Los Altos, Calif.: Lange, 1986.

22. Sweetwood, H.M. *Clinical Electrocardiography for Nurses*. Rockville, Md.: Aspen Systems Corp., 1983.

23. Swiryn, S., McDonough, T., and Hueter, D.C. Sinus node function and dysfunction. *Med. Clin. N. Am.* 68:935, 1984.

24. Watanabe, Y., Drefifus, L., and Sodeman, W. Sr. Arrhythmias: Mechanisms and pathogenesis. In W.A. Sodeman, Jr., and T.M. Sodeman (eds.), *Pathologic Physiology: Mechanisms of Disease* (7th ed.). Philadelphia: W.B. Saunders, 1985.

25. Wellens, H.J. The wide QRS tachycardia. *Ann. Intern. Med.* 104:879, 1986.

26. Weller, D.M., and Moore, J. Mechanism of arrhythmias: Enhanced automaticity and reentry. *Critical Care Nurse* 9(5):42, 46, 47, 1989.

27. Winkle, R.A. Cellular basis of cardiac arrhythmias. In R.A. Winkle (ed.), *Cardiac Arrhythmias: Current Diagnosis and Practical Management*. Menlo Park, Calif.: Addison-Wesley, 1983.

28. Zipes, D.P. Cardiac arrhythmias. In W.N. Kelley, (ed.). *Textbook of Internal Medicine*. Philadelphia: J.B. Lippincott, 1989.

# chapter 24

Barbara L. Bullock

# Compromised Pumping Ability of the Heart

## Chapter Outline

## Learning Objectives

1. Differentiate between cardiac and circulatory failure.
2. Describe preload and afterload.
3. Discuss compensatory mechanisms of cardiac failure.
4. Describe cause and effect of dilatation of the heart chambers.
5. List the underlying factors that can precipitate heart failure.
6. Compare the pathophysiology of right and left heart failure.
7. Describe the basis for the clinical manifestations of left heart failure.
8. Describe the basis for the clinical manifestations of right heart failure.
9. Discuss radiologic changes in right and left heart failure.
10. Identify the purposes of the Swan-Ganz catheter in monitoring congestive heart failure.
11. Identify blood tests used to aid in the diagnosis of congestive heart failure.
12. Discuss pathophysiology of cardiogenic shock.
13. Discuss the mechanisms of compensated shock.
14. Identify clinical signs and symptoms of cardiogenic shock.
15. Discuss irreversible or decompensated shock.
16. Define *cardiomyopathy*.
17. Differentiate primary and secondary cardiomyopathies.
18. Describe congestive, restrictive, and hypertrophic cardiomyopathies.

# CONGESTIVE HEART FAILURE

Heart failure refers to a constellation of signs and symptoms that result from the heart's inability to pump enough blood to meet the body's metabolic demands. The pump, itself, is impaired and unable to supply adequate blood to meet the cellular needs. Cardiac failure is one type of circulatory failure, a term that also includes hypoperfusion resulting from extracardiac conditions, such as hypovolemia, peripheral vasodilatation, and inadequate oxygenation of hemoglobin (Box 24-1).

The clinical result of heart failure includes circulatory overload or congestive heart failure (CHF). This is a clinical syndrome characterized by abnormal retention of sodium and water resulting from renal compensation for the decreased cardiac output. Circulatory overload is enhanced by the resulting excess blood volume and increased venous return.

The causes of heart failure are varied and include intrinsic myocardial disease, malformation or injury, and secondary abnormalities (Table 24-1). Myocardial failure is often the cause of death in terminal illness of noncardiac etiology.

## Pathophysiology of Heart Failure

The onset of heart failure may be acute or insidious. It is often associated with systolic or diastolic overloading and with myocardial weakness. As the physiologic stress on the heart muscle reaches a critical level, the contractility of the muscle is reduced and cardiac output declines, but venous input to the ventricles remains the same or becomes increased. The systemic responses to the decreasing cardiac output are predictable and include: (1) reflex increase in sympathetic activity; (2) release of renin from the juxtaglomerular cells of the kidneys; (3) anaerobic

**TABLE 24-1.**

INTRINSIC AND SECONDARY CAUSES OF HEART FAILURE

| INTRINSIC* | SECONDARY |
|---|---|
| Cardiomyopathy | Pulmonary embolism |
| Myocardial infarction | Anemia |
| Myocarditis | Thyrotoxicosis |
| Ischemic heart disease | Systemic hypertension |
| Congenital heart defects | Arteriovenous shunts |
| Pericarditis/cardiac tamponade | Blood volume excess |
| | Metabolic/respiratory acidosis |
| | Drug toxicity |
| | Cardiac dysrhythmias |

*Intrinsic refers to myocardial, endocardial, and pericardial disease, and congenital malformations that increase ventricular volume load and ischemia or infarction of the ventricular myocardium.

metabolism by affected cells; and (4) increased extraction of oxygen by the peripheral cells. The responses of the heart to increased volume of blood in the ventricles are also predictable and include short-term and long-term mechanisms.

In *acute* or *short-term mechanisms*, as the end-diastolic fiber length increases, the ventricular muscle responds with dilatation and an increased force of contraction (Starling's law). In *long-term mechanisms*, ventricular hypertrophy increases the ability of the heart muscle to contract and push its volume into the circulation. The pathology of the predisposing condition determines whether heart failure is acute or insidious in onset because compensation often occurs for long periods before the clinical manifestations of heart failure develop.

An example of long-term compensation is that which results from systemic hypertension. Because the ventricles must pump against increased pressure (increased

**BOX 24-1.**

CLASSIFICATION OF CIRCULATORY FAILURE AND CIRCULATORY OVERLOAD

I. Circulatory failure
   A. Heart (cardiac) failure
   B. Noncardiac (peripheral) circulatory failure
      1. Decrease return of blood to heart, inadequate blood volume
      2. Increased capacity of vascular bed
      3. Peripheral vascular abnormalities or disease
      4. Inadequate oxyhemoglobin
II. Circulatory congestion
   A. Cardiac circulatory overload
      1. Heart (cardiac) failure
   B. Noncardiac circulatory overload
      1. Increase in blood volume
      2. Increase in venous return and/or decrease in peripheral vascular resistance

Source: J. W. Hurst, et al., eds. The Heart (7th ed.). New York: McGraw-Hill, 1990.

afterload), the ventricular myocardium hypertrophies, the heart pumps with more force, and the heart rate is often elevated. These mechanisms may maintain normal cardiac output for years prior to the onset of failure. Symptoms of CHF signal that the pump can no longer keep up with cellular demands. Gradually, the manifestations of heart failure become apparent.

An example of acute onset of heart failure is an extensive myocardial infarction (MI), which causes direct impairment of cardiac contractility, a sudden decrease in cardiac output, and insufficient available time for the development of hypertrophy (see Chap. 25).

### Sympathetic Response to Heart Failure

A decrease in cardiac output results in decreased blood pressure, which causes a reflex stimulation of the sympathetic nervous system (SNS). The SNS causes an increase in the rate and force of contraction of the ventricles through the conduction system and through an increase in ventricular irritability. It also results in vasoconstriction of the arterioles throughout the body.

The SNS activity is mediated through epinephrine and norepinephrine (see Chap. 26). Epinephrine mostly increases the rate and force of cardiac contractions, while norepinephrine functions mainly in arteriolar vasoconstriction.

### Renin-Angiotensin-Aldosterone System

When blood pressure decreases, the decline is perceived by the renal juxtaglomerular cells, which release renin. Renin acts on angiotensinogen, a plasma protein produced by the liver, to form angiotensin I. Angiotensin I is converted to angiotensin II by an enzyme present mostly in the lungs (Figure 24-1). Angiotensin II is a potent vasoconstrictor that constricts renal arterioles, stimulates the thirst center in the brain, and stimulates the secretion of aldosterone by the adrenal glands.[4] These actions cause vasoconstriction, which leads to increased blood pressure and expansion of the blood volume through the aldosterone effect of sodium preservation. The renin-angiotensin aldosterone system constantly functions to maintain fluid volume and blood pressure. The end product, angiotensin II, is rapidly destroyed by angiotensinase, a term used for a number of different blood and tissue enzymes.[4]

### Anaerobic Metabolism

When cells do not receive adequate circulation or oxygen, metabolism decreases and alternative methods are used to produce energy. The major alternative method is the anaerobic production of adenosine triphosphate, which is an inefficient process but accomplishes the pur-

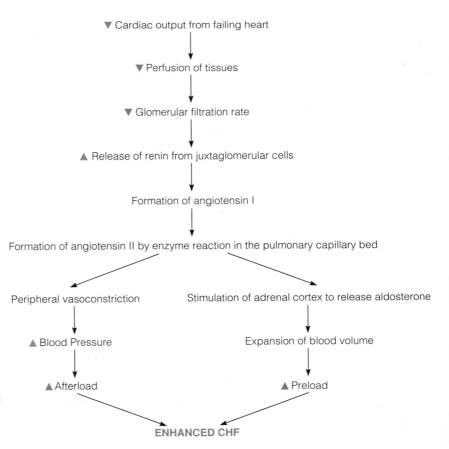

▼ Cardiac output from failing heart

▼ Perfusion of tissues

▼ Glomerular filtration rate

▲ Release of renin from juxtaglomerular cells

Formation of angiotensin I

Formation of angiotensin II by enzyme reaction in the pulmonary capillary bed

Peripheral vasoconstriction       Stimulation of adrenal cortex to release aldosterone

▲ Blood Pressure       Expansion of blood volume

▲ Afterload       ▲ Preload

**ENHANCED CHF**

**FIGURE 24–1.**
Renin-angiotensin-aldosterone (RAA) system in CHF. Note the positive feedback created as the body attempts to adjust to decreased cardiac output.

pose of keeping cells alive for a limited time. The unfortunate byproduct of producing energy is the absence of oxygen in the liberation of metabolic acids, especially lactic acid. This serves to depress cell function and produce a metabolic acidosis (see Chap. 9). This compensatory mechanism is activated only in severe circulatory failure and shock (see Chap. 11).

### Oxygen Extraction from the Red Blood Cells

Oxygen extraction from the red blood cells to the tissues increases when the circulation is inadequate and perfusion is diminished. Normally, about 30% of oxygen is extracted from red blood cells by the peripheral tissue but greater amounts can be extracted during periods of poor perfusion. Unfortunately, this mechanism is not very useful to the myocardial tissue because myocardial muscle normally extracts 65% to 75% of the oxygen it receives.[4]

### Frank-Starling Law of the Heart

When the heart is not pumping all of its contents out, increased amounts of blood are left within the organ. This residual volume increases diastolic fiber length. The inherent compensatory mechanism is an increase in the force of recoil so that the heart responds with increased stroke work and volume[14] (see Chap. 22). In the failing heart, diastolic fiber length is continually increased, causing the heart to enlarge. With activation of the renin-angiotensin-aldosterone (RAA) system, blood volume is increased, adding to this diastolic preload (see Figure 24-1).

### Hypertrophy of the Myocardium

When increased stress is placed on any chamber of the heart, hypertrophy can result. This physiologic myocardial response is due to chronically increased workload. The individual myocardial muscle cells increase in size but not in number. Hypertrophy probably results when the wall tension of the chamber must continuously increase on systole to eject the contents of the chamber. Ventricular hypertrophy is more common than atrial hypertrophy and provides for compensatory adaptation to a chronically increased workload.

Hypertrophy may be classified as *concentric* or *eccentric*. Concentric hypertrophy reveals a thickened ventricular wall without apparent enlargement of the heart.[8] This often occurs with aortic stenosis and sometimes with systemic hypertension.

Eccentric hypertrophy exhibits a proportionate increase in the wall size and diameter of the ventricle.[2,8] This type of hypertrophy often occurs in conditions associated with increased preload. Hypertrophy maintains

or increases contractility until heart failure ensues. The stimulus for hypertrophy is unknown but it is thought that increased systolic wall tension causes synthesis of sarcomeres parallel to existing sarcomeres.[8] The compensatory hypertrophy in persons with chronic pressure or volume overload can bring the systolic wall tension (pressure) to normal but the diastolic wall tension may remain abnormal when there is volume overload.[8] Hypertrophy, especially concentric hypertrophy, reduces the compliance of the ventricle so that elastic recoil and relaxation may both be impaired.[8] In eccentric hypertrophy, there is myocyte elongation which leads to a spherical shape of the heart.[14] Figure 24-2 shows the changes in left ventricular configuration depending upon the basic mechanism producing the hypertrophy. In a standard chest radiograph, these changes may be noted and become more pronounced as there is a progression of heart failure.

Hypertrophy increases the myocardial requirement for oxygen. This is supplied by the coronary arteries, and energy is produced by an increasing number of mitochondria which proliferate early in the process of developing hypertrophy.[14] As long as the oxygen supply from the coronary arteries and the mitochondrial production of adenosine triphosphate keeps up with the enlarging muscle, the ventricle will pump very efficiently. When an imbalance between oxygen supply and demand occurs, ischemia and cardiac dysfunction result.

### Dilatation of the Heart

Dilatation refers to enlargement of cardiac chambers. It often occurs because of increased volume of blood that enters the heart. The ventricles are always dilated in acute CHF. Dilatation often coincides with hypertrophy, especially if the stressful event causing the failure is chronic, such as chronic systemic hypertension.

Radiographic enlargement of the cardiac shadow characterizes heart failure. In the normal heart, increased input to the ventricle results in increased ventricular force of contraction but no permanent enlargement occurs. As the cardiac reserve fails, the ventricle is unable to pump out all of its contents and thus enlarges. The cardiac reserve is the ability of the heart to increase its output under stress.

Dilatation imposes a mechanical disadvantage on the ventricles. As ventricular volume increases, a large portion of the mechanical energy of contraction is expended in imparting tension to the fibers and a smaller portion for fiber recoil or shortening. An example of this concept can be illustrated by comparing the contractile power of two left ventricles. If one ventricle had twice the diameter of another, it would take four times the contractile power to produce the same systolic pressure in the larger ventricle.[8,13]

**FIGURE 24–2.**

Typical left ventricular pressure—volume relationships under basal conditions for a normal person (panel A) and for patients with compensated (early) and decompensated (late) congestive heart failure (CHF) due to left ventricular volume overload [mitral regurgitation (MR); panel B], pressure overload [aortic stenosis (AS); panel C], and ischemic heart disease after myocardial infarction or idiopathic congestive cardiomyopathy (panel D). The loops progress in a counterclockwise direction as they trace the phases of the cardiac cycle. In panel A, normal ventricular systolic ejection occurs from aortic opening (AO) to aortic closure (AC), whereas diastolic filling begins at mitral opening (MO) and terminates just before mitral closure (MC). The stroke volume (SV) for compensated CHF is normal (70 mL) and for decompensated CHF, it is reduced (40 mL), but the forward SV is similar to that in the other CHF examples (70 and 40 mL). The remaining SV is ejected into the left atrium. Left ventricular filling pressure (LVFP) occurs at mitral valve closure and in the examples shown is 18 mm Hg for compensated and 35 mm Hg for decompensated CHF. The upper limit of normal is 12 mm Hg. If heart rate (HR) is normal for compensated CHF (75 beats per minute) and comparably elevated for each example of decompensated CHF (95 beats per minute), it is clear that cardiac output (HR × forward SVj) is exactly normal in compensated and equivalently depressed in decompensated CHF. However, there are marked differences between the six CHF examples with respect to the ejection fraction (EF), the percent of end-diastolic volume ejected during systole, and the chamber volumes at end-systole (ESV) and end-diastole (EDV). This is due to the particular pattern of cardiac compensatory mechanism (hyperthropy and dilatation) activated by each of the examples of CHF depicted in panels B, C, and D. Diastolic stiffness can be estimated from the ratio of change in pressure to the change in volume (P, V) at different points during diastole. (Source: W.N. Kelley, *Textbook of Internal Medicine*. Philadelphia: J.B. Lippincott, 1989.)

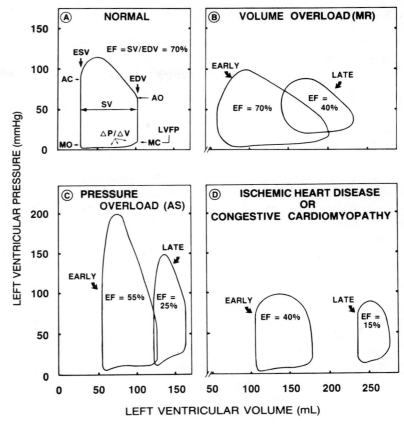

A heart that is greatly dilated also works at a metabolic disadvantage because its need for oxygen is increased. More blood to the myocardium is required, which may not be supplied by the coronary arteries.

Dilatation is characteristic of cardiomyopathy in which separation of the trabeculae carneae may occur together with fibrosis of the myocardium. Usually, the greater the dilatation, the more ineffective the cardiac contraction. Ineffective left ventricular contraction is often called *hypokinesis of the left ventricle*.

In persons with valvular insufficiency, septal defects, or other abnormal communications, the diastolic inflow to one or both ventricles is permanently augmented. In such conditions, dilatation of cardiac chambers occurs to maintain normal or near normal circulation even if a defect is quite large (see Chap. 25).

## Summary of Compensatory Mechanisms

The compensatory mechanisms described above may preserve the life of the individual but they usually aggravate the underlying condition.

Sympathetic regulation tends to preserve circulation to the brain and heart but it increases the cardiac workload by increasing the afterload, which may depress the effectiveness of cardiac contraction. Activation of the RAA system also increases afterload because of the peripheral vasoconstriction produced. The aldosterone effect increases blood volume and thus increases preload. Anaerobic metabolism causes metabolic acidosis, which depresses myocardial contractility. The Frank-Starling effect increases the energy requirements of the myocardium. Hypertrophy increases the oxygen need of each myocardial muscle cell, which is a problem if the blood flow is reduced from coronary artery disease.

The *cardiac reserve* is accomplished by increasing the stroke volume and increasing the heart rate. The normal heart can increase its output four to five times normal under conditions of stress.[4] As heart failure ensues, the reserve falls so that the individual may first have symptoms of heart failure when placed under significant stress. Later in the course of the disease, symptoms develop when only minor stress is encountered. Heart failure manifestations at rest indicate that there is no cardiac reserve for any stressful situation at all.

## Classification of Heart Failure

Heart failure has been classified as left-sided and right-sided on the basis of clinical manifestations. It has further been divided into forward and backward effects to explain its low-output and venous congestion components. In some cases, the forward or low-output syndrome dominates, while in others, the congestive phenomenon is the major manifestation. In reality, both features are present in heart failure just as both left-sided and right-sided effects necessarily must be present. Biventricular failure refers to failure of both ventricles. Usually right heart failure (RHF) follows left heart failure (LHF). This discussion divides LHF and RHF into separate entities. However, the reader must keep in mind that the heart and lungs are interconnected; what affects one side of the heart eventually affects the other (Figure 24-3).

## Left Heart Failure

Left heart failure occurs when the output of the left ventricle is less than the total volume of blood received from the right side of the heart through the pulmonary circulation. As a result, the pulmonary circuit becomes congested with blood that cannot be moved forward and the systemic blood pressure falls.

### Causes

The most common cause of predominantly left ventricular failure is a myocardial infarction (MI). Other causes include systemic hypertension, aortic stenosis or insufficiency, and cardiomyopathy. Mitral stenosis and mitral insufficiency also cause the symptoms of LHF (Figure 24-4).[8]

### Pathophysiology

Because the left ventricle cannot pump out all of its blood, blood dams back to the left atrium into the four pulmonary veins and the pulmonary capillary bed (PCB). As the volume of blood in the lungs increases, the pulmonary vessels enlarge. The pressure of blood in the PCB increases. When it reaches a certain critical point (approximately 25 to 28 mm Hg), fluid passes across the pulmonary capillary membrane into the interstitial spaces around the alveoli and finally into the alveoli (Fig-

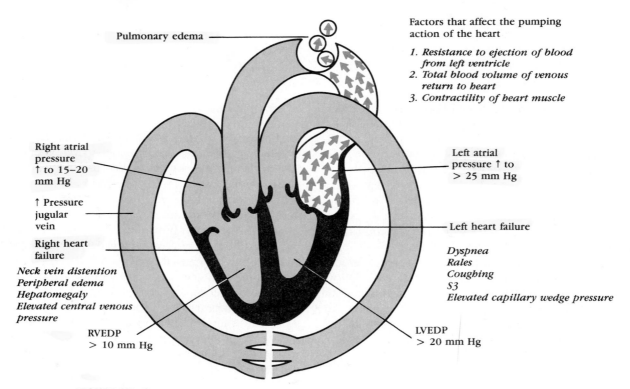

Pulmonary edema

**Factors that affect the pumping action of the heart**

1. *Resistance to ejection of blood from left ventricle*
2. *Total blood volume of venous return to heart*
3. *Contractility of heart muscle*

**Right atrial pressure** ↑ to 15–20 mm Hg

↑ Pressure jugular vein

**Right heart failure**

*Neck vein distention*
*Peripheral edema*
*Hepatomegaly*
*Elevated central venous pressure*

RVEDP > 10 mm Hg

**Left atrial pressure** ↑ to > 25 mm Hg

**Left heart failure**

*Dyspnea*
*Rales*
*Coughing*
*S3*
*Elevated capillary wedge pressure*

LVEDP > 20 mm Hg

**FIGURE 24-3.**
Biventricular failure usually results when left ventricular failure occurs, with elevated pulmonary pressures and subsequent elevation of the right-sided pressures leading to right-sided failure. (Adapted from C. Kenner, C. Guzzetta, and B. Dossey, *Critical Care Nursing: Body, Mind, Spirit* (2nd ed.). Boston: Little, Brown, 1985.)

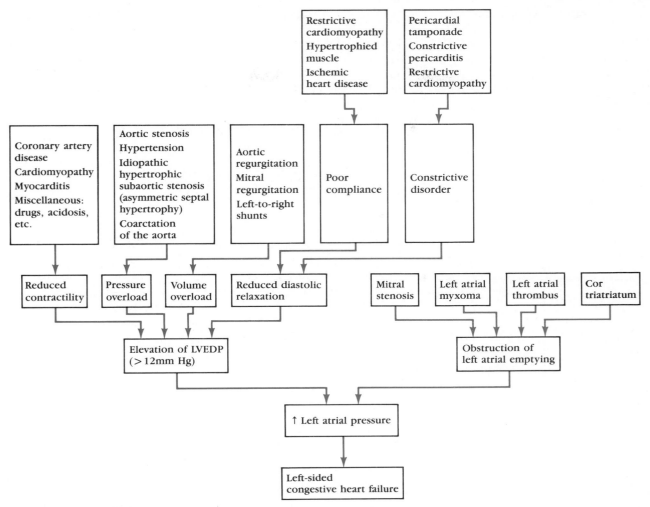

**FIGURE 24–4.**
Various pathologic conditions may ultimately cause an elevation in left atrial pressure and thereby precipitate left-sided congestive heart failure. In general, the rise in left atrial pressure can be attributed either to mechanical obstructions that interfere with diastolic emptying of the left atrium or to those clinical syndromes that produce an elevation in left ventricular end-diastolic pressure (LVEDP). (© Scientific American, Inc. All rights reserved. From *Scientific American Medicine*, Figure 3, Section 1, Subsection II.)

ure 24-5). Actual alveolar pulmonary edema occurs when the rate of fluid transudation exceeds the ability of the plentiful lymphatic drainage to remove it from the interstitial spaces.[8] Acute pulmonary edema (APE) results as the alveoli fill with fluid; this impairs gas exchange, which can be life-threatening. Higher PCB pressures may cause microhemorrhages in the sacs or rust-colored sputum due to the presence of hemosiderin-laden alveolar macrophages.[2,7,10] The presence of large amounts of these hemosiderin-laden macrophages (heart failure cells) is often indicative of longstanding cases of pulmonary congestion, as with mitral stenosis.[2]

These phenomena just described are the congestive phenomena of LHF that result from the volume overload

of the left ventricle. They are also called the *backward effects of LHF.*

The left ventricle also cannot pump its normal stroke volume out to the aorta. Thus, the systemic blood pressure decreases. This decrease is sensed by the baroreceptors that cause a reflex stimulation of the SNS. The result of SNS stimulation is increased heart rate and peripheral vasoconstriction. The RAA system is stimulated, leading to further vasoconstriction, together with sodium and water retention (see Figure 24-5).

The phenomena described above result from the inherent compensatory mechanisms of the body to preserve blood volume and pressure even at the expense of organs and tissues. The vasoconstriction helps to

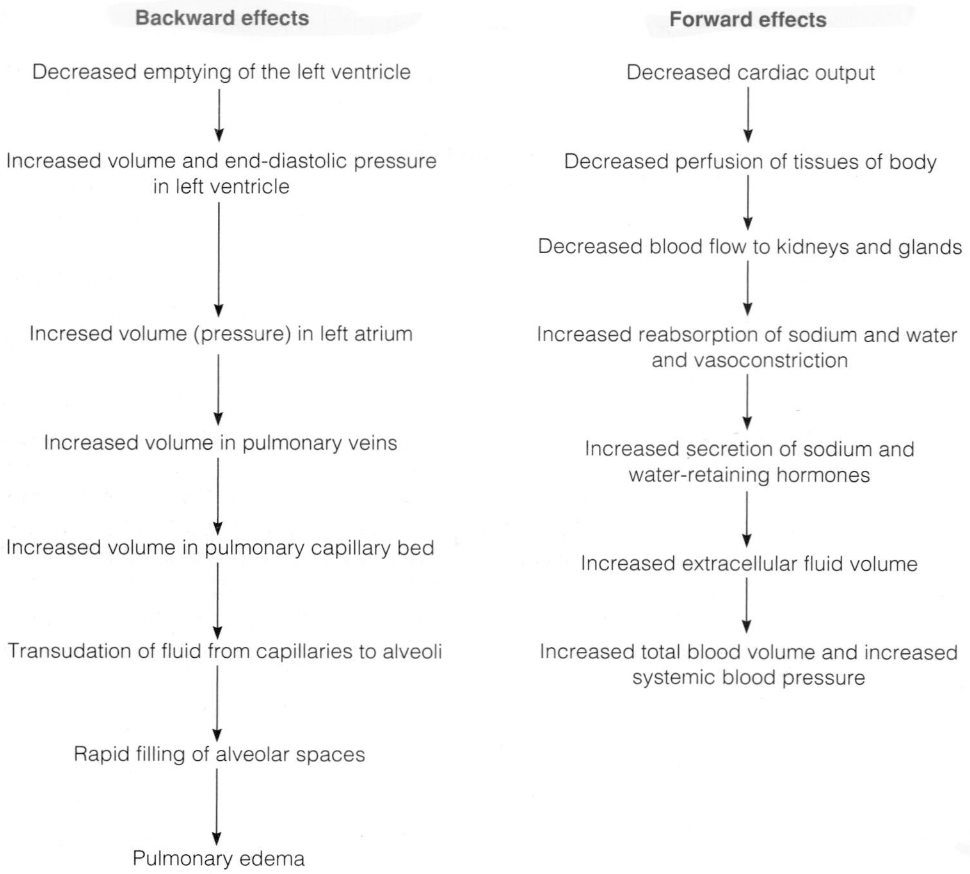

**Backward effects**

Decreased emptying of the left ventricle

↓

Increased volume and end-diastolic pressure in left ventricle

↓

Incresed volume (pressure) in left atrium

↓

Increased volume in pulmonary veins

↓

Increased volume in pulmonary capillary bed

↓

Transudation of fluid from capillaries to alveoli

↓

Rapid filling of alveolar spaces

↓

Pulmonary edema

**Forward effects**

Decreased cardiac output

↓

Decreased perfusion of tissues of body

↓

Decreased blood flow to kidneys and glands

↓

Increased reabsorption of sodium and water and vasoconstriction

↓

Increased secretion of sodium and water-retaining hormones

↓

Increased extracellular fluid volume

↓

Increased total blood volume and increased systemic blood pressure

**FIGURE 24–5.**
Highly schematic representation of the pathophysiology of left heart failure.

centralize blood volume while the aldosterone mechanism increases blood volume through sodium retention. These are the main manifestations of the *forward effects of LHF.*

Chronic LHF often occurs in mitral valve disease and it may progressively occur in cardiomyopathy and postmyocardial infarction. In the last two conditions, pulmonary congestion may be evidenced but APE does not occur unless additional stress increases the cardiac demand. Individuals with mitral stenosis, for example, have been shown to have a pulmonary pressure greater than 30 mm Hg without symptoms of APE. This is mainly due to increased lymphatic absorption of interstitial pulmonary fluid as previously described. In conditions of sudden onset, however, this level would cause acute pulmonary congestion.

### Signs and Symptoms

In the early stages of LHF, *dyspnea* is exhibited when the cardiac reserve is exceeded. As fluid begins to accumulate in the PCB, the formation of interstitial edema causes a defect in oxygenation.[12] The oxygen saturation of blood decreases, causing the chemoreceptors to stimu-

late the respiratory center. The respiratory rate increases at first during exercise and later even at rest. Shortness of breath on exertion (dyspnea on exertion, DOE) is a common and relatively early symptom. The person may complain of breathlessness when walking or after eating a heavy meal.[10]

Because of decreased cardiac output and decreased oxygen saturation of the blood, hypoxia of the body tissues occurs, which results in easy fatigue, weakness, and dizziness. Dizziness is the result of hypoxia to the brain. As failure and hypoxia worsen, disorientation, confusion, and ultimately unconsciousness can occur. Loss of potassium induced by increased levels of aldosterone also causes muscle weakness. Aldosterone conserves sodium at the expense of potassium and is often called the potassium-wasting hormone.

Inability to breathe in a supine position is called *orthopnea.* In chronic LHF, interstitial and alveolar pulmonary edema may be present all of the time; the upright position is assumed so fluid gravitates to the bases of the lungs.

Auscultation of the heart reveals an S3 gallop and a paradoxic split of the second sound on expiration. A *pulsus alternans*, characterized by alternating weaker and stronger pulsations in the peripheral arteries, often occurs and indicates a poorly functioning ventricle.

*Paroxysmal nocturnal dyspnea* refers to the onset of acute episodes of dyspnea at night. The cause of this condition is unknown but it is thought to result from improved cardiac performance at night during recumbency. This causes increased reabsorption of fluid that has accumulated in the lower half of the body into the systemic veins, where it is returned to the heart. The increased fluid returns to and overloads the left ventricle, causing acute pulmonary congestion until the individual assumes the orthopneic position. Acute breathlessness and a feeling of smothering are described.[9] This particular breathing difficulty is considered to be a very specific symptom of LHF.[10]

*Cardiac asthma* is the term used to describe wheezing due to bronchospasm induced by heart failure.[10] The bronchioles may react to the increased fluid in the alveoli, constrict, and produce the characteristic wheezing.

*Pulmonary edema* is an acute, life-threatening condition that usually results from LHF and may also result from abnormal permeability of the alveolocapillary membrane. Signs and symptoms of APE include dyspnea of sudden onset, basal rales, gasping respirations, extreme anxiety, rapid weak pulse, increased venous pressure, and decreased urinary output. The skin is cool and moist to the touch, ashen-gray, or cyanotic. A cough accompanied by expectoration of frothy white, pink-tinged, or bloody sputum may be present. Most attacks gradually subside in 1 to 3 hours, usually with treatment but they may progress rapidly to shock and death[9] (see Chap. 31).

## Right Heart Failure

Right heart failure occurs when the output of the right ventricle is less than the input from the systemic venous circuit. As a result, the systemic venous circuit is congested and output to the lungs decreases.

### Causes

The major cause of RHF is LHF; the right ventricle fails because of the excessive pulmonary pressures generated by failure of the left heart. Other causes include chronic obstructive lung disease, pulmonary embolus, right ventricular infarction, and congenital heart defects, especially those that involve pulmonary overloading and pulmonary hypertension (Figure 24-6). Right heart failure that results from lung disease is called *cor pulmonale*.

### Pathophysiology

In RHF, the right ventricle cannot pump all of its contents forward so blood dams back from the right ventricle to the right atrium causing an increased pressure in the systemic venous circuit. The increased volume and pressure are transmitted to distensible organs, such as the liver and spleen. Increased pressure in the peritoneal vessels leads to transudation of fluid into the peritoneal cavity. Increased pressure at the capillary line causes fluid to move into the interstitial space and systemic peripheral edema results (Figure 24-7). The cardinal signs of RHF are jugular venous distention, hepatomegaly, splenomegaly, and peripheral, dependent edema. These are considered the *backward* or *congestive* effects of RHF.

The right ventricle also cannot maintain its output to the lungs. This results in a decreased pulmonary circulation and decreased return to the left side of the heart. These *forward effects of RHF* cause all of the forward effects of LHF (see Figure 24-7).

### Signs and Symptoms

The signs and symptoms of RHF reflect both forward and backward effects. Dependent, pitting edema is characteristic and may be noted in the sternum or sacrum of a bedridden person, as well as the feet and legs of a person in the sitting position.

Enlargement of the spleen and liver can cause pressure on surrounding organs, respiratory impingement, and organ dysfunction. Inadequate deactivation of aldosterone by the liver may lead to additional fluid retention. Jaundice and coagulation problems may result with severe, longstanding, decompensated RHF. Ascites also occurs when RHF is severe and may cause respiratory embarrassment and abdominal pressure. Pleural effusions also may appear due to the increased capillary pressure.

Jugular venous distention occurs and can be measured at the bedside. It is measured in centimeters when the head is elevated to a 30-degree, 45-degree, or a 90-degree angle (Figure 24-8).

With pure RHF (that not precipitated by LHF), the pulmonary symptoms are minimal to absent, whereas engorgement of the venous and portal systems is significant.[2] The peripheral edema may be massive and gradually affect most of the tissues of the body, a condition termed *anasarca*. When RHF is due to lung disease, the underlying lung problem will present its symptoms, as well as the cardiac dysfunction.

## Biventricular Congestive Heart Failure

As stated previously, CHF usually affects both the left and right sides. The manifestations may be more low-output or congestive but they affect almost all of the organs and

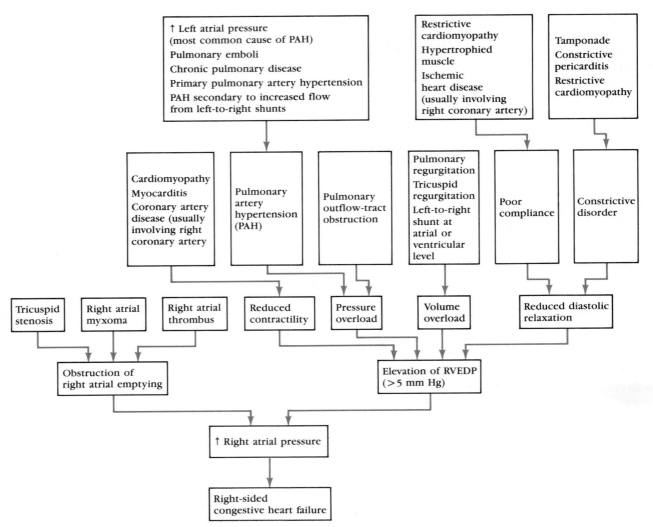

**FIGURE 24–6.**
Various pathways may lead to an increase in right atrial pressure and consequently provoke right-sided congestive heart failure. Elevation of right atrial pressure can be induced either by mechanisms that cause an increase in the right ventricular end-diastolic pressure (RVEDP) or by lesions that obstruct blood flow from the right atrium. The most common cause of right ventricular failure is left ventricular failure, which produces a rise in left atrial pressure. This, in turn, leads to pulmonary artery hypertension, which imposes a pressure overload on the right ventricle and may trigger right ventricular failure. (© 1987, Scientific American, Inc. All rights reserved. From *Scientific American Medicine,* Figure 4, Section 1, Subsection II.)

tissues of the body. Table 24-2 summarizes the clinical abnormalities of CHF.

## Diagnosis of Congestive Heart Failure

### Radiologic Changes

Radiologic evidence of pulmonary congestion usually precedes the development of audible rales in LHF. Cardiac enlargement is noted by an increased size of the left ventricular shadow. The left ventricle extends past the midclavicular line and fluid effusion may be present throughout the lung fields (Figure 24-9). In RHF, the right ventricular shadow can be seen extending out from the right sternal border. Pulmonary markings may be decreased due to decreased pulmonary circulation (Figure 24-10).[10]

### Hemodynamic Monitoring

The balloon-tipped flow-directed catheter (Swan-Ganz) is an effective monitoring system for assessing pulmonary and systemic circulations. The Swan-Ganz catheter

**Backward effects**

Decreased emptying of the right ventricle

↓

Increased volume and end-diastolic pressure
in the right ventricle

↓

Increased volume (pressure) in right atrium

↓

Increased volume and pressure in the great veins

↓

Increased volume in the systemic venous circulation

↓

Increased volume in distensible organs
(hepatomegaly, splenomegaly)

↓

Increased pressure at capillary line

↓

Peripheral, dependent edema and serous effusion

**Forward effects**

Decreased volume from the
right ventricle to the lungs

↓

Decreased return to left atrium and
subsequent decreased cardiac output

↓

All the forward effects of left heart failure

↓

Expansion of blood volume
and vasoconstriction

**FIGURE 24–7.**
Highly schematic illustration of the
pathophysiology of right heart
failure.

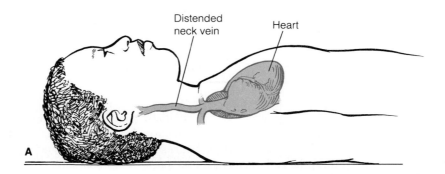

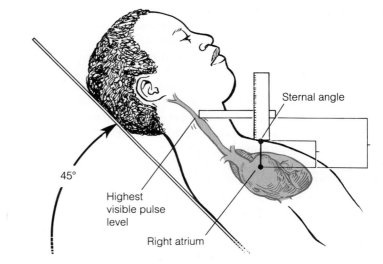

**FIGURE 24–8.**
Measuring jugular venous pressure. **A.**
Neck veins are normally distended when
the person is in the supine position. **B.** Place
the person at 45° angle in which position the
sternal angle is approximately 5 cm above
the right atrium. Place ruler on sternal angle
and measure the distance in centimeters
from the sternal angle to the horizontal level
of the highest visible pulse of the distended
neck vein. Value obtained by this measurement plus 5 cm (distance from sternal angle
to right atrium) provides an approximate
measure of CVP.

**TABLE 24–2.**

CLINICAL ABNORMALITIES IN CONGESTIVE HEART FAILURE

| ABNORMALITY | ORGAN/TISSUE | SYMPTOMS AND SIGNS |
|---|---|---|
| Low output (reduced regional blood flows) | Kidneys | Salt and water retention; azotemia; hyponatremia; impaired drug excretion |
| | Skeletal muscle | Fatigue; tiredness; decreased aerobic capacity; lactic acidemia; tachypnea from somatic afferent nerve stimulation |
| | Skin | Cold, pale, cyanotic, sweaty extremities; impaired heat loss |
| | Brain | Sleep reversal; Cheyne-Stokes respiration; reduced central ventilatory drive; confusion; stupor (late) |
| | Gut | Early satiety; postprandial discomfort |
| | Liver | Centrilobular necrosis (rare) |
| Congestion (increased pulmonary and systemic venous pressures) | Lungs | Shortness of breath (dyspnea) on exertion, when recumbent (orthopnea), awakening the patient from sleep (paroxysmal nocturnal dyspnea); pulmonary edema; tachypnea; rales; pleural effusions; redistribution of blood flow from base to apex of lungs; ventilation-perfusion mismatch; hypoxemia |
| | Jugular veins | Distension; prominent v waves |
| | Skin | Dependent pitting edema |
| | Liver | Enlargement; tenderness; ascites; reduced drug metabolism; splenomegaly (late) |
| | Kidney | Proteinuria; hypoalbuminemia |
| | Gut | Ascites; poor absorption; anorexia; protein and lymphocyte loss; constant fullness |
| | Skeletal muscle | Fatigue |

Source: W. N. Kelley, Textbook of Internal Medicine. Philadelphia: J. B. Lippincott, 1989.

is threaded into the pulmonary artery where it finally halts in a vessel slightly smaller than the inflated balloon tip, blocking the flow of blood from the right ventricle.[11] A pressure reading at this time reflects the diastolic pressures of the left ventricle if there is no concomitant mitral valve disease. This pulmonary artery wedge pressure reflects its pressures because of the continuous circuit to the left heart. Thus pressure measurements reflect the left ventricular end-diastolic pressure (LVEDP) (Figure 24-11).

The end-diastolic volume, normally 70 mL per m² of body surface, is elevated in the failing heart. Because an increase in end-diastolic volume is often associated with an increase in end-diastolic pressure (EDP), the EDP can be used as an indicator of ventricular function. The EDP of the left ventricle is usually 12 mm Hg or less and in the right ventricle 5 mm Hg or less. A high LVEDP can be the result of increased left ventricular volume or reduced left ventricular compliance or both. In the absence of increased pulmonary vascular resistance and mitral valve

disease, mean pulmonary capillary wedge pressure and pulmonary artery diastolic pressure reflect LVEDP. When the balloon tip is deflated, the catheter tip usually locates in a branch of the main pulmonary artery.[11] The Swan-Ganz catheter also measures central venous pressure (right atrial pressure) and pulmonary artery pressure. Most Swan-Ganz catheters also can be used to measure cardiac output by the thermodilution method, in which a computer analyzes a temperature differential between two points on the catheter. The normal cardiac output is approximately 4 to 8 liters per minute. The level of decreased cardiac output in persons with CHF helps to determine the necessary treatment. Levels of 2.2 to 3.0 liters per minute or below may indicate cardiogenic shock, depending on the size and age of the individual.

## Arterial Blood Gases

The normal arterial and venous blood gases are presented in Table 24-3. Hypoxemia (decreased partial pres-

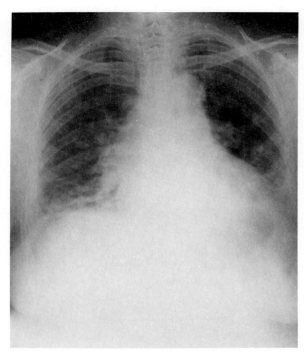

**FIGURE 24–9.**
Radiologic changes in LHF. Note left ventricular enlargement and fluid effusion in lung fields.

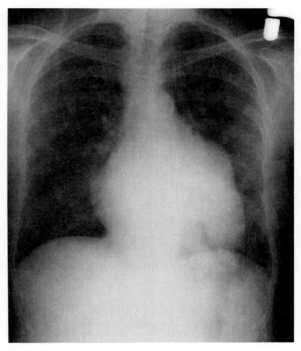

**FIGURE 24–10.**
Radiologic changes in RHF. Note right ventricular shadow extending out from the right sternal border.

sure of oxygen or $PO_2$) is often the only change that is noted with CHF. Oxygen saturation often remains normal until decompensation is severe. The partial pressure of carbon dioxide ($PCO_2$) may be low due to hyperventilation. In end-stage CHF, the $PCO_2$ may be elevated.

### Other Laboratory Tests

*Serum sodium* levels are often low in CHF even though body sodium levels are almost always elevated. This lab picture results from the retention of sodium and water described in Chapter 8. *Serum potassium* may be decreased due to the aldosterone effect and the administration of potassium-depleting diuretics (see Chap. 8).

## CARDIOGENIC SHOCK

### Causes of Cardiogenic Shock

Heart failure may lead to cardiogenic shock with a low-output component, the congestive phenomena, or both. The most common cause of cardiogenic shock is MI; however, cardiomyopathy, dysrhythmias, cardiac tamponade, pulmonary embolism, or any factor that can depress myocardial function may precipitate this syndrome.

Cardiogenic shock always carries a grave prognosis. If it develops after MI, mortality is approximately 60% to 80%, which correlates well with the amount of ventricular mass lost.[5] A 30% to 40% loss of left ventricular mass by infarctions, both new and old, is often correlated with cardiogenic shock[6] (see Chap. 11).

### Pathophysiology of Cardiogenic Shock

Cardiogenic shock results from decreased ability of the left or right ventricle to maintain adequate cardiac output. This results in decreased systolic blood pressure with reduced peripheral perfusion manifested by cold, clammy skin, diaphoresis, tachycardia, mental confusion, and decreased urinary output. The cold, clammy skin and tachycardia result from sympathetic stimulation. The effects of SNS stimulation increase the taxation on an already overtaxed heart but enhance cerebral and coronary blood flow. It markedly decreases renal perfusion and increases the risk for acute renal failure (see Chap. 35).

Anaerobic metabolism begins in peripheral cells as vital oxygen deprivation occurs. The effect of this energy production is to keep cells viable but the production of

A.  Catheter advanced to right atrium, balloon is inflated. Pressure is low, usually 2–5 mm Hg.

B.  Catheter is floated to right ventricle with the balloon inflated. Wave-forms indicate a systolic pressure of 25–30 mm Hg and a diastolic pressure of 0–5 mm Hg.

C.  As the catheter moves into the pulmonary artery, the systolic pressure remains the same but the diastolic pressure elevates to 10–15 mm Hg.

D.  The balloon is deflated and the catheter is moved until it can be wedged in a smaller vessel. When the balloon is inflated, the pressure recorded is that pressure in front of the catheter. It is an approximate measure of the left ventricular end diastolic pressure.

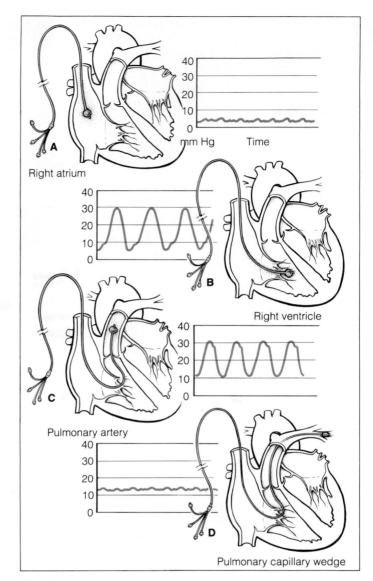

**FIGURE 24–11.**
Insertion of a flow-directed cardiac catheter.

**TABLE 24–3.**
ARTERIAL AND VENOUS BLOOD GAS STUDIES
(NORMAL VALUES IN HEALTHY ADULTS)

|  | ARTERIAL BLOOD | MIXED VENOUS BLOOD |
|---|---|---|
| pH | 7.40* (7.35–7.45) | 7.36* (7.30–7.41) |
| $PO_2$ | 80–100 mm Hg | 35–40 mm Hg |
| $O_2Sa$ | 95% | 70–75% |
| $PCO_2$ | 35–45 mm Hg | 41–51 mm Hg |
| $HCO_3$ | 22–26 mEq/L | 22–26 mEq/L |
| Base excess | −2 to +2 | −2 to +2 |

*Indicates the mean.

lactic acid as a byproduct leads to metabolic acidosis (see Chap. 9). Acidosis depresses cardiac function and further depression may result from a *myocardial depressant factor* released from the pancreas in shock situations.[3]

Cardiogenic shock is often described in stages. If the compensatory mechanisms can restore arterial pressure and urinary output, it is termed *compensated shock*. If the underlying cause of the shock is not corrected, the response of the body to poor tissue perfusion results in continuation of the shock state, which is called *progressive shock*. When arteriolar tone is finally destroyed and peripheral pooling occurs, death becomes inevitable. This condition is called *irreversible* or *decompensated shock*. Pooling is enhanced by loss of arteriolar tone prior to loss of venular tone, which encourages fluid movement into the interstitial spaces. Anaerobic energy production and lactic acidosis eventually cause cellular failure and death.

## Diagnosis of Cardiogenic Shock

Diagnosis of cardiogenic shock is often one of exclusion. Sometimes hypovolemic shock must be ruled out. Physical examination reveals gallop rhythms, sometimes venous engorgement, and effects of acute hypotension. The ECG often shows cardiac dysrhythmias and evidence of MI. The Swan-Ganz catheter reveals elevated pulmonary wedge pressures and decreased cardiac output.[5]

## DISEASES AFFECTING MYOCARDIAL CONTRACTILITY

The term *cardiomyopathy* refers to a group of myocardial diseases that primarily affect the pumping ability of the heart (Figure 24-12). *Myocarditis* is the word used for myocardial disease associated with inflammation of the myocardium.

## Cardiomyopathy

*Primary* or *idiopathic myocardial disease* refers to conditions affecting the ventricular muscle that have no known origin. *Secondary* cardiomyopathy designates conditions in which the causative factors are known. The cardiomyopathies have been classified as congestive, restrictive, and hypertrophic.[13]

### Congestive or Dilated Cardiomyopathy

Congestive or dilated cardiomyopathy is usually of unknown etiology but it has been described in association with beriberi, thyrotoxicosis, alcoholism, childbirth or the postpartum period, diabetes mellitus, drug toxicity (especially from daunorubicin), cobalt therapy, and

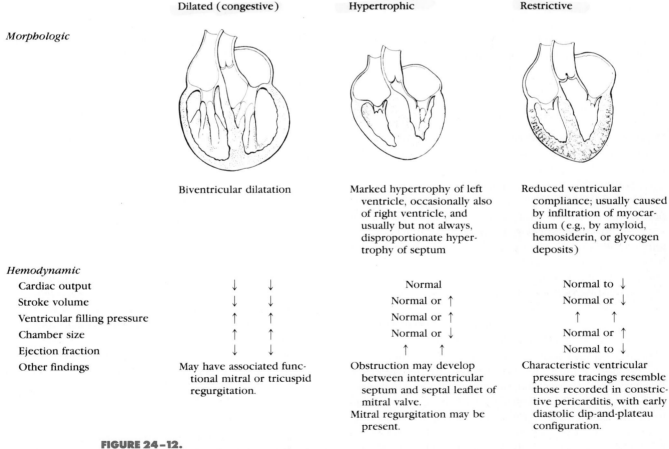

| | Dilated (congestive) | | Hypertrophic | Restrictive |
|---|---|---|---|---|
| *Morphologic* | Biventricular dilatation | | Marked hypertrophy of left ventricle, occasionally also of right ventricle, and usually but not always, disproportionate hypertrophy of septum | Reduced ventricular compliance; usually caused by infiltration of myocardium (e.g., by amyloid, hemosiderin, or glycogen deposits) |
| *Hemodynamic* | | | | |
| Cardiac output | ↓ | ↓ | Normal | Normal to ↓ |
| Stroke volume | ↓ | ↓ | Normal or ↑ | Normal or ↓ |
| Ventricular filling pressure | ↑ | ↑ | Normal or ↑ | ↑  ↑ |
| Chamber size | ↑ | ↑ | Normal or ↓ | Normal or ↑ |
| Ejection fraction | ↓ | ↓ | ↑  ↑ | Normal to ↓ |
| Other findings | May have associated functional mitral or tricuspid regurgitation. | | Obstruction may develop between interventricular septum and septal leaflet of mitral valve. Mitral regurgitation may be present. | Characteristic ventricular pressure tracings resemble those recorded in constrictive pericarditis, with early diastolic dip-and-plateau configuration. |

**FIGURE 24-12.**
Morphologic and hemodynamic characteristics of the cardiomyopathies. (Source: © 1987, Scientific American Inc. All rights reserved from *Scientific American Medicine*, Table 1, Section 1, Subsection XIV.)

certain neuromuscular disorders. The striking effect of this type of cardiomyopathy is immense cardiomegaly. The enlargement is a combination of dilatation and hypertrophy of the heart. This dilatation leads to a hypokinetic myocardium with the usual onset of biventricular CHF. Symptoms include exertional dyspnea, fatigue, paroxysmal nocturnal dyspnea, and pulmonary edema with symptoms of RHF late in the course of the disease. Atrial and ventricular gallops may be noted on auscultation. Peripheral edema and hepatomegaly are signs of RHF.

### Restrictive Cardiomyopathy

Restrictive cardiomyopathy describes the clinical picture of constrictive pericarditis, the underlying cause of which is actually myocardial. The etiology is generally unknown but it has been described in association with such diverse conditions as amyloidosis, hemosiderosis, and glycogen storage disease. The myocardial muscle becomes infiltrated with abnormal substances that apparently cause dysfunction of the ventricle.

Congestive and restrictive cardiomyopathies are mostly differentiated on the basis of the presence or absence of cardiomegaly. Symptoms of biventricular failure are common. Ventricular filling is impeded and the EDP of the ventricles usually becomes exceedingly high. The prognosis for survival is poor and death often results from CHF.

### Hypertrophic Cardiomyopathy

Hypertrophic cardiomyopathy usually refers to an asymmetric increase in ventricular muscle mass. It has also been termed *idiopathic hypertrophic subaortic stenosis* and *hypertrophic obstructive cardiomyopathy.*[1]

The etiology of this condition is unknown. Familial occurrence is noted with no predominance for either sex. Certain studies support a genetic abnormality of protein synthesis.[1] The pathologic features include greater hypertrophy of the ventricular septum than of the ventricular chambers. Small or normal ventricular chamber size and disorganization of septal muscle cells, especially of the myofibrils, may occur.

Other significant abnormalities associated with this condition include fibrous plaque on the endocardium, abnormal septal arteries, and mitral valve insufficiency.[13]

Because of the septal hypertrophy, the left ventricular cavity is misshapen and, on contraction, the hypertrophied septum causes obstruction to the flow of blood from the ventricle. Any condition that enhances contractility increases the degree of obstruction. The associated left ventricular hypertrophy causes impairment of ventricular filling during diastole and reduced ventricular compliance.[1]

The signs and symptoms are mainly those of LHF, including exertional dyspnea, angina, periods of syncope, and orthopnea. Right-sided effects occur later in the course of the disease. The prognosis is generally better than in the previous types.

## Myocarditis

Inflammation of the myocardium may result from an infectious process or from radiation therapy or chemical agents. Viruses, especially the coxsackieviruses, have been implicated in the etiology. Myocarditis is often a self-limiting condition that is manifested by tachycardia, symptoms of heart failure, and gallop rhythm on auscultation. Many types of myocarditis resolve with bed rest, fluid restriction, and limited drug therapy. In a small percentage of affected persons, the disease is progressive and leads to all of the manifestations of dilated, congestive myocardiopathy.

## REFERENCES

1. Bristow, M.R., and O'Connell, J.B. Myocardial diseases. In W.N. Kelley (ed.), *Textbook of Internal Medicine.* Philadelphia: J.B. Lippincott, 1989.
2. Cotran, R.S., Kumar, V., and Robbins, S.L. *Robbins' Pathologic Basis of Disease* (4th ed.). Philadelphia: W.B. Saunders, 1989.
3. Ferguson, D.W., and Abboud, F.M. The pathophysiology, recognition, and management of shock. In J.W. Hurst et al. (eds.), *The Heart* (7th ed.). New York: McGraw-Hill, 1990.
4. Guyton, A.C. *Textbook of Medical Physiology* (8th ed.). Philadelphia: W.B. Saunders, 1990.
5. Houston, M.C., Thompson, W.L., and Robertson, D. Shock: Diagnosis and management. *Arch. Intern. Med.* 144:1433, 1984.
6. Leier, C.V. Approach to the patient with hypotension and shock. In W.N. Kelley (ed.), *Textbook of Internal Medicine.* Philadelphia: J.B. Lippincott, 1989.
7. Saul, S. Heart. In V.A. LiVolsi et al. (eds.), *Pathology* (2nd ed.). Media, Penn.: Harwal, 1989.
8. Schlant, R.C., and Sonnerblick, E.H. Pathophysiology of heart failure. In J.W. Hurst et al. (eds.), *The Heart* (7th ed.). New York: McGraw-Hill, 1990.
9. Sokolow, M., and McIllroy, M.B. *Clinical Cardiology* (4th ed.). Los Altos, Calif.: Lange, 1986.
10. Spann, J.F., and Hurst, J.W. The recognition and management of heart failure. In J.W. Hurst et al. (eds.), *The Heart* (7th ed.). New York: McGraw-Hill, 1990.
11. Swan, H.J. Monitoring the seriously ill patient. In J.W. Hurst et al. (eds.), *The Heart* (7th ed.). New York: McGraw-Hill, 1990.
12. Wallace, A.G. and Waugh, R.A. Pathophysiology of cardiovascular diseases. In L.H. Smith and S.O. Thier (eds.), *Pathophysiology: The Biological Principles of Disease* (2nd ed.). Philadelphia: W.B. Saunders, 1985.

**13.** Wenger, N.K., Abelman, W.H., and Roberts, W.C. Cardio-myopathy. In J.W. Hurst et al. (eds.), *The Heart* (7th ed.). New York: McGraw-Hill, 1990.

**14.** Zelis, R., and Sinoway, L.I. Pathophysiology of heart failure. In W.N. Kelley (ed.), *Textbook of Internal Medicine*. Philadelphia: J.B. Lippincott, 1989.

*chapter* # 25

Barbara L. Bullock

# Alterations in Specific Structures in the Heart

## *Chapter Outline*

## *Learning Objectives*

1. Describe the following diagnostic procedures: coronary arteriogram, thallium scan, exercise electrocardiogram, multigated blood pool scan, cardiac catheterization, and echocardiography.

2. Differentiate the pathologic and clinical manifestations of angina and myocardial infarction.

3. Describe the development of an atherosclerotic plaque in a coronary artery.

4. Identify the most common sites of coronary artery lesions.

5. Discuss the risk factors for coronary atherogenesis.

6. Describe the process of healing after a myocardial infarction.

7. List and explain the significance of the characteristic electrocardiogram changes of angina and myocardial infarction.

*(continued)*

## Learning Objectives (continued)

8. Describe briefly why heart pain occurs and why it radiates to other areas.

9. Explain how a myocardial infarction impairs myocardial contractility.

10. Differentiate the significant changes of each of the cardiac enzymes.

11. Describe at least four common complications of myocardial infarction.

12. Relate the pathophysiologic consequences of acute rheumatic fever to chronic valvular disease.

13. State the major pathophysiology and compensatory mechanisms that are used in mitral stenosis, mitral insufficiency, mitral valve prolapse, aortic stenosis, and aortic regurgitation.

14. Describe the clinical manifestations of mitral stenosis, mitral insufficiency, mitral valve prolapse, aortic stenosis, and aortic regurgitation.

15. Describe how pulmonary hypertension can develop from mitral stenosis and from congenital heart defects.

16. Describe briefly the major characteristics of cardiac murmurs produced by valvular defects.

17. Identify the pathophysiologic alterations in and clinical manifestations of infective endocarditis.

18. State the pathophysiologic alterations in and clinical manifestations of pericarditis.

19. Describe the embryologic events leading to cardiac structure.

20. Differentiate the consequences of left-to-right and right-to-left shunts.

21. Identify the pathophysiologic results of these common congenital defects: patent ductus arteriosus (PDA), atrial and ventricular septal defects (VSDs), tetralogy of Fallot, transposition of the great vessels, and coarctation of the aorta.

## CORONARY ARTERY DISEASE: ISCHEMIC HEART DISEASE

Cardiovascular disease (CVD) is the leading cause of death and disability in the United States.[18] One of every three men and one of every 10 women can expect to develop CVD before age 60 years.[18] Overall, CVD mortality has declined by 39% from a peak in the 1960s. The death rate in the United States has been falling at a rate of 2% to 3% per year, mainly due to declining mortality from CVD.[18] Improved CVD mortality figures may reflect widespread application of cardiopulmonary resuscitation, better medical control of emergencies, control of hypertension, lower cholesterol diets, or numerous other factors.[26] *Coronary heart disease* (CHD), a term used interchangeably with the term *coronary artery disease* (CAD), causes about 800,000 new heart attacks and about 450,000 recurrent heart attacks each year. Men have a higher incidence than women and at an earlier age.[13] Coronary heart disease is the leading cause of death in American adults, causing more than one fourth of deaths in persons over age 35 years.[13] More than half of these deaths are sudden, out-of-hospital fatalities.[13]

Coronary artery disease is almost totally caused by atherosclerosis of the coronary arteries, a fact that has led to widespread research into the cause of atherosclerosis. There are numerous theories of the pathogenesis of atherosclerosis. Most agree that it begins early in life and progresses over decades (see Chap. 27). Many factors probably interact to accelerate the atherogenic process. These have been identified as risk factors in epidemiologic studies since they seem to reflect an increase in the probability of a person developing coronary atherosclerosis but do not predict the severity or extent of an atherosclerotic lesion.[26]

## Risk Factors

The probability for developing CAD is determined by certain risk factors. These have been labeled as risk factors that cannot be altered and those than can be changed by lifestyle changes. Table 25-1 lists the major factors that are described below.

### Alterable Risk Factors

Diet is a main factor in the development of CAD. In the United States, the intake has been increasingly geared toward consumption of a high-fat, high-carbohydrate diet. This American diet has resulted in generally high serum plasma cholesterol levels. Coronary risk is directly re-

**TABLE 25–1.**
RISK FACTORS FOR CORONARY ARTERY DISEASE

| ALTERABLE | UNALTERABLE |
|---|---|
| Diet | Age |
| Smoking | Sex |
| Hypertension | Race |
| Stress | Genetic heritage |
| Sedentary living | |
| Diabetes mellitus | |
| Alcohol | |

lated to serum cholesterol: the higher the plasma cholesterol, the greater the risk.[26] Those who have plasma cholesterol levels below 175 mg per dL have less than half the risk of myocardial infarction (MI) than those with levels of 250 mg per dL.[26] Foods high in saturated fat content are readily used by the liver to make cholesterol. Table 25-2 lists the various forms and risks of serum cholesterol levels (see Chap. 42). The low density lipoprotein (LDL) form of cholesterol is associated with an increased risk of CAD, while the high density lipoprotein (HDL) form tends to exert a protective effect in preventing CAD. Factors such as exercise, age (children and premenopausal women), and diet cause increases in HDL levels and apparently decrease the risk of CAD.[26] The current recommendation of the National Cholesterol Education Program is to restrict total fat intake to 30% or less of total calories. Widespread public education has led many convenience food vendors to offer foods with a decreased fat content. The changing diet may be a major factor in the declining mortality figures for CAD. A small percentage of cases of hyperlipidemia are due to a hereditary disorder. These cases should be diagnosed at an early age and can be treated with diet restrictions and lipid-lowering drugs.

*Cigarette smoking* has been labeled the single most preventable cause of premature death in the United States.[18] Current evidence indicates that the risk of CAD decreases after quitting so that after 1 year the risk is similar to that of nonsmokers.[18] Risk of cerebrovascular accident is also decreased after quitting, perhaps due to decreased fibrinogen levels, which are usually elevated in smokers. Smoking is addictive and probably synergistic to other risk factors.[26] It decreases HDL and increases LDL cholesterol and alters oxygen transport in the myocardium.[26] Because of the oxygen uptake problem, smokers have a much increased risk of cardiac dysrhythmias and sudden death.[18] Overall, smoking has declined from 50% to 30% in men and 34% to 24% among women over the past 20 years, which probably also has contributed to the declining mortality from CAD.[18]

Hypertension, described in Chapter 26, is a significant risk factor for CAD that can be decreased with antihypertensive drugs, diet, and exercise. The risk of CAD is related especially to the elevation of the systolic pressure, especially in men over age 50 years and in the elderly population.[18,26]

Stress or behavioral factors have always been correlated to an increased incidence of CAD. The type A behavior pattern, characterized by competitiveness, impatience, aggressiveness, time urgency, and so on, has yet to be convincingly documented as causative in CAD.[18]

**TABLE 25–2.**
SERUM CHOLESTEROL AND CAD RISKS

| TYPES OF LIPIDS | SOURCE | FUNCTIONS AND CAD RISKS |
| --- | --- | --- |
| Chylomicron | 80–95% triglyceride (TG) | Low risk, little association with CAD; largest lipoprotein, transports triglycerides to fat and muscle and liver |
| Very low density lipoprotein (VLDL) | 45–65% TG 25% cholesterol | Synthesized by liver, primarily transports triglycerides to tissue capillaries and fat and muscle cells |
| Intermediate density lipoprotein (IDL) | 45% cholesterol | Lipoprotein remnants that remain when triglycerides are removed from VLDL |
| Low density lipoprotein (LDL) | 70% cholesterol | Major cholesterol transport; uptake of LDL in arteries can result in the development of atherosclerosis; high levels seen with familial hyperlipoproteinemias, smokers, diabetics; often elevated in obese individuals |
| High density lipoprotein (HDL) | 25% cholesterol | Carrier that removes cholesterol from tissues and transports it to the liver for catabolism and excretion; levels are increased in premenopausal women, athletes, moderate alcohol drinkers |

*Summarized from R. S. Cotran, V. Kumar, and S. L. Robbins, Robbins' Pathologic Basis of Disease (4th ed.). Philadelphia: W.B. Saunders, 1989.*

Stressful life events, job problems, limited social support, and lifestyle changes have all been associated with increased CAD, although the mechanism is unknown.[26] These psychosocial factors may also be associated with other risk factors, such as diet and smoking.

Sedentary living has been implicated in increased CAD risk with some of the newer studies suggesting decreased risk with regular, moderate, or vigorous physical activity.[26] Controlled studies are difficult to attain but all of the correlates of moderate exercise with its attendant psychological and physical improvement seem to have a positive effect on decreasing CAD.

Diabetes mellitus causes alteration in carbohydrate and fat metabolism and increases the frequency of coronary and other atherosclerotic diseases. Keeping the body weight and blood sugar levels under control decreases the onset of CAD.

Although alcohol has not been shown to cause an increase in serum cholesterol, it is positively correlated with high blood pressure. Some studies have shown that one to two drinks per day can increase serum HDL. The danger in recommending this as medical therapy is that alcohol consumption is correlated with increased smoking behavior, alcoholism, obesity, and other systemic problems.[26]

### *Unalterable Risk Factors*

Increased age is associated with increased CAD. All forms of atherosclerotic disease increase with age.

Sex differences favor an increased incidence in men at an earlier age. Female hormones may be protective but if the woman is diabetic, is a cigarette smoker, or takes oral contraceptives, her incidence increases. As men and women become elderly, the frequency of CAD nearly equals.

Racial differences have been studied with little conclusive evidence of differences when the other risk factors are ruled out. Blacks have an equal incidence of CAD but a higher incidence of hypertension, while Orientals have a somewhat lower incidence due, in part it is assumed, to diet.[2]

Genetic heritage is a strong factor in the development of CAD. History taking in the young person suffering from acute MI will often reveal a close family member with early CAD. Despite controlling the other risk factors, the risk is definitely increased when heart disease "runs in the family." Persons with a family history of premature CAD (before age 55 years) in first degree relatives have two to five times the risk of those without this history.[18] This risk is further increased with the presence of other risk factors in the individual and in the family.

### *Pathogenesis of Coronary Artery Disease*

The lesions of coronary atherosclerosis develop progressively in much the same manner as those of atheroscle-rosis of the other major arteries (see Chap. 27). The initial change occurs early in life and consists of a fatty streak that may develop into a fibrous plaque or atheroma. This atheromatous plaque is white, becomes elevated, and partially occludes the lumen of the artery. The core of the plaque becomes necrotic, and hemorrhage and calcification may result. Thrombosis on or around the plaque may also occur, partially or completely occluding the lumen of the vessel (Figure 25-1).

Lesions do not usually cause symptoms until the atherosclerotic process is well advanced, occluding 60% or more of the vascular supply to an area. Sometimes total occlusion of a vessel does not cause ischemia to a sup-

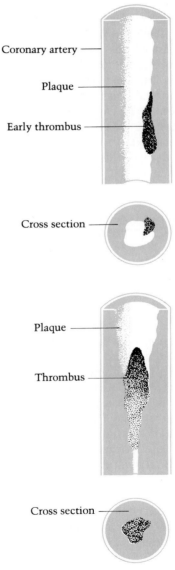

**FIGURE 25-1.**
The arterial thrombus most frequently begins at areas of luminal narrowing caused by atherosclerotic plaques. The chief components are platelets, followed by platelets and fibrin. (Source: C. Kenner, C. Guzzetta, and B. Dossey, *Critical Care Nursing: Body, Mind, Spirit.* Boston: Little, Brown, 1981.)

plied area because of the development of collateral circulation.

Atherosclerotic plaques tend to appear at bifurcations, curvatures, and tapering of arteries. The right and left main coronary arteries branch sharply off the aorta and thus become a prime target for the development of atheromas. The vessels then bifurcate and taper rapidly so that these areas also can become affected quickly.

As the coronary artery lumen narrows with increasing plaque formation, resistance to blood flow increases and myocardial muscle blood supply is compromised. As was noted in Chapter 22, normal myocardial oxygen uptake is quite efficient, taking 60% to 75% of the oxygen supplied for use by myocardial muscle. As the amount of blood flow through the vessel decreases, oxygen uptake cannot increase significantly, resulting in compromise of the oxygen supply to the tissues. When this compromise causes myocardial ischemia, angina pectoris results. Further compromise or lack of blood supply may cause necrosis of the myocardial muscle.

A considerable latent period usually exists between the onset of arterial lumen narrowing and symptomatic disease. This can be two to four decades, with symptoms beginning when the lumen is obstructed over 75%. The final event that produces infarction may be sudden and involve hemorrhage into an atherosclerotic plaque, thrombosis on an established plaque, or coronary artery spasm. Figure 25-2 shows a schematic representation of the multiple mechanisms leading to clinical CHD. Complications that can occur in atherosclerotic plaques are further described in Chapter 27.

## Angina Pectoris or Myocardial Ischemia

Myocardial ischemia is manifested by angina pectoris, which is a squeezing, substernal pain described as a feeling of tightness or fullness. The pain results from an imbalance between myocardial oxygen supply and demand. In other words, insufficient oxygen is supplied to the myocardial cell for it to function effectively.[23] This condition is almost always related to atherosclerotic narrowing of the coronary arteries. For a long time, as blood flow decreases, the myocardium avoids ischemia through autoregulation of coronary blood flow. This is probably a result of smooth muscle relaxation of the arterioles in response to release of adenosine, a powerful vasodilator of the coronary vasculature. This vasodilation decreases resistance in the coronary arteriolar bed, making the reduced supply of blood flow more easily to the myocardial muscle.[5] When this mechanism fails to meet the metabolic needs of the myocardium, ischemia results, causing pain. The pain is intermittent and often is relieved on rest or the taking of a vasodilator, such as nitroglycerin. This type of ischemia suggests that the changes are reversible and cellular function can be restored with restoration of

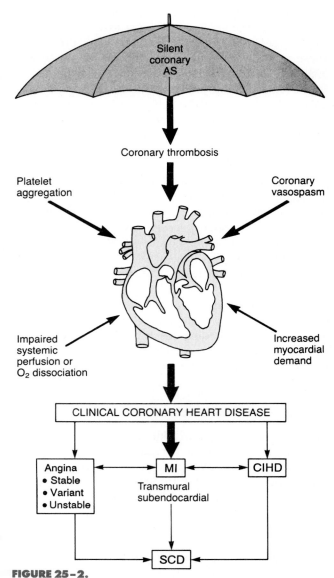

**FIGURE 25-2.**
A schematic representation of the multiple mechanisms leading to clinical coronary heart disease and the interrelationships of the various clinical patterns. CIHD = chronic ischemic heart disease; SCD = sudden cardiac death. (Source: R. Cotran, V. Kumar, S. Robbins, *Robbins Pathologic Basis of Disease*. Philadelphia: W.B. Saunders, 1989.)

oxygen to the affected muscle. Anaerobic metabolism is used to produce adenosine triphosphate during oxygen insufficiency but the resulting accumulation of lactic acid impairs left ventricular function. This results in decreased strength of cardiac contraction and impaired wall motion. The degree of impairment depends on the size of the ischemic area and the general contractility of the left ventricular myocardium. Depression of left ventricular function may lead to a temporary decrease in stroke volume and changes in systemic blood pressure.

The heart is unique in that it can be manipulated or operated on without pain; however, ischemia of cardiac muscle causes intense pain. The cause of this pain is not fully understood but ischemic myocardial muscle releases acidic substances (lactic acid) that may then stimulate the nerve endings in the muscle, conducting pain through the sympathetic nerves to the middle cervical ganglia and through the thoracic ganglia to the spinal cord. The referred nature of the pain (to the left or right arm or neck) probably has to do with interconnections in the sympathetic nerves. These nerve fibers enter the cord all the way from C3 to T5.[10] When ischemia is very severe, cardiac pain may be described as crushing and substernal. The source of pain also is not entirely understood but may be from sensory nerve endings from the heart to the pericardium that reflect pain sensation to the great vessels.[10]

The ischemic episodes causing the chest pain of angina pectoris usually subside in minutes if the imbalance is corrected. Ischemia is totally reversible, and a return to normal metabolic, functional, and hemodynamic balance occurs.

## Clinical Manifestations

The clinical features of angina pectoris are related to the pain and the persons's physiologic response to it. Anginal pain is typically described as substernal, a feeling of tightness or fullness, or oppression. It may radiate down one or both arms or into the neck and jaws.

Characteristically, the person becomes immobile and also may exhibit pallor, profuse perspiration, and dyspnea. The dyspnea may be a compensatory result of temporary cardiac failure induced by left ventricular hypokinesis (see Chap. 24). It also may result from anxiety that is produced by the onset of pain.

Classically, angina is precipitated by activity (physical or emotional stress) and is relieved within minutes by rest or the administration of a coronary vasodilator, such as nitroglycerin. During the anginal attack, typical electrocardiographic changes occur, including T wave inversion and ST segment depression (Figure 25-3). It also indicates the general cardiac area involved and, to some extent, the amount of myocardium in jeopardy (Table 25-3). Approximately 50% to 70% of persons with angina pectoris who have had no previous MI have a normal resting electrocardiogram (ECG). Changes, either symptomatic or asymptomatic, may be produced when the in-

dividual is placed on a treadmill and monitored during exercise stress. Levels of cardiac enzymes in blood drawn during or after an anginal attack are usually normal. This finding helps to differentiate angina from MI.

## Diagnostic Tests

The ECG, cardiac enzymes, and other routine tests may be performed to differentiate angina pectoris from a MI or cardiomyopathy.[1] Other tests are also used for differential diagnosis and to determine the degree of cardiac impairment. These include the exercise ECG, myocardial imaging, and cardiac catheterization with a coronary arteriogram. Establishing that the cause of chest pain is angina rather than another condition is extremely important. Major therapeutic decisions depend on the diagnosis.

## Exercise ECG or Graded Exercise Test

The exercise test with a treadmill or stationary bicycle allows for the evaluation of exercise-induced symptoms and electrocardiographic changes. Exercise-induced ST segment displacement is the only reliable electrocardiographic change of diagnostic significance in myocardial ischemia.[3] Exercise is conducted according to a controlled program so that the heart rate increases progressively, or until 85% of the individual's maximum heart rate is achieved.

Exercise testing helps to evaluate the severity of CAD. For example, a person who becomes hypotensive with marked ST abnormalities during exercise has a poorer prognosis than one who maintains a good cardiac output with no significant ST changes. Exercise testing may be used to screen apparently healthy individuals. In a study of 3000 healthy men aged 30 to 79 years, 6% exhibited a positive response to submaximal treadmill testing.[3] A 4.6 times greater risk of heart attack than in the general population is reported for persons who have abnormal results of exercise tests.[3]

## Nuclear Cardiology

Nuclear cardiology techniques detect, define, and quantify irradiation that emanates from cardiac structures to determine myocardial metabolism, perfusion, and viability.[27] The procedures are basically noninvasive and involve the injection of short-lived radionuclides.

One of the more common procedures uses thallium 201 radionuclide tracer. This substance is able to substitute for ionic potassium so it rapidly accumulates in viable myocardial cells.[27] The nuclear camera records an image of thallium distribution in the myocardium after injection of the tracer. Thallium may be injected at peak exercise or at rest. With normal myocardial perfusion, the radioisotope is distributed equally throughout the myo-

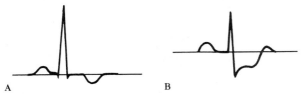

**FIGURE 25-3.**
A. Inversion of T wave; B. Depression of ST segment.

**TABLE 25–3.**

CORRELATION BETWEEN ECG LOCATION OF ISCHEMIC CHANGES AND AREA OF
MYOCARDIUM AND CORONARY ARTERY INVOLVED

| ECG LEADS REFLECTING ISCHEMIC CHANGES | AREA OF MYOCARDIUM INVOLVED | CORONARY ARTERY |
|---|---|---|
| II, III, AVF | Inferior | Right coronary artery |
| $V_1$, $V_2$ (reciprocal changes) | Posterior | Right coronary artery |
| $V_2$–$V_4$ | Anteroseptal | Left anterior descending branch of left coronary artery |
| $V_3$–$V_5$ | Anterior | Left anterior descending branch of left coronary artery |
| I, AVL | High lateral | Marginal branch of circumflex artery or diagonal branch of left coronary artery |
| $V_5$, $V_6$ | Apical | Usually left anterior descending branch of left coronary artery; may be posterior descending branch of right coronary artery |

cardium. If coronary blood flow is significantly decreased, thallium fails to localize in that segment of the myocardium. This is called a *perfusion defect* or *cold spot*, which is a negative image. Positioning of the individual is crucial in localizing defects, especially if the areas affected are small.

Multigated blood pool imaging supplies information about size, contraction pattern, and ejection fraction of the left ventricle. Exercise stress can be added to assess ventricular performance. Ergometer bicycles are often used. Some are built into exercise tables so either the supine or upright position can be used. The normal response to exercise stress is an absolute increase of at least 5% in the ejection fraction.[27]

## Coronary Arteriography

The coronary arteriogram is the most specific test for diagnosing the presence, location, and extent of coronary artery atherosclerosis. The procedure involves injecting a radiopaque substance into each coronary artery, followed by sequential radiographs of up to 12 per second. In cineangiography, dye is injected and its movement through the vessels is followed. The picture obtained usually is more detailed than that with cinematography but cinematography provides a dynamic picture. The arteriogram reveals: (1) the location of lesions, (2) the degree of obstruction, (3) the status of vessels distant to a point of obstruction, and (4) the presence of collateral circulation. The decision to perform coronary artery bypass surgery is usually made on the basis of the results of coronary arteriograms.

Stenosis is commonly graded after viewing two or three projections as follows: (1) a 50% reduction in diameter is equivalent to a 75% reduction in cross-sectional area; (2) a 75% reduction in diameter is equal to a 90% reduction in cross-sectional area; or (3) 100% reduction as total occlusion.[8] Because of differences in techniques, *cross-sectional reduction* (the measurements indicated above) is not equivalent to the *diameter method* of classification, therefore, choice of reporting is crucial in interpreting results of the test.

During coronary arteriography, contrast material can also be injected into the left ventricle. This permits visualization of left ventricular wall motion and chamber size. Pressure readings and oxygen saturations also give valuable information.

## Unstable or Preinfarctional Angina

As atherosclerotic disease progresses in the coronary arteries, symptoms of pain may become more severe and occur with increasing frequency. An impending MI is often heralded by increasing severity of anginal attacks. The ECG often shows continual signs of ischemia and injury.

## Myocardial Infarction

### Pathophysiology

Myocardial infarction, or ischemic necrosis of the myocardium, results from prolonged ischemia to the myocar-

**TABLE 25–4.**
ARTERIAL MYOCARDIAL LESION AND AREA OF INFARCTION

| CORONARY ARTERY AFFECTED | PERCENTAGE OF CASES | AREAS OF INFARCTION |
|---|---|---|
| Left anterior descending | 40–50 | Anterior left ventricle; anterior interventricular septum |
| Right coronary artery | 30–40 | Posterior wall of left ventricle; posterior interventricular septum |
| Left circumflex | 15–20 | Lateral wall of left ventricle |

*Summarized from R. S. Cotran, V. Kumar, and S. L. Robbins, Robbins' Pathologic Basis of Disease (4th ed.) Philadelphia: W.B. Saunders, 1989.*

dium with irreversible cell damage and muscle death. The time between onset of ischemia and myocardial muscle death is approximately 15 to 20 minutes, although this varies with the individual and the vessel that is occluded. Myocardial infarction almost always occurs in the left ventricle and often significantly depresses left ventricular function. The larger the infarcted area, the greater the loss of contractility. Functionally, MI causes the following: (1) reduced contractility with abnormal wall motion; (2) altered left ventricular compliance; (3) reduced stroke volume; (4) reduced ejection fraction; and (5) elevated left ventricular end-diastolic pressure (LVEDP).

Alterations in function depend not only on the size but on the location of an infarct. An anterior left ventricular infarct often results from occlusion of the left anterior descending coronary artery. Posterior left ventricular infarcts often arise from right coronary artery obstruction, while lateral wall infarcts usually arise from circumflex artery obstruction (Table 25-4). This distribution varies because of individual differences in coronary artery supply. The infarct is also described in terms of where it occurs on the myocardial surface. Figure 25-4 illustrates the commonly used terms for different types of infarcts based on their location in the ventricular wall. The *transmural infarct* extends from endocardium to epicardium. The *subendocardial* type is located on the endocardial surface, while the *subepicardial* occurs on the epicardial surface. *Intramural infarction* is often seen in patchy areas of the myocardium and is usually associated with longstanding angina pectoris. The relative frequency of different types of MIs according to arterial involvement has been documented as follows: left anterior descending artery, 40% to 50%; right coronary artery, 30% to 40%; and left circumflex artery, 15% to 20%.[2]

All acute MIs have a central area of necrosis or infarction that is surrounded by an area of injury; the area of injury is surrounded by a ring of ischemia (Figure 25-5). Each of these emits characteristic electrocardiographic patterns that help to localize and determine the extent of the infarct on the 12-lead recording.

When myocardial muscle cells die, they liberate the

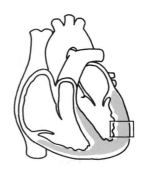

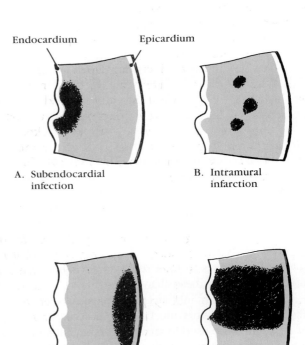

Endocardium          Epicardium

A. Subendocardial infection

B. Intramural infarction

C. Subepicardial infarction

D. Transmural infarction

**FIGURE 25–4.**
Names of various types of infarctions based on their location in the ventricular wall. (Adapted from C. Kenner, C. Guzzetta, and B. Dossey, *Critical Care Nursing: Body, Mind, and Spirit* (2nd ed.). Boston: Little, Brown, 1985.)

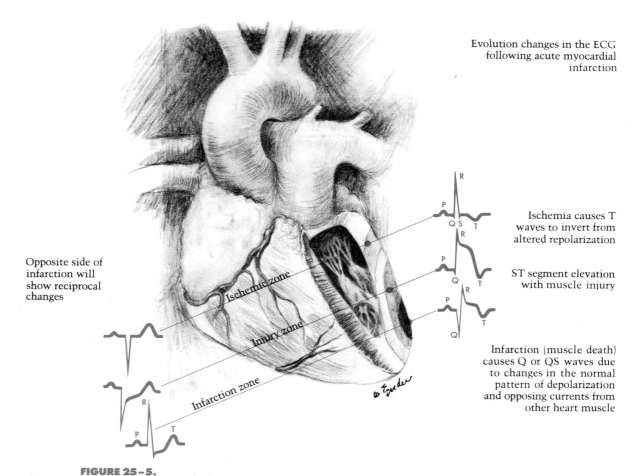

Evolution changes in the ECG
following acute myocardial
infarction

Opposite side of
infarction will
show reciprocal
changes

Ischemic zone

Injury zone

Infarction zone

Ischemia causes T
waves to invert from
altered repolarization

ST segment elevation
with muscle injury

Infarction (muscle death)
causes Q or QS waves due
to changes in the normal
pattern of depolarization
and opposing currents from
other heart muscle

**FIGURE 25–5.**
The effects of cardiac ischemia, injury, and infarction. (Source: C. Kenner, C. Guzzetta, and B. Dossey, *Critical Care Nursing: Body, Mind, Spirit* (2nd ed.). Boston: Little, Brown, 1985.)

intramyocardial cellular enzymes. These enzymes can be used to date an infarct and partially to judge its severity.[22]

Because the affected myocardial muscle is dead, tissue does not regenerate after an infarction. Healing requires the formation of scar tissue that replaces the necrotic myocardial muscle. This involves a series of morphologic changes from no apparent cellular change in the first 6 hours to total replacement by scar tissue. Table 25-5 outlines these changes.

Scar tissue may inhibit contractility. As contractility fails, the compensatory mechanisms described in Chapter 24 begin to be used in an attempt to maintain cardiac output. Arteriolar vascular constriction, heart rate increase, and renal retention of sodium and water all help to regulate cardiac output. Ventricular dilatation is commonly seen. If a large amount of scar tissue is present, contractility may be greatly compromised and congestive heart failure or cardiogenic shock may ensue.

*Right ventricular infarction* is uncommon but may occur with occlusion of the right coronary artery. The

**TABLE 25–5.**
MORPHOLOGIC CHANGES OF TRANSMURAL MYOCARDIAL INFARCTION

| TIME POSTINFARCT | MORPHOLOGIC APPEARANCE |
|---|---|
| 0–6 h | Usually inapparent |
| 6–12 h | Pallor of affected area |
| 18–24 h | Pale, gray-brown |
| 2–4 d | Necrotic focus with hyperemic border, central portion yellow-brown and soft |
| 4–10 d | Yellow-gray to bright yellow (fatty change); central necrotic area, often contains areas of hemorrhage; margins intensely red and highly vascularized |
| 10–14 d | Progressive replacement of necrotic muscle by fibrous, vascularized scar tissue |
| Up to 6 wk | Usually total replacement by scar tissue |

*Summarized from R. S. Cotran, V. Kumar, and S. L. Robbins, Robbins' Pathologic Basis of Disease (4th ed.). Philadelphia: W.B. Saunders, 1989.*

central venous pressure may be elevated markedly if acute right ventricular failure develops. Low right ventricular output causing shock often responds well to vigorous fluid therapy. Infusions raise both right and left ventricular filling pressures.[9]

The clinical manifestations of MI depend on the severity of the infarct, the previous physical condition of the individual, and whether earlier infarcts have occurred. They may reflect changes in the autonomic nervous system. The location of the infarct may affect symptoms, including magnitude and location of pain. The manifestations can range from sudden death due to dysrhythmias or ventricular rupture to no symptoms whatsoever. Acute, substernal, radiating chest pain is often described. Areas of radiation follow nerve channels described in Chapter 51. Diaphoresis, dyspnea, nausea and vomiting, extreme anxiety, and any type of dysrhythmia may be noted. Often the clinical features reveal associated complications (see p. 506–507).

Diagnosis of MI is made on physical examination as well as specific diagnostic tests. Absence of typical symptoms cause 12 to 30 percent of MIs to go unrecognized.[12] Of these atypical symptoms, respiratory difficulties are the most common. The response of most individuals is to deny the possibility that an MI is occurring.

## Diagnostic Tests

Laboratory studies are often very helpful in the diagnosis of acute MI. The complete blood count often reveals an elevated leukocyte count; the sedimentation rate and cardiac enzyme levels elevate because of cellular damage. Cardiac enzymes, normally present in myocardial muscle, are available in abnormally large amounts in the blood as a result of cellular death. These enzymes include creatinine phosphokinase, serum glutamic oxaloacetic transaminase, and lactic dehydrogenase (Figure 25-6). Their values elevate and return to normal in a characteristic pattern after a MI (Table 25-6). Because the enzymes are present in other tissues, coexisting disease can produce misleading enzyme elevations. Isoenzymes provide more specific accuracy. The isoenzyme creatinine phosphokinase-MB is usually considered diagnostic of MI, especially in the presence of increased levels of lactic dehydrogenase$_1$.

Electrocardiographic changes of acute MI consist of pronounced Q waves and ST elevation. These changes are reflected in the leads overlying the area of injury, so that the infarction can be generally localized by the ECG. In the acute phase, only ST segment and T wave changes are seen. Over 36 to 48 hours, Q wave changes develop. In the early phase, the ECG diagnosis is probable acute MI, which changes to acute MI when Q waves are added to the ST and T wave changes. Over time, the ST segment and T wave changes return to normal but the Q wave persists as evidence of an old infarction and can be used to localize the defect throughout the person's life.

Bedside techniques to measure pulmonary artery pressures and cardiac output are invaluable in evaluating left ventricular function after MI. Insertion of the pulmonary artery balloon-tipped thermodilution catheter intravenously through the right heart into the pulmonary artery allows for continuous monitoring of pulmonary artery pressures. When the balloon on the catheter is inflated, the pressure monitored is called the pulmonary artery wedge pressure (PAWP). It reflects left ventricular function. The catheter also permits periodic calculations of cardiac output. An MI that results in significant alteration of left ventricular contractility leads to increased left ventricular end-diastolic pressure (LVEDP). This is reflected as increased PAWP and decreased cardiac output (See Chap. 24).

## Myocardial Infarction Imaging

*Technetium pyrophosphate myocardial imaging* has proved to be a sensitive indicator of acute myocardial damage. After infarction, there is an efflux of calcium out of damaged cells. Technetium pyrophosphate combines with the calcium and shows up as a *hot spot*. Normally, intravenously injected technetium is not visualized in the myocardium when images are taken. This procedure is most beneficial in determining the presence of MI in the acute situation but its usefulness is limited to specific instances.[27] *Multigated blood pool scan* is another procedure that uses pyrophosphate, which has an affinity for red blood cells (RBCs). Twenty minutes after pyrophosphate is injected, technetium is injected and attaches to the pyrophosphate-tagged RBCs. The pooling or accumulation of blood in the heart allows technetium to be visualized by a special nuclear camera. The computerized camera allows many images to be taken during the cardiac cycle. The computer calculates several measurements that include end-diastolic volume, end-systolic volume, ejection fraction, and stroke volume. This pro-

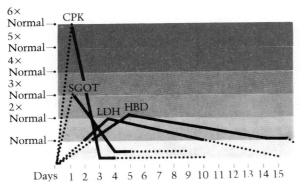

**FIGURE 25-6.**
Time sequence of serum enzyme elevations in acute myocardial infarction. (Source: C. Kenner, C. Guzzetta, and B. Dossey, *Critical Care Nursing: Body, Mind, and Spirit* (2nd ed.). Boston: Little, Brown, 1985.)

**TABLE 25–6.**
SERUM ENZYME CHANGES IN MYOCARDIAL INFARCTION

| ENZYME | ELEVATES | PEAKS | PERIOD OF ELEVATION | SITE OF FORMATION |
|---|---|---|---|---|
| **CPK** (creatinine phosphokinase) | 4–8 h | 12–36 h | 72 h | |
| Isoenzymes | | | | |
| CPK I (BB) | 0 | 0 | 0 | Produced mostly by brain |
| CPK II (MB) | 4–8 h | 12–36 h | 72 h | Produced mostly by heart |
| CPK III (MM) | 0 | 0 | 0 | Produced mostly by skeletal muscle |
| **SGOT** (serum glutamic oxaloacetic transaminase); **also called aspartate aminotransferase (AST)** | 6–12 h | 36–48 h | 4–6 d | Mostly heart, liver, muscles, erythrocytes |
| **LDH** (lactic dehydrogenase) | 12–24 h | 24–96 h | 8–14 d | Heart, liver, muscles, erythrocytes |
| Isoenzymes LDH1 | 12–24 h | 24–96 h | 8–14 d | Produced mostly by heart and erythrocytes |
| LDH2 | 0 | 0 | 0 | Produced mostly by mononuclear phagocyte system |
| LDH3 | 0 | 0 | 0 | Produced mostly by lungs and tissues |
| LDH4 | 0 | 0 | 0 | Produced by placenta, kidneys, pancreas |
| LDH5 | 0 | 0 | 0 | Produced by liver and skeletal muscle |

cedure is particularly beneficial in evaluating the effects of infarction on myocardial function.

## Complications of Myocardial Infarction

*DYSRHYTHMIAS.*    The most common complication (90%) of acute MI is a disturbance in cardiac rhythm. Myocardial infarction, itself, produces numerous predisposing factors to account for this high frequency, including: (1) tissue ischemia; (2) hypoxemia; (3) sympathetic and parasympathetic nervous system influences; (4) lactic acidosis;, (5) hemodynamic abnormalities; (6) drug toxicity; and (7) electrolyte imbalance. The basic mechanisms for cardiac rhythm abnormalities are abnormal *automaticity*, abnormal *conduction*, or both together (see Chap. 23). The most common dysrhythmias associated with MI are listed in Table 25-7. Dysrhythmias may cause a decline in cardiac output, an increase in cardiac irritability, and further compromise of myocardial perfusion. The most common cause of death outside of the hospital in individuals with MI is probably ventricular fibrillation.

*CONGESTIVE HEART FAILURE AND CARDIO-GENIC SHOCK.*    Congestive heart failure is a state of circulatory congestion produced by myocardial dysfunction. Myocardial infarction compromises myocardial function by reducing contractility and producing abnormal wall motion. As the ability of the ventricle to empty becomes less effective, stroke volume falls and residual volume increases. The fall in stroke volume elicits compensatory mechanisms to maintain cardiac output (see Chap. 24).

Cardiogenic shock results from profound left ven-

**TABLE 25–7.**
COMMON DYSRHYTHMIAS AFTER MYOCARDIAL INFARCTION

| TYPE OF DYSRHYTHMIA | EXAMPLES |
|---|---|
| Ventricular | Premature ventricular contractions (PVCs) Ventricular tachycardia Ventricular fibrillation |
| Atrial | Premature atrial contractions Atrial flutter Atrial fibrillation |
| Conduction defects | Bundle branch block, right or left Second-degree heart block Third-degree or complete heart block |
| Sinus | Sinus tachycardia Sinus bradycardia Sinus dysrhythmia |

**TABLE 25–8.**

A CLINICAL CLASSIFICATION OF HEART FAILURE AFTER ACUTE
MYOCARDIAL INFARCTION

| CLASS | DESCRIPTION | OUTCOME |
|---|---|---|
| I | No pulmonary congestion; no hypoperfusion | 1–3% mortality |
| II | Pulmonary congestion; no hypoperfusion | 9–11% mortality |
| III | Peripheral hypoperfusion without congestion | 18–23% mortality |
| IV | Both hypoperfusion and pulmonary congestion | 51–60% mortality |

*Summarized from J. E. Zimmerman and W. A. Knaus, Outcome prediction in adult intensive care, in W. C. Shoemaker et al., eds. Textbook of Critical Care. Philadelphia: W.B. Saunders, 1989.*

tricular failure, usually from a massive MI. This pump failure shock follows MI in 10% to 15% of cases; mortality is approximately 80%.[2] The Forrester classification of heart failure after acute MI is helpful in determining prognosis and treatment[28] (Table 25-8).

*THROMBOEMBOLISM.* Mural thrombi are common in postmortem examinations of individuals who die of MI. In a study of 924 fatalities due to acute MI, 44% had mural thrombi attached to the endocardium.[2] These thrombi are usually associated with large infarcts and, therefore, probably occur more frequently in nonsurvivors than survivors. Mural thrombi adhere to the endocardium overlying an infarcted area. Fragments, however, can produce systemic arterial embolization. Autopsy studies reveal that 10% of individuals who die of MI also have arterial emboli to the brain, kidneys, spleen, or mesentery.

Almost all pulmonary emboli originate in the veins of the lower extremities. Bed rest and heart failure predispose an individual to venous thrombosis and pulmonary embolism. Both occur in those with acute MI. When prolonged bed rest was standard therapy for all cases of MI, the rate of pulmonary embolus was 20%. With early mobilization and widespread use of prophylactic anticoagulation therapy, pulmonary embolus has become a rare cause of death as a complication of MI.

*PERICARDITIS.* This syndrome associated with MI was first described by Dressler and is often called Dressler's syndrome. It usually occurs after a transmural infarction but may follow subepicardial infarction. It is less common than in previous years since the discontinuation of treatment of MI with warfarin.[24] A pericardial friction rub occurs in about 10% of individuals after transmural infarction. Pericarditis is usually transient, appearing in the first week after infarction. The chest pain of acute pericarditis develops suddenly, and is severe and constant over the anterior chest. The pain worsens with inspiration and is usually associated with tachycardia, low-grade fever, and a transient, triphasic, pericardial friction rub.[24]

*MYOCARDIAL RUPTURE.* Rupture of the free wall of the left ventricle accounts for 15% to 20% of deaths in the hospital due to acute MI.[12] It causes immediate cardiac tamponade and death. Rupture of the interventricular septum is less common, occurs with extensive myocardial damage, and produces a ventricular septal defect. Rupture of the papillary muscle is an uncommon complication of MI and is more common with right coronary artery occlusions.[11] The rupture of the posteromedial papillary muscle follows infarction related to right coronary artery occulsion.

*VENTRICULAR ANEURYSM.* This event is a late complication of MI that involves thinning, ballooning, and hypokinesis of the left ventricular wall after a transmural infarction. The aneurysm often creates a paroxysmal motion of the ventricular wall with ballooning out of the aneurysmal segment on ventricular contraction. The dysfunctional area often becomes filled with necrotic debris and clot, and sometimes is rimmed by a calcium ring. The debris or clot may fragment and travel into the systemic arterial circulation.[12] Occasionally, these aneurysms rupture, causing tamponade and death, but usually the problems that result are due to declining ventricular contractility or embolization. The end result of embolization relates to sudden interruption of blood supply to any systemic artery (see Chap. 27).

## VALVULAR DISEASE

Valvular disease, such as stenosis or insufficiency, may interfere with valve functions and the flow of blood through the heart. In valvular stenosis, the valve orifice (opening) narrows and the valve leaflets (cusps) become fused together in such a way that the valve cannot open freely. This narrowing of the opening causes obstruction of blood flow. As a result, the chamber behind the affected valve must build up more pressure to overcome resistance. The muscle fibers in that chamber must thicken to do more work to push the blood through the narrowed opening. Gradually, the muscle hypertrophies in response to the added workload. With valvular insufficiency (regurgitation), the valve cannot close completely. The incomplete closure usually results from scarring and retraction of the valve leaflets. As a result, blood is permitted to flow backward (retrograde) through the opening. The heart chamber, which receives the additional retrograde flow, is then forced to pump the added regurgitant volume together with the volume being received. As a response to the increased volume present in the chamber behind the regurgitant valve, the muscle fibers lengthen or stretch. This dilatation of muscle fiber increases the surface area to accommodate the additional volume. Both hypertrophy and dilatation are compensatory mechanisms that occur in the presence of specific valvular defects.

When stenosis and regurgitation occur simultaneously, the defect is called a mixed lesion, and usually is a feature of advanced disease. In the clinical setting, the lesions are classified in terms of the predominant mechanical load that is placed on the heart. This leads to the classification of valvular defects. Stenosis can be predominant or "pure," as can regurgitation, or the lesions can be mixed. In addition to having a mixed lesion on one valve, there may be disease on another valve at the same time. This is known as combined valvular disease, which may present a rather complex clinical picture depending on the number of valves involved and the types of lesions.[25]

## Diagnostic Tests

### Chest Radiography

The chest radiograph (roentgenogram) is used to recognize abnormalities in cardiac size and to identify certain valvular lesions that cause cardiac failure. The cardiac silhouette enlarges, for instance, in the presence of aortic regurgitation (insufficiency) because of the dilatation of the chamber and hypertrophy of the muscle. Cardiac failure as a sequela of mitral stenosis, for example, can be seen on chest films as accumulation of fluid in the interlobular spaces of the lung, the result of blood damming back into the pulmonary area.

### Electrocardiography

The ECG, which records the electrical current produced by the excitable cells of the myocardium, is useful in diagnosing atrial, ventricular, or biventricular hypertrophy related to valvular disease. Chamber hypertrophy usually causes an increase in amplitude of the QRS complex, and characteristic ST and T wave changes.

The ECG can also be useful evaluating acute pericarditis (see pp. 519–521). The ST segments may be elevated or depressed in many leads; T wave inversion may or may not accompany these changes. In addition, if pericardial effusion is present, there may be low voltage in both the QRS complex and T wave in all leads.

### Echocardiography

Echocardiography uses sound waves to identify intracardiac structures based on the principle of sonic reflection.[6] When a sound wave passes through a medium such as blood, it is reflected backward (echoed), when it comes in contact with a medium of different density or elasticity, such as the muscle of the heart. Intracardiac structures have different densities, which are referred to as interfaces. In echocardiography, an ultrasound wave (beam) is transmitted from the transducer to the cardiac interfaces. These waves are reflected back to the transducer as an echo. The sonic energy is then transformed into electrical energy that can be displayed in graphic form (Figure 25-7). The recording depends on the transducer's angle and on the intracardiac structures that lie within the beam's pathway.[6]

Used as a noninvasive tool at the bedside, echocardiography is employed to assess valvular motion and pumping action of the heart, and to measure cardiac chamber size. Because it assesses valvular motion, the echocardiogram can be used to diagnose such valvular abnormalities as stenosis, regurgitation, mitral valve prolapse, and ruptured chordae tendineae. Fluid inside the pericardial membrane (pericardial effusion) can also be detected. In addition, echocardiography is useful in the assessment of abnormal thickening of the ventricular walls and septum or abnormal dilatation of the cardiac chambers.

### Cardiac Catheterization

Cardiac catheterization is an invasive diagnostic procedure that can yield important information regarding the chambers of the heart. A catheter is passed either to the right or left side of the heart; pressure and oxygen are recorded throughout the process. Left heart catheterization assesses the function of the left ventricle and aorta and the mitral and aortic valves. Right heart catheterization assesses the function of the right atrium and ventricle and the tricuspid and pulmonic valves.

In right heart catheterization, the catheter is normally inserted into the antecubital or saphenous vein and guided sequentially into the right atrium, right ventricle, pulmonary artery, and pulmonary arterial wedge position. With left heart catheterization, the catheter is inserted into the femoral or brachial artery and is advanced retrograde through the aorta into the left ventricle. Another method of insertion is the transseptal approach. This is accomplished by inserting a long, curved needle through a catheter positioned in the right atrium to puncture the intact interatrial septum. This approach is not

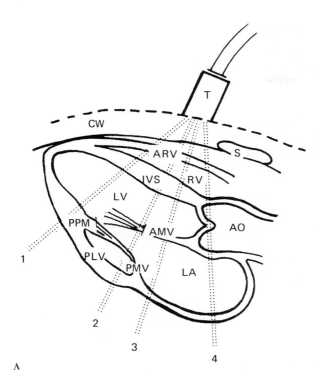

commonly used but may be employed when mitral disease is suspected.[8]

Once a catheter is in place in either the left or right heart, the chambers may be visualized by injecting a radiopaque substance (dye) through the catheter into the specific chamber under investigation. This is known as cardiac angiography. During the injection of the dye, abnormalities in valvular motion, such as stenosis or regurgitation, may be detected.

Cardiac catheterization is also useful in determining pressure differences between chambers, as in valvular stenosis in which a pressure gradient may be present. This procedure helps to assess the severity of the disease process and to determine whether surgical intervention is necessary. Quantitative measurements of volumes, pressures, ejection fraction, and cardiac output are recorded.

Because it is invasive, the procedure has inherent risks. Right heart catheterization is rarely associated with morbidity or mortality. However, left heart catheterization can produce serious complications.[8] These include cardiac perforation, major dysrhythmias, hypotension, hemorrhage, vascular thrombosis, acute MI, and cerebral embolism, as well as death.

## *Acute Rheumatic Fever: A Major Cause of Valvular Disease*

Rheumatic fever is an inflammatory disease that occurs in susceptible persons after untreated pharyngeal infection with group A beta-hemolytic *Streptococcus*. It appears to be an individual immune reaction to the streptococcal organism. The disease causes inflammation of the joints, heart, skin, and nervous system.[14] The attack rate of rheumatic fever is 1% to 3% in individuals with untreated streptococcal sore throat. Effective treatment with penicillin virtually eliminates the disease. The most common age of onset is 5 to 15 years, and frequency is greatest in areas of crowded, substandard living conditions. Recurrent attacks of rheumatic fever are common in susceptible, untreated individuals, and carry a greater risk of valvular disease with each recurrence.

### *Pathophysiology*

The joints are affected with an exudative synovitis with associated subcutaneous nodules. A characteristic acute carditis is noted with the diagnostic lesion, the *Aschoff body*, present in the myocardium. *Verrucae*, which are small, warty vegetations produced by fibrin or ground substance, appear on the valve leaflets. These apparently cause inflammation and exudation, leading to interadherence of the leaflets (Figure 25-8). These also may develop in a line on the chordae tendineae and produce scarring and shortening of these structures over a long time.

**FIGURE 25-7.**
**A.** Schematic representation of the course of the ultrasonic beam to achieve the echo represented in **B.** CW = chest wall; T = transducer; S = sternum; ARV = anterior right ventricular wall; RV = right ventricle; IVS = interventricular septum; LV = left ventricle; PPM = posterior papillary muscle; AMV = antior mitral valve leaflet; AO = aorta; PLV = posterior left ventricular wall; PMV = posterior mitral valve leaflet; LA = left atrium. B. Schematic representation of an echocardiogram from the four transducer positions. RS = right side of interventricular septum; LS = left side of interventricular septum; EN = endocardium; EP = epicardium; PER = pericardium; PLA = posterior left atrial wall; AV = aortic valve cusps. (Reprinted with permission from H. Feigenbaum, Clinical application of echocardiography. *Prog Cardiovasc Dis* 14:531, 1972, Grune and Stratton, Inc., Publishers.)

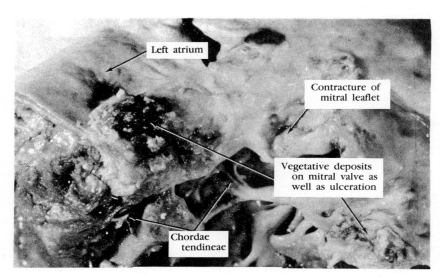

**FIGURE 25–8.**
Mitral valve viewed from above showing vegetative deposits, ulceration of valve leaflets, and fusion of commussisures. (Reprinted from J. Kernicki, B. Bullock, and J. Mathews, *Cardiovascular Nursing*. New York: G.B. Putnam, 1971.)

During the acute phase of disease, the valves and endocardial surface are inflamed and edematous. Nervous system involvement is manifested by Sydenhams' chorea, which is rapid, jerky, involuntary movements of the arms and legs, and emotional instability.[2,14] No diagnostic central nervous system lesion has been found to explain this manifestation.

### Clinical Manifestations

Onset of the disease may be acute or subacute. The acute form causes migratory polyarthritis, which refers to joint inflammation that moves from joint to joint. Subcutaneous nodules appear over the extensor surfaces of joints, such as the wrist or elbows.[14] Fever is characteristic. Tachycardia out of proportion to the level of the fever may be associated with mitral or aortic murmurs, cardiac enlargement, and congestive heart failure. Chorea is uncommon and may begin up to 3 months after the streptococcal infection.

Erythema marginatum may be noted, and is described as a pink, erythematous rash on the trunk and extremities. It often appears in concentric circles that fade and enlarge in minutes to hours. Rheumatic arteritis, pneumonitis, and pleuritis are other relatively rare manifestations of the disease.

Chronic rheumatic carditis may occur and run a fatal course over a few months. Fortunately, it is rare and cardiac involvement is subsequently expressed through valvular defects, often years after the initial disease.

Laboratory tests are not diagnostic, but the antistreptolysin O titer is increased after streptococcal infection. The erythrocyte sedimentation rate is increased, indicating an inflammatory process. Most cases of rheumatic fever abate within 12 weeks. The onset in later years of valvular dysfunction is hard to predict but treatment of later streptococcal infections, thus preventing rheumatic

fever, has led to few reported cases of valvular stenosis or regurgitation in the United States. Significant numbers of cases still are reported from the Middle East, Southeast Asia, and developing countries.

## Mitral Stenosis

Stenosis of the mitral valve causes impairment of blood flow from the left atrium to the left ventricle (Figure 25-9). The impairment is due to an abnormality in the structure of the valve leaflets that prevents the valve from opening completely in diastole. The most common cause of mitral stenosis is scarring after rheumatic endocarditis. In pure mitral stenosis (without regurgitation), about one half of patients describe a history of known rheumatic fever.[20]

### Pathophysiology and Compensatory Mechanisms

The basic alteration in mitral stenosis is decreased blood flow from the left atrium to the left ventricle. As a result of the rheumatic process, the commissures (junctional areas between the leaflets) become fibrous and fused, the chordae become shortened, and the valve becomes funnel-shaped. As the valve becomes more stenotic, the leaflets thicken with scar tissue and become calcified at the valve ring and at the leaflet margins. There are rarely any symptoms until the mitral valve orifice decreases in size from the normal 4 to 6 cm to 1.5 to 2.5 cm.[20] As the orifice further decreases in size, pulmonary symptoms appear. Mitral valve orifice (opening) size correlates relatively well with symptoms. Since the size usually decreases very gradually over years, symptoms are often first noted in the fourth or fifth decade of life.

In the normal heart, there is no functional pressure

gradient between the left atrium and left ventricle in diastole. A pressure gradient is the difference in pressure in two chambers when the valve dividing them is open. In mitral stenosis, the gradient is determined by the size of the mitral valve orifice and the flow across the valve. The flow is determined by the duration of diastole (during which filling occurs) and by cardiac output.[20] The stenotic mitral valve does not permit increases in blood flow, therefore, left atrial pressure must increase to discharge its contents into the left ventricle. Because of the constant increase in left atrial volume and pressure, the left atrium dilates and hypertrophies. As the atrium size increases, the risk for developing various atrial dysrhythmias also increases. Atrial fibrillation commonly develops, further compromising the blood flow to the ventricle because of ineffective atrial contraction. Constant increased pressure and volume in the left atrium cause an increase in pressure in the pulmonary veins and capillary bed. If the pressure in the pulmonary capillaries becomes greater than the plasma oncotic pressure, fluid passes into the interstitial spaces. Lymphatic circulation increases at least fourfold to keep the interstitial fluid drained and prevent alveolar pulmonary edema. Fluid in the alveoli is a late manifestation of mitral stenosis.

Chronic elevation of left atrial pressure causes the onset of pulmonary hypertension. Pulmonary hypertension results from chronic elevation of pulmonary capillary pressure. This excessive pulmonary pressure can rise to nearly systemic values, causing an increased pressure load against which the right ventricle must pump. Chronic pulmonary edema (congestion) in the interstitial spaces occurs, and right ventricular failure is the result (see Chap. 24). The classic manifestations of mitral stenosis include pulmonary congestion and all the signs of right heart failure.[20]

## Clinical Manifestations

Dyspnea as a result of the pulmonary congestion is the most common symptom. Dyspnea is increased by any condition that increases heart rate, such as exercise, stress, fever, or atrial fibrillation with a rapid ventricular response. Paroxysmal nocturnal dyspnea may be reported by persons with some degree of right heart failure. Fatigue is also common and is related to both pulmonary hypertension and right ventricular failure. Hemoptysis may occur as a result of pulmonary venous hypertension and, in rare cases, may be massive.[20] Palpitations may be reported, especially in the presence of atrial fibrillation. Palpation of the precordium may reveal a parasternal lift with the development of right ventricular hypertrophy.[20]

Auscultation reveals: (1) a loud first heart sound, (2) an opening snap, and (3) a diastolic rumble (Figure 25-10). The loud first heart sound is due to closure of the mitral valve apparatus when it remains deep in the left ventricle at the time of contraction. Changes in leaflet

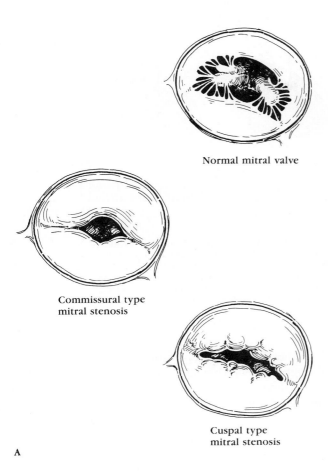

Normal mitral valve

Commissural type
mitral stenosis

Cuspal type
mitral stenosis

A

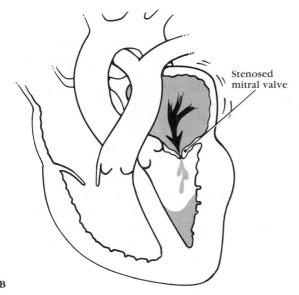

B

**FIGURE 25-9.**
**A.** The mitral valve (viewed from the atrium) demonstrating the normal valve in the closed position as well as commissural type mitral stenosis, in which fusion leads to adherence of leaflets of normal thickness and cuspal mitral stenosis caused by stiff, fibrocalcific leaflets. (Source: N.K. Wenger, W. Hurst, and M. McIntyre, *Cardiolgy for Nurses.* St. Louis: Mosby, 1980.) **B.** Mitral stenosis as viewed during atrial contraction.

Stenosed
mitral valve

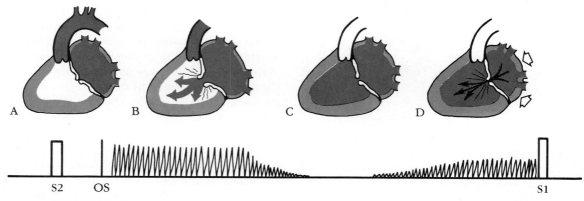

**FIGURE 25-10.**

Hemodynamic basis for the auscultatory findings of mitral stensis. **A.** Aortic valve closes second heart sound (S2) is generated. **B.** Mitral valve opens and opening snap (OS) occurs, early diastolic component is generated. **C.** Flow from left atrium to left ventricle diminishes and murmur decreases in mid-diastole. **D.** Atrial systole increases flow across mitral valve, resulting in presystolic increase in intensity of murmur. Ventricular systole then causes closure of thickened mitral valve resulting in loud first heart sound (S1) (Source: R. Judge, G. Zuidema, and F. Fitzgerald, *Clinical Diagnosis.* Boston: Little, Brown, 1982.)

mobility also contribute to the production of the loud first heart sound.[18] The opening snap heard on auscultation is thought to result from the sudden snapping of fused commissures of the valve into the ventricle. It also may be due to calcification of the valve leaflets.

The diastolic rumble of mitral stenosis is a loud, long murmur that begins just after the opening snap and has a decrescendo pattern. It results from the movement of the valve leaflets toward the closed position in mid-diastole, despite the continuing blood flow across the mitral valve produced by the pressure gradient.[20]

### Diagnostic Tests

The appearance of the cardiac silhouette in mitral stenosis on chest film is characteristic. In the posteroanterior view, the left heart border is straightened, the pulmonary artery is enlarged, and there is a double density due to left atrial enlargement. In the lateral view, the enlarged left atrium and right ventricle are seen.

The ECG characteristically shows a broad, notched P wave in lead II, called *P mitrale*. This probably reflects atrial enlargement. As many as 40% of persons with mitral stenosis develop atrial fibrillation.[20] As pulmonary hypertension develops, right ventricular hypertrophy may be noted.

Loss of posterior leaflet movement, left atrial enlargement, changes suggestive of pulmonary hypertension, and right ventricular enlargement may be seen on the echocardiogram. If mitral stenosis is complicated by the presence of mitral valve incompetence, left ventricular enlargement is also noted on the echocardiogram.[2]

Direct measurements of a gradient across the mitral valve cannot be made by conventional means but can be assessed by simultaneous measurement of the PAWP and left ventricular diastolic pressure. Correlation of the pressure gradient with cardiac output, heart rate, and diastolic filling time provides the examiner with data to calculate the mitral valve area.[25]

### Course and Complications

The uninterrupted course of mitral stenosis is long and progresses toward total disability and death. Atrial fibrillation adds an additional burden to the already compromised hemodynamics. Systemic emboli complicate the course of mitral stenosis and relate to onset of atrial fibrillation. Pulmonary hypertension is associated with permanent vascular changes and the development of right heart failure. Fatigue is a major complaint and is often associated with peripheral edema, ascites, liver enlargement, and an enlarged right ventricle.

## Mitral Regurgitation or Insufficiency

Mitral regurgitation is described as the backflow of blood from the left ventricle across the mitral valve to the left atrium during ventricular systole. Regurgitation occurs when the mitral valve fails to close completely. The most common causes of mitral regurgitation are mitral valve prolapse, CAD, and rheumatic valve disease.[20]

### Pathophysiology and Compensatory Mechanisms

The pathophysiology of mitral insufficiency depends on the underlying cause. Displacement of the leaflets of the mitral valve in mitral valve prolapse prevents closure of the valve and allows blood flow back into the left atrium (see p. 514). Rupture of the papillary muscles after MI can produce a marked mitral insufficiency. The same rheumatic processes that lead to mitral stenosis contribute to the production of mitral regurgitation. When changes on the valve leaflets and chordae cause the leaflets to stay in a closed position, stenosis results. When the changes cause the valve to stay in the open position, regurgitation results. The scarring and retraction of the mitral leaflets extend from one leaflet to another, crossing one or more commissures.

In mitral regurgitation, cardiac output is divided into regurgitant and systemic flows (Figure 25-11). The amount of regurgitant flow is determined by the degree of mitral valve incompetence and the resistance to flow through the aortic valve. Regurgitant flow increases proportionately to mitral valve orifice size. Any factor that increases resistance at the aortic valve, such as aortic stenosis, decreases systemic flow and increases regurgitant flow.

The left ventricle responds to the increased volume from the left atrium with dilatation and hypertrophy so sufficient systemic cardiac output is maintained.[18] The regurgitant volume entering the left atrium gradually increases and the left atrium gradually dilates, sometimes being termed of *aneurysmal* size to accommodate the increased volume. As a result of left atrial enlargement, the valve anulus stretches and displaces the posterior leaflet of the mitral valve, which leads to further mitral regurgitation. As mitral regurgitation progresses, contractility of the left ventricle decreases, leading to a decrease in systemic flow and onset of left ventricular failure.

### Clinical Manifestations

Many people with mitral regurgitation have no symptoms for several years but acute onset causes symptoms immediately. When symptoms do appear, dyspnea and fatigue are common. They are due to a decreased cardiac output and increased pulmonary venous pressure. Other common symptoms include orthopnea, paroxysmal nocturnal dyspnea, and palpitations.

The person with mitral regurgitation usually can better tolerate the onset of atrial fibrillation than one with mitral stenosis. Atrial fibrillation occurs in about 75% of persons with chronic mitral regurgitation.

The individual's general appearance is normal but signs of congestive heart failure may develop when the problem has been present for a long while. In chronic mitral regurgitation, the apex impulse is often displaced laterally and is larger than normal. This finding is related to left ventricular dilatation. The systolic murmur characteristic of mitral regurgitation is almost always present.[20] The murmur is loud, high pitched, holosystolic (of constant intensity throughout systole), and heard best at the apex (Figure 25-12). The murmur may radiate to the axilla or back. The first heart sound is usually diminished

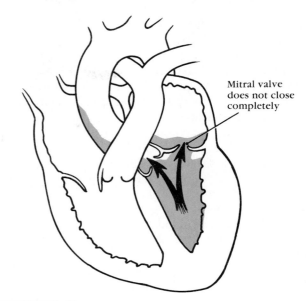

**FIGURE 25–11.**
View of mitral insufficiency during systole.

in mitral regurgitation. A third heart sound that is associated with the rapid phase of ventricular filling may also be present. If present, the third heart sound indicates some degree of cardiac decompensation.

### Diagnostic Tests

Left atrial and ventricular enlargement are frequent findings on chest films in those who have mitral regurgitation. As in mitral stenosis, the left atrium may be greatly enlarged. Pulmonary venous changes may be noted on chest films but their occurrence is less frequent than in mitral stenosis.[20]

The usual electrocardiographic findings of chronic mitral regurgitation are atrial and ventricular hypertrophy. Atrial fibrillation is common. Right ventricular hypertrophy, however, is less common in mitral regurgitation than in mitral stenosis.[20]

Cardiac catheterization provides data to describe the amount of mitral regurgitation and the pumping ability of the left ventricle. The amount of mitral regurgitation can be measured quantitatively during catheterization. The ejection fraction is measured and is useful in determining the pumping ability of the left ventricle. Cardiac output is usually decreased in symptomatic individuals.

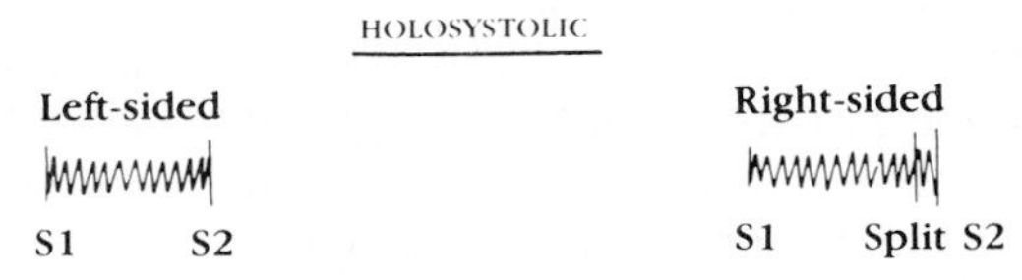

HOLOSYSTOLIC

Left-sided

S1    S2

Right-sided

S1    Split S2

**FIGURE 25–12.**
Holosystolic mitral regurgitation murmur.

## Mixed Mitral Stenosis and Regurgitation

A mitral valve that has both fused commissures and structures that fail to close properly exhibits a mixture of mitral stenosis and regurgitation. Most mixed mitral lesions are rheumatic in origin. The course of these mixed lesions depends on which one is predominant. If the degree of stenosis is greater than the degree of incompetence, there is a smaller amount of backflow of blood across the mitral valve during systole and a smaller amount of forward flow of blood across the valve in diastole. If incompetence is greater than stenosis, there is more backflow of blood across the valve in systole and more forward flow of blood across the valve in diastole.[25]

Dyspnea is the most common symptom and may be of acute onset when atrial fibrillation ensues. Palpitations are also common and are frequently related to rapid atrial dysrhythmias. The heart is usually enlarged. The first heart sound may be loud and there may be an opening snap. Often, a third heart sound is present in addition to, or instead of, the opening snap. The characteristic pansystolic murmur of mitral regurgitation and the diastolic murmurs of mitral stenosis are usually present.[25] Pulmonary congestion in mixed stenosis and regurgitation may lead to pulmonary edema, especially with the onset of atrial fibrillation.

## Mitral Valve Prolapse

Mitral valve prolapse is a common condition caused by posterior displacement of the posterior cusp of the mitral valve. It is probably a congenital abnormality of the valve tissues in which the large posterior leaflet bulges back into the left atrium during systole.[25] As the ballooning of the leaflet into the left atrium continues, the chordae and papillary muscles become stressed. Contraction of the papillary muscles decreases and mitral regurgitation occurs. The amount of this regurgitation is usually hemodynamically insignificant but may produce symptoms. More frequently, the symptoms produced are the result of an atrial dysrhythmia.

Most persons with mitral valve prolapse are completely free of symptoms. For this reason, it is commonly diagnosed during a routine physical examination. A nonanginal type of chest pain may be present with palpitations, fatigue, and dyspnea.

Mitral valve prolapse is most commonly diagnosed in women in the second to fourth decade of life.[20,21] There may be a familial tendency toward development of the condition. Auscultation at the apex reveals a late systolic murmur that is crescendo, loud, and musical. The murmur may be preceded by one or more clicks in systole.

Mitral valve prolapse is associated with extracardiac defects, including bony abnormalities such as scoliosis, pectus excavatum, pectus carinatum, and kyphosis.

A normal cardiac shadow is usually evident on radiographs. The ECG often reveals several dysrhythmias, especially sinus dysrhythmias, atrial fibrillation, premature ventricular contractions, and ventricular tachycardia. Other ECG changes include ST-T wave abnormalities and prolongation of the QT interval. The echocardiogram is useful in diagnosis and helps to determine the presence and amount of insufficiency.

Complications are rare but may include bacterial endocarditis or acute mitral insufficiency from chordae rupturing or stretching.

## Aortic Stenosis

Among the several causes of aortic stenosis are rheumatic heart disease, congenital aortic stenosis with a bicuspid or a unicuspid valve, degenerative calcific disease of the elderly, and idiopathic hypertrophic subaortic stenosis.[19] The most frequent cause in those under 30 years of age is a congenital stenotic aortic valve. Between 30 and 70 years of age, rheumatic heart disease is the usual underlying cause. However, in individuals over 70 years of age, the degenerative calcific type is predominant.

### Pathophysiology and Compensatory Mechanisms

Significant narrowing of the valve orifice leads to a decrease in blood flow from the left ventricle to the aorta. The obstruction of outflow from the left ventricle leads also to strain or pressure load on the left ventricle that occurs as the left ventricle tries to push blood through the narrowed opening (Figure 25-13). This resistance to ejection is reflected by an increase in pressure in the left ventricle to force more blood through the stenotic valve during systole.

A systolic pressure gradient develops between the left ventricle and aorta and is called an *aortic valve gradient*. These hemodynamic consequences are not manifested until the valve orifice, which is normally 2.6 to 3.5 cm², has narrowed to approximately one third of normal. The left ventricle is capable of compensating for increasing pressure demands through myocardial hypertrophy. This mechanism allows for increasing systolic pressures to maintain an adequate systemic blood pressure. The increased muscle mass requires increased oxygen supply that may or may not be supplied by the

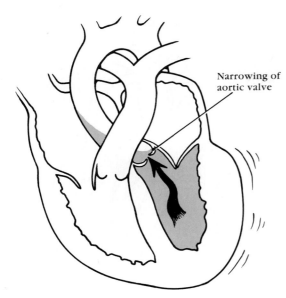

**FIGURE 25–13.**
View of aortic stenosis during systole.

coronary arteries. If the stenosis becomes increasingly severe, the persistent pressure overload (strain) leads to myocardial failure. Hypertrophy is a long-term compensatory mechanism that maintains systolic blood pressure at or slightly below normal levels.

## Clinical Manifestations

The classic clinical manifestations that accompany severe aortic stenosis are chest pain, syncope, and heart failure. Chest pain and syncope are related to reduced cardiac output, increased perfusion needs, and decreased perfusion of the coronary arteries and brain. Congestive heart failure results from the inability of the left ventricle to keep pace with the demands placed upon it. Once heart failure ensues, the course of the condition is rapidly debilitating.

Chest pain is usually manifested after physical exertion as a result of inability of the heart to increase coronary blood flow.[25] This type of angina can occur in up to 70% of persons with severe aortic stenosis.[19]

Syncopal episodes, "grey outs" or periods of confusion associated with severe aortic stenosis, are dangerous signs. Without surgical intervention, the prognosis is poor.

The chronic strain imposed on the left ventricle eventually leads to heart failure and may terminate in pulmonary edema. Left ventricular failure is the cause of death in over one half of those who have severe stenosis.

Auscultation may reveal a paradoxic splitting of the second heart sound, which is due to aortic valve closure following that of the pulmonic valve. In addition, a dia-

mond-shaped (crescendo-decrescendo) systolic ejection murmur begins after the first heart sound, increases in intensity to reach a plateau toward the middle of the ejection period, and fades progressively to end just before the aortic valve closes (Figure 25-14). An ejection click may also occur during systole as the calcified stiff valve leaflets try to open.

## Diagnostic Tests

A chest film may show apical bulging if hypertrophy is present. Calcification of the valve ring may be seen. In the presence of left ventricular failure, pulmonary vascular enlargement may be noted.

Electrocardiographic abnormalities include left ventricular hypertrophy and strain. Left ventricular hypertrophy produces changes in the amplitude of the QRS complex and ST segment displacement (strain pattern) in the precordial leads particularly.[19] Conduction system disturbances, such as heart block, may be manifested.

The echocardiogram is useful in assessing valve structure and motion, as well as in providing information regarding ventricular function. Changes in the thickness, calcification, and mobility of the aortic valve can be recorded, and ventricular wall thickness can be evaluated.

Cardiac catheterization is useful in determining the systolic gradient across the valve, as well as the valve orifice size. The gradient may be as much as 100 mm Hg which means, for example, that to attain a systemic sys-

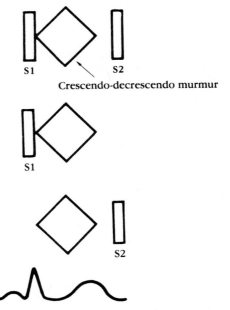

**FIGURE 25–14.**
Diagrammatic depiction of a crescendo-decrescendo murmur. Note the relationship of the sound to the ECG recording below. The examiner should concentrate on each component the S1 is followed by a sound of increasing intensity that stops just prior to S2.

tolic pressure of 100 mm Hg, the left ventricle must attain a systolic pressure of 200 mm Hg.

## Aortic Regurgitation, Insufficiency, or Incompetence

Aortic regurgitation is incomplete closure of the aortic valve. It can occur as a chronic or acute lesion. Causes of chronic lesions include rheumatic fever, syphilis, hypertension, connective tissue disorders, and atherosclerosis.[19] The acute lesion can result from a dissecting aneurysm of the aorta, infectious endocarditis, and, occasionally, rheumatic fever.

### Pathophysiology and Compensatory Mechanisms

The pathologic process in aortic regurgitation differs with each cause. For example, with rheumatic aortic insufficiency, fibrosis and unequal contracture of the leaflets lead to malalignment of the leaflets.[19] Perforation or destruction of one or more of the leaflets with infectious endocarditis may occur. In syphilitic aortic regurgitation, dilatation of the ascending aorta stretches the individual leaflets, rendering them too short to close completely during diastole. Dissecting aortic aneurysm dilates the valve ring and prevents aortic closure.[19]

The hemodynamic alterations of aortic insufficiency depend on the etiology of the process, the size of the leak, the diastolic pressure gradient across the valve, and the duration of diastole.[19] During systole, blood is ejected out of the left ventricle through the aortic valve and into the aorta but some of it flows back into the ventricle during diastole when the pressure in the aorta exceeds that in the left ventricle. Similarly, during diastole, blood flows into the ventricle from the left atrium (Figure 25-15). The left ventricle then becomes volume-overloaded by receiving blood from the left atrium through the regurgitant valve. An increase in the left ventricular end-diastolic volume results.

If the increase in end-diastolic volume in the left ventricle occurs over a long period of time (chronically), the left ventricle gradually dilates as a compensatory mechanism. In other words, the myocardial fibers stretch to increase the surface area to accommodate this extra volume. This dilatation permits the left ventricle to eject a larger stroke volume (Frank-Starling's law) to maintain the cardiac output.

Longstanding hypertrophy is associated in this case with dilatation and often results in myocardial fibrosis so that cardiac muscle cells become unable to resume their normal shape after surgical replacement of the diseased valve.[25] As a result, left ventricle failure and acute pulmonary edema may ensue.

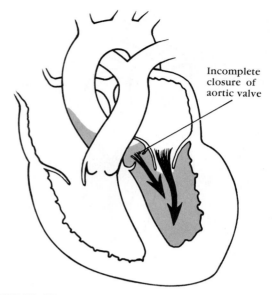

**FIGURE 25-15.**
View of aortic insufficiency during early ventricular diastole.

In *acute aortic regurgitation*, the time factor does not permit the compensatory mechanisms to develop. The volume overload in this case is so sudden that acute dilatation occurs and the left ventricle cannot maintain stroke volume and cardiac output. In acute aortic regurgitation, there is a sudden increase in the LVEDP. This is reflected to the pulmonary capillary bed, causing pulmonary edema. Death often rapidly ensues unless heroic measures are instituted.

### Clinical Manifestations

In chronic aortic insufficiency with the compensatory mechanisms functioning, symptoms may not develop for many years. Palpitations may be described, especially when the person lies on the left side. A prominent apical impulse and an observable left ventricular lift on the precordium are often noted.[19] The onset of heart failure is indicated by increasing fatigue, dyspnea, chest pain, orthopnea, paroxysmal nocturnal dyspnea, and pulmonary edema.

Auscultatory findings depend on the severity of the regurgitation. In mild regurgitation, a decrescendo diastolic murmur begins shortly after S2 and ends before S1 (Figure 25-16). With moderate regurgitation, there may be another type of murmur called an *Austin Flint murmur*, which is a diastolic rumble heard at the apex. It is caused by premature closure of the mitral valve during rapid filling of the ventricles and corresponds to the severity of aortic regurgitation.

The diastolic murmur of acute aortic regurgitation differs from those heard in chronic aortic regurgitation. The diastolic murmur can be cooing or coarsely vibrat-

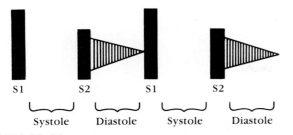

**FIGURE 25–16.**
Diastolic murmur of aortic regurgitation.

ing. The first heart sound may be diminished or absent because of the premature closure of the mitral valve.[19]

In severe regurgitation, the amplitude of the pulse increases markedly when it is palpated. This is noted as a sudden sharp pulse followed by a rapid collapse of the diastolic pulse, and is referred to as a *water-hammer* or *Corrigan's pulse.* A widening of the pulse pressure reflects inability of the aortic valve to exert its influence to maintain the aortic diastolic blood pressure.[19,25] The ECG reflects left ventricular hypertrophy, especially in the precordial leads, and the echocardiogram reflects the increased chamber dimensions that may occur in later stages.[6] Cardiac catheterization documents the severity and extent of aortic regurgitation and makes quantitative measurements of left ventricular function.

Once symptoms develop in both the acute and chronic forms, deterioration is fairly swift and, if left untreated, the severe condition eventually leads to heart failure and death.

## Mixed Aortic Stenosis and Regurgitation

When aortic stenosis and regurgitation are both present, the condition is referred to as a mixed lesion. It has been reported that the majority of individuals with aortic valve disease have mixed lesions. Either stenosis or regurgitation usually predominates over the other hemodynamically.

## INFECTIVE ENDOCARDITIS

Infective endocarditis affects the lining of the heart and is caused by an invading microorganism. The causative agents include bacteria, fungi, rickettsiae, and, rarely, viruses and parasites.[25] Infective endocarditis has been described by a variety of terms: (1) subacute bacterial endocarditis (SBE); (2) acute bacterial endocarditis (ABE); (3) prosthetic valve endocarditis; (4) native valve endocarditis; and others.[4] Subacute and acute bacterial endocarditis are included in this discussion.

The invading organism of SBE is usually of low virulence and the process can develop gradually over weeks and months.[4] The disease usually affects an already damaged heart, such as one with congenital or rheumatic heart disease. The most common causative organism is the *Streptococcus viridans*. Acute bacterial endocarditis often occurs in persons with a normal heart but can affect damaged hearts. Because the organism is of high virulence, the process usually progresses very rapidly. The most common organism is *Staphylococcus aureus*.

The organisms traveling in the bloodstream attach to the endocardial lining of a normal heart or to the area of defect of an abnormal heart. After attaching themselves, the organisms become enmeshed in deposits of fibrin and platelets, with vegetations occurring on the leaflets of the valves. These vegetations vary in size, shape, and color and may become quite friable depending on the invading organisms (Figure 25-17).[4] Acute bacterial endocarditis often produces large friable vegetations that embolize and produce embolic abscesses; SBE produces smaller vegetations that also embolize and lodge in the microcirculation and spleen. Some precipitating factors for ABE are drug abuse and cardiac surgery; SBE often results after dental work or through instrumental manipulation of the upper respiratory tract.

The clinical manifestations of infective endocarditis include fever, hematuria, splenomegaly, petechiae, Osler's nodes, and anemia. Cardiac murmurs are common. The fever and its related symptomatology are dependent on the type of infection. With acute ABE, the fever has a rapid onset with spikes to high elevations that are accompanied by shaking chills.[4] In SBE, the fever is usually low grade, intermittent with elevations, and without chills. In addition, complaints of weakness, fatigue, night sweats, anorexia, and arthralgias, and exhibition of splenomegaly are common. In both types of infective endocarditis, there may be Osler's nodes, which are painful, tender, red, subcutaneous nodules in the pads of the fingers; Janeway's lesions, which are flat, small, irregular, nontender, red spots on the palms and soles; and Roth's spots, which are retinal hemorrhages that have a white or yellow center surrounded by a red, irregular halo.[4]

The vegetations produced by the infectious process settle on the cardiac valves and invade the leaflets. These vegetations prevent normal alignment of the cusps and may, therefore, cause incomplete closure or regurgitation, leading to cardiac murmurs. The murmurs produced correspond to the affected valve. For example, with mitral insufficiency, a systolic murmur results, and with aortic insufficiency, the murmur is an early diastolic murmur.

If the vegetations grow and infiltrate the downstream side of the valve, small fragments may break off as blood is pushed through the valve orifice. These fragments, if located on the left side of the heart, may embolize to the cerebral and systemic circulations and, if on the right side, may embolize to the lungs. In addition, heart failure may ensue with severe hemodynamic alterations that occur from severe valvular regurgitation.[4]

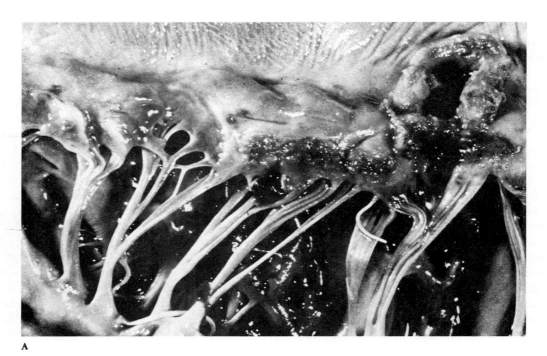

A

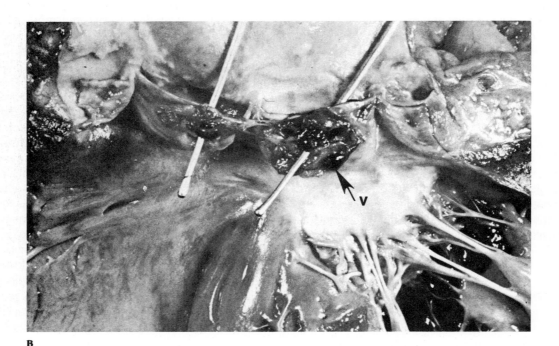

B

**FIGURE 25–17.**
Infective endocarditis. **A.** The vegetations are massive, crumbly, and hemorrhagic. Top and to the right the valve has been perforated by the infective process. **B.** The aortic valve cusps are distorted and perforated. Vegetations (V) are present on the ventricular aspect of the valve (Source: R. Cawson, A. McCracken, and P. Marcus, *Pathologic Mechanisms and Human Disease*. St Louis: Mosby, 1982.)

The diagnosis of infective endocarditis is based on positive blood cultures, which are present in the majority of cases. Also, a normocytic, normochromic anemia and an elevated sedimentation rate may be noted.

Treatment is aimed at identifying the causative microorganism followed by antibiotic therapy strong enough to penetrate the vegetation and reach the microorganism and kill it. Recovery from untreated infective endocarditis is rare and death often results.[4]

# PERICARDITIS

The pericardium is the fibrous sac surrounding the heart that protects the heart and secretes a lubricant for cardiac movement. It also prevents dilatation of the chambers of the heart during exercise and hypervolemia, and contains the heart in a fixed position. In addition, it provides a barrier to infections from the lungs and pleural cavities. Pericarditis is an inflammation of the pericardium that may be caused secondarily to many conditions including open heart surgery (the leading cause), uremia, MI, viral or bacterial infections, tumors, anticoagulants, or trauma.[24]

## Acute Pericarditis

In acute pericarditis, serous, serofibrinous, or purulent exudates form on the epicardial and pericardial surfaces.[2] The nature of the exudates depends on the underlying cause. The volume of the exudates also varies. Small volumes usually do not encroach on cardiac function but larger volumes restrict cardiac input and produce a cardiac tamponade which is described below.

Some of the clinical manifestations include pain, pericardial friction rub, electrocardiographic changes, pericardial effusion with cardiac tamponade, and a paradoxic pulse. The pain can be described as severe, sharp, and aching. It is usually precordial or substernal, and it may radiate to the left or right shoulder, arms, and elbows. On occasion, pain may spread to the jaw, throat, and ears. It may be intensified by deep breathing, sneezing, coughing, moving, or changing position. The pain may be relieved when the person sits up and leans forward. Acute pericarditis is often confused with the pain of myocardial ischemia, which may lead to misdiagnosis.[25]

In addition to pain, one of the most important physical signs of pericarditis is a friction rub that is heard best at the apex and at the lower left sternal border. It is an intermittent, transitory sound that imitates the sound of sandpaper rubbing together. This loud, "to and fro," leathery sound may disappear on one day and reappear on the next.

Acute pericarditis can produce the following changes on ECG: (1) ST elevation occurs in two or three standard limb leads and precordial leads $V_2$ through $V_6$; (2) reciprocal depressions occur in AVR and $V_1$; and (3) several days to weeks after the early stage, the ST segments return to normal and the T waves invert. Low voltage is characteristic and no Q waves develop; this helps to distinguish acute pericarditis from an acute MI.

## Pericardial Effusion, Hemopericardium, and Purulent Pericarditis

Pericardial effusion may develop in cases of acute pericarditis. This is fluid that accumulates between the pericardium and myocardium. Pericardial effusion refers to a collection of noninflammatory fluids in the pericardial sac. This fluid may be serous, serosanguineous, chylous, or, rarely, of other compositions, such as cholesterol.[2] Serous effusions are seen in congestive heart failure and hypoproteinemia, such as that due to liver failure. Serosanguineous effusions result from blunt chest trauma, especially postcardiopulmonary resuscitation. Chylous effusions contain lipid droplets, being seen especially with conditions causing lymphatic obstruction.[2] Hemopericardium refers to accumulation of blood in the pericardial sac. Purulent pericarditis with pus or inflammatory exudate is not considered to be an effusion but large volumes of bacterial, mycotic, or parasite-laden fluid can accumulate and produce a reddened, granular, inflammatory reaction.[2] If the fluid accumulates rapidly, it can cause cardiac compression. With pericardial effusion, the heart sounds are faint and apical impulse may disappear. The chest film shows enlargement of the cardiac silhouette. The heart may appear as a "water bottle" configuration (Figure 25-18). The echocardiogram detects the presence of pericardial fluid.

When fluid accumulates rapidly or in an amount large enough to impair cardiac function, the condition is referred to as cardiac tamponade. The amount of fluid that can cause tamponade varies according to the rate of fluid accumulation. In rapid accumulation of fluid, 250 mL may produce significant obstruction. When an effusion develops slowly, 1000 mL or more may accumulate before significant symptoms develop. As fluid collects in the pericardium, the pressure rises in the pericardial cavity to a level equal to the pressures in the heart during diastole. The first structures to be compressed are the right atrium and ventricle because they have the lowest diastolic pressures. This compression causes increased venous pressure with decreased right atrial filling. Jugular venous distention and systemic venous congestion with edema and hepatomegaly result. There is also a decrease in diastolic filling of the ventricles, which leads to decreases in stroke volume and cardiac output. This can be a life-threatening complication of pericarditis, and death may result from circulatory collapse.[25]

A characteristic sign of cardiac tamponade is *pulsus*

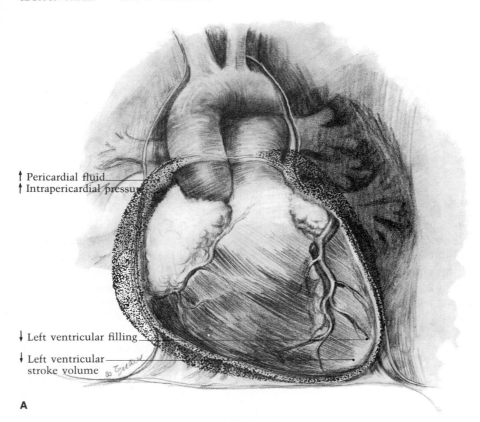

↑ Pericardial fluid
↑ Intrapericardial pressure

↓ Left ventricular filling

↓ Left ventricular
   stroke volume

**A**

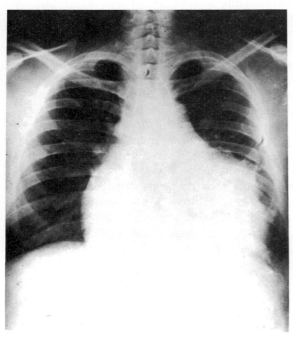

**B**

**FIGURE 25-18.**

**A.** Pericardial effusion and cardiac tamponade. The following hemodynamic effects may result after pericardial effusion: (1) accumulation of pericardial fluid resulting in intrapericardial pressure, (2) elevation of right atrial pressure, (3) elevation of left ventricular end-diastolic pressure, (4) reductions in left ventricular end-diastolic volume and cardiac output, and (5) elevated venous pressure. **B.** Chest film of an individual with a large pericardial effusion that resulted in pericardial tamponade. (Source: C. Kenner, C. Guzzetta, and B. Dossey, *Critical Care Nursing: Body, Mind, Spirit* (2nd ed.). Boston: Little, Brown, 1985.)

*paradoxus.* This is a large inspiratory reduction in arterial pressure that can be heard with a stethoscope. In pulsus paradoxus, the systolic blood pressure drops more than 10 mm Hg during inspiration. If the tamponade is severe, pulsus paradoxus may be palpated as a weakness or disappearance in the arterial pressure during inspiration.

## Chronic Constrictive Pericarditis

Chronic constrictive pericarditis results from the healing of acute pericarditis and formation of granular tissue that gradually contracts to form a firm scar surrounding the heart. This scar causes constriction of the heart and, therefore, interferes with filling of the ventricles. This complication is similar to the physiologic abnormality that results from cardiac tamponade except that it develops slowly over weeks to months.

Clinical manifestations of chronic constrictive pericarditis are weakness, fatigue, weight loss, anorexia, and edema. Individuals may complain of abdominal discomfort due to systemic venous congestion. This discomfort is due to hepatic congestion and swelling of the abdomen. A characteristic sign of constrictive pericarditis is jugular neck vein distention, which is indicative of elevated venous pressure.

The echocardiogram may show pericardial thickening and paradoxic septal motion in constrictive pericarditis. Also noted on the echocardiogram is that the left ventricular wall moves distinctly outward in early diastole, after which there is little or no change.[24] The chest film may be diagnostic when calcification appears in the pericardium.

## CONGENITAL HEART DISEASE

Congenital cardiovascular disease is an abnormality of structure or function of the heart, circulatory system, or both. The abnormalities usually result from an alteration or failure of development of a structure within the heart. The condition causes a shunting or obstructive defect, or both. A cardiovascular shunt refers to blood flow through an abnormal communication between the chambers of the heart or between the pulmonary and systemic circulations. An obstructive defect causes increased intraventricular or interatrial pressures.

The frequency of congenital cardiovascular malformations is difficult to determine because many are asymptomatic and not diagnosed in infancy. Prolapses of the bicuspid aortic and mitral valves are common asymptomatic congenital defects. It is estimated that approximately 0.8% of live births are complicated by a cardiovascular malformation.[17]

The etiology of congenital heart disease is variable and appears to result from multifactorial interactions between genetic and environmental systems. A causative factor usually cannot be identified. Some environmental insults include viral infection (especially rubella) in the first 8 weeks of pregnancy, and drug and alcohol abuse. Maternal lupus erythematosus has been implicated as a major risk factor. Hereditary factors may be involved in such conditions as atrial septal defect (ASD), patent ductus arteriosus (PDA), and coarctation of the aorta. Some lesions are more prevalent in women (ASD, PDA), and some in males (coarctation of the aorta, congenital aortic stenosis). Extracardiac anomalies occur in approximately 25% of infants with significant cardiac anomalies.[7] Preterm infants often have persistence of the ductus arteriosus, a structure that normally closes at birth. Stillborn infants have a very high frequency of complex cardiac anomalies.

## Embryology

To understand the congenital heart defects, one must understand the development of the heart. The heart develops from a straight cardiac tube, which appears in the first month of gestation. This forms a primitive atrium and ventricle, followed rapidly by a large truncus arteriosus. The tube doubles over on itself during the second month of gestation to form two parallel pumping systems, each having two chambers and a great artery (the truncus arteriosus). As a consequence of this doubling, the heart begins to situate in the left side of the chest. An *endocardial cushion* develops within the common chamber and is the first of the structures to divide the chambers of the heart. From the endocardial cushion, the mitral and tricuspid orifices develop. The large truncus divides into the aorta and pulmonary arteries. Rotation of the truncus coils the aortopulmonary septum and creates the normal spiral relationship between the aorta and pulmonary artery. The truncus arteriosus is connected to the dorsal aorta by six pairs of aortic arches that appear and disappear at different times during the formation of the heart and vessels. Abnormalities of the regression of the arch system in a number of sites can produce a wide variety of arch abnormalities. The major septa of the heart are formed between the 27th and 37th days of development.[15]

In addition to formation of heart and vessel structures, changes occur in the fetal circulation that enable the newborn to survive in the extrauterine environment. During fetal growth, the placenta performs the duties of respiration, excretion, and nourishment for the fetus. There are three essential structures: the *ductus venosus*, a vessel that connects the umbilical vein to the inferior vena cava; the *foramen ovale*, an opening in the interatrial septum; and the *ductus arteriosus*, a vessel that joins the main pulmonary artery and the distal aortic arch.

During fetal life, the blood passes from the placenta along the umbilical vein through the ductus venosus and into the inferior vena cava, where it is mixed with venous return from the lower extremities. It enters the right atrium and is mainly channeled through the foramen ovale, a one-way valve, into the left atrium where it is channeled to the rest of the body to provide oxygen and nutrients to all of the tissues. Blood flow from the head and upper extremities returns to the superior vena cava, is channeled into the right ventricle, and is pumped out the pulmonary artery. Because of the nonfunctioning, nonexpanded lungs, the resistance to blood flow into the lungs is higher and blood shunts through the ductus arteriosus into the descending aorta (Figure 25-19). Because of the resistance of the lungs, the pressures in the right ventricle and thus those in the right atrium are elevated, causing a right-to-left shunt of blood across the foramen ovale into the left atrium.

Birth changes are as follows: the infant cries and expands its lungs, the resistance in the pulmonary circulation decreases, and the pressure lowers in the right side of the heart. With dilatation of the pulmonary vessels and lowered pulmonary arterial pressure, the flow is diminished through the ductus arteriosus and it gradually closes, usually becoming a thin ligamentlike structure within 6 to 8 weeks after birth. Clamping the umbilical cord leads to clotting of blood in the umbilical vein and ductus venosus; the latter occludes within 1 to 5 days to become a ligament also. The increased systemic resistance created with clamping of the umbilical arteries is transmitted to the left atrium. This, in conjunction with increased venous return from the lungs, causes the pressure in that chamber to exceed right atrial pressure, thus tending to create a left-to-right flow through the foramen ovale. The foramen ovale acts as a one-way valve, and the tendency toward reversal of flow causes the flap of the valve to close. Closure is followed by gradual, permanent obliteration of the opening by fibrous adherence of the flap to the interatrial septum within 6 to 8 months (see also Chap. 4).

## Consequences of Congenital Heart Disease

### Left-to-Right Shunt

Because blood flows along the path of least resistance from higher to lower pressures, most congenital defects having an abnormal communication between chambers or vessels end up with a left-to-right shunt. A portion of blood returned to the left heart is diverted back into the pulmonary circuit before it can reach the systemic capil-

laries. This often causes increased volume in the right heart and subsequently, in the pulmonary circuit. Most atrial septal defects (ASDs) and ventricular septal defects (VSDs) as well as patent ductus arteriosus (PDA) result in a left-to-right shunt. The result is pulmonary overloading and eventually, pulmonary hypertension and congestion. *Pulmonary hypertension* results from increased pressures in the pulmonary vascular bed usually produced by a large left-to-right shunt. The pulmonary vasculature begins to undergo changes that eventually destroy the ability of the pulmonary arterioles to deliver blood to the pulmonary capillaries.[17] The amount of pulmonary resistance can be estimated from data obtained at cardiac catheterization. Significant pulmonary hypertension indicates permanent damage and a poor prognosis. Prevention of pulmonary overloading early in life through surgical correction or palliation must be instituted to prevent this dread complication. The systemic circulation also may become impaired if the shunt is large. The result may be right ventricular failure due to the continual volume and pressure that the right ventricle is required to pump.

### Right-to-Left Shunt

This type of shunt occurs when desaturated, systemic, venous blood is diverted to the left side of the heart without passing through the capillaries of the lungs. For this condition to occur, there must be a communication from the right heart to the left heart, and the pressures in the right heart must exceed those of the left. The common signs and symptoms include cyanosis, polycythemia, clubbing, squatting, and failure to thrive. When cyanosis is present, the shunt is large, with about one third of the arterial hemoglobin being unsaturated. Polycythemia is the normal reaction of the body to the lack of oxygen. The kidneys release erythropoietin, which stimulates the release of more RBCs. The increased numbers of RBCs increase blood viscosity. Clubbing also occurs with long-term polycythemia and cyanosis. The ends of the phalanges become bulbous and the nails curved. The cause of clubbing may be dilatation and engorgement of the local capillaries in an attempt to gain oxygen. The child may assume a squatting position, which may be a way of centralizing the available oxygen. Failure to thrive and growth retardation may be related to tissue hypoxia and poor nutrient absorption.

### Congestive Heart Failure

One child in five with any type of congenital heart defect will develop CHF.[17] It often develops early in life in the severe defects with significant shunting. In small ASDs or VSDs, congestive heart failure, if seen, develops after years of pulmonary hypertension from the left-to-right

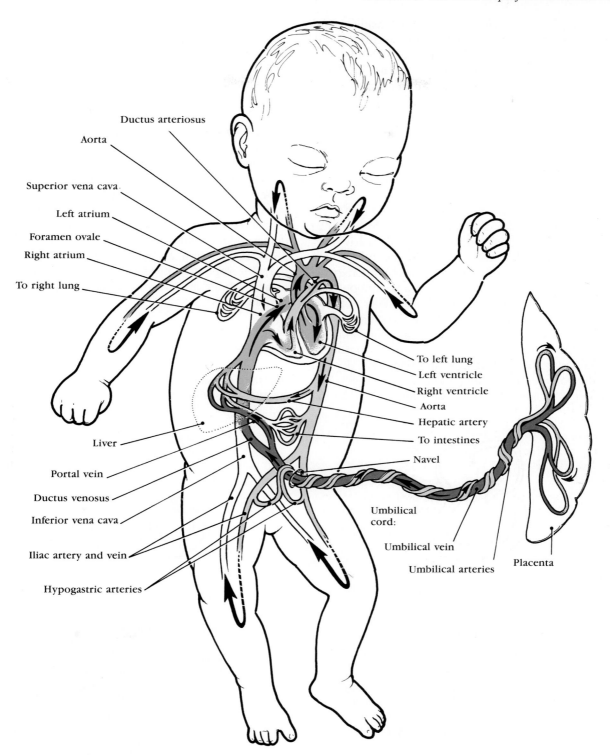

Ductus arteriosus

Aorta

Superior vena cava

Left atrium

Foramen ovale

Right atrium

To right lung

Liver

Portal vein

Ductus venosus

Inferior vena cava

Iliac artery and vein

Hypogastric arteries

To left lung

Left ventricle

Right ventricle

Aorta

Hepatic artery

To intestines

Navel

Umbilical cord:

Umbilical vein

Umbilical arteries

Placenta

**FIGURE 25–19.**
Diagrammatic illustration of fetal circulation. Arrows show the direction of blood flow.

shunt. In infants, CHF may be fulminant or insidious and may be associated with respiratory tract infections.[17] It is manifested by difficulty breathing and rapid grunting respirations.[17] Symptoms of right heart failure are less common and usually seen in association with pulmonary hypertension or cyanosis.

## *Patent Ductus Arteriosus*

When the embryonic PDA fails to close after birth, it persists as a shunt between the pulmonary artery and the aorta. It often occurs as an isolated defect and is the second most common defect in infants and children.[17] The patent ductus often does not manifest in the early postnatal days, but within about 2 weeks the blood flow through the ductus from the aorta to the pulmonary artery first produces a systolic and then a continuous machinerylike murmur, indicating a constant flow of blood through the shunt. The result of this condition is increased volume and pressure in the pulmonary system, basically short-circuiting one fourth to three fourths of left ventricular output. The signs and symptoms depend upon the volume of the shunt and often are absent. The condition is usually discovered on routine physical examination when the murmur is detected. Other symptoms include pulmonary congestion and manifestations of heart failure.

## *Atrial Septal Defects*

Congenital ASDs are very common and result from failure of the atrial septum to close. There are various forms: *ostium primum, persistent atrioventricular communis*, and *ostium secundum*. Figure 25-20 shows the embryologic development of the atrial septum. Figure 25-21 shows the location of the common types of ASDs.

Clinical manifestations depend upon the size of the defect and the volume of shunted blood. The majority of ASDs are asymptomatic but right ventricular hypertrophy, frequent respiratory infections, feeding difficulties, dyspnea, fatigability, and growth retardation may develop with larger defects.

## *Ventricular Septal Defects*

VSDs are considered to be the most common congenital heart lesions and account for 8% to 20% of congenital

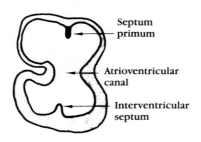

A

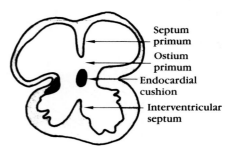

B

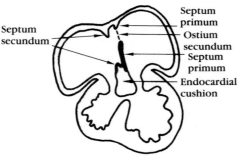

C

D

**FIGURE 25-20.**

Schematic illustration of the embryological development of the atrial septum. **A.** Septum primum beginning to divide the fetal single atrium. **B.** Development of the endocardial cushion that will form a portion of the atrioventricular valves. **C.** Two septi, the septum primum and the osteo secundum, basically divide the atria into two chambers. **D.** The septum secundum forms as an incomplete structure, the septum primum remains as a flap valve. Right to left flow of blood in fetal circulation keeps this foramen ovale open. When the flow of blood changes to a left to right shunt, the flap valve over the foramen ovale closes, anatomically dividing the chambers. (Reprinted from J. Kernicki, B. Bullock, and J. Matthews, *Cardiovascular Nursing*. New York: G.P. Putnam, 1971).

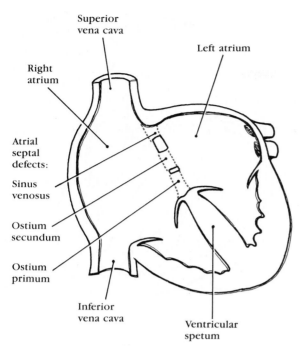

**FIGURE 25-21.**
Location of the common types of atrial septal defects.

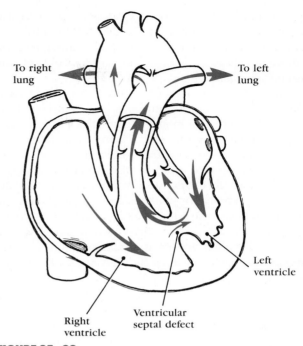

**FIGURE 25-22.**
Blood flow in a ventricular septal defect.

heart disease. The ventricular septum grows in a cephalad (headward) fashion and fuses at the endocardial cushion. It begins as a muscular septum with a membranous portion at the point of closure.[15] The shunt of blood in a VSD is almost always left-to-right from the high pressure in the left ventricle to the low pressure in the right ventricle (Figure 25-22). The shunt produces a holosystolic murmur of a high grade, often creating a palpable thrill on the chest wall. In a large shunt, there is significant overloading of the right ventricle and pulmonary circulation. In the small defect, the shunt of blood is much smaller and may be occluded during part of ventricular systole by the contraction of the muscular septum.

The clinical manifestations of VSDs depend upon the amount of pulmonary overloading and right ventricular strain. In some cases (as many as 10% to 30%), the defect apparently closes spontaneously and a preexisting murmur then disappears. Pulmonary hypertension and right ventricular failure are signs of poor prognosis without surgical intervention. The defect may progress to a cyanotic condition if the right ventricular pressures become high enough to reverse the shunt to right-to-left.

## Tetralogy of Fallot

This condition was first described by Fallot in 1888. It is the primary cause of cyanotic heart disease and is more common in males than females. It involves the combination of pulmonary stenosis, VSD, dextroposition of the

aortic root, and hypertrophy of the right ventricle (Figure 25-23). The degree of pulmonary stenosis is responsible for the volume and direction of the shunt. It increases right ventricular pressure, causing shunting of blood from the right ventricle to the left through the ven-

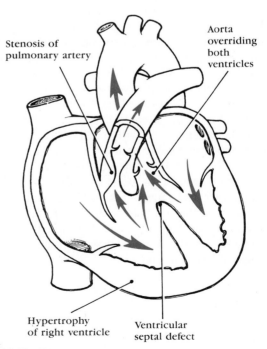

**FIGURE 25-23.**
Blood flow in tetralogy of Fallot.

tricular septal defect. Pulmonary stenosis also decreases pulmonary blood flow and the available blood for oxygenation. Direct pumping of blood to the aorta from the right ventricle causes direct access of venous blood to the systemic circulation.

Cyanosis may be severe and deepens during exertion, pulmonary infection, and dyspnea. Clubbing of the fingers also depends upon the degree of cyanosis. The oxygen saturation in the arterial system may be 80% or lower, while venous oxygen saturation may be below 60% (normal 75% to 80%). Polycythemia is compensatory and causes increased blood volume and elevated hematocrit. Cerebral anoxia may cause periods of dizziness and convulsions. Squatting is often a habitual response. Stunting of growth is characteristic when there is severe cyanosis. Complications of the condition include cerebral embolism, subacute bacterial endocarditis, and brain damage from hypoxia.

## Transposition of the Great Vessels

In the fourth week of gestation, the common truncus arteriosus is divided into the pulmonary artery and the aorta. The two vessels rotate so that the pulmonary artery lies anterior and in the right ventricle and the aorta arises posterior and in the left ventricle, thus providing for normal blood flow. In transposition, this rotation does not occur and the aorta arises anteriorly from the right ventricle and the pulmonary artery arises posteriorly from the left ventricle. Blood is pumped from the right ventricle through the aorta to the systemic system, and returns through the cavae to the right atrium. Blood from the left ventricle passes through the pulmonary artery to the lungs and returns through the pulmonary veins to the left atrium (Figure 25-24). These two closed circuits are obviously incompatible with life.

Other defects usually associated with this condition include ASDs, VSDs, and enlarged bronchial arteries to carry blood from the aorta to the lungs. In some cases, the ductus arteriosus remains patent and the foramen ovale remains open due to the increase in right atrial pressure. The clinical manifestations depend upon the amount of intermixing of blood from the associated life-sustaining defects. Cyanosis may be severe or minimal to absent; it is intensified with exertion. Dyspnea is common, and congestive heart failure frequently occurs in early infancy. Death within the first year is common without surgical intervention.

## Coarctation of the Aorta

The aortic arch develops between the fifth and seventh weeks of gestation. The area of the aorta near the ductus arteriosus may develop improperly, leaving a restricted

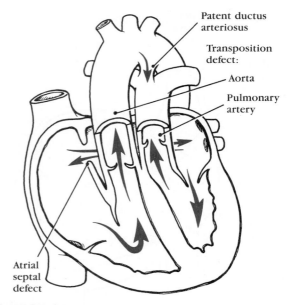

**FIGURE 25–24.**
Blood flow in transposition of the great vessels.

lumen proximal to, at, or distal to the insertion of the ductus.[15,17] Postductal coarctation obstructs blood flow beyond the left subclavian artery so the blood pressure in the upper extremities is much higher than in the lower extremities (Figure 25-25). No cyanosis is evident because the ductus closes at birth. The symptoms result from high blood pressure and decreased circulation to the lower extremities. Headaches, dizziness, epistaxis, and intermittent claudication, coolness, or pallor in the lower extremities may be noted. Preductal or ductal co-

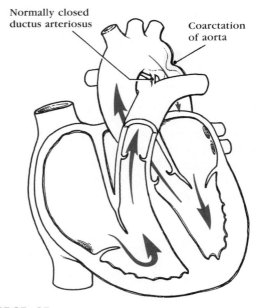

**FIGURE 25–25.**
Postductal coarctation of the aorta.

arctation usually results in persistent patency of the ductus with blood shunting from the pulmonary artery to the aorta. The result is cyanosis of the lower extremities. In either case, congestive heart failure may result, especially after 5 years of age.[17]

## Other Defects

Less common congenital heart diseases include *total anomalous pulmonary venous connection*, with the pulmonary veins connected to the right atrium; *truncus arteriosus*, in which the embryonic truncus fails to divide into the aorta and pulmonary arteries; the *endocardial cushion defect*, in which the valves and septi fail to form adequately and may result in a one-chambered heart; and numerous others. *Isolated pulmonic stenosis* is a relatively common congenital anomaly and produces symptoms when it is severe. *Bicuspid aortic valve* refers to development of the aortic valve with only two cusps. This defect is very common and usually asymptomatic. *Mitral valve prolapse*, discussed on page 514, results when the posterior leaflet of the mitral valve is abnormally large and inferiorly placed. It causes abnormal cardiac hemodynamics, which can include mitral insufficiency and various cardiac dysrhythmias. This condition is very common, especially in women, and is frequently asymptomatic.

## REFERENCES

1. Bristow, M.R., and O'Connell, J.B. Myocardial disease. In W.N. Kelley (ed.), *Textbook of Internal Medicine*. Philadelphia: J.B. Lippincott, 1989.
2. Cotran, R.S., Kumar, V., and Robbins, S.L. *Robbins' Pathologic Basis of Disease* (4th ed.). Philadelphia: W.B. Saunders, 1989.
3. DeBusk, R.F. Technique of exercise testing. In J.W. Hurst et al. (eds.), *The Heart* (7th ed.). New York: McGraw-Hill, 1990.
4. Durack, D.T. Infective and noninfective endocarditis. In J.W. Hurst et al. (eds.), *The Heart* (7th ed.). New York: McGraw-Hill, 1990.
5. Factor, S.M. Pathophysiology of myocardial ischemia. In J.W. Hurst et al. (eds.), *The Heart* (7th ed.). New York: McGraw-Hill, 1990.
6. Felner, J.M. Echocardiography. In J.W. Hurst et al. (eds.), *The Heart* (7th ed.). New York: McGraw-Hill, 1990.
7. Fink, B.W. *Congenital Heart Disease: A Deductive Approach to Its Diagnosis* (2nd ed.). Chicago: Yearbook, 1985.
8. Franch, R.H., King, S.B., and Douglas, J.S. Techniques of cardiac catheterization including coronary arteriography. In J.W. Hurst et al. (eds.), *The Heart* (7th ed.). New York: McGraw-Hill, 1990.
9. Geft, I.L., et al. ST elevation in leads $V_1$ to $V_5$ may be caused by right coronary occlusion and right ventricular infarction. *Am. J. Cardiol.* 53:991, 1984.
10. Guyton, A.C. *Textbook of Medical Physiology* (8th ed.). Philadelphia: W.B. Saunders, 1990.
11. Healy, B.P. Pathology of coronary atherosclerosis. In J.W. Hurst et al. (eds.), *The Heart* (7th ed.). New York: McGraw-Hill, 1990.
12. Hurst, J.W., et al. Atherosclerotic coronary heart disease. In J.W. Hurst et al. (eds.), *The Heart* (7th ed.). New York: McGraw-Hill, 1990.
13. Kannel, W.B., and Thorn, T.J. Incidence, prevalence, and mortality of cardiovascular diseases. In J.W. Hurst et al. (eds.), *The Heart* (7th ed.). New York: McGraw-Hill, 1990.
14. Kaplan, E.L. Acute rheumatic fever. In J.W. Hurst et al. (eds.), *The Heart* (7th ed.). New York: McGraw-Hill, 1990.
15. Langman, J. *Medical Embryology: Human Development—Normal and Abnormal* (2nd ed.). Baltimore: Williams & Wilkins, 1969.
16. Limacher, M.C., et al. Detection of coronary artery disease with exercise two-dimensional echocardiography. *Circulation* 67:1211, 1983.
17. Nugent, E.W., Plauth, W.H., Edwards, J.E., and Williams, W.H. The pathology, abnormal physiology, clinical recognition, and medical and surgical treatment of congenital heart disease. In J.W. Hurst et al. (eds.), *The Heart* (7th ed.). New York: McGraw-Hill, 1990.
18. Oberman, A. Epidemiology and prevention of cardiovascular disease. In W.N. Kelley (ed.), *Textbook of Internal Medicine*. Philadelphia: J.B. Lippincott, 1989.
19. Rackley, C.E., Edwards, J.E., Wallace, R.B., and Katz, N.M. Aortic valve disease. In J.W. Hurst et al. (eds.), *The Heart* (7th ed.). New York: McGraw-Hill, 1990.
20. Rackley, C.E., Edwards, J.E., and Karp, R.B. Mitral valve disease. In J.W. Hurst et al. (eds.), *The Heart* (7th ed.). New York: McGraw-Hill, 1990.
21. Rahimtoola, S.H. Valvular heart disease. In W.N. Kelley (ed.), *Textbook of Internal Medicine*. Philadelphia: J.B. Lippincott, 1989.
22. Roberts, R. Acute myocardial infarction. In W.N. Kelley (ed.), *Textbook of Internal Medicine*. Philadelphia: J.B. Lippincott, 1989.
23. Roberts, R. Ischemic heart disease. In W.N. Kelley (ed.), *Textbook of Internal Medicine*. Philadelphia: J.B. Lippincott, 1989.
24. Shabetai, R. Diseases of the pericardium. In J.W. Hurst et al. (eds.), *The Heart* (7th ed.). New York: McGraw-Hill, 1990.
25. Sokolow, M., and McIlroy, M.B. *Clinical Cardiology* (4th ed.). Los Altos, Calif.: Lange, 1986.
26. Wenger, N.K., and Sclant, N.C. Prevention of coronary atherosclerosis. In J.W. Hurst et al. (eds.), *The Heart* (7th ed.). New York: McGraw-Hill, 1990.
27. Zaret, B.L., and Berges, H.J. Nuclear cardiology. In J.W. Hurst et al. (eds.), *The Heart* (7th ed.). New York: McGraw-Hill, 1990.
28. Zimmerman, J.E., and Knaus, W.A. Outcome prediction in adult intensive care. In W.C. Shoemaker et al. (eds.), *Textbook of Critical Care*. Philadelphia: W.B. Saunders, 1989.

# Hypertension

## Chapter Outline

## Learning Objectives

1. Define *hypertension* as it relates to different age groups.
2. Compare the definitions of borderline, mild to moderate, labile, benign, and malignant hypertension.
3. List and briefly describe the factors that related to the cause of hypertension.
4. Describe briefly the significance of serum lipoproteins.
5. Explain how blood pressure levels are normally maintained in the arterial system.
6. Describe the abnormal renin theory in the production of essential hypertension.
7. Compare the pathophysiology of essential and secondary hypertension.
8. List the typical symptoms of hypertension.
9. Explain the four major morbid sequelae of hypertensive disease.
10. List the diagnostic tests used in hypertensive disease.

---

Hypertension is the most common disease in the United States and is a direct risk factor for and contributor to myocardial infarction, congestive heart failure, and cerebrovascular accidents.[5] The etiology of the disorder is poorly understood, treatment is lifelong, and the condition is generally asymptomatic until complications develop. The frequency of sudden death is markedly increased among hypertensive persons.

## DEFINITIONS

*Hypertension* is defined as abnormal elevation of the systolic arterial blood pressure (BP). Levels that are considered to be hypertensive vary with age. Blood pressure levels fluctuate within certain limits depending on body position, age, and stress (Table 26-1). Borderline hypertension in adults is considered to be consistent readings between 140/90 and 160/95, with readings above 160/95 definitely hypertensive.[4] Hypertension is also frequently classified as mild, moderate, or severe on the basis of the diastolic pressure. Mild hypertension has a diastolic pressure in the range of 90 to 95; moderate, 95 to 100; and severe, 110 or greater. The diagnosis is made by high readings (> 140/90) on three separate occasions after 20 minutes or more of rest.[12] Sustained hypertension occurs when the BP remains elevated over hours or days.[14] Persons who have occasional elevation of BP have labile hypertension.

The most common feature of hypertension is a mixed elevation of systolic and diastolic BPs. Occasionally, the diastolic pressure is elevated without a signifi-

**TABLE 26-1.**
HYPERTENSION AS IT RELATES TO DIFFERENT
AGE GROUPS

| AGE GROUP | NORMAL | HYPERTENSIVE |
| --- | --- | --- |
| Infants | 80/40 | 90/60 |
| Children 7–11 y | 100/160 | 120/80 |
| Teenagers 12–17 y | 115/70 | 130/80 |
| Adults | | |
| 20–45 y | 120–125/75–80 | 135/90 |
| 45–65 y | 135–140/85 | 140/90–160/95 |
| Over 65 y | 150/85 | 160/90 (borderline) |

**TABLE 26-2.**
CAUSES OF HYPERTENSION

| TYPES OF HYPERTENSION | CAUSES |
| --- | --- |
| Essential, idiopathic, or primary | Related to obesity, hypercholesterolemia, atherosclerosis, high-sodium diet, diabetes, stress, type A personality, familial history, smoking, and lack of exercise |
| Secondary | Renovascular<br>  Parenchymal disease, such as acute and chronic glomerulonephritis<br>  Narrowing, stenosis of renal artery—due to atherosclerosis or congenital fibroplasia<br>Cushing's disease or syndrome<br>  May be due to increased secretion of glucocorticoids as result of adrenal disease or pituitary dysfunction<br>Primary aldosteronism<br>  Increased aldosterone secretion, often a result of adrenal tumor<br>Pheochromocytoma<br>  Tumor of adrenal medulla causing increased secretion of adrenal catecholamines<br>Coarctation of the aorta<br>  Congenital constriction of aorta usually at the level of the ductus arteriosus with increased blood pressure above the constriction and decreased pressure below the constriction |

cant increase in systolic pressure. This indicates an increase in peripheral vascular resistance (PVR) and is most frequent in young persons. Increase in systolic pressure without diastolic elevation may occur in elderly persons, those with hyperdynamic circulation (eg, hyperthyroidism), or persons with aortic insufficiency. It is called *isolated systolic hypertension.*

Other definitive terms include *essential* (idiopathic) *hypertension,* which has no specific etiologic basis, and *secondary hypertension,* which is due to a known cause (Table 26-2). Benign and malignant hypertension refer to the course of the disease, and either may result from essential or secondary hypertension. Benign hypertension is a misnomer because it causes permanent damage, even though it has a gradual onset and begins with BP levels only slightly above normal. It is chronic with secondary effects that are not clinically evident for a long time.[11] Malignant hypertension is rapidly progressive, uncontrollable BP elevation that causes rapid onset of end organ complications, including renal failure, cerebrovascular accident, retinal hemorrhages, congestive heart failure, and encephalopathy.

## ETIOLOGY OF HYPERTENSION

### Age

There is a positive relationship between age and the frequency of hypertension with the prevalence increasing as the individual ages. As much as 50% of the population over age 50 years may be hypertensive.[3] Hypertension in those below age 35 years markedly increases the frequency of heart disease or coronary artery disease (CAD) and premature death.

### Sex

Overall, men have a higher frequency than women. However, at middle age and beyond, the prevalence begins to change, and disease in women exceeds that in men at the older ages (over age 65 years).

### Race

Blacks have at least twice the frequency of hypertension as whites.[15] The consequences of the disease are usually more severe in blacks. For example, at diastolic levels of 115 or over, mortality for black men is 3.3 times that of similarly hypertensive white men and 5.6 times that of white women.[3]

### Heredity

Genetic influences play a role in the development of hypertension. Prevalence of the disease is clustered in families. For example, if both parents have essential hypertension, prevalence in offspring is one out of two. One hypertensive parent produces a one in three frequency while normotensive parents produce a one in 20 frequency in their children.[14]

## Lifestyle

The relationship between hypertension and factors such as education, income, diet, and aspects of lifestyle have been studied with inconclusive results. Low income, low educational levels, and stressful lives or occupations seem to be related to greater frequency of hypertension. Family history of the disease has always been considered a risk factor. However, this relationship may be related more to lifestyle than to a straight genetic link, especially with respect to essential hypertension. Obesity is considered to be a major risk factor. When weight reduction is achieved, BP often returns to the normal range. Cigarette smoking is implicated as a high risk factor for both hypertension and CAD. Dietary intake of saturated fats is thought to be a major factor in the development of high serum cholesterol levels. Hypercholesteremia and hyperglycemia are both major factors in the development of atherosclerosis, which is closely associated with hypertension. The lipoproteins responsible for hypercholesteremia have been studied in terms of atherogenesis.

### Serum Lipoproteins

Five families of lipoproteins have been identified: (1) chylomicron, (2) very-low-density lipoprotein, (3) intermediate-density lipoprotein, (4) low-density lipoprotein, and (5) high-density lipoprotein.[1]

Each group performs different functions in the body. Chylomicrons transport most of the dietary substances, and very-low-density lipoproteins carry most of the triglycerides. Much of the plasma cholesterol is carried by low-density lipoproteins; high-density lipoproteins apparently serves as a reservoir for lipoproteins involved in triglyceride transport and in the esterification of cholesterol. The level of high-density lipoprotein is usually higher in women than in men and may encourage the storage of cholesterol in the liver in women.[1] High-density lipoprotein levels are often increased in athletic individuals. Figure 26-1 shows the composition of the major lipoproteins. Research continues into the role of high-density lipoprotein in protection from CAD.

## Diabetes Mellitus

The relationship between diabetes mellitus and hypertension is obscure but the statistics support a definite link between hypertension and CAD. The main cause of death in diabetes mellitus is cardiovascular disease, especially with early onset and poor control of the diabetic condition. Hypertension associated with diabetes causes increased mortality. Mortality in diabetics without hypertension is 2.47 times that of healthy subjects. That of hypertensive diabetics (BP 150/95) is 13.52 times normal. This difference in mortality declines with age. Therefore, at age 50 years, hypertensive diabetics have 2.96 times normal mortality compared to nonhypertensive diabetics, who have 2.21 times normal mortality for age.[3]

## Secondary Hypertension

As described earlier, hypertension can develop secondary to known diseases (see Table 26–2). When the causative factor is treated, the BP may return to normal.

## PATHOPHYSIOLOGY

## Blood Pressure Determinants

To understand the pathophysiology of hypertension, a review of normal arterial pressure determinants is necessary. Blood pressure is normally maintained within rather narrow limits. During sleep, however, it may fall

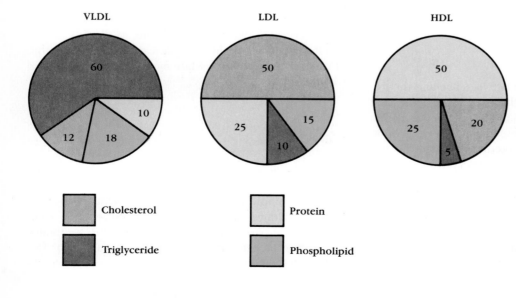

**FIGURE 26–1.**
Contents of the three major lipoproteins in percentages. VLDL = very low-density lipoproteins; LDL = low-density lipoproteins; HDL = high density lipoproteins. (Source: S. Kaufman, and S. Papper, *Review of Pathophysiology.* Boston: Little, Brown, 1983.)

to 60/40 mm Hg or less; during exercise, marked increases may be noted that often correspond to changes in heart rate and cardiac output (CO).

Total peripheral resistance (TPR) is an important factor in the regulation of arterial BP. It is the sum of all resistances offered by the vascular beds of the body. These vary with different organs but the systemic peripheral resistance has the greatest effect on the mean arterial BP. Very small changes in arteriolar diameter, also called the precapillary sphincter diameter, cause significant effects on both systemic arterial pressure and blood flow. Mean arterial pressure (MAP) can be calculated by using the following formula:[2]

$$CO \times TPR = MAP.$$

Another simple measurement may be calculated by adding the diastolic pressure and one third of the pulse pressure (which is the difference between systolic and diastolic pressures). For example, if the BP is 160/100, then $100 + 1/3(60) = 20 + 100 = 120$ (MAP). The normal MAP is from 70 to 100 mm Hg.[6]

Arterial pressure is maintained by: (1) the CO which is the main determining factor for systolic BP and is determined by the volume pumped from the heart; (2) blood volume, which is the amount of blood in the vascular tree that can be pumped; and (3) peripheral resistance, which is mainly determined by the caliber of the arterioles.[10] When they are more constricted, it takes more pressure to pump blood through them, and conversely, less pressure when they are dilated.

Aortic impedance is another factor that affects systolic and diastolic pressure. It is regulated by the aortic valve and the elasticity of the aortic wall. Each time the heart pumps, it meets some resistance from the aortic valve and the distension of the aortic wall. If the wall is stiff or thickened, it will offer more resistance to CO.[4]

Other factors have an influence on arterial pressure through affecting CO and peripheral resistance. The sympathetic nervous system (SNS) causes increased PVR and increased cardiac contractility which, in turn, increase the BP. The SNS also influences the renin-angiotensin-aldosterone (RAA) system, which causes arteriolar constriction through the release of angiotensin II and increased blood volume through the liberation of aldosterone (see below).

## *Compensatory Mechanisms for Increased Afterload*

In hypertension, there is usually an elevation of the afterload (resistance) against which the ventricle must empty. A higher afterload requires the ventricle to develop more pressure to empty its contents. Consistent increase in workload requires thicker heart muscle, so the ventricular muscle hypertrophies.[4] This hypertrophy is concentric, with enlargement occurring from the epicardium to the endocardium (Figure 26-2). The chamber size does not increase so that the heart does not appear enlarged on radiographs but the increased muscle mass may increase the weight of the heart significantly. Hypertrophy can be demonstrated ECG by increased amplitude of the R waves of the precordial leads (see Chap. 23). The increased muscle mass increases the myocardial need for oxygen and usually reduces the compliance of the ventricle. Together with a muscle mass needing more oxygen to sustain its increased workload is an acceleration of coronary atherosclerosis from the hypertensive process. This then reduces myocardial blood flow and increases the risk of cardiac ischemia and infarction.[4]

## *Essential Hypertension*

There is no real agreement as to the etiology of essential hypertension; 90% of all hypertension has no definite identifiable cause. It is known that arterioles offer abnormally increased resistance to blood flow. This increases PVR, causes a decreased capillary flow, and results in increased resistance against which the heart must pump. Numerous theories have been offered to explain hypertension, including: (1) changes in the arteriolar bed itself, causing chronically increased resistance; (2) abnormally increased tone of the SNS from the vasomotor centers causing increased PVR; (3) increased blood volume resulting from renal or hormonal dysfunction; and (4) a genetic increase in arteriolar thickening causing the abnormal PVR. It is more likely of multifactorial etiology.[5,14,15]

One theory that has been studied extensively is the abnormal renin theory. It has been demonstrated that when blood flow to the kidneys is decreased, the juxtaglomerular cells release renin (a proteolytic enzyme), which reacts with angiotensinogen (a plasma protein formed by the liver) to form angiotensin I, which is then converted to angiotensin II in the lungs. Angiotensin I elaborated in an intermediate step of the process exhibits no physiologic activity but angiotensin II is a potent vasoconstrictor. The target for angiotensin II effect is the arterioles. Circulating angiotensin II also stimulates aldosterone secretion which, in turn, increases blood volume by conserving sodium and water (Figure 26-3). Renin synthesis is increased by sodium deprivation and decreased by sodium overloading. Angiotensin II, the end product of the cascade, besides it vasoconstrictive and aldosterone effects, increases the activity of the SNS and inhibits sodium excretion.[4]

Increased serum renin levels are not present in every form of hypertension but they correlate well with some types, especially the accelerated or malignant form.[12] Renin levels are ascertained from peripheral or renal venous blood. The renin studies can help deter-

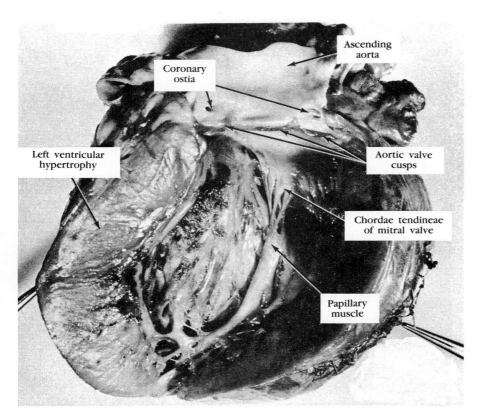

**FIGURE 26-2.**
Marked thickening of the left ventricular myocardium showing a normal aorta and medial leaflet of the mitral valve. (Reprinted from J. Kernicki, B. Bullock, and J. Matthews, *Cardiovascular Nursing.* New York, G.P. Putnam, 1971.)

Labels on figure: Ascending aorta; Coronary ostia; Aortic valve cusps; Left ventricular hypertrophy; Chordae tendineae of mitral valve; Papillary muscle

mine if a renal artery lesion is the cause of the hypertension. The renal vein blood allows more accurate sampling and the ratio of renin activity in blood samples drawn from each renal vein is determined. A renal vein renin ratio of 1.5 or greater on the stenotic side is abnormal and generally indicates a significant renal artery stenosis.[7] High-renin essential hypertension is often associated with high plasma norepinephrine levels.[16] High-renin hypertension is more common in whites than blacks and the condition may respond to beta-blocker medication as the initial therapy. Blacks usually have a lower plasma renin level and are more responsive to diuretic therapy. In conditions of accelerated malignant hypertension or hypertensive encephalopathy, there is usually an elevated plasma renin activity which may respond to a converting enzyme inhibitor such as captopril.[5,16]

## Secondary Hypertension

Secondary hypertension develops from a specific underlying cause (see Table 26–2). Approximately 5% to 10% of cases of hypertension are due to secondary causes.[10]

*Renovascular hypertension* has been studied extensively. It results from atherosclerotic or fibrous dysplastic stenosis of one or both renal arteries.[5,7] The resultant decrease in renal perfusion causes activation of the renin-angiotensin-aldosterone system. The degree of hypertension is closely related to the amount of renal ischemia produced by the obstruction. Serum renin levels are usually elevated but the amount of aldosterone secreted in relation to the amount of angiotensin II present is inappropriately increased for no known reason.[4] The result of this type of hypertension is a marked increase in PVR and CO with very high levels of systemic BP.

*Renal parenchymal disease,* such as glomerulonephritis and renal failure, often causes a renin-dependent or sodium-dependent type of hypertension. The pathophysiology varies depending on the extent of renal insufficiency and type of renal disease. Hypervolemia with normal PVR may appear, or normal or diminished circulation with a very increased PVR or both increased volume and PVR may result.[8]

*Cushing's disease* is a disease of the adrenal cortex that causes an increase in blood volume and pressure. Excess adrenocorticotropic hormone with bilateral adrenal hyperplasia accounts for about two thirds of the disease.[9]

*Primary aldosteronism* is caused by aldosterone excess from an adenoma of the adrenal gland and accounts for less than 1% of persons with hypertension.[4] High BP that results from increased production of aldosterone is a classic example of volume-related hypertension. The major criterion for the diagnosis of this condition is excess aldosterone in the presence of low plasma renin activity. Plasma renin is not a good screening test because

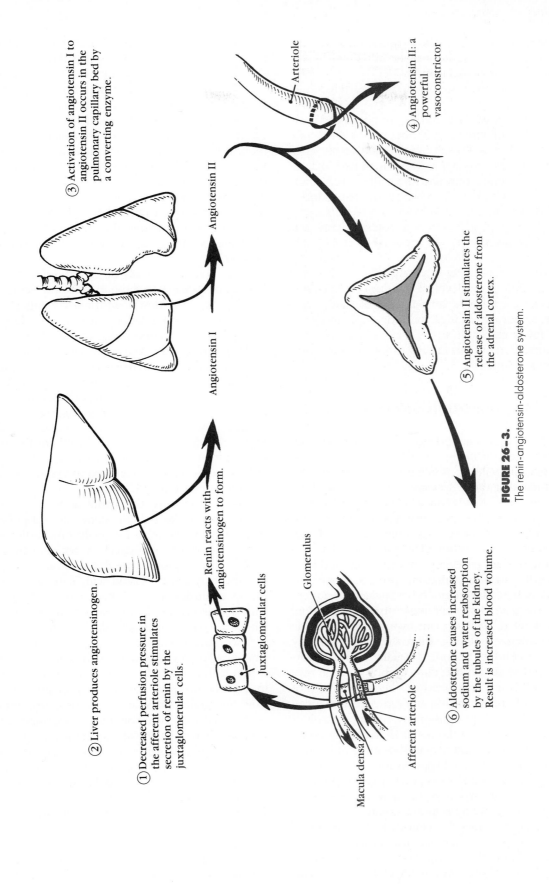

③ Activation of angiotensin I to angiotensin II occurs in the pulmonary capillary bed by a converting enzyme.

Angiotensin II

Arteriole

④ Angiotensin II: a powerful vasoconstrictor

② Liver produces angiotensinogen.

① Decreased perfusion pressure in the afferent arteriole stimulates the secretion of renin by the juxtaglomerular cells.

Angiotensin I

Renin reacts with angiotensinogen to form.

Juxtaglomerular cells

Glomerulus

Macula densa

Afferent arteriole

⑤ Angiotensin II stimulates the release of aldosterone from the adrenal cortex.

⑥ Aldosterone causes increased sodium and water reabsorption by the tubules of the kidney. Result is increased blood volume.

**FIGURE 26–3.**
The renin–angiotensin–aldosterone system.

approximately 30% of essential hypertension patients have subnormal plasma renin activity.[7] Although hyper-aldosteronism promotes salt and water retention, the ultimate mechanism that sustains the hypertension is unknown.

*Pheochromocytoma* is a secreting tumor of chromaf-fin cells, usually of the adrenal medulla. This tumor causes hypertension as a result of increased secretion of epinephrine and norepinephrine. Epinephrine mainly increases cardiac contractility and rate while norepineph-rine mainly increases PVR. The hypertension produced by a pheochromocytoma is usually severe and runs a very malignant course.[4] Surgery offers a potential cure but should be undertaken only when the BP is completely controlled.

*Coarctation of the aorta* is a congenital constriction of the aorta, often at the level of the ductus arteriosus. This produces a syndrome of markedly elevated pres-sures in the upper extremities and a decrease in perfu-sion of the lower extremities (see Chap. 25). Sometimes the PRA is increased but this finding is not consistent and PVR may not be elevated.[4]

## Clinical Manifestations of Hypertension

Hypertension is often categorized as mild or moderate; severe, accelerated, or malignant; labile; or isolated sys-tolic hypertension. Mild or moderate hypertension is of-ten asymptomatic or vague symptoms may be described. It is frequently discovered on a screening BP check. When mild or moderate hypertension is sustained, there is a great possibility of target organ damage. This is de-scribed further in this section. The presence of family history; arterial bruits, especially carotid, renal, and fem-oral; and cardiac signs or symptoms provide a basis for further studies. If a cause cannot be delineated, treatment measures are begun to prevent target organ dysfunction. Severe, accelerated, or malignant hypertension often is seen in the emergency setting where the BP is extremely high and the diastolic pressure is usually over 125 mm Hg.[7] Very rapid renal, cardiac, and cerebral damage may occur if the BP is not controlled quickly. Assessment of the status of end-organ function and rapid treatment can be lifesaving.[15] Labile hypertension is a common result of stress or other disease conditions. It is characterized by wide fluctuations in BP. Assessment should be much like that for mild or moderate hypertension, especially to make sure that there is no evidence of target organ dam-age. Isolated systolic hypertension may be associated with many disease conditions and is common in the el-derly individual. It carries the same risks for cardiovas-cular damage as mild or moderate hypertension.[7]

When symptoms do occur, hypertension is usually far advanced. The classic symptoms of headache, epi-staxis, dizziness, and tinnitus thought to be associated with high BP are no more common in hypertensive than in normotensive individuals. Unsteadiness, waking head-ache, blurred vision, depression, and nocturia have been shown to be increased in untreated hypertension.[7]

Changes in the retina (retinopathy) provide some objective clues to the clinical course of the disease. The Keith-Wagener-Barker funduscopic classification in-dicates a I rating for minimal arteriolar narrowing; II for more significant narrowing and arteriovenous nicking; III for flame-shaped hemorrhages and cotton wool exu-dates; and IV for the above changes with papilledema. Retinopathy has been shown in studies to be associated with 5-year survival rates of 85% for Group I, 50% for Group II, 13% for Group III, and 0% for Group IV.[7] Pap-illedema is always associated with malignant hyper-tension.[7,12]

The pathologic triad of hypertension was first de-scribed by Richard Brighton in 1863 and George Johnson in 1873. Brighton described the following: (1) the sym-metrically contracted kidneys with fibrotic lesions in the nephrons, and (2) concentric hypertrophy of the left ven-tricle. Johnson described arteriolar hyaline sclerosis of the systemic vessels. These have been accepted as the pathologic sequelae of hypertension, regardless of the cause. Untreated hypertension damages the small arteri-oles which, in turn, causes *target organ dysfunction*. The organs most acutely affected by vascular damage are the brain, eyes, kidneys, and heart. Problems that may result in the target organs are summarized in Table 26-3. The effects on the target organs are the result of prolonged elevation of systemic BP.

The BP remains consistently above the normal level for the age of the person. Many affected persons com-plain of angina pectoris, especially on exertion or during stressful situations. Headache is occasionally described, especially an occipital type that may be present on wak-ing and may be associated with nausea, vomiting, and mental confusion. Renal dysfunction may be the first sign with nocturia or hematuria. Symptoms of left ventricular failure are common, especially dyspnea on exertion.

Accelerated (malignant) hypertension is a state in which end organ damage from the disease occurs rapidly within a short time. It is manifested by a rapid increase in diastolic pressure (130 mm Hg or greater). This is a true emergency, causing symptoms of hypertensive en-cephalopathy: nausea, vomiting, restlessness, blurred vi-sion, and headache. Renal damage is inevitable. Left ven-tricular failure, seizures, or coma may develop. Death often ensues without immediate, appropriate treatment.

Four major morbid sequelae are associated with hy-pertensive disease: (1) stroke, (2) myocardial infarction, (3) renal failure, and (4) encephalopathy.[13]

### Stroke

Vascular lesions may cause either a hemorrhagic or ischemic stroke. The increasing pressures may cause dilatation of the small, sometimes nonelastic, and aged

**TABLE 26-3.**
HYPERTENSIVE EFFECTS ON TARGET ORGANS

| ORGAN | EFFECT | MANIFESTED BY |
|---|---|---|
| Heart | Myocardial infarction | ECG changes; enzyme elevations |
| | Congestive failure | Decreased cardiac output; S3 or summation gallop auscultated; cardiomegaly on radiograph |
| | Myocardial hypertrophy | Increased voltage R wave in $V_3$–$V_6$; increased frequency of angina; left ventricular strain, manifested by ST and T wave changes |
| | Dysrhythmias | Usually ventricular dysrhythmias or conduction defects |
| Eyes | Blurred or impaired vision | Nicking arteries and veins; hemorrhages and exudates on visual examination |
| | Encephalopathy | Papilledema |
| Brain | Cerebrovascular accident | Severe occipital headache, paralysis, speech difficulties, coma |
| | Encephalopathy | Rapid development of confusion, agitation, convulsions, death |
| Kidneys | Renal insufficiency | Nocturia, proteinuria, elevated blood urea nitrogen, creatinine |
| | Renal failure | Fluid overload, accumulation of metabolites, metabolic acidosis |

vessels. This, in turn, causes breaks in the vessel and hemorrhage into the brain parenchyma. The dilatations of the smaller intracerebral arteries are called *Charcot-Bouchard microaneurysms*. These microaneurysms may rupture and cause signs of intracerebral hemorrhage. In the process of aneurysm formation, the vessels undergo some repair, which eventually leads to thickening and tortuosity of the endothelium.

Ischemic infarcts often occur from associated atherosclerosis of the extracranial vessels (carotids and vertebrals). The thickened endothelium of the small vessels decreases or obstructs the blood flow to an area.

### *Myocardial Infarction*

Myocardial infarction may result from atherosclerosis of the coronary arteries or from the same type of hyaline sclerosis previously described in relation to arterioles of the brain. It is believed that hypertension accelerates atherosclerosis because it causes injury to the endothelium, which increases lipid accumulation and atheroma formation.[13] The associated left ventricular hypertrophy increases the risk for developing a myocardial infarction. All of these factors lead to a much increased incidence of congestive heart failure.[7,15]

### *Renal Failure*

Renal failure from primary hypertension frequently results from progressive damage to the arcuate arteries and the afferent arterioles. Progressive hyaline sclerosis leads to ischemic death of nephrons and to fibrosis, which leads to contracted kidneys. With significant loss of nephrons, renal failure ensues. This process is markedly accelerated with fibroid necrosis of the larger arteries when it is associated with malignant hypertension[8] (see Chap. 35).

### *Encephalopathy*

This ominous manifestation results from leakage of water and electrolytes from the brain capillaries into the tissues of the brain. The leakage produces cerebral edema and is often associated with papilledema (optic disk swelling). Encephalopathy is most common in malignant hypertension or when a hypertensive state assumes a malignant pattern. It may be heralded by severe headache, confusion, or lethargy followed by agitation, convulsions, or coma, and frequently death.[7]

## *DIAGNOSIS OF HYPERTENSION*

Unlike many other diseases, hypertension is usually asymptomatic and the disease may not be recognized for years unless the person seeks medical attention for another health problem or has a routine BP reading. Correct and accurate measurement of BP is the key element in making the diagnosis. Blood pressure should be measured after at least 5 to 20 minutes of rest in a quiet, familiar environment. Several positions are usually rec-ommended to attain the most accurate readings: right and left arms with the person sitting, right arm with the person supine, and right leg with the person prone. As noted in Chapter 22, arterial BP is determined by CO and resistance to blood flow. The higher pressure is the sys-tolic pressure and the lower pressure is the diastolic. An error factor of a few millimeters for both systolic and diastolic pressures is accepted because they are indirect measures.

Examination for vascular insufficiency, including pe-ripheral pulses, is essential. Evidence of cardiac involve-ment may be revealed by gallop rhythms on auscultation or displacement of the point of maximal impulse, indi-cating cardiomegaly. Changes in the vascular bed of the eyes may be noted on ophthalmic examination.

A complete health history should be taken, including family history, age at onset of hypertension, presence of risk factors, diet, symptoms of atherosclerotic disease, and symptoms relating to hypertension. Tests, including an electrocardiogram, intravenous pyelogram, blood urea, and creatinine level, provide supportive objective data. An electroencephalogram may also be indicated. All of the tests are to determine presence and extent of target organ damage.

The prognosis for uncontrolled hypertension is dis-mal. Statistics of premature death correlate with levels of BP elevation. The risk of cerebrovascular accident, for ex-ample, is five times higher for hypertensive than for nor-motensive individuals. Better case finding and proper treatment have improved the outlook for victims of sys-temic hypertension.

## REFERENCES

1.  Brown, M.S., and Goldstein, J.L. A receptor-mediated path-way for cholesterol homeostasis. *Science* 232:33, 1986.

2.  Calvin, J.E., and Sibbald, W.J. Applied cardiovascular physi-ology in the critically ill with special reference to diastole and ventricular interaction. In W.A. Schoemaker (ed.), *Textbook of Critical Care*. Philadelphia: W.B. Saunders, 1989.

3.  Cotran, R.S., Kumar, V., and Robbins, S.L. *Robbins' Patho-logic Basis of Disease* (4th ed.). Philadelphia: W.B. Saun-ders, 1989.

4.  Dustan, H.P. Systemic hypertension. In J.W. Hurst et al. (eds.), *The Heart* (7th ed.). New York: McGraw-Hill, 1990.

5.  Fishman, M.C., et al. *Medicine* (2nd ed.). Philadelphia: J.B. Lippincott, 1985.

6.  Ganong, W.F. *Review of Medical Physiology* (15th ed.). Los Altos, Calif.: Appleton & Lange, 1991.

7.  Hall, W.D., Wollam, G., and Tuttle, E. Diagnostic evaluation of the patient with hypertension. In J.W. Hurst et al. (eds.), *The Heart* (7th ed.). New York: McGraw-Hill, 1990.

8.  Kelleher, S.P., and Schrier, R.W. The kidney in hyperten-sion. In R.W. Schrier (ed.), *Renal and Electrolyte Disorders* (3rd ed.). Boston: Little, Brown, 1986.

9.  Krieger, D.T. Physiopathology of Cushing's disease. *En-docr. Rev.* 4:22, 1983.

10.  Phillips, K. Arterial hypertension. In C. Richard (ed.), *Com-prehensive Nephrology Nursing*. Boston: Little, Brown, 1986.

11.  Saul, S.H. Heart. In V.A. LiVolsi et al. (eds.), *Pathology* (2nd ed.). Media, Penn.: Harwal, 1989.

12.  Sokolow, M. Heart and great vessels. In M.A. Krupp, M.J. Chalton, and L.M. Tierney (eds.), *Current Medical Diag-nosis and Treatment 1986*. Los Altos, Calif.: Lange, 1986.

13.  Sokolow, M., and McIlroy, M.B. *Clinical Cardiology* (4th ed.). Los Altos, Calif.: Lange, 1986.

14.  Wallace, A.G., and Waugh, R.A. Hypertension. In L.H. Smith and S.O. Thier (eds.), *Pathophysiology: The Biological Prin-ciples of Disease* (2nd ed.). Philadelphia: W.B. Saunders, 1985.

15.  Weinberger, M.H. Systemic hypertension. In W.N. Kelley (ed.), *Textbook of Internal Medicine*. Philadelphia: J.B. Lip-pincott, 1989.

16.  Wollam, G., and Hall, W. Treatment of systemic hyperten-sion. In J.W. Hurst et al. (eds.), *The Heart* (7th ed.). New York: McGraw-Hill, 1990.

# Alterations in Systemic Circulation

## Learning Objectives

1. Define *atherosclerosis* and *arteriolosclerosis*.
2. Discuss the process of atheroma formation.
3. Describe the factors that make an atherosclerotic lesion complicated.
4. Describe the clinical effects of atherosclerosis in the abdominal aorta; aortoiliac, femoral, carotid, and cerebral arteries; and renal and mesenteric arteries.
5. Describe the pathologic process of atherosclerotic occlusive disease.
6. Describe the differences in the pain of intermittent claudication, rest pain, ulceration, and gangrene.
7. Describe the etiology, site, signs, and symptoms of the major types of aneurysms.
8. Discuss Raynaud's phenomenon and Raynaud's disease.
9. Explain the mechanism behind the typical color changes in Raynaud's disease.
10. Describe thromboangiitis obliterans (Buerger's disease).
11. Enumerate the signs and symptoms of arterial insufficiency to a limb.
12. List the three major predisposing factors in venous thrombosis.
13. Differentiate the types of thrombophlebitis.
14. Compare superficial and deep thrombophlebitis with respect to signs, symptoms, and complications.
15. Describe the mechanism that causes chronic venous insufficiency.
16. Describe the etiology of varicose veins.
17. List at least three contributing factors in the development of varicosities.
18. Describe the pathology of venous insufficiency.
19. Identify the skin changes that may be associated with venous insufficiency.
20. Define *lymphedema, lymphangitis,* and *lymphadenitis.*
21. Differentiate primary and secondary lymphedema.
22. Describe the following diagnostic procedures that are useful in detecting peripheral vascular disease: arteriography, Doppler ultrasound, translumbar aortography, and peripheral arteriography.

*Peripheral vascular disease* is a term that in its broadest sense applies to disease of any of the blood vessels outside of the heart and to disease of the lymph vessels. It is a general term that generally is used to describe a group of disorders that exhibit thickening and loss of elasticity of the walls of the arteries. Included in this group are atherosclerosis, arteriolosclerosis, and Monckeberg's medial calcific sclerosis. Many of the changes in the vessels are closely related to advancing age but the onset of changes is accelerated, probably by diet and other environmental factors.

## *PATHOLOGIC PROCESSES OF ARTERIES*

### *Arteritis*

*Arteritis* is a general term for inflammation of the artery. The process can be infectious or it may be due to some generalized systemic disease. Takayasu's disease causes inflammation of the aorta and upper branches, especially in Oriental women.[13] Polyarteritis nodosa is a vasculitis of the medium-sized arteries of middle-aged men. It tends to affect the branchings and bifurcations of arteries with an inflammatory process that may lead to weakening of the wall and aneurysms.[3] This condition is often thought to be a connective tissue disorder but the etiology is unknown. The symptoms vary with the location of the lesions.

### *Atherosclerosis*

Atherosclerosis is a disease of the large and medium-sized arteries that begins as a fibrofatty plaque on the intimal surface of the vessel (Figure 27-1). It usually causes no symptoms until the impeded arterial blood flow causes ischemia or infarction of the affected organ.

Many factors have been studied in the development of atherosclerosis. While not totally explanatory for every case, these factors have been correlated statistically to atherosclerotic plaque development (Table 27-1). All of the factors correlate, with many of them usually interacting to cause the pathology. Table 27-2 shows the proposed cellular mechanisms of the atherogenic risk factors. Most of the statistics regarding atherosclerosis are related to myocardial infarction mortality, so the actual frequency of extracardiac occlusive or nonocclusive atherosclerotic disease can only be surmised.

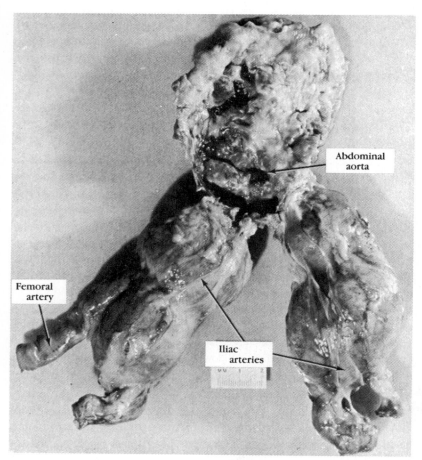

**FIGURE 27-1.**
Opened abdominal aortal showing diffuse atherosclerotic plaques with ulceration. There are aneurysms of both common iliac arteries. (Reprinted from J. Kernicki, B. Bullock, and J. Matthews, *Cardiovascular Nursing.* New York: G.P. Putnam, 1971.)

Abdominal aorta

Femoral artery

Iliac arteries

## TABLE 27-1.
### FACTORS IMPLICATED IN THE DEVELOPMENT OF ATHEROSCLEROSIS

| FACTOR | RELATIONSHIP TO DISEASE |
| --- | --- |
| Age | Increased frequency with advancing age |
| Weight | Probably related to diet; obesity correlates with increased frequency of myocardial infarction |
| Heredity | Increased frequency at early age within certain families points to familial predisposition that also may reflect dietary habits |
| Diet | Diet high in saturated fats with frequency of hyperlipidemia increases ischemic heart disease |
| Sex | Significantly increased in males until age 75 years or greater, when it approaches equality |
| Diabetes mellitus | Almost twofold increase as compared to nondiabetics; also relates to obesity |
| Cigarette smoking | Correlates with number of cigarettes smoked and decreases when smoking stops |
| Hypertension | Correlates with degree of hypertension; diastolic pressure the most important figure |
| Occupation or lifestyle | Behavior pattern (type A or B personality) inconclusive but risk appears to be twofold with type A personality |

## TABLE 27-2.
### PROPOSED CELLULAR MECHANISMS OF ATHEROGENIC RISK FACTORS

| RISK FACTOR | CELLULAR MECHANISM |
| --- | --- |
| Elevated serum cholesterol | Increases LDL, which damages endothelium<br>Increases passage of cholesterol carried by LDL, especially when HDL is low, leading to increased proliferation of smooth muscle cells |
| Hypertension | Increases endothelial permeability through increased artery wall tension, endothelial damage from angiotensin, platelet adherence with release of vasoactive agents, and hemodynamic stress |
| Cigarette smoking | Damages arterial cell membrane through circulating carbon monoxide, and platelet adherence (vasopressin)<br>Lipid mobilization (catecholamines) |

*HDL = high-density lipoprotein; LDL = low-density lipoprotein.*
*Source: C.E. Kaufman and S. Papper, Review of Pathophysiology. Boston: Little, Brown, 1983.*

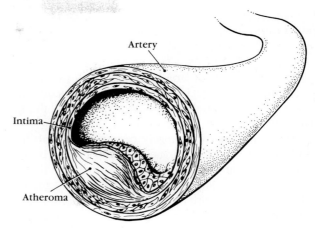

**FIGURE 27-2.**
Schematic of an atheromatous plaque. A central area of necrosis and hemorrhage into the area both impinge on the lumen of the vessels.

## Pathology

The possible precursor of the lesion of atherosclerosis is the fatty streak that often develops within the first decade of life.[1,15] This streak is composed of lipid material that is deposited on the intima of arteries. When the atherosclerotic lesion forms, it is often referred to as an atheroma or an atheromatous plaque. It is composed of fatty and fibrofatty material that is white to yellow. It protrudes into the artery and may combine with other localized atheromas to form a large mass.[10] As shown in Figure 27-2, plaques have essentially three components: (1) cells of smooth muscle, macrophages, and other leukocytes; (2) connective tissue with collagen, elastic fibers, and proteoglycans; and (3) lipid deposits both intracellularly and extracellularly.[1] The center of the plaque becomes necrotic and contains cellular debris, lipid-laden "foam cells," calcium, cholesterol crystals, and a mass of lipid material.[1] The smooth muscle cells form on the surface and make a fibrous cap. Atherosclerotic lesions differ in different areas of the body and in different individuals. Coronary artery lesions, for example, are very fibrous, and in longstanding lesions, the fibrosis may convert the atheroma to a scar.[1]

Complicated plaques are labeled this when they have become significantly calcified, ulcerated or thrombosed, undergo a hemorrhage, or cause a weakened medial wall.[1] The calcium can account for a stiff, brittle artery that does not accommodate well the dynamic flow of blood through it. Ulceration on the surface may dislodge the debris within the plaque and cause embolization to a smaller artery. Thrombosis is very common and occurs with initiation of the intrinsic clotting cascade, gradual accumulation of blood cells, and, finally, obstruction of the lumen of the vessel. Thrombi are also frequently incorporated into the plaque; the thrombosis gradually grows until the lumen is occluded and the blood supply stopped. Hemorrhage results from disruption of thin-walled capillaries that provide blood to the plaque.[1] The hematoma may occlude the lumen or be localized in the plaque. Medial atrophy accounts for the association of atherosclerosis and aneurysm formation.[1] It may be due to disruption of medial blood supply or the calcium infiltration of the endothelium and, to some extent, the medial layer.

The atheroma alone rarely causes arterial obstruction but does so when thrombosis and hemorrhage of the plaque occur (see Figure 27-2). Sometimes the atheromatous lesion causes medial weakening and aneurysmal dilatation of the artery.[10] Calcification of longstanding lesions is common and contributes to stiff, noncompliant vessels.

Because atherosclerosis can be induced in most animals by feeding them a diet high in cholesterol and because the disease process rarely occurs in humans unless the cholesterol level is greater than 160 mg per dL, hyperlipidemia can be considered as a major causative factor. The lipid in the atheroma is derived from serum lipoproteins.[10]

Even though any vessel in the body may be affected by atherosclerosis, the aorta and coronary, carotid, and iliac arteries are involved with the greatest frequency. The abdominal aorta is involved more frequently than the thoracic, and the lesions tend to locate at ostia and bifurcations.[1] A wide range of clinical effects may result from the ischemia and infarction of specific areas.[15] Table 27-3 summarizes some of the common clinical and pathologic effects.

Embolization from a thrombosed atheroma causes the characteristic signs of arterial occlusion: (1) diminished or absent pulses; (2) skin pallor, cyanosis, or both; (3) pain; and (4) muscle weakness. A large embolus may arise from a thrombosed atheroma in the descending aorta and may travel to the terminal aorta. If the embolus occludes the iliac arteries and terminal aorta, it is known as a *saddle embolus*. Its source is usually the heart, either from a subendocardial infarction or from mitral valve disease.

## Atherosclerotic Occlusive Disease of the Lower Extremity

### Pathogenesis

Gradual occlusion of an atherosclerotic terminal aorta or of other large vessels can cause symptoms and signs of ischemia to the part supplied. If the terminal aorta is affected, clinical manifestations include intermittent claudication, loss of peripheral hair, shiny skin, and impotence. Atherosclerotic occlusive disease other than coronary artery disease most commonly affects the terminal portion of the aorta and the large and medium arteries, especially those of the lower extremities. It predominantly occurs in men between ages 50 and 70 years. The prevalence and severity of this disorder are increased if the individual suffers from concomitant diabetes mellitus.

When a large artery is obstructed, the pressure in the smaller arteries distal to the obstruction decreases and blood flow declines. As the main arterial trunk progressively becomes narrowed, collateral circulation develops to maintain blood flow.

This may provide circulation to the limb for an extended time.[12] Limb-threatening arterial insufficiency may result as the lesion progresses, leading to gangrene if the cellular deprivation of oxygen is critical enough to cause cell death.[12]

### Pain

Various types of pain are described that are related to the degree of impairment of circulatory supply. Intermittent claudication is an aching, persistent, cramplike, squeez-

**TABLE 27–3.**

CLINICAL AND PATHOLOGIC EFFECTS OF ATHEROSCLEROSIS IN DIFFERENT ANATOMIC SITES

| SITE | CLINICAL AND PATHOLOGIC EFFECTS |
| --- | --- |
| Abdominal/terminal aorta | Ischemic effects in lower extremities; gangrene of toes, feet; effects of fusiform abdominal aneurysm; embolism of atherosclerotic debris to smaller arteries |
| Aortoiliac and femoral arteries | Intermittent claudication; gangrene of toes, feet; aneurysm formation in iliac arteries |
| Coronary arteries | Angina pectoris; conduction disturbances; myocardial infarction |
| Carotid and vertebral arteries | Transient ischemic attacks; cerebrovascular accident (CVA) or stroke |
| Renal artery | Hypertension; renal ischemia (hematuria, proteinuria) |
| Mesenteric arteries | Intestinal ischemia (ileus, bowel perforation with peritonitis) |

ing pain that occurs after a certain amount of exercise of the affected extremity.[4] It is relieved by rest without change of position and occurs in almost all persons at some stage of the disease. It is frequently the first symptom noticed and often begins in the arch of the foot or calf of the leg.

Rest pain is usually localized in the digits. It is described as a severe ache or a gnawing pain, often occurring at night and persisting for hours at a time. Rest pain is caused by severe ischemia of tissues and sensory nerve terminals. It may herald the onset of gangrene.[12] It is aggravated by elevation of the extremity and often relieved by dependency.

Pain of ischemic neuropathy usually occurs late in the course of progressive disease with severe ischemia. This severe pain is often associated with various types of paresthesia. It may be described as a lightening, shock-like sensation that usually occurs in both the foot and leg and follows the distribution of the peripheral sensory nerves. The pain of ulceration and gangrene is usually localized to the areas adjacent to ulcers or gangrenous tissue. It is severe, persistent, and frequently worse at night. The pain is described as an aching sensation and sometimes may be associated with sharp, severe stabs of pain.

### Coldness or Cold Sensitivity

Coldness or sensitivity to cold is a frequent symptom of occlusive disease. Complaints of coldness in the digits of the feet with exposure to a cold environment may be associated with color changes such as blanching or cyanosis.

### Impaired Arterial Pulsations

Pulsation in the posterior tibial and dorsalis pedis arteries is impaired or absent in the majority of lower-extremity occlusions. Impairment of pulsations in the popliteal and femoral arteries is less frequent.

### Color Changes

Affected extremities may be of a normal color; however, in advanced disease, cyanosis or an abnormal red color called *rubor* may be seen, particularly when the extremity is placed in a dependent position. Postural color changes are often asymmetric, and affected extremities or digits become abnormally blanched after being elevated for a few minutes. When the extremity is placed in a dependent position, a delay of 5 to 60 seconds may be required for color to return to the skin. The part first becomes abnormally red and then gradually the rubor lessens. The rubor is due to maximal dilatation of the arterioles and capillaries of the part.[7]

### Ulceration and Gangrene

These lesions may occur spontaneously on an ischemic extremity or they may result from trauma, such as pressure on the toenails from shoes. In the absence of diabetes mellitus, gangrene is rare unless there is some traumatic event.[8] Bruises, nicks, or cuts in the skin; freezing; burning; or application of strong, irritating medicines or chemicals may cause the initial injury that will not heal. It is usually confined to one extremity at a time. The lesion may be manifested by small spots on a digit or it may involve a whole extremity.

Ulcers may develop on the tips of digits, between the toes, or at the base of the flexor surface of the toes. The area around the ulcer is painful and may be swollen or exhibit redness at the margin. Secondary infections are common and lead to abscess formation, cellulitis, and spread of infection. Gangrene and ulceration related to diabetes are discussed in Chapter 39.

### Edema

Edema of the feet and legs may occur when there is severe obstruction. It is most evident when the legs are in a dependent position. The edema is not as dominant as that seen with venous occlusions (see p. 547). Associated ischemic skin lesions, capillary atony, deep venous thrombosis, and lymphangitis contribute to the edema.

### Sexual Dysfunction

Occlusive disease of the terminal aorta can decrease the blood supply to the vascular tree supplying penile circulation. The problem of inability to attain or maintain an erection is reported, especially in cases of total occlusion of the terminal aorta.[12]

### Other Changes

As a result of moderate to severe chronic ischemia, small scars, depressions, or pitting may form on the tips of the pedal digits. Nail growth is slow and nails may become thickened and deformed. They also may be paper-thin. The digits or an entire foot may appear shrunken and the muscles atrophy. Therefore, the calf or thigh may decrease in size.

### Superficial Thrombophlebitis

At some stage of the disease, superficial nonvaricose veins are involved in a type of thrombophlebitis. This occurs in approximately 40% of persons with atherosclerotic occlusive disease. The smaller veins are usually involved with lesions or are red, raised, indurated, tender, cordlike veins that measure approximately 0.5 to 3.0 cm long. The lesions usually cause permanent occlusion of the veins but the redness and symptoms of thrombophle-bitis subside, usually in 1 to 3 weeks after onset.

## Atherosclerotic Occlusive Disease of the Upper Extremity

Just as atherosclerosis is the major cause of lower extremity occlusion, it also is the main cause of brachiocephalic, carotid, and subclavian artery occlusion. Lesions tend to be located at the bifurcations of the arch vessels and the common carotid arteries.[8] The proximal left subclavian artery is the most frequently affected, excluding the common carotid artery occlusions which are described in Chapter 50. Upper extremity ischemia is very uncommon due, in part, to the *subclavian steal*. This phenomenon refers to cerebral ischemia that results from a flow off of blood from the circle of Willis back through the affected side vertebral artery to the ischemic arm. The steal is invariably produced by exercising the arm and diversion of cerebral flow retrograde to the arm.[8] The syndrome usually presents with the typical picture of transient ischemic attacks or other central nervous system dysfunction. Diagnostic studies, especially using Doppler techniques, will demonstrate obstruction to blood flow.

## Aortic Aneurysms

An aneurysm is a localized dilation of the wall of an artery. It develops at a site of weakness of the medial layer of the artery. The majority of aneurysms are atherosclerotic but they may result from congenital defects, infections such as syphilis, and trauma.

Fusiform aneurysms produce circumferential dilatation of the vessel. The wall balloons out on all sides (Figure 27-3). As the process is occurring, the aneurysmal sac

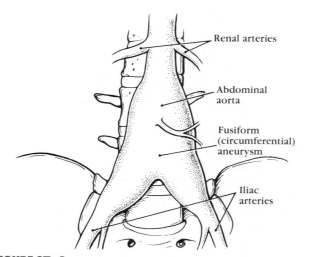

**FIGURE 27-3.**
Fusiform aneurysm of the aorta.

fills with necrotic debris and thrombus. Calcium infiltrates the area. The sac dilates because of a weakened medial layer. The dangers of this type of aneurysm include rupture, embolization to a peripheral artery, pressure on surrounding structures, and obstruction of blood flow to organs supplied by the tributary arteries.

### Abdominal Aortic Aneurysms

Almost all abdominal aortic aneurysms are atherosclerotic and most arise at a level below the branchings of the renal arteries. They often extend to and include the iliac arteries (see Figure 27-3).[8] Clinical manifestations are usually nonexistent. Occasionally, the person discovers a pulsatile abdominal mass. More frequently, the aneurysm is discovered when a physical examination is performed for some other reason, such as vague abdominal symptoms or poor peripheral circulation. Pain of recent onset may herald an expanding aneurysm with impending rupture.[8]

Rupture may cause the initial symptoms with bleeding frequently occurring into the retroperitoneal space. In such instances, exsanguination is generally prevented due to the location of the hemorrhage. The initial symptoms of this type of hemorrhage include abdominal pain and symptoms of hemorrhagic shock. Pressure from a large or enlarging abdominal aortic aneurysms on surrounding abdominal organs, together with lack of blood supply to the intestines, can precipitate ileus or intestinal obstruction.

Physical examination reveals a pulsatile abdominal mass. This is almost a diagnostic finding. Due to intra-aneurysmal clot, the size of the aneurysm may not be appreciated on angiographic studies.[8]

### Thoracic Aneurysms

Thoracic aortic aneurysms may be caused by atherosclerosis, necrosis of the medial arterial layer, and syphilis. Atherosclerotic aneurysms are usually fusiform and may be located in the ascending, arch, or descending segments (Figure 27-4). Aneurysms that result from medial necrosis and syphilis are discussed in the following sections.

Most thoracic aneurysms are asymptomatic and are detected incidentally on chest radiograph.[8] The most common clinical manifestation of thoracic aneurysms is deep, aching pain. This may be associated with erosion of the ribs or may be an indication that the aneurysm is expanding and that rupture may be imminent.[8] Compression of respiratory structures and of the recurrent laryngeal nerve may cause dyspnea, hoarseness, and coughing. Rupture as the initial manifestation is usually fatal.

### Dissecting Aneurysms

Dissecting aneurysms are not true aneurysms and are often called *dissecting hematomas*. An intimal tear and de-

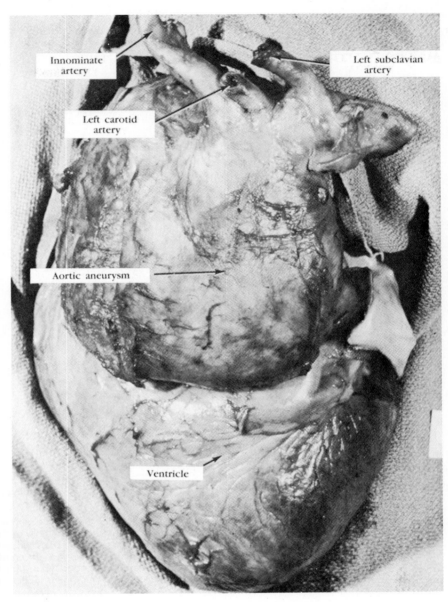

**FIGURE 27-4.**
External view of the heart showing aneurysmal dilation of the ascending aorta and involvement of the arch. (Reprinted from J. Kernicki, B. Bullock, and J. Matthews, *Cardiovascular Nursing.* New York: G.P. Putnam, 1971.)

generation of the medial layer allow blood to separate the intimal layer from the adventitial layer (Figure 27-5). Weakening of the medial layer appears to be essential in the production of dissection.[6] Aortic dissection most frequently occurs in the ascending aorta.[6,8] Eighty percent of individuals with this problem also have systemic hypertension. It also may be associated with the hereditary disorder called *Marfan's syndrome.*

Marfan's syndrome is characterized by degeneration of the elastic fibers of the aortic media, usually beginning at the aortic root and spreading segmentally throughout the aorta. Physical examination reveals long arms and legs, thin hands and feet, lax ligaments, and deformities of the thoracic cage.[1]

The clinical manifestations of dissection often present a striking change in appearance. External rupture may lead to exsanguination but more frequently, the process involves dissection from the initial point away from the heart. As it dissects through the aortic segment, it often causes obstruction to vessels branching off the aorta. If it occurs across the arch of the aorta, color changes and cerebral ischemia may be noted suddenly. Aortic regurgitation may result if the dissection occurs through the aortic valve. The affected person usually complains of the sudden onset of severe chest pain that radiates to the back, abdomen, and hips.[2,16]

Mortality of dissecting hematomas is very high. In the initial 24 hours after dissection, it is 35% and continues high in the first and second weeks. Two of the main factors that determine the mortality are the place of origin of dissection and whether or not the process is self-limiting.[8]

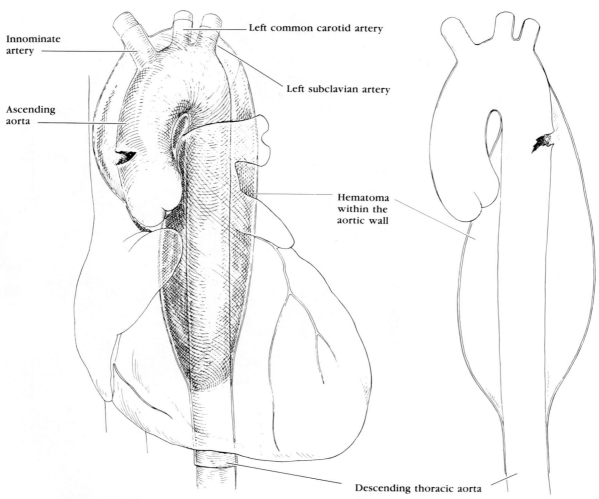

**FIGURE 27-5.**
Aortic dissection most often involves an intimal tear in the proximal ascending aorta or the proximal descending thoracic aorta. The dissection may propagate proximally or distally or in both directions. Regardless of the site of the tear, aortic dissections are best classified as those that involve the ascending aorta (type A, left) and those that are limited to the descending aorta (type B, right). Type A dissection may or may not also involve the descending aorta. (Copyright 1987, Scientific American, Inc. All rights reserved. From *Scientific American Medicine*, Figure 1, Section 1, Subsection XII.)

### *Saccular Aneurysms*

Saccular aneurysms are frequently associated with syphilis or congenital malformations rather than atherosclerosis. They are characterized by an outpouching on one side of an artery (Figure 27-6). Common congenital saccular aneurysms are described as *berry aneurysms* when they occur on the arteries of the circle of Willis. The danger of the intracerebral aneurysms is intracranial rupture and bleeding, which often has a fatal outcome (see Chap. 50).

Saccular syphilitic aneurysms most frequently arise on the ascending and descending thoracic aorta. These can compress the mediastinal structures, cause pressure on the surrounding skeletal structures, thrombose, or rupture. Syphilitic or leutic aneurysms are rarely re-

ported in the United States because of improved treatment and measures to control syphilis.

One of the most common aneurysms is the *false aneurysm* that may form at a surgical site for arterial repair. These have been reported after revascularization surgeries, such as aorto-iliac bypass, of the lower extremities and repair of arteries damaged by trauma. This aneurysm may erode into a surrounding structure and rupture, causing grave effects.[4]

### *Monckeberg's Sclerosis (Medial Calcific Sclerosis)*

This type of arterial hardening causes focal calcification of the medial layer, especially in the medium-sized arter-

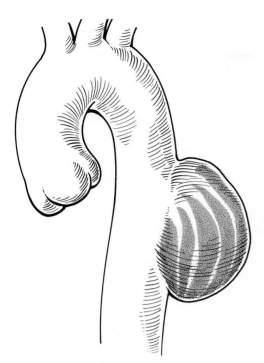

**FIGURE 27–6.**
Saccular aneurysm of the descending aorta.

ies. This condition is rare under age 50 years and is often asymptomatic even in aged individuals.[1] The vessels most commonly affected are the femoral, tibial, radial, and ulnar arteries.[1] In some cases, atherosclerosis is associated with the calcification process but the process is not atherosclerotic.

## Arteriolosclerosis

*Arteriolosclerosis,* as its name implies, involves degeneration of the intima and media of small arteries and arterioles. When this affects the kidney, hypertension results, but hypertension often is the initiator of the condition (see Chap. 26). It also may occur in the peripheral arteries and arterioles of the aged, and is often considered to be a part of the aging process.

## Arteriospastic Disorders

The terminology for the arteriospastic disorder of Raynaud's is conflicting.[1,7,9,12] In some literature, it is all termed *Raynaud's syndrome.*[12] Other literature makes a clear distinction between Raynaud's phenomenon and Raynaud's disease.[1,11] The clinical picture is almost the same except for the underlying etiology. In this discussion, *Raynaud's phenomenon* and *Raynaud's disease* will be used.

*Raynaud's phenomenon* is defined as an episode of constriction of the small arteries or arterioles of the extremities, resulting in intermittent pallor and cyanosis of the skin of the extremities. After an episode of constriction, hyperemia may produce rubor. Raynaud's phenomenon may occur in association with several conditions and diseases. Thus, it is a vasospastic disorder that produces temporary changes in skin color and is secondary to some underlying disorder.[1] A large group of seemingly unrelated conditions may have this as one of their features (Table 27-4). The link with connective tissue disease, especially scleroderma, is notable in that Raynaud's phenomenon may precede the skin changes by months or years.[11]

*Raynaud's disease* occurs predominantly in women and heredity may play a role in its development. Onset of symptoms usually begins between ages 20 and 40

**TABLE 27–4.**
MECHANISTIC CLASSIFICATION OF
RAYNAUD'S PHENOMENON

**Vasospastic**
Primary (idiopathic) Raynaud's phenomenon
Drug-induced
  β-Adrenergic blockers
  Ergot
  Methysergide
Pheochromocytoma
Variant angina
Migraine

**Structural**
Vibration syndrome
Arteriosclerosis
Thromboangiitis obliterans
Cold injury (frostbite, pernio, immersion foot)
Neurovascular compression (thoracic outlet syndrome, carpal tunnel syndrome, crutch pressure)
Chemotherapy (bleomycin, vinblastine)
Polyvinyl chloride disease
Connective tissue disease
  Systemic sclerosis
  Systemic lupus erythematosus
  Overlap syndrome
  Polymyositis/dermatomyositis
  Rheumatoid arthritis

**Hemorrheologic**
Cryoglobulinemia
Cryofibrinogenemia
Cold agglutinin disease
Paraproteinemia (plasma cell dyscrasia)
Polycythemia (essential thrombocythemia, polycythemia vera)

Source: W.N. Kelley, *Textbook of Internal Medicine. Philadelphia: J.B. Lippincott, 1989.*

years. Because investigators rarely are able to examine sections of the blood vessels in cases of early Raynaud's disease, little is known of the pathologic changes in the initial stages. In advanced stages, the intima of the digital arteries is thickened.

The typical clinical picture of Raynaud's disease is color changes on exposure to cold. At first, only the tips of the fingers are involved but later, the more proximal parts also exhibit color changes. All of the fingers of both hands usually undergo color changes that include pallor, cyanosis, and rubor. The sequential change from pallor to cyanosis and finally to rubor is characteristic.

Pallor is caused by spasm of the arterioles and possibly the venules. During this time, blood flow into the capillaries is decreased or absent, causing the affected part to appear dead white. Cyanosis results from capillary dilatation, which occurs later in the course of the disease. Blood flow becomes sluggish with extraction of more oxygen. Rubor indicates excessive hyperemia due to reactive vasodilatation. Exposure to emotional or thermal (cold) stimuli initiate vasoconstriction with subsequent color changes in the digits. Pain characterizes advanced disease, often associated with ulceration on the tips of the digits. paresthesia such as numbness, tingling, throbbing, and a dull ache may be present. During an actual attack, coldness of the digits is evident, sensory acuity is decreased, and the involved digits may swell. Table 27-5 compares the clinical features of primary Raynaud's phenomenon with that picture associated with connective tissue disease.

## Thromboangiitis or Buerger's Disease

Buerger's disease affects the small and medium-sized arteries and medium-sized, mostly superficial, veins of the extremities. It is mainly seen in young men between ages 20 and 35 years but the frequency is increasing in women. It is almost invariably a disease that affects individuals who use tobacco. It frequently results in arterial occlusion, causing ischemia and gangrene to the extremities. The nonatherosclerotic lesion consists of microabscesses that have a central focus of polymorphonuclear leukocytes usually surrounded by mononuclear cells.[1] Histopathologic evidence indicates that Buerger's disease has some of the characteristics of a collagen or autoimmune disease.

Clinical manifestations include frequent coexisting migratory phlebitis, early tenderness over the involved vessels, upper extremity involvement, absence of heart disease, marked early venospasm, and generally a low serum cholesterol concentration.

Pathologically, the disease has the following outstanding characteristics:

1. Thromboangiitis is primarily a disease of the blood vessels of the extremities. It involves the lower extremities more severely than the upper extremities.
2. The disease almost always develops in medium-sized or small arteries. Arteries commonly involved are the posterior tibial, anterior tibial, radial, ulnar, plantar, palmar, and digital. Larger arteries, such as the femoral and brachial, are affected late and only when the disease is se-

**TABLE 27-5.**
CLINICAL FEATURES HELPFUL IN DISTINGUISHING PRIMARY RAYNAUD'S PHENOMENON FROM RAYNAUD'S PHENOMENON OF EARLY CONNECTIVE TISSUE DISEASE

| FEATURE | PRIMARY RAYNAUD'S PHENOMENON | RAYNAUD'S PHENOMENON SECONDARY TO CONNECTIVE TISSUE DISEASE |
|---|---|---|
| Sex | Overwhelmingly female | Male or female |
| Age of onset | Menarche | Mid-20s and later |
| Extent of involvement | Usually all digits | Frequently a single digit to start |
| Frequency of attacks* | Usually >10/d | Usually 0–5/d |
| Symptoms | Mild to moderate | Moderate to severe |
| Symptoms also precipitated by emotional stress | Yes | Rarely |
| Evidence of ischemic injury (eg, ulcers or loss of finger pulp) | No | Yes |
| Finger edema | Rare | Common |
| Periungual erythema | Rare | Common |
| Evidence of other vasomotor syndromes (eg, migraine or livedo reticularis) | Yes | No |

*Frequency of attacks is somewhat variable and depends on climate.
Source: W.N. Kelley, Textbook of Internal Medicine. Philadelphia: J.B. Lippincott, 1989.

vere. Small and medium-sized veins are affected less commonly and large veins, rarely.

3. The lesions are focal or segmental and not diffuse.
4. The lesions appear to be of different ages but, in general, the disease throughout a single affected segment seems to be of essentially the same age.
5. The disease produces occlusions of the vessels, followed by development of collateral and anastomotic vessels.[1,7,12]

The gross characteristics of the vessels affected by thromboangiitis obliterans vary depending on the age of the lesions at the time they are examined. The vessels appear contracted at the site of destruction. The occluded segments are indurated but not brittle. The arteries are more frequently obliterated than their accompanying veins. In the diseased vessel, the occlusion may extend for variable lengths and then stop abruptly. Occlusions may occur at two different levels in the same vessel, and between these sites the vessel may be completely patent.

The most striking physiologic change is the impairment of arterial blood flow. Blood flow through peripheral arteries in the extremities is reduced, particularly in more distal portions. Another factor that contributes to ischemia is arteriolar spasm. The degree of spasm varies among individuals and perhaps with the stage of disease.

The degree of arterial insufficiency in the affected extremities depends on two factors: (1) the amount of arterial occlusive disease, and (2) the tone of the arterioles, which may vary from normal to moderate or severe spasm.

Venous obstruction, the result of thrombophlebitis, may be an associated factor in the circulatory disturbance in thromboangiitis obliterans. The obstruction is often minor because the venous circulation has a great capacity to develop collateral circulation. In some cases, venous obstruction contributes to malnutrition of capillaries and a tendency to develop edema in the affected extremity if it remains in a dependent position for a long time.

Dependent rubor is caused by the presence of numerous dilated capillaries in skin that contain blood of high oxygen content.[7] Rubor is seen in thromboangiitis that is associated with chronic and moderately severe arterial insufficiency. One explanation, supported by studies of the oxygen content of venous blood, is that capillaries suffer from malnutrition and become atonic, and their capacity to interchange oxygen and other metabolic products is impaired.

## PATHOLOGIC PROCESSES OF VEINS

The veins have walls that contract or relax, an intact endothelium to prevent clotting, and valves that promote blood flow to the heart.[5] Normally, the valves of the larger veins and communicating veins prevent retrograde flow of blood in the superficial and deep veins, which promotes the forward flow of blood (see Chap. 22).[5]

## Obstructive Disease of Veins

Obstructive lesions of the veins may be permanent or temporary, partial or complete. Obstruction to some portion of the main trunk causes the distal large veins to become dilated, with incompetent valves. The small veins and venules may be damaged permanently as a result of pressure, stretching, hypoxemia, and malnutrition. Permanent impairment in interchange of fluid may result from disruption of small vessels. Damaged venous capillaries may function normally when the person is in a recumbent position but show inadequacy in a standing position. This inadequacy is due to increased hydrostatic pressure and sometimes to associated incompetent valves.

### Venous Thrombosis

Lesions in veins may produce localized thrombi in small veins or extensive thrombi in the larger veins. Venous thrombosis may develop as a result of an inflammatory or traumatic lesion of the endothelium of the vein wall. In the majority of cases, however, there is no evidence of either. An inflammatory reaction may develop in the wall of the vein as a reaction to primary thrombosis, so that phlebitis may ensue several hours after the thrombus is formed.

Lesions of the endothelium, relative stasis of venous blood flow, and hypercoagulability of blood are the three factors that precipitate venous thrombosis. One or a combination of these factors may produce a thrombus. A thrombus develops as a result of slowed flow in the venous bloodstream and is associated with platelet aggregation. After several days and after development of a secondary reaction in the wall of the thrombosed vein, a sudden proximal extension may protrude from the end of the original organizing thrombus. Emboli may develop at this time from the proximal extension, or the new clot may stick and become organized. Emboli may be small or large, and tend to lodge in the vessels of the pulmonary circulation (see Chap. 31).[1]

A thrombus organizes from its outer margins centrally. In some veins, the entire thrombus becomes organized with complete and permanent occlusion of the lumen. In a large thrombus, involution usually occurs by a process of partial fibrosis and partial lysis, which is probably due to the action of naturally occurring fibrinolysins in the blood. In most cases, the center disappears and a varying portion of the periphery may organize on a fibrous ring. In other instances, bands of fibrous tissue extend across the old lumen of the vein and divide it into many small lumina. The result is usually some restoration of function of the vein but the lumen is partially obstructed by the remaining fibrous tissue and decrease of its circular diameter.[12]

The degree of inflammatory reaction in the different

layers of the veins varies. In some persons, the thrombus causes minimal reaction, while in others an intense reaction extends throughout all layers. Inflammatory cells, leukocytes, lymphocytes, and fibroblasts accumulate and cause congestion of capillaries in and around the venous wall. Venous thrombosis causes obstruction to venous blood flow and relates to the size and location of the involved vein. If it occurs in superficial veins and in short segments, collateral circulation will compensate. This may also be true in obstruction of the saphenous vein of the leg or a larger vein of the arm (eg, median basilic or cephalic) because of the numerous anastomoses that occur. Collateral channels may become evident even after obstruction of the superior or inferior vena cava.[12]

When thrombosis occurs in the iliofemoral or axillary veins, the collateral circulation compensates only partially and venous pressure increases in the veins distal to the thrombosis. This increased pressure results in distention of all veins and even venules of the limb. The increased pressure in the venules and capillaries causes intense congestion of these areas. Pressure changes inhibit normal resorption of fluid and electrolytes from the tissues in the venous end of the capillaries. Edema of the affected limb then develops.

## Thrombophlebitis and Phlebothrombosis

Thrombophlebitis refers to an inflamed vein as a result of a thrombus. Phlebothrombosis is probably the same entity but does not exhibit a marked inflammatory component. Thrombosis in a vein ultimately causes inflammatory changes.[1]

*Idiopathic thrombophlebitis* is a recurrent condition that produces segmental lesions in the small and medium-sized veins. The thrombus may be recanalized and the luman restored but more frequently the vein becomes completely obliterated. *Suppurative thrombophlebitis* differs in that it usually results from bacterial invasion. The wall of the vein becomes markedly inflamed and leukocytes infiltrate the area. Bacteria within the thrombus and portions of the endothelium ultimately lead to abscesses. The abscesses may rupture into the bloodstream. *Chemical thrombophlebitis* may result from venous irritation from drugs (eg, antibiotics or potassium) or other chemicals that gain access to the venous circulation. The thrombus becomes adherent and completely organized, resulting in a vein that is contracted, fibrotic, and cordlike.

The symptoms and signs of thrombophlebitis develop acutely and usually persist for 1 to 3 weeks. In small or medium-sized veins, acute thrombophlebitis rarely produces systemic reactions. With involvement of the larger vessels, temperature may rise to as high as 102°F

(39°C). Thrombosis of superficial veins often involves redness, pain, tenderness, and localized edema.

Thrombophlebitis of the deep veins of the legs produces calf pain and tenderness in the calf muscles. Enlargement of the calf and a positive Homans' sign may result. Homans' sign refers to pain in the calf muscle when the foot is dorsiflexed. Thrombosis of the iliofemoral vein usually produces a typical, acute, clinical picture. Moderate to severe pain in the thigh and groin with diffuse pain throughout the limb is described. Superficial veins may be prominent and distended in an enlarged limb. The skin of the leg and thigh may be slightly cyanotic. Thrombosis is manifested by impaired or absent pulses from associated arterial spasm. Fever and tachycardia may also be associated. Pitting edema is characteristic with onset a few days after the obstruction ensues. As the edema becomes chronic, it may be associated with skin changes and brawny edema (thick, hardened skin with nonpitting edema).

Thrombosis of the axillary and subclavian veins produces a clinical picture similar to that of iliofemoral thrombosis. The axillary vein becomes tender, prominent, and enlarged with pitting edema in the forearm and hand. Superficial veins of the entire arm are prominent and those of the pectoral region on the affected side may be distended.

## Venous Insufficiency and Stasis

Chronic venous insufficiency results from stasis of venous blood flow, especially of the iliofemoral veins. Old iliofemoral thrombophlebitis leaves behind a thickened, inelastic vein wall, damaged venous valves, and a partially or sometimes completely obstructed lumen. In the lower extremity ,the three groups of veins—deep, communicating, and superficial—normally have thin, elastic walls and segmentally spaced valves of the bicuspid type. Venous flow against gravity in the lower limbs is possible by action of the calf muscle and the competent valves. Muscular compression of the elastic veins forces blood upward and the valves prevent retrograde flow. This mechanism fails in chronic venous insufficiency, usually because of incompetent valves. The result is venous hypertension in the affected system.[5]

Ambulatory venous pressure is high and this upsets the normal equilibrium of capillary fluid exchange, causing congestion and edema. Stasis also results from the high ambulatory pressures, as manifested by changes in the skin and subcutaneous tissues around the distal one third of the leg and around the ankle. Changes that may occur include edema, hyperpigmentation, dermatitis, induration, stasis cellulitis, and ultimately, venostasis ulcers (Figure 27-7). The amount of edema varies according to length of dependency of the affected limb. There is characteristically a light brown pigmentation in white skin

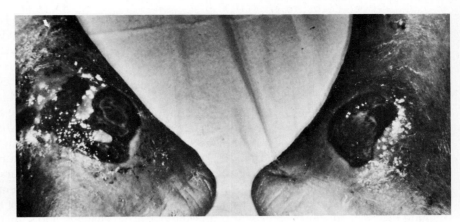

**FIGURE 27-7.**
Bilateral stasis ulcers of the ankles with surrounding dermatitis. (Source: R. Judge, G. Zuidema, and F. Fitzgerald, *Clinical Diagnosis*. Boston: Little, Brown, 1982.)

with a darker pigmentation in black skin. The edema is brawny and often feels hard to the touch. Pain may or may not be present. A dull ache in the affected leg may develop after the individual has been standing for variable periods. Pain is usually described as being more severe when standing still rather than when walking. The pain usually disappears within 5 to 30 minutes after assuming a recumbent position with the leg elevated. Nocturnal muscular cramps may be reported.

## Varicose Veins

Varicose veins are dilated, elongated, and tortuous superficial veins of the lower extremities.[12] They are produced by incompetent valves and increased intraluminal pressure[14] (Figure 27-8). Varicosities probably develop because of an inherent weakness in the structure of the vein. Superficial veins dilate when normal resistance against intraluminal pressure is lacking. Primary varicose veins may develop from hereditary predisposition, pregnancy, standing for a long time, and marked obesity. Prolonged periods of standing favor development of varicosities because of the high gravitational pressure within the veins. Obesity tends to place external pressure on the veins, especially the iliofemoral veins. It is estimated that 10% to 20% of the general population have varicose veins, with women affected four times more often than men.[1]

Deep thrombophlebitis often gives rise to secondary varicosities. Loss of valve sufficiency produces unusual strain on the superficial veins. A frequent finding is the presence of localized dilations just distal to the venous valves. Valve incompetency is due primarily to extreme dilatation in the affected veins, which causes separation of the valve cusps. In primary varicose veins, the incompetency tends to progress downward in the saphenous main channel and in its tributaries. In secondary varicose veins, which arise because of deep vein insufficiency, the incompetency tends to progress upward from incompetent perforating veins in the lower one third of the leg.[7]

Varicose veins can lead to chronic venous insufficiency. In the early stages, localized pain and heat may be noticed after prolonged standing. Persistent edema may develop, together with trophic skin changes and stasis ulcers. The stasis ulcers heal slowly and often become infected.

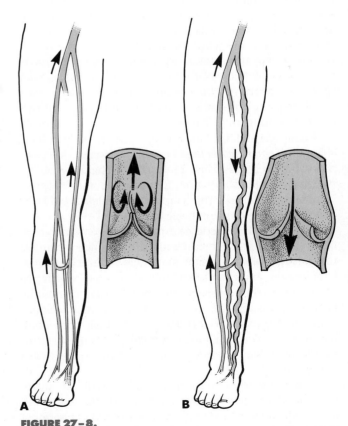

**FIGURE 27-8.**
Varicose veins. (**A**) Normal vein with competent valves. (**B**) Incompetent valve with tortuous, dilated segment.

Diagnosis of venous insufficiency can be made by assessment of physical findings and, occasionally, phlebography. *Phlebography* involves injecting radiopaque material into the venous system and taking radiographs of the injected area. It is performed to localize deep vein thrombosis or to evaluate varicosities.

## PATHOLOGIC PROCESSES OF THE LYMPHATIC SYSTEM

The lymphatic system serves the essential function of draining excess fluids and proteins from the interstitial space. It provides the only means for returning plasma proteins that have leaked into this space to the general circulation. Whenever tissue fluid levels increase, lymphatic drainage also increases.

In this way, lymphatic flow is an essential method for control of tissue fluid volume. Venous obstruction and congestive heart failure have been identified as factors that can alter capillary pressure and produce edema. When fluids continually escape into the interstitial spaces, edema may not be noted because of compensation by the lymphatic system.

Obstruction of the lymph vessels interferes with this control mechanism and may precipitate or contribute to edema. Numerous factors may cause lymphedema and are categorized as inflammatory or noninflammatory. *Lymphangitis* is the word for inflammation of the lymph vessels, usually by bacterial organisms. *Lymphadenitis* refers to inflammation of the lymph nodes. *Lymphedema* specifies edema resulting from lymphatic obstruction.[6]

Primary or idiopathic lymphedema is rare. Milroy's disease, a congenital lymphedema noticeable at birth, is usually caused by faulty development of lymphatic channels. *Lymphedema praecox* affects females predominantly between ages 9 and 25 years. It is characterized by swelling of one foot or both feet that becomes progressive and unremitting. The lymphatic channels are dilated due to incompetent lymph valves.

Secondary lymphedema is much more common than the primary form. Obstruction of the lymph channels may result from malignant metastatic infiltration of the lymph nodes and channels. Hodgkin's disease, which primarily affects the lymphatic system, also may obstruct the channels. Inflammation or infection of the channels may result in fibrosis and obstruction. A final, very common cause of lymphedema is the surgical removal or irradiation of lymph nodes to prevent the spread of a malignancy.

Lymphedema is essentially the result of stasis. Chronic stasis often leads to *brawny* edema, which describes the appearance of the skin subjected to continual stretch. The skin becomes thick, hardened, infiltrated with plasma proteins, and often "orange-peel" in appearance. The edema is different from cardiac edema in that it does not pit on digital pressure.

Inflammatory lymphedema usually occurs after an acute infection of the lymphatic system. Lymphangitis is characterized by painful red streaks following the lymph vessels, which may eventually involve the lymph nodes as well. The agent that most commonly causes lymphangitis is beta-hemolytic *Streptococcus* but any virulent pathogen may initiate it. Systemic effects include a marked temperature elevation, malaise, and chills. Localized edema occurs and may become progressive if attacks are recurrent. *Chronic lymphangitis* may follow, causing fibrosis of the affected area, further edema, skin changes, and sometimes ulcerations.

Diagnosis of lymphedema is primarily to differentiate it from edema of venous origin. Lymphangiography involves injecting radiopaque dye into the affected lymph vessel and monitoring its passage radiologically. This procedure may localize the source of the obstruction.

## DIAGNOSTIC PROCEDURES FOR VASCULAR LESIONS

### Physical Examination

Diagnosis of vascular system problems is usually based on the signs and symptoms of arterial occlusion or of venous insufficiency. Palpation of the peripheral pulses is important in estimating blood flow in the peripheral arterial circuit. Systolic bruits over the abdominal area and femoral artery are common and, in association with other signs, may indicate peripheral arterial disease. Bruits refer to sounds produced in the blood vessels, usually only audible if some factor is obstructing blood flow. Tenderness to palpation or tenderness with the inflation of a blood pressure cuff over the calf or thigh (Lowenberg's cuff sign) gives high suspicion for deep vein thrombosis. Pain on dorsiflexion of the foot with stretching of the gastrocnemius muscle (Homans' sign) also may be present.[12] Ankle edema, especially unilateral, may be seen. Many procedures may be performed to diagnose vascular lesions.

### Doppler Ultrasound

This procedure involves the use of a Doppler recorder to hear flow over the larger veins. Flow is normally increased by distal compression of the vein and decreased by the Valsalva maneuver, and varies with respiration. Lack of flow sound may indicate venous thrombosis. Arterial lesions also may be evaluated by Doppler studies. The proximal and distal pressures of the suspected lesion are auscultated to determine the pressure gradient. The

Doppler flowmeter is used at the ankle to compare arterial pressure there with brachial systolic pressure.

## Angiography

Angiography involves the use of a contrast material of high opacity to outline the great vessels, particularly the aorta and its branches. The contrast material may be injected into an artery, vein, or chamber of the heart.

In individuals with symptoms of obstruction involving the superior vena cava, angiography shows the site and extent of obstruction and may give other important data about it. Angiography also may be of great value in studying known aneurysms of the thoracic aorta.

Specific procedures used to visualize special vessels include. (1) translumbar aortography, which is performed mainly to study aorto-iliofemoral thrombo-occlusive disease; (2) renal arteriography; (3) visceral arteriography; and (4) inferior venacavography, especially to identify caval thrombosis.

### Translumbar Aortography

In the presence of severe atherosclerosis, the translumbar puncture method of aortography may be preferable because of the hazards of retrograde catheterization from a femoral artery: injuring the arterial wall and embolization from a dislodged thrombus or plaque, perforations, and aggravation of thrombus formation. Because atherosclerotic occlusive disease of the lower extremities involves many segments of the vascular system, it is important to evaluate inflow proximal to the diseased artery. Translumbar aortography carries the main risk of retroperitoneal bleeding from direct puncture of the aorta. Careful assessment of blood coagulation and blood pressure are necessary prior to performing this procedure. Aortography can detail the entire peripheral arterial system. Renal arteries can be evaluated for stenosis by injecting dye at the level of these arteries.

### Peripheral Arteriography

Femoral arteriography can be performed when aortic visualization is unnecessary and when the lesion is limited to the leg. This approach also may be used to pass a catheter retrograde up the aorta to the desired position for dye injection. The clinical usefulness of this procedure is in the precise localization of atherosclerotic disease, and sometimes in thromboangiitis obliterans and aneurysms. This method may be used to selectively inject dye into any aortic tributary by moving the catheter to the ostium of the selected artery and injecting dye. The risk of bleeding is less than in other approaches and can be more quickly assessed.

## REFERENCES

1. Cotran, R.S., Kumar, V., and Robbins, S.L. *Robbins' Pathologic Basis of Disease* (4th ed.). Philadelphia: W.B. Saunders, 1989.
2. Erskine, J.M. Blood vessels and lymphatics. In M.A. Krupp, M.J. Chalton, and L.M. Tierney (eds.), *Current Medical Diagnosis and Treatment*. Los Altos, Calif.: Lange, 1986.
3. Fishman, M.C. *Medicine* (2nd ed.). Philadelphia: J.B. Lippincott, 1985.
4. Glover, J.L. Aneurysms and occlusive diseases of the aorta and veins. In W.N. Kelley (ed.), *Textbook of Internal Medicine*. Philadelphia: J.B. Lippincott, 1989.
5. Glover, J.L. Diseases of the veins. In W.N. Kelley (ed.), *Textbook of Internal Medicine*. Philadelphia: J.B. Lippincott, 1989.
6. Glover, J.L. Miscellaneous vascular problems. In W.N. Kelley (ed.), *Textbook of Internal Medicine*. Philadelphia: J.B. Lippincott, 1989.
7. Juergens, J.L., Fairbairn, J.E., II, and Spittell, J.A., Jr. *Peripheral Vascular Diseases* (5th ed.). Philadelphia: W.B. Saunders, 1986.
8. Lindsay, J., DeBakey, M.E., and Beall, A.C. Diseases of the aorta. In J.W. Hurst et al. (eds.), *The Heart* (7th ed.). New York: McGraw-Hill, 1990.
9. Rivers, S.P., and Porter, J.M. Raynaud's syndrome, upper extremity vasospastic disorders, and small artery occlusive disease. In S.E. Wilson et al. (eds.), *Vascular Surgery: Principles and Practice*. New York: McGraw-Hill, 1987.
10. Ross, R. Factors influencing atherogenesis. In J.W. Hurst et al. (eds.), *The Heart* (7th ed.). New York: McGraw-Hill, 1990.
11. Seibol, J.R. Management of Raynaud's phenomenon and scleroderma. In W.N. Kelley (ed.), *Textbook of Internal Medicine*. Philadelphia: J.B. Lippincott, 1989.
12. Smith, R.B., and Perdue, G.D. Diseases of the peripheral arteries. In J.W. Hurst et al. (eds.), *The Heart* (7th ed.). New York: McGraw-Hill, 1990.
13. Sokolow, M., and McIlroy, M.B. *Clinical Cardiology* (4th ed.). Los Altos, Calif.: Lange, 1986.
14. Tomaszewski, J.E. Vascular system. In V.A. LiVolsi et al. (eds.), *Pathology* (2nd ed.). Media, Penn.: Harwal, 1989.
15. Wallace, A.G., and Waugh, R.A. Pathophysiology of cardiovascular disease. In L.H. Smith and S.O. Thier (eds.), *Pathophysiology: The Biological Principles of Disease* (2nd ed.). Philadelphia: W.B. Saunders, 1985.
16. White, R.A. Diagnosis and therapy of emergent vascular diseases. In W.A. Shoemaker et al. (eds.), *Textbook of Critical Care*. Philadelphia: W.B. Saunders, 1989.

## UNIT BIBLIOGRAPHY

Alboni, P., Parparella, N., Cappato, R., Baggioni, F., Scarfo, S., Percoco, F., and Tomasi, A. Intrinsic electrophysiologic properties of reentrant supraventricular tachycardia involving bypass tracts. *Am. J. Cardiol.* 58:226, 1986.

Alpert, M.A., and Flaker, G.C. Arrhythmias associated with sinus node dysfunction. *J.A.M.A.* 250:2160, 1983.

Akhtar, M. Management of ventricular tachycardias. *J.A.M.A* 247:671, 1982.

Arnsdorf, M.F. Basic understanding of electrophysiologic actions of arrhythmic drugs. *Med. Clin. N. Am.* 68:1247, 1984.

Baker, J.D. Assessment of peripheral arterial occlusive disease. *Crit. Care Clin. N. Am.* 3:493, 1991.

Boucher, C.A., Brewster, D.C., Darling, R.C., et al. Determination of cardiac risk by dipyridamole-thallium imaging before peripheral vascular surgery. *N. Engl. J. Med.* 312:389, 1985.

Braunwald, E. Heart failure. In J. Wilson et al. (eds.). Harrison's Principles of Internal Medicine (2nd ed.). New York: McGraw-Hill, 1991.

Chang, S. *Echocardiography: Techniques and Interpretation.* Philadelphia: Lea & Febiger, 1981.

Chung, E.K. *Principles of Cardiac Arrhythmias.* Baltimore: Williams & Wilkins, 1982.

Chase, K.M. Use vectors to round out an EKG. *RN* 49:18, 1986.

Childers, R. Classification of cardiac dysrhythmias. *Med. Clin. N. Am.* 60:3, 1976.

Commerford, P.J., and Llioyd, E.A. Arrhythmias in patients with drug toxicity, electrolyte imbalance, & endocrine disturbances. *Med. Clin. N. Am.* 68:1051, 1984.

Conner, R. The electrocardiographic diagnosis of posterior M.I. *Crit. Care Nurse* 5:20, 1986.

Conner, R.P. Coronary artery anatomy: The electrographic & clinical correlations. *Crit. Care Nurse* 3:68, 1983.

Conover, M.B. VT or SVT? *Crit. Care Nurse* 9:2, 1989.

Cotran, R., Kumar, V., and Robbins, S. *Robbin's Pathologic Basis of Disease* (4th ed.). Philadelphia: W.B. Saunders, 1989.

Davis, M.J. *Pathology of Cardiac Valves.* Woburn, Mass.: Butterworths, 1980.

Dawber, T.R. *The Framingham Study Series: Commonwealth Fund.* Cambridge, Mass.: Harvard University Press, 1980.

deFaire, U., and Theorell, T. *Life Stress and Coronary Heart Disease.* St. Louis: Warren Green, 1982.

Doroghazi, R.M., and Slater, E.E. *Aortic Dissection.* New York: McGraw-Hill, 1983.

Dubin, D. *Rapid Interpretation of EKGs* (7th ed.). Tampa: Cover Publishing Co., 1984.

Duke, D.M. Intraventricular conduction block. *Crit. Care Nurse* 4:30, 1982.

Feigenbaum, H. *Echocardiography* (3rd ed.). Philadelphia: Lea & Febiger, 1981.

Fink, B.W. *Congenital Heart Disease: A Deductive Approach to Its Diagnosis* (2nd ed.). Chicago: Year Book, 1985.

Finklemeier, B.A., and Salinger, M.H. The atrial electrocardiogram: Its diagnostic use following cardiac surgery. *Critical Care Quarterly* 4:42, 1984.

Fortuin, N.J. Echocardiography: How it works. *Med. Times* 108: 120, 1980.

Fowler, N.O. *Cardiac Diagnosis and Treatment* (3rd ed.). Hagerstown, Md.: Harper & Row, 1980, 186.

Friedman, S.A. *Vascular Diseases: A Concise Guide to Diagnosis, Management, Pathogenesis and Prevention.* Littleton, Mass.: Wright-PSG Publishing, 1982.

Genest, J., et al. *Hypertension: Physiopathology and Treatment* (2nd ed.). New York: McGraw-Hill, 1983.

Goldberger, E. *Textbook of Clinical Cardiology.* St. Louis: Mosby, 1982.

Gomes, J.C., and El-Sherif, N. Atrioventricular block: Mecha-

nism, clinical presentation, & therapy. *Med. Clin. N. Am.* 68:1247, 1984.

Hurst, J.W., et al. *The Heart* (4th ed.). New York: McGraw-Hill, 1990.

Juergens, J.L., et al. *Peripheral Vascular Disease* (6th ed.). Philadelphia: W.B. Saunders, 1986.

Kallenberg, C.G.M., Wouda, A.A., and The, T.H. The systemic involvement and immunologic findings in patients presenting with Raynaud's phenomenon. *Am. J. Med.* 69:675, 1980.

Killip, T. Arrhythmias in myocardial infarction. *Med. Clin. N. Am.* 60:233, 1976.

Langman, J. *Medical Embryology: Human Development— Normal and Abnormal* (2nd ed.). Baltimore: Williams & Wilkins, 1969.

Little, R. *Physiology of the Heart and Circulation* (3rd ed.). Chicago: Year Book, 1986.

Marcus, M.L. *The Coronary Circulation in Health and Disease.* New York: McGraw-Hill, 1983.

Mason, D.T. *Congestive Heart Failure: Mechanisms, Evaluation and Treatment.* New York: Yorke, 1976.

Melstein, S., Sharma, A., and Klein, G. Electrophysiologic profile of asymptomatic Wolff-Parkinson-White pattern. *Am. J. Cardiol.* 57:1097, 1986.

Meyerburg, R.J. Electrocardiography. In J. Wilson et al. (eds.). *Harrison's Principles of Internal Medicine* (12th ed.). New York: McGraw-Hill, 1991.

Plauth, W.H., et al. Congenital Heart Disease. In J.W. Hurst, (ed.), *The Heart* (6th ed.). New York: McGraw-Hill, 1986.

Porterfield, J.G., Porterfield, L., and Brown, S. Sudden cardiac death. *Focus on Critical Care* 13:23, 1986.

Rackley, C.E., et al. Aortic Valve Disease. In J.W. Hurst et al. (eds.), *The Heart* (7th ed.). New York: McGraw-Hill, 1990.

Ross, J.H. Reentrant supraventricular tachycardia. *Crit. Care Nurse* 4:30, 1984.

Scheicht, S. Basic electrocardiography: Leads, axes, arrhythmias. *Clinical Symposia* 35:2, 1983.

Scorde, K.A. Taming the cardiac monitor (Part 1). *Nursing* 12:59, 1982.

Scorde, K.A. Taming the cardiac monitor (Part 2). *Nursing;* 12:61, 1982.

Shamroth, L. *The Disorders of Cardiac Rhythm* (2nd ed.). St. Louis: Blackwell/Mosby, 1980.

Shoenberg, B.S. *Precursors of Stroke: Etiologic, Preventive and Therapeutic Implications.* New York: Oxford University Press, 1982.

Silverman, M.D., et al. *Electrocardiography: Basic Concepts and Clinical Application.* New York: McGraw-Hill, 1983.

Sodeman, W., and Sodeman, W. *Pathologic Physiology* (2nd ed.). Philadelphia: W.B. Saunders, 1986.

Sokolow, M., and McIlroy, M.B. *Clinical Cardiology* (4th ed.). Los Altos, Calif.: Lange, 1986.

Summers, G. The clinical and hemodynamic presentation of the shock patient. *Crit. Care Nurs. Clin. N. Am.* 2:2, 1990.

Visant, M., and Spence, M. *Common Sense Approach to Coronary Care* (4th ed.). St. Louis: C.V. Mosby, 1985.

Wilson, J.E. *Vascular Surgery: Principles and Practice.* New York: McGraw-Hill, 1987.

# RESPIRATION

This unit is divided into four chapters; each deals with aspects of the pulmonary system. Chapter 28 discusses the normal anatomy and physiology of the pulmonary system. It is a review that provides the basis for the material in Chapters 29, 30, and 31, which cover various aspects of pathophysiology of the pulmonary system.

Diseases of the pulmonary system have been categorized as restrictive, obstructive, and other alterations. There is necessarily some overlap among these categories but an attempt has been made to classify them according to functional impairments. The chapters contain discussion of pathologic, clinical, and diagnostic aspects of pulmonary disease.

The reader is encouraged to use the learning objectives as study guides and to supplement the material with references listed in the unit bibliography.

# Normal Respiratory Function

## *Learning Objectives*

1. Describe the normal basic pulmonary anatomy.
2. Describe the action of the pulmonary pumping mechanism.
3. Identify the mechanisms of nervous control in the respiratory tract.
4. Compare the concepts of compliance and elastance in the normally functioning pulmonary system.
5. Describe the importance of the anatomic dead space in pulmonary function.
6. Identify the major muscles of respiration and their function.
7. Compare tissue resistance and airway resistance.
8. Relate the concept of work of breathing to oxygen consumption and carbon dioxide production.
9. Describe the major patterns of airway resistance.
10. Describe the anatomy and dynamics of pulmonary perfusion.
11. Compare normal ventilation and perfusion from the apex to the base of the lung.

12. List factors that alter ventilation and perfusion.
13. List the normal pressures in the heart and pulmonary vascular system.
14. Relate the oxyhemoglobin dissociation curve to tissue oxygenation.
15. Outline the pattern of normal gas exchange.
16. Describe the function of surfactant in the alveoli.
17. Describe the function of alpha₁-antitrypsin in the lungs.
18. Identify deposition sites of particulates in the airway.
19. List the major protective reflexes of the lungs.
20. Explain the function of the mucociliary transport system in the defense of the lungs.
21. Trace the clearance of particulates from the alveoli.
22. Distinguish between humoral and cell-mediated immunity in the lungs.
23. Describe the role of the macrophages in the lungs.
24. Explain the probable activity of interferon.

To delineate clearly the pathophysiology of respiratory diseases, this chapter reviews the anatomy and physiology of the pulmonary system and includes an indepth discussion of the following essential concepts: compliance, elastance, resistance, ventilation, perfusion, diffusion, and alveolar airway clearance in health. A description of pulmonary function tests (PFTs) is also included.

To live is to breathe. Between a newborn's first breath and the last expiration is a lifetime of respiration. Breathing is the only bodily function that occurs automatically and can be controlled voluntarily as well. It is also the only bodily function that immediately interacts with the environment, whatever it may be: a fresh ocean breeze, stale cigarette smoke, noxious automobile exhaust, a damp cellar, or a dusty workplace. Normally, breathing occurs below the level of consciousness, rhythmically and inconspicuously, unless some kind of physical stress interferes, such as breathlessness after running, swimming, or climbing a mountain, or when the lungs are impaired by diseases, such as asthma, emphysema, bronchitis, pneumonia, or fibrosis.

The human body must adapt itself continually to an unfriendly environment. The lungs especially are constantly attacked by irritants, gases, and microorganisms. Consequently, the respiratory apparatus has developed an elaborate defense system to protect itself and the body from these inhalants.

The main function of the lungs is to take oxygen from the air and deliver it across the alveolar-capillary membrane to the hemoglobin. It is transported on hemoglobin by circulating blood to the tissues. At the tissue line, it diffuses across the cellular membrane to the mitochondria to aid in producing energy to support the metabolic processes of life. As a result of these metabolic processes, carbon dioxide is produced that is transported back to the lungs and expelled into the environmental air.

## ANATOMY OF THE PULMONARY TREE

### Airways

Air normally enters the body through the nose or the mouth. Here and in the pharynx it is warmed, moistened, and filtered. Even though air has been filtered in the upper respiratory tract, it is not sterile when it reaches the lower respiratory tract. Much debris remains, as evidenced by autopsies of the lungs of cigarette smokers or those exposed to heavy air pollution.

The air passes through the larynx and into the respiratory tree, which is a series of successively smaller, branching tubes (Figure 28-1). Immediately below the larynx is the trachea, which divides at a point called the carina into the right and left main stem bronchi. The right main stem bronchus is shorter and wider than the left,

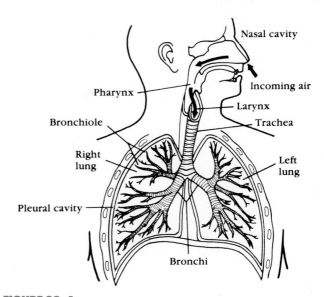

**FIGURE 28–1.**
Respiratory system. (Source: H.A. Braun, F.W. Cheney, Jr., and C.P. Loehnen, *Introduction to Repsiratory Physiology* (2nd ed.). Boston: Little, Brown, 1980.)

coming off the trachea in a nearly straight line (Figure 28-2). This explains why aspirated objects and fluids lodge more frequently in the right lung than in the left. It also makes suctioning of the left main stem bronchus difficult.

The right and left main stem bronchi divide into the lobar bronchi, which divide into the segmental bronchi. The segmental bronchi then divide into the terminal

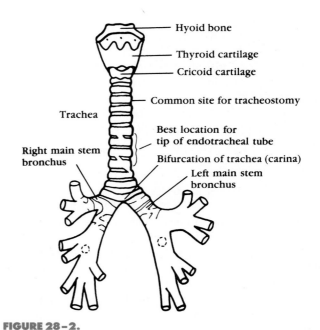

**FIGURE 28–2.**
Tracheobronchial divisions. (Source: H.A. Braun, F.W. Cheney, Jr., and C.P. Loehnen, *Introduction to Repsiratory Physiology* (2nd ed.). Boston: Little, Brown, 1980.)

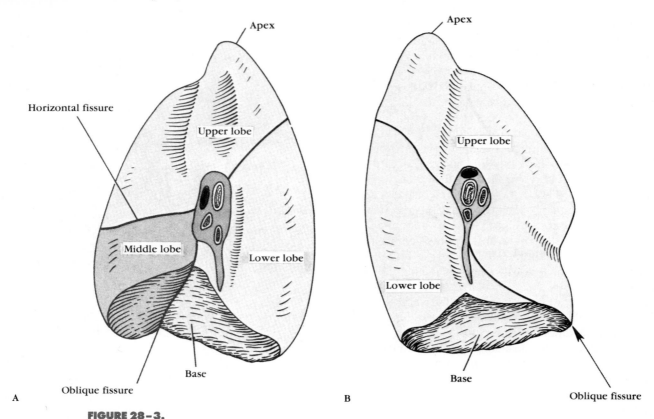

**FIGURE 28-3.**
**A.** Lateral and medial surfaces of right lung. **B.** Lateral and medial surfaces of left lung. (Source: R.S. Snell, *Clinical Anatomy for Medical Students* (2nd ed.). Boston: Little, Brown, 1981.)

bronchioles. The diameter of each of these successive segments is smaller than the last but the number of airways in the smaller segments is greater than in the larger ones, providing a broader surface area. This anatomic division, called the *generations of bronchi* ends at approximately the 16th generation from the trachea. The lower airway divisions are called bronchi down to the smallest division that contains cartilage. Thereafter, they become bronchioles. The terminal bronchioles branch into the respiratory bronchioles, which open into alveolar ducts and are completely surrounded by alveoli where gas exchange takes place (see pp. 568–572).

## Anatomy of the Lungs

The lungs lie in the thoracic cavity, separated from each other by the mediastinum. The lungs are cone-shaped with the narrow ends, or *apices*, directed upward and the wide *bases* at the lower portion. Each lung is composed of lobes: three on the right and two on the left (Figure 28-3). The lobes are divided into smaller compartments called *lobules*. The lobules are further divided into smaller segments and terminate finally in the alveolar sacs.

Surrounding the lungs is the pleural membrane,

which provides a covering over the lungs and lines the thoracic wall. The layer overlying the lung parenchyma is called the *visceral pleura* and the outer layer is the *parietal pleura* (Figure 28-4). Between these layers is a thin film of serous fluid that allows the visceral layer to move on the parietal layer without friction during normal ven-

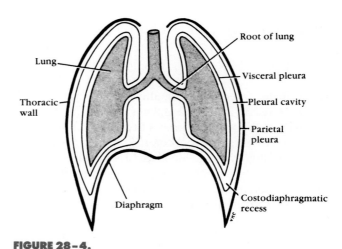

**FIGURE 28-4.**
Position of visceral and parietal pleura with the pleural space. (Source: R.S. Snell, *Clinical Anatomy for Medical Students* (2nd ed.). Boston: Little, Brown, 1981.)

tilation. Fluid between these two slick surfaces causes movement like two pieces of wet glass, friction free, but the presence of negative pressure causes the surfaces to adhere tightly to each other. The pleurae glide easily over each other but cannot easily be pulled apart. Between the layers is a potential space called the *intrapleural* or *pleural* space.

## Parenchyma of the Lungs

The alveolar ducts, the final generation, are totally lined with alveoli (Figure 28-5). Respiratory exchange of gas (diffusion) takes place only in the alveoli. Therefore, these structures are designated collectively as the respiratory zone of the lungs. Because of their tiny size and large numbers, the alveoli have a volume of about 2500 mL in the adult. They have a diffusing area (surface area) about the size of a tennis court (approximately 70 m²). Each terminal bronchiole supplies its own unit called the *acinus*, consisting of several respiratory bronchioles, each with alveoli arising from its walls. The alveoli in the acinus do not have separate connections with the terminal bronchiole but are of various shapes and are interconnected, resembling a long corridor with adjacent rooms (the alveoli) on each side.

The individual alveolus is one layer of cells thick and is built on a structure of elastin and muscle fibers. Each alveolus communicates with the pulmonary capillary bed to move gases by diffusion across the *alveolocapillary interspace* (Figure 28-6). Interconnecting the alveoli are tiny openings called the *pores of Kohn* (Figure 28-7), which allow air to circulate among the alveoli so within a second or less after inspiration all alveoli in an acinus have the same gas concentration. In young children, the pores of Kohn are few in number and poorly

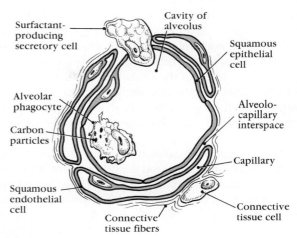

**FIGURE 28-6.**
Representation of single alveolus with surrounding capillaries and other cells. Note alveolocapillary interspace.

developed but with age these structures increase in number and size.

The pores of Kohn are helpful in the event of obstruction of a small airway. In a process called *collateral ventilation*, if an airway smaller than a lobar bronchiole is obstructed, the alveoli that the airway normally supplies can continue to be ventilated by the pores of Kohn.[7] Collateral ventilation appears to be more effective in adults than in young children.

## PULMONARY CIRCULATION

The lung has two blood supplies: the *bronchial* and *pulmonary circulations*. The first consists of the bronchial

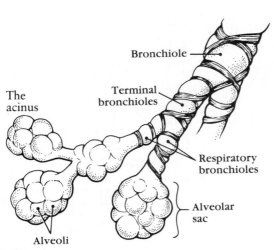

**FIGURE 28-5.**
Termination of the generations of respiratory tubes in alveolar sacs and individual alveoli.

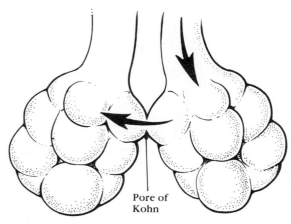

**FIGURE 28-7.**
Schematic demonstration of collateral communication between the alveoli through pore of Kohn.

arteries, which arise in the thoracic aorta and upper intercostal arteries. As a part of the systemic blood supply, these arteries nourish the trachea and bronchi to the level of the respiratory bronchioles. After forming capillary plexuses, some of the bronchial circulation returns through a pulmonary vein to the left atrium, while some empties into the bronchial vein that terminates in the azygos vein which, in turn, empties into the superior vena cava.

The bronchial circulation supplies the lung's supporting tissues, its nerves, and the outer layers of the pulmonary arteries and veins. Normally, it supplies neither the alveolar walls and ducts, nor the respiratory bronchioles. In the event of interruption of the pulmonary circulation, the bronchial circulation can support the metabolic needs of these tissues but the tissues lose the ability to participate in gas exchange.

The second blood supply to the lungs is the pulmonary circulation. From the pulmonary artery, the lungs normally receive the entire output of the right ventricle, approximately 70 cc of blood. Imagine this volume spread over the surface area of the lung (70 m²), and one can see how rapidly diffusion of gases with blood can take place. This blood circulates through the pulmonary capillary bed and then returns to the left heart by way of the pulmonary veins (Figure 28-8).

## MAJOR MUSCLES OF VENTILATION

The major muscle of ventilation, which enlarges the chest cavity, is the *diaphragm*. Innervated by the phrenic nerves, this flat, dome-shaped muscle lowers approximately 1 cm in quiet respiration. In forced inspiration, it may descend as much as 10 cm. This diaphragmatic movement temporarily compresses the abdominal contents. Consequently, the movement of the diaphragm can be impeded by abnormalities in the abdominal cavity, such as ascites and hepatomegaly. If abdominal pain is present, diaphragmatic action is reduced because of the *splinting effect*, a voluntary limitation of ventilatory movements.

The thoracic cavity is further enlarged by an upward and outward motion of the lower ribs accomplished by the *external intercostal muscles*. The upper ribs also move outward. The ribs are attached to the vertebrae in such a way that they rotate on an axis as they are moved by these muscles.

While inspiration normally is an active effort, expiration is a passive one in which the muscles relax and allow the lungs and chest wall structures to return to resting size. The pressure in the thorax gradually rises and air moves out of the lungs.

The *internal intercostal muscles* are used in forced

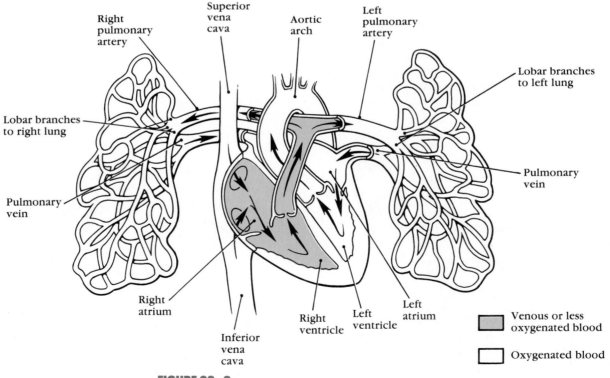

**FIGURE 28–8.**
Circulation from the right heart to the lungs to the left heart.

expiration to stiffen the intercostal spaces during straining. The *muscles of the abdominal wall* are also powerful aids to forced expiration. Normally, they are used only to generate the explosive pressure that is necessary for coughing. They also contract at the end of forced inspiration in synchrony with glottic closure to limit and stop the inspiration abruptly. The *accessory muscles*, scalene and sternomastoid, are used during labored breathing to raise the first two ribs and sternum and increase the size of the thoracic cavity.

## NERVOUS CONTROL OF RESPIRATION

### Nerve Supply

The major nerve supply to the diaphragm is through the two *phrenic nerves*. Each half of the diaphragm is innervated by one of these nerves, which originate mainly from the fourth cervical nerve of the respective side. The 11th cranial nerve, the accessory, innervates most of the larynx and pharynx.

Bronchial smooth muscle is innervated by both *parasympathetic (vagus) and sympathetic nerve supply*. Increased vagal influence causes bronchoconstriction, while increased sympathetic stimulation causes bronchodilation. Any factor that decreases the caliber of the airway (bronchoconstriction) increases resistance and work of breathing, whereas increased caliber of the airway (bronchodilation) has the opposite effect.[16]

The vagus nerve also transmits the appropriate signal to limit inspiration when an overstretch signal is received from the lungs. This reflex, called the *Hering-Breuer reflex*, serves as a protective mechanism to limit lung inflation.

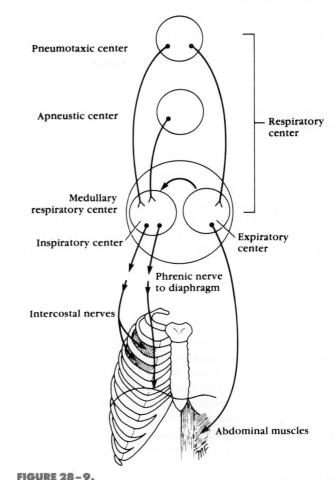

**FIGURE 28–9.**
The medullary inspiratory and expiratory centers. (Source: R.S. Snell, *Clinical Histology for Medical Students*. Boston: Little, Brown, 1984.)

### Respiratory Centers

The nervous system adjusts alveolar ventilation to the demands of the body. This occurs through the *respiratory centers* that are located in the medulla oblongata and the pons. Normally, these areas of the brain regulate ventilatory rate and depth through the chemical signals of carbon dioxide and hydrogen ion levels.

### Central Chemoreceptors

Respiratory neurons located in the medulla oblongata are the major chemosensitive areas (chemoreceptors). Figure 28-9 shows separate areas responsible for inspiration and expiration. The major stimulus for the *inspiratory area* is the carbon dioxide concentration of the

blood. This area also transmits input from the peripheral chemoreceptors. The regular rhythm of the ventilatory effort is generated in the inspiratory area. The effort continues below the conscious level, although the conscious control of breathing always overrides the unconscious.

The *expiratory area* is located in a separate part of the medulla but is usually not active unless there is some respiratory distress. When pulmonary ventilation becomes excessive, the expiratory muscles are activated to aid the expiratory effort. How the interaction occurs between the inspiratory and expiratory areas is not known.[9]

The *pneumotaxic center* is located in the pons and participates continually in the inspiratory effort through directly limiting the tidal volume of air inspired. Activation of this center increases rate of respiration while decreased stimulation decreases the respiratory rate. Another center in the pons, the *apneustic center*, functions in some brain pathology to cause excessive inflation of the lungs with occasional expiratory efforts.

## Peripheral Chemoreceptors

Decreased oxygen tension levels in arterial blood are sensed by the peripheral chemoreceptors of the carotid bodies and aortic arch (Figure 28-10). The hypoxic stimulus, described as 30 mm Hg oxygen tension less than normal for the person, is transmitted to the respiratory center. It results primarily in stimulation of inspiratory neurons and effects an increased respiratory rate through the phrenic nerve. The peripheral chemoreceptors are also sensitive to changes in carbon dioxide and hydrogen but the direct effect of the central respiratory center overrides the sensitivity from the peripheral receptors.[11]

## COMPLIANCE AND ELASTANCE

To understand pulmonary pathology, it is important to understand the concepts of *compliance* and *elastance*, also called *elasticity*. Generally, it can be said that the respiratory system behaves like a pump with a flow-resistive mechanism. The pumping part of the mechanism can be thought of as two separate components: the lungs and the chest wall with its associated structures.

*Compliance* is a measurement of distensibility or how easily a tissue is stretched. In other words, the fewer elastic forces to be overcome to stretch a substance, the more compliant it is. Compliance is measured and recorded by the amount of volume change that results from

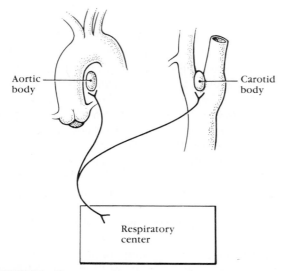

**FIGURE 28-10.**
Decreased oxygen tension causes stimulation of the respiratory center and an increased respiratory rate.

Aortic body

Carotid body

Respiratory center

pressure applied. Compare the blowing up of an old balloon with that of a new one.

Less pressure is needed to make a large volume change in the old balloon while more pressure is required to make a smaller volume change in the new one. Compliance is, thus, important because the more compliant a tissue is, the less pressure is required to stretch it. Using delta ($\Delta$) as a symbol for change, compliance is expressed as follows:

$$C = \frac{V \text{ (liters) } (\Delta \text{ volume})}{P \text{ (cm water) } (\Delta \text{ pressure})}$$

Using the balloon analogy, one can discover which balloon is more compliant if arbitrary numbers are assigned as follows:

| Old Balloon | New Balloon |
|---|---|
| Small pressure needed:  1 | Large pressure needed:  10 |
| Large volume change:   10 | Small volume change:      3 |
| $C = \dfrac{10}{1}$ | $C = \dfrac{3}{10}$ |
| $C = 10$ | $C = 0.30$ |

From these figures, one finds that the old balloon is much more compliant or more easily stretched than the new one. Therefore, it has fewer elastic forces to oppose the stretch than the new balloon.

*Elastance* is the opposite of compliance. Compliance refers to the forces promoting expansion of the lung, while elastic forces are those promoting the return to the normal resting position or original shape. Compliance and elastance are closely related in pulmonary dynamics. The lungs inherently tend to be elastic, so without normal aids to expansion, they will tend to collapse. Compliance refers to the amount of force necessary to produce the volume change or stretch. The amount depends on the elastic forces at work. A highly compliant rubber band, for example, has few elastic forces, while a less compliant (thicker) rubber band has more.[3] The thick rubber band takes more work to stretch it and returns much more readily to its original shape than the thin one. Therefore, the thick rubber band is less compliant and more elastant than the thin one. The following formula is used to calculate elastance:

$$E = \frac{\Delta \text{ pressure (P)}}{\Delta \text{ volume (V)}}$$

The chest wall also has the properties of elastance and compliance but they differ from those of the lungs. To illustrate this difference, one can imagine that the lungs and chest wall could be separated but remain as living and moving structures retaining all of their properties. Each of the two structures could be separated from the pull of the other and could seek its own resting size at an equilibrium between elastance and compliance. In the case of the chest wall freed from the lungs, it would seek a much larger resting size than when it was attached to the lungs. Without the inward pull of the lungs, the chest wall would be abnormally large.

On the other hand, the lungs separated from the chest wall would tend to relax to a much smaller size than when they rested against the chest wall. They have more elastic recoil than might be expected from the amount of elastin and fiber they contain. This is because of a meshlike network, the structure of which itself increases elastic recoil. This arrangement is termed *nylon stocking elasticity*.

Taking the properties of the lungs and chest wall together, it can be seen that elastance of the lungs prevents overdistention of the thorax, while chest wall compliance prevents collapse of the lungs. Contraction of the diaphragm, discussed earlier, lowers that muscle and increases the size of the thoracic cage. All of this creates a negative intrapleural pressure, causing air to move from the atmosphere to the lungs. Relaxation of the diaphragm, a passive process, causes the muscle to move to its resting position, intrapleural pressure to increase, and air to move from the lungs to the atmosphere. These properties account for the fact that expiration is normally a passive process, while inspiration is an active process.

Many diseases alter the compliance and elastance of either the lungs or chest wall but disease need not affect *both* properties of either structure. In general, bronchopulmonary diseases affect lung compliance, while chest wall obesity and diseases of the thoracic skeleton or respiratory nerves affect chest wall compliance. Alveolar edema and atelectasis reduce compliance by reducing the number of inflated alveoli.

Compliance of the lung is increased by emphysema and is somewhat increased in the aged person. Usually, dynamic measurements of compliance are used rather than estimates of elastance, and changes are referred to as *decreased* or *increased* compliance. In the case of pulmonary fibrosis, where there is increased fibrous tissue and stiffening of the lung tissues, compliance is reduced. More pressure than usual is needed to stretch this lung and chest wall system. The total compliance of this lung and chest wall system is then less than normal. The following is a method for calculating *total compliance*:

Normal total compliance = 0.1 L (BTPS)/cm $H_2O$ (during quiet breathing), where *BTPS/cm* $H_2O$ refers to the fact that the measurement is calculated at body temperature, at ambient pressure, and with water vapor saturation.[11]

If a person is being mechanically ventilated, measurements of compliance provide useful objective assessment data. *Dynamic lung compliance* calculated in this way is not entirely accurate because the true calculation requires static conditions. It is accurate enough to be a useful tool for assessing gross changes in total compliance, however. The following method is used to calculate dynamic compliance:

$$\text{Effective dynamic compliance} = \frac{\text{expired tidal volume (mL)}}{\text{inspiratory pressure (cm } H_2O)}$$

The measurement of compliance may be even more useful if related to lung volume. Compliance per lung volume is called *specific compliance*. Decreased specific compliance means that the lung tissue has become more rigid and, in severe cases, the pressures needed to expand the lungs adequately over time are more than the person can produce or maintain. This results in hypoventilation. Many disorders, including obstructions, pulmonary edema, and pneumonia, may decrease both compliance and lung volume. Specific compliance is also related to lung size and is reduced by 50% in pneumonectomy.

## THE MECHANICS OF BREATHING

As stated previously, a particular pressure is necessary to cause a change in the volume of the lungs. Volume can be changed by either a high pressure from outside the body forcing air in or a negative pressure from inside the body causing air to move into the lungs. Normally, humans breathe by using negative pressure.

### Phases of Ventilation

The phases of ventilation involve the movement of the diaphragm and the other respiratory muscles (Figure 28–11). As the diaphragm descends, it enlarges the intrapleural space, which causes a negative intrapulmonary pressure. The air then flows into the lungs to equalize the pressure. The subatmospheric or negative pressure, which is necessary for air to flow into the lungs, is achieved by enlarging the lung and chest cavity. When the chest and lungs enlarge, the pressure inside the thorax is lower than it was before the enlargement. At the end of active effort, the diaphragm relaxes and moves upward, which increases intrapulmonary pressure to above atmospheric level. The air moves passively out of the lungs. The elastic recoil of the lung tissue moves the lung to their resting or unstretched state.

Thus, inspiration is an active process initiated by the contraction of the diaphragm and the outward pull by the intercostals. Air moves from greater to less pressure. Expiration is a passive process that occurs when the respiratory muscles relax and the intrapulmonic pressure increases above the atmospheric level. Even when the system is relaxed, the lungs are continually pulling in and

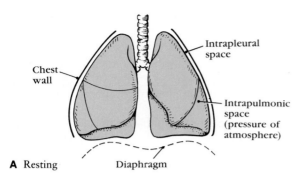

**A** Resting

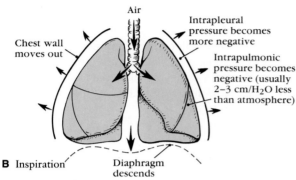

**B** Inspiration

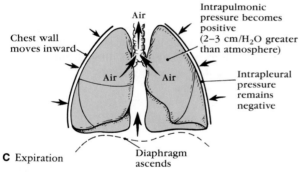

**C** Expiration

**FIGURE 28-11.**
Phases of ventilation. **A.** No movement of air (resting). **B.** Air moves from the environment to the intrapulmonic space (inspiration). **C.** Air moves from the intrapulmonic space to the environment (expiration).

attempting to return to their smaller relaxed size. This process creates a negative intrapleural pressure and explains one of the reasons that air is pulled into the chest when the chest wall is punctured.[13]

## Changes in Airway Size

The size of the airways is also affected by the process of ventilation. The airways are attached to and supported by the lung parenchyma. Since the lungs expand to fill a larger space on inspiration, all of these structures, including the airways and alveolar ducts, are pulled to a larger size. The size of the airways and alveolar ducts is reduced as lung volume decreases during expiration. During

quiet ventilation, some of the smaller airways close during expiration. Because of the effects of gravity, airway closure is more pronounced in the supine position.

## Airway Resistance

During respiration, the volume of the thorax and consequently of the airways is changing. Airways offer resistance to airflow, the amount of which directly affects the amount of pressure needed to move air in and out of the lungs.

Pressure-flow relationships may be quite complex even in simple straight tubes. Because the respiratory tree is a series of branching tubes of varying sizes, the relationships become more complex.

The amount of pressure lost because of friction depends on the flow pattern of the air. The two major air flow patterns are laminar and turbulent (Figure 28-12). In laminar (or streamline) flow, the gas in the airways is like very thin cylinders moving inside each other. The cylinder on the outside moves slowly and each inner cylinder of air moves progressively faster. Gas density has no influence on the velocity of this type of flow. Basically, the gas flows along a straight line with little friction to the molecules. When airway caliber changes, however, the laminar pattern is altered. Additional pressure may be required to reaccelerate the gas and to reestablish a laminar flow pattern. Laminar flow occurs more readily in the small peripheral airways, which are generally straight and smooth.

When flow rates are high or when airways are partially obstructed or collapsed, airflow becomes turbulent. In normal lungs, turbulent flow occurs in the large central airways because of molecular collision and resistance at the sides of the tubes. In turbulent flow, gas density becomes important. The pressure difference for a given flow is reduced by lowering gas density. Much of the airflow in the lungs is probably transitional between turbulent and laminar.[15] The work required for maintaining turbulent airflow is greater than that required to maintain laminar flow.[12]

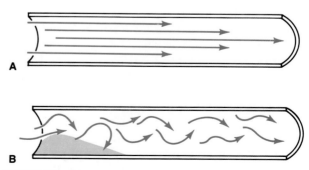

**FIGURE 28-12.**
**A.** Schematic representation of laminar gas flow. **B.** Representation of turbulent gas flow.

Change in airway width greatly alters resistance. When airways widen, resistance is greatly diminished and air flows through easily. When airways narrow, resistance is increased and air moves through them with much more difficulty. It takes more pressure to move air through a narrow airway than a wide one. In the area of the lung where flow is laminar, if airway radius is reduced by one half, resistance is increased by 16 times.[15] This fact has great importance for individuals whose airways are narrowed by bronchospasm or pressure from tumors or infectious processes, as increased airway resistance increases the work of breathing.

Since airways normally widen on inspiration and narrow on expiration, resistance is generally greater on expiration than on inspiration. This normal change in resistance helps to explain why air becomes trapped on expiration in asthma or chronic lung disease.

Although there are many extremely small peripheral airways, they are so tiny that they make little difference in the resistance factors that can be measured. It is postulated that the initial changes of chronic lung disease occur in these airways where they cannot be measured.[21] These airways make up areas called silent zones where diseases can be present without detection.

In normal respiration in the upright position, the bases of the lungs tend to ventilate better than the apices. This has been demonstrated by having a person inhale radioactive xenon gas and monitoring its diffusion with a radiation camera. During the inspiratory phase, the bases undergo a larger change in volume and have a smaller resting volume than the apices. In the supine position, this difference disappears and the ventilations become the same. In abnormalities such as pulmonary edema, the apices tend to ventilate better and the smaller airways in the bases often close.[21]

Airway resistance can be altered by many factors. A sigh or deep inspiration usually reduces resistance, while forced expiration even in the healthy individual increases it. Airway compression is the usual cause of increased resistance during forced expiration; this factor is markedly enhanced in persons with diseased or weakened airway walls.[15] The presence of mucus, or inflammation of the airway, as well as endotracheal intubation, will increase resistance to airflow.

Measurements of resistance are the *forced expiratory volume* in one second (FEV$_1$) and forced vital capacity (FVC) (see p. 576).

## Tissue Resistance

In addition to airway resistance, there is some resistance in the lung and chest wall tissues called *tissue resistance*. Although the frictional resistance of tissue movement cannot be measured directly, it can be calculated. In the healthy, young, adult man, tissue resistance is about 20%

of total pulmonary resistance. Tissue resistance is rarely increased to the point of being limiting by itself. It is increased in pulmonary sarcoidosis, pulmonary fibrosis, diffuse carcinomatosis, asthma, and kyphoscoliosis. Tissue resistance may be particularly high where movement of the thoracic cage is severely limited, as in neurologic disease, musculoskeletal disease, or deformity of the chest structures.

## THE WORK OF BREATHING

The act of breathing requires muscular work to overcome the elastic forces of the lungs and chest wall. Work is also needed to overcome airway and tissue resistance. Initial work is minimal at normal breathing frequency but increases significantly at high breathing frequencies. Resistive work is minimized with a slow, deep respiratory pattern and increases with respiratory frequency. The opposite is true of elastic work. Two thirds of the work of breathing is against elastic forces, prompting the lungs to return to the resting position. Slow, deep breathing greatly increases the work necessary to overcome elastic forces. When the work forces are summarized, respiratory work is the least at a frequency of 14 breaths per minute.

The work of breathing, as described earlier, is proportional to the pressure change times the volume change. Volume change is the amount of air moved in and out with each breath called *tidal volume*. The pressure change is that pressure needed to overcome the *elastic* and *resistive* forces. During quiet breathing, 65% of the work done overcomes elastic forces and 35% overcomes frictional resistance.[12] The elastic forces are mainly the elastic recoil of the chest wall and lungs themselves. Resistive forces are mainly those of airway and tissue resistance.[11]

Respiratory pathology usually alters breathing patterns. The pattern finally adopted by the individual will be the one that requires the least work, although it always requires more work than the normal pattern. For example, if flow resistance increases, the breathing may be slow and deep. If compliance is reduced, a rapid, shallow pattern of breathing may be adopted.

The work of breathing, as in other body work, consumes oxygen. Normally, at rest, respiration accounts for less than 5% of the total metabolic rate. This increases moderately with normal ventilatory changes but with significant respiratory pathology, the work of breathing may increase many times.[11] In advanced disease states, the oxygen cost of ventilation can be 25% to 30% of the total metabolic rate. In this situation, the ventilatory effort may cost the person more oxygen than it delivers and may produce more carbon dioxide than can be eliminated. This progressive process, without appropriate intervention, continues until respiratory failure ensues.

# SUBSTANCES IMPORTANT IN ALVEOLAR EXPANSION

## Surfactant

Surfactant, a phospholipid made up of dipalmitoyl-lecithin, is synthesized in the type II or granular pneumocytes lining the alveolus and is secreted to form a film across the alveolar surface. Surfactant provides surface stability and prevents collapse of the alveolar structures, despite their extreme smallness.[8]

*Surface tension* is the force required to tear liquid apart at the surface where fluid interfaces with air. In the lungs, instead of water surrounded by air, there are millions of air bubbles (alveoli), each with an air-liquid interface. Surface tension can be illustrated by blowing soap bubbles. The pressure required to blow the bubble causes it to distend, but when the pressure is released, the surface tension causes the bubble to collapse.

A deficiency of surfactant results in an increase in the surface tension in the alveolus during expiration that leads to collapse or atelectasis of the alveoli. Amounts of surfactant in the lungs vary according to the diameter of the alveoli. As the alveoli inflate, the surfactant spreads out over the surface of the alveolar membrane. As the alveoli empty, the surfactant layer becomes thicker in relation to the decreased space. Smaller alveoli have a thicker layer while larger alveoli have a thinner layer. This promotes expansion and stability of the alveoli.[9]

To be effective, it is necessary that the surfactant layer be replenished continually. The half-life of pulmonary lecithin is 14 hours, which suggests that active synthesis must continually take place in the type II cells of the alveoli. Normal ventilation seems to be the most important factor in the replenishment of surfactant, which probably is due to the need for oxygen in the production of this substance. Hypoventilation may lead to atelectasis due to diminished renewal of surfactant. A sigh or a deep breath normally provides renewal of surfactant. In hypoventilation, a decreased supply of oxygen with decreased synthesis of surfactant leads to decreased surface tension in the alveoli. The result is widespread collapse of the alveoli.

Surfactant also acts as a waterproof material and may prevent the transudation of fluid across the alveolar capillary membrane during the respiratory cycle. Fluid exudation from capillary to alveolus has been shown to result from a decrease in the surfactant levels. Therefore, surfactant helps keep the alveoli dry. The absence of surfactant leads to a tendency to pull fluid into the alveoli, causing severe pulmonary edema.

Without surfactant, the surface tension of the alveoli would be fixed. Greater pressure would be necessary to keep an alveolus open because its volume and radius would decrease on expiration. Atelectasis would regularly occur at low lung volumes due to collapse of small alveoli. Large inspiratory pressures would be required to reopen the alveoli. The point of collapse is referred to as the *critical closing pressure*; the pressure necessary to open a collapsed alveolus must be enough to overcome surface tension. Without surfactant, each breath would require as much work as the first breath at birth.

Disorders that involve destruction, inactivation, or insufficient production of surfactant cause marked changes in pressure-volume relationships, even without changes in lung or chest wall tissues. Possibly the best known instance of surfactant deficiency is in the *infant respiratory distress syndrome*, also called *hyaline membrane disease*, although the presence of the membrane seems to be secondary to the pathology rather than the cause of the disease. The condition is closely associated with prematurity and appears to be caused by immaturity of the type II cells and deficiency of surfactant synthesis. Further discussion of a similar problem, adult respiratory distress syndrome, appears in Chapter 29.

## Alpha₁-antitrypsin

In the search for the cause of emphysema, clinicians noted that some families had a high frequency of the disease and that the onset was at an early age. The correlation between the absence of alpha₁-antitrypsin (a glycoprotein synthesized by the liver) and familial early-onset emphysema was first studied in 1962 when the level of alpha₁-antitrypsin was found to be genetically controlled.[6] The *homozygous* state is linked with early onset of panlobular emphysema. The *heterozygous* or intermediate state may have greater susceptibility to emphysema, particularly in the presence of repeated inflammatory reactions (see Chapter 3).

Produced by the liver, the primary function of alpha₁-antitrypsin is to inhibit proteolytic enzymes including elastase, collagenase, trypsin, and chymotrypsin. Deficiency of the enzyme decreases the protective action and tips the balance in favor of the proteolytic enzymes and leads to tissue destruction.[14] A widely accepted hypothesis (protease-antiprotease mechanism) for the tissue destruction states that leukocytes and macrophages release proteases, mainly elastases, in the inflammatory response (Figure 28-13). That these proteases are capable of producing emphysema has been well-established in animal research.[5,10] Proteases are neutralized by alpha₁-antitrypsin. Without this inhibitor, these enzymes attack and destroy the alveolar membrane. The protease-antiprotease hypothesis is supported in studies of cigarette smoking. Smokers have increased numbers of neutrophils in the alveoli, and the condensates of smoke stimulate the release of their elastases into the alveoli. Decreased antielastase activity in these individuals results from inhibition of alpha₁-antitrypsin activity by oxidants in cigarette smoke and other factors, resulting in disease

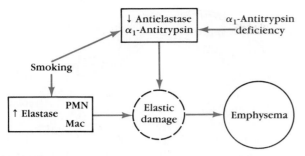

**FIGURE 28–13.**
Protease-antiprotease mechanism of emphysema. PMN = polymorphonuclear leukocytes; Mac = alveolar macrophages. (Source: R.S. Cotran, V. Kumar, and S.L. Robbins, *Robbins Pathologic Basis of Disease* (4th ed.). Philadelphia: W.B. Saunders, 1989.)

in spite of normal levels of alpha$_1$-antitrypsin. Research related to the role of protease-antiprotease imbalance in the development of emphysema in the alpha$_1$-antitrypsin sufficient individual (the most common form of emphysema) is hampered by the fact that the process occurs over 30 to 40 years.[22]

## DEFENSES OF THE AIRWAYS AND LUNGS

### Mucociliary Transport or the Mucociliary Escalator System

The mucociliary escalator system or *mucous blanket*, provides the major defense of the respiratory tract against disease. The components of this system include the goblet cells, which secrete mucus; the ciliated epithelial cells; and mucus, itself.

The *ciliated epithelial cells* of the respiratory tract clear the airways by moving fluid forward (Figure 28-14). These cells line the entire respiratory tract with the exception of the anterior one third of the nose, part of the pharynx, and the alveoli. The surface of each ciliated cell contains about 200 cilia. The cilia move in a continuous wave to carry mucus and debris up the airway to the larynx.

From an upright position, the cilia sweep forward about 30 to 35 degrees and then bend to make their recovery (Figure 28-14B). Comroe[4] likened the movement to strokes of the oars of a boat. Each cilium makes a forceful, fast effector stroke forward, followed by a less forceful, slower stroke backward to get in position again. There is precise timing and coordination of the strokes of a row of cilia; together they move as a wave. Beating in sequential waves as high as 1000 cycles per minute, cilia move mucus up the airway. Because the beat is rapid, the mucous layer does not have time to recoil between beats.

A mucous blanket, made up primarily of the secretions of goblet cells that line the airways and mucus-secreting glands located in the larger ciliated bronchi, moves forward on the cilia. Cells in the alveoli may also contribute secretions to the mucous blanket. The rate of secretion of these cells is difficult to estimate because of resorption and expectoration of mucus. The mucous blanket consists of two layers: the *sol layer*, which surrounds the cilia, and the *gel (surface) layer*. The less viscous sol layer provides a medium in which the cilia can move. With power strokes, the tips of the cilia strike the bottom of the gel layer and propel it toward the mouth to either be swallowed or expectorated.[12] Smoking a cigarette paralyzes the cilia for approximately 30 minutes. Chronic smoking leads to loss of cilia.

The mucous layers retain a constant depth, and the rate of transport of mucus increases rapidly as the mucus moves toward the trachea. Some mucus is resorbed in the large airways to maintain a constant depth with little removed by evaporation because inspired air is virtually 100% saturated with moisture by the time it reaches the pharynx. Mucociliary transport is known to be altered by depressed ciliary activity, changes in the property of mucus, and injury to the respiratory epithelium cells.

*Mucus* is produced primarily by the goblet or mucus-secreting cells that lie along the tracheobronchial tree. In the healthy person, these cells produce an estimated 100 mL of mucus per day, continually humidifying and protecting the respiratory passages. Disease such as chronic bronchitis can increase mucus production to 200 mL or more per day. The mucous covering of the epithe-

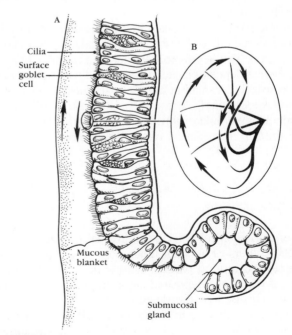

**FIGURE 28–14.**
**A.** The mucociliary escalator. **B.** Conceptual scheme of ciliary movement allowing forward motion to move viscous gel layer and backward motion to take place entirely within more fluid sol layer.

lium in the respiratory passages is normally uninterrupted. Adhesive properties of mucus allow particles that
bind particulates to adhere so that they can move out of
the respiratory tract. Respiratory tract mucus has been
likened to well-engineered paint, which flows easily
when brushed rapidly. But when the brushing ceases, it
sticks to the wall to which it was applied.[12] Mucus is normally composed of water, electrolytes, and several types
of mucopolysaccharides, which account for its viscosity.

## Alveolar Clearance

Mucociliary transport, lymphatic drainage, blood flow,
and phagocytosis all contribute to creating a sterile environment within the alveoli. Macrophage activity is the
principal *alveolar* defense against particulates. These alveolar macrophages regularly scavenge the surface of the
epithelium, digesting foreign material (represented schematically in Figure 28-15).

   Surface tension may play a part in removing particulates from the lungs. Particulates move from an area of
low surface tension to an area of higher surface tension.
Therefore, particulates may move from the environment
of alveolar surfactant to the higher surface tension of the
respiratory bronchioles and up the mucus escalator to
the pharynx.[12]

   Some particulates are removed to perivascular, peribronchial, and hilar lymph nodes. The lymphatics probably transport the particulates engulfed in macrophages.
It is not clear to what extent blood flow is responsible for
alveolar clearance.

   Some particulates remain in the lungs for protracted
periods, while others stay for an intermediate period and
are cleared. This seems to depend on a number of factors, such as deposition site, nature of the particulate, and
host resistance. A small number of particulates remain in
the lungs indefinitely. Those such as asbestos, silica, and
carbon may stimulate fibroblast proliferation and over
time, this can create severe restrictive pulmonary disease.

## Deposition of Particulates
## in the Airways

Under normal conditions, an individual inspires 10,000
to 12,000 liters of air daily. Each liter of urban air may
have several million particles suspended in it, the majority of which are deposited along the respiratory tract
and are cleansed by the defenses of the lung. Particles
smaller than 0.5 $\mu$m in diameter usually remain suspended in inhaled air and are expelled from the lungs
during expiration.

   The first site of deposition of particulates in the airway is the nose (Figure 28-16). Particulates larger than

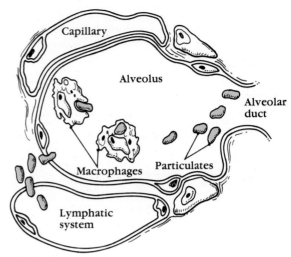

**FIGURE 28–15.**

Alveolar clearance effected by macrophage ingestion of particulate matter, particles traveling in the alveolar duct, lymphatic clearance of particulate matter, blood flow clearance, and carriage of
particulates within the macrophages.

10 $\mu$m in diameter are filtered out in the nares or trapped
in the nasal mucosa. It is the inertia of large particles that
determines deposition at these sites. Their large mass
and high linear velocity force them to rain out in the nasal mucosa. Together with being filtered, the warming
and moistening of air in the nose allows the defense
mechanisms of the lower respiratory tract to function
more effectively.

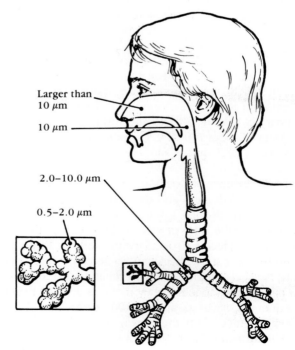

**FIGURE 28–16.**

Deposition of particulates in the airways depends on their size.

As the inhaled air flows over the tonsils and adenoids, particulates are deposited by impaction. These structures are ideally located in the airway to entrap debris that passes over them. In addition to mechanical defense, the tonsils and adenoids may function in the immunologic reaction. Farther along the respiratory tract, linear velocity of air decreases as the surface area increases, which allows particulates in the range of 2 to 10 $\mu$m to be deposited on the mucociliary blanket by sedimentation.

Particulates smaller than 2 $\mu$m reach the alveoli by gravitational forces and, to a lesser extent, by Brownian movement, which describes the random movement of molecules due to thermal energy. The particulates are removed primarily by mucociliary transport and phagocytosis. Smaller particles may present more of a threat to the lungs than larger ones because they penetrate more deeply and remain longer in the tissue.

Together with size, the aerodynamic properties of particulates and deposition sites must be considered. Asbestos particles up to 300 $\mu$m have been shown to reach the lung periphery where, because of their aerodynamic properties rather than their size, they behave as particles of about 1 $\mu$m.[15] This explains why asbestos often severely damages the distal portions of the lung.

## Reflexes of the Airways

The respiratory tract is equipped with reflexes that rid it of debris and protect it from inhaled foreign substances. As is true of other mechanisms, hypoactivity or hyperactivity of these reflexes creates conditions that are detrimental to the host.

The *sneeze reflex* is one of the defenses against irritant materials. Particulates or irritants stimulate sensory receptors of the trigeminal nerves, resulting in the sneeze response. The sneeze is characterized by a deep inspiration, followed by a violent expiratory blast through the nose.

The *cough reflex* is important in clearing the trachea and large bronchi of foreign matter. Irritants cause different impulses to be carried by the vagus nerve to the medulla. Conscious control can also initiate the cough mechanism. The cough reflex initiates a deep inspiration. The glottis then closes, the diaphragm relaxes, and the muscles contract against the closed glottis. Maximum intrathoracic and interairway pressures are produced that cause the trachea to narrow. When the glottis opens, the large pressure differential between the airways and the atmosphere, coupled with tracheal narrowing, create airflow through the trachea at velocities as high as 75 to 100 miles an hour.[9] This is very effective in propelling secretions toward the mouth. While the cough is more effective in clearing the major airways, it also may help clear the peripheral airways through a milking action created

by the high intrathoracic pressures. This may deliver secretions from the peripheral airways to the main bronchi for expulsion by coughing.

Together with other mechanisms, reflex *bronchoconstriction* protects the upper and lower airways from mechanical and chemical irritants. Both cough and reflex bronchoconstriction are initiated in the subepithelium of the airways by receptors sensitive to irritants. For example, when the receptors are exposed to dust, the reflex narrowing of the airways, along with cough, increases the linear velocity of airflow and assists in the removal of dust from the airways. Reflex bronchoconstriction also protects the alveoli from harmful fumes and prevents gases from entering the pulmonary circulation.

Removal of gases from the inspired air depends on their solubility in water. Highly soluble gases, such as sulfur dioxide and acetone, are removed in the upper respiratory tract. Less soluble gases, such as nitrous oxide and ozone, reach the peripheral lungs. This accounts for the observation that sulfur dioxide inhalation results in bronchitis while nitrous oxide inhalation may lead to pulmonary edema. The protection offered by reflex bronchoconstriction is dose-related and time-related, which means that if exposure to the toxic fumes is brief or of low concentration, reflex bronchoconstriction may protect the lungs.

## DEFENSES AGAINST INFECTION

## Defense Against Microbial Agents

Invasion of the lungs by microbial agents presents special problems in defense. Microorganisms have the ability to replicate themselves and, conceivably, one organism could multiply and completely permeate lung tissue. The defenders against infectious agents must act quickly to kill the organisms before they have sufficient opportunity to multiply, which can be in minutes to hours.

Under normal circumstances, the alveolar macrophage system is the primary bactericidal mechanism for clearing infectious agents from the lungs.[10] The *alveolar macrophages* ingest bacteria at such a rapid rate that the majority are destroyed in situ. The rate of bacterial killing in the lungs exceeds the rate at which the bacteria are transported out of the lungs. This has been demonstrated by radioactive tracer-labeled bacteria. In 24 hours, 30% to 40% of the radioactivity is cleared but nearly all bacteria are killed. This is known as *net bacterial lung clearance*. Three factors contribute to this process: (1) physical transport of bacteria out of the lung; (2) in situ bacterial killing; and (3) bacterial multiplication.[17]

The rate of bactericidal activity by the macrophages is influenced by different bacterial strains. For example, *Staphylococcus aureus* is removed at a faster rate than *Proteus mirabilis*. Some organisms are readily inactivated by phagocytosis while others appear resistant to this process. *Klebsiella pneumonia* and *Pseudomonas aeruginosa* are slowly killed in the lungs, resulting in a net increase, rather than a net clearance, of these organisms.[17]

Conditions in the metabolic environment, such as hypoxia, acidosis, and high levels of cortisol, slow net bacterial lung clearance. Ethyl alcohol and tobacco smoke have been shown to depress clearance but all organisms are not depressed equally. For example, alcohol completely suppresses the killing of *P. mirabilis* but not of *S. aureus* or *Staphylococcus albus*. This selective action on the alveolar macrophages has important clinical ramifications. In chronic obstructive lung disease, mixed flora are constantly present in the respiratory tract. Yet, one predominant organism will be responsible for lung infection when it occurs.

Acute viral infections predispose the host to bacterial infections in the lungs. Viruses appear to interfere with alveolar macrophages and suppress their bactericidal ability. The greatest susceptibility appears between the sixth and 10th day after the acute viral infection, during which time superimposed bacterial pneumonias frequently develop.

The dynamics of different responses to bacteria, fluctuations in host resistance, and environmental changes may permit one or another organism to multiply at any given time.[1] All of these factors influence the fate of the microorganism, whether it remains in a localized area or is disseminated throughout the body.

## Immunologic Defense

Closely associated with the macrophage system is the *immunologic defense of the lungs*. The cells involved in the specific immune response are described in Chapter 14. These include the T lymphocytes (thymic-dependent) and B lymphocytes (bone marrow-derived), which in a complex, interacting pattern provide immunity and defend the body against foreign invasion.

Specialized B lymphocytes become immunoglobulin-secreting plasma cells that assist the macrophages in inactivating infectious material. This action is called the *humoral response* and involves five classes of immunoglobulins: IgG, IgM, IgA, IgD, and IgE. The first three classes are important in the control of infectious diseases. Both IgM and IgG provide the primary and secondary antibody responses against pathogens by facilitating opsonization and phagocytosis of bacteria.

Two types of IgA have been identified: *secretory* and *serum*. Secretory IgA is the major immunoglobulin on the surfaces of the mucous membranes. On the respiratory mucosa, IgA protects the lungs against viral and bacterial invasion. It may inhibit the ability of the organisms to adhere to the mucosal surfaces. Persons with chronic bronchitis often have low levels of IgA, which apparently results in a high frequency of recurrent pulmonary infections.[18]

The T lymphocytes provide for cell-mediated immunity. They play a major role in attracting macrophages to the site of an infection. Tuberculosis is an excellent prototype for understanding this response. Inhaled tuberculosis bacilli travel from the lungs to the lymph nodes, where the macrophages engulf, process, and concentrate the antigens of the bacilli. A few T lymphocytes bearing receptors for tuberculin antigens react with the bacillus and undergo multiplication. These T cells circulate back to the lungs and release chemical mediators that induce macrophages and other leukocytes to kill the bacteria. The presence of *Pneumocystis carinii* pneumonia is found only in the immunocompromised host, especially in the acquired immune deficiency syndrome (AIDS). *P. carinii* has emerged as the leading opportunistic pathogen in persons with AIDS who have depressed T cell function.[20]

Humoral and cell-mediated immunity function together to protect the body from infection. Both are essential for maximum defense.

## Interferon

Interferon is a protein that inhibits viral replication. It appears to be produced and regulated within the cells. Cells react to viruses by producing interferon, which causes unaffected surrounding cells to synthesize another protein that protects the cells by preventing viral replication. All cells seem to produce interferon when exposed to a virus but viruses differ in their ability to act as interferon inducers. It is thought that lymphocytes assist the host to counteract viruses, and these lymphocytes have the ability to produce interferon. Because of this, it has been suggested that interferon may be the mediator of the cellular immune response with certain viruses.[1]

Interferon may also be important in protecting the organism against bacteria and tumors. It has been used experimentally in the treatment of cancer and in viral infections in immunosuppressed individuals.

## NORMAL GAS EXCHANGE

Oxygen makes up about 21% of the atmospheric air and most of the remaining 79% is nitrogen. Carbon dioxide in the atmosphere is only a minute percentage (approximately 0.02%) and minuscule amounts of other trace gases, such as argon, neon, and helium, are present.

## Oxygen Transport to the Tissues

The oxygen tension, or partial pressure of oxygen at sea level, is equal to the barometric pressure of 760 mm Hg multiplied by the fraction of oxygen in dry air (20.93%), which equals 159 mm Hg. As the inspired air is warmed and humidifed in the upper airways, however, it is diluted by water vapor, and this causes the oxygen tension to fall to 149.3 mm Hg. The inspired air is then further diluted by carbon dioxide in the lower airways and alveoli. Factors that lower inspired oxygen concentration or that raise alveolar carbon dioxide levels also lower alveolar oxygen levels and hence lower arterial blood oxygen tension, which may reduce the delivery of oxygen to the tissues. Table 28-1 displays the blood gas pattern seen when normal arterial blood is drawn for analysis.

Oxygen is delivered by a linked chain of transfers from the atmosphere to the alveoli to the blood and then to the tissues and cells of the body. It diffuses from areas of higher partial pressure to areas of lower pressure. It is transported initially from the air of the atmosphere to the larger airways by movements of the diaphragm and chest wall that cyclically lower the intrathoracic pressure. This results in air moving in and out of the lungs (*ventilation*) and then being delivered by the smaller peripheral airways to the alveoli (*distribution*). Air then crosses the alveolar-capillary membrane (*diffusion*) and is carried in the plasma, bound chemically to hemoglobin. During *perfusion*, blood is delivered through the pulmonary capillary system past the alveoli for the purpose of gas exchange. At the capillary level, it diffuses into the tissue fluid surrounding the cells and then to the cells themselves, where it is metabolized.

Oxygen is essential for cellular metabolism and the cells have no capability to store it. Without constant delivery of oxygen, tissue hypoxia and anaerobic metabolism result. *Tissue hypoxia* is defined as inadequate critical oxygen tension to meet the needs of the cell. *Critical oxygen tension* is that cellular oxygen tension which causes mitochondrial dysfunction.[19]

Tissue hypoxia is not synonymous with *arterial hypoxemia*, which refers to decreased oxygen tension in the arterial blood. Tissue hypoxia and arterial hypoxemia may exist simultaneously or independently of each other. Arterial hypoxemia can be measured by measuring arterial blood gas. Tissue hypoxia cannot be directly measured but is assessed on the basis of clinical signs and symptoms.

The relationship between arterial and tissue oxygenation is explained in large part by the relationship between hemoglobin and oxygen. Oxygen and carbon dioxide diffuse across a membrane along a gradient from higher pressure to lower pressure. Most of the oxygen is transported to the body cells in chemical combination with hemoglobin. *Hemoglobin* is a complex spheric molecule that is made up of four heme groups, each of which is enfolded in a chain of amino acids. Each heme group can combine with an oxygen molecule, which gives hemoglobin the capability of carrying four oxygen molecules per hemoglobin molecule. Hemoglobin combined with oxygen is called *oxyhemoglobin* while oxygen-free hemoglobin is called *reduced* hemoglobin (see Chap. 19).

In the adult, normal hemoglobin levels range from 12 to 16 g per dL of blood. It has been found that 1 g of hemoglobin fully saturated can carry 1.34 mL of oxygen. Each milliliter of blood with an oxygen tension of 100 mm Hg can carry about 0.03 mL of dissolved oxygen. This means that 100 mL of blood with a hemoglobin of 15 g and 100% saturation has an oxygen content of about 20.4 mL of oxygen, which is expressed as *volumes percent*. A very small percentage of oxygen is carried dissolved in the plasma but hemoglobin is by far the most important method of oxygen transport in the blood.

## *Oxyhemoglobin Dissociation Curve*

The relationship between oxygen and hemoglobin is nonlinear. The affinity of hemoglobin for oxygen has been plotted on an oxyhemoglobin dissociation curve, an S-shaped curve (Figure 28-17). It is derived by plotting oxyhemoglobin saturation (the percentage of hemoglobin that has combined with oxygen) against the oxygen tension (mm Hg) to which it is exposed. Because oxyhemoglobin dissociation is readily reversible, the curve reflects the ease with which hemoglobin gives up oxygen, as well as the ease with which it takes up oxygen. This is important because, to a large extent, oxygen delivery to the tissues depends on the ease with which hemoglobin gives up its oxygen once it reaches the tissues.

In studying the oxyhemoglobin dissociation curve, it is readily apparent that it is initially very steep and then flattens. The upper portion of the curve is flat, showing that when the oxygen tension ($PO_2$) is 70 mm Hg or above, hemoglobin becomes nearly fully saturated. When the available oxygen begins to fall below 60 mm Hg, the degree of saturation also falls rapidly. Note in Figure

**TABLE 28-1.**
ARTERIAL BLOOD GAS VALUES

| SUBSTANCE | VALUES |
|---|---|
| Oxygen | |
| Tension ($pO_2$) | 75–100 mm Hg breathing room air |
| Saturation ($SAO_2$) | 96–100% of capacity |
| Carbon dioxide | |
| Tension ($pCO_2$) | 35–45 mm Hg |
| pH | 7.35–7.45 |
| Bicarbonate ($HCO_{3-}$) | 22–26 mEq/L |
| Carbonic acid ($H_2CO_3$) | 1.05–1.35 mEq/L (always 3% of $PCO_2$) |
| Base excess/deficit | +2/−2 |

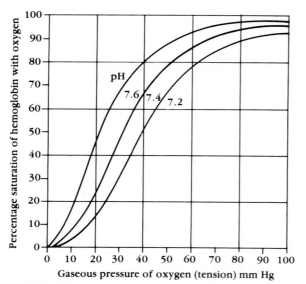

**FIGURE 28–17.**
The oxyhemoglobin dissociation curve.

28-18 that when the $PO_2$ falls to 40 mm Hg, the saturation of hemoglobin is 75%, or approximately the level of venous blood. At 20 mm Hg $PO_2$, the saturation is 35%, which will not sustain life.

Many factors alter the affinity of hemoglobin for oxygen. An increase in hemoglobin affinity for oxygen makes the curve shift to the left and oxygen is given up less readily to the tissues. Alkalemia, hypothermia, and hypocarbia are among factors that can cause a leftward shift. Conversely, acidemia, hypercarbia, and hyperthermia reduce the affinity of hemoglobin for oxygen and cause, by inference, increased oxygen availability to the tissues, noted on the curve as a shift to the right. This is a desirable situation permitting the $O_2$ demands of a person with increased metabolism to be more easily met. Figure 28-18 shows the effects of pH, $pCO_2$, and body temperature on the affinity of hemoglobin for oxygen.

The factors that affect tissue oxygenation are summarized in Box 28-1. Oxygen content of arterial blood is determined by a combination of alveolar oxygenation,

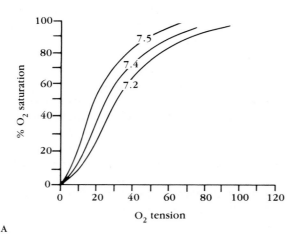

A

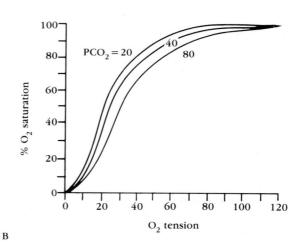

B

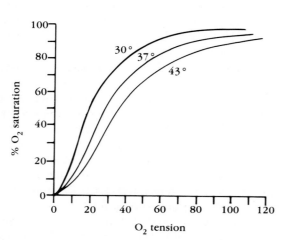

C

**FIGURE 28–18.**
Effects of (**A.**) pH, (**B.**) $pCO_2$, and (**C.**) temperature on oxyhemoglobin dissociation curve.

## BOX 28-1.
### FACTORS THAT AFFECT TISSUE OXYGENATION

Oxygen tension arterial blood
Hemoglobin content
Hemoglobin saturation
Blood flow to tissues
Diffusion of oxygen to tissues
Diffusion of carbon dioxide
Arterial pH
Body temperature

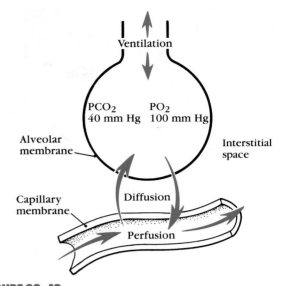

## FIGURE 28-19.
Movement of gases across the alveolocapillary membrane due to ventilation, diffusion, and perfusion.

hemoglobin level and quality, and hemoglobin affinity for oxygen. Oxygen delivery to the tissues depends on the status of the cardiovascular system and regional perfusion. At the tissue level, oxygenation depends on vascularity, diffusion characteristics, and intracellular mechanisms.

## Carbon Dioxide Transport

Carbon dioxide is the product of metabolic combustion and travels the pathway opposite to oxygen, along pressure gradients from tissues to blood to alveoli to airways and then out to the atmosphere. Total amounts of oxygen consumed and carbon dioxide produced are *not* determined by the quantity of ventilation but by the actual *metabolic demands* of the cells. The body at rest requires about 250 cc of oxygen per minute and produces about 200 cc of carbon dioxide per minute as a result of its continuing metabolic cellular requirements. Heavy exercise may increase the production of carbon dioxide up to 20 times this volume.

The normal match between ventilation and perfusion serves the ultimate purpose of supplying oxygen and eliminating carbon dioxide from the cells and eventually from the body. Alveolar ventilation is about 4 liters of air per minute. Cardiac output and resulting tissue perfusion is about 5 liters of blood per minute.

Because carbon dioxide diffuses about 20 times more readily than oxygen, tissue carbon dioxide diffuses rapidly into the venous end of the capillaries with a gradient of less than 1 mm Hg. Venous blood entering the lungs with a $PCO_2$ of 46 mm Hg readily transfers carbon dioxide into the alveoli (Figure 28-19).

With normal alveolar ventilation, alveolar carbon dioxide ($PaCO_2$) of 40 mm Hg is in equilibrium with the resulting arterial carbon dioxide ($PaCO_2$) of 40mm Hg. The levels of both alveolar and arterial carbon dioxide are directly and inversely proportional to the volume of alveolar ventilation (Va). Thus, in alveolar hypoventilation, halving the alveolar ventilation from 4 to 2 liters per minute doubles the $PaCO_2$ from 40 to 80 mm Hg. In hyperventilation, doubling the alveolar ventilation from 4 to 8 liters a minute halves the $PaCO_2$ to 20 mm Hg.[8,9]

Blood carries carbon dioxide in three different forms: (1) 5% or less is transported to the lungs in the *plasma* as *dissolved carbon dioxide*; (2) nearly 70% diffuses into the red blood cells (RBCs) and is carried in the form of *bicarbonate*; and (3) approximately 25% is carried in the RBCs bound to the hemoglobin.[13]

Figure 28-20 illustrates the reaction of carbon dioxide as it is carried dissolved in the RBCs. It is important to note that this is a reversible reaction that occurs rapidly at the tissue level where carbon dioxide is picked up and in the lungs where it is released. Most carbon dioxide diffuses into the RBCs where it is catalyzed in a reaction with carbonic anhydrase and water to form carbonic acid. This carbonic acid immediately dissociates into hydrogen ions ($H^+$) and bicarbonate ions ($HCO_3^-$) that can diffuse back into the plasma or may stay in combination with a positive ion in the RBCs. The excess hydrogen ion formed in this reaction usually binds with the hemoglobin molecule to form hydrogen hemoglobin. If significant amounts of ($HCO_3^-$) diffuse into the plasma, a negative ion is drawn into the RBCs to equalize the electrochemical gradient. This ion is usually chloride and the mechanism of its movement is called the *chloride shift*.[9] This process can provide bicarbonate to the plasma when the pH is decreased. Normally, in the lungs a reverse process occurs very rapidly. Hydrogen is released from hemoglobin and recombines with bicarbonate to form carbonic acid, which dissociates into carbon dioxide and water. Carbon dioxide diffuses out of the RBCs into the alveoli and is blown off in the exhaled air.

Carbon dioxide may react directly with hemoglobin and be carried in a loose chemical bond on the hemoglo-

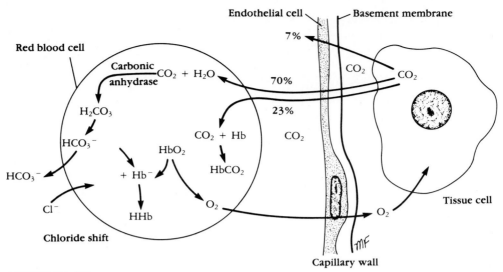

**FIGURE 28–20.**
Methods of carbon dioxide transport in the red blood cell (RBC). Seventy percent of $CO_2$ is combined with $H_2O$ to form carbonic acid and bicarbonate, 23 percent is carried in combination with Hb and 7 percent is carried in the plasma. (Source: R.S. Snell, *Clinical Histology for Medical Students*. Boston: Little, Brown, 1984.)

bin molecule. This is referred to as *carbaminohemoglobin* and accounts for about 25% of the carriage of carbon dioxide to the lungs. In the pulmonary capillary bed, carbon dioxide is simply released to the alveoli and blown off in exhaled air.

## Ventilation-Perfusion Relationships

Arterial oxygenation is affected not only by ventilation but by the *blood supply to the lungs*. Abnormalities in pulmonary blood flow (perfusion) or in relationships between ventilation and perfusion (Va/Q ratio) alter arterial oxygen tension and subsequently, oxygenation of body tissues.

Oxygen and carbon dioxide are exchanged as blood circulates through the pulmonary capillary bed. The capillaries are arranged so each is adjacent to an alveolus. The capillaries are very small, approximating the size of a RBC. The capillary wall and alveolar wall are each only one cell thick so the diffusing membrane is very thin. Gases, therefore, diffuse across the membrane with little difficulty (Figure 28-21).

Each RBC stays in the pulmonary capillary bed about 1 second and exchanges gases with two or three alveoli during this time. Approximately 70 mL of blood is normally exchanging gases at a given moment in the pulmonary capillary bed of an adult, in contrast to the large volume of air that is moved by the alveoli with each breath. This is an important, if temporary, safeguard against oxygen lack. Storing oxygen, even for a few moments, guards against the extra oxygen needs encountered during breath holding.[21]

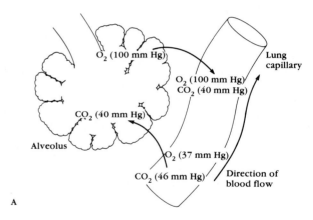

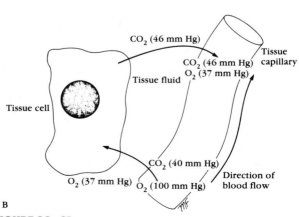

**FIGURE 28–21.**
**A.** Representation of gas exchange at alveolus. **B.** Representation of gas exchange at tissue level. (Source: R.S. Snell, *Clinical Histology for Medical Students*. Boston: Little, Brown, 1984.)

In addition to moving blood to the blood-gas barrier for gas exchange, the pulmonary circulation also provides a reservoir for blood, filters small thrombi from the blood, and traps white blood cells.

Generally, the pulmonary circulation is a low-pressure system with pressures much lower than the systemic circulation. The normal mean pulmonary artery pressure is 14 mm Hg. Since the mean left atrial pressure of the heart is about 5 mm Hg, the driving pressure across the pulmonary bed is only about 9 mm Hg.

Pressure in the pulmonary artery or in the pulmonary capillary bed may be increased by pathology but an increase in one does not necessarily mean a corresponding increase in the other. The pulmonary and systemic circulations are compared in Table 28-2. Table 28-3 lists the normal pressures within the heart and the pulmonary circulation.

Both acidemia and hypoxemia can stimulate constriction of the pulmonary arteries and, thus, increase resistance in the pulmonary capillary bed. Either of these conditions causes vasoconstriction alone; together they provide a synergistic effect. Once this vasoconstriction occurs and persists for some time, it may cause an adverse effect on the right ventricle because of increased work needed to pump blood into the constricted pulmonary vasculature. Over time, this may lead to right ventricular hypertrophy and subsequent right ventricular failure.

**TABLE 28–3.**

## APPROXIMATE NORMAL PRESSURES IN THE HEART AND PULMONARY CIRCUIT

| LOCATION | PRESSURE (mm Hg) | | |
|---|---|---|---|
| | Systolic | Diastolic | Mean |
| Superior vena cava | | | 6–10 |
| Inferior vena cava | | | 6–10 |
| Right atrium | | | 2–5 |
| Right ventricle | 25 | 0–5 | |
| Pulmonary artery | 25 | 10 | |
| Pulmonary capillary bed | | | 8–12 |
| Left atrium | | | 5–10 |
| Left ventricle | 120 | 0–10 | |
| Aorta | 120 | 80 | |
| Systemic arteriole | | | 30 |

Approximately 10% to 20% of the total blood volume is present in the pulmonary vascular bed at any given time. The bed is capable of accepting several times this amount, which allows it to accommodate variations in cardiac output or blood volume. The distensibility of the bed is accomplished both by dilating pulmonary vessels and by opening closed or unused vessels. Distention of the pulmonary vascular bed reduces pulmonary vascular

**TABLE 28–2.**

## DIFFERENCES BETWEEN PULMONARY AND SYSTEMIC CIRCULATIONS

| FACTOR | PULMONARY | SYSTEMIC |
|---|---|---|
| Pressures | Low (pulmonary artery mean 14 mm Hg) | High (aortic mean 100 mm Hg) |
| Pressure changes | Symmetric and of low magnitude within lungs | Asymmetric and of great magnitude depending on system supplied (eg, renal arteriole pressure much higher than hepatic circulation) |
| Pressure determined by | Arteriolar/alveolar gradient and/or arteriolar/venular gradient | Arteriolar/venular gradient |
| Vascular resistance | One-tenth of that of systemic circulation; can decrease resistance as pulmonary pressure rises | Resistance 10 times that of pulmonary circulation; less ability to lower resistance when pressure rises |
| Capillary support | Capillaries surrounded by gas-filled alveoli; collapse or distend depending upon pressure in and around | Capillaries surrounded by tissue; less tendency to collapse or distend |
| Directing blood flow | System rarely directs blood between regions | Regulates and distributes blood to specific areas throughout body |

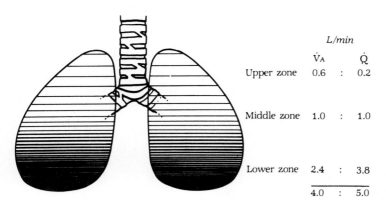

| | L/min | |
|---|---|---|
| | $\dot{V}_A$ | $\dot{Q}$ |
| Upper zone | 0.6 : | 0.2 |
| Middle zone | 1.0 : | 1.0 |
| Lower zone | 2.4 : | 3.8 |
| | 4.0 : | 5.0 |

**FIGURE 28-22.**
V/Q in different zones of the upright lung showing marked variation in values in different areas. In the upright individual, upper segments are relatively hypoperfused and V/Q is high. Lower segments are relatively hypoventilated; V/Q is low. (Source: H.A. Braun, F.W. Cheney, and C.P. Loehnen, *Introduction to Respiratory Physiology* (2nd ed.). Boston: Little, Brown, 1980.)

resistance until its capacity is reached. Then as increases in blood flow cannot be accommodated, pulmonary vascular resistance increases.

Perfusion changes more rapidly from the top to the bottom of the upright lungs than does ventilation. Therefore, the ventilation-perfusion ratio decreases down the lungs (Figure 28-22). If the individual is in the upright position, pulmonary blood flow increases linearly from top to bottom due to gravitational forces. At the apex, the pulmonary arterial pressure is just sufficient to raise minimal amounts of blood to the top of the lungs and perfuse the apices. Capillary pressure is very low. If blood volume is reduced for some reason, such as systemic loss or pulmonary capillary destruction, apical perfusion may decrease or cease altogether.[21]

Blood flow to the lungs changes with exercise and position. With exercise, all areas of the lung receive increased blood flow. When a person lies down, flow from apices to bases becomes uniform.

The concept of regional differences in ventilation has important ramifications for the person with asymmetric lung pathology. An example might be the person whose left lung appears to be radiographically *whited out* by a process such as pneumonia. To maximize ventilation, perfusion, and gas exchange, the person should not be positioned on the left side. Instead, the person should be turned onto his or her right side or back to capitalize on the abilities of the unaffected lung. Arterial blood gas values can be significantly affected with this type of positioning.

As previously mentioned, the perfusion gradient down the lung exceeds the ventilation gradient. To state a Va/Q ratio, ventilation and perfusion must be expressed in the same units. For example, blood flow of 4 liters per minute and ventilation of 5 liters per minute in the average adult male results in a Va/Q ratio of about 0.8:1.0 or 0.8. In the healthy person, the deviation from a ratio of 1 is largely due to anatomic dead space. Normally, a portion of the air inspired does not come in contact with the alveoli and does not participate in gas exchange. This *anatomic dead space* usually remains relatively constant but *alveolar dead space* (where alveolar gas does not

participate in blood-gas exchange) may be significantly altered in pathologic states. The Va/Q ratio is altered in conditions in which alveolar *dead space ventilation* and thus physiologic dead space ventilation are increased. A higher than normal amount of inspired gas is wasted, with the result that a lower than normal amount of inspired gas is exchanged with the blood. To compensate for this wasted ventilation and to maintain normal PaO$_2$ and PaCO$_2$, total ventilation must increase. This moves more inspired gas per minute to improve exchange with blood. If the body is incapable of increasing ventilation and blood flow enough to maintain adequate gas exchange, carbon dioxide retention and hypoxemia may result. In any case, the work of breathing is increased. If the body is incapable of altering ventilation and blood flow to meet this need, altered blood gases, decreased cellular oxygenation, and clinical symptoms occur.[13]

The opposite of dead space ventilation is *shunting*. All cardiopulmonary and pulmonary disease leads to problems with dead space ventilation, or shunting, or both. Shunting refers to an area that is perfused but not ventilated (Figure 28-23). A small amount of shunting (less than 2.5% of cardiac output) is normal; it occurs because not all blood is exchanged at the alveolocapillary line. This accounts for the fact that normal oxygen saturation of hemoglobin in arterial blood gases is 96% to 100%. Pathologic amounts of shunting may be caused by such problems of nonventilation as atelectasis and pneumonia (see Chap. 29).

In shunting, the Va/Q is decreased. Blood returning from the affected areas of the lung mixes with blood returning from the oxygenated areas. This lowers the total level of oxygen in the arterial blood, resulting in a lowered PaO$_2$.[11]

If shunting is not severe, the body can compensate for the amount of carbon dioxide that is not excreted by the shunted areas. Hyperventilation of the unaffected areas can blow off enough carbon dioxide to compensate. Oxygen exchange cannot be compensated for so readily because carbon dioxide is much more diffusible than oxygen. If compensation occurs, it leads to a blood gas pattern of normal PaCO$_2$ with hypoxemia. If the body

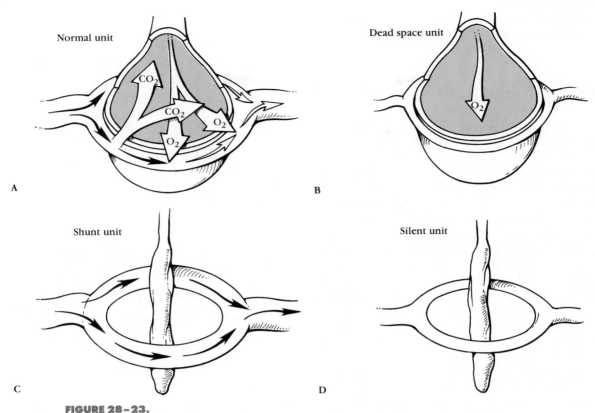

**FIGURE 28-23.**
**A.** Schematic representation of normal alveolar-capillary unit. **B.** Representation of ventilation without perfusion. **C.** Representation of perfusion without ventilation. **D.** Representation of neither perfusion nor ventilation.

is unable to compensate adequately for the carbon dioxide exchange, blood gases show acidemia, hypoxemia, and hypercapnia. A compromised pulmonary or cardiovascular system could lead to loss of ability to compensate for the demands of shunting or other abnormalities.

Both shunt and dead space defects are often referred to as Va/Q mismatching. All other factors being equal, the lung with a Va/Q mismatch is not able to exchange as much oxygen and carbon dioxide as the lung with a normal Va/Q ratio.

## RESPIRATORY REGULATION OF ACID-BASE EQUILIBRIUM

As is described in Chapter 9, the major blood buffers are hemoglobin, the plasma proteins, and the carbonic acid-bicarbonate system. Any increase in carbon dioxide concentration in the blood causes a shift in its pH toward the acidic side; any decrease causes it to shift toward the alkaline side. Therefore, the amount of carbon dioxide present in the blood affects the pH significantly. Carbon dioxide, usually in the form of carbonic acid ($H_2CO_3$), is closely regulated by the physiologic buffer system of the lungs.

If the metabolic rate increases, the rate of carbon dioxide formation increases. Conversely, if the rate of metabolism decreases, the formation of carbon dioxide also decreases. Alveolar ventilation changes according to nervous control of respiration through the *chemoreceptors* in the medulla. These chemoreceptors are extremely sensitive to minute changes in the carbon dioxide level and stimulate an increase or decrease in the respiratory rate. If the blood pH declines to 7.0, alveolar ventilation may increase up to five times above the resting value. An increase in pH to above 7.5 may decrease alveolar ventilation to one half the normal value. Thus, the respiratory rate and depth of respiration physiologically can retain or blow off excess carbon dioxide according to the pH of blood.

The two major alterations in acid-base balance related to pulmonary function are *respiratory acidosis* and *alkalosis*. Respiratory acidosis is always due to some factor that compromises ventilation. Thus, hypoventilation leads to retained carbon dioxide and causes an excess of carbonic acid in the blood. The excess carbon dioxide or hydrogen ion is a powerful stimulus for the central chemoreceptor in the medulla oblongata, which initiates a response increasing respiratory rate and depth.

Respiratory alkalosis results from hyperventilation,

which blows off carbon dioxide, leading to decreased carbonic acid and a shift of the pH to alkaline.

## PULMONARY FUNCTION TESTING

Pulmonary function tests measure many variables, including lung volume. They are important tools in the diagnosis and evaluation of pulmonary status. Spirometric tests have the limitations of recognizing abnormalities only when they are relatively diffuse. Therefore, results of these studies may be normal in early disease states or in localized, rather than diffuse, conditions. When results of a PFT are abnormal, other clinical data must be collected prior to making an accurate diagnosis.[2] The effectiveness of spirometry also is totally dependent on the ability and cooperation of the persons being tested. Pulmonary function study results are evaluated in relation to predicted normals. Tables of norms based on age, sex, and size are used to predict normal values for each person. The tables are not totally reliable because of individual differences among persons.

Pulmonary function tests provide a yardstick in establishing the amount of disability in the course of pulmonary disease. They are used in many settings to diagnose and manage patients with pulmonary or cardiac disability and in epidemiologic surveys for industrial hazards or community disease risks.

Lung contents can be divided into four capacities or compartments, each of which is made up of two or more volumes. Figure 28-24 illustrates how the spirometer is used and the "average" values for the various tests. The *lung volumes* usually are measured as follows:

1. *Tidal volume (Vt)* is the volume of gas moved in and out of the lungs with each breath. The normal Vt ( ± 500 mL) is only a small percentage of the amount of air that the lungs are capable of moving.
2. *Expiratory reserve volume (ERV)* is the additional amount of gas or air that can be forcefully exhaled after a normal expiration is complete ( ± 1200 mL).
3. *Residual volume (RV)* is the amount of air remaining in the lungs after a forced expiration ( ± 1200 mL).
4. *Inspiratory reserve volume (IRV)* is the maximum volume of air that can be inhaled after a normal resting inspiration ( ± 3100 mL).

The *lung capacities* are as follows:

1. *Total lung capacity (TLC)* is the maximum volume of gas that the lungs can hold. All of this gas is not available for exchange because it includes dead space gas. The TLC equals the IRV plus the Vt plus the ERV plus the RV (TLC = IRV + Vt + ERV + RV). Given the figures above, the TLC equals approximately 6000 mL of air.
2. *Functional residual capacity (FRC)* refers to the volume of gas remaining in the lungs at the end of a spontaneous expiration and includes the ERV and the RV (FRC = ERV

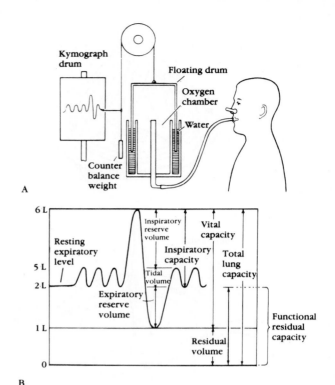

**FIGURE 28-24.**
**A.** Structure of the spirometer used for direct measurement of lung volumes. **B.** Components of lung volume. (Source: E.E. Selkurt, *Basic Physiology for the Health Sciences*, (2nd ed.). Boston: Little, Brown, 1982.)

+ RV). The FRC decreases in conditions such as obesity that affect the chest wall mass. With an increased FRC, it would take more change in the ventilatory rate or more time to reduce a given high carbon dioxide level than with a normal FRC. The FRC equals approximately 2400 mL of air.
3. *Vital capacity (VC)* can be measured either as expiratory or inspiratory. *Expiratory* VC is the maximum volume of gas that can be exhaled after the deepest possible inspiration. Usually expiratory VC equals *inspiratory VC*, which is the maximum amount of gas that can be inhaled after the fullest possible expiration. *Total vital capacity*, therefore, equals IRV plus Vt plus ERV (VC = IRV + Vt + ERV). It equals about 5000 cc in men. In severe obstructive pulmonary disease, the inspiratory VC may be much greater than the expiratory. The VC increases with height, usually is greater in men, and is roughly proportional to lean body weight in young adults. It decreases slightly in the supine position due to the splinting of posterior rib movement and reduced diaphragmatic action. On quiet breathing, the lungs are roughly one third inflated in the supine position and one half inflated in the upright position.
4. *Inspiratory capacity (IC)* is the maximum volume of air that can be inhaled from a resting position. It equals the Vt plus the IRV (IC = Vt + IRV). A reference value for IC is approximately 3600 mL of air.

The RV, TLC, VC, and FRC are not anatomically fixed but depend on elastic characteristics and muscle forces. Increased age changes all lung volumes and capacities by decreasing the elastic recoil. The resting position (at the end of quiet expiration) shifts in the direction of inspiration. Therefore, with age, the RV and FRC increase slightly and the VC decreases. This decrease is partially due to stiffening of the thoracic cage and decreased chest mobility.

Besides lung volumes, the *forced expiratory vital capacity* (FVC) can yield much information in persons with chronic obstructive disease. As shown in Figure 28-25A, the amount of air that can be forced out of the lungs on expiration is measured first at 1 second and then the time it takes to complete the expiratory effort. The 1-second measurement is called the forced expiratory volume in one second ($FEV_1$). The shape of the curve is important in indicating abnormalities. Generally, in obstructive disease, expiration takes much longer than normal and is less complete because of premature airway closure and subsequent air trapping (Figure 28-25B). In restrictive disease, the shape of the curve may be normal but compressed due to the smaller chest volume without changes in the actual air flow (Figure 28-25C). The volume obtained by the $FEV_1$ is placed over the FVC to get a ratio or percentage. Normally, the $FEV_1$/FVC is 80%, which means that 80% of the total volume can be expired in the first second. Generally, in restrictive lung disease, both FVC and $FEV_1$ are reduced. In contrast, obstructive disease tends to reduce the $FEV_1$ much more than the FVC. Mixed restrictive and obstructive patterns are not uncommon and the $FEV_1$ may also be affected by changes in airway resistance, elastic recoil, and in lung compliance.

*Alveolar ventilation* or the amount of gas actually reaching the exchange area refers to the Vt minus the dead space. This is calculated as follows: Va = (Vt − Vd) · f, where *Va* is alveolar ventilation in 1 minute; the dot indicates that it is a timed measurement; and *f* equals respiratory frequency. Dead space is usually estimated from standard tables but it can be approximated to equal an adult's ideal weight in pounds.

*Minute ventilation* is the total amount of air entering or leaving the body per minute. It is calculated by multiplying the Vt by the respiratory rate. It includes the anatomic dead space. The formula for this calculation is as follows: Ve = Vt × R.

# REFERENCES

1. Bellanti, J.A. *Immunology III*. Philadelphia: W.B. Saunders, 1985.
2. Braun, H.A., Cheney, F.W., and Loehnen, C.P. *Introduction to Respiratory Physiology* (2nd ed.). Boston: Little, Brown, 1980.
3. Burrows, B., Knudson, R., and Kettel, L. *Respiratory Disorders, A Pathophysiologic Approach* (2nd ed.). Chicago: Yearbook, 1983.
4. Comroe, J.H. *Physiology of Respiration* (2nd ed.). Chicago: Yearbook, 1974.
5. Cotran, R.S., Kumar, V., and Robbins, S.L. *Robbins' Patho-*

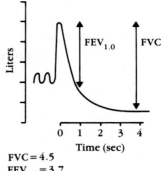

FVC = 4.5
$FEV_{1.0}$ = 3.7
$\dfrac{FEV_{1.0}}{FVC}$ % = 82

A

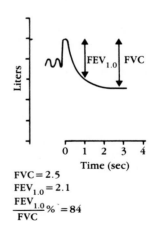

FVC = 3.2
$FEV_{1.0}$ = 1.7
$\dfrac{FEV_{1.0}}{FVC}$ % = 53

B

FVC = 2.5
$FEV_{1.0}$ = 2.1
$\dfrac{FEV_{1.0}}{FVC}$ % = 84

C

**FIGURE 28–25.**
Patterns of forced expiration: **A.** Normal; **B.** Obstructive; **C.** Restrictive. (Source: H.A. Braun, F.W. Cheney, Jr., and C.P. Loehnen, *Introduction to Respiratory Physiology* (2nd ed.). Boston: Little, Brown, 1980.)

*logic Basis of Disease* (4th ed.). Philadelphia: W.B. Saunders, 1989.

6. Eriksson, S. Alpha₁-antitrypsin deficiency: Lessons learned from the bedside to the gene and back again. *Chest* 90:181, 1989.

7. Farzan, S. *A Concise Handbook of Respiratory Diseases* (2nd ed.). Reston, Va.: Reston, 1985.

8. Ganong, W.F. *Review of Medical Physiology* (14th ed.). Los Altos, Calif.: Lange, 1989.

9. Guyton, A.C. *Textbook of Medical Physiology* (8th ed.). Philadelphia: W.B. Saunders, 1990.

10. Kuhn, C., and Askin, F.B. Lung and mediastinum. In J.M. Kissane (ed.), *Anderson's Pathology* (9th ed.). St. Louis: C.V. Mosby, 1990.

11. Levitsky, M.G. *Pulmonary Physiology* (2nd ed.). New York: McGraw-Hill, 1986.

12. Martin, D., and Youtesy, J. *Respiratory Anatomy and Physiology*. St. Louis: C.V. Mosby, 1988.

13. Nunn, J.F. *Applied Respiratory Physiology* (3rd ed.). London: Butterworths, 1987.

14. Scoggin, C. Hereditary lung diseases. In W.N. Kelley (ed.), *Textbook of Internal Medicine*. Philadelphia: J.B. Lippincott, 1989.

15. Seaton, A., Seaton, D., and Leitch, A. *Crofton and Douglas's Respiratory Diseases* (4th ed.). Oxford: Blackwell Scientific, 1989.

16. Selkurt, E. *Physiology* (5th ed.). Boston: Little, Brown, 1984.

17. Toews, G. Pulmonary clearance of infectious agents. In J.E. Pennington (ed.), *Respiratory Infections: Diagnosis and Management* (2nd ed.). New York: Raven Press, 1989.

18. Unanue, E.R., and Benacerraf, B. *Textbook of Immunology* (2nd ed.). Baltimore: Williams & Wilkins, 1984.

19. Walter, J.B. *An Introduction to the Principles of Disease* (2nd ed.). Philadelphia: W.B. Saunders, 1982.

20. Walzer, P. Pneumocystis carinii infections. In W.N. Kelley (ed.), *Textbook of Internal Medicine*. Philadelphia: J.B. Lippincott, 1989.

21. West, J. *Respiratory Physiology: The Essentials* (4th ed.). Baltimore: Williams & Wilkins, 1990.

22. Wewers, M. Pathogenesis of emphysema: Assessment of basic science concepts through clinical investigation. *Chest* 90:190, 1989.

# chapter 29

Darlene H. Renfroe

# Restrictive Alterations in Pulmonary Function

## Chapter Outline

## Learning Objectives

1. Describe compression and absorption atelectasis.
2. Discuss the role of surfactant in the development of atelectasis.
3. Discuss ventilation-perfusion abnormalities in atelectasis.
4. List the organisms and the areas that they affect in upper respiratory tract infections.
5. Discuss the pathophysiology of pneumococcal pneumonia.
6. List the cause of tuberculosis and the role of individual susceptibility in acquiring the disease.
7. Describe the pathophysiology of primary and reinfection tuberculosis.
8. List two causes of aspiration pneumonia and describe the danger of each.
9. Describe in detail the pathophysiology of alveolar and interstitial pulmonary edema.
10. Discuss how restrictive pulmonary disease can occur in a person having a simple rib fracture.
11. Describe the hemodynamics of flail chest abnormality.
12. List and describe disease-induced pleural effusion.
13. Outline the clinical manifestations of pleural effusion.
14. Describe tension pneumothorax.
15. Review central nervous system control of respiration.
16. Indicate how a head injury may affect respiration.
17. Describe the pulmonary problems that may occur with Guillain-Barré syndrome.
18. Describe the onset of respiratory failure in Duchenne muscular dystrophy.
19. Outline the ways in which silicosis and asbestosis can cause a restrictive process.
20. Indicate how particulate matter is cleared in coal worker's pneumoconiosis.
21. Relate the development of pulmonary fibrosis to emphysematous changes in the pneumoconioses.
22. Indicate two chest deformities that may cause restrictive pulmonary disease.
23. Explain why restrictive pulmonary disease can occur in obese individuals, especially those afflicted by the Pickwickian syndrome.
24. Define the role of surfactant in the development of idiopathic respiratory distress syndrome of newborns.
25. Describe in detail the pathophysiology of the adult respiratory distress syndrome.

**TABLE 29-1.**
RESTRICTIVE DISEASES

| CATEGORY | EXAMPLES | PATHOGENESIS | ASSESSMENT OF FINDINGS |
|---|---|---|---|
| Respiratory center depression | Narcotic and barbiturate dependence | Direct depression of respiratory center | Respiratory rate: < 12/min; associated signs of hypoventilation |
| | Central nervous system lesions, head trauma | Injury to or impingement on respiratory centers | Hyper- or hypoventilation; cerebral edema and its signs |
| Neuromuscular | Guillain-Barré syndrome | Acute toxic polyneuritis; intercostal paralysis leads to diaphragmatic breathing; vagal and SNS paralysis lead to reduced ability of bronchioles to constrict, dilate, react to irritants | Reduced negative inspiratory pressure, $V_T$, $V_C$, compliance, breath sounds; hypoxemia, hypercapnia |
| | Duchenne muscular dystrophy | Genetic; thoracoscoliosis; paralysis of intercostals, abdominal muscles, diaphragm, accessory muscles | Pulmonary symptoms appear late; reduced IC, ERV, $V_C$, $V_T$, FRC, compliance $PO_2$; elevated $PCO_2$; abnormal respiratory patterns |
| Restriction of thoracic excursion | | | |
| Thoracic deformity | Kyphoscoliosis, pectus excavatum | Deformity of chest compresses lung tissue and limits thoracic excursion | Reduced breath sounds in affected areas, probably with rales; reduced compliance, TLC, $V_C$, ERV; signs of hypoventilation, hypoxemia, increased work of breathing |
| Traumatic chest wall instability | Flail chest | Fracture of a group of ribs leads to unstable chest wall; reduced intrathoracic pressure on inspiration pulls area in and causes pressure on parenchyma; this increases work of breathing and hypoventilation | Obvious flail, unequal chest excursion, bruising, skin injuries, localized pain on inspiration, dyspnea, reduced breath sounds with rales and rhonchi; reduced compliance, ERV, TLC, $V_C$, $PO_2$ |
| Obesity | Obesity hypoventilation syndrome (Pickwickian syndrome) | Excess abdominal adipose tissue impinges on thoracic space and diaphragmatic excursion; reduced respiratory drive; increased weight of chest restricts thoracic excursion | Somnolence, twitching, periodic respirations, polycythemia, right ventricular hypertrophy/failure; reduced compliance, ERV, TLC, $V_C$, $PO_2$; elevated $PCO_2$; distant breath sounds |
| Pleural disorders | Pleural effusion | Accumulation of fluid in pleural space secondary to altered hydrostatic or oncotic forces | Unequal chest expansion; dullness and reduced breath sounds in affected area; may be constant chest discomfort; dyspnea if amount of fluid large; if over 250 mL, shows on radiographs; if large, bulging of intercostal space |
| | Pneumothorax | Accumulation of air in pleural space with proportional lung collapse | Hyperresonance; reduced breath sounds; tracheal deviation away from pneumothorax; tachycardia; unequal chest expansion; breath sounds reduced or absent; shows on radiographs |
| Disorders of lung parenchyma | Pulmonary fibrosis | Many possible causes: occupational sarcoid, etc. | Reduced compliance, hypoxemia, hypercapnia, and their consequences |
| | Tuberculosis | Bacterial invasion leads to scarring, reduced compliance, and reduced lung function | Visible on films; positive skin test, sputum; malaise, weight loss, fatigue, evening fever with night sweats, cough, hemoptysis |
| | Atelectasis | Obstruction of bronchioles, shrunken airless alveoli; reduced compliance; right-to-left shunting | Dyspnea, tachycardia, cough, fever, decreased chest wall expansion, hypoxemia, radiologic evidence |

(continued)

**TABLE 29–1.**
RESTRICTIVE DISEASES *(Continued)*

| CATEGORY | EXAMPLES | PATHOGENESIS | ASSESSMENT OF FINDINGS |
|---|---|---|---|
| | Adult respiratory distress syndrome (ARDS) | Widespread atelectasis; loss of surfactant; interstitial edema, formation of hyaline membrane. | Dyspnea, tachypnea, grunting, labored respirations, hypoxemia, occasional hypercapnia, cyanosis; radiographs show bilateral patchy infiltrates |
| | Pulmonary edema | Increased pulmonary capillary pressure leads to interstitial and alveolar edema | Hypoxemia, tachypnea; signs of congestive heart failure, radiologic butterfly infiltrates, rales |
| | Aspiration pneumonia | Chemical irritant from aspirant leads to bronchoconstriction, necrosis, and fibrosis of airways | Hypoxemia, signs of ARDS, wheezing, tachypnea, tachycardia |
| | Pneumoconiosis | Inhalation of pollutants, results in scarring, fibrosis, and secondary emphysema | Slow developing pulmonary signs of dyspnea, hypoxemia, hypercapnia, cor pulmonale |
| | Bacterial pneumonia | Virulent bacteria, especially pneumococcal; inflammatory exudate with congestion and edema; poor ventilation in consolidated areas | Rapidly developing fever, chest pain, cough, blood-streaked or rusty-colored sputum; responds well to antibiotic treatment |
| | Viral pneumonia | Rapid onset of inflammation of alveoli and terminal and respiratory bronchioles; secondary bacterial infection common | Respiratory distress with or without fever; much more severe in children with fever, dehydration, and respiratory failure, especially under 2 y of age |

Restrictive pulmonary disease is an abnormal condition that causes a decrease in total lung capacity (TLC) and vital capacity. It involves difficulty in the inspiratory phase of respiration. In this chapter, several conditions are considered, some of which do not precisely fit the above definition but that may lead to significant restriction. Table 29-1 classifies the conditions and their pathogenesis.

## ATELECTASIS

Atelectasis is a very common, acute, restrictive disease that involves the collapse of previously expanded lung tissue or incomplete expansion at birth. It is usually described as a shrunken, airless state of the alveoli.

The two major alterations that occur with atelectasis are compression of lung tissue from a source outside the alveoli and absorption of gas from the alveoli. *Compression atelectasis* may be produced by such conditions as pneumothorax, pleural effusion, and tumors within the thorax (Figure 29-1A). *Absorption atelectasis* occurs when secretions, pus, or mucosal edema in the bronchi and bronchioles obstruct these airways and prevent the movement of air into the alveoli (Figure 29-1B). The air trapped in the alveoli is absorbed and the alveolar sacs collapse. Stasis of secretions in the larger airways, the most common cause of obstruction, provides an excellent medium for bacterial growth and stasis pneumonia. Breath-

ing 100% oxygen will result in more rapid collapse of alveoli since pure oxygen is more readily absorbed than the normal mixture of gases.

Atelectasis is a common postoperative complication due to retained secretions. After surgery, the patient's protective cough response decrease due to medications and pain. An ineffective cough reflex, which diminishes the tidal volume, and decreased sigh mechanism lead to inadequate alveolar expansion. Increased viscosity of sputum results with a tendency for secretions to gravitate to the dependent areas.

Adults are susceptible to atelectasis, particularly in the right middle lobe, which is most vulnerable because of the angle of convergence of its bronchus with the right main bronchus. The right middle lobe also seems to have increased susceptibility to bacterial pneumonia, which tends to flourish in copious pooled secretions.

As noted in Chapter 28, the natural tendency of the lungs is to collapse. In other words, elastic forces are constantly trying to force the lung tissue inward. These forces are opposed by the negative intrapleural forces and chest wall expansion. When airflow into the alveoli is obstructed, alveolar sacs collapse and produce little or no surfactant. Surfactant, due to its short half-life, must be constantly replenished and this requires normal ventilation. To offset the tendency to collapse, collateral communication often occurs through the pores of Kohn. The amount of communication partly depends on the overall

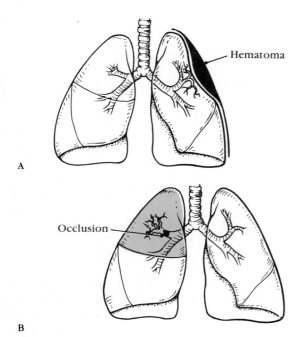

**FIGURE 29–1.**
**A.** Compression of lung tissue by hematoma. **B.** Right upper lobe atelectasis caused by bronchial occlusion.

degree of inflation of the lungs (Figure 29-2). Eventually airways to adjacent alveoli will also be obstructed and this collateral becomes ineffective.

Initially, perfusion to the collapsed airways is not affected so blood shunts by the ineffective alveoli and is not oxygenated. This results in a *perfusion-without-ventilation* shunt or a direct right-to-left shunt across the lungs (Figure 29-3). Therefore, if atelectasis is significant, hypoxemia will also be significant.

One can readily see that the process of atelectasis may occur in many situations, including the obstructive conditions in which a portion of lung tissue is hyperinflated and adjacent sections are collapsed. Clinical manifestations depend on the amount of atelectasis. Rales in the bases and/or diminished breath sounds are common in postoperative atelectasis. A mild case may produce no symptoms but as it progresses or becomes more widespread, dyspnea, tachycardia, cough, fever, and disturbances in chest wall expansion may occur. Blood gas analysis shows hypoxemia when significant atelectasis is present. Hypercapnia and decreased pH may herald a progression toward respiratory failure (see Chap. 31).

## INFECTIOUS DISEASE OF THE RESPIRATORY TRACT

Infectious processes can involve either the upper or lower respiratory tract or both. They may be caused by viruses, bacteria, rickettsia, fungi, or protozoa, and be mild, self-limited, or very debilitating.

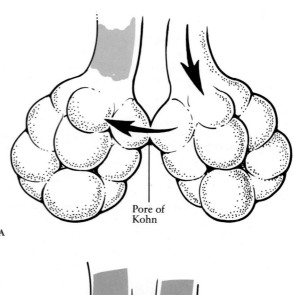

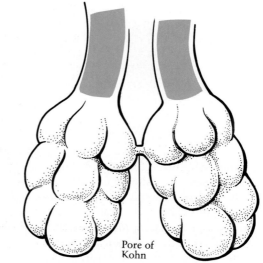

**FIGURE 29–2.**
**A.** Demonstration of collateral circulation between the alveoli through pores of Kohn. **B.** Atelectasis occuring with obstruction to both bronchioles.

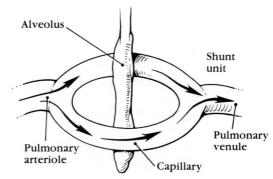

**FIGURE 29–3.**
Demonstration of a right-to-left shunt across the pulmonary bed.

## Upper Respiratory Tract Infection

The upper respiratory tract warms, humidifies, and filters the air. In this process, it is exposed to a wide variety of pathogens that may lodge and grow in various areas depending on the susceptibility of the host. Pathogens may lodge in the nose, pharynx (particularly the tonsils), larynx, or trachea, and may proliferate if the defenses of the host are depressed. The spread of the infection depends on the resistance mounted by the host and on the virulence of the organism. Figure 29-4 shows the defensive anatomy and physiology of the upper respiratory tract, including the mucociliary blanket, which normally provides a very efficient cleansing mechanism for expelling foreign material.

An example of an upper respiratory tract infection is the sore throat (nasopharyngitis) which, if caused by the bacteria beta-hemolytic streptococci, leads to suppuration in the nasopharynx and tonsils that may spread to the sinuses. Susceptible individuals may later develop a reaction to the organism that is manifested as rheumatic fever (see Chap. 25).

Viruses also cause pathology of the upper respiratory tract. Influenza, for example, is characterized by an acute inflammation of the nasopharynx, trachea, and bronchioles and leads to edema, congestion, and necrosis of these structures. The common cold is characterized by an acute inflammation of the nasopharynx, pharynx, larynx, and trachea, resulting in swelling of the mucous membranes and mucopurulent serous exudate. The purulence is due to secondary bacterial infection.

## Lower Respiratory Tract Infection

Infectious processes of the lower respiratory tract can be caused by any of the pathogens that affect the upper respiratory tract. These lead to a variety of pathologic and clinical features depending on host resistance and virulence of the organism.

### Bacterial Pneumonia

Bacterial pneumonia is a common infection that is life-threatening for many of our population, especially the aged, chronically ill, and immunosuppressed. This threat has been drastically reduced by antimicrobial preparations, which have decreased the death rate, shortened the course of the disease, and prevented many serious complications, such as empyema. However, pneumonia remains a common cause of death and is the most common cause among the infectious diseases.[11] Pneumonias

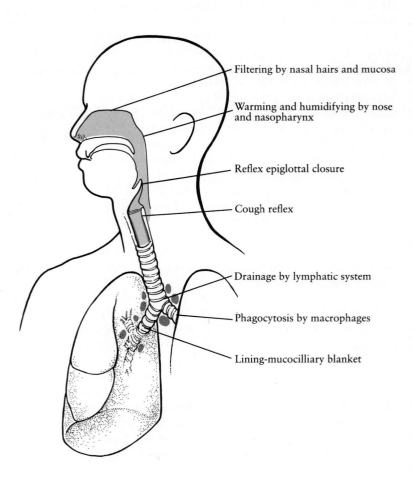

Filtering by nasal hairs and mucosa

Warming and humidifying by nose and nasopharynx

Reflex epiglottal closure

Cough reflex

Drainage by lymphatic system

Phagocytosis by macrophages

Lining-mucocilliary blanket

**FIGURE 29-4.**
Defense of the respiratory tract.

can be classified as either *hospital-acquired* or *community-acquired*. Pneumonia is considered to be hospital-acquired (nosocomial) if the onset is 48 hours or more after the person's admission to the hospital. Community-acquired pneumonia is typically treated on an outpatient basis.

For bacteria to invade the lung successfully, there must be an alteration in net bacterial lung clearance. This alteration may occur as a result of decreased bactericidal ability of the alveolar macrophages, the extreme virulence of the bacteria, or increased susceptibility of the host to infection. Normally, the bactericidal activity of macrophages is extremely important in supplementing the mucociliary escalator system in removing pathogens.

*Pneumococcal pneumonia (Streptococcus pneumoniae)*, once considered synonymous with bacterial pneumonia, is still the most common bacterial pneumonia. It is responsible for 40% to 80% or more of community-acquired pneumonias.[11] It follows an orderly sequence in the lung; its severity depends greatly on host resistance, medical intervention, or both. While infection may develop in healthy persons, underlying factors (eg, malnutrition, alcoholism, aging) seem to increase risk. Pathophysiologically, an initial, acute, inflammatory response occurs that brings excess water and plasma proteins to the dependent areas of the lower lobes. Red blood cells, fibrin, and polymorphonuclear leukocytes (PMNs) infiltrate the alveoli. The bacteria are contained within segments of pulmonary lobes by this cellular recruitment, causing leukocytes and fibrin to consolidate within the involved area.

The inflammatory exudate progresses through stages including *hyperemia* and *red* and *gray hepatization*, and finally terminates in resolution. Hyperemia, also called the stage of congestion, is characterized by engorgement of the alveolar spaces with fluid and hemorrhagic exudate. The outpouring of edema fluid provides a rich medium for proliferation and rapid spread of the organism through the lobe.[17] In the stage of red hepatization, the exudate coagulates, resulting in a red appearance of affected lung tissue, which demonstrates the consistency of liver tissue.

The stage of gray hepatization occurs when the number of red cells in the exudate decreases and they are replaced by increased numbers of neutrophils which infiltrate the alveoli, causing the tissue to become solid and grayish.[1,8] During resolution, PMN leukocytes are replaced by macrophages that are highly phagocytic and destroy the organisms. The exudate liquefies and is coughed up or absorbed.

The filling of alveoli with exudate (consolidation) causes them to become airless. Sustained perfusion with poor ventilation occurs in the consolidated area but this rarely is severe enough to cause a true hypoxemic picture. The infection resolves as exudate is lysed and resorbed by the neutrophils and macrophages. The lymphatics carry exudate away from the site of infection, resulting in restoration of both structure and function of the lung. In some cases, resolution does not occur and the exudate is converted to fibrous tissue, rendering the affected alveoli functionless.[8]

The clinical manifestations of pneumococcal pneumonia include fever, tachypnea, cough, pleuritic chest pain, and production of rusty-colored or blood-streaked sputum. Pneumonia in the elderly individual seldom exhibits these classic findings, and the person may experience lethargy, confusion, and deterioration of a preexisting disease.[10] Complications include pleural involvement with empyema and pleuritis, lung abscess, and bacteremia.[8]

Bacterial pneumonia also may result from other bacteria, including species of *Staphylococcus*, *Streptococcus*, *Klebsiella*, *Pseudomonas*, and *Escherichia coli*. At times, these organisms are opportunistic and lead to additional infection or disease in an already debilitated person. Such imposed conditions often are complicated by abscess formation, empyema, and pleural effusion.

It has been estimated that as many as 15% of deaths in hospitalized persons are due to nosocomial pneumonia. Fifty to sixty percent of all hospital-acquired pneumonias are due to gram-negative bacilli (GNB). Intubation, both short-term for surgery and long-term for respiratory failure, is the single most important factor in the development of nosocomial pneumonia. Antibiotic treatment, predisposing the individual to "super infections" with gram-negative bacilli and gastric alkalinization with either antacid or histamine-2 blockers, resulting in gastric colonization with gram-negative bacilli, are also important risk factors of severe nosocomial pneumonia. Surgery, obesity, concurrent disease, and advanced age also increase the risk.[12]

## Legionella Pneumonia (Legionnaires' Disease)

During a 1976 American Legion convention in Philadelphia, 182 persons developed a strange type of pneumonia resulting in the death of 29 people. By January 1977, the bacterium which caused the outbreak had been identified. *Legionella pneumophila* is a fussy organism that refuses to grow unless its precise requirements are met but proliferates when conditions are right. Initially, it was thought to be a new bacterium but previously unclassified organisms were subsequently recognized to belong to the same family. Legionella pneumonia often occurs in minor sporadic epidemics probably arising by spread from contaminated water such as that from the air conditioning cooling tower of a public building. The disorder is not spread from person to person. Although the disease may be subclinical, symptoms that appear after a 2 to 10 day incubation include flulike complaints, a dry nonproductive cough, and headache that may be severe.

An elevated temperature is common and may be associated with a relative bradycardia. Diagnosis is often difficult in a nonepidemic setting.[4]

### Pneumocystis Carinii Pneumonia

*Pneumocystis carinii* pneumonia (PCP) is the most common pulmonary infection in persons with acquired immune deficiency syndrome (AIDS). It ultimately occurrs in 60% to 80%. The death rate from an acute episode of PCP is 15% to 20%. *P. carinii* is typically classified as a protozoa. The clinical features of PCP include fever, cough, dyspnea, and hypoxemia. Pathologically, there is intraalveolar inflammation that results in a decreased diffusion capacity leading to an early arterial hypoxemia. In 25% of those with PCP, the disease progresses to respiratory failure with an alarming 90% mortality rate.[3]

### Histoplasmosis Capsulatum Pneumonia

Histoplasmosis is caused by the fungus *histoplasmosis capsulatum*, which is released into the air when soil containing the spores is disturbed and inhaled. The organism thrives on bat or bird feces, placing persons who explore caves or work with chickens or pigeons at risk of exposure. Such exposures result in acute disease, which is typically benign. Chronic disease seems related to the presence of preexisting lung and presents symptoms very difficult to distinguish from tuberculosis. Disseminated histoplasmosis mainly affects the immunosuppressed, making it a complication of AIDS. Weight loss, malaise, and fever are common symptoms, and chronic pulmonary fibrosis may occur.[14]

### Mycoplasmal Pneumonia

Mycoplasmal organisms are smaller than bacteria but are not classified as viruses. *Mycoplasma pneumoniae* is a common cause of upper respiratory tract infections, with pneumonia occurring in less than 10% of infected subjects.[14] It normally affects younger individuals with a fibrinous pleurisy and interstitial pneumonia. The disease tends to be self-limited and is rare after age 45 years.[8] However, adulthood does not prevent the disease and it should be considered even in the elderly who have contact with children.

### Viral Pneumonia

Viral pneumonias are frequently mild and self-limited in adults but may be rapidly proliferative and fatal in children. The pediatric diseases include bronchiolitis and pneumonia. Epidemics of this viral infection occur in winter and often affect children under 2 years of age.[8,17] In adults, viral pneumonias may affect the alveolar epithelial cells or the bronchioles. The course may be very rapid, causing an acute clinical picture of respiratory distress with or without fever. A major concern with virus infection is that the terminal and respiratory bronchioles may become damaged and then become susceptible to secondary bacterial invasion that spreads to the surrounding alveoli. The common types of viruses are the influenza, adenovirus, chicken-pox virus, and respiratory syncytial virus.

### Tuberculosis

Tuberculosis (TB) is caused by *Mycobacterium tuberculosis*, which is classified as an acid-fast bacillus because of its staining property. This disease is most common in malnourished and aged persons, and its spread is closely related to host resistance. Frequency of the disease decreased every year from 1953 to 1985 when the decline stopped. Since then, a gradual increase in incidence has been seen, especially in nonwhites, urban poor, and the elderly. In association with human immune deficiency virus, TB is a frequent cause of morbidity. TB is transmitted by droplets from persons with an active tuberculous process. The portal of entry is usually the respiratory system but may be the skin or gastrointestinal tract.

Respiratory transmission begins with inhalation of the mycobacteria. Because of their small size, the organisms are deposited in the lung periphery, usually in the lower part of the upper lobe or the upper part of the lower lobe (Figure 29-5). In primary infection, the mycobacteria become surrounded by PMN leukocytes and inflammation results. After a few days, macrophages replace the PMN leukocytes. Some mycobacterial organisms are carried off by the lymphatics to the hilar lymph nodes. The combination of the initial lesion and lymph node involvement is called the *Ghon complex* but this rarely results in spread to other body organs.

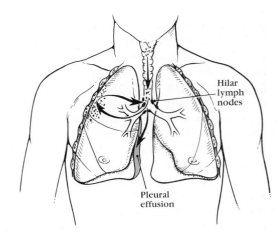

**FIGURE 29-5.**
Tuberculosis organisms are usually deposited in the lung periphery, either in the lower part of the upper lobe or the upper part of the lower lobe. Arrows indicate entrance, deposition, spread to hilar lymph nodes, and pleural effusion.

Macrophages called *epithelioid cells* engulf the mycobacteria. These cells join together to form giant cells that ring the foreign cell. Within the giant cell, caseous necrosis develops, probably a result of acquired hypersensitivity to the organism. Caseous necrosis has a characteristic granular, cheesy appearance. The area surrounding the central core of necrosis is ringed with sensitized T lymphocytes. Fibrosis and calcification develop as the lesion ages, resulting finally in a *granuloma*, which is called a *tubercle*. Collagenous scar tissue encapsulates the tubercle, effectively separating the organisms from the body. The organisms may or may not be killed in the process but sensitized T lymphocytes develop to enhance the bactericidal ability of the macrophages. This results in cell-mediated immunity that usually lasts through life and can be demonstrated by administering purified protein derivative of the bacilli. A positive inflammatory wheal response indicates the presence of memory T cells for the mycobacteria.

After initial exposure, 5% of individuals who inhale the mycobacteria develop clinical tuberculosis. The clinical manifestations vary and include night fever, cough, and symptoms of airway obstruction from hilar node involvement. The disease may spread involving the meninges, kidneys, bones, or other structures. In a small number of individuals, the actual disease develops years after the initial exposure. Mycobacteria that are not destroyed by alveolar defenses lie dormant until a decrease in host resistance allows the original focus to become a source of progressive disease. This *postprimary*, or *reinfection (secondary) tuberculosis* is most frequent in persons who have developed a secondary immunodeficiency, especially from cancer, cirrhosis of the liver, diabetes mellitus, AIDS, or steroid therapy.

## ASPIRATION PNEUMONIA

Aspiration usually refers to the inhalation of gastric contents, food, water, or blood into the tracheobronchial system. Aspiration pneumonia results when the material is propelled into the alveolar system, and most frequently occurs after vomiting or near-drowning.

*Aspiration of gastric contents* is relatively common and is especially associated with impaired consciousness, which includes such conditions as cardiac arrest, seizure, alcoholic intoxication, stroke, and general anesthesia. The gastric contents are very acidic, having a pH of less than three. Aspiration of this material results in chemical irritation and destruction of the mucosa of the tracheobronchial tree. In the lungs, areas of hemorrhage and edema occur, especially in dependent portions.

The severity of the response depends on the person's physiologic status and the quantity and acidity of the aspirant. Nosocomial cases of aspiration are more likely to contain gram-negative bacteria, particularly if the person

is intubated or has received histamine-2 blockers or antacids. Persons receiving nasogastric tube feeding are at particular risk of aspiration.

After aspiration, respiratory distress usually begins abruptly with evidence of bronchospasm, dyspnea, tachycardia, and cyanosis. Severe hypoxemia frequently occurs and may precipitate the adult respiratory distress syndrome (ARDS).[4]

Aspirated foodstuffs may be diagnosed by their content or appearance. Lipid-laden macrophages, for example, indicate that fats have been aspirated and have caused an acute or chronic pneumonia. Foods may cause mechanical obstruction of the airway or chemical irritation of the mucosal lining, especially if they are mixed with acid gastric secretions.

In *drowning* or *near-drowning*, aspiration of water usually causes intense laryngospasm, which is not enough to protect the alveoli from fluid. The result of near-drowning is severe hypoxemia and acidosis. Sea water aspiration may lead to secondary pulmonary edema because of the high sodium content of the water.[5] The close relationship between near-drowning and the ARDS may, in part, be due to washing out of surfactant from the alveolar linings.

## PULMONARY EDEMA

The pulmonary vascular system has a great capacity to accommodate amounts of blood up to three times its normal volume but at a critical pressure point fluid moves across the alveolocapillary line, and pulmonary edema occurs. Pulmonary edema is simply an accumulation of fluid in the tissues (interstitium and alveoli of the lungs).

Understanding the mechanism by which pulmonary edema occurs is enhanced by the understanding of *Starling's equation*. Hydrostatic and osmotic pressures are the major forces that affect movement of water across the capillary membrane (see Chap. 8). The normal hydrostatic pressure in the pulmonary capillaries is approximately 7 to 10 mm Hg. The plasma oncotic pressure is approximately 25 mm Hg. Therefore, the alveoli tend to stay "dry" because the pressures oppose fluid movement into the interstitium and alveoli.[6]

Pulmonary edema fluid is distributed positionally. Normally, when a person is in the upright position, the hydrostatic pressures are higher in the lung bases than at the apices.[6] Acute pulmonary edema may show bizarre patterns of distribution because of variations in the transmission of pleural pressures in different areas of the lungs. However, in chronic pulmonary edema, the fluid tends to accumulate at the lung bases.

Hydrostatic pressure in the pulmonary bed must increase to a level of approximately 25 to 30 mm Hg for pulmonary edema to occur when capillary permeability is normal and the alveolar system is intact. Lymphatic drainage of a few milliliters per hour is usually sufficient to drain any excess protein and fluid that does not move back into the capillary. Lymphatics are probably sparse in the alveolar regions and more plentiful in the peribronchial and perivascular spaces but these can increase lymph-carrying capacity sixfold to tenfold, so that a sustained increase in hydrostatic pressure can be compensated for by increased lymphatic drainage.[18]

The most common cause of pulmonary edema is left ventricular failure. This is discussed in more detail in Chapter 24. Left ventricular failure may be due to such pathology as acute myocardial infarction, hypertension, or mitral valve disease. Pulmonary edema may also result from acute inflammation, poisoning with certain gases (especially chlorine and nitrogen peroxide), pulmonary aspiration of gastric juice, excessive volume overload, some cases of cerebral damage, and smoke inhalation (Table 29-2). The mechanisms for producing edema are different but all result in increased interstitial or alveolar fluid (Figure 29-6).

In the case of pulmonary edema from acute inflammation, the result is alveolar damage, which leads to increased permeability and fluid exudation into the alveoli. In cerebral damage, the reaction of the body is to increase sympathetic nervous system stimulation, resulting in diversion of blood to the lungs, which increases the hydrostatic pressure and causes edema. Fluid overloading is rare with a normal heart but occurs when the fluid volume exceeds the heart's ability to pump it all. Smoke

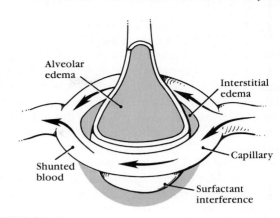

**FIGURE 29-6.**

Schematic representation of interstitial alveolar edema, right-to-left shunting, alveolar edema, and surfactant interference.

inhalation may be injurious due to chemical pneumonitis from the fumes, gases, and particulate matter.[18] Intraalveolar hemorrhage, congested, edematous alveoli, and interstitial edema may all result from this type of injury.

Pulmonary edema due to heart failure occurs when the left side of the heart is no longer able to accept all of the output sent to it from the right side of the heart. As a result, a small amount of blood is dammed back into the pulmonary circulation with each beat of the heart. Gradually, the amount of accumulated blood exceeds the distensible capacity of the pulmonary vasculature. The excess blood in the pulmonary tree increases pulmonary capillary hydrostatic pressure. This pressure increase is

**TABLE 29-2.**
CAUSES OF PULMONARY EDEMA

| CAUSE | CONDITION |
| --- | --- |
| Left ventricular failure (increased pulmonary capillary pressure) | Myocardial infarction, mitral valve disease, cardiomyopathy, mitral stenosis, arrhythmias |
| Alveolar damage and increased capillary permeability | Acute inflammation, sepsis, inhalation of poisonous gases, smoke fumes and particulates, aspiration of toxic fluids |
| Drug-induced injury | Oxygen radicals produced by chemotherapeutic agents; alveolocapillary cytotoxicity due to heroin, oxygen toxicity; allergic reactions causing increased alveolocapillary permeability by antibiotics, inhalants, and iodinated radiocontrast media, for example; hydrochlorothiazide and tocolytic induced, mechanism unknown |
| High altitude | Mechanism unknown, diffuse pulmonary edema |
| Post head injury | Autonomic nervous system stimulation, volume diverted to heart and lungs |
| Fluid overloading | Massive transfusions, intravenous fluids, electrolyte (especially sodium) imbalance |
| Lymphatic obstruction/insufficiency | Diffused carcinomatous infiltration lymphatic channels, silicosis, lymphangitis |
| Decreased colloid osmotic pressure | Hypoalbuminemia from liver, kidney, wasting diseases |

most severe in the dependent areas of the lungs, accounting for increased fluid buildup in the bases.

Pulmonary blood pressure is also raised by reflex vasoconstriction of the pulmonary vessels that occurs in response to hypoxemia, which may result from the decreased cardiac output. As pressure in the pulmonary circulation increases, fluid is forced into the pulmonary interstitial spaces. This phenomenon is known as *transudation*.

Pulmonary edema actually occurs in two stages (Figure 29-7). The first stage is *interstitial edema*, in which fluid accumulates in the peribronchial and perivascular spaces. The lymphatics attempt to decrease this fluid by widening their lumina and increasing the rate of flow. Some widening of the alveolar walls may also occur at this stage. Interstitial pulmonary edema widens the distance between the alveoli and pulmonary capillaries but has little effect on gaseous exchange in the early stages.

The second stage occurs when interstitial hydrostatic pressure is so high that it pushes fluid into the alveoli, resulting in *alveolar edema*. The alveoli fill one at a time, diluting surfactant with the incoming fluid. This reduces the surface tension in the alveoli and predisposes them to collapse. Some alveoli may be compressed by surrounding edematous alveoli, while others are not aerated because the airways that supply them are filled with fluid. When no oxygen is present in the alveoli, right-to-left shunting occurs. Sometimes the shunt may be as large as 50%, resulting in severe hypoxemia and later, hypercapnia. This ventilation-perfusion (V/Q) abnormality is called a *shunt unit* (see Figure 29-6).

The symptoms of pulmonary edema are directly attributable to its pathophysiology. The onset of symptoms may be sudden or gradual. If pulmonary edema is mild and develops slowly, the major symptoms are wheezing, paroxysmal nocturnal dyspnea, and dry cough. When it is

fully developed, there is dyspnea, orthopnea, wheezing, and productive cough. The person expectorates profuse amounts of sputum that initially may be white and frothy but this becomes pink-tinged or bright red. The pink-tinged fluid results from microvascular leaking of red blood cells. Bloody, frothy sputum comes from pulmonary capillaries that have ruptured under high pressure if the underlying cause is heart failure.[7] Hemoptysis (bloody sputum) also may occur with severe alveolocapillary damage due to toxins, smoke, and so on.

The elastic work of breathing is greatly increased because the accumulated interstitial fluid causes lung stiffening and loss of compliance. This, together with hypoxemia, leads to a pattern of rapid, shallow breathing. The lungs fill with fluid, which causes moist bubbling, rales, and wheezing. Abnormal heart sounds are common due to heart failure. Chest roentgenograms show cardiomegaly and the fluid accumulation appears as confluent patchy opacifications that are concentrated centrally in the lungs, having the appearance of a butterfly or bat's wing.[18] Arterial blood gases reflect the degree of hypoxemia, hypercapnia, or both.

## TRAUMATIC INJURIES OF THE CHEST WALL

Traumatic injuries of the chest wall are common results of automobile accidents or other injuries. The injuries may be simple, such as a rib fracture, or as serious as flail chest abnormality.

The most common chest wall injury is *simple rib fracture*. Because it causes inspiratory pain, there is voluntary splinting, which results in restricted tidal volume and an increased respiratory rate. The victim voluntarily inhibits the urge to cough. The young, previously healthy

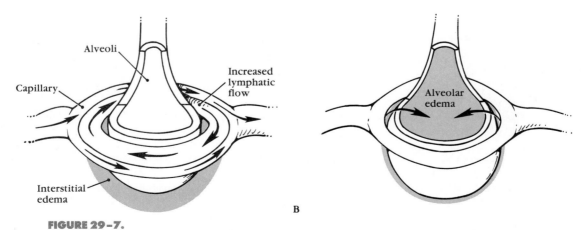

**FIGURE 29-7.**
Illustration of stages of pulmonary edema. **A.** Interstitial pulmonary edema and increased lymphatic flow. **B.** Alveolar pulmonary edema.

person usually tolerates a fractured rib well but a person with underlying pulmonary disease or the aged individual may develop impaired clearance of secretions, atelectasis, pneumonia, or even respiratory failure. The condition is further aggravated if the chest is strapped and narcotic analgesics are used. Chest strapping limits the ability to take a deep breath and, thus, enhances the risk for atelectasis and pneumonia. Compliance and all measurements of lung volume are reduced. The respiratory drive and the cough reflex may be depressed by administration of narcotic analgesics.

If several adjacent ribs in an area are fractured, the stability of that area of chest wall may be lost (Figure 29-8). As a result, on inspiration the intrathoracic pressure is lowered and that area of the chest wall is sucked in. The underlying lung tissue does not expand and gas exchange becomes impaired. Compliance is reduced. When the victim exhales, the affected area of the chest is elevated somewhat because of the increased intrathoracic pressure, creating a paradoxic movement during the ventilatory cycle.

This injury increases the work of breathing and impairs ventilatory efficiency. The more the person works to maintain adequate ventilation, the more paradoxic the respiratory motion. In severe cases, a pendulum movement of the mediastinum may occur with each breath, putting pressure on the otherwise unaffected lung. The paradoxic motion may increase central venous pressure while decreasing venous return to the heart, resulting in decreased blood pressure. Normal breathing is impaired and coughing is impossible, resulting in hypoventilation, hypoxemia, and even respiratory failure. Clinical manifestations of *flail chest* abnormality include the obvious signs of chest wall trauma, "flail" movement with unequal chest excursion, severe dyspnea, pain especially on inspiration, rales, or reduced breath sounds. Chest radiographs show evidence of fractured ribs and blood gases indicate the degree of hypoxemia.

## PLEURAL EFFUSION

Pleural fluid is normally produced in quantities just sufficient to lubricate the surfaces of the visceral and parietal pleura to provide a smooth sliding surface. This small amount of fluid is continually replenished and reabsorbed, maintaining a constant amount in the pleural space.

Pleural fluid accumulation or effusion may result from disease or trauma. Conditions that may lead to fluid accumulation include neoplasms, infections, thromboemboli, and cardiovascular and immunologic defects. Thoracic trauma may cause bleeding into the pleural space.

Pleural effusions are frequently categorized as transudates and exudates. Generally, inflammatory diseases and those of tissue destruction produce exudates with a specific gravity of above 1.017 and a high concentration of protein and lactic dehydrogenase (LDH). Transudates, which are produced by diseases such as congestive heart failure, show lower values for these components with protein below 3.5 g per dL and LDH below 200 units.[1]

The accumulation of pleural transudates is sometimes referred to as *hydrothorax*. If the effusion contains purulent material, it is called *empyema*. If empyema ultimately leads to fibrous fusing of the lung and chest wall, it is called *fibrothorax*. If the pleural fluid contains blood, it is called *hemothorax*.

Fluid in the intrapleural space occupies space and displaces lung tissue by reducing the amount of lung expansion possible by direct pressure on the tissue, resulting in compression atelectasis (Figure 29-9). It may cause a mediastinal shift, which puts pressure on the opposite lung as well. Compliance decreases, altering ventilation and perfusion on the affected side. When fluid is removed from the pleural space, lung tissue reexpands, allowing ventilation and perfusion to return to normal.

Clinical manifestations depend on the rate of effusion. A hemothorax from a ruptured thoracic aneurysm,

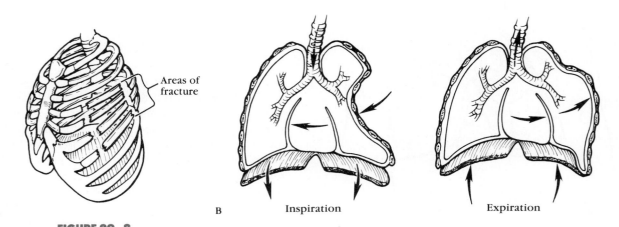

**FIGURE 29-8.**
**A.** Chest wall injury that can produce flail chest abnormality. **B.** Physiology of flail chest abnormality resulting in paradoxical breathing.

A

B                Inspiration

Expiration

Areas of fracture

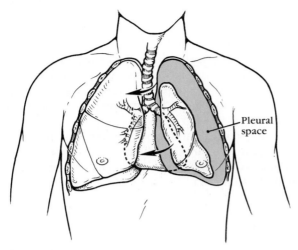

**FIGURE 29–9.**
Pleural effusion. Fluid has collected in the pleural space and displace lung tissue. Also note shift of fluid into the mediastinum and torsion of the bronchus.

for example, causes rapid accumulation of blood, as well as dramatic signs and symptoms of blood loss and a mediastinal shift. In a slower process, 2000 mL of fluid in the pleural space may accumulate before dyspnea is noted. Common symptoms relate to the amount of pulmonary embarrassment and include dyspnea, blood gas abnormalities, cyanosis, and jugular vein distention.

## PNEUMOTHORAX

Pneumothorax occurs when air enters the pleural space (Figure 29-10). Once this takes place, lung tissue is displaced in much the same way as if fluid had entered the space.

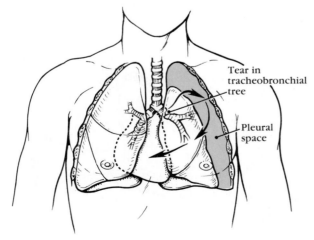

**FIGURE 29–10.**
Pneumothorax. Tear in the tracheobronchial tree has caused air to move into the pleural space; the lung collapses, and the mediastinum shifts to the unaffected side.

Air may enter the pleural space from an opening in the chest wall or from the lungs themselves. Some of the causes of pneumothorax from the lungs include puncture by a fractured rib, spontaneous rupture of a superficial bleb, and rupture of a bleb during vigorous mechanical ventilation. Tracheobronchial rupture due to trauma may also cause pneumothorax. Surgical pneumothorax occurs as a part of every thoracotomy. *Spontaneous pneumothorax* may occur secondary to disease, such as emphysema, when a bleb on the surface of the lung ruptures and releases air into the pleural spaces. Primary spontaneous pneumothorax may occur in healthy, young adults with no preexisting lung disease.

Pressure in the potential intrapleural space is normally lower or more negative than intraalveolar pressure. Therefore, if there is a break in either the integrity of the lung through the visceral pleura or the chest wall through the parietal pleura, air rushes to the area of lowest pressure, the pleural space. This continues as long as the air leak is present. Sometimes air leaks into the pleural space on inspiration but the tissue seals itself on expiration and outward leakage does not occur. This results in *tension pneumothorax*, which is a life-threatening condition of air buildup in the space, with displacement of and pressure on the structures within the mediastinum. This displacement to the opposite side affects the other lung and may impede the venous return to the heart.

Clinical signs of a significant pneumothorax may include dyspnea and chest pain of sudden onset. The trachea may deviate toward the unaffected side, and vesicular or bronchial breath sounds on the affected side may be reduced. Arterial blood gases may reveal acute hypoxemia at the outset. The degree of all of the clinical signs depends on the extent of the pneumothorax. Symptoms of tension pneumothorax include increasing respiratory distress and cyanosis, bulging sternum, distended neck veins, elevated central venous pressure, and hypotension.

## CENTRAL NERVOUS SYSTEM DEPRESSION

The respiratory center is made up of groups of nerve cells that are scattered through the reticular formation in the medulla oblongata. This center is responsible for respiratory rhythm. Although this structure is the major respiratory control, the pons coordinates breathing. The respiratory neural structure in the pons is called the *pneumotaxic center*. Stimulation of this center increases respiratory frequency, while depression slows respiration. The apneustic center also modifies the respiratory pattern. Cranial or cerebral trauma or central nervous system lesions, such as malignancies, brain abscesses, and other conditions may result in injury to or impingement on the mediators of respiration and result in alterations of respiratory patterns.

If head injury affects the pneumotaxic center in the medulla, it may alter the rate, rhythm, and depth of respiration. Apnea may also occur. If central nervous system depression results because of trauma or disease, it frequently leads to decreased ventilatory drive, decreased responsiveness to ventilatory stimuli, and absence of the sigh mechanism. The result is a restrictive pathology that decreases total lung capacity.[15]

Increasing intracranial pressure may lead to pressure on the respiratory center and change in breathing patterns, but more common is hypoxemia in obtunded individuals due to the acute restrictive disease. The airway reflexes are depressed, increasing the risk of obstruction and aspiration.

## NEUROMUSCULAR DISEASES

Many types of neuromuscular diseases may cause impairment of the respiratory system. The most common are summarized in Table 29-3. These can lead to an acute or chronic restrictive pulmonary process.

### Guillain-Barré Syndrome

Guillain-Barré syndrome (acute inflammatory demyelinating polyradiculoneuropathy, Landry's syndrome), which is named after the two persons who originally described it, is an acute toxic polyneuritis. Typically, in its early stages, it is mistaken for a flu syndrome. As it progresses, it is accompanied by varying degrees of muscular weakness and paralysis. This condition appears in some cases to result from an individual hypersensitivity response to a particular type of virus (see Chap. 53). It has been described as occurring after a wide variety of conditions, such as upper respiratory tract infection, mononucleosis, or it may have no antecedent event.[1] The respiratory muscles typically become involved and death, if it occurs, is most frequently due to respiratory complications.

The pulmonary problems in Guillain-Barré syndrome are threefold. First, paralysis of the internal and external intercostal muscles reduces functional breathing ability. Breathing then becomes entirely diaphragmatic, leading to reduced tidal volume, hypoxemia, and hypercapnia. Second, there is paralysis of the preganglionic fibers of the vagus nerve and of the postganglionic fibers of the sympathetic nervous system. Vagal paralysis causes loss of the normal protective mechanisms that respond to bronchial irritation, foreign bodies, and so on. The reflex bronchoconstriction is also lost. Paralysis of the sympathetic postganglionic fibers causes loss of bronchodilation. Third, the gag reflex is diminished or absent.

Pathologically, segmental loss of myelin sheath in the peripheral nerves may occur. Other body areas are also affected by paralysis but this is not life-threatening. Even though the syndrome may last for a few weeks, recovery may be complete if respirations are adequately supported during the acute stage.

Clinical manifestations include the rapid onset of symmetric weakness beginning in the legs and moving upward. The muscles are flaccid and sensory changes may or may not be present.

Muscles of the pharynx and larynx may lead to impaired swallowing and gag reflexes. Cough reflex is depressed and superimposed respiratory infection frequently occurs. Functional return is variable and usually progresses in a reverse pattern with respiratory improvement occurring first, followed by functional improvement beginning in the upper extremities and finally in the lower extremities. Various types of residual impairment have been described.

### Duchenne Muscular Dystrophy

The most common, rapidly progressive type of muscular dystrophy is Duchenne muscular dystrophy (DMD). Two types of the disease are described according to its progression: one form progresses rapidly and the other more slowly. Both forms of DMD are hereditary, being X-linked recessive. Women are the carriers and their sons tend to manifest the disorder (see Chap. 44).

Muscular weakness results, leading to difficulty walking in the early years of life. Thoracoscoliosis and respiratory muscle weakness then progress rapidly. The muscles seem to weaken in this order: intercostals, abdominals, diaphragm, and accessory muscles of respira-

**TABLE 29-3.**
NEUROMUSCULAR DISEASES EXHIBITING
RESPIRATORY INSUFFICIENCY

| DISEASE | EXAMPLE |
|---|---|
| Spinal cord disease | Trauma:<br>quadriplegia<br>paraplegia<br>Poliomyelitis |
| Motor nerve disease | Acute inflammatory demyelinating<br>polyradiculoneuropathy<br>Guillain-Barré syndrome<br>Landry's ascending paralysis<br>Tick-bite paralysis<br>Porphyria |
| Myoneural junction disease | Myasthenia gravis<br>Myasthenic syndrome |
| Muscle-wasting disease | Muscular dystrophy<br>Congenital myotonia |
| Infectious disease | Tetanus |

tion. Despite this respiratory impairment, studies show that alveolar hypoventilation occurs only as an acute or terminal event. As the severity of respiratory involvement increases, many patients are left with the use of only the accessory muscles of respiration. As a result, they may display unusual breathing patterns such as frog breathing, gulping air, head bobbing, and pursed-lip breathing. The final acute respiratory failure is often triggered by an acute respiratory infection.[5]

## RESPIRATORY DISEASES CAUSED BY EXPOSURE TO ORGANIC AND INORGANIC DUSTS

Many organic and inorganic dusts have been identified as being injurious to the lungs. The group of diseases caused by these dusts are collectively called the *pneumoconioses.*

### Silicosis

Silicosis is the oldest and most widespread of the industrial diseases. It results from inhalation of silicon dioxide (silica), the most abundant compound in the earth's crust. Workers with high silica exposure include stone masons, potters, sand blasters, and foundry workers.

The main characteristic of silicosis is fibrosis, which is manifested initially as hard nodules of about 1 mm in diameter in lung parenchyma that increase in size and coalesce as the disease progresses. It usually takes 20 years or more of exposure for silicosis to development interstitial fibrosis and respiratory insufficiency.[8]

Silicosis causes defects in the immune response, both humoral and cellular.[8] The reason for the defects is not known. It is believed that the silica particles cause lysis of the macrophages that ingest them.[8] Immune response may then be responsible for the development of the fibrotic lesion. Among the industrial inhalants, silica is particularly dangerous because of its effect on macrophages, allowing the fibrotic lesions to proceed unchecked. This causes a very severe restrictive pulmonary disease. Silicotic patients have an increased susceptibility to tuberculosis.

### Coal Workers' Pneumoconiosis (Black Lung Disease)

The efficiency of alveolar clearing of coal dust was first demonstrated by Davies.[2] He found that although miners may inhale 100 to 150 gm of dust per year, only 0.5 g could be recovered at autopsy.

Most coal dust (carbon and silica) is removed by the alveolar macrophages with the remainder accumulating in the macrophages. Over time, the dustladen macrophages gather at the perivascular structures and local fibrosis ensues. Early in the disease, the process is manifested as a restrictive process with progressive fibrosis. As the disease progresses, the respiratory bronchioles dilate as a result of traction created by the contracting fibrous tissue. Centrilobular emphysema ensues from the dilatation and destruction of the respiratory bronchioles. The walls of the bronchioles break down, forming single spaces. If exposure to coal dust continues, centrilobular emphysema may occur throughout the lungs. Panlobular or primary emphysema characterized by destruction of the alveoli rather than the more central respiratory bronchioles is not observed in relationship to dust inhalation.

A small percentage of those afflicted with simple pneumoconiosis due to silica or coal dust develop a more complicated form of the disease characterized by massive pulmonary fibrosis and chronic restrictive pulmonary disease. While it is generally accepted that simple pneumoconiosis is related to the quantity and composition of dust retained in the lungs, the etiology of complicated pneumoconiosis is not as clear. It has been suggested that the process involves an immunologic mechanism and that it results in the development of massive fibrotic lesions. In the past, the recovery of the tuberculosis bacillus from the lungs of miners with complicated pneumoconiosis led researchers to conclude that the bacillus was the mediator of the immunologic defense. This theory has not been substantiated and the pathogenesis of the condition remains obscure.

### Byssinosis (Brown Lung Disease)

Bronchoconstriction also occurs due to hypersensitivity to inorganic and organic dusts. An example is byssinosis, which results from long-term exposure to cotton dust. Cotton dust extracts have been shown to cause bronchoconstriction; it is now believed that exposure leads to a discharge of naturally produced histamine, leading to bronchospasm. When histamine stores are depleted, reactivity to cotton dust decreases, which explains the dynamics of byssinosis.

Textile workers experienced chest tightness, low-grade fever, and dyspnea. The symptoms were more pronounced on Monday after a weekend away from the factory. Hence, the syndrome became known as *Monday fever.* Later in the week, the symptoms gradually disappeared. Researchers demonstrated that the textile workers had decreased ventilatory capacities and increased airway resistance during the Monday workday.

Eventually, the worker may complain of chest tightness on subsequent days of the week until symptoms may be accompanied by permanent incapacity. More work in the areas of epidemiology and the mechanisms of bronchial inflammation are necessary before byssinosis will be fully understood.[14]

## Asbestosis

Occupational exposure to asbestos has occurred in the mining, manufacturing, and application occupations. The main use of asbestos is in cement products for construction but it is also used in insulation and fireproofing. The most important health-related effects from asbestos exposure are pulmonary fibrosis and tumors.

The minerals known as asbestos vary considerably in length and diameter. Chrystotile is a type of serpentine fiber with a curly configuration able to shear into many small fibrils. It accounts for 95% of the asbestos in the world. All other forms of asbestos are amphiboles, straight fibers that do not shear. Crocidolite, an amphibole, can penetrate deep into the lung and is implicated in the development of mesothelioma, a cancer of the pleura with a grim prognosis.[9]

Particles of asbestos may be cleared by the mucociliary escalator system or, if deposited deep within the lung parenchyma, may be partially or completely engulfed by alveolar macrophages.[6] Some of the fibers may be removed through lymphatic circulation.

Diffuse pulmonary fibrosis resulting from asbestos exposure is termed *asbestosis* (white lung). The fibrosis initially affects the alveolar walls and gradually involves the interstitium. Prominent symptoms include exertional dyspnea, severe nonproductive cough, clubbing of the fingers, and, ultimately, symptoms of respiratory failure.[6] Rales and restriction of lung inflation are common clinical findings. Pleural changes may be associated and include hyaline plaques that undergo calcification. Recurrent exudative pleural effusions may also be associated.

Although it is uncertain whether asbestos acting alone can cause lung cancer in nonsmokers, asbestos and smoking appear to combine in a multiplicative fashion to produce lung cancer.[9]

## PULMONARY FIBROSIS

Pulmonary fibrosis is a chronic restrictive condition that involves diffuse fibrosis of the lung tissue and results in severe loss of compliance with lung stiffness. As indicated above, fibrosis is frequently due to occupational exposure to substances, such as coal dusts. In cases where the cause is unknown, the disease may be referred to as the *Hamman-Rich syndrome* or preferably, *idiopathic pulmonary fibrosis*.[16] *Sarcoidosis* is another disease that includes among its features a severe, diffuse, pulmonary fibrosis. Severely decreased compliance and diffusing capacity may lead to hypoxemia and cor pulmonale. The cause of sarcoidosis is unknown.

## THORACIC DEFORMITY

Many chest deformities are not severe enough to compromise pulmonary status. Severe deformities do compress lung tissue in one or more areas of the chest, however, and may limit thoracic excursion. Severe *kyphoscoliosis*, in which the body is essentially twisted over to one side, is one example. Another is *pectus excavatum* or funnel chest, in which the lower end of the sternum is caved in because of attachment to the spine by thick fibrous bands. *Pectus carinatum* (pigeon breast)) causes abnormal prominence of the sternum, and the rib structure may limit respiratory movement. Many other deformities also restrict pulmonary status.

In general, severe thoracic deformities compress portions of lung tissue and limit chest expansion, leading to areas of small lung volume and atelectasis. Compliance, TLC, and other volume measurements are reduced. The pulmonary vascular bed in the affected areas is also reduced, resulting in increased work of breathing, alveolar hypoventilation, and the consequences of hypoxemia.

Because of the wide variety of deformities and their effects on pulmonary status, the pulmonary function of each affected person must be assessed carefully. Generally, the effect of pectus excavatum is not severe, while the effect of kyphoscoliosis varies from mild to very severe.

## SLEEP-RELATED BREATHING DISORDERS

The normal effects of sleep on breathing vary according to the stages of sleep (see Chap. 6). During rapid eye movement (REM) sleep, an increased rate and even paradoxical breathing frequently occurs. During nonrapid eye movement (NREM), the rate of breathing may decrease and the rhythm may become irregular.[5]

### Sleep Apnea Syndrome

Sleep apnea is classified as *central*, when airflow ceases due to absence of ventilatory efforts, *obstructive*, when there are chest and abdominal movements with no airflow, or *mixed*, when there is initial loss of ventilatory effort followed by ventilatory efforts without air flow.[5] The pathophysiologic effects depend on the duration and frequency of the apneic episodes. Figure 29-11 illustrates the pathogenesis of the syndrome.

### Obesity Hypoventilation Syndrome

The obesity hypoventilation syndrome is recognized as a part of the spectrum of sleep-related breathing disor-

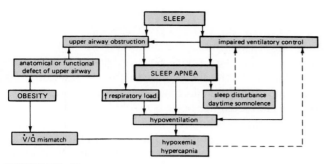

**FIGURE 29–11.**

Schematic demonstration of pathogenesis of sleep apnea syndrome. Note that the abnormalities of both the upper airway and ventilatory control mechanisms are involved. (Source: S. Farzan, *A Concise Handbook of Respiratory Disease* [2nd ed.]. Reston, VA: Reston Publ, 1985.)

ders.[5] Severe obesity may result in restricted ventilation, especially in the supine position. Obesity hypoventilation syndrome (once referred to as *Pickwickian syndrome*) is related to morbid obesity and presents a picture of hypoventilation, somnolence, severe hypoxemia, polycythemia, and cor pulmonale.[5] The term comes from Charles Dickens's description of Joe, a fat boy notorious for falling asleep in *Posthumous Papers of the Pickwick Club*.

Severe obesity causes pulmonary restriction by two means. First, the extreme excess of adipose tissue in the abdomen tends to force the thoracic contents up into the chest and, thus, restricts diaphragmatic excursion. Second, the weight of the chest wall greatly increases the amount of work required to move the chest for inspiration. This is especially true for a woman with pendulous breasts. Severe obesity results in reduced compliance, expiratory reserve volume, TLC, and vital capacity, with all of these reductions due to a great increase in the work of breathing and great susceptibility to respiratory infections. Arterial blood gas studies reveal hypercapnia and hypoxemia.

Obesity alone does not provide an adequate explanation of the disorder since some massively obese persons have the syndrome and some do not. Severely affected individuals have depression of the ventilatory drive and may experience apneic episodes due to upper airway obstruction during sleep. Somnolence is characteristic and may be related to sleep deprivation that occurs as a result of frequent awakenings after the airway-obstructive episodes. Figure 29-12 shows the development of the syndrome.

When hospitalized or immobilized, these obese individuals are prone to develop deep vein thrombosis and pulmonary edema due to their immobility, polycythemia, obesity, and heart failure.

## IDIOPATHIC RESPIRATORY DISTRESS SYNDROME OF THE NEWBORN

Idiopathic respiratory distress syndrome (IRDS) of the newborn is the most clearly understood abnormality that involves surfactant deficiency. The surfactant layer develops late in fetal life, at about the 28th to the 32nd week.

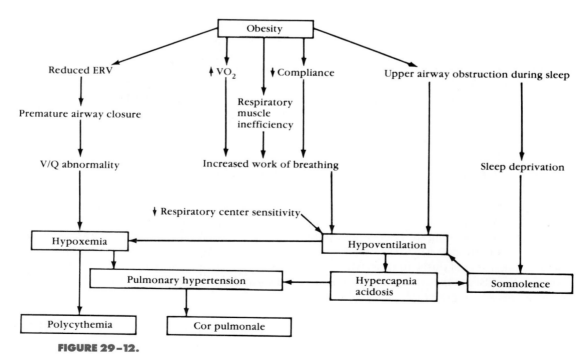

**FIGURE 29–12.**

Pathogenesis and pathophysiology of obesity hypoventilation syndrome. (Source: S. Farzan, *A Concise Handbook of Respiratory Disease*. Reston, VA: Reston Publ, 1978.)

Infants born before the 28th week are at a greater risk for developing acute respiratory distress. This is still a major cause of death in premature infants. The severity of the respiratory distress and the mortality are related to gestational age at birth.

The pathology of IRDS includes inadequate pulmonary expansion and diffuse atelectasis, which is of a primary type because the lungs have never been expanded. Pulmonary vascular resistance increases because of high pulmonary arterial pressures, presumably due to increased pulmonary arteriolar resistance. The resulting increased pressure creates a higher than normal pressure on the right side of the heart. This high pressure perpetuates fetal circulation by keeping the foramen ovale and the ductus arteriosus patent. The IRDS, or hyaline membrane disease, is characterized by large right-to-left shunting that accentuates hypoxemia and hypercapnia in later stages and is increased by hypoxemia, which leads to increased right heart pressures. Ischemic injury in the lung fields causes fluid to leak into interstitial and alveolar spaces and the hyaline membrane to form. Vascular engorgement occurs, the lymphatics dilate, and cellular debris lines the alveoli, with evidence of degenerating epithelial and endothelial cells in the alveolocapillary membrane. The hyaline membranes are apparently composed of plasma, fibrin, necrotic epithelial cells, and amniotic fluid, and contribute to the respiratory distress.[8] Atelectasis is extensive with widespread infiltration of the pulmonary tissue (Figure 29-13).[5]

Clinical manifestations include dyspnea from the first moments of life and rapid, shallow respirations. The lower ribs retract on inspiration and an expiratory grunt usually is heard.

Hypoxemia is characteristic, and an elevated $PCO_2$ with respiratory or metabolic acidosis may complicate the picture.

Treatment measures are improving the prognosis in this condition. Continuous positive airway pressure is used with good results to improve oxygenation, and replacement of surfactant appears to be of benefit. The condition still carries a high mortality rate.

# ADULT RESPIRATORY DISTRESS SYNDROME (ARDS)

ARDS is a condition characterized by severe hypoxemia and progressive loss of lung compliance. It causes severe restrictive disease. It has been known by a number of other names, including shock lung, traumatic wet lung, capillary leak syndrome, postperfusion lung, congestive atelectasis, and posttraumatic pulmonary insufficiency.

This syndrome is never a primary disease but occurs secondary to some other insult to the body. General etiologic factors have been identified and classified as to the mechanism of causation (Table 29-4). The following categories are described: (1) reduced perfusion, (2) increased capillary permeability, (3) direct tissue and capillary insults, and (4) others, with obscure mechanisms. The evolution of the process has been divided into three phases:

1. Injury phase: alveolar capillary and epithelial injury with increased permeability and edema
2. Reparative/proliferative phase: indicated by type II cell regeneration along with interstitial inflammation
3. Fibrotic phase: interstitial collagen accumulation and alteration of the alveolar capillary network.[13]

In the injury phase, the effects of ARDS are similar despite the initiating underlying condition (Figure 29-14). The insult leads to capillary congestion and consequent alteration of capillary permeability. Endothelial cell damage occurs, as does malfunction of the type II pneumocytes. The activity of these cells decreases, which results in decreased production of surfactant. Fluid leaks into the pulmonary interstitium and eventually into the alveoli. This causes stiffening of the lungs (loss of compliance) and dilution of surfactant. The altered compliance and diluted surfactant work together to lead to widespread atelectasis, which causes hypoxemia. In addition, there may be pulmonary interstitial edema and hemorrhage, the formation of alveolar exudate or hyaline membrane, and a predisposition to secondary pulmonary infection. Widespread atelectasis leads to an in-

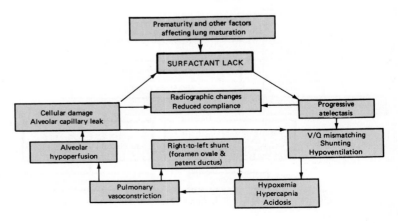

**FIGURE 29-13.**
Pathogenesis and pathophysiology of respiratory distress syndrome of the newborn. The central abnormality is the lack of surfactant. Note several vicious cycles in the scheme. (Source: S. Farzan, *A Concise Handbook of Respiratory Disease* [2nd ed.]. Reston, VA: Reston Publ, 1985.)

**TABLE 29-4.**
UNDERLYING CAUSES THAT CAN PRECIPITATE ADULT RESPIRATORY DISTRESS SYNDROME (ARDS)

**Reduced Perfusion**

Cardiogenic shock

Trauma

Major burns

Fat embolus

Hemorrhage

Severe hypovolemia

**Increased Capillary Permeability**

Sepsis

Pneumonia

Noxious fume or smoke inhalation

Reactions to drugs

Venoms or toxins

Immune complex diseases

Overtransfusion of crystalloids

Uremia

**Direct Tissue and Capillary Insults**

Aspiration of gastrointestinal contents

Rapid decompression

Near-drowning

Oxygen toxicity

Hypoxemia

Fluid overload

Starvation

**Other Mechanisms, Not Well Understood**

High-altitude reactions

Sudden changes in intrathoracic pressure

Central nervous system injuries

Narcotic overdose

Cardiopulmonary bypass

creased right-to-left shunt across the pulmonary capillary bed, causing critical hypoxemia. In the reparative phase, the major manifestations are much like an acute pneumonia with major problems with oxygen saturation and poor pulmonary compliance. New infections may result from life support measures and must be diagnosed and treated. In the fibrotic phase, the goal of treatment is to prevent permanent damage. Most survivors of ARDS have resolution of the fibrosing condition.[1,5]

A special pulmonary pathophysiologic process has been described in individuals exposed to high levels of oxygen for more than 24 to 36 hours. Continuous breathing of high concentrations of oxygen leads to *oxygen toxicity*, with diffuse parenchymal damage resulting in inter-

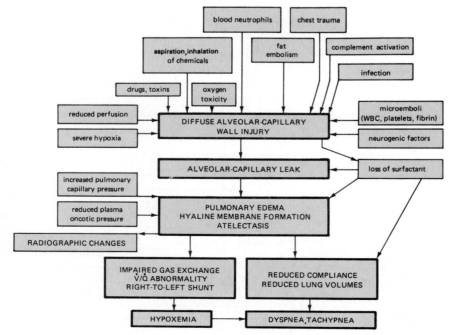

**FIGURE 29-14.**

Pathogenesis and pathophysiology of adult respiratory distress syndrome. (Source: S. Farzan, *A Concise Handbook of Respiratory Disease* [2nd ed.]. Reston, VA: Reston Publ, 1985.)

ference with the production of surfactant and formation of hemorrhagic exudate, with fibrin in the alveoli, alveolar ducts, and respiratory bronchioles. The earliest change is thickening of interstitial spaces with fluid containing fibrin, PMN leukocytes, and macrophages. Two special processes explain the resulting dysfunction. First, breathing pure oxygen results in absorption of the gas from the alveoli. Nitrogen, normally present in atmospheric gas, is not present under these circumstances and, therefore, does not exert its function of keeping the alveoli expanded. The result is alveolar collapse. Second, oxygen has a toxic effect on the surfactant-producing cells so that this vital substance is not produced in adequate quantities. Without adequate surfactant, the alveoli collapse and fluid exudes from the capillaries to the alveolar sacs.

The results of ARDS are progressive hypoxemia and reduced lung compliance, despite the administration of high levels of oxygen. Any individual whose oxygen tension decreases while receiving high concentrations of oxygen should be considered a prime candidate for ARDS.

Those at a high risk for ARDS should be observed for onset of the condition throughout the first 96 hours after insult. No previous history of lung disease may be obtained but persons with previous lung pathology are somewhat more susceptible to development of ARDS. Obvious observable symptoms include extreme dyspnea, tachypnea and grunting, and labored respirations that occur late in the phenomenon. Therefore, the arterial blood gases of persons who develop the disease indicate decreasing $PO_2$ despite oxygen therapy. If the arterial $PO_2$ is not correctable to above 50 when a person is receiving 100% oxygen, there should be a high index of suspicion for this condition. Usually, clinical deterioration is rapid and progressive. Hemoptysis and cyanosis may or may not occur. The hypoxemia and increased work of breathing may initially lead to metabolic acidosis. As respiratory muscles tire, respiratory acidosis occurs. Chest films show progressive, patchy, bilateral infiltrates. The prognosis for affected individuals is improving with the use of positive end-expiratory pressure on volume-cycled ventilators but it still remains at or above 50%. However, if the underlying cause is treatable or self-limiting and treatment is initiated at an early stage, a higher survival rate can be expected.[14]

## REFERENCES

1. Cotran, R.S., Kumar, V., and Robbins, S.L. *Robbins' Pathologic Basis of Disease* (4th ed.). Philadelphia: W.B. Saunders, 1989.
2. Davies, C.N. A comparison between inhaled dust and the dust recovered from human lungs. *Health Phys.* 10:129, 1964.
3. Edelson, J., and Hyland, R. The pulmonary complications of the acquired immunodeficiency syndrome (AIDS). In D. Simmons (ed.), *Current Pulmonology, Vol. 11.* Chicago: Yearbook 1990.
4. Edelstein, P., and Meyer, R. Legionella pneumonias. In J.E. Pennington (ed.), *Respiratory Infections: Diagnosis and Management* (2nd ed.). New York: Raven Press, 1989.
5. Farzan, S.A. *A Concise Handbook of Respiratory Diseases* (2nd ed.). Reston, Va.: Reston, 1985.
6. Fishman, A.P. *Pulmonary Diseases and Disorders* (2nd ed.). New York: McGraw-Hill, 1988.
7. Hurst, J.W. The physician's approach to the patient: Goals and cardiac appraisal. In J.W. Hurst et al. (eds.), *The Heart* (7th ed.). New York: McGraw-Hill, 1990.
8. Kuhn, C., and Askin, F.B. Lung and mediastinum. In J.M. Kissane (ed.), *Anderson's Pathology* (9th ed.). St. Louis: Mosby, 1990.
9. Mossman, B., and Gee, J. Asbestos-related diseases. *N. Engl. J. Med.* 320:1721, 1989.
10. Niederman, M.S., and Fein, A.M. Pneumonia in the elderly. *Clin. Geriatr. Med.* 2:241, 1986.
11. Pachon, J., Prados, D., Capote, F., Cuello, J., Garnacho, J., and Verano, A. Severe community-acquired pneumonia: Etiology, prognosis, and treatment. *Am. Rev. Respir. Dis.* 142:369, 1990.
12. Pennington, J. Hospital-acquired pneumonias. In J.E. Pennington (ed.), *Respiratory Infections: Diagnosis and Management* (2nd ed.). New York: Raven Press, 1989.
13. Rinaldo, J. Adult respiratory distress syndrome. In W. Shoemaker et al. (eds.), *Textbook of Critical Care* (2nd ed.). Philadelphia: W.B. Saunders, 1989.
14. Seaton, A., Seaton, D., and Leitch, A. *Crofton and Douglas's Respiratory Diseases* (4th ed.). Oxford: Blackwell, 1989.
15. Shapiro, B.A., et al. *Clinical Application of Respiratory Care* (3rd ed.). Chicago: Yearbook, 1985.
16. Sodeman, W.A., and Sodeman, T.M. *Sodeman's Pathologic Physiology* (7th ed.). Philadelphia: W.B. Saunders, 1985.
17. Stauffer, J.L., and Carbone, J.E. Pulmonary diseases. In M.A. Krupp and M.J. Chatton (eds.), *Current Medical Diagnosis and Treatment 1990.* Los Altos, Calif.: Lange, 1990.
18. West, J.B. *Pulmonary Pathophysiology: The Essentials* (3rd ed.). Baltimore: Williams & Wilkins, 1987.

# chapter 30

Darlene H. Renfroe

# Obstructive Alterations in Pulmonary Function

## Chapter Outline

▶ **Acute Obstructive Airway Disease**
  **Acute Bronchitis**
  **Asthma**
    Pathophysiologic Mechanisms
    Clinical Manifestations

▶ **Chronic Obstructive Pulmonary Disease**
  **Bronchiectasis**
  **Cystic Fibrosis (Mucoviscidosis)**

**Chronic Bronchitis**
**Pulmonary Emphysema**
  Pathophysiology
  Clinical Manifestations

## Learning Objectives

1. Define *obstructive pulmonary disease*.
2. Differentiate between acute and chronic bronchitis.
3. Describe the pathophysiology of an acute asthmatic attack.
4. Describe the symptoms that result from bronchoconstriction.
5. Discuss pulsus paradoxus.
6. Compare the conditions that are classified as chronic obstructive pulmonary disease.
7. Explain the pathology of bronchiectasis.
8. Describe the signs and symptoms of bronchiectasis.
9. Discuss the basis for the development of cystic fibrosis.
10. List the criteria used in diagnosing cystic fibrosis.
11. List at least two risk factors in the development of chronic bronchitis.

12. Describe the pathophysiology of chronic bronchitis.
13. Differentiate chronic bronchitis from emphysema on the basis of pathologic and clinical features.
14. Relate similarities of chronic bronchitis and emphysema.
15. Describe the interrelationships of all the obstructive pulmonary diseases.
16. Describe the pathology of the different types of emphysema.
17. Discuss the pathophysiologic course of emphysema.
18. Define *hypoxia*, *hypoxemia*, and *hypercapnia*.
19. Explain why polycythemia occurs with chronic obstructive pulmonary disease.
20. Differentiate between compensated and uncompensated respiratory acidosis.

In general, obstructive pulmonary conditions obstruct airflow within the lungs, leading to less resistance to inspiration and more resistance to expiration. This results in prolongation of the expiratory phase of respiration. Many conditions can obstruct airflow; the more prominent ones are detailed in this chapter.

## ACUTE OBSTRUCTIVE AIRWAY DISEASE

The classification of an acute obstructive airway disease is dependent on the episodic nature of the condition. The

two major entities in this classification are *acute bronchitis* and *asthma*. In both, the obstruction is intermittent and reversible.

## Acute Bronchitis

Acute bronchitis is a common condition caused by infection and inhalants that results in inflammation of the mucosal lining of the tracheobronchial tree. The most common infectious causes of acute bronchitis include influenza viruses, adenoviruses, rhinoviruses, and the organism *Mycoplasma pneumoniae*. Increased mucus secretion, bronchial swelling, and dysfunction of the cilia lead to increased resistance to expiratory airflow, usually resulting in some air trapping on expiration.

Bronchitis causes cough and production of large amounts of usually purulent mucus with associated wheezing if there is significant air obstruction. Coughing that produces purulent material may indicate a superimposed bacterial infection if the underlying etiology was viral. Once the stimulus for bronchitis is treated or removed, bronchial swelling decreases and the airways return to normal.

## Asthma

Asthma is an episodic, acute airway obstruction that results from stimuli that would not elicit such a response in healthy individuals. It has been defined as a disorder characterized by recurrent paroxysms of wheezing and dyspnea that are not attributable to underlying cardiac disease or other disease. This means that the person with asthma has a tendency toward bronchospasm as a response to a variety of stimuli. An estimated 5% of the population of the industrialized world is affected by asthma.[2] The common characteristics of all asthmatic reactions are hyperresponsiveness and an inflammatory response in the airways. Between acute attacks, the lungs are usually normal or relatively normal.

While asthma is characterized by wheezing, not all wheezing is asthma. Unilateral localized wheezing may be caused by aspiration of foreign bodies or by a tumor. Other causes include pulmonary emboli, infections, left ventricular failure, cystic fibrosis, immunologic deficiency, and viral respiratory illnesses. Wheezing is always a significant sign that should be investigated.

### Pathophysiologic Mechanisms

The causes of asthma may be divided into two major categories: extrinsic and intrinsic.

*Extrinsic (allergic) asthma* commonly affects the child or young teenager who frequently relates a personal or family history of allergy, hives, rashes, and eczema. Results of skin tests are usually positive for specific allergens, indicating the probability that extrinsic asthma is allergic.

Childhood asthma attacks are usually self-limited and frequently are precipitated by exposure to specific antigens. A major allergen is the mite found in house dust. Seasonal asthma suggests pollen allergies. It is not uncommon for the person who "outgrows" asthma in childhood to develop other allergic manifestations in adulthood. Usually, the asthmatic attacks decrease in severity and frequency as the person matures. However, the more severe the childhood asthma, the less likely it is to remit in adulthood.

The pathophysiology of asthma attacks is related to the release of chemical mediators in an IgE-mast cell interaction (see Chap. 16). This results in constriction of the bronchial smooth muscle, increased bronchial secretion from the goblet cells, and mucosal swelling, all of which lead to significant narrowing of the air passages.[5] It is basically an IgE-associated immune reaction in which the allergen evokes immediate production of histamine and other chemicals by the target organ, which is the lung. The acute respiratory obstruction, resistance to airflow, and turbulence of airflow are due to the following three responses: (1) bronchospasm, which involves rhythmic squeezing of the airways by the muscle bands surrounding them; (2) production of abnormally large amounts of thick mucus; and (3) the inflammatory response, including increased capillary permeability and mucosal edema (Figure 30-1).

Allergy alone as a basis for the attacks is rare, and many mechanisms may be involved. Exercise, infection, and emotional upset are factors that often amplify the symptoms. Whatever the mechanisms, once bronchospasm is induced by one agent, the airway response to superimposed stimuli is greatly enhanced. For example, if a person with a subclinical response to pollen becomes emotionally upset, the airway response to the emotions

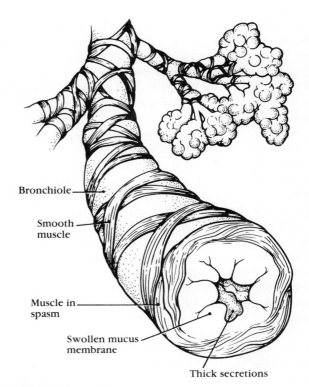

Bronchiole

Smooth muscle

Muscle in spasm

Swollen mucus membrane

Thick secretions

**FIGURE 30–1.**
Bronchial asthma. The bronchiole is obstructed on expiration, particularly by muscle spasm, edema of the mucosa, and thick secretions.

may be greatly magnified because of the pollen sensitivity already established. It is important to note that without a tendency toward bronchospasm, emotions, pollen, or other substances will not produce asthma. Recent research supports the idea that asthma is a syndrome rather than a specific disease. As such, there may be a number of pathologic mechanisms resulting in a common response: bronchoconstriction.[11]

*Intrinsic asthma* usually affects adults, including those who did not have asthma or allergy prior to middle adulthood. The family history for allergy, eczema, hives, and rashes is usually negative. Attacks are most often related to infection of the respiratory tract or to exercise; emotion, allergy, and other factors also may play a part.

In either type, respiratory infection may be a major precipitator of a severe asthma attack. Both bacterial and viral infections may precipitate the attack but viruses seem to be more important in this respect.

## Clinical Manifestations

The signs and symptoms of an asthmatic attack are closely related to the status of the airways. The only certainties about the manifestations of asthma are its variability and unpredictability. Bronchospasm leads to both obstruction of the airways and air trapping. Air trapping is probably due to the acute increase in expiratory flow resistance, which means that the inspired air simply cannot be exhaled in the time available before metabolic demands trigger another inspiration. As a result, a portion of each breath is retained. The hyperinflated alveoli exert lateral traction on the bronchiolar walls so that inspiratory airway diameter is further increased. This may aid slightly in gas exchange but it requires more inspiratory energy to overcome the tension of the already stretched elastic tissue.

The pressure of the trapped air tends to flatten the diaphragm's ability to function as the major organ of respiration and may oppose expansion of the lower chest. The costal fibers that are attached to the lower ribs are pulled into a horizontal, rather than upright, position. They can no longer move up and out so the lower chest cannot expand normally. With the flat, fixed diaphragm, the accessory muscles are called on to enlarge the chest with each inspiration. This increases energy cost and also causes increased inflation of the apices rather than the bases. Figure 30-2 shows characteristic pulmonary function studies before, during, and after an acute asthmatic attack.

Wheezing, a common sign, can be likened to pulling on the opening of a balloon full of air to make it squeak. The smaller the opening past which the air is rushing, the more squeaking occurs. In the chest, wheezing results from air squeezing past the greatly narrowed airways. Narrowing is caused by bronchospasm plus muco-

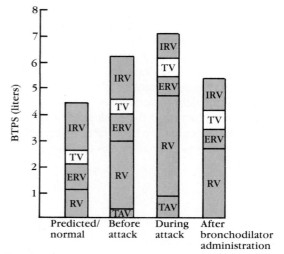

**FIGURE 30-2.**
Pulmonary function before, during, and after an asthma attack. The normal values are indicated as predicted values: inspiratory reserve volume (IRV), tidal volume (TV), expiratory reserve volume (ERV). Before the attack, there is a small volume of trapped air (TAV) with a larger than usual residual volume (RV). During the attack, the residual volume increases dramatically. After bronchodilator therapy, the trapped air volume and residual volume decrease markedly.

sal edema and obstructive secretions. Since the airways are normally smaller on expiration, expiratory wheezing occurs first. As the attack progresses, wheezing is both inspiratory and expiratory. Wheezes are *adventitious lung sounds*, which are musical, louder than the underlying sounds, and continuous. They are often described as *expiratory* or *inspiratory* to indicate the phase of respiration in which they are loudest.[5]

Pulsus paradoxus, or paradoxic pulse, is an objective measure of bronchospasm in a severe attack. The amplitude of the arterial pulse normally decreases with inspiration and is produced by the pooling of blood in the pulmonary vessels. Due to respiratory distress in the asthmatic attack, the amount of pooling apparently increases.

The paradoxic pulse is an exaggeration of normal with a fall of arterial blood pressure more than 10 mm Hg on inspiration.[13] It is measured by pumping up the blood pressure cuff to above the systolic pressure and lowering the pressure very slowly while the person breathes quickly. If a paradoxic pulse is present, Korotkoff's sounds become audible first during expiration and then during all phases of respiration.[5] The point at which all beats are equally loud is recorded as the bottom of the paradoxic pulse. Paradoxic pulse is recorded as follows: 140 − 120 / 60.

The point at which beats can be heard on expiration = 140. The point at which all beats are equally loud = 120, and the diastolic pressure = 60. Therefore, the pulsus paradoxus is 20. The normal is less than 8 mm Hg. Assessment of pulsus paradoxus can help to evaluate the severity of airway obstruction.[5]

Fatigue is a major problem in an acute asthma attack. The increased work of breathing leads to increased oxygen consumption until a point is reached at which the individual begins to tire and is no longer able to hyperventilate enough to meet the increased oxygen need. The degree of hypoventilation that results can be accurately assessed by monitoring arterial carbon dioxide levels, which may indicate the onset of respiratory failure.

A large amount of yellow or green sputum is produced by the bronchial mucosa in an asthma attack. It tends to be thick and obstructive due to its volume and the associated bronchoconstriction and dehydration. Inflammation is responsible for mucosal edema, which may be due to infection, a common precipitator of the attack.

Once the attack has subsided and underlying precipitators have cleared, the lungs usually return to normal. There is, however, a significant relationship between asthma and the development of chronic obstructive lung disease (COLD) later in life. Table 30-1 summarizes the symptoms of asthma and the underlying pathophysiology.

Acute, severe attacks of asthma, sometimes referred to as *status asthmaticus*, may occur unpredictably but are commonly provoked by a viral infection. Typically, breathlessness builds until the affected person cannot do anything other than breathe. Anxiety, extreme orthopnea, loud wheezing, sweating, tachycardia, and obvious increased work of breathing develop. A paradoxic pulse with a decrease in systolic pressure on inspiration as much as 50 to 60 mm Hg is an indication of a severe attack. Tachycardia, paradoxic pulse, and altered blood gases are the best indicators of severity and prognosis. Onset of respiratory failure may be signaled by cyanosis, decreased wheezing with progressive hypoventilation, and decreased levels of consciousness.[9] Currently, treatment usually brings relief of these symptoms but some individuals may require mechanical ventilation and some will die of cardiopulmonary arrest during the attack.[10]

## CHRONIC OBSTRUCTIVE PULMONARY DISEASE

Chronic obstructive pulmonary disease (COPD) is the fifth leading cause of death in the United States; mortality has nearly tripled in the last 30 years.[8] The age-adjusted death rate for COPD has been increasing while rates for the leading causes of death have decreased. Mortality from COPD is inversely related to education and income. In the short-term future, COPD is expected to decrease in men and increase in women due to the history of increased smoking by women begun in the 1950s.[7] Additionally, disability due to COPD is enormous, causing an estimated 250 million hours lost from work annually.[8]

Chronic obstructive lung diseases are similar to asthma in that expiratory airflow is obstructed and exacerbations and remissions are common. The acute and chronic obstructive diseases differ in that the lung tissues do not return to normal between exacerbations in chronic conditions. Instead, pulmonary damage is a slowly progressive process.

The abbreviations *COPD* and *COLD* refer to a group of conditions associated with chronic obstruction to airflow within the lungs. Usually they refer to emphysema or chronic bronchitis but they may include inflammation of the small bronchi, bronchiectasis, and cystic fibrosis. Asthma, considered in this chapter as an acute obstructive condition, is also often grouped with the chronic conditions. Of these diseases, the obstruction of chronic bronchitis, bronchiectasis, and cystic fibrosis chiefly results from secretions while that in emphysema is anatomic. Pneumoconiosis is often classified with chronic obstruc-

**TABLE 30-1.**

SYMPTOMS OF ASTHMA AND UNDERLYING PATHOPHYSIOLOGY

| SYMPTOMS | PATHOPHYSIOLOGY |
| --- | --- |
| Dyspnea; orthopnea; coughing; wheezing; chest tightness; elevated paradoxic pulse; reduced breath sounds; hyperresonance | Bronchospasm; air trapping; diphragmatic flattening |
| Tachycardia; labored breathing; air hunger; intercostal retractions | Increased work of breathing; fatigue; increased oxygen consumption |
| Thick, sticky sputum; poor skin turgor; other signs of dehydration | Increased sputum production; dehydration |
| Thick green or yellow sputum | Infection |
| Bronchospasm, eosinophilia, if allergy present | Inflammation |
| Apprehension/panic | Anxiety |

tive diseases, however, because of its underlying pathogenesis, it is discussed in Chapter 29.

## Bronchiectasis

Bronchiectasis is a chronic disease of the bronchi and
bronchioles, characterized by irreversible dilatation of
the bronchial tree and associated with chronic infection
and inflammation of these passageways. It is usually preceded by respiratory infection, especially bronchopneu-
monia, that causes the bronchial mucosa to be replaced
by fibrous scar tissue. This process leads to destruction
of the bronchi and permanent dilatation of the bronchi
and bronchioles, which allows the areas affected to be
targets for a chronic, smoldering infection (Figure 30-3).

This disease affects all ages and both sexes, often
with onset in childhood. Usually the initiating event is an
infection, such as pneumonia or bronchitis. It is not
known whether the condition begins as an infection or if
it is due to abnormal structure of the bronchial walls.[5] It
frequently is asymptomatic but may progress until it is
disabling or life-threatening.

The lower lobes are the most vulnerable and usually
are filled with a yellow-green, infected material that may
spread to the pleural cavity. It may or may not be associated with an acute inflammatory exudate with bronchial
ulceration or abscess.[4]

The common symptoms are cough and symptoms of
infection. The person raises large amounts of mucopurulent sputum and occasionally experiences hemoptysis.

## Cystic Fibrosis (Mucoviscidosis)

Cystic fibrosis is a hereditary disorder in which large
quantities of viscous material are secreted. It affects the
sweat glands, bronchi, pancreas, and mucus-secreting

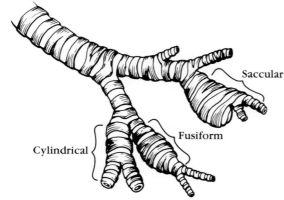

**FIGURE 30-3.**
Various types of bronchiectasis; the morphology varies.

glands of the small intestine (see Chap. 39). It may arise
shortly after birth, in childhood, and in early adulthood.

The pathologic features include a high concentration
of sodium and chloride in the sweat, and abnormal mucus secretion and elimination. Secretion of tenacious mucus throughout the airways produces airway obstruction
that leads to various combinations of atelectasis, pneumonia, bronchitis, emphysema, and other respiratory
conditions. Secondary bacterial infection is common.

Associated pancreatic insufficiency causes abnormal
stools, malnutrition, and abdominal distention. Intestinal
obstruction is common in the neonate.

The clinical manifestations are variable, with some
individuals having mainly gastrointestinal symptoms and
others developing severe pulmonary problems. All of the
manifestations relate to inability to handle excessive secretions. Pulmonary signs and symptoms are very common and include chronic cough, persistent lung infections, and cor pulmonale.

To diagnose the disease, at least three of the following four criteria are essential:[4] (1) increased sodium and
chloride in the sweat; (2) deficient pancreatic enzymes in
the gastrointestinal secretions; (3) chronic pulmonary infections, especially with opportunistic organisms such as
*Pseudomonas aeruginosa* and *Staphylococcus aureus*;
and (4) family history of the problem. The prognosis is
variable with survival past age 20 years increasing. Gastrointestinal and pulmonary problems are encountered
throughout life.

## Chronic Bronchitis

Continued bronchial inflammation and progressive increase in productive cough and dyspnea not attributable
to specific causes are classic features of *chronic bronchitis*. The term has usually been applied to persons who
have a productive cough on most days for at least 3 consecutive months in 2 successive years. Usually, the inflammation and cough are responses of the bronchial mucosa
to chronic irritation from cigarette smoking, atmospheric
pollution, or infections.[8]

Pathophysiologically, thickening and rigidity of the
bronchial mucosa result from vasodilatation, congestion,
and edema. The mucosal areas may be infiltrated with
lymphocytes, macrophages, and polymorphonuclear leukocytes. Excessive secretion plus narrowing of the passageways causes obstruction first to maximal expiration
and later to maximal inspiratory airflow.[13] Bacteria, especially *Hemophilus influenzae* and *Streptococcus pneumoniae*, are often cultured from the airways.[8]

This bronchitis is closely related to emphysema but
is usually defined as an abnormality that involves excessive secretion of mucus and bronchial inflammation,
while emphysema involves degeneration of the alveolar
parenchyma. Bronchitis may lead to the following: (1) in-

creased airway resistance with or without emphysematous changes; (2) right heart failure (cor pulmonale); and (3) dysplasia of the respiratory epithelial cells, which may undergo malignant change.[4]

The clinical manifestations include cyanosis, copious production of sputum, mild degrees of hyperinflation, marked hypercapnia, and severe hypoxemia. Heart failure with manifestations of right-sided failure occurs as the disease progresses. These manifestations include jugular venous distention, cardiac enlargement, liver engorgement, and peripheral edema. Bronchitic persons have often been called "blue bloaters" because of the presence of marked cyanosis and edema. The clinical picture varies depending on the amount of associated emphysema. Table 30-2 compares the clinical and physiologic features of the two conditions. Bronchitis and em-

physema rarely occur in isolation from each other. Some mixture of clinical signs and symptoms is usually present.

## Pulmonary Emphysema

Emphysema is the most common chronic pulmonary disease and is frequently classified with chronic bronchitis because of the simultaneous occurrence of the two conditions. In anatomic terms, emphysema involves the portion of lungs distal to a terminal bronchiole (*acinus*) where gas exchange takes place. Emphysema results in permanent, abnormal enlargement of the acinus with associated destructive changes.[4] It may be classified as *vesicular* when it involves the spaces distal to the terminal bronchioles and *interlobular* or *interstitial*, when it af-

**TABLE 30–2.**
FEATURES THAT DISTINGUISH BRONCHIAL AND EMPHYSEMATOUS TYPES OF CHRONIC OBSTRUCTIVE LUNG DISEASE

| | BRONCHIAL | EMPHYSEMATOUS |
|---|---|---|
| **Clinical Features** | | |
| History | Often recurrent chest infections | Often only insidious dyspnea |
| Chest exam | Noisy chest, slight overdistention | Quiet chest, marked overdistention |
| Sputum | Frequently copious and purulent | Usually scanty and mucoid |
| Weight loss | Absent or slight | Often marked |
| Chronic cor pulmonale | Common | Infrequent |
| Roentgenogram | Often evidence of old inflammatory disease | Often attenuated vessels and radiolucency |
| General appearance | "Blue bloater" | "Pink puffer" |
| **Physiologic Tests** | | |
| Lung volumes | | |
|   Total lung capacity (TLC) | Normal or slightly decreased | Increased |
|   Residual volume (RV) | Moderately increased | Markedly increased |
|   RV/TLC | High | High |
| Long compliance | | |
|   Static | Normal or low | High |
|   Dynamic | Very low | Normal or low |
| Airway resistance | | |
|   Expiratory | Very high | High |
|   Inspiratory | High | Normal |
| Diffusing capacity | Variable | Low |
| Chronic hypoxemia | Often severe | Usually mild |
| Chronic hypercapnia | Common | Unusual |
| Pulmonary hypertension | Often severe | Usually mild |
| Cardiac output | Normal | Often low |

Source: B. Burrows et al., Respiratory Insufficiency (2nd ed.). Chicago: Yearbook, 1983.

fects the tissue between the air spaces.[8] The common term *pulmonary emphysema* usually designates the vesicular type.

## Pathophysiology

Emphysema seems to be due to many separate injuries that occur over a long time. Prevalence and severity are greatest in elderly individuals. The elastin and fiber network of the alveoli and airways is broken down. The alveoli enlarge and many of their walls are destroyed. Alveolar destruction leads to the formation of larger than normal air spaces (pools), which greatly reduce the alveolar diffusing surface. Once the process begins, it progresses slowly and inconsistently. Alveolar destruction also undermines the support structure for the airways, making them more vulnerable to expiratory collapse. There may be associated airway inflammation and consequent increase in mucus production, although many persons with emphysema produce little or no sputum.

The exact mechanism of injury is yet to be determined. Ischemia may cause alveolar breakdown, although specific vascular lesions have not been found. Repeated injuries from smoking, infection, and air pollution often lead to emphysema but the exact mechanism of injury has not been identified. Most, but not all, of those affected are cigarette smokers.

Specific types of emphysema have been shown to be related to a deficiency in the enzyme alpha₁-antitrypsin, which inhibits the proteases of elastase and collagenase. These proteases are normally major contributors to tissue destruction during the inflammatory process. Without the inhibition of alpha₁-antitrypsin, the destruction or digestion of pulmonary tissue occurs more at the bases than at the apices of the lungs. This circumstance leads to the onset of severe obstructive lung disease early in adult life, often before age 40 years.[12,14] The onset of hypoxia and cor pulmonale in these persons heralds a poor prognosis.

The types of emphysema have been classified according to the area of lung affected; that is, classification is anatomic, and may describe lobules or acini (Tables 30-3 and 30-4). Many types of emphysema can only be classified with certainty by autopsy report. Pulmonary interstitial emphysema is an associated condition that involves overdistention of the alveoli and dissection of air into the perivascular spaces. The dissection may continue into the mediastinum causing *pneumomediastinum*, or into the pleural cavity causing *pneumothorax*. Figure 30-4 illustrates the appearance of alveoli in the main types of emphysema.

Emphysema has a major effect on compliance and elasticity. The major abnormality is loss of *elastic recoil*.[8] Because alveolar walls are destroyed, fibrous and muscle

tissues are lost, making the lungs more distensible. Even in severe disease, inspiratory airway resistance tends to be normal. Air trapping occurs because of loss of elastic recoil, which increases airway size on inspiration and causes collapse of the small airways on expiration. Thus, a minor obstruction on inspiration is a serious obstruction on expiration. If expiration is forced, a sharp rise in pressure on the airways leads to compression of the bronchi and bronchioles. The resultant distention eventually leads to disruption in the alveolar walls and surrounding musculoelastic tissue around the small airways. Figure 30-5 illustrates the difference between normal alveoli and distended alveoli of emphysema. The loss of gas-exchanging surface with associated vascular changes results in decreased diffusion capacities.[8]

**TABLE 30-3.**
## CLASSIFICATION OF EMPHYSEMA

| CLASSIFICATION | DESCRIPTION |
|---|---|
| Diffuse or generalized | Lobules or acini through affected lung |
| Focal | Associated with focal dust deposition (eg, coal dust) |
| Irregular | Associated with shrinkage of fibrotic scars, usually from old disease |
| Obstructive | Accompanied by demonstrable bronchial obstruction |
| Bulla | Emphysematous space of more than 1 cm in an inflated lung; may occur in any type of emphysema |

**TABLE 30-4.**
## LOBULAR AND ACINAR TERMINOLOGY OF EMPHYSEMA

| LOBULES | ACINI |
|---|---|
| Panlobular: all lung affected; diffuse throughout lung | Panacinar: whole acinus affected; diffuse throughout lung |
| Centrilobular: spaces around central bronchioles affected; usually affects apices | Centriacinar: area around alveolar ducts affected; usually affects apices |
| Periseptal: occurs at periphery of lobule; less common than above types | Periacinar: occurs at periphery of acinus; less common than above types |
| Irregular: scarring throughout the acinus irregularly | |

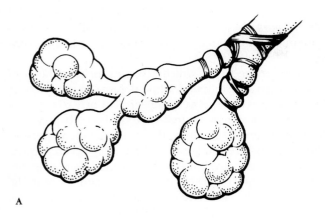

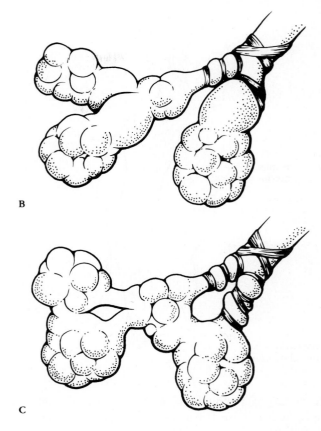

**FIGURE 30–4.**
Alterations in alveolar structure. **A.** Normal respiratory bronchioles and alveoli. **B.** Centrilobular emphysema—dilation of the respiratory bronchioles. **C.** Panlobular emphysema—destruction of the alveolar walls.

## Clinical Manifestations

The clinical manifestations of emphysema are usually absent in the early stages and very insidious in onset. They may overlap with those of bronchitis. The person with emphysema has often been called the "pink puffer" on

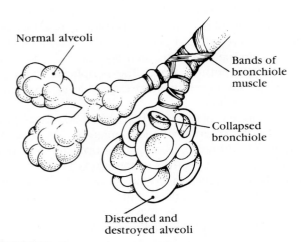

**FIGURE 30–5.**
Distended and destroyed alveoli versus normal ones.

the basis of appearance. Dyspnea is characteristic. In the early stages, it occurs with exertion and later progresses to dyspnea at rest. Severe hyperinflation of the lungs may lead to an increased anteroposterior chest diameter, resulting in the typical barrel chest. Dorsal kyphosis, prominent anterior chest, and elevated ribs all contribute to this appearance (Figure 30-6). The accessory muscles are used to raise the thorax on inspiration and the abdominal muscles are developed to force air out actively. As a result, the expiratory cycle is prolonged. Pulmonary function tests show a prolonged $FEV_1$ with decreased vital capacity, despite an increase in total lung capacity. Respiratory sounds are frequently very quiet unless a superimposed infection accounts for expiratory wheezes and rales.

Chronic bronchitis and emphysema coexist in the majority of persons with COPD. Figure 30-7 shows how the clinical manifestations of chronic bronchitis and emphysema overlap. The majority of persons exhibit manifestations of both conditions.

*Hypoxia* is a very common result of emphysema. It is defined as inadequate delivery of oxygen to satisfy the metabolic requirements of the organs and cells of the body. Direct measurement of oxygen in the tissue is impossible so hypoxia is usually diagnosed by its end-organ

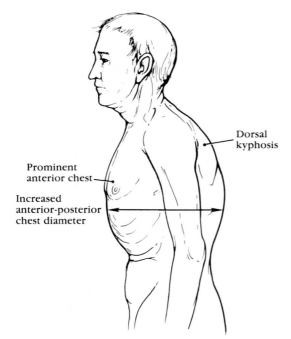

**FIGURE 30–6.**
Barrel chest of emphysema.

effects. Hypoxia of the brain, for example, causes clinical signs, such as mental changes, stupor, and coma. *Hypoxemia* is defined as reduced levels of oxygen in the blood. Blood gas levels are measured directly, and normal oxygen tension in the arterial blood is 80 to 100 mm Hg. A value of 55 to 60 mm Hg or lower for oxygen indicates hypoxemia.[1]

As a response to prolonged hypoxia, the individual may develop cyanosis, clubbing, and polycythemia. Clinically, evident cyanosis is a late and unreliable sign of hypoxemia. It does not occur unless reduced hemoglobin

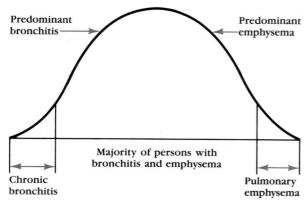

**FIGURE 30–7.**
The overlay of clinical manifestations of chronic bronchitis and emphysema in chronic obstructive pulmonary disease. (Source: D. Mahler, P. Barlow, and R. Mathay, Chronic obstructive pulmonary diseases. *Clin Geriatric Med* 2:2 May 1986.)

is more than 5 g per 100 mL of capillary blood. In the anemic person, cyanosis may not occur at all. In the polycythemic, cyanosis may be present despite adequate oxygen levels.

The human brain, which accounts for about 20% of total oxygen consumption while comprising only about 2% of body weight, is very sensitive to hypoxia. Therefore, cerebral symptoms may be induced by hypoxemia. A small degree results in restlessness, change in personality, and impaired judgment. Moderately severe hypoxemia causes impaired motor function and confusion. Severe hypoxemia, at levels between 20 and 30 mm Hg, often causes delirium and coma. If persistent and severe, it can cause permanent cortical damage.

Chronic hypoxemia causes a release of renal erythropoietic factor, which reacts with a plasma protein to form erythropoietin. This substance stimulates increased production of red blood cells and blood volume increase (see Chap. 19). The resulting *polycythemia* characteristically develops in patients having COPD and leads to increased blood viscosity, which further impedes oxygenation of the tissues. The oxygen-hemoglobin dissociation curve shifts to the right with hypoxemia, allowing for increased release of oxygen to the tissues. Table 30-5 summarizes the general effects of hypoxemia.

*Hypercapnia* (retention of carbon dioxide) is also common with COPD when the disease becomes severe, usually when $FEV_1$ is less than 1 liter.[10] It results from hypoventilation mostly due to an uneven match-up of ventilation and perfusion in the lungs. At normal ventilatory rates, inadequate carbon dioxide is excreted and carbon dioxide is retained. Increasing $PCO_2$ levels leads to increased ventilation due to the central chemoreceptor in the medulla. When pulmonary disease is severe, ventilation changes do not usually return $PCO_2$ levels to normal. In other words, the work of breathing becomes too great to sustain the high ventilatory rate.[6]

Hypercapnia becomes chronic and depresses the receptiveness of the medullary chemoreceptor. The person may lose most of the stimuli for breathing from the central chemoreceptor and depend on the peripheral chemoreceptors on the aortic arch and carotid sinuses to stimulate a ventilatory drive. The peripheral chemoreceptors are stimulated by hypoxemia of less than 60 mm Hg oxygen tension.

The normal pH change that would accompany the retention of carbon dioxide is counteracted by renal retention of bicarbonate, leading to a normal or near normal pH (see Chap. 9). This adaptation is protective and assists the body function, even though the $PCO_2$ remains excessively high. The adjusted pH reflects *compensated respiratory acidosis*. Table 30-6 shows examples of compensated and uncompensated respiratory acidosis.

Any of the chronic lung diseases may lead to respiratory failure, which is discussed further in Chapter 31.

**TABLE 30–5.**

PHYSIOLOGICAL EFFECTS OF HYPOXEMIA

| PaO$_2$ (mm Hg) | FUNCTION | ABNOR-MALITY | SIGN OR SYMPTOM |
|---|---|---|---|
| <60 | Heart rate | ↑ | Tachycardia |
| | Respiratory rate | ↑ | Tachypnea |
| | Na+ and H$_2$O excretion | ↑ | Edema |
| <55 | Cardiac output | ↑ | Bounding pulses |
| | Arrhythmias | ↑ | Tachyarrhythmias<br>Bradyarrhythmias |
| | Mentation | ↓ | Somnolence<br>Confusion<br>Pinpoint pupils |
| | Red blood cell mass | ↑ | Plethora<br>Erythrocythemia<br>Thromboemboli |
| | PA pressure | ↑ | ↑ JVP<br>Edema<br>RV S$_4$<br>Hepatomegaly<br>Abnormal ECG* |
| <30 | Cardiac output | ↓ | Cyanosis<br>↓ Pulse pressure<br>Shock |
| | Metabolism | ↓ | Lactic acidosis |

*ECG findings of cor pulmonale.
*RAE, RVE, rightward shift in ventricular or atrial vectors.*
Source: W.N. Kelley, Textbook of Internal Medicine. *Philadelphia: J.B. Lippincott, 1989.*

**TABLE 30–6.**

COMPARATIVE VALUES FOR COMPENSATED AND UNCOMPENSATED RESPIRATORY ACIDOSIS

| ARTERIAL BLOOD GAS COMPONENTS | NORMAL VALUES | COMPENSATED RESPIRATORY ACIDOSIS (AN EXAMPLE) | UNCOMPENSATED RESPIRATORY ACIDOSIS (AN EXAMPLE) |
|---|---|---|---|
| pH | 7.35–7.45 | 7.35 | 7.22 |
| PCO$_2$ | 35–45 mm Hg | 54 mm Hg | 74 mm Hg |
| PO$_2$ | 80–100 mm Hg | 62 mm Hg | 40 mm Hg |
| O$_2$ saturation | 95–100% | 83% | 69% |
| HCO$_3$ | 22–26 mEq/L | 32 mEq/L | 28 mEq/L |
| H$_2$CO$_3$ | 1.05–1.35 mEq/L | 1.8 mEq/L | 2.9 mEq/L |

## REFERENCES

1. Albert, R.K. Approach to the patient with cyanosis and/or hypoxemia. In W.N. Kelley (ed.), *Textbook of Internal Medicine.* Philadelphia: J.B. Lippincott, 1989.

2. Barnes, P. A new approach to the treatment of asthma. *N. Engl. J. Med.* 321:1517, 1989.

3. Braman, S.S., and Davis, S.M. Wheezing in the aged: Asthma and other causes. *Clin. Geriatr. Med.* 2:269, 1986.

4. Cotran, R.S., Kumar, V., and Robbins, S.L. *Robbins' Pathologic Basis of Disease* (4th ed.). Philadelphia: W.B. Saunders, 1989.

5. Farzan, S.A. *A Concise Handbook of Respiratory Diseases* (2nd ed.). Reston, Va.: Reston, 1985.

6. Guyton, A.C. *Textbook of Medical Physiology* (8th ed.). Philadelphia: W.B. Saunders, 1990.

7. Higgins, M., and Thom, T. Incidence, prevalence, and mortality: Intra- and intercountry differences. In M. Hensley

and N. Saunders (eds.), *Clinical Epidemiology of Chronic Obstructive Pulmonary Disease*. New York: Marcel Dekker, 1989.

8. Kuhn, C., and Askin, F.B. Lung and mediastinum. In J.M. Kissane (ed.), *Anderson's Pathology* (9th ed.). St. Louis: Mosby, 1990.

9. Pare, P., and Montaner, J. Asthma. In W.N. Kelley (ed.), *Textbook of Internal Medicine*. Philadelphia: J.B. Lippincott, 1989.

10. Seaton, A., Seaton, D., and Leitch, A. *Crofton and Douglas's Respiratory Diseases* (4th ed.). Oxford: Blackwell, 1989.

11. Snapper, J. Inflammation and airway function: The asthma syndrome. *Am. Rev. Respir. Dis.* 141:531, 1990.

12. Sodeman, W.A., and Sodeman, T.M. *Sodeman's Pathologic Physiology* (7th ed.). Philadelphia: W.B. Saunders, 1985.

13. Stauffer, J.L., and Carbone, J.E. Pulmonary diseases. In M.A. Krupp and M.J. Chatton (eds.), *Current Medical Diagnosis and Treatment 1990*. Los Altos, Calif.: Lange, 1990.

14. Wewers, M. Pathogenesis of emphysema: Assessment of basic science concepts through clinical investigation. *Chest* 90:190, 1989.

# chapter **31**

Darlene H. Renfroe

# Other Alterations Affecting the Pulmonary System

## Learning Objectives

1. Describe the ventilation-perfusion abnormality that occurs with pulmonary embolus.
2. Discuss the underlying risk factors for the development of pulmonary embolus.
3. List and describe three conditions that favor thrombus formation in the deep veins.
4. Describe the clinical manifestations that may occur in the process of pulmonary embolization.
5. Explain briefly how resolution of emboli occurs.
6. Describe the development of pulmonary hypertension.
7. Define *cor pulmonale*.
8. Define *rhinitis, pharyngitis, sinusitis,* and *laryngitis*.
9. Explain briefly the dangers of laryngeal edema.
10. Classify and briefly describe cancer of the larynx.
11. Define *hamartoma* of the lungs.

12. Discuss some factors that predispose to the onset of malignancy in the lung.
13. Describe the pathology, major clinical manifestations, and prognosis of four major types of intrapulmonary malignancy.
14. List the most common sites of metastasis of lung cancer.
15. Differentiate between respiratory insufficiency and respiratory failure.
16. Explain how adaptation can occur in chronic respiratory insufficiency.
17. List the criteria for diagnosing respiratory failure and the other factors that should be taken into account.
18. Describe the clinical manifestations of respiratory failure.
19. Define *carbon dioxide narcosis*.
20. Discuss the prognoses in acute and chronic respiratory failure.

Several of the pulmonary disease processes do not easily lend themselves to strict classification as restrictive or obstructive. This chapter discusses some of these conditions, including pulmonary embolus, tumors of the lung, and respiratory insufficiency and failure. Respiratory failure may result from many intrapulmonary and extrapulmonary diseases. It is frequently the cause of death in chronic pulmonary disease.

As discussed in Chapter 28, the normal ratio of alveolar ventilation (4 liters/minute) to volume of blood flow in the pulmonary capillaries (V/Q̇) is about 0.8 because cardiac output averages about 5 liters per minute. A decrease of alveolar ventilation in relation to perfusion occurs in any part of the lung where airways are obstructed by secretions (bronchitis), expiratory dynamic collapse (emphysema), or muscular spasm (asthma), or where alveoli are collapsed (atelectasis) or are filled with fluid (pulmonary edema). These conditions cause increased venous blood flow past nonventilated alveoli. The oxygen-poor mixture is added to the arterial blood and the result is hypoxemia. As stated previously, hypoxemia resulting from underventilated alveoli is, in essence, a form of right-to-left shunting of venous blood past the alveoli (see Chap. 29).

Another type of ventilation-perfusion abnormality is the reduction of perfusion in relation to ventilation. This occurs most frequently when pulmonary emboli obliterate arteriolar blood supply but may occur when cardiac output is reduced because of congestive heart failure. In these examples, ventilated but nonperfused alveoli increase the physiologic dead space because a significant number of alveoli receive inspired air but do not participate in the exchange of oxygen or carbon dioxide.

In conditions in which hypoxemia is the result of a ventilation-perfusion abnormality, the pressure of carbon dioxide ($PCO_2$) often is normal or low, since compensatory hyperventilation is able to lower the more easily diffusible $PCO_2$. Thus, the clinical pattern of ventilation-perfusion inequality is often one of hypoxemia with hyperventilation, lowered $PCO_2$, and even respiratory alkalosis. This picture is directly related to the degree of the ventilation-perfusion defect and eventually may result in hypoxemia, hypercapnia, and respiratory acidosis.

## PULMONARY EMBOLUS

A pulmonary embolus is defined as an occlusion of one or more pulmonary vessels by matter that has traveled from a source outside the lung. Any foreign material freely traveling in the systemic venous system must finally terminate in the pulmonary vascular bed. For example, if a clot in a small vein dislodges, it travels through progressively larger vessels until it reaches the right ventricle, where it is pumped by the pulmonary artery to the lungs. The usual cause of pulmonary embolus is a thrombus from the deep veins of the legs or pelvis that dislodges and travels with the flow of blood to the lungs. It may also result from a fat embolus, amniotic fluid embolus, air embolus, particulate matter injected intravenously, or rarely, gas, parasites, or foreign objects.

Pulmonary embolus is probably the third most common acute cause of death in the United States but the diagnosis is often missed.[5] It is thought that many persons have thrombi in the venous system that may actually embolize but may be diagnosed as a pulmonary infection, pleurisy, or not diagnosed at all. Pulmonary emboli rarely strike the young or healthy but occur in a high-risk group that includes bedridden persons, the obese, the elderly, and those with a history of prior emboli or thrombosis. Persons who suffer from congestive heart failure, who undergo abdominal or pelvic surgery, or who have sustained trauma to the legs are also at high risk. The risk factors are cumulative: the more factors present, the greater the risk of developing pulmonary emboli.

## Sequence of Events in Pulmonary Embolization

The right lung is more frequently involved in the embolic process than the left with the degree of obstruction related to the size of the embolus. It has been shown in some studies that the physiologic consequences of pulmonary embolus are greater than can be explained by the degree of occlusion alone. A large embolus may cause infarction of the lung parenchyma but this is not directly related to the size of the embolus because the bronchial arteries continue to nourish the lung tissue.[7]

As stated before, most pulmonary emboli are the result of thrombi that dislodge from the deep veins of the legs and pelvis. Phlebothrombosis is the most common type of deep vein thrombosis and frequently occurs in immobilized or obese persons and in those who have sustained surgical or accidental trauma (see Chap. 27).

For a thrombus of this nature to form, an abnormality must be present because clotting rarely occurs when blood flow and vascular integrity are normal. Three conditions, known as Virchow's triad, have been described that favor clot formation: (1) venostasis, (2) endothelial disruption of the vessel lining, and (3) hypercoagulability.

Local concentration of coagulation factors, together with an injury to the venous wall, may provide a place for clots to form. As the flow of blood slows or stops over the injured area, the clot begins to form and extends or propagates itself up the vein (Figure 31-1). It may then retract and pull away from the vessel wall and become a free-floating embolus. Vagal stimulation or minor physical exertion may immediately precede embolization. Small fragments of the clot may break off and produce several areas of embolization on the lungs. Multiple embolization of the pulmonary capillary bed is more common than occlusion of the main pulmonary artery or its branches.

Once the blood clot lodges in the pulmonary capillary bed, it obstructs blood flow beyond the point of the obstruction. Perfusion in the pulmonary capillary bed stops. If large areas are affected, there may be infarction of the lung tissue, which occurs in perhaps 5% to 10% of cases with infarcts of various sizes. The newly formed infarct becomes hemorrhagic but later is filled with scar tissue.[5]

A wide variety of pathophysiologic responses to a pulmonary embolus occurs, depending on the size of the embolus and the ability of the host to compensate. Small obstructions to the blood supply usually create no hemodynamic changes and are called *silent pulmonary em-*

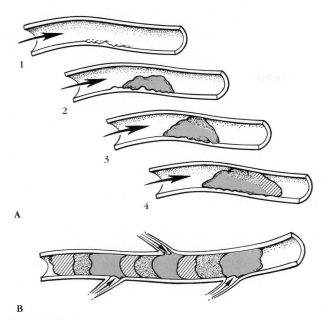

**FIGURE 31-1.**
**A.** Sequence of clot formation on area of intimal damage.
**B.** Propagation of clot up the length of the vein wall may lead to pulmonary embolus.

*boli.* Larger obstructions may cause increased resistance to pulmonary blood flow, which may lead to right ventricular failure (cor pulmonale). Studies show that more than 50% of the pulmonary vasculature must be obstructed to cause significant increase in pressure in the pulmonary artery.[13] However, in individuals with preexisting lung disease, increased pulmonary artery pressure leading to cor pulmonale may occur with much less vasculature obstructed. Vasoconstriction in the smaller pulmonary arterial vessels is apparently common and may be due to the liberation of vasoactive substances, such as serotonin. Vasoconstriction enhances the risk for pulmonary ischemia and infarction.

The increase in pulmonary artery pressure leads to an increased workload for the right side of the heart in pumping blood into the pulmonary circulation. Tachycardia results and progresses to signs of right ventricular failure, including jugular venous distention, hepatomegaly, and peripheral edema. A large saddle embolus obstructing the main pulmonary artery at its bifurcation to the right and left branches leads to acute cor pulmonale, severe shock, and often, sudden death.[7] Bronchoconstriction due to release of various chemical mediators, such as thromboxanes, prostaglandins, serotonin, and histamine, may produce an asthmalike picture causing initial misdiagnosis.[2]

The process of embolization may be continuous, with small emboli being released from a thrombotic focus over months or years. Often undiagnosed, this process may lead to pulmonary embarrassment.

The lungs are capable of clearing emboli more rapidly than any other organ. The pulmonary endothelium is rich in both plasmin activator and heparin.[10] Resolution of the pulmonary embolus occurs by absorption and fibrosis. Activation of the intrinsic fibrinolytic system may restore the pulmonary circulation within a few hours or days.[9] This may begin as early as a few hours after a small embolic episode. Fibrous replacement converts infarcted lung tissue to scar tissue. Clots are partly or totally dissolved by the fibrinolytic system. Residual material, resistant to fibrinolytic attack, may organize and become small, scarred areas.

## Clinical Manifestations

The signs and symptoms of pulmonary embolus vary greatly and depend on both the amount of lung tissue affected and the state of health of the heart and lungs prior to the event (Box 31-1).

The embolus may be clinically silent with no manifestations at all. The most frequent symptom is the sudden onset of mild, moderate, or severe dyspnea that may occur transiently. Tachypnea that persists is suggestive of pulmonary embolus. Fever and cough, sometimes with associated hemoptysis, often occur. Pain may be absent,

**BOX 31-1.**
SIGNS AND SYMPTOMS OF PULMONARY EMBOLUS

Initial manifestations
  May be clinically absent
  Dyspnea of sudden onset
  Cough
  Fever
  Pain—pleuritic or deep and crushing
  Hemoptysis
  Tachypnea
  Anxiety, apprehension, restlessness
  Palpitations
  Weakness
  Diaphoresis
  Nausea and vomiting
  Shock
Physical examination findings
  Splinting of involved side
  Cyanosis
  Distended neck veins
  Area of dullness over involved side
  Tachycardia
  S3 or S4 gallop
  Atrial fibrillation, right bundle branch block
  Right axis deviation on 12-lead
  Rales
  Localized decreased breath sounds
  Localized wheezing
  Chest film may be normal or show patchy areas of infiltration
Lung scan and pulmonary arteriogram definitive
Arterial blood gases frequently show hypoxemia and hypercapnia

mild, or severe, and may be manifested as pleural pain or deep, crushing, substernal pain mimicking that of myocardial infarction. The pain often occurs with pulmonary infarction and may be oppressive and substernal. Anxiety, apprehension, and restlessness are common responses to hypoxemia. Palpitations and weakness associated with profuse perspiration, nausea, and vomiting often are present. If embolization is massive, cardiovascular collapse may result, leading to sudden shock, seizures, or cardiopulmonary arrest.

Clinical signs of pulmonary embolus may include splinting of the involved side, cyanosis, distended neck veins, tachycardia with an increased pulmonic sound, or an S3 or S4 gallop. Rales, wheezing, and decreased breath sounds in the affected areas are frequent findings.

Definitive diagnosis is often difficult. Chest radiograph often appears normal and any abnormalities may be general, such as elevated diaphragm, atelectasis, or pleural effusion. The serum enzyme lactic dehydrogenase level is often elevated. Arterial blood gases may show hypoxemia, hypocapnia, and respiratory alkalosis due to the marked tachypnea. Hypoxemia correlates well with the extent of the area occluded.

Radioisotope lung scan shows perfusion defects in areas of the lung and supports the diagnosis. A pulmonary arteriogram is occasionally performed to provide visualization of the vessels of the pulmonary tree.

### Fat Embolization

Fractures of the long bones are the major source of emboli composed of fat particles. The origin appears to be the bone marrow, and the particles enter the bloodstream through the ruptured veins 12 to 24 hours postfracture. Fat also may be mobilized from the injured site and may form large globules in the plasma.[9] Alveolar edema often occurs, exhibiting a clinical picture much like the adult respiratory distress syndrome. The person begins to exhibit marked respiratory distress, fever, and tachycardia, and sometimes multiple petechiae over the thorax and upper extremities.[8]

## PULMONARY HYPERTENSION

Pulmonary hypertension can result from heart disease, lung disease, or both. It refers to an increase in pulmonary artery pressure, which increases the workload of the right ventricle. Significant pulmonary vascular obliteration must be present for pulmonary arterial pressure to be elevated because there is normally a large reserve in the pulmonary capillary bed.

As a rule, pulmonary hypertension involves progressive disease either of the pulmonary vessels or of the lung parenchyma. The medial layer of the pulmonary arteries usually hypertrophies, and the system loses its ability to adapt to stress factors, such as increased blood flow or hypoxia. Hypoxic vasoconstriction is a cause and a result of pulmonary hypertension.[9]

As the process becomes persistent, end-diastolic pressure in the right ventricle becomes elevated. The right ventricle hypertrophies and further increases its systolic pressure. In the early stages, symptoms of right ventricular failure or *cor pulmonale* (heart failure resulting from lung disease) occur only during periods of increased stress. As it progresses, cor pulmonale is present all of the time, manifested by jugular venous distention, hepatomegaly, and peripheral edema.

The pulmonary artery pressure, which is normally approximately 25/10 mm Hg, is elevated to above approximately 40/15 mm Hg and may be much higher as the disease progresses. At a certain critical point, the right ventricle cannot compensate for the increased pressure, and intractable cardiac failure occurs.

Death from chronic respiratory disease may be due to heart failure or respiratory failure. Nearly all persons with these diseases exhibit some symptoms of right ventricular failure, also called chronic cor pulmonale.

Other conditions besides chronic obstructive lung disease may cause pulmonary hypertension. Congenital cardiac left-to-right shunts that overload the pulmonary vascular system can eventually cause pulmonary hypertension. Also, some valvular conditions, particularly mitral stenosis, cause increased volume and pressure in the pulmonary vascular bed. Any condition in which hypoxia is sustained may cause vasoconstriction and ultimately, pulmonary hypertension. Left-sided heart failure of long-standing duration and pulmonary emboli also may cause this condition.

## UPPER RESPIRATORY TRACT ALTERATIONS

Alterations in the upper respiratory tract (URT) are very common, usually self-limiting conditions that include rhinitis, pharyngitis, sinusitis, and laryngitis. Cancer of the larynx is a more serious disease that may affect the URT.

*Rhinitis* refers to inflammation of the nasal cavities, resulting in a persistent nasal discharge caused by secretory hyperactivity of the submucosal glands of the nasal cavities. The etiology of rhinitis is commonly viral, bacterial, or allergic. The viral form is recognized as the common cold. Allergies or exposure to irritants injure the normal cilia of the nasal mucosa. Bacterial growth often occurs after an initial viral attack.

*Pharyngitis* usually results from viral or bacterial invasion of the pharynx that causes a sore throat. The appearance of the throat varies depending on the causative agent. Tonsils are often affected and become reddened and swollen, and exude a suppurative discharge. Most pharyngitis is relatively innocuous but untreated streptococcal infections may have systemic effects in some persons. These effects may be manifested as scarlet fever, rheumatic fever, rheumatic heart disease, or glomerulonephritis. Other organisms such as the *Corynebacterium diphtheriae* and *Hemophilus influenzae* may cause grave effects.

*Sinusitis* is an inflammation of the sinus cavities that often spreads from a rhinitis infection to the sinuses. The most common organisms causing this condition are group A *Streptococcus pyogenes, Staphylococcus aureus*, and *H. influenzae*. The infection usually causes localized pain in the frontal, maxillary, ethmoid, or sphenoid sinuses (Figure 31-2). A purulent exudate indicates bacterial infection that, when severe, is associated with the constitutional symptoms of fever, chills, pain in the sinuses, and nasal obstruction. Chronic disease may be indicated by a postnasal discharge and tenderness over the sinus cavity.

*Laryngitis* often occurs in persons who overuse the voice in singing or other vocal activities. It may also be due to any organism that may affect the URT. It affects both vocal cords and is manifested by cough and hoarseness with loss of the voice. Laryngitis may also be chronic, precipitated by overusing tobacco, straining the voice, or inhaling toxic gases. Rarely, this condition causes *laryngeal edema* and obstruction to airflow. Complete obstruction causes asphyxia while incomplete obstruction causes laryngeal stridor and acute respiratory distress.

## CARCINOMA OF THE LARYNX

*Polyps* of the vocal cords are not usually premalignant but the *laryngeal papilloma* is a true neoplasm that has the potential of undergoing malignant transformation. Most affected persons are or have been heavy tobacco smokers.

Most cancers of the larynx arise on the vocal cords and are clinically manifested by hoarseness. This malignancy is closely associated with chronic laryngitis and smoking. Its frequency is greatest in men after the fourth decade.

Clinical manifestations of cancers of the larynx include pain, a palpable lump, dysphagia, and, occasionally, respiratory distress. The tumor, being a relatively slow-growing malignancy of the squamous epithelium, is curable in the early stages.

## LUNG TUMORS

Tumors of the lung may be benign or malignant. The majority are malignant and have an unremitting, progressive course leading ultimately to a poor prognosis. The only benign tumor that is discussed in this section is the ha-

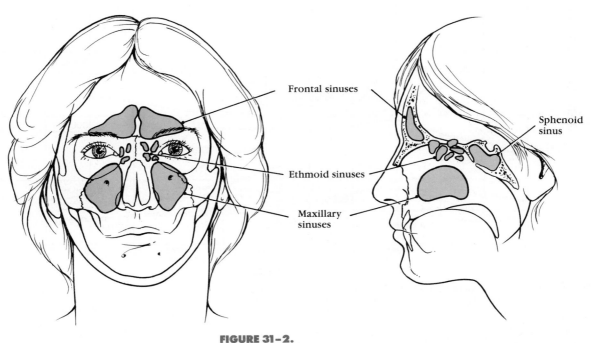

**FIGURE 31–2.**
Location of paranasal sinuses.

martoma because it is frequently difficult to differentiate it from a malignancy. The malignant tumors are described according to histologic classification and pathogenesis.

## Benign Tumors

The *hamartoma* is not a true neoplasm but is a congenital anomaly that frequently leads to tumorlike lesions containing connective tissue, cartilage, and bronchial epithelium in the bronchi or lung tissue.[9] The lesions are encapsulated, firm, and grayish-white with a rough, nodular surface. They appear on chest films on the periphery of the lung, in the subpleural area, and endobronchially, making them difficult to distinguish from malignant tumors. These uncommon lung tumors rarely cause any clinical symptoms but must be differentiated from malignancy.

## Malignant Tumors

### Factors Predisposing to Malignancy

Cigarette smoking, air pollution, and industrial chemicals seem to account for the increasing frequency of bronchogenic carcinoma. Statistical evidence supports the relationship between cigarette smoking and certain types of lung cancer. The death rate from lung cancer is twice as high in urban areas as in rural areas, implicating air pollution as an etiologic factor (see Chaps. 17 and 18). Figure 31-3 shows the phenomenal increase in lung cancer deaths since 1930.[4] Lung cancer mortality has increased by 15% overall from 1979 to 1986—by 7% among men and 44% among women,[4] proving prophetic the words of former Health, Education, and Welfare Secretary Califano: "Women who smoke like men, die like men who smoke."[14] Lung cancer has now overtaken breast cancer as the leading cause of cancer death in women.[12] Lung cancer *alone* is responsible for an increased cancer mor-

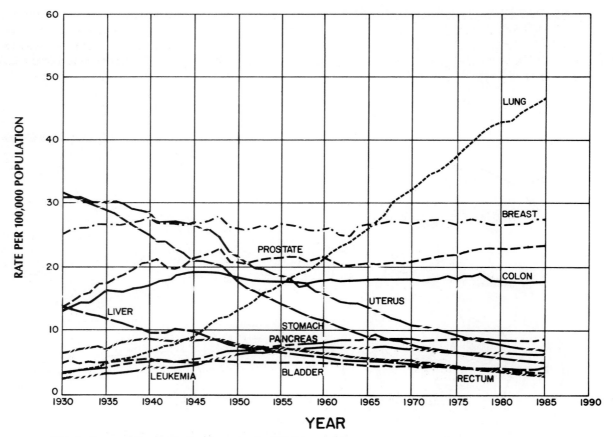

*Rate for the population standardized for age on the 1970 U.S. population.
Sources of Data: National Center for Health Statistics and Bureau of the Census, United States.
Note: Rates are for both sexes combined except breast and uterus female population only and prostate male population only.

**FIGURE 31-3.**
Cancer death rates by site, United States 1930–85. (Source: National Center for Health Statistics and Bureau of the Census, United States.)

tality rate from 1950 to 1985. Excluding lung cancer, cancer mortality has actually been falling by 13%.[15] Reducing cigarette smoking is clearly the single most important means of reducing lung cancer in the United States. Although other factors are associated with lung cancer, each of these agents is potentiated by cigarette smoking. For example, 85% of deaths from lung cancer associated with radon exposure in the home are due to a combination of radon *and* cigarette smoke.[4]

Certain occupations apparently predispose persons to lung cancer. Asbestos workers have about a 10 times greater risk of developing the disease than the general population. More startling, an asbestos worker who smokes has a 90 times greater risk of developing lung cancer than the general population. Other industrial agents that increase risk are uranium, chromate, arsenic, and iron.

Studies suggest a correlation between chronic bronchitis and bronchogenic carcinoma with the differences in mortality from lung cancer reported among countries being related to varying frequency of chronic bronchitis.[5] The excess mucus secretion characteristic of chronic bronchitis may interfere with the bronchial epithelial cells, making them likely to undergo malignant change. Also, the bronchial mucosa, which is chronically inflamed, exhibits depressed ciliary activity, and airway cleansing is decreased.[9]

## Gross Appearance of Pulmonary Malignancy

Although variability may occur, the appearance of pulmonary carcinoma may be one of three types: (1) *hilar, infiltrating form*, which causes a large tumor mass that presses on the bronchi; (2) *peripheral* or *nodular form*, which may appear as a single tumor or multiple nodular masses through the lung; or (3) *diffuse type*, which looks very much like pneumonia and may be difficult to see grossly.[9] Squamous cell and small cell carcinomas tend to be centrally located, hilar infiltrating; adenocarcinoma and large cell are more commonly peripheral.

## Microscopic Appearance of Pulmonary Malignancy

There are four major types of pulmonary neoplasms which account for about 95% of lung cancers. The relative frequency of each type varies considerably at different research centers. This is due to several different classification guidelines and histopathologists' difficulty in analysis of small biopsy material obtained from fiberoptic bronchoscopy.[11] Some sources classify cancer as simply small-cell and nonsmall-cell since the behavior and treatment of the two types is so different.[6]

The *squamous cell carcinoma* is the most common morphologic type of bronchogenic carcinoma. It causes 45% to 60% of lung malignancies. The cell type may be well-differentiated but more frequently, it is undifferentiated and quite pleomorphic in appearance. It tends to have large, well-outlined areas of tumor growth arising from the bronchi.[5] These invade surrounding tissue in the early stages of the disease but later metastasize readily to the lymph nodes, brain, bone, adrenal glands, and liver. This tumor type has a very high correlation with heavy cigarette smoking, occurring almost exclusively in smokers. The 2-year prognosis is poor, with less than 50% survival but it is the best of the four major types.

*Adenocarcinoma* of the lungs, accounting for about 30% of lung tumors, appears to be increasing, especially among women, in whom this tumor represents 40% of the total.[3] One theory for this is that as cigarette smokers switch to lower tar and nicotine filtered cigarettes, they compensate by inhaling more deeply, increasing the risk of this peripherally located tumor.[16] A greater proportion of women than men tend to compensate after switching by inhaling more deeply and smoking more cigarettes per day.[1] This carcinoma also appears in nonsmokers. Although the tumor is comparably slow-growing, its tendency for early invasion of lymphatics and blood vessels produces its low survival rate.[3] The overall 2-year prognosis is poor with only about 20% survival.

*Large-cell, undifferentiated, or giant-cell carcinoma* is distinct from the previous two tumors in that the cells involved are large and very anaplastic. The cells do not secrete hormones and also do not tend to grow at the same rate as the small-cell type. The tumor is most frequently located in the peripheral areas of the lungs. These tumors account for about 15% of lung cancers. The overall prognosis remains very poor with only about 12% survival for 2 years.

The *small-cell (oat-cell) carcinoma* consists of small, dark cells located between the cells of the mucosal surfaces. They are characterized by rapid growth and early metastasis through the lymphatic system and blood. This disease is rare in the peripheral areas and frequently exhibits large, obstructive growths in the main bronchi.[9] These small-cell carcinomas often secrete substances like those normally found in other areas of the body, including adrenocorticotropic hormone and antidiuretic hormone. The result of adrenocorticotropic hormone secretion is Cushing's syndrome, leading to obesity, osteoporosis, hypokalemia, alkalosis, and other problems. Secretion of antidiuretic hormone leads to retention of water, hyponatremia, renal sodium loss, anorexia, nausea, and lethargy. The prognosis in this malignancy is the worst of lung cancers with only 3% to 5% survival rate for 2 years. The median survival rate after diagnosis is 3 months. Small-cell accounts for almost 25% of lung cancers.[11] Small-cell carcinomas also occur almost exclusively in cigarette smokers.

The propensity for metastasis at differing rates is very common with lung cancer. Over one half of afflicted persons (perhaps as many as 75%) have metastasis at the time of diagnosis.[9] The spread commonly occurs to the pleura, mediastinum, lymph nodes, liver, bone, brain, and adrenal glands.

The clinical manifestations of carcinoma of the lung are difficult to classify. Most individuals are asymptomatic for a long time or may develop signs of metastasis. The most common symptoms of the primary tumor are cough and expectoration of bloody sputum. Since most persons with lung cancer are heavy smokers, they tend to dismiss the symptoms as routine. Hemoptysis may be severe. Lymph node enlargement may cause encroachment on the superior vena cava, obstruction, and dramatic signs and symptoms. Chest pain, dyspnea, and hoarseness may be present. Often the first symptoms are those caused by distant spread of the malignancy and include superior vena caval obstruction, recurrent nerve paralysis, bone lesions, neurologic symptoms, and others. Radiologic evidence on a routine chest film is frequently the first sign. However, by the time a lung tumor is radiologically evident, it has usually invaded surrounding structures. Sputum cytology and bronchoscopy help to confirm the diagnosis.

# RESPIRATORY FAILURE

## *Respiratory Insufficiency*

Respiratory insufficiency is said to occur when the lungs are not able to exchange adequate amounts of carbon dioxide and oxygen to carry out the normal activities of daily living. In chronic respiratory insufficiency, the body gradually adapts to the pulmonary dysfunction. This process of adaptation includes hyperventilation; use of accessory muscles to breathe; circulatory changes to adjust the oxygen delivery to vital organs; and renal compensation to maintain the blood pH.[7] In *acute respiratory insufficiency*, hypoxemia and hypercapnia become severe and the compensatory mechanisms instituted by the body do not adjust the oxygen and carbon dioxide levels sufficiently to supply the body's needs. Inadequate tissue oxygen and severe respiratory acidosis occur without immediate treatment.

## *Respiratory Failure*

Respiratory failure is the inability of the lungs to meet the basic demands for tissue oxygenation at rest. Respi-

---

**BOX 31–2.**
CLASSIFICATION OF ACUTE RESPIRATORY FAILURE

A. Ventilatory failure
   1. Drug overdose
   2. Anesthetic agents
   3. Ventilatory depression in postoperative patient
   4. Stroke and other central nervous system problems
   5. Flail chest
   6. Cord injury above C4

B. Respiratory failure
   1. Postoperative or posttraumatic states
   2. Hemorrhage shock states
   3. Head injury
   4. Septic shock
   5. Multiple vital organ failure
   6. Pulmonary embolism
   7. Chronic obstructive lung disease
   8. Viral and bacterial pneumonia
   9. Interstitial pneumonitis

C. Direct injury
   1. Lung trauma: contusion, intrapulmonary hemorrhage, blunt or penetrating chest wounds
   2. Aspiration pneumonia
   3. Smoke inhalation
   4. Thoracotomy and pulmonary disease

D. Cardiac failure
   1. Fluid overload
   2. Acute exacerbation of chronic congestive heart failure with or without fluid overload
   3. Acute myocardial infarction with pulmonary edema

Source: W. Shoemaker, Textbook of Critical Care (2nd ed.). Philadelphia: W.B. Saunders, 1989.

**TABLE 31-1.**
PRECIPITATING FACTORS THAT MAY RESULT IN THE DEVELOPMENT OF
RESPIRATORY FAILURE

| FACTOR | EXAMPLE |
| --- | --- |
| Pulmonary infection, especially in presence of chronic obstructive pulmonary disease | Bacterial pneumonia<br>Viral pneumonia<br>Fungal pneumonia |
| Trauma | Automobile accident<br>Gunshot/knife wound<br>Burns |
| Infection | Sepsis<br>Wound infection |
| Cardiovascular event | Myocardial infarction<br>Aortic aneurysm<br>Pulmonary embolism |
| Allergic reaction | Transfusion reaction<br>Drug allergy<br>Bee sting or other venom |
| Pulmonary aspiration | Vomitus<br>Near drowning |
| Surgical procedure | Abdominal or thoracic surgery |
| Drug reaction | Overdose barbiturates or narcotics<br>Anesthetic reaction |
| Mechanical factor | Pneumothorax<br>Pleural effusion<br>Abdominal distention |
| Iatrogenic factor | Endotracheal intubation/failure of clearance of tracheobronchial secretions |
| Neuromuscular disorders | Guillain Barré syndrome<br>Multiple sclerosis<br>Muscular dystrophy |

ratory failure can occur as a result of a wide variety of intrapulmonary or nonpulmonary disorders (Box 31-2). Table 31-1 indicates that certain precipitating factors may cause the exacerbation of preexisting respiratory insufficiency.

The definitive diagnosis of respiratory failure depends on the arterial blood gases. A $PO_2$ of less than 50 mm Hg and a $PCO_2$ of greater than 50 mm Hg often are accepted as determining values.[7] These are related also to the patient's age, past history, and overall condition. Acute deterioration of blood gases in the person with chronic lung disease indicates failing compensation and respiratory failure.[7] The disorder may exist with hypoxemia as the predominant problem or with a combination of hypoxemia and hypercapnia.

As respiratory failure ensues, the $PCO_2$ begins to accumulate and leads to significant respiratory acidosis, indicating the inability of the lungs to eliminate the excess carbon dioxide. The normal chemoreceptors for carbon dioxide may become inoperative, and the hypoxic stimulus may be the stimulus for the respiratory effort. Oxygen should be administered with caution to these patients.

The clinical manifestations are dependent on the underlying cause but especially involve the resulting oxygen-carbon dioxide imbalance.[7] Dyspnea may not occur if there is depression of the respiratory center, so the respiratory rate may be very rapid or slow. Hypoxemia leads to inadequate tissue perfusion with varying degrees of cyanosis, depending on the amount of right-to-left shunting. This would be seen especially with severe atelectasis or adult respiratory distress syndrome (see Chap. 29). Hypercapnia refers to $PCO_2$ levels above 45 mm Hg. It indicates inadequate alveolar ventilation and the inability to release carbon dioxide. The symptoms, which are often associated with hypoxemia, include increased pulse and blood pressure, dizziness, headache, mental clouding and central nervous system depression, muscle twitching, and tremor.

*Carbon dioxide narcosis*, which occurs as levels of carbon dioxide progressively increase, leads to loss of consciousness, dilation of cerebral blood vessels, increased blood flow to the brain, increased intracranial pressure, and constriction of the pulmonary vessels.[7] Respiratory acidosis is frequent and may develop rapidly or slowly, depending on renal compensation.

The prognosis of acute or chronic respiratory failure

depends on the underlying causative mechanisms and whether or not lung function can improve. Respiratory failure is frequently the cause of death in pulmonary conditions.

## REFERENCES

1. Augustine, A., Harris, R., and Wynder, E. Compensation as a risk factor for lung cancer in smokers who switch from nonfilter to filter cigarettes. *Am. J. Public Health* 79:188, 1989.

2. Braman, S.S., and Davis, S.M. Wheezing in the aged: Asthma and other causes. *Clin. Geriatr. Med.* 2:269, 1986.

3. Bruderman, I. Bronchogenic carcinoma. In G. Baum and E. Wolinsky (eds.), *Textbook of Pulmonary Diseases* (4th ed.). Boston: Little, Brown, 1989.

4. Centers for Disease Control. Chronic disease reports: Deaths from lung cancer—United States, 1986. *Morbidity and Mortality Weekly Report* 38:501, 1989.

5. Cotran, R.S., Kumar, V., and Robbins, S.L. *Robbins' Pathologic Basis of Disease* (4th ed.). Philadelphia: W.B. Saunders, 1989.

6. Engelking, C. The language of staging. *Am. J. Nurs.* 87:1434, 1987.

7. Farzan, S.A. *A Concise Handbook of Respiratory Diseases* (2nd ed.). Reston, Va.: Reston, 1985.

8. Flenley, D. *Respiratory Medicine* (2nd ed.). London: Bailliere Tindal, 1990.

9. Kuhn, C., and Askin, F.B. Lung and mediastinum. In J.M. Kissane (ed.), *Anderson's Pathology* (9th ed.). St. Louis: Mosby, 1990.

10. Nunn, J.F. *Applied Respiratory Physiology* (3rd ed.). London: Butterworths, 1987.

11. Seaton, A., Seaton, D., and Leitch, A. *Crofton and Douglas's Respiratory Diseases* (4th ed.). Oxford: Blackwell, 1989.

12. Silverberg, E., Boring, C., and Squires, T. Cancer statistics, 1990. *CA* 40(1):9, 1990.

13. Sodeman, W.A., and Sodeman, T.M. *Sodeman's Pathologic Physiology* (7th ed.). Philadelphia: W.B. Saunders, 1985.

14. U.S. Department of Health, Education and Welfare. Public Health Service: Smoking and health: A report of the surgeon general. Department of Health, Education and Welfare, Public Health Service, Office on Smoking and Health. DHEW Pub. No. (PHS) 79–50066. Washington, D.C.: Government Printing Office, 1979.

15. Warner, K. Smoking and health: A 25-year perspective. *Am. J. Public Health* 79:141, 1989.

16. Wynder, E., Goodman, M., and Hoffman, D. Lung cancer etiology: Challenges of the future. In M. Mass, D. Kaufman, J. Siegfried, V. Stelle, and S. Nesnow (eds.), *Carcinogenesis—A Comprehensive Survey. Volume B: Cancer of the Respiratory Tract: Predisposing Factors*. New York: Raven Press, 1985.

## UNIT BIBLIOGRAPHY

Anderson, J. Dust in the lungs. *American Lung Association Bulletin* 66(4):7, 1980.

Augustine, A., Harris, R., and Wynder, E. Compensation as a risk factor for lung cancer in smokers who switch from nonfilter to filter cigarettes. *Am. J. Public Health* 79:188, 1989.

Barnes, P. A new approach to the treatment of asthma. *N. Engl. J. Med.* 321:1517, 1989.

Bellanti, J.A. *Immunology III*. Philadelphia: W.B. Saunders, 1985.

Belshe, R. Viral respiratory disease in the intensive care unit. *Heart Lung* 15:222, 1986.

Biggs, C. The cancer that can cost a patient his voice. *RN* 50(4):44, 1987.

Braman, S.S., and Davis, S.M. Wheezing in the aged: Asthma and other causes. *Clin. Geriatr. Med.* 2:269, 1986.

Brandstetter, R., Reddy, G., Bhalla, A., and Fulco, R. Idiopathic pulmonary fibrosis presenting as bilateral, ill-defined pulmonary densities. *Heart Lung* 13:671, 1984.

Braun, H.A., Cheney, F.W., and Loehnen, C.P. *Introduction to Respiratory Physiology* (2nd ed.). Boston: Little, Brown, 1980.

Braun, M.M., et al. Increasing incidence of tuberculosis in a prison inmate population. *JAMA* 261:393, 1989.

Braun, S.R. *Concise Textbook of Pulmonary Medicine*. New York: Elsevier, 1989.

Brown, L.H. Pulmonary oxygen toxicity. *Focus on Critical Care* 17(1):68, 1990.

Bruderman, I. Bronchogenic carcinoma. In G. Baum and E. Wolinsky (eds.), *Textbook of Pulmonary Diseases* (4th ed.). Boston: Little, Brown, 1989.

Burrows, B., Knudson, R., and Kettel, L. *Respiratory Disorders, A Pathophysiologic Approach* (2nd ed.). Chicago: Yearbook, 1983.

Carroll, P.F. What you can learn from pulmonary function tests. *RN* 49(7):24, 1986.

Caruthers, D.D. Infectious pneumonia in the elderly. *Am. J. Nurs.* 90(2):56, 1990.

Centers for Disease Control. Chronic disease reports: Deaths from lung cancer—United States, 1986. *Morbidity and Mortality Weekly Report* 38:501, 1989.

Cherniack, R., and Cherniack, L. *Respiration in Health and Disease* (3rd ed.). Philadelphia: W.B. Saunders, 1983.

Churg, A., and Green, F. *Pathology of Occupational Lung Disease*. New York: Igaku-Shoin, 1988.

Clark, T. *Clinical Investigation of Respiratory Disease*. London: Chapman and Hall, 1981.

Coleman, D. TB: The disease that's not dead yet. *RN* 47(9):49, 1984.

Coleman, D. Pneumonia: Where nursing care really counts. *RN* 49:22, 1986.

Comroe, J.H. *Physiology of Respiration* (2nd ed.). Chicago: Yearbook, 1974.

Connor, P., Berg, P., Flaherty, N., Klem, B., Lawton, R., and Tremblay, M. Two stages of care for pleural effusion. *RN* 52(2):30, 1989.

Cotran, R.S., Kumar, V., and Robbins, S.L. *Robbins' Pathologic Basis of Disease* (4th ed.). Philadelphia: W.B. Saunders, 1989.

Council on Scientific Affairs. A physician's guide to asbestos-related diseases. *J.A.M.A.* 252:2593, 1984.

Crystal, R.G., et al. The alpha$_1$-antitrypsin gene and its mutations. *Chest* 95:196, 1989.

Davies, C.N. A comparison between inhaled dust and the

dust recovered from human lungs. *Health Phys.* 10:129, 1964.

Engelking, C. The language of staging. *Am. J. Nurs.* 87:1434, 1987.

Eriksson, S. Alpha₁-antitrypsin deficiency: Lessons learned from the bedside to the gene and back again. *Chest* 90:181, 1989.

Eubanks, D., and Bone, R. *Comprehensive Respiratory Care: A Learning System.* St. Louis: Mosby, 1985.

Farzan, S.A. *A Concise Handbook of Respiratory Diseases* (2nd ed.). Reston, Va.: Reston, 1985.

Fischbein, A., and Rohl, A. Pleural mesothelioma and neighborhood asbestos exposure. *JAMA* 252:86, 1984.

Fishman, A.P. *Pulmonary Diseases and Disorders* (2nd ed.). New York: McGraw-Hill, 1988.

Flenley, D. *Respiratory Medicine* (2nd ed.). London: Bailliere Tindal, 1990.

Fry, J., White, R., and Whitfield, M. *Respiratory Disorders.* Edinburgh, United Kingdom: Churchill Livingstone, 1984.

Ganong, W.F. *Review of Medical Physiology* (14th ed.). Los Altos, Calif.: Lange, 1989.

Gee, J.B. *Occupational Lung Disease.* New York: Churchill Livingstone, 1984.

Goetter, W.E. The pathophysiology of asthma: Extrinsic influences other than immunologic. *Clin. Chest Med.* 5:589, 1984.

Greifzu, S., Crebase, C., and Winnick, B. Lung cancer: By the time it's detected, it may be too late. *RN* 50(5):52, 1987.

Grzybowski, S. *Tuberculosis and Its Prevention.* St. Louis: Warren H. Green, 1983.

Guenter, C.A., and Welch, M.H. (eds.). *Pulmonary Medicine* (2nd ed.). Philadelphia: J.B. Lippincott, 1982.

Guyton, A.C. *Textbook of Medical Physiology* (8th ed.). Philadelphia: W.B. Saunders, 1991.

Hahn, K. Slow-teaching the COPD patient. *Nurs. 87* 17(4):34, 1987.

Hensley, M., and Saunders, N. *Clinical Epidemiology of Chronic Obstructive Pulmonary Disease.* New York: Marcel Dekker, 1989.

Holgate, S.T., et al. *The Role of Inflammatory Processes in Airway Hyperresponsiveness.* Oxford: Blackwell, 1989.

Hoyt, K.S. Chest trauma: When the patient looks bad, act fast. And when he looks good, act fast. *Nurs. 83* 13(5):34, 1983.

Ioli, J.G. Giving surfactant to premature infants. *Am. J. Nurs.* 90(3):59, 1990.

Janson-Bjerklie, S. Status asthmaticus. *Am. J. Nurs.* 90(9):52, 1990.

Keller, C., Solomon, J., and Reyes, A. *Respiratory Nursing Care.* Englewood Cliffs, N.J.: Prentice-Hall, 1984.

Kelley, W.N. *Textbook of Internal Medicine.* Philadelphia: J.B. Lippincott, 1989.

Kissane, J.M. *Anderson's Pathology* (9th ed.). St. Louis: Mosby, 1990.

Komshian, S., Chandrasekar, P., and Levine, D. Adenovirus pneumonia in healthy adults. *Heart Lung* 16:146, 1987.

Krokosky, N. Black lung and silicosis. *Am. J. Nurs.* 85:883, 1985.

Krupp, M.A., and Chatton, M.J. *Current Medical Diagnosis and Treatment 1990.* Los Altos, Calif.: Lange, 1990.

Levitsky, M.G. *Pulmonary Physiology* (2nd ed.). New York: McGraw-Hill, 1986.

Madsen, L.A. Tuberculosis today. *RN* 53(3):44, 1990.

Martin, D., and Youtesy, J. *Respiratory Anatomy and Physiology.* St. Louis: Mosby, 1988.

Martin, R.A. AIDS with disseminated histoplasmosis. *J. Fam. Pract.* 29:628, 1989.

Martin, R.J. *Cardiorespiratory Disorders During Sleep* (2nd ed.). Mt. Kisco, N.Y.: Future, 1990.

Mass, M., Kaufman, D., Siegfried, J., Stelle, V., and Nesnow, S. *Carcinogenesis—A Comprehensive Survey. Volume 8: Cancer of the Respiratory Tract: Predisposing Factors.* New York: Raven Press, 1985.

McMahan, B.E. Why deep vein thrombosis is so dangerous. *RN* 50(1):20, 1987.

Mines, A.H. *Respiratory Physiology* (2nd ed.). New York: Raven Press, 1986.

Mossman, B., and Gee, J. Asbestos-related diseases. *N. Engl. J. Med.* 320:1721, 1989.

Niederman, M.S., and Fein, A.M. Pneumonia in the elderly. *Clin. Geriatr. Med.* 2:241, 1986.

Notkins, A., and Oldstone, B.A. *Concepts in Viral Pathogenesis.* New York: Springer-Verlag, 1984.

Nunn, J.F. *Applied Respiratory Physiology* (3rd ed.). London: Butterworths, 1987.

Pachon, J., Prados, D., Capote, F., Cuello, J., Garnacho, J., and Verano, A. Severe community-acquired pneumonia: Etiology, prognosis, and treatment. *Am. Rev. Respir. Dis.* 142:369, 1990.

Pennington, J. *Respiratory Infections: Diagnosis and Management* (2nd ed.). New York: Raven Press, 1989.

Rieder, H., Cauthen, G., Kelly, G., Bloch, A., and Snider, D. Tuberculosis in the United States. *JAMA* 262:385, 1989.

Roitt, I. *Essential Immunology* (6th ed.). Oxford: Blackwell, 1988.

Roitt, I., Brostoff, J., and Male, D. *Immunology* (2nd ed.). St. Louis: Mosby, 1989.

Romanski, S.O. Interpreting ABGs in four easy steps. *Nurs. 86* 16(9):58, 1986.

Schluttenhofeer, N. The special challenge of empyemas. *Nurs. 84* 14(12):57, 1984.

Seaton, A., Seaton, D., and Leitch, A. *Crofton and Douglas's Respiratory Diseases* (4th ed.). Oxford: Blackwell, 1989.

Selkurt, E. *Physiology* (5th ed.). Boston: Little, Brown, 1984.

Shaman, D. Silicosis: The occupational disease that shouldn't exist. *American Lung Association Bulletin* 69(2):6, 1983.

Shapiro, B.A., et al. *Clinical Application of Blood Gases* (4th ed.). Chicago: Yearbook, 1989.

Shapiro, B.A., et al. *Clinical Application of Respiratory Care* (3rd ed.). Chicago: Yearbook, 1985.

Shoemaker, W., et al. *Textbook of Critical Care* (2nd ed.). Philadelphia: W.B. Saunders, 1989.

Shovein, J.T., Land, L.P., Richter, G., and Leedom, C.L. Near-drowning. *Am. J. Nurs.* 89:680, 1989.

Silverberg, E., Boring, C., and Squires, T. Cancer statistics, 1990. *CA* 40(1):9, 1990.

Slonim, N.B., and Hamilton, L.H. *Respiratory Physiology* (5th ed.). St. Louis: Mosby, 1987.

Snapper, J. Inflammation and airway function: The asthma syndrome. *Am. Rev. Respir. Dis.* 141:531, 1990.

Sodeman, W.A., and Sodeman, T.M. *Sodeman's Pathologic Physiology* (7th ed.). Philadelphia: W.B. Saunders, 1985.

Stratton, C. Bacterial pneumonias—An overview with emphasis

on pathogenesis, diagnosis, and treatment. *Heart Lung* 15:226, 1986.

Stratton, M.B. Ventilation-perfusion scintigraphy in diagnosis of pulmonary thromboembolism. *Focus on Critical Care* 17: 287, 1990.

Surveyer, J. Smoke inhalation injuries. *Heart Lung* 9:825, 1980.

Tafuro, P., Digamon-Beltran, M., and Cunha, B. Approach to hospital-acquired pneumonias. *Heart Lung* 13:482, 1984.

Thurlbeck, W.M. *Pathology of the Lung*. New York: Thieme, 1988.

U.S. Department of Health, Education and Welfare. Public Health Service: Smoking and health: A report of the surgeon general. Department of Health, Education and Welfare, Public Health Service, Office on Smoking and Health. DHEW Pub. No. (PHS) 79–50066. Washington, D.C.: Government Printing Office, 1979.

Unanue, E.R., and Benacerraf, B. *Textbook of Immunology* (2nd ed.). Baltimore: Williams & Wilkins, 1984.

Walter, J.B. *An Introduction to the Principles of Disease* (2nd ed.). Philadelphia: W.B. Saunders, 1982.

Walter, J.B. *Pathology of Human Disease*. Philadelphia: Lea & Febiger, 1989.

Warner, K. Smoking and health: A 25-year perspective. *Am. J. Public Health* 79:141, 1989.

Weaver, T., and Millman, R. Broken sleep. *Am. J. Nurs.* 86:146, 1986.

Wegmann, J., and Forshee, T. Malignant pleural effusions: Pertinent issues. *Heart Lung* 12:533, 1983.

Weinberger, S. *Principles of Pulmonary Medicine*. Philadelphia: W.B. Saunders, 1986.

Weinberger, S., Schwartzstein, R., and Weiss, J. Hypercapnia. *N. Engl. J. Med.* 321:1223, 1989.

West, J.B. *Pulmonary Pathophysiology: The Essentials* (3rd ed.). Baltimore: Williams & Wilkins, 1987.

West, J.B. *Respiratory Physiology: The Essentials* (4th ed.). Baltimore: Williams & Wilkins, 1990.

West, J.B. *Ventilation/Blood Flow and Gas Exchange* (4th ed.). Oxford: Blackwell, 1985.

Wewers, M. Pathogenesis of emphysema: Assessment of basic science concepts through clinical investigation. *Chest* 90: 190, 1989.

Whitcomb, M. *The Lung: Normal and Diseased*. St. Louis: Mosby, 1982.

Williams, M. *Essentials of Pulmonary Medicine*. Philadelphia: W.B. Saunders, 1982.

Woodin, L.M. Your patient with pneumothorax. *Nurs. 82* 12(11):50, 1982.

unit

10

# URINARY EXCRETION

The urinary system maintains the appropriate concentration of electrolytes and water in the blood and eliminates many waste products. Chapter 32 explains normal renal function and provides a basis for the subsequent chapters that discuss different forms of renal pathology. Chapter 33 details the immunologic, infectious, and toxic alterations that can affect renal function. Chapter 34 describes the common causes of micturition dysfunction and genitourinary obstruction with emphasis on the formation of different types of calculi. Benign prostatic hyperplasia and renal and bladder tumors are included. Chapter 35 describes renal failure, its causes, and clinical course.

The reader is encouraged to use the learning objectives to provide a systematic method for study. The extensive bibliography provides a current and historical perspective on general and specific aspects of renal function and dysfunction.

# Normal Renal and Urinary Excretory Function

## Chapter Outline

## Learning Objectives

1. Describe the location and size of the kidneys.
2. Explain the internal structure of the kidneys, including the lobes, lobules, cortex, medulla, and renal pelvis.
3. Identify the structures of the renal corpuscle.
4. Relate the main layers of the glomerular membrane, including the epithelial, glomerular basement membrane, and endothelial layers, to the formation of ultrafiltrate.
5. Describe the juxtaglomerular apparatus.
6. Identify the various parts of the nephron.
7. Describe the blood supply to the kidneys.
8. Describe in detail the mechanisms responsible for urine formation, including glomerular filtration, tubular reabsorption, and secretion.
9. Define *filtration, filtrate, tubular reabsorption, transport maximum*, and *secretion*.
10. Describe the pressures responsible for filtration.
11. Calculate the net filtration pressure and relate it to the glomerular filtration rate.
12. Describe active transport of glucose ions and protein from the proximal convoluted tubules.

13. Explain the passive transport of water and ions from the proximal convoluted tubules.
14. Describe hypotonic and hypertonic urine formation and explain the countercurrent mechanism in the loop of Henle.
15. Discuss antidiuretic hormone and its relationship to water regulation in the distal convoluted tubules and collecting tubules.
16. Discuss the secretion of PAH and potassium.
17. Explain the secretion of hydrogen ions and its relationship to acid-base balance.
18. Discuss the functions of the kidney in erythrocyte production, vitamin D₃ activation, and gluconeogenesis.
19. Explain renal regulation of the renin-angiotensin-aldosterone system.
20. Explain the physical characteristics of urine.
21. Describe the structure and purpose of the ureters.
22. Explain the micturition reflex.
23. Differentiate between the female and male urethras.

For the body to maintain a steady state, the renal system must function normally. This system not only is important in removing waste products from the blood, it maintains sufficient amounts of water and electrolytes in the blood. Urine is produced by the kidneys and is transported to the ureters, which empty into the bladder. Urine is excreted from the body through the urethra.

## ANATOMY OF THE KIDNEYS

### Macroscopic Anatomy

The kidneys are bean-shaped, reddish-brown organs that are located retroperitoneally on either side of the vertebral column, extending from the 12th thoracic vertebra to the third lumbar vertebra. Each kidney is approximately 11.0 cm in length, 5.0 to 7.0 cm in diameter, and 2.5 cm in thickness. The right kidney is slightly lower than the left because the liver is located above it (Figure 32-1).

Surrounding the kidneys is a layer of adipose tissue, or perirenal fat, that helps protect and support them. A fibrous layer of connective tissue called *renal fascia* encapsulates and anchors the kidneys in place in the abdomen.

Located externally at the concave portion of the kidney is a notch called the hilum. Structures at the hilum of each kidney are the renal artery and vein, lymphatics, nerves, and renal pelvis (Figure 32-2). The renal pelvis is the funnel-shaped extension of the upper ureter that provides a passageway for urine to the bladder.[9]

Internally, the kidneys are composed of the cortex and the medulla. The cortex, the outer portion, lies under the renal fascia. Substantial portions of the inner medullary layer are separated by cortical substances that are called renal columns or columns of Bertin.[3] Also, originating in the cortex and extending into the medulla are the uriniferous tubules, which are made up of the parenchymal (functioning) units of the kidneys, the nephrons. The medulla, the inner portion of the kidney, contains an estimated 8 to 18 *renal pyramids,* so-called because they are triangular. They are striated due to the collecting ducts, nephrons, and blood vessels of which they are composed. The apex of each pyramid is called the papilla. Below the papillae is a large cavity called the renal pelvis, which is interrupted by cuplike extensions

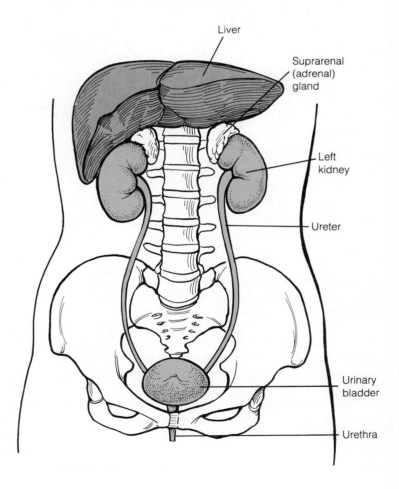

**FIGURE 32–1.**
Posterior abdominal wall showing kidneys and ureters in situ. (Adapted from R.S. Snell, *Clinical Histology for Medical Students.* Boston: Little, Brown, 1984.)

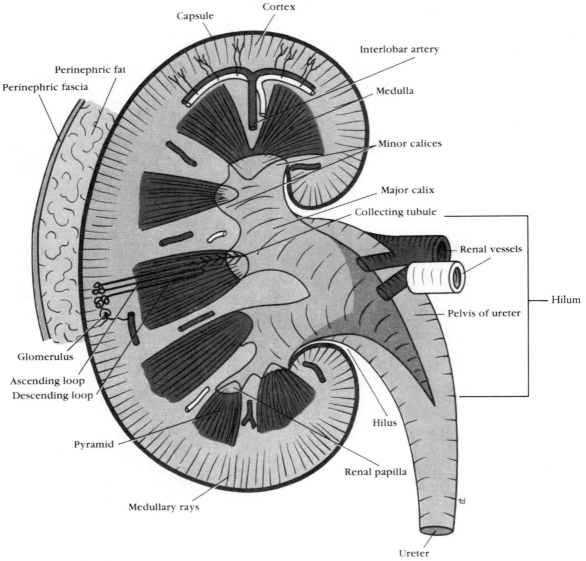

**FIGURE 32–2.**
Longitudinal section through kidney, showing cortex, medulla, pyramids, renal papillae, and calices. Note also perinephric fascia and fat and their relation to renal capsule. (Source: R. Snell, *Clinical Anatomy for Medical Students* [2nd ed.]. Boston: Little, Brown, 1981.)

called the minor and major calices. These structures are lined with transitional epithelium. The minor calices (approximately 10 in number) have openings that collect urine from the collecting ducts of the pyramids and empty urine into the major calices (approximately three in number) and then into the renal pelvis, where it is excreted from the kidneys to the ureters (see Figure 32-2).

The human kidney has up to 18 lobes, each of which are made up of cortical tissue and a conical medullary pyramid. Each pyramid of the kidney corresponds to a single lobe.[3] The lobes are well-defined structures with a number of lobules that make them up. The lobules are the parts of the kidney whose nephrons drain into common collecting tubules.[3]

## Microscopic Anatomy: The Nephron

It is estimated that a pair of kidneys contains 2.5 million nephrons. The nephron is a unique and complex structure. It is composed of Bowman's capsule, the proximal convoluted tubule (PCT), the loop of Henle, and the distal convoluted tubule (DCT). Many distal tubules empty into one collecting tubule or duct.

Bowman's capsule is a cuplike structure that sur-

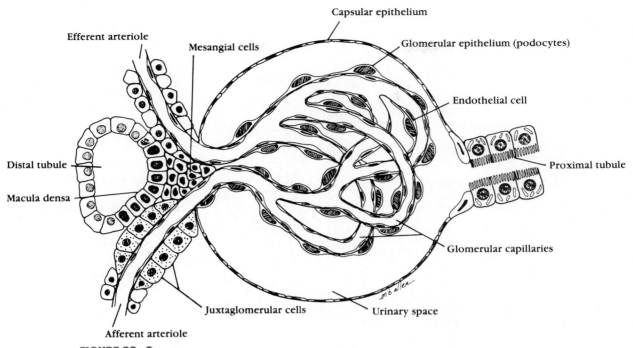

**FIGURE 32-3.**
Bowman's capsule with the glomerulus within. (Source: M. Borysenko, et al., *Functional Histology* [2nd ed.]. Boston: Little, Brown, 1984.)

rounds a capillary network called the glomerulus; the two together are called the *renal corpuscle.* The renal corpuscle has been likened to a fist (glomerulus) pushed into a balloon (Bowman's capsule).[9] There is an inherent space between the two structures where ultrafiltrate is received from the blood through the membrane of the glomerulus (Figure 32-3).

The membrane of the glomerular capillaries is composed of three main layers: epithelial, glomerular basement membrane (GBM), and endothelial. The main function of the glomerular membrane is to form glomerular filtrate, a solution-like plasma but without plasma proteins (see pp. 628–630). This is the initial step in urine formation.

Nephrons are classified as either cortical or juxtamedullary (Figure 32-4). The glomeruli of the cortical nephrons are in the outer two thirds of the cortex. The tubules of the cortical nephrons lie mainly within the cortex. The remaining one third of the cortical area consists of glomeruli of the juxtamedullary nephrons, which contain a long loop of Henle that extends deep into the medulla.

Lining the inner layer of Bowman's capsule, adjacent to the glomerulus, is a thin layer of epithelial cells called podocytes. These podocytes have projections called pedicles (foot processes) that cover the GBM. Between the pedicles are narrow regions called slit pores (filtration slits), through which proteins with a molecular weight of less than 50,000 can pass.[4] Because plasma proteins have a slightly higher molecular weight they normally cannot cross the GBM. Because of the location, numbers, and arrangement of slit pores, there is a large surface area that allows for rapid filtration of fluid. Diseases that affect the foot processes allow plasma proteins and sometimes cells to pass into the glomerular filtrate (see Chap. 33).

Adjacent to the layer of epithelial cells is the GBM, which consists of a continuous meshwork of fibrillae that contain mucopolysaccharides. This meshwork prevents large proteins and molecules from passing into Bowman's capsule, a function that prevents protein loss in the urine.

The inner layer of the glomerular capillary is composed of endothelial cells. This layer consists of thousands of pores (fenestrations) that line the glomerulus and aid in membrane permeability. The glomerular filtrate passes through three layers before it arrives in Bowman's capsule but each layer is several hundred times more permeable than the usual capillary membrane.[5]

Once the glomerular filtrate passes through the glomeruli into Bowman's capsule, it enters the PCT, which is located in the cortex and is approximately 14 mm long. Cuboidal epithelial cells line the PCT. On the luminal surface of these cells is a brush border of microvilli that increases the surface area available for secretion and absorption of fluids and solutes. Also located in the PCT cells are mitochondria. More than 65% to 80% of the glomerular filtrate is resorbed in the PCT and the remaining 20% to 35% proceeds to the loop of Henle.

The two major portions of the loop of Henle are the

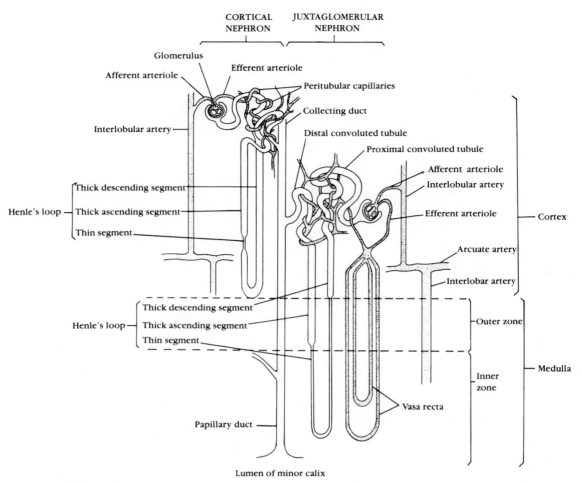

CORTICAL
NEPHRON

JUXTAGLOMERULAR
NEPHRON

**FIGURE 32–4.**

Structure of cortical and medullary nephrons. Blood supply to the nephron. The vasa recta is shown schematically; this capillary structure normally surrounds Henle's loop. (Source: M. Borysenko, et al., *Functional Histology* [2nd ed.]. Boston: Little, Brown, 1984.)

descending and ascending limbs (see Figure 32-4). The thickened descending limb begins in the cortex. As it dips into the medulla, it becomes thinner and varies in length from 4.5 to 10.0 mm.[2]

The descending limb loops and makes a tight hairpin turn upward, where it becomes thin and is called the thin portion of the ascending limb. The main function of both limbs of the loop of Henle is to concentrate urine. Once urine passes through the limbs, it proceeds to the DCT, which is located in the renal cortex.

The DCT is lined with cuboidal cells containing mitochondria and fewer microvilli than are present in the PCT. As the cuboidal cells change to columnar cells, the area becomes very dense, thus forming the macula densa (see Figure 32-4).

The macula densa lies in close contact with the vascular component of the juxtaglomerular apparatus (Figure 32-5). Located within the apparatus are juxtaglomerular cells that produce the enzyme renin, which trans-

forms angiotensinogen to angiotensin I (see Chap. 26). The macula densa cells also contribute to the control of the glomerular filtration rate (GFR).[9]

The main function of the DCT is to transport electrolytes and water. Two or more DCTs join together to form the collecting duct, which conducts the formed urine. The collecting ducts are lined with cuboidal cells, contain few mitochondria, and terminate in the renal medulla.

Urine is transported from the collecting duct to a papillary collecting duct, which opens into the minor calix. Urine is then excreted from the minor to the major calices and into the renal pelvis, ureters, bladder, and urethra.

## Blood Supply to the Kidneys

In a resting state, it is estimated that the kidneys receive 20% to 25% of cardiac output, which is more than 1000

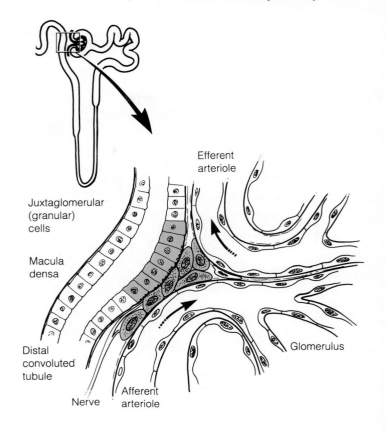

**FIGURE 32-5.**
The relationship of the juxtaglomerular apparatus, the distal convoluted tubule, and the glomerulus.

mL per minute. Thus, by way of the aorta, blood enters the hilum of the kidney by a renal artery, which branches into segmental arteries and then interlobar arteries that run between the pyramids of the medulla (Figures 32-4 and 32-6). At the junction between the cortex and medulla (corticomedullary junction), the interlobar arteries convert to arcuate arteries that penetrate the cortex and branch into smaller arteries called interlobular arteries, thus giving rise to the afferent arterioles. The afferent arterioles subdivide into a tuft of capillaries called a glomerulus. Blood leaves the glomerulus by the efferent arteriole and forms a second network of capillaries called the peritubular capillary network that mainly encircles the convoluted tubules (proximal and distal). The arrangement of capillaries between these arterioles is unique because it allows a higher pressure to be maintained in the glomerulus. Also, the efferent arterioles are smaller in diameter than the afferent arterioles, again causing higher glomerular pressure due to increased vascular resistance.

The deeper-lying (juxtamedullary) glomeruli also break up into the peritubular network but have a set of capillaries penetrating the medulla. These thin-walled vessels are in close proximity to the thin ascending and descending loops of Henle and are referred to as the vasa recta (see Figure 32-4). The vasa recta aid in concentrating urine.

The interlobular veins are formed from the peri-

tubular capillary network and empty into the arcuate veins and then the interlobar veins, and converge to form the renal vein. Blood from the renal vein leaves the kidneys and drains into the inferior vena cava.

## *Innervation of the Kidneys*

Nerve fibers reach the kidneys through the renal plexus, which extends along the renal artery. The kidneys are innervated mostly by the sympathetic division of the autonomic nervous system but smaller numbers of parasympathetic fibers are also present.[3] The nerve supply generally follows the distribution of the arterial vessels in the renal parenchyma. The nerve supply comes mostly from the celiac plexus, and the mesenteric, upper splanchnic, and thoracic nerves.[4] The sympathetic nerves, when stimulated, constrict the afferent arteriole and cause an increase in blood pressure. The parasympathetic system has important effects on the ureters and urinary bladder but no noted effects on the kidneys per se.[9]

## *PHYSIOLOGY OF THE KIDNEYS*

The kidneys function to maintain a constant plasma concentration of substances by removing some from the

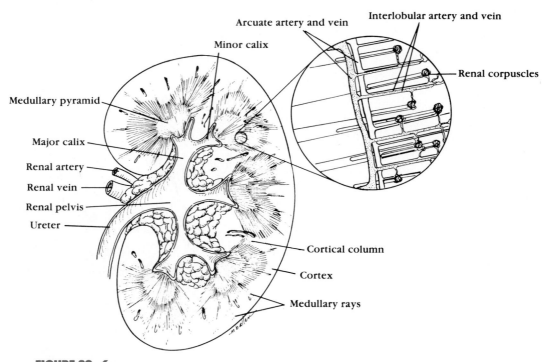

**FIGURE 32–6.**
Hemisected kidney with vascular distribution. (Source: M. Borysenko, et al., *Functional Histology* [2nd ed.]. Boston: Little, Brown, 1984.)

blood and adding some back to it (Box 32-1).[9] The functions are essential to maintain life, even though the kidneys do not regulate all inorganic or organic substances. The kidneys have a large reserve in renal function due to large numbers of nephrons.

The critical functions of blood pressure regulation, erythropoietin production, 1,25 dihydroxyvitamin $D_3$ secretion, and gluconeogenesis are discussed after the discussion of balancing body water and inorganic ions. The kidneys use three major mechanisms to maintain a balance that alters the composition of urine to keep the composition of plasma within strict limits. These mechanisms are glomerular filtration, tubular reabsorption,

and tubular secretion. Figure 32-7 provides a reference for the major functions of each portion of the nephron.

## Glomerular Filtration

Filtration, the initial step in urine formation, is the result of pressures that force fluids and solutes through a membrane. The filtration process occurs between the layers of the glomerulus and Bowman's capsule. The resulting fluid is *glomerular filtrate*, a relatively protein-free solution.

Approximately 125 mL per minute, or 180 liters per

---

**BOX 32–1.**
FUNCTIONS OF THE KIDNEYS

1. Regulation of water and electrolyte balance
2. Removal of metabolic waste products from the blood and their excretion in the urine
3. Removal of foreign chemicals from the blood and their excretion in the urine
4. Regulation of arterial blood pressure by altering both sodium excretion and the secretion of renin and possibly other vasoactive substances
5. Secretion of erythropoietin
6. Secretion of 1,25-dihydroxyvitamin $D_3$
7. Gluconeogenesis

Source: A.J. Vander, Renal Physiology. New York: McGraw-Hill, 1991.

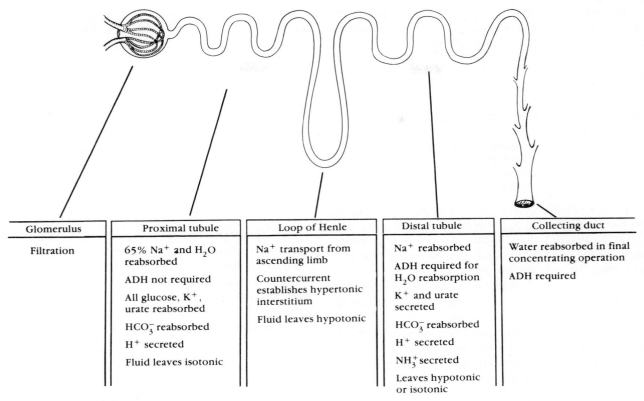

| Glomerulus | Proximal tubule | Loop of Henle | Distal tubule | Collecting duct |
|---|---|---|---|---|
| Filtration | 65% $Na^+$ and $H_2O$ reabsorbed<br><br>ADH not required<br><br>All glucose, $K^+$, urate reabsorbed<br><br>$HCO_3^-$ reabsorbed<br><br>$H^+$ secreted<br><br>Fluid leaves isotonic | $Na^+$ transport from ascending limb<br><br>Countercurrent establishes hypertonic interstitium<br><br>Fluid leaves hypotonic | $Na^+$ reabsorbed<br><br>ADH required for $H_2O$ reabsorption<br><br>$K^+$ and urate secreted<br><br>$HCO_3^-$ reabsorbed<br><br>$H^+$ secreted<br><br>$NH_3^+$ secreted<br><br>Leaves hypotonic or isotonic | Water reabsorbed in final concentrating operation<br><br>ADH required |

**FIGURE 32–7.**
Major functions of each portion of the nephron. (Source: S. Papper, *Clinical Nephrology* [2nd ed.]. Boston: Little, Brown, 1978.)

day, of glomerular filtrate is produced. Normally, urine output equals approximately 1 to 2 liters per day, which means that the tubules are responsible for reabsorbing approximately 179 liters. The measurement of the large quantity of glomerular filtrate each minute is called the *glomerular filtration rate*.

The quantity of filtrate and the filtration process are dependent on several factors. Various pressures contribute to the outward flow of filtrate into Bowman's capsule and retention of fluid within the glomerulus. The *hydrostatic pressure* is a simple outward force created by the systemic blood pressure. The *colloid osmotic pressure* or *oncotic pressure* is the inward force or pressure that holds fluid within the glomerulus (Figure 32-8).

The pressure that is chiefly responsible for filtration is the *glomerular hydrostatic pressure* ($P_{GC}$). This pressure forces filtrate out of the glomerulus into Bowman's capsule and normally is approximately 60 mm Hg. If the hydrostatic pressure decreases to 50 mm Hg, filtration usually does not take place.

Working in opposition to the hydrostatic pressure is the *capsular hydrostatic pressure* ($P_{BC}$) in Bowman's capsule, which is normally estimated to be about 18 mm Hg. This pressure is exerted by the walls of Bowman's capsule and the fluid in the renal tubule. Increased capsular pressure causes the GFR to decrease.[5]

The other pressure that works in opposition to the glomerular pressure is the *blood colloidal osmotic pressure (COP)*, normally about 30 mm Hg. Because blood contains more protein than filtrate does, the colloidal property constantly exerts an inward force.

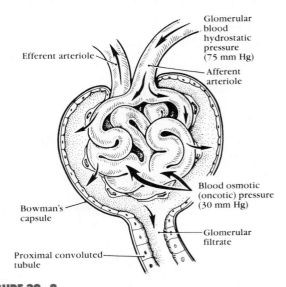

**FIGURE 32–8.**
Schematic representation of the relationship between hydrostatic pressure and colloid osmotic pressure.

The net result of all these pressures—glomerular, capsular, and colloidal osmotic—is the *net filtration pressure* (NFP). The NFP can be calculated as follows:

$$\text{NFR} = \underset{\substack{\text{forces inducing}\\ \text{filtration}}}{P_{GC}} - \underset{\substack{\text{forces opposing}\\ \text{filtration}}}{(P_{BC} + \pi_{GC})}$$

where  $P_{GC}$ = glomerular capillary hydrostatic or hydraulic pressure;

$P_{BC}$ = hydrostatic or hydraulic pressure in Bowman's capsule; and

$\pi_{GC}$ = oncotic or colloid osmotic pressure in glomerular-capillary plasma[9]

As an example, if the $P_{GC}$ is 60 mm Hg, the $P_{BC}$ is 18, and the $\pi_{GC}$ is 32, the NFP will be 10 mm Hg (60 −[18 + 32] = 10). If 1 mm Hg effective filtration pressure produces a GFR of 12.5 mL per minute from both kidneys, then 10 mm Hg produces 125 mL per minute, which is a normal rate. Many factors can change the GFR. Increased hydrostatic pressure or decreased COP can increase the GFR (Figure 32-9).

Sympathetic nervous system stimulation results in vasoconstriction of the afferent and efferent arterioles, which affects the NFP. Because constriction of the afferent arterioles is usually greater that that of the efferent arterioles with sympathetic stimulation, the result is a decrease in $P_{GC}$ and GFR.

### Renal Clearance

Renal clearance refers to the volume of plasma from which a substance is completely cleared by the kidneys per unit time.[9] Measuring the clearance of substances is extremely useful in the evaluation of renal function. It has been used successfully to evaluate the GFR. A polysaccharide called *inulin* is freely filtered at the glomerulus and not reabsorbed in any way in the tubules. It can, therefore, be used to determine the GFR. It must be administered intravenously at a constant rate for several hours. The GFR can be calculated by the following formula:

$$\text{GFR} = \frac{U_{In}V \; (\text{urine inulin} \times \text{urine volume})}{P_{In} \; (\text{plasma inulin})}$$

where: urine inulin is multiplied times the volume of urine over a specified time; and plasma inulin concentration is maintained constant at 4 mg/L. An example cited in Vander[9] may clarify this concept

$$\text{GFR} = \frac{360 \text{ mg/L} \times 0.2 \text{ L/2 hr}}{4 \text{ mg/L}} = 18 \text{ L/2 hr} = 150 \text{ mL/min}$$

In clinical practice, estimating the GFR from inulin is inconvenient so an endogenous substance, creatinine, is used to estimate it. Creatinine is almost totally excreted. Using it to calculate GFR usually overestimates the true value but the value is very close to actual GFR. It can be calculated by collecting a 24-hour urine and obtaining a blood sample.[9] The formula then becomes:

$$\text{Estimated GFR} = \frac{U_{cr}V}{P_{cr}}$$

where $U_{cr}$ = amount of creatinine in mg/dL excreted in the urine in 24 hours; V = volume of urine in mL/min. Total volume is divided by 1440 minutes (24 hours); and $P_{cr}$ = serum creatinine in mg/dL. An example might be:

$$
\begin{aligned}
U_{cr} &= 104 \text{ mg/dL}\\
V &= 1800 \text{ mL/24 hr} = 75 \text{ mL/hr} = 1.25 \text{ mL/min}\\
P_{cr} &= 1.0 \text{ mg/dL}\\
\text{GFR} &= \frac{104 \times 1.25}{1.0} = \frac{130}{1.0} = 130 \text{ mL/min}
\end{aligned}
$$

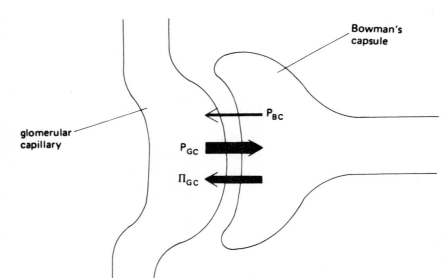

**FIGURE 32-9.**

Net filtration pressure in the renal corpuscle equals glomerular-capillary hydraulic pressure (Pgc) minus Bowman's capsule hydraulic pressure (Pbc) minus glomerular-capilllary oncotic pressure (gc). (Source: A.J. Vander, *Renal Physiology* [4th ed.]. New York: McGraw-Hill, 1991.)

## Reabsorption: Tubules

As described in the previous section, approximately 179 liters of filtrate of the 180 liters filtered per day are reabsorbed in the tubules. The kidneys are able to change the composition of urine by excreting different concentrations of substances.[5] This is achieved by reabsorption and secretion. For example, when a person ingests a large volume of water, the resulting urine is very dilute. In a dehydrated state, the urine output is markedly decreased and urine becomes very concentrated. *Tubular reabsorption*, the second step of urine formation, requires movement of solutes between the filtrate and blood of the surrounding vasa recta and peritubular capillaries.

## Reabsorption in the Proximal Convoluted Tubules

In the *proximal convoluted tubules*, tubular reabsorption is accomplished by active and passive transport (diffusion or osmosis). Approximately 70% of glomerular filtrate is resorbed in the PCT. Ions are transported by active and passive transport. Some ions passively follow the active transport of other ions.[5]

### Active Transport

Active transport is the movement of molecules against a concentration gradient and requires an expenditure of energy. It causes movement of substances from PCT to plasma. The PCT are able to carry on active transport because of their epithelial cells that contain mitochondria. These cells also have a brush border that increases the surface area for reabsorption and secretion. Some of the substances that are moved actively include glucose, many electrolytes, amino acids, proteins, and vitamins.[8]

*Glucose* is actively transported from the tubules into the plasma and normally none appears in the urine. Glucose apparently binds with, and is dependent upon, the same sodium carrier in the brush border that transports sodium ions through this membrane.[5,9] This transport is related to a mechanism called *transport maximum* ($T_M$) in which there is a maximum amount of substance that can be reabsorbed at any time.[2] If the plasma glucose level exceeds the *threshold* of approximately 175 mg per dL, glucose appears in the urine (glycosuria) because the transport mechanism has become saturated with glucose and must leave it in the tubules so that it is excreted in the urine. The $T_M$ varies with different individuals, especially if there is a chronic increase in glucose load, as often happens in diabetes mellitus (see Chap. 39).

*Sodium* and *potassium* are actively transported from the tubules into the plasma of the peritubular capillaries by way of the basal channels of the epithelial cells. Because sodium and potassium are positive ions, they set up an electronegative cytoplasm in the epithelial cells. This allows negative ions, such as chloride and phosphate, to follow the positive ions.[5]

*Proteins* are reabsorbed in the PCT through the energy-dependent process of endocytosis.[9] The proteins attach to the membrane of the brush border of the PCT, are ingested by the tubular cells, and are broken down into amino acids, which are transported into the plasma. If permeability of the glomerular membrane increases, large protein molecules can leak into the filtrate, causing proteinuria.

### Passive Transport

Passive transport, including osmosis and diffusion, involves the movement of substances across a membrane without the expenditure of energy. It is accomplished by the established electrical gradient of positive ions, mainly sodium, allowing negative ions and water to diffuse across the tubular membrane.

Water is removed from the tubules as the result of the *isosmotic process*, which maintains equal osmotic pressures of fluid inside the tubules and in the plasma. When the solutes are actively reabsorbed into the plasma, the concentration of solute in the tubules decreases and the concentration in the peritubular capillaries increases, causing water to move into the peritubular capillary. Approximately 70% of water is reabsorbed by passive transport in the PCT. The role of the kidneys in controlling osmolality of the plasma through the transport of water is critical in maintaining fluid balance. The excretion of excess water or conservation of water maintains the plasma osmolarity at a fixed specific gravity of 1.010. This regulation is greatly influenced by antidiuretic hormone (ADH) in the distal convoluted and collecting tubules (see Chap. 36).

*Chloride* and *bicarbonate* apparently diffuse across the tubular membrane into the peritubular capillaries. In the PCT, their diffusion occurs because of an electrochemical gradient created by positive ions.

## Functions of the Loop of Henle

The main function of the loop of Henle is to concentrate urine. For this concentration to occur, the countercurrent mechanism is used. The two components of this mechanism are the countercurrent multiplier and the countercurrent exchanger. The concept of the countercurrent multiplier system was proposed by Drs. Kuhn and Ruffel in 1942. The hypothesis states that a small difference in osmotic concentration between fluids flowing in opposite directions in two parallel tubes connected in a hairpin fashion can be multiplied many times along the length of the tubes.[1] The nephrons involved in renal concentration are the juxtamedullary nephrons whose loops of Henle extend into the medulla of the kidney. These loops are surrounded by vessels of the vasa recta. Both the loops of Henle and the juxtamedullary capillary system (vasa recta) work together to concentrate urine. In 20% to 30% of the nephrons, the loops of Henle extend into the medulla and are surrounded by the vasa recta. Reabsorption through the vessels of the vasa recta is partly responsible for operating the mechanism that concentrates urine.[10]

## Countercurrent Multiplier Effect

In the PCT, tubular fluid is neither concentrated nor diluted because reabsorption is due to water permeability of tubular epithelium.[1] As fluid progresses down the descending limb of the loop of Henle, it is still isotonic to plasma. The excretion of excess solutes (concentrated urine) requires a hyperosmolality of the medullary interstitial fluid. This hyperosmolality is greater in the long segments of the loop of Henle and may increase to as much as 1200 mOsm per liter at the turn of the loop. Sodium and chloride are transported from the thin segment (descending and loop portions) into the medullary interstitium. Current research indicates that this movement occurs when the interstitial concentration of urea is high, causing water to move into the interstitial area. Approximately half of the medullary osmolarity is determined by urea.[9] The sodium and chloride concentration becomes increased in the thin segment, and these ions probably diffuse passively out of this area and into the interstitium.[1] Urea is poorly absorbed by the vasa recta and becomes trapped in the medullary interstitium. It is partly reabsorbed by ascending limbs of the loop of Henle.

As sodium, chloride, potassium, and water move up the ascending limb (thick portion), sodium, chloride, and potassium are transported out of the tubule into the interstitium. Thus, the distal tubule receives a hypotonic fluid.[1] Water is not removed because the ascending limb is nearly impermeable to it. Because this process continuously concentrates the filtrate with sodium chloride and urea in the section of the loop of Henle that is located in the medulla, it is called the *countercurrent multiplier*. As fluid moves up the ascending loop, sodium is transported out and the filtrate becomes more dilute. As the filtrate passes to the distal and collecting tubules, water is reabsorbed under the influence of ADH, resulting in the final regulation of the specific gravity of the urine. Figure 32-10 summarizes the process for countercurrent multiplication.

Urea is also exchanged by this mechanism and excess is excreted in the urine. Urea is produced through degradation of amino acids, and the amount formed usually depends on the protein intake in the diet and the ability of the liver to convert ammonia to urea. Normally,

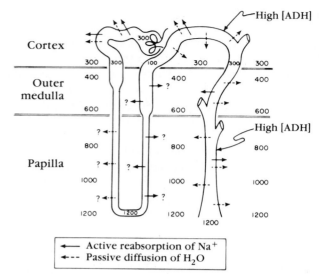

### FIGURE 32-10.

Operation of the countercurrent mechanism in a normal human during antidiuresis. The numbers refer to the osmolality (mOsm/Kg $H_2O$) of either intratubular or interstitial fluid. Solid arrows denote active reabsorption of $Na^+$ (its accompanying anions, mainly $Cl^-$, being reabsorbed passively); dashed arrows denote passive reabsorption of water. The question marks in the loops of Henle indicate that it is not yet known (1) how much $H_2O$ is reabsorbed from descending limbs, (2) whether soluted transport out of thin ascending limbs is active or passive, and (3) whether $Na^+$ or $Cl^-$ is actively reabsorbed from thick ascending limbs. The number of arrows in each nephron segment signifies semiquantitatively the amounts of solute transported relative to water. For example, in ascending limbs of Henle, solute is reabsorbed to the virtual, but not complete, exclusion of water, since renal membranes are not absolutely impervious to water. (Source: H. Valtin, *Renal Function: Mechanisms Preserving Fluid and Solute Balance in Health* [2nd ed.]. Boston: Little, Brown, 1983.)

the body produces 25 to 30 g of urea each day but maintains only 8 to 20 mg per dL in the plasma. Approximately half of the urea that is filtered remains in the interstitial fluid of the medulla. The ascending thin limb of the loop of Henle is permeable to urea but the DCT and collecting ducts are not. Therefore, urea remaining in the tubules at this point is excreted.

## Countercurrent Exchanger

As discussed above, the vasa recta are important in carrying out the countercurrent mechanism. The vasa recta run parallel to the loops of Henle. Due to the hairpin loops, blood entering the system follows the same gradients as those produced in the loops. The looped vessels do not create the gradient but they do protect it.[9] Blood enters the descending limbs of the vasa recta with a solute concentration of approximately 300 mOsm per liter. At this point, sodium, chloride, and urea diffuse from the interstitial fluid into the blood, thus creating a higher osmolality in the blood, which causes water to move back into the blood. At the tip of the U in each of the vasa recta, osmolality can reach 1200 mOsm per liter for a maximum concentration, which is also the concentration of surrounding interstitium.

As blood ascends the vasa recta, water returns to the blood, and sodium, chloride, and urea move back by diffusion into the interstitial fluid. When blood leaves the medulla, its osmolality is slightly higher than that of blood that enters the vasa recta.[1] This mechanism provides a precise balance between the countercurrent systems and prevents sodium from accumulating in the interstitium.[10] This entire action by the vasa recta is called the *countercurrent exchange mechanism.*

## Clinical Considerations in Urine Concentration

In any form of renal disease, the inability to achieve maximal urinary concentration occurs early.[9] The medullary gradient is almost invariably affected, and conditions such as changes in renal blood flow will alter the gradient by carrying away too much or too little water or solute.[9] Osmotic diuresis can wash out the gradient and prevent concentration of the urine.

The concentration of urine is usually measured by specific gravity which, by usual measurement methods, measures urine density, not concentration. Urine osmolarity may be quite different from the specific gravity. An example is protein in the urine, which causes an increased specific gravity with no significant change in osmolarity.[9]

The osmolarity of urine may be increased due to increased concentrations of urea, creatinine, uric acid, potassium, and other substances. Due to the effect of aldosterone, there may be small amounts of sodium in the urine even when the urine appears maximally concentrated.[9]

## Distal Convoluted Tubules and Collecting Tubules

### Sodium, Chloride, and Potassium Reabsorption

The DCT and collecting tubules reabsorb sodium in smaller amounts than in the loop of Henle, depending on the amount of aldosterone in the blood. The release of aldosterone stimulated by serum potassium concentration and the renin-angiotensin-aldosterone system affects sodium reabsorption at the DCT. Both potassium and angiotensin II apparently are necessary for aldosterone biosynthesis[6] (see Chap. 37).

The final urine product normally contains less than 1% of total filtered sodium and chloride.[9] Sodium is reabsorbed by primary active transport. Chloride reabsorption is both passive (following sodium) and active. Active chloride transport is usually with bicarbonate ion and may involve reabsorption of chloride in deficiency states with loss of bicarbonate or the reverse.[9]

An increase in serum potassium from increased intake provides a direct stimulus for the release of aldosterone. Aldosterone then causes retention of sodium ion and urinary excretion of potassium. This is an important mechanism in maintaining the serum concentration of potassium.[6]

## Water Reabsorption

Water is regulated in the DCT and collecting tubules by the production of *antidiuretic hormone (vasopressin).* This hormone is produced by the hypothalamus and stored and released by the posterior pituitary gland. It is secreted by the posterior pituitary when the osmoreceptors in the anterior hypothalamus respond to an increase in the osmolarity of the plasma (see Chap. 36). The hormone directly regulates the permeability of the membranes of the renal epithelial cells. This occurs by binding to receptors in the membranes of the collecting duct.

If amounts of ADH in the blood are increased, water is osmotically moved from the tubules into the capillaries by increasing the permeability of the tubular membrane to water. This results in more concentrated urine and adds water to the plasma. Without ADH, the permeability is decreased, causing water to stay in the tubules, which results in very dilute urine.

## Secretion: Tubules and Collecting Ducts

Secretion, the final step to urine formation, is the movement of fluid and solute from the blood back into the glomerular filtrate, usually requiring an expenditure of energy to cross the electrochemical gradient. Active and a few passive secretory mechanisms are present at various points in the tubules.

## Substances That Are Secreted

### Para-Aminohippurate (PAH)

Artificially injected organic acids such as para-aminohippurate (PAH) are secreted in the PCT by way of carrier sites. When the plasma PAH concentration is low, almost all of it is secreted into the tubules and very little remains in the blood. The flow of plasma through the kidneys is always slightly greater than the clearance of PAH. Therefore, by knowing the PAH clearance, one can calculate effective renal plasma flow (ERPF).[5] By knowing the hematocrit and knowing that the average PAH clearance is 630 mL per minute, one can calculate the ERPF by the following formula: PAH (1—Hct) = ERPF, for example, 630(1.0—0.43) = 1158 mL per minute.

## Hydrogen Ions

Hydrogen ions (H$^+$) are secreted in the PCT, DCT, and collecting tubules. The number of H$^+$ secreted is dependent on the pH of the extracellular fluid and the amount of buffer in the glomerular filtrate. The normal pH of urine varies from 4.5 to 8.0 depending on dietary intake and metabolism. If the urine pH decreases to 4.4, secretion becomes inhibited.

When the hydrogen ion concentration is high in extracellular fluid (plasma), large quantities of hydrogen are secreted. Low concentrations cause small amounts of H$^+$ secretion.

When ammonia (NH$_{3+}$) is passively secreted by the tubules, it can combine with the actively secreted hydrogen, forming ammonium (NH$_{4+}$). Hence, NH$_4$ is secreted into the filtrate and sodium (Na$^+$) is replaced. The exchange of Na$^+$ and H$^+$ causes Na$^+$ to move into the renal capillaries and combine with bicarbonate ion to form sodium bicarbonate. This is one way the renal cells maintain acid-base balance and buffer excess H$^+$ (see Chap. 9). A special enzyme, carbonic anhydrase, in the renal cells is necessary in this process and causes water and carbon dioxide to combine, resulting in the formation of carbonic acid (H$_2$CO$_3$). When H$_2$CO$_3$ dissociates, it forms hydrogen and bicarbonate ions (H$^+$ + HCO$_{3-}$). The hydrogen ions are then exchanged for sodium in the cell. This ammonia-ammonium mechanism is especially important when excess acid loads continually bombard the kidneys, such as with chronic respiratory insufficiency.

## Potassium

Potassium ions are transported with sodium from the proximal tubules to the peritubular capillaries and more is reabsorbed in the distal tubules. This means that less than 10% of potassium in the glomerular filtrate actually arrives at the distal tubules.[9] Excretion of excess potassium requires active secretion of potassium from the capillaries into the cortical and collecting ducts. This is partly under the control of aldosterone. The reabsorption of sodium leaves a negative electrochemical gradient in the tubules. Electrochemical neutrality must be maintained, so positive potassium takes the place of sodium. Excess potassium is ingested in the normal diet, up to several hundred mEq per day. The secretion method for potassium excretion is essential to maintain the normal serum value of 3.5 to 5.0 mEq per liter. Levels of 7.0 mEq per liter or higher may precipitate cardiac dysrhythmias and death (see Chap. 8). Figure 32-11 shows pathways by which excess potassium intake leads to increased excretion. When a person is on a very low potassium diet or is potassium depleted, the cortical collecting duct does not secrete potassium.[9] The medullary collecting duct also reabsorbs some potassium. This is the only mechanism for the conservation of potassium, causing its value to be depleted rather easily in dietary deficiency or when osmotic diuretics are administered.

## Blood Pressure Regulation by the Kidneys

The regulation of arterial blood pressure by the kidneys involves sodium retention and excretion, as well as the *renin-angiotensin-aldosterone system*, which is a combination of the enzyme renin and its activity with the hormone aldosterone and its activity. Sodium effects on blood volume and blood pressure are discussed in Chapter 26.

Located in each kidney are special cells called *juxtaglomerular cells*, which make up the juxtaglomerular apparatus. This apparatus produces *renin*, an enzyme, and secretes it into the blood. The stimulus for this secretion is decreased perfusion pressure in the afferent arteriole. Renin then causes angiotensinogen, a plasma protein, to split and produce *angiotensin I*, a polypeptide that is transformed into *angiotensin II* in the lungs. Angiotensin II causes vasoconstriction throughout the body and stimulates the adrenal cortex to release *aldosterone*. With the release of aldosterone, sodium is transported from the tubules to the blood, passively followed by water. Thus, blood volume and blood pressure are increased. Increasing the volume of blood circulation causes the renal cells to receive increased amounts of oxygen. Vasoconstriction increases the peripheral resistance and blood pressure.

The release of renin is the primary initiator of the mechanism for blood pressure control. Its release is basically dependent upon four interrelated mechanisms:

1. Intrarenal baroreceptors that respond to stretch and vary renin secretion inversely to the degree of stretch. Thus, when blood volume (and thus blood pressure) decreases, more renin is released from the granular juxtaglomerular cells.[9]
2. Sodium or chloride receptors in the macula densa respond to increased concentrations by inhibiting renin release and to decreased concentrations by stimulating release.[9]
3. Renal sympathetic nerves, besides causing a decrease in renal blood flow resulting in baroreceptor and macula densa response, cause direct stimulation of the juxtaglomerular cells and renin release.[9]
4. Angiotensin II directly inhibits renin secretion, which is a negative feedback process that controls its own production.[9]

Other factors such as ADH, potassium, and calcium also can affect renin release.

The kidney functions as a critical part of blood pres-

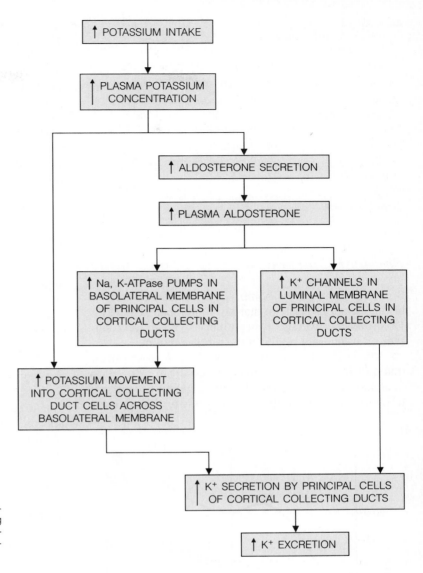

**FIGURE 32–11.**
Pathways by which an increased potassium intake induces increased potassium excretion by increasing the potassium secretion of principal cells in the cortical collecting duct. (Source: A.J. Vander, *Renal Physiology* [4th ed.]. New York: McGraw-Hill, 1991.)

sure regulation through chemical mediators and blood volume. Alterations to kidney function often have profound effects on the arterial blood pressure.

## *Erythropoietin Secretion*

The hormone erythropoietin has been identified as a major factor in the control of erythrocyte production (see Chap. 19). The location of cells that secrete this hormone has not been precisely identified but the stimulus for its secretion is hypoxia to the renal cells.[9] Erythropoietin directly stimulates the bone marrow to cause erythrocyte production. Without this hormone, anemia results and is usually very severe. Chronic hypoxia, such as that seen with COPD, causes increased erythrocyte production and erythrocytosis.

## *Secretion of 1,25 Dihydroxyvitamin D3*

Vitamin $D_3$ is either formed by ultraviolet light effects on the skin or it is ingested in certain foods. It is inactive and undergoes several changes before it can stimulate active absorption of calcium by the intestine.[9] The changes are through hydroxylation in the liver and kidneys. The effects of vitamin $D_3$ on calcium balance and bone reabsorption are discussed in detail in Chapter 45.

## *Gluconeogenesis in the Kidneys*

The kidneys have been shown to be gluconeogenic organs in cases of prolonged fasting.[9] They can synthesize glucose from amino acids and release it into the bloodstream.[9]

## BOX 32-2.
### PHYSICAL CHARACTERISTICS OF URINE

| | |
|---|---|
| pH | 4.6–8.0 |
| Amount | 600–2500 mL/24 h |
| Color | Amber or straw-colored and clear |
| Specific gravity | 1.003–1.030 |
| Protein | 0–0.1 g/24 h |
| Glucose | 0–0.3 g/24 h |
| RBCs | 1–2/microscopic slide |
| Urobilinogen | 0–4 mg/24 h |

Source: J. Wallach, Interpretation of Diagnostic Tests (4th ed.). Boston: Little, Brown, 1984.

## Physical Characteristics of Urine

Box 32-2 summarizes some specific characteristics of urine. Variations relate to diet and fluid intake. Figure 32-12 shows the average concentrations of different substances at different points of the tubular system.

The color of urine varies according to how concentrated or dilute it is. It normally ranges from pale yellow to amber, which is the result of the pigment urochrome. It often varies with the specific gravity, being more deeply colored when the specific gravity is increased. The urine may become discolored from certain disease conditions or from foods or medicines. The most common change is dark or bright red urine from bleeding along the upper or lower urinary tract. Dark yellow urine may be associated with increased concentration of conjugated bilirubin in the blood. Drugs such as phenazopyridine and phenytoin can produce a pink, red, or red-brown urine. Severe pseudomonas infection, especially of the entire urinary tract, may produce a blue-green or green, often cloudy, urine.

## ACCESSORY URINARY STRUCTURES AND BLADDER

When urine is excreted from the kidneys, it is transported from the renal pelvis to the ureters by peristaltic wave contractions. It is emptied into the bladder, which releases it into the urethra.

### Ureters

The ureters vary in length from 25 to 30 cm and are approximately 1.25 cm wide. They enter the bladder at oblique angles. They are composed of three layers of smooth muscle, including an inner layer of longitudinal muscle, a middle layer of circular muscle, and an outer layer that is a fibrous coat. The ureters also are lined with a layer that is composed of mucous membrane. This layer, because of mucous secretion, cannot be permeated by the constituents of urine (Figure 32-13).

The ureters are innervated by both sympathetic and parasympathetic nerves. Each has an intramural plexus of nerve fibers that extend along its entire length.[5] As urine is formed, it collects in the renal pelvis, and as pressure increases, a peristaltic contraction moves down the ureter to force urine toward the bladder. The peristaltic movement allows contractions to occur at a rate of once every 10 seconds to once every 2 to 3 minutes.[5] These cause a spurting action by which urine fills the bladder.

### Bladder

When empty, the bladder is like a deflated balloon. When filled with urine, it rises into the abdomen and becomes pear-shaped. The bladder is located behind the symphysis pubis. It is composed of several layers: mucosa, submucosa, detrusor muscle, and serous layer. The mucosal layer, which contains *transitional epithelium*, in combination with the rugae (multiple folds in the mucosa) allows the bladder to stretch during urinary filling.[3] The submucosa contains connective tissue that connects the

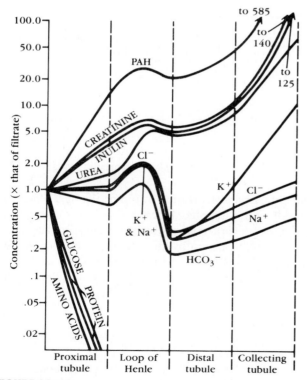

**FIGURE 32-12.**
Composite figure showing average concentrations of different substances at different points in the tubular system. (Source: A.C. Guyton, *Textbook of Medical Physiology* [7th ed.]. Philadelphia: W.B. Saunders, 1986.)

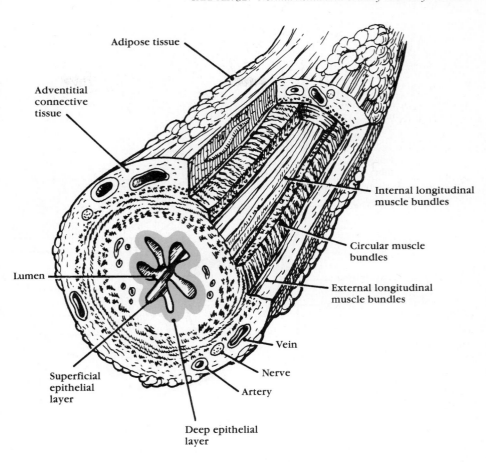

**FIGURE 32–13.**
Structure of the ureter, including smooth muscle layers, outer connective tissue, and blood and nerve supply.

mucous and muscular layers. The serous layer coats the superior portion of the bladder and is formed by the peritoneum. The detrusor muscle is composed of longitudinal and circular muscles, allowing for contractility. The contractions of the detrusor muscle of the bladder can increase its pressure as high as 40 to 60 mm Hg. This muscle is, therefore, the one that causes bladder emptying.[5,7]

An area called the *trigone* is located at the base of the bladder and is formed by the two ureters and the urethra. Between the bladder and the urethra is an *internal urethral sphincter*; below it is an *external urethral sphincter*. These sphincters are formed by circular muscles and, when stimulated, allow urine to pass from the bladder into the urethra (Figure 32-14).

The principal nerve supply to the bladder is through the sacral plexus, which mainly connects with spinal cord segments S2 to S4.[5,7] Sensory fibers respond to stretch of the bladder walls. The motor nerve fibers are mainly parasympathetic. Sympathetic fibers connect with the lumbar portion. The pudendal nerves supply the external sphincter.[5]

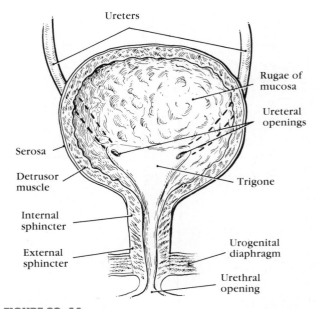

**FIGURE 32–14.**
Structure of the bladder and its internal and external urethral sphincters.

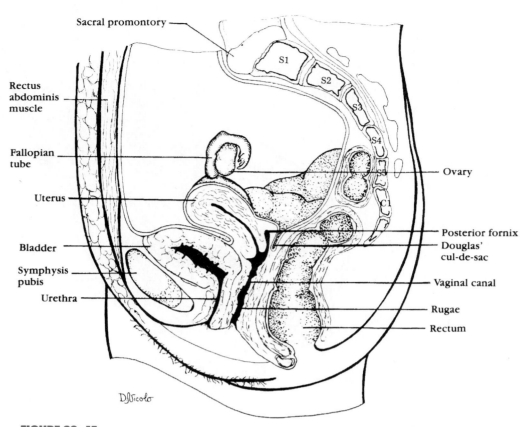

**FIGURE 32–15.**

Structure of the female genitourinary anatomy. (Source: M.A. Miller and D.A. Brooten, *The Child-bearing Family: A Nursing Perspective* [2nd ed.]. Boston: Little, Brown, 1983.)

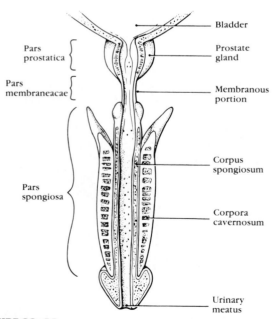

**FIGURE 32–16.**

Structure of the male genitourinary anatomy.

## Micturition Reflex

Micturition (voiding) is the result of a spinal reflex from the sacral portion of the spinal cord. Stretch receptors become stimulated when there is 150 to 300 mL of urine in the bladder. The bladder pressure increases with increased filling and the parasympathetic nerves become stimulated. This causes the micturition reflex, which results in contraction of the detrusor muscle and relaxation of the internal sphincter. Urination proceeds unless it is stopped by voluntary contraction of the external sphincter, which is under cerebral control. The cerebral centers keep the micturition reflex partly inhibited until micturition is desired. The higher centers can inhibit the reflex by continual tonic contraction of the external sphincter. The centers also can facilitate the reflex by relaxing the external sphincter.[5,7]

## Urethra

The urethra, located at the apex of the bladder, is the final excretory passageway for urine. The urethral opening to the exterior is the urinary meatus.

The female urethra is located posteriorly to the symphysis pubis and anteriorly to the vagina. The urethra is approximately 3.75 cm long and is composed of smooth muscle (Figure 32-15).

When the male urethra leaves the bladder, it passes through the prostate gland, then between a membrane portion extending from the prostate to the corpus spongiosum of the penis. Finally, the urethra passes through the corpus spongiosum and terminates at the urinary meatus. The male urethra is approximately 20 cm long and transports both urine and semen (Figure 32-16).

## REFERENCES

1. Berl, T. and Schrier, R.W. Disorders of water metabolism. In R.W. Schrier, *Renal and Electrolyte Disorders* (3rd ed.). Boston: Little, Brown, 1986.

2. Brenner, B.M. and Rector, F.C. *The Kidney* (3rd ed.). Philadelphia: Ardmore, 1986.

3. Cormack, D.H. *Ham's Histology* (9th ed.). Philadelphia: J.B. Lippincott, 1987.

4. DeWardener, H.E. *The Kidney: An Outline of Normal and Abnormal Function* (5th ed.). Edinburgh: Churchill-Livingstone, 1985.

5. Guyton, A.C. *Textbook of Medical Physiology* (8th ed.). Philadelphia: W.B. Saunders, 1990.

6. Linas, S.L. and Schrier, R.W. Disorders of the renin-angiotensin-aldosterone system. In R.W. Schrier, *Renal and Electrolyte Disorders* (3rd ed.). Boston: Little, Brown, 1986.

7. Stafford, S. Disorders of micturition. In R.W. Schrier and C.W. Gottschalk, *Diseases of the Kidney* (4th ed.). Boston: Little, Brown, 1988.

8. Valtin, H. *Renal Function: Mechanisms Preserving Fluid and Solute Balance in Health* (2nd ed.). Boston: Little, Brown, 1983.

9. Vander, A.J. *Renal Physiology* (4th ed.). New York: McGraw-Hill, 1991.

10. Vick, R.L. *Contemporary Medical Physiology*. Menlo Park, Calif.: Addison-Wesley, 1984.

# Immunologic, Infectious, Toxic, and Other Alterations in Function

## Chapter Outline

## Learning Objectives

1. List the major organisms that can cause cystitis.
2. Differentiate between hemorrhagic and suppurative cystitis.
3. Explain the normal protection against infection in the male and female urinary systems.
4. Describe vesicoureteral reflux.
5. Differentiate between acute and chronic pyelonephritis, pathologically and clinically.
6. Describe antiglomerular basement membrane disease using Goodpasture's syndrome as a model.
7. Explain the significance of crescents in renal pathology.
8. Describe the etiology, pathology, clinical manifestations, and prognosis for poststreptococcal glomerulonephritis.
9. Describe briefly the pathology of rapidly progressive glomerulonephritis.
10. List the major types of primary and secondary glomerular disease.
11. Define *nephrosis*.
12. Explain why persons with nephrotic disease also have hyperlipidemia.
13. Describe the development of edema in nephrotic disease.
14. Describe the relationships among idiopathic nephrotic syndromes, minimal change disease, focal glomerulosclerosis, membranous glomerulopathy, and membrane proliferative glomerulonephritis.
15. Describe how aspirin, phenacetin, codeine, and caffeine can cause nephritis.
16. Outline the mechanisms by which hyperuricemia, hypercalcemia, and hypokalemia can cause tubular or parenchymal alterations.
17. Review the immunologic mechanisms that can cause tubulointerstitial alterations.
18. Describe the mechanisms that can result in renal tubular acidosis.
19. Explain briefly polycystic disease of the kidneys.

Many factors can affect the genitourinary system and can cause relatively innocuous problems or progressive conditions that lead to renal failure. The most common genitourinary disease is infection of the bladder mucosa that may ascend to the pelvis of the kidney. Other conditions that can cause renal dysfunction include immune complex or antiglomerular basement membrane (anti-GBM) antibody disease, toxic injury, and congenital malformations.

## INFECTIONS OF THE GENITOURINARY TRACT

Urinary tract infections (UTI) are diagnosed by culture of the causative microorganism. Active infection is usually considered to be present when more than 100,000 bacteria per mL of urine appear in a clean-voided specimen. The most common cause of UTI is *Escherichia coli*, an aerobic organism present in large numbers in the lower intestinal area. It causes about 80% of infections acquired outside the hospital.[10] Infections also may be caused by other organisms, such as *Klebsiella, Proteus,* and *Staphylococcus* species, especially in the presence of an indwelling catheter. Recurrent infections are more often caused by these organisms. Hospital-acquired infections often result from the presence of an indwelling urethral catheter and are found in persons receiving antimicrobial agents. These persons often develop infections with resistant bacteria.[10]

## Cystitis

Inflammation of the bladder is more common in women than men because of the proximity of the urethral opening and vagina to the anal area. Normally, the urethra contains diphtheroids and *Streptococcus* and *Staphylococcus* organisms. Gram-negative organisms may gain access to the bladder during sexual intercourse, after urethral trauma, or as a result of poor hygiene. Normally, these organisms are rapidly expelled by voiding because urine is acidic and flushes away excess bacteria. In men, prostatic secretions have antibacterial properties.

Risk factors for cystitis include sexual intercourse, pregnancy, neurogenic bladder, kidney disease, obstructive conditions, and diabetes mellitus. The most dangerous sequel of cystitis is pyelonephritis, which is thought to result from organisms in the bladder that have ascended to the renal pelvis (see p. 642). Vesicoureteral reflux increases the risk of pyelonephritis from cystitis (Figure 33-1). This condition occurs in children who have abnormalities of the bladder or urinary tract that allow urine to reflux from the bladder to the renal pelvis.

The pathology of cystitis varies. If bloody urine is present, it is called hemorrhagic cystitis; this is a frequent

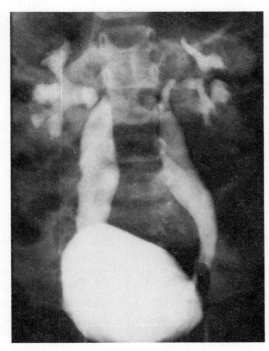

**FIGURE 33–1.**
Grade 4 vesicoureteral reflux in a 2-year-old. (Source: S. Papper, *Clinical Nephrology* [2nd ed.]. Boston: Little, Brown, 1978.)

sequel of chemotherapy or radiation therapy over the bladder area. Suppurative cystitis occurs when suppurative exudate accumulates on the endothelial lining of the bladder (Figure 33-2). The exudate is composed of polymorphonuclear (PMN) leukocytes in early stages

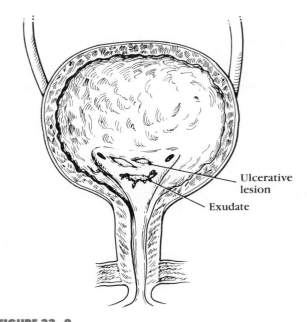

**FIGURE 33–2.**
Suppurative cystitis with ulceration of the bladder mucosa and suppurative exudate on the lining of the bladder.

but mononuclear infiltrates appear if the condition progresses to chronic cystitis. Ulcerations may be present in either the acute or chronic stage.

Clinical manifestations include significant bacteriuria in 60% to 70% of cases. Some persons may have symptomatic cystitis that cannot be diagnosed by culture.[1] Dysuria, frequency, urgency, and suprapubic pain are classic symptoms.[1] Any individual who has an indwelling catheter for a long time has a high risk for developing cystitis with organisms that become resistant to therapy.

## Pyelonephritis

Inflammation of the renal pelvis is called pyelonephritis, which is mainly caused by bacterial kidney infection.[9] Because the genitourinary system is continuous from the urethra to the bladder to the kidneys, ascending infection from the bladder is the most common cause of pyelonephritis.[10] In addition to ascending infection, pyelonephritis may be caused by septicemia (hematogenous) or vesicoureteral reflux, or the cause may be unknown. As with cystitis, the infection most frequently is caused by gram-negative bacteria. Two forms of pyelonephritis have been described: acute and chronic.

### Acute Pyelonephritis

Acute pyelonephritis (APN) usually occurs suddenly with onset of fever, chills, nausea, vomiting, diarrhea, and pain at the costovertebral angle. It may follow a symptomatic or asymptomatic bladder infection or it may result from vesicoureteral reflux. Occasionally, APN is initiated by a bloodborne, virulent organism but this route of infection almost always signifies the presence of other kidney injury.

Pathologically, APN gives rise to abscesses on the cortical surface of the kidney, which often surround the glomeruli. Glomerular damage is rare but the tubules may rupture. The infection also may follow urinary tract obstruction, with suppurative exudate filling the renal pelvis. Healing usually involves replacement of affected areas of the cortical surface by scar tissue.

Clinical manifestations of APN include the sudden onset of high fever and chills, with marked tenderness on deep pressure of one or both costovertebral areas. Leukocytosis and pyuria with leukocytic casts are common. In the acute phase, some hematuria may be present but it usually does not persist after the acute manifestations have subsided. The symptoms of APN subside with or without treatment but pyuria may persist for weeks or months. Uncomplicated APN generally responds well to treatment but a high percentage of recurrence is common.[1]

### Chronic Pyelonephritis

Chronic pyelonephritis (CPN) is difficult to diagnose except when a history of UTIs, pyuria, and bacteriuria can be elicited. Chronic pyelonephritis may follow obstructive conditions, such as congenital anomalies or renal calculi. It is often the cause of renal insufficiency in vesicoureteral reflux. Chronic pyelonephritis is a common cause of chronic renal failure, found in 11% to 20% of persons having chronic renal dialysis for end-stage renal disease (see Chap. 35).[1]

Pathologically, the kidneys are scarred and irregular, and the calices and renal pelvis are deformed. Gradual atrophy and destruction of the tubules lead to impairment of function that results in chronic renal failure.[9] Chronic pyelonephritis has been reported to follow vascular and hypertensive conditions that affect the glomeruli.

The clinical manifestations of CPN vary, sometimes manifesting recurrent episodes of APN or gradual onset of renal insufficiency and failure. Mild proteinuria with lymphocytes and plasma cells is characteristic. While CPN has been linked to bacterial infections, not all affected persons relate a history of UTI. Damage may result from asymptomatic bacterial infection.[1]

## NEPHRITIC GLOMERULAR DISEASE

Glomerular injury is the most common cause of chronic renal failure, with immunologically induced glomerulonephritis (GN) causing one half of the cases of endstage renal failure.[1] Glomerular injury may result from chemicals, irradiation, hypoxemia, and other agents, as well as from immunologically mediated disorders. Table 33-1 lists the most common forms of glomerular diseases. These forms may be primary or secondary. Primary glomerular disease is often idiopathic or immunologically mediated, while secondary forms result from systemic or hereditary diseases. Two major immunologic mechanisms have been described: (1) anti-GBM disease and (2) immune complex glomerular disease.

### Antiglomerular Basement Membrane (Anti-GBM) Disease

In anti-GBM disease, antibodies form that destroy the GBM and cause a rapidly progressive glomerulonephritis (RPGN) (see p. 645). It may also involve antibodies that form against the alveolar basement membrane (Goodpasture's syndrome).

### Goodpasture's Syndrome

This rare autoimmune disorder affects young men (age 18 to 35 years) more frequently than women and begins

### TABLE 33–1.
## GLOMERULAR DISEASES

### Primary Glomerulonephritis

Acute diffuse proliferative glomerulonephritis (GN)
  Poststreptococcal
  Nonpoststreptococcal
Crescentic (rapidly progressive) GN
Membranous GN
Lipoid nephrosis (minimal change disease)
Focal segmental glomerulosclerosis
Membranoproliferative GN
IgA nephropathy
Focal proliferative GN
Chronic GN

### Systemic Diseases

Systemic lupus erythematosus
Diabetes mellitus
Amyloidosis
Goodpasture's syndrome
Polyarteritis nodosa
Wegener's granulomatosis
Henoch-Schonlein purpura
Bacterial endocarditis

### Hereditary Disorders

Alport's syndrome
Fabry's disease

Source: *R. S. Cotran, V. Kumar, and S. L. Robbins,* Robbins' Pathologic Basis of Disease *(4th ed.). Philadelphia: W.B. Saunders, 1989.*

The prognosis for this condition is improving, and depends upon the severity of pulmonary and renal involvement. Twenty-five to thirty-five percent of affected persons die during initial hospitalization with a 50% 2-year mortality rate.[12] Treatment with steroids has induced remissions. Renal failure and uremia have been controlled by hemodialysis. Pulmonary hemorrhage usually decreases after bilateral nephrectomy.

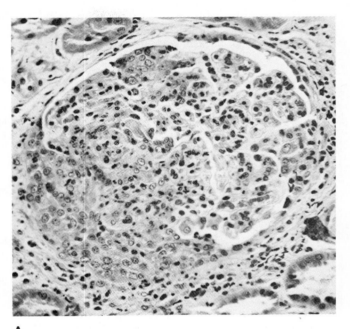

**A**

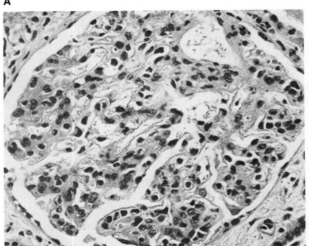

**B**

### FIGURE 33–3.
Crescent formation in acute glomerulonephritis. **A.** Acute exudative glomerulonephritis. Hypercellularity is due to a tremendous increase in the number of polymorphonuclear neutrophils within the capillary loops, together with epithelial cell proliferation (crescents) at the 12, 3, and 7 o'clock positions. **B.** Acute exudative glomerulonephritis showing a large crescent (Source: J. Metcoff, *Acute Glomerulonephritis.* Boston: Little, Brown, 1967.)

abruptly, often preceded by a flulike illness or exposure to hydrocarbon fumes.[5] It may progress rapidly, causing severe and sometimes fatal hemoptysis, or it may exhibit long remissions. More than 90% of affected individuals exhibit anti-GBM antibodies, usually of the IgG class.[5,12] Pathologically, the glomeruli may have nearly normal configuration or they may exhibit focal or necrotizing proliferations called *crescents*. These characteristic lesions of severe renal disease involve massive proliferation of epithelial cells in crescent-shaped masses within the glomeruli (Figure 33-3). Deposits of fibrin, complement fragments, and immunoglobulins may be present within the crescents. Anti-GBM antibodies may be bound to the alveolar basement membrane. These antibodies can cause alveolar damage and intrapulmonary and extrapulmonary hemorrhage that may be massive and life-threatening.

Clinical features include hematura, red cell casts, proteinuria, and nephrosis.[5] Pulmonary bleeding often recurs in episodes and may be fatal even without evidence of renal disease.[5] Rapidly progressive or insidious renal failure may result.

**TABLE 33-2.**

CLASSIFICATION OF IMMUNOPATHOGENETIC MECHANISMS OF
GLOMERULAR DISEASE

| MECHANISM | CLINICAL PROTOTYPE |
|---|---|
| Antitissue antibody-mediated disease<br>  Antibody to "native" glomerular<br>  basement membrane glycoprotein<br>  antigens | |
|     Exogenous | Antilymphocyte serum treatment |
|     Endogenous | Goodpasture's syndrome and some forms of<br>idiopathic crescentic glomerulonephritis |
| Antibody to other "native" glomeru-<br>lar antigens (in situ immune complex<br>disease) | |
|     Exogenous | None known |
|     Endogenous | ? Membranous glomerulopathy |
| Antibody to "planted" glomerular<br>antigens | |
|     Exogenous | None known |
|     Endogenous | ? Systemic lupus erythematosus, ? drugs,<br>? poststreptococcal, ? glomerulonephritis |
| Circulating immune complex-<br>mediated disease | |
|   Endogenous antigen | Systemic lupus erythematosus, neoplasia-<br>associated glomerular disease |
|   Exogenous antigen | |
|     Nonreplicating | Serum sickness |
|     Replicating | Bacterial, viral, protozoal glomerulonephritis |
| Disease associated with activation of<br>alternative complement pathway | Pneumococcal glomerulonephritis, mem-<br>branoproliferative glomerulonephritis<br>(type II) |
|   Cell-mediated disease | ? Minimal change disease (lipoid nephrosis),<br>? allograft glomerulopathy |

Source: R. W. Schrier (ed.), Renal and Electrolyte Disorders (3rd ed.). Boston: Little, Brown, 1986.

## Immune Complex Glomerular Disease

Many types of glomerular damage are caused by antigen–antibody complexes precipitated in the glomeruli. These complexes have been classified in many ways. Table 33-2 shows exogenous and endogenous mechanisms. Antigen–antibody responses to infectious agents are frequent causes of immune complex disease but the condition can be associated with many types of autoimmune disease, malignancies, and even thyroiditis. The most common exogenous type is poststreptococcal glomerulonephritis (PSGN) but nonstreptococcal forms are being identified in increasing numbers.[1]

### Poststreptococcal Glomerulonephritis

Group A, beta-hemolytic streptococci have been shown to possess nephrotoxic surface proteins. Glomerulonephritis develops 1 to 2 weeks after an infection with this organism. Nasopharyngeal infection is the usual source but occasionally it may be a streptococcal skin infection. Development of PSGN requires an individual sensitivity

to beta-hemolytic streptococci, as is evidenced by the fact that no active infection can be demonstrated by blood or urine cultures. Increased antistreptolysin or other streptococcal exoenzyme titers and depressed serum complement levels are common.

Pathologically, enlarged hypercellular glomeruli can be demonstrated, with proliferation of cells on the epithelial side of the GBM. Infiltration of the area with PMN leukocytes and monocytes is followed by interstitial edema and inflammation. "Humps" can be seen on the epithelial side of the GBM, which probably represent precipitated antigen-antibody complexes. Increased permeability of the GBM results in loss of red blood cells and protein in the urine. A decrease in glomerular filtration rate (GFR) leads to retention of sodium and water. Hypocomplementemia is frequently associated with and results from large amounts of precipitated complement in the complexes.

The clinical manifestations of PSGN include the acute onset of edema, oliguria, proteinuria (usually less than 3 g/day), anemia, and a characteristic cocoa-colored urine with red blood cell casts. Hypertension is usual and probably results from fluid retention. A markedly elevated antistreptolysin O titer indicates the presence of circulating antibody to the hemolysin streptolysin O, which is usually elevated within 2 months after an attack. Other streptococcal exoenzymes include DNAse, beta-hyaluronidase, and NADase. These titers are often increased and are measured by the streptozyme test, a combination of tests that is used to screen individuals for recent streptococcal infection. The erythrocyte sedimentation rate is usually increased, indicating inflammation.

The disease occurs most frequently in children, most of whom totally recover within a week and then exhibit immunity to further infection. Occasionally, PSGN converts to either a rapidly or slowly progressive form of GN. In either case, renal failure results. Adults who develop PSGN have a higher frequency of persistent proteinuria, hematuria, and renal failure than children.[7]

### Nonstreptococcal Glomerulonephritis

Besides the *Streptococcus* organisms, other bacteria, viruses, and parasites have been implicated in the etiology of acute GN. These also presumably cause the precipitation of immune complexes and lead to a variety of lesions, including crescentic GN and proliferative GN.[5,7] As with PSGN, this type of GN occurs after infection and usually responds well to treatment.

### Rapidly Progressive Glomerulonephritis

Rapidly progressive GN leads to renal failure over weeks to months. It may occur as a complication of acute or subacute infectious disease, from multisystem disease such as systemic lupus erythematosus, or from Goodpasture's syndrome. It also may occur as an idiopathic or primary condition (Box 33-1).

Pathologically, characteristic capillary proliferation with crescents involves more than 70% of the glomeruli. Gaps or discontinuities of the GBM also may be associated with the crescents. Anti-GBM antibodies or deposits of immunoglobulins may be demonstrated on the glomerulus. Circulating antibodies are not usually detected unless the condition is associated with a specific process for which antibody production can be demonstrated.

---

**BOX 33-1.**
CAUSES OF RAPIDLY PROGRESSIVE
GLOMERULONEPHRITIS

Postacute or subacute infections
  Beta-hemolytic streptococci
  Bacteria, viruses, parasites
Idiopathic or primary
Multisystem or autoimmune disease

---

The idiopathic form of disease is common and may be identified by enlarged, pale kidneys with cellular proliferation in Bowman's space. Crescents form very rapidly, and distort and compress the capillary lumina with fibrin deposition throughout.[1] The GBM is disrupted; interstitial edema with infiltration of leukocytes leads to degenerative changes of the tubules. Crescent formation indicates severe glomerular disease (see Figure 33-3) Widespread crescent formation indicates a bleak prognosis with over 90% of persons developing chronic renal failure.[7]

Clinical manifestations include a rapid, progressive diminution in renal function, severe oliguria, or anuria with irreversible renal failure in weeks or months.[7] Hypertension, proteinuria, and hematuria are common.

### Chronic Glomerulonephritis

Chronic glomerulonephritis (CGN) is an insidiously developing, progressive dysfunction that usually terminates in end-stage renal failure after years of increasing renal insufficiency. It may result from any type of glomerular disease, and exhibits both the nephrotic and nephritic syndromes. Figure 33-4 indicates the variety of primary glomerular diseases that may lead to CGN.

Pathologically, the glomeruli become scarred and may become totally obliterated. The tubules are atrophic. The glomeruli and renal capsule become infiltrated with lymphocytes and plasma cells. Hyalinization of the glomeruli leads to obliteration of the pathology of the original disease. Vascular sclerosis of arteries and arterioles probably contributes to the arterial hypertension that is almost always associated with this disease.

The progression of the condition is related to the underlying disorder but it almost always continues relentlessly to uremia. Proteinuria, hypertension, and azotemia are common with later manifestations of uremia (see Chap. 35).

## NEPHROTIC GLOMERULAR DISEASE

Nephrosis refers to the sequelae of albuminuria that is usually greater than 3.5 g per day. The result of the urinary loss of large amounts of albumin is hypoalbuminemia. A serum albumin level of less than 3 g per dL results in generalized body edema. Hyperlipidemia results from hepatic lipoprotein synthesis, which is stimulated by the decreased serum protein levels. The excess lipids formed are mostly cholesterol in the early stages; in late stages triglycerides also become elevated.[1]

The loss of protein results from increased permeability of the GBM, which allows plasma proteins to escape into the urine (Figure 33-5). The resulting hypoalbuminemia causes decreased colloid osmotic pressure

Percentage of patients progressing to
chronic glomerulonephritis

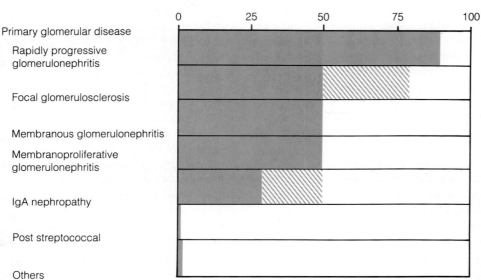

Primary glomerular disease

Rapidly progressive
glomerulonephritis

Focal glomerulosclerosis

Membranous glomerulonephritis

Membranoproliferative
glomerulonephritis

IgA nephropathy

Post streptococcal

Others

**FIGURE 33–4.**
Primary glomerular diseases leading to chronic glomerulonephritis (GN). The thickness of the arrows reflects the approximate proportion of patients in each group progressing to chronic GN. Poststreptococcal (1–2%) rapidly progressive (crescentic; 90%); membranous (50%); focal glomerulosclerosis (50–80%); MPGN (50%); IgA nephropathy (30–50%). (Adapted from: R.S. Cotran, V. Kumar, and S.L. Robbins, *Robbins' Pathologic Basis of Disease* [4th ed.]. Philadelphia: W.B. Saunders, 1989.)

and systemic edema (anasarca). Loss of other proteins may lead to decreased levels of immunoglobulins and anticoagulant factors. The latter is thought to account for an increased incidence of thromboembolic events.[1]

Nephrosis may result from GN or from unknown causes (Box 33-2). Several of the more common idiopathic syndromes are discussed in this section.

## *Minimal Change Disease (Lipoid Nephrosis)*

Lipoid nephrosis is the most common nephrosis in children between ages 2 and 8 years. It results in decreased GFR and loss or binding together of adjacent glomerular foot processes. The epithelial cells of the GBM form

pedicles or projections called *foot processes*. Normally, these structures are involved with preventing large protein and fat molecules from escaping into the urine. Loss or binding of these structures allows the leakage of albumin and fat particles into the urine. No antibodies have been demonstrated in this condition but a relationship with respiratory infections or routine immunization has led to the theory that it is a hypersensitivity reaction.

Because it also responds to steroid therapy and is associated with other atopic diseases, it is thought to involve T cells (see Chap. 16).[1]

The disease is named for its pathologic features, which show few changes except that the adjacent glomerular foot processes bind together and allow plasma proteins and fats to pass into the urine. The kidneys appear edematous and pale.

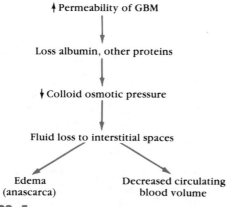

↑ Permeability of GBM

↓

Loss albumin, other proteins

↓

↓ Colloid osmotic pressure

↓

Fluid loss to interstitial spaces

Edema                    Decreased circulating
(anascarca)              blood volume

**FIGURE 33–5.**
Development of edema in nephrosis.

**BOX 33–2.**
CAUSES OF NEPHROTIC DISEASE

Idiopathic or primary
  Minimal change disease or lipoid nephrosis
  Focal glomerulosclerosis
  Membranous glomerulopathy
  Membranoproliferative, mesangiocapillary, or lobular glomerulonephritis
Secondary to glomerulonephritis
  Poststreptococcal
  Autoimmune diseases
  Diabetes mellitus
  Postinfectious: viral, bacterial, parasitic
  Hypersensitivity reaction to drugs or stings

The clinical course is variable, usually including massive proteinuria without hypertension or hematuria. It is characterized by periods of remissions and exacerbations and 90% 10-year survival.[4] In a few persons it progresses to focal glomerulosclerosis and then to renal failure.

## Focal Segmental Glomerulosclerosis

Focal segmental glomerulosclerosis (FSG) involves sclerosis and hyalinization of some of the juxtamedullary glomeruli. Deposits of IgM and C3 fragments are seen on immunofluorescence of the segmental sclerosing lesions. Idiopathic FSG accounts for 10% and 15% of cases of nephrotic syndrome in children and adults, respectively.[1] Secondary FSG may occur as a complication of nonglomerular renal diseases, such as diabetic nephropathy. A progressive decline in GFR with increasing albuminuria and hypoalbuminemia occur, and renal failure finally results.

## Membranous Nephropathy

Membrane nephropathy (membranous glomerulonephritis) is most common in young and middle-aged adults. Protein is deposited uniformly in the outer glomerular capillary wall, with the deposits usually containing IgG and complement.[1] Capillary thickening with basement membrane projections account for the loss of protein in urine. The kidneys usually are large, swollen, and pale. If nephrosis with edema and hypoalbuminemia occurs, the disease generally progresses to renal failure. Hematuria and mild hypertension may be present. This disease is usually idiopathic but it may develop in association with systemic lupus erythematosus, exposure to inorganic (gold or mercury) or organic (penicillamine, captopril) drugs, solid tumors, or some infections. It may progress with increasing renal impairment or it may show a spontaneous and complete remission.

## Membranoproliferative Glomerulonephritis

In membranoproliferative glomerulonephritis (mesangiocapillary or tubular GN), the basement membrane thickens and mesangial cells proliferate. The disease apparently does not occur after a streptococcal infection but does account for 5% to 10% of cases of idiopathic nephrosis in children and adults.[1] Abnormalities of the immune system seem to account for circulating immune complexes. In some persons, *hypocomplementemia*, especially of the C3 component, occurs.

Clinical manifestations include any of the manifestations of the nephrotic syndrome. The disease assumes several forms but tends to be slowly progressive and unremitting. About 50% of affected persons develop chronic renal failure within 10 years.[1,5]

## TUBULAR AND INTERSTITIAL DISEASES

Histologic and functional abnormalities of the renal tubules and parenchyma can be caused by many factors. When the etiology is infectious, the term *pyelonephritis* is usually used to describe the process (see p. 642). Nonbacterial factors such as toxins, metabolic imbalances, and immunologic derangements can cause impairment of concentrating ability, metabolic acidosis, and loss of sodium, chloride, potassium, and water. Tables 33-3 and 33-4 describe some of the congenital and acquired tubular disorders.

## Toxic Mechanisms

The renal tubules and parenchyma sustain damage from nephrotoxic substances because of the large quantities of renal blood flow and the concentration of the substances in the tubules. The most common toxic substances are pharmaceutic agents, including phenacetin, aspirin, certain antibiotics, and diuretics. *Chronic analgesia nephritis* is a common cause of renal insufficiency in some countries, such as Australia and New Zealand, and occurs most frequently when mixtures of aspirin, caffeine, phenacetin, and codeine are ingested. The mechanism may include inhibition of prostaglandins' vasodilatory effect by aspirin, which may lead to renal ischemia.[1] Phenacetin may have a directly toxic effect on the vasa recta or may cause papillary necrosis. The result is fibrosis, necrosis, and calcification of the papillary areas.

The papillae of the kidneys have necrotic areas and calcification fragments. Entire papillae may be sloughed off and excreted in the urine. Headache, anemia, gastrointestinal symptoms, and hypertension also may occur. The kidneys first lose the ability to concentrate urine; severe renal insufficiency leads to azotemia and electrolyte imbalance. If the drugs are discontinued, renal function tends to improve over time.

Hypersensitivity reactions to antibiotics and furosemide or other thiazide diuretics usually begin about 15 days after exposure to the drug. The reactions are characterized by fever, eosinophilia, hematuria, sterile pyuria, proteinuria, and skin rash.[1] Cortical tubulointerstitial nephritis occurs secondary to the papillary necrosis.[1] Oliguria and azotemia develop transiently, or acute renal

**TABLE 33–3.**
EFFECTS OF CONGENITAL TUBULAR DISORDERS ON RENAL FUNCTION

| DISORDER | ALTERED FUNCTION |
| --- | --- |
| **Single Tubular Defect** | |
| Nephrogenic diabetes insipidus | Decreased reabsorption of water |
| Renal glycosuria | Decreased reabsorption of glucose<br>Few tubules (normal $Tm_G$)<br>Most tubules (decreased $Tm_G$) |
| Vitamin D-resistant rickets (familial) (? tubular disorder) | Decreased reabsorption of phosphate |
| Bartter's syndrome | Decreased reabsorption of potassium, ? decreased reabsorption of sodium |
| Cystinuria | Decreased reabsorption of selected amino acids (associated jejunal defect) |
| Hartnup disease | Decreased reabsorption of amino acids other than those in cystinuria or proline or glycine (associated jejunal defect) |
| **Tubular Defects** | |
| Idiopathic Fanconi's syndrome | Decreased reabsorption of glucose, amino acids, and phosphate (and potassium and bicarbonate in some) |
| Renal tubular acidosis | Proximal tubule<br>  Decreased reabsorption of bicarbonate<br>Distal tubule<br>  Decreased excretion of hydrogen ion |

Source: S. Pepper, Clinical Nephrology (2nd ed.). Boston: Little, Brown, 1978.

failure may develop. When the drug is discontinued, recovery usually is complete.

## Metabolic Imbalances

Abnormal body metabolism may lead to the production of metabolites that are toxic to the renal tubules. The three imbalances that most frequently cause renal dysfunction are: hyperuricemia, hypercalcemia, and hypokalemia.

### Hyperuricemia

The most common cause of hyperuricemia is gout (see Chap. 45). Gouty nephropathy results from prolonged elevations of the serum uric acid level. Crystalline deposits of uric acid are left in the tubules, especially the distal tubules and collecting ducts. The result is intrarenal obstruction with inflammation and fibrosis of the tubules. Nephropathy is characterized by insidious renal insufficiency with proteinuria and decreased renal concentrating ability. The precipitated urate bodies induce a *tophus*, which is the urate bodies surrounded by mononuclear giant cells. Tophi commonly occur in the ear, the patellar bursae, and around connective tissues. In the kidney, they tend to be deposited in the medulla or pyramids and evoke a typical inflammatory reaction.[1] This may result in tubular destruction and scarring.

Acute uric acid nephropathy has been reported after the administration of cytotoxic drugs in the therapy of certain leukemias and lymphomas. Volume depletion, such as after severe vomiting, can contribute to the process. Uric acid crystals precipitate in the collecting ducts, leading to partial or total tubule obstruction. The obstruction can result in acute renal failure. Uric acid nephrolithiasis occurs in about 15% of persons with uncontrolled gout and chronic hyperuricemia (see Chap. 34).

### Hypercalcemia

Any condition that causes an increase in circulating calcium can result in increased frequency of calcium stones, obstruction, and nephropathy (see Chap. 34). Deposits of calcium often precipitate in the parenchyma of the kidneys. Intracellular accumulation of calcium can disrupt the cell processes, causing cell death and consequent obstruction of nephrons by cell debris.

### Hypokalemia

When moderate or severe hypokalemia persists for several weeks, it can lead to a functional decrease in concentrating ability. Chronic hypokalemia may occur with

**TABLE 33–4.**
SELECTED ACQUIRED TUBULAR DISORDERS

| DISORDER | PRIMARY CONDITIONS |
|---|---|
| **Single Tubular Defect** | |
| Acquired nephrogenic diabetes insipidus | Hypercalcemic nephrocalcinosis |
| | Hypokalemic nephropathy |
| | Sickle cell disease |
| | Interstitial nephritis |
| | Medullary cystic disease |
| | Medullary sponge kidney |
| | Multiple myeloma |
| | Postobstructive nephropathy |
| | Drugs (lithium, demeclocycline, methoxyflurane, glybenclamide, ? isophosphamide, ? propoxyphene, ? colchicine) |
| Renal salt wasting | Medullary cystic disease |
| | Medullary sponge kidney |
| | Interstitial nephritis |
| | Postobstructive nephropathy |
| **Numerous Tubular Defects** | |
| Acquired Fanconi's syndrome | Cystinosis |
| | Galactosemia |
| | Glycogen storage disease |
| | Lowe's syndrome |
| | Luder-Sheldon syndrome |
| | Heavy metals: cadmium, copper (Wilson's disease), mercury, lead |
| | Multiple myeloma |
| | Light-chain nephropathy |
| | Outdated tetracycline |
| **Secondary Renal Tubular Acidosis** | |
| Proximal tubule | Fanconi's syndrome (all causes) |
| | Hereditary fructose intolerance |
| | Hyperglobulinemia |
| | Amyloid |
| | Renal transplantation |
| Distal tubule | Hypercalciuria |
| | Hyperglobulinemia |
| | Medullary sponge kidney |
| | Amyloid |
| | Renal transplantation |
| | Interstitial nephritis |
| | Drugs (amphotericin B, lithium) |
| | Toluene "sniffing" |

Source: S. Papper, Clinical Nephrology (2nd ed.). Boston: Little, Brown, 1978.

gastrointestinal diseases and adrenal hyperfunction, and with long-term diuretic therapy. Function usually returns to normal when potassium levels are restored.

## Immune Mechanisms Affecting the Tubulointerstitial Areas

Allergic drug reactions may cause acute interstitial nephritis. Antibodies to the tubules have been demonstrated by immunofluorescent studies.

Immune mechanisms may cause a reaction to the renal tubular cells, which frequently occurs in transplant rejections. Also, immune antibodies similar to those causing GN may affect the renal tubules.[1]

## Renal Tubular Acidosis

Renal tubular acidosis (RTA) refers to a group of disorders, either primary renal or systemic, characterized by defective secretion of hydrogen ions with normal glo-

## TABLE 33–5.
### CAUSES OF RENAL TUBULAR ACIDOSIS

| DISTAL (TYPE I) | PROXIMAL (TYPE II) |
|---|---|
| Hypokalemic or normokalemic | Primary (idiopathic) |
| Primary (idiopathic) | Cystinosis |
| Hypercalcemia | Wilson's disease |
| Nephrocalcinosis | Lead toxicity |
| Multiple myeloma | Cadmium toxicity |
| Hepatic cirrhosis | Mercury toxicity |
| Lupus erythematosus | Amyloidosis |
| Amphotericin B | Multiple myeloma |
| Lithium | Nephrotic syndrome |
| Toluene | Early renal transplant injury |
| Renal transplant rejection | Medullary cystic disease |
| Medullary sponge kidney | Outdated tetracycline |
| Hyperkalemic | |
| Hypoaldosteronism | |
| Obstructive nephropathy | |
| Sickle cell nephropathy | |
| Lupus erythematosus | |

Source: R. W. Schrier, Renal and Electrolyte Disorders (3rd ed.). Boston: Little, Brown, 1986.

merular filtration. It may be the result of failure to secrete hydrogen ion in the collecting duct or failure to resorb bicarbonate in the proximal tubule.[6] The result is metabolic acidosis. Numerous conditions can produce RTA (Table 33-5). Renal tubular acidosis is often described in terms of type I, which is that produced by distal tubule failure, or type II, where the dysfunction is in the proximal tubule. Type I RTA is caused by impaired distal tubular hydrogen ion secretion and decreased bicarbonate regeneration.[8] The daily accumulation of acid exhausts the serum buffers and eventually bone calcium is used to buffer the serum.[8] Because of the inability to secrete hydrogen, the urine pH remains high. Type II RTA involves

impairment at the proximal tubule with a resultant loss of bicarbonate. A hyperchloremic metabolic acidosis and alkaline urine result. If the distal tubule is not affected, the serum bicarbonate will fall to about 14 mEq per liter, at which point secretion of hydrogen occurs and the acid base balance is preserved.[8] Table 33-6 compares the clinical features of the two types of RTA.

## CONGENITAL DISORDERS LEADING TO RENAL DYSFUNCTION

Renal malformations are very common at birth but may not manifest significant clinical problems until adult life. Congenital renal disease most frequently results from a developmental defect arising during gestation rather than having a hereditary basis. An exception to this is polycystic disease, which is clearly hereditary.[1]

Renal malformations may result from failure of renal development (renal agenesis or hypoplasia), displacement of the kidneys (abdominal or pelvic), or renal cysts. Developmental malformations account for about 20% of chronic renal failure in children.

*Autosomal dominant polycystic kidney disease,* which accounts for 6% to 12% of renal transplantations or chronic dialysis, is an inherited condition, autosomal dominant. It affects both kidneys, and renal function usually begins to deteriorate after the third decade of life. The kidneys appear to be largely infiltrated with cysts that encroach upon the calices and renal pelvis.[1] Clinical manifestations may include recurrent UTIs, hypertension, abdominal or flank pain, hematuria, and proteinuria.[1,2,11] It is often asymptomatic for years and is difficult to diagnose. Persons with polycystic kidney disease also tend to have other congenital anomalies, such as cystic disease of the liver and intracranial berry aneurysms.[1,3]

## TABLE 33–6.
### CLINICAL FEATURES OF RENAL TUBULAR ACIDOSIS (RTA)

| PROXIMAL RTA (DISORDERED RECLAMATION) | DISTAL RTA (DISORDERED REGENERATION) |
|---|---|
| Defect in H+ secretion causing: | Defect in H+ secretion causing: |
| Sodium bicarbonaturia | Hyperchloremic metabolic acidosis |
| Hyperchloremic metabolic acidosis | Cellular (bone) H+ buffering |
| High (>6) urine pH | Hypercalciuria/hyperphosphaturia |
| Contracted extracellular volume (ECV) | Nephrolithiasis/calcinosis |
| Hypokalemia | Natriuresis/contracted ECV |
| Acid-base balance (and low urine pH) | Kaliuresis/hypokalemia |
| at new steady state of metabolic | Always positive H+ balance (urine |
| acidosis | pH >6) |
| Treatment: Hydrochlorothiazide and KCl | Treatment: K+, HCO₃ |

Source: R. S. Muther, J. M. Barry, and W. M. Bennett, Manual of Nephrology, Philadelphia: Dekker, 1990.

# REFERENCES

1. Cotran, R.S., Kumar, V., and Robbins, S.L. *Robbins' Pathologic Basis of Disease* (4th ed.). Philadelphia: W.B. Saunders, 1989.
2. Fishman, M.C., et al. *Medicine* (2nd ed.). Philadelphia: J.B. Lippincott, 1986.
3. Gardner, K.D. Cystic diseases of the kidney. In W.N. Kelley (ed.), *Textbook of Internal Medicine*. Philadelphia: J.B. Lippincott, 1989.
4. Glascock, R.J., and Brenner, B.M. The major glomerulopathies. In J. Wilson et al. (eds.), *Harrison's Principles of Internal Medicine* (12th ed.). New York: McGraw-Hill, 1991.
5. Glascock, R.J. Clinical, immunologic, and pathologic aspects of human glomerular diseases. In R.W. Schrier (ed.), *Renal and Electrolytes Disorders* (3rd ed.). Boston: Little, Brown, 1986.
6. Kaehy, W.D., and Gabow, P.A. Pathogenesis and management of metabolic acidosis and alkalosis. In R.W. Schrier (ed.), *Renal and Electrolyte Disorders* (3rd ed.). Boston: Little, Brown, 1986.
7. Knutson, D.W., and Abt, A.B. Immune-mediated glomerulopathies. In W.N. Kelley (ed.), *Textbook of Internal Medicine*. Philadelphia: J.B. Lippincott, 1989.
8. Muther, R.S., Barry, J.M., and Bennett, W.M. *Manual of Nephrology*. Philadelphia: B.C. Dekker, 1990.
9. Rubin, R.H., Tolkoff-Rubin, N.E., and Cotran, R.S. Urinary tract infection, pyelonephritis, and reflux nephropathy. In B.M. Brenner and F.C. Rector (eds.), *The Kidney* (3rd ed.). Philadelphia: Ardmore, 1986.
10. Toye, B., and Ronald, A. Approach to infections of the genitourinary tract including perinephric abscess and prostatitis. In W.N. Kelley (ed.), *Textbook of Internal Medicine*. Philadelphia: J.B. Lippincott, 1989.
11. Vick, R.L. *Contemporary Medical Physiology*. Menlo Park, Calif.: Addison-Wesley, 1984.
12. Walters, L.C. Miscellaneous and alveolar-filling lung diseases. In W.N. Kelley (ed.), *Textbook of Internal Medicine*. Philadelphia: J.B. Lippincott, 1989.

# Disorders of Micturition and Obstruction of the Genitourinary Tract

## Learning Objectives

1. Compare obstructive and irritative mechanisms of voiding dysfunction.
2. Review the micturition reflex and relate dysfunction to voiding patterns.
3. Describe the patterns and etiologies of incontinence.
4. Define *benign prostatic hyperplasia.*
5. Discuss the pathogenesis of benign prostatic hyperplasia (BPH), including hormonal (testosterone, estrogen, dihydrotestosterone) influences.
6. Discuss the pathology of BPH.
7. List the symptoms and complications of BPH.
8. Define *urolithiasis* and *nephrolithiasis.*
9. Describe the composition of renal calculi.
10. Explain the factors that may cause stone formation.
11. Define *staghorn calculi.*
12. Discuss the factors that may contribute to the production of calcium stones.
13. Explain the factors that contribute to the production of uric acid stones.
14. Identify the major cause of cystine stones.
15. Discuss the formation of struvite stones.
16. Discuss the pathogenesis of renal cell carcinoma.
17. List the signs and symptoms associated with renal malignancy.
18. Identify the staging mechanism for renal cell carcinoma.
19. Describe the histology of Wilms' tumor.
20. Discuss the etiologic factors that contribute to carcinoma of the bladder.
21. Identify the clinical manifestations of bladder cancer.

# DISORDERS OF MICTURITION

Voiding difficulties, including difficulty initiating a stream, painful urination, and incontinence, are among the most common problems that are brought to medical attention. It is thought that a vast number of voiding problems are not diagnosed due to the embarrassing nature of the problem. Some of these problems, such as stress incontinence, are intermittent. They usually occur in response to a sudden increase in bladder pressure without an adequate pressure increase in the sphincter control by the bladder.

In reviewing the micturition reflex, one can note that the cerebral centers inhibit or facilitate the reflex voluntarily when urination is either suppressed or desired. Emptying of the bladder is at least partly due to contractions of the detrusor muscle of the bladder (see Chap. 32). Voiding then requires an intact central nervous system, functional sphincter and bladder muscles, as well as an unobstructed pathway to the external portion of the body. Female voiding is at lower intrabladder pressure than for males due to the short, straight, female urethra. The neurologic connections to accomplish micturition are complex. Disturbance of any of these connections produces a disorder of micturition.[10]

## Interference With Emptying of the Bladder

Difficulty starting and maintaining a urinary stream is a common symptom of benign prostatic hyperplasia (BPH). Urinary symptoms are the presenting complaint of most men with this condition (see p. 654). The difficulty in urination may be associated with uninhibited bladder contractions, which result in dribbling incontinence or difficulty in stopping the urinary stream.[11] Individuals who have had prostatic surgery, prostatitis, or denervation injury also may have this problem.

Acute inflammation of the bladder or of the vulva and vagina in females may be associated with urinary retention due to incomplete bladder emptying.[10] The presence of edema at the urethra increases outflow resistance. Chronic infections can cause urethral scarring and subsequent stenosis. Inflammation or hypersensitivity of the urethra produces a low voiding flow rate and raised voiding pressure, together with symptoms of frequency, nocturia, and urgency.[10] Surgical procedures for stress incontinence may result in difficulty in bladder emptying.

Bladder overdistention can be caused by repressing the urge to void or after surgical procedures when a catheter is not used to drain the bladder. The bladder muscle may become overdistended; as a result, it becomes poorly contractile. Incomplete emptying is common after suprasacral spinal cord injury or lesion. When reflex activity is initially lost, then reflex voiding is not coordinated with sphincter function.[11]

## Interference With Urine Storage in the Bladder

### Frequency

Frequency refers to voiding more than every 2 hours. Persons affected often complain of urgency (intense need to void), dysuria (discomfort or pain on voiding), or incontinence (involuntary voiding). These symptoms are often called irritative symptoms.[11]

### Incontinence

Urinary incontinence is a very common health problem in the adult population, especially in the elderly group. Recent data indicate a 10% to 20% incidence of significant urinary incontinence in community-dwelling elderly.[9] The problem is more common in women and is associated with cognitive and functional impairment.[9] It can be divided into overlapping categories of stress incontinence, overflow incontinence, or total incontinence (Table 34-1).[11]

*Stress urinary incontinence* refers to the loss of urine on physical effort, such as sneezing, coughing, or running.[12] It occurs most frequently in women, affecting 5% to 15% of this population. The cause is not known but it results from decreased urethral resistance related to multiple childbirth, estrogen deprivation, congenital bladder neck malformation, surgical procedures for prolapse, denervation of sphincter muscles, or multiple bladder infections.[13,14] In men, the most common cause is postsurgical procedures for BPH or denervation injuries. Loss of urine occurs when the pressure in the bladder exceeds that generated by the urinary sphincter muscle.[13]

*Urgency incontinence* is often associated with stress incontinence in that leakage of urine occurs because of inability to delay voiding after bladder fullness is perceived.[9] It is associated with sphincter dysfunction but also may be associated with detrusor muscle motor or sensory instability. This type of incontinence may occur temporarily with bladder infections, stones, or tumors, or it may be continuous, such as with central nervous system disorders.[4] Lesions in the frontal lobes, internal capsule, and reticular formation of the pons and cerebellum affect voiding function variably according to the severity of the lesion.[10] Spinal cord lesions above the sacral area usually produce a hyperreflexic detrusor muscle with uncoordinated sphincter activity, making control of urinary output very difficult. Lesions below the sacral root tend to produce an acontractile bladder.[10] Pelvic plexus injuries may result from pelvic surgeries, and the bladder impairment may be incomplete and unpredictable.[9]

**TABLE 34-1.**

BASIC TYPES AND CAUSES OF PERSISTENT URINARY INCONTINENCE

| TYPE | DEFINITION | COMMON CAUSE |
|------|------------|--------------|
| Stress | Involuntary loss of urine (usually small amounts) simultaneously with increases in intraabdominal pressure (eg, cough, laugh, or exercise) | Weakness and laxity of pelvic floor musculature<br>Bladder outlet or urethral sphincter weakness |
| Urge | Leakage of urine (usually larger volumes) because of inability to delay voiding after sensation of bladder fullness is perceived | Detrusor motor and/or sensory instability, isolated or associated with one or more of the following: local genitourinary condition such as cystitis, urethritis, tumors, stones, and outflow obstruction<br>Central nervous system disorders such as stroke, dementia, parkinsonism |
| Overflow | Leakage of urine (usually small amounts) resulting from mechanical forces on an overdistended bladder or from other effects of urinary retention on bladder and sphincter function | Anatomic obstruction by prostate, stricture, cystocele<br>Acontractile bladder associated with diabetes mellitus or spinal cord injury<br>Neurogenic (detrusor-sphincter dyssynergy), associated with multiple sclerosis and other suprasacral spinal cord lesions |
| Functional | Urinary leakage associated with inability to toilet because of impairment of cognitive and/or physical functioning, psychological unwillingness, or environmental barriers | Severe dementia and other neurologic disorders<br>Psychological factors such as depression, anger, and hostility |

Source: W. N. Kelley, Textbook of Internal Medicine. *Philadelphia: J. B. Lippincott, 1989.*

*Overflow incontinence* may be associated with the previous two types or it may be noted by the loss of small amounts of urine when the bladder is full.[9] It also may occur in association with neurologic disorders, especially the neurogenic bladder of diabetes mellitus.[4] Strictures or BPH may impede the flow of urine, resulting in small amounts of dribbling when the bladder is distended and the muscles contract.

*Total incontinence* occurs when there is no conscious control of voiding behavior. It occurs with severe central nervous system disorders and occasionally with severe psychologic dysfunction.[9,11] Loss of urine occurs reflexively, much like that seen in infants. Constant dribbling of urine is unusual but normal bladder filling and distention stimulate bladder contractions with smaller than normal urine volumes. The desire to void, if noted, occurs immediately before uncontrolled bladder emptying. Return to normal voiding patterns can occur when the neurologic or psychologic status improves.

## OBSTRUCTION OF THE GENITOURINARY TRACT

Obstructive disorders may cause considerable renal dysfunction, including hemorrhage and renal failure, if they are left untreated. The principal obstructive conditions are prostatic hyperplasia, renal calculi, and renal tumors.

### Benign Prostatic Hyperplasia

Benign prostatic hyperplasia affects the majority of men over age 50 years. In years past, the word *hypertrophy* was used, which was misleading because the increase in the size of the prostate gland is due to hyperplastic proliferation of glandular and cellular tissue (Figure 34-1).

Normally, the prostate gland weighs 20 g, surrounds the urethra, and consists of four lobes. By age 70 years, the prostate may weigh from 60 to as much as 200 g.[7]

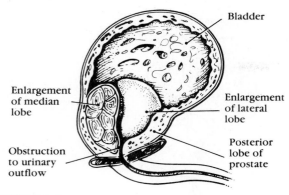

**FIGURE 34-1.**
Enlargement of median and lateral lobes of the prostate gland. Note the obstruction to urinary outflow.

Further discussion of prostatic diseases is found in Chapter 55.

## Pathogenesis

The cause of BPH is unknown but it is believed to result from an imbalance between the male and female sex hormones that occurs with advancing age. Normally, testosterone is the main androgen in the blood and forms two metabolites: dihydrotestosterone and 17β-estradiol. Dihydrotestosterone metabolizes to 3α-androstanediol (Figure 34-2). Dihydrotestosterone is responsible for mediating many of the actions of testosterone. Estradiol is a steroid that possesses estrogenic properties and acts with androgens for many physiologic activities. It can act independently and cause the opposite effect of androgens. Testosterone metabolites and estradiol have been shown to act together to produce prostatic hyperplasia in the dog.[8]

*THE RELATIONSHIP OF AGE TO TESTOSTERONE AND ESTROGEN.* In a man older than age 60 years, the plasma testosterone level decreases but BPH can occur, possibly due to increased estradiol levels which may sensitize the prostate gland to growth promotion from dihydrotestosterone.[7] The plasma levels of estradiol and dihydrotestosterone apparently do not cause BPH but their effect in the prostate may initiate the process.

In the plasma, testosterone binds to two proteins: globulin and albumin. A small percentage of free hormones is in balance with a protein-bound steroid and is able to enter the cells. Within the cells, testosterone is converted by a 5α-reductase enzyme to dihydrotestosterone. It is then bound to a specific androgen receptor protein, and the hormone receptor complex changes before entering the nucleus.[2,8] Study of both BPH and carcinoma of the prostate gland has demonstrated these specific receptor complexes in both stromal and glandular compo-

nents. They are responsive to estradiol and dihydrotestosterone stimulation.[3,7,8]

Figure 34-3 shows the possible roles of these receptors in the pathogenesis of BPH.

Estrogen levels increase in men with aging, and the estrogen binds to specific receptors in the cytoplasm and thus goes into the nucleus as a hormone-receptor complex. Dihydrotestosterone is apparently the hormonal mediator in BPH partly because of decreased catabolism of the molecule and partly because of increased intracellular binding of the molecule. Therefore, prostate growth is accelerated because of increased estrogen, which increases the level of the androgen receptor in the gland.[3,7]

*PATHOGENESIS OF BPH.* Hyperplasia usually occurs in the median and lateral lobes, with the posterior lobe generally not affected. Seventy-five percent of prostatic carcinomas arise in the posterior lobe[7] (see Chap. 55). In BPH, the lobes vary in size and are separated from each other by stroma, including connective tissue and smooth muscle fibers. Enlargement of the lateral lobes compresses the urethra, while enlargement of the medial lobe actually obstructs urine outflow by obstructing the urethral orifice (Figure 34-4).

Hyperplasia, which may be fibromuscular or glandular, results in proliferation of cells, beginning in the periurethral region and causing a smooth and regular appear-

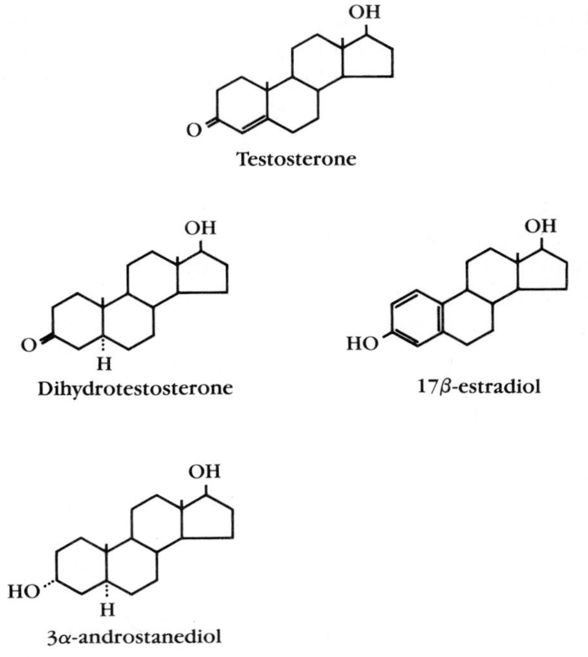

**Testosterone**

**Dihydrotestosterone**

**17β-estradiol**

**3α-androstanediol**

**FIGURE 34-2.**
Plasma testosterone serves as a precursor for two other type of steroid hormones: 5α reduced androgens (dihydrotestosterone and 3-α-androstanediol) and 17-β-estradiol (Source: J.D. Wilson. The pathogenesis of benign prostatic hyperplasia. *Am J Med* 65:745, 1980.)

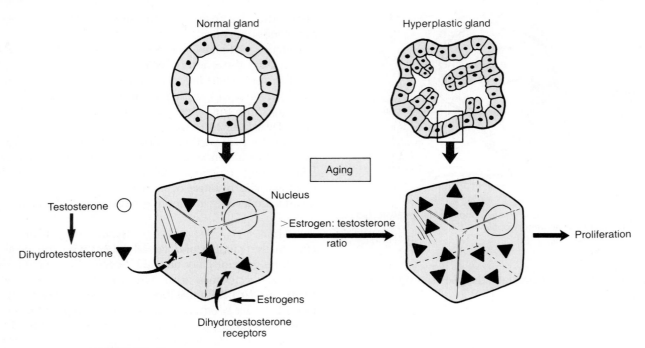

**FIGURE 34-3.**
Diagrammatic representation of the possible roles of estrogen, testosterone, and the dihydrotestosterone receptors in the pathogenesis of nodular prostatic hyperplasia. (Source: R. Cotran, V. Kumar, and S.L. Robbins, *Robbins' Pathologic Basis of Disease* [4th ed.]. Philadelphia: W.B. Saunders, 1989.)

ance of the gland. Located in the adjacent prostatic tissue are areas of ischemia and necrosis encircled by margins of squamous metaplasia. A capsule can be formed surgically between the hyperplastic area and normal tissue. As the periurethral lobes enlarge, the normal tissue and the urethra are compressed.

### Clinical Manifestations

When hyperplasia causes significant obstruction, frequency of urination, decrease in force and size of stream, hesitancy, straining to urinate, difficulty in starting and stopping the stream, and inability to empty the bladder are noted. Urinary obstruction complications that may arise from BPH include hydroureter, acute urinary retention of sudden onset, acute renal failure, hematuria, calculi, cystitis, reflux, urinary tract infection, and thickening of the bladder muscles.

### Renal Calculi

Calculi can form in various areas of the renal system. Crystallization in the renal pelvis or calices is called nephrolithiasis. Urolithiasis refers to stones anywhere in the urinary tract. The stones may be composed of calcium salts, uric acid, oxalate, cystine, xanthine, and struvite.[7]

Symptoms of urolithiasis may vary from hematuria or oliguria to renal colic. Hematuria results from the dam-

age done by the stone in the urinary tract. Oliguria may result when the stone obstructs the flow of urine.[7] Renal colic results from spasms as calculi are passed, causing flank pain that radiates to the abdomen and groin.

Urinary stones or calculi are common in the United States with an annual incidence of seven to 21 cases per 10,000 population.[7] The frequency is higher in men, in persons leading a sedentary lifestyle, and in families with a history of stones. The average age for the occurrence of

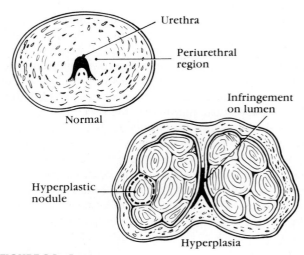

**FIGURE 34-4.**
Relationship to the urethra of normal and hyperplastic prostate. Note infringement on the lumen in the latter.

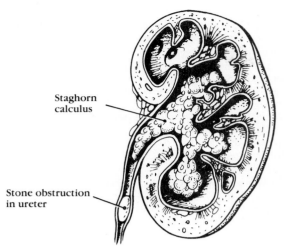

**FIGURE 34–5.**
Staghorn calculus obstructing the entire renal pelvis.

renal stones is between 20 and 30 years but they can occur at any age.[7]

## Structure and Composition

Calculi vary in shape and size; some are as small as grains of sand and others entirely filling the renal pelvis (staghorn calculi) (Figures 34-5 and 34-6). They also vary in color, texture, and composition. Stones may be either unilateral or bilateral and may be single or multiple.

Stones contain an organic matrix (framework) and crystalloids, such as calcium, oxalate, phosphate, urate, uric acid, or cystine. The matrix is a mucoprotein that is reabsorbed by the epithelium of the tubule and then released into the lumen of the tubule, resulting in a site (*nidus*) for stone propagation. Growth of preformed crystal on a site or nidus is called *metastability*.[1,7]

## Factors That May Cause Stone Formation

Stone formation may result from alteration in urine pH, decrease in inhibitors, and supersaturation of urine. Not all of these factors have to be present for urolithiasis to occur. The urine almost always shows an increase in concentration of the stones' constituents. Calculi may occur in the absence of these constituents, and other individuals may have hypercalciuria, hyperoxaluria, or hyperuricosuria without forming stones.[7]

*ALTERATIONS IN pH.* Crystalloids' solubility is affected by alterations in pH that cause them to leave the urine and attach to the matrix, resulting in crystallization. Stones that form in an acid urine contain uric acid, cystine, oxalate, or xanthine. In alkaline urine, most stones contain calcium phosphate or struvite. Persistent use of medications containing aluminum hydroxide, calcium carbonate, ascorbic acid, and sodium bicarbonate affect urinary pH and thus increase the risk of stone formation.

*DECREASE IN INHIBITORS.* A decrease in inhibitors (magnesium, sodium, pyrophosphate, urea, citrate, amino acids, and trace metals) may cause stone formation. The stone must be stable to grow to a size that is clinically significant. Urine contains inhibitors for cal-

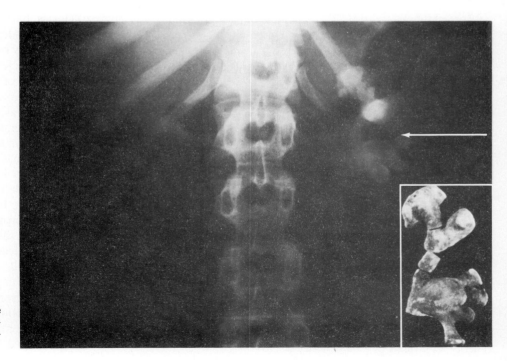

**FIGURE 34–6.**
Radiologic appearance of a large staghorn calculus. Arrow shows location of stone. Insert pictures actual appearance on removal.

cium oxalate and calcium phosphate but not for uric acid, cystine, or struvite.[5] It was concluded in one study that calculi may result from alterations in several urine components, resulting in abnormal formation or abnormal accumulation of crystals.[5]

*SUPERSATURATION OF URINE.*  The main cause of stone formation is breakdown of the balance between conservation of water and excretion of materials that are poorly soluble. When urine becomes saturated with certain materials, crystals may form, aggregating to create a stone.[6] As the insoluble material accumulates, urine reaches a critical point at which it can no longer keep the material in solution. This point is called the *upper limit of metastability*, at which time stone growth occurs. Urine pH affects the formation of stones as some precipitate in acid urine while others require alkaline urine.[7]

## Types of Stones

Even though many stones are composed of mixtures of substances, they usually have distinctive characteristics. The majority contain calcium but uric acid, oxalate, cystine, struvite, and xanthine also may predominate. Table 34-2 lists the main types of renal stones.

*CALCIUM STONES.*  Calcium stones are often formed in the presence of hypercalciuria or hypercalcemia (Box 34-1). Hypercalciuria occurs with increased excretion of urinary calcium. Calcium stones are radiopaque, white to grey, and usually small and soft. Normally, the calcium level in urine is approximately 75 to

### BOX 34–1.
### CAUSES OF HYPERCALCEMIA AND HYPERCALCIURIA

Increased bone resorption
  Hyperparathyroidism—primary and ectopic
  Metastatic tumors
  Multiple myeloma, lymphoma, leukemia (produce bone-resorbing activity)
  Nonmetastatic tumors (produce prostaglandin)
  Immobilization osteoporosis
  Hyperglucocorticoidism
  Hyperthyroidism
  Paget's disease
Increased intestinal absorption of calcium
  Sarcoidosis
  Berylliosis
  Absorptive hypercalciuria
  Vitamin D excess
  Infantile hypercalciuria
Increased calcium intake—milk-alkali syndrome
Renal wasting of calcium
  Fanconi's syndrome
  Renal tubular acidosis
  Hypermineralocorticoidism
  Renal hypercalciuria

Source: N. A. Kurtzman, Pathophysiology of the Kidney (1st ed.). Springfield, IL: Charles C. Thomas Publisher, 1977; Table 28–II.

175 mg per 24 hours. Hypercalciuria occurs when urinary excretion exceeds 250 mg per 24 hours in women and 300 mg per 24 hours in men.[6] Hypercalcemia occurs when the serum calcium exceeds 5 mEq per liter in adults. Calcium is excreted in the urine in increased amounts or it may precipitate into the kidney substance (nephrocalcinosis).

Hypercalciurias have been classified according to cause as absorptive, resorptive, and renal. These classifications overlap and may be continuums of the same type conditions.[5] Despite these limitations, the classifications may clarify the source of the excess calcium and stone formation. *Absorptive hypercalciuria* results from exaggerated absorption of calcium from the bowel due to an increased rate of conversion of vitamin D that often occurs with hyperparathyroidism. The condition has also been noted with normal levels of serum calcium and phosphorus, normal to low levels of parathyroid hormone, and increased filter loads of calcium. Another explanation for absorptive hypercalciuria is that when the amount of calcium absorption from the gut increases, the serum level increases, thus, reducing parathyroid hormone secretion, which leads to an increased filter load of calcium in the glomeruli.

*Resorptive hypercalciuria* results when calcium is removed or reabsorbed from the bone. This can occur in persons who are immobilized, for example, after spinal cord injury. Five to ten percent of persons who are immobilized for prolonged periods of time develop renal

### TABLE 34–2.
### TYPES OF RENAL STONES

| TYPE | PERCENT OF ALL STONES |
|---|---|
| Calcium oxalate (phosphate)<br>  Idiopathic hypercalciuria (50%)<br>  Hypercalcemia and hypercalciuria (10%)<br>  Hyperoxaluria (5%)<br>    Enteric (4.5%)<br>    Primary (0.5%)<br>  Hyperuricosuria (20%)<br>  No known metabolic abnormality (25%) | 75 |
| Struvite (Mg; $NH_3$; Ca; $PO_4$)<br>  Renal infection | 10–15 |
| Uric acid<br>  Associated with hyperuricemia<br>  Associated with hyperuricosuria<br>  Idiopathic (50%) | 6 |
| Cystine | 1–2 |
| Others or unknown | ±10 |

Source: R. S. Cotran, V. Kumar, and S. L. Robbins, Robbins' Pathologic Basis of Disease (4th ed.). Philadelphia: WB Saunders, 1989.

calculi.[4] Stones resulting from reabsorption abnormality develop over a long time.

A *renal defect* causing hypercalciuria is the result of a tubular defect causing a calcium leak. An example of this defect is renal tubular acidosis in which the distal convoluted tubule and collecting duct are not able to maintain acid urine (see Chap. 33). Calcium is not as soluble in alkaline urine and may precipitate to form stones. In renal tubular acidosis, stones may also be the result of low levels of urinary citrate, an inhibitor of calcium.

Several disorders of calcium metabolism result in hypercalcemia, including Paget's disease, multiple myeloma, and primary hyperparathyroidism. Calcium deposits in the renal parenchyma (nephrocalcinosis) and renal calculi are common in these conditions.[7]

Seventy-five percent of all calcium-containing stones are composed of calcium oxalate.[7] Oxalates are present in certain green leafy vegetables but stones are rarely due to excess consumption of these foods. Stones can be caused from intestinal diseases, increased amounts of ethylene glycol, hereditary disorders, and renal insufficiency.[6] Hyperoxaluria may occur after intestinal bypass surgery and with Crohn's disease. Oxalate, the product of glycine metabolism, is produced from glyoxylate or glycolate.

*URIC ACID STONES.* Calculi composed of uric acid cause approximately 10% of all kidney stones in persons living in the United States.[5] These stones are yellow to brown, smooth and soft, and are formed in acid urine. Both urine supersaturated with uric acid and decreased urinary pH contribute to their formation. The urinary concentration of free uric acid determines the probability of stone formation. Normal total uric acid excretion is about 500 mg per 24 hours. If the urinary pH increases from five to six, for example, the amount of free acid decreases and crystal formation does not occur.[6] Persons with uric acid stones excrete less urinary ammonia than normal, and acid urine results.

Hypovolemia, due to dehydration or other causes, contributes to stone formation because of the concentrated uric acid and low urinary pH that result. Diseases such as the leukemias cause cell necrosis resulting in hyperuricosuria because purines convert mostly to uric acids. Massive hyperuricosuria is fairly common after chemotherapy of certain tumors.

Uric acid stones are usually radiolucent and may be of any size from small, gravellike particles to staghorn that fill the renal pelvis.[4] Renal function declines rapidly with the larger, space-occupying stones. Their size may be reduced with medical intervention.

*CYSTINE STONES.* Cystine stones are formed in acid urine and are white or yellow, small and soft. They are characterized by hexagonal crystals that eventually form staghorn calculi. They usually do not occur in adults unless cystine excretion exceeds 300 mg per day. However, affected persons often excrete 600 to 1800 mg per day.[7] Cystinuria is due to an inherited renal tubular defect affecting the absorption of the urine amino acids, including cystine, which is the least soluble.

*STRUVITE OR MAGNESIUM AMMONIUM PHOSPHATE STONES.* Struvite stones are the result of urinary tract infection, most commonly with bacteria of the *Proteus* species. They may form after bladder catheterization and cystoscopy. Long-term antibiotic therapy may predispose the individual to *Proteus* infection. Struvite stones are more frequent in women and tend to be recurrent.[1]

The causative bacteria contain the enzyme urease, which splits urea into ammonia and causes elevated urinary pH (Figure 34-7). The organisms are often called *urea-splitters*. Staghorn calculi fill the renal pelvis and are difficult to treat. Sometimes nephrectomy must be performed to relieve the obstruction.

## Renal Tumors

Tumors of the renal system can cause damage to the renal parenchyma whether they are benign or malignant. A renal tumor is usually larger when found by palpation than when it is discovered on a routine radiologic examination. Symptoms are usually late in developing and may include complaints of dull pain in the flank area or hematuria. Renal tumors are classified as benign or malignant and also according to their area of involvement (Table 34-3).

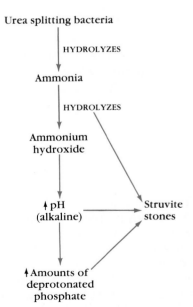

**FIGURE 34-7.**
Formation of struvite stones.

**TABLE 34–3.**
CLASSIFICATION OF RENAL TUMORS

**Tumors of the Renal Parenchyma**

Benign
  Cortical (tubular) adenoma; solid; cystic
  Fibroma
  Lipoma
  Myxoma
  Angioma
  Lymphangioma
  Hemangiopericytoma
  Leiomyoma
  Mixed tumor with combination of above elements (eg, angiomyolipoma, myxolipoma)
  Dysontogenetic rests
    Adrenal cortical rests
    Chondral and osseous rests
    Dermoid cysts
    Endometrioma
Malignant
  Adenocarcinoma (tubular) (Grawitz's tumor, hypernephroma)
  Wilms' tumor
  Fibrosarcoma
  Liposarcoma
  Leiomyosarcoma
  Angiosarcoma and other compounded sarcomas
  Metastatic tumors

**Tumors of the Renal Pelvis**

Papilloma
Papillary transitional cell (epidermoid) or squamous cell carcinoma
Nonpapillary transitional cell (epidermoid) squamous cell carcinoma
Mucous adenocarcinoma

**Tumors of the Renal Capsule**

Fibroma
Lipoma
Angioma
Leiomyoma
Myxoma
Tumors with combinations of the above elements and their malignant counterpart

**Tumors of the Paranephric Tissue**

Tumors of type found in renal capsule
Extraosseous osteogenic sarcoma

Source: A. Allen, The Kidney: Medical and Surgical Diseases (2nd ed.). New York: Grune & Stratton, 1962.

## Benign Tumors

*Cortical adenomas* are usually found during postmortem examination of elderly people and are the most prevalent benign tumors of the kidneys. They are usually not larger than 3 cm in diameter and do not produce symptoms unless they enlarge.

These adenomas are believed to originate from the tubular epithelium and may be responsible for painless hematuria. They may be difficult to distinguish histologically from small, well-differentiated renal cell carcinomas.[7]

*Hemangiomas* are rare and can result in massive hematuria, causing renal colic as blood clots pass through the ureters. These tumors have thin-walled sinuses and are usually present in the renal medulla or pelvis. They generally occur singly and are unilateral.

*Lipomas* are rare and originate mainly from the paranephric fat. These tumors, which are usually small in diameter, may develop in the parenchyma, renal capsule, and paranephric tissue.

*Juxtaglomerular cell tumors* are renin-secreting tumors that originate from the juxtaglomerular apparatus

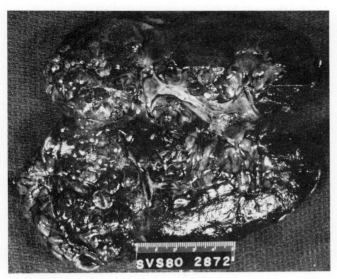

**FIGURE 34-8.**
Renal carcinoma showing enlargement and infiltration of the kidney parenchyma.

and are associated with high blood pressure. Histologically, various shapes and sizes of granules are seen in the cytoplasm of these tumors.[7]

*Oncocytomas* are large, encapsulated, benign tumors composed of large eosinophilic cells.[7] Biopsy is essential to differentiate these tumors from renal cell carcinomas.

## Malignant Tumors

*RENAL CELL CARCINOMAS.* Renal carcinomas usually occur between ages 50 and 70 years, are most common in men, and account for 85% to 89% of tumors of the kidney. A higher percentage of renal adenocarcinomas is reported among users of tobacco products. Renal carcinomas or cysts often occur in association with von Hippel-Lindau disease, which is a hereditary defect involving angiomas of the retina and cerebellum.[7]

Renal carcinomas arise from tubular epithelium and can occur anywhere in the kidney. They vary in size from a few to several centimeters and their weight may be in kilograms (Figure 34-8). The tumors may proliferate throughout the kidneys to the ureters, invading the hilum, to the renal vein and the inferior vena cava. Their color varies from white to yellow to gray.[7]

The tumor margins are usually clearly defined and cause pressure on the renal parenchyma. The tumors often spread or bulge into the renal calices and may extend to the ureter. They characteristically invade the venous system and spread by vascular metastases to the lungs, bone, lymph nodes, liver, and brain. Metastases may occur to almost any organ. Morphologically, the cells may be very anaplastic, giant cells, or clear cells, or they may be more well-differentiated.

Another characteristic of renal cell carcinoma is that the abnormal cells produce hormones or hormonelike substances such as erythropoietin, parathyroidlike hormone, renin, gonadotropins, or glucocorticosteroids.[7] The results of these secretions produce *paraneoplastic syndromes* that may be the first manifestations of disease and lead to diagnosis of the tumor.

The behavior of the tumors is unpredictable with rapid growth and metastases being followed by years of slow growth. Metastases may resolve after nephrectomy.

Symptoms are variable with microscopic or macroscopic hematuria being the most consistent feature. Other symptoms include flank pain, fever, weight loss, and tumor mass that may be palpated. The combination of hematuria, flank pain, and palpable mass is labeled "the classic triad" and represents a poor prognosis.[1]

Regardless of type and pattern, there is significant consistency in the staging of renal cell tumors (Table 34-4). Prognosis is based on several factors that include staging, the number of metastases, cell type, and size and weight of the tumor.

*WILMS' TUMOR.* Wilms' tumor is a malignant tumor that accounts for 6% to 30% of abdominal tumors in

**TABLE 34-4.**
STAGING OF RENAL CELL CANCERS

| STAGE | EXTENT OF DISEASE | 5-YEAR SURVIVAL |
|---|---|---|
| I | Tumor confined within kidney capsule | 60%–75% |
| II | Tumor invasion through renal capsule but confined within fascia | 47%–65% |
| III | Involvement of regional lymph nodes, ipsilateral renal vein, or vena cava | 25%–50% without regional lymph node involvement<br>5%–15% with regional lymph node involvement |
| IV | Distant metastases | < 5% |

Source: Summarized from B.M. Brenner, E.L. Milford, J.L. Seiffer, Urinary tract obstruction. In J.D. Wilson et al. (eds.). Harrison's Principles of Internal Medicine (12th ed.). New York: McGraw-Hill, 1991.

**TABLE 34-5.**
WILMS' TUMOR STUDY: STAGING OF TUMORS OF THE KIDNEY

| STAGE | DESCRIPTION |
|---|---|
| I | Tumor limited to kidney and completely resected |
| II | Tumor extending beyond kidney but completely resected |
| III | Residual nonhematogenous tumor confined to abdomen |
| IV | Hematogenous metastasis |
| V | Bilateral renal involvement either initially or subsequently |

Source: M. Forland, Nephrology (2nd ed.). Garden City, NJ: Medical Examination, 1983.

children, usually occurring between 2 and 4 years of age.[7] By the time the tumor is discovered, a very large abdominal mass is often palpable. Other symptoms that may develop include microscopic hematuria, pain, fever, vomiting, and hypertension due to renal ischemia. Pulmonary metastasis is often present at the time of diagnosis.

Wilms' tumor is gray to yellow, circular, with a fibrous capsule, and frequently has solid, cystic, and hemorrhagic areas. Histologically, it contains proliferating embryonic connective tissue with dense nuclei. The glomeruli are primitive with a poorly formed Bowman's capsule, and they lack a basement membrane.[1] At first, the tumor is surrounded by a dense capsule and grows by pushing the renal parenchyma out of its path. When the capsule ruptures, metastasis to the lungs, lymphatic system, liver, and brain occurs rapidly.

Numerous factors determine the prognosis for this tumor but of great importance is the stage at the time of diagnosis. The National Wilms' Tumor Study has adopted the staging system seen in Table 34-5. Long-term survival rates have improved to 90% with treatment by chemotherapy, radiotherapy, and surgery.[7]

*TUMORS OF THE RENAL PELVIS.* Of the malignant tumors of the kidneys, those of the renal pelvis account for 5% to 10%. Their frequency is increased in persons with analgesia-induced nephropathy but the precise carcinogen is unknown.[7] Infiltration of the pelvic wall and renal calices is common, as is renal vein involvement. Five-year survival rates are from 10% to 70%, depending upon the spread of the tumor.[7]

## Tumors of the Bladder

Bladder cancer is the sixth most common malignancy in the United States with 40,000 new cases annually and about 11,000 deaths.[7] Most tumors of the bladder are malignant with an increased number being reported each year. There is a prolonged period of progressively atypi-

**TABLE 34-6.**
GRADING AND STAGING OF BLADDER CARCINOMAS

| GRADE | EXTENT OF DISEASE |
|---|---|
| I | The tumor cells are well differentiated and resemble normal transitional cells. Usually papillary, cauliflower-like structure; noninvasive. |
| II | Tumor cells are still transitional but exhibit variability in cell size and shape. May be papillary or flat, invasive or noninvasive. |
| III | Very anaplastic tumors, flat or fungating, necrotic, ulcerative, deeply invasive. |

| STAGE | PATHOLOGY | 5-YEAR SURVIVAL |
|---|---|---|
| Stage 0 | Carcinoma is limited to the mucosa. | 30–80% |
| Stage A | Carcinoma invades the lamina propria but not the muscularis. | |
| Stage B$_1$ | Carcinoma invades superficial muscle layer. | |
| Stage B$_2$ | Carcinoma invades deep muscle. | |
| Stage C | Carcinoma invades perivesical region. | 10–30% |
| Stage D$_1$ | Carcinoma exhibits regional metastases. | |
| Stage D$_2$ | Carcinoma exhibits distant metastases. | |

Summarized from: R.S. Cotran, V. Kumar, D. Robbins. Robbins' Pathologic Basis of Disease (4th ed.). Philadelphia: W.B. Saunders, 1989.

cal cells that precedes the appearance of these neoplasms. Carcinoma of the bladder usually affects the transitional epithelium and may be classified as transitional cell papilloma, invasive or noninvasive transitional cell carcinoma, or other forms such as squamous cell or adenocarcinoma.[1]

Bladder cancer occurs much more frequently in industrialized countries and is definitely associated with dyes and pigments used in textile, printing, plastic, rubber, and cable industries.[7] The risk is two to four times greater among tobacco users and in persons who abuse analgesics. The parasite, *Schistosoma haematobium*, in the bladder probably accounts for the very high frequency in Egypt. Certain metabolites, such as L-tryptophan, and certain drugs, such as cyclophosphamide, have been linked to an increased risk of cancer.

A general grading and staging system for bladder tumors is indicated in Table 34-6. The papillary lesions are usually grade I, whereas the grade III are usually invasive in nature.

The usual presentation of bladder cancer is gross or microscopic hematuria that usually causes no pain. Dysuria, urinary frequency, or urgency may accompany the hematuria.[1] Other symptoms are rare until late in the course of the disease. Long-term survival depends on early diagnosis and adequate treatment.

## REFERENCES

1. Anderson, W.A.D., and Scotti, T.M. *Synopsis of Pathology* (12th ed.). St. Louis: Mosby, 1990.
2. Bartsch, G., Mikuz, G., Dietz, D., and Rohr, H.P. Morphometry in the abnormal growth of the prostate. In J.M. Fitz-patrick and R.J. Krane (eds.), *The Prostate*. New York: Churchill-Livingstone, 1989.
3. Brendler, C.B. Benign disorders of the prostate. In W.N. Kelley (ed.), *Textbook of Internal Medicine*. Philadelphia: J.B. Lippincott, 1989.
4. Coe, F.L. Nephrolithiasis: Causes, classification and management. *Hosp. Pract.* 16:33, 1981.
5. Coe, F.L., and Favus, M.J. Disorders of stone formation. In B.M. Brenner and C.C. Rector (eds.), *The Kidney* (3rd ed.). Philadelphia: Ardmore, 1986.
6. Coe, F.L., and Favus, M.J. Nephrolithiasis. In J.D. Wilson (ed.), *Principles of Internal Medicine* (12th ed.). New York: McGraw-Hill, 1991.
7. Cotran, R.S., Kumar, V., and Robbins, S.L. *Robbins' Pathologic Basis of Disease* (4th ed.). Philadelphia: W.B. Saunders, 1989.
8. Chanadian, R. Hormone receptors in the prostate. In J.M. Fitzpatrick and R.J. Krane *The Prostate*. New York: Churchill-Livingstone, 1989.
9. Ouslander, J.G. Incontinence. In W.N. Kelley (ed.), *Textbook of Internal Medicine*. Philadelphia: J.B. Lippincott, 1989.
10. Shah, P.J.R. Pathophysiology of voiding disorders. In J.O. Drife, P. Hilton, and S.L. Stanton (eds.), *Micturition*. New York: Springer Verlag, 1990.
11. Stafford, S.J. Disorders of micturition. In R.W. Schrier and C.W. Gottschalk (eds.), *Diseases of the Kidney* (4th ed.). Boston: Little, Brown, 1988.
12. Stanton, S.L. Stress urinary incontinence. *1990 Neurobiology of Incontinence*. Wiley, Chichester: Ciba Foundation Symposium, 1990.
13. Swash, M. The neurogenic hypothesis of stress incontinence. *1990 Neurobiology of Incontinence*. Wiley, Chichester: Ciba Foundation Symposium, 1990.
14. Warrell, D.W. Pathophysiology of genuine stress incontinence. In J.O. Drife, P. Hilton, and S.L. Stanton (eds.), *Micturition*. New York: Springer-Verlag, 1990.

# Renal Failure and Uremia

## Chapter Outline

## Learning Objectives

1. Define *acute renal failure (ARF)*.
2. Define *azotemia* and *oliguria*.
3. Describe prerenal, renal, and postrenal causes of ARF.
4. Discuss the two major causes of acute tubular necrosis (ATN).
5. List some of the drugs that can cause nephrotoxic renal failure.
6. Describe the pathologic features of nephrotoxic and ischemic ATN.
7. Discuss the three mechanisms that have been proposed to explain glomerular filtration rate reduction in ARF.
8. Discuss arterial vasoconstriction and prostaglandins in relation to oliguria.
9. Differentiate among the three stages of ARF.
10. Discuss the pathogenesis of water imbalance, hyponatremia, hyperkalemia, metabolic acidosis, anemia, and elevated levels of creatinine, phosphate, and urea during the oliguric stage of ARF.
11. Identify the clinical manifestations characteristic of the diuretic phase of ARF.
12. Define *chronic renal failure (CRF)*.
13. Discuss the causes and stages of CRF.
14. Discuss the intact nephron theory and its relation to CRF.
15. Discuss fluid imbalances in CRF.
16. Define *hyposthenuria, polyuria,* and *isosthenuria*.
17. Explain how hyponatremia and hypernatremia can occur in CRF.
18. Identify causes of hyperkalemia and hypokalemia in CRF.
19. Discuss the causation of metabolic acidosis in CRF.
20. Explain the relation of metabolic acidosis to osteodystrophy in CRF.
21. Discuss hyperparathyroidism and vitamin D metabolism in relation to bone disease in CRF.
22. Explain the factors leading to anemia in CRF.
23. Define *uremia*.
24. List symptoms and causes of the altered neurologic system in relation to uremia.
25. Identify causes of hypertension in relation to uremia.
26. Discuss cardiopulmonary effects of uremia.
27. Discuss gastrointestinal abnormalities in relation to uremia, including ulcerations, oral changes, and bleeding.
28. Define *osteomalacia, osteitis fibrosa, soft-tissue metastatic calcification,* and *osteosclerosis*.
29. Discuss dermatologic alterations in relation to uremia.

Renal failure occurs when the kidneys are unable to remove accumulated metabolites from the blood. The process causes alterations in electrolyte, acid-base, and water balance, as well as the accumulation of substances that normally are totally excreted by the body. Renal failure describes the process of cessation of renal function. It can occur abruptly, as in acute renal failure (ARF), or over a long period, as in chronic renal failure (CRF). This chapter details the effects of both processes.

## ACUTE RENAL FAILURE

ARF is a clinical syndrome in which the kidneys are unable to excrete the waste products of metabolism, usually because of renal hypoperfusion. The syndrome usually has an abrupt onset. It may lead to *azotemia,* which is the accumulation of nitrogenous waste products in the blood, and to *oliguria,* in which urine output is less than 400 mL/24 h. About 40% of ARF is nonoliguric.

ARF can result from different causes. These have been divided into the major categories of *prerenal functional, intrarenal structural,* and *postrenal obstructive* (Box 35-1).

### Causes

ARF is broadly defined as any condition that causes sudden suppression of kidney function.[4] It is related to a number of factors, including ischemic disorders, nephrotoxic disorders, diseases of the small blood vessels, dis-

---

**BOX 35–1.**
ETIOLOGY OF ACUTE RENAL FAILURE

**Prerenal Functional**

Hypotension

Extrarenal sodium loss
  Gastrointestinal loss (vomiting, diarrhea, nasogastric suction, intestinal fistula, acute bleeding)
  Skin loss (heat exposure, burns, inflammatory diseases)

Renal sodium loss
  Extrinsic (osmotic diuresis, diuretic administration, mineralocorticoid deficiency)
  Intrinsic (salt-wasting nephropathy)

Third-space fluid accumulation
  Generalized edematous disorders (congestive heart failure, cirrhosis, nephrotic syndrome)
  Gastrointestinal (pancreatitis, peritonitis)
  Miscellaneous (crush injury, skeletal fracture)

Hepatorenal syndrome

Drug-induced
  Nonsteroidal antiinflammatory drugs or aspirin
  Angiotensin-converting enzyme inhibitor

**Intrarenal Structural**

Ischemic acute tubular necrosis

Nephrotoxic acute tubular necrosis
  Antibiotics (aminoglycosides, amphotericin B)
  Heavy metals (cisplatin)
  Radiocontrast agents
  Endogenous toxins (myoglobin, hemoglobin, myeloma light chains)

Vascular processes
  Atheroembolic disease
  Renal artery occlusion
  Vasculitis

Acute glomerulonephritis

Acute tubulointerstitial nephritis

**Postrenal Obstructive**

Intrarenal
  Acute uric acid nephropathy
  Drugs (methotrexate)

Extrarenal

Source: W. N. Kelley, Textbook of Internal Medicine. *Philadelphia: J. B. Lippincott, 1989.*

eases of the major blood vessels, and acute interstitial nephritis.[21] The most common causes are ischemia and nephrotoxicity.

Prerenal functional disease refers to any condition that diminishes renal perfusion pressure, such as hypovolemia and shock. Acute azotemia is caused by hypotension, hypovolemia, and decreased renal perfusion. This may be acutely reversed by immediate intervention. Hepatorenal syndrome is renal failure that occurs in the patient with hepatic failure. It often occurs in association with a gastrointestinal hemorrhage, dehydration, excessive diuresis, or massive paracentesis (see Chap.43).[11]

Intrarenal ARF results from acute parenchymal changes that damage the nephrons. Many conditions can cause parenchymal damage, including acute glomerulonephritis, vascular diseases, interstitial nephritis, and acute tubular necrosis (ATN). *Acute intrinsic renal failure,* or *vasomotor nephropathy,* can be induced by renal hypoperfusion and ischemia, nephrotoxins, and other mechanisms. It also is called ATN, which is a syndrome of abrupt and sustained decline of glomerular filtration rate (GRF) (see below).

The postrenal obstructive category includes any condition that obstructs excretion of normally elaborated urine. The most common intrarenal causes of postrenal ARF are uric acid crystal precipitation and methotrexate toxicity.[11] The extrarenal causes of obstructive ARF are much more common, and include benign prostatic hyperplasia, renal calculi, or any condition that obstructs urine flow.

## Pathogenesis

ARF results in a severe reduction in GFR. Several mechsms have been proposed in the alteration of GFR, such as the *back-leak theory,* the *tubular obstruction theory,* and the *primary filtration failure theory.*

The back-leak theory of increased permeability proposes that the lack of urine output is caused by disruption of tubular epithelium rather than GFR. Therefore, substances are reabsorbed from the tubular lumen and interstitium into the peritubular circulation. In experimental models of ARF, tubular damage was demonstrated anatomically after administration of nephrotoxic substances.[6] Tubular alterations are inconsistent and may be minor in ATN. The role that they play in decreasing GFR is unknown.[18]

Tubular obstruction by intraluminal casts, debris, or interstitial edema may cause a decrease in GFR because of the increased hydrostatic pressure in Bowman's capsule. Demonstration of acute obstruction with casts within 1 week of onset is usual, but patency usually returns in 2 weeks. Pressures fall to normal levels at 2 weeks.[6] The tubular debris may be the result or the cause of the failed filtration.[18]

Filtration failure theories relate to a decrease in renal blood flow (RBF) that leads to increased renovascular resistance. Afferent arteriolar vasoconstriction initially may cause a 60% to 80% decrease in renal cortical blood flow.[18] Later restoration of RBF does not improve the glomerular filtration pressure or renal function. In the initial stage, RBF is definitely decreased. In the established phase, the GFR decreases out of proportion to RBF. Loss of renal autoregulation seems to be the major occurrence, and may be related to the renin-angiotensin-aldosterone system or other phenomena.

## Acute Tubular Necrosis

ATN is the term given to ARF caused by destruction of tubular epithelial cells.[8] It is a major pathologic finding in ARF.

### Etiology

The two most common causes of ATN are ischemia and exposure to nephrotoxic agents (Box 35-2). Ischemia is the most frequent cause, with its duration determining the extent of damage and the prognosis for return of uri-

---

**BOX 35-2.**
ISCHEMIA AND NEPHROTOXINS THAT ARE IMPLICATED IN ACUTE TUBULAR NECROSIS

**Ischemia**
Severe congestive heart failure: Cardiogenic shock
Hemorrhagic, septic, neurogenic shock
Burns
Dehydration
Hepatic failure with ascites
Complications of pregnancy: Toxemia

**Nephrotoxins**
Antibiotics such as gentamicin
Antibacterials such as sulfonamides
Diuretics such as furosemide
Antineoplastic drugs such as methotrexate
Contrast media, especially those containing iodine
Organic solvents such as carbon tetrachloride
Hemoglobin/myoglobin products
Fungicides such as amphotericin B
Heavy metals such as gold therapy
Anesthetic agents such as methoxyflurane
Antitubercular drugs such as isoniazid
Narcotic analgesics such as heroin
Antigout drugs such as colchicine
Anti–heavy metal poisoning agent such as calcium edetate disodium

nary function. According to one study, ischemia present for 25 minutes or less caused mild and reversible damage.[5] Others showed that 2 hours of ischemia caused severe and irreversible damage.[10] ATN most frequently appears after an episode of shock, usually subsequent to conditions such as sepsis, burns, crushing injuries, and peripheral circulatory collapse.[8] It seldom occurs as a result of massive hemorrhage alone. Another form of ischemic ATN results from hemolysis or skeletal muscle breakdown. There is precipitation of hemoglobin and myoglobin in the blood and urine. These substances are toxic to the tubules, but they are almost always associated with dehydration and oxygen lack.[8]

*Nephrotoxic agents* destroy tubular cells by direct cellular toxic effects, lysis of red blood cells (RBCs), intravascular coagulation, precipitation of oxalate and uric acid crystals, and tissue hypoxia.[18] Factors that promote nephrotoxicity of agents include the hydration status, preexisting renal disease, and the person's age.

As one ages, the number of nephrons decreases, so that drugs become more concentrated in the tubules. People over age 75 who are exposed to nephrotoxic drugs have a much higher frequency of nephrotoxicity than those between ages 16 and 30.[16]

Antibiotics, including the aminoglycosides, penicillins, cephalosporins, tetracyclines, amphotericin B, and sulfonamides, are probably the principal cause of renal disruption.[19] Radiographic contrast materials that contain iodine, solvents, heavy metals, and pigments of hemoglobin and myoglobin also can cause ATN.[14]

## Pathology

In the *ischemic type of ATN,* patchy necrosis occurs in the tubules (Figure 35-1A). The main area of necrosis is in the straight portion of the proximal tubules, but lesions also occur in the distal tubules.

If severe injury has been sustained, injury to the basement membrane occurs, and exposes the tubular lumen to the interstitial space. The mitochondria in the epithelium have been noted to be swollen when viewed through the electron microscope.[21] The areas that have no lesions have dilated tubules and flattened epithelium. Damage to the brush border of the proximal tubule cells also results.[8]

A characteristic finding of ischemic ATN is blockage of tubule lumina by casts. Other abnormalities include leukocytes in the vasa recta, dilation of Bowman's spaces of the glomeruli, interstitial edema, and inflammatory cells in the interstitium. The glomeruli appear to be normal.[21]

In the *nephrotoxic type of ATN,* a more uniform appearance is characteristic (Figure 35-1B). Lesions are located in the proximal tubules, but may occur in the basement membrane and distal tubules when severe injury has been sustained. Less basement membrane dis-

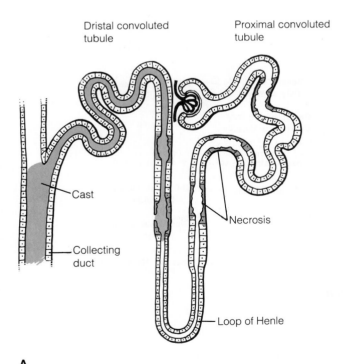

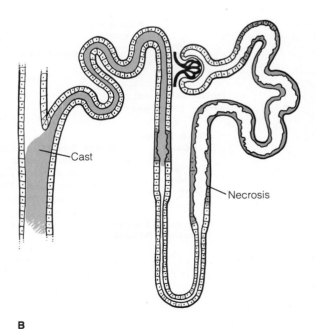

**A**                                                              **B**

**FIGURE 35–1.**

**A.** Patchy ischemic necrosis of the proximal tubules. **B.** Characteristic nephrotoxic injury of large segments of proximal tubule.

ruption usually occurs with nephrotoxic ATN than with ischemic ATN.[10]

Casts, which are debris from cells, obstruct the distal tubules, and necrosis is present in all nephrons. Interstitial edema, leukocytes in the vasa recta, and inflammatory cells in the interstitium are characteristic.

## Pathophysiology

*Oliguria* is a cardinal feature of the early stages of ARF with vascular or tubular etiology. Not all forms of ARF exhibit oliguria, but progressive azotemia occurs because of the impaired renal function. The possible mechanisms for the production of oliguria are shown in Figure 35-2 and are described below.

Research suggests that *tubular factors* are the primary sources in the pathogenesis of renal insufficiency (Figure 35-3).[5] If oliguria is caused by a tubular abnormality, it is believed to be the result either of backleakage or intratubular obstruction, as described below.

*Tubular obstruction* is believed to be caused by casts, debris, or interstitial edema. Tubular obstruction occurs as a result of tubular ischemia, which causes swelling and necrosis of the cells of the tubules. The necrotic cells are sloughed off, causing obstruction to the tubules and increased pressure in Bowman's capsule. This pressure opposes the glomerular hydrostatic pressure and results in a decreased GFR.[14] Oliguria results, often progressing to anuria. Together with output de-

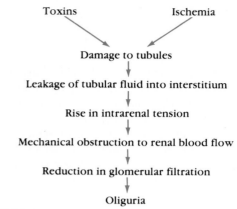

**FIGURE 35-3.**

Chain of events that lead to oliguria in acute renal failure. (From R. Heptinstall, *Pathology of the Kidney* [3rd ed.]. Boston: Little, Brown, 1983.)

cline, there is dysfunction in the ability to excrete urea, creatinine, potassium, sodium, and water (see Chap. 32).

Oliguria also may result from *vascular changes,* especially renal artery vasoconstriction. In early stages of ARF, renal vasoconstriction occurs in the renal cortex, resulting in ischemia and a reduction in GFR, and leading to oliguria. The renin-angiotensin-aldosterone system may contribute to the vasoconstriction and oliguria. Renin is released when plasma volume is low. The secretion of renin causes conversion of angiotensinogen to angio-

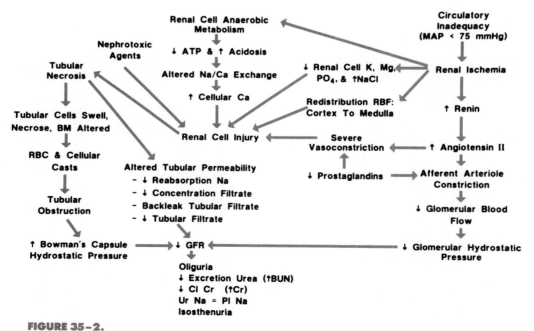

**FIGURE 35-2.**

Schema of pathophysiology of ATN. BM, basement membrane; Cr, creatinine; Cl, clearance; MAP, mean arterial pressure; RBF, renal blood flow; Ur, urine; Pl, plasma; GFR, glomerular filtration rate; RBC, red blood cells; ATP, adenosine triphosphate; K, potassium; Mg, magnesium; PO4, phosphate; Na, sodium; NaCl, sodium chloride; Ca, calcium; BUN, blood urea nitrogen. (From L. Lancaster. Renal response to shock. *Crit. Care Clin. North Am.* 2:221, 1990.)

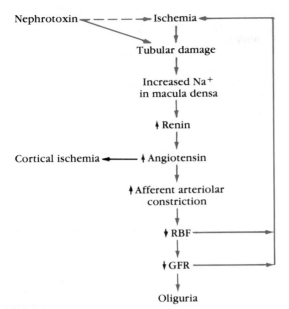

**FIGURE 35-4.**
The possible role of the renin-angiotensin-aldosterone system in the development and maintenance of oliguria (and cortical ischemia) in acute tubular necrosis. (From S. Papper, *Clinical Nephrology* [2nd ed.]. Boston: Little, Brown, 1978.)

tensin, finally leading to vasoconstriction. Thus the afferent arteriole constricts, which leads to decreased GFR and oliguria (Figure 35-4). The arterial vasoconstriction also may be enhanced by the loss of the vasodilator effects of some of the prostaglandins.[8] Early in the course of renal vasoconstriction, autoregulation, partly through the effect of prostaglandin release, retains blood flow through the kidneys and prevents tubular necrosis. As the constriction continues, this mechanism may be lost (Figure 35-5).

## Stages of ARF

The course of ARF can vary tremendously among persons with different physiologic problems. The three stages of ARF are (1) initiating, (2) maintenance, and (3) recovery.

The *initiating stage* is the initial or inciting event that causes necrosis of the convoluted tubules. The course of ARF is related to the magnitude of the inciting insult, the period of hypotension, and the length of time the hemodynamics are altered.[8]

The *maintenance stage* is characterized by oliguria and electrolyte imbalances.[8] If urine production ceases (anuria), bilateral renal obstruction may be the cause. The urine specific gravity often remains at about 1.010, which is the same as plasma. The RBF decreases with a marked decrease in GFR. As the GFR decreases, the fluid and electrolyte balance becomes greatly altered. Water imbalance may occur because of exogenous administration of fluids during the early critical stage. Excess body

water also may be related to fat catabolism, with demonstration of mild to moderate hyponatremia. As much as 300 mL of water per day may result from protein and fat catabolism.[21] The hyponatremia that occurs during the oliguric phase is mainly due to the dilution of extracellular fluid, but it also may be due to gastrointestinal disturbances, such as vomiting and diarrhea. Hyperkalemia often occurs during the maintenance stage, which is mostly due to decreased renal excretion, but may be related to excessive breakdown of muscle protein. Sometimes metabolic acidosis is associated because of inappropriate excretion of hydrogen by the kidneys (see Chap. 9). If ARF persists for 2 to 3 days, nearly all persons develop moderate to severe anemia because of suppressed erythropoiesis (probably caused by lack of erythropoietin and uremic toxins). Elevations of creatinine, phosphate, and urea result from breakdown of muscle protein and inability to excrete metabolites. With the increase of urea and other nitrogenous wastes in the blood, *azotemia* progresses.

The *recovery stage* is characterized by gradual increase of urine output. Diuresis may begin as early as 24 hours after the onset of ARF, or it may begin much later. The increased output, as much as 6 L/d, does not indicate total return of renal function. Tubular function remains altered, which is indicated by large amounts of sodium and potassium lost in urine. Serum urea, creatinine, and other accumulated substances act as osmotic diuretics. They also continue to rise during the first days of diuresis. Dehydration may occur as a result of the inability to conserve water. Laboratory values indicate a progression

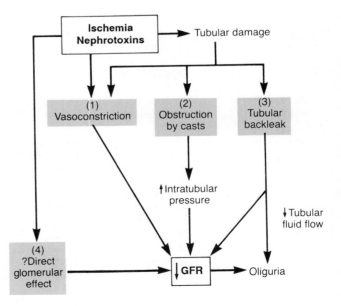

**FIGURE 35-5.**
Possible pathogenetic mechanisms in acute renal failure. (From R.S. Cotran, V. Kumar, and S.L. Robbins, *Robbins' Pathologic Basis of Disease* [4th ed.]. Philadelphia: W.B. Saunders, 1989.)

toward normal levels and increased production of RBCs. Wide fluctuations in fluid and electrolyte balance are common during this stage. Recovery is gradual, with GFR, RBF, and tubular function improvement over 6 to 12 months. The ability to concentrate urine appropriately is the final stage of recovery.[14]

### Prognosis

The prognosis for ARF depends on the underlying cause, the onset and severity of the disease, and medical intervention. Mortality varies from 10% to 75%, with the highest risks being in the traumatized, postoperative, and aged populations.[11]

## CHRONIC RENAL FAILURE

CRF is an irreversible condition characterized by diminished functioning of the nephrons, which results in decreased GFR, RBF, tubular function, and resorption ability. Renal impairment is progressive, and leads to *end-stage renal disease* (ESRD) (Table 35-1).

Numerous conditions that cause CRF primarily affect the renal parenchyma (Box 35-3). Regardless of the cause, the result is damage to the nephrons and glomeruli. This damage may be diffused throughout both kidneys, or it may be focal. Progressive loss of nephrons leads to greater dysfunction with more difficulty in maintaining an adequate fluid and electrolyte balance. Systemic effects occur in all of the organs of the body. The progression toward *uremia* (urine in the blood) usually is gradual, being controlled by diet and fluid restrictions for long periods (Figure 35-6). When the kidneys can no longer maintain the fluid and electrolyte balance, dialysis therapy becomes necessary.

**BOX 35-3.**
CAUSES OF CHRONIC RENAL FAILURE

**Glomerulopathies**

*Primary glomerular diseases*
Focal and segmental glomerulosclerosis
Membranous nephropathy
Membranoproliferative glomerulonephritis
IgA nephropathy
Idiopathic crescentic glomerulonephritis
Other

*Secondary glomerular diseases*
Diabetes mellitus
Amyloidosis
Postinfectious glomerulonephritis
Heroin-abuse nephropathy
Collagen vascular diseases (systemic lupus erythematosus, systemic sclerosis, polyarteritis nodosa, Wegener's granulomatosis)
Sickle cell glomerulopathy

**Tubulointerstitial Renal Diseases**

Nephrotoxic (antibiotics, nonsteroidal antiflammatory agents, heavy metals, diuretics)
Analgesic nephropathy
Reflux/chronic pyelonephritis
Hypercalcemia nephropathy/nephrocalcinosis
Renal tuberculosis
Myeloma kidney
Lymphoma/leukemia (with infiltration)
Multisystem disorders (sarcoidosis, Sjögren's syndrome)

**Hereditary Diseases**

Polycystic kidney diseases
Alport syndrome
Medullary cystic disease
Fabry disease

**Vascular Diseases**

Renal artery obstruction
Hypertensive nephrosclerosis
Chronic radiation nephritis

**Obstructive Nephropathy**

Prostatic diseases
Nephrolithiasis
Retroperitoneal fibrosis/tumor
Congenital
Other

Source: W. N. Kelley, Textbook of Internal Medicine. *Philadelphia: J. B. Lippincott, 1989.*

**TABLE 35-1.**
STAGES OF CHRONIC RENAL FAILURE

| STAGE | DESCRIPTION |
|---|---|
| 1. Decreased renal reserve | Homeostasis maintained; no symptoms; residual renal reserve 40% of normal |
| 2. Renal insufficiency | Decreased ability to maintain homeostasis; mild azotemia and anemia; may be unable to concentrate urine and conserve H$_2$O; residual renal function 15%–40% of normal; GFR decreases to 20 mL/min (normal 100–120 mL/min) |
| 3. Renal failure | Azotemia and anemia severer; nocturia, electrolyte and fluid disorders; residual renal function 5%–15% of normal |
| 4. Uremia (end-stage renal disease) | No homeostasis; becomes symptomatic in many systems, residual renal function less than 5% of normal |

GFR, glomerular filtration rate.

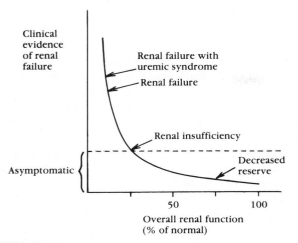

**FIGURE 35–6.**
The relation of clinical manifestations to renl function. (From S. Papper, *Clinical Nephrology* [2nd ed.]. Boston: Little, Brown, 1978.)

## Pathophysiology

The intact nephron theory aids in explaining the pathophysiology of CRF. Experiments support an *orderliness* of impaired renal function in the diseased kidney, which means that total nephron units are lost.[13] This finding lends support to the theory that the manifested net renal function is the result of a decreased number of correctly functioning nephrons, rather than being reflective of the number of diseased nephrons. A crucial feature of this theory is that the balance between the glomeruli and tubules must be maintained. As the nephrons receive more filtrate, they also must be able to reabsorb more to maintain the steady state (Figure 35-7).

When renal failure occurs, it eventually affects all of the body systems through the inability of the kidney to perform its metabolic functions and to clear toxins from the blood. These problems are discussed in the next section.

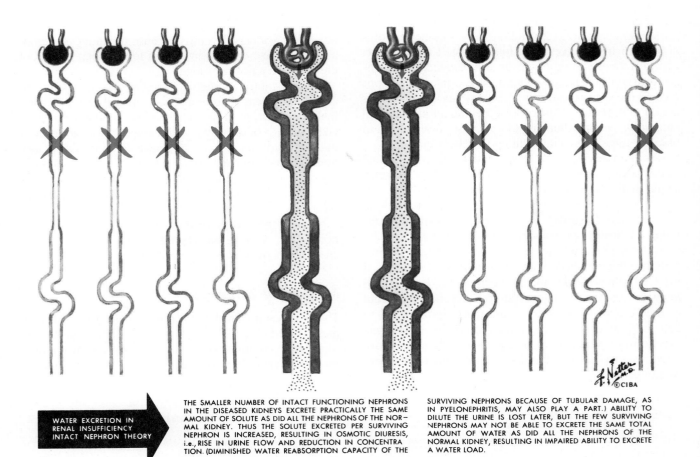

WATER EXCRETION IN RENAL INSUFFICIENCY INTACT NEPHRON THEORY

THE SMALLER NUMBER OF INTACT FUNCTIONING NEPHRONS IN THE DISEASED KIDNEYS EXCRETE PRACTICALLY THE SAME AMOUNT OF SOLUTE AS DID ALL THE NEPHRONS OF THE NORMAL KIDNEY. THUS THE SOLUTE EXCRETED PER SURVIVING NEPHRON IS INCREASED, RESULTING IN OSMOTIC DIURESIS, i.e., RISE IN URINE FLOW AND REDUCTION IN CONCENTRATION. (DIMINISHED WATER REABSORPTION CAPACITY OF THE SURVIVING NEPHRONS BECAUSE OF TUBULAR DAMAGE, AS IN PYELONEPHRITIS, MAY ALSO PLAY A PART.) ABILITY TO DILUTE THE URINE IS LOST LATER, BUT THE FEW SURVIVING NEPHRONS MAY NOT BE ABLE TO EXCRETE THE SAME TOTAL AMOUNT OF WATER AS DID ALL THE NEPHRONS OF THE NORMAL KIDNEY, RESULTING IN IMPAIRED ABILITY TO EXCRETE A WATER LOAD.

**FIGURE 35–7.**
Water excretion in renal insufficiency. (From CIBA Pharmaceutical Company. © 1973, Division of CIBA-GEIGY Corp. Illustrated by Frank H. Netter, M.D.)

# Physiologic Problems Caused by CRF

## Fluid Imbalance

Early in CRF, when the kidneys lose renal function, they are unable to concentrate urine appropriately (*hyposthenuria*), and this results in excess water loss (*polyuria*). Hyposthenuria is not only related to the diminished number of nephrons, but is due to the increased solute load per nephron. The increased solute (urea) load results because the intact nephrons that carry the solute and water for those nephrons are no longer functioning properly. Osmotic diuresis may result, causing the person to become dehydrated.

As greater numbers of nephrons become dysfunctional, an inability to dilute urine (*isosthenuria*) results. This term refers to urine and plasma having the same osmolality—about 1.010. Fluid overload with water and sodium retention may result when the GFR decreases to less than 5 mL/min.[1]

## Sodium Imbalance

Maintaining sodium balance is a serious problem, in that the nephrons may excrete as little as 20 to 30 mEq of sodium daily or up to 200 mEq/d. The varying amounts of sodium lost are believed to be related to the intact nephron theory. In other words, the damaged nephrons are unable to exchange sodium, so the intact nephrons receive the excess, causing an excess amount to be excreted in the urine. This increased elimination is accompanied by osmotic diuresis, which causes a reduction in blood volume and GFR, resulting in dehydration.

Sodium loss may be enhanced by gastrointestinal disturbances, especially vomiting and diarrhea, that may aggravate the hyponatremia and dehydration.

In severe CRF, sodium balance can be maintained even though flexibility in adjusting to sodium levels is lost. A healthy person can reduce urinary excretion of sodium practically to zero, or increase it to above 500 mEq/d when faced with sodium deficit or excess. If the GFR of a person with CRF decreases to less than 25 to 30 mL/min, obligatory sodium excretion of about 25 mEq/d may occur, with maximum excretion of 150 to 200 mEq. If water intake is restricted, hypernatremia may result. If water intake is excessive, dilutional hyponatremia may occur, often associated with edema and weight gain.[1,12]

## Potassium Imbalance

Hyperkalemia is seldom a problem in CRF before ESRD (stage 4) if water balance is maintained and metabolic acidosis is controlled. Potassium balance is believed to be the result of the adaptations made to the increased potassium presented to each functioning nephron. The mechanism for maintaining potassium balance is not understood, but may be related to enhanced aldosterone secretion. As long as urine output is maintained, the potassium level usually is maintained. Hyperkalemia may result, however, from excessive intake of potassium, certain medications, hypercatabolic illness (infection), or hyponatremia. In acute acidosis, either metabolic or respiratory, the serum potassium level rises. For every 0.1 decrease of pH unit, the serum potassium increases by about 0.6 mEq/L (see Chaps. 8 and 9).[22] It also is characteristic in uremia or ESRD.

Hypokalemia also can occur in association with a number of factors, including poor intake, diuretic therapy, hyperaldosteronism, vomiting, and excessive diarrhea.[1,9] In tubular renal disease, the nephrons may fail to resorb potassium, leading to increased potassium excretion. Hypokalemia causes a functional inability of the nephron to concentrate urine. It also increases the renal excretion of ammonium to promote potassium conservation.[9] The result is metabolic alkalosis, a characteristic feature of hypokalemia (see Chap. 9).

## Acid-Base Imbalance

Metabolic acidosis develops because the kidneys are unable to excrete enough hydrogen ion to keep the pH of the blood in a normal range.

Renal tubule dysfunction leads to progressive inability to excrete hydrogen ion. In general, the decreased hydrogen excretion is proportional to the decreased GFR.[1] Acids, continually being formed by metabolism in the body, are not filtered as effectively through the glomerular basement membrane, the production of ammonia decreases, and the tubular cell is dysfunctional. Failure to form bicarbonate also may contribute to this imbalance.

Part of the excess serum hydrogen is buffered by the bone salts. As a result, chronic metabolic acidosis increases the possibility of osteodystrophy (Figure 35-8).[1]

## Magnesium Imbalance

The magnesium level is normal in early CRF, but progressive reduction in urinary excretion may cause accumulation. A combination of decreased excretion and high intake of magnesium may result in cardiac or respiratory arrest.[15]

## Phosphorus and Calcium Imbalance

Calcium and phosphorus levels normally are maintained by the parathyroid hormone, which causes renal reabsorption of calcium by the kidneys, mobilization of calcium from bone, and depression of tubular reabsorption

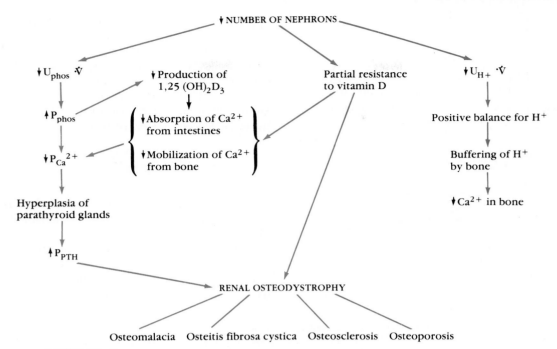

**FIGURE 35-8.**

Possible pathways by which chronic renal failure leads to hyperparathyroidism and osteodystrophy. The various forms of defective bone formation may coexist in the same person. $U_{phos}$. V, urinary excretion of phosphate; UH + V, urinary excretion of hydrogen ions, $P_{phos}$, plasma concentration of parathyroid hormone; 1,25 $(OH)_2D_3$, 1.25 dihydroxyvitamin $D_3$. (From H. Valtin, *Renal Dysfunction*. Boston: Little, Brown, 1979.)

of phosphorus. When the renal function deteriorates to 20% to 25% of normal, hyperphosphatemia and hypocalcemia occur, leading to secondary hyperparathyroidism.[15] This secondary hyperparathyroidism also is associated with altered vitamin D metabolism. When prolonged, it results in renal osteodystrophy (see Chap. 38).

Activated vitamin D normally is responsible for enhancing calcium absorption in the gastrointestinal tract and increasing reabsorption of calcium from bone. When CRF is present, hypocalcemia develops because of decreased absorption of calcium.[1] Figure 35-8 summarizes the development of renal osteodystrophy in CRF.

## Anemia

A decreased hemoglobin in patients with CRF is the result of several factors: (1) short life span of RBCs because of altered plasma; (2) increased loss of RBCs because of gastrointestinal ulceration, dialysis, and blood taken for laboratory analysis; (3) reduced erythropoietin because of decreased renal formation and inhibition from uremia; (4) folate deficiency when the person is undergoing dialysis; (5) iron deficiency; and (6) elevated levels of parathyroid hormone, which stimulates fibrous tissue or osteitis fibrosis, taking up bone marrow space and causing

decreased production by the marrow.[2] The normocytic, normochromic anemia, with hematocrit in the range of 15% to 30%, usually is proportionate to the degree of azotemia.[1]

## Bleeding Disorders

Bleeding disorders are common in CRF, and are mainly due to thrombocytopenia or platelet dysfunction. As the nitrogenous wastes accumulate, there is increased risk of hemorrhage. Bleeding often is manifest by purpura, which is characterized by hemorrhage into the skin. Factor VIII deficiency also may play a role in the bleeding disorder.[1]

## Urea and Creatinine Alterations

Urea, a by-product of protein metabolism, accumulates as the uremic stage develops. The blood urea nitrogen level is not an adequate indicator of renal disease because it is elevated whenever the GFR decreases and with an increased protein intake. Serum creatinine level is a better indicator of renal dysfunction because urinary excretion of creatinine equals the amount produced in the body. Therefore, the GFR can be estimated by changes in

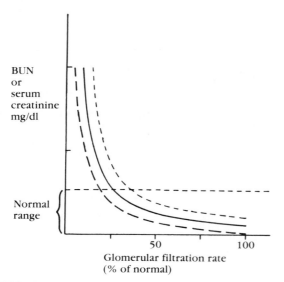

**FIGURE 35–9.**
The relation of blood urea nitrogen, or serum creatine concentration to glomerular filtration rate. The broken lines indicate that there is a family of curves rather than a single one for all. (From S. Papper, *Clinical Nephrology* [2nd ed.]. Boston: Little, Brown, 1978.)

the serum creatinine level (Figure 35-9). With normal renal function, an increase of serum creatinine from 1 to 2 mg/dL represents a fall of GFR from 120 to 60 mL/min. With severe renal failure, plasma creatinine stabilizes at about 10 mg/dL.[5]

### Carbohydrate Intolerance

Carbohydrate intolerance can occur in persons with CRF, and may be due to impaired degradation of insulin by diseased kidneys and decreased uptake of hepatic glucose. Hyperglycemia correlates with the extent of renal failure, and is probably due to insulin resistance, since insulin levels are normal or increased.[1]

## UREMIC SYNDROME

As renal failure progresses, it eventually becomes symptomatic, and the steady state is not maintained. This condition represents stage 4 of CRF, or uremia (see Table 35-1). Uremia is defined as symptomatic renal failure associated with metabolic events and complications.[17] The symptoms are described according to the effects they have on all body systems (Figure 35-10).

### Neurologic System

*Peripheral neuropathy*, an early symptom of uremia, begins in the lower extremities. Affected persons gradually develop a delayed sensory and motor response, burning sensations, and numbness in the feet and legs. Even in the absence of peripheral neuropathy, evidence of auto-

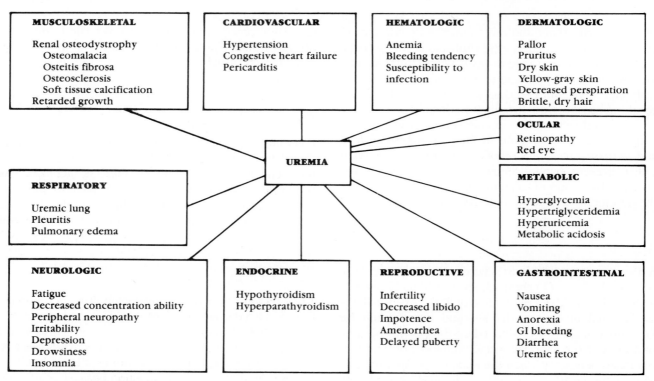

**FIGURE 35–10.**
Systemic effects of uremia. (From S. Lewis, Pathophysiology of chronic renal failure. *Nurs. Clin. North Am.* 16:38, 1981.)

nomic dysfunction—for example, hypotension or impotence—may be present.[3] Peripheral neuropathy may be generalized or in isolated areas, usually manifesting as symmetric and both motor and sensory. Restless leg syndrome or constant leg motion is present in 40% of cases.[1] Complaints of a crawling sensation, prickling, and pruritus are common. A specific uremic neurotoxin has not been identified.[3]

As renal failure progresses, central nervous system (CNS) effects vary, and include drowsiness, inability to concentrate, poor memory, hallucinations, seizures, and coma. The alterations are believed to be related to the accumulation of uremic toxins, to deficiency of ionized calcium in spinal fluid with retention of potassium and phosphates, to hypertensive crises, and to altered fluid loads.[5] The CNS disorders that persist, in both untreated and dialyzed persons, are called *uremic encephalopathy*.[3]

Dialysis dementia is a progressive and frequently fatal neurologic disease that affects some persons on long-term hemodialysis. The cause of the condition is unclear, but it has been linked with aluminum intoxication and, in the growing child, exposure of developing brain tissue to uremia. Personality changes, dementia, seizures, and death may result. Electroencephalographic changes are common.[3]

## Cardiovascular System

Hypertension, present in most persons with uremia, may result from fluid overloading but usually is related to vascular changes (nephrosclerosis) or increased renin secretion.[5]

Fluid overloading is the result of sodium and water imbalance. Vascular changes include accelerated atherosclerosis and narrowing of the arterioles. *Hyperreninemia* often is noted. Cardiovascular disease accounts for more than 50% of all deaths from CRF.[17]

Fibrinous pericarditis may develop in ESRD, and may be associated with an excess of pericardial fluid and fibrin formation on the epicardial surface.[1] The fluid can cause cardiac restriction and even tamponade. Fibrinous pericarditis may be asymptomatic, associated with substernal pain, or symptomatic of cardiac tamponade. Cardiomyopathy with patchy degeneration of muscle fibers may occur. Pericarditis may be due to the uremia, and associated with elevated serum urea and creatinine levels. It also may result after dialysis, arising acutely with elevated temperature and pain. Persons who do not comply with routine dialysis therapy tend to have a high frequency of pericarditis.[17]

Congestive heart failure may develop as a result of salt and fluid overloading, together with the characteristic hypertension. Pulmonary edema may be characterized by the uremic lung.

## Respiratory System

The *uremic lung* noted on radiologic examination characteristically exhibits "bat wings" and involves perihilar congestion. The term is a misnomer because the syndrome is not always present with uremia. An end-stage pattern has been noted, which resembles the respiratory distress syndrome and is related to high serum urea levels. Pneumonia also is a major threat in CRF because the uremic environment depresses the immune response.

## Gastrointestinal System

The most common gastrointestinal symptoms are nausea, vomiting, hiccups, and anorexia. Their cause is not well understood, but they are related to the degree of uremia and may improve if hydration is maintained. Ulcers, called *uremic stomatitis*, may form in the oral mucosa. These probably form from the production of ammonium by bacteria ureases from high levels of salivary urea.[1] Uremic fetor, or urine breath, occurs when the salivary urea is broken down to ammonia, causing an unpleasant metallic taste. The oral mucosa often is dry and the tongue is yellow-brown. Gastritis, peptic ulcer disease, esophagitis, and colitis are common localizations of gastrointestinal lesions.[8] Gastrointestinal bleeding is a complication that may result from ulcerations and capillary fragility.

## Musculoskeletal System

The effects of altered levels of calcium and phosphorus are shown in Figure 35-8. The resulting faulty bone metabolism, called *renal osteodystrophy*, is caused by a combination of hyperparathyroidism, calcium and phosphorus alterations, and decreased synthesis of the active form of vitamin D. Several resulting bone lesions include osteomalacia, osteitis fibrosa, soft-tissue calcification, and osteosclerosis.

Hyperparathyroidism is a response to serum containing decreased ionized calcium. The causes of decreased calcium include phosphate retention, altered vitamin D metabolism, altered feedback with calcium and parathyroid hormone (PTH), and other factors. Phosphate retention is a consequence of decreased renal function and higher levels of PTH. Phosphaturia results at the expense of high PTH levels. Phosphate retention also leads to hypocalcemia and increased PTH levels. Calcium feedback is altered, and excessive levels of calcium are required to suppress PTH in persons with uremia.[7]

*Osteomalacia* is the result of poor tissue use of vitamin D that causes accumulation of osteoid material after calcification has ceased. *Osteitis fibrosa* occurs when fibrous tissue replaces bone tissue. It may result from secondary hyperparathyroidism. Soft-tissue *metastatic calcification* is the deposition of calcium and phosphate crystals in the synovial tissues and soft tissues, especially the eyes, joints, muscles, and lungs. *Osteosclerosis*, believed to be similar to soft-tissue calcification, is due to bone redistribution and remodeling. This lesion causes enhanced bone density, mainly affecting the face, skull, and spine.

Renal osteodystrophy causes an enhanced tendency to spontaneous fractures. Many of the complications of this condition can be prevented by using phosphate-binding agents, administering activated vitamin D, and supplementing dietary calcium.[15]

## Hematologic Alterations

The hematologic effects of uremia include a normocytic, normochromic anemia, and altered hemostasis (see Chaps. 19 and 21). Anemia results from lack of erythropoietin response to hypoxia and obliteration of erythropoietin production sites. Hemolysis of RBCs is common; it is related to a decreased survival time of erythrocytes in uremic plasma. Uremic plasma interferes with the ability of the erythrocyte membrane to pump sodium out, leading to swelling and hemolysis of RBCs. Dialysis also may cause hemolysis by mechanical destruction or reaction to the dialysate.[5] Increased frequency of hepatitis is associated with the need for blood transfusions and dialysis therapy. Coagulation defects are caused by platelet defects, and occur in most persons with uremia. Abnormal bleeding results, causing a wide range of problems, including epistaxis, purpura, and frank hemorrhage.[2] Depressed immune response leads to a high frequency of infection and inhibition of phagocytosis.[20]

## Dermatologic Alterations

Skin pallor results from anemia, and there also is a characteristic sallow, yellow pigmentation. Retention of pigmented urochromes results in their deposition in the subcutaneous fat. Dryness of the skin is caused by atrophy of the sweat glands and dehydration. Uremic itching or pruritus is unexplained but possibly related to excess PTH, skin deposits, or peripheral neuropathy. Uremic frost may occur in advanced uremia when the urea deposits are excreted in sweat and crystallize. Soft-tissue calcification results from secondary hyperparathyroidism, which leads to chalky plaques being deposited under the skin.[17] Other organ and system alterations also occur, as noted in Figure 35-10.

## REFERENCES

1. Alfrey, A.C. Chronic renal failure: Manifestations and pathogenesis. In R.W. Schrier (ed.), *Renal and Electrolyte Disorders* (3rd ed.). Boston: Little, Brown, 1986.
2. Anagnostou, A., and Kurtzman, M.A. Hematologic consequences of renal failure. In B.M. Brenner and F.C. Rector (eds.), *The Kidney* (3rd ed.). Philadelphia: Ardmore, 1986.
3. Arieff, A.I. Neurologic manifestations of uremia. In B.M. Brenner and F.C. Rector (eds.), *The Kidney* (3rd ed.). Philadelphia: Ardmore, 1986.
4. Bastl, C.P., Rudnick, M.R., and Narino, D.G. Assessment of renal function: Characteristics of the functional and organic forms of acute renal failure. In B.M. Brenner and F.C. Rector (eds.), *The Kidney* (3rd ed.). Philadelphia: Ardmore, 1986.
5. Brenner, B.M., and Rector, F.C. (eds.). *The Kidney* (3rd ed.). Philadelphia: Ardmore, 1986.
6. Brezis, M., Rosen, S., and Epstein, F.H. Acute renal failure. In B.M. Brenner and F.C. Rector (eds.), *The Kidney* (3rd ed.). Philadelphia: Ardmore, 1986.
7. Coburn, J.W., and Slatopolsky, E. Vitamin D, parathyroid hormone, and renal osteodystrophy. In B.M. Brenner and F.C. Rector (eds.), *The Kidney* (3rd ed.). Philadelphia: Ardmore, 1986.
8. Cotran, R., Kumar, V., and Robbins, S.L. *Robbins' Pathologic Basis of Disease* (4th ed.). Philadelphia: W.B. Saunders, 1989.
9. Gabow, P.A., and Peterson, L.N. Disorders of potassium metabolism. In R.W. Schrier (ed.), *Renal and Electrolyte disorders* (3rd ed.). Boston: Little, Brown, 1986.
10. Harris, R.C., Meyer, T.W., and Brenner, B.M. Nephron adaptation to renal injury. In B.M. Brenner and F.C. Rector (eds.), *The Kidney* (3rd ed.). Philadelphia: Ardmore, 1986.
11. Humes, H.D., and Messana, J.M. Approach to the patient with acute renal failure. In W.N. Kelley (ed.), *Textbook of Internal Medicine*. Philadelphia: J.B. Lippincott, 1989.
12. Innerarity, S.A. Electrolyte emergencies in the critically ill renal patient. *Crit. Care Clin. North Am.* 2(1):89, 1990.
13. Knochel, J.P. The biochemistry of renal failure. In G. Eknoyan and J.P. Knochel (eds.), *The Systemic Consequences of Renal Failure*. Orlando, Fla.: Grune & Stratton, 1984.
14. Lancaster, L. Renal response to shock. *Crit. Care Clin. North Am.* 2(2):221, 1990.
15. Massry, S.G. Disorders of divalent ion metabolism. In G. Eknoyan and J.P. Knochel (eds.), *The Systemic Consequences of Renal Failure*. Orlando, Fla.: Grune & Stratton, 1984.
16. Minaken, K.L., and Rowe, J.W. Disorders of fluid and osmolality regulation. In W.N. Kelley (ed.), *Textbook of Internal Medicine*. Philadelphia: J.B. Lippincott, 1989.
17. Mujais, S.K., Sabatini, S., and Kurtzman, N.A. Pathophysiology of uremia. In B.M. Brenner and F.C. Rector (eds.), *The Kidney* (3rd ed.). Philadelphia: Ardmore, 1986.
18. Oken, D.E., Wolfert, A.J., and Gehr, T.W. The pathophysiology and differential diagnosis of acute renal failure. In W.C. Shoemaker et al. (eds.), *Textbook of Critical Care* (2nd ed.). Philadelphia: W.B. Saunders, 1989.

**19.** Richard, C.J. *Comprehensive Nephrology Nursing.* Boston: Little, Brown, 1986.

**20.** Saxton, C.R., and Smith, J.W. The immune system and infections. In G. Eknoyan and J.P. Knochel (eds.), *The Systemic Consequences of Renal Failure.* Orlando, Fla.: Grune & Stratton, 1984.

**21.** Schrier, R.W. *Renal and Electrolyte Disorders* (3rd ed.). Boston: Little, Brown, 1986.

**22.** Ziyadeh, F.N., and Agus, Z.S. Approach to the patient with chronic renal failure. In W.N. Kelley (ed.), *Textbook of Internal Medicine.* Philadelphia: J.B. Lippincott, 1989.

## UNIT BIBLIOGRAPHY

Abuelo, J.G. *Renal Pathophysiology.* Baltimore: Williams & Wilkins, 1989.

Anderton, J.L., and Thomson, D. *Nephrology.* New York: Churchill-Livingstone, 1988.

Andreucci, V.E. *Acute Renal Failure: Pathophysiology, Prevention and Treatment.* Boston: Kluwer, 1984.

Bach, P.H., and Locks, E.A. *Nephrotoxicity In Vitro and In Vivo.* New York: Plenum, 1989.

Blandy, J.P., and Moors, J. *Urology for Nurses.* Boston: Blackwell, 1989.

Brenner, B.M., and Lazarus, J.M. *Acute Renal Failure.* Philadelphia: W.B. Saunders, 1983.

Brenner, B.M., and Rector, F.C. (eds.). *The Kidney* (3rd ed.). Philadelphia: Ardmore, 1986.

Burgio, K.L., Pearce, K.L., and Lucca, A.J. *Staying Dry: A Practical Guide to Bladder Control.* Baltimore: Johns Hopkins University Press, 1989.

Cattell, W.R. *Clinical Renal Imaging.* New York: Wiley, 1989.

Catto, G.R., and Rower, W.A. *Nephrology in Clinical Practice.* Baltimore: Arnold, 1988.

Davison, A.M. *Nephrology.* London: Heinemann, 1988.

DeWardener, H.E. *The Kidney: An Outline of Normal and Abnormal Function* (5th ed.). Edinburgh: Churchill-Livingstone, 1985.

Drife, J.O., Hilton, P., and Stanton, S.L. *Micturition.* New York: Springer-Verlag, 1990.

Evans, D.B., and Henderson, R.G. *Lecture Notes on Nephrology.* Boston: Blackwell, 1985.

Fitzpatrick, J.M., and Kram, R.J. *The Prostate.* New York: Churchill-Livingstone, 1989.

Freeman, R.M., and Malvern, J. *The Unstable Bladder.* Boston: Wright, 1989.

Gabriel, R. *Postgraduate Nephrology* (3rd ed.). Boston: Butterworth, 1985.

Gabriel, R. *Renal Medicine* (3rd ed.). Philadelphia: Bailliaere-Tindall, 1988.

Gonick, H.C., and Buckalew, V.M. *Renal Tubular Disorders: Pathophysiology, Diagnosis and Management.* New York: Dekker, 1985.

Heptinstall, R.H. Acute renal failure. In R.H. Heptinstall (ed.), *Pathology of the Kidney* (3rd ed.). Boston: Little, Brown, 1983.

Jelter, K.F. *Nursing for Continence.* Philadelphia: W.B. Saunders, 1990.

Kinne, R.K. *Renal Biochemistry Cells, Membranes, Molecules.* Amsterdam, N.Y.: Elsevier, 1985.

Leaf, A., and Cotran, R. *Renal Pathophysiology* (2nd ed.). New York: Oxford University Press, 1985.

Mandelstan, D. *Understanding Incontinence: A Guide to the Nature and Management of a Very Common Complaint.* London: Disabled Living Foundation, Chapmans Hall, 1989.

Massry, S.G. *Textbook of Nephrology* (2nd ed.). Baltimore: Williams & Wilkins, 1989.

Muther, R.S., Barry, J.M., and Bennett, W.M. *Manual of Nephrology.* Philadelphia: Dekker, 1990.

*1990 Neurobiology of Incontinence.* Wiley, Chichester: Ciba Foundation Symposium 151.

O'Rourke, R.A. *The Heart and Renal Disease.* New York: Churchill-Livingstone, 1984.

Rodman, M., and Smith, D. *Pharmacology and Drug Therapy in Nursing* (2nd ed.). Philadelphia: J.B. Lippincott, 1984.

Rose, B.D. *Pathophysiology of Renal Disease* (2nd ed.). New York: McGraw-Hill, 1987.

Schrier, R.W. *Manual of Nephrology* (3rd ed.). Boston: Little, Brown, 1990.

Schrier, R.W. *Renal and Electrolyte Disorders* (3rd ed.). Boston: Little, Brown, 1986.

Schrier, R.W., and Gottschalk, C.W. *Diseases of the Kidney* (4th ed.). Boston: Little, Brown, 1988.

Seldin, D.W., and Giebisch, G. *The Kidney—Physiology and Pathophysiology.* New York: Raven, 1985.

Stone, W.J., and Rabin, P.L. *End-Stage Renal Disease.* New York: Academic, 1983.

Sweny, P., Farrington, K., and Moorhead, J. *The Kidney and Its Disorders.* Boston: Blackwell, 1989.

Tischer, C., and Brenner, B.M. *Renal Pathology with Clinical and Functional Correlations.* Philadelphia: J.B. Lippincott, 1989.

Uldall, R. *Renal Nursing* (3rd ed.). Boston: Blackwell, 1988.

Ulrich, B.T. *Nephrology Nursing.* Norwalk, Conn.: Appleton & Lange, 1989.

Vander, A.J. *Renal Physiology* (4th ed.). New York: McGraw-Hill, 1991.

# ENDOCRINE REGULATION

The endocrine system is a complex system that coordinates and maintains the steady state through secretion of hormones. The secretion of hormones usually is activated by other hormones, neural influences, or both and follows a closely regulated feedback mechanism. Chapter 36 describes pituitary function and explains how alterations can affect other body functions. Chapter 37 details the activity of the adrenal gland, its role in the stress response, and major alterations in function. Chapter 38 follows normal thyroid activity, with discussion of hyperthyroidism, hypothyroidism, and thyroid cancer. Parathyroid function also is included in this chapter. Chapter 39 discusses the normal endocrine secretion activities of the pancreas (exocrine activities are discussed in Chapter 42). Diabetes mellitus, pancreatitis, carcinoma of the pancreas, and cystic fibrosis are major pathologies presented in this chapter.

The reader is encouraged to use the learning objectives at the beginning of each chapter to organize the study of this unit. The unit bibliography is helpful in providing direction for further study.

# Pituitary Regulation and Alterations in Function

*Learning Objectives*

1. Describe the basic structure and function of hormones.
2. Differentiate the structure and function of the adenohypophysis and the neurohypophysis.
3. Identify the area called the pars intermedia.
4. List and describe the functions of the hormones of the adenohypophysis.

5. Describe the functions of the two hormones of the neurohypophysis.
6. Draw the feedback method of control between the hypothalamus and pituitary.

(continued)

## Learning Objectives (continued)

7. Briefly outline the vascular supply to the pituitary and hypothalamus.
8. List at least four known hormones released by the hypothalamus.
9. Differentiate clearly between specific pituitary hormones and secretions of the target gland.
10. List and describe the effects of growth hormone.
11. Describe the physiologic effects of antidiuretic hormone (ADH).
12. Explain the different factors that cause the release of ADH.
13. Briefly describe the effects of oxytocin on uterine contractility and lactation.
14. Explain the mechanical and hormonal effects of pituitary malfunction.
15. Briefly describe conditions that cause enlargement of the sella turcica and their effects.
16. List some causes of deficiency conditions of the anterior pituitary.
17. Define *panhypopituitarism*.
18. Explain how deficiencies in single pituitary hormones affect the metabolism of the entire organism.
19. Describe Sheehan's syndrome.
20. Describe the results of hypersecretion of single pituitary hormones.
21. Differentiate between gigantism and acromegaly.
22. Define and explain *ADH deficiency* (diabetes insipidus).
23. Clearly explain the syndrome of inappropriate ADH secretion (SIADH).
24. List at least six causative factors of SIADH.
25. Relate pituitary tumors to hyperpituitarism and hypopituitarism.
26. List at least three clinical manifestations of pituitary tumors.

The human organism contains complex systems of communication that coordinate and maintain a steady state essential to its functions. Through these systems the body monitors the activities and needs of each of its parts and responds accordingly to maintain normalcy.

Through these systems of communication, it is possible for one cell to influence the functions of other adjacent and distant cells. When studying the mechanisms of the endocrine glands, it is imperative to consider the impact of neural control, while also examining the endocrine glands themselves.

Research in the past two decades has determined that the neurologic and endocrine systems and their functions are multiple, complex, and closely interrelated.[7,8] This interrelation is clearly evident in both normal physiology and disease pathophysiology. Neuroendocrinology investigates the pathway mechanisms of neural control and endocrine secretions.[17]

Endocrine cells primarily secrete hormones into the bloodstream. Hormones may act directly on specific organs, or may have more generalized effects on different and widespread tissues of the body. Each component of the endocrine system has specific functions, coordinating with other cells to create an environment conducive to survival of the total organism. Figure 36-1 shows the anatomy and location of the endocrine glands.

Many of the endocrine glands have neural input that controls their flow and secretory activity, while endocrine function, in turn, regulates many functions within the nervous system.[8] Thus, the balance of neuroendocrine function is intricate and precise. Neural influence of endocrine function is maintained by three mechanisms: (1) input to neurons that secrete hypothalamic hormones, (2) the intermediate lobe of the pituitary, and (3) autonomic innervation of glands (such as the pancreatic islets that are not directly controlled by trophic hormones).[7]

This chapter describes the characteristics of hormones and clarifies their effects on target cells. The major focus is on the pituitary gland, its anatomic structure and physiologic function, its role within the complex communication system for maintaining a steady state, its relation to the overall endocrine system, and pathologic manifestations of functional imbalance.

## HORMONES

The word hormone stems from the Greek root *ormaino,* which means "to excite, arouse, set in motion." Hormones are chemical substances that exert a physiologic effect on other cells. The capacity to synthesize these substances is not limited to endocrine organs, but may be a characteristic of peripheral tissues or even of precursors in the bloodstream.

Secretion of a given hormone usually is activated by hormonal or neural influences on specific target cells by feedback mechanisms. Secreted hormones that act selectively on other specific target cells to regulate and maintain normal function are called *trophic hormones.* Hormones affect function in four broad physiologic areas: (1) reproduction, (2) growth and development, (3) maintenance of the internal environment of the organism, and (4) regulation of available energy.[8] Hormonal action can be both diffuse and complex, as well as limited and tissue-specific.

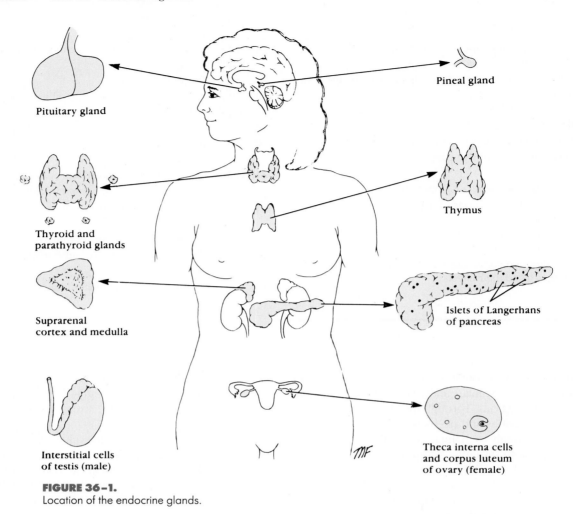

**FIGURE 36–1.**
Location of the endocrine glands.

The action of hormones in endocrine tissues may occur in one of four modes: endocrine, neural, paracrine, and autocrine.[7,8,12,17] Classically, *endocrine* influence is carried out by hormonal messengers that are secreted into and carried by circulating body fluids. *Neural* communication occurs when chemical messengers transmit cell-to-cell communication across synaptic junctions. *Paracrine* influence is the result of messenger hormones acting locally by diffusion onto contiguous cells. *Autocrine* influence occurs when the messenger hormones are able to modify the secretory activity of the cells that produced them. Figure 36-2 shows the modes of hormone action.

Hormones also are classified according to chemical structure. The basic types are steroids, derivatives of tyrosine (amines), and protein-based hormones.

*Steroid hormones* are derived from a basic precursor, cholesterol. Steroids are lipids, and can move through the cell membranes of target tissues to exert their action by affecting the cytoplasm or nucleus. Steroids enter the cell, bind with a cytoplasmic receptor, and then enter the nucleus to form messenger ribonucleic

acid (RNA). This promotes translation at the ribosomes to form new proteins.[9]

The amines, or derivatives of the amino acid tyrosine, enter the cell through specific cell membrane receptors and combine with a nuclear receptor. These synthesize proteins, and include the thyroid hormones, epinephrine, and norepinephrine.[19]

The proteins, or peptides, are classified according to whether they have long or short chains. The short chains are peptides, and the more complex long chains are proteins. Peptide linkage is a major way by which amino acids are joined to form proteins. The average protein has about 400 amino acids.[9] Most protein hormones bind directly with nuclear deoxyribonucleic acid (DNA).

Table 36-1 lists the major endocrine hormones as to type, target tissue, and action. The actions of hormones are highly selective because of binding of specific receptor sites in target tissue. Some, such as epinephrine and glucagon, act on cell membrane receptors, whereas the lipid-soluble steroids act on intracellular nuclear and cytoplasmic receptors.

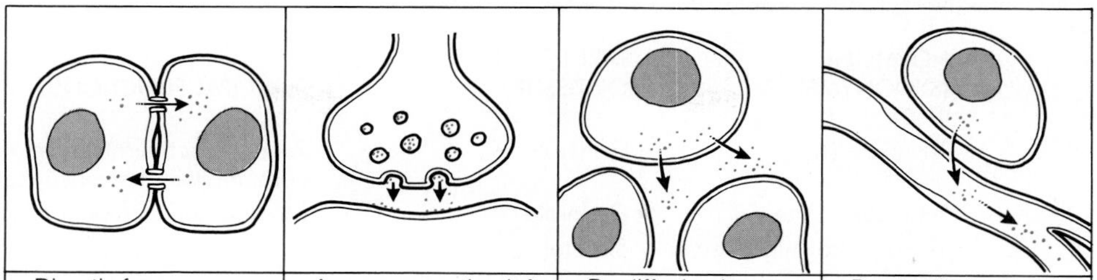

| | Gap Junction | Synapse | Paracrine | Endocrine |
|---|---|---|---|---|
| Method of transmission: | Directly from cell to cell | Across synaptic cleft | By diffusion in interstitial fluid | By circulating body fluids |
| Area of action: | Local | Local | Locally diffuse | General |
| Specific to: | Anatomic location | Anatomic location and receptors | Receptors | Receptors |

**FIGURE 36-2.**
Intercellular communication by chemical mediators.

**TABLE 36-1.**
GENERAL ENDOCRINE GLANDS AND THEIR HORMONES

| GLAND | HORMONE (SYNONYMS) | TARGET ORGAN OR TISSUE | PRINCIPAL FUNCTIONS |
|---|---|---|---|
| Pituitary (hypophysis cerebri) | | | |
| Adenohypophysis | Somatotropin (growth hormone, somatotropic hormone) | General | Accelerates rate of body growth, particularly growth of bone and muscle; exerts anabolic effect on calcium, phosphorus, and nitrogen metabolism; affects metabolism of carbohydrate and lipid; elevates skeletal and cardiac muscle glycogen content |
| | Thyrotropin (thyrotropic hormone, thyroid-stimulating hormone) | Thyroid | Synthesis and secretion of thyroid hormones |
| | Corticotropin (adrenocorticotropin, adrenocorticotropic hormone) | Adrenal cortex | Synthesis and secretion of adrenal cortical steroids |
| | Follicle-stimulating hormone | Ovaries, testes | Stimulates growth of ovarian follicle in female, spermatogenesis in male |
| | Luteinizing hormone (interstitial cell–stimulating hormone) | Ovaries, testes | Stimulates development of corpus luteum after ovulation and progesterone synthesis therein; in male, stimulates development of interstitial tissue of testes and secretion of androgen |
| | Prolactin (luteotropic hormone, luteotropin lactogenic hormone, mammotropin) | Mammary glands | Proliferation of tissue; initiation of milk secretion |
| Pars intermedia | $\alpha$-melanocyte-stimulating hormone and $\beta$-stimulating hormone (intermedin) | Expand melanophores in lower vertebrates | Insignificant in humans |
| Neurohypophysis | Antidiuretic hormone (vasopressin) | Renal tubules | Facilitates water absorption |
| | | Arterioles | Produces vasoconstriction, hence, exerts a pressor effect |
| | Oxytocin | Smooth muscle, especially of uterus | Contraction, parturition |

(continued)

**TABLE 36-1. (continued)**

GENERAL ENDOCRINE GLANDS AND THEIR HORMONES

| GLAND | HORMONE (SYNONYMS) | TARGET ORGAN OR TISSUE | PRINCIPAL FUNCTIONS |
|---|---|---|---|
| Thyroid | Thyroxine ($T_4$) | General | $T_3$ and $T_4$ accelerate the metabolic rate and oxygen consumption of all bodily tissues |
| | Triiodothyronine ($T_3$) | General | Metabolism of calcium and phosphorus |
| | Thyrocalcitonin (same as parathyroid calcitonin) | Skeleton | |
| Parathyroid | Parathormone | Skeleton, kidneys, gastrointestinal tract | Metabolism of calcium and phosphorus |
| | Calcitonin | Skeleton | Metabolism of calcium and phosphorus |
| Endocrine pancreas | Insulin | General | Regulates carbohydrate metabolism, stimulates protein synthesis |
| | Glucagon, pancreatic | Liver | Stimulates hepatic gluconeogenesis, glucogenolysis |
| | | Adipose tissue | Stimulates lipogenesis |
| Adrenal cortex | Adrenal cortical steroids (eg, cortisol) | General | Metabolism of carbohydrate |
| | Aldosterone | Renal tubules | Metabolism of electrolytes and water |
| Adrenal medulla | Epinephrine | Heart muscle, smooth muscle, arterioles | Accelerates heart rate; causes arteriolar vasoconstriction, hence, pressor response; stimulates contraction of most smooth muscle |
| | | Liver, skeletal muscle | Stimulates glycogenolysis |
| | | Adipose tissue | Stimulates lipolysis |
| | Norepinephrine | Arterioles | Causes arteriolar vasoconstriction, hence, pressor response |
| Testes | Testosterone | Accessory sex organs | Stimulates normal growth, development, and functions |
| | | General | Stimulates maturation of secondary sex characteristics |
| Ovaries | Estrone, estradiol | Accessory sex organs | Stimulates normal growth, development, and cyclic functions |
| | | Mammary glands | Development of system of ducts |
| | | General | Stimulates maturation of secondary sex characteristics |
| | Progesterone (from corpus luteum) | Uterus | Prepares endometrium for implantation of fertilized ovum |
| | | Mammary glands | Development of alveolar system |

Source: *Adapted from D. Jensen, The Principles of Physiology (2nd ed.). New York: Appleton-Century-Crofts. Reprinted by permission of Appleton & Lange, Simon & Schuster Professional Information Group, 25 Van Zant St., E. Norwalk, CT 06855.*

## MORPHOLOGY OF THE PITUITARY GLAND

### Gross Anatomy

The human adult pituitary is about 1 cm long, 1.0 to 1.5 cm wide, and 0.5 cm thick. It is round or ovoid, and weighs about 0.5 g. Because of its position beneath the hypothalamus of the diencephalon, it also is called the *hypophysis*, taken from the Greek roots *ypo*, meaning "under," and *phyo* meaning "to grow." The gland rests in a small depression (hypophyseal fossa) of the sphenoid bone called the *sella turcica*. It is covered by a tough membrane, diaphragma sellae, through which passes the structure joining the pituitary to the hypothalamus, the hypophyseothalamic stalk. This structure also is called the infundibular stalk. Because disorders of the hypothalamus often are expressed as those of pituitary secretion, one must appreciate the functional and anatomic relation of the hypothalamus to the pituitary gland.[3]

Anatomically and physiologically, the pituitary is divided into regions that function as distinct and different endocrine organs. The anterior lobe is called the *adenohypophysis,* and is subdivided into two regions: (1) the pars tuberalis, made up of a small mass of tissue running up along the infundibulum and surrounding the stalk, and (2) the pars distalis, which forms the bulk of the anterior lobe. The posterior lobe is called the *neuro-*

*hypophysis,* and includes three regions: (1) neural lobe, (2) infundibular stalk, and (3) median eminence of the tuber cinereum, which forms the attachment with the hypothalamus (Figure 36-3). The intermediate lobe (pars intermedia) lies between the anterior and posterior lobes, and often is considered separate and distinct. Because it is poorly developed in the adult human, its function is questionable. The only known secretion of the intermediate lobe is melanocyte-stimulating hormone (MSH), which is synthesized from a large prohormone that also is a precursor of corticotropin.[16] These hormones do not seem to be of major importance in skin pigmentation in humans.

The pituitary develops from a common germ layer, the ectoderm, but originates from two distinctly different embryologic anatomic sources. The adenohypophysis derives from an upward diverticulum of the ectodermal layer of the roof of the mouth or pharyngeal epithelium

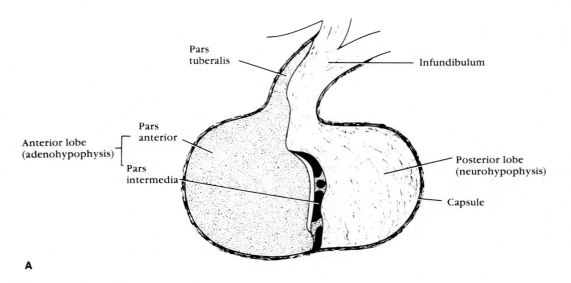

**A.**

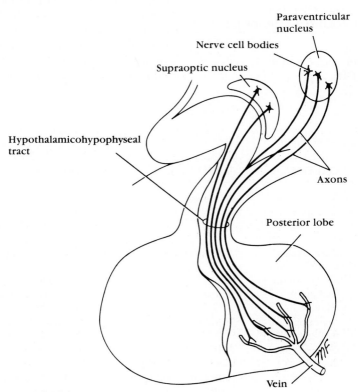

**B.**

**FIGURE 36–3.**
**A.** Divisions of the hypophysis. **B.** The hypothalamohypophyseal tract.

known as Rathke's pouch. The neurohypophysis originates as a downward ectodermal diverticulum from the hypothalamic portion of the diencephalon. These two lobes come together to form the hypophysis. Whereas Rathke's pouch loses its connection with the pharyngeal membrane, the neurohypophysis retains neural tract connections with the hypothalamus. These neural fiber connections are crucial in the secretory functions of the neurohypophysis.

The functioning pituitary remains connected to the hypothalamus through the neural tracts of the infundibular stalk and by an elaborate vascular system. These neural and vascular pathways are essential to the function of the pituitary, which is the bridging of the nervous system with the endocrine system.[16]

## Histology

### Adenohypophysis

Traditionally, anterior pituitary cells were classified on the basis of their staining properties. Many of these cells contain secretory granules, but some are sparsely granulated or considered to be agranular. This classification has been replaced by the development of assays to measure the levels of hormones in the blood. Radioimmunoassays are highly successful in measuring the levels of specific hormones. The ideal test is probably the demonstration of hormone action on target tissues.[19]

The following are the recognized anterior pituitary cell types[5]:

1. Somatotropes originally were called acidophilic cells and secrete growth hormone (GH).

2. Lactotropes or mammotropes also are acidophilic and secrete prolactin (PRL).
3. Thyrotropes are basophilic-staining cells that secrete thyroid-stimulating hormone (TSH).
4. Gonadotropes are basophilic-staining cells associated with the lactotropes and secrete luteinizing hormone (LH) and follicle-stimulating hormone (FSH).
5. Corticotropes may exhibit basophilic characteristic or be relatively agranular (chromophobic); they secrete adrenocorticotropic hormone (ACTH).
6. Other cell types include 15% to 20% of the anterior pituitary cells, which are either nonsecretory or primitive and whose function is unknown.

Table 36-2 summarizes these cell types with respect to hormones secreted.

The foregoing discussion represents an attempt to simplify cellular–hormonal relations; however, it is recognized that in actual fact, no simple one-to-one interaction exists. A review of Table 36-2 shows that in at least two instances, two hormones are secreted by the same type of cell. In other instances, secretion of a given hormone may be stimulated by many factors. Stress, for example, has been shown to increase the secretion of ACTH and TSH.

### Neurohypophysis

The neurohypophysis contains neuroglial cells and cells known as *pituicytes*. The pituicytes serve no endocrine function, but act as supporting structures for the terminal nerve fibers and tracts of the hypothalamus. The bulk of the posterior lobe consists of the hypothalamicohypophyseal tract. This tract consists of a bundle of nonmyelinated nerve fibers whose cell bodies are located in the supraoptic nucleus of the hypothalamus near the optic

## TABLE 36-2.
ANTERIOR PITUITARY CELL TYPES

| HORMONE | CELL TYPE | TARGET ORGAN | FUNCTION |
|---|---|---|---|
| Somatotropic hormone, growth hormone | Somatotrope Acidophil | All tissues | Increases rate of protein synthesis in all cells; decreases rate of carbohydrate use throughout body; increases mobilization of fats and use of fats for energy |
| Adrenocorticotropic hormone | Corticotrope Basophil, large chromophobe | Adrenal cortex | Regulates secretion of cortisol and corticosteroids; enhances production of adrenal androgens |
| Prolactin | Lactotrope Acidophil | Breasts | Produces lactation; stimulates development of alevolar secretory system |
| Thyroid-stimulating hormone | Thyrotrope Basophil | Thyroid | Increases all known activities of thyroid glandular cells |
| Gonadotropic hormones: follicle-stimulating hormone, luteinizing hormone | Gonadotrope Basophil | Follicles of ovaries, interstitial cells of Leydig in testes, seminiferous tubules of testes | Regulates spermatogenesis; regulates maturation of ovarian follicle and ovulation production of testosterone |

chiasma, and in the paraventricular nucleus in the wall of the third ventricle.

Axons from these cell bodies traverse the hypophyseal stalk to terminate in the posterior lobe in proximity with the vessels that make up the capillary plexus. The neurohypophysis stores and releases two hormones, *oxytocin* and *antidiuretic hormone* (ADH) (the latter also is known as vasopressin). These hormones are synthesized by the hypothalamus and carried to the posterior pituitary through the system described earlier.

## Pars Intermedia

The intermediate lobe lies between the adenohypophysis and the neurohypophysis. As previously noted, this lobe, which has a major role in pigmentation and coloration in lower animal species, apparently has little effect on the normal skin pigmentation of humans.[3,4] The pigmentary changes encountered in several endocrine diseases, such as the abnormal pallor of hypopituitarism and the hypopigmentation of adrenal insufficiency, are attributed to changes in circulating ACTH. Because ACTH has a common 13–amino acid sequence with MSH, it has melanocyte-stimulating activity.

## RELATION OF THE PITUITARY TO THE HYPOTHALAMUS

Although the pituitary has been called the "master gland," it is now known that most of its functions are controlled by the hypothalamus. Secretion of pituitary hormones is activated by signals from the hypothalamus through a complex humoral and neural communication system.

## Hypothalamic Secretion of Releasing and Release-Inhibiting Factors

Through feedback and other mechanisms of communication, specialized neurons in the hypothalamus are stimulated to synthesize and secrete substances called releasing and inhibiting hormones. The function of these agents is to regulate the secretion of pituitary hormones, which, in turn, control the secretion of hormones of the target endocrine glands. Figure 36-4 shows the target organs of the pituitary hormones.

The hypothalamus secretes a corresponding releasing hormone or factor for each anterior pituitary hor-

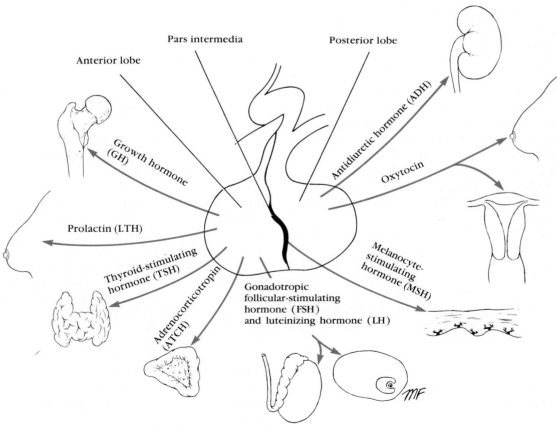

**FIGURE 36–4.**
Diagram showing the target organs of pituitary hormones.

**TABLE 36–3.**
ANTERIOR PITUITARY HORMONES AND THEIR ASSOCIATED RELEASING
HORMONES

| ANTERIOR PITUITARY HORMONE | RELEASING HORMONE |
|---|---|
| Thyroid-stimulating hormone | Thyrotropin-releasing hormone |
| Luteinizing hormone | Luteinizing hormone–releasing hormone |
| Follicle-stimulating hormone | Luteinizing hormone–releasing hormone |
| Adrenocorticotropin hormone | Corticotropin-releasing hormone |
| Growth hormone | Growth hormone–releasing hormone |
| Prolactin | Prolactin-releasing hormone (no single hormone identified) |

mone. In addition, the hypothalamus exerts dual influence, as PRL and GH also have inhibiting hormones secreted (Table 36-3). Dopamine, which exerts the dominant influence, is the inhibiting hormone secreted for PRL. Somatostatin is the inhibiting hormone for GH.

An inverse relation exists between the blood level of hormones of the target organs and the stimulation of synthesis and secretion of the related pituitary hormones. The mechanism of control occurs through a negative feedback system that involves the hypothalamus, anterior pituitary, and trophic, or target, gland (Figure 36-5). Figure 36-5B shows the specific mechanism for the regulation of ACTH secretion.

When the circulating plasma concentration level of any given target organ hormone is elevated above body need, the hypothalamus senses this imbalance and suppresses the secretion of the corresponding releasing hormone. Accordingly, the anterior pituitary responds by decreasing hormone secretion, thereby decreasing the stimulus to the target gland hormone. Conversely, when the circulating plasma level concentration of a target organ hormone falls below some critical level, the hypothalamus secretes a releasing hormone, triggering hormone secretion from the anterior pituitary gland, which in turn stimulates the target organ hormones. Through this feedback system, hormone balance is carefully regulated and controlled.

Because the neuroendocrine regulation of hormonal balance is extremely sensitive, other influences on the body's internal and external environment may produce changes in circulating hormone levels during periods of extreme states. Emotion, trauma, and diurnal changes create hormonal and other variations.

## Hypothalamic-Pituitary Neural and Circulatory Structures

To clearly understand the influence of the hypothalamus on the pituitary, it is necessary to understand the neural and circulatory structure essential to their interrelation. As stated earlier, each lobe of the pituitary functions as a distinct and different endocrine gland. Therefore, the structural relation of each with the hypothalamus is different. The modes of transmission of signals from the hypothalamus are through neural connections for the neurohypophysis and through a complex vascular portal system for the adenohypophysis.

### Adenohypophysis

The adenohypophysis secretes or fails to secrete its hormones into the circulation as a result of signals from the hypothalamus that arrive by the hypothalamicohypophyseal portal system. This communication system uses two capillary plexuses organized in series within the structures. Branches of the internal carotid and posterior communicating arteries of the circle of Willis give origin to the superior hypophyseal arteries. These arteries immediately branch to form a network of fenestrated capillaries called the *primary plexus,* located on the ventral side of the hypothalamus (Figure 36-6). Some capillary loops also penetrate into the median eminence, and serve the dual functions of supplying nerve cells around the base of the hypothalamus and of receiving regulating factors secreted by hypothalamic cells.

The primary plexus drains into the sinusoidal hypophyseal portal vessels that carry blood down the infundibular stalk to the anterior pituitary. After reaching the adenohypophysis, the vessels again form a capillary network called the *secondary plexus.* These vessels maintain the cells of the anterior pituitary and deliver the regulatory factors from the hypothalamus to each cell. Vessels of the secondary plexus drain into the anterior hypophyseal veins. From here, hormones ultimately are transported to their target glands. The system begins and ends in capillaries and is called the *hypothalamicohypophyseal portal system.*[9]

Anterior pituitary function is achieved through neural as well as vascular communication. The anterior pitu-

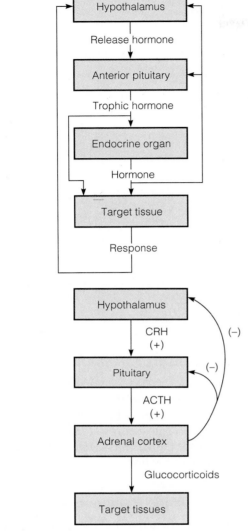

**A**

**B**

**FIGURE 36–5.**
**A.** Possible mechanism of a negative feedback system for maintaining hormone balance. **B.** Negative feedback mechanism regulating ACTH secretion. The hypothalamus secretes corticotropin releasing hormone, which stimulates release of ACTH by the pituitary. ACTH stimulates glucocorticoid secretion by the adrenal cortex. Glucocorticoids have a negative feedback on the pituitary and on the hypothalamus. Negative feedback mechanism regulating ACTH secretion. The hypothalamus secretes corticotropin releasing hormone, which stimulates release of ACTH by the pituitary. ACTH stimulates glucocorticoid secretion by the adrenal cortex. Glucocorticoids have a negative feedback on the pituitary and on the hypothalamus.

blood passes through the primary plexus, which extends into the median eminence. Significant numbers of nerve fibers terminate in the vicinity of these capillaries. These nerve fibers release neurosecretory products that are carried through the capillary sinusoids of the anterior lobe through hypophyseal portal vessels to effect release of anterior pituitary hormones.[9]

Neural signals may arise from external stimuli such as heat or cold or from internal stimuli such as emotion. Other neural stimuli that exert an influence but are as yet poorly understood include sleep-related and diurnal or circadian rhythms.

Another unique feature of the pituitary gland is that the blood-brain barrier is incomplete in the area in which the major plexus of the portal system originates. Endothelial fenestrations provide access for hormone molecules to the hypothalamus and pituitary. This allows for the feedback regulation of pituitary function described below.[3]

### Neurohypophysis

The neurohypophysis, unlike the adenohypophysis, contains no cells with secretory granules. Embryologically, the posterior pituitary arises essentially as an invagination from the hypothalamus and retains neural tract connections from this area.

Cell bodies located in the supraoptic nucleus of the hypothalamus synthesize ADH. Synthesis of oxytocin, the second hormone secreted by the posterior lobe, takes place in the paraventricular nucleus.[9]

The neurosecretory process occurs in the following sequence. Hormone biosynthesis takes place within the cell bodies of the supraoptic or paraventricular regions of the hypothalamus in the form of hormonally inactive precursors. The active hormone is thought to be cleaved from the precursors during the 1 to 2 hours in which they are transported down the axons of the neuron fibers to the posterior pituitary. By-products of this cleavage are the proteins *neurophysins.* The posterior pituitary contains two distinct neurophysins that provide specific carriers essential for the transport of ADH and oxytocin.[3] Hormones are stored in the posterior pituitary until release is triggered by the hypothalamus. Because neurosecretory cells retain their capacity to conduct electrical impulses, stimuli from the cell bodies in the hypothalamus are conducted down the axons of the neurosecretory fibers to trigger hormone release.

### FUNCTIONS OF THE ANTERIOR PITUITARY

The adenohypophysis secretes at least six hormones, four of which directly control the functioning of specific target glands—the thyroid, adrenals, and gonads. Hormones

itary, however, is poorly supplied with neural tracts from the hypothalamus. It has no secretomotor nerve fibers and only sparse vasomotor fibers.

The following is a summation of the probable mechanism through which neural transmissions take place. The unusual vascular system of the pituitary facilitates transmission of signals from the central nervous system (CNS) to the adenohypophysis. As discussed previously, before reaching secretory cells of the gland, arterial

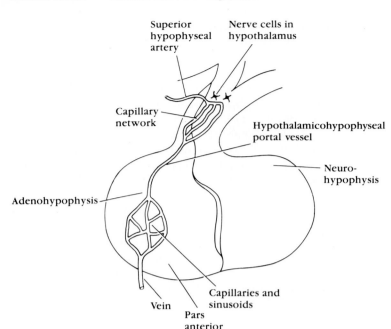

**FIGURE 36-6.**
The hypothalamicohypophyseal portal system.

that control the functioning of target glands are called *trophic* from the Greek *trophos,* meaning "to nourish," or *tropos,* meaning "to turn toward." The six peptide hormones secreted by the anterior pituitary are (1) GH, also called somatotropin; (2) ACTH, also called corticotropin; (3) TSH, also called thyrotropin; (4) FSH; (5) LH; and (6) PRL, also called lactogenic hormone (Figure 36-7) (see Table 36-1).

All anterior pituitary hormones except GH and PRL regulate the functions of other endocrine glands and are, therefore, trophic hormones. GH, ACTH, and PRL are polypeptides, whereas TSH, LH, and FSH are glycoproteins. GH stimulates the secretion of the somatomedins from the liver. These small proteins act as intermediaries in the action of GH itself.

As discussed earlier, secretion of pituitary hormones is regulated by hypothalamic release of release hormones. These include thyrotropin-releasing hormone, growth hormone—releasing hormone, corticotropin-releasing factor, and luteinizing hormone—releasing hormone, also called gonadotropin-releasing hormone. In addition, two release-inhibiting substances are liberated by the hypothalamus. These are growth hormone release-inhibiting hormone, also called somatostatin, and prolactin-inhibiting factor.

Release factors are liberated by neurosecretion, which is the release of a substance from nerve endings directly into the bloodstream. Liberated release hormones are carried to the sinuses of the anterior pituitary. Within the adenohypophysis, the release hormones act on the gland's cells to control their secretions. The mechanisms that trigger synthesis and release of the hormones include feedback as well as various other stimuli in the internal and external environments.

## Anterior Pituitary Hormonal Function

### Thyroid-Stimulating Hormone

The physiologic role of TSH is to activate synthesis and secretion of the hormones of the thyroid to maintain the size of the gland and its rate of blood flow (see Chap. 38). The pathologic problems that result from derangements in TSH secretion are the same as those of hypersecretion and hyposecretion of the thyroid hormones.

### Adrenocorticotropic Hormone

The physiologic role of ACTH is to regulate synthesis and secretion of adrenal steroids by adrenal cortical tissue. It also maintains the size and blood flow of the adrenal cortex. Excessive secretions of the cortex result in enlargement of the gland, and absence or marked diminution results in atrophy. Pathologic problems that stem from imbalance in ACTH secretion are equivalent to those caused by hypersecretion or hyposecretion of adrenal hormones (see Chap. 37).

### Follicle-Stimulating Hormone

In men, the target organs for FSH are the testes, where the hormone directly stimulates the germinal epithelium of the seminiferous tubules to activate and facilitate the rate of spermatogenesis. For optimal effects, it appears to require the concomitant presence of LH. Sometimes these hormones are used to treat infertility in both men and women.

In women, the target organs for FSH are the ovaries; FSH is essential for the normal cyclic growth of the

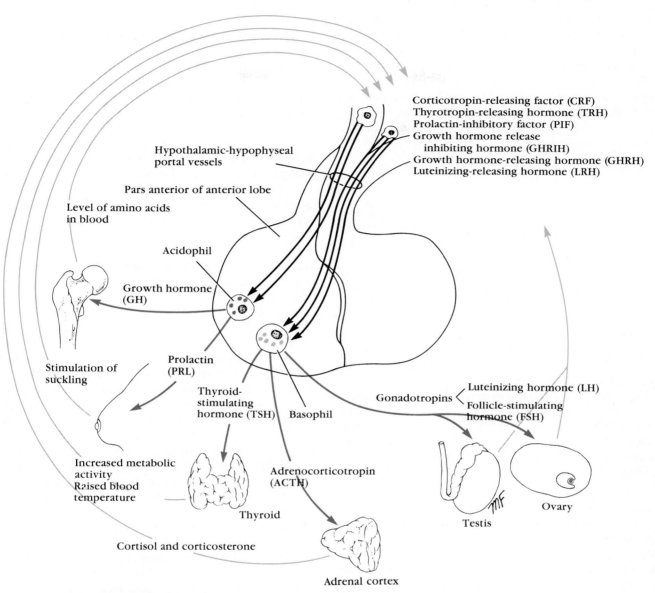

**FIGURE 36–7.**
The mechanisms involved in controlling the activities of the pars anterior of the anterior lobe of the pituitary gland. Note the important feedback mechanisms.

ovarian follicle. It is responsible for the development and growth of a large number of graafian follicles and for an increased ovarian weight.

The gonadotropins stimulate the synthesis of testosterone in men and estradiol and progesterone in women. As with other anterior lobe hormones, secretion is triggered from the hypothalamus and is mediated by feedback mechanisms. Therefore, increased circulation levels of androgens and estrogens inhibit FSH secretions (see Unit 16).[5]

### Luteinizing Hormone

Target organs for LH in men are the testes, where it stimulates the growth and secretory activity of the testicu-

lar interstitial cells (Leydig's cells). This action stimulates the synthesis and secretions of the male androgen testosterone.

The female target organs are the ovaries, where LH is essential for ovulation. Action of the hormone readies the ovarian follicle and forms the corpus luteum from the ruptured follicle. As noted previously, the presence of FSH is required to accomplish these functions.[4]

### Prolactin

The predominant physiologic roles for PRL are in breast development and lactation. The hormone acts in synergy with estrogen to promote growth and development of the female mammary glands; therefore, it is said to have a dual role in lactation. It acts with estrogen to prepare the mammary glands for lactation and then initiates secretion of the nutrients of these glands. PRL secretion increases during pregnancy, reaching a peak with delivery. The secretion is regulated by a release-inhibiting factor. Release also may be initiated by suckling. The initiation and adequacy of secretion show physiologic variations associated with sleep, stress, and other stimuli, similar to other pituitary hormones.

## Growth Hormone

GH is the only hormone secreted by the anterior pituitary that has no specific target organ. All cells of the human body may be considered target cells for this hormone.

GH, or somatotropin, is regulated by release hormones from the hypothalamus and by somatomedin, a substance synthesized in the liver. Because growth is a complex phenomenon, many other factors play a role in the rate and mode of growth. Action of GH is influenced by other hormones, such as thyroid hormone, insulin, the steroids, and androgens. It also is influenced by nutritional status, exercise, stress, diurnal variations, and sleep. Secretion of GH is suppressed by an inhibiting factor (somatostatin). GH varies from the other hormones in that it is species-specific. It has recently been synthesized from *Escherichia coli* through recombinant DNA technology. This type of GH can be used to treat deficiency.[3] Effects of GH may be summarized as follows.

*EFFECTS ON GROWTH OF BONE AND CARTILAGE.*    GH exerts an indirect rather than direct effect on the growth of bone and cartilage. It stimulates growth of these structures by promoting the synthesis of several proteins that are collectively called somatomedin. These proteins are known to be formed in the liver and probably in the muscle and kidneys also. Somatomedin acts directly on the bone and cartilage to promote growth. It is essential to the depositing of chondroid sulfate and collagen.[9] Because the formation of cartilage is accelerated and the epiphyseal plates widen, additional matrix is formed at the ends of long bones. Through this mechanism, linear structure is increased. After the epiphyses close, linear growth is no longer possible. Therefore, excessive GH after adolescence results in thickening of bones and tissues.

*EFFECTS ON PROTEIN METABOLISM.*    GH facilitates the transport of amino acids through the cell membrane. This increase in amino acid concentrations in the cells is thought to be partially responsible for increased protein synthesis. It also is believed to exert a direct effect on ribosomes to make them produce greater numbers of protein molecules.[9] As a result of these mechanisms, it creates a positive nitrogen and phosphorous balance and is, therefore, an anabolic protein hormone.

*EFFECTS ON RNA FORMATION.*    GH stimulates the transcription process in the nucleus, causing increased formation of RNA. This, in turn, promotes growth by promoting protein synthesis.

*DECREASED CATABOLISM OF PROTEIN.*    In addition to an increase in protein synthesis, a decrease in the breakdown of cell proteins occurs. The reduction is believed to result from GH's ability to mobilize free fatty acids from adipose tissue to supply energy. This response acts as a protein-sparer as well as a carbohydrate-sparer.[9]

*EFFECTS ON ELECTROLYTE BALANCE.*    GH increases gastrointestinal absorption of calcium and reduces sodium and potassium excretion.[4]

*EFFECTS ON FAT AND GLUCOSE METABOLISM.*    GH exerts a strong influence in stimulating fat catabolism in adipose tissue. This action results in the production of large amounts of acetylcoenzyme A, which acts as a ready source of energy and has the effect of reducing the use of glucose for energy (glucose-sparing). In the presence of excessive quantities of GH, several potential problems may develop from this action. The response may result in increased ketone levels in the blood (ketogenic effect) or in increased concentration of liver lipids (fatty liver). The glucose-sparing effect of fat catabolism results in storage of increased amounts of glucose in the cells as glycogen. When cellular capacity becomes saturated, circulating blood levels of glucose are elevated (diabetogenic effect), resulting in increased demand for insulin. If this effect persists long enough, the beta cells of the islets of Langerhans are exhausted and diabetes mellitus results.[5] GH is not the only anterior pituitary hormone that increases blood glucose levels, however; ACTH, TSH, and PRL all have this capacity.

Two additional facts seem important to the understanding of GH. First, GH fails to cause growth if carbohydrate is lacking. Second, secretion of GH is increased during episodes of hypoglycemia *except* those that occur in adult hypopituitarism.

All of this information indicates that GH has many functions other than those of stimulating and supporting growth in the developing child. Although secretion and the subsequent physiologic effects are most pronounced during the early developing years, secretion and release are essential to many bodily functions throughout life.

## Circadian Patterns of Anterior Pituitary Secretions

The secretions of the pituitary are cyclic, and can be demonstrated on a regular rhythmical basis called *circadian* or *diurnal rhythm*. Secretion of GH and PRL is greatest in the early hours of sleep; ACTH regulates cortisol secretion, reaching maximum between 2 AM and 4 PM, causing peak levels at about 8 AM; TSH reaches a maximum level between 8 PM and midnight. Loss of diurnal rhythm can be an early diagnostic feature of hypothalamic or pituitary dysfunction. Measurement of hormone levels and supplemental replacement should be governed by the susceptibility of the pituitary at different times.[4,16]

## FUNCTIONS OF THE NEUROHYPOPHYSIS

Unlike the adenohypophysis, the neurohypophysis does not function as an endocrine gland. Posterior pituitary hormones are synthesized in the hypothalamus and stored in the posterior lobe to await the signal from the hypothalamus for release.

Cell bodies located in the supraoptic nuclei of the hypothalamus are considered to be largely responsible for synthesis of ADH, whereas cell bodies located in the paraventricular nuclei synthesize oxytocin. It is recognized, however, that both supraoptic and paraventricular nuclear cell bodies synthesize some amount of both of the hormones secreted by the neurohypophysis (Figure 36-8).

Synthesis and secretion of posterior lobe hormones takes place in a two-step process.[16] In the first step, a hormonally inactive precursor is synthesized in the specified cells of the hypothalamus. This precursor is transported by way of secretory granules down the neuron fibers of the hypothalamicohypophyseal tract. The actual hormone is believed to be separated from the precursor during the period in which the granules traverse the axons of this tract to reach the posterior lobe. Hormones are then stored in the posterior pituitary until appropriate stimulus for secretion is initiated by the hypothalamus. Be-

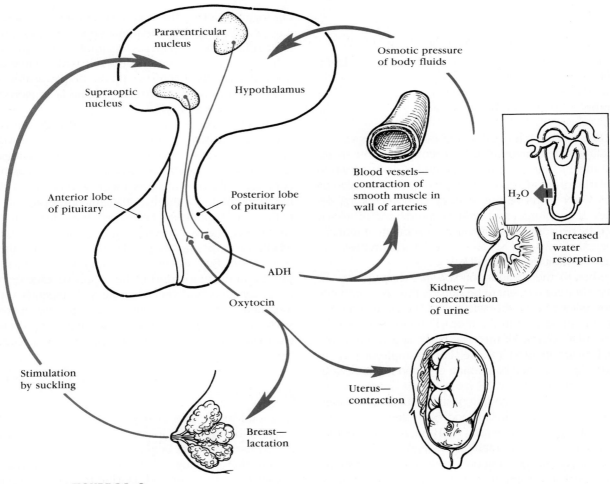

**FIGURE 36–8.**
Schematic drawing of the mechanisms involved in controlling the activities of the posterior lobe of the pituitary gland.

cause neurosecretory cells and fibers also have the capacity to conduct electrical impulses, action potentials initiated by stimulus to cell bodies of the hypothalamus are conducted down the axons of the neuron fibers to stimulate release of the hormones.

## Physiologic Action of ADH

The kidneys are the specific target organs of ADH. In the presence of ADH, the distal tubules and collecting ducts of the nephrons become more permeable to water, causing increased water reabsorption. This results in decreased concentration (osmotic pressure) of the extracellular fluid (plasma). In the absence of ADH, tubules and collecting ducts of the nephrons are almost impermeable, and little or no water is reabsorbed.[9]

In addition, ADH has a vasopressor effect when administered in large doses and may cause hypertension. The effect is caused by direct action of ADH on smooth muscles in the vascular wall. It may improve systemic fluid volume by reducing the size of the vascular bed.

## Regulation of ADH by the Hypothalamus

Increased osmolarity of plasma and decreased circulating vascular volume are the major physiologic stimuli for initiating ADH secretion. Both osmoreceptors and volume receptors influence the hypothalamus to initiate the signal for release of ADH.[9]

*Osmoreceptors* located in the hypothalamus consist of small vesicles surrounded by a semipermeable membrane in which nerve endings are embedded. Increased osmolarity of plasma in the vicinity of the hypothalamus causes water to move out of these osmoreceptors, decreases their volume, and reduces the degree of stretch sensed by neurons. This response presumably stimulates the hypothalamus and initiates the electrical impulse that signals for pituitary release of ADH.

Although the location of *volume receptors* is unknown, they are thought to be outside the CNS, probably predominantly in the thoracic cavity. The circulating vascular volume sensed in the thoracic region, rather than the vascular volume of the total body, apparently is the crucial factor in ADH release. For example, a shift in blood volume, caused by pooling of blood in the periphery, is accompanied by ADH release, as is change from a supine to a sitting or standing position. Exposure to high temperatures, which shifts blood from deeper to more superficial regions, increases ADH secretion, whereas exposure to cold temperatures, which shifts blood from superficial to deeper regions, reduces its secretions. Positive-pressure respiration, which decreases blood volume in the great veins of the thorax, also results in ADH release.

## Other Factors That Regulate ADH Secretion and Release

As previously noted, feedback mechanisms protect blood osmolarity and volume balance through influence on ADH secretion. When all factors are in balance, uniform secretion of ADH maintains the fluid balance. When body fluids are depleted or osmotic pressure rises, appropriate mechanisms are activated and ADH is released. This stimulates the kidneys to reabsorb more water, which restores blood volume or reduces osmotic pressure, and balance is achieved. The state of balance inhibits release of ADH until further need arises (see Figure 36-8).

Other factors that may influence ADH secretion include trauma, pain, anxiety, and drugs such as nicotine, morphine, and tranquilizers. Alcohol inhibits secretion, which partially accounts for the diuresis associated with excess intake of alcohol.

## Oxytocin

### Effects on the Uterus

Oxytocin stimulates the contraction of smooth muscle in a number of organs in the human body. A major physiologic role of this hormone is to stimulate smooth-muscle cells in the pregnant uterus. It is released in large quantities during the expulsive phase of parturition. The mechanism by which oxytocin release is triggered has been described as follows.

When labor begins, the tissues of the uterine cervix and vagina distend and become stretched. This stretch reflex initiates afferent impulses to the hypothalamus and stimulates the synthesis of oxytocin in cell bodies of the paraventricular nucleus. Oxytocin then migrates down the nerve fibers of the hypothalamicohypophyseal stalk to the neurohypophysis. From there it is released into the circulation and is carried by the blood to the uterus, where it acts on smooth-muscle cells to reinforce uterine contraction. Because greatest amounts of oxytocin are present in the blood during the expulsive stage of labor, it appears that the quantity released depends on the forcefulness of uterine contractions and the degree of stretch of cervical and vaginal tissues. It is recognized that oxytocin may be one of the factors that precipitate labor.[16]

### Effects on Lactation

A second major role of oxytocin is to eject milk from lactating breasts. Milk formed by cells of the breasts is stored until suckling begins. For about 30 seconds to 1 minute after suckling is initiated, no milk is ejected. This is called the latent period. During this period, suckling stimuli to the nipple initiate signals that are transmitted to neuron cell bodies in the paraventricular and supraoptic nuclei to initiate posterior pituitary release of oxytocin. Circulating blood transports oxytocin to the breasts, where it initiates contraction of myoepithelial cells to force milk out of the alveoli into the ducts and lacteal sinuses opening to the nipple.[9] Because epinephrine inhibits oxytocin secretion, emotion, anxiety, and pain can inhibit oxytocin release and, thus, lactation.

### Effects on Fertilization

In lower animals, distention and stretch of vaginal and cervical tissues during copulation increases the secretion of oxytocin. Uterine contractions experienced during orgasm have been attributed in part to this increased secretion. It also has been postulated that oxytocin facilitates fertilization by causing the uterus to propel semen upward through the fallopian tubes. It is unknown if this process occurs in the human female.[9]

## INTRODUCTION TO PITUITARY PATHOLOGY

Malfunctions of the pituitary gland result from one or more of the following: (1) invasive or impinging tumors of the pituitary or hypothalamus; (2) vascular infarction within the gland; (3) mechanical damage from trauma or surgery; (4) inflammatory processes; (5) genetic or familial predisposition; (6) developmental and structural anomalies of the gland itself; (7) feedback from prolonged malfunction of one or more of its target glands; (8) autoimmune responses; and (9) idiopathic origin.[2–4]

Symptoms of pituitary malfunction may be precipitated by changes in hormonal balance or by purely mechanical forces. For example, tumors of the pituitary cause malfunction because of pressure from their space-occupying properties, destruction of tissue, and contributions to hypersecretion as a result of tumor cell secretory capacity. More advanced or larger lesions may impinge on surrounding tissues, such as the optic chiasma or the area of the third ventricle, producing visual disorders, headaches, or other neurologic changes.[4] Vascular and tumor infarctions, structural and developmental anomalies or inflammatory processes, and autoimmune responses influence functioning by compromising or destroying tissue. Feedback from malfunction of a target gland can result in hyperplasia of the pituitary gland.

Because the pituitary is a crucial link in the production of several hormones, abnormalities of the gland often alter normal hormone secretion. Pressure or tissue destruction may compromise function and result in problems associated with hyposecretion. Conversely, because many tumors of the pituitary secrete hormones, the presence of these lesions may result in symptoms stemming from hypersecretion.

Factors that influence hormone secretions of the pituitary inevitably influence functions of the specific endocrine gland, depending on the hormone. For example, conditions that stimulate hyperfunctioning of the pituitary initiate excessive activation of the target organs, whereas suppression or destruction of pituitary tissue with loss of hormone secretions results in hypofunction of target organs.

For convenience, pituitary pathology may be categorized as disorders of the adenohypophysis or the neurohypophysis. They may be subdivided further as disorders of hyperfunctioning or hypofunctioning. Because the anterior and posterior lobes of the pituitary operate as distinct and separate functional units, malfunctions of each differ characteristically.

## PATHOLOGY OF THE ANTERIOR PITUITARY

Four types of anterior pituitary disorders usually are described: (1) enlargement of the sella turcica with or without evidence of a space-occupying lesion, (2) visual disorders, (3) hypopituitary hormone secretion, and (4) hyperpituitary hormone secretion.[3] Hormone deficiencies resulting in malfunction may be classified as primary, secondary, or tertiary: Primary deficiencies are the result of disease of the target gland; secondary deficiencies result from pituitary lesions or disorders; tertiary deficiencies result from hypothalamic disorders.[3]

Evaluation of persons with pituitary diseases may include physical examination and radiologic, neuroophthalmic, and endocrine diagnostic studies. The types of tests used and the extent of testing depend on the symptoms. Radiologic studies include plain skull films, computed tomographic scans, pneumoencephalography, and arteriography. Neuroophthalmic evaluation is done by formal visual field examination using tangent screening. Endocrine studies include plasma levels and urinary excretion levels of each of the pituitary and target gland hormones. Radioimmunoassay is an important advance in diagnosing endocrine problems, using antibodies that are specific for certain chemical groups. The accuracy of assay results depends on the specificity of the antibody and its ability to bind the hormone.[1] Other assays include protein binding and radioreceptor assays that use proteins to bind to the hormones.

Chemical assays and free hormone levels are other methods of determining certain hormone concentrations. Free hormone can be assessed directly or by measuring bound hormone and calculating the free level. Plasma or urinary levels indicate marked excess or deficiency. To evaluate the results, the normal circadian pattern, stress reaction, and other factors must be taken into consideration. Urine measurements are much more effective for steroid hormones than for protein-derived hormones because the metabolites of the former are excreted in urine. Dynamic testing assesses the ability of the gland to respond to stimulation. Hormones that stimulate a response may be administered, or suppressive drugs or substances may be given. Many other tests provide indirect information, including levels of blood sugar, serum calcium, and serum potassium.[1]

## Enlargement of the Sella Turcica

An increase in the size of the sella turcica often results from erosion of this structure caused by pressure from lesions in the pituitary region. Enlargement may be caused by pituitary adenomas, craniopharyngiomas, meningiomas, epithelial cysts, granulomas, malignant tumors of primary origin, or metastasis from carcinoma of the breast. Enlargement may result from nontumorous enlargement of the sella, called *empty sella syndrome*. Sella enlargement also may result from primary hypothyroidism or hypogonadism, which may be attributed to hyperplasia of the thyrotropes or gonadotropes, as it is accompanied by elevated thyrotropin or gonadotropin levels.[3] This is most frequent in children.

Endocrine evaluation for an enlarged sella turcica should include assessment of thyroid and adrenal hormone levels together with basal gonadotropin levels. Basal PRL levels are important, since more than one-half of pituitary tumors secrete PRL.

### Empty Sella Syndrome

The empty sella syndrome is classified as primary or secondary, according to its underlying cause. Primary, or idiopathic, sella syndrome results from an abnormally large opening through which the hypophyseal stalk passes. This often is a developmental defect. With increased intracranial pressure, the arachnoid membrane tends to herniate through the opening, creating a sac filled with cerebrospinal fluid. This compresses the pituitary gland against the wall of the sella turcica, creating the appearance of an empty sella (Figure 36-9). The condition also may occur as a consequence of necrosis of a pituitary adenoma or of Sheehan's syndrome, which are discussed on page 697. Empty sella can develop secondary to spontaneous infarctions or regression of a tumor. The secondary variant of the syndrome results from ablation of the gland by irradiation or surgery.

Radiographically, the sella may appear enlarged or normal in size. The primary disease seldom is manifested as pituitary hypofunction. When hypofunction occurs, it usually is evidenced by depressed GH and gonadotropin secretion.

About 90% of persons with primary sella syndrome are female. It most often is asymptomatic.[11] It is diagnosed most often in obese, hypertensive, middle-aged women who have borne many children. The tendency for

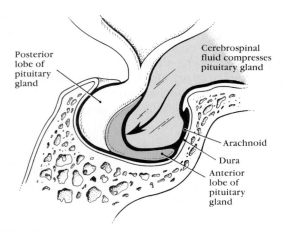

**FIGURE 36–9.**
Empty sella syndrome.

the pituitary to enlarge during pregnancy and regress afterward may be the basis of pathogenesis. Headache is a common symptom. Visual field defects are rare but do occur in persons who have infarction of a pituitary tumor with subsequent development of empty sella or when the optic chiasma prolapses into the sella.

## Hypopituitarism

Hypopituitarism (panhypopituitarism) may be initiated by extremely low secretion of hypophyseal hormone, or by pituitary or hypothalamic disease.[17] Panhypopituitarism refers to the failure of all cell types in the pituitary gland. Surgical hypophysectomy (removal of the pituitary) causes dramatic clinical features of both anterior and posterior hormone deficiency.[5] The most common processes are Sheehan's pituitary necrosis, nonsecreting adenomas, and craniopharyngioma.[18] Other causes include cysts, inflammation of the pituitary as a result of diabetes, meningitis, sarcoidosis, tuberculosis, syphilis, metastatic cancer, and granulomas that may be nonspecific. Anterior pituitary hormone deficit may occur singly or in various combinations of several deficits. The speed of onset and extent of hormone deficiency depend on the nature and size of the precipitating cause. Onset may be acute and life-threatening, as in acute adrenocortical insufficiency. More often, however, onset is slow, and may occur over a period of months or years. Clinical signs and symptoms seldom manifest until at least 75% of the anterior lobe is destroyed.[2]

In adults, the clinical features of panhypopituitarism may include absence of axillary and pubic hair, genital and breast atrophy, skin pallor, pallor of nipples, fine skin wrinkling (especially of the face), intolerance to cold, premature aging, poor muscle development, amenorrhea in premenopausal women, loss of previously normal libido and potency in men, and several endocrine deficiencies. Shortness of stature may be evident if onset occurs before puberty. If hypothyroidism is marked, overweight is common. Reduced visual acuity, optic atrophy, and hemianopsia may occur if there is suprasellar expansion of a lesion or mass.

Diagnosis is made on the basis of history and physical examination, neuroophthalmic examination, and plasma immunoassay. Treatment consists of hormone replacement to reestablish function. Thyroid replacement, cortisone, or hydrocortisone may be used as indicated. In women, diethylstilbestrol or preparations of conjugated estrogens (Premarin) help to maintain secondary sex characteristics, while androgens or testosterone can restore libido and potency in men.

## Deficiency of Single Anterior Pituitary Hormones

### Prolactin Deficiency

Postpartum failure to lactate is the only symptom of clinical significance in deficient PRL secretion. This condition has classically been associated with the postpartum pituitary necrosis that results from hemorrhage and shock during delivery (Sheehan's syndrome).

### Gonadotropin Deficiency

As previously stated, hypogonadism is the most common pituitary deficiency among adults. Its occurrence in the premenopausal woman is manifested by amenorrhea, atrophy of the breasts and uterus, and cornification of the vaginal orifice. A man experiences testicular atrophy associated with decreases in libido, potency, beard growth, and muscle tone. When onset of the deficiency occurs before puberty, the manifestations include eunuchoid appearance, lack of development of secondary sex characteristics, and infertility. Men fail to develop facial hair, an adult male voice, and normal genitalia. Women fail to manifest normal breast development and onset of menses. Both sexes may exhibit absence of axillary and pubic hair. The most common tumors responsible for the syndrome are the craniopharyngioma and chromophobe adenoma.[3,5]

Fröhlich's syndrome is a severe gonadotropin deficiency that usually affects prepubertal boys. It includes obesity and hypogonadism associated with diabetes insipidus, retardation, and visual problems, all of which are related to hypothalamic rather than pituitary dysfunction. The obesity is probably the result of hypothalamic-induced overeating.[15]

### Thyrotropin Deficiency

Hypothalamic or pituitary hypothyroidism exhibits some symptoms in common with primary hypothyroidism but usually is less severe. Isolated TSH deficiency is rare, however, and symptoms of other anterior lobe hormone deficiency usually are present concomitantly. This factor distinguishes pituitary from primary hypothyroidism. In pituitary hypothyroidism, fine wrinkling of the skin and loss of secondary sex characteristics, which are related to gonadal insufficiency, are distinguishing characteristics. Menstrual history is significant, since menorrhagia is common in primary hypothyroidism, whereas amenorrhea is expected in the pituitary form.[4]

### ACTH Deficiency

Deficiency of ACTH is the most serious of the endocrine deficiencies in persons with pituitary disease.[4] Like pituitary hypothyroidism, ACTH deficiency usually is associated with deficiency of other pituitary hormones; this can be a characteristic that distinguishes pituitary origin from adrenal origin of disease. Symptoms include poor response to stress, nausea, vomiting, hyperthermia, and collapse. Decreased skin and nipple pigmentation is exhibited, which also distinguishes pituitary hypoadrenalism from primary adrenal disease (see Chap. 37).

### GH Deficiency

GH deficiency results from pituitary insufficiency of GH that affects children in the formative years. It is caused by a suprasellar cyst or craniopharyngioma, resulting in hypothalamic or pituitary hypofunction. Genetic transmission of GH deficiency accounts for about 10% of pituitary dwarfism, and results from an autosomal recessive trait.[4] It often is associated with evidence of sella turcica destruction seen radiographically. It also can be caused by ischemic necrosis and inflammatory changes.

Deficiency of GH is considered in children whose proportional short stature (below the third percentile) is far below that of their normal counterparts (Figure 36-10).[4] Other characteristics include delayed sexual development associated with bright rather than dull mentality. Most children with this condition exhibit excess subcutaneous fat, poorly developed muscles, thin hair, and underdeveloped nails. In some cases, an appearance of premature aging is evident, with dry, wrinkled skin.

The characteristics of anatomic symmetry without gross deformity and normal mentality distinguish the person with GH deficiency from one with *cretinism* resulting from thyroid deficiency.[2]

### Sheehan's Syndrome

Sheehan's syndrome, or postpartum pituitary necrosis, was first described as pituitary necrosis occurring postpartally after a delivery complicated by hemorrhage and shock. In the course of pregnancy, the pituitary gland en-

Inches

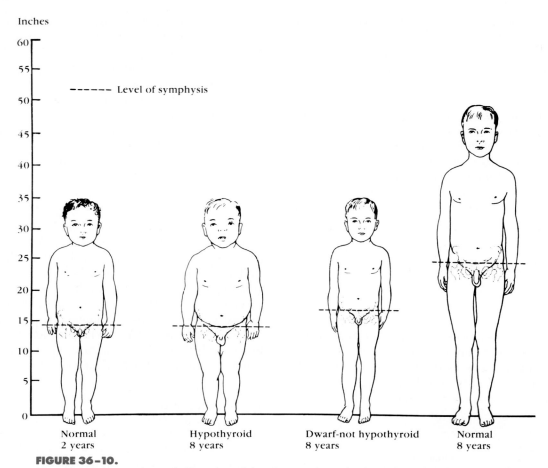

**FIGURE 36-10.**
Normal and abnormal growth. Hypothyroid dwarfs retain their infantile proportions, whereas dwarfs of the constitutional type and, to a lesser extent, the hypopituitary type have proportions characteristic of their chronologic age. (From L. Wilkins, *The Diagnosis and Treatment of Endocrine Disorders in Childhood and Adolescence* (3rd ed.). Springfield, Ill.: C. C. Thomas, 1966.)

larges and develops increased circulation. In the event of acute blood loss, which sometimes accompanies labor and delivery, sudden systematic hypotension can precipitate ischemia and destruction of the anterior lobe.[2] The result is hypofunction of the gland. There may be a lag of months or years between the intrapartum incident and full development of symptoms. Characteristic symptoms are common to a variety of pathologic processes that destroy a significant proportion of pituitary function. Therefore, the syndrome may be produced by any destructive lesion of the pituitary.

Symptoms depend on the degree of impairment of pituitary function relative to the extent of tissue destruction. These initially include evidence of increased intracranial pressure, headache, visual deficits, stiff neck, papilledema, and convulsions, later followed by symptoms of hormone deficiency, including gonadal, thyroidal, and adrenal effects.[3]

Table 36-4 depicts the causes of hypopituitarism. Evaluation and diagnosis are by physical examination, neuroophthalmic evaluation, and measurement of baseline hormone levels.

## Hyperpituitarism

Pituitary hypersecretion normally involves overproduction of only a single hormone except in certain hormone-secreting tumors.[4] It often is due to a decreased feedback signal when there is hypofunction of a target gland. The pituitary responds to the decreased hormone level by increasing stimulating hormone production. Pituitary adenomas also may secrete primarily one type of hormone. These almost exclusively involve the somatotropic (GH), lactotropic (PRL), or corticotropic (ACTH) cells.[4]

### Hyperprolactinemia

Women with PRL-secreting adenomas may exhibit galactorrhea, amenorrhea, or depressed libido. Some exhibit

## TABLE 36-4.
PITUITARY LESIONS CAUSING HYPOPITUITARISM

**Tumors**

Pituitary adenoma
Craniopharyngioma
Metastatic carcinoma
Primary pituitary carcinoma
Meningioma

**Pituitary Infarction**

Pituitary apoplexy (pituitary tumor)
Postpartum pituitary necrosis (Sheehan's syndrome)
Diabetes mellitus
Shock
Sickle cell anemia (crisis)
Infections (malaria, epidemic hemorrhagic fever)
Cavernous sinus thrombosis
Vasculitis (temporal arteritis, Takayasu's arteritis)
Trauma (stalk section or sella fracture)

**Infiltrative Diseases**

Sarcoidosis
Tuberculosis
Leukemia
Lymphoma
Hemochromatosis
Autoimmune hypophysitis

**Miscellaneous**

Hypophysectomy
Radiation necrosis
Carotid artery aneurysm
Pituitary abscess
Congenital anomalies (hypoplasia, aplasia)

*Source: W.N. Kelley, Textbook of Internal Medicine. Philadelphia: J.B. Lippincott, 1989.*

evidence of decreased estrogens and hirsutism (excessive hair growth in inappropriate places), which are believed to be the result of depression of ovarian function or stimulation of adrenal androgen function. Men with PRL-secreting adenomas do not exhibit galactorrhea because of lack of development of acini in the male breasts. These lesions in men usually occur only as space-occupying lesions with hypogonadism. The hypogonadism apparently occurs because of a defect in endogenous gonadotropin-releasing hormone.[5] Diagnosis and evaluation are by radiologic studies and studies of basal PRL level.

## Hypersecretion of ACTH

Excess secretion of ACTH by the pituitary gland results in *Cushing's disease*. Excess ACTH stimulates excess cortisol, which alters the distribution of fat, blood glucose, and many other conditions. When the excess cortisol is due to adrenal overproduction, the condition is called *Cushing's syndrome*. Manifestations of Cushing's syndrome are detailed in Chap. 37. Cushing's disease of pituitary origin is most frequently due to a basophil ACTH-secreting adenoma of the gland. Excess ACTH causes hyperplasia and hyperfunction of the adrenal cortex.

## Hypersecretion of GH

Hypersecretion of GH that occurs before puberty results in gigantism. This pituitary abnormality has been defined as height exceeding 80 inches in adults or exceeding three standard deviations above the mean for age in children. The disorder is the result of oversecretion of GH by a pituitary adenoma in a growing child before closure of the epiphyses. Before epiphyseal closure, growth is linear and symmetric. Hypogonadism often is associated and leads to delayed epiphyseal closure and a more prolonged growth period.[5]

Clinical features of gigantism include symmetric growth of stature to enormous proportions, sometimes reaching 8 to 9 ft in height (Figure 36-11). Growth is symmetric because both epiphyseal and oppositional bone growth occur concurrently. Affected people also may develop the distortions that are characteristic of acromegaly. Cardiac hypertrophy often is associated with mild hypertension that eventually may lead to cardiac failure.[5] Thyroid enlargement and adrenocortical hyperplasia occasionally occur. Early in the course of the disease, people with gigantism may be unusually strong, but osteoporosis and muscle weakness are characteristic in later stages.[3,5]

Acromegaly occurs when GH-secreting tumors of the pituitary develop after puberty and after fusion of the epiphyses. After epiphyseal closure, linear growth of bones is no longer possible. Tissues thicken and growth takes place in the acral areas (hands, feet, nose, and mandible).[3] The clinical signs and symptoms associated with acromegaly result from (1) the local effects produced by tumor growth on other pituitary hormones, producing hypopituitarism; (2) the effects of tumor growth on extrasellar CNS structures; and (3) the effects of hypersecretion of GH.[13,14]

Somatotropic adenomas are predominantly responsible for these tumors. Growth of the tumor ultimately may destroy normal cells. As a consequence, hypopituitarism may develop as the disease progresses. Both sexes are affected equally, and the condition most often is detected in the third or fourth decade of life. The disease progresses slowly and insidiously and often goes undetected for years. Affected persons may first notice progressive increase in ring, shoe, hat, and glove sizes. The skull and head increase in size, and the fingers and hands become broad and spadelike. Increased growth of subcutaneous connective tissue of the face leads to coarsen-

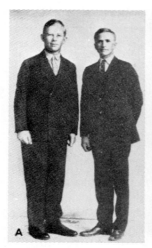
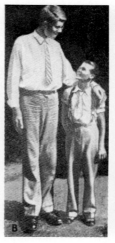
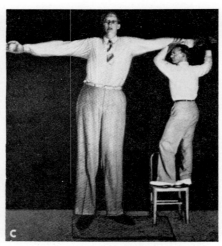

**FIGURE 36–11.**

One of the most notable examples of growth hormone excess in the human was Robert Wadlow, later known as the "Alton Giant." Although he weighed only 9 lb at birth, he soon began to grown excessively, and by 6 months of age weighed 30 lb. At 1 year, he had reached a weight of 62 lb. Growth continued through his life. Shortly before his death, at age 22, from cellulitis of the feet, he was 8 ft 11 in tall and weighed 475 lb, according to the careful measurements of Dr. C. M. Charles. **A.** Age 9 years: height 6 ft 1 in (shown with his father). **B.** Age 13 years: height 7 ft 2 in (shown with a friend of the same age). **C.** Age 20 years: height 8 ft 6 in, weight 430 lb. (**A** and **B**, from F. Fadner, *Biography of Robert Wadlow*, 1944. Courtesy of Bruce Humphries, Publishers. **C**, Courtesy of Drs. C. M. Charles and C. M. MacBryde.)

ing of the features (Figure 36-12). The face assumes a thick, fleshy appearance. The lips are thickened and enlarged, and have accentuated skin folds. The ears and nose become enlarged because of hypertrophy of the cartilages. There is overgrowth of the supraorbital ridge and the cheeks become prominent. Overgrowth of the maxilla results in lengthening of the face, and alveolar bone growth results in separations of the teeth. Overgrowth of the mandible results in prognathism (jaw projection). Hypertrophy of the costal cartilage leads to an increased circumference of the chest. Absorption of bone is rapid and osteoporosis occurs. Acromegalic arthritis develops from proliferation of joint cartilage, and affects joints of the long bones and the spine. Long bones thicken and become massive. There often is bowing of the legs. The skin becomes thickened, and hirsutism occurs in females. The tongue enlarges and may protrude from the mouth. The lungs, liver, spleen, kidneys, and intestines enlarge twofold to fivefold. Hypertension, coronary artery atherosclerosis, and marked cardiomegaly occur. Congestive heart failure often develops. The gonads enlarge but their function is subnormal. The adrenals, thyroid, and parathyroid become enlarged.[3]

The typical physical picture is one of a big, burly person with forward carriage of the head, prognathism, kyphosis, bowlegs, prominent forehead, thickened chest, and husky, cavernous voice. Many men develop impotence and women develop amenorrhea. Growth of the adenoma apparently impinges on the normal cells and induces insufficiency of other hormones.

Diagnosis is by assessment of physical characteristics, serial radiographs, and photographs. Laboratory immunoassay of plasma GH levels and response to glucose stimulation during a glucose tolerance test can help in diagnosis. People normally suppress GH after ingestion of 100 g of glucose, but the acromegalic may show increased levels.[13]

## PATHOLOGY OF THE POSTERIOR PITUITARY

Pathologic conditions stemming from lesions of the neurohypophysis are rare. Posterior lobe pathology is almost always related to primary disease or other processes outside the gland itself. The posterior lobe releases two hormones, ADH and oxytocin, which are synthesized and secreted by the hypothalamus.

## ADH Deficiency

A deficiency in ADH release causes the condition known as *diabetes insipidus.* The underlying causes of ADH deficiency have been categorized as follows: (1) neoplastic or inflammatory processes that impinge on the hypothalamoneurohypophyseal axis, such as adenomas, metastatic carcinoma, abscesses, meningitis, tuberculosis, and sarcoidosis; (2) surgical or irradiation injury to the hy-

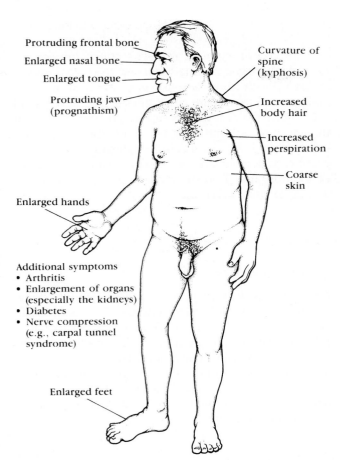

**FIGURE 36–12.**
Composite of all symptoms of acromegaly. (From M. Beyers and S. Dudas (eds.), *The Clinical Practice of Medical Surgical Nursing* [2nd ed.]. Boston: Little, Brown, 1984.)

Protruding frontal bone

Enlarged nasal bone

Enlarged tongue

Protruding jaw (prognathism)

Enlarged hands

Additional symptoms
• Arthritis
• Enlargement of organs (especially the kidneys)
• Diabetes
• Nerve compression (e.g., carpal tunnel syndrome)

Enlarged feet

Curvature of spine (kyphosis)

Increased body hair

Increased perspiration

Coarse skin

pothalamoneurohypophyseal axis, such as hypophysectomy; (3) severe head injuries; and (4) idiopathic influences. Rarely, the syndrome is familial, and inherited as a mendelian dominant.[2,18]

Lack of ADH causes a failure of the distal and collecting ducts of the nephrons to reabsorb water. Water is lost through a dilute, low osmolality urine despite hyperosmolality in the serum and extracellular fluid.[6] The resulting clinical features of diabetes insipidus include polyuria, excessive thirst, and polydipsia. Polyuria causes a rise in serum osmolarity that stimulates the thirst center. Normal function of the thirst center ensures that polydipsia will replace water lost through polyuria.[18] Symptoms usually are sudden in onset and pronounced, with urine output reaching 10 or more liters in a 24-hour period. Urine is pale, and its concentration is very dilute.

Diagnosis is on the basis of clinical manifestations, dehydration tests, and response to vasopressin administration. Treatment is administration of ADH (vasopressin), usually by nasal spray.

## Syndrome of Inappropriate ADH Secretion

The syndrome of inappropriate ADH secretion (SIADH) is the persistent release of ADH unrelated to plasma osmolarity or volume deficit. The normal feedback inhibition of the posterior pituitary is hypoactive or inactive, causing continued release of ADH. The result is excessive reabsorption of water in the renal system and excessive retention of water with expansion of fluid volume. Fluid overload, hyponatremia, and hemodilution result.

The syndrome may occur from a stimulus either inside the hypothalamicohypophyseal system or from an outside source (Box 36-1). It may occur as a result of a

**BOX 36–1.**
## CAUSES OF SIADH

Cancer
  Oat cell carcinoma of lung
  Carcinoma of pancreas
  Lymphosarcoma, reticulum cell sarcoma, Hodgkin's disease
  Carcinoma of duodenum
  Thymoma
Nonmalignant pulmonary disease
  Tuberculosis
  Lung abscess
  Pneumonia
Central nervous system disorders
  Skull fracture
  Subdural hematoma
  Subarachnoid hemorrhage
  Cerebrovascular thrombosis
  Cerebral atrophy
  Acute encephalitis
  Tuberculous meningitis
  Purulent meningitis
  Guillain-Barré syndrome
  Lupus erythematosus
  Acute intermittent porphyria
  Physical or emotional stress
  Pain
Drugs
  Chlorpropamide
  Vincristine
  Cyclophosphamide
  Carbamazepine
  Oxytocin
  General anesthetics
  Narcotics
  Barbiturates
  Thiazide antidepressants
  Tricyclic antidepressants
Miscellaneous
  Hypothyroidism
  Positive-pressure respiration

Source: *Reproduced with permission from E. Braunwald et al., Harrison's Principles of Internal Medicine (11th ed.). Copyright ©1987. McGraw-Hill Book Company.*

tumor of the hypothalamus or hypophysis that impinges on tissues that control secretions. SIADH also may result from a paraneoplastic syndrome in which nonendocrine tumors demonstrate inappropriate secretion of ADH.[10] Oat cell bronchogenic carcinoma is the most common ADH-secreting lesion causing SIADH. Other conditions capable of this ectopic secretion include carcinoma of the pancreas, lymphoma, bronchogenic tuberculosis, Hodgkin's disease, and thymoma. Disorders and trauma of the CNS, such as subdural hematoma and infection, may be the basis of malfunction. Conditions such as stress, pain, and hypovolemia may cause the physiologic release of ADH in the absence of a hypertonic plasma.[18] Diagnosis is made on the basis of serum sodium levels and the clinical picture of hypervolemia. It should be suspected in any person with hyponatremia who has hypertonic urine.

Management includes fluid restriction, diuretics, assessment of sodium balance, assessment for evidence of congestive heart failure, and treatment for the underlying cause of the syndrome. No drugs are available that effectively suppress ADH.

## TUMORS OF THE PITUITARY

### Adenomas

More than 90% of all pituitary neoplasms are adenomas. Pituitary tumors account for 6% to 18% of all brain tumors, only 10% to 20% of which are nonfunctioning.[5] Pituitary adenomas may be classified according to predominant cell type. They also may be classified according to their secretory qualities. They may interfere with pituitary functions by virtue of their space-occupying properties or by secretions of various hormones. In general, problems stemming from the space-occupying factor are the result of destruction or suppression of surrounding tissue. Those stemming from secretory properties result in hypersecretion or hyperfunction. All lesions may produce CNS symptoms or visual problems because of their space-occupying properties, depending on the size and location of the lesion.

The growth pattern of adenomas is variable and unrelated to hormone secretion. The tumors often become apparent clinically because of their compressive effect or impingement on adjoining structures. Pituitary adenomas are almost always benign but may exhibit aggressive growth so that surgical removal is impossible.[5]

Pituitary adenomas may cause neurologic or endocrinologic clinical signs and symptoms, including visual or neurologic deficits, headaches, or impaired gonadal function. The tumors may be discovered accidentally on review of skull films.[5] Growth disturbances such as acromegaly or gigantism may be the major sign of a GH-secreting adenoma. PRL-secreting hormones cause gonadal dysfunction, and ACTH-secreting adenomas may produce Cushing's disease.

*Craniopharyngiomas (Rathke's pouch tumors)* are tumors of congenital origin derived from remnants of Rathke's pouch. These lesions commonly occur in young children and usually are cystic, although some are solid. They normally are well encapsulated and benign, although some become malignant. Many contain sufficient calcification to be visualized on radiographs. They may reach considerable size (8–10 cm in diameter). Because of location, they frequently compress the optic nerve, leading to visual impairment.[4,5]

## Malignant Tumors

### Primary Lesions

Although they are rare, primary malignant lesions do occur in the anterior lobe of the pituitary. They occasionally arise in preexisting benign adenomas or craniopharyngiomas. Characteristically, they are fast-growing and rapidly exhibit clinical manifestations. They also are massive and extensively invade nearby structures; distant metastasis may occur, especially to the liver. The histologic distinction between rapidly growing adenoma and carcinoma often is difficult.[2]

### Secondary Lesions

Neoplastic metastasis to the pituitary is rare. It may occur with carcinoma of the breast, lung, or thyroid.

## REFERENCES

1. Baxter, J.D. Principles of endocrinology. In J.B. Wyngaarden and L.H. Smith (eds.), *Cecil's Textbook of Medicine* (18th ed.). Philadelphia: W.B. Saunders, 1988.
2. Cotran, R.S., Kumar, V., and Robbins, S.L. *Robbins' Pathologic Basis of Disease* (4th ed.). Philadelphia: W.B. Saunders, 1989.
3. Daniels, G.H., and Martin, J.B. Neuroendocrine regulation of the anterior pituitary and hypothalamus. In J.D. Wilson et al. (eds.), *Harrison's Principles of Internal Medicine* (12th ed.). New York: McGraw-Hill, 1991.
4. Daughaday, W.H. The anterior pituitary. In J.D. Wilson and D.W. Foster (eds.), *Williams' Textbook of Endocrinology* (7th ed.). Philadelphia: W.B. Saunders, 1985.
5. Frohman, L.A. The anterior pituitary. In J.B. Wyngaarden and L.H. Smith (eds.), *Cecil's Textbook of Medicine* (18th ed.). Philadelphia: W.B. Saunders, 1988.
6. Germon, K. Fluid and electrolyte problems associated with diabetes insipidus and syndrome of inappropriate antidiuretic syndrome. *Nurs. Clin. North Am.* 22(4):785–796, 1987.
7. Greenspan, F.S. (ed.). *Basic and Clinical Endocrinology* (3rd ed.). Norwalk, Conn.: Appleton & Lange, 1991.

8. Griffin, J.E., and Ojeda, S.R. Organization of the endocrine system. In J.E. Griffin and S.R. Ojeda (eds.), *Textbook of Endocrine Physiology*. New York: Oxford University Press, 1988.

9. Guyton, A. *Textbook of Medical Physiology* (8th ed.). Philadelphia: W.B. Saunders, 1990.

10. Ihde, D.C. Paraneoplastic syndromes. *Hosp. Pract.* [Off] 22(8):105–124, 1987.

11. Kannan, C.R. *The Pituitary Gland (Vol. 1)*. New York: Plenum, 1987.

12. Lloyd, R.V. *Endocrine Pathology*. New York: Springer-Verlag, 1990.

13. Mendelsohn, G. *Diagnosis and Pathology of Endocrine Diseases*. Philadelphia: J.B. Lippincott, 1988.

14. Molitch, M.E. Acromegaly. In R. Collu, G.M. Brown, and G.R. Van Loon (eds.), *Clinical Neuroendocrinology*. Boston: Blackwell, 1988.

15. Olefsky, J.M. Obesity. In J.D. Wilson et al. (eds.), *Harrison's Principles of Internal Medicine* (12th ed.). New York: McGraw-Hill, 1991.

16. Reichlin, S. Neuroendocrinology. In J.D. Wilson and D.W. Foster (eds.), *Williams' Textbook of Endocrinology* (7th ed.). Philadelphia: W.B. Saunders, 1985.

17. Slaunwhite, W.R. *Fundamentals of Endocrinology*. New York: Dekker, 1988.

18. Streeten, D.H.P., Moses, A.M., and Miller, M. Disorders of the neurohypophysis. In J.D. Wilson et al (eds.), *Harrison's Principles of Internal Medicine* (12th ed.). New York: McGraw-Hill, 1991.

19. Wilson, J.D. Hormones and hormone action. In J.D. Wilson et al. (eds.), *Harrison's Principles of Internal Medicine* (12th ed.). New York: McGraw-Hill, 1991.

# Adrenal Mechanisms and Alterations

*Learning Objectives*

1. Discuss the normal anatomy of the adrenal gland.
2. Describe the mechanisms of regulating adrenocortical hormone secretions.
3. Identify the pattern of synthesis of each of the major hormones of the adrenal cortex.
4. Outline the physiologic effects of mineralocorticoids, glucocorticoids, and androgen hormones.
5. Identify the process that results in Cushing's syndrome.
6. Define *Cushing's syndrome* and its major clinical manifestations.
7. Differentiate between primary and secondary aldosteronism.
8. Describe the pathologic process and resulting physical changes of the adrenogenital syndromes.
9. Outline the clinical manifestations of primary adrenocortical insufficiency.
10. Compare primary and secondary adrenocortical insufficiency.
11. Discuss the clinical features of adrenal crisis.
12. Describe catecholamine biosynthesis and storage.
13. Describe the etiology of pheochromocytoma.
14. Outline the major clinical features of pheochromocytoma.
15. Discuss multiple endocrine neoplasia syndrome and its relation to pheochromocytoma.

The adrenal cortex and adrenal medulla and their associated hormones probably developed as protection from immediate stress or injury and against prolonged food and water deprivation.[9] One of the primary functions of the adrenal glands remains protection of the body against both acute and chronic forms of stress.[9] The adrenal cortex and the adrenal medulla share adjacent sites but have no similar functions. The hormonal anatomy and physiology of both of these structures are discussed in this chapter. Altered states of function also are included.

## ANATOMY OF THE ADRENAL GLANDS

The adrenal, or suprarenal, glands are located retroperitoneally at the superior pole of each kidney. Although structurally connected, the adrenal cortex and adrenal medulla are separate organs in both tissue origin and physiologic function.

The adrenals are rather flat, with the right gland having a pyramidal appearance and the left a curved, semilunar shape (Figure 37-1). A thick, fibrous capsule surrounds the glands, and peritoneal fasciae, independent of the kidneys, provide support. The usual weight of each gland in a healthy adult is between 3 and 6 g, and the adrenals tend to be slightly heavier in males.

Arterial blood supply is from the renal, or inferior, phrenic arteries or directly from the abdominal aorta. Once inside the glands, the vessels break up into sinusoids and drain medially into the glands. Venous drainage is different for the right and left glands. The right adrenal empties venous blood directly into the vena cava, whereas the left empties into the left renal vein (see Figure 37-1). Nervous innervation is both sympathetic and parasympathetic. Nerves enter through the cortex and progress to the medulla.

The golden yellow adrenal cortex encompasses the medulla, which is more medially located. Three distinct

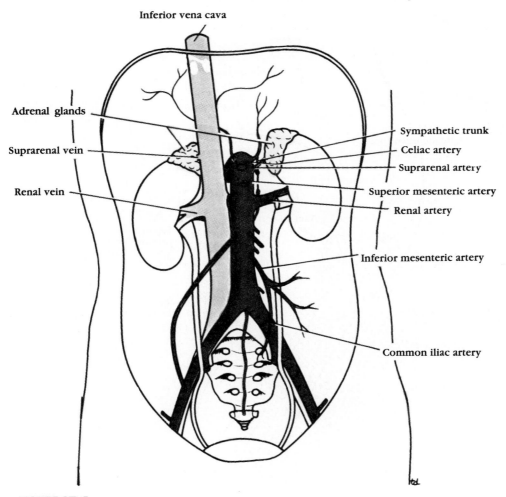

**FIGURE 37-1.**
Position of the adrenal glands on the kidneys. (From R.S. Snell, *Clinical Anatomy for Medical Students* [2nd ed.]. Boston: Little, Brown, 1981.)

layers compose the cortex. The first is the *zona glomerulosa,* composed of a thin layer of irregularly shaped cuboidal cells. Immediately beneath is the second layer, the *zona fasciculata.* Cuboidal cells of this layer run in long strands and are separated by the sinusoidal spaces. The third layer of the cortex, the *zona reticularis,* is composed of groups of cells of irregular shape (Figure 37-2). Both the zona fasciculata and the zona reticularis are regulated so closely by adrenocorticotropic hormone (ACTH) that deficiency or excess alters their structure and function. During periods of adrenal inactivity, when ACTH is deficient, the cells of the zonae fasciculata and reticularis atrophy and become filled with vacuoles, but during periods of active function, when ACTH is present in large or excess amounts, hyperplasia and hyperactivity result.[24]

The adrenal medulla lies central to and is surrounded by the adrenal cortex. It is flat and gray, and composed of sheets of irregularly shaped masses of cells with small nuclei. The cells are surrounded by sinusoidal blood vessels.

## THE ADRENAL CORTEX

### Adrenocortical Hormones

The adrenal cortex is responsible for secreting three major groups of steroid hormones. The *mineralocorticoids* and *glucocorticoids* are the two most important of these, with the third and less significant being the *androgens.* The major glucocorticoid is *cortisol,* which is se-

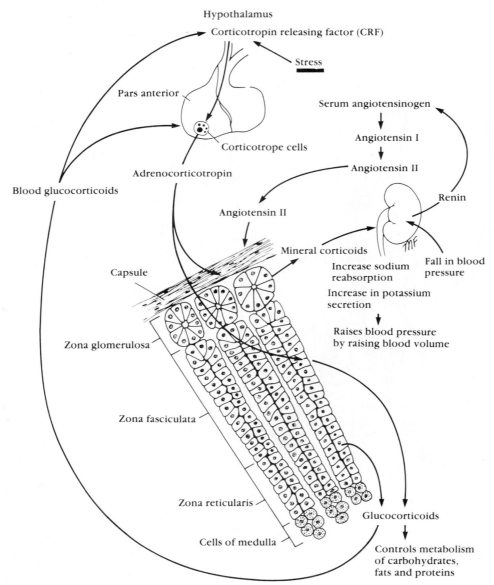

**FIGURE 37-2.**
Mechanisms involved in the control of mineralocorticoid secretion and glucocorticoid secretion of the adrenal cortex.

creted mostly by the zona fasciculata. The major mineralocorticoid is *aldosterone,* which is secreted by the zona glomerulosa almost independently of ACTH influence; ACTH is necessary only to maintain the viability of the glomerulosa cells. Androgens are produced by the cells of the zona fasciculata and probably the zona reticularis.

## Control of Secretion

Regulation of adrenocortical hormone secretion is accomplished mainly through ACTH, which exerts direct control over the glucocorticoids and sex steroids. Aldosterone secretion is primarily controlled by the renin-angiotensin-aldosterone system and by serum potassium and serum sodium levels (see Figure 37-2).

## Adrenocorticotropic Hormone

ACTH is produced by the anterior pituitary gland. Its release is controlled by corticotropin-releasing factor (CRF), which is produced by the hypothalamus. The amount of circulating ACTH normally is controlled by three factors: (1) circulating levels of cortisol, (2) individual biorhythms, and (3) stress. These factors, together with states of dysfunction, stimulate CRF to release ACTH into the bloodstream.

## Feedback System of Cortisol-ACTH Levels

When circulating levels of cortisol (the principal glucocorticoid) decrease, ACTH acts directly on the adrenal cortex to stimulate production. Increased secretion of cortisol occurs within a few minutes after ACTH initiates production of the hormone. Low levels of ACTH result in decreased hormone biosynthesis and in decreased renal blood flow. Thus, circulating levels of cortisol respond directly to a feedback system with ACTH. Decreased cortisol levels result in stimulation of ACTH, whereas elevated levels cause decreased release of ACTH (see Chap. 36).

## Biorhythms: Effects on ACTH Secretion

Individual biorhythms, or *circadian* or *diurnal rhythms,* affect the normal circulating levels of ACTH. The pattern is related to sleep periods, and may be altered by changes in daily activity.[26] In the hours before and just after waking, ACTH levels reach the highest peak of the 24-hour day. The levels decrease continually during the remainder of the day. In relation to this, cortisol levels rise at about the same times as the ACTH levels and also decline

as the day progresses. The plasma cortisol concentration usually is highest on awakening in the morning, falls later during the day, and reaches the lowest levels during the first 2 hours of sleep.[26] From this point, cortisol gradually returns to its maximum level before the period of waking. Although the basic pattern of biorhythms is similar for all humans, wide variations can occur in any individual.

## Effects of Stress on ACTH Secretion

Any physical or emotional stress increases the secretion of ACTH, resulting in increased production and secretion of cortisol (see Chap. 6). Stresses that may initiate this reaction include illness, hypotension, and exposure to extreme cold. The mechanism behind this is thought to be related to the ability of the glucocorticoids to provide the body with the materials needed for energy. These materials include amino acids, protein, fatty acids, glucose, sodium, and water, levels of all of which increase in a stressful situation.[1]

Specific stress responses of the body occur with the stages of the general adaptation syndrome (GAS) as defined by Selye. Corticotropin-releasing hormone and ACTH often are referred to as the "stress hormones," and are routinely measured as indicators of levels of stress and coping ability.[18] During the initial stages of the alarm phase of the GAS, acute release of epinephrine produces characteristic catecholamine effects. This is followed by changes that resemble adrenocortical insufficiency, such as decreased blood pressure, decreased serum glucose and serum sodium levels, and increased serum potassium levels. The period of insufficiency is followed by a period of active adrenocortical function that continues until a stable baseline has been reestablished. Stable levels of hormone production occur during the resistance phase. If the stage of exhaustion is reached, adrenocortical hormone insufficiency may once again be encountered.

## Renin-Angiotensin-Aldosterone System

The renin-angiotensin-aldosterone system is the major influence over the production of aldosterone by the zona glomerulosa. The enzymelike substance renin is released from the juxtaglomerular apparatus in the nephrons of the kidneys in response to changes in perfusion pressure and solute delivery in the renal distal tubules. Through a complex process of hydrolysis, renin undergoes chemical changes to become angiotensin II, which exerts a strong control over the regulation of aldosterone secretion (see Figure 37-2). The mechanism by which this is accomplished is not completely understood. It is known that the action is rapid, and that the production of aldosterone stops when angiotensin II is removed. The renin-angiotensin-aldosterone system does not influence cortisol production or secretion.

## Effect of Electrolytes on Aldosterone Secretion

The electrolyte with the major influence on aldosterone secretion is potassium. When serum potassium levels are elevated, aldosterone secretion increases. An increase in potassium of less than 1 mEq/L triples aldosterone secretion. It also appears that potassium affects the release of renin, exerting an indirect stimulus on aldosterone synthesis.[25] Lowered levels of potassium decrease the rate of aldosterone release.

Sodium functions by similar, but reverse, principles. Decreased sodium levels stimulate aldosterone secretion, and increased sodium concentrations inhibit aldosterone secretion.

## Adrenocortical Hormone Biosynthesis

Adrenocortical hormone, or steroid, biosynthesis uses cholesterol as the initial basis of its hormones (Figure 37-3). Cholesterol is obtained from both blood and the adrenal cortex. Within the cortex, during normal states of activity, cholesterol is stored in lipid droplets in the cytoplasm of the cells. Although the adrenal cortex is capable of synthesizing cholesterol for steroid production, most is taken from the cholesterol stores in the cortex that were obtained from cholesterol circulating in the bloodstream. During periods when the cortex is not being stimulated by one of the regulating mechanisms, available cholesterol remains in storage, and the production of steroid hormones is minimal.[25]

Stimulation from any of the adrenal regulators begins the process of steroid biosynthesis. Cholesterol undergoes many chemical and enzymatic conversions in the process of manufacturing steroids. In this series of changes, the one step through which all steroids must pass is the conversion of cholesterol to pregnenolone.[25] At this point, the production of the major hormones occurs by different and individual mechanisms.

## Transport of Steroid Hormones

After steroid biosynthesis, the steroid hormones are released into the bloodstream to be carried to the tissue cells. In the blood they bind to specific proteins known as

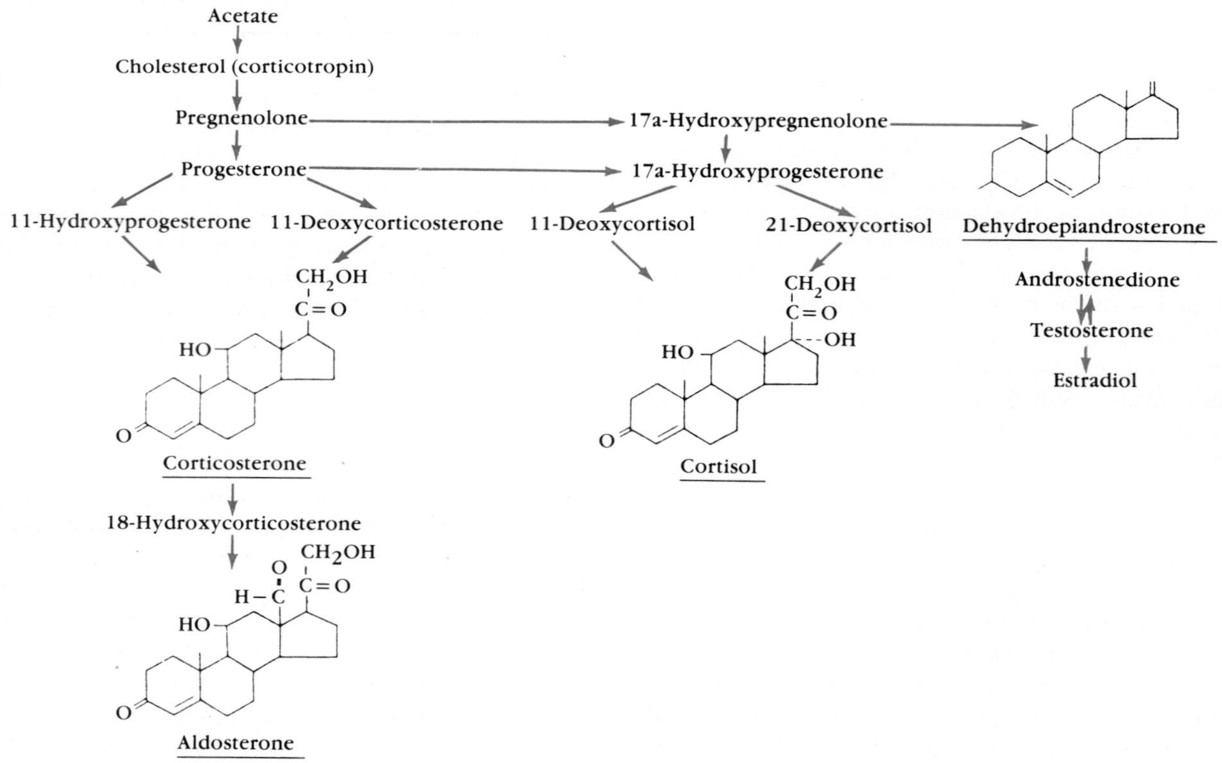

**FIGURE 37-3.**

Formation of adrenocortical hormones. (From D. Jensen, *The Principles of Physiology* [2nd ed.]. New York: Appleton-Century-Crofts, 1980.)

transcortins, or *corticosteroid-binding globulins,* which have an affinity for all major steroids. Binding causes inactivation of the steroid hormones, excretion of the steroid by the kidneys, and prevention of excess tissue uptake. At the target site, the steroids are released to exert their physiologic action.

## Physiologic Actions of Mineralocorticoids

The principal mineralocorticoid that exerts a physiologic action is aldosterone. Almost all mineralocorticoid activity is produced by this steroid, but cortisol contributes slightly. The single most important action of aldosterone is sodium retention. Because of this action and its resultant effect on intracellular and extracellular fluid volume, aldosterone has a profound effect on fluid balance.

Sodium retention results in a simultaneous loss of potassium by excretion in the urine. This exchange of ions takes place in the distal renal tubules. Together with sodium, water is retained. Thus, higher circulating levels of aldosterone cause sodium retention, increased plasma volume, and higher blood pressure; decreased circulating levels have opposite effects. Any excess or deficit in normal circulating aldosterone can lead to a variety of basic electrolyte disturbances with resultant effects on body functions.

In addition to the tubules, aldosterone acts on other tissues to retain sodium. Salivary and sweat glands are influenced to conserve sodium in extreme heat. Absorption of sodium by the intestinal mucosa prevents excess loss in fecal waste. Aldosterone also conserves sodium by influencing the exchange of intracellular and extracellular water.

## Physiologic Actions of Glucocorticoids

Glucocorticoids are named for their ability to regulate serum glucose levels by several mechanisms. Their effect is not as pronounced or prolonged as that of the regulating ability of insulin. In looking at the total picture of the effects of glucocorticoid activity, the primary action in the tissues is *catabolic,* with increased breakdown of proteins and increased excretion of nitrogen. In the liver, *anabolic* actions occur, such as increased amino acid uptake and increased synthesis of ribonucleic acid and protein.

The activities generated by the glucocorticoids are accomplished by the production and secretion of cortisol. Cortisol is important in the control and metabolism of carbohydrates, lipids, and proteins; also, it assists in metabolic reactions to stress. In nonstressful situations, cortisol has no demonstrable functions.[20] In greater than physiologic amounts, the effect of cortisol in inflammation and allergies is vital.

The action of cortisol on carbohydrate metabolism may be primarily viewed by its two major effects on glucose production and use. The first major effect of cortisol is to increase the amount of glucose released by enhancing the ability of the liver for gluconeogenesis (glucose production). This is accomplished by stimulating adipose tissue to release free fatty acids, the gluconeogenic substrate needed by the liver. The second major action of cortisol is to decrease the use of glucose by the tissues. In muscle, adipose, and lymphatic tissues, uptake and metabolism are reduced. Through these actions—increased gluconeogenesis and the inhibition of glucose use by tissues—serum glucose concentrations are increased.

By stimulating the release of fatty acids from tissue stores into the plasma, lipids in the form of free fatty acids are made available for energy use. This ability to mobilize fat stores is one of the factors that cause a metabolic alteration in times of stress or deprivation from the use of glucose to the use of fatty acids for energy.[5] It is not understood how cortisol initiates the mobilization of fatty acids, or why fat deposits are removed from one area of the body and deposited in another, as may easily be seen in adrenocortical dysfunction.

The effects of cortisol on protein are twofold. First, it decreases protein stores in all tissues of the body except the liver. This is carried out by preventing the synthesis of protein and by breaking down protein stores in the cells into amino acids. Second, protein synthesis in the liver is stimulated. Amino acids are released into the liver from cell protein catabolism, thereby increasing the amount of amino acids available to the liver for protein synthesis.

The mechanism by which cortisol responds to stress is not understood, yet it is recognized as being almost essential for survival of the human organism. Any extreme physical or emotional stress may initiate the response, including severe trauma, emotional upset, chronic or debilitating diseases, infection, or extreme temperatures (Figure 37-4).

Administration of glucocorticoids—specifically cortisol—in larger than normal amounts decreases the inflammatory response to infection or injury. Each step of the inflammatory process is blocked by steroids. Cortisol reduces the passage of water into and out of the cell. Also, allergic processes are stopped with the administration of cortisol, which alters the inflammatory process that occurs in response to any allergen. The mechanism by which the components of the inflammatory process are blocked is not understood, but it is thought to be related to the ability of the glucocorticoids to stabilize cell membranes and prevent rupture of the lysosomes.

Cortisol affects the blood cells in a variable manner. The circulating levels of eosinophils and lymphocytes

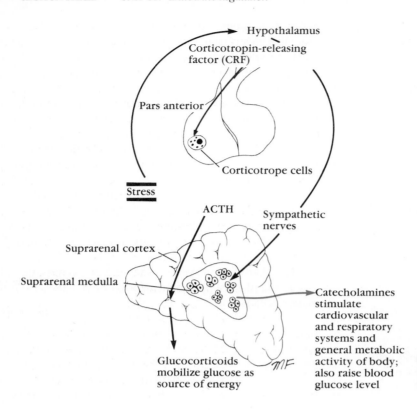

**FIGURE 37–4.**
The effects of stress on the activities of the adrenal gland.

are decreased, and red blood cell and platelet production is increased. Because of the decreased lymphocyte level, humoral immunity is decreased and infection may occur.[5]

## *Physiologic Actions of Androgens*

Adrenal androgens, or male sex hormones, produced in the adrenal cortex have little physiologic significance in the healthy adult. Some of the androgens produced are converted to testosterone, the major male sex hormone; hypersecretion of the cortex can cause the appearance of dramatic masculinizing changes as a result of the androgens.

## *ALTERED ADRENOCORTICAL FUNCTION*

### *Adrenocortical Hyperfunction*

#### *Cushing's Syndrome*

The term *Cushing's syndrome* refers to the clinical manifestations that result from excess glucose production caused by hypersecretion of cortisol from the adrenal cortex. Although clinically similar, three separate factors may cause Cushing's syndrome: (1) adrenal neoplasms, (2) hypersecretion of ACTH by the anterior pituitary (this condition is called *Cushing's disease*), and (3) ectopic ACTH syndrome.[26]

The growth of adrenocortical cells into a tumor that secretes cortisol causes cellular growth and additional secretion of cortisol. As cortisol secretion increases, it is no longer controlled by ACTH. Cortisol secretion by the neoplasm eventually exceeds that of normal adrenocortical cells, at which point the normal cells may cease producing cortisol altogether. Cortisol-secreting tumors of the adrenal glands seldom secrete excessive androgenic hormones.

In pituitary-dependent Cushing's disease, cortisol oversecretion is caused by excessive release of ACTH from the anterior pituitary gland.[1] This causes increased secretion and release of both cortisol and androgenic hormones. Some authors classify all forms of conditions that involve excessive cortisol secretion as Cushing's syndrome.[7,15,17]

The third form of Cushing's syndrome occurs from excess production of ACTH by a neoplasm not located in the adrenal gland. This particular form often occurs in persons afflicted with oat cell carcinoma of the lung.[21] Other malignant neoplasms may secrete ACTH, causing this peculiar paraneoplastic syndrome. In addition to hypersecretion of cortisol, persons with Cushing's syndrome exhibit the absence of circadian rhythm changes in the release of ACTH and cortisol.

With increased cortisol secretion there is an increased rate of gluconeogenesis, resulting in elevated serum glucose levels. The islet cells of the pancreas eventually are unable to produce sufficient amounts of insulin, and diabetes mellitus results.[5] Loss of protein occurs almost everywhere in the body except the liver. In the muscular system, protein loss results in decreased strength and muscle wasting. Humoral immunity is reduced, decreasing the threshold to infection. Skin tissues lose collagen and become very thin, tearing and bruising easily. In the bones, osteoporosis can cause weakness and actual bone fractures. Hyperpigmentation may be seen, and is due to the melanostimulating properties of ACTH.

The clinical signs and symptoms vary only slightly with the cause of the disease. Although scattered in the population, Cushing's syndrome is more frequently seen in women, especially those of childbearing age.[23] Androgens are responsible for a few of the bodily changes, but most of the abnormalities are direct results of hypercortisolism. The three classic manifestations are truncal obesity, purple striae, and round facial features. The frequency of different clinical effects is noted in Table 37-1.

Truncal obesity results from the mobilization of fat in the lower parts of the body to the trunk, causing the abdomen to be greatly protuberant, even as the extremities become thin and wasted. Many persons with Cushing's syndrome cannot rise from a squatting position without assistance. The enlarged abdomen is characteristic, and may be an extension of thoracic accumulation of fat, the buffalo torso. Fat accumulation around the neck

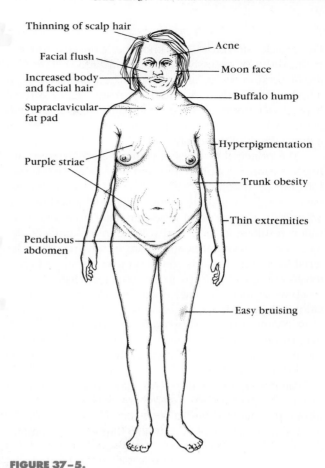

**FIGURE 37-5.**
A composite of symptoms in Cushing's disease. (From M. Beyers and S. Dudas [eds.], *The Clinical Practice of Medical Surgical Nursing.* Boston: Little, Brown, 1984.)

and cervical area is termed the *buffalo hump.* Purple striae appear on the abdomen as a result of the stretching of the abdominal skin when the fat cells are being deposited. They are purple as a result of the collagen deficit in the skin tissues. Round and full facial features, often called moon facies, also result from the hypercortisolism (Figure 37-5).

Other manifestations also occur. Excessive androgen secretion results in excess hair growth, often on the face, which is especially prominent in women. Androgen hormones may cause acne and oligomenorrhea. Extreme androgen excess may result in coarsening of the voice, recession of the hairline, and hypertrophy of the clitoris. Psychiatric disturbances may surface, with personality alterations or more severe changes. Polyuria may result from hyperglycemia. Varying degrees of hypertension are exhibited, often with the development of left ventricular hypertrophy. The mortality of Cushing's syndrome is 50% or greater unless treatment is initiated. Death usually results from severe infection.

When Cushing's syndrome occurs in children, growth ceases. If treatment is not begun before the epiphyses of the bones have sealed, short stature is permanent.[26]

**TABLE 37-1.**
CLINICAL EFFECTS OF CUSHING'S SYNDROME AND THEIR FREQUENCY

| EFFECTS | FREQUENCY (%) |
|---|---|
| Obesity | 94 |
| Facial plethora | 84 |
| Hirsutism | 82 |
| Menstrual disorders | 76 |
| Hypertension | 72 |
| Muscle weakness | 58 |
| Back pain | 58 |
| Striae | 52 |
| Acne | 40 |
| Psychologic symptoms | 40 |
| Bruising | 36 |
| Congestive heart failure | 22 |
| Edema | 18 |
| Renal calculi | 16 |
| Headache | 14 |
| Polyuria/polydipsia | 10 |
| Hyperpigmentation | 6 |

Source: *Reproduced with permission from P. Felig et al. Endocrinology and Metabolism. Copyright © 1981, McGraw-Hill Book Company.*

## Primary Aldosteronism

Primary aldosteronism, also known as *Conn's syndrome*, is the result of excessive and uncontrolled secretion of the mineralocorticoid aldosterone. The usual cause is an adrenocortical adenoma; rarely, it results from adrenal hyperplasia. Because aldosterone conserves sodium and wastes potassium, the clinical features of this disorder are a direct result of those functions.

The principal features of primary aldosteronism are hypertension, hypernatremia, and hypokalemia.[22] Therefore, this condition may be suspected in any hypertensive patient who concurrently exhibits hypokalemia (less than 3.5 mEq/L). Conservation of sodium leads to retention of water, resulting in increased volume in the extracellular and vascular compartments, which in turn results in arterial hypertension. This condition may resemble hypertension originating from cardiovascular disease.

Loss of potassium may produce a variety of manifestations, depending on the severity of the depletion. The most common result is muscle cramps and weakness. It may progress to tetany and even muscle paralysis because of hypokalemia. Changes in the pattern of cardiac conduction may develop.

Alterations in renal function are apparent because this is the primary site of sodium conservation. Polydipsia, polyuria, and nocturia occur in response to the sodium-induced increased fluid volume and volume-dependent hypertension.

## Secondary Aldosteronism

Secondary aldosteronism results from stimulation of aldosterone secretion from outside the adrenal cortex, usually by the renin-angiotensin-aldosterone system. Almost any factor that decreases the blood supply to the kidneys results in increased plasma renin levels. Thus the mechanism is somewhat compensatory: increased renin levels lead to increased aldosterone secretion and sodium conservation; water retention results from sodium conservation, leading to increased blood flow to vital organs. Edema occurs only in the presence of preexisting or underlying cardiovascular disease. Secondary aldosteronism leads to a combination of elevated plasma renin and aldosterone levels.[2]

## Adrenogenital Syndromes

The adrenogenital syndromes are the result of adrenocortical overproduction of androgens, caused by tumor or adrenocortical hyperplasia. In all of the adrenogenital syndromes, the ultimate result is the same—virilization. The age and sex of the affected person determine the nature and severity of the disorder. The most common causes of adrenogenital syndromes include congenital adrenal hyperplasia, "postpubertal" adrenal hyperplasia, adrenal adenoma, and adrenal carcinomas.[13]

Androgens ultimately are converted to the male hormone testosterone. Testosterone is extremely potent, and only small amounts are required to produce bodily changes. In men, masculinizing effects are masked by the production of testosterone from the testes. It is in children and women that virilization becomes most apparent.

Young boys begin to develop secondary sex characteristics, regardless of their age at the time of onset. Females respond to androgen stimulation with hirsutism, clitoral hypertrophy, and other masculinizing effects (Figure 37-6).

## Congenital Adrenal Hyperplasia

One of the most common adrenogenital syndromes, congenital adrenal hyperplasia results from a congenital deficiency in the enzymes that causes adrenocortical biosynthesis. It occurs most often in the pediatric age-group.[12] There is not an absence of the enzymes, but an error in metabolism pathways of steroid production. The appearance of clinical manifestations depends on the point at which synthesis of cortisol, aldosterone, and androgens is blocked. There may be clinical signs and symptoms either of glucocorticoid or mineralocorticoid deficiency or excess. Also, androgen excess and virilization or sexual ambiguity and infantism may occur. For example, in the most frequently encountered of these conditions, a defect in 21-hydroxylase, excessive androgen production in the female fetus may cause the external genitalia to resemble those of a male, while internal structures—uterus, ovaries, and fallopian tubes—are normal and functional. Male children have the infant Hercules appearance.[14]

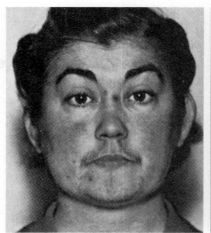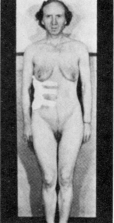

A                                                      B

**FIGURE 37-6.**
Adrenogenital syndromes of the female. A. Hirsutism. B. Masculinizing of the female. (From J.D. Wilson and D.W. Foster, *Williams' Textbook of Endocrinology* [7th ed.]. Philadelphia: W.B. Saunders, 1985.)

## Adrenocortical Hypofunction

### Primary Adrenocortical Insufficiency

Also known as *Addison's disease,* primary adrenocortical hypofunction results from insufficient secretion of adrenocortical hormones because of insidious and profound destruction in the adrenal glands. It is not a common disorder, and becomes evident only if 90% of the functioning adrenocortical cells have been destroyed.[2] The two major causes of adrenal destruction that result in this condition are idiopathic atrophy (80%) and tuberculosis (20%). In regions where tuberculosis is poorly controlled, the frequency of Addison's disease is high.

Idiopathic atrophy has been attributed to an autoimmune disorder, with adrenal autoantibodies present in many affected people.[16] Primary adrenocortical failure, associated with organ-specific immunity, results from progressive destruction of both adrenals by an autoimmune process.[2,8] Further, autoimmune failure may be an isolated problem, or may appear as part of an autoimmune alteration in several endocrine glands, including the ovaries, parathyroids, thyroid, and B cells of the pancreas.[8] The principal feature of autoimmune adrenal failure results from lymphatic infiltration of the adrenal cortex. As a result, the adrenal glands atrophy and the capsule thickens.

Adrenocortical insufficiency primarily results from deficient cortisol secretion and, in some cases, deficient aldosterone and androgen production.[23] Clinical manifestations depend on the degree of hormonal deficiency. Changes in the skin are the most dramatic; they occur in about 98% of affected people, and help to diagnose the primary (adrenocortical) insufficiency.[2] Skin color changes result from increased ACTH production, which is uninhibited by steroid response from the adrenal cortex. Areas of hyperpigmentation become visible because the pituitary increases the production of ACTH in an attempt to compensate, and ACTH also has melanostimulating properties. These darkened areas are especially visible in the body areas most exposed to light, pressure areas, hand creases, and buccal mucosa.[14] Areas of vitiligo (pale patches surrounded by excess pigmentation) also are apparent. Muscle weakness and fatigue commonly occur.

Many people experience hypotension as a result of volume depletion. Sodium and potassium retention result in depletion of extracellular volume, which in turn causes decreased cardiac output and decreased blood pressure.[11] Hypoglycemia also can result from the decrease in gluconeogenesis caused by the reduction in cortisol levels. Nausea, vomiting, weight loss, and diarrhea are the most common gastrointestinal disturbances. Other body changes include loss of hair, decreased sexual function, and mental disturbances ranging from mild neuroses to deep depressions.[11] Because the symptoms often are vague and the disease onset insidious, the potential for adrenocortical insufficiency should be evaluated in any person who is seriously ill without a specific identifiable cause.[25]

It has been reported with increasing frequency that other physiologic disorders may be associated with primary adrenocortical insufficiency. This association has been called *Schmidt's syndrome,* which refers to autoimmune endocrine failure together with polyglandular failure.[26] Disorders that may be associated include gonadal failure, thyroid dysfunction, diabetes mellitus, hypoparathyroidism, and pernicious anemia.

### Adrenal Crisis

Adrenal crisis (Addisonian crisis, acute adrenal insufficiency) usually occurs because of a sudden decrease or absence of adrenocortical hormones, and most commonly is due to stress.[8] It may affect people with both treated and undiagnosed Addison's disease in which the individuals are exposed to major stresses, such as trauma, infection, surgery, or severe illness. Affected people may develop severe dehydration caused by nausea and vomiting. Weakness, confusion, and hypovolemic shock also are associated.[26] Immediate intervention is necessary or death will rapidly ensue. The cause of the crisis is not understood, but it may be due to primary disease in the adrenal gland itself, such as hemorrhage, infection, or infarction.[19]

### Secondary Adrenocortical Insufficiency

Secondary adrenocortical insufficiency results from decreased cortisol secretion because of atrophy of the adrenal cortex. The disorder is a result of decreased ACTH secretion caused by pituitary or hypothalamic disease or by therapeutic pharmacologic doses of glucocorticoids. Mineralocorticoid secretion usually is not affected. Clinically, the features may resemble those of primary insufficiency, except for the absence of hyperpigmentation. The most common cause of secondary adrenocortical insufficiency is acute withdrawal of exogenous steroid therapy.[17] When a person is receiving steroid therapy, slow tapering off is required to allow the adrenal glands to return to active production of their own corticosteroids.

## THE ADRENAL MEDULLA

### Catecholamines

The most important human catecholamines are epinephrine, norepinephrine, and dopamine, which are synthesized in the brain, sympathetic nerve endings, and chromaffin tissues. The adrenal medulla produces and secretes the catecholamines epinephrine (adrenalin) and norepinephrine (noradrenalin) from the chromaffin cells of the medulla. As related to these two catecholamines, the adrenal medulla functions as part of the autonomic nervous system.[14] These cells stain readily with chromium salts and secrete adrenalin. Adrenal medullary secretion is about 80% epinephrine and 20% norepinephrine.[5]

Epinephrine exerts its greatest effect on the heart, increasing both rate and contractility. It is a potent mediator of the metabolic rate. Norepinephrine, on the other hand, is secreted by both the adrenal medulla and the sympathetic nerve terminals. It exerts its greatest influence on the arterioles, causing vasoconstriction that leads to increased blood pressure. Stimulation of the sympathetic nervous system (SNS) causes both direct SNS effects and release of the adrenal medullary hormones.

## Catecholamine Biosynthesis and Storage

The precursor for catecholamine biosynthesis is tyrosine. Through hydroxylation, decarboxylation, and methylation, tyrosine yields norepinephrine and, ultimately, epinephrine (Figure 37-7). The sequence of the process is as follows[6,25]:

tyrosine → dihydroxyphenylaline (dopa)
    → dopamine (DA)
    → norepinephrine (NE) → epinephrine (E).

It is thought that the tyrosine hydroxylase reaction is probably the factor that controls the rate of catecholamine production.

Catecholamine is stored by subcellular particles, called granules, which are present in most adrenomedullary cells in the chromaffin granules.

## Catecholamine Secretion

Catecholamines may be released with acetylcholine stimulation of calcium passage into the chromaffin granules and subsequent liberation into the extracellular fluid. As the adrenal medulla produces the major portion of circulating epinephrine, a small amount is released into the bloodstream almost continuously. Norepinephrine is primarily produced by the sympathetic ganglion cells. Release of large amounts of catecholamines occurs after SNS stimulation. Other substances and conditions that may stimulate the release of epinephrine and norepinephrine include serotonin, bradykinin, exercise, hypovolemia, glucagon, and hypoglycemia.[7] Catecholamines participate in metabolic processes together with insulin

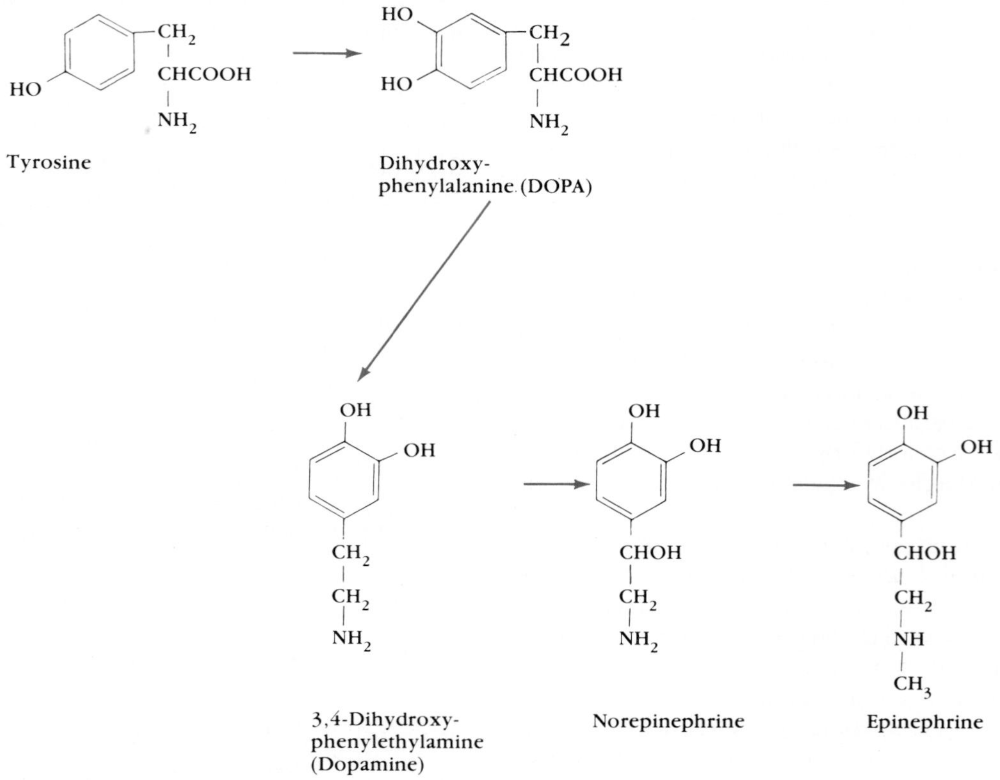

**FIGURE 37-7.**
Steps in the synthesis of norepinephrine and epinephrine from tyrosine. (From I. Danishefsky, *Biochemistry for Medical Science*. Boston: Little, Brown, 1980.)

and glucagon.[26] The action of the catecholamines is opposite that of insulin and similar to that of glucagon, such that it is the interaction that is important.

Extremely stressful situations cause a massive release of epinephrine and norepinephrine, which results in the fight-or-flight reaction. This enables the body to react effectively to any severe hazard or threat to survival. Physiologic response to this massive release of epinephrine includes increased blood pressure and heart rate, pupil dilatation, decreased peristalsis, and circulatory constriction in all major organ systems except the muscular and cardiovascular. The response to norepinephrine stimulation is similar, but with the major action being increased arterial blood pressure, a result of vigorous vasoconstriction. These responses are apparently normal catecholamine actions that are accelerated to meet the unusual and immediate cellular demands.[25]

## Altered Function of the Adrenal Medulla

The only significant disorders of altered function of the adrenal are neoplasms. The gland itself is not considered necessary for life because the body has other sources of catecholamines. The presence of a *pheochromocytoma* in the adrenal medulla produces apparent states of hyperfunction of the adrenomedullary catecholamines.

### Pheochromocytoma

Pheochromocytomas are rare tumors of the adrenal medulla whose primary clinical manifestation is hypertension. Pheochromocytomas originate in the chromaffin cells of the medulla.

During fetal life, the chromaffin cells are widespread in the developing body, and their function is associated with the sympathetic ganglia. After birth, most of these cells disappear. Those that remain cluster in the adrenal medulla.[6] Although more than 95% of all functioning chromaffin tumors are located in the adrenal medulla, others have been found in common extraadrenal sites, including areas near the kidney and heart, and within the cranial vault.[4]

Pheochromocytomas occur in either sex, usually between ages 25 and 50 years. Children seldom are affected. It is not uncommon for this disorder to affect more than one member of the same family. The tumors usually are benign and bilateral, but a small percentage are malignant with metastasis. Most tumors are well encapsulated and extremely vascular. Because of their high vascularity, rupture can cause massive hemorrhage that can be fatal.[6] Sometimes the actual tumors may be palpable.

The pheochromocytoma produces and secretes excessive quantities of epinephrine and norepinephrine into the bloodstream, resulting in clinical manifestations of catecholamine excess. Therefore, the affected person remains in an accelerated state of response similar to the fight-or-flight reaction. Symptoms may occur spontaneously, or may be induced with increased physical or emotional activity or stress.[7]

The primary finding is systemic arterial hypertension. Elevated blood pressure may be sustained or intermittent, mild or malignant, depending on the rate and amount of catecholamine secreted. These persons also may exhibit clinical signs and symptoms of headache, pallor, palpitations, and sweating because of the direct effects of the elevated blood pressure and increased epinephrine and norepinephrine.[3] Most pheochromocytomas secrete a greater amount of norepinephrine, which is then responsible for the hypertension.[6] Together with this, the smaller amounts of epinephrine produced are responsible for the myocardial side effects. Sustained elevation of catecholamine secretion can lead to cardiomegaly, left ventricular failure, cardiomyopathy, and, ultimately, death caused by heart failure. Cardiac dysrhythmias also may be observed. Other metabolic effects include excessive perspiration, palpitations, headaches, hyperventilation, and flushing. Increased frequency of neurofibromatosis, a familial disorder, has been associated with pheochromocytoma.

### Multiple Endocrine Neoplasia

Pheochromocytomas also may be associated with a disorder known as multiple endocrine neoplasia syndrome (see Chap. 39). This complicated group of disorders is termed multiple because of the multicentricity and bilateral growth of the tumors, as well as the involvement of several glands.[7] One of the important aspects concerning the association of symptoms is that 85% of persons with either familial or sporadic pheochromocytomas who also have medullarthyroid carcinomas are normotensive, whereas more than 60% of persons with familial or sporadic pheochromocytomas not associated with medullary carcinoma have chronic hypertension.[26]

## REFERENCES

1. Carrieri, V.K., Lindsey, A.M., and West, C.M. *Pathophysiological Phenomena in Nursing: Human Responses to Illness*. Philadelphia: W.B. Saunders, 1986.
2. Cotran, R.S., Kumar, V., and Robbins, S.L. *Robbins' Pathologic Basis of Disease* (4th ed.). Philadelphia: W.B. Saunders, 1989.
3. DeQuattro, V., Myers, M., and Campese, V.M. Pheochromocytoma: Diagnosis and therapy. In L.J. DeGroot (ed.), *Endocrinology* (2nd ed.). Philadelphia: W.B. Saunders, 1989.
4. Goldfien, A. Adrenal medulla. In F.S. Greenspan (ed.), *Basic and Clinical Endocrinology* (3rd ed.). Norwalk, Conn.: Appleton & Lange, 1991.
5. Guyton, A. *Textbook of Medical Physiology* (8th ed.). Philadelphia: W.B. Saunders, 1990.

6. Harris, R.B., and Dela Roca, R.R. Pheochromocytoma: A medical review. *Heart Lung* 13(1):73, 1984.

7. Jubiz, W. *Endocrinology: A Logical Approach for Clinicians* (2nd ed.). New York: McGraw-Hill, 1985.

8. Kannan, C.R. Addison's disease. In C.R. Kannan (ed.), *The Adrenal Gland* (Vol. 2). New York: Plenum Medical, 1987.

9. Kaplan, N.M. The adrenal glands. In J.E. Griffin and S.R. Ojeda (eds.), *Textbook of Endocrine Physiology*. New York: Oxford University Press, 1988.

10. Kohler, P.O. Diseases of the hypothalamus and anterior pituitary. In E. Braunwald et al. (eds.), *Harrison's Principles of Internal Medicine* (11th ed.). New York: McGraw-Hill, 1987.

11. Larson, C.A. The critical path of adrenocortical insufficiency. *Nursing84* 14(10):66, 1984.

12. Lloyd, R.V. Adrenal gland. In R.V. Lloyd (ed.), *Endocrine Pathology*. New York: Springer-Verlag, 1990.

13. Longcope, C. Adrenogenital syndrome. *Hosp. Med.* 20:4, 1984.

14. Marsden, P., and McCullagh, A.G. *Endocrinology*. Littleton, Mass.: PSG Publishing Co., 1985.

15. Mazzaferri, E.L. *Textbook of Endocrinology* (3rd ed.). New Hyde Park, N.Y.: Medical Examination, 1986.

16. Mendelsohn, G. Pathology of the adrenal gland. In G. Mendelsohn (ed.), *Diagnosis and Pathology of the Endocrine Diseases*. Philadelphia: J.B. Lippincott, 1988.

17. Metz, R., and Larson, E.B. *Blue Book of Endocrinology*. Philadelphia: W.B. Saunders, 1985.

18. Reus, V.I., and Collu, R. Endocrine effects of stress. In R. Collu, G.M. Brown, and G.R. Van Loon (eds.), *Clinical Neuroendocrinology*. Boston: Blackwell, 1988.

19. Richelin, S.D. Neuroendocrinology. In J.D. Wilson and D.W. Foster (eds.), *Williams' Textbook of Endocrinology* (7th ed.). Philadelphia: W.B. Saunders, 1985.

20. Slaunwhite, W.R. Fuel metabolism. In W.R. Slaunwhite (ed.), *Fundamentals of Endocrinology*. New York: Marcel Dekker, 1988.

21. Sodeman, W.A., and Sodeman, T.M. *Sodeman's Pathologic Physiology: Mechanisms of Disease* (7th ed.). Philadelphia: W.B. Saunders, 1985.

22. Thompson, N.W. Conn's syndrome: Primary aldosteronism. In S.R. Freisen and N.W. Thompson (eds.), *Surgical Endocrinology: Clinical Syndromes* (2nd ed.). Philadelphia: J.B. Lippincott, 1990.

23. Tuck, M.L., and Stern, N. Adrenal disease. In J.M. Hershman (ed.), *Endocrine Pathophysiology: A Patient-Oriented Approach*. Philadelphia: Lea & Febiger, 1988.

24. Tyrell, J.B., Aron, D.C., and Forsham, P.H. Glucocorticoids and adrenal androgens. In F.S. Greenspan (ed.), *Basic and Clinical Endocrinology* (3rd ed.). Norwalk, Conn.: Appleton & Lange, 1991.

25. Williams, G.H., and Dluhy, R.G. Diseases of the adrenal cortex. In E. Braunwald et al. (eds.), *Harrison's Principles of Internal Medicine* (11th ed.). New York: McGraw-Hill, 1987.

26. Wilson, J.D., and Foster, D.W. (eds.). *Williams' Textbook of Endocrinology* (7th ed.). Philadelphia: W.B. Saunders, 1985.

# chapter 38

Camille Stern

# Thyroid and Parathyroid Functions and Alterations

## Learning Objectives

1. Describe the normal anatomy of the thyroid gland.
2. Explain the process by which the thyroid hormones are formed.
3. Identify the function of the iodide pump.
4. Describe the mechanism for releasing and transporting the thyroid hormones.
5. Describe the function of calcitonin.
6. Describe the effects of the thyroid hormones on metabolic processes, carbohydrate metabolism, and vitamin metabolism.
7. Define *goiter*.
8. Identify the clinical manifestations of hyperthyroidism.
9. Outline the autoimmune component of Graves' disease.
10. Relate the signs and symptoms of Graves' disease to underlying pathophysiology.
11. Differentiate between toxic multinodular goiter and toxic adenoma.
12. Identify the clinical manifestations of hypothyroidism.
13. Identify the cause of cretinism.
14. Describe the physical changes and underlying causes of adult hypothyroidism.
15. Compare thyrotoxic crisis and myxedema coma.
16. Identify the common element in chronic autoimmune thyroiditis.

(continued)

17. Differentiate the etiology and symptoms of each of the thyroid carcinomas.
18. Describe the normal anatomy and function of the parathyroid glands.

19. Describe hypoparathyroidism.
20. Identify the two major causes of hyperparathyroidism.
21. Compare the effects of primary, secondary, and tertiary hyperparathyroidism.

---

The thyroid gland is primarily responsible for controlling the rate of metabolic processes in the body. The parathyroid glands control calcium levels and bone resorption. These two glands are related by proximity and, as recently discovered, by function. In this chapter, normal structure and physiology are explored and the major disorders of these glands examined.

## ANATOMY OF THE THYROID GLAND

The primary function of the thyroid gland, the second largest endocrine gland in the human body, is to regulate and control the rate of metabolism. The thyroid is located in the anterior neck, between the larynx and the trachea (Figure 38-1). In the normal thyroid, two lobes lie slightly lateral to the trachea, one on either side, and are connected by a thin band of tissue known as an isthmus. The isthmus lies just below the cricoid cartilage of the trachea. Characteristically, the superior portion of each lobe is somewhat pointed, whereas the inferior portion is rounded and blunt.

The thyroid is reddish and beefy in appearance and has a rubbery texture on palpation. In the average adult, the gland weighs 20 to 30 g. It is enclosed in two layers of connective tissue, with the outer layer being continuous with the cervical fascia of the neck and the inner layer of connective tissue closely adhering to the gland itself.

Thyroid tissue originally develops from the oral epithelium. In an adult, the foramen cecum, a depression on the dorsum of the tongue, points to the location from which thyroid tissue evolved. Rarely, the duct that connects the thyroid and the foramen cecum, known as the *thyroglossal duct,* may remain.

Blood supply to the thyroid arises from two main pairs of arteries. Branching from the external carotid arteries, the superior thyroid arteries enter and supply the upper portions of the lobes. The inferior thyroid arteries, arising from the subclavian arteries, supply the lower portion of the lobes. An estimated 4 to 6 L of blood per hour circulate through the thyroid.

Nervous system control is accomplished primarily from the second to fifth thoracic spinal nerves and through the superior and middle ganglia of the thoraco-lumbar nervous system controls. Cervical ganglia provide the thyroid with adrenergic stimulation, and the vagus nerve provides cholinergic stimulation.

The body of the thyroid is composed of a mass of tiny follicles that are all about equal in size (Figure 38-2). These follicles, or sacs, are each, in effect, separately functioning glands the size of a pinhead. The iodine-accumulating function of each follicle is directly proportional to its individual surface area.[23] Although the sacs do not have outside openings, rich vascular, lymph, and nervous networks surround them, exchanging iodine for hormones. The follicles have a single-layer epithelial lining, and an amorphous, secretory fluid, colloid, fills each sac. The primary component of colloid is a large protein molecule called *thyroglobulin,* from which the thyroid hormones are released.

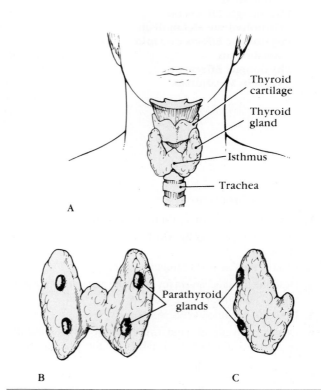

**FIGURE 38–1.**
The thyroid gland. **A.** Anterior view. **B.** Posterior view showing parathyroid gland. **C.** Lateral view.

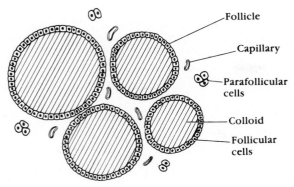

**FIGURE 38–2.**
Follicles of thyroid gland showing colloid filling each sac.

Another distinct cell type in the thyroid gland is the *parafollicular* cell. It has an ovoid and irregular shape, and may be scattered among the other, more numerous thyroid cells.

## PHYSIOLOGY OF THE THYROID GLAND

### Thyroid Iodide Pump

Iodide is essential to the normal function of the thyroid gland. When iodide enters the body through eating or drinking, it is rapidly absorbed into the bloodstream from the gastrointestinal tract within about an hour. Circulating in the blood, iodide is competed for by the thyroid and the kidneys. About two-thirds of the iodide circulating in the bloodstream is excreted in the urine, and the remaining one-third is selectively removed from the blood by the thyroid.

Removal of iodide from the circulation is accomplished by means of an iodide pump or trap. Thyroid-stimulating hormone (TSH) enhances and is most influential in the iodide transport, although other factors also affect the mechanism.[23] The iodide pump normally is able to concentrate iodide to about 25 times greater than the concentration in the blood, but at those times when the thyroid gland becomes maximally active, the concentration can increase to as high as 350 times greater than blood concentration.[5] Once iodide is taken into the thyroid cell, it is oxidized to iodine.[13]

To prevent a basic iodine deficiency, sufficient intake of iodine is necessary. Ingested quantities of iodine vary, depending on the natural content in the soil and water in any given environment and on the intake of iodine-enriched salt and foods. Ordinary table salt contains 1 part sodium iodide to 100,000 parts of sodium chloride.

## Structure and Storage of Thyroid Hormones

The thyroid iodide trap is an active, energy-requiring mechanism. At the beginning of this process, iodine is removed from the circulation in the form of sodium or potassium iodide. It then passes through the follicular cells and into the colloid. The thyroglobulin molecules in the colloid contain an active amino acid, tyrosine, which combines with the iodine in the process of forming the thyroid hormones.

Iodine ions must first undergo a change to an active, elemental form of iodine. This occurs under the influence of the enzyme *peroxidase*. Once iodine is in a simple form, it is able to combine with the tyrosine ring. Active iodine attaches itself to the 3 position of the tyrosine ring to form the molecule *monoiodotyrosine* (MIT). After the formation of MIT, the 5 position of the tyrosine ring becomes iodized. This structure becomes *diiodotyrosine* (DIT) (Figure 38-3).

Two separate combinations of these molecules form the two main thyroid hormones. When two DIT molecules fuse in a coupling reaction, thyroxine ($T_4$) is formed. The fusion of molecules of MIT and DIT form triiodothyronine ($T_3$). Nearly 10 times more $T_4$ than $T_3$ is secreted from the thyroid gland, but as it circulates, some of the $T_4$ deiodinates, making 2 to 3 times as much available to the tissues. $T_3$ is three to five times more active than $T_4$, but the duration of $T_4$ is three to five times longer. The $T_3$ hormone results in increased total ribonucleic acid (RNA) synthesis in some tissues, and specific messenger RNA synthesis increases in others.[20] The overall effect of both hormones is similar, and their functions appear to be identical (see below).[13]

These thyroid hormones are stored in the follicular colloid as part of the thyroglobulin molecule. The thyroid gland is unique in its ability to store hormones in the thyroglobulin molecule. Colloid in the normal thyroid is primarily composed of thyroglobulin molecules. In effect, this is a storage mechanism, which functions if synthesis of the thyroid hormones should cease.

## Release and Transport of Thyroid Hormones

The thyroid hormones are regulated through an extremely complex interaction. The hypothalamus, pituitary, and thyroid glands are part of the interaction, which is further controlled by higher centers in the brain. The major regulator of thyroid hormone secretion is TSH, or thyrotropin, which is a glycoprotein hormone secreted by the anterior pituitary gland. It is thought to be responsive to slight changes in thyroid hormone levels.[17] The release of TSH is mediated by the thyroid-releasing hormone (TRH) from the hypothalamus. This hormone stimu-

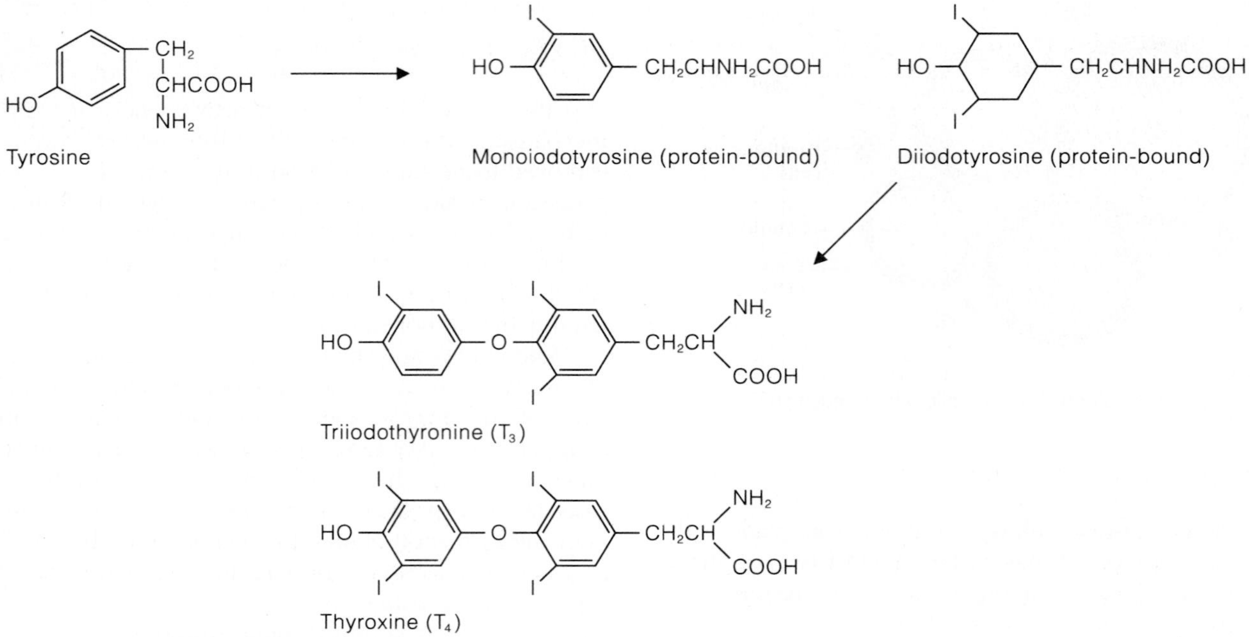

Tyrosine

Monoiodotyrosine (protein-bound)

Diiodotyrosine (protein-bound)

Triiodothyronine (T₃)

Thyroxine (T₄)

**FIGURE 38-3.**
Tyrosine and compounds formed by its iodination in the thyroid gland, including the thyroid hormones triiodothyronine and thyroxine.

lates the synthesis and release of TSH. Thyroid hormones inhibit these functions, thereby exerting influence on the feedback regulation of TSH secretion. The relation of TRH, TSH, and the thyroid hormones exists as a feedback system (Figure 38-4). Whenever $T_3$ and $T_4$ levels become too low in the circulating bloodstream, TRH triggers the release of TSH to increase the secretion of $T_3$ and $T_4$. It accomplishes this by increasing all of the known activities of the thyroid gland cells.[5] As the blood levels of $T_3$ and $T_4$ begin to rise, the anterior pituitary decreases secretion of TSH, thereby decreasing the rate of thyroid hormone production. TSH stimulates an increase in the size and

number of the follicular cells, thereby increasing their ability to absorb iodide.[8] It also increases the breakdown of thyroglobulin, releasing $T_4$ and $T_3$ from the thyroid gland. Through these mechanisms, adequate levels of hormones are maintained in the bloodstream at all times.

When the hormones are needed, an enzymatic reaction splits the thyroglobulin molecule and frees the hormones for entry into the bloodstream. In the blood, $T_4$ and $T_3$ immediately combine with circulating plasma proteins. The affinity of circulating hormones and proteins is so great that the hormones are released to the tissue cells slowly. As the hormones enter the cells, both $T_4$ and $T_3$

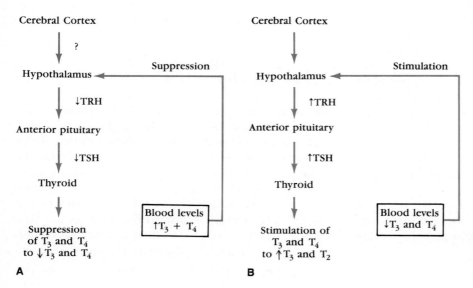

**FIGURE 38-4.**
Feedback system of thyroid hormone secretion. **A.** Suppression to decrease levels. **B.** Stimulation to increase levels.

bind with intracellular proteins, where they are again stored. They are then inside tissue cells and are available to nourish those cells. The hormones have a direct effect on the mitochondria of the cells, resulting in an increased total number and an increased concentration of oxidative enzymes.[8,13] Through these actions, the hormones directly influence cell metabolism and metabolic rate. The thyroid hormones are used within several days to several weeks.

## CALCITONIN: FORMATION AND FUNCTION

In the 1960s, another thyroid hormone, calcitonin, was discovered. Its formation and mechanisms of action are so different that it must be considered separately from $T_4$ and $T_3$. Calcitonin is a large polypeptide that contains 32 amino acids. It is synthesized in the parafollicular, or C, cells of the interstitial tissue between the follicular cells of the thyroid.[5]

Calcitonin has a direct effect on bone tissue by counteracting hypercalcemia. Increased serum calcium levels stimulate the release of this hormone from the thyroid gland. Once released, it inhibits bone reabsorption, thus inhibiting the rate of release of calcium from bone tissue to plasma. This process causes a reduction in blood calcium levels. The action of calcitonin is essentially the reverse action of the parathyroid hormone. Whereas the action of parathyroid hormone is long-acting and continually maintains constant levels of circulating calcium, calcitonin only begins to act when there is excess calcium in the blood. It does not block parathyroid hormone or prevent its release. Calcitonin merely exerts an opposite action on both bone and kidneys. Bone reabsorption by osteoclasts is inhibited, and in response to calcitonin, the loop of Henle allows calcium to be filtered out and excreted in urine.

## FUNCTION OF THE THYROID HORMONES

### Physiologic Effects on Metabolic Processes

Because the thyroid hormones are carried to all body tissues, their effects are widespread and varied. They exert influence over all major body systems, as well as the most intricate of cell functions. Their major influence is to increase basal metabolic rate (BMR), which is heat production and energy expenditure in the body. A test to measure BMR is actually a measurement of oxygen consumption. Several nonthyroid factors can affect the usefulness of this test.

The BMR rises during periods of increased hormone production and secretion, thus increasing energy expenditure and heat production. When this occurs, the effect of calorigenesis—the use of food for energy—also is increased. Calorigenesis increases the consumption of oxygen by the body.

### Physiologic Effects on Protein Metabolism

The thyroid hormones increase protein synthesis, and thus are essential for normal growth and development in children and young adults. They also stimulate the synthesis of many enzymes and hormones.[20] When fat and carbohydrate stores have been depleted, proteins may be used for energy. This protein depletion results in a negative nitrogen balance. It is not clear whether this is a direct result of the thyroid hormone or caused by a negative caloric balance.[23] Releasing proteins also releases amino acids, making them available for energy, and increases the rate of gluconeogenesis.

### Physiologic Effects on Carbohydrate Metabolism

Thyroid hormones affect virtually every function of carbohydrate metabolism. They are responsible for increasing the rate of gluconeogenesis, rapid cellular uptake of glucose, increasing intestinal absorption of glucose and galactose, and increasing the rate of glucose uptake by adipose tissue.

Especially in carbohydrate metabolism, thyroid hormones are interactive with or dependent on other hormones. Insulin secretion is increased, which also enhances carbohydrate metabolism.

### Physiologic Effects on Lipid Metabolism

Thyroid hormones essentially stimulate all aspects of lipid or fatty metabolism. The major result of their influence is depletion of fat storage, especially of lipids. This leads to increased plasma concentration levels of free fatty acids. Serum cholesterol, however, is lowered by the action of thyroid hormones, probably because of increased intestinal excretion and conversion of cholesterol into bile acids.

### Physiologic Effects on Vitamin Metabolism

Because thyroid hormones increase the rate of metabolic processes, they increase the physiologic need for vitamins. Because many vitamins contain enzymes or coenzymes, increased secretion of thyroid hormones causes depletion of vitamins because of the liberation of enzymes, unless the intake of vitamins by ingestion is increased.

## ALTERED THYROID FUNCTION

### Goiter

The presence of a goiter, or enlarged thyroid gland, is not necessarily indicative of thyroid dysfunction, but may demonstrate insufficient iodine intake.[13] Goiters may appear in states of hypofunction as well as hyperfunction.[13] The gland enlarges in an attempt to produce sufficient amounts of thyroid hormones. Various types of disorders can alter the size and state of the thyroid (Figure 38-5). Without the presence of identifiable clinical manifestations, an enlarged thyroid gland is referred to as a *nontoxic goiter*.

### Hyperthyroidism

Hyperthyroidism, also known as *thyrotoxicosis*, is characterized by increased $T_3$ and $T_4$ production, often 5 to 15 times normal rates, resulting in an excess amount of thyroid hormones that are circulated to the tissues. Hyperthyroidism may be related entirely to disease of the thyroid, or it may originate from outside the thyroid. Exogenous hyperthyroidism is most commonly caused by self-medication with thyroid hormone drugs.[21] In years past, thyroid was prescribed for weight loss through increased BMR, and still is taken for weight loss, even though the side effects can be severe. Hyperthyroidism

may be permanent or temporary, mild or severe. The severity of the disease may be affected by the person's age, duration of hyperthyroid function, and presence of other disease processes in any other organ systems. Thirty to 40% of all cases of thyrotoxicosis occur in people over age 60.[10] It is much more common in women than in men, with an estimated incidence rate of 2 to 3 per 1000 women.[21]

Because of the increased amount of thyroid hormones reaching the cells, all metabolic activities are accelerated. Thus, BMR rises, energy expenditure is increased, and heat production rises.

### Clinical Manifestations

The clinical manifestations of hyperthyroidism are varied, and may arise in any major organ system (Figure 38-6). One of the primary features is a palpable goiter or growth of a preexisting goiter. The skin becomes flushed, warm, and moist. Hair tends to be fine and breaks easily; in some instances, hair is lost. Nails of the fingers and toes break easily and often separate from the beds.

Hyperthyroidism often causes a stare. This is due to upper eyelid retraction, and frequently occurs with thyrotoxicosis. Movements of the eyelids are jerky and irregular. Most people with hyperthyroidism develop some *exophthalmos*, protrusion of the eyeballs that may cause difficulty in closing the eyelids. The causes of exophthalmos are edematous swelling of the retroorbital tissues and degenerative changes in the muscles that control the eye.[5]

Cardiovascular system changes are pronounced because of the increased metabolic demands on the heart. Pronounced tachycardia always is present, even during sleep. Systolic blood pressure often rises.[15] Palpitations occur because of the increased force of cardiac contrac-

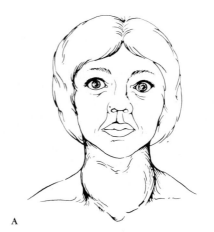
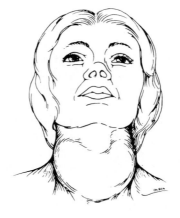
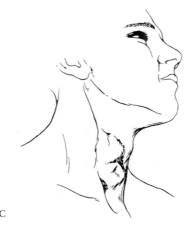

A                    B                    C

**FIGURE 38-5.**
Thyroid abnormalities. **A.** Diffuse toxic goiter (Graves' disease) with exophthalmos. **B.** Diffuse nontoxic goiter. **C.** Nodular goiter. (From R.D. Judge, G.D. Zuidema, and F.T. Fitzgerald [eds.], *Clinical Diagnosis* [4th ed.]. Boston: Little, Brown, 1982.)

**PHYSIOLOGY**

**TRH** = thyrotropin-releasing
hormone
**TSH** = thyroid-stimulating
hormone
$T_3$ = triiodothyronine
$T_4$ = thyroxine

**PATHOPHYSIOLOGY**
Diffuse enlargement of the thyroid
Graves' disease
Activity similar to that of thyroid-stimulating hormone
Choriocarcinoma
Hydatidiform mole
Hepatoma (rare)
Pituitary adenoma secreting thyroid-stimulating hormone
Nodular, enlarged thyroid
Graves' disease
Toxic multinodular goiter (Plummer's disease)
Toxic uninodular goiter (functional thyroid adenoma)
Tender, enlarged thyroid
Subacute thyroiditis
Hashimoto's thyroiditis (occasionally tender)
Irradiation thyroiditis
Iodine thyroiditis (jodbasedow) (occasionally tender)
Nonpalpable thyroid
Factitious hyperthyroidism—excessive ingestion of thyroid hormone
Struma ovarii
Metastatic thyroid carcinoma
Normal gland (may be nonpalpable)

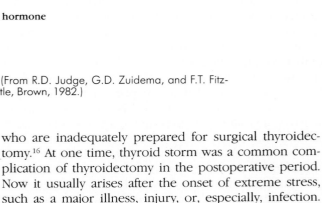

**FIGURE 38-6.**

Hyperthyroidism: Physiology and pathophysiology. (From R.D. Judge, G.D. Zuidema, and F.T. Fitzgerald [eds.], *Clinical Diagnosis* [4th ed.]. Boston: Little, Brown, 1982.)

tions. Atrial or supraventricular dysrhythmias are not uncommon. Most people who have no underlying or preexisting cardiac failure can maintain the increased rate of cardiovascular function required. Hyperthyroidism eventually may precipitate congestive heart failure, however.

Changes in nervous system function are indicated by increasing restlessness and nervousness, decreased attention span, and the need to be almost constantly in motion, even though fatigue occurs rapidly. Afflicted people also become emotionally labile, having bursts of temper and rapid mood changes.

In the gastrointestinal system, increased appetite is apparent, but there usually is associated weight loss. Increased food intake may be insufficient to meet the increased metabolic demands, and there also may be complaints of nausea, vomiting, or diarrhea. The affected person usually is thin, even emaciated.

Other systemic changes may become apparent. Dyspnea occurs during periods of increased physical activity. Mild polyuria, heat intolerance, excessive perspiration, and increased susceptibility to infection may be manifested.

### Thyroid Storm

Thyrotoxic crisis, or thyroid storm, is an uncommon but life-threatening complication of hyperthyroidism. It may occur in people with untreated hyperthyroidism or those

who are inadequately prepared for surgical thyroidectomy.[16] At one time, thyroid storm was a common complication of thyroidectomy in the postoperative period. Now it usually arises after the onset of extreme stress, such as a major illness, injury, or, especially, infection. Other medical causes include trauma, diabetic ketoacidosis, toxemia of pregnancy or labor, and premature discontinuation of antithyroid therapy.[9]

The symptoms of thyroid storm result from a sudden increase in thyroid hormone levels in the bloodstream, resulting in a marked increase in all of the clinical manifestations of hyperthyroidism. The hallmark is considered to be uncontrolled fever of 100° to 106°F. Other hypermetabolic symptoms include profuse diaphoresis, shock, vomiting, and dehydration. Central nervous system symptoms also may be exacerbated, including hyperkinesis, anxiety, and confusion.[16] The physiologic effects of the hypermetabolic processes are so devastating to the body tissues that those in crisis must receive immediate intervention or death rapidly ensues. Treatment should include aggressive antithyroid drug therapy and measures to reduce the high fever.

### Graves' Disease

The most common and well-known form of hyperthyroidism is Graves' disease, also known as exophthalmic goiter, diffuse toxic goiter, Basedow's disease, and primary hyperthyroidism. It is not simply a disease of the thyroid, but a multisystem syndrome that may include major manifestations of hyperthyroidism, diffuse thyroid enlargement, infiltrative ophthalmopathy, infiltrative dermopathy, and generalized lymphoid hyperplasia. These features may occur individually or in any combination.

Graves' disease may occur at any age but primarily strikes those between ages 30 and 50. Women have the disease more frequently than men, and more than one member of the same family often is affected.

It is now accepted that there is an autoimmune component to this disease. The T lymphocytes become sensitized to antigens within the thyroid gland and stimulate the B lymphocytes to synthesize antibodies to these antigens.[4] In the 1950s, a substance was discovered in the serum of many people with Graves' disease. It was an immunoglobulin G1, later called *long-acting thyroid stimulator*. This antibody is now referred to as thyroid-stimulating immunoglobulin.[4] It has all of the functions of TSH, but the effects are longer lasting and are not subject to the control of rising levels of thyroid hormones in the blood. In nearly every person with untreated Graves' disease, this antibody is detected. More recently a thyroid-stimulating autoantibody has been found to be the functional analogue to TSH, binding so strongly to TSH-receptor sites that it can prevent the binding of TSH.[22] Because the autoantibody is not under feedback control, thyroid hypersecretion results. The exact mechanism is not clearly understood.

Heredity and genetic factors also are accepted contributors to the development of Graves' disease. This form of hyperthyroidism frequently occurs in more than one family member, and may affect several generations of the same family. Thus genetic and autoimmune components are of major influence. It also has been suggested that severe emotional stress may be a factor, since the disease frequently arises after severe emotional or physical trauma.

The outstanding clinical features of Graves' disease are diffuse and palpable goiter, unilateral or bilateral exophthalmos, pretibial myxedema, and signs of hypermetabolism, or thyrotoxicosis.[13,23] The onset of symptoms usually is gradual. Complaints of nervousness, irritability, fatigue, heat intolerance, and weight loss are common. These symptoms are a result of the increased metabolic rate.

The thyroid gland is enlarged to two to three times the normal size in most cases. It may, however, be massively enlarged or remain near normal size. Enlargement usually is symmetric, and the surface is smooth.

Exophthalmos, the most common ocular change, normally is accompanied by periorbital edema. The person has a characteristic bulging, wide-eyed stare. The eye musculature often is so affected that the cornea and sclera are damaged because of an inability to close the eyes. In most cases, exophthalmos gradually disappears

with treatment of the hyperthyroidism. Infiltrative ophthalmopathy is a more serious and extensive involvement, and may cause permanent changes in eye function. It also may cause especially difficult problems in treatment.

Infiltrative dermopathy, commonly called *pretibial myxedema*, is a rare but dramatic manifestation that affects the pretibial area of one or both legs, causing a barklike appearance of the skin. Localized edema and swelling of the skin and subcutaneous tissues occur. Hyaluronic acid accumulates in the interstitial spaces and, combining with water, forms edema that is boggy and nonpitting. Persons having pretibial myxedema have a profound immunologic disruption, and it is thought that these dermatologic changes are a direct result of that immunologic reaction.[13]

## Toxic Multinodular Goiter

In some people with a longstanding history of nontoxic goiter, hyperthyroidism may appear insidiously. This disorder is known as toxic multinodular goiter, or *Plummer's disease*. Women over age 50 most frequently are affected. The origin of the mechanism that causes nontoxic goiter to become toxic is not known.

The clinical manifestations are mild in comparison to Graves' disease. Thyrotoxicosis signs are less prominent, and serum thyroxine levels are only marginally elevated. Cardiovascular symptoms are the most pronounced. Atrial fibrillation, tachycardia, and congestive heart failure may develop. Also apparent are muscle weakening and fatigue. It often is difficult to diagnose toxic multinodular goiter because of its slow onset. The signs and symptoms may be attributed to lethargy and aging.

## Toxic Adenoma

Toxic adenoma is a less common form of hyperthyroidism. It usually results from the development of a follicular adenoma. These adenomas are subdivided according to the size of the follicles into macrofollicular, microfollicular, and embryonal varieties.[23] It may occur in pairs or triplets. The function of the adenoma may be more or less than that of normal thyroid gland tissue, but it secretes thyroid hormone without the stimulation of TSH.

As the adenoma grows, it begins to take over the function of normal thyroid tissue. Without intervention, complete atrophy and suppression of the remainder of the thyroid gland eventually occurs.[23] The adenoma must reach the size of 2 to 3 cm before it is capable of producing a state of hyperthyroidism. The lesion may undergo necrosis and hemorrhage of its center. If this occurs, symptoms of thyrotoxicosis recede, and the remainder of the thyroid gland tissue resumes normal functioning.

Most persons affected with toxic adenoma are in the 30- to 40-year age range and usually have a history of a lump in the neck that has been growing slowly for many years. Clinical features are not pronounced; cardiovascular symptoms are probably the most prominent.

## Hypothyroidism

Hypothyroidism is the result of a deficiency of thyroid hormone, leading to a decreased rate of body metabolism and a general slowing down of body processes. Any of the following factors may contribute to the onset of hypothyroidism: hypothalamic dysfunction, TRH or TSH deficiency, pituitary disorders, specific idiopathies, thyroid deficiencies, and thyroid destruction.[2] The degree of dysfunction is related to the relative amount of hormone deficiency in the tissues. Hypothyroidism is fairly common, and is recognized as an underdiagnosed health problem, particularly in the elderly.[12]

### Clinical Manifestations

Changes in the skin occur with hypothyroidism when hyaluronic acid binds with water. The combination produces the characteristic baggy, full, edematous skin. Edema is most apparent in the face, hands, and feet. The skin is pale, cool, and dry. Wounds or breaks in the skin heal slowly.

Cardiovascular symptoms may closely resemble those of congestive heart failure. Cardiac output is decreased, as are heart rate and circulating blood volume. Peripheral vascular resistance is increased, ultimately resulting in decreased flow of blood to the tissues. The term *myxedema heart* refers to the clinical picture of an enlarged heart, with electrocardiographic and serum enzyme changes.

The gastrointestinal tract, together with other body functions, slows down under the influence of a hypothyroid state. Most persons have a decreased appetite and, contrary to popular belief, only a slight increase in weight. Decreased peristalsis leads to an accumulation of gas and complaints of constipation.

Hypothyroid effect on the nervous system also decreases function. Thinking and movement begin to slow down. Mental dullness often is apparent. Personality changes may occur, resulting in severe depression or extreme agitation and anxiety. Movements are slow and disorganized, causing the appearance of clumsiness.

Other body system changes also result from hypothyroidism. Muscle pains are common, and strength decreases. Reduced renal blood flow and glomerular filtration contribute to the cardiovascular changes. Anemia and changes in clotting factors occur. In both sexes, hypothyroidism decreases sexual drive.

Exactly the opposite of hyperthyroidism, hypothyroidism causes decreased thyroid function and reduced energy metabolism, resulting in a lower metabolic rate.

Protein synthesis and degradation are reduced, resulting in retarded growth of bone and muscle tissue. Glucose absorption from the stomach and intestines is delayed, resulting in delayed insulin time. As with protein, the synthesis and degradation of lipids are decreased. The net result is a decreased rate of energy metabolism.

### Cretinism

Thyroid hormone deficiency during embryonic and neonatal life results in a state known as cretinism in infants and young children. This deficiency is not readily apparent at birth, and it may take several weeks to several months before hypothyroidism is discovered. The infant becomes sluggish and falls behind the normal rate of growth and development. Mental retardation and delayed growth patterns are characteristic.

Cretins are dwarflike. Their arms and legs are short in relation to the trunk (Figure 38-7). The face of a cretin is broad and puffy, and the teeth usually are malformed; the skin is coarse and dry with sparse hair. The abdomen is protuberant, which often results in umbilical hernias.

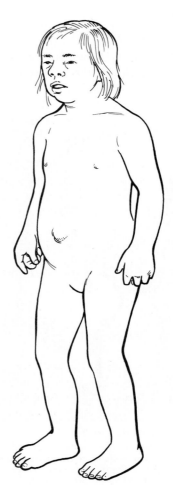

**FIGURE 38-7.**
Cretinism caused by hypothyroidism.

Early recognition and treatment reverse the effects of hypothyroidism in an infant, preventing the onset and development of cretinism.

## Endemic Goiter

The term endemic goiter refers to an enlargement of the thyroid gland to twice normal size or larger in at least 10% of the area population.[7] In some areas of the world, an iodine deficiency exists in the environment to the degree that goiters may be common among the people dwelling in that region. The term *endemic goiter* refers to such an area and population. The Great Lakes region of the United States and mountainous areas of other countries, such as the Swiss Alps, are noted for iodine deficiency of their soil and water (Figure 38-8).

Because of the lack of iodine, the thyroid cannot synthesize $T_4$ and $T_3$, resulting in decreased serum levels of thyroid hormones. Secretion of TSH is increased, and the thyroid gland becomes hyperplastic, leading to the formation of a goiter that is the attempt by the gland to produce thyroid hormones.

## Adult Hypothyroidism

Severe hypothyroidism in the adult often is called *myxedema*. Its onset is slow and may not be recognized for many years. Primary adult hypothyroidism results from the loss or destruction of thyroid gland tissue. This may be caused by an autoimmune or disease process within the thyroid or removal of the gland, or it may occur after treatment for Graves' disease. Secondary hypothyroidism results from pituitary TSH insufficiency, usually because of a lesion in the pituitary gland.

Early symptoms of adult hypothyroidism are fatigue and lethargy. A goiter may be present, which indicates an attempt to compensate for the deficiency.[13] Marked sensitivity to cold temperatures occurs, as well as gradual slowing of mental and physical function. These progress through the course of the disease. The skin, hair, and nails become dry, with the hair and nails becoming brittle and breaking easily. The muscles and joints are stiff and aching, especially in the morning after waking. Slight weight gain often is noted despite decreased appetite.

As the clinical signs and symptoms continue to develop, the full picture of myxedema may appear (Figure 38-9). Thickness, especially in the face, hands, and feet, becomes apparent, caused by the same process that results in pretibial myxedema in the person with Graves' disease. The voice becomes hoarse and the tongue thickens. The body temperature is lower than normal, resulting in mild hypothermia. Finally, mental and physical lethargy progress to extremes. If untreated, this process will continue for many years.

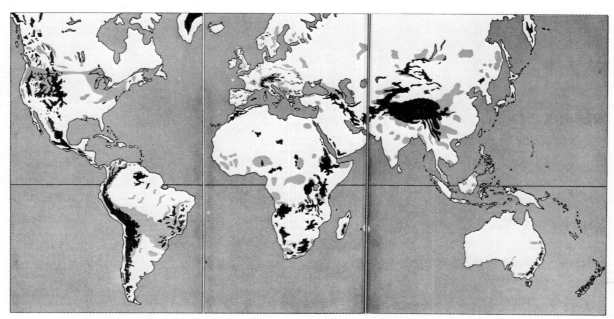

**FIGURE 38-8.**

Regions of endemic goiter and the mountainous terrain with which it often is associated were mapped by the World Health Organization. Areas where iodine-deficiency goiter is endemic are shown in gray. Populations near sea-coasts are seldom affected because of the iodine content of seafood. Not all inland areas are equally affected; the geology and remoteness of mountainous regions (solid black) make them most susceptible. (Illustration by Robin Ingle. From "Endemic Goiter" by Bruce Gillie. © 1974 by Scientific American Inc. June 1971, Vol. 2246.)

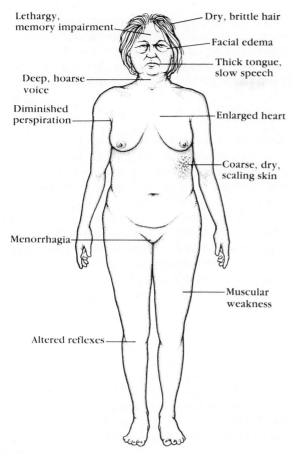

Lethargy, memory impairment

Dry, brittle hair

Facial edema

Thick tongue, slow speech

Deep, hoarse voice

Diminished perspiration

Enlarged heart

Coarse, dry, scaling skin

Menorrhagia

Muscular weakness

Altered reflexes

**FIGURE 38–9.**
A composite of the symptoms of myxedema. (From M. Beyers and S. Dudas, *The Clinical Practice of Medical Surgical Nursing* [2nd ed.]. Boston: Little, Brown, 1984.)

## Sick Euthyroid Syndrome

A clinical condition that may occur in acutely or chronically ill people has been called the sick euthyroid syndrome.[17,23] The common finding is depressed $T_3$ and $T_4$ levels, deficient enough to be well within the definition of hypothyroidism. Sick euthyroid syndrome is distinct from primary hypothyroidism, however, in that the TSH levels are not elevated. The TSH response to TRH may be slightly elevated but not above the normal range.[17]

Sick euthyroid syndrome is rather common in intensive care units after a variety of illnesses and disorders such as surgery, myocardial infarction, renal insufficiency, ketoacidosis, cirrhosis, thermal injury, and other critical problems.[17] Therefore, it is important that this problem be differentiated from true thyroid disease as quickly as possible.

## Myxedema Coma

Myxedema coma is a medical emergency in persons with hypothyroidism. The comatose state is the most severe expression of profound hypothyroid function.[15,18] It usually occurs during the winter months, and affects mostly elderly myxedematous persons. Any stress, such as extreme cold, trauma, infection, central nervous system depressants, or physical stress, may precipitate this crisis. Myxedema coma also may occur as the end stage of adult hypothyroidism.[14] Lethargy progresses to coma, with hypotension and hypothermia on examination. Hypothermia is considered the most characteristic symptom. The coma results from a continuous slowing of the vital centers; the respiratory center becomes more depressed, cardiac output continues to drop, and cerebral hypoxia increases as a result. Other changes include hypotension, bradycardia, hypoventilation with respiratory acidosis, and carbon dioxide narcosis, together with various fluid and electrolyte disorders.[9] Without intervention, the mortality is as much as 50%.

Although myxedema coma is quite rare now, its frequency may increase in the future because of the increasing use of radioiodine for the treatment of Graves' disease. Reaction to radioiodine may result in permanent hypothyroidism.[4]

## Chronic Autoimmune Thyroiditis

The chronic autoimmune form of thyroiditis, also known as *Hashimoto's disease*, primarily occurs in women aged 30 to 50, but it may occur at any age and is thought to be a major cause of hypothyroidism in children.[23] The two most characteristic findings are a large, palpable goiter and high levels of circulating autoantibodies.

The goiter results from defects of hormone biosynthesis in the thyroid. Because of the failure to produce adequate hormone levels, the pituitary produces TSH abundantly. The result is a goiter without clinical evidence of thyrotoxicosis. Chronic autoimmune thyroiditis may lead to hyperthyroidism, but usually results in thyroid hypofunction.

The thyroid gland enlarges very gradually. The goiter becomes firm and rubbery and usually is minimally tender, although extreme pain can occur. When left untreated, the gland will continue to enlarge over the years.

There often is a family history of chronic autoimmune thyroiditis, or a history of family members with Graves' disease, nontoxic goiter, or primary hypothyroidism. Also, families may show an increased frequency for other autoimmune disorders, such as rheumatoid arthritis and pernicious anemia.

## Nontoxic Goiter

Sometimes the thyroid gland enlarges without evidence of alterations in rate of body metabolism. This is termed a *nontoxic*, or simple, goiter. It commonly occurs at puberty, during adolescence, or during pregnancy. This disorder occurs in 10% of all North American women.[13]

Several causes may be responsible for the goiter, such as iodine deficiency or genetic enzymatic defects. They result in a decreased rate of production of thyroid hormones, which in turn results in increased secretion of TSH from the pituitary. Hyperplasia of thyroid tissue occurs in compensation, and in mild cases, there usually is no clinical evidence of alteration in function. If thyroid hypertrophy is severe, there may be signs of hyperthyroidism. The only clinical evidence usually is the enlarged, palpable thyroid.

## Malignant Thyroid Tumors

Carcinoma of the thyroid gland is not common, and accounts for only a small percentage of the total number of diagnoses of cancer. No existing evidence supports a familial tendency or predisposition to thyroid carcinoma other than the parafollicular type. It has been shown that radiation therapy in childhood dramatically increases the risk of at least two forms of thyroid carcinoma.

### Papillary Carcinoma

Papillary carcinoma originates in the papillary cells of the thyroid, and is the most common type of thyroid cancer, accounting for about 70% to 80% of all thyroid cancers.[19] It is most frequent in children and young adults and especially affects women. Radiation exposure in childhood contributes to the causation of this cancer. It is a slow-growing cancer, and may remain in the gland for many years. The first indication may be a palpable node in the thyroid or enlarged lymph nodes in the neck region. Metastasis can occur through the lymphatics to other areas of the thyroid or, in some cases, to the lungs.

### Follicular Carcinoma

Follicular carcinoma, as the name implies, originates in the follicular cells, and accounts for 10% to 20% of thyroid carcinomas.[19] It affects an older population, usually over age 40; it occurs in women two to three times more frequently than in men. Childhood exposure to radiation increases the risk of this cancer. The initial feature is an asymptomatic thyroid nodule that exhibits slow patterns of growth. This tumor is more invasive than the papillary carcinoma, and may spread through the area blood vessels. Common sites of metastasis are the lungs and bones.

### Anaplastic Carcinoma

Anaplastic carcinoma is a highly malignant form, and accounts for about 10% of thyroid cancers. The tumors usually arise in the seventh to eighth decade of life.[3] It is slightly more common in women than in men. Metastasis occurs rapidly, first to the surrounding areas and then to all parts of the body. The person initially may complain

of a mass in the region of the thyroid. As the cancer involves structures adjacent to the thyroid, hoarseness, stridor, and difficulty swallowing may occur. Tracheal deviation and tumor ulceration may develop.[8] Life expectancy after diagnosis usually is only several months.

### Parafollicular Carcinoma

Parafollicular, or medullary, carcinoma is unique among the thyroid cancers. Only a small number of cases are related to this type. It affects women more than men and is most common in those past age 50. Parafollicular carcinoma also metastasizes quickly, often to distant sites of the body, such as the lungs, bones, and liver. Its distinctive feature is its ability to secrete calcitonin because of its origin in the parafollicular cells.[19] This carcinoma frequently has familial tendencies, and may be associated with multiple endocrine neoplasia (see Chap. 37).

## THE PARATHYROID GLANDS

### Anatomy

The parathyroid glands, four in number, lie posterior and adjacent to the thyroid gland. There is one parathyroid gland in each superior and inferior lateral area of the thyroid. Each gland is small, about the size of a pea, and their combined total weight is about 120 mg. The glands are reddish brown or yellowish brown, and each is enclosed in a small fibrous capsule (see Figure 38-1).

There are two cell types in the parathyroid gland—the *oxyphil cell* and the *chief*, or principal, *cell*. Oxyphil cells are slightly larger but are not actually engaged in the secretion of hormones and do not have a known function.[3] Chief cells are responsible for producing and secreting parathyroid hormone (Figure 38-10).

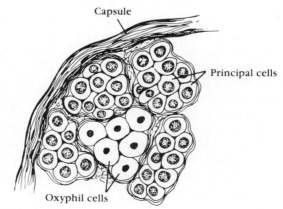

**FIGURE 38-10.**

Parathyroid glands. The cells are arranged in cords by loose connective tissue. The principal cells are predominant in number. Oxyphil cells are recognized by their smaller, more condensed nuclei and larger relative cytoplasmic volume. (From M. Borysenko, et al. *Functional Histology* [2nd ed.]. Boston: Little, Brown, 1984.)

## *Function*

The parathyroid glands regulate the serum levels of calcium in the body and control the rate of bone metabolism. Vitamin D and calcitonin also affect calcium metabolism. The parathyroid glands secrete *parathyroid hormone* (*parathormone* or *PTH*). Secretion of this hormone is not under the control of the pituitary gland, but is directly regulated by a negative feedback system of the circulating blood levels of calcium. Therefore, as calcium levels fall, more PTH is secreted; as calcium levels rise, hormone secretion is reduced. Almost any factor that reduces serum calcium levels stimulates the release of PTH (Figure 38-11A).[13]

Vitamin D is obtained through dietary ingestion of foods with a high content of the vitamin and through synthesis in the skin. Foods that contain vitamin D include milk products and fish-liver oils. Many vitamin D-enriched foods also are available. Vitamin D synthesized in the skin is known as calciferol, and is activated on direct exposure to sunlight. Vitamin D is essential for calcium absorption from the intestinal tract into the bloodstream. It also increases retention of calcium and phosphorus and controls the mineralization of bone matrix. Thus, it is important in controlling and maintaining circulating levels of calcium.[13]

*Calcitonin*, or thyrocalcitonin, which is produced and secreted by the parafollicular cells of the thyroid gland, opposes the action of PTH and lowers blood calcium levels. Serum calcium levels are decreased when

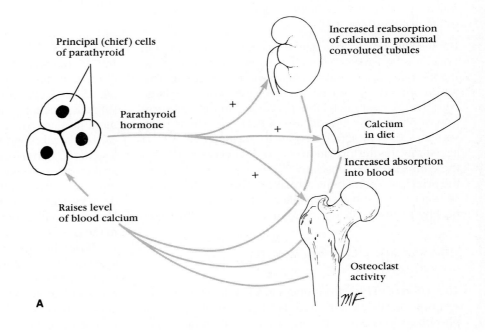

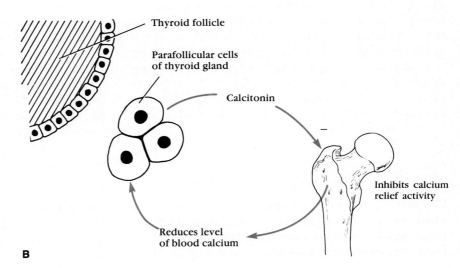

**FIGURE 38-11.**
**A.** Regulation of the parathyroid gland.
**B.** Regulation of calcitonin secretion by the parafollicular cells of the thyroid gland.

calcium circulating in the blood is transferred back to the bones (Figure 38-11B). Although the physiologic role of calcitonin is not clear, and almost certainly minor, calcitonin secretion is stimulated by a rise in serum calcium.[6]

To maintain calcium levels, PTH acts on bones, kidneys, and intestines to resorb calcium. Some of calcium's most important effects are (1) to increase plasma calcium concentration and decrease plasma phosphate concentration; (2) to increase urinary excretion of phosphate but decrease urinary excretion of calcium; (3) to increase the rate of skeletal remodeling and the net rate of bone reabsorption; (4) to increase the number of osteoblasts and osteoclasts on bone surfaces; (5) to cause an initial increase in calcium entry into the cells of its target tissues; (6) to alter the acid-base balance of the body; and (7) to increase gastrointestinal absorption of calcium.[23]

### Effect of Parathyroid Hormone on Bone Reabsorption

Because the greatest storage of calcium in the body is in bone, it is here that PTH has its greatest effect on increasing the rate of metabolic breakdown of bone tissue. This action primarily is exerted on osteoclasts, which are large cells with several nuclei that participate in the reabsorption of bone.[5] After the release of PTH, osteoclasts reabsorb an area of mineralized bone to release calcium. PTH also stimulates the formation of new osteoclasts and delays the conversion of osteoclasts into osteoblasts, which are the principal cells of bone formation. The overall strength of bone is not substantially altered by this process in a healthy person with normally functioning parathyroids.

### Effect of Parathyroid Hormone on Kidney Reabsorption

The action of PTH on the kidneys involves increased reabsorption of calcium ions and decreased reabsorption of phosphate ions. These actions occur at different sites in the kidneys and by different mechanisms. Decreased reabsorption of phosphate is due to the effect of PTH directly on tubular absorption, and the increase in calcium reabsorption is due to a direct effect on the distal convoluted tubule. In early research, the effect of PTH on the tubular absorption of phosphate was considered the primary and most important role. Now, it is recognized that this action is secondary to the hormone's role in bone reabsorption of calcium.

### Effect of Parathyroid Hormone on Intestinal Reabsorption

PTH also influences the reabsorption of calcium from the small intestine. It is necessary for activated vitamin D to be present for this process to occur. Reabsorption of calcium from the intestines also increases absorption of calcium phosphate, thus decreasing the amount of phosphate elimination.

## ALTERED FUNCTION OF THE PARATHYROID GLAND

### Hypoparathyroidism

Hypoparathyroidism results when insufficient amounts of PTH are secreted, or when the hormone fails to act at the tissue level. Without circulating PTH, calcium is not resorbed from bone, kidneys, or intestines. The result is a decreased serum concentration of calcium. This in turn causes increased neuromuscular excitability and the symptoms of tetany. Therefore, all of the clinical manifestations result from decreased levels of serum calcium concentration.

### Clinical Manifestations

In 70% of cases of hypoparathyroidism, tetany becomes the major clinical manifestation.[23] It begins with numbness and tingling of the extremities and progresses to stiffness, cramps, and spasms. Carpal spasms are common, and are the most prominent symptoms. If serum calcium levels continue to fall, the neuromuscular manifestations become more severe and pronounced. Laryngeal muscles are susceptible to spasms, and death by asphyxiation can result if intervention is not immediate. At the very least, wheezing caused by bronchospasm occurs. Hypocalcemia seldom presents as an acute crisis, except in the postoperative period.[1]

When hypoparathyroidism exists for several months to several years, other physical changes may become apparent. Nails become brittle and may atrophy, and horizontal ridges are apparent on the surface. These persons often experience alopecia in patches on the head and almost complete loss of eyebrows. The skin becomes coarse and dry with patches of brownish pigment. Papilledema often is present, and may occur with increased intracranial pressure. The electrocardiogram of hypocalcemia may show a lengthening of the Q-T interval. Serum calcium levels fall and remain subnormal. Sometimes personality changes and psychiatric symptoms occur, such as emotional lability, extreme irritability and anxiety, depression, and delirium. Convulsions and grand mal seizures may occur.

Three clinical signs are used to diagnose tetany and hypoparathyroidism. (1) The first test is for a positive Chvostek's sign. A quick tap or light blow over the parotid gland near the ear produces twitching of the facial muscles, especially the upper lip, nose, and eye. (2) Trousseau's sign is elicited by occluding blood supply to the arm for 3 minutes. The result is positive when carpopedal spasms occur (Figure 38-12). (3) Erb's sign is

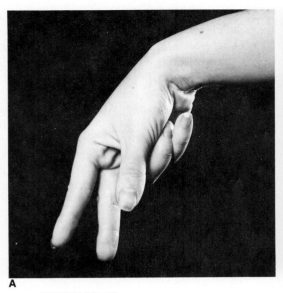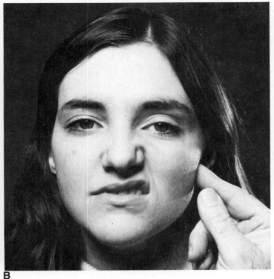

**FIGURE 38–12.**
Diagnostic signs of hypoparathyroidism. **A.** Carpopedal spasm in Trousseau's sign. **B.** Facial muscle contraction in Chvostek's sign. (From M. Beyers and S. Dudas, *The Clinical Practice of Medical Surgical Nursing* [2nd ed.]. Boston: Little, Brown, 1984.)

considered positive when a 6-mV current produces a motor response. Specific positive responses to any of these clinical signs usually is considered diagnostic.

### Idiopathic Hypoparathyroidism

Idiopathic hypoparathyroidism is relatively uncommon. The course of dysfunction is variable. It may be congenital or acquired, mild or severe, transient or lifelong. The congenital form is related to defective or absent parathyroid glands. Children are most commonly diagnosed, with females being affected twice as often as males. It is widely suspected that an autoimmune state may be related to the idiopathic form. The symptoms, including tetany, usually are severe.

### Postoperative Hypoparathyroidism

More common than the idiopathic form, hypoparathyroidism may be related to damage or removal of the parathyroid glands during thyroid surgery. Removing the thyroid gland without detaching the parathyroids is the most frequent cause. Any surgery that involves manipulation of the structures of the throat, such as radical neck dissection, can result in clinical features of hypoparathyroidism.

With damage or partial removal, the remaining parathyroid tissue usually is able to compensate. Thus, the loss of PTH is transient. Complete removal of the glands would result in total loss of parathyroid function, and severe hypocalcemia would rapidly follow.

### Pseudohypoparathyroidism

Pseudohypoparathyroidism, also known as *Albright's hereditary osteodystrophy*, is a form of hypoactive functioning that is familial in origin. It is widely believed to be transmitted by an X-linked dominant gene. Hypocalcemia and hypophosphatemia are characteristic of this disorder. The parathyroid glands are normal in size or slightly enlarged, and there is no deficit in circulating levels of PTH. Women are affected twice as frequently as men.

These persons have developmental skeletal abnormalities and usually exhibit a mild to moderate degree of mental retardation. They are short and stocky, often less than 5 ft tall, and usually obese. The face is very round because of structural abnormalities in the development of the facial and cranial bones. The metacarpal bones are short and stubby. There normally is some degree of widespread subcutaneous soft-tissue ossification and calcification.

*Pseudopseudohypoparathyroidism* is similar to pseudohypoparathyroidism. The major difference between it and pseudohypoparathyroidism is that the levels of serum calcium and phosphates are normal. Familial tendencies also exist with this disorder.

### Hyperparathyroidism

The frequency of hyperparathyroidism, which is much more common than hypoparathyroidism, appears to be continually increasing. The specific etiology of any form of hyperparathyroid function is not well understood. Hypersecretion of PTH results in elevated serum calcium levels and excessive secretion of phosphorus by the kidneys. In most cases, a single benign adenoma is the cause. It also is thought that a history of longstanding hypocalcemia may contribute to the predisposition of hyperparathyroidism. The three forms of hyperfunction of the parathyroid glands usually are recognized as primary, secondary, and tertiary.

## Primary Hyperparathyroidism

Primary hyperparathyroidism is characterized by hypercalcemia that results from failure of the normal feedback mechanism to decrease secretion of PTH. The three most common causes are parathyroid adenomas, hyperplasia of all four parathyroid glands, or some form of parathyroid carcinoma.[12] As the serum calcium concentrations rise, parathyroid secretion is no longer reduced and calcium levels continue to increase.

The clinical manifestations are variable and nonspecific. Some people experience mild symptoms, whereas others have severe symptoms. The most common manifestation is from renal calculi in the genitourinary system, which probably result from precipitation of calcium and phosphate in the kidneys.[3]

Other variable symptoms include renal symptoms, skeletal changes, and hypercalcemia. In addition to the formation of renal stones, hematuria may be noted. Gastrointestinal complaints include anorexia, nausea, vomiting, and constipation, as well as generalized abdominal pain.[15] Changes within the skeletal system are diverse. Sometimes new bone is laid as quickly as calcium is reabsorbed, and the person has only mild complaints of vague skeletal pains. At other times, various bone diseases such as osteoporosis or osteomalacia may result.

## Secondary Hyperparathyroidism

In secondary hyperparathyroidism, levels of circulating PTH are high, perhaps initiated by a variety of causes that result in a low serum calcium concentration. Although renal disease is the most common cause of secondary hyperparathyroidism, causes may include low-calcium diet, pregnancy or lactation, rickets, and osteomalacia. In the Western world, the usual cause is renal failure. Low calcium levels cause the parathyroid glands to become hyperplastic to compensate for the condition that initially caused the low calcium levels. After compensation attempts, calcium may remain low or may attain normal levels (see Chap. 35).

## Tertiary Hyperparathyroidism

Tertiary hyperparathyroidism results from previously developed, longstanding secondary hyperparathyroidism, which eventually leads to elevated serum calcium levels.[11] Autonomous secretion of PTH continues without regard for serum calcium levels. In most instances, adenomas have developed in the already-hyperplastic parathyroid glands after the onset of secondary hyperparathyroidism.[12] This condition is accompanied by abnormally high calcium levels. Tertiary hyperparathyroidism often is described in persons with renal failure who develop hypercalcemia.

*Renal osteodystrophy*, which may occur with tertiary hyperparathyroidism, arises in persons with chronic renal failure who develop hyperphosphatemia.[6] Parathyroid hyperfunction then occurs and increases serum calcium concentrations (see Chap. 35). Metastatic calcifications in the soft tissues, such as the eyes, lungs, and joints, may occur.[3]

## REFERENCES

1. Bybee, D.E. Saving lives in parathyroid crises. *Emerg. Med.* 19(15):62, 1987.
2. Clinical highlights: Causes of hypothyroidism. *Hosp. Med.* 20(1):163, 1984.
3. Cotran, R., Kumar, V., and Robbins, S.L. *Robbins' Pathologic Basis of Disease* (4th ed.). Philadelphia: W.B. Saunders, 1989.
4. Greenspan, F.S., and Rapoport, B. Thyroid gland. In F.S. Greenspan (ed.), *Basic and Clinical Endocrinology* (3rd ed.). Norwalk, Conn.: Appleton & Lange, 1991.
5. Guyton, A.C. *Textbook of Medical Physiology* (8th ed.). Philadelphia: W.B. Saunders, 1990.
6. Hahn, T.J. Calcium, phosphate, magnesium, and bone: Physiology and disorders. In J.M. Hershman (ed.), *Endocrine Pathophysiology: A Patient-Oriented Approach* (3rd ed.). Philadelphia: Lea & Febiger, 1988.
7. Hershman, J.M. Thyroid disease. In J.M. Hershman (ed.), *Endocrine Pathophysiology: A Patient-Oriented Approach* (3rd ed.). Philadelphia: Lea & Febiger, 1988.
8. Jubiz, W. *Endocrinology: A Logical Approach for Clinicians* (2nd ed.). New York: McGraw-Hill, 1985.
9. Klein, I.L., and Levey, G.S. Thyroid storm and myxedema coma. *Emerg. Med.* 5(4):33, 1984.
10. Leebaw, W.F., and Morley, J.E. Effects of aging on normal and abnormal function. *Consultant* 24(7):165, 1984.
11. Lloyd, R.V. Parathyroid glands. In R.V. Lloyd (ed.), *Endocrine Pathology*. New York: Springer-Verlag, 1990.
12. Marsden, P., and McCullagh, A.G. *Endocrinology*. Littleton, Mass.: PSG, 1985.
13. Mazzaferri, E.L. *Textbook of Endocrinology* (3rd ed.). New Hyde Park, N.Y.: Medical Examination, 1986.
14. McMillan, J.Y. Preventing myxedema coma in the hypothyroid patient. *Dimens. Crit. Care Nurs.* 7(3):136, 1988.
15. Metz, R., and Larson, E.B. *Blue Book of Endocrinology*. Philadelphia: W.B. Saunders, 1985.
16. Patient Care Highlights. Is your patient in thyroid storm? *Patient Care* 18(5):191, 1984.
17. Streck, W.F., and Lockwood, D.H. *Endocrine Diagnosis: Clinical and Laboratory Approach*. Boston: Little, Brown, 1983.
18. Urbanic, R.C., and Mazzaferri, E.L. Thyrotoxic crisis and myxedema. *Heart Lung* 7:435, 1978.
19. Utiger, R. Approach to the patient with a thyroid nodule. In

W.N. Kelley (ed.), *Textbook of Internal Medicine*. Philadelphia: J.B. Lippincott, 1989.

20. Utiger, R. Control of thyroid hormone synthesis. In W.N. Kelley (ed.), *Textbook of Internal Medicine*. Philadelphia: J.B. Lippincott, 1989.

21. Utiger, R. Diseases of the thyroid gland. In W.N. Kelley (ed.), *Textbook of Internal Medicine*. Philadelphia: J.B. Lippincott, 1989.

22. Volpe, R. Autoimmune thyroid disease. *Hosp. Pract.* 19(1): 141, 148, 1984.

23. Wilson, J.D., and Foster, D.W. (eds.). *Williams' Textbook of Endocrinology* (7th ed.). Philadelphia: W.B. Saunders, 1985.

# Normal and Altered Functions of the Pancreas

## Learning Objectives

1. Describe the anatomy of the pancreas, its size, shape, parts, ducts, and cells.
2. Explain the physiologic regulation of insulin secretion.
3. Describe the metabolic effects of insulin.
4. Explain the actions of glucagon and somatostatin, and their effects on metabolism.
5. Discuss the frequency and etiology of diabetes mellitus.
6. Differentiate between the types of diabetes.
7. Relate the stages or degrees of abnormality of diabetes.
8. Explain the pathophysiology of diabetes.
9. Relate the clinical manifestations of diabetes to the pathophysiologic changes.
10. Explain the pathophysiology of complications of diabetes mellitus.
11. Differentiate ketoacidosis; hyperglycemic, hyperosmolar, nonketotic coma; and lactic acidosis.
12. Outline the physiologic responses to hypoglycemia.
13. Identify tests used in the diagnosis and evaluation of diabetes mellitus.
14. Explain the pathophysiology of pancreatic islet cell diseases: hyperinsulinism, Zollinger–Ellison syndrome (gastrioma), and multiple endocrine neoplasia (Werner's syndrome).
15. Discuss the frequency and etiology of acute pancreatitis.
16. Describe the chemical and pathologic changes characteristic of pancreatitis.
17. Relate the clinical manifestations of acute pancreatitis to the histologic alterations.
18. Discuss the complications of acute pancreatitis.
19. Relate laboratory findings of acute pancreatitis.
20. Compare clinical manifestations and complications of acute and chronic pancreatitis.
21. Discuss the frequency, etiology, types, and clinical course of carcinoma of the pancreas.
22. Discuss the frequency and genetics of cystic fibrosis.
23. Describe the pathophysiologic changes that occur in various body systems in cystic fibrosis.
24. Relate the clinical manifestations of cystic fibrosis to the pathophysiologic changes.
25. Discuss laboratory and diagnostic findings related to cystic fibrosis.

This chapter describes the anatomy, physiology, pathology, and alterations in function of the pancreas. The pancreas consists of both exocrine and endocrine portions. It is important in the digestion and metabolism of food, and much of its anatomic structure serves gastrointestinal function. The most frequent disorders of the exocrine pancreas are cystic fibrosis, pancreatitis, and tumors. Special cells in the islets of Langerhans influence metabolism through the secretion of insulin and glucagon. Diabetes mellitus is the most common disorder associated with pancreatic islet dysfunction of the endocrine portion, and is a leading cause of death in the United States.

## ANATOMY AND PHYSIOLOGY

The pancreas is an elongated retroperitoneal gland that lies in the upper portion of the posterior abdominal wall. It resembles a fish, with its head and neck lying in the C-shaped curve of the duodenum, its body extending horizontally behind the stomach, and its tail touching the spleen (Figure 39-1). The head is at the level of the second lumbar vertebra, makes up about 30% of the gland, and lies within the concavity of the duodenum. The neck, the narrowed portion between the head and the body, joins to the body, which accounts for the largest portion of the gland. The tail tapers off from the body. The pancreas is firm, and has a characteristic lobular appearance with a light yellow and slightly pink coloration.

In the adult, the total length of the pancreas varies between 12 and 20 cm, with a width of 3 to 5 cm and a maximal thickness of 2 to 3 cm. Its weight is between 60 and 140 g.

The exocrine portion of the pancreas forms the largest mass (about 80%) of the gland and is composed of small groups of *acini* (grapelike formations) in which digestive enzymes and large volumes of sodium bicarbonate are synthesized and transported. Major enzymes secreted include trypsin, chymotrypsin, peptidases, amylases, lipases, phospholipases, and elastase. Trypsin is critical in enzyme activity because it activates other enzymes. Exocrine secretion varies from 1.5 to 3.0 L daily, depending on demands of intestinal volume and contents.

The acini form a network of larger ducts that eventually drain into the major secretory ducts of Wirsung and Santorini. The duct of Wirsung extends from the surface of the tail of the pancreas to the duodenum at the ampulla of Vater, usually alongside the common bile duct. It empties into the duodenum at the same place as

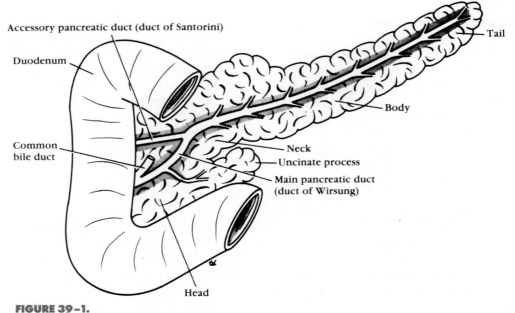

**FIGURE 39–1.**

Parts of the pancreas. (From R.S. Snell, *Clinical Anatomy for Medical Students* [2nd ed.]. Boston: Little, Brown, 1981.)

the common bile duct, the duodenal papilla. In most cases, the sphincter of Oddi surrounds both ducts. In one third of cases, the duct of Wirsung and the common bile duct form a common channel before terminating at the ampulla of Vater. The accessory duct of Santorini exits from the main duct near the neck of the pancreas and enters the duodenum about 2 cm above the main duct.

The endocrine portion of the pancreas, the islets of Langerhans, is embedded between exocrine units like small islands. The islets contain four types of cells: the *alpha* (A), *beta* (B), *delta,* and *pancreatic polypeptide* (PP or F) cells (Figures 39-2 and 39-3). These types compose 20%, 70%, 5% to 10%, and 1% to 2% of islet cell population, respectively. All of these cells empty their secretions into the bloodstream. Alpha cells secrete *glucagon,* beta cells secrete *insulin,* and delta cells contain secretory granules that secrete gastrin or *somatostatin.* The PP cells have small dark granules, and are present on the islets and the exocrine pancreas. The PP cells secrete a unique pancreatic polypeptide that causes gastrointestinal effects of gallbladder contraction and inhibition of pancreatic enzyme secretion. No metabolic effects by *pancreatic polypeptide* on glucose, fat, or amino acids have been established. Studies have revealed elevated basal and postprandial PP in lean people who have non–insulin-dependent diabetes mellitus.[22] Although there are as many as 2 million islets, 20 to 300 $\mu$ in diameter, the endocrine portion composes only about 1% of the weight of the pancreas.

## Physiologic Regulation of Insulin Secretion

The main function of the endocrine portion of the pancreas is to secrete *insulin,* a hormone essential for normal carbohydrate metabolism. Insulin also influences the metabolism of fats and proteins. Therefore, it is a prime anabolic hormone and integrates the major metabolic fuels (see Figure 39-3).

Insulin consists of two amino acid chains and is synthesized from a biologically inactive precursor, *proinsulin,* by the beta cells. Study indicates that proinsulin itself is derived from an even larger polypeptide, *preproinsulin.*[18] The average adult pancreas secretes an estimated 35 to 50 units of insulin daily.

Carbohydrates (primarily glucose), fats, and proteins influence insulin output during meals. Insulin is the only known hormone that reduces the circulating glucose levels. Although numerous physiologic factors may alter insulin secretion, output is regulated mainly by blood glucose level through a negative feedback mechanism (Figure 39-4). When the glucose in the blood that is perfusing the pancreas exceeds about 100 mg/dL, an immediate beta cell response extrudes the granule's contents from the beta cell. When blood glucose levels fall, the rate of insulin secretion also decreases. The release of insulin is biphasic. Glucose prompts both an immediate and a sustained release as more insulin is synthesized. The feedback mechanism is rapid-acting, with insulin levels reaching 10 to 20 times the basal rate with blood

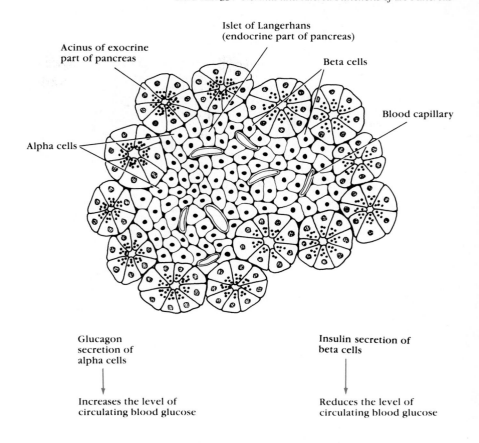

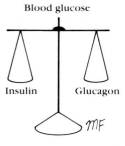

**FIGURE 39–2.**
Regulation of the secretion of insulin and glucagon from the cells of the islets of Langerhans.

glucose levels of 300 to 400 mg/dL. The cessation of secretion is equally rapid, occurring within minutes after restoration of blood glucose to fasting level.[8]

Amino acids also can stimulate insulin secretion in varying degrees. The most potent stimulants are arginine, lysine, and phenylalanine. Insulin in turn promotes transport of the amino acids into the tissue cells.

Fats, although weak stimulators of insulin release, promote sufficient amounts to prevent ketoacidosis. Oral ingestion of fat triggers release of gastrointestinal hormones that augment insulin secretion.

Although insulin secretion is mostly considered in terms of response to nutrients, measurable amounts are secreted at a low basal rate between meals and during prolonged fasting. The gastrointestinal hormones secretin, cholecystokinin, gastrin, and gastric-inhibiting pep-

tide, which are released by the gastrointestinal tract after a meal, stimulate pancreatic insulin release. These hormones, released during digestion, cause an anticipatory increase in blood insulin preparatory for the glucose and amino acids absorbed from the meal.

Other hormones that either directly increase the secretion of insulin or potentiate glucose stimulation of insulin are glucagon, cortisol, growth hormone, progesterone, and estrogen. Prolonged increased amounts of these hormones can lead to exhaustion of the beta cells and diabetes. The hormone glucagon, which is synthesized in the pancreatic alpha cells, affects hepatic glucose production and is important in the pathophysiology of diabetes (see pp. 742–756). High pharmacologic doses of corticosteroids also may induce diabetes, especially in people who have a tendency toward diabetes.

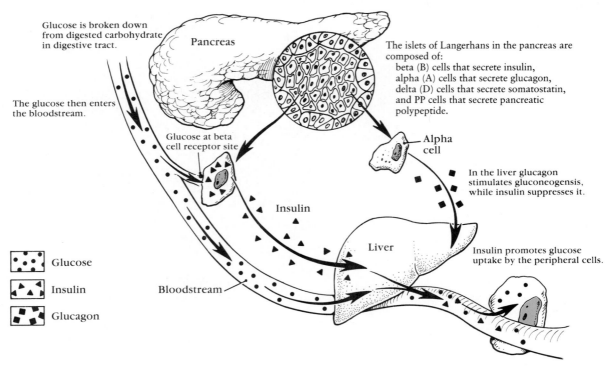

Glucose is broken down from digested carbohydrate in the digestive tract.

Pancreas

The islets of Langerhans in the pancreas are composed of:
beta (B) cells that secrete insulin,
alpha (A) cells that secrete glucagon,
delta (D) cells that secrete somatostatin,
and PP cells that secrete pancreatic polypeptide.

The glucose then enters the bloodstream.

Glucose at beta cell receptor site

Alpha cell

In the liver glucagon stimulates gluconeogensis, while insulin suppresses it.

Insulin

Glucose

Insulin

Liver

Insulin promotes glucose uptake by the peripheral cells.

Glucagon

Bloodstream

**FIGURE 39–3.**
Secretions of islets of Langerhans. (From *Patient Care* 3:17, 1982. © 1982, *Patient Care*, Oradell, NJ.)

The autonomic nervous system plays a major role in modulating insulin secretion between meals, during times when there is no intake, and in response to stressors. Norepinephrine and acetylcholine, transmitters of the autonomic nervous system, and the adrenomedullary hormone epinephrine influence secretions of alpha, beta, and delta cells of the islets of Langerhans. The alpha-adrenergic activities of the sympathomimetic amines (epinephrine and norepinephrine) inhibit insulin secretion. Although catecholamine stimulation of beta-adrenergic sites increases insulin secretion, the alpha-adrenergic action of epinephrine predominates.

Other factors, primarily pharmacologic, that stimulate insulin secretion include sulfonylurea drugs and theophyline. In contrast, beta receptor—blocking agents and diazoxide inhibit secretion (Table 39-1).

## Effect of Insulin on Facilitated Diffusion

Insulin is an influential hormone that affects the biochemical function of every organ in the body. Its most important action is to accelerate the transport of glucose across most cell membranes in the body. In the absence of insulin, the rate of transport of glucose into body cells is about one-fourth normal; when an excess is secreted, the rate may increase to five times normal. Figure 39-5 shows the carrier-mediated transport of the inside of the membrane and its release transport by means of a carrier

mechanism called *facilitated diffusion,* or carrier transport. Insulin influences this transport of glucose into the cell by combining with a receptor protein in the cell membrane. A direct action on the cell membrane is implied, since glucose transport occurs within seconds or minutes. Once the glucose concentration inside the cell is equal to that on the outside, additional glucose is not transferred into the cell. Insulin is especially effective in facilitating transport of glucose in skeletal and adipose tissue, the liver, and the heart. Adipose and skeletal tissues alone make up 65% of body weight.

Insulin does not enhance glucose transport into the brain, erythrocytes, leukocytes, intestinal mucosa, or epithelium of the kidneys. The brain continues to function normally when insulin deficiency causes hyperglycemia. In erythrocytes and leukocytes, the level of free glucose is close to that in plasma. These cells do not suffer from insulin deficiency, but they cannot survive glucose deficiency.

## Metabolic Effects of Insulin

Insulin stimulates reactions that involve fats, carbohydrates, and proteins. Insulin affects *carbohydrate metabolism* by increasing the rate of glucose metabolism, decreasing blood glucose concentration, and increasing glycogen stores in the muscle and liver. Insulin affects *fat metabolism* by increasing the rate of glucose transport

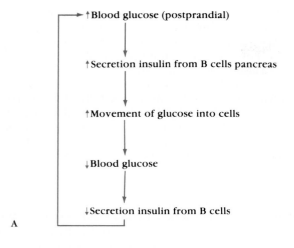

A

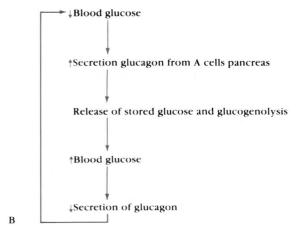

B

**FIGURE 39–4.**
Negative feedback system of (**A**) insulin and (**B**) glucagon.

into fat cells, forming lipids from fatty acids, and promoting storage in adipose tissue. Insulin affects *protein metabolism* and increases the quantity of protein by increasing translation of the messenger ribonucleic acid (RNA) code in the ribosomes to form more protein, and by enhancing transcription of deoxyribonucleic acid (DNA) to form more RNA, thereby resulting in additional protein synthesis.

Insulin's diverse effects are integrated so that it is the prime synthesis and storage hormone in metabolism. Its actions are focused on three metabolically important target tissues—*liver, adipose tissue*, and *muscle*; they are summarized in Table 39-2 and in the following discussion.

## Liver

The liver is the major site for synthesis of glycogen, lipids, and protein, and is the major endogenous source of glucose. Insulin is secreted by the pancreas into the portal system and enters the systemic circulation through the liver. The role of the liver with respect to insulin and carbohydrate homeostasis is unique because of the following aspects:

1.  Insulin promotes glycogen storage by inhibiting the action of an enzyme, phosphorylase, responsible for breakdown of liver glycogen and release of glucose into circulation.
2.  Insulin also promotes glycogen synthesis by increasing the action of enzymes necessary for formation of glycogen.
3.  Insulin is not necessary for transport of glucose into the liver because the liver cells are freely permeable to glu-

**TABLE 39–1.**
FACTORS THAT AFFECT INSULIN SECRETION

| INCREASES | DECREASES |
|---|---|
| Glucose | Epinephrine |
| Glucagon | Norepinephrine |
| Cortisol | Somatostatin |
| Amino acids | Hypokalemia |
| Growth hormone | Fasting (except in diabetes) |
| Secretin, gastric-inhibitory peptide, possibly other hormones of small intestine | Nervous impulses by way of sympathetic nervous system |
| Nervous impulses—especially oral and pharyngeal mucosa by way of vagus nerve | Diazoxide[a] |
| Sulfonylureas[a] | Beta receptor–blocking agents[a] |
| Alpha receptor–blocking agents[a] | |
| Beta receptor–stimulating agents[a] | |
| Theophylline[a] | |

[a] *Pharmacologic agents.*
Source: *Reprinted with permission from J. O'Hara and C. Warfield, The diabetic neuropathies. Hosp. Prac. November 1984, Vol. 19, No. 11, p. 436.*

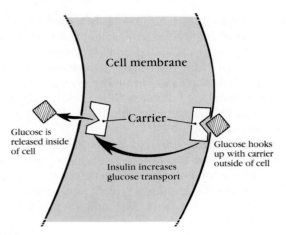

**FIGURE 39-5.**
Insulin increases glucose transport by facilitated diffusion, a passive process.

cose. The uptake is increased by glucokinase, an enzyme that is responsible for "trapping" glucose inside liver cells so that the intracellular concentration is roughly equal to the plasma concentration.

4. In the basal state, glucose is continuously released from the liver at a rate of 2.0 to 3.5 mg/kg/min (200–3350 g/d).[23] The ability of the liver to release free glucose derives from its capability for glycogenolysis and gluconeogenesis and from its possession of an enzyme that promotes further breakdown of glycogen into glucose. This process is critical during prolonged fasting, when glucose is oxidized minimally in most tissues and is used almost exclusively by the brain. Once glucose is in the free form, it readily diffuses into the circulating blood and the liver cell membrane.

5. In the basal state, between meals, when blood glucose level falls and the pancreas secretes less insulin, glycogen synthesis and storage are halted.

6. The concentration of insulin in portal blood is more than two times greater than that in peripheral blood. This concentration is due to the secretion of insulin by the pancreas directly into the portal system.[25]

7. Absorbed hexoses have direct access to the liver through the portal vein before circulating to peripheral tissues. Because of the previously mentioned characteristics, the

liver is important in buffering blood glucose. When there is an excess of insulin or glucose, the hepatic cells take up large quantities of glucose, which are deposited as glycogen as well as being converted to fat. About 60% of glucose ingested in a meal is stored in this manner.[8] When there is an absence of insulin or the blood glucose concentration falls too low, the hepatic cells release quantities of glucose into the blood by breaking down stored glycogen (glycogenolysis) and forming new glucose (gluconeogenesis). Thus insulin enables the organism to maintain a stable blood glucose balance.

### Adipose Tissue

Maintenance of energy balance is a major role of adipose tissue. It is the only tissue that can store a variable amount of "fuel" in the form of fat. The oxidation of 1 g of fat yields 9 calories. Unlike the liver cell, the fat cell (adipocyte) membrane is capable of excluding glucose. Adipose tissue does not release glucose but can release free fatty acids and certain amino acids. Insulin greatly enhances the transport of glucose into fat cells and promotes fat storage in adipose tissue.

The metabolism of glucose within fat cells occurs in several steps:

1. Glucose is rapidly phosphorylated within the fat cell.
2. Glucose is further metabolized to 2-carbon fragments (acetylcoenzyme A), which are converted to fatty acids.
3. A larger portion is degraded by glycolysis into alpha-glycerophosphate. The latter readily combines with free fatty acids to form triglycerides, the primary storage form of fat within the adipose cell.

Insulin promotes fat storage by (1) inhibiting the action of the enzyme lipase within the fat cell, which results in inhibition of both lipolysis and release of fatty acids into the circulation; and (2) promoting glucose transport into the cell. Through its action on glucose metabolism, insulin provides the precursors necessary for combining and storing fatty acids as triglycerides.

Fatty acids and all of the lipid components of plasma greatly increase in the absence of insulin. High lipid con-

**TABLE 39-2.**
TARGET SITES AND METABOLIC ACTIONS OF INSULIN

| SUBSTANCE | LIVER | ADIPOSE CELL | MUSCLE |
|---|---|---|---|
| Carbohydrate | Glycogen synthesis<br>Gluconeogenesis<br>Glycogenolysis | Glucose transport<br>Glycerol synthesis | Glucose transport<br>Glycolysis<br>Glycogen synthesis |
| Fat | Lipogenesis | Triglycerides<br>Fatty acid synthesis<br>Promotes storage | |
| Protein | Proteolysis for<br>gluconeogenesis | | Amino acid uptake<br>Protein synthesis<br>Protein anabolism |

centrations in the plasma, especially cholesterol, increase the risk of developing atherosclerosis.

## Muscle

As in adipose tissue, insulin increases transport of glucose across the membrane into muscle cells through facilitated diffusion. Once in the cell, the glucose is metabolized completely to carbon dioxide or, if oxygen is limited, lactic acid. After the glucose molecule that enters the cell is phosphorylated, it is used for energy or stored as glycogen. Unlike the liver, muscle cannot release glucose from stored glycogen into the body fluids because it lacks the necessary enzyme, glucose phosphatase, to convert glycogen into glucose. Little glucose is stored in the form of triglyceride.

Quantitatively, muscle cell consumption of glucose is small during a resting state. Muscle tissue uses mostly fatty acids for energy because the normal resting muscle membrane is almost impermeable to glucose except in the presence of insulin. During exercise, glucose use greatly increases. This usage of glucose requires smaller amounts of insulin because exercising muscle fibers are more permeable to glucose in the absence of insulin. The contraction process itself increases permeability of fibers. Muscles also use large amounts of glucose in the first few hours after a meal. Food intake increases the blood glucose level, which stimulates the secretion of large amounts of insulin and the transport of glucose into muscle cells.[8]

In summary, insulin is primarily a storage hormone. Its diverse metabolic actions on various target tissues demonstrate the integrated and synergistic effect it has on the metabolism of fats, carbohydrates, and protein. Each molecule of glucose that enters a cell is immediately phosphorylated. Adipose tissue and muscle take up glucose only under the influence of insulin, phosphorylate it, and either store it in the form of glycogen or convert it to triglycerides (fatty acids). At the same time, the presence of free fatty acids impedes glucose oxidation and decreases the release of amino acids from muscle for hepatic gluconeogenesis. Glucose uptake by muscle is also stimulated, providing fuel to replace fatty acids whose release from adipose tissue is inhibited by insulin. Fat accumulation also is increased by release of fatty acids at the adipose cell from lipoproteins that arrive by way of the circulation from the liver and gastrointestinal tract. The antilipolytic action of insulin on the adipose cell increases fat storage, and thereby inhibits gluconeogenesis in the liver by depriving the liver of fatty acids and cofactors used in gluconeogenesis.

## Physiology of Glucagon

Glucagon, a hormone secreted by the alpha cells of the islets of Langerhans, is important in regulating carbohydrate metabolism. The action of glucagon is opposite to that of insulin, and its secretion results in an increase in blood glucose concentration. The major effects of glucagon are stimulation of *glycogenolysis* and *gluconeogenesis* (see Figure 39-3). It also promotes proteolysis and ketogenesis.

Glucagon is potent, and causes glycogenolysis in the liver, which quickly increases blood glucose. Only 1 g/kg of glucagon can elevate the blood sugar about 20% within minutes. The hormone can continue to increase blood glucose levels, even after the glycogen level in cells has been exhausted, by increasing gluconeogenesis in liver cells.[4]

Glucagon secretion is regulated by blood glucose concentration. Changes in blood glucose levels have the opposite effect on glucagon secretion from that on insulin secretion. A decrease in the level of blood glucose increases glucagon secretion. In almost every instance, glucagon has a metabolic effect directly opposite that of insulin: insulin promotes storage of glycogen in liver and muscle, glucagon inhibits it; insulin inhibits glycogenolysis, glucagon promotes it; insulin inhibits lipolysis, glucagon stimulates it. Thus a negative feedback system with opposing action of insulin and glucagon maintains blood glucose levels (see Figure 39-4). Glucagon secretion is increased by exercise, starvation, insulin lack, and amino acid ingestion. It is important in maintaining glucose levels during fasting, exercise, and stressful situations. It helps to protect the body against hypoglycemia.

## Somatostatin

Somatostatin, a hormone excreted by the delta cells of the pancreas, is essential in the metabolism of fats, carbohydrates, and proteins. It acts as a neural agent by inhibiting secretions of insulin and glucagon and other non-islet hormones, and is different from hypothalamic somatostatin, which inhibits growth hormone release. Although not a neurotransmitter, its actions are opposite to those of acetylcholine. The release of somatostatin is stimulated by epinephrine. Somatostatin also is widely present in the central nervous system, primarily the hypothalamus. Smaller amounts have been noted in the cells of the thyroid and gastrointestinal tract. The precise mechanism of somatostatin in metabolic processes is not clearly defined, but it is postulated that it may be important in regulating insulin and glucagon secretion.[25]

## Regulation of Blood Glucose

In the healthy person, the blood glucose ranges between 60 and 100 mg/dL in the fasting state. This concentration rises to 120 to 140 mg/dL after a meal. The feedback system returns the concentration to normal within about 2 hours after the last absorption of carbohydrates.

The blood glucose level is vital in maintaining nutritional balance in the brain, retinae, and germinal epithelium of the gonads because glucose is the only nutrient that can be used to supply adequate energy. More than one-half of all glucose formed by gluconeogenesis during the interdigesting period is used by the brain.[4]

The liver acts as a reservoir and buffering system for glucose. The liver stores sufficient glycogen to maintain a normal blood sugar for 12 to 24 hours. When blood glucose levels are high, almost two thirds of the glucose is stored; when blood glucose concentration falls below normal, the stored glucose is released to maintain the blood level. When the blood glucose level is high (eg, after meals), insulin secretion is increased to return the concentration to normal.

The glucagon feedback system assists in maintaining the range of glucose concentration by stimulating glycogenolysis and gluconeogenesis. Under normal circumstances, the insulin feedback mechanism is the most important, but in starvation states or excessive use of glucose during stress and exercise, the glucagon system becomes important.

Stimulation of the sympathetic nervous system causes a rise in blood glucose level. The release of the catecholamines epinephrine and norepinephrine stimulates glycogenolysis in the liver, resulting in rapid release of glucose into the circulation.

Growth hormone and cortisol increase blood glucose levels less rapidly than the insulin–glucagon system. Both hormones decrease use of glucose in peripheral cells. Cortisol also stimulates gluconeogenesis, thereby resulting in an increased blood glucose level. Growth hormone and glucocorticoids are secreted during periods of hypoglycemia, and decrease the rate of glucose use by most cells of the body. These hormones are less powerful in regulating blood glucose than insulin and glucagon, and require hours rather than minutes to effect a change in the serum glucose.

## DIABETES MELLITUS

Diabetes is a metabolic disorder characterized by a relative or absolute lack of the hormone insulin, or insulin resistance, or both, which results in impaired use of carbohydrates and altered metabolism of fats and protein. The word *diabetes*, from the Greek meaning "a siphon," suggests excessive urine formation; the word *mellitus*, from the Greek meaning "honey," suggests sweetness.

### History

Writings about diabetes go back more than 3000 years, to the Ebers papyrus, in which afflicted people were described as passing frequent and large amounts of urine. Ayur Veda described the sweetness of the urine and noted that ants were attracted to it. He wrote of weakness, emaciation, polyuria, and carbuncles in affected people. Aretaeus, a first-century Greek physician, is credited with naming the disorder. He described the disease as a "melting down of the flesh and limbs into urine." Lipemia of diabetic blood was noted by Helmunt sometime between AD 1573 and 1664. The first diagnostic sign of the disease was established by Thomas Willis in the seventeenth century, when he tasted the urine of his patients and noted its sweetness. A French physician, Michel Chevreul, discovered that the sweetness was caused by sugar. In 1869, Langerhans, while a medical student, described the group of cells in the pancreas that produce insulin. Elliot Joslin was prescribing dietary restrictions long before the discovery of insulin. In 1921, Banting and Best were able to purify islet cell tissues from dogs, and obtained a drop in blood sugar when the tissue was injected into diabetic animals. Within 6 months, insulin was administered to humans, and the "rapid melting" and "speedy death" described by Aretaeus were alleviated.

In 1936, long-acting insulins were introduced, protamine being added to prolong the action and zinc being added for stability. In 1942, Hagedorn modified the PZI (protamine zinc insulin) and produced the first intermediate-acting insulin, NPH (neutral protamine Hagedorn). Globin and lente insulins soon followed. In 1955, oral hypoglycemic agents were introduced. Insulin has been further purified, and biosynthetic human insulin has been developed through recombinant DNA techniques.

### Classification

In 1979, the National Diabetes Data Group and National Institutes of Health, endorsed by the World Health Organization and the American Diabetes Association, outlined a classification of diabetes (Box 39-1).[15] Most cases consist of one of two variants: *type I, insulin-dependent diabetes mellitus (IDDM)* and *type II, non–insulin-dependent diabetes mellitus (NIDDM)* (Table 39-3).

Type I diabetes, previously called juvenile-onset diabetes, has an onset before age 30 in people who are not obese. Only 10% of these persons have a positive family history of a diabetic parent or sibling, although there may be a family history of the disease. Plasma insulin levels are low, and respond little or not at all to insulin stimulators such as glucose and oral hypoglycemics. These persons are ketosis-prone and require exogenous insulin. The pancreas contains little or no endogenous insulin, and the overall beta cell mass is reduced. Ability to synthesize insulin is evident at birth, but the level falls with time. About one third experience a "honeymoon" period, a remission characterized by temporary restoration of insulin secretion, which is reflected in C-peptide re-

## BOX 39-1.
### CLASSIFICATION OF DIABETES MELLITUS AND OTHER TYPES OF GLUCOSE INTOLERANCE

1. Insulin-dependent, type I
2. Non–insulin-dependent (NIDDM), type II
   Nonobese NIDDM
   Obese NIDDM
3. Secondary: Other types, including diabetes mellitus associated with certain conditions and syndromes that may be (a) pancreatic disease, (b) hormonal, (c) drug- or chemical-induced, (d) insulin receptor abnormalities, (e) certain genetic syndromes, or (f) other.
4. Impaired glucose tolerance (IGT). Previously called chemical, latent, or subclinical diabetes.
   Nonobese IGT
   Obese IGT
5. Gestational diabetes
6. Normal glucose tolerance but risk classes
   Previous abnormality of glucose tolerance
   Potential abnormality of glucose tolerance

## TABLE 39-3.
### COMPARISON OF TYPES I AND II DIABETES

| VARIABLES | TYPE I | TYPE II |
|---|---|---|
| Heredity | HLA-linked | No HLA association |
| Gene location | Chromosome 6 | Chromosome 11 |
| Age of onset | Frequency before age 20; most commonly preadolescence; can occur after age 30 | Usually after age 30; can occur before age 30 |
| Onset | Abrupt | Insidious |
| Body weight | Thin | Usually obese (80%) |
| Symptoms | Polyuria, polydipsia, polyphagia, weight loss, weakness, fatigue | Polyuria, polydipsia, polyphagia, vulvovaginitis, often asymptomatic |
| Control | Wide fluctuations of blood sugar in relation to growth, diet, insulin, and exercise | Stable, usually easily controlled |
| Exogenous insulin | Needed by all | May be needed during stress or initial management |
| Oral hypoglycemics | Not useful | May be useful in 30%–40% of cases |
| Beta cells of pancreas | Destruction or inability of cells to secrete insulin | Secrete inadequate or varying amounts of insulin |
| Ketoacidosis | Most prevalent first 5 years of known diabetes and in teenage years | Uncommon except with stress, infection |
| Insulin reactions | Frequent | Uncommon |
| Seasonal distribution | Increased onset during fall and winter | No known association |

lease (measure of residual beta cell secretory capacity). This period is followed by a relapse within weeks or months.

Type II diabetes, previously called adult-onset diabetes, usually occurs after age 30, and about 70% to 80% of affected people are obese. This type accounts for about 80% of total cases of diabetes. In contrast to IDDM, patients with NIDDM have a positive history of diabetes in the immediate family. At birth, these people synthesize insulin, but the level falls as they age and beta cell function deteriorates. Insulin resistance also may occur, together with relative insulin deficiency. Persons with NIDDM are not ketosis-prone. *Maturity-onset diabetes in young people (MODY)* is a rare form of type II diabetes. In these persons, diabetes is mild, ketosis-resistant, and non–insulin-dependent and occurs before age 25. It affects children as young as 10 years, and there is an autosomal dominant inheritance pattern.

Type I and type II disease constitute the majority of diabetic cases. Diabetes also can occur in association with other conditions and syndromes such as pancreatic disease, Cushing's syndrome, insulin-receptor abnormalities, genetic syndromes, and hormone- or drug-induced disorders. Gestational diabetes occurs only during pregnancy. Pregnancy may be a diabetogenic condition. Women demonstrate varying degrees of glucose intolerance related to metabolic effects of hormones secreted during pregnancy. Clinical manifestations may be evident in people who have a predisposition for diabetes. Impaired glucose tolerance is a clinical class that includes those whose glucose tolerance tests are abnormal. They are asymptomatic but are recognized as being at higher risk for diabetes than the general population (see Box 39-1 and Table 39-3).

## Stages

Diabetes also can be classified by degree or stage of abnormality, based on measurable carbohydrate tolerance and presence or absence of hyperglycemia. Classifications are outlined in Table 39-4, using the American Diabetes Association terminology. The separation of stages is arbitrary. A person may remain in one stage, progress to another, or revert to a prior one. Progression or regression of carbohydrate intolerance may occur slowly, never occur, or occur rapidly.

## Frequency and Etiology

Diabetes is a common disorder of the endocrine system, with more than 2 million affected people in the United States alone. Because carbohydrate intolerance is decreased in the elderly, disease frequently increases in later years. Various theories have been offered to explain the genesis of diabetes. Multifactorial causes such as genetic, metabolic, microbiologic, and immunologic etiologies have been cited for the variants of the disease.[3] Abnormalities may occur in the *beta cell* (inadequate insulin secretion, abnormal insulin), *plasma* (abnormal binding, destruction), and *target cell* (cell membrane or intracellular abnormalities).

The frequency varies among different populations, and the prevalence is difficult to quantify because the criteria for the diagnosis of NIDDM have varied over the years. In the United States, the frequency is between 2% and 4% with IDDM, constituting 7% to 10% of the cases.[18]

## Insulin-Dependent Diabetes, Type I

Current thinking leans toward beta cell destruction and absence or severe lack of insulin in the causation of IDDM. Genetic predisposition to beta cell destruction, infection, autoimmunity, and environmental factors have been postulated as causative mechanisms.[4,23] Figure 39-6 shows the interrelation of these factors.

**TABLE 39-4.**
STAGES OF DIABETES

| DETERMINANT | PREDIABETES | SUBCLINICAL DIABETES | LATENT | OVERT |
|---|---|---|---|---|
| Fasting blood sugar | Normal | Normal | Normal or abnormal | Abnormal |
| Glucose tolerance test | Normal | Normal; abnormal during pregnancy stress | Abnormal | Abnormal |
| Delayed or decreased response to glucose | + | + + | + + + | + + + + |
| Symptoms | None | None | None | Present |
| Vascular changes | + | + | + + | + + + |

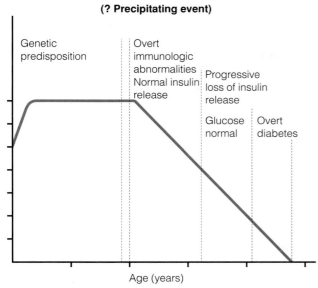

**(? Precipitating event)**

Genetic predisposition

Overt immunologic abnormalities

Normal insulin release

Progressive loss of insulin release

Glucose normal

Overt diabetes

Age (years)

**FIGURE 39–6.**

Stages in the development of type I diabetes mellitus. The stages of diabetes are listed from left to right, and hypothetical beta-cell mass is plotted against age. (From G.E. Eisenbarth, Type I diabetes—a chronic autoimmune disease. *N. Engl. J. Med.* 314:1360, 1986.)

## Infection and Autoimmunity

No specific environmental factor has been identified in the pathogenesis of IDDM, but viral agents are highly suspected. Many types of infections have been reported to precede the onset of diabetes mellitus. These include mumps, rubella, varicella, measles, influenza, coxsackievirus, cytomegalovirus, and viral and, occasionally, bacterial pneumonias. In addition, the number of cases diagnosed increases during autumn and winter, when viral infections are most frequent. This temporal association of onset of IDDM with an infection may be related to genetic susceptibility of beta cells to viruses and other toxic agents. A specific genetic marker has been located. At least one of the susceptibility genes for type I diabetes resides on the histocompatibility region of chromosome 6 (HLA-D). About 80% of persons with IDDM are HLA-positive.[3,5]

The exact role of viruses is not established, but investigations have implicated either virus-induced injury of the beta cell and autoimmunity against the islet cell, or breakdown of beta cell mass caused by prior autoimmune reactions of unknown origin.[24] Autoimmunity is evident in the onset of type I diabetes. Specific human leukocyte antigen (HLA) types are more common in IDDM, especially in children. These children tend to have high levels of islet cell antibodies (ICAs), lymphocytes, monocytes, and eosinophils. The ICAs have been found in the islets of recent-onset IDDM. In addition, sensitized T cells reactive against beta cells have been identified.[4] These findings are strengthened by the association of other autoimmune disorders (eg, Addison's disease, pernicious anemia, and thyroid disease) with IDDM. The person with NIDDM lacks this antigenic tendency.

In summary, the pathogenesis of IDDM is most frequently related to a combination of environmental (probably viral), genetic (HLA-linked), and immunologic factors, with viral-induced injury occasionally being a component of autoimmunity.

## Non–Insulin-Dependent Diabetes Mellitus, Type II

The pathogenesis of NIDDM, in which the lack of insulin is not severe, has been explained as a consequence of various causative factors. The following is a summary of several theories that have been offered.

### Alteration of Insulin Secretion

The changes of NIDDM may not be due to an actual reduction in beta cell mass and insulin production, but to either an inadequate or a delayed initial-phase response to the glucose load. Second-phase responses are within normal ranges or elevated. Even though the second-phase secretion reverts plasma glucose to basal levels, postprandial hyperglycemia results. This alteration is demonstrated in NIDDM when the rise in plasma insulin is delayed after oral glucose intake, when peak insulin level is reached after the glucose peak, and when diabetic blood glucose curves in healthy, nondiabetic people (simulated by computer-programmed glucose infusions) are compared with those of people with NIDDM. The latter secrete less insulin than age-, sex-, and weight-matched healthy subjects. Similar findings of impaired insulin secretion have been noted in prediabetics.[3]

### Insulin Resistance

Insulin resistance, a common characteristic in NIDDM, is a major factor in pathogenesis. It exists when a specific quantity of insulin produces less than the normal anticipated biologic effect at target sites. Insulin resistance and hyperinsulinemia are associated with obesity.

Insulin resistance can be attributed to three principal causes: (1) an *abnormal beta cell secretory product*, such as abnormal insulin molecule or incomplete conversion of proinsulin to insulin; (2) *circulating insulin antagonists*, such as antiinsulin antibodies, antiinsulin-receptor antibodies, or elevated levels of opposing regulatory hormones (eg, growth hormone, cortisol, glucagon, or catecholamines); and (3) *receptor defects in target tissues* (decrease in receptors in a variety of cells).[18] Alterations are demonstrated when the insulin requirements are increased during infection, stress, or endocrine disorders. Most persons with NIDDM are both insulin-deficient and insulin-resistant. Both insulin deficiency and insulin resistance contribute to the hyperglycemia of NIDDM.

### Heredity

For centuries, it has been noted that diabetes "runs in families" because about 40% of people who develop the disease have a positive family history. A genetic component is accepted in the etiology. The human insulin-receptor gene is believed to have a role in insulin resistance, and glucose intolerance is believed to contribute to the disorder.[20] Family histories, twin studies, and studies of histocompatibility of antigens confirm this.[1,18] Although evidence supports the role of genetic factors in both IDDM and NIDDM, the pattern of inheritance has not been established. The *recessive gene theory* holds that diabetes is transmitted as a recessive genetic characteristic that is present in about 20% of the population. The theory of *multifactorial inheritance* holds that diabetes results from an interaction between several different genes and environmental factors.[18] Both IDDM and NIDDM exhibit genetic differences. Studies of identical twins and first-generation relatives of diabetics reflect a concordance rate (both twins affected) in IDDM of less than 50%, but a concordance rate approaching 100% for twins with NIDDM.[1,18] Therefore, genetic factors play a greater role in the occurrence of NIDDM than of IDDM.

### Age

Except for IDDM, increasing age is related to a decline in glucose tolerance and an increase in insulin resistance with an increased prevalence of diabetes. The frequency rises sharply after age 40, probably reflecting a general change in glucose tolerance. The blood glucose is low in childhood and rises progressively; after age 70, about 15% of the population may show a mild abnormal glucose tolerance. The separation between diabetes and nondiabetes may present a problem if tolerance is not adjusted for age. This increasing frequency has been explained as a decrease in body function that occurs in all body cells with senescence.

### Body Weight

About 80% of persons with NIDDM are obese, and the frequency of diabetes in obese people is greater than in the general population. The interrelation occurs because obesity is associated with insulin insensitivity in target tissues (muscle, liver, and adipose cells). It is well known that blood levels of insulin are higher in an obese person and take longer to return to the fasting state. Obesity acts as a diabetogenic factor because the accompanying insulin resistance increases the need for insulin. Because the obese are resistant to the effects of insulin, in practice,

the obese diabetic responds poorly to treatment with insulin. Weight loss increases glucose tolerance.

### Sex

Diabetes is more frequent in women than in men. Between ages 40 and 60, women diabetics outnumber men almost 2:1. In Japan, Malaya, and India, diabetes is 50% to 100% more common in men. In the West Indies, the sex distribution is equal, but black women with diabetes outnumber black men with diabetes. The reason for increased occurrence in women may be related to the late effects of high parity, which may not be manifested until after age 45.

### Diet

Certain factors implicate diet as a possible causative factor in the onset of diabetes. The frequency is great in wealthier communities in the United States. The effects of high-carbohydrate and high-fat diets in the causation of NIDDM have been studied extensively. Modification of dietary intake of carbohydrates minimizes hyperglycemia in this population, and limitation of saturated fat intake may delay the onset of atherosclerosis.

Numerous theories—none mutually exclusive—explain the variants of diabetes. In many cases, there is no single biochemical cause of the disorder, and it can be described only in terms of impairment of insulin secretory response resulting from multifactorial causes. Similarly, it is difficult to separate factors that are the result of disease and those that cause disease.

### Pregnancy

During pregnancy, alterations in carbohydrate metabolism occur. To provide for the energy requirements of the fetus, fasting hypoglycemia and increased lypolysis occur. The workload of the pancreas and tissue insensitivity to insulin increase. The clinical picture may resemble that of NIDDM.

### Stress

Any form of stress with the neuroendocrine response increases gluconeogenesis and glycogenolysis. Infection, life changes, and various environmental factors can be stressors that induce or worsen a diabetic state.

## Introduction to the Pathology of Diabetes

Few diseases have as many widespread and systemic lesions as those that are associated with diabetes. Changes occur in the pancreas, blood vessels, kidneys, and eyes. In classic IDDM, the number of islet cells is reduced, degranulation of beta cells and fibrosis of the islets may occur, and there may be lymphocytic infiltration. In NIDDM, the number of islets usually is normal, the degree of beta cell granulation is somewhat reduced or may be normal, and hyaline deposits may be observed.

## Pathology of the Pancreas

*HYALIN.* A frequent pancreatic lesion is hyalinization of the islets. Hyalin, an eosinophilic, glassy, translucent material, may infiltrate small areas or the entire islet. It may have the fibrillar structure characteristic of amyloid.[3] Progressive accumulation of the deposits reduces beta cell mass. Hyalinization occurs in IDDM but is more common in NIDDM, and correlates with the duration of the disease. It may occur in nondiabetics.

*FIBROSIS.* Thickening of the capsule and islets by fibrous connective tissue is a common change, and the islet cells may be replaced by collagen tissue. This change is correlated with the duration of diabetes; it also occurs in nondiabetics who have pronounced atherosclerotic changes and in people with other types of pancreatic lesions.

*DEGRANULATION OF BETA CELLS.* A reduction in beta cells is a consistent finding, and is most frequent in IDDM. The amount of beta cell granulation correlates with the amount of extractable pancreatic insulin.

*VACUOLATION.* Beta granules are replaced by distended, foamy, watery, vacuolated beta cells. Glycogen accumulation is related to the level and duration of hyperglycemia, and is reversible.

*LEUKOCYTIC INFILTRATIONS.* Eosinophils and lymphocytes infiltrate the islets in an inflammatory type of reaction that is referred to as insulitis. The inflammatory infiltrates are considered a type of immunologic reaction.

*HYPERTROPHY AND HYPERPLASIA OF ISLETS.* These processes occur infrequently except in the children of diabetic mothers and mothers with a latent diabetic tendency. The mother's hyperglycemia causes fetal hyperglycemia and compensatory fetal islet hyperplasia.

## Vascular System Pathology

Vascular lesions are a hallmark of diabetes and are probably related to hyperlipidemia. Electron microscopic studies have revealed microangiopathy (thickening of the walls of the arterioles, capillaries, and venules) in the kidneys, retinae, and neural and epidermal vascular beds.

Atherosclerosis, characterized by fatty intimal plaque and intimal fibrosis, appears mostly in the large vessels. Lipid deposits, called *atheromas* or *plaque*, are laid down on the intimal surfaces. Lipids (cholesterol, triglycerides, phospholipids) circulating in plasma as large molecules combine with proteins and are called lipoproteins. Low-density lipoprotein carries about 75% of circulating cholesterol, whereas high-density lipoprotein carries about 15% to 20%. Investigations have revealed an inverse correlation of high-density lipoprotein with atherosclerosis (see Chap. 25).[6] Fibroblasts and calcium may be deposited, and calcified plaques develop in the vessels. The hyperlipidemia characteristic of diabetes also relates to the high frequency of hypertension in diabetes.

The atherosclerosis is the major factor in the high frequency of myocardial infarction, cerebrovascular accidents, and gangrene of the extremities in diabetes. Coronary atherosclerosis is up to five times more prevalent than in the general population, and myocardial infarction is the most common cause of death.[19] Atherosclerosis is most prevalent in diabetic women, including those who are premenopausal. Atherosclerosis develops within a few years of the onset of the disease. People who have had diabetes for 10 to 15 years, whatever the age of onset, usually have significant atherosclerosis.[3]

The principal clinical manifestations of peripheral arterial disease are ischemic lesions of the feet and the lower extremities. In addition, neurotrophic changes cause loss of sensation, which may decrease attention to small injuries that become infected. A small break may lead to cellulitis, lymphangitis, infection, and necrosis of tissue (Figure 39-7). The arterioles also thicken and microcirculation is impaired.

## Pathology of the Kidneys

The kidneys usually are affected in diabetes. The predominant renal changes are three lesions of the glomeruli: *nodular glomerulosclerosis, diffuse glomerulosclerosis,* and *exudative lesions.* About 20% of deaths in diabetes under age 40 can be related to kidney failure.

*NODULAR GLOMERULOSCLEROSIS.* Nodular glomerulosclerosis (Kimmelstiel–Wilson lesion, a specific lesion of diabetes) appears as a round hyalin mass in the glomerulus, and results in focal thickening of the basement membrane. The mass is located in the periphery of the glomerulus and often is surrounded by capillary loops. It occurs in 25% of those with long-term diabetes.[3]

*DIFFUSE GLOMERULOSCLEROSIS.* Diffuse glomerulosclerosis involves overall thickening of the basement membrane of the glomerular capillaries, together with increased deposits of matrix in the mesangial portion. This condition is the most common form of ne-

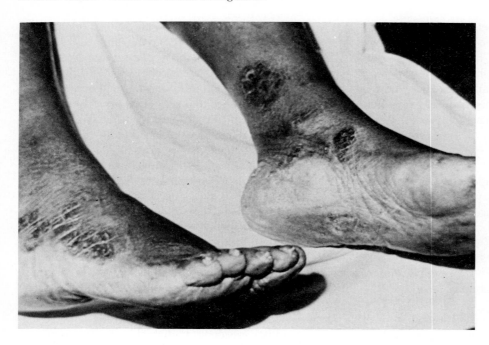

**FIGURE 39-7.**
Atherosclerosis and venostasis of lower legs. (Courtesy of Dr. Walter C. Grundy, pathologist.)

phropathy and leads to proteinuria, which initially is intermittent and then persistent. Sclerosis eventually may involve the entire glomerular bed and cause renal failure.[3]

*EXUDATIVE LESIONS.*  Exudative lesions in the kidneys take two forms. Glassy, brightly eosinophilic, crescentic deposits that hang into the uriniferous space are called capsular drops. Similar deposits are called fibrin caps when they occur on the outer surface of the glomerular capillaries. The capsular drops are diagnostic of diabetes.[3]

*OTHER LESIONS.*  Other common renal lesions affect the vascular supply, renal pelvis, and medulla. Atherosclerosis and arteriolosclerosis of the renal artery or arterioles are common and may be related to hypertension. Pyelonephritis usually is a bacterial ascending infection of the kidneys, which occurs most frequently in diabetics. *Necrotizing renal papillitis*, or renal medullary necrosis, involves unilateral or bilateral necrosis of the renal pyramids, which may result in sloughing of necrotic papillae in urine.

## Pathology of the Eye

*RETINOPATHY.*  Diabetic retinopathy, the inclusive term for several retinal changes related to diabetes, is a leading cause of blindness in the United States. Duration of disease is a variable in its development. Whether visual handicap occurs depends on whether the macula are involved. This condition is rare before the growth-spurt years and develops slowly, corresponding to the duration

of the disease. Retinopathy follows alterations in blood flow through the retinae and has various manifestations: thickening of retinal capillaries, microangiopathies, and microaneurysms, which are discrete saccular dilatations or outpouchings of vessels (Figure 39-8). The microaneurysms are asymptomatic; they are seen as discrete, dark red, circular spots near retinal vessels, and are diagnostic of diabetes mellitus.

Hemorrhages usually are present in the macular area between the superior and inferior temporal vessels and resemble red blotches. If located in the area of the fovea, they can destroy central vision. Exudates occur as a result of abnormal porosity of the retinal vessels and seepage of fluid into the retinae. Soft exudates, called cotton-wool spots, are large, fluffy, and gray-white, and may resolve in several weeks. More commonly hard exudates are yellow, with discrete sharp edges that may coalesce, take longer to develop, and produce retinal degeneration. Venous changes include enlarged, irregular veins, sometimes resembling strings of sausages.

*LESIONS OF THE VITREOUS.*  Lesions of the vitreous are a serious complication, and include neovascularization, or formation of new vessels, and fibrous tissue in the fundus. In time, atrophy of new vessels and contraction of fibrous tissue affect central and peripheral vision. Changes between fibrovascular tissue and the vitreous may lead to hemorrhage and retinal detachment.

*CATARACTS.*  Accumulation of sorbital (polyhydroxy alcohol formed from glucose) in the lens causes cataracts. Opacities of the lens are common in diabetics, usually are of gradual onset, and are similar to senile

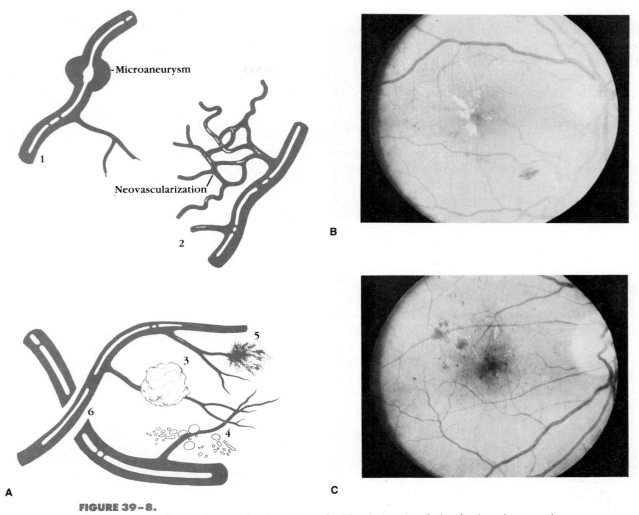

**FIGURE 39–8.**

Characteristic diabetic changes in the retina. **A.** Blood vessels of the fundus shown with (1) microaneurysms, (2) new vessel formation (neovascularization), (3) soft exudates, (4) hard exudates, (5) hemorrhages, and (6) arteriovenous nicking. **B.** Diabetic retinopathy with hard exudates. **C.** Deep retinal hemorrhage. (From R. Judge, G. Zuidema, and F. Fitzgerald [eds.], *Clinical Diagnosis* [4th ed.]. Boston: Little, Brown, 1982.)

cataracts. Transitory lens changes caused by dehydration also occur in diabetics.

## Nervous System Pathology

Neurons are vulnerable to the ketoacidosis of uncontrolled diabetes and the hypoglycemia of insulin reactions. Neuropathy may involve the peripheral nerves, brain, spinal cord, cranial nerves, or autonomic nervous system. The relation between metabolic aspects of disease and diabetic neuropathy remains unknown. Failure of affected people to improve with management of hyperglycemia supports the proposed relation between peripheral neuropathy and a process independent of glucose and insulin metabolism. A correlation has been found between duration of disease and diabetic control.[3] Earlier research focused on abnormalities of myelinated nerve fibers caused by a metabolic defect that affects Schwann cells and myelin. More recently *myo*-inositol, an alcohol sugar present in normal nerves and essential in axonal function, has been implicated. Experimental studies reflect a correlation between nerve *myo*-inositol and metabolic control. Glycosylation of nerve myelin also may be a factor in neuropathy.[3,17]

*Polyneuropathy*, characterized by myelin degeneration and eventual irreversible injury to axons, is caused by an accumulation of abnormal metabolites and by depletion of substances necessary for nerve cell conduction. The associated sensory loss and motor weakness usually occur first and most severely in the feet.

*Mononeuropathy* is probably related to ischemia and infarction of the vessels that supply the nerves. Manifestations of nervous system involvement include pain, paresthesia, decreased proprioceptive sensations, motor impairment, and muscle weakness and atrophy.

Alterations in the autonomic nervous system may

lead to nocturia and atony of the bladder, postural hypotension, and delayed gastric emptying. Disturbances in neural innervation of the pelvic organs lead to sexual impotence in men and orgasmic difficulties in women.

Because of peripheral arterial ischemic disease and neurotrophic changes, the feet of diabetics are more susceptible to infection because of loss of sensation. A pathologic condition may not be noticed and may progress rapidly.

*Charcot's joint*, or neuropathic joint disease, develops because of the trauma and stress of joint motion. Relaxation of supporting structures of the joint leads to cartilage degeneration, disorganization, and collapse of bones. Neuropathic joint disease usually involves the feet.

Various classifications of neuropathies have been proposed. These often are based on anatomic and clinical features (Tables 39-5 and 39-6).

## Skin Changes

Frequently an indicator of diabetes, the skin of the diabetic is structurally different from that of the nondiabetic. Dryness is due to dehydration and occurs in poorly controlled diabetes. Poor skin turgor may be related to protein wasting and dehydration. Impaired granulocyte function and decreased circulation lead to skin changes and also may contribute to infection.

*NECROBIOSIS LIPOIDICA EPIDERMIS.* Most frequent on the shins, this lesion usually develops after diabetes has been present for years. It begins as a papule that progresses to a soft, yellow, ulcerated plaque. Histologically, the lesion consists of collagen surrounded by an inflammatory infiltrate composed of lipid-laden macrophages.[11]

*DIABETIC DERMOPATHY.* Dermopathy, or shin spots, is seen microscopically as atrophy of the epidermis and fibrosis of the dermis. These hemorrhagic-like areas are brown, scaly, round patches, and look as though the person has been struck time and time again in the shins. There is no associated pain or ulceration.[11]

*INFECTIONS.* Bacterial infections are more frequent in diabetics than in nondiabetics. Infections that arise from acne may expand and progress into cellulitis. Furuncles and carbuncles are of serious concern. Dermatophytosis (athlete's foot) is common, and although relatively harmless in the nondiabetic, it may lead to serious infection and loss of a foot in the diabetic. Monilial infections occur in the diabetic, often in the genitalia and groin and under the breasts. The high moisture, the glucose content of the skin, and chafing support the growth of *Candida albicans*, especially in an obese person. Severity of infections may be worsened by reduction of circulation and nerve degeneration.

**TABLE 39-6.**

DISTRIBUTION AND CLINICAL FEATURES OF DIABETIC AUTONOMIC NEUROPATHIES

| SYSTEM | FEATURES |
| --- | --- |
| Cardiovascular | Diminished cardiac beat-to-beat variation; orthostatic hypotension; diminished sympathetic cardiac drive |
| Genitourinary | Erectile impotence; retrograde ejaculation; neurogenic bladder; female sexual dysfunction |
| Gastrointestinal | Decreased gastric motility, gastroparesis; nocturnal (diabetic) diarrhea; constipation; fecal incontinence |
| Miscellaneous | Abnormal pupil reactivity; sweating disturbances; impaired adrenergic glucose counterregulation; vasomotor instability |

Source: *Reprinted with permission from J. O'Hara and C. Warfield, The diabetic neuropathies. Hosp. Pract. November 1984, Vol. 19, No. 40.*

**TABLE 39-5.**

CLASSIFICATION OF DIABETIC NEUROPATHIES ON ANATOMIC BASIS

| STRUCTURE | LESION | CLINICAL FEATURES |
| --- | --- | --- |
| Nerve terminals | Polyneuropathy | Glove and stocking sensory loss, distal painless ulceration, mild peripheral weakness, edema of Charcot's joints, distal reflex loss |
| Mixed spinal or cranial nerve | Mononeuropathies | Pain, weakness, sensory loss; may be spinal or cranial |
| Nerve root | Radiculopathy | Pain or sensory loss in root distribution |
| Nerve terminal(?) or muscle? | Amyotrophy | Pain in anterior thigh, buttocks, or hips; muscle weakness |
| Sympathetic ganglion | Automatic | Postural hypotension, impotence, gastropathy, bladder atony |

Source: *Reprinted with permission from S. Locke, "The peripheral nervous system in diabetes mellitus." Diabetes 13:307, 1964.*

*LIPODYSTROPHY.* Lipodystrophy is characterized by general or partial loss of body fat and may be caused by insulin injections. Scar and lipoma-like accumulations beneath the skin form large bumps (lipohypertrophy) with repeated injection of insulin. These sites tend to become fibrous and insensitive, and insulin is absorbed poorly from these areas.

The use of single-peak insulin, a chemically pure form of insulin, is thought to decrease the extent of lipodystrophy. Rotating injection sites and administering insulin in deep subcutaneous tissue at room temperature also help to prevent lipodystrophy.

*XANTHOMAS.* Firm, yellowish pink nodules develop under the epidermis of knees and elbows and on the periorbital areas and buttocks as a result of the hyperlipemia of diabetes. The lesions may be as large as 5 mm, and the papule is surrounded by an inflammatory-type halo. Although these nodules are not limited to persons with diabetes, they signify high serum triglyceride levels and disappear with return of triglycerides to normal.

## Hepatic Fatty Changes

In longstanding diabetes, fatty changes develop and the size of the liver increases. Infiltration of fat causes it to appear yellowish, and glycogen vacuoles may be present in nuclei of the cells. These liver changes are related to elevated serum lipid levels.

## Muscle Changes

Degenerative changes occur in striated muscle in persons who have longstanding, poorly controlled diabetes. The pathology is probably related to microangiopathy and neuronal degeneration. Diabetic amyotrophy, a syndrome of muscle weakness, pain, and atrophy, occurs in the elderly, especially in men. The disorder usually is limited to the psoas and quadriceps muscles.

## Clinical Manifestations and Complications

Most diabetics have polydipsia, polyuria, polyphagia, weight loss, and weakness. Many also have infections. A hyperglycemic person is at risk for infection because neutrophil functions are handicapped by high glucose levels. Infection is a leading cause of morbidity and mortality. Prominent pathogens are *Staphylococcus aureus* and *Candida albicans*. *Candida* secrets a protein that diminishes phagocytosis by the host.[9]

The predominant pathophysiology of diabetes is due to (1) impaired use of glucose by cells; (2) increased mobilization, abnormal metabolism, and deposition of fats; and (3) depletion of protein in body tissues. The manifestations occur from insulin deprivation, which results in *hyperglycemia* (blood glucose as high as 200–1000 mg/dL) because of the impaired uptake of glucose, especially into muscle and adipose tissue, and increased gluconeogenesis and glycogenolysis by the liver. These factors, together with increased dietary intake of carbohydrate, result in an increased blood sugar level.

With hyperglycemia, osmotic pressure of the plasma increases, fluid shifts to the intravascular compartment, and cells become dehydrated. When the blood glucose level reaches about 160 to 180 mg/mL, the renal tubules cannot resorb all of the glucose filtered by the glomeruli, and glycosuria occurs. When the blood glucose level reaches 300 to 400 mg/mL, a common occurrence in untreated diabetes, a person may lose as much as 100 g of glucose into the urine each day. The renal excretion of glucose requires accompanying water and produces osmotic diuresis, *polyuria*. Excessive urination also increases loss of water, potassium, sodium, and chloride, resulting in extracellular fluid depletion and compensatory intracellular dehydration. As sodium and potassium are lost, electrolyte imbalance, weakness, fatigue, and malaise occur. Loss of water causes an increase in serum osmolality, which stimulates the thirst center in the hypothalamus and the body's response of *polydipsia*. With the loss of large quantities of glucose and semistarvation of the cells, there is a compensatory increase in hunger, *polyphagia*. As the level of insulin, an anabolic hormone, decreases, protein and fat catabolism increase, resulting in the release of ketones, nitrogen, and potassium into the circulation. Weight loss is common, especially in IDDM.

## Diabetic Ketoacidosis

The metabolic result of lack of insulin and severe dehydration is ketoacidosis. With the stress response, there is increased secretion of counterregulatory hormones, including cortisocatecholamines and glucagon, which further increase glucose production. The signs and symptoms are pronounced manifestations of uncontrolled diabetes. Polyuria, polydipsia, polyphagia, weakness, and anorexia, plus nausea, vomiting, and abdominal pain occur in increasing severity. Ketonemia, gastric dilatation, and decreased peristalsis from potassium loss contribute to nausea and vomiting. The gastrointestinal symptoms and tender abdomen may mimic a surgical emergency. Ketonuria increases electrolyte loss.

The most important pathogenic element in ketoacidosis is marked decrease in insulin production that leads to hyperglycemia, glycosuria, and progressive metabolic acidosis. Without insulin, glucose cannot enter the cells, and a form of intracellular starvation occurs. Glucose accumulates in the blood, increasing osmolality and pulling water from the cells into the intravascular compartment. The body enters a catabolic state, and there is a shift from carbohydrate to protein and fat metabolism. Fats are broken down (lipolysis) for energy faster than they can be metabolized. The ketone acids (acetoacetic and beta-hydroxybutyric acids) are strong, and dissociate to yield hydrogen ions, consequently causing a drop in pH. At a plasma pH of 7.2, a person's respiratory center is stimulated to prevent further decline in pH, and breathing becomes deep and rapid (Kussmaul respiration). The acetone formed during ketosis is volatile and is blown off during expiration, giving the breath a sweet or fruity odor. When acidosis depresses their action, ketones are not well metabolized, so that acidosis and catabolism are enhanced. Hypovolemia and increased blood viscosity also may cause systemic thrombi or emboli, a myocardial infarction, or a cerebrovascular accident.

Protein catabolism results in the breakdown of amino acids and electrolytes from muscle tissue. The liver, the primary site for glucose synthesis, converts amino acids to glucose, perpetuating the hyperglycemic and acidotic states. The metabolic derangement also is increased by the presence of glucoregulatory hormones during diabetic ketoacidosis. The antagonistic activity exhibited by these hormones promotes gluconeogenesis and worsens the hyperglycemia.

When the lungs are no longer able to maintain pH by blowing off carbon dioxide, plasma carbonic acid levels rise and acidosis progresses. Further decrease in pH, accompanied by hyperosmolality, dehydration, hypotension, and tissue breakdown, contributes to depression of cerebral function and eventually leads to coma and death (Figure 39-9). Persons with NIDDM seldom develop ketoacidosis.

## Hyperglycemic, Hyperosmolar, Nonketotic Coma

Hyperglycemic, hyperosmolar, nonketotic (HHNK) coma has been recognized with increasing frequency. This variation in hyperglycemic diabetic coma is characterized by extreme hyperglycemia (800–2000 mg/dL) and hyperosmolality (greater than 350 mOsm/kg), mild or undetectable ketonuria, and absence of acidosis. The syndrome occurs almost exclusively in older people and in persons with mild diabetes that does not require insulin.

The mechanism of HHNK is best understood by considering the principles of osmolality. Without insulin to

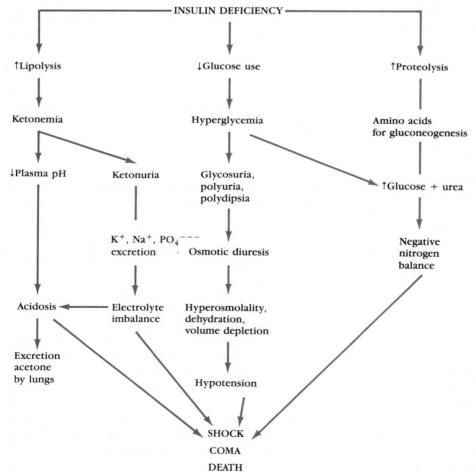

**FIGURE 39-9.**
Pathogenesis of ketoacidosis.

lower blood glucose, the blood becomes more concentrated because glucose is a large molecule that does not easily pass cell walls and draws large amounts of water. The profound hyperglycemia is largely responsible for the increased plasma osmolality that causes an osmotic diuresis. The intracellular fluid is drawn out to help equalize the increasing osmotic pressure of blood hypertonic with sugar. Water in the intracellular fluid moves from cells into the bloodstream, leaving cells dehydrated and shrunken. Dehydration stimulates secretion of the glucoregulatory hormones glucagon, cortisol, and epinephrine. If hypokalemia also occurs, it decreases insulin secretion. These two events cause further hyperglycemia.

Fluid intake initially balances the fluid lost to glycosuria. Later, intake is insufficient and dehydration ensues. The person gradually becomes more obtunded and cannot respond to thirst. Without treatment with insulin and fluids, the process becomes self-perpetuating. Hyperosmolality leads to hemoconcentration and is conducive to thrombus formation. Fluid losses lead to hypovolemia and shock. If these are not corrected, death may result.

Similarities exist between HHNK and ketotic coma. In both, a shortage of insulin and a defect in use of glucose result in hyperglycemia, osmotic diuresis, and dehydration. Elevation of urea nitrogen levels usually occurs in both, although the causes may be different. Metabolic acidosis occurs in both, but less frequently in the hyperosmolar disorder.

The major difference is that large quantities of ketone bodies are produced in ketotic coma but not in HHNK coma. No insulin is secreted in ketotic coma, but some residual ability to secrete insulin remains in HHNK coma. The small quantities of circulating insulin probably prevent the mobilization of fat from tissues and the release of ketone bodies. The lesser elevation of plasma growth hormone and cortisol levels in HHNK coma also accounts for decreased ketone bodies.

The signs and symptoms of HHNK are polyphagia, polydipsia, polyuria, glycosuria, dehydration, abdominal discomfort, hyperpyrexia, hyperventilation, electrolyte imbalance, central nervous system dysfunction, postural hypotension, and shock. Impaired mental status is related to dehydration or electrolyte imbalance. The skin has decreased turgor, mucous membranes are dry, and the eyes are sunken and soft. Some degree of renal impairment occurs in many affected persons.

The onset of HHNK may be triggered by an acute illness or surgery as well as by stressful events, for example pancreatic disease, myocardial infarction, hemodialysis, renal dialysis, severe burns, and hyperalimentation. A number of drugs (corticosteroids, diuretics, diphenylhydantoin, and immunosuppressive agents) also may induce the syndrome.

The laboratory results are similar to those of ketoacidosis, except that the glucose levels usually are higher (often greater than 1000 mg/dL) and serum osmolalities also are more elevated (greater than 350 mOsm/kg $H_2O$). Bicarbonate concentrations and pH often are normal but may decrease as the syndrome progresses. There usually is no ketoacidosis in classic cases, but lactic acidosis may result from hypovolemic shock. Plasma acetone is absent or slightly elevated; creatinine and blood urea nitrogen levels become elevated with renal impairment. Compared with ketoacidosis, there is less elevation of the plasma free fatty acids, growth hormone, and cortisol. The prognosis in HHNK coma is not as good as in diabetic ketoacidosis, and death often is attributed to the underlying or associated disease that precipitated the coma.

### Lactic Acidosis

When anaerobic glycolysis in the body produces more lactic acid than can be used or converted to glucose, lactic acidosis occurs. It frequently occurs with sustained hypoxia or hypotension (eg, shock, septicemia, hemorrhage, renal insufficiency, and starvation). Lactic acidosis may develop in diabetics as a spontaneous syndrome or in association with diabetic ketoacidosis or HHNK coma when marked hypoperfusion occurs.

Lactic acidosis should be suspected in any stuporous or comatose person in metabolic acidosis. Diagnosis is confirmed by a plasma lactate level in excess of 7 mmol/L, with a low plasma bicarbonate level, absence of ketosis, and an anion gap produced by the excess lactate.

### Insulin Reactions

Hypoglycemia is a rather frequent metabolic complication of diabetes, although it is largely a consequence of insulin therapy. Most diabetics who take insulin experience a hypoglycemic reaction at some time. Reactions result from (1) an overdose of insulin, (2) inadequate food intake, (3) increased amounts of exercise, and (4) nutritional and fluid imbalances caused by nausea and vomiting.

The symptoms of hypoglycemia reflect glucose deprivation to the brain. The following physiologic responses occur: (1) epinephrine release (sweating, shakiness, nervousness, headache, palpitations, and increased blood pressure, heart rate, and respirations); (2) parasympathetic nervous system response (hunger, nausea, eructation); and (3) cerebral function decline (bizarre behavior, dulled sensorium, lethargy, convulsions, coma). Clinical signs and symptoms may not correlate with blood glucose level. They may occur when the glucose level drops rapidly from a very high to a still-elevated level.

The adrenergic response results in increased liver glycogenolysis to raise blood glucose concentration and stimulation of the reticular activating system to a state of wakefulness and alertness. If the liver glycogen supply is exhausted and glucose is not replaced, convulsions and permanent brain damage result.

Hypoglycemia also can occur independently of insulin. The following conditions can cause low blood glucose levels: severe *liver disease*, which impairs glycogen uptake and release; *adrenocortical insufficiency*, in which the glucocorticoids (cortisol and cortisone) are unavailable to stimulate gluconeogenesis; and *islet cell tumors*, which overproduce insulin. Some medications, such as salicylates, oral antidiabetic agents, propranolol, monoamine oxidase inhibitors, and certain sulfonamides, contribute to hypoglycemia. Alcohol (ethanol) has long been recognized as an agent that can induce hypoglycemia. It also potentiates the effects of insulin and oral antidiabetic agents.

### Somogyi Effect

Somogyi described a syndrome of chronic hypoglycemia in persons who receive large amounts of insulin. The syndrome may be caused by increased sensitivity to insulin. It occurs more frequently in children and type I diabetics.

Some people have wide variations in blood sugar level that occur when insulin dosage is increased to control elevated levels. The exogenous insulin produces hypoglycemia. These people often have nocturnal hypoglycemia, followed by hormone-mediated hyperglycemia in the morning. Epinephrine, adrenal corticosteroids, and growth hormone are secreted as part of the body's response to the excessive action of insulin. Epinephrine spurs glycogenolysis in the liver, corticosteroids stimulate gluconeogenesis in the liver, and hyperglycemia occurs. The blood sugar usually is elevated, but periods of severe hypoglycemia may be experienced. If this *rebound hypo-hyperglycemia* is suspected, the insulin dose is slowly reduced, divided into smaller doses, or administered at different times. Table 39-7 offers a comparison between hypoglycemia and different types of coma in diabetes.

## Clinical Course

The course of diabetes may be insidious or abrupt. The ketosis-prone insulin-dependent type that usually affects younger people sometimes undergoes transient remission after onset, called a honeymoon period, which may last a few weeks to a few months; then glucose intolerance becomes unstable or brittle. The person is sensitive to changes in exogenous insulin, dietary deviations, growth spurts, unusual physical activity, infection, and stress, and is vulnerable to hypoglycemia and ketoacidosis.

Maturity-onset, nonketosis-prone diabetes may have few, if any, symptoms, and follows an insidious course.

**TABLE 39-7.**
COMPARISON OF HYPOGLYCEMIA, DIABETIC KETOACIDOSIS, LACTIC ACIDOSIS, AND HYPERGLYCEMIC HYPEROSMOLAR NONKETOTIC COMA

| VARIABLES | HYPOGLYCEMIA | DKA | LACTIC ACIDOSIS | HHNK |
|---|---|---|---|---|
| Physical response | Trembly, weak; difficulty talking | Nausea, vomiting; polyuria; polyphagia; polydipsia; headache | Similar to DKA (varied, depending on factors contributing to development) | Similar to DKA |
| Mental status | Anxious, confused; behavioral changes | Irritable; comatose | Acute changes in state of consciousness; stuporous; comatose | Similar to DKA; stuporous; focal motor seizures |
| Blood pressure | Normal | Low | Low | Low |
| Skin | Cold, moist, pale | Hot, flushed, dry | Pallid, dry | Very dry |
| Mucous membranes | Normal | Very dry | Dry | Extremely dry |
| Respiration | Normal | Hyperventilation | Hyperventilation | Normal |
| Urine sugar | 0–2+ | 4+ | 0–2+ | 4+ |
| Urine acetone | 0 | 4+ | 0–2+ | 0–1+ |
| Blood sugar | 40 mg or less | 300–800+ mg | 80–200 mg | 800–2000 mg |
| Serum ketones | 0 | 4+ | 0–2+ | 0–2+ |
| Blood $CO_2$ | 24–30 | 5–16 or less | 5–16 | 18–24 |
| Plasma lactic acid | Normal | Normal | High | Normal |
| Plasma pH | 7.4 | 7.1–7.3 | 6.8–7.2 | 7.4 |

*DKA, diabetic ketoacidosis; HHNK, hyperglycemic hyperosmolar nonketotic coma.*

Thus the person with nonketosis-prone NIDDM usually does not experience the acute metabolic syndrome, but suffers from other complications.

## Laboratory Findings

Numerous laboratory tests are performed to diagnose and follow the course of diabetes mellitus.

### Fasting Blood Sugar

Normal test values rule out significant diabetic problems but do not completely exclude diabetes, since only about 30% to 40% of cases can be diagnosed with a fasting blood sugar. The fasting blood sugar (FBS) should be measured in the early morning, at least 8 hours after a meal. Normal values are 65 to 100 mg/dL using a method specific for glucose, or 80 to 120 mg/dL using a method that measures all blood sugars and reducing substances. A FBS above 120 mg/dL should be further investigated with a glucose tolerance test.

### Two-Hour Postprandial Blood Sugar

Values may range from 200 to 2000 mg/dL, depending on duration and severity of the diabetes. Glucose levels seldom are elevated 2 hours after carbohydrate intake in nondiabetics.

### Glucose Tolerance Test

The glucose tolerance test (GTT) is based on the principle that a nondiabetic person can absorb a test amount of glucose from circulation at a faster rate than a diabetic. As demonstrated in Figure 39-10, when a nondiabetic fasting person ingests 1 g glucose per kilogram of body weight, the blood glucose rises to peak levels of 150 to

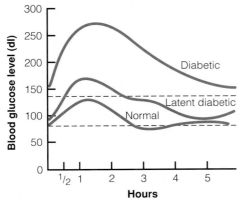

**FIGURE 39–10.**
Glucose tolerance curves.

160 mg/dL and falls to normal within 2 to 3 hours. The urine usually remains free of glucose.

In the diabetic, the blood sugar peak levels are much higher, and the return to fasting levels is delayed 5 to 6 hours because of a lack of insulin response to the glucose.

### Glycosylated Hemoglobin

About 5% of hemoglobin in the red cells usually is a variety called hemoglobin $A_{1c}$. Glycosylated hemoglobin ($HbA_{1c}$) is formed slowly and irreversibly from glucose and hemoglobin throughout the 120-day life span of the red blood cell. The process occurs through a nonenzymatic process that results in attachment of glucose to protein hemoglobin. The higher the blood glucose level, the more $HbA_{1c}$ is present in the red cell. In nondiabetic adults, the level of $HbA_{1c}$ is 2.2 to 4.8; in children, it is 1.8 to 4.0. Good diabetic control should maintain a level of 2.5 to 6.0. A value above 8.0 reflects poor control.

This test decreases the problem of spurious results for blood glucose because it depends little on cooperation, stress, exercise, food intake, and renal threshold. Also, $HbA_{1c}$ is useful in monitoring how well diabetics control blood glucose at home and in differentiating noncompliance from an acute illness that results in elevated blood glucose. As a diagnostic tool, it is not as discriminating in identifying borderline diabetes as glucose tolerance or fasting blood sugar. Glycosylation of a large number of proteins is being investigated in various laboratories.[25]

### Urine Glucose

In normal kidneys, the glucose filtered through the glomeruli from the blood is resorbed in the proximal tubules. The renal tubules have a maximum absorptive capacity (renal threshold) of about 160 to 180 mg/dL of blood. At blood levels greater than this, sugar is spilled into the urine and can be detected by screening methods. Glucose may appear in the urine at normal blood levels in people without diabetes if the ability of the renal tubules to absorb glucose is impaired. Many diabetics, especially those with a history of atherosclerosis, may have a higher renal threshold, which prevents the appearance of glucose in urine until the blood level is quite high.

### Urine Ketones

Ketonuria refers to the loss of ketone bodies, such as acetone, beta-hydroxybutyric acid, and acetoacetic acid, in the urine. This reflects the abnormal oxidation of fats and may occur in diabetes, glycogen storage disease, starvation, and high-fat diets. Ketones occasionally are present with fever or other conditions that increase metabolic requirements. Accumulation of acidic ketones in the blood leads to metabolic acidosis and an acetone smell to the breath.

### Volume of Urine in a 24-Hour Period

A nondiabetic person secretes an average of 1200 to 1800 mL of urine in 24 hours, whereas the uncontrolled diabetic excretes 2000 or more milliliters in 24 hours.

## PANCREATIC ISLET CELL DISORDERS

Syndromes associated with hyperfunction of the islets of Langerhans may be caused by (1) diffuse hyperplasia of the islets, (2) adenomas, and (3) malignant islet tumors.

## Hyperinsulinism

When hyperplasia or tumors (insulinomas) of the beta cells occur, enough insulin may be secreted to induce hypoglycemia. Most islet cell tumors are benign, but a small percentage are metastasizing malignant tumors. Most persons with insulinomas are women, and the median age at diagnosis is 50 years with the exception of multiple endocrine neoplasia syndrome, in which the median age at diagnosis is in the 20s.[21]

The insulin-producing adenomas, or insulinomas, vary from minute lesions to large masses. They occur singly or scattered throughout the pancreas, and usually appear as encapsulated firm nodules that are distributed throughout the pancreas and compress the surrounding tissue. Histologically, they do not differ from the normal islet cell.[3]

Hyperinsulinism also may be caused by hyperplasia of the pancreatic islets, an alteration that occurs in infants born of diabetic mothers. The infant responds to the elevated blood sugar levels of the mother by producing increased numbers of cells and an increase in size of the cells. After delivery, the increased secretion causes serious episodes of hypoglycemia.

Postprandial hypoglycemia may occur in persons who have undergone surgical procedures such as gastrectomy, gastrojejunostomy, and vagotomy. Rapid emptying of gastric contents may lower glucose levels far more rapidly than insulin levels and produce hyperinsulinism and hypoglycemia.[21]

## Zollinger–Ellison Syndrome

A syndrome described by Zollinger and Ellison is a clinical condition of peptic ulceration associated with a non–beta-cell islet tumor (see Chap. 41). It is characterized by large amounts of gastric secretion of hydrochloric acid and pepsin. The stimulus for the hypersecretion is attributed to gastrin; hence the tumor also is known as a gastrinoma. Although most of the tumors occur in the pancreas, about one-tenth are located in the duodenum or duodenal wall.

About one fourth of persons with Zollinger–Ellison syndrome have a hereditary form of peptic ulcer disease. The syndrome most frequently occurs between ages 30 and 65 and affects men more than women.

Various types of islet cells have been implicated as the causative agents. Gastrin-producing delta cells have been found in tumors and hyperplastic tissue, but it is still unclear whether these cells are the distinct agents responsible for gastrinomas.[3]

Microscopically, the tumors resemble islet cells or cancerous tumors. About 60% of gastrinomas are malignant and metastasize to regional lymph nodes. There may be metastasis to bones, mediastinum, and skin. Morbidity and mortality usually are attributed to the effects of the secretion of gastrin from the tumor and its metastases, and to complications of ulcer disease such as bleeding and perforation. The tremendous gastric hypersecretion leads to intractable ulcers. The site of the ulcers is similar to that of peptic ulcers. Likewise, symptoms are similar but more progressive and less responsive to treatment. The high acidity of the small intestine causes inactivation of pancreatic lipase; this precipitates bile salts and causes fluid and electrolyte imbalance. Large volumes of acid gastric juices promote diarrhea. As a result, many affected persons develop malabsorption syndromes. Alteration in the intestinal mucosa from acidity affects absorption of nutrients. *Steatorrhea* (excessive secretion of sebum or fat in feces) may occur from the mucosal defects that interfere with transport of fats and other nutrients across the mucosa. Also, acid inactivates pancreatic lipase and decreases bile acids, which contribute to fat malsorption. Calcitonin levels also are elevated. This elevation is attributed to stimulation of calcitonin release from the thyroid by gastrin.

## Werner's Syndrome

Werner's syndrome is familial with an autosomal dominant pattern of transmission with incomplete penetrance. Clinical features resemble early senescence, and it is referred to as adult progeria. Multiple adenomas are present in the parathyroid glands, pituitary, and pancreas. The disorder often is associated with peptic ulcer and gastric hypersecretion (Zollinger–Ellison syndrome). Both Zollinger–Ellison and Werner's syndromes have been found in some families, implying that the syndromes are variants of the same mutant gene. Some of the tumors are malignant, and the term *multiple endocrine neoplasia (MEN)* has replaced the term *multiple endocrine adenomatosis* previously used.

The major syndromes that are caused by multiple endocrine hyperfunction are MEN. Several of the conditions are familial with an autosomal dominant pattern. There are three types of MEN syndromes:

1. Type I (MEN I, Werner's syndrome) includes tumors or hyperplasia of the parathyroids, thyroid, pancreatic islet cells, pituitary, and adrenal cortex. The clinical manifestations vary, depending on the systems involved. More than one half of those affected have adenomas of two or more endocrine glands, and three or more glands are involved in one fifth of these persons. It is proposed that the fundamental defect is due to an excess of a circulating growth factor.[14]
2. Type II (MEN IIa, Sipple's syndrome) includes pheochromocytoma, medullary thyroid carcinoma, and parathyroid hyperplasia (see Chaps. 37 and 38).
3. Type IIb or MEN III (mucosal neuroma syndrome) includes medullary thyroid carcinoma and pheochromocytoma, but may be accompanied by distinct dysmorphic features such as neuromas of the lips, buccal mucosa, tongue, and gastrointestinal tract.

Clinical manifestations of MEN include intractable peptic ulcers, hyperparathyroidism, hyperinsulinism, Cushing's syndrome, and hypertension related to pheochromocytoma.[3]

# PANCREATITIS

## Acute Pancreatitis

Pancreatitis, or inflammation of the pancreas, is characterized by hemorrhage, necrosis, and suppuration of pancreatic parenchyma. Pathologic changes occur in varying degrees of severity and are caused by escape of active lytic pancreatic enzymes into the glandular parenchyma.

### Frequency and Etiology

This condition accounts for about 1 out of every 500 medical and surgical hospital admissions. Acute pancreatitis occurs most frequently in middle life and more in women than in men. Two major causes, *alcoholism* and biliary tract disease, especially *cholelithiasis* (gallstones), are responsible for 50% to 90% of cases. Factors in the etiology of pancreatitis are listed in Box 39-2. In men, pancreatitis often is associated with high consumption of alcohol, but the condition develops only after years of alcohol abuse. Gallstones have been demonstrated in the feces of 40% to 60% of patients with acute pancreatitis.[3]

Pancreatitis also may occur as a result of surgical trauma, particularly that involving the pancreas and ad-

**BOX 39-2.**
FACTORS IN THE ETIOLOGY OF PANCREATITIS

Alcoholism
Biliary tract disease
Postoperative (abdominal, nonabdominal)
Postendoscopic retrograde cholangiopancreatography
Trauma (abdominal injury)
Metabolic (hyperlipidemia, uremia, renal failure, after renal transplantation, hypercalcemia, pregnancy, cystic fibrosis, kwashiorkor)
Vascular (shock, lupus erythematosus, thrombocytopenic purpura, polyarteritis, athermatous embolism)
Drugs
  Association
    Immunosuppressive—corticosteroids, L-asparaginase, azathioprine
    Diuretics—thiazides, furosemide, ethacrynic acid
    Estrogens, oral contraceptives
    Antibiotics—tetracyclines, sulfonamides
  Possible association
    Acetaminophen
    Isoniazid, rifampin
    Propoxyphene
    Valproic acid, procainamide
    Anticoagulants
Infections (mumps, viral hepatitis, coxsackievirus, echovirus, *Ascaris*, *Mycoplasma*)
Mechanical (ampulla of Vater tumor, Crohn's disease, diverticula, pancreas divisum)
Penetrating duodenal ulcer
Hereditary pancreatitis
Idiopathic

joining organs. Other possible causes are metabolic (hyperparathyroidism, pregnancy, uremia, and kidney transplantation), certain drugs (opiates, thiazides, steroids, oral contraceptives, and sulfonamides), vascular disease, infection, and nutritional and hereditary factors.

## Pathology

The chemical and pathologic changes characteristic of pancreatitis reflect the destructive effects of pancreatic enzymes. What triggers the activation of enzymes and the exact role of the pancreatic enzymes is speculated to be autodigestion.

The major histologic alterations in pancreatitis are (1) *necrosis of fat (lipolysis)*, (2) *proteolytic destruction of pancreatic parenchyma (proteolysis)*, (3) necrosis of blood vessels with *hemorrhage*, and (4) *inflammation*.

The exocrine pancreas secretes more than 20 enzymes. The proteolytic enzymes are secreted in a proenzyme or inactive form that prevents autodigestion of the pancreas. Trypsin plays a major role because it activates the major proteolytic enzymes involved in autodigestion (Figure 39-11). Trypsin normally is secreted from the pancreas in the form of trypsinogen and is activated in the duodenum (see Chap. 42). The major initiating pathology is premature activation of trypsinogen in the pancreas. Significant amounts of trypsin, chymotrypsin, and elastase have been detected in the diseased pancreas.

Elastase exists in high concentrations in granules of acinous cells, and is present in pancreatic secretions as an inactive precursor. When activated by trypsin, it causes elastic fibers of blood vessels and ducts to dissolve. Hemorrhage caused by breakdown of elastic fibers of the vessels may be minor or extreme, varying from red blood cells and fibrin clots to large masses of blood over large areas. Prekallikrein is converted to kallikrein by trypsin. Kallikrein leads to the release of bradykinin and kallidin (a plasma kinin), which further increase vasodilatation and vascular permeability. Phospholipase A acts on phospholipids, with a resultant release of compounds that have strong cytotoxic effects and damage cell membranes and the ductal system, leading to necrosis. There are inhibitors in the plasma or in the pancreas itself that can quickly inactivate the proteolytic enzymes. Whether deficiencies in the inhibitors are factors in pancreatic disease is unknown.

A leukocytic reaction appears around the areas of hemorrhage and necrosis. Secondary bacterial invasion may produce a suppurative necrosis or abscess. Milder lesions may be absorbed, or they may calcify or become fibrotic when they are more severe. When fluid is walled off by fibrous tissue during the inflammatory process, a pancreatic cyst known as a pseudocyst is formed.

Several theories are offered to explain the mechanisms and sequence of events leading to activation of enzymes within the pancreas rather than the intestinal lumen.

According to the *duct obstruction theory*, obstruction of the common channel causes a reflux of bile that results in activation of pancreatic enzymes. The main

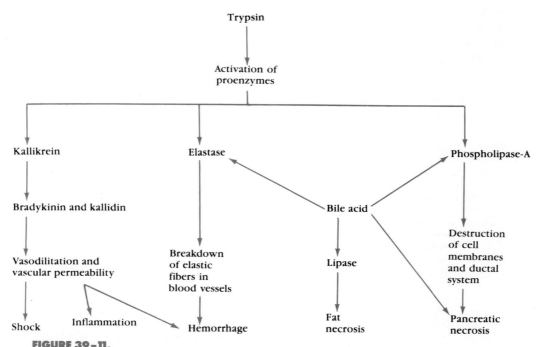

**FIGURE 39-11.**
Pathogenesis of acute pancreatitis. (Adapted from L.H. Smith and S.O. Thier, *Pathophysiology: The Biologic Principles of Disease* [2nd ed.]. Philadelphia: W.B. Saunders, 1985.)

pancreatic duct joins the common bile duct in two thirds of normal people.[3] Many persons with pancreatitis have no common channel, and the respective ducts join the duodenum separately. Bile reflux frequently occurs with pancreatitis, however, and it is believed to be active in the inflammatory process. Duodenal reflux may occur if the sphincter of Oddi is damaged by disease. Impacted gallstones in the common duct or duodenal papilla also could dilate and obstruct the sphincter. Rupture of the ducts occurs from active pancreatic secretion in the presence of ductal obstruction of any cause and consequent tearing of cell membranes, permitting activated enzymes to leak back into the gland.[1]

*Alcohol-induced* changes are major factors in the pathogenesis of pancreatitis. Alcohol is a stimulator of pancreatic secretions and also causes duodenal edema of the ampulla of Vater, obstructing flow of secretions. Long-term alcohol ingestion increases the protein concentration of secretions, which leads to formation of protein plugs in the ducts and subsequent obstruction by the precipitates, resulting in degeneration and fibrosis of acini cells. Alcohol may decrease the tone of the sphincter of Oddi and cause duodenal reflux. Another factor that predisposes alcoholics to pancreatitis may be the elevated serum triglyceride levels that occur after a meal.[7]

*Hyperlipidemia* is known to be associated with pancreatitis. Experimental studies indicate that lipolysis of triglycerides by pancreatic lipase in the pancreas leads to high concentration of free fatty acids in tissues. Animal studies indicate that these free fatty acids can initiate pancreatic injury.[3,7]

*Hypercalcemia* is thought to be a factor in activating trypsinogen and in the subsequent development of acute pancreatitis. An association of pancreatitis with parathyroid adenomas and carcinomas has been noted.

*Acinar cell injury* caused by viruses, endotoxins, toxic chemicals, ischemia, or trauma may precipitate activation and release of pancreatic enzymes. This theory is postulated for pancreatitis not caused by alcoholism or biliary disease.[3]

## Clinical Manifestations

There are no precise clinical features that distinguish pancreatitis from other disorders. *Abdominal pain* and *tenderness* are present in almost all cases of acute pancreatitis and frequently occur in chronic pancreatitis. The pain usually has no prodromal symptoms and often occurs after a large meal or an episode of heavy alcoholic consumption. It usually is severe, and may reach full intensity in a matter of minutes or gradually over several hours. Pain is frequently localized in the epigastrium, becoming more severe to the right or left of the epigastrium or generalized throughout the upper abdomen. Pancreatic pain usually is steady, boring, and penetrating. Unlike the pain of biliary colic, it radiates straight through to the back in about one half of affected people. Affected persons are restless, and may seek relief by flexing the spine, by bending forward and flexing the knees against the chest, or by lying on one side with knees flexed. Characteristically, the pain of acute pancreatitis lasts for hours and days rather than a few minutes or a few hours.

The pain of pancreatitis is related to ductal swelling, extravasation of plasma and red cells, and release of digested proteins and lipids into surrounding tissue. The pancreatic capsule is stretched by the edema, exudate, red cells, and digestive products. These substances seep out of the gland into the mesentery, causing a peritonitis that stimulates the sensory nerves and causes intense pain in back and flanks when the gland is damaged extensively. During an acute attack, the pain is generalized over the abdomen because of peritoneal irritation and release of kinins. Large doses of narcotics are avoided because they may induce spasm of the sphincter of Oddi, which aggravates the pancreatitis and increases pain. As pain increases with the spread of intraperitoneal and retroperitoneal inflammation, local or diffuse paralytic ileus may occur. Peripheral vascular collapse and shock may develop rapidly. The stretching of the gland also may cause nausea and vomiting. Vomiting and abdominal distention also are related to intestinal hypomotility and chemical peritonitis.

Other nonspecific findings include hypotension, tachycardia, and shock. Bowel sounds usually are diminished. A pancreatic pseudocyst may be palpable in the upper abdomen. In severe necrotizing pancreatitis, discoloration of the flanks (Grey Turner's sign) or around the umbilicus (Cullen's sign) may be noted. A history of a prior attack of pancreatitis may be a valuable indicator if clinical manifestations are related to pancreatitis.

The extensive injury to tissue, necrosis, and inflammation produce fever in about two thirds of cases of acute pancreatitis. Fever is due to absorption of pyrogens into the circulation, but persistent high fever or temperature spikes imply pancreatic abscess or other septic complications.[23]

## Complications

CARDIOVASCULAR COMPLICATIONS. With massive exudation of plasma into the retroperitoneal space and in cases of hemorrhage, there is a drop in blood pressure and a rise in pulse. Activation of the proteolytic enzyme kallikrein liberates bradykinin and kallidin, which are vasoactive peptides. The result is marked peripheral vasodilatation, which further reduces blood pressure. Accumulation of fluid in the small bowel, a third-space shift, causes additional loss of fluid and leads to systemic hypotension and shock.

The decrease in intravascular volume together with hypotension diminishes urine output, and acute tubular necrosis of the kidneys may result. Myocardial and cerebral ischemia also may occur.[23]

*COAGULATION DEFECTS.* Although not a frequent feature of the disease, hypercoagulability of blood caused by elevations in levels of platelets, factor VIII, fibrinogen, and possible factor V may occur.

*ILEUS.* The large and small bowel may dilate in a general response to inflammation of the peritoneum. The gut may contain air and fluid, contributing to hypovolemia.

*PULMONARY–PLEURAL COMPLICATIONS.* Acute pancreatitis frequently is accompanied by a pleural effusion. The fluid may be hemorrhagic. This pleural effusion apparently is caused by the retroperitoneal transudation of fluid, with markedly elevated secretion of amylase into the pleural cavity from the inflamed, swollen pancreas.

*GASTROINTESTINAL BLEEDING.* This may occur in association with a pseudocyst or abscess, mucosal bleeding of the duodenum caused by adjacent inflammation from the pancreas, or esophageal or gastric varices related to splenic or portal vein thrombosis.[27] Gastritis and esophagitis in alcoholics may be a source of hemorrhage in pancreatitis.

*HYPOCALCEMIA.* Sharp falls in serum calcium levels may occur in acute pancreatitis, related to extensive lipolysis of peripancreatic mesenteric and fatty tissues, releasing free fatty acids that combine with calcium to form soaps. The parathyroids do not rapidly compensate for the abrupt lowering of calcium by the mechanism of soap formation. Neuromuscular irritability and tetany result from severe hypocalcemia.

*ACIDOSIS.* Lactic acidosis may result from the central hypovolemia, or ketosis occasionally occurs when there is extensive destruction of the gland.

*HYPERLIPIDEMIA.* High levels of serum lipids often are noted during attacks of pancreatitis, especially in persons with alcoholic pancreatitis and in those with preexisting elevated triglyceride levels. The plasma may have a creamy appearance.

*PSEUDOCYSTS.* Inflammatory pseudocysts are a frequent complication during recovery from an episode of severe acute pancreatitis. The cysts are non–epithelium-lined cavities that contain plasma, blood, pancreatic products, and inflammatory exudate. They are solitary, and measure 5 to 10 cm in diameter. They occur as a result of destruction of tissue and obstruction in the ductal system. Pancreatic juice may collect in them and leak into the peritoneal cavity. If large, pseudocysts may impinge on neighboring structures such as the portal vein, causing *acute portal hypertension*, and on the bile duct, causing *jaundice*. Sometimes the cysts rupture and cause generalized peritonitis.[23]

The formation of inflammatory pseudocysts may be associated with pancreatic ascites, which develops from a direct communication between the pseudocyst and the peritoneal cavity.

*PANCREATIC ABSCESS.* One of the most serious complications of acute pancreatitis is a pancreatic abscess, a collection of purulent and necrotic tissue. It occurs if an episode of pancreatitis is severe enough to cause parenchymal necrosis and if the pancreatic and retroperitoneal tissues become secondarily infected. There usually are several foci of infection rather than a discrete abscess that can be easily drained. Pancreatic abscesses may develop in pancreatitis of various causes; however, most occur in association with alcohol abuse. They account for about 3% to 4% of all cases of pancreatitis. Fistulization into an adjacent structure with massive bleeding may occur.

*JAUNDICE.* Mild jaundice is common in acute pancreatitis. The swelling of the head of the pancreas impinges on the common bile duct that passes through it. If the bile duct is compressed by pseudocysts or stones, jaundice may be more severe.

## Diagnostic Tests

The cardinal findings of acute pancreatitis are increases in *serum amylase* and *lipase* activities. Serum amylase values usually exceed 200 Somogyi units; normal levels are 60 to 180 Somogyi units/dL. The amylase-creatinine clearance ratio is increased, and isoamylase determination reflects increased *p*-isoamylase. There does not appear to be a correlation between elevation of amylase and severity of disease.

Serum lipase activity parallels that of serum amylase, and abnormal levels persist for a longer time. Normal serum lipase values depend on the laboratory procedure used, but usually are below 1.5 U/mL. The increased activities occur shortly after onset of disease, almost always within the first 24 hours, and may remain high for weeks.

*Leukocytosis* with increased polymorphonuclear leukocytes and a shift to the left is frequent. The white blood counts range from 9000 to 20,000 but occasionally rise to 50,000 mm³. The *hematocrit* may be elevated from loss of serum into the peritoneal spaces with resultant hemoconcentration.

*Hyperglycemia* is related to various factors such as increased glucagon, decreased insulin, and increased glucocorticoid and catecholamine levels. *Hyperlipemia* often occurs, and may predate the onset of overt pancreatitis. Levels of *serum calcium* and *magnesium* decrease, especially in persons having fat necrosis. Blood calcium levels may fall and remain down for 7 to 10 days. Hypocalcemia is an indicator of severe pancreatitis.

*Ultrasonic examination* of the pancreas in severe pancreatitis may help to confirm a clinical impression, assess degree of resolution of inflammation, and reveal dilatation of common bile duct secondary to obstruction and presence of gallstones. *Computed tomographic scan* may be performed if unexplained abdominal pain suggests either pancreatitis or pancreatic carcinoma. Scans also may be used in prolonged pancreatitis or recurrent pancreatitis to rule out a pseudocyst or interductal calculi. *Roentgenograms* may be obtained to rule out a perforation and exclude other diagnoses.

## Chronic Pancreatitis

Manifestations of chronic pancreatitis are similar to those of acute pancreatitis except for their chronicity and recurrence. This disorder occurs in the same type person who is prone to developing acute pancreatitis. The person usually is an alcohol abuser and less frequently has biliary disease. Nonalcoholic tropical pancreatitis and hereditary or familial pancreatitis are forms of chronic pancreatitis that are relatively rare. If bouts recur, a pancreatic insufficiency may result, even though the pancreas has considerable functional reserve.

In chronic pancreatitis, histologic changes persist even after the causative agent has been removed. In the United States, the most common cause of chronic pancreatitis is alcohol abuse. The pathologic changes are characterized by the deposition of protein plugs in the pancreatic ductules. An inflammatory process is set up, and fibrous tissue is deposited. Eventually there is intraductal calcification and marked parenchymal destruction, with only a few islet cells and some acinar tissue remaining.

Exocrine pancreatic insufficiency is manifested by steatorrhea (excess fat in the stools), azotorrhea (excess nitrogenous material in the feces), and weight loss. Microscopically, the stool exhibits fat globules and striated meat fibers that indicate impaired digestion of fats and proteins. Endocrine pancreatic insufficiency may lead to diabetes mellitus. Abdominal pain is a serious problem in chronic pancreatitis, and may be responsible for severe weight loss, malnutrition, and general debility. During early stages of the disease, the person may be asymptomatic between attacks.

The predominant complications of chronic pancreatitis that are associated with abdominal pain are pancreatic pseudocyst, stricture and obstruction of the common bile duct or pancreatic duct, and, occasionally, carcinoma of the pancreas.

# CARCINOMA OF THE PANCREAS

Carcinoma of the pancreas occurs mainly in the exocrine portion of the gland in the ductal epithelium. Pancreatic cancers have a poor prognosis, causing about 5% of all neoplastic deaths in the United States.[3] A significant increase in frequency has been attributed to smoking, consumption of alcoholic beverages, and consumption of fat. Increased risk also has been associated with disease of the gallbladder and bile duct (extrahepatic). Chemists and people exposed to industrial agents also are at higher risk for pancreatic cancer. Most tumors occur in people over age 60; they seldom occur before age 40.

Clinical symptoms of cancer of the pancreas depend on its site of origin and manifestations of metastasis. Tumors of the head of the pancreas tend to obstruct the bile duct and duodenum, and lead to early symptoms of obstructive jaundice; carcinoma of the body and tail are less easily recognized clinically, and become apparent only when adjacent structures are involved or when metastatic dissemination produces symptoms.

Most carcinomas of the pancreas grow in well-differentiated glandular patterns and are *adenocarcinomas*. About 10% assume an *adenosquamous* pattern or an uncommon pattern of extreme anaplasia with *giant cell* formation. About 0.5% arise in cysts, and are called *cystadenocarcinoma*. An *acinar cell carcinoma* occasionally occurs in children.[2,3]

## Carcinoma of the Head of the Pancreas

Tumors of the head of the pancreas are fairly small lesions with poorly defined margins. They often impinge on the common bile duct and pancreatic duct, causing atrophy of the pancreas. The tumors usually extend to the duodenum and cause compression and crowding of the common bile duct and ampulla of Vater, with distention of the gallbladder.

Carcinoma of the head of the pancreas usually is not a widely disseminated lesion because it produces biliary duct obstruction and jaundice at an early date. Affected persons usually die of hepatobiliary dysfunction before the tumor has become widely disseminated.

## Carcinoma of the Body and Tail of the Pancreas

These tumors usually are large, and invade the entire tail and body of the pancreas; they may even be palpable in a thin person. They spread more extensively than tumors of the head, and crowd the vertebral column, spread into the retroperitoneal spaces, and may even invade the spleen, adrenals, colon, or stomach. Metastases spread by way of the splenic vein, which lies on the margins of the organ, to surrounding nodes and the liver. The liver may be enlarged two to three times its normal size.[3]

## Clinical Manifestations

The clinical manifestations are those that relate to the encroachment of the pancreas on surrounding organs. Dull epigastric abdominal pain, which may radiate to the back; weight loss with anorexia; and jaundice are among the few characteristic signs or symptoms that point to a diagnosis of pancreatic cancer. Anorexia occasionally is accompanied by a curious aversion to meats and a metallic taste in the mouth.[2] Jaundice occurs in 80% to 90% of persons with carcinoma of the head of the pancreas, and occurs in 10% to 40% of those with tumors of the body and tail.[7] Large tumors that arise from the head of the pancreas often encase the common bile duct. Jaundice is accompanied by pruritus. Weight loss and jaundice often are accompanied by a distended gallbladder.

Nausea, vomiting, weakness, fatigue, diarrhea, and dyspepsia also are fairly common. Vomiting may indicate gastric or duodenal encroachment or peritoneal metastasis. Hematemesis and melena indicate invasion of the tumor into duodenal or gastric organs that are vascular. About one fourth of persons with pancreatic cancer have a palpable abdominal mass when examined and often complain of both constipation and diarrhea. Emotional disturbances may be noted. Thrombophlebitis and diabetes mellitus are other clinical features. An abdominal bruit may be auscultated in the periumbilical area and left upper quadrant because of compression of the splenic artery by a tumor.

## Clinical Course

Carcinomas of the pancreas progress insidiously, and probably are present for months and perhaps years before symptoms appear. Major symptoms include weight loss, abdominal pain, back pain, anorexia, nausea, vomiting, generalized malaise, and weakness. Pain occurs in advanced stages of the disease. Jaundice is present in about one half of those with carcinoma of the head of the pancreas.[2]

Laboratory procedures are important in providing clues to the presence of these cancers in their early stages.

About 80% to 90% have elevated levels of carcinoembryonic antigen. Measurement of this antigen may be helpful in following the course of pancreatic cancer, with titers of greater than 20 mg/mL usually being associated with metastases. As with obstructive jaundice, serum bilirubin levels increase, stools become clay-colored, and urine urobilinogen levels fall. Alkaline phosphatase levels are elevated.[2]

Ultrasonography can assist in localizing tumors and differentiating them from cysts. A computed tomographic scan and magnetic resonance imaging of the pancreas are helpful in confirming presence of tumor. Percutaneous needle biopsy is useful in diagnosing when tumors are localized.

Spontaneously appearing phlebothrombosis, also called migratory thrombophlebitis, is noted in carcinoma of the pancreas (Trousseau's sign). Trousseau diagnosed his own fatal disease when he developed migratory thrombophlebitis. Thromboses appear and disappear in other forms of cancer, but the two highest correlations are in pancreatic and pulmonary neoplasms. The thromboses are attributed to confinement to bed and surgical treatment. Thromboplastic factors have been identified in the serum that lead to a hypercoagulable state because of thromboplastic properties of the necrotic products of the tumor.[3]

## CYSTIC FIBROSIS

Cystic fibrosis (CF), formerly referred to as mucoviscidosis or fibrocystic disease of the pancreas, is a systemic disease of infancy or childhood. Alterations in the secretory process of the exocrine (mucus-producing) glands result in several complications, especially in the pulmonary system and gastrointestinal tract.

## Frequency

CF has clearly been recognized as a disease entity only since the late 1930s. Historical notes tell of the midwife licking the forehead of the newborn to identify any salty taste. It is now considered to be a common inherited condition and the most fatal genetic disease in Caucasians. The incidence is about 1 in 2000 in Caucasian populations. Black and Oriental races seldom are affected. There is no difference in sex distribution.

CF is transmitted by the autosomal recessive mode of inheritance. The CF gene is located on the long arm of chromosome 7.[16] Chromosome number and structure are normal. Clinical manifestations are only evident in homozygotes. Carriers of the gene (heterozygotes) show no symptoms of the disease. About 5% of the Caucasian population carry the CF gene. More children with this disease are surviving to adulthood, marrying, and reproducing; therefore, genetic risks are now being considered. Affected people transmit the gene to all of their offspring, but the children cannot develop the disease (homozygote) unless both parents are carriers.

## Pathogenesis

CF is a disorder of secretory epithelia of the airways, sweat glands, pancreas, and other organs. Because of the defective gene, abnormalities occur in regulation of transport proteins across the epithelium from blood to lumen. This alteration affects Cl transport, and is manifested by a decrease in fluid and salt secretion.[10,12] Mucus abnormalities are apparent, but the glands themselves are normal until cellular changes related to the disease process occur. Elevation in sweat chloride levels seems to be the only consistent biochemical alteration (Figure 39-12).

The anatomic changes of CF are thought to result from obstruction of exocrine ducts by thick, heavy, dehydrated mucus. Abnormalities have been reported in autonomic nervous system function, related to reduction of cell membrane beta-adrenergic receptors on leukocytes. Higher levels of calcium have been found in cells and certain mucous glands of persons with CF, particularly the salivary glands.[14] Both intracellular calcium and autonomic nervous system activity influence secretory processes of glands and have been cited as factors in the pathogenesis of CF.

CF is a generalized disorder that affects many body organs. The organs most frequently involved in CF are the lungs, pancreas, intestine, liver, reproductive tract, and sweat and tear glands (see Figure 39-12).

### Gastrointestinal Tract

The extent of changes is related to whether secretions are carried to the gastrointestinal tract from cells with narrow

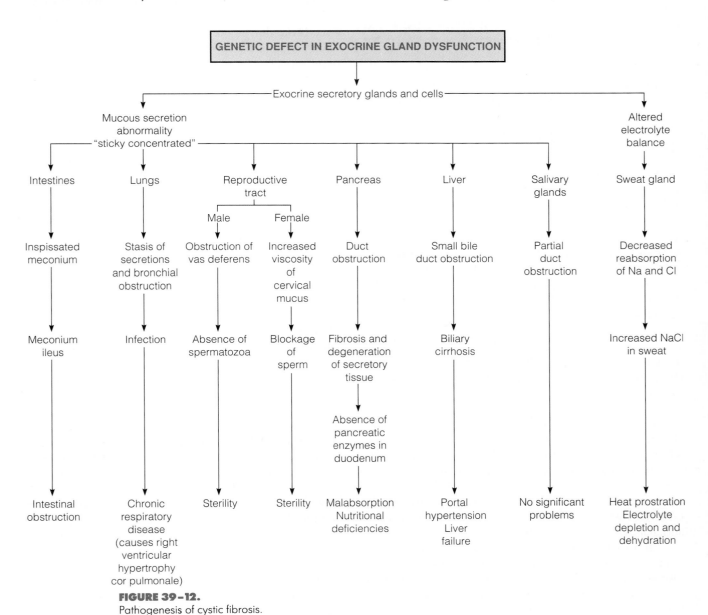

**FIGURE 39-12.**
Pathogenesis of cystic fibrosis.

necks, such as the goblet cells; from wide-mouthed ducts, such as glands in the duodenum; or from narrow ducts, such as those in the pancreas, liver, and salivary glands. The thick, tenacious secretions tend to cause more problems in longer, narrow ducts with resultant changes in tissues and alterations of function. The greatest alterations in structure and function occur in the pancreas.

*STRUCTURAL CHANGES IN THE PANCREAS.*    Abnormalities in the pancreas occur in about 85% of affected people. These changes are evident microscopically and macroscopically as early as the neonatal period. The changes are variable, and depend on the age of onset and severity of disease. They may consist of accumulation of mucus or, as the disease progresses, blockage of the collecting ducts, damage to acinar tissue, fibrosis and duct dilatation, and degeneration of the parenchyma. The ducts may be replaced by fat and fibrous tissue and converted into cysts. These changes in appearance are the bases for the designation fibrocystic disease of the pancreas.

Pathologic changes begin during fetal life, and frequently are severe enough by birth to prevent exocrine secretions from reaching the duodenum. The development of diabetes mellitus in some older people is suggestive of impairment of the blood supply by progressive fibrosis.

Functional changes occur as a result of structural alterations. There is a lack of enzymes (trypsin, amylase, lipase) in the duodenum, and as a result, proteins are not completely digested and nitrogen is excreted in the stools; starch is not completely broken down and appears as granules; fats are largely undigested and are excreted in the stools in excessive amounts. The stools are large and oily, and have a pungent odor caused in part by breakdown products of protein produced by bacteria in the intestine.

*LIVER.*    Blockage of the bile duct by mucus and mononuclear periportal cell infiltration leads to cirrhosis and portal hypertension. Esophageal varices and splenomegaly may result.

*INTESTINE.*    Absence of pancreatic enzymes and altered gastrointestinal mucus secretions produce thick tenacious plugs of viscid mucus that obstruct the lumen of the small intestine, causing meconium ileus.

*SALIVARY GLANDS.*    The salivary glands frequently undergo histologic changes such as dilatation of ducts and glandular atrophy and fibrosis.

Pathologic changes also occur in other glands. Plugging occurs in the bile ducts, leading to fibrosis and liver dysfunction. CF is an important cause of hepatic cirrhosis and portal hypertension in adolescents and young adults.

## Respiratory System

Pulmonary changes occur in almost all affected persons and usually are the primary determinants of the ultimate outcome of the disease. Both upper and lower respiratory tracts are involved because of the presence of mucus-secreting glands and cells. The lungs are structurally normal at birth, but problems begin in the small bronchioles, where the thick, tenacious mucus collects and provides a medium for bacterial growth. The most common organisms are *Staphylococcus aureus, Haemophilus influenzae*, and *Pseudomonas aeruginosa*. The mucoid form of the last is especially troublesome.

Infection alters the integrity of the bronchial epithelium and invades the peribronchial tissues. Bronchiectasis develops in the terminal bronchioles. Trapping of air produces an overinflated barrel-shaped chest. Mucopurulent exudates also are present in the upper respiratory tract. Nasal polyps occur with increased frequency, and often are associated with sinus infections. Pulmonary hypertension results from thickened arterioles, which, together with the obstructive bronchial disease, leads to right ventricular hypertrophy and cor pulmonale.

## Reproductive System

Abnormalities include atresia or obstruction of the vas deferens and epididymis in the male. Spermatogenesis is decreased or absent.

In the female, mucus-producing glands of the cervix also may produce viscid mucus that blocks the entry of sperm. The frequency of cervical polyps is increased.

## Sweat Glands

Although there is a high electrolyte content of the sweat and an alteration in resorption of sodium chloride in the sweat ducts, no structural abnormalities are noted in the ducts.

## Clinical Manifestations

In recent years, new genetic markers have been identified that make it possible to diagnose CF prenatally and to detect carriers in families with a history of CF.[16] Because CF affects several organ systems in varying degrees, sometimes it is difficult to recognize. Most persons are diagnosed in early childhood because of symptoms related to the respiratory and gastrointestinal systems. An early manifestation of CF is meconium ileus in the newborn, which blocks the small intestine with thick, tenacious, puttylike meconium. The degree varies from a delay in passing meconium (meconium plug syndrome) to an obvious intestinal obstruction, usually in the area of the ileocecal valve, that may be accompanied by atresia, volvulus, or perforation and peritonitis. Prolapse of the rectum related to chronic constipation is a common complication in children with untreated CF.

In the classic case, the child is examined after 1 month of life because of respiratory symptoms, failure to thrive, and foul-smelling, bulky, greasy stools. Any one or all characteristics may be noted. In some cases, symptoms are not apparent until several years have passed. Many infants have a dry, repetitive cough that occurs in an attempt to remove the sticky secretion. Vomiting may follow a bout of coughing. Classic progression of chest infection occurs, with increased coughing and sputum, development of barrel chest, finger-clubbing, dyspnea, and cyanosis. Sputum is thick, sticky, and difficult to expectorate. In the early stages, it is yellow, particularly if due to *S. aureus*. With the mucoid strain, *P. aeruginosa*, sputum is greenish and slimy.

Microscopic examination of the stool reveals the presence of numerous fat globules. Many children compensate for stool losses with a voracious appetite, but they lose weight, exhibit tissue wasting, and fail to grow. In geographic areas where humidity is high, babies with CF may develop dehydration and electrolyte imbalance because of salt loss. Bleeding disorders may occur as a result of vitamin K deficiency from malabsorption.

Uncommonly, the disorder may be diagnosed during adolescence or adulthood. Diagnosis is difficult, as the sweat test is less reliable in these age-groups than in younger ones. Persons affected with CF who have not had severe chest infection may have abdominal problems, diabetes, or liver disease.

## Laboratory and Diagnostic Findings

Criteria for diagnosis of CF include increased electrolyte concentration of sweat, absence of pancreatic enzymes, impaired fat absorption, chronic pulmonary involvement, and family history of the disorder.

The *sweat test* is the simplest and most reliable method to confirm the diagnosis. Up to age 20, a level of more than 60 mEq/L of sweat chloride is diagnostic of CF. Values between 50 and 60 mEq/L are highly suggestive. The sweat test is repeated if results are questionable or if they are negative and clinical manifestations are strongly suggestive of CF. Reliable sweat tests are difficult to obtain in the first 3 to 4 weeks of life because the sweat glands are not yet well developed functionally.

Roentgenograms reveal changes in respiratory and gastrointestinal systems. Chest films reveal slightly increased diameter of upper chest, with overaerated lungs, widespread consolidation, and fibrotic changes. There may be areas of lobar or segmental collapse.

Changes in radiologic patterns of the small intestine

are noted in CF as in other malabsorptive diseases. Fibrosis abnormalities also are evident in barium studies of the duodenum.

*Pancreatic deficiency* is noted on examination of duodenal contents for pancreatic enzyme (trypsin and chymotrypsin) activity. Trypsin is absent in about 80% of affected people. Chemical examination of feces reveals marked steatorrhea. Normal stools should not contain more than 4 g of fat per day. Stools of children with CF often contain 15 to 30 g/d.

## REFERENCES

1. Barnett, A.H. Diabetes in identical twins: A study of 200 pairs. *Diabetologia* 20:57, 1981.
2. Cello, J.P. Carcinoma of the pancreas. In J.B. Wyngaarden and L.H. Smith (eds.), *Cecil's Textbook of Medicine* (18th ed.). Philadelphia: W.B. Saunders, 1988.
3. Cotran, R.S., Kumar, V., and Robbins, S.L. *Robbins' Pathologic Basis of Disease* (4th ed.). Philadelphia: W.B. Saunders, 1989.
4. Doniach, D. Etiology of type I diabetes mellitus: Heterogeneity and immunologic events leading to clinical onset. *Annu. Rev. Med.* 23:13, 1983.
5. Foster, D.W. Diabetes mellitus. In J.D. Wilson et al. (eds.), *Harrison's Principles of Internal Medicine* (12th ed.). New York: McGraw-Hill, 1991.
6. Ganda, O.P. Pathogenesis of macrovascular disease including the influence of lipids. In A. Marble et al. (eds.), *Joslin's Diabetes Mellitus* (12th ed.). Philadelphia: Lea & Febiger, 1985.
7. Greenberger, N.J., Toskes, P.P., and Isselbacher, K.I. Acute and chronic pancreatitis. In J.D. Wilson et al. (eds.), *Harrison's Principles of Internal Medicine* (12th ed.). New York: McGraw-Hill, 1991.
8. Guyton, A.C. *Textbook of Medical Physiology* (8th ed.). Philadelphia: W.B. Saunders, 1990.
9. Hostetter, M.K. Handicaps to host defense: Effects of hyperglycemia on C3 and *Candida albicans*. *Diabetes* 39:271, 1990.
10. Jetten, A.M., Yankaskas, J.R., Stutts, M.J., et al. Persistence of abnormal chloride conductance regulation in transformed cystic fibrosis epithelia. *Science* 244:1472, 1989.
11. Kozak, G.P., and Krall, L.P. Disorders of the skin. In A. Marble et al. (eds.), *Joslin's Diabetes Mellitus* (12th ed.). Philadelphia: Lea & Febiger, 1985.
12. Levitan, I.B. The basic defect in cystic fibrosis. *Science* 244:1423, 1989.
13. Locke, S., and Tarsy, D. The nervous system and diabetes. In A. Marble et al. (eds.), *Joslin's Diabetes Mellitus* (12th ed.). Philadelphia: Lea & Febiger, 1985.
14. Loeb, J.N. Polyglandular disorders. In J. Wyngaarden and L.H. Smith (eds.), *Cecil's Textbook of Medicine* (18th ed.). Philadelphia: W.B. Saunders, 1988.
15. National Diabetes Data Group. Classification and diagnosis of diabetes mellitus and other categories of glucose intolerance. *Diabetes* 28:1039, 1979.

16. O'Connell, D.M., Leppert, M., Park, A., et al. Three additional polymorphisms in the met gene and D758 locus: Use in prenatal diagnosis of cystic fibrosis. *J. Pediatrics* 111:490, 1987.

17. O'Hare, J.A., and Warfield, C.A. The diabetic neuropathies. *Hosp. Pract.* 19:40, 1984.

18. Olefski, J.M. Diabetes mellitus. In J. Wyngaarden and L.H. Smith (eds.), *Cecil's Textbook of Medicine* (18th ed.). Philadelphia: W.B. Saunders, 1988.

19. Osterby, R. Basement membrane morphology in diabetes mellitus. In M. Ellenberg and H. Rifkin (eds.), *Diabetes Mellitus: Theory and Practice* (3rd ed.). New Hyde Park, N.Y.: Medical Examination, 1983.

20. Seino, S., Seino, M., and Bell, G.I. Human insulin-receptor gene. *Diabetes* 39:243, 1990.

21. Service, F.J. Hypoglycemic disorders. In J. Wyngaarden and L.H. Smith (eds.), *Cecil's Textbook of Medicine* (18th ed.). Philadelphia: W.B. Saunders, 1988.

22. Service, J., et al. Pancreatic polypeptide A for lean non-insulin-dependent diabetes mellitus? *Diabetes Care* 8:July-August, 1985.

23. Smith, L.H., and Thier, S.O. (eds.). *Pathophysiology: The Biologic Principles of Disease* (2nd ed.). Philadelphia: W.B. Saunders, 1985.

24. Srikanta, S. Type I diabetes mellitus in monozygotic twins: Chronic progressive beta cell dysfunction. *Ann. Intern. Med.* 99:320, 1983.

25. Unger, R.H., and Foster, D.W. Diabetes mellitus. In J.D. Wilson and D.W. Foster (eds.), *Williams' Textbook of Endocrinology* (7th ed.). Philadelphia: W.B. Saunders, 1985.

## UNIT BIBLIOGRAPHY

Anderson, J.R. *Muir's Textbook of Pathology*. London: Edward Arnold, 1985.

Anderson, R.A., et al. Effect of exercise (running) on serum glucose, insulin, glucagon and chromium excretion. *Diabetes* 31:212, 1982.

Barrett, E.J., and Defronzo, R.A. Diabetic ketoacidosis: Diagnosis and treatment. *Hosp. Pract.* 19:89, 1984.

Biesbroeck, J.J., et al. Abnormal composition of high density lipoproteins in non-insulin-dependent diabetes. *Diabetes* 31:126, 1982.

Bogardus, C., et al. Effects of physical training and diet therapy on carbohydrate metabolism in patients with glucose intolerance and non-insulin-dependent diabetes mellitus. *Diabetes* 33:311, 1984.

Burch, W.M. *Endocrinology for the House Officer* (2nd ed.). Baltimore: Williams & Wilkins, 1988.

Cahill, G.F., and McDevitt, H.O. Insulin-dependent diabetes mellitus: The initial lesion. *N. Engl. J. Med.* 304:1454, 1981.

Calloway, C. When the problem involves magnesium, calcium, or phosphate. *RN* 50(5):30, 1987.

Carter Center of Emory University. Closing the gap: The problem of diabetes mellitus in the United States. *Diabetes Care* 8:391, 1985.

Chambers, J.K. Metabolic bone disorders: Imbalances of calcium and phosphorus. *Nurs. Clin. North Am.* 22:861, 1987.

Chernow, B., Wiley, S., and Zaloga, G. Critical care endocrinology. In W. Shoemaker et al. (eds.), *Textbook of Critical Care* (2nd ed.). Philadelphia: W.B. Saunders, 1989.

Cotran, R.S., Kumar, V., and Robbins, S.L. *Robbins' Pathologic Basis of Disease* (4th ed.). Philadelphia: W.B. Saunders, 1989.

Dillon, R.S. *Handbook of Endocrinology* (2nd ed.). Philadelphia: Lea & Febiger, 1980.

DiMagno, E.P. Answers to questions on acute pancreatitis. *Hosp. Med.* 19:91, 1983.

Featherston, W.E., and Ram, C.V.S. Secondary causes of hypertension: Health and cost benefits of making these diagnoses. *Consultant* 27:109, 1987.

Feek, C., and Edwards, C. *Endocrine and Metabolic Disease*. New York: Springer-Verlag, 1988.

Few, B.J. Corticosteroids and respiratory distress syndrome. *Maternal-Child Nurs.* 13:17, 1988.

Gann, D.S., and Lilly, M.P. The neuroendocrine response to multiple trauma. *World J. Surg.* 7:101, 1983.

Geelhoed, G.B., and Chernow, B. *Endocrine Aspects of Acute Illness*. New York: Churchill Livingstone, 1985.

Guyton, A.C. *Textbook of Medical Physiology* (8th ed.). Philadelphia: W.B. Saunders, 1990.

Hall, R., and Kobberling, J. *Thyroid Disorders Associated with Iodine Deficiency and Excess*. New York: Raven Press, 1984.

Harper, J. Use of steroids in cerebral edema: Therapeutic implications. *Heart Lung* 17:70, 1988.

Holmes, E.W. Endocrinology, metabolism, and genetics. In W.N. Kelley (ed.), *Textbook of Internal Medicine*. Philadelphia: J.B. Lippincott, 1989.

Jubiz, W. *Endocrinology: A Logical Approach for Clinicians* (2nd ed.). New York: McGraw-Hill, 1985.

Lancaster, L.E. Renal and endocrine regulation of water and electrolyte balance. *Nurs. Clin. North Am.* 22:761, 1987.

Laycock, J.F., and Wise, P.H. *Essential Endocrinology*. New York: Oxford University Press, 1983.

Longcope, C. Adrenogenital syndrome. *Hosp. Med.* 20:79, 1985.

Marsden, P., and McCullagh, A.G. *Endocrinology*. Littleton, Mass.: PSG Publishing Co., 1985.

Martin, C.R. *Endocrine Physiology*. New York: Oxford University Press, 1985.

Mazzaferri, E.L. *Textbook of Endocrinology* (3rd ed.). New Hyde Park, N.Y.: Medical Examination, 1986.

Metz, R., and Larson, E.B. *Blue Book of Endocrinology*. Philadelphia: W.B. Saunders, 1985.

Mishell, D.R., and Davajon, V. *Infertility, Contraception, and Reproductive Endocrinology*. Oradell, N.J.: Medical Economics Books, 1986.

Mohan, V., et al. High prevalence of maturity-onset diabetes of the young (MODY) among Indians. *Diabetes Care* 8:171, 1985.

Moore-Ede, M.C., Sulzman, F.M., and Fuller, C.A. *The Clocks That Time Us: Physiology of the Circadian Timing System*. Cambridge, Mass.: Harvard University Press, 1982.

Pittman, C.S., and Menefee, J.K. Pathophysiology of Graves' disease. *Hosp. Pract.* 22:147, 1987.

Plowman, P.N. *Endocrinology and Metabolic Diseases*. New York: Medical Examination, 1987.

Poyss, A.S. Assessment and nursing diagnosis in fluid and electrolyte disorders. *Nurs. Clin. North Am.* 22:773, 1987.

Sarsany, S.L. Thyroid storm. *RN* 51:46, 1988.

Service, F.J. Hypoglycemic disorders. In J. Wyngaarden and L.H. Smith (eds.), *Cecil's Textbook of Medicine* (18th ed.). Philadelphia: W.B. Saunders, 1988.

Shearman, R.P. *Clinical Reproductive Endocrinology.* New York: Churchill Livingstone, 1985.

Skelton, C.W. Use of glycosylated hemoglobins in the long-term management of diabetes. *Nurse Pract.* 11:42, 1986.

Smith, L.E., and Thier, S.O. (eds.). *Pathophysiology: The Biological Principles of Disease* (2nd ed.). Philadelphia: W.B. Saunders, 1985.

Sodeman, W.A., and Sodeman, T.M. *Sodeman's Pathologic Physiology: Mechanisms of Disease* (7th ed.). Philadelphia: W.B. Saunders, 1985.

Srikanta, S., et al. Autoimmunity to insulin, beta cell dysfunction, and development of insulin-dependent diabetes mellitus. *Diabetes* 35:139, 1986.

Tucker, S.M., Canobbio, M.M., Paquette, E.V., and Wells, M.F. Hyperthyroidism: Thyroid crisis. *J. Emerg. Nurs.* 15:352, 1989.

Ward, W.K., et al. Pathophysiology of insulin secretion in non-insulin-dependent diabetes mellitus. *Diabetes Care* 7:491, 1984.

Wilson, J.D. et al. (eds.). *Harrison's Textbook of Internal Medicine* (12th ed.). New York: McGraw-Hill, 1991.

Wilson, J.D., and Foster, D.W. (eds.). *Williams' Textbook of Endocrinology* (8th ed.). Philadelphia: W.B. Saunders, 1990.

Wyngaarden, J.B., and Smith, L.H. (eds.). *Cecil's Textbook of Medicine* (18th ed.). Philadelphia: W.B. Saunders, 1988.

Normal Function of the Gastrointestinal System

Alterations in Gastrointestinal Function

Normal Hepatobiliary and Pancreatic Exocrine Function

Alterations in Hepatobiliary Function

# DIGESTION, ABSORPTION, AND USE OF FOOD

**K**nowledge of the anatomic and functional activities of the entire gastrointestinal system is essential for the understanding of the pathologies of part or all of the system. Digestion, absorption, and use of food require the participation of all of the gastrointestinal organs, including the liver and pancreas. Alterations can occur at any point in the system and affect the entire system. Chapter 40 describes the normal activities of the gastrointestinal system, including the oral cavity, stomach, intestines, and other components. Chapter 42 includes the normal liver and pancreatic exocrine functions. Chapter 41 details alterations in the gastrointestinal system, and Chapter 43 explains alterations in hepatobiliary function. Pancreatic alterations are covered in detail in Chapter 39.

The reader is encouraged to use the learning objectives as study guides for chapter content. The unit bibliography also gives current resources for further study.

# Normal Function of the Gastrointestinal System

## Learning Objectives

1. Differentiate appetite, hunger, and satiety.
2. Describe the function of salivary ptyalin.
3. Briefly define *functional syncytium* as applied to the gastrointestinal system.
4. Locate and describe the functional significance of the sphincters in the gastrointestinal tract.
5. Locate and clearly describe the function of the gastric glands.
6. Explain the important characteristics of chyme as it moves into the small intestine.
7. Describe the appearance and function of the intestinal microvilli.
8. Locate the blood supply, nerve supply, and lymphatic drainage of the gastrointestinal system.
9. Relate the importance of oral secretions to digestion.
10. Describe swallowing.
11. Clearly delineate the purposes of all of the gastric secretions in digestion.
12. Describe the relation of nervous and hormonal mechanisms in digestion.
13. Briefly outline the cephalic, gastric, and intestinal phases of gastric secretions.
14. Define and list examples of *secretagogues*.
15. Explain the mechanisms that cause emesis.
16. Describe how the intestines inhibit gastric secretions.
17. Describe specifically where nutrients are absorbed in the small intestine.
18. Relate the mechanisms necessary for the absorption of carbohydrates, proteins, and fats.
19. Briefly list the form and mechanism for the absorption of nutrients, vitamins, and minerals.
20. Describe defecation.
21. Briefly explain the role of the large intestine in regulating water balance.

Normal functioning of the human body depends on an intact digestive system. In the broadest sense, the gastrointestinal tract is a tubular structure called the *alimentary canal,* which extends from the pharynx to the anus. Throughout this tubular structure ingested food is processed, digested, and absorbed. The nutrients absorbed may be further processed by accessory organs, used for energy, or stored for later energy.

For digestion to occur, the vital functions of motility, secretion, and absorption must proceed in a regulated manner. Finally, by participating in the excretion of waste products, the gastrointestinal system helps to keep the host in a balanced state. In the adult, the steady state normally provides for a balanced body weight, so that ingested nutrients are used and weight remains stable.

## APPETITE, HUNGER, AND SATIETY

Appetite refers to a desire for specific types of food.[7] Learned patterns of behavior alter the appetite, creating a desire for food beyond the needs of the body. Hunger refers to the desire for food that results from the manifest need for energy. Satisfaction of hunger is called satiety.

The hunger center is in the *hypothalamus,* as is the *satiety center,* but the two are in separate locations.[7] The feeling of hunger frequently is generated by rhythmic contractions of the stomach, which may cause a painful sensation called hunger pangs. Stimulation from the hunger center is related to the nutritional status of the body. Especially important in this process is the concentration of glucose in the blood. A decreased concentration of blood glucose intensifies the hunger response. Serum fat levels and amino acids also affect satiety. Distention of the gastrointestinal tract suppresses the hunger center through inhibitory signals, probably from sensory signals by the vagal nerves.[7]

The *appetite center* is more subtly controlled by the cortical areas, and is stimulated by sight, touch, and smell. Even thoughts of food can stimulate the appetite center. Alterations of appetite for specific foods are conditioned by culture, environment, and socioeconomic circumstances.

## ANATOMY OF THE GASTROINTESTINAL TRACT

The activity of the gastrointestinal tract is carried out through a continuous structure that begins with the oral cavity and terminates with the anal sphincter (Figure 40-1).

### Oral Cavity

The lips, tongue, cheeks, teeth, taste buds, and salivary glands are associated with the oral cavity, and contribute to the preparation of food for eventual absorption. This preparation includes reducing food particles to manageable size, stimulating salivary glands to increase saliva secretion, and moving food to the appropriate position for swallowing. Table 40-1 summarizes the oral structures and their participation in preparing food for digestion.

The submandibular, parotid, and sublingual salivary glands continuously secrete *saliva,* which contains large amounts of water and small amounts of sodium, chloride, bicarbonate, urea, and a few other solutes (Figure 40-2). Saliva also contains *ptyalin* (salivary amylase), an enzyme that digests starches. The average amounts of salivary secretion range from 1000 to 1500 mL/d. Stimulation for this secretion is relayed to the medulla by the parasympathetic fibers of the facial, trigeminal, glossopharyngeal, and vagus nerves. Efferent parasympathetic stimulation leads to increased secretion of saliva. Stimulation of the sympathetic system causes localized vasoconstriction and a decrease in salivary secretion.

### Pharynx

The pharynx is an important structure for swallowing. It actively moves food into the esophagus, while closing and sealing off the trachea. Once the swallowing reflex is initiated by voluntary movement of food to the back of the mouth, swallowing continues as a reflex activity.

### Esophagus

The esophagus provides a passageway for food from the pharynx to the stomach. An *upper esophageal sphincter* prevents food or fluid movement into the posterior pharynx and trachea. It is a muscular, pliable tube that is easily affected by intrathoracic or intraabdominal pressures or volumes. The esophagus is lined with a mucosal layer composed of squamous epithelium.[4] Glands along its length secrete mucus to lubricate the bolus of food passing through.

The construction of the smooth muscle of the esophagus and other structures in the alimentary canal has been described as a *functional syncytium* because the smooth-muscle fibers lie close to one another. This construction allows for waves of muscular contraction called *peristalsis.*[7]

About 5 cm above the esophageal entry to the stomach is a narrowed area called the *gastroesophageal, cardiac,* or *lower esophageal sphincter* (see Figure 40-1). A sphincter is an opening that has an extra amount of muscle surrounding it. The gastroesophageal sphincter cannot be identified on anatomic dissection, but it acts as a sphincter. It normally remains constricted but relaxes when a peristaltic wave is conducted through it, allowing food to pass to the stomach. The gastroesophageal

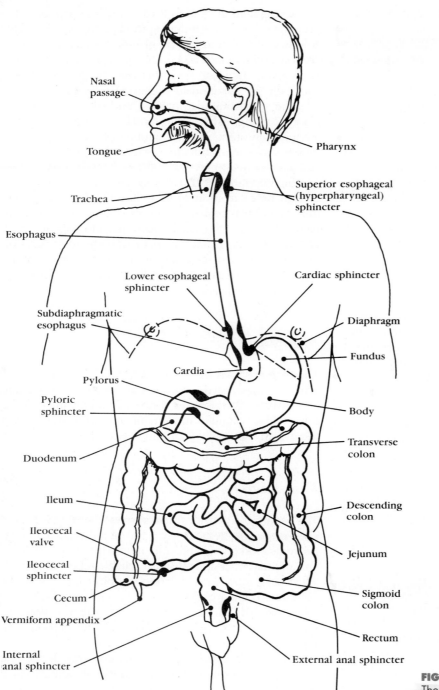

**FIGURE 40–1.**
The digestive system.

sphincter seems to prevent acid reflux into the esophagus (Table 40-2).

## Stomach

The stomach is a pear-shaped, hollow, distensible organ whose parts consist of the cardia, fundus, body, antrum, and pylorus (Figure 40-3). Figure 40-3 also shows the position of the greater and lesser curvatures of the stomach.

The upper portion of the stomach is continuous with the esophagus, and lies close to the diaphragm; the lower portion is continuous with the duodenum through the lower pyloric sphincter.

The interior lining of the stomach lies in mucosal folds called *rugae*. Within the mucosal folds are glands that secrete gastric juices. Gastric juice is composed of secretions from four major cell types: (1) *chief,* (2) *parietal,* (3) *mucus-producing,* and (4) *gastrin-producing (G cells)* (Figure 40-4). The chief cells secrete the pro-

**TABLE 40–1.**
PARTICIPATION OF THE ORAL STRUCTURES
IN DIGESTION

| STRUCTURE | PROCESS |
|---|---|
| Teeth | Reduce food to sizes appropriate for swallowing; break down dense particles |
| Tongue | Places food in proper position for swallowing; mixes secretions to moisten food |
| Salivary glands | Moisten and lubricate foods in the mouth; add ptyalin enzyme for digestion of starches |
| Muscles of mastication, or chewing | Provide movement for the grinding of food to smaller particles; provide more surface area for the digestive enzymes to act |

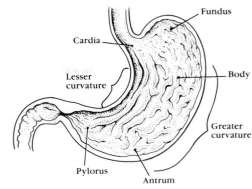

**FIGURE 40–3.**
Segments of the stomach. Note the greater and lesser curvatures.

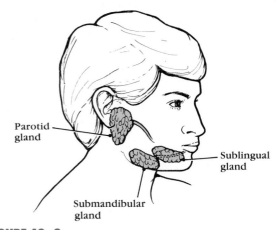

**FIGURE 40–2.**
Salivary glands.

**TABLE 40–2.**
SPHINCTER FUNCTION

| SPHINCTER | FUNCTION |
|---|---|
| Upper esophageal | Presents expulsion of food into posterior pharynx |
| Lower esophageal | Transports food bolus from esophagus to stomach and prevents gastric reflux into upper esophagus |
| Pyloric | Coordinates organized emptying of stomach and prevents reflux of duodenal contents |
| Ileocecal | Prevents retrograde expulsion of intestinal contents |
| Anal | Inhibits expulsion of colonic contents unless voluntary relaxation is established |

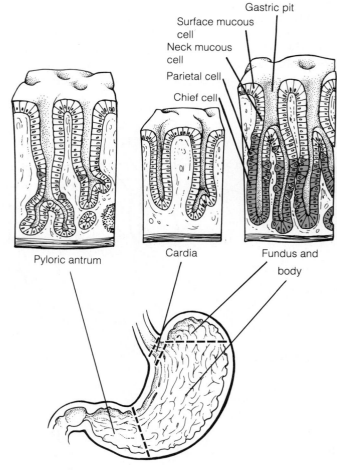

**FIGURE 40–4.**
Four anatomic and three histologic regions of the stomach. The depths of the gastric pits and the glandular composition are different in the various areas of the stomach. (Adapted from C.M. Fenoglio-Preiser, et al., *Gastrointestinal Pathology: An Atlas and Text.* New York: Raven, 1989.)

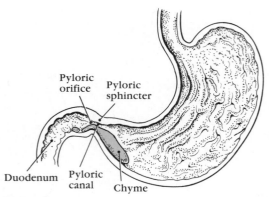

**FIGURE 40–5.**

Movement of chyme through the pyloric sphincter.

enzyme *pepsinogen,* which, when activated, digests proteins. The parietal cells secrete *hydrochloric acid,* which has a pH of about 0.8. It is thought that these cells also secrete the intrinsic factor, a glycoprotein that binds with vitamin B₁₂ and makes it available for absorption in the small intestine.[7] Mucous cells constantly secrete a thin mucus film that is produced by gastric surface epithelial cells.[4] Mucous neck cells are located in the middle and upper portions of gastric glands, and have as their major

function regeneration of mucus-secreting cells.[4] When stimulated, G cells release gastrin into the bloodstream.[4]

About 1500 to 3000 mL of gastric juice is secreted daily, and mixes with the food entering the stomach. The combination of food and gastric juice makes a semiliquid mass called *chyme,* which is propelled into the small intestine through the pyloric sphincter (Figure 40-5).

The nervous supply to the stomach is through the intrinsic and the autonomic nervous systems. The intrinsic system begins in the esophagus and continues all the way to the anus. The layers involved in this system include the *myenteric* and the *submucosal plexuses*. These control the tone of the bowel, rhythmic contractions, and the velocity of excitation of the gut. The autonomic nervous system increases excitation through the parasympathetic branches, especially in the esophagus, stomach, large intestine, and anal region. The main function of the sympathetic portion of the autonomic nervous system is to inhibit activity of the gastrointestinal system.

The arterial blood supply to the stomach comes mainly from the celiac artery. Venous blood is drained through the gastric veins, which connect to and terminate in the portal vein (Figure 40-6). The stomach has profuse lymphatic drainage through lymphatic vessels and nodes (Figure 40-7).

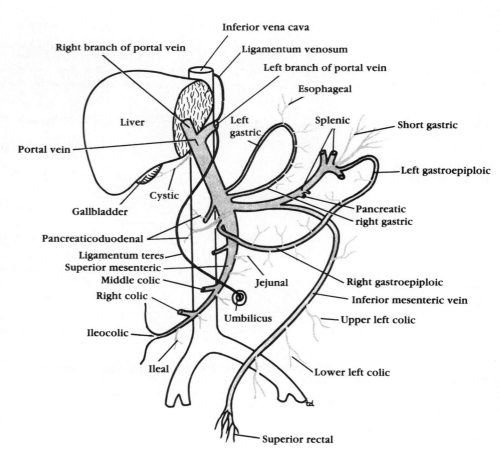

**FIGURE 40–6.**

Venous drainage of the stomach and small intestine. (Source: R.S. Snell, *Clinical Anatomy for Medical Students* [2nd ed.]. Boston: Little, Brown, 1981.)

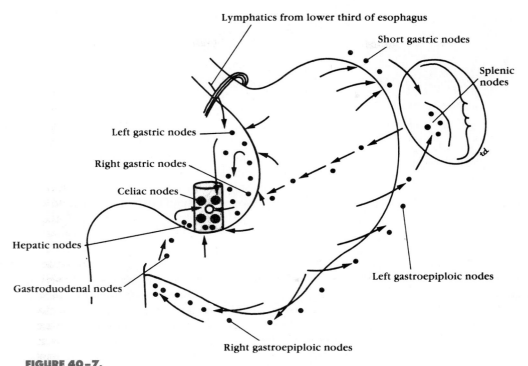

**FIGURE 40-7.**
Lymphatic drainage of the stomach. (From R.S. Snell, *Clinical Anatomy for Medical Students* (2nd ed.). Boston: Little, Brown, 1981.)

## Small Intestine

The small intestine extends from the pylorus to the ileocecal valve. It is about 12 ft long in the living human. In the cadaver, it is longer because the muscles of the intestinal wall are relaxed.[4,15] The small intestine is divided into sections: *duodenum, jejunum,* and *ileum* (see Figure 40-2). Absorption and secretion occur throughout the length of the small intestine (Table 40-3).

The intestinal wall is composed of four layers: mucosa, submucosa, muscularis, and serosa (Figure 40-8). Fingerlike folds of the mucosa, called *villi,* project into the lumen of the interior of the intestines and increase the absorptive surface by about 600-fold (Figure 40-9).

The *crypts of Lieberkuhn* are pitlike structures that lie in grooves between the villi, and are composed of absorptive cells and mucus-producing goblet cells. The absorptive cells are columnar, and have a brush border on the luminal side. These cells have a marked power for regeneration and differentiate from intestinal epithelial cells into absorptive cells. An intestinal epithelial cell lives about 5 days, after which it is shed into the intestinal secretions.[15]

Blood circulation to the small intestine occurs through the gastroduodenal, superior pancreaticoduodenal, and celiac arteries. Venous drainage is through the superior mesenteric vein, which empties into the portal vein and travels to the liver (see Figure 40-6). The entire small intestine is richly supplied with lymphatic vessels.

The intestinal cells form large quantities of secretions that have a neutral pH. These secretions contain enzymes that function to a limited extent in the breakdown of nutrients. Another important secretion is cholecystokinin, which is secreted from the mucosa and absorbed into the bloodstream and stimulates the gallbladder and

**TABLE 40-3.**
PRINCIPAL SITES OF ABSORPTION

| NUTRIENT | ABSORPTIVE SITE |
| --- | --- |
| Carbohydrates | Jejunum |
| Protein | Jejunum |
| Fat | Jejunum |
| Water | Jejunum; also duodenum, ileum, and colon |
| Fat-soluble vitamins— A, D, E, K | Duodenum |
| Vitamin $B_{12}$ | Terminal ileum |
| Other water-soluble vitamins | Duodenum |
| Iron | Duodenum |
| Calcium | Duodenum |
| Sodium | Jejunum by passive diffusion; ileum and colon by active transport |
| Potassium | Jejunum and ileum |
| Magnesium | Distal ileum |

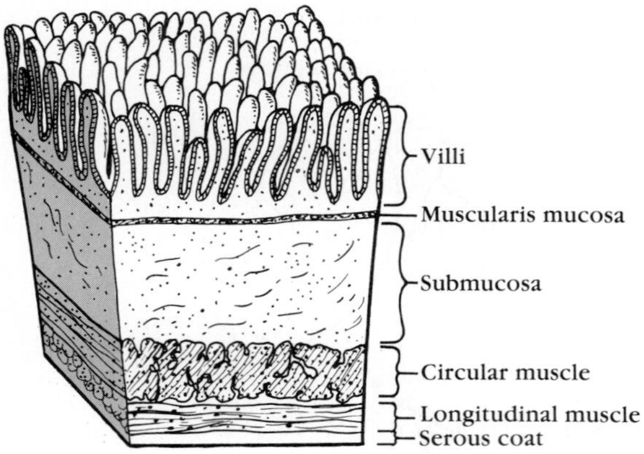

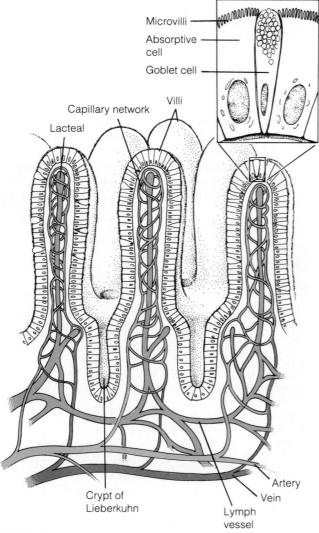

**FIGURE 40–8.**
Layers of the intestinal wall.

pancreas (see Chap. 42). At one time, it was thought that two hormones, cholecystokinin and pancreozymin, were secreted by the mucosa of the upper small intestine. These were found to be the same hormone, now called cholecystokinin.

The liver, gallbladder, and pancreas, considered in greater detail in Chap. 42, are essential organs in the promotion of digestion. Chyme entering the small intestine stimulates cholecystokinin by distending the small intestine. This hormone, in turn, stimulates the pancreas to release its enzymatic secretions into the duodenum. The stimulation from cholecystokinin causes the gallbladder to contract and push bile into the small intestine.

## Large Intestine

The large intestine begins with the end of the ileum at the ileocecal valve (Figure 40-10). The area of meeting is called the cecum. A small structure extends from the cecum called the *vermiform appendix,* which is a relatively nonfunctional pouch. The colon portion of the large intestine is subdivided into the ascending, transverse, descending, and sigmoid areas. The large intestine itself begins with the cecum, contains the colon, and terminates in the rectum and anal canal.

The number of mucus-secreting goblet cells is increased in the large intestine. The mucous material secreted is important in preventing trauma to the bowel, providing material that causes feces to form a mass, and protecting the bowel against resident bacteria. Most of the liquid and electrolytes from the semiliquid material of the small intestine are absorbed in the large intestine, especially in the ascending and transverse colon. Feces usually consist of about three-fourths water and one-

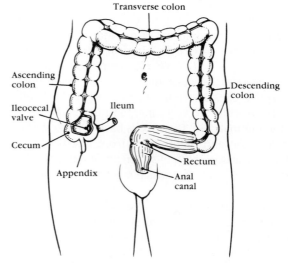

**FIGURE 40–10.**
Segments of the large intestine.

**FIGURE 40–9.**
Structure of the intestinal villi.

fourth solid matter, of which about 30% is dead bacteria. The brown color of fecal material produced by breakdown products (simpler pigments) of bilirubin.

The rectum is about 20 cm of the final descending portion of the large intestine and terminates in the anal canal. It is separated from the sigmoid colon by an external sphincter, the *sphincter ani,* which opens to the outside of the body.

The blood supply to the large intestine is profuse, and arises from branches of the superior and inferior mesenteric arteries (Figure 40-11). Venous drainage is mainly through the mesenteric veins, terminating in the portal veins (see Figure 40-6). This system is important in the pathology of portal hypertension because increased portal pressure is reflected in the veins surrounding the esophagus and anal canal (see Chap. 43). The entire large intestine is supplied with an extensive lymphatic drainage system of vessels and nodes.

## PHYSIOLOGY OF THE DIGESTIVE SYSTEM

Digestion takes substances in one form and breaks them down into molecules that are small enough to pass through the intestinal wall to the blood and lymphatic system. This activity requires chemical secretions and mechanical movements, all working together in a coordinated manner. The molecules may be moved by simple diffusion, active transport, or facilitated diffusion (see Chap. 1). *Motility, secretion,* and *absorption* work together to effect digestion.

## *Oral Secretions and Movement of Food to the Stomach*

The major digestive secretion of the salivary glands is the enzyme *ptyalin,* which breaks down starches. This amylase, or carbohydrate digester, is active not only in the mouth, but continues its function in the stomach. The action continues until the digestive secretions of the stomach begin to alter the chyme. It is estimated that 30% to 40% of starches are broken down by ptyalin.

Saliva contains water, mucus, and other substances. It liquefies and lubricates ingested food. The amount of saliva secreted is regulated by the parasympathetic nervous pathways. Increased secretion occurs in response to irritation of stomach mucosa, which initiates a reflex increase in salivation.

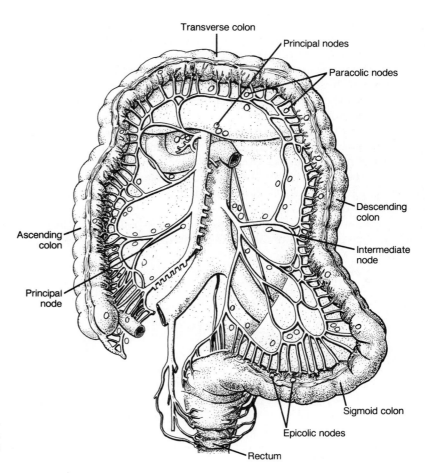

**FIGURE 40-11.**
Diagram of the blood supply and lymphatic drainage of the large intestine. (From C.M. Fenoglio-Preiser et al., *Gastrointestinal Pathology: An Atlas and Text.* New York: Raven, 1989.)

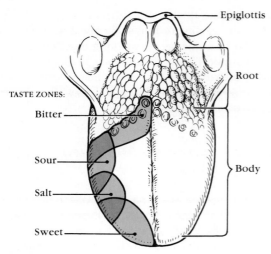

**FIGURE 40-12.**
The tongue and areas of taste.

The movements of the tongue are important to position the *bolus* of ingested food, which has been reduced to smaller sizes by the teeth, into proper alignment for swallowing. The taste buds, scattered over the mucous membrane of the tongue surface, carry sensory input through the seventh and ninth cranial nerves to the brain, where taste is interpreted. Perception of taste is a complex process, with various areas of the tongue being sensitive to different tastes. Figure 40-12 shows the areas of the tongue that respond to sweet, sour, salty, and bitter tastes. The major motor nerve of the tongue is the hypoglossal, which is closely aligned with the vagus nerve. It innervates the extrinsic and intrinsic muscles to move the tongue into various positions.

Swallowing is the key event in the initiation of digestion because it increases esophageal peristaltic motion, decreases pressure in the lower esophagus, and initiates the gastroenteric reflex. This reflex increases small-bowel motility and assists in moving nutrients along the alimentary canal.

Swallowing, or deglutition, is initiated when the tongue moves a bolus of food to the pharynx. The crico-

pharyngeal sphincter relaxes for 1 second or less and the *primary peristaltic wave* is initiated. This wave begins in the pharynx and spreads to the esophagus.[7] The respiratory passages are closed to prevent food from moving into them. The bolus of food then passes through the pharynx to the esophagus in about 1 second (Figure 40-13). The respiratory passages reopen and breathing resumes.

As food passes into the esophagus, peristalsis and pressure changes move it toward the stomach. Peristalsis, which occurs throughout the gastrointestinal tract, is a series of sequential muscular movements. The primary wave moves down the esophagus and *secondary peristalsis* continues until all of the food is in the stomach.[7] The syncytium of the entire system allows for wavelike movements of the smooth muscle. As the food moves toward the lower esophageal or gastroesophageal sphincter, the wave of peristalsis causes the normally constricted area to relax, and the food moves into the stomach. The peristaltic waves are initiated by vagal reflexes from the esophagus to the medulla oblongata back to the esophagus.[7] These are termed *vagal central* and *local pathways*.[11]

## Gastric Motility and Secretion

The fundus of the stomach increases its volume as it fills with food, and by its distensibility maintains a low intragastric pressure. The antrum is responsible for mixing food through contraction waves that push the food (now chyme) toward the pylorus.

### Gastric Motility and Emptying

Solids must be broken down to less than a millimeter in size before they can pass through the pyloric sphincter. Gastric motility patterns occur in phases: phase I occurs 1.5 to 2 hours after meals, when gastric contractions decrease to one every 4 to 5 minutes; phase II is a 30-minute span of irregular contractions; this is followed

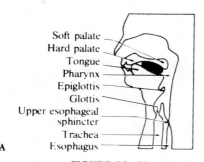
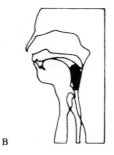
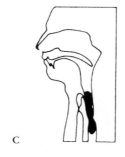
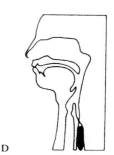

Soft palate
Hard palate
Tongue
Pharynx
Epiglottis
Glottis
Upper esophageal sphincter
Trachea
Esophagus

A        B        C        D

**FIGURE 40-13.**
Passage of a food bolus from the mouth through the pharynx and upper esophagus during swallowing. (From E.E. Selkurt, *Physiology* [5th ed.]. Boston: Little, Brown, 1984.)

by phase III, which is 5 to 15 minutes of sweeping contractions.[11] Hunger pangs may be experienced during phases II or III. Contractile movements in the full stomach are of three types: (1) peristaltic waves, (2) contractions of the antrum, and (3) contractions of the fundus and body.

Peristaltic activity in the stomach arises from a pacemaker located high on the greater curvature of the stomach. Electrical slow waves are propagated through the longitudinal muscle layer to the pylorus. This cyclical wave, also called the *basic electrical rhythm,* of partial depolarization and repolarization occurs in humans about three times per minute.[5,11]

## Gastric Secretion

The glands of the stomach secrete 1500 to 3000 mL of gastric juice per day. Secretory activity follows a regular daily pattern, with the least secretion occurring in the early morning. The amount of gastric secretion also varies with individual dietary habits, other stimuli that provoke secretions, and the strength of the inhibitory mechanisms.

Gastric juice contains mucus, intrinsic factor, hydrochloric acid, pepsinogen, and the electrolytes sodium, potassium, magnesium, chloride, and bicarbonate. Certain other enzymes, such as gastric lipase, urease, lysozyme, and carbonic anhydrase, also are present in the secretions. The three types of cells that make up the gastric glands secrete mucus, pepsinogen, and hydrochloric acid (see Figure 40-4).

The parietal cells in the fundus and body of the stomach secrete *hydrochloric acid* as a highly concentrated juice with a pH of about 0.8. A suggested mechanism for the formation of hydrochloric acid is shown in Figure 40-14. The theory relating hydrochloric acid secretion to bicarbonate replenishment in the blood is supported by the observation that each hydrogen ion secreted is matched by bicarbonate that is returned to the blood. This means that the amount of bicarbonate entering the blood during the gastric secretory phase is directly proportional to the amount of acid secreted. Carbon dioxide enters the cell or is formed in the cell during metabolism, reacts with water catalyst by using carbonic anhydrase, and forms carbonic acid. This carbonic acid then dissociates to bicarbonate and hydrogen. The hydrogen ion enters the parietal cell canaliculi by active transport, whereas bicarbonate is diffused back into the blood. The chloride ion also is actively transported from blood to the canaliculi.[3,14] Only during periods of relative gastric inactivity is adequate carbon dioxide produced to make a small amount of hydrochloric acid. During digestion, the parietal cell takes its needed carbon dioxide from the circulating blood. This elevates the venous pH after eating, which has been called the *postprandial alkaline tide.* The urine also becomes more alkaline.[5,11]

*Pepsin* is the main proteolytic enzyme of gastric juice. It is secreted by the chief cells of the gastric glands in the form of pepsinogen. It has no digestive activity until it is activated into pepsin, which occurs in the presence of hydrochloric acid and previously activated pepsin. Pepsin is most active in a highly acid medium. It functions optimally in a pH of 2.0 and is almost inactive in secretions with a pH greater than 5.0.

*Mucus* is produced by the columnar cells of the surface epithelium. The surface of the stomach mucosa has a continuous layer of columnar epithelial cells that secretes large amounts of viscous and alkaline mucus to coat the mucosa and create a protective sheet. The epithelial lining of the stomach has remarkable properties of repair and can reproduce itself in 36 to 48 hours. The mucous cells secrete a thin mucus, and the amount of this secretion varies with vagal stimulation and irritation. This additional line of defense lubricates the passage of food, absorbs pepsin, and washes away noxious substances. Failure to secrete mucus in adequate quantities to protect the underlying mucosa increases the susceptibility of the mucosa to the action of hydrochloric acid and pepsin.[7]

*Gastric juices* contain small quantities of the enzymes gastric lipase, gastric amylase, gastric urease, gelatinase, carbonic anhydrase, and lysozyme. Gastric lipase acts primarily on butterfat and has little effect on other fats, which require bile for their digestion. Gastric amylase has a minor role in digesting starch. Gastric urease, formed by the bacteria that contaminate the gastric mucosa, splits urea to produce ammonia. Gelatinase helps to liquefy some of the proteoglycans in meats.[7] Carbonic anhydrase, present in the epithelial cells and in high concentrations in parietal cells, is thought to be produced by the disintegration of desquamated epithelial cells and is essential in forming hydrochloric acid. Lysozyme is a carbohydrate-splitting enzyme present in small amounts in the gastric juice. Its cellular origin is not known.

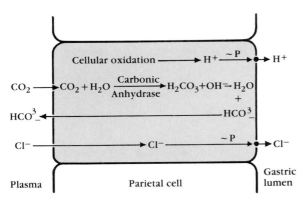

**FIGURE 40-14.**
A possible mechanism for the gastric secretion of hydrochloric acid. (From E.E. Selkurt, *Basic Physiology for the Health Sciences* [2nd ed.]. Boston: Little, Brown, 1982.)

## Formation of Chyme

Gastric motility is governed by the peristaltic waves that occur every 15 to 25 seconds and mix ingested food with gastric secretions. The result of this movement and mixing is the thin, highly acidic liquid chyme. Chyme is moved into the small intestine mostly because of the higher pressure gradients in the stomach that exceed the duodenal pressure. The acidity and amount of chyme entering the duodenum help to regulate the duodenal and pancreatic secretions.

## Nervous and Hormonal Influences

Digestion also is regulated by nervous and hormonal mechanisms. Innervation through the vagus nerve excites stomach excretion directly by stimulating the gastric glands. Distention of the stomach wall activates local reflexes to stimulate gastric secretion. The local reflexes elicit autonomic nervous system activity and cause the release of the hormone gastrin. This hormone is absorbed into the bloodstream and stimulates the gastric secretory glands to cause a marked increase in gastric acid secretion. Gastric secretion is thought to occur in three phases: *cephalic, gastric,* and *intestinal* (Figure 40-15).

The cephalic phase prepares the stomach for food and digestion. It is under nervous control, and initiated by stimuli such as the sight, smell, or thought of food. Impulses from receptors such as the retinae, taste buds, and olfactory glands travel to the cerebral cortex, and the motor fibers of the vagi of the stomach stimulate the glands of the stomach to secrete juice rich in hydrochloric acid and gastrin.[11]

The *gastric phase* is initiated when food enters the stomach. Gastrin is released by acetylcholine stimulation of the gastrin-producing cells. The process is triggered by distention of the stomach caused by food and by exposure of the mucosa to substances called *secretagogues.* Examples of secretagogues are caffeine and alcohol. Gastrin is absorbed in the blood and stimulates acid and pepsin secretion from parietal and chief cells, which produce about two thirds of the total gastric secretions.[7,11] Food in the stomach initiates local reflexes in the intramural plexus of the stomach, and vasovagal reflexes induce parasympathetic stimulation to increase the secretion. The rate of secretion in response to gastrin continues for several hours while food remains in the stomach. Both the gastrin and vagal mechanisms are important in gastric secretion. Gastrin also has extragastric action, including the stimulation of insulin and release of calcitonin. It causes muscle contraction of the lower esophageal sphincter, small intestine, colon, and gallbladder. It inhibits smooth-muscle contraction of the pyloric, ileocecal, and Oddi sphincters.[11]

The *intestinal phase* of gastric secretion is less active than the cephalic or gastric phases, but once initiated, it may last for 8 to 10 hours while food remains in the duodenum. This phase is not well understood, but it begins with the entrance of acidic chyme into the small intestine, which leads to an increase in gastrin secretion.[11]

The intestines also inhibit gastric secretion when there are partially digested proteins, acid, fat, or hypertonic solutions in the duodenum. Distention, caused by the presence of food, initiates the *enterogastric reflex,* which slows the influence of the vagus nerve. The purpose of the enterogastric reflex appears to be to delay stomach emptying until some emptying can occur in the small intestine. Intestinal hormones, especially secretin and cholecystokinin, oppose the stimulatory effects of

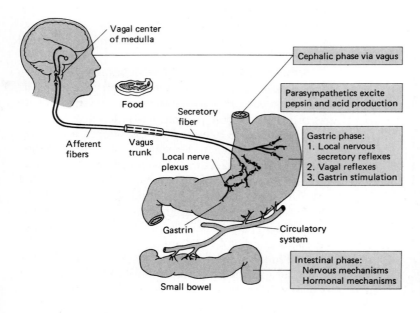

**FIGURE 40-15.**

The phases of gastric secretion and their regulation. (From A.C. Guyton, *Textbook of Medical Physiology* [7th ed.]. Philadelphia: W.B. Saunders, 1986.)

gastrin and slow the movement of chyme from the stomach to the small intestine.[7] This inhibitory feedback prevents excessive acid secretion and protects the intestinal mucosa from injury. During the interdigestive phase, while no digestion is occurring in the gastrointestinal tract, the stomach secretes only a few milliliters of gastric juice per hour. Secretions in the stomach normally follow a steady, dynamic course regulated by both nervous and hormonal factors that foster structural and functional integrity in the mucosa. Pathologic conditions, drugs and chemicals, or surgery can disrupt the balance between secretion and inhibition.

The best-known chemical stimulant of gastric secretion is *histamine*, which is released from surface mast cells during an antigen–antibody reaction. Although less potent than gastrin, histamine causes the parietal cells to secrete large amounts of gastric juice. Large amounts of endogenous histamine may be present in the gastric mucosa, and during active secretion, small amounts are present in gastric juice and urine. Physical or emotional stress increases the release of histamine.

## Other Influences on Gastric Secretion and Motility

Caffeine and nicotine are secretagogues that increase the amount and acidity of gastric secretion. Alcohol has been found to stimulate only the amount of gastrin secretion. Aspirin, alcohol, and bile salts alter the permeability of the epithelial barrier and allow back-diffusion of hydrochloric acid, which may result in injury to tissue and blood vessels. Aspirin produces changes in the gastric mucosa and decreases the total output of mucus, which reduces its protective effect on the gastric mucosa. It has been observed that prolonged administration of large quantities of corticotropic and adrenal steroids increases gastric secretion, which favors the development or recurrence of peptic ulcers.[10,14] The frequency may not be quite as significant as previously reported. A number of studies have reported a slight increase in frequency of peptic ulcers in patients treated with adrenocortical steroid drugs.[6] Nonsteroidal antiinflammatory drugs (NSAIDs) have been implicated in acute gastric injury with erosive and hemorrhagic gastritis. Of the NSAIDs studied, aspirin has been shown to cause both acute and chronic injury.[16] Parasympathetic agents such as acetylcholine, reserpine, and pilocarpine also are secretory stimulants. Insulin, through its hypoglycemic effects, excites the vagus nerve and increases gastric gland activity.

Belladonna and its alkaloids atropine and hyoscine depress secretions by reducing vagal stimulation. Synthetic anticholinergic drugs, such as propantheline bromide (Probanthine), are used to control gastric activity and secretion.

Emotional disruptions have long been recognized as

exerting an important influence on the secretory and motor functions of the stomach. Studies seem to indicate that prolonged anxiety, guilt, conflict, hostility, and resentment lead to engorgement of the gastric mucosa and increased secretion. The significant decrease in gastric secretion after complete vagotomy suggests that hypersecretion is caused by excessive stimulation of the vagus nerve.[16]

## Emesis

Emesis is a complex reflex triggered by the central nervous system, and involves a sequential and coordinated contraction of many muscles. The central nervous system has a diffuse group of neurons located on the dorsal surface of the floor of the fourth ventricle called the *chemoreceptive trigger zone*. This zone is not a discrete anatomic structure, but disruption of neural pathways in this area abolishes this response. These neurons sense the presence of chemicals such as morphine or other stimuli in the blood and activate the vomiting center in the medulla. This vomiting center also can be directly activated by the stomach during gastrointestinal irritation by way of the sympathetic and vagal afferent neurons.[2] Varied conditions can stimulate the emesis response, and individuals are unique in their propensity for emesis. It may be associated with a pathologic condition, or it may be a response to stress, offensive odors, or other conditions of daily life (Box 40-1).

Activation of the vomiting center causes active con-

### BOX 40-1.
### STIMULI FOR EMESIS RESPONSE

Drugs
Toxins
Pregnancy
Motion
Alcohol consumption
Radiation therapy
Ketosis
Pain
Psychogenic conditions
Infections
Anesthesia
Acute head injury
Increased intracranial pressure
Brain tumors
Migraine headache
Overdistention of gastrointestinal tract
Obstruction of gastrointestinal tract
Vestibular disease
Fever

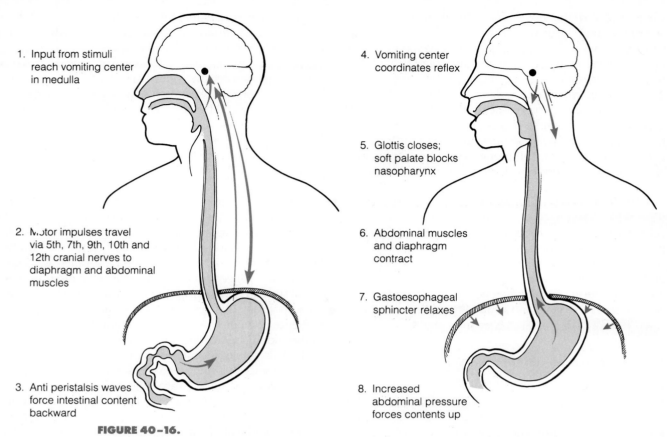

1.  Input from stimuli
    reach vomiting center
    in medulla

2.  Motor impulses travel
    via 5th, 7th, 9th, 10th and
    12th cranial nerves to
    diaphragm and abdominal
    muscles

3.  Anti peristalsis waves
    force intestinal content
    backward

4.  Vomiting center
    coordinates reflex

5.  Glottis closes;
    soft palate blocks
    nasopharynx

6.  Abdominal muscles
    and diaphragm
    contract

7.  Gastoesophageal
    sphincter relaxes

8.  Increased
    abdominal pressure
    forces contents up

**FIGURE 40–16.**
Emesis response. 1. Antiperistalsis is the first stage. Antiperistaltic waves travel backward from the intestine or stomach. 2. Vomiting itself involves closure of the glottis, lifting the soft palate to close the nares, and contraction of the diaphragm and abdominal muscles. The result of this is relaxation of the gastroesophageal sphincter, allowing expulsion of gastric contents through the esophagus.

traction of the somatic muscles, with inhibition of gastric tone, opening of the esophageal sphincters, and closing of the glottis. This muscular activation is accomplished through the motor pathways from the fifth, seventh, ninth, tenth, and twelfth cranial nerves. Figure 40-16 summarizes the physiology of the emesis response.

A person experiences the emesis response within its three components of nausea, retching, and expulsion. These components can occur in sequence, but nausea and retching often occur without expulsion. The person commonly experiences the perception of nausea at the onset of this response. Other associated symptoms include pallor, cold sweats, and hypotension caused by sympathetic nervous system stimulation. Nausea and the accompanying sensations often diminish after expulsion of the stomach contents.[2]

## Secretion and Absorption in the Small Intestine

The major nutrients are mostly absorbed in the small intestine, with the simpler substances usually being ab-

sorbed in the first portion of the small bowel. Substances that require greater hydrolysis and simplification are absorbed at later points in the small intestine. Table 40-3 shows the specific absorption sites of major nutrients. The anatomic structure, previously detailed, provides the mechanism for this to occur. In the small intestine, secretions are received from the pancreas and liver and supplemented by intestinal secretions. *Secretions of the small intestine* include enzymes, hormones, and mucus. These substances, listed in Tables 40-4 and 40-5, include secretions from the pancreas and liver. The major effects of all of the enzymes and hormones are detailed in the tables.

All of the secretions work together to digest carbohydrates, proteins, and fats. Absorption depends on the proper hydrolysis of nutrients by secretions that increase the movement from the intestinal lumen to the bloodstream. Biliary secretions include bile salts, lipids, water, electrolytes, and bilirubin. Of these, bilirubin is a waste product that gives color to the feces. Bile salts exert a detergent-like effect on fat and emulsify it. The pancreatic secretions contain enzymes and large amounts of bicarbonate and water. Formation of pancreatic and biliary secretions is detailed in Chapter 42.

**TABLE 40–4.**
DIGESTIVE ENZYMES

| ENZYME | SOURCE | SUBSTRATE | PRODUCTS | REMARKS |
|---|---|---|---|---|
| Ptyalin | Salivary glands | Starch | Smaller carbohydrates | |
| Pepsin | Chief cells of stomach mucosa | Protein (nonspecific) | Polypeptides | Activated by hydrochloric acid |
| Gastric lipase | Stomach mucosa | Triglycerides (lipids) | Glycerides and fatty acids | |
| Enterokinase | Duodenal mucosa | Trypsinogen | Trypsin | Activates or converts trypsinogen to trypsin; trypsinogen hydrolyzed to expose active site |
| Trypsin | Pancreas | Protein and polypeptides | Smaller polypeptides | Converts chymotrypsinogen to chymotrypsin |
| Chymotrypsin | Pancreas | Proteins and polypeptides (different specificity than trypsin) | Smaller polypeptides | |
| Nuclease | Pancreas | Nucleic acids | Nucleotides (base + sugar + $PO_4$) | |
| Carboxypeptidase | Pancreas | Polypeptides | Smaller polypeptides | Cleaves carboxy terminal end |
| Pancreatic lipase | Pancreas | Lipids, especially triglycerides | Glycerides, free fatty acids, glycerol | Very potent |
| Pancreatic amylase | Pancreas | Starch | 2 disaccharide units = maltose | Very potent |
| Aminopeptidase | Intestinal glands | Polypeptides | Smaller peptides | |
| Dipeptidase | Intestine | Dipeptides | 2 amino acids | |
| Maltase | Intestine | Maltose | 2 glucose | |
| Lactase | Intestine | Lactose | 1 glucose, 1 galactose | |
| Sucrase | Intestine | Sucrose | 1 glucose, 1 fructose | |
| Nucleotidase | Intestine | Nucleotides | Nucleosides and phosphates (base + sugar) | |
| Nucleosidase | Intestine | Nucleosides | Base and sugar | |
| Intestinal lipase | Intestine | Fats | Glycerides, fatty acids, glycerol | |

Note: *Enzymes act on one another during and after digestion, but it is only after digestion (after their substrates are removed) that they have any marked effect on one another.*

The chyme that enters the duodenum is highly acidic because it was mixed with large amounts of hydrochloric acid in the stomach. All of the intestinal enzymes work best in an alkaline medium, which requires chyme to be neutralized and alkalinized. The amount of the alkaline pancreatic secretion is closely correlated with the pH of the chyme entering the small intestine.

Chemical and mechanical digestion require that food be changed into the forms that can be moved by absorption through the mucosal lining cells to the blood and lymph vessels. The diffusible forms include monosaccharides, amino acids, fatty acids, glycerol, and glycerides.[7] Figure 40-17 shows schematically where materials are absorbed in the entire gastrointestinal system. Nearly all of the nutrients are absorbed in the small intestine, and 90% of all absorption occurs here.

### Carbohydrate Absorption

Carbohydrates are ingested primarily as disaccharides, starches, and polysaccharides. Polysaccharides are hydrolyzed into their component disaccharides by the action of ptyalin and the gastric, intestinal, and pancreatic amylases. Intact disaccharides can be passively absorbed by the small intestine, but relatively few are absorbed in this manner. Most are first split into monosaccharides by en-

**TABLE 40–5.**
HORMONES OF DIGESTION

| HORMONE | SOURCE | AGENTS THAT STIMULATE PRODUCTION | ACTION |
|---|---|---|---|
| Gastrin | Gastric mucosa (primarily pylorus) | Distention of stomach and some protein derivatives | Stimulates production of hydrochloric acid |
| Enterogastrone | Mucosa of small intestine and duodenum | Fats, sugars, or acids in intestine | Inhibits gastric secretion and mobility |
| Secretin | Duodenal mucosa | Polypeptides, acids, etc., in intestine (duodenum) | Stimulates pancreas to produce a watery, enzyme-poor juice, with high $HCO_3^-$ content |
| Cholecystokinin | Duodenal mucosa | Fats in duodenum | Stimulates pancreas to produce enzyme-rich juice and stimulates gallbladder to contract and release bile |

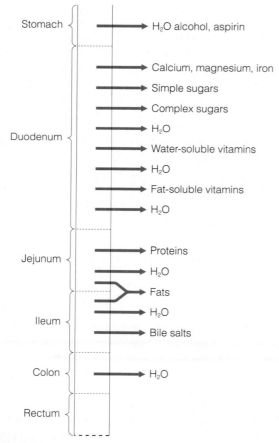

**FIGURE 40–17.**
Schematic representation of absorption of nutrients in the digestive tract.

zymes located in the intestinal microvilli. These monosaccharides are then actively absorbed into the blood capillaries of the villi. Absorption occurs against a concentration gradient and apparently requires active transport, although the method by which this occurs is obscure. It is known that sodium increases cellular permeability to glucose, so that glucose transport is related to sodium transport.

### Protein Absorption

Protein absorption mostly occurs in the duodenum and jejunum. As a result of gastric pepsin and pancreatic enzymes, 70% of protein ingested in the diet is presented to the intestinal absorptive membrane in the form of small peptides, and 30% is in the form of amino acids. The amino acids are immediately absorbed, but only a small amount of peptide is absorbed intact. Most of the peptides are reduced by peptidases in the microvilli to amino acids, and absorption rapidly follows. The sodium transport mechanism also probably provides for amino acid transport. Many amino acids apparently need pyridoxine, a component of vitamin $B_6$, to aid in transport.

### Fat Absorption

Dietary fat mainly consists of long-chain triglycerides, which are hydrolyzed intraluminally into fatty acids and monoglycerides. Hydrolysis occurs in the jejunum through the action of lipase. The most important lipase is secreted from the pancreas.[7] Bile salts and fatty acids aggregate to form *micelles*, which are water-soluble structures. A major function of bile salts is to make fat globules fragmentable by agitating them in the small bowel.[7] These fragments attach themselves to the surface of the epithelial cells. The fatty acids leave the micelles and enter the cell by diffusion, while the bile salts are released to return to chyme to aid in the absorption of more fats. When the fats in the duodenum and upper jejunum have been removed, bile salts are resorbed and eventually returned to the liver. Lipids are resynthesized into triglycerides in the endoplasmic reticulum of intestinal epithelial cells. Molecules of triglycerides then organize into minute fat droplets, which contain small amounts of phospholipid and cholesterol and protein-coated surface. These droplets, called *chylomicrons*, then pass out of the base of the epithelial cells and enter either the bloodstream or the lymphatic system. About 80% to 90% of all fatty acids enter the bloodstream in the form of chylomicrons. Small amounts of fats are not digested and are excreted in the feces.

## Water Absorption

About 8 L of water per day are absorbed from the small intestine into the portal blood entirely by diffusion.[7] The greatest amount of this absorption occurs in the jejunum. Water crosses the intestinal cell membrane by passing through the pores of this membrane. The rate of absorption is great and probably is enhanced by glucose and oxygen. Therefore, active transport may increase water absorption through shifting of other ions.

## Electrolyte Absorption

Additional water is absorbed in the large intestine. Electrolytes, like water, must cross the intestinal cell membrane by passing through its pores or by using a membrane carrier. Like water, electrolytes are primarily absorbed into the portal blood rather than into the lymphatic system, and the absorption rate is greater in the proximal than in the distal portion of the small bowel. Monovalent electrolytes, such as sodium, chloride, potassium, nitrate, and bicarbonate, are more easily absorbed than polyvalent electrolytes, such as calcium, magnesium, and sulfate.

Most of the *sodium* is absorbed in the jejunum, with less being absorbed in the ileum and the colon. The mechanism for this is active transport of sodium from the epithelial cells into the intercellular spaces. This requires a carrier and energy. Increased sodium concentration in the intercellular spaces creates an osmotic gradient for water, which follows the sodium passively. Both sodium and water are finally absorbed into the capillaries of the villi.[7]

*Chloride* passively moves through the membranes of the duodenum and jejunum. It is actively transported in the large bowel, where it is exchanged in close relation to bicarbonate ions, which are used to neutralize any acid products in the large intestine.

*Potassium* can be passively or actively absorbed through the intestinal mucosa.[5,7] Most absorption occurs in the jejunum and ileum through a system not clearly identified.

*Calcium* is absorbed by active transport throughout the small intestine, but most actively in the duodenum. The solubility of calcium salts is increased in duodenal acid, rather than in the more alkaline medium lower in the intestines. The rate of calcium absorption is altered by the level of parathyroid hormone in the blood (see Chap. 38). Vitamin D is important in stimulating the rate of intestinal absorption; it is activated by a specific process in the kidneys and then increases calcium absorption.

*Magnesium* absorption and regulation are tied to both calcium and potassium balance; however, the specific stimuli for magnesium absorption is not well delineated.[1] The distal small bowel is the primary site for magnesium absorption. Because this area often is affected by bowel resection and inflammatory bowel disease, persons with these problems must have supplemental dietary intake. Alcoholism also disrupts magnesium intestinal absorption, and kidney excretion is accelerated.[9]

Most *iron* is absorbed in its ferrous form in the duodenum. An acid medium facilitates iron absorption. Iron uptake is an active process, and is facilitated by *ascorbic acid*, which reduces the ferric to the ferrous form. The rate of absorption is extremely slow, but increases with iron deficiency and decreases with excessive dietary intake of iron.

The *vitamins* are primarily absorbed in the proximal intestine, except for vitamin $B_{12}$, which is absorbed in the ileum. Most vitamins are passively absorbed. Some are stored in the body, and some have to be replenished on a regular basis. Vitamin $B_{12}$ forms a complex with the intrinsic factor that, in the ileum, is bound to a specific, unknown receptor in the mucosa and, finally, is absorbed into the blood.

## Secretion, Absorption, and Excretion in the Large Intestine

The function of the large intestine (colon) is mainly to absorb water, but it also is vital in synthesizing vitamin K and some B complex vitamins and in forming and excreting feces.[13] Electrical activity within the colon is more irregular than in the small intestine. Structurally, the colon has no smooth-muscle gap junctions and does not function as a syncytium. Contraction and motility in the colon depend on the individual integration of groups of smooth muscles by neural mechanisms. Proximal colon motility is antiperistaltic to augment water removal from the feces.[8]

The movements of the large intestine are part of the peristaltic activity initiated by the ingestion of food. The final movement of the large intestine is *mass peristalsis,* which drives digested waste material into the rectum. This usually occurs three to four times a day. The glands of the lining of the large intestine secrete mucus that lubricates the material and protects the lining of the bowel.

Active bacteria in the bowel ferment any remaining carbohydrates and release hydrogen, carbon dioxide, and methane gas, and break proteins down into amino acids. This activity gives fecal material its odor.

Water (1800–3000 mL) is absorbed daily in the large intestine, along with a few electrolytes. This absorption regulates the consistency of the feces and provides for final water balance in the gastrointestinal system.

Defecation is the process of emptying the rectum, and is initiated by distention of rectal walls. The external sphincter is under voluntary control and relaxes when intraabdominal and intrathoracic pressures increase, pushing the fecal material out of the body. Increased rectal and intraabdominal pressures may increase the vagal tone and reflexively decrease the heart rate.

## REFERENCES

1. Altura, B.M. Magnesium. *Ischemic Heart Disease and Magnesium* 1:57, 1988.
2. Carpenter, D.O. Emesis. In S.G. Schultz, *Handbook of Physiology: The Gastrointestinal System* (Vol. 1, Part 1). Bethesda, Md.: American Physiological Society, 1989.
3. Dharmsathaphorn, K. Transport of water and electrolytes in the gastrointestinal tract. In M.H. Maxwell, C.R. Kleeman, and R.G. Narins, *Clinical Disorders of Fluid and Electrolyte Balance* (4th ed.). New York: McGraw-Hill, 1987.
4. Fenoglio-Preiser, C.M., Lantz, P.E., Listrom, M.B., et al. *Gastrointestinal Pathology: An Atlas and Text.* New York: Raven, 1989.
5. Ganong, W.F. *Review of Medical Physiology* (12th ed.). Los Altos, Calif.: Lange, 1985.
6. Greenberger, N.J. *Gastrointestinal Disorders: A Pathophysiologic Approach* (3rd ed.). Chicago: Yearbook, 1986.
7. Guyton, A.C. *Textbook of Medical Physiology* (8th ed.). Philadelphia: W.B. Saunders, 1990.
8. Livingston, E.H., and Passaro, E.P. Postoperative ileus. *Digestive Diseases and Sciences* 35:121, 1990.
9. Metheny, N. *Fluid and Electrolyte Balance.* Philadelphia: J.B. Lippincott, 1987.
10. Morson, B.C., Dawson, I.M., Day, D.W., et al. *Morson and Dawson's Gastro Intestinal Pathology.* Oxford: Blackwell, 1990.
11. Nord, H.A., and Sodeman, W.A. The stomach. In W.A. Sodeman and T.M. Sodeman, *Sodeman's Pathologic Physiology* (7th ed.). Philadelphia: W.B. Saunders, 1985.
12. Shearman, D.J., and Finlayson, N.D. *Diseases of the Gastrointestinal Tract and Liver.* Edinburgh: Churchill Livingstone, 1989.
13. Sodeman, W.A., and Watson, D.W. The large intestine. In W.A. Sodeman and T.M. Sodeman, *Sodeman's Pathologic Physiology* (7th ed.). Philadelphia: W.B. Saunders, 1985.
14. Spiro, H.M. *Clinical Gastroenterology* (3rd ed.). New York: Macmillan, 1986.
15. Watson, D.W., and Sodeman, W.A. The small intestine. In W.A. Sodeman and T.M. Sodeman, *Sodeman's Pathologic Physiology* (7th ed.). Philadelphia: W.B. Saunders, 1985.
16. Yardley, J.H. Gastritis. In H. Goldman, H.D. Appelman, and N. Kaufman, *Gastrointestinal Pathology.* Baltimore: Williams & Wilkins, 1988.

# Alterations in Gastrointestinal Function

## Chapter Outline

## Learning Objectives

1. List the major sources of inflammation of the gums.
2. Describe the anatomic and functional changes that occur with achalasia.
3. Outline the mechanism for mucosal damage that occurs with esophagitis.
4. List at least two diagnostic procedures that demonstrate reflux.
5. Describe pathophysiologically a rolling hiatal hernia and a sliding hiatal hernia.
6. Differentiate between acute and chronic gastritis.
7. Differentiate the types of peptic ulcerations according to underlying etiology, symptomatology, and relationship to malignancy.
8. Briefly describe the pathology of gastric carcinoma.
9. Describe the pathologic changes that result in malabsorption in celiac enteropathy and tropical sprue.
10. Discuss nausea, vomiting, and diarrhea in terms of etiology and physiologic effects.
11. Differentiate regional enteritis and ulcerative colitis on the basis of etiology, pathology, symptomatology, and course of the disease.
12. Define *adynamic* or *paralytic ileus*.
13. Explain the ischemia/infarction bowel syndrome.
14. Distinguish between paralytic ileus and bowel obstruction.
15. Define *reducible, incarcerated*, and *strangulated hernias*.
16. Describe Hirschsprung's disease.
17. Explain why diverticula are common in elderly persons.
18. List some common conditions that can cause hemorrhoids.
19. List some ways that the American diet may cause carcinoma of the colon.
20. Differentiate the pathology and symptomatology of carcinoma arising in different areas of the colon.

## DISEASES OF THE ORAL CAVITY

### Alterations in the Gums and Teeth

The gums, or *gingiva*, are subject to localized inflammatory diseases, and they may react to other systemic diseases or drug therapy. *Gingivitis*, an inflammation of the borders surrounding the teeth, may result in pain, bleeding, and destruction of gingival tissue. When this inflammation spreads to the underlying tissues, bones, or roots of the teeth, it is called *peridontitis*. This destructive disease may result in purulent drainage and loss of teeth.

Overgrowth of the gingiva occurs in persons having long-term treatment with phenytoin (Dilantin). Hormonal and metabolic conditions may cause an increased inflammatory response, with enlarged gingiva noted especially at puberty, during pregnancy, and with conditions such as leukemia and thrombocytopenia.

### Changes in the Oral Mucosa

Changes in the oral mucosa often reflect systemic changes in the body. A variety of conditions may cause these mucosal changes, and the manifestations vary. For example, in scarlet fever the tongue becomes bright red (strawberry tongue), whereas in a *Candida albicans* infection (thrush), localized white lesions of the oral mucosa occur.

Tumors of the oral mucosa are uncommon and are much like skin tumors, except that many of the oral growths are benign rather than malignant lesions.[2] The salivary glands may also develop benign or malignant tumorous growths.

## ESOPHAGEAL ALTERATIONS

Many conditions affect esophageal motility and secretion, but only the major alterations are reviewed in this section.

### Achalasia

*Achalasia* is an uncommon disorder of esophageal motility that is characterized by a combination of decreased peristalsis and constriction of the lower esophageal sphincter (Figure 41-1A). Degeneration of the myenteric ganglion cells in the esophagus and alteration in vagal tone apparently are the precipitating causes. The esophagus becomes distended and may retain several liters of fluid.

This condition becomes chronic and slowly progressive, causing dysphagia, vomiting, nausea, and weight loss. Pain occurs in about one third of the cases.[16] Lung changes, regurgitation, and infections due to unusual organisms (eg, mycobacteria) are probably related to repeated episodes of nocturnal aspiration. The degree of swallowing difficulty in the early stages is increased by stress and anxiety. Increasing dysphagia results, and finally even liquids become difficult to swallow.

Diagnostic tests usually include a barium swallow, which reflects a normally functioning pharynx and cricoesophageal sphincter. However, after a few centimeters, peristaltic action stops or decreases to ineffectual motions. The distended, nonemptying lower esophagus is easily identified as a pouch that narrows into the esophagogastric junction (Figure 41-1B). Although the lower esophageal sphincter does not open in response

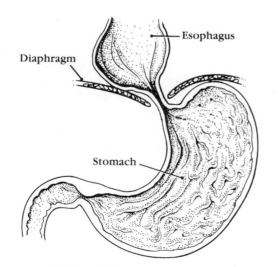

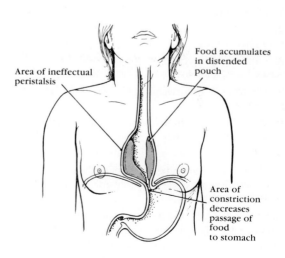

**FIGURE 41-1.**
(**A.**) Location and appearance of achalatic esophagus. (**B.**) Nonemptying or poorly emptying lower esophagus resulting from achalasia.

to swallowing, it may open slightly as food moves into the area and allow some contents to pass through. Frequent follow-up examinations are required because these persons have a statistical increase in frequency of esophageal carcinoma. Surgical intervention may be required to decrease the amount of obstruction.

## Esophageal Diverticulum

An *esophageal diverticulum* is an outpouching of the esophagus at any level that can result in trapped food and complaints of dysphagia and regurgitation. It may be caused by a congenital weakness of the esophageal wall, by high pressure developing proximal to an esophageal spasm, or by a hyperactive upper esophageal sphincter.[10] In the pharyngeal portion of the esophagus, it is called *Zenker's pouch* or *diverticulum*.[10] Other diverticula may develop following esophageal or tracheal infection.

## Gastroesophageal Reflux and Esophagitis

*Gastroesophageal reflux* is the movement of gastric contents into the esophagus. Normally, pressure on the lower esophageal sphincter prevents backflow, or secondary peristalsis moves gastric contents from the esophageal mucosa before damage occurs. An incompetent lower esophageal sphincter is believed to be the primary cause of reflux esophagitis. Other causes of include prolonged gastric intubation, ingestion of corrosive chemicals, uremia, infections, mucosal alterations, and systemic diseases such as systemic lupus erythematosus.[2] Frequent regurgitation through the gastroesophageal junction causes substernal pain. The reflux may be accentuated by postural changes, such as assuming a supine position. Pulmonary aspiration is a common complication when the condition is severe.[8]

*Esophagitis*, inflammation of the esophageal mucosa, most frequently results from gastroesophageal reflux due to prolonged vomiting or an incompetent lower esophageal sphincter. Mucosal damage is related to the contact time between the esophageal mucosa and gastric contents, as well as the acidity and quantity of gastric secretions.

Gastric hydrochloric acid alters the pH of the esophagus and permits mucosal protein to be denatured. The pepsin in the gastric secretion has proteolytic properties that are enhanced when the pH is around 2.0. The combination of pepsin and hydrochloric acid increases the capability for damage. Often, an increase in bile salts is associated with gastroesophageal reflux and enhances the effect of the hydrogen ion on the mucosa. This reflux has been shown to cause an inflammation that penetrates

to the muscularis layer, resulting in motor dysfunction and decreased esophageal clearance. The results are increased esophageal contact time, more muscle damage, and increased amounts of reflux (Figure 41-2).[10,16]

The most common symptoms of esophageal inflammation include heartburn, retrosternal discomfort, and the regurgitation of sour, bitter material. These symptoms are frequently precipitated by ingestion of large amounts of fatty or spicy foods or alcohol. Symptoms correlate with the amount and acidity of reflux. Dysphagia for both solids and liquids increases when severe obstruction occurs. Permanent strictures may develop that make food passage difficult. Irritation of the mucosa may cause bleeding and eventually produce an iron-deficiency anemia. Nocturnal reflux of material into the pharynx may lead to aspiration into the lungs. Reflux may occur in the upright or supine positions, or both.[10]

Diagnosis is difficult but may be based on clinical, radiographic, and endoscopic appearances. The most effective tests are measurement of pH in the esophagus and biopsy to demonstrate inflammatory changes.[16] Scintiscans, which involve swallowing a radionucleotide, can demonstrate reflux by measuring the radioactivity of the esophagus in serial scans.

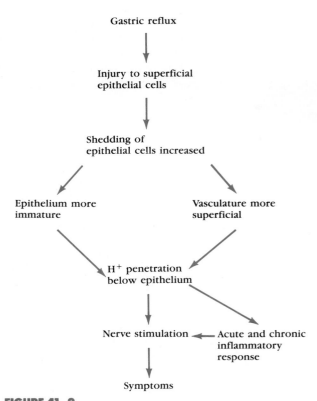

**FIGURE 41–2.**
Possible mechanism for symptoms of reflux esophagitis. (Source: C.E. Kaufman and S. Papper. *Review of Pathophysiology.* Boston: Little, Brown, 1983.)

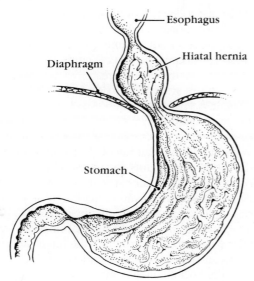

**FIGURE 41–3.**
Location and appearance of hiatal hernia.

## Hiatal Hernia

A *hiatal hernia* is a condition in which part of the stomach protrudes through the opening of the diaphragm (Figure 41-3). This condition may be continuous or occur sporadically. The continuous type is called a *rolling paraesophageal hernia* and occurs in fewer than 10% of persons with this condition. Part or all of the stomach and even intestines may herniate, causing dyspnea, severe pain, and often gastric ulceration.[16] The sporadic type, or *sliding hernia*, accounts for 80% to 90% of hiatal hernias and occurs with changes in position or with increased peristalsis. The stomach is forced through the opening of the diaphragm when the person lies down, and moves back to its normal position when the person stands upright. This type of hernia may be associated with a congenitally short esophagus or may be secondary to postgastritis scarring.

Many persons with a hiatal hernia exhibit no symptoms. Symptoms such as heartburn, gastric regurgitation, dysphagia, and indigestion are accentuated when in the supine position postprandially, and after overeating, physical exertion, or sudden changes of posture.

Radiographs will reveal a hernia. A test to determine the presence of gastroesophageal reflux, the acid-perfusion study, involves instilling hydrochloric acid into the stomach. When reflux does not occur, the hiatal hernia is considered to be of little clinical importance, and the person usually remains asymptomatic. Surgery is usually recommended with the continuous type of hernia, and it involves fixing the stomach to the abdominal wall by suture (gastropexy).[16]

## Esophageal Varices

This condition is closely related to portal hypertension and involves protrusion of the esophageal veins into the esophageal lumen (Figure 41-4). The distended, thin-walled veins become subject to rupture, a catastrophic event that may occur spontaneously or after a sudden increase in intraabdominal pressure such as occurs with vomiting (see Chap. 43).[9]

Rupture of these vessels creates a very large amount of bleeding into the gastrointestinal system and usually leads to large-volume hematemesis. A first bleeding event results in 40% mortality; subsequent episodes are equally catastrophic.[2]

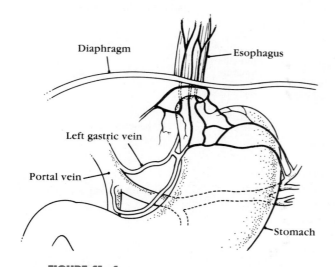

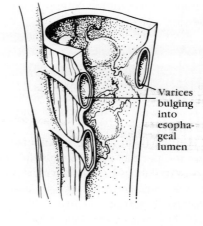

**FIGURE 41–4.**
**(A.)** Venous plexus around the esophagus. **(B.)** Dilated venous channels from portal hypertension. These varices bulge into the lumen of the esophagus and rupture easily.

## Carcinoma of the Esophagus

Approximately 5% to 10% of malignancies of the gastrointestinal tract arise in the esophagus, with a marked variability in incidence depending on country of origin. Turkey and eastern China, for example, have rates of 20% to 25%.[16] These malignancies usually remain asymptomatic until they become surgically unresectable. This type of malignancy usually occurs after age 50 years and occurs more often in men. A strong correlation between heavy alcohol intake, cigarette smoking, and esophageal carcinoma has been recorded.[11]

The squamous cell carcinoma is the most common morphologic form. The malignancy may grow around the esophagus at the level of the diaphragm, impinging on the lumen or the tube, or it may cause a bulky, ulcerating tumor mass. Most tumors are located in the middle and lower one-third of the esophagus.

This disease is usually asymptomatic for long periods, with the earliest complaint being a mild dysphagia that becomes progressively worse. Postprandial regurgitation may motivate the person to seek medical assistance. Weight loss is a common complaint; hematemesis and guaiac-positive stools are relatively uncommon. Invasion of surrounding structures may result in back pain, and pressure on respiratory structures may cause varying degrees of respiratory distress.

Definitive diagnosis is through esophagoscopy with biopsy of the tumor mass. Other diagnostic measures, such as barium swallow, chest film, and blood tests, give additional information. Prognosis for this malignancy is very poor, with only about 3% surviving for 5 years.[2,16]

## ALTERATIONS IN THE STOMACH AND DUODENUM

### Gastritis

*Gastritis* is a general term for an inflammation of the gastric mucosa. It may occur with excessive or completely absent gastric acid secretion. The classification into *acute* and *chronic gastritis* describes the onset and course of the disease. Chronic gastritis may be associated with gastric mucosal atrophy, achlorhydria, and peptic ulceration.

### Acute Gastritis

Acute gastritis causes transient inflammation of the gastric mucosa, mucosal hemorrhages, and erosion into the mucosal lining. It is frequently associated with alcoholism, aspirin ingestion, smoking, and severely stressful conditions such as trauma, burns, central nervous system damage, chemotherapy, and radiation therapy. Hydrochloric acid is present in gastritis, but its secretion does not have to be excessive.[22] Erosion of the gastric mucosa can result in a massive gastric hemorrhage. Therefore, acute gastritis may be associated with discomfort or serious outcome.

### Gastric Erosions

Gastric erosions or stress ulcers occur after a major insult to the body. Causes include hypovolemic or septic shock, peritonitis, serious brain injury, drug ingestion (usually aspirin or NSAIDs), or major burn injury.[16] Gastric ulcerations after brain damage are called *Cushing's ulcers*; those after burn injury are called *Curling's ulcers*. Ulceration can usually be attributed to ischemia.

When gastric erosions occur, they are multiple and superficial, and are present in large areas of the gastric mucosa. Superficial erosions and discrete ulcers form, especially in the fundus. An *erosion* is a superficial mucosa defect of the stomach that does not penetrate the muscularis layer. An *acute peptic ulcer* penetrates the muscularis layer. Such injury permits damage by continual activation of pepsinogen. Gastric acid secretion is sometimes increased, and the erosions often localize in the acid-secreting portion of the stomach. Two mechanisms for production of stress ulcers have been proposed: (1) mucosal ischemia, which relates to lack of blood supply to the gastric mucosa during the poststress period and results from a sympathetic vasoconstrictive action; and (2) enhanced back-diffusion of hydrogen ions due to increased sensitivity of the disrupted gastric mucosa to hydrochloric acid and pepsin. The surface mucosal cells are disrupted, and stimulation of the myenteric plexus leads to hypersecretion of gastric acid and pepsinogen.[15] Histamine is also released from damaged cells, and its effects increase the damage (Figure 41-5).

*Lipid mediators* play a role in either amplifying or delaying ulcerative repair that has been triggered by another factor.[19] In ischemic injury, platelet-activating factor or prostaglandins may promote gastric ulceration (Figure 41-6). The role of cortisone and aspirin in causing ulceration may be through lipid mediators.[19]

The major clinical manifestation of gastric erosions or ulceration is massive, painless, gastric bleeding with an onset 2 to 15 days after the original insult.[16] This bleeding, from multiple sites in the gastric mucosa, is very difficult to control. Because of the danger of bleeding after acute stress, preventive measures are routinely used to decrease hydrogen ion secretion and to neutralize gastric acid.

### Peptic Ulcer Disease (PUD)

*Peptic ulcers* (peptic ulcer disease, or PUD) are ulcerative conditions of the gastrointestinal tract that result from

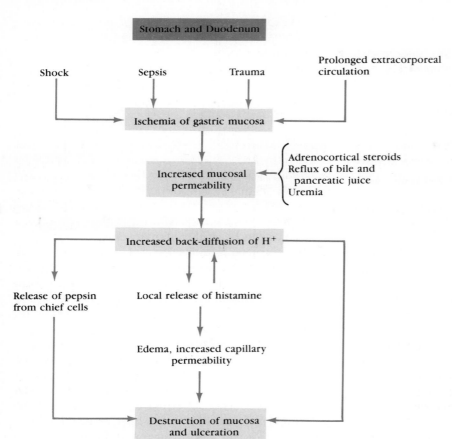

**FIGURE 41–5.**
Events postulated to occur in the production of stress ulcers. (Source: N.J. Greenberger, *Gastrointestinal Disorders: A Pathophysiologic Approach* [3rd ed.]. Chicago: Yearbook, 1986.)

acid-pepsin imbalance. They are thought to develop when the aggressive proteolytic activities of the gastric secretions are greater than their normal protective abilities. An increase in acid and pepsin from any cause may produce ulcerations if the protective mechanisms are not ade-

quate. Major factors that alter the mucosal barrier include the failure to regenerate the mucous epithelium at a sufficient rate, a decrease in quantity and quality of mucus, and a poor local mucosal blood flow. It has been suggested that vascular occlusion of small nutrient vessels in the mucosa or submucosa causes localized necrosis and subsequent ulcer formation. Peptic activity alone is not responsible for ulcerations; individual susceptibility is necessary.

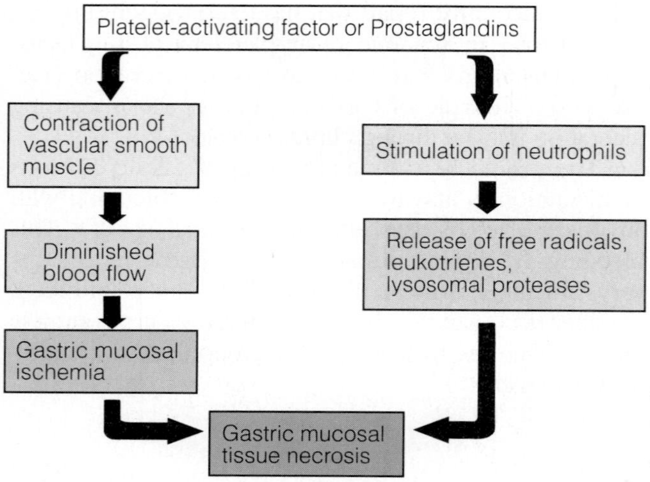

The most frequent site for peptic ulcers is the pyloric region of the duodenum, but lesions also occur in the greater curvature of the stomach (Figure 41-7). Duodenal ulcers comprise 80% of all peptic ulcers. Ulcerative conditions affect approximately 10% to 15% of the general population. Table 41-1 explains differential features of PUD.

## Gastric Ulcers

The primary problem with gastric ulcers appears to be decreased resistance of the gastric mucosa to ingested substances. The level of hydrochloric acid secretion is usually normal or reduced. True *achlorhydria*, or lack of hydrochloric acid secretion, is rare with these ulcers and usually indicates a gastric carcinoma. Because gastric ulcers often occur in conjunction with gastric atrophy, the secretions may contain mostly water and small amounts

**FIGURE 41–6.**
Platelet-activating factor or prostaglandins can promote gastric ulceration through ischemia or through the production of free radicals or other tissue toxic substances.

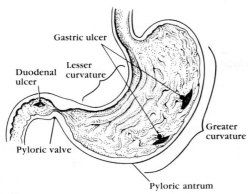

**FIGURE 41–7.**
Common locations of gastric and duodenal ulcers.

of mucus. The intrinsic factor may not be secreted, causing decreased absorption of vitamin $B_{12}$ and pernicious anemia (see Chap. 19).

Pathologically, gastric ulcers are often associated with atrophy of the gastric glands. Gastritis always surrounds the ulcerated area. The classic ulcer has a sharply punched-out appearance with a smooth, clean base. The mucosa surrounding it is often edematous. Bleeding may occur if the ulceration erodes through a vessel. Malignant gastric ulcers exhibit a shaggy, necrotic base, as opposed to the smooth base of nonmalignant ulcers. Gastric ulcers transform into malignancy frequently enough to call them premalignant and to encourage frequent follow-up.

Gastric ulcers can be diagnosed by barium swallow

**TABLE 41–1.**
DIFFERENTIAL FEATURES OF PEPTIC ULCER DISEASE (PUD)

| TYPE OF LESIONS | FREQUENCY | PATHOPHYSIOLOGY | CLINICAL FEATURES | COURSE |
|---|---|---|---|---|
| Duodenal ulcer | Men:women, 3:1<br>Peak frequency 5th–6th decades<br>Prevalence 10%–12% | Normal to increased parietal cell mass<br>Normal to increased gastric acid secretion<br>Normal to mildly elevated circulating gastrin levels<br>Excessive gastrin response to meals; excessive parietal cell sensitivity<br>Genetic factors—familial tendency, frequent blood group O, nonsecretor<br>Positive associations—chronic obstructive lung disease, hepatic cirrhosis, pancreatic insufficiency, hyperparathyroidism<br>Located in duodenal bulb, pyloric channel, postbulbar area | Pain: rhythmicity, periodicity, chronicity<br>Pain-food-relief-pain pattern | Remissions and exacerbations for 10–25 years after onset. "Once an ulcer, always an ulcer." Seasonal trend (spring and fall). |
| Gastric ulcer | Men:women, 3–4:1<br>Peak frequency 6th–7th decades<br><br>Duodenal ulcer: gastric ulcer 4:1 | Normal to decreased parietal cell mass<br>Normal to decreased gastric acid secretion (not achlorhydria)<br>Normal to elevated circulating gastrin level<br>Presence of gastritis<br>Abnormal gastric mucosal barrier<br>Abnormal pyloric function, bile reflux<br>Ulcerogenic drugs | Pain-food-relief-pain pattern, or food-pain pattern<br><br>Weight loss, anorexia | Remissions and exacerbations less than in duodenal ulcer; high recurrence rate. No seasonal trend. |
| Gastric erosions or stress ulcer | No sex difference<br>Related to severe stress, sepsis, burns, trauma, head injuries | Head injuries—marked gastric acid hypersecretion<br>Others—gastric mucosal ischemia, acid back-diffusion, acute gastritis | Bleeding frequent in recognized cases; may be severe, persistent (actual frequency unknown) | Half of those who bleed require surgery. |

(upper gastrointestinal series) and direct endoscopy. Biopsy and routine cytology studies can be performed with endoscopy. Gastric analysis usually reveals a lower than normal output of hydrochloric acid, but the large overlap of values among different persons makes this an obsolete test for gastric ulcers except in diagnosing Zollinger—Ellison syndrome.[16] Benign ulcers frequently localize on the greater curvature of the stomach and are usually smaller than malignant lesions. If there is associated achlorhydria, the ulcers are almost always malignant.

The most common symptom with gastric ulcer disease is epigastric pain. The pain may or may not be relieved by eating or it may be precipitated when food is ingested. Gastric ulcers that localize in the pyloric area often relay symptoms of duodenal ulcers. Nausea, vomiting, and weight loss are common. Hemorrhage occurs in approximately 25% of these persons and is often profound. Perforation of the ulcer into the peritoneal cavity is less frequent than with duodenal ulcer. Healing and recurrence are common, with lack of healing or failure to decrease in size suggesting gastric malignancy. Healing, with a decrease in the size of the ulcer by 50%, should occur in 3 months of initiating therapy.[8,16]

### Zollinger–Ellison Syndrome (ZES)

This disease is usually the result of a gastrin-secreting tumor of the pancreas (see Chap. 39). It can be a primary gastrinoma of the stomach or intestines. Serum gastrin levels are markedly elevated, and large amounts of hydrochloric acid are produced. The tumors of ZES are malignant and produce ulceration in any portion of the stomach or duodenum. The ulcerations have a high probability of hemorrhage and rupture.[16]

### Duodenal Ulcers

Numerous causes and predisposing factors in combination upset the balance between the protective mechanism and the acid-pepsin proteolytic action in the duodenal wall. Duodenal ulcers occur in the presence of acid, but hyperacidity is not always a significant component. Persons with excess acid secretion may also have excess secretion of gastrin or gastrinlike substances from the duodenal wall, as well as from the parietal cells. Evidence that the disease has a strong family history and occurs among the type O blood group supports a theory of genetic weakness.[2] Elevated serum pepsinogen level is under study as a significant indicator of predisposition to duodenal ulcer. The genetic trait for hypersecretion of pepsinogen is autosomal dominant and may be a marker for predisposition to duodenal ulcers.[2]

The emotional factors that increase gastric secretions and influence the pathogenesis of duodenal ulcerations often precipitate the onset or recurrence of symptoms. Studies have been conducted to identify an "ulcer personality," but the findings have not been conclusive.[18] Numerous instances have been reported where the disease has been reactivated when the affected person suffers undue stress, anxiety, or fatigue.[2] Endocrine factors, such as estrogen and the adrenal steroids, also may contribute to the formation of ulcerations.

Duodenal ulcers are usually deep, with a sharp line of demarcation from uninvolved tissue. Most of these ulcerations occur in the first portion of the duodenum, close to the pylorus. Disruption of the integrity of the mucosal wall caused by the acid-pepsin imbalance penetrates the entire thickness of the mucosal membrane, including the muscularis mucosa. Healing requires the formation of granulation tissue and scar. Secretory cellular functions are lost in the area of scarring. A typical duodenal ulcer is a round or oval-shaped, indurated, with a funnel-shaped lesion that extends into the muscularis layer. It is frequently located within 1 to 3 cm of the pyloric junction, on either the anterior or posterior wall.

Acute ulcerations may develop on chronic ulcers, and perforations through the duodenal wall in active ulcers result in spilling of gastric or duodenal contents into the peritoneum and peritonitis. Erosion of an artery or a vein at the base of the lesion may cause a hemorrhage. The amount of bleeding depends on the vessel involved, and the effects are related to the rapidity and amount of blood loss. Scar formation may cause deformity, shortening, and stiffening of the duodenum, which may interfere with normal emptying of the stomach. Actual obstruction may result from stenosis, spasm, edema, and inflammation.

Clinical manifestations of duodenal ulcerations include a documented pattern of remissions and exacerbations over varying periods of time. An attack is frequently triggered by stress, and exacerbations have been observed to occur most frequently in the fall and spring seasons. A definite pain-food-relief pattern is characteristic of duodenal ulcer. Pain usually develops 90 minutes to 3 hours after eating, often waking the person at night. This pain is immediately relieved by food or antacids. Pain on awakening in the early morning is rare, and is thought to be due to decreased gastric secretions.[8] The pain is usually described as steady, boring, burning, aching, or hungerlike, and is localized in the midepigastrium, the right epigastric area, and sometimes in the back. The pain mechanism in duodenal ulcers is thought to be related to irritation of exposed sensory nerve endings by hydrochloric acid. It may result from increased motility or spasm of the muscles at the ulcer site. In rare cases, no pain is described, and the ulcer is discovered when complications arise.

Other gastrointestinal symptoms include heartburn

and regurgitation of sour juice into the back of the mouth. Anorexia is not a usual complaint because the individual seeks relief of pain through eating. A duodenal ulcer may rupture because of erosion through the duodenal wall, and this leads to contamination of the peritoneal cavity. As in gastric ulcer disease, hemorrhage may lead to profound blood loss and hypovolemic shock; a slowly bleeding ulcer may be detected by guaiac-positive stools. Localized tenderness around the epigastric area is the only common finding on physical examination.

Diagnosis of duodenal ulcer requires a reliable and accurate history of the characteristic pain. Radiologic and fluoroscopic examinations with barium swallow demonstrate ulcer craters and niches as well as outlet deformities. Gastric endoscopy, direct visualization of the gastric mucosa through a lighted scope, is useful in revealing lesions too small or superficial to be seen on radiographs. Tissue for histologic studies may also be taken during the procedure. Gastric juice analysis may be helpful in persons who do not have typical duodenal ulcer disease to determine the cycle of hydrochloric acid and pepsin secretion. Basal acid output and maximal histamine stimulation analysis may be performed. Basal acid output measures the acidity of gastric secretions without a known or intentional stimulation. Achlorhydria after histamine stimulation demonstrates loss of secretory function and almost never occurs with duodenal ulcerations.

A 12-hour nocturnal test provides information regarding secretion during a prolonged basal state. Nocturnal levels of hydrochloric acid and pepsin are frequently higher in persons with duodenal ulcers than in those with gastric ulcers. With Zollinger—Ellison syndrome, very high levels of gastric acid secretion are measured (see Chap. 39).

All of the therapeutic approaches for duodenal ulcer disease are directed toward relieving pain, promoting healing, and preventing complications. The histamine antagonist drugs that reduce gastric acidity promote healing in a significant number of cases, evidence that supports excess gastric acid as a cause.[3] Helping the person recognize lifestyle and personal factors that precipitate symptoms may enhance compliance with therapy and thus help prevent recurrence of the disease.

### Complications of PUD

Hemorrhage occurs in 15% to 20% of cases of PUD. It may be manifested by melena (occult blood in the stools) or hematemesis and hemorrhagic shock. Ulcers located posteriorly are more likely to bleed than those in other locations, and the bleed is often arterial and massive.[3] Other complications include perforation of the wall, which is most common with duodenal ulcer disease and causes abdominal pain and peritonitis. Penetration of the ulcer into surrounding structures is relatively uncom-

mon, but may affect the pancreas, liver, and abdominal wall. Symptoms of penetration are those of damage to the affected area.

The inlet and outlet of the stomach may become obstructed; this is most common in the pyloric area. Obstruction may cause severe pain, vomiting, weight loss, and anorexia. The ulcer may be intractable, with frequent recurrence or lack of response to therapy. Other complications, especially obstruction and penetration, may lead to intractable ulcers. When ulcers continue despite therapy, Zollinger—Ellison syndrome must be ruled out.

## Gastric Carcinoma

Of all malignancies of the stomach, 90% to 95% are classified as carcinomas. The frequency of gastric carcinoma has been declining steadily over the past few decades in the United States, but in several countries, especially Japan, Iceland, and Finland, it is high. However, its occurrence appears to be declining in the high-risk countries as well.[16] Gastric cancer generally occurs between the ages of 60 and 65 years of age. Survival rates are poor, with less than 5% to 15% surviving for 5 years after diagnosis. Early diagnosis has improved the mortality figures, so that if the lesion is confined to the mucosa and submucosa, 5-year survival improves to 60% to 90%.[16]

Environmental factors evidently play a large part in the origin of gastric cancer, although the significance of each factor generally is not known. These factors include diet, socioeconomic class, occupation, and urban residence.[2] Diet has been implicated in gastric carcinoma, especially with regard to the nitrates that are used as food preservatives. These convert to nitrites, which convert to nitrosamine, a well-known carcinogen.[18] Genetic or hereditary linkage is supported by an increased risk among families and the preponderance of occurrence in persons with blood group A. Gastric carcinoma also is associated with atrophic gastritis or polyps of the stomach.

Pathologically, these carcinomas may arise anywhere on the mucosal surface. They begin as *in situ* (localized) lesions that progress to lesions called *early gastric carcinoma (EGC)*. These lesions are limited to the mucosa and submucosa. Early spread to regional lymph nodes may occur. As the lesions progress, they may infiltrate the wall or protrude as bulky masses into the outlet of the stomach.[16] Ulceration may occur, with a shaggy, necrotic-appearing base. A diffuse form of carcinoma, the *leather-bottle stomach*, causes thickening of the entire stomach. Distant metastasis is frequent, most often to the liver, lungs, ovaries, and peritoneum. These metastases are often already established at the time of diagnosis.

The clinical manifestations are often vague and nonspecific, including early satiety, loss of appetite, weight loss, abdominal pain, vomiting, and change in bowel habits. Anemia and guaiac-positive stools may be discovered. Bleeding may result from vascular erosion as the tumor ulcerates. Pain in gastric carcinoma may mimic ulcer pain or be related to partial outlet obstruction. Massive hemorrhage may cause hemorrhagic shock.

The only definitive diagnostic test is gastric biopsy, usually obtained through gastric endoscopy. Other studies may be helpful, such as barium swallow, blood work, and additional tests to demonstrate a mass in the gastric area.

## ALTERATIONS IN THE SMALL INTESTINE

Most nutrient absorption occurs in the small intestine. Any alteration of the integrity of the small bowel can result in malabsorption or maldigestion or both, whether the source is motor or mucosal. The common conditions of vomiting, diarrhea, and enteritis can also result in fluid, electrolyte, and nutritional imbalances.

*Malabsorption* refers to inadequate absorption of ingested nutrients and water. *Maldigestion* is the inability to absorb foodstuffs because they have been broken down inadequately. Box 41-1 outlines some of the major causes of malabsorption. Many disorders can cause malabsorption through differing mechanisms, and the categories are not entirely separate. The more common conditions are discussed in this section. Table 41-2 summarizes the laboratory tests most commonly used to detect malabsorption.[20]

## Vomiting and Diarrhea

Because 3 to 6 liters of gastrointestinal secretions are placed in the gastrointestinal lumen every day, excessive vomiting or diarrhea can lead to volume depletion and electrolyte abnormalities.[14] Triggers of gastrointestinal losses can be bacteria, viruses, drug reactions, toxins, and excessive use of laxatives and enemas, along with many other conditions.

Vomiting is usually preceded by nausea. Many clinical

## BOX 41-1.
### CAUSES OF MALABSORPTION

Incomplete Digestion of Nutrients
  *Primary*—deficient production of pancreatic enzymes
    Chronic relapsing pancreatitis
    Cancer of the pancreas
    Cystic fibrosis
    Extensive pancreatic resection
  *Secondary*—defective use of pancreatic enzymes
    Post-Billroth II
    Zollinger–Ellison syndrome
Deficiency of Conjugated Bile Salts
  Severe liver disease
  Extrahepatic biliary tract obstruction
Abnormal Loss of Nutrients or Bile Salts
  Ileal resection
  Ileectomy
  Ileal bypass
  Severe disease of the terminal ileum
Abnormal Bacterial Overgrowth in the Small Bowel
  Surgically created blind loops
  Fistulas—enteroenteric, enterocolic, gastrojejunocolic
  Chronic intestinal obstruction due to adhesions or strictures
  Small bowel diverticula
  Motor abnormalities except scleroderma
Drug-induced Precipitation or Sequestration
  Neomycin
  Calcium carbonate
  Cholestyramine
Inadequate Mechanical Mixing of Chyme with Digestive Enzymes
  Post-Billroth II
  Post-total gastrectomy

Abnormalities of the Absorptive Surface
  *Biochemical or genetic*
    Disaccharidase deficiency
    Abetalipoproteinemia
    Primary vitamin $B_{12}$ malsorption
    Cystinuria
    Hartnup disease
    Celiac sprue
  *Inflammatory or infective disorders*
    Tropical sprue
    Regional enteritis
    Eosinophilic enteritis
    Infectious enteritis
Lack of Absorptive Surface
  Intestinal resection
  Gastroileostomy
Lymphatic Obstruction
  Whipple's disease
  Intestinal lymphangiectasia
  Lymphoma
Cardiovascular Disorders
  Mesenteric vascular insufficiency
  Congestive heart failure
  Constrictive pericarditis
Endocrine and Metabolic Disorders
  Diabetes mellitus
Hypoparathyroidism
Adrenal insufficiency
Hyperthyroidism
Carcinoid syndrome

*(Summarized from N.J. Greenberger and K.J. Isselbacher. Disorders of absorption. In J.D. Wilson et al., Harrison's Principles of Internal Medicine [12th ed.]. New York: McGraw-Hill, 1991.)*

**TABLE 41–2.**
LABORATORY TESTS SPECIFIC TO THE DETECTION OF MALSORPTION

| TEST | NORMAL FINDING | MEANING OF ABNORMAL FINDINGS |
|---|---|---|
| Fecal fat balance: quantitative determination of stool fat | 6 g (or fewer) of fatty acids extracted from stool in 24 hours | More than 6 g/24 hours—clinically significant steatorrhea |
| D-xylose tolerance test | 5 g (or more) D-xylose excreted by kidneys in 5 hours; or 25 mg (or more) D-xylose/dL of blood in 1–2 hours | Decreased values in diseases of intestinal mucosa and in intestinal stasis; values normal in pancreatic insufficiency |
| Schilling test | Greater than 7% of radioactive vitamin $B_{12}$ excreted in urine/24 hours | Decreased value can indicate (1) lack of intrinsic factor, (2) competition with bacteria, (3) disease of ileum |
| With administration of intrinsic factor | | Decreased—(2) or (3) above |
| After 2 weeks of antimicrobial therapy | | Decreased—(1) or (3) above |
| Serum carotene | 70–290 ng/mL | Decreased with malsorption and also perhaps due to dietary insufficiency or hepatic disease |
| $^{14}C$ triolein absorption (break test) | More than 3.5% of $^{14}CO_2$ appears in breath/hour (6 hr) | Correlates with chemical stool fat |

*(Values from J. Wallach, Interpretation of Laboratory Tests [4th ed.]. Boston: Little, Brown, 1986.)*

states have nausea and vomiting as common manifestations, but the precise mechanisms that trigger vomiting are poorly understood[4] (see Chap. 40). The main categories associated with nausea and vomiting include (1) acute abdominal emergencies such as intestinal obstruction of appendicitis; (2) chronic indigestion such as ulcer disease or food intolerance; (3) acute systemic infections of viral, bacterial, or parasitic nature; (4) central nervous system disorders associated with increased intracranial pressure of inner ear disorders; (5) acute myocardial infarction or congestive heart failure; (6) endocrine disorders such as diabetic ketoacidosis; (7) side effects of drugs and chemicals; and (8) psychogenic vomiting due to stress of psychic disturbances.[4]

Vomiting and diarrhea often are components of an acute disease condition such as viral or bacterial infection. Vomiting may be the primary symptom, or both vomiting and diarrhea may be seen. The process may be accompanied by elevated body temperature, joint aching, and shaking chills. The condition may be self-limiting, or it may require fluid, electrolyte, and antibiotic therapy. At high risk are elderly persons and young children, because they have less fluid in reserve and can suffer rapid depletion of fluid and electrolyte balance (see Chap. 8).

Diarrhea can be classified as *osmotic, secretory*, or of *mixed origin* (Box 41-2). Osmotic diarrhea occurs when there is a poorly absorbable solute in the alimentary tract. It contains large quantities of water and potassium. Copious osmotic diarrhea can lead to rapid fluid and potassium depletion. Secretory diarrhea results when the normal secretory processes are stimulated and electrolytes and water are not absorbed. Depletion of electrolytes including sodium, bicarbonate, and potassium occurs along with the water loss. Diarrhea of mixed origin may be due to rapid intestinal transit, and the underlying cause may be difficult to identify.[8]

## Enteritis

Enteritis, or *gastroenteritis*, is an inflammatory process of the stomach or small intestine. It may be caused by viruses, bacteria, or allergic reactions. It may be caused by the ingestion of contaminated food, especially food contaminated by staphlococci, which produce a toxin that reacts with the small intestine mucosa. Dysentery caused by bacteria affects the colon. The pathologic process has varying manifestations that result in abdominal cramping, diarrhea, and vomiting.

A fluid and electrolyte imbalance often results from enteritis. Parasites may localize in the gastrointestinal tract or invade the circulation. Eosinophilic enteritis is uncommon but may result from an allergy. It is manifested by the accumulation of eosinophils in the gut

**BOX 41–2.**
CLASSIFICATION AND CAUSES OF DIARRHEA

---

## Osmotic Diarrhea
*Surgical*
    Gastric: rapid gastric emptying; pyloroplasty; gastroenterostomy; antrectomy
    Intestinal: resection or bypass of jejunum and proximal ileum
*Disease with histopathologic lesions*
    Mucosal: celiac (nontropical) sprue, collagenous sprue; tropical sprue; dermatitis herpeti-
    formis and other cutaneous diseases; nutritional (protein calorie malnutrition or *kwashior-*
    *kor;* marasmus)
    Submucosal (obstructive): Whipple's disease; lymphoma; intestinal lymphangiectasia;
    amyloidosis
    Inflammatory: granulomatous enterocolitis; ulcerative colitis
    Infectious or parasitic disease: postgastroenteritis; *Giardia lamblia;* coccidia; *Endolimax*
    *nana; Strongyloides stercoralis; Capillaria philippinensis*
*Biochemical mucosal disease*
    Membrane digestive defects: lactase deficiency (alactasia, congenital lactose intolerance
    with lactosuria, prematurity, diarrhea of breastfed newborns, adult primary lactase defi-
    ciency); sucrase-isomaltase deficiency; sucrase deficiency; enterokinase deficiency
    Membrane transport defects: glucose-galactose malabsorption; congenital chloridorrhea
*Immune deficiency states*
    Specific immunoglobulin deficiency: IgA deficiency with normal villi; IgA deficiency with ce-
    liac sprue type flat mucosa; IgA deficiency with ataxia-telangiectasia; IgA and IgM defi-
    ciency with nodular lymphoid hyperplasia
    General immunoglobulin deficiency (acquired): decreased IgA, IgM, IgG
    Immunoglobulin metabolism abnormality: IgA heavy-chain disease
*Drug-induced*
    Osmotic cathartics: sorbitol, lactulose; sodium sulfate purge; antacids
    Other: colchicine; neomycin; para-aminosalicylic acid; phenformin; lincomycin; tetracycline

## Secretory Diarrhea
*Exogenous: enteric infections*
    Toxigenic diarrhea: *Vibriocholerae; Escherichia coli* strains; *Shigella dysenteriae I; Staphylo-*
    *coccus aureus* strains; *Clostridium perfringens; Pseudomonas aeruginosa*
    Invasive diarrhea: shigella strains; salmonella strains; *Escherichia coli* strains; *Entamoeba*
    *histolytica*
*Endogenous*
    Secretagogues and inhibitors of absorption
        Deconjugated and dehydroxylated bile salts
            Acting on small intestine and colon: bacterial overgrowth; surgical (vagotomy-pyloro-
            plasty; intestinal blind loop); anatomic defects (small bowel diverticula; stricture; fis-
            tula; blind loop); inflammatory bowel disease; hypomotility (diabetic autonomic neu-
            ropathy; scleroderma; submucosal disease)
            Acting on colon: surgical (ileal resection; ileal bypass); inflammatory bowel disease
            involving distal ileum
        Hydroxy fatty acids, steatorrhea
            Surgical: post-gastric surgery
            Pancreatic insufficiency
            Small intestinal mucosal disease
            Methionine malabsorption (metabolized to hydroxybutyrate)
    Neoplasms: villous adenoma; ganglioneuroma; medullary carcinoma of the thyroid; pan-
    creatic islet cell tumors (Zollinger–Ellison syndrome, watery diarrhea hypokalemia achlor-
    hydria syndrome)
    Defective electrolyte transport: colectomy

## Diarrhea of Mixed Origin
*Hypermotility*
    Exogenous: cholinergic drugs
    Endogenous: hypocalcemia; hyperthyroidism; hypoadrenalism; hypopituitarism; carcinoid
    syndrome

---

*(Source: N.J. Greenberger, Gastrointestinal Disorders: A Pathophysiologic Approach [3rd ed.]. Chicago: Year-book, 1986.)*

wall.[21] In general, enteritis causes inflammatory changes in the intestinal mucosa that return to normal when the precipitator is removed.

## Celiac Disease

### Celiac Enteropathy (Nontropical Sprue)

*Celiac enteropathy* has many names and is thought to be related to gluten intolerance. Its frequency is greater in women than in men, and the onset of symptoms usually occurs in young adulthood.

Histopathologic changes in the absorptive surface in response to exposure to the protein gluten or its breakdown products, found mostly in wheat, are responsible for the manifestations of a general malabsorption syndrome. The mechanism underlying this reaction is not known, but the data supports a hypersensitivity reaction to gluten and its derivative gliadin.[2]

Gluten proteins have been shown to have antigenic properties, and circulating antibodies to dietary gluten have been demonstrated in persons with active celiac enteropathy. The lamina propria of affected mucosa contains mononuclear leukocytes and plasma cells. In some cases, serum levels of IgA are elevated and levels of IgM are depressed. Antibodies cannot be demonstrated in all cases, however, and there is a poor correlation between the level of the antibodies and the severity of the disease.[2] Corticosteroid therapy has been shown to improve both intestinal absorption and histologic appearance.

Regardless of cause, the pathologic changes are characteristic. The villi are flattened or absent, and the epithelium is disorganized and consists of cuboidal rather than the normal columnar cells. The brush border is thickened, and the lamina propria is infiltrated with inflammatory cells. Cytoplasmic changes include membrane disruption and rounded mitochondria. All of these changes result in malabsorption, with impaired uptake and transport of nutrients.[2]

Clinical features include frequent, foul-smelling, steatorrheic stools (ie, the stools have a fatty or greasy appearance). Loss of body weight and malabsorption of fat-soluble vitamins are common. Severe muscle-wasting and hypoproteinemia may occur.

Treatment measures support the theory of gluten hypersensitivity, since a dramatic or delayed remission of symptoms occurs when barley, wheat, rye, and oats are removed from the diet. Restoration of the normal mucosal epithelium occurs, and malabsorption decreases.

### Tropical Sprue

*Tropical sprue* differs in etiology from celiac enteropathy but is usually characterized by identical mucosal changes in the small intestine. It probably results from nutritional and bacterial alterations and occurs with the greatest frequency in certain tropical areas. It may be caused by *Escherichia coli* bacteria. Symptoms may not arise for months or years after exposure.[2] Because the mucosal lesions result in malabsorption, the clinical picture closely resembles that of celiac enteropathy. Treatment with folic acid is restorative in some cases, and antibiotics may be helpful.

## Regional Enteritis: Crohn's Disease

*Crohn's disease* is an idiopathic, chronic, inflammatory bowel disease that may affect any segment of the gastrointestinal tract, although it most commonly affects the terminal ileum or colon.[2] The frequency of this chronic inflammatory disease is equal in men and women, is slightly higher in members of the Jewish race, and exhibits a familial predisposition. Onset is most common between the ages of 15 and 20, with a secondary peak between 55 and 60 years. It is much more frequent in the United States, Britain, and Scandinavia than in Japan, Russia, and South America.[2] Crohn's disease and ulcerative colitis have many etiologic similarities and commonly are grouped as *inflammatory bowel disease (IBD)*. The origins may be infectious, immunologic, psychosomatic, dietary, hormonal, or unknown. Viruses continue to be studied as major possible causative factors. The immunologic features of the diseases may be primary or secondary responses to the viral organism.[2] Ulcerative colitis is described in more detail on page 804.

Gross inspection of the affected bowel discloses shallow, longitudinal mucosal ulcers; long or short areas of stricture; and a cobblestone appearance of the mucosa (Figure 41-8). The cobblestone appearance results from interconnecting fissures that cut deeply into the intestinal

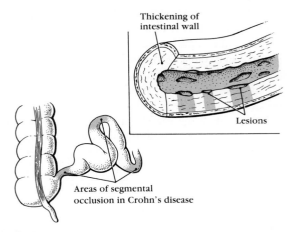

**FIGURE 41-8.**

Crohn's disease showing segmental areas of occlusion and transmural involvement of intestinal wall.

wall and create islands of mucosa elevated by the existing transmural (full-wall thickness) inflammation and its accompanying edema. The bowel wall becomes congested, thickened, and rigid, with adhesions involving the periintestinal fat.[1] Areas of involvement are localized and interrupted by areas of normal gut. Sometimes, several segments of bowel are affected and are separated by normal bowel. These segments are called *skip lesions* and produce chronic partial intestinal obstruction.[17] Fistulas to other parts of the gastrointestinal tract or other adjacent structures may be present.

Microscopically, all layers of the intestinal wall, particularly the submucosa, are edematous and infiltrated with aggregations of lymphocytes and macrophages.[2] Characteristic noncaseating granulomas, which have large mononuclear phagocytes and multinucleated giant cells, form in the bowel wall and often are present in the regional lymph nodes. Dilated lymphatic channels and lymphoid deposits occur at all levels of bowel involvement. The inflammatory changes cause functional disruption of the mucosa, producing malabsorption, especially of bile salts and vitamin $B_{12}$, which are normally absorbed in the jejunum and ileum. Fluid imbalances occur when large segments of ileum are affected. The strictures and fistulas that occur with this disease predispose the intestine to bacterial overgrowth and abscess formation. Bowel obstruction and peritonitis may result from the strictures and abscesses.

The clinical manifestations of Crohn's disease vary. Diarrhea is a dominant symptom and is often accompanied by fever and right lower quadrant or abdominal pain. The apparent linkage with stress and personality factors has been studied extensively with depression and dependency being seen as typical personality patterns. The clinical manifestations are variable, usually beginning with insidious onset of malaise and diarrhea. As the disease progresses, weight loss, occult blood in the feces, and nausea and vomiting occur. Obstruction and ileus may occur. Fistulas develop in 10% to 15% of cases, and peritonitis may result from rupture of the fistulous connection. A significant correlation of this disease with several autoimmune diseases and with adenocarcinoma of the small bowel exists. Chronic debilitation may finally require bowel resection.

Diagnosis of regional enteritis is based on the clinical history, physical examination (which may reveal a right lower quadrant mass), and characteristic radiograph. The string sign is commonly noted on radiologic studies (Figure 41-9).

## ALTERATIONS IN THE LARGE INTESTINE

### Adynamic or Paralytic Ileus

The word *ileus* has come to refer to a functional obstruction of the bowel. It may occur in the small or large in-

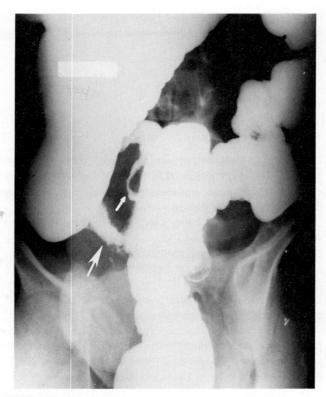

**FIGURE 41-9.**

Crohn's disease. Radiograph of colon showing a wide fistula (*large arrow*) between cecum and sigmoid colon and an irregularly narrowed distal ileum (*small arrow*). This is called the "string sign." (Source: J.H. Stein [ed.], *Internal Medicine.* Boston: Little, Brown, 1983.)

testine and is often classified as physiologic or paralytic. Lack of propulsive peristalsis makes the bowel unable to move contents downward, which leads to absence of bowel sounds and bowel distention.

Peristalsis becomes diminished or absent due in part to a triggering of the sympathetic inhibitory reflex by a noxious stimulus such as anesthesia, any peritoneal injury, interruption of nerve supply, abdominal injury or surgical manipulation, intestinal ischemia, electrolyte (especially potassium) disturbances, and retroperitoneal pathology.[13] A true ileus can be described as *adynamic*, having absent propulsive motor activity.[21]

The result of ileus is distention of the bowel with gas and fluid. The process is similar to actual bowel obstruction. Colonic bacteria may contribute to the abdominal distention and cause marked alterations of fluid and electrolyte balance. Loss of potassium leads to further intestinal atony. Vomiting and hypotension can cause alteration in the acid-base balance. As fluid shifts to the intestinal area, central blood volume decreases and distention increases.[21] If there is associated mesenteric ischemia, necrosis and rupture of the bowel may occur, causing peritonitis. Clinical findings include abdominal distention, decreased or absent bowel sounds, and signs of dehydration and shock. Symptoms are those of a rapidly progressive colonic obstruction with perforation of the bowel if the individual is not treated by colonoscopic deflation (through an intestinal drainage tube) or surgery.[15]

## Intestinal Ischemia and Infarction

*Ischemia* occurs when tissue demand for oxygen exceeds the supply and toxic metabolites accumulate. Ischemia is particularly prevalent in highly vascular systems such as the mesentery that supplies the intestines. Intestinal ischemia can result from any condition that interferes with blood supply to the mesentery (Figure 41-10). If ischemia or infarction is prolonged, the following events occur in the intestine: (1) the epithelial cells in the intestinal villi detach from the basement membrane; (2) subepithelial blebs of tissue protrude in the villi and, after an hour of continuous oxygen deprivation, the villi have no viable epithelial surface; (3) absorption and processing of nutrients is impaired; (4) the mucosal layer becomes necrotic and is shed into the stool as bloody diarrhea; (5) perforation of the intestine is promoted, leading to peritonitis; and (6) because the mucosal barrier is lost, intestinal bacteria can enter the bloodstream and cause bacteremia.

Symptoms of intestinal ischemia and infarction can be chronic or acute. Atherosclerotic ischemia may create an anginalike, cramping, abdominal pain which becomes worse after meals and then dissipates. Vasospasm and emboli produce an acute, severe abdominal pain with associated vomiting or diarrhea or both. Abdominal distention and tenderness are usually present. Bowel sounds may be loud and high-pitched (*borborygmi*) from an increase in rate and force of peristalsis. Hypotension may occur due to displacement of intravascular volume into the intestinal lumen. Prompt diagnosis can prevent shock, peritonitis, or sepsis. Surgery and antibiotics can help salvage the area of intestinal damage.[7]

## Intestinal Obstruction

*Intestinal obstruction* is blockage of the lumen of the bowel by an actual mechanical obstruction. Figure 41-11

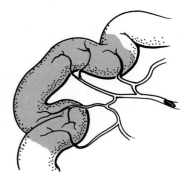

**FIGURE 41–10.**
Mesenteric occlusion causing intestinal ischemia.

illustrates some of the causes, which include foreign bodies, volvulus, adhesions, intussusception, hernias, infarction, and neoplasms.

After blockage occurs, gas and air are the primary bowel distenders, and distention occurs proximal to the area of blockage. As the process continues, gastric, biliary, and pancreatic secretions pool. Water, electrolytes, and serum proteins also begin to accumulate in the area. Pooling and bowel distention decrease the circulating blood volume due to a *third-space shift* that moves water into the area proximal to the obstruction and thus decreases plasma volume. Bowel wall edema also interferes with the blood supply to the bowel tissue and depresses normal sodium transport in the mucosa (Figure 41-12).

Strangulation of a bowel segment may cause necrosis, perforation, and loss of fluid and blood into the inactive bowel. Impairment of blood supply leads at first to increased peristalsis and bacterial invasion of the tissue, and finally causes necrosis and peritonitis when intestinal contents are released into the peritoneal cavity. Stasis of the intestinal contents provides an area for increased growth of organisms, with toxins being released into the tissues, further disrupting the intestinal cellular dynamics. Loss of fluids and electrolytes is a major problem and results in decreased systemic circulating fluid volume due to the shift from the vascular to the intestinal lumen.

Clinical manifestations include the acute onset of severe, cramping pain that correlates roughly to the area or level of obstruction. Pain may decrease in severity as the distention of the bowel and abdomen increases, which is probably due to impaired motility in the edematous intestine. Increases in the rate and force of peristalsis cause borborygmi in the early period, but these may progress to a silent bowel as the condition persists. Vomiting is almost always present and may be bilious or feculent (having the appearance of feces) depending on the level of the obstruction. Diarrhea may occur if obstruction is not complete.

Hypovolemic shock is the result of a shift of fluid greater than 10% of body weight. Septicemic shock may also result from contamination of the peritoneum when the bowel ruptures. Sepsis and hypovolemic shock produce a life-threatening clinical picture that must be treated aggressively.

Tenderness, rigidity, and fever usually indicate peritonitis. Leukocytosis and elevation of serum amylase level are also common. Distention of the bowel may be noted radiologically, but is not conclusive evidence of the cause or exact level of obstruction.

## Hernias

A *hernia* is a defect in the abdominal wall. It may occur in the scrotal or inguinal area or in the abdominal wall

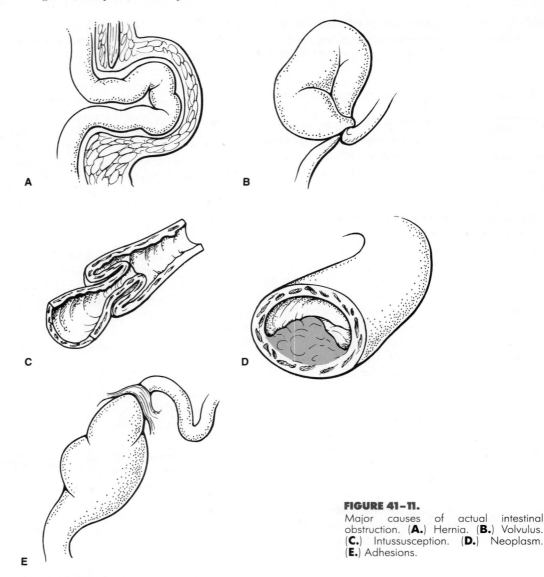

**FIGURE 41–11.**
Major causes of actual intestinal obstruction. (**A.**) Hernia. (**B.**) Volvulus. (**C.**) Intussusception. (**D.**) Neoplasm. (**E.**) Adhesions.

or diaphragm (Figure 41-13). Incisional hernias occur in an area weakened by surgical incision. Whatever the cause, the defect allows abdominal structures (eg, peritoneum, fat, bowel, or bladder) to fill the area, producing a sac filled with the material. Abdominal contents usually move into the defect when abdominal pressure increases. If the bulging of the sac is intermittent, the hernia is called *reducible*. *Incarcerated hernias* contain abdominal contents all the time, and *strangulated hernias* cause necrosis of the abdominal contents due to lack of blood supply. Necrosis of the bowel then leads to all the clinical manifestations of intestinal obstruction.

## Hirschsprung's Disease

*Hirschsprung's disease*, also called *congenital megacolon*, is usually manifested in early infancy and is caused by congenital absence of parasympathetic ganglion cells in the submucosal and intramuscular plexuses. Consequently, the bowel becomes greatly dilated, with no peristaltic action in the aganglionic area. The area most frequently affected is the rectosigmoid.

Hirschsprung's disease is a congenital disorder with much higher frequency in boys than in girls. When manifested in early infancy, abdominal distention, constipation, and vomiting occur. Occasionally, this condition is diagnosed in young adults who describe a lifelong problem with constipation.

*Megacolon*, or enlargement of the colon, may also be produced by any process that inhibits bowel evacuation. Among such processes are psychogenic megacolon, which results from ignoring the urge to defecate, some neurologic disorders, fecal impaction, and chronic depression.

The clinical manifestations depend on the degree of aganglionosis or bowel distention. The person is often

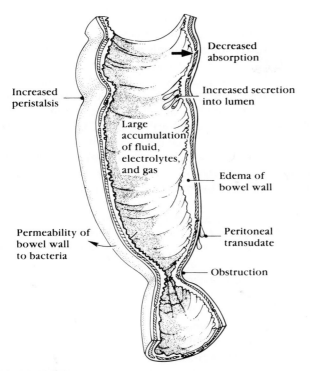

**FIGURE 41-12.**
Pathophysiology of intestinal obstruction and peritonitis. (Source: P.A. Jones, C.F. Dunbar, and M.M. Jirovec, *Medical-Surgical Nursing.* New York: McGraw-Hill, 1978.)

poorly nourished and anemic, and rarely produces fecal material. The congenital type is often associated with other anomalies such as Down syndrome.

## Diverticula

Diverticula are multiple saclike protrusions of the mucosa along the gastrointestinal tract. Although the terms are loosely used, a *true diverticulum* has all layers of the bowel in its walls, whereas a *false diverticulum* occurs in a weak area of the muscularis of the bowel.

An example of true diverticular disease is *Meckel's diverticulum*, which occurs in 1% to 2% of the population. This sac, located 1 to 3 feet proximal to the ileocecal junction, is formed by the persistence of a mesenteric structure that normally closes in fetal life. It may be lined with ileal mucosa or contain other types of gastrointestinal mucosal cells. Meckel's diverticulum is usuall asymptomatic, but it may cause symptoms that mimic acute appendicitis, Crohn's disease, or pelvic inflammatory disease.[3] Gastrointestinal bleeding and intestinal obstruction may complicate the condition.[3] False colonic diverticula are common and usually occur in the sigmoid colon.

Because of their frequency in elderly persons, it is thought that diverticula are related to the blood supply

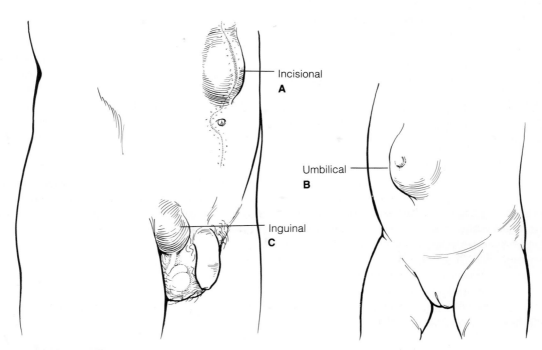

**FIGURE 41-13.**
Types of hernias. (**A.**) Incisional hernia. (**B.**) Inguinal hernia. (**C.**) Umbilical hernia.

or nutrition of the bowel in the elderly.[2] Lack of dietary fiber or roughage and decreased fecal bulk also have been correlated with this process.

*Diverticulosis* refers to the presence of diverticula in the colon that are rarely symptomatic. *Diverticulitis* is inflammation in or around a diverticular sac that results in retention of undigested food and bacteria in the sac. This forms a hard mass called a *fecalith*.[12] Colonic obstruction, fistulas, and abscesses can result. Rupture of the infected material into the peritoneal cavity may lead to peritonitis.

The clinical manifestations of symptomatic diverticular disease vary. Constipation is frequently reported. Fibrosis in the area may develop and cause obstruction by adhesions. The complaint of lower, left-sided abdominal pain may be associated with the signs of peritonitis, including guarding, fever, abdominal rigidity, and rebound tenderness. Radiographs and sigmoidoscopy may not indicate the extent of the problem. Surgery may be performed if the process causes obstruction or perforation.

## Hemorrhoids

*Hemorrhoids* are dilatations of the venous plexus that surround the rectal and anal areas. These dilatations are very common and develop in susceptible persons due to persistently increased pressure in the hemorrhoidal venous plexus. Hemorrhoids are often related to other types of abnormalities, especially varicose veins. Predisposition may result from constipation or pregnancy. Bleeding hemorrhoids may be a dangerous outcome of portal hypertension (see Chap. 43).

The dilated venous sacs protrude into the anal and rectal canals where they become exposed; thromboses, ulcerations, and bleeding then develop. Hemorrhoids may be painful and irritating. Bright red bleeding during defecation or with increased intraabdominal pressure is common. Usually blood loss is insignificant, but chronic anemia may be an outcome. Bleeding in association with portal hypertension may be profound and even life-threatening.[9]

## Ulcerative Colitis

*Ulcerative colitis* is primarily an inflammatory disease of the mucous membrane of the colon. The disease may be confined to the rectum, or it may affect segments of the colon or even the entire colon. The bowel fills with a bloody, mucoid secretion that produces a characteristic cramping pain, rectal urgency, and diarrhea.

Pathologically, ulcerative colitis usually begins in the rectal area and extends along the colon. Microscopic inflammatory ulcerated areas may be adjacent to healing areas, but the process is continuous, without the skip lesions characteristic of Crohn's disease.[2] In the *acute phase* the colon mucosa is hyperemic and edematous, and the usual secretions are absent. Small mucosal hemorrhages are evident, and abscesses form into small ulcerations. The mucosa tends to slough off and is lost in the feces. The ulcerations are confined to the mucosa and submucosa, and coalescence of the ulcers can denude large areas of the involved colon.[2] As the disease enters the *chronic phase*, the ulcerations become fibrotic, and thickening of the bowel wall results. Obstruction of the bowel rarely occurs from the fibrous thickening.[2]

Complications of ulcerative colitis include intestinal obstruction, dehydration, and major fluid and electrolyte imbalances. Malabsorption is common, and loss of blood in the stools may cause chronic iron-deficiency anemia. There is a significant relationship between ulcerative colitis and cancer of the colon. Ten percent to 15% of persons who have ulcerative colitis for more than 10 years will develop colon carcinoma.

The etiology of ulcerative colitis is unknown, but a genetic basis has been suggested because the disease occurs with increased frequency in some families. Its peak occurrence is between ages 15 and 35, and it is much more common in whites than in other races.[6] Agents such as viruses and microorganisms are implicated, and the disease may be associated with autoimmunity. The plasma serum in some persons with the disease has been shown to have an antibody to the colonic epithelial cells. Remissions and exacerbations are common and often can be directly related to major psychological stresses.[6] Many of the etiologic factors of Crohn's disease are also common to ulcerative colitis.

Clinical manifestations vary. The classic symptoms including cramping abdominal pain, bloody diarrhea, fever, and weight loss. About 60% of cases are classified as mild disease, and these individuals have less bleeding and diarrhea than in severe disease.[2] Laboratory findings include anemia, leukocytosis, hypoalbuminemia, electrolyte imbalance, and increased serum alkaline phosphatase. Despite their evident pathologic differences, ulcerative colitis and regional enteritis may be confused clinically. Table 41-3 shows the major differences between them.

Diagnosis of ulcerative colitis is made on the basis of the clinical features, results of barium enema, and sigmoidoscopic appearance of the mucosa. Biopsy and cultures are essential to exclude carcinoma and bacterial diarrhea.

## Polyps

A *polyp* in the large intestine is a benign growth that protrudes into the lumen. Polyps are divided into two major categories, *adenomatous* and *hyperplastic*.

Adenomatous polyps are true neoplasms. The growths begin in the mucosa deep within the crypts of the colonic mucosal glands.[18] The polypoidal cells continue to divide

**TABLE 41-3.**
MAJOR DIFFERENCES BETWEEN ULCERATIVE COLITIS AND CROHN'S DISEASE

| VARIABLE | ULCERATIVE COLITIS | CROHN'S DISEASE |
| --- | --- | --- |
| Extent of disease | Mucosa | Entire wall |
| Ulceration | Extensive, superficial | Patchy, deep |
| Mesentery | Normal | Thickened |
| Lymph nodes | Normal | Diseased |
| Granulomata | Absent | Present (25%–75%) |
| Distribution[a] | Symmetric | Eccentric |
| Skip areas | Never[b] | Common |
| Diseased rectum | Always[b] | 10%–20% |
| Small intestine disease | Never[b] | Usual |
| Results of surgery | Cure | Frequent recurrence |

[a] Radiologically, the entire circumference of the colon is involved in ulcerative colitis, whereas in Crohn's disease only one side may be diseased.
[b] The words "always" and "never" should not be used to describe biological processes, but here they are probably appropriate.
(Source: B.N. Brooke et al., Crohn's Disease: Aetiology, Clinical Manifestations and Management, 1977. Reprinted by permission of Macmillan, England.)

and become hyperplastic growths. When reproductive control is lost throughout the mucosal crypt, a neoplasm results. Polyps are very common in the general population. They rarely exceed 5 mm in diameter. These growths may be discovered by routine sigmoidoscopy or barium enema. They may bleed, causing bright red feces. The major clinical significance of hyperplastic polyps is that they have potential to become neoplastic or adenomatous.

Adenomatous polyps may be benign or malignant, and it is difficult to determine the difference unless they have obviously invaded the surrounding mucosa. Smaller growths are called *tubular* or *glandular polyps*, and the larger growths are called *villous adenomas*. Twenty-five percent to 50% of villous adenomas harbor carcinomas. Some researchers view the development as a sequence of events from controlled hyperplasia through a series of stages that terminate in carcinoma [2]. Polyps are usually surgically excised because they have such a close relationship with carcinoma of the colon.

## Colorectal Carcinoma

Colorectal carcinoma is second only to lung cancer in causes of death from cancer in the United States. When colon and rectal cancer are detected and treated in early localized stages, there is a 5-year survival rate of 80% to 90%.[1] Factors that predispose a person to colorectal cancer are heredity, fat intake, inflammatory bowel disease, homosexuality, and polyposis of the colon.[5] It is common in both men and women; it occurs at all ages, but the frequency is greatest during the fifth, sixth, and seventh decades. Prevalence is highest in northwest Europe and North America and lowest in South America, Africa, and Asia.

Investigations into causes of colorectal carcinoma have led to the study of animal fat in the diet, anaerobic bacteria of the large bowel, and fiber content of the diet.[4] Each of these factors may partially explain the disease's geographic distribution. The fiber aspect is interesting in that increased bulk in the diet decreases the transit time and also the time of contact between food and bowel. In the average American diet, the transit time may be as much as 4 to 5 days compared to 30 to 35 hours in African blacks. Since the American diet is much lower in fiber than the black African diet, colonic cancer is much more prevalent in America.[2] Based on the above observations, Table 41-4 lists nine recommendations for lowering the risk of colorectal cancer. These recommendations focus on ways to reduce production of carcinogens specific to the colon.

About 60% to 70% of these carcinomas arise in the rectum, rectosigmoid area, or sigmoid colon.[2] The type of the growth depends on the area of origin. Left-sided carcinoma tends to grow around the bowel, encircling it and leading to early obstruction. On the right side, the tumors tend to be bulky, polypoid, fungating masses. Either type may penetrate the bowel and cause abscess, peritonitis, invasion of surrounding organs, or bleeding. These tumors tend to grow slowly, and they remain asymptomatic for long periods of time. Ninety-five percent of carcinomas of the colon are adenocarcinomas that secrete mucin, a substance that aids in extending the malignancy.[2] Metastasis may occur to the liver, lungs, bones, or lymphatic system.

Clinical manifestations depend on the location of the tumor. The person may have melena, diarrhea, and constipation; these are the most frequent manifestations of left-sided lesions. Right-sided tumors often cause weakness, malaise, and weight loss. Pain is rare with either

**TABLE 41-4.**

RECOMMENDATIONS FOR LOWERING THE RISK OF COLON AND RECTAL CANCER

| ACTION | MECHANISMS |
|---|---|
| 1. Regular exercise | Increase intestinal motility |
| 2. Lower total fat intake (20%–25% of calories) | Lower total bile acid and fatty acid flux with promoting and cytotoxic actions |
| 3. Increase proportion of monounsaturated fats (olive oil, special rapeseed oils) | Lower total bile acid flux |
| 4. Increase intake of fish and fish oils | Protective effect of omega-3 fatty acids (prostaglandin synthetases and metabolism) |
| 5. Have optimal intake of bran cereals, whole grain bread, unrefined rice | Avoids constipation, nonneoplastic intestinal diseases antecedent to neoplasia. Optimal amount gives daily stool of about 200 g |
| 6. Have optimal intake of yellow-green and brassica vegetables (cauliflower, Brussels sprouts, broccoli) | Specific mechanisms not clear; provides micronutrients and bulk, replacing harmful, more energy-dense foods |
| 7. Have optimal intake of calcium-rich foods (some vegetables, but especially low- or nonfat yogurt or milk) | Controls intestinal cell duplication rates |
| 8. Avoid excessive intake of alcoholic beverages | Lower cell turnover rates in rectum |
| 9. Lower intake of highly fried or broiled, browned foods | Possible lower intake of intestine-specific carcinogens |

(Source: R.R. Frentzel-Beyme, Colorectal Cancer. Berlin: Springer–Verlag, 1989.)

type and, if present, may result from contractions of the bowel related to partial obstruction of the colon or nerve involvement. The tumor mass is often palpated on physical examination. Obstruction of the bowel may be the first sign of the disease. At the time of diagnosis, some extension of the tumor often has occurred, but because this malignancy grows slowly, it is considered to be highly curable with early diagnosis and surgical treatment.

Diagnosis requires the standard techniques of proctoscopy, barium enema, radionucleotide scanning, and determination of levels of tumor antigens. Colon cancers produce a wide variety of tumor antigens, the carcinoembryonic antigen (CEA) being the most well known. The test for CEA is positive in nearly all cases with widespread metastases. The usefulness of the CEA test is being evaluated because normal levels do not rule out malignancy; however, it can gauge the effectiveness of therapy. "Normal" levels of CEA are less than 2.5 ng/mL, but they may be elevated in nonmalignant inflammatory disease, especially of the gastrointestinal tract.[20]

Prognosis with colorectal carcinoma depends on the extent of bowel involvement, the presence or absence of spread, differentiation of the lesion, and the location of the lesion within the colon. It is frequently staged by the TNM (tumor, node, metastasis) system as follows:[2]

TIS: Carcinoma *in situ*

$T_1$: No involvement of the muscle wall, may be polypoid or papillary

$T_2$: Involvement of the muscle wall

$T_3$: All layers of wall involved with extension to adjacent structures

$T_4$: Same as $T_3$ with evidence of fistulas

$T_5$: Tumor spread beyond the immediate adjacent area

N: Number of lymphatic nodes involved

M: Evidence of metastasis

## REFERENCES

1. *Cancer Facts and Figures, 1990.* New York: American Cancer Society, 1989.

2. Cotran, R.S., Kumar, V., and Robbins, S.L. *Robbins' Pathologic Basis of disease* (4th ed.). Philadelphia: W.B. Saunders, 1989.

3. Fenoglio-Preiser, C.M., Lantz, P.E., Listrom, M.B., Davis, M., and Rilke, F.O. *Gastrointestinal Pathology: An Atlas and Text.* New York: Raven Press, 1989.

4. Friedman, L.S. and Isselbacher, K.J. Anorexia, nausea and vomiting. In J.D. Wilson et al. (eds.), *Harrison's Principles of Internal Medicine* (12th ed.). New York: McGraw-Hill, 1991.

5. Frentzel-Beyme, R.R. Acquired conditions of increased risk of colorectal cancer. In H.K. Seitz, U.A. Simanowski, and

N.A. Wright, *Colorectal Cancer: From Pathogenesis to Prevention*. Berlin: Springer-Verlag, 1989.

6. Glickman, R.M. Inflammatory bowel disease. In J.D. Wilson et al. (eds.), *Harrison's Principles of Internal Medicine* (12th ed.). New York: McGraw-Hill, 1991.

7. Gottlieb, J.E., Menashe, P.I., and Cruz, E. Gastrointestinal complications in critically ill patients. *Am. J. Gastroenterology* 81:4, 1986.

8. Greenberger, N.J. *Gastrointestinal Disorders: A Pathophysiologic Approach* (3rd ed.). Chicago: Yearbook, 1986.

9. Grozmann, I. Portal hypertension. In I.M. Arias, W.B. Jacoby, A. Popper, D. Schachter, and D.A. Shafritz, *The Liver: Biology and Pathobiology* (2nd ed.). New York: Raven Press, 1988.

10. Hamilton, S.R. Diseases of the esophagus. In H. Goldman, H.D. Appelman, and W. Kaufman, *Gastrointestinal Pathology*. Baltimore: Williams & Wilkins, 1988.

11. Kissane, J.M. *Anderson's Pathology* (9th ed.). St. Louis: Mosby, 1991.

12. LaMont, J.T., and Isselbacher, K.J. Disease of the small and large intestine. In J.D. Wilson et al. (eds.), *Harrison's Principles of Internal Medicine* (12th ed.). New York: McGraw-Hill, 1991.

13. Livingston, E.H., and Passaro, E.P. Postoperative ileus. *Digestive Diseases and Sciences* 35(1):121–132, 1990.

14. Metheny, N. *Fluid and Electrolyte Balance*. Philadelphia: J.B. Lippincott, 1987.

15. Morson, B.C., Dawson, I.M., Day, D.W., Jass, J.R., Price, A.B., and Williams, G.T. *Morson and Dawson's Gastrointestinal Pathology*. Oxford: Blackwell, 1990.

16. Shearman, D.J., and Finlayson, N.D. *Diseases of the Gastrointestinal Tract and Liver*. Edinburgh: Churchill-Livingstone, 1989.

17. Sodeman, W.A., and Watson, D.W. The large intestine. In W.A. Sodeman and T.M. Sodeman, *Sodeman's Pathologic Physiology* (7th ed.). Philadelphia: W.B. Saunders, 1985.

18. Spiro, H.M. *Clinical Gastroenterology* (3rd ed.). New York: Macmillan, 1985.

19. Wallace, J.L. Lipid mediators of inflammation in gastric ulcer. *Am. J. Physiol.* 11:G1-G9, 1990.

20. Wallach, J. *Interpretation of Diagnostic Tests* (4th ed.). Boston: Little, Brown, 1986.

21. Watson, D.W., and Sodeman, W.A. The small intestine. In W.A. Sodeman and T.M. Sodeman, *Sodeman's Pathologic Physiology* (7th ed.). Philadelphia: W.B. Saunders, 1985.

22. Yardley, J.H. Gastritis. In H. Goldman, H.D. Appelman, and N. Kaufman, *Gastrointestinal Pathology*. Baltimore: Williams & Wilkins, 1988.

# Normal Hepatobiliary and Pancreatic Exocrine Function

## Chapter Outline

## Learning Objectives

1. Locate the anatomic structures vital to the function of the liver lobule.
2. Describe the structure of the liver sinusoids.
3. Identify the cells of the mononuclear phagocyte system in the sinusoids of the liver.
4. Explain the purpose of the dual blood supply to the liver.
5. Describe the role of the liver in protein synthesis and metabolism.
6. Review the relationship of albumin to the colloid osmotic pressure.
7. Identify the factors necessary for capillary fluid dynamics.
8. State the relationship of protein, ammonia, and urea in the liver.
9. Describe the functions of the plasma proteins produced by the liver.
10. Explain why the lymphatic system is important in plasma protein absorption.
11. Outline the role of the liver in fat synthesis and metabolism.
12. Describe how the liver functions in carbohydrate metabolism.
13. Define *proteolysis, deamination*, and *transamination*.
14. Describe the oxidative and conjugative reactions that affect drug and hormone metabolism.
15. Explain specifically the effect of alcohol on liver function.
16. Define *hepatotoxin*.
17. Describe the process for the conjugation of bilirubin.
18. List and briefly describe the activities of each of the components of bile.
19. List and describe the major liver function tests.
20. Differentiate briefly between the constituents of liver and gallbladder bile.
21. Describe the hormonal and nervous factors that cause the emptying of the gallbladder.
22. Differentiate between endocrine and exocrine secretions of the pancreas.
23. Delineate specifically the actions of the major enzymes in pancreatic secretions.

Knowledge of the anatomic and functional activities of the liver is essential to an understanding of the alterations of the liver in pathologic states. Liver function involves the secretion of bile and the formation of many essential substances. The effects of these activities on all the metabolic processes of other organs are crucial to maintaining a steady balance in the body. Basic reviews of liver anatomy and physiology and the accessory functions of the gallbladder and pancreas are included in this chapter. The reader is referred to the comprehensive materials listed in the unit bibliography for additional information.

## ANATOMY OF THE LIVER

The liver is a large, glandular organ weighing approximately 1.5 kg in the adult. It is composed of two major divisions, the right and left lobes. The right lobe contains two lobes called the *quadrate* and *caudate* lobes. The many units within the lobes that perform the functions of the liver are called the *lobules*. The structure of the liver and the blood flow through the lobules are illustrated in Figure 42-1. An admixture of venous and arterial blood is carried into the *sinusoids*, which are the capillaries of the liver. These provide both oxygen and nutrients to the liver.

The lobules process many substances in the *hepatocytes*, the parenchymal cells of the liver. The venous blood supply, carried by a branch of the portal vein, moves highly concentrated foodstuffs, including fats, carbohydrates, and proteins that have been absorbed from the small intestine. The arterial blood supply contains high concentrations of oxygen. The lobules are composed of sinusoids, rows of cuboidal hepatocytes, bile capillaries, and branches of the hepatic artery and portal vein (Figure 42-2). The sinusoids and surrounding hepatocytes provide a processing plant for the raw materials delivered to the liver from the small intestine.

The sinusoids are lined with cells of the mononuclear phagocyte system, which are called *Kupffer cells*. These cells trap foreign material and function mainly in phagocytosis. The porous endothelial lining allows plasma proteins to pass from the sinusoid to a narrow space around the hepatocyte, which is called the *space of Disse*.[11] This space connects with the lymphatic system and allows drainage of plasma proteins and excess fluid.

Within the liver lobules are *canaliculi*, the receptacles for bile produced by the hepatocytes. A meshwork of bile ducts forms from the canaliculi and terminates eventually in the common bile duct, which empties into the duodenum during digestion. The gallbladder receives bile from the liver and then stores, concentrates, and releases it into the common bile duct under appropriate stimulation (see p. 817).

Blood is supplied to the liver through divisions of the hepatic artery and portal vein, which pass through the complex sinusoidal network to form venules and veins. These terminate in the hepatic vein, which empties into the inferior vena cava (see Figure 42-1). The physiologic tasks that must be performed by the liver require access to a large quantity of the circulation. About 30% of cardiac output flows through the liver each minute, making this organ a large reservoir for blood. Even with its large volume and flow, the pressure in the portal system remains low. The liver can distend and increase its volume by a great margin before portal pressure increases.[1]

## PHYSIOLOGY OF THE LIVER

### General Information

The liver performs a wide variety of vital, life-sustaining functions. The hepatocyte is responsible for maintaining these functions through its numerous organelles. It is important in the synthesis and metabolism of protein, carbohydrates, and fats, and also performs the essential function of phagocytosis, which occurs constantly while blood passes through the liver. Many foreign substances, such as pharmacologic agents, are biotransformed as they pass through the liver. The production and excretion of bile, together with the processing of bilirubin into a form that can be excreted, are essential liver functions. Enzymes necessary to carry out many activities are also synthesized by the liver. Many hormones are biotransformed or inactivated by the liver, which also stores many vitamins and minerals. The major functions of the liver are discussed in the following section.

### Protein Synthesis and Metabolism

*Proteins* are nitrogen-containing constituents of all cells and tissues in the body and are present in all body fluids except bile and urine. Proteins are essential to the formation of the cell, as well as to synthesis of enzymes, hormones, immunoglobulins, and blood cells. All proteins are in a state of constant turnover, making the task of maintaining body functions an awesome one.

The primary function of protein metabolism is to synthesize proteins. Unlike fats and carbohydrates, proteins are not stored, and the size of the amino acid pool is the result of the actual turnover of body proteins and amino acids from exogenous or dietary sources. Protein synthesis depends on the availability of amino acids in the pool at any given time. The ratio of available amino acids is of extreme importance because every protein is made up of specific amino acids in absolute sequences. If one of these amino acids is absent, synthesis of a specific protein is not possible.

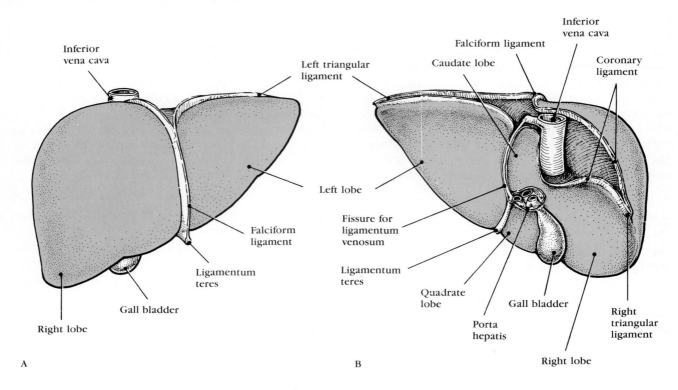

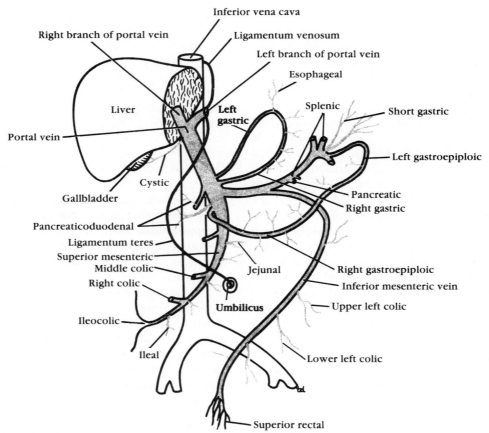

**FIGURE 42–1.**

Macroscopic appearance of the liver. (**A.**) Lobes of the liver. (**B.**) Posterior surface showing gallbladder and inferior vena cava. (**C.**) Blood flow to the liver from the portal vein. (Source: R.S. Snell, *Clinical Anatomy for Medical Students* [2nd ed.]. Boston: Little, Brown, 1981.)

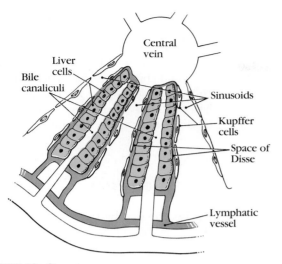

**FIGURE 42–2.**
Liver lobule showing Kupffer cells and the space of Disse through which lymphatic material can flow.

## Synthesis of Amino Acids

Of the many amino acids that make up human proteins, 10 cannot be synthesized in adequate amounts to meet the body's metabolic needs. These have been termed *essential amino acids (EAAs)* and are available through dietary intake. The EAAs are not all required in the same amounts but in a ratio, so that foods containing proteins with the correct proportion of EAAs have a high biologic value. Egg albumin is considered to have a nearly perfect mixture; therefore, all other proteins are compared to that mixture. If one EAA is lacking in the diet, a negative nitrogen balance results. That is, when one or more essential amino acids are missing from the diet, nitrogen excretion exceeds nitrogen intake. The result is the same as if the total protein intake were inadequate. Loss of body protein occurs and usually is manifested as muscle wasting.[13]

The liver takes up amino acids from the nutrient-rich portal blood and converts them to various proteins. The amino acids are relatively strong acids. They rarely accumulate in the bloodstream because of protein synthesis and because they are excreted by the kidneys. Most amino acids are actively transported through the cell membranes and then converted into cellular proteins, a transformation that requires an enzymatic reaction. These cellular proteins can be broken down rapidly to form amino acids that can be transported out of the cells to the bloodstream.[1] The amount of amino acids in blood remains fairly constant, but may vary slightly with diet and the individual person. After the cells have reached their capacity for storing proteins, the excess amino acids can be degraded and used as energy, or changed into fat or glycogen and stored.[7]

## Amino Acid (AA) Metabolism

The liver is the major site of amino acid metabolism, and the process–called *deamination of amino acids*–results in the formation of ammonia. Deamination of AAs is required before they can be used for energy or for conversion to fats or carbohydrates.[7] Large amounts of ammonia are formed from amino acids and from bacterial action in the large bowel. The liver normally removes 80% of ammonia as blood passes through the portal system.[12] The liver then converts the ammonia to urea, which is more readily excreted by the kidneys than is ammonia. The conversion of ammonia to urea is an important mechanism of the liver and results in biotransformation and removal of ammonia from the body. Nearly all urea is produced in the liver; this substance is much less toxic to the central nervous system than is ammonia.

## Plasma Proteins

The *plasma proteins* are large molecules that circulate for the most part in the bloodstream and are mainly synthesized by the liver. All of the albumin, the most abundant plasma protein, is made in the liver. It serves many bodily functions, including binding many substances such as bilirubin and barbiturates in the plasma. Albumin is the principal protein necessary for maintaining colloid osmotic pressure (COP) (see Chap. 8). It also binds hydrogen ions and alters serum pH.

When the amino acid levels in blood are decreased, the plasma proteins are split to make new amino acids. Equilibrium is thus maintained between plasma proteins and amino acids. Decreased levels of amino acids stimulate the liver to increase its production of plasma proteins. It is estimated that approximately 400 g of protein is synthesized daily.[7] Significant liver damage leads to hypoproteinemia, which markedly disrupts COP and amino acid levels. The concentration of plasma proteins normally remains at a constant ratio, with more albumin in plasma than globulin. The globulins compose about 15% of plasma proteins and are the protein group to which antibodies produced by B lymphocytes belong (see Chap. 14).[7]

The liver also synthesizes the majority of the plasma proteins necessary to coagulate blood. Of these, prothrombin and fibrinogen are the most abundant; however, all the proteins of coagulation are important (see Chap. 21). For prothrombin formation, the liver uses vitamin K, the absorption of which depends on the production of bile. Fibrinogen is a large-molecule protein formed entirely by the liver and is in the cascade of coagulation.

All of the plasma proteins participate in the production of the colloid osmotic pressure throughout the capillaries of the body. The *plasma colloid osmotic pressure (PCOP)* retains or pulls fluid into the intravascular area.

Because the plasma proteins are too large to cross the capillary membrane, they remain in increased concentrations at the capillary line and produce an osmotic pressure or pull. This has been described as an inward pressure or force. The level of the PCOP remains constant at the arteriolar, capillary, and venular sections of the capillary, and provides the major force encouraging fluid to return to the capillary and the intravascular area.

Plasma proteins are not easily lost in interstitial spaces because of their size. When leaked into the interstitial area, the only route for return to the bloodstream is through the profuse lymphatic drainage in the interstitial compartment. The lymphatic vessels empty into the lymphatic and thoracic ducts, which empty directly into the superior vena cava.

## Fat or Lipid Metabolism

The liver forms almost all of the lipoproteins, which contain mixtures of triglycerides, phospholipids, and cholesterol, as well as protein. These are in the form of *high-density lipoproteins (HDL), low density lipoproteins (LDL),* and *very low-density lipoproteins (VLDL),* which are discussed below. Cholesterol is used to form bile salts, which are important in the absorption of fats in the small intestine. Cholesterol is also used to form steroid hormones.

Ninety-five percent of the fat ingested daily in the American diet is in the form of triglycerides, which contain both saturated and unsaturated fatty acids. The liver can convert carbohydrates or proteins to fat. Insulin promotes the movement of glucose into the cell and conversion to fat storage molecules occurs if the glucose is not used for energy.

### Lipid Transport

Knowledge of how lipids are transported and of the significance of lipoprotein types enhances the understanding of fat deposits in the body. The largest source of lipids is dietary fats. These are carried in the forms of chylomicrons, VLDLs, remnants of cholestryl esters and triglycerides, low-density lipoproteins (LDLs), and HDLs. The VLDLs interact with the lipoprotein lipase enzyme, which contributes to the formation of LDLs and eventually establishes a cycle by which LDLs deliver cholesterol to extrahepatic cells. The VLDLs are produced when the liver converts excess carbohydrate to fatty acids and, through another conversion process, forms triglycerides that are the core of the VLDLs. The LDL is the form of most of the total cholesterol of the plasma. This is important in the pathway for the synthesis of steroid hormones as well as in supplying cholesterol to other cells of the body. The HDLs pick up cholesterol, which then reacts with a plasma enzyme, leading again to the formation of LDLs (Figure 42-3).

In the obese person, when an excess of carbohydrate, fat, or protein reaches the cells, it can be converted to energy, fat stores, and cholesterol. Fat is broken down to acetate, which, when not needed for energy, is metabolized into fat or adipose stores. Energy production for the most part requires oxygen, whereas synthesis of fat does not.

## Carbohydrate Metabolism

Carbohydrate may be released by the liver in its usable form, glucose, after it has been stored in the form of glycogen. About 5% to 7% of normal liver weight is stored glycogen. When blood glucose increases above normal, glycogenesis is stimulated. *Glycogenesis* is the formation of glycogen from carbohydrate sources, especially glucose. Conversely, when the blood sugar level falls below normal, glycogenolysis is stimulated. *Glycogenolysis* is the breakdown of glycogen into glucose.

The liver maintains normal blood glucose levels. After a high-carbohydrate meal, an increased amount of carbohydrate is delivered to the liver, where it is stored and released when the blood glucose begins to drop. The pancreatic hormone glucagon is very important in initiating the release of glucose by the liver.

In the process called *gluconeogenesis,* the liver synthesizes glucose from noncarbohydrate substances, especially proteins. Glucose needs that cannot be met from glycogen stores or exogenous sources must be met through this process. This process is critically important for cells that cannot use fat for metabolism—the blood cells and the cells of the kidney medulla. The cells of the central nervous system use glucose preferentially but can adapt to fatty acid oxidation in the form of ketones in 2 to 4 days. During fasting, such as between meals and during sleep, the carbon skeleton of amino acids is converted to glucose for energy.

## Phagocytosis

The sinusoids of the liver are lined with Kupffer cells, which pick up and destroy foreign material circulating through the liver. The portal vein, which circulates the venous blood from the intestine to the liver, carries a higher concentration of toxins and bacteria than other venous blood because these substances are absorbed when nutrients are absorbed from the intestine. The Kupffer cells are highly phagocytic and can remove 99% of bacteria in portal venous blood.[7]

If the level of bacteria or foreign material in the sinusoids increases, the Kupffer cells become active, proliferate, and destroy the foreign material. This activity is

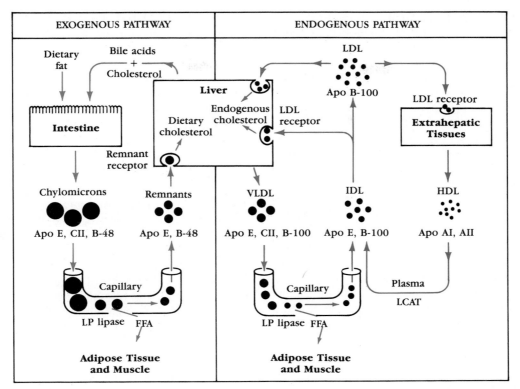

**FIGURE 42-3.**
Model for plasma triglyceride and cholesterol transport in humans. VLDL = very low-density lipoprotein; IDL = intermediate-density lipoprotein; LDL = low-density lipoprotein; HDL = high-density lipoprotein; and LCAT = lecithin cholesterol acyltransferase (catalyzes reaction). (Source: E. Braunwald, et al. *Harrisons' Principles of Internal Medicine* [11th ed.]. New York: McGraw-Hill, 1987.)

crucial to preventing the spread of pathogens to the systemic circulation.

## *Biotransformation of Foreign Substances*

Destruction, biotransformation, and inactivation of foreign substances are carried out in the hepatocytes, and substances are changed to acceptable forms for excretion. Many of the endocrine secretions are inactivated in the liver, and many pharmacologic agents are biotransformed there. Some substances are conjugated in the same way as bilirubin, with glucuronic acid, whereas others may be inactivated by proteolysis, deamination, or oxidation. *Proteolysis* refers to the breakdown of proteins into simpler substances. *Deamination* means the removal of amino acids and may involve transamination or transfer of this group to another acceptor substance. Oxidative deamination causes the release of the amino radical.[5,8]

The oxidative and conjugative reactions promote the biodegradation or excretion of foreign substances. It has been found that many drugs affect the reactions of other drugs or hormones. These interactions, whether they involve speeding up or slowing down the reactions, occur in hepatocytes. An example is the metabolism of warfarin (Coumadin), the effects of which can be potentiated by aspirin. Phenobarbital increases the activity of drug-metabolizing enzymes and hastens the inactivation of warfarin and other agents. Many endogenous hormones, especially corticosterone and aldosterone, are inactivated and conjugated for excretion by the liver. Estrogens impair the secretory activity of the hepatocytes and may alter the results of liver function tests.

Acute alcohol intoxication inhibits drug metabolism by the liver. The chronic alcoholic, however, metabolizes drugs quickly and has an increased tolerance to them, unless there is associated liver failure, which appears to cause decreased drug tolerance. Many drug interactions with alcohol vary according to whether the person is acutely intoxicated or sober. Acute intoxication often significantly potentiates the activity of central nervous system depressants, antihypertensives, antidiabetics, anticoagulants, and antiinflammatory agents.[10]

Substances that are directly toxic to liver cells are called *hepatotoxins*. One drug that is a known hepatotoxin in excessive dosages is acetaminophen (Tylenol), which causes centrilobular necrosis due to the exhaustion of the glutathione to which it is normally conjugated.

If a glutathione precursor is given in response to an overdose, the liver will be protected from permanent injury. If no treatment is given, the rate of liver failure after overdose is very high and often fatal.

Most liver damage resulting from foreign substances is due to hypersensitivity reactions by hepatic cells after exposure to drugs. Some drugs cause jaundice; a notable example is chlorpromazine, which causes cholestasis within the liver. Several other drugs can cause parenchymal necrosis; isoniazid (INH) and halothane anesthetic are typical examples.[10]

## Bile Synthesis

Bile is formed by the liver and stored and concentrated by the gallbladder. The liver secretes 250 to 1500 mL of bile per day.[1] The hepatocytes make bile, which is a liquid material normally composed of bilirubin, plasma electrolytes, water, bile salts, bicarbonate, cholesterol, fatty acids, and lecithin.

### Bilirubin

Bilirubin is a waste product that is excreted from the body only in the form of conjugated bilirubin. Most bilirubin is released in the breakdown of red blood cells. The red blood cell gives off hemoglobin, which further breaks into its component parts, heme and globin. The globin portion is a protein that probably returns to the intracellular amino acid pool. The heme portion is broken down further into bilirubin and iron. The iron is either stored in the form of ferritin or used to produce new hemoglobin. Except for the iron in the hemoglobin, most iron in the body is stored by the liver in the form of ferritin. When iron is released from the heme of the red blood cell, it combines with apoferritin, a protein synthesized by the liver, and becomes ferritin or storage iron.[7]

Bilirubin undergoes several reactions and ends up being bound to albumin, on which it travels to the liver. It is called *unconjugated, fat-soluble*, or *indirect bilirubin* because it cannot be excreted in bile or through the kidneys. In the liver it is converted on the smooth endoplasmic reticulum to a water-soluble form when it combines with *glucuronic acid* through the intervention of the enzyme *glucuronyl transferase*.[8] In this water-soluble or conjugated form it can be secreted into bile and excreted by the intestine or, in special circumstances, by the kidneys. In the intestine, the intestinal bacteria change the excreted bilirubin to *urobilinogen*. Some of this material is resorbed and reexcreted by the liver. Most of the bilirubin is converted to *stercobilinogen*, which is oxidized to *stercobilin* before being excreted in the feces.[7] Stercobilin and other bile pigments impart the brown color to the feces. Figure 42-4 outlines the process of hemoglobin breakdown and the resulting fate of bilirubin.

In summary, bilirubin must be converted to a conjugated, water-soluble form to cross the cell membrane of the hepatocytes and be excreted in bile. In bile duct obstruction, conjugated bilirubin can cross the membrane of the glomeruli and be excreted by the kidneys. Excess bilirubin in the blood leads to the condition called *jaundice* (see Chap. 43).

### Bile Salts

The bile salts function as detergents and break fat particles into smaller sizes. They aid in making fat more soluble by forming special complexes called *micelles*, which are soluble in the intestinal mucosa. Bile salts are formed by the liver with cholesterol precursors; large amounts can be formed and secreted during periods of increased need. The bile salts are also essential for the absorption of the fat-soluble vitamins A, D, E, and K.

### Other Components of Bile

The electrolytes in bile are to some extent reabsorbed through the gallbladder mucosa because of the concentrating process that occurs in that organ. Substances that are not absorbed become highly concentrated in the gallbladder bile. For example, liver bile contains about 0.04 g/dL of bilirubin, whereas gallbladder bile contains about 0.3 g/dL. Much of the water in bile is absorbed through the gallbladder mucosa. Reabsorption of water, electrolytes, and free cholesterol in the secreted bile occurs in the small intestine. Cholesterol is excreted through the formation of bile salts and directly in the bile. Imbalance can cause excessive cholesterol in bile and may predispose a person to gallstone formation (see Chap. 43).

## MAJOR LIVER FUNCTION TESTS

The major liver function tests provide an index of hepatic function and are helpful in establishing a differential diagnosis in intrahepatic and extrahepatic pathology. The tests discussed below are summarized in Table 42-1.

### Serum Enzymes

*Alkaline phosphatase* of the serum is an enzyme that is produced in the liver, kidneys, bone, and other areas, and is excreted in bile. Serum levels are elevated in conditions that increase calcium deposits in bone–viral hepatitis, obstructive jaundice, malignancies, and many other conditions. Serum levels may be decreased in hypopara-

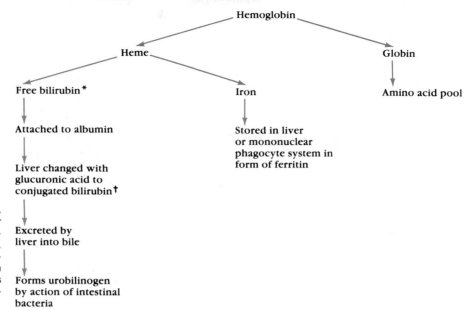

**FIGURE 42–4.**
Fate of hemoglobin. Free unconjugated, indirect bilirubin persists until the liver changes its form. This bilirubin is lipid soluble, water insoluble, and nonexcretable (*). Conjugated, direct or bilirubin glucuronide is the form after conjugation with glucuronic acid. Conjugated bilirubin is water soluble, fat insoluble, and excretable (†).

thyroidism, pernicious anemia, hypothyroidism, and a few other conditions.

*Serum glutamic oxaloacetic transaminase (SGOT)*, also called *aspartate aminotransferase (AST)*, is an enzyme that is produced and concentrated in skeletal muscle, cardiac muscle, and liver. It catalyzes certain deamination processes. The AST-SGOT level is increased in acute myocardial infarction, liver disease, muscular diseases, pancreatitis, and other conditions.

*Serum glutamic pyruvic transaminase (SGPT)*, also called *alanine aminotransferase (ALT)*, is present in high concentrations in the liver and to a lesser extent, the heart and skeletal muscle. Levels increase with all types of hepatic injury.

*Lactic dehydrogenase (LDH)* is present in large quantities in liver tissue. Its level is elevated significantly in liver damage and also with cardiac and muscular damage. The level is increased with pulmonary embolus, certain malignancies, pernicious anemia, and others. The LDH isoenzymes are isolated into concentrations of isoenzymes 1 through 5; specific isoenzymes are concentrated in different organs. Isoenzyme LDH-5 is the most specific to liver disease, expecially hepatitis.

*γ-glutamyltranspeptidase (GGT)* is present throughout the hepatobiliary system and is a sensitive indicator of biliary tract disease. Its levels correlate with alkaline phosphatase levels and elevations are nonspecific.[9]

## Bilirubin

Bilirubin is measured as a total value and in its conjugated and unconjugated fractions. These evaluations measure the ability of the liver to conjugate and excrete bilirubin in the intestine. A high level of unconjugated bilirubin with a normal or high level of conjugated bilirubin usually indicates significant intrahepatic cellular damage, but this may also occur with hemolytic jaundice. An increase in conjugated bilirubin and a normal or slight increase in unconjugated bilirubin level, especially in the presence of dark urine and light stools, are almost conclusive evidence of biliary obstruction.

## Plasma Proteins

*Albumin*, the most abundant plasma protein, maintains the PCOP, synthesizes specific amino acids, and binds certain molecules for transport from area to another. Albumin levels are evaluated by a process called *electrophoresis*. Decreased serum albumin, or hypoalbuminemia, results from severe hepatocellular dysfunction. The result of hypoalbuminemia is alteration of COP, leading to systemic edema.

*Fibrinogen* levels are important in determining the potential for normal blood coagulation. Depletion of this protein occurs in *disseminated intravascular coagulation* with precipitation of fibrin in the small vessels and rapid depletion of the clotting factors (see Chap. 21). Deficiency also is noted in conditions that can cause fibrinolysis, such as hemorrhage, burns, poisoning, and cirrhosis.

The *globulins* are important in the production of antibodies (see Chap. 14). They also act with albumin to maintain intravascular colloid osmotic pressure. Alterations of globulin levels occur with immunosuppression and with chronic inflammations. Elevation or suppres-

**TABLE 42–1.**
MAJOR LIVER FUNCTION TESTS

| TEST | NORMAL LEVEL | ABNORMALITIES[a] |
|---|---|---|
| Alkaline phosphatase | 2–5 BU/mL | I Biliary obstruction<br>I Early drug toxicity<br>I Cholestatic hepatitis<br>I Extrahepatic inflammatory condition |
| Aspartate amino transferase (AST) (formerly called SGOT) | 5–40 U/mL | I Acute myocardial infarction<br>I Liver damage and most liver disease<br>I Muscle, pancreas, brain, lung, bowel damage<br>D Some severe liver disease<br>D Diabetic ketoacidosis |
| Alanine amino transferase (ALT) (formerly called SGPT) | 5–35 U/mL | I Markedly in liver necrosis and acute hepatitis<br>I Slightly in myocardial infarction<br>I Pulmonary, renal, pancreatic injury<br>I Slightly in cirrhosis and chronic liver disease |
| Lactic dehydrogenase (LDH) | 200–680 U/mL | I Cardiac injury<br>I Hepatitis, especially LDH isoenzyme 5<br>I Malignant tumors<br>I Muscle, pulmonary, and renal disease |
| Bilirubin<br>  Total<br>    Direct<br>    Indirect | <br>0.2–0.9 mg/dL<br>0.1–0.4 mg/dL<br>0.1–0.5 mg/dL | <br>I Hepatocellular necrosis or damage<br>I Cholestasis due to obstruction<br>I Hemolytic anemia |
| Serum Ammonia | 80–110 ug/dL | I Liver failure |
| Plasma proteins<br>  Total<br>    Albumin<br>    Globulin | <br>6–8 g/dL<br>3.5–5.5 g/dL<br>1.5–3.0 g/dL | <br>D Severe liver disease<br>D Pyelonephritis and nephrosis<br>D Malnutrition and protein lack<br>D Chronic inflammation |
| Fibrinogen | 0.2–0.4 g/dL | D Disseminated intravascular coagulation<br>D Congenital afibrinogenemia<br>D With depletion of other coagulation factors<br>D With major alteration of hemodynamics in body (eg, circulatory shock) |
| Prothrombin time | 11–16 seconds (control); 80%–100% of control | I (Prolonged) severe liver disease, especially cirrhosis<br>I Fibrinogen deficiency<br>I Warfarin therapy<br>I Biliary destruction |
| Partial thromboplastin time | 22–37 seconds | I (Prolonged) in bleeding disorders, especially of the intrinsic pathway<br>I Heparin therapy<br>I Cirrhosis and severe liver disease |
| Urine bilirubin | Absent/24 degrees | I Biliary obstruction<br>I Cirrhosis<br>I Hepatitis |
| Urine urobilinogen | 0–4 mg/24 degrees | D Biliary obstruction<br>I Hemolysis<br>Normal or cirrhosis |
| Bromsulphalein (BSP) excretion | 5% retention after 45 min | I Fever<br>I All types liver disease<br>I Specific drugs (eg, morphine)<br>I Acute cholecystitis<br>I GI bleeding |
| Liver scans<br>  Colloidal | <br>Uptake of colloid by Kupffer cells | <br>Demonstrates large defects; false negative result with small defects |
|   Rose bengal | Uptake of dye by hepatocytes | Area of reduced intake, "hole" in neoplastic or inflammatory cells |
|   Gallium | Little uptake of dye by normal cells | Uptake by neoplastic and inflammatory cells |
| Liver biopsy | Normal hepatocytes | Specific pathology of any material sampled; diagnostic of cirrhosis, malignancy, hepatitis, and so forth |
| Computed tomography | Normal integrity on image of intraabdominal organs | Fluid collections in liver differentiated from tumors; gallbladder or duct enlargement seen |

[a] I = test results are increased in these conditions; D = test results are decreased in these conditions.

sion of globulin levels is not a specific sign of liver disease.

Another protein that is measured in liver function screening is *prothrombin*. The prothrombin time (PT) reflects the presence of prothrombin, fibrinogen, and other factors. A prolonged PT indicates a deficiency of prothrombin and the other clotting factors or impaired uptake of vitamin K. The test measures the factors of the extrinsic system and the common pathway of both extrinsic and intrinsic systems (see Chap. 21). The *partial thromboplastin time (PTT)* measures factors concerned in the intrinsic clotting pathway and the common pathway, and is a good screening test for bleeding disorders. The other clotting factors can be separately measured, and their levels may be altered in liver dysfunction.

## Urine Urobilinogen

Small amounts of bilirubin are usually excreted in the urine in the form of urobilinogen. Conjugated bilirubin may be present in urine when an excessive amount is not being cleared from the plasma. This finding is common in obstructive biliary tract disease and severe cirrhosis of the liver (see Chap. 43).

## Bromsulphalein Excretion

This test measures the ability of the liver to remove a dye from the circulation. Liver injury is probable when more than 10% of injected dye remains in circulation after 45 minutes.

## Liver Scanning (Scintiscans)

Scans are performed to determine the position, shape, size, and structure of the liver. They involve injecting radiopharmaceutical isotopes, which are taken up by hepatocytes, Kupffer cells, or neoplasms. Several scanning procedures are used, with some isotopes concentrating in neoplasms or in areas of inflammation, and others concentrating in the hepatocytes. Areas of abscess or tumor produce a void in the scan.

When reading the liver scan, one looks for areas of increased or no uptake, depending on the isotope used. Agents that are excreted in the bile can be followed for bile duct obstruction, whereas those having affinity for mononuclear phagocytes are concentrated in the spleen. Changes in the liver scan can also assist in following the course of cirrhosis. Persons with early hepatomegaly have even distribution of the radiopharmaceutical agent. As the disease progresses, the left lobe of the liver enlarges, the right lobe becomes smaller, and the spleen

takes up increased amounts. As liver failure progresses there may be a spotty appearance due to the fibrosis dividing the lobules.

## Liver Biopsy

Liver biopsy is performed to make a precise diagnosis of liver disease. It can be beneficial in the diagnosis of hepatitis, cirrhosis, and, sometimes, primary neoplasms. It may be performed as open biopsy during a surgical procedure or as a needle biopsy using a percutaneous intercostal approach. In the latter, the material aspirated from the needle is examined histologically for abnormalities. Accurate placement of the needle is imperative for precise diagnosis. Care must be exerted to prevent laceration of the liver and consequent hemorrhage.

## Computed Tomography

The computed tomography (CT) scan is a popular procedure because it provides a radiologic image of the abdominal organs without the need to inject dyes or isotopes. In the initial evaluation of liver disease, CT scans help to differentiate fluid-filled from tumor-filled lesions. The appearance of the surrounding organs and ducts can also be assessed. It is a sensitive scan for determining metastases of primary malignancies, but less so for fluid-filled bile ducts.[8]

## THE GALLBLADDER

The *gallbladder* is a saclike organ that is attached to the inferior portion of the liver. It receives bile from the liver that has been diverted from the common bile duct (Figure 42-5). The liver secretes about 700 mL of bile each day. It flows continuously through the bile duct to the intestine. This flow, called *choleresis*, is increased after meals.[2] The gallbladder's maximum volume is 40 to 70 mL, but its bile is 5 to 10 times more concentrated than that of the liver. Approximately 90% of the water content of gallbladder bile is continually absorbed by the mucosa. Its electrolyte composition includes an increased concentration of potassium and calcium and a decreased amount of chloride and bicarbonate as compared to liver bile.[5,7] The gallbladder is composed of folds and rugae and can increase its size to accommodate incoming bile.

The gallbladder empties its bile into the common bile duct when a stimulus is received. The major stimulus for this is *cholecystokinin (CCK)*, a hormone secreted from the duodenal mucosa when fat-containing foods arrive in that area. The CCK causes bile to move into the

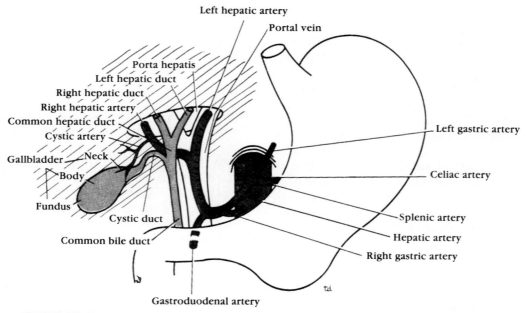

**FIGURE 42–5.**
Appearance and location of gallbladder. (Source: R.S. Snell, *Clinical Anatomy for Medical Students* [2nd ed.]. Boston: Little, Brown, 1981.)

intestine by causing contractions of the gallbladder and relaxation of the sphincter of Oddi.[2] The gallbladder also receives stimulation from the autonomic nervous system. The parasympathetic division is the major mediator for contraction of the gallbladder, whereas stimulation of the sympathetic division causes relaxation of the organ.

Alterations in function of the gallbladder are discussed in Chapter 43. Gallstones and inflammation of the gallbladder are common causes of abdominal pain.

## EXOCRINE PANCREATIC FUNCTION

The *pancreas* is a large organ that lies behind the stomach and extends between the spleen and the duodenum. It is composed of a head, a body, and a tail, which contain the acinar cells and the cells of the islets of Langerhans (Figure 42-6). The exocrine acinar cells secrete digestive juices, whereas the endocrine islet cells secrete hormones that are essential in glucose metabolism. The exocrine functions, or those related to digestion, involve the secretion of pancreatic juice into a system of ducts that empty into the pancreatic duct and, in turn, the ampulla of Vater. Pathologic alterations in the pancreas are discussed in Chapter 39.

### Exocrine Pancreatic Secretion

The cells of the pancreas that secrete pancreatic juice are *acinar cells*. The secretion is composed of an alkaline component and enzymes necessary for digesting proteins, fats, and carbohydrates. The alkaline component contains sufficient bicarbonate ion to give the pancreatic juice a pH of about 8. The pancreas normally secretes about 1500 mL of fluid daily.[4] The enzymes are made by the acinar cells and stored until stimulated for release. The enzymes contained in the secretion are (1) *amylase*, which hydrolyzes carbohydrates to disaccharides; (2) *pancreatic lipase*, which hydrolyzes fats to yield glycerol and fatty acids; and (3) the *preproteolytic enzymes*, mainly trypsinogen and chymotrypsinogen, which, when activated, hydrolyze proteins to amino acids. Table 42-2 summarizes the enzymes and proenzymes of pancreatic secretions.

### Nervous and Hormonal Regulation of Pancreatic Secretions

Nervous stimulation of the pancreas is mainly through the vagus nerve, which transmits impulses to the pancreas during the cephalic and gastric phases of digestion. This results in the secretion of enzymes by the acinar cells. The nervous influences also affect the secretion of the endocrine islet cells.

The hormonal mechanisms are mainly mediated through *secretin* and *cholecystokinin (CCK)*. When chyme containing fat or amino acids comes into contact with the mucosal cells of the duodenum, the hormone is released,

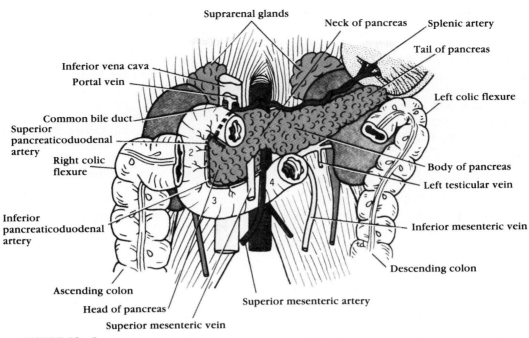

**FIGURE 42–6.**
Appearance and location of the pancreas. (Source: R.S. Snell, *Clinical Anatomy for Medical Students* [2nd ed.]. Boston: Little, Brown, 1981.)

causing the pancreas to secrete large amounts of fluids with large amounts of bicarbonate and few or no enzymes. This alkaline secretion neutralizes the highly acid gastric juice emptied into the duodenum from the stomach, stops the activity of gastrin, and provides an alkalinity of about pH 7, which is optimal for pancreatic enzyme activity. Cholecystokinin also is released from the intestinal mucosa in the presence of food, and it increases the secretion of pancreatic enzymes from the acinar cells.

Distention of the intestinal wall by food is the apparent stimulus for the release of CCK.

Pancreatic polypeptide (PP) is gastrointestinal hormone found in the *endocrine cells* of the pancreas. It is released after meals due to vagal and cholecystokinin stimulation. Pancreatic polypeptide is thought to be involved in the regulation of exocrine pancreatic secretion, gallbladder emptying, and migrating the contractions within the gut.[6]

**TABLE 42–2.**
ENZYMES OF PANCREATIC SECRETION

| PROENZYME | ENZYME | ACTIVATOR |
|---|---|---|
| Trypsinogen | Trypsin | Enterokinase, $Ca^{++}$, trypsin |
| Chymotrypsinogen | Chymotrypsin | Trypsin |
| Procarboxypeptidase A | Carboxypeptidase A | Trypsin |
| Procarboxypeptidase B | Carboxypeptidase B | Trypsin |
| Proelastase | Elastase | Trypsin |
| Proelastomucase | Elastomucase | Trypsin |
|  | Amylase | Chloride |
|  | Lipase | Emulsifying agents |
|  | Esterase | Bile salts |
| Prophospholipase A | Phospholipase A | Bile salts |
|  |  | Trypsin |
|  | Cholesterol esterase | Bile salts |

(Adapted from W. Ganong, *Review of Medical Physiology* [12th ed.]. Los Altos, CA: Lange, 1985.)

## Protein Digestion

Trypsinogen is converted to the active enzyme trypsin in an alkaline medium through the action of *enterokinase*, which is released by the intestinal mucosa when it comes into contact with chyme. Trypsin then activates other trypsinogen molecules and triggers the conversion of chymotrypsinogen into chymotrypsin. These proteolytic enzymes can split proteins into amino acids for absorption in the intestine.

The two most important protective mechanisms to prevent digestion of the pancreas by the enzymes it secretes are (1) synthesis of enzymes in an inactive form and (2) the presence of a *trypsin inhibitor* that is secreted by the same cells that secrete the pancreatic enzymes. This trypsin inhibitor is stored in the cytoplasm of the cells surrounding the enzyme granules and prevents the activation of trypsin, thus preventing activation of the other proteolytic enzymes. When the pancreas becomes damaged or when a duct is blocked, pancreatic secretions accumulate. It is hypothesized that the trypsin inhibitor is overwhelmed and the pancreatic enzymes become activated to cause acute pancreatitis.[7]

## Fat Digestion

Pancreatic lipase is an important ingredient for fat breakdown. There are several forms of pancreatic lipase that apparently are activated by trypsin.[12] It works with the bile salts and helps to break fats into fatty acids and glycerol.

## Carbohydrate Digestion

Pancreatic amylase hydrolyzes starches, glycogen, and other carbohydrates into disaccharides. It does not break plant cellulose down into simpler substances.

## REFERENCES

1. Arias, I.M., Jakoby, W.B., Popper, H., Schachter, D., and Shafritz, D.A. *The Liver: Biology and Pathobiology* (2nd ed.). New York: Raven Press, 1988.
2. Bolt, R.J. Pathophysiology of gallbladder disease. In W.A. Sodeman and T.M. Sodeman, *Sodeman's Pathologic Physiology* (7th ed.). Philadelphia: W.B. Saunders, 1985.
3. Fenogliio-Preiser, C.M., Lantz, P.E., Listrom, M.B., Davis, M., and Rilke, F.O. *Gastrointestinal Pathology: An Atlas and Text.* New York: Raven Press, 1989.
4. Ganong, W.F. *Review of Medical Physiology* (12th ed.). Los Altos, CA: Lange, 1985.
5. Greenberger, N.J., and Wenship, D.H. *Gastrointestinal Disorders: A Pathologic Approach* (3rd ed.). Chicago: Yearbook, 1986.
6. Greenberger, N.J., and Toskes, P.P. Approach to the patient with pancreatic disease. In J. Wilson, et al. (eds.), *Harrison's Principles of Internal Medicine* (12th ed.). New York: McGraw-Hill, 1991.
7. Guyton, A.C. *Textbook of Medical Physiology* (8th ed.). Philadelphia: W.B. Saunders, 1990.
8. Iber, F.L., and Lathan, P.S. Normal and pathologic physiology of the liver. In W.A. Sodeman and T.M. Sodeman, *Sodeman's Pathologic Physiology* (7th ed.). Philadelphia: W.B. Saunders, 1985.
9. Podolsky, D.K., and Isselbacher, K.J. Diagnostic tests in liver disease. In J.D. Wilson, et al. (eds.), *Harrison's Textbook of Internal Medicine* (12th ed.). New York: McGraw-Hill, 1991.
10. Rodman, M.J., and Smith, R.W. *Clinical Pharmacology in Nursing.* Philadelphia: J.B. Lippincott, 1984.
11. Saul, S.H. Liver. In V.A. LiVolsi, et al., *Pathology* (2nd ed.). Media, PA: Harwal, 1989.
12. Snodgrass, P.J. Pathophysiology of the pancreas. In W.A. Sodeman and T.M. Sodeman, *Sodeman's Pathologic Physiology* (7th ed.). Philadelphia: W.B. Saunders, 1985.
13. Zakim, D. Pathophysiology of liver disease. In L.H. Smith and S.O. Thier (eds.), *Pathophysiology: The Biological Principles of Disease* (2nd ed.). Philadelphia: W.B. Saunders, 1985.

# Alterations in Hepatobiliary Function

## Learning Objectives

1. Define *jaundice* and describe its etiology and physiologic effects.
2. Explain how ascites can result from liver failure.
3. Describe the pathologic appearance of fatty liver.
4. Define *portal hypertension*.
5. Relate esophageal varices to portal hypertension.
6. Define *hepatorenal syndrome*.
7. List the physiologic changes of liver failure.
8. Describe how hepatic encephalopathy and coma can result from liver failure.
9. Explain the major pathologic features of cirrhosis of the liver.
10. Define *alcoholic hepatitis*.
11. Discuss a major contributor to benign liver tumors.
12. Differentiate between primary and metastatic carcinoma of the liver.
13. Discuss the etiology, incubation, pathology, and clinical features of hepatitis A and B.
14. Describe the various stages of hepatitis B infection.
15. Define *cholelithiasis* and *cholecystitis*.
16. List the major constituents of biliary tract stones.
17. Describe the clinical manifestations of biliary obstruction.

The liver has a wide range of intricate metabolic functions (see Chap. 42). Its large, functional reserve accounts for the lack of clinical signs of dysfunction until large portions of the organ are greatly diseased or damaged. It is estimated that 10% of liver function is necessary to sustain life. This chapter organizes liver and gallbladder dysfunction into the general effects of alterations and how these effects are related to specific diseases. Common alterations in liver and gallbladder function are discussed.

## GENERAL CONSIDERATIONS IN LIVER DYSFUNCTION

### Jaundice

Jaundice, or *icterus*, is the yellowish or greenish hue imparted to a person's skin by a disturbed flow of bile or bilirubin (bile pigment). Bilirubin may accumulate in unconjugated or conjugated form, staining the skin, sclerae, and all the tissues of the body. The major types of jaundice result from impairment of uptake, conjugation, or secretion of bilirubin; excessive destruction of red blood cells; and obstructive conditions.[4] The most common causes are impairment of bilirubin metabolism, lysis of red blood cells, and obstruction of the bile ducts or liver cells.

## Impairment of Uptake, Conjugation, or Secretion of Bilirubin

Neonatal jaundice may occur when there is a deficiency of glucuronyl transferase, an enzyme necessary for the conjugation of bilirubin with glucuronic acid. Frequently occurring in premature infants, this impairment has been successfully treated with phenobarbital, which stimulates the essential enzymatic reaction. Improvement usually occurs within days to weeks. The *Crigler—Najjar syndrome* is a related condition in which glucuronyl transferase activity is congenitally absent and unconjugated bilirubin accumulates and crosses the blood-brain barrier. The result is *kernicterus*, the deposition of pigment in the basal ganglia of the brain, which causes brain damage. Kernicterus only occurs in premature or newborn infants because the blood-brain barrier will develop impermeability to bilirubin in early infancy.

Impaired uptake of bilirubin that interferes with its conjugation may cause jaundice. Decreased uptake by the hepatic cells is probably due to lack of sufficient glucuronyl transferase to effect the release of the unconjugated bilirubin from the albumin on which it has been carried. This is usually a benign, familial condition, called *Gilbert's syndrome*, and occurs in up to 7% of men.[4,9] It creates significant jaundice when stress increases both the metabolism of bilirubin and the need for conjugation. It is probably the result of more than one genetic error, possibly autosomal dominant.[4]

Another benign, familial jaundice condition is the *Dubin-Johnson syndrome*, which is characterized by excessive conjugated hyperbilirubinemia and a grossly pigmented liver. The defect is an inability to transport conjugated bilirubin in the bile for excretion.[4] Most persons with this condition are asymptomatic.

## Excessive Destruction of Red Blood Cells

Excessive destruction of red blood cells causes jaundice through hemolysis. The red blood cells break down into hemoglobin and red cell fragments. Hemoglobin is processed further to heme and globin, releasing free, unconjugated bilirubin into the plasma. Hemolysis can occur with blood transfusion reactions, after cardiopulmonary bypass, in sickle cell anemia, in marrow or splenic destruction of red blood cells, and with some pharmacologic agents. The blood transfusion reaction involves an antigen—antibody reaction to the donor red cells. The red cells are destroyed in an acute hemolytic reaction.

In sickle cell anemia, abnormal hemoglobin and a fragile cell membrane lead to hemolysis and an increase in the amount of free unconjugated bilirubin in plasma. The precipitating cause of hemolysis is usually hypoxemia, leading to sickling of the red cell and fragmentation as it passes through tight spaces (see Chap. 19). The liver retains the capability to conjugate bilirubin, but it becomes overwhelmed with the free bilirubin and cannot conjugate all that is sent to it.

Bone marrow disease leads to destruction of red blood cells before they leave the marrow. This can be caused by thalassemia or by some pharmacologic agents. Levels of either unconjugated and conjugated bilirubin or both may be elevated. Generally classified as bone marrow developmental problems, or defective erythropoiesis, are conditions in which the erythrocytes, poorly manufactured, are fragile and have a short life span. These cells hemolyze as they pass through the pulp of the spleen and other tight spaces. The result is that an excess of unconjugated bilirubin reaches the liver for conjugation.

Many drugs can cause hemolysis from drug-induced, defective erythropoiesis or as a side effect. Hemolysis usually results from a hypersensitivity reaction to the drug. Some examples of implicated drugs are listed in Table 43-1.

Thalassemias are a group of congenital diseases in which defective synthesis of hemoglobin leads to an increased propensity for hemolysis (see Chap. 19).

## Obstructive Jaundice

Two major types of obstructive jaundice have been described: (1) *intrahepatic block*, or failure of the hepatocytes to function; and (2) *posthepatic block*, which commonly results from cholestasis as a result of cholecystitis or cholelithiasis.

Intrahepatic obstruction frequently occurs with hepatitis and hepatocellular failure from cirrhotic fibrosis or hepatic scarring. Some pharmaceutic agents, such as oral contraceptives and chlorpropamide (Diabinese), have been shown to cause intracellular damage and blockage in certain persons.

Extrahepatic obstructive conditions in adults include gallstones, malignancies of intrahepatic or extrahepatic source, surgical obstruction of the ampulla of Vater, and others. Obstruction in infancy most commonly results from congenital atresia of the biliary tree.[10] The obstruction limits the excretion of bilirubin in the bile, and an excess of conjugated bilirubin accumulates.[4]

The physiologic effects of obstruction depend on the ability of the liver to conjugate and excrete bilirubin. When the source of jaundice is hepatocellular failure, in-

**TABLE 43–1.**
MAJOR HEPATIC DRUG REACTIONS AND SOME IMPLICATED AGENTS

| TISSUE REACTION | EXAMPLES |
| --- | --- |
| Microvesicular fat | Tetracycline<br>Salicylates |
| Macrovesicular fat | Methotrexate<br>Perhexiline<br>Ethanol |
| Cholestasis (with or without hepatocellular injury) | Chlorpromazine<br>Sex steroids, including oral contraceptives |
| Centrilobular necrosis | Acetaminophen<br>Halothane |
| Massive necrosis | Halothane<br>Acetaminophen<br>Alpha-methyldopa |
| Hepatitis, acute to chronic | Isoniazid<br>Oxyphenisatin<br>Alpha-methyldopa<br>Nitrofurantoin<br>Phenytoin<br>Cinchophen |
| Fibrosis-cirrhosis | Methotrexate<br>Cinchophen<br>Amiodarone |
| Granuloma formation | Sulfonamides<br>Alpha-methyldopa<br>Quinidine<br>Phenylbutazone<br>Hydralazine<br>Allopurinol |
| Veno-occlusive disease | Cytotoxic drugs |
| Hepatic or portal vein thrombosis | Estrogens, including oral contraceptives |
| Focal nodular hyperplasia | ?c-17 alkylated steroids, including oral contraceptives |
| Adenoma | Oral contraceptives |
| Hepatocellular carcinoma | ?Anabolic steroids, oral contraceptives |

(Source: R.S. Cotran, V. Kumar, and S. Robbins, Robbins' Pathologic Basis of Disease [4th ed.]. Philadelphia: W.B. Saunders, 1989.)

creased serum levels of unconjugated bilirubin often result due to failure of hepatocytes to produce conjugated bilirubin. Extrahepatic obstruction causes increased levels of conjugated bilirubin with excretion of bilirubin in the urine. As the liver becomes engorged with bilirubin, the activity of the hepatocytes diminishes, and the serum unconjugated and conjugated bilirubin levels increase.

Determining whether jaundice is caused by conjugated or unconjugated bilirubin is important in establishing the source and sometimes the severity of the causative condition. Deposition of pigments in the skin leads to the yellowish or greenish discoloration, which may be most noticeable in the sclerae of the eyes. In neonates, increased bilirubin levels may lead to kernicterus and neurologic impairment. In adults, the degree of jaundice often correlates with the severity of liver dysfunction. As-

sessment of the degree of jaundice is difficult in dark-skinned individuals, but intense yellowish discoloration can be seen in the sclerae.

## Ascites

*Ascites* is the accumulation of fluid in the peritoneal cavity. It is usually a direct result of increasing portal pressure or decreasing plasma protein levels or both. Sodium retention as a result of aldosterone retention and excessive lymphatic flow may add to the amount of ascitic fluid. Figure 43-1 illustrates the factors that can contribute to the development of ascites.

Portal hypertension, or increased pressure in the portal venous system, can occur because of an intrahe-

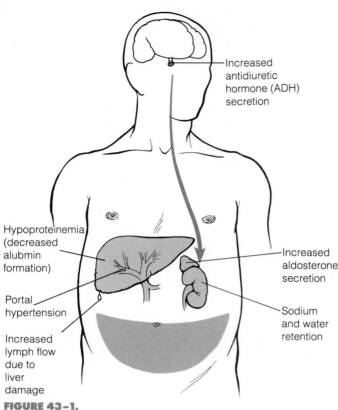

- Increased antidiuretic hormone (ADH) secretion
- Hypoproteinemia (decreased alubmin formation)
- Portal hypertension
- Increased lymph flow due to liver damage
- Increased aldosterone secretion
- Sodium and water retention

**FIGURE 43–1.**
Factors contributing to the development of ascites.

patic block to blood flow through the liver. The resultant increase in capillary pressure leads to disruption of the normal osmotic force at the capillary line, pushing fluid into the peritoneal cavity.

Decreased plasma proteins, especially albumin, lead to a reduction in the plasma colloid osmotic pressure (PCOP), which decreases the inward forces or reabsorption pressures, further encouraging fluid to pass into the peritoneal space. Albumin synthesis is depressed in conditions of liver failure.

Ascitic fluid, or transudate, contains large quantities of albumin, the loss of which results in further hypoalbuminemia. Complicating this process is a decrease or depletion of central blood volume as the amount of ascitic fluid increases. As a compensatory mechanism, the body increases the secretion of aldosterone from the adrenal cortex, which leads to retention of sodium and water. The retention indirectly provides more available fluid and increased ascites.

Antidiuretic hormone (ADH), which is synthesized by the hypothalamus and released by the posterior pituitary, also is secreted in greater quantities when the central blood volume is depleted. Increases in renal tubular water reabsorption and blood volume result.

It is probable that elevated intrasinusoidal pressure within the liver associated with cirrhosis leads to an increase in the lymphatic flow. Lymph fluid may ooze from

the hepatic surface and cause increases in the amount of ascitic fluid and in its protein concentration.[4]

Ascites is a self-defeating condition in which the compensatory efforts of the body end up making the condition worse. Without intervention, the course progressively degenerates, leading to greater ascites. Ascites causes abdominal swelling that is noted as increased girth. The extra intraabdominal fluid may cause pressure on the diaphragm and respiratory difficulties. Ascitic fluid may be removed by peritoneal tapping, but it frequently reaccumulates rapidly. The associated hypoproteinemia may lead to further ascites together with production of generalized edema, or *anasarca*. The edema results mostly from a decrease in the PCOP generated from the decreased albumin levels, which encourages fluid exudation into all of the interstitial compartments.

## Fatty Liver

*Fatty liver* refers to the infiltration of hepatocytes by fat or lipid material. This infiltration by itself usually does not significantly disrupt the physiologic processes of the cells, but over time the fatty cells become surrounded by fibrous tissue that separates the liver lobules. The pathologic appearance may be either micronodular or macronodular. Micronodular infiltration can only be seen with a high-intensity microscope, but macronodular lobules have fat infiltration and fibrosis that are visible grossly.

Several factors influence the deposition of fat. A diet high in fat may overwhelm the metabolic activity of the liver, leading to increased triglyceride stores. A diet with too little protein, or starvation, leads to mobilization of fatty acids from adipose tissue. Fatty acids then travel to the liver and infiltrate the hepatocyte (see Chap. 10 for effects of starvation). Alcoholism leads to fat accumulation in the parenchymal cells of the liver and distention of the cytoplasm with fat. In certain areas, the infiltrated cells undergo fibrosis, which increases the likelihood of portal hypertension.

Alcohol is thought to be a direct hepatotoxin. Large amounts of alcohol have been demonstrated to increase accumulation of lipids within the cells, resulting in a liver that weighs 2.0 to 2.5 kg (normal weight is about 1.5 kg) and appears soft and greasy when cut.[4] Alcohol may affect the conversion of fatty acids to lipoproteins in the liver, but the mechanism for its induction is not precisely known. In addition, alcoholism usually results in nutritional inadequacy, which promotes fatty infiltration of the liver.

## Clotting Disturbances

Because the liver produces many of the major clotting factors, liver dysfunction of 60% or more leads to depletion of these factors and a tendency to bleed. A decrease in the uptake of vitamin K into hepatocytes leads to defective synthesis of factors II (prothrombin), VII (proconvertin), IX (Christmas factor), and X (Stuart—Prower factor).[13] Vitamin K deficiency may result from fat malabsorption when bile amounts are inadequate. The major clotting dysfunction results from depressed production of prothrombin, and other clotting factors may also be depressed.

Deficiency in clotting factors is one of the earliest signs of liver failure. They are usually altered before elevation of bilirubin levels of hypoalbuminemia. The platelet count may be inadequate as a result of hypersplenism, which is a frequent companion of liver failure. Hypersplenism results from congestion caused by the portal hypertension.[4] In liver failure, an increased risk of hemorrhage is always present when it is associated with esophageal varices, and the bleeding is very difficult to control with the attendant clotting disturbances.

## Portal Hypertension and Esophageal Varices

Obstruction of blood flow through the liver results in increased pressure in the portal venous system. The term *portal hypertension* refers to high pressures in the portal vein and its tributaries. The main cause of this condition is cirrhosis of the liver, but the various causative conditions have been divided into the following categories:

▶ *Posthepatic*, which results from increased pressure in the inferior vena cava and venous return to the heart. It may be produced by severe right-sided heart failure, constrictive pericarditis, or hepatic veno-occlusive disease.

▶ *Intrahepatic*, which results from blockage to blood flow within the liver. The main cause is cirrhosis of the liver, but other conditions such as fatty change, biliary tuberculosis, and idiopathic portal hypertension may be at fault.

▶ *Prehepatic*, which results from blockage of blood flow to the liver, as may be seen in portal vein thrombosis, splenomegaly, or arteriovenous fistula.[4]

Meeting resistance in the portal vein, blood seeks collateral channels around the high pressure areas or through the obstructed liver. In the portal system, the vessels most susceptible to the high pressure are the esophageal and the hemorrhoidal veins (Figure 43-2). The esophageal veins protrude into the lumen of the esophagus and become thin-walled varices that look like bulging bags on the inner surface of the esophagus.

Esophageal varices can become irritated by gastric acidity or by spasmotic vomiting. Alcohol and other irritants can cause chemical breakdown of the walls of the varices. Any of these situations can result in rupture and massive upper gastrointestinal hemorrhage. The two main factors that encourage hemorrhage are depressed formation of clotting factors and high portal pressures.

Continued vomiting after the first bleeding event usually results in additional bleeding. Rupture of esophageal varices may result in exsanguination and death if not treated immediately. Rectal hemorrhoids also may rupture and bleed under pressure, causing a massive amount of bright red bleeding from the rectum. Anything that can cause increased motility of the lower gastrointestinal tract can increase the risk of hemorrhage from this area.

Collateral channels develop because of the high portal pressure and provide a route for direct shunting of blood from the portal veins to the inferior vena cava, thus bypassing the liver. The shunted blood contains large amounts of ammonia that may precipitate onset of hepatic encephalopathy. The blood-borne bacteria absorbed from the small intestine and normally processed and biotransformed in the liver are also shunted directly into the systemic circulation. Toxic substances may bypass the liver without being metabolized and may accumulate in the body with deleterious effects on the nervous system.

Bleeding from esophageal varices, duodenal ulcers, or other sources may precipitate jaundice and production of ammonia due to the processing and absorption of products of the red blood cell in the intestine. These developments may lead to increased risk of encephalopathy, which, with the bleeding event, is often life-threatening (see below).

## Hepatorenal Syndrome

In liver failure, the development of associated renal failure indicates a very poor prognosis. The hepatorenal syndrome seems to leave the kidneys almost normal morphologically but functionally impaired. It is diagnosed in persons developing acute renal failure in the presence of significant hepatic disease; frequently it is precipitated by clinical deterioration such as a gastrointestinal bleeding episode or the onset of hepatic coma.[4] The term *hepatorenal syndrome* should not be used for conditions that produce damage to both the liver and kidneys.

Hepatorenal syndrome begins suddenly, with decreased urinary output and elevated serum urea nitrogen and creatinine levels. It is accompanied by elevated blood ammonia level and increasing jaundice, probably due to the failure of bilirubin to be excreted in the urine. At autopsy, no permanent morphologic change can be demonstrated in the kidneys. The syndrome seems to be an evolutionary process of functional impairment of the kidneys resulting from liver failure. The kidney dysfunction markedly improves with restoration of liver function.[4]

## Liver Failure

*Liver failure* refers to a constellation of clinical manifestations that are the ultimate outcome of many types of

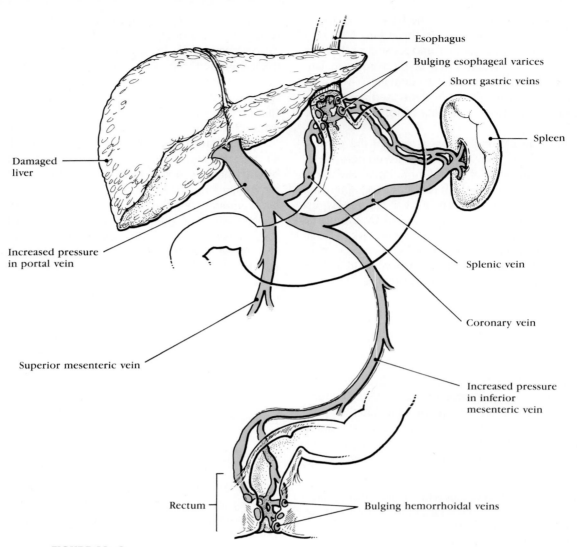

**FIGURE 43–2.**

Appearance of esophageal varices and dilated hemorrhoidal veins resulting from portal hypertension.

liver disease (Figure 43-3). The liver has a large reserve, and approximately 80% of its parenchyma can be destroyed before clinical signs of liver failure are evident. Cirrhosis and chronic active hepatitis are the most common causes of liver failure. Chemicals and drugs, such as carbon tetrachloride and halothane, can cause massive liver necrosis. Reye's syndrome, fatty liver of alcoholism, and antibiotics such as tetracycline can cause functional insufficiency.[4] These conditions cause liver damage that leads to a number of characteristic physiologic changes, including the following: (1) jaundice, with increased conjugated and unconjugated bilirubin levels; (2) coagulopathy due to malabsorption of vitamin K and reduced synthesis of clotting factors II, V, VII, IX, and X; (3) changes in neurologic status with hepatic encephalopathy and coma; (4) hypogonadism and gynecomastia due to imbalance of androgen-estrogen levels; (5) palmar erythema with vasodilation in the palms of the hands and feet due to hyperestrogenism; (6) spider angiomas of the skin, probably related to clotting disturbances or hyperestrogenism or both; (7) fetor hepaticus, a peculiar musty odor of the breath often associated with high serum ammonia levels; and (8) ascites and edema related to portal hypertension and hypoalbuminemia.[4]

The characteristic wasting of liver disease is manifested by muscular atrophy, weight loss, and loss of plasma proteins and clotting factors. Liver failure frequently causes death from cirrhosis; recovery depends on the amount of liver damage sustained.

## Hepatic Encephalopathy and Coma

*Hepatic encephalopathy* refers to an alteration in the neurologic status in persons with significant liver disease. Its onset may be gradual, but more frequently it is pre-

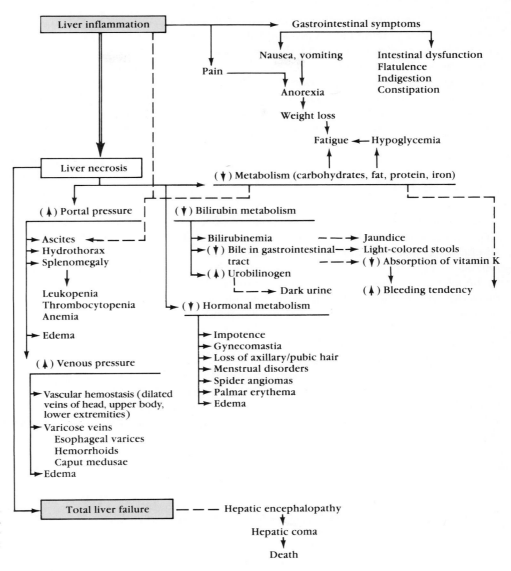

**FIGURE 43–3.**
Progression of liver cell failure. (Source: W.J. Phipps, B.C. Long, and N.F. Woods, *Medical-Surgical Nursing* [2nd ed.]. St. Louis: Mosby, 1983.)

cipitated by a major hemodynamic insult in the marginally compensated individual suffering from cirrhosis of the liver. Conditions that may precipitate encephalopathy include bleeding from esophageal varices; ingestion of narcotics or barbiturates, or anesthetics; excessive protein intake; electrolyte imbalance; and hemodynamic alterations such as hypovolemia or shock. Anything that can increase the metabolic demands placed on the borderline liver can precipitate liver failure with resultant encephalopathy and coma.

Hepatic encephalopathy occurs because the liver is no longer able to remove neuroactive metabolites from the blood. These metabolites inhibit normal neural functioning by acting as false neurotransmitters. Onset is related to the inability of the liver to metabolize nitrogenous products absorbed from the intestine. These nitrogenous products may include dietary protein or proteins released in gastrointestinal bleeding episodes. Serum ammonia levels are often elevated in encephalopathy, and

other substances probably produce the clinical syndrome as well.[9]

Hepatic encephalopathy has been described in terms of phases that vary in length and may progress insidiously from one level to the next. The earliest phase of encephalopathy is characterized by psychiatric and behavioral changes. Subtle impairment of intellectual abilities is also noted. In the next phase, the person experiences confusion, delusion, and eventual diminished consciousness. As the condition progresses, a phase having the distinct neurologic patterns of hyperreflexia and asterixis occurs. *Asterixis* is a peculiar "flapping tremor" that can be elicited by dorsiflexion of the hands. Violent, abusive behavior, accompanied by changes on the electroencephalogram (EEG), is frequent. The characteristic EEG changes of symmetrical, high-voltage, slow-wave patterns occur 1 to 3 times per second and are imposed on a relatively normal reading.

Progression of encephalopathy to coma results in absence of the flapping tremor and depression or decline of the wave forms on the EEG. A positive Babinski's sign and hyperactive reflexes occur with the onset of the comatose phase. Persons exhibiting recurrent or progressive forms of this condition have been found to have distinctive changes in the brain tissue, with proliferation of the astrocytes and patchy cortical necrosis. When these changes occur, areas of permanent damage result.[4]

## Drug-Related Liver Damage

Drug reactions are responsible for a number of toxic effects on the human body. (See Table 43-1 for a list of several drugs that can cause hepatotoxic effects.) Hepatotoxicity can result from formation of toxic metabolites as the liver is biotransforming the drug, or from a drug metabolite converting an intracellular protein into an immunogenic molecule. The damage sustained depends on dosage and individual hypersensitivity. Table 43-2 indicates some mechanisms that cause drug-induced hepatotoxicity. Some drugs affect a significant number of persons and the damage occurs in a relatively short period of time. Many drugs cause problems only due to hypersensitivity reactions, and these may not be manifested for weeks to months after initiating therapy. The pathology depends on the amount and location of injury.[4]

## Reye's Syndrome

Reye's syndrome (RS) is an acute illness that occurs most frequently in children between the ages of 6 months and 15 years.[4] The onset of symptoms begins about 3 to 5 days after a viral illness such as varicella. In nearly every case, the viral fever has been treated with aspirin. The initial symptoms are lethargy progressing to coma, with increased serum bilirubin, aminotransferases, and ammonia.[4] Pathologically, there is massive infiltration of the liver parenchyma with fat (steatosis). Liver and brain mitochondria are swollen and cerebral edema occurs in all cases.[4,12] The amount of cerebral edema corresponds to the severity of the neurological dysfunction. Fatality rates vary from 10% to 40% depending upon early diagnosis and accurate reporting.[12] The incidence of RS is declining with education of adults to not treat febrile illness with aspirin.[4,10]

## CIRRHOSIS OF THE LIVER

Cirrhosis is a general term for a condition that destroys the normal architecture of the liver lobules. It has the following important structural features: (1) destruction of liver parenchyma, (2) separation of the lobules by fibrous tissue, (3) formation of structurally abnormal nodules, and (4) abnormal vascular architecture.[4,10] Cirrhosis

**TABLE 43–2.**
MECHANISMS OF DRUG-INDUCED HEPATOTOXICITY

|  | DIRECT | INDIRECT |
|---|---|---|
| Mechanism of liver injury | Protoplasmic poison | Interference with hepatic secretory or excretory processes without parenchymal damage. Hepatic necrosis produced by competition or binding with essential metabolites; inhibition of specific enzyme functions |
| Time interval between exposure and liver damage | Brief | Latent period (1–4 wk) to sensitization |
| Toxicity | Dose dependent | Independent of dose |
| Reproducible in experimental animals | Common | Infrequent |
| Frequency | High | Low |
| Hepatic lesions | Distinct liver cell necrosis | Variable; hepatitislike; cholestasis; mixed |
| Rash, fever, eosinophilia, arthralgia | Unusual | High frequency |
| Examples | CC14, CHC13, phosphorus | Chlorpromazine, chlorpropamide, chlorothiazide |

(Source: Reproduced with permission from N.J. Greenberger, Gastrointestinal Disorders: A Pathophysiologic Approach [3rd ed.]. Copyright © 1986 by Yearbook Medical Publishers, Chicago.)

is classified according to its causative agent and the resultant pathologic configurations. The major classifications are *biliary, postnecrotic*, and *alcoholic*. A significant percentage of cases throughout the world are of unknown mechanism and have been called *cryptogenic cirrhosis*.[4]

## Biliary Cirrhosis

Biliary cirrhosis may be due to an intrahepatic block that obstructs the excretion of bile or it may occur secondary to obstruction of the bile ducts. The ultimate outcome differs with each type.

Intrahepatic biliary stasis is considered to result from two major mechanisms. *Primary intrahepatic stasis* is caused by autoimmune destruction of interlobular bile ducts. This type is most frequent in women over age 40 years, suggesting an endocrine contribution. Specific and nonspecific immunologic abnormalities have been implicated based on the demonstration of antibodies and impaired T lymphocyte function.[4,12] *Secondary biliary cirrhosis* results from obstruction of the hepatic or common bile duct and produces stasis of bile in the liver. This excess bile may lead to progressive fibrosis, parenchymal cell destruction, and regenerative nodules. The last is an apparent reaction of the interlobular bile ducts to the increased amounts of bile within them. Injury, inflammation, and scarring result from stasis of bile in the lobular compartments.[4] Both intrahepatic and extrahepatic biliary cirrhosis show evidence of fibrosis that surrounds hepatocytes and separates the lobules. Scarring and injury are located in close proximity to the interlobular bile ducts.

The clinical course is usually more severe in the primary than the secondary type because surgical intervention usually relieves the biliary stasis in the latter. Jaundice may be severe with either type and is associated with bilirubinemia and clay-colored stools. Results of liver function tests are abnormal, with alkaline phosphatase and cholesterol levels often becoming markedly elevated. Serum cholesterol is often elevated with this condition, and when it exceeds 450 mg/dL, *cutaneous xanthomas* (nodular swellings filled with cholesterol and tissue macrophages) may develop. Levels of both conjugated and unconjugated bilirubin may rise. With increasing liver damage, the signs of hepatocellular failure may appear.

## Postnecrotic Cirrhosis

Postnecrotic cirrhosis follows massive liver necrosis and involves the destruction of lobules and even lobes of the liver. It may occur after hepatitis or after exposure to hepatotoxins such as carbon tetrachloride and certain drugs. After the onset of disease or injury, a period of time passes during which the liver attempts to regenerate. The liver may become small and composed of large nodules separated by fibrous bands or scars. The nodules become infiltrated with lymphocytes. The liver architecture is distorted due to cell loss and attempts at parenchymal regeneration.[13]

Early clinical manifestations include an enlarged, tender liver that later becomes shrunken and nodular. Signs of portal hypertension are often present, and many problems of liver dysfunction complicate the condition. This type of cirrhosis is suspected in persons who have no history of excessive alcohol ingestion but who have signs of chronic liver disease. Abnormal results of liver function tests are the rule, and liver biopsy determines the underlying pathology. This condition also may be associated with an altered immune system, often with increased immunoglobulins, positive antinuclear antigen tests, and positive lupus erythematosus (LE) cell preparations.

## Alcoholic (Laënnec's) Cirrhosis

Laënnec's cirrhosis, also called *alcoholic liver disease (ALD)*, has been shown to be caused by chronic alcoholism, often following a pattern of fatty liver, alcoholic hepatitis, and finally, alcoholic cirrhosis.[4] At least 10% to 20% of persons who are chronic alcoholics have clinical or morphologic evidence of cirrhosis. Significant frequency of the disease is noted in highly civilized countries, among all economic classes, and in all races.

Alcohol has been shown to be a hepatotoxin. It induces metabolic changes within the liver that lead to fat infiltration of the hepatocytes and scarring between the lobules. Alcoholic liver disease usually follows long-term ingestion of more than 80 g/day of ethanol. This amount is found in eight 12-ounce beers, 1 liter of wine, or a half-pint of 80-proof whiskey.[5] In susceptible persons, as little as 40 to 60 g/day for males and 20 g/day for females can produce ALD.[5] There is usually a close association between poor diet and long-term alcohol abuse.

The phases of ALD are usually described as progressing from *alcoholic steatosis* to *alcoholic hepatitis* to *alcoholic cirrhosis*. The steatosis is the fatty liver, which is caused by increased liver synthesis of triglycerides and fatty acids, decreased fatty acid oxidation, and decreased formation and release of lipoproteins.[4] The alcoholic steatosis may be asymptomatic or it may be associated with malaise, anorexia, nausea, liver tenderness and enlargement, jaundice, or even sudden death.[4]

When alcoholic hepatitis ensues, there is the onset of acute liver cell necrosis. Inflammatory cell infiltrates and inclusions called *Mallory's bodies*, or alcoholic hyalin, may lead to pericellular and perivenular (around the cells and veins) fibrosis.[4,12] The liver becomes enlarged, and hepatocytes degenerate and become infiltrated by leukocytes and lymphocytes. Mallory's bodies produce sclerosing hyaline necrosis.[4,9] The early disease has an inflammatory character that decreases as the cirrhotic process progresses to the destruction of heptatocytes. Infiltrating fibroblasts and collagen formation lead to early scar formation. Acute exacerbations of alcoholic hepatitis cause inflammation and further damage to the liver parenchyma.

As alcoholic cirrhosis ensues, the liver capsule becomes firm to the touch, and regenerative nodules form, resulting in a hobnail appearance. As the pathology progresses, the liver shrinks and becomes finely nodular in appearance. The nodules are surrounded by evenly spaced, grayish connective tissue.[4] The liver pathology is usually associated with enlargement of the spleen.

The physiologic results of Laënnec's cirrhosis depend on the amount of inflammation, degeneration, infiltration of cells by fat, and scarring. Liver cell degeneration may lead to portal hypertension and ascites. Jaundice and esophageal varices often occur later in the disease. All of the complications associated with liver dysfunction may occur, depending on the degree of parenchymal damage. Some of the more common complications are clotting disorders, hypoproteinemia, biliary obstruction, and gastrointestinal bleeding.

Clinically, cirrhosis of this type is an insidious condition causing abnormal liver function tests, fluid retention, ascites, and esophageal varices (Figure 43-4). With abstinence from alcohol, results of liver function tests may return nearly to normal, but excessive ingestion of alcohol or continued poor diet may lead to decompensation. Alcoholic hepatitis recurs, leading to bouts of decompensation and finally to liver failure. It has been shown that 50% of persons with significant cirrhosis of the liver die of the disease within five years. Disease progression can be markedly altered by abstinence from alcohol. Death may be due to liver failure, infection, gastrointestinal bleeding, or hepatocellular carcinoma, which appears in 3% to 6% of cases.[4]

## TUMORS OF THE LIVER

Tumors of the liver that cause functional impairment and hepatomegaly are almost always malignant. The rare benign tumors are often classed as angiomas or adenomas.

### Benign Hepatic Tumors

Most hepatocellular tumors are *adenomas* that occur in women and are related to oral contraceptive use.[12] They cause a well-circumscribed, tan to white mass and may have a diameter of 5 to 15 cm.[12] These tumors may be discovered following complaints of abdominal pain and do not recur after excision.

*Focal nodular hyperplasia*, thought to be a hamartomatous malformation, also occurs mainly in young women who have taken oral contraceptives for a long period of time. Bile duct hamartomas and adenomas are small masses in the ductal structures. Sometimes the gross appearance of multiple hamartomatous malformations may simulate metastatic carcinoma or other conditions, but they do not cause symptoms.[4,12]

*Hemangiomas* of the liver are very common, reddish-purple lesions about 2 to 4 cm in size. These rarely are symptomatic but occur in about 1% of routine autopsies.[12]

### Primary Malignancies

Primary carcinoma of the liver is relatively rare and may arise within the hepatocytes or the biliary canaliculi, or it may be of mixed type. Hepatocellular carcinoma (HCC) accounts for 80% to 90% of primary malignancies of the liver.[4]

A study of the epidemiology of primary liver tumors shows that they may be related to diet and other types of liver disease, especially hepatitis. In the United States, the prevalence of primary liver carcinoma is less than 3%, whereas in some parts of Africa this malignancy may rep-

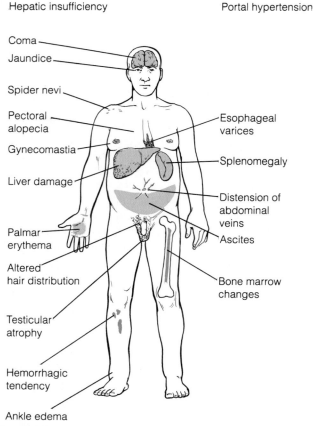

Hepatic insufficiency                Portal hypertension

Coma
Jaundice
Spider nevi
Pectoral alopecia
Gynecomastia
Liver damage
Palmar erythema
Altered hair distribution
Testicular atrophy
Hemorrhagic tendency
Ankle edema

Esophageal varices
Splenomegaly
Distension of abdominal veins
Ascites
Bone marrow changes

**FIGURE 43–4.**
Clinical effects of cirrhosis of the liver.

resent 50% of all cancers in men and 20% in women. Some of the influences that may contribute to its occurrence include (1) carcinogenic agents in food, (2) cirrhosis of the liver, (3) viral infections of the liver, and (4) parasitic liver infections.[4] Viruses, especially the hepatitis B virus (HBV), can account for the difference in frequency of liver cancers in the United States and Africa. In Africa, markers for HBV are almost invariably present.[12]

Pathologically, the growth may be limited to one area, occur in numerous nodules, or occur as infiltrates on the surface of the liver.[9] The tumors may secrete different substances, especially bile products. Usually the growth rate is very rapid, metastasizes early, and terminates in gastrointestinal hemorrhaging, liver failure, and death.

Physiologically, these tumors interfere with the normal function of the hepatocytes, but they often create no difficulty until they are far advanced. Biliary obstruction with jaundice, portal hypertension with ascites, and different sorts of metabolic disturbances related to the functional impairment of hepatocytes result. Metabolic disturbances include hypoalbuminemia, hypoglycemia, and bleeding problems.

Clinically, the affected person exhibits signs of debilitation, weight loss, and cachexia. Typical complaints are of abdominal pain and bloating. Early manifestations may resemble cirrhosis. Jaundice, ascites, and other signs of liver failure are often related to progression of the condition and frequently are seen in the terminal state.[4] Tumors of the liver are rarely considered to be resectable. Precise diagnosis is made by biopsy, but liver and computed tomography (CT) scans are helpful. Ultrasound examination is used to detect small, space-occupying lesions.[12] Arteriography is then employed to detect small hepatocellular carcinomas or intrahepatic metastases.[11] Alterations in liver function tests reflect the degree of disruption of normal function.

## Metastatic Carcinoma

The liver is very frequently the site of metastases of malignancies arising in other areas of the body, especially those of the pulmonary tract, breast, and gastrointestinal tract. Other types of malignancies metastasize less readily to the liver.

Physiologically, the liver is vulnerable to metastatic carcinoma because of the large volume of blood it receives each minute, the high nutrient level of its blood, and the large reserve of lymphatic drainage. Metastases usually widely involve the liver and disrupt its function. Results of liver function tests are frequently abnormal, especially alkaline phosphatase, serum enzymes, and Bromsulphalein (BSP) retention. The level of carcinoembryonic antigen (CEA) in the serum, which is increased in many malignancies, is also increased with many liver malignancies and metastases. Serum levels

correlate to some extent with tumor size and degree of metastasis, and levels decrease markedly after successful treatment.

The clinical course depends on the rapidity of growth of the metastatic lesion and the site of the primary malignancy. The nutritional status of the affected person declines rapidly, with marked cachexia, muscule wasting, and hepatomegaly. Obstruction of bile flow may lead to jaundice, and all of the other dysfunctions of liver disease may be present depending on the amount of liver involvement.

The prognosis for persons with liver metastasis is poor due to the lack of response to treatment and the impossibility of resecting the tumor surgically. Five-year survival has been reported to be less than 5%.

## VIRAL HEPATITIS

*Hepatitis* refers to inflammation and injury of the liver. It is a reaction of the liver to a variety of conditions, specifically viruses, drugs, and alcohol. This section details acute hepatitis resulting from viral infection.

*Acute viral hepatitis* is an infectious disease that is caused by a number of different strains of viruses. Hepatitis A and hepatitis B have been identified and described in detail. These organisms are distinguished by their antigenic properties, but both types are transmissible, and the complications that may result can inflict permanent liver damage. Non-A, non-B hepatitis and delta agent hepatitis have been identified, but study has been hampered by inability to precisely identify the virus or a specific antibody response.[1] Any of the agents causing hepatitis can produce a chronic, active hepatitis syndrome that may lead to hepatic failure.

## Hepatitis A

Hepatitis A (HAV) infection results most frequently from fecal-oral contamination with the hepatitis A virus. In rare cases it is transmitted through blood contamination. It frequently occurs in crowded, unsanitary living conditions, has no sex predilection, and is often epidemic in children or young adults. It has been called the "dormitory disease," because epidemics may break out and infect large numbers of students living close together. This infection may also be transmitted by contaminated, inadequately cooked shellfish. Contaminated water has also been implicated as carrying the organism.

After exposure, an incubation period of 2 to 6 weeks occurs before clinical signs are evident. In children the disease is usually *anicteric* (without jaundice), and diarrhea, nausea, and malaise are the predominant symptoms. In adults, the disease is more severe, usually with the onset of jaundice following a flulike syndrome. The clinical course is usually described in three phases: *prodromal, icteric*, and *recovery*. The prodromal phase is the period of time when the person first becomes symptomatic with anorexia, nausea, vomiting, and the flulike symptoms. It usually precedes jaundice by 1 to 2 weeks. Chronic infection or a fulminant course leading to liver failure is rare.[1] The course is rather predictable. The incubation period is about 3 to 4 weeks, and fecal shedding of infective virions precedes the onset of jaundice by 1 to 2 weeks.[1] As jaundice begins, serum IgM levels begin to rise, followed by an elevation in IgG levels that may last for decades. The liver enzymes alanine aminotransferase (ALT) or aspartate aminotransferase (AST) also rise, indicating hepatocellular necrosis. The jaundice remains present and the transaminases typically remain elevated up to 8 weeks after exposure.[1] The jaundiced or *icteric* phase is usually caused by conjugated hyperbilirubinemia (bilirubin > 2.5 mg/dL), causing the urine to become dark, whereas the stools may become lighter due to cholestasis (stasis of bile in the liver).[4] The icteric phase clears slowly, and usually complete recovery of the liver parenchyma results. It is probable that lifetime immunity results from HAV infection.[2] In areas such as Costa Rica, where the disease is endemic, 90% of the population have anti-HA antibodies by their teenage years.[2,4] The disease does not induce a carrier state and does not produce a chronic state.

## Hepatitis B

Hepatitis B (HBV) results most frequently from blood transfusion or needle virus contamination, but it also may be transmitted orally and venereally. It is estimated that there are over 200 million carriers of HBV worldwide.[1] Populations at high risk for hepatitis B are those exposed to needle contamination, including persons receiving many blood transfusions, personnel and persons in renal dialysis units, and drug addicts. Also at high risk are the sexual partners of affected persons, male homosexuals, children with Down syndrome, and persons taking immunosuppressive medications. Families or other close contacts of any of these individuals may also be at higher risk due to contact with body secretions. Hepatitis B vaccinations are available and are recommended for health care workers who have contact with blood.

Viral hepatitis is difficult to identify in the elderly because it presents with nonspecific symptoms such as fatigue, malaise, and diarrhea. Hepatic failure secondary to viral hepatitis is also more common in the elderly, and their response to the hepatitis B vaccine diminishes.[6]

Hepatitis B has a longer incubation period than hepatitis A, averaging 6 weeks, but clinical manifestations can occur up to 6 months after exposure. The hepatitis B organism can be identified by the presence of the *Australian antigen (AA)*, which is present in the bloodstream of infected individuals but lacks the critical core of the HBV. Therefore, the AA is not infective, but it is a diagnostic hallmark of HBV. Levels of this and several other antigens begin to rise several weeks before symptoms appear.

The *Dane particle* is the identified virion of hepatitis B. It is composed of two coats, or shells, and probably is the intact hepatitis B virus. The particle core is synthesized within the nucleus of the hepatocyte and is composed of HBV core, DNA, and antigen.[4] An associated antigen, the *hepatitis B surface antigen (HBsAg)*, may contain several related antigens that may be used to differentiate hepatitis B from other hepatitis. The first viral antigen to appear is the HBsAg. Another antigen (HBeAg) becomes detectable at about 6 weeks, but it is rapidly cleared from the serum.[1] If it persists beyond 11 weeks, it indicates a high risk of chronic hepatitis. When HBsAg clears from the serum, it indicates clearance of the virus.[1] Through laboratory studies, the hepatitis B virus has been classified as a DNA virus, which means that it uses deoxyribonucleic acid for replication.[4]

Pathologically, HAV and HBV look much alike. Hepatocellular injury and necrosis is usually surrounded by inflammatory cells, mainly lymphocytes and macrophages. The regeneration of hepatocytes begins very early in the disease; and multinucleate hepatocytes, increased mitotic figures, and hepatocyte thickening indicate regeneration.[4] The necrotic pattern may be spotty, confluent (groups of hepatocytes), or massive when most of the liver is affected. In general, there is evidence of (1) liver cell injury and scarring, (2) regeneration of liver cells, and (3) proliferation of inflammatory cells including Kupffer cells.

The clinical syndrome of HBV is unpredictable and can include any of the various syndromes listed below: (1) carrier states, either healthy carrier without evidence of disease or with chronic hepatitis; (2) acute, icteric, or nonicteric hepatitis; (3) chronic persistent or chronic active hepatitis; or (4) fulminant hepatitis with massive or submassive hepatic necrosis. The HBV also has been shown to be related to the development of hepatocellular carcinoma.[4]

*CARRIERS.*   "Healthy" carriers can transmit the disease even though they have no evidence of infection themselves. Individuals who are immune deficient for any number of reasons are more likely carriers than other individuals. Children who receive the virus during childbirth are usually carriers.[4]

*ACUTE HEPATITIS.*   With HBV the incubation time varies from 30 to 180 days after exposure. During the preicteric phase, rash, fever, and joint pain occur. The icteric phase may be present in only 50% of cases.[1] Other liver symptoms such as prolonged prothrombin time and hepatic tenderness may be present. HBV is often not diagnosed due to lack of specific symptoms.

*CHRONIC HEPATITIS.* Chronic persistent hepatitis is a smoldering infection that may not disrupt liver function severely. Chronic active hepatitis progresses very rapidly to progressive liver damage, leading to cirrhosis, hepatic failure, and death.[4] Approximately 5% of HBV infections become chronic, and two-thirds of these infections are chronic active hepatitis.[4]

*FULMINANT HEPATITIS.* This form of HBV infection progresses very rapidly from onset to fulminant liver failure and death in 2 to 3 weeks. It can result from other causative agents, but viral hepatitis accounts for 50% to 65% of all cases.[4]

## Delta Hepatitis

Delta hepatitis (HDV) is produced by a defective RNA virus distinct from all others. Its onset is abrupt, with symptoms similar to hepatitis B. The delta agent and B virus often coinfect, or the delta may be opportunistic when the HBV is present.[2] The organism is thought to have a direct cytopathic effect on hepatocytes.[1] It is transmitted by blood, serous body fluids, contaminated needles, and blood transfusions. A carrier state may persist with HDV or with the combination of HBV and HDV.

The diagnosis is often overlooked or called an exacerbation of chronic hepatitis B. Delta hepatitis is a common and serious cause of fulminant hepatitis, with 25% to 50% of fulminant HBV thought to relate to the delta agent. Delta agent is a defective virus that requires HBV to multiply.[2]

## Non-A, Non-B Hepatitis

This disease is caused by at least three unidentified agents distinct from the HAV and HBV. These viruses can produce an infection similar to HAV or HBV, but they can induce an active, carrier, chronic, or fulminant state.[4] The incubation period varies from 14 to 180 days, with epidemics being reported in India and Africa.[2] It is most common in young adult men.[2,4] It is often transmitted through blood transfusions, and as many as 60% of these progress to chronic hepatitis.[4] Epidemic forms are commonly transmitted through sewage-contaminated drinking water.[1,4] The epidemic form seems to be less virulent than the parenteral transfusion form. Chronicity in non-A, non-B hepatitis may result and symptoms may progress to cirrhosis. The usual pattern is one of improvement within 2 to 3 years.

# GALLBLADDER DISEASE

## Cholecystitis and Cholelithiasis

The most common disorders of the gallbladder are *cholecystitis* (inflammation) and *cholelithiasis* (gallstones). Inflammation of the gallbladder is the second most frequent cause of abdominal pain that requires abdominal surgery, the first being appendicitis. Dietary factors, including high fat intake, have long been associated with cholecystitis.

Cholelithiasis refers to biliary tract stones, most of which form in the gallbladder itself. Their major constituents are *cholesterol* and *pigment*, and they often contain mixtures of components of bile. Stones composed primarily of cholesterol account for 80% of gallstones in the United States. Gallstones occur in an estimated 20 million Americans per year, with considerable differences based on race and socioeconomics. Ten percent to 15% of adults in the United States have cholelithiasis, and 50% of these persons are asymptomatic. There is a dramatic increase in frequency among American Indians and Swedish individuals. Some predisposing factors include middle age, female sex, obesity, and possibly multiparity. Pregnancy, oral contraceptives, and estrogen therapy may be contributors.

## Clinical Manifestations

The clinical manifestations of gallstones arise when the stones migrate to and obstruct the common bile duct. The obstruction causes pain and blocks bile excretion. Visceral pain is precipitated by biliary contractions and is termed *biliary colic*. This pain is not colicky, but is usually perceived as a steady, severe aching or pressure in the epigastrium.[3]

Obstruction of the bile duct is followed by acute cholecystitis that may be due to increased pressure and ischemia in the gallbladder or to chemical irritation of the organ caused by prolonged exposure to concentrated bile. Primary bacterial infection may cause cholecystitis, but in up to 80% of cases, obstructive stones in the bile duct are present. Therefore, it is thought that bacterial contamination may either be secondary to the stasis or may result from severe infection such as septicemia. Pancreatic reflux may occur and cause irritation by contact of pancreatic enzymes with the mucosa of the bile duct.

Acute cholecystitis may cause complications with abscesses and/or perforation of the gallbladder. Chronic cholecystitis usually is associated with stones in the biliary ducts and is manifested by intolerance to fatty food, nausea and vomiting, and pain after eating.

## Diagnosis

The simplest diagnostic sign is nonvisualization of the gallbladder on oral or intravenous cholecystogram. The white blood cell count may be elevated to 10,000 to 15,000 mm³. Bilirubin level is often increased, causing jaundice. The pain of cholecystitis may mimic myocardial infarction, peptic ulcer, or intestinal obstruction, among other conditions.

# REFERENCES

1. Bain, V.G., Alexander, G.J., and Eddleston, A.L. Immuno-pathogenesis of viral hepatitis. In S.R. Targan and F. Shan-ahan, *Immunology and Immunopathology of the Liver and Gastrointestinal Tract*. New York: Igaku-Shoin, 1990.

2. Benenson, A.S. *Control of Communicable Diseases in Man* (14th ed.). Washington, D.C.: American Public Health Association, 1985.

3. Bolt, R.J. Pathophysiology of gallbladder disease. In W.A. Sodeman and T.M. Sodeman, *Sodeman's Pathologic Physiology* (7th ed.). Philadelphia: W.B. Saunders, 1985.

4. Cotran, R.S., Kumar, V., and Robbins, S.L. *Robbins' Pathologic Basis of Disease* (4th ed.). Philadelphia: W.B. Saunders, 1989.

5. Crabb, D.W., and Lumeng, L. Alcoholic liver disease. In W.N. Kelley, *Textbook of Internal Medicine*. Philadelphia: J.B. Lippincott, 1989.

6. Dam, J.V., and Zeldis, J.B. Hepatic diseases in the elderly. *Gastroenterology Clin. of No. Amer.* 19(2):193, 1990.

7. Dienstag, J.L., Wands, J.R., and Isselbacher, K.J. Acute hepatitis. In J.D. Wilson, et al. (eds.), *Harrison's Textbook of Internal Medicine* (12th ed.). New York: McGraw-Hill, 1991.

8. Felig, P., Hanel, R.J., and Smith, L.H. Metabolism. In L.H. Smith and S.O. Thier, *Pathophysiology: The Biological Principles of Disease* (2nd ed.). Philadelphia: W.B. Saunders, 1985.

9. Greenberger, N.J., and Winship, D.H. *Gastrointestinal Disorders: A Pathophysiologic Approach* (3rd ed.). Chicago: Yearbook, 1986.

10. Iber, F.L., and Lathan, P.S. Normal and pathologic physiology of the liver. In W.A. Sodeman and T.M. Sodeman, *Sodeman's Pathologic Physiology* (7th ed.). Philadelphia: W.B. Saunders, 1985.

11. Ohtomo, K., and Itai, Y. Early diagnosis of hepatocellular carcinoma. In J.T. Ferrucci and D.G. Mathieu, *Advances in Hepatobiliary Radiology*. St. Louis: Mosby, 1990.

12. Saul, S.H. Liver. In V.A. LiVolsi, et al., *Pathology* (2nd ed.). Media, Penn.: Harwal Publ., 1989.

13. Zakim, D. Pathophysiology of liver disease. In L.H. Smith and S.O. Thier, *Pathophysiology: The Biological Principles of Disease* (2nd ed.). Philadelphia: W.B. Saunders, 1985.

# UNIT BIBLIOGRAPHY

Anderson, J.R. *Muir's Textbook of Pathology* (12th ed.). London: Arnold, 1985.

Arias, I.M., Jakoby, W.B., Popper, H., Schachter, D., and Shafritz, D.A. *The Liver: Biology and Pathobiology* (2nd ed.). New York: Raven Press, 1988.

Berk, J.E. *Bockus' Gastroenterology* (4th ed.). Philadelphia: W.B. Saunders, 1985.

Brown, M.S., and Goldstein, J.L. A receptor-mediated pathway for cholesterol homeostasis. *Science* 232(4):34, 1986.

Cohen, S. *Clinical Gastroenterology, a Problem-Oriented Approach*. New York: Wiley, 1983.

Cotran, R.S., Kumar, V., and Robbins, S. *Robbins' Pathologic Basis of Disease* (4th ed.). Philadelphia: W.B. Saunders, 1989.

Dam, J.V., and Zeldis, J.B. Hepatic diseases in the elderly. *Gastroenterology Clin. of No. Amer.* 19(2):43, 1990.

Daorken, H.J. *Gastroenterology, Pathophysiology and Clinical Application*. Boston: Butterworths, 1982.

Eastwood, G.L. *Core Textbook of Gastroenterology*. Philadelphia: J.B. Lippincott, 1984.

Eisen, H.N. *Immunology* (2nd ed.). New York: Harper & Row, 1980.

Elias, E., and Hawkins, C. *Lecture Notes on Gastroenterology*. Boston: Blackwell, 1985.

Farmer, R.G., Achkar, E., and Fleshler, B. *Clinical Gastroenterology*. New York: Raven Press, 1983.

Fenoglio-Preiser, C.M., Lantz, P.E., Listrom, M.B., Davis, M., and Rilke, F.O. *Gastrointestinal Pathology: An Atlas and Text*. New York: Raven Press, 1989.

Ferguson, G.C. *Pathophysiology, Mechanisms and Expressions*. Philadelphia: W.B. Saunders, 1984.

Ferrucci, J.T., and Mathieu, D.G. *Advances in Hepatobiliary Radiology*. St. Louis: Mosby, 1990.

Golden, A., Powell, D., and Jennings, C.D. *Pathology: Understanding Human Disease* (2nd ed.). Baltimore: Williams & Wilkins, 1985.

Goldman, H., Appelman, H.D., and Kaufman, N. *Gastrointestinal Pathology*. Baltimore: Williams & Wilkins, 1988.

Greenberger, N.J., and Winship, D.H. *Gastrointestinal Disorders: A Pathophysiologic Approach* (3rd ed.). Chicago: Yearbook, 1986.

Guyton, A.C. *Textbook of Medical Physiology* (7th ed.). Philadelphia: W.B. Saunders, 1986.

Kaufman, C.E., and Papper, S. *Review of Pathophysiology*. Boston: Little, Brown, 1983.

Kennan, C.R. *Gastroenterology, a Problem-Oriented Approach*. New Hyde Park, N.Y.: Medical Examination, 1986.

Kissane, J.M. *Anderson's Pathology* (9th ed.). St. Louis: Mosby, 1991.

Lamphter, T., and Robin, A. Upper GI hemorrhage: Emergency evaluation and management. *Am. J. Nurs.* 81:1814, 1981.

Morson, B.C., Dawson, I.M., Day, D.W., Jass, J.R., Price, A.B., and Williams, G.T. *Morson and Dawson's Gastrointestinal Pathology*. Oxford: Blackwell, 1990.

Netter, F.H. *The CIBA Collection of Medical Illustrations: Digestive System* (Vol. 3). New York: CIBA Pharmaceutical Products, 1957.

Nursing grand rounds: Gastric bypass for morbid obesity. *Nurs. 81* 2:54, 1981.

Poli, G., Cheeseman, K.H., Dianzani, M.U., and Slater, T.F. *Free Radicals in the Pathogenesis of Liver Injury*. New York: Oxford, 1988.

Rozman, K., and Hanninen, O. *Gastrointestinal Toxicology*. Amsterdam: Elsevier, 1986.

Seitz, H.K., Simonowski, U.A., and Wright, N.A. *Colorectal Cancer From Pathogenesis to Prevention*. Berlin: Springer Verlag, 1989.

Shaninpour, N. The adult patient with bleeding esophageal varices. *Nurs. Clin. North Am.* 12:331, 1977.

Shearman, D.J., and Finlayson, N.D. *Diseases of the Gastrointestinal Tract and Liver*. Edinburgh: Churchill-Livingstone, 1989.

Sheldon, H. *Boyd's Introduction to the Study of Disease* (9th ed.). Philadelphia: Lea & Febiger, 1984.

Shiff, L. *Diseases of the Liver* (4th ed.). Philadelphia: J.B. Lippincott, 1975.

Sleisenger, M.H., and Fordtran, J.S. *Gastrointestinal Disease: Pathophysiology, Diagnosis and Management* (3rd ed.). Philadelphia: W.B. Saunders, 1983.

Sodeman, W., Jr., and Sodeman, W.A. *Pathologic Physiology: Mechanisms of Disease* (7th ed.). Philadelphia: W.B. Saunders, 1986.

Spiro, H.M. *Clinical Gastroenterology* (3rd ed.). New York: Macmillan, 1983.

Targan, S.R., and Shanahan, F. *Immunology and Immunopathology of the Liver and Gastrointestinal Tract*. New York: Igaku-Shoin, 1990.

Wallach, J. *Interpretation of Diagnostic Tests* (4th ed.). Boston: Little, Brown, 1986.

Watanabe, S., Wolff, M., and Sommers, S.C. *Digestive Disease Pathology*. New York: Macmillan, 1988.

Zakim, D., and Boyer, T.D. *Hepatology: A Textbook of Liver Disease* (2nd ed.). Philadelphia: W.B. Saunders, 1990.

**Normal and Altered Functions of the Muscular System**

**Normal and Altered Structure and
Function of the Skeletal System**

# MUSCULOSKELETAL FUNCTION

The musculoskeletal system provides for the framework and for voluntary movement of the body. The muscular system is described in Chapter 44, beginning with the appearance of the muscle cell and progressing to the process of muscle contraction. Smooth-muscle physiology is contrasted to that of skeletal muscle, and cardiac muscle structure is reviewed. A short discussion of exercise as it affects muscle physiology is included. Common primary muscle abnormalities are described.

Chapter 45 describes the architectural framework of the body, especially in relationship to the formation and composition of bone. Detailed anatomic information concerning specific bones is listed in the anatomy texts in the Unit bibliography. The important disease processes of bone are covered, as are traumatic bone and joint injuries. Pathophysiology of the disease processes and bone healing is included.

As with each unit, the reader is encouraged to use the learning objectives as study guides for chapter content. The bibliography lists a number of excellent resources for further research.

# Normal and Altered Functions of the Muscular System

## Chapter Outline

## Learning Objectives

1. Describe the anatomic components of striated muscle tissue.
2. Define *actin* and *myosin* and describe their interactions.
3. Discuss the functions of the organelles of the muscle cell.
4. Briefly describe the neuromuscular or myoneural junction.
5. Explain the *sliding filament theory*.
6. Explain the contraction of a muscle from the generation of an action potential to the return to the resting stage.
7. Describe four mechanisms by which energy is provided to the muscle cell.
8. List and briefly describe how exercise affects muscle physiology.

9. Compare the anatomy of smooth muscle to that of striated muscle.
10. Differentiate the two types of action potential in smooth muscle.
11. Describe the functional difference between *visceral* and *multiunit smooth muscle*.
12. Differentiate briefly the anatomy of cardiac muscle and that of striated muscle.
13. Describe common problems in muscles: cramps, twitches, fasciculations, fibrillation, tetany, myoclonus, and tics.
14. Differentiate between *adaptive* and *maladaptive muscular hypertrophy*.
15. Describe at least four causes of muscular atrophy.

(continued)

**16.** Classify the major types of muscular dystrophy.
**17.** Describe the pathology and clinical course of Duchenne muscular dystrophy.

**18.** List the laboratory and diagnostic findings that are helpful in the diagnosis of muscular dystrophy.

The muscles of the body are well-adapted to the work they must perform. Coordination of skeletal muscle provides humans with functional abilities ranging from gross motor activities to fine, precise mobility. Involuntary muscle coordination includes the regular contractions of the heart muscle, gastrointestinal peristalsis, and other essential functions. From the moment of conception, the human body is programmed to perform with coordination for many years. When alterations in muscular function occur, the entire body is affected.

## ANATOMY OF STRIATED MUSCLE

Striated muscle forms the voluntary or skeletal muscular system. Cardiac muscle, which is involuntary, is also striated muscle. Skeletal striated muscle is the predominant type of muscle in the human body. The muscles are arranged in regular bundles surrounded by a sheath of connective tissue called *epimysium*. This structure binds muscles to each other and to other structures, while allowing some freedom of movement.

## Description of Muscle Cells

A single muscle is composed of hundreds to thousands of muscle fibers. Muscle fibers are bundles of long, multinucleated cells in which the oval-shaped nuclei are close to the cell membrane.[7] Bundles of fibers called *fascicles* are embedded in a web of connective tissue called the *perimysium* (Figure 44-1). Each of the muscle fibers is bounded by a network of delicate tissue called *endomysium*. This tissue contains an extensive supply of capillaries and nerve fibers, and provides support for the blood vessels and nerves that are adjacent to the muscle fibers.[7] Muscle cells have a reddish appearance due to the presence of the myoglobin pigment, an oxygen depot in muscles. The muscles that must maintain activity for periods of time usually contain more myoglobin than others.

Skeletal muscle fibers, whose diameter ranges between 10 and 100 $\mu$, may extend the entire length of the muscle unit or may be joined by connective tissue. Muscle is *striated* when regularly bands of alternating light and dark appear along the muscle fiber. Interfaces of actin and myosin project this gridlike appearance.

The muscle cell contains sarcoplasm and its many myofibrils, numerous mitochondria, sarcoplasmic reticulum, a T-tubule system, numerous sarcoplasmic inclusions, and nuclei very close to the cell membrane. The cell membrane is called the *sarcolemma* (see Figure 44-1).

## Myofibrils, Actin, and Myosin

The myofibrils are the contractile units of the muscle. Each myofibril is composed of repeating units called *sarcomeres,* which are composed of contractile proteins actin and myosin (Figure 44-2). This structure is the functional unit of skeletal and cardiac muscle. Actin is a thin filament and has two proteins—troponin and tropomyosin—associated with it.[6] The myosin filaments, about 1500 per fibril, are thicker and have projections known as *cross-bridges* that extend outward toward the actin molecule.

Actin and myosin, lying beside each other, partially overlap, causing the myofibril to exhibit alternate light and dark bands when viewed under polarized light in unstained preparations. The light bands containing only actin filaments are called *I bands*, and the dark bands containing myosin filaments and part of the actin filaments are called *A bands*. In the middle of the light band is a dark line called the *Z line*. Between the Z lines is the smallest contractile apparatus, the sarcomere (see Figure 44-2).[10]

## Organelles of the Muscle Cell

Inside the cell is *sarcoplasm*, which is the cytoplasm of the muscle cell. In addition to myofibrils, the cell contains structural and chemical parts common to all cells (Figure 44-3). Especially important are the mitochondria, sarcoplasmic reticulum, T tubules, electrolytes, and water. Large quantities of potassium, magnesium, and phosphates are present, together with enzymatic proteins, bicarbonate, sulfate, and small amounts of sodium, chloride, and calcium.

Mitochondria, present in enormous numbers, provide a major source of energy for contraction. Energy is produced through a supply of adenosine triphosphate

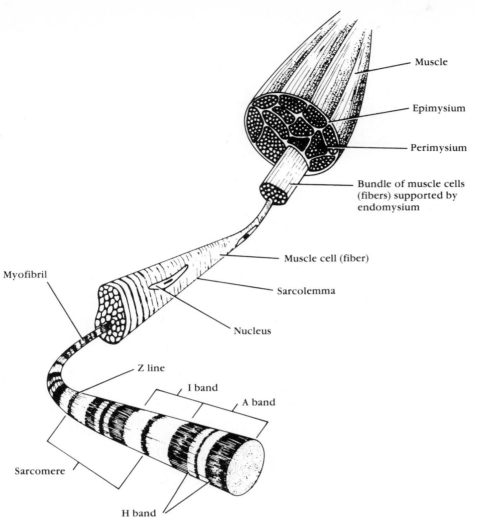

**FIGURE 44–1.**
Structure of striated muscle. (Source: R.S. Snell, *Clinical Histology for Medical Students.* Boston: Little, Brown, 1984.)

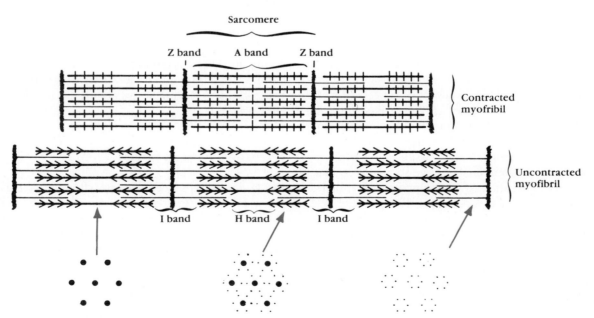

**FIGURE 44–2.**
Portions of contracted and uncontracted myofibrils. The I bands diminish in length in the contracted myofibrils. The punctuated arrays represent an ultrastructural view of the relationships of thick (myosin) and thin (actin) filaments in cross-section through different areas of the sarcomere. A sarcomere is the distance between successive Z bands. (Source: M. Borysenko, et al., *Functional Histology* [2nd ed.]. Boston: Little, Brown, 1984.)

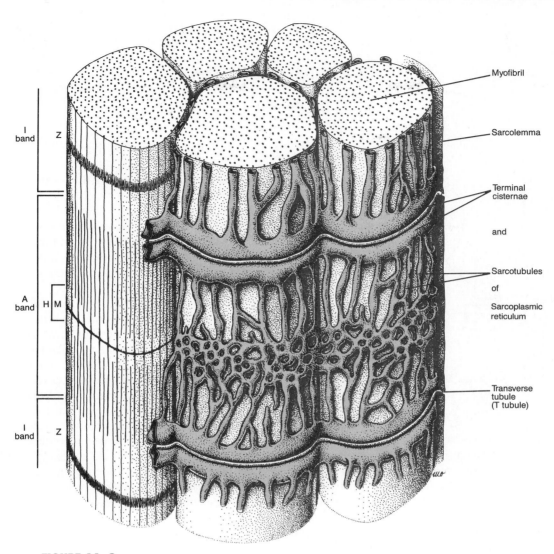

**FIGURE 44–3.**

Part of a mammalian skeletal muscle fiber, illustrating the sarcoplasmic reticulum surrounding its myo-fibrils. In mammalian skeletal muscle, two transverse (T) tubules supply a sarcomere. Each T tubule is situated at the junction between an A and an I band, where it is associated with two terminal cisternae of sarcoplasmic reticulum. Terminal cisternae connect with sarcotubules located around the A band, and these anastomose to form a network in the central region of the A band. The triple structure seen in cross-section where terminal cisternae from adjacent sarcomere flank a transverse tubule is called a *triad*. (Courtesy of C.P. Leblond; Source: D.H. Cormack, *Ham's Histology* [9th ed.]. Philadelphia: J.B. Lippincott, 1987.)

(ATP), which is mostly formed by the extraction of energy from nutrients and oxygen (see pp. 843–844).

The sarcoplasmic reticulum (SR) is similar to the endoplasmic reticulum of other cells. Its major function appears to be to transport calcium into the sarcomere unit to initiate muscle contraction. The SR is composed of tubules running longitudinally and parallel to the myo-fibrils. The tubules terminate in closed sacs at the end of each sarcomere (terminal cisternae). This allows for communication during depolarization and contraction. The SR is highly developed in skeletal muscle but is less well developed in cardiac muscle cells. In smooth muscle, SR is poorly developed with narrow tubules of reticulum beneath which are many vesicles called *caveolae*.[7,10] The transverse-tubule (T-tubule) system is closely associated with the SR. It is composed of tubules that extend across the sarcoplasm but open to and communicate with the exterior of the muscle cell (see Figure 44-3).

## Neuromuscular or Myoneural Junction

Each skeletal muscle fiber is normally innervated by a motor nerve. The nerve fiber branches at its end to form a motor end plate or myoneural junction that indents the surface of the muscle fiber membrane (Figure 44-4). The

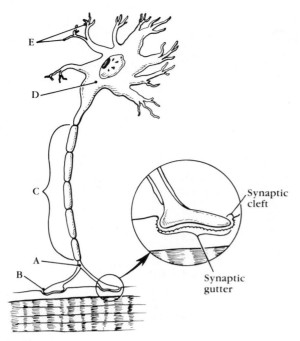

**FIGURE 44–4.**
Myoneural or neuromuscular junction. **A.** Terminal branching of nerve fibers for the end plate. **B.** Junction of axon terminal and muscle cell membrane. **C.** Axon. **D.** Nerve cell. **E.** Dendrites.

neuromuscular junction is a type of synapse, a junction of excitable cells that allows a signal to be transmitted from one cell to the next.[6] The junction of the axon terminal with the muscle fiber includes the following structures: (1) the synaptic gutter, the indentation of the fiber membrane where the axon terminal comes in close contact with the fiber; and (2) the synaptic cleft, the small space between the axon and the muscle. Within the axon terminal are synaptic vesicles that contain acetylcholine, the excitatory chemical transmitter. Cholinesterase is present on the surface of the folds of the synaptic gutter and destroys acetylcholine immediately after the response is initiated.

## PHYSIOLOGY OF STRIATED MUSCLE

### Generation of an Action Potential

For a skeletal muscle to contract, a stimulus from the nervous system must be present. When this stimulus arrives from the nerve axon to the myoneural junction, acetylcholine is released into the synaptic gutter space. This neurotransmitter causes the muscle cell membrane to become very permeable to positive ions in the cleft. The channels allow for the movement of sodium, potassium, and calcium.[6] Sodium is the main ion that rushes into the muscle fiber, causing a rise in membrane potential or generation of end-plate potential. The action potential

thus generated passes down the sarcolemma, depolarizing the T-tubule system and causing the release of calcium ions from the SR. Calcium ions, thus released, strongly bind with troponin-tropomyosin, and the sliding of actin on myosin occurs. This initiates the contractile phase.

### Sliding Filament Theory

The basis of muscular contraction is the movement or sliding of actin on myosin, which results in shortening of the entire sarcomere unit. Actin and myosin have been shown to have a strong affinity for each other that is inhibited by the proteins troponin and tropomyosin. The structure of myosin facilitates cross-linkages with actin, completing the system needed to perform the muscular contraction.

Pure actin filaments bind strongly with myosin when they are the presence of magnesium ions and ATP, which exist in abundance in the myofibrils. When troponin and tropomyosin are added to the thin filaments, binding between actin and myosin is inhibited. When the muscle is at rest, troponin and tropomyosin cover the actin filaments so that they cannot bind with myosin. Initiation of the contractile process requires that troponin and tropomyosin be inhibited. Calcium ions, released from the SR, bind to sites on troponin molecules. This binding causes the troponin molecule to change shape, which pulls on the tropomyosin strands, moving them to the side and uncovering the cross-bridge binding sites on the actin molecules.[10] Adenosine triphosphate interacts at the site, splits, and activates myosin. Myosin binds to actin creating a cross-bridge that moves the thin (actin) filaments toward the center. The cross-bridge is broken by the binding on a new ATP molecule. Splitting of this molecule causes the binding to reform at a different place on the actin molecule. This power stroke pulls the actin on the myosin in a step-by-step process described as a ratchetlike movement by Huxley in 1954.[8] The ATP is essential to provide energy through splitting for the cross-bridge movement and to break the myosin-actin connection, which allows the cross-bridge on myosin to return to its original position.

### The "Walk-Along" Mechanism

The mechanism by which the cross-bridges on myosin interact with actin is not completely understood. The cross-bridges attach to and disengage from active sites on the actin filament in a "walk-along" fashion (Figure 44-5).[6] The attachment causes dragging of the actin filament (sliding of actin on myosin). After this power stroke, the sites are disengaged and attach to the next active site, pulling the actin filament step by step toward the center

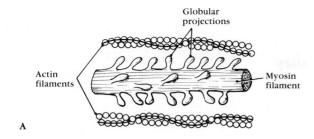

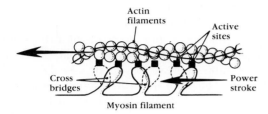

**FIGURE 44–5.**
"Walk-along" mechanism for muscle contraction. **A.** The relationship between the myosin filament with its globular projections and the actin filaments. **B.** The hinges of the myosin filament attach to successive active sites on the actin filaments.

of the myosin filament. The cross-bridges theoretically operate independently of each other, so that if more cross-bridges are in contact with the actin filament, the force of the contraction is greater.[6]

## Return to Muscle Relaxation

Calcium must be returned to the tubules of the SR so that troponin and tropomyosin can resume their inhibitory function. This is accomplished by an active calcium pump in the walls of the SR. This pump also can concentrate calcium within the tubules, creating a low level of calcium in the myofibrils. As calcium leaves troponin, it returns to its original configuration, which then allows tropomyosin strands to recover the actin-binding sites.[10] Without a communication between actin and myosin, the sarcomere unit extends, and the muscle relaxes. Figure 44-6 summarizes the processes of muscle contraction and relaxation.

Significant amounts of ATP are required to operate the calcium pump. In addition, the sodium pump is required to restore sodium-potassium balance and water balance within the cell. This active process is described in Chapter 1.

## Energy Requirements of Muscle Contraction

Four physiologic reactions are available to provide energy for muscle contraction: (1) use of the limited supply of ATP stores within the cell; (2) conversion of high-energy stores from phosphocreatine (creatine phosphate); (3) generation of ATP through anaerobic glycolysis; and (4) oxidative metabolism of acetyl CoA.

### Stored ATP

Adenosine triphosphate is a high-energy compound that is supplied mostly through an oxidative process. The ATP existing in the resting muscle cell is rapidly depleted during muscular contraction. Continued demand for energy

Stimulus from nerve axon to myoneural junction

Acetylcholine release in synaptic gutter

Increased permeability of muscle cell membrane to sodium

Rise in membrane potential (action potential generation)

Transmission of action potential through T tubules

Release of calcium from sarcoplasmic reticulum

Binding of calcium with troponin-tropomyosin

Sliding of actin on myosin with shortening of sarcomere unit

Contraction of the muscle fiber

Calcium pump moves calcium back to sarcoplasmic reticulum

Unbinding of troponin-tropomyosin

Inhibition of actin and myosin

Lengthening of sarcomere unit

Relaxation of muscle fiber

**FIGURE 44–6.**
Summary of the processes of muscle contraction and relaxation.

is met by donation of phosphate from phosphocreatine stores and by anaerobic production of ATP. As exercise is sustained, the increased blood flow to muscle allows for the aerobic production of more ATP.

### Phosphocreatine (Creatine Phosphate)

Muscle has a small store of creatine phosphate that can rapidly donate its phosphate to produce ATP and energy. This process occurs very rapidly, but the stores of creatine phosphate are rapidly depleted. Resynthesis in the resting muscle occurs with metabolism of food.

### Anaerobic Metabolism

Anaerobic metabolism provides ATP when the cellular supply of oxygen is insufficient to produce enough to meet the energy requirements of the cell. In the muscular system, it is often used when the skeletal muscles are taxed, as in athletic exertion. Without the adequate oxygen supply, pyruvate does not enter the citric acid cycle to yield carbon dioxide and water, but rather is reduced to lactic acid. The net ATP formed is much less than with oxygen, but it allows the muscle cells to continue their activity for a short period of time.

### Aerobic Production of ATP

As exercise is sustained, blood flow to the area is increased and a new steady state of muscle metabolism is achieved through the initiation of aerobic production of needed ATP.

Once the intense level of activity has stopped, the body consumes excess amounts of oxygen, as evidenced by the labored breathing of runners after a long-distance race. The intake of oxygen oxidizes the excess lactic acid and also aids in the metabolism that replenishes supplies of ATP and creatine phosphate. The amount of excess oxygen required to recover from the intense activity is directly related to the energy demands of the body. The amount of oxygen needed is called the *oxygen debt*.

At rest the skeletal muscle uses mostly fatty acids for energy production. During exercise the uptake of glucose and fat increases. It is estimated that 90% of carbon dioxide is produced through the use of fat.[6]

## Circulatory Adjustments to Exercise

Exercise performance depends on the ability of the circulatory system to compensate for increased needs. Blood flow to the muscles is increased by opening capillary beds not open at rest. The stimuli for this phenomenon are probably tissue hypoxia and release of local vasodilator agents. Exercise increases cardiac output and heart rate, whereas vasodilation decreases systemic vascular resistance.

Dynamic exercise (isotonic) results in increases in systolic blood pressure, heart rate and stroke volume, and normal or depressed diastolic pressure. This type of exercise includes jogging, running, walking, and playing tennis. Sympathetic nervous system stimulation produces vasoconstriction in other vascular beds such as the kidneys, gastrointestinal tract. Increased metabolic activity increases the body temperature so that heat loss is initiated. The two main methods of heat loss are through cutaneous vasodilation with radiation from the skin and sweating with evaporation.[13]

In static (isometric) exercise, muscle contractions create tensions but do not move a load. Isometric exercise results in elevation of both systolic and diastolic blood pressures, increased systemic vascular resistance, and a modest increase in cardiac output and heart rate. Static exercise principally increases cardiac afterload stress by increasing systemic vascular resistance, whereas dynamic exercise increases the preload stress by increasing venous return and cardiac output.[13]

Muscles vary according to the work required of them. The speed of contraction is matched to the function endowed on the corresponding muscle. Eye muscles, for example, provide fine, precise movement and react swiftly, whereas large muscles, such as those necessary to maintain posture, react slowly. The larger, slower muscles have smaller fibers and more capillaries and mitochondria than do faster-moving muscles.[6] They are often called *red muscles* because they contain large quantities of myoglobin, an iron-containing protein similar to hemoglobin in red blood cells.[6] Muscle fibers have been classified into three basic types: (1) slow, or type I, which contain large amounts of myoglobin and provide for muscular endurance activities; (2) fast-oxidative-glycolytic, or type IIa; and (3) fast-glycolytic, or type IIb. Types IIa and IIb use slightly different energy sources and are adapted for rapid and powerful muscle contractions as in sprinting and jumping.[6,13]

*Muscle tone* is the term applied to the tautness of healthy muscle tissue at rest. This tone is maintained by spinal cord impulses and decreases as neuron excitability decreases or is lost. When tone is lost, the muscle is said to be *flaccid*. Increased excitability of the lower motor unit reflex arc may cause *spasticity* or *rigidity* (see Chaps. 48 and 54).

Exercise training over a period of weeks to months increases the number and size of mitochondria in the muscle cells; the level of mitochondrial enzyme activity; the capacity of muscle to oxidize fat, carbohydrate, and ketones; myoglobin levels; and the capacity to generate ATP.[6] The net effect is to increase the capability of muscles to extract oxygen and to increase aerobic capability at any given workload. The results on the cardiovascular system are decreases in heart rate, blood pressure, and systemic vascular resistance, and increased stroke volume at any submaximal workload.[6]

## ANATOMY OF SMOOTH MUSCLE

The anatomy of smooth muscle differs somewhat from that of striated muscle, but the greatest difference between the two is functional. The smooth-muscle cell is long and spindle-shaped, and has a single nucleus near the center of the cell. A sarcolemma surrounds the fiber, beneath which are many vesicles, or caveolae. These may function like SR storing calcium.[10] Smooth-muscle fibers lack the characteristic striations of skeletal fibers and vary markedly in length. The lack of striations probably is due to a poorly developed SR and T-tubule system. Two distinct groups of smooth muscle have been identified: visceral and multiunit (Figure 44-7). The three different filaments described for smooth muscle are the thin (actin), thick (myosin), and intermediate (dense bodies) filaments, which are neither actin nor myosin and run continuously through the fiber.[6]

## Visceral (Unitary) Smooth Muscle

Visceral smooth muscle is present in the walls of the hollow visceral organs, such as the uterus, gut, and bile ducts. The cells are closely aligned and form large sheets of tissue. Because of the close proximity of cells, an action potential spreads cell to cell along the muscle until the entire muscle mass is stimulated. These muscles respond to innervation from the autonomic nervous system to increase or decrease the rate of activity, but it is a slow response to this stimulation. When one portion of visceral muscle tissue is stimulated, the action potential is conducted throughout by direct electrical conduction.[6]

## Multiunit Smooth Muscle

Multiunit smooth muscle is present in the ciliary muscles of the eye and in the piloerector muscles of the skin that can cause a goose-flesh appearance. This type of smooth muscle is composed of independent muscle fibers that are individually innervated. They contract more rapidly than the visceral smooth muscle.

## PHYSIOLOGY OF SMOOTH MUSCLE

Four properties distinguish smooth-muscle contractions from other types: (1) the contractile process is relatively slow, with contractions lasting for long periods of time; (2) energy expended during the long contractions is far less than that of striated muscle; (3) in certain circumstances, such as childbirth, the strength of contractions can be very forceful; and (4) slow relaxation follows the slow contraction.

In visceral smooth muscle, electrical excitation proceeds from one muscle fiber to the next due to tight junctions that allow the impulse to pass from muscle cell to muscle cell; this is a *syncytial effect*.

## Action Potentials in Smooth Muscle

### Spike Potential

Action potentials develop differently in visceral smooth-muscle tissue. The spike potential, similar to that of striated muscle, can be elicited by (1) electrical stimulation; (2) hormone action; (3) nerve fibers; and (4) spontaneous generation in the muscle fiber itself.[6] A typical spike action potential can be recorded much like that in skeletal muscle.

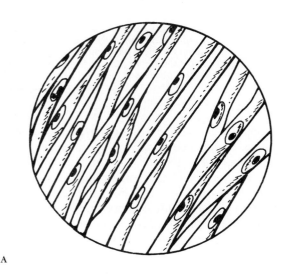

A

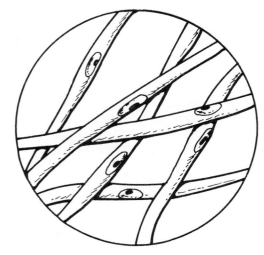

B

**FIGURE 44–7.**
**A.** Visceral smooth muscle as present in the walls of hollow visceral organs. Note close arrangement of fibers. **B.** Multiunit cells as present in ciliary muscles of the eyes, for example. Note loose arrangement of fibers.

## Slow-Wave Potential

The second type of action potential is the slow-wave potential. Some smooth muscle is self-excitatory, needing no apparent external stimulation. This is evidenced by rhythmic peristaltic waves. The slow waves apparently contribute to the action potential, a type of pacemaker wave.

Action potentials also may involve *plateaus*, long periods of depolarization, prolonged contraction, and slow repolarization. Prolonged contractions occur in the ureters, the vascular system, and the uterus.[6] Waves of contraction, called *peristalsis*, occur along the gastrointestinal tract. These are inhibited by stimulation of the sympathetic nervous system (SNS) and augmented by stimulation of the parasympathetic nervous system (see Chap. 48).[7]

## Smooth-Muscle Tone

Smooth-muscle tone describes the ability of fibers to maintain the long-term contraction that occurs in the peristaltic type of contraction. The smooth muscles of the arterioles exhibit continuous variable degrees of contraction that respond to changing autonomic nervous stimulation. These may also be responsive to local tissue factors or circulating hormones.

## Neuromuscular Junctions of Smooth Muscle

Two types of neuromuscular junctions are present in the innervation of smooth muscle: (1) the *contact type*, in which the nerve fibers come into direct contact with the muscle cells; and (2) the *diffuse type*, which occurs when nerve fibers never come into direct contact with the smooth-muscle fibers. The contraction may be initiated by nerve impulses (through transmitter substances), chemical agents, changes in the muscle itself, and even local stretch or distention.

Smooth muscle has one nerve supply for inhibition and another for excitation. The transmitters for inhibition and excitation, acetylcholine and epinephrine, are secreted by the autonomic nervous system. The response to the chemical transmitters varies, but generally, if acetylcholine excites an organ, norepinephrine acts as an inhibitor and vice versa.

## ANATOMY OF CARDIAC MUSCLE

Before advances in microscopic technology, cardiac muscle cells were thought to form a morphologic *syncytium*. *Syn* refers to being together; *cyte* means cell. Light

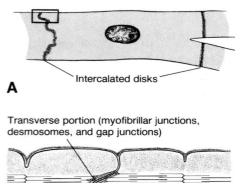

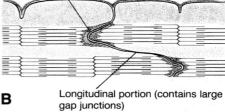

**FIGURE 44-8.**
**A.** Diagram of a cardiac muscle cell with intercalated disks at either end. **B.** Boxed-in area in A as seen in the electron microscope, showing the cell junctions in the two different portions of an intercalated disk. The longitudinal portions possess large gap junctions, and the transverse portions possess small gap junctions. (Source: D.H. Cormack, *Ham's Histology* [9th ed.]. Philadelphia: J.B. Lippincott, 1987.)

microscopy reveals cardiac tissue to have cross-striations with unique dark bands encircling the fibers at random sites. Seemingly, the cells are incomplete and branch into one another, forming a continuous mass of protoplasm. Electron microscopy, however, reveals that cardiac muscle cells are net-like in appearance, with fibers running together, spreading apart, and again running together in no apparent pattern. The dark bands that can be seen with the light microscope are abutting bands of tissue encircling the cardiac fibers (Figure 44-8). They are called *intercalated disks* and are located at the sites of the Z bands. The disks represent areas where membranes of adjacent cells approach each other. Functionally, these disks allow a wave of depolarization to pass unhindered from one cell to the next. Although each cardiac fiber branches and anastomoses with other fibers, a plasma membrane actually encases each fiber. Each cell has a single, centrally located nucleus. An abundance of elongated mitochondria are present close to the myofibrils in cardiac tissue. As in skeletal cells, myofibrils and the contractile proteins (actin and myosin) are present.

Structural differences between skeletal and cardiac tissue are apparent. A sarcoplasmic reticulum is present in cardiac muscle, but it is very rudimentary in comparison to that of skeletal muscle. The T tubules are 5 times larger in cardiac tissue than in skeletal tissue and are lined with mucopolysaccharide filaments. These filaments seem to trap calcium ions that are used by the sarcoplasm once an action potential has been initiated. Because *terminal cisternae* of skeletal tissue are missing in cardiac tissue, scientists believe that the T tubules act as reservoirs for calcium in cardiac muscle, as the terminal cisternae do in skeletal tissue.

Myocardial muscle fibers are structured in such a way that the atria and ventricles, when normal and intact, react individually as syncytial units. The specialized conductive units—the sinoatrial (SA) node, atrioventricular (AV) node, bundle of His, and Purkinje fibers—work in concert to cause cardiac contraction. The physiology of cardiac contraction is described in detail in Chapter 22.

## ALTERATIONS IN MUSCLES OF THE BODY

### Common Problems in Muscles

#### Cramps

Cramps, or spasms, are frequent occurrences in the skeletal muscles. They may be idiopathic or associated with motor system disease, metabolic disease (eg, uremia), tetanus, and electrolyte depletion, especially of sodium, potassium, and calcium. Muscle cramps are often reported at night or during rest and may be due to lowered blood sugar levels at night. Dehydration also may cause cramping, especially if associated with sodium depletion. Cramps are involuntary spasms of specific muscle groups in which the muscles become taut and painful. They may occur in the calf, thigh, hip, or any other major muscle group. Visible fasciculations may also occur before and after cramps.[9,13]

#### Strain

Various degrees of muscle damage may be diagnosed as strain, which usually results from overuse. Strains usually occur at the most susceptible part of the muscle-tendon unit and may be very painful or associated with tendinitis. Strains may cause an inflammation of the affected muscle, causing the tissue to swell and become erythematous and hot to the touch.

#### Injury

Direct trauma may cause a hematoma in a muscle, which is identified by localized tenderness, swelling, and pain on movement. Large hematomas can cause damage to the muscle. Muscle tears may result from inadequate warm-up prior to participating in rigorous sports. Mild tears will heal with rest and splinting, but severe cases may require surgical repair.[14] The most common locations for these tears are in the quadriceps of sprinters, the hamstrings and biceps of weight lifters, and in the gastrocnemius in tennis players.[14]

### Twitches, Fasciculations, and Fibrillations

These reactions are the result of spontaneous discharge of motor units and single muscle fibers. Twitches occurring at rest may be idiopathic or associated with motor neuron disease and peripheral neuropathies.

Fasciculations are involuntary contractions of a single motor unit. They may occur in healthy persons and cause visible dimpling or twitching of the skin. Fasciculations may occur rhythmically, starting and stopping for no apparent reason. Those during contraction of a muscle indicate excessive irritation and may occur years after poliomyelitis or a degenerative nervous system disease. The molecular pathogenesis is not fully understood but apparently involves hypersensitivity of the neuronal membrane to acetylcholine.[12] Continuous fasciculations, called *myokymia*, of unknown etiology may involve all of the voluntary muscles. They may be abolished or alleviated by curare, succinylcholine, and diphenylhydantoin.[12] Fasciculation is often confused with fibrillation, which results from the contraction of single muscle fibers. It occurs when the motor unit of the axon is destroyed. The fibers contract rhythmically, often up to 3 to 10 times per second. As denervation continues, the muscle fibers atrophy and fibrillation stops.[6]

### Tetany

Tetany, a spasmotic condition, most frequently results from hypocalcemia and hypomagnesemia. It is probably due to unstable depolarization of the distal segments of the motor nerves.[6] Hyperventilation may precipitate tetany by lowering serum carbon dioxide level, which reduces the level of ionized calcium.

### Myoclonus

Myoclonus is a sudden, unexpected contraction of a single muscle or group of muscles that involves the limbs more than the trunk. This disorder has many causes, from idiopathic benign (sleep) jerks to central nervous system disease.[6]

### Tics

Tics differ from myoclonus in that they are sudden, behavior-related, repetitive movements that may be a form of learned behavior or occur as a part of Tourette's syndrome. In the latter, tics may be accompanied by involuntary vocalizations.[12]

### Other Motor Disorders

Many motor disorders and disturbances, such as fatigue of the muscles, are benign. Others represent severe central nervous system dysfunction, such as convulsions. Those related to central nervous system dysfunction are described in Unit 15.

## Hypertrophy

Hypertrophy, the enlargement of individual muscle fibers, is an adaptive condition of the cells that results from an increased demand for work. The cardiac and skeletal muscle cells apparently cannot regenerate to adapt to a need for increased function. Although research evidence is conflicting, they are thought to adapt by enlarging individual fibers.[13] Nutrients such as ATP, creatine phosphate, and glycogen increase in concentration within the cell when there is need for increased work.

Most hypertrophy is considered to be adaptive in that it results when resistance is continually applied to the muscle walls. A weight lifter or athlete increases the workload through specific muscles that increase size and strength up to a physiologic limit.

Cardiac hypertrophy is a common adaptation for arterial hypertension, aortic valvular stenosis, and coarctation of the aorta. Hypertrophy increases the force of the cardiac contraction, which can maintain cardiac output for long periods of time. Initially, this is considered to be an adaptive mechanism, but it may become maladaptive if the nutritional needs of the hypertrophied ventricle outstrip the blood supply from the coronary arteries.

## Atrophy

Atrophy refers to the decrease in muscle mass due to diminution in size of the myofibrils. Atrophic muscles can result from such diverse factors as aging, immobilization, chronic ischemia, malnutrition, and denervation.[4] Muscle atrophy can occur very rapidly with one half of the final decrease being 4 to 6 days when the muscle is immobilized in a shortened position.[13] *Disuse atrophy* describes wasting of muscle tissue due to lack of muscle stress; an example is atrophic changes occurring after a bone fracture and treatment with casting. In one study, after a mean casting period of 131 days, leg size was reduced by 12% in the casted leg.[13]

Ischemia causes an inadequate blood supply, so that the oxygen and nutrients required for cellular maintenance are diminished. Eventually, ischemic changes may result in infarction of the tissue.

Denervation causes atrophic muscular changes that become irreversible. Loss of normal neural stimulation and reduction of muscle tone seem to be the major factors in these changes, rather than lack of weight bearing. If a muscle cell is reinnervated within 3 to 4 months, full function can be restored. After this time, some of the muscle fibers become permanently atrophied, and after 2 years muscle function is rarely restored (see Chap. 52).

Atrophy of muscle tissue may also occur in malnutrition or in wasting diseases such as cancer and cirrhosis of the liver. The muscle does not receive adequate nutrition, and consequently protein wasting occurs.

## Rigor Mortis

Rigor mortis is a state of muscular contraction that occurs approximately 2 to 4 hours after somatic death. It results from nonproduction of ATP, which is necessary to break the cross-bridges and promote lengthening of the sarcomere unit.[10] The contracture becomes intense, and the joints become fixed into immovable positions. This state continues for approximately 15 to 25 hours, after which gradual autolysis of muscle protein causes the onset of muscle and tissue flaccidity.[6]

## PATHOLOGIC PROCESSES AFFECTING THE SKELETAL MUSCLES

*Myopathies* is the general term given to diseases intrinsic to muscles. The category includes inherited muscular dystrophies, inherited and acquired metabolic myopathies, and inflammatory myopathies. Box 44-1 lists the major categories of neurogenic and myopathic disease of muscle. Following is a brief review of the more common myopathies and rhabdomyosarcoma.

## Muscular Dystrophies

The muscular dystrophies are genetically determined, progressive diseases of specific muscle groups. The syndromes are classified mainly by the distribution of involved muscles. Classification may also be based on pattern of inheritance, age of onset, and speed of progression.[4] Several members of the same family may be affected, with males predominating and females carrying the genetic abnormality. Muscle fiber necrosis is a major pathologic finding in muscular dystrophy. Studies imply that intracellular calcium overload is an essential factor because it activates proteases and impairs mitochondrial function.[3,15]

### Duchenne Muscular Dystrophy

This genetic recessive disorder occurs almost exclusively in males. Recent advances in molecular biology have identified the defective gene on the short arm of the X chromosome.[4,11] The affected gene fails to direct the production of dystrophin, the protein that controls the

## MAJOR CATEGORIES OF NEUROGENIC AND MYOPATHIC DISEASE OF MUSCLE

**NEUROGENIC DISEASE**
Myasthenic syndromes
  Myasthenia gravis
  Lambert–Eaton syndrome
  Congenital myasthenia
Denervation atrophy
**MYOPATHIC DISEASE**
Inflammatory myopathies
  Polymyositis-dermatomyositis
  Myositis associated with collagen vascular disease
Muscular dystrophies
  Duchenne or Becker
  Limb girdle
  Facioscapulohumeral
  Myotonic dystrophy
Inherited metabolic and congenital
  McArdle's syndrome
  Mitochondrial myopathies
  Nemaline myopathy
  Hyper- or hypokalemic periodic paralysis
  Central core disease
  Centronuclear or myotubular myopathy
  Congenital fiber—type disproportion
Acquired metabolic and toxic
  Steroid-induced
  Hypothyroid and thyrotoxic
  Alcohol
  Chloroquine
  Epsilon-aminocaproic acid
  D-Penicillamine
  Procainamide

(Source: R.S. Cotran, V. Kumar, and S.L. Robbins. Robbins Pathologic Basis of Disease [4th ed.]. Philadelphia: W.B. Saunders 1989.)

calcium release necessary for muscle fiber contraction.[11] Duchenne dystrophy is characterized by early development of motor difficulties, inability to walk, symmetric weakness of the arms, and enlargement of the muscles of the calves. Intellectual impairment is common.

Pathologically, calcium accumulates in muscle fibers. Associated with this is activation of the *complement* cascade demonstrated in muscle fibers undergoing necrosis.[3] Nonnecrotic fibers do not demonstrate a positive reaction for complement, but excess calcium has been demonstrated in nonnecrotic muscle fibers.[3]

The disease characteristically begins with lower extremity weakness that progresses upward and finally affects the head and chest muscles. The characteristic pseudohypertrophy of calf muscles is due to infiltration of the fibers with fatty deposits. The muscle becomes significantly weakened. Weakness of the back muscles results in lordosis. Respiratory or cardiac failure often causes death.

Prognosis in this disease is very poor, with death usually occurring before the age of 20. Before that time, increasing disabilities require much medical assistance.

## Adult Forms of Muscular Dystrophy

Adult forms of muscular dystrophy, such as the Becker's, limb-girdle, facioscapulohumeral, and myotonic forms, have a later onset and differ somewhat in the pattern of muscle involvement, heredity, and rate of progression.

## Laboratory and Diagnostic Tests

Most persons with any form of muscular dystrophy have elevated levels of enzymes normally present in the muscles. These include creatine phosphokinase (CPK), lactic dehydrogenase (LDH), glutamic transaminase, and glucose phosphate isomerase. All of these findings indicate abnormal muscle plasma membranes.[4] Lymphocyte abnormalities also have been described. Electromyography reveals weak electrical currents present in the muscle cell. Muscle biopsies are abnormal due to the presence of fatty tissue deposits in the cell.

## Myasthenia Gravis

Myasthenia gravis is a disease related to the inability of the neuromuscular junctions to transmit nerve impulses to the muscle cells effectively (see Chap. 54).

## Inflammatory Myopathies

*Polymyositis* and *dermatomyositis* are rare inflammatory myopathies of autoimmune or viral origin.[2,5] Clinically the onset is usually in adulthood with proximal limb and neck weakness associated with muscle pain. Muscle necrosis is patchy, and inflammation becomes chronic. In dermatomyositis, cutaneous manifestations of papules, erythematous patches over the joints, and erythema of the face and neck are associated with the muscle weakness.[5] Progression of the weakness in both polymyositis and dermatomyositis often affects the heart and pulmonary systems. Laboratory findings include elevation of the transaminases and myoglobinemia in those who have lost considerable muscle mass.[2,5]

*Fibrositis-fibromyalgia syndrome* is a common condition of musculoskeletal pain without evidence of arthritis.[1] It occurs predominantly in women of childbearing age with the following major complaints: musculoskeletal pain, stiffness, and easy fatigability. The stiffness tends to improve with movement, and a sleep disturbance is often described. Muscle biopsies are inconclusive, but decreased ATP and creatine phosphate in areas of described tenderness have been noted. The most commonly related feature is a disturbance of stage 4 (non-REM) sleep.[1] Continuing research may clarify this common condition.

## Inherited Metabolic and Congenital Myopathies

These diverse myopathies, often found in infants, affect muscle tone and produce weakness. In the inherited McArdle's syndrome, for example, the problem is in the glycolytic pathways for the production of energy. The mitochondrial myopathies exhibit varying pathologies of the mitochondria and a wide range of effects. The congenital myopathies often present as a "floppy infant" who has other associated developmental diseases.[4] The reader is referred to a comprehensive text of neuromuscular disorders for further discussion.

## Acquired Metabolic and Toxic Myopathies

Acquired metabolic myopathies are often secondary to disorders of the endocrine system. Many endocrine dysfunctions can cause weakness and fatigability, although they usually respond to appropriate endocrine management.[11] Nutritional and vitamin deficiency may lead to myopathy, especially protein deficiency and lack of Vitamins D and E.

Toxic myopathies are related to certain drugs and chemicals. Focal, localized myopathies are related to the injection of narcotic analgesics, especially pentazocine and meperidine.[11] Penicillamine, cimetidine, procainamide, and other drugs have been shown to produce weakness, myositis, and even muscle fiber necrosis. In most cases the mechanism of toxicity to the muscles is poorly understood.[11] Corticosteroid therapy causes steroid-induced muscle weakness, and differentiating it from the initial condition being treated can be difficult.

Excessive alcohol use can produce a severe rhabdomyolysis (breakdown of striated muscle), which can affect the skeletal and heart muscle.[4] Renal failure may result when there is significant elevation of the myoglobin in the urine.

## Rhabdomyosarcoma

Rhabdomyosarcoma is a malignant tumor of striated muscle. It occurs most commonly in children and adolescents, and may affect the striated muscles of the extremities, head, or neck. This type of sarcoma is very invasive, with extremely anaplastic cells.[4] Five-year survival is 30% to 40%; treatment includes resection, radiation therapy, and chemotherapy.

## REFERENCES

1. Bennett, R.M. The fibrositis-fibromyalgia syndrome. In H.R. Schumacher, *Primer on the Rheumatic Diseases* (9th ed.). Atlanta: Arthritis Foundation, 1988.
2. Bradley, W.G. and Tandan, R. Dermatomyositis and polymyositis. In J. Wilson et al., *Harrison's Principles of Internal Medicine* (12th ed.). New York: McGraw-Hill, 1991.
3. Cornelia, F. Muscle fiber degeneration and necrosis in muscular dystrophy and other muscle disease: Cytochemical and immunocytochemical data. *Ann. Neurol.* 12:694, 1984.
4. Cotran, R.S., Kumar, V., and Robbins, S.L. *Pathologic Basis of Disease* (4th ed.). Philadelphia: W.B. Saunders, 1989.
5. Cronin, M.E., Miller, F.W., and Plotz, P.H. Polymyositis and dermatomyositis. In H.R. Schumacher, *Primer on the Rheumatic Diseases* (9th ed.). Atlanta: Arthritis Foundation, 1988.
6. Guyton, A.C. *Textbook of Medical Physiology* (8th ed.). Philadelphia: W.B. Saunders, 1990.
7. Ham, A.W., and Cormack, D.H. *Histology* (8th ed.). Philadelphia: J.B. Lippincott, 1987.
8. Huxley, H.E. The double array of filaments in cross-striated muscle. *J. Biophys. Biochem. Cytol.* 3:631, 1957.
9. Kaufman, C.E., and Solomon, P. *Review of Pathophysiology.* Boston: Little, Brown, 1983.
10. McClintic, J.R. *Physiology of the Human Body* (3rd ed.). New York: Wiley, 1985.
11. Mendell, J.R., and Griggs, R.C. Muscular dystrophy and other chronic myopathies. In J. Wilson et al., *Harrison's Principles of Internal Medicine* (12th ed.). New York: McGraw-Hill, 1991.
12. Plum, F., and Posner, J. Neurology. In L.H. Smith and S.O. Thier (eds.), *Pathophysiology: The Biological Principles of Disease* (2nd ed.). Philadelphia: W.B. Saunders, 1985.
13. Pollock, M.L., Wilmore, J.H., and Fox, S.M. *Exercise in Health and Disease.* Philadelphia: W.B. Saunders, 1984.
14. Pullman, S., and Mooar, P. Sports and occupational injuries. In H.R. Schumacher, *Primer on the Rheumatic Diseases* (9th ed.). Atlanta: Arthritis Foundation, 1988.
15. Uchino, M., et al. Structural proteins of the opaque muscle fibers in Duchenne muscular dystrophy. *Neurology*, 35(9): 1364, 1985.

# Normal and Altered Structure and Function of the Skeletal System

## Chapter Outline

## Learning Objectives

1. Differentiate between *intramembranous* and *endochondral ossification* in bone formation.
2. Describe the blood supply to a bone, including the nutrient and periosteal arteries.
3. Describe epiphyseal growth.
4. Name the factors that retard and accelerate bone growth.
5. Explain the calcium-parathyroid feedback mechanism.
6. Discuss the feedback mechanism for calcitonin and calcium.
7. Describe the relationships among bone formation, sex hormones, and age.
8. Discuss the effects of weight bearing on bone structure.
9. Differentiate among the three classifications of joints.
10. Describe the structures of tendons, ligaments, and bursae.
11. Define *complete, comminuted, compression, depressed, stress,* and *avulsion fractures.*
12. Describe the process of fracture healing.
13. Differentiate among *delayed union, nonunion,* and *malunion.*
14. List the symptoms of anterior compartmental syndrome.
15. Describe the clinical syndrome of osteogenesis imperfecta.
16. Describe fibrous dysplasia and Paget's disease of bone.
17. Discuss the skeletal manifestations of the hormone condition in von Recklinghausen's disease.
18. Identify the usual pathogenesis of rickets or osteomalacia.
19. Compare rickets and scurvy with regard to etiology and physical findings.
20. Describe the pathology of avascular necrosis of the head of the femur.
21. Describe the course of osteomyelitis from beginning infection to the chronic stage.
22. Describe the physical changes of scoliosis.
23. List some causes of a congenitally dislocated hip.
24. Describe the joint pathology of rheumatoid arthritis.
25. Discuss how rheumatoid arthritis affects other systems such as heart, lungs, eyes, and nerves.
26. Describe the metabolic disorder responsible for gout.
27. Describe bursitis and its principal causes.
28. Describe basic differences between benign and malignant bone tumors.
29. Compare and contrast the sarcomas of cartilaginous origin with those of osteogenic origin with respect to symptoms, gross pathology, survival, and frequency.
30. Discuss the skeletal involvement and symptoms of multiple myeloma.

# NORMAL STRUCTURE AND FUNCTION OF BONE

The framework of the human body is the skeletal system. This system of more than 206 bones protects internal organs, provides for support and movement through its muscle attachments, serves as a storehouse for mineral supply, and produces blood cells. A living, dynamic tissue, bone contains a blood, nerves, and lymph supplies, and provides for the constant movement of calcium, phosphorus, and other minerals into and out of the bloodstream.

Bone is a collagenous protein that is partially composed of complex calcium salts. The organic matrix of bone, called the *osteoid*, is made up primarily of collagen (protein), some polysaccharides, and lipids. The salts, which consist of calcium carbonate ($CaCO_3$), and calcium phosphate ($Ca_3[PO_4]_2$), form a substance that is a hard crystalline salt. The matrix supplies tensile strength (resistance to being pulled apart), whereas the mineral deposits provide compressive strength (resistance to being crumbled). This combination gives bone the tensile strength of white oak and a compressive strength greater than granite.

## Bone Formation

### Cellular Components

Bone tissue is constantly being formed and reformed. This modeling is facilitated by three types of cells. *Osteoblasts* are formed from osteogenic cells present in the endosteum, periosteum, and epiphyseal plates of long bones. These are bone-forming cells that synthesize the collagenous matrix osteoid in the process of ossification. Osteoid is a protein substance that becomes calcified to produce hard bone. Osteoblasts also help control the calcification of bone. Alkaline phosphatase, which is thought to aid in the mineralization process, is produced by osteoblasts.[10] Osteoblasts synthesize osteocalcin and osteonectin, both of which bind to calcium and have a local effect on calcification of bone.[18] When the matrix surrounding the osteoblasts becomes calcified, the cells are called *osteocytes. Osteoclasts* are cells of monocyte-macrophage origin whose primary function is the reabsorption of bone. These cells produce acids that make the bone salts soluble and then digest the organic matrix.[6]

### Intramembranous Ossification

Bone formation begins in early fetal life. The fetal skeleton is composed mostly of hyaline cartilage that undergoes ossification. The swapping of the cartilaginous material with bone, begun *in utero*, continues until after puberty. There are two main types of bone formation: intramembranous and endochondral. The more simple and direct type is intramembranous ossification, which occurs in the flat bones of the face and skull. In the cartilaginous fetal structure, osteoblasts secrete organic material that calcifies; from this center of ossification, small bone spicules build up an interlacing network on which more bone is developed. Eventually, the osteoblasts are trapped in small spaces called *lacunae* and become osteocytes. The spongy bone developed is then covered by layers of compact bone.

## Endochondral Ossification

The process by which the long bones of the body are formed is called *endochondral ossification* (Figure 45-1). The "baby skeleton," which is cartilage, is transformed into bone by ossification, which begins in the center of the shaft (diaphysis) and in each end (epiphysis) of the bone. This formation spreads, and with it the destruction of cartilage, until only two thin strips are left at either end of the bone (the epiphyseal plate). These strips remain until bone growth and maturation are completed. As spongy bone is formed within, marrow is formed in the spaces and the marrow cavity develops in the center of the bone. The osteoblasts on the outside form layers of hard, compact bone. The perichondrium, which is the layer surrounding the early cartilage, becomes the periosteum, and as more layers of compact bone are laid circumferentially, osteoclasts make the marrow, or medullary cavity, larger to support the larger bone.

## Bone Structure

### Microscopic Structure

Bone has three structural forms: cortical or compact (hard surface area), cancellous or spongy, and medullary (inner core). Whenever bone matrix is laid down rapidly and haphazardly, as occurs after fractures and in fetal growth, the resultant immature form is termed *woven bone*. The microscopic structure of compact bone consists of numerous, parallel, longitudinal canals (haversian canals), which contain blood vessels, lymphatics, and nerves (Figure 45-2). Around each canal are several layers, or rings, of bone called *lamellae*. Connecting the haversian canals with the lamellae are the minute canals (canaliculi) that carry oxygen and nutrients to the bone cells. Each canal with its contents and surrounding lamellae makes up a *haversian system* or *osteon*. Directly under the periosteum and surrounding the medullary canal, several thicknesses of lamellae are laid down surrounding the entire shaft with hard thickness. The haversian systems run parallel to each other and longitudi-

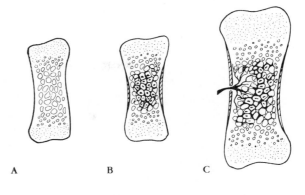

A          B          C

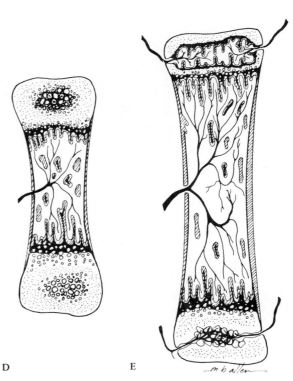

D                    E

## FIGURE 45-1.

Some major events in the formation of a long bone by endochondral ossification. **A.** Hyaline cartilage model; hypertrophy of central chondrocytes. **B.** Hypertrophied chondrocytes begin to die due to initiation of matrix calcification; formation of the bone collar. **C.** Invasion of blood vessels and pluripotential osteoprogenitor cells; resorption of calcified cartilage matrix to form exposed surfaces for bone tissue apposition in primary center of ossification. **D.** Growth of bone formation of marrow cavity by cartilage proliferation at epiphyseal ends; bone tissue apposition at calcified cartilage surfaces and resorption in diaphyseal cavity; initiation of secondary center of ossification above; and elongation of bone collar. **E.** Further growth of bone; formation and development of secondary center of ossification above, leaving cartilaginous epiphyseal plate separating epiphysis from diaphysis; appearance of additional secondary center of ossification below; growth in girth of bone by concomitant bone tissue apposition on outer diaphyseal surface and resorption from inner surface. Black = calcified cartilage; black arborizations = blood vessels; parallel diagonal lines = bone tissue. (Source: M. Borysenko, et al., *Functional Histology* [2nd ed.]. Boston: Little, Brown, 1984.)

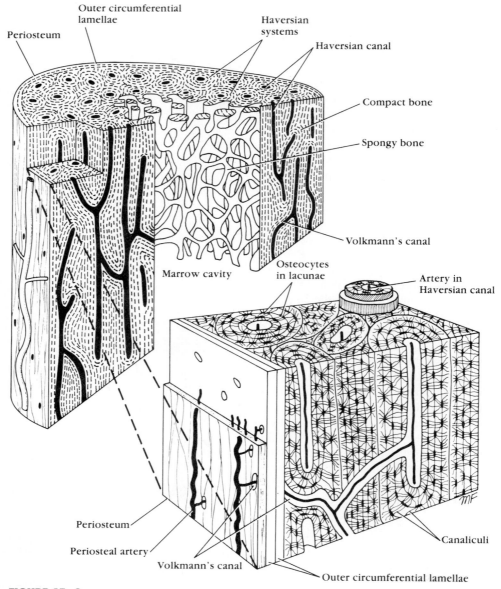

**FIGURE 45–2.**

Compact bone tissue in histologic section. (Source: R.S. Snell, *Clinical Histology for Medical Students*. Boston: Little, Brown, 1984.)

nally, from metaphysis to metaphysis, and are connected transversely by tubes called *Volkmann's canals*. Blood vessels from the periosteum enter the bone and pass through these canals to enter and leave the haversian system.

### Cancellous and Medullary Bone

Cancellous bone is present in flat bones and in the ends of long bones. It is a collection of *trabeculae*, or beams of bone, which gives it a spongy appearance and adds strength due to the many interlacing parts (Figure 45-3). The spaces in between these trabeculae are filled with bone marrow. The red marrow actively participates in the formation of red blood cells, and is present in the adult in the cancellous bone of the ribs, sternum, vertebrae, and pelvis. Red marrow is present in many bones in infants and is gradually converted to yellow marrow composed of fat cells. Most long bones of the adult contain yellow marrow rather than red. Medullary bone is simply a continuation of cancellous bone and is the central area filled with marrow, blood, and lymph vessels.

### Nerve and Blood Supply

Because bone is a living tissue, nutrients must be supplied and waste material removed. Total bone blood flow has been estimated at from 200 to 400 mL per minute.[9]

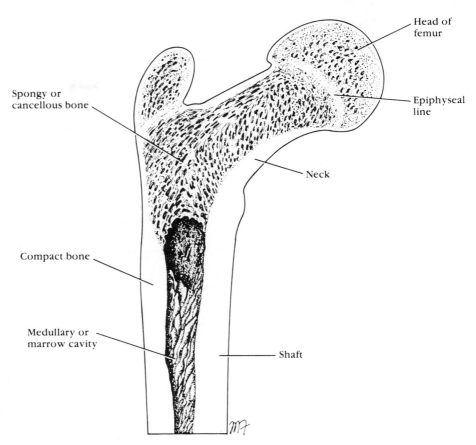

Head of femur

Epiphyseal line

Spongy or cancellous bone

Neck

Compact bone

Medullary or marrow cavity

Shaft

**FIGURE 45–3.**
Bone structure. Note the differences in the three forms of bone structure: spongy, compact, and medullary. (Source: R.S. Snell, *Clinical Histology for Medical Students*. Boston: Little, Brown, 1984.)

Small bones usually have a single artery and vein entering them, and large bones have several. The chief artery, which enters near the middle of the shaft of long bones, is called the *principal nutrient artery* (see Figure 45-1E). After piercing the shaft and reaching the medullary canal, it branches into ascending and descending branches and ends in sinusoidal capillaries. The artery and its branches supply the marrow and cortex, as well as the haversian systems.

Nerve supply to bone is sparse and present mainly in the outer layer, the periosteum. It consists of both afferent (sensory) and sympathetic fibers, with the autonomic fibers accompanying and controlling the dilatation of bone blood vessels.

## Types of Bones

Most commonly, bones are classified as long, short, flat, and irregular. Table 45-1 defines common anatomic terms.

### Long Bones

Long bones are the bones of the extremities and are elongated in shape. Each one consists of the following:

two epiphyses, or ends, which are knobby areas containing cancellous bone; the diaphysis, which composes the shaft or long portion; and the metaphysis, which contains the epiphyseal plate and newly formed bone. In the adult, the metaphysis and epiphysis are continuous.

The outer and inner surfaces of bone are covered with specialized connective tissue. The dense, white, fibrous membrane wrapping the outside is called the *periosteum* and is composed of two layers. The outer layer, or fibrous layer, has relatively few cells and is made up of fibrous tissue. The inner layer of the periosteum is very vascular and has an osteogenic function. Lining the marrow and haversian cavities as well as the spaces of spongy bone is a membrane called the *endosteum*. In addition to supplying a site of attachment for tendons and ligaments, the periosteum is richly supplied with nerves and blood vessels that are important in nourishing the bone. Long bones form most of the appendicular skeleton, such as the femur, humerus, and phalanges (Figure 45-4).

### Short Bones

Short bones, such as those in the wrist, are cube-shaped and consist of cancellous bone enclosed in a thin case of compact bone. These often are combined with other short bones.

**TABLE 45-1.**

ANATOMIC TERMS IN COMMON USE FOR BONES

| TERM | DEFINITION |
|---|---|
| Process | General term for any bony prominence |
| Spine or spinous process | Sharp prominence |
| Tubercle | Rounded prominence on a bone |
| Tuberosity | Protuberance on a bone |
| Trochanter | Large process (eg, below the neck of the femur) |
| Crest | Ridge or linear prominence (eg, iliac crest) |
| Condyle | Rounded protruding mass that carries an articular surface (eg, knuckle) |
| Head | The top, beginning, or most prominent part (eg, enlargement beyond the constricted part as in the femoral head) |
| Sinus | Cavity within a bone |
| Foramen | Hole or opening in a bone |
| Axial skeleton | The 80 bones composing the skull, vertebral column, sternum, and ribs |
| Appendicular skeleton | The 126 lower bones composing the upper and lower extremities |
| Proximal | Near the origin of the limb |
| Distal | Away from the origin of the limb |
| Medial | Nearer to the midline of the body |
| Lateral | Farther from the midline of the body |

## Flat Bones

The bones of the skull, ribs, scapulae, and sternum are examples of flat bones. Their function is largely protective. They consist of two plates of hard compact bone covering a thin layer of cancellous bone. These bones, especially the ribs and sternum, are important sites for blood formation.

## Irregular Bones

Bones that are irregular in shape are similar in composition to the short bones. The vertebrae and the ossicles of the ears are examples of irregular bones.

## Bone Growth and Factors Affecting Bone Growth

### Location of Bone Growth

The epiphyses of a long bone are separated from the shaft by the epiphyseal plate, which is responsible for the longitudinal growth of bone. On the distal side of this plate, osteoblasts are constantly secreting the bone matrix, which immediately becomes ossified, increasing the length of the bone. At the same time, on the proximal side of the epiphyseal plate, new cartilage is being formed. During puberty, ossification exceeds cartilage formation. Gradually the cartilaginous epiphyseal plate becomes completely ossified, and linear bone growth ceases. Epiphyseal closure occurs about 3 years earlier in women than it does in men, in whom bone length ceases to increase at about age 20 years.[9]

As bones grow longitudinally, they also increase in circumference. Osteoblasts on the inner surface of the periosteum deposit layers of new bone, while osteoclasts in the area next to the medullary cavity make the canal larger to fit the larger bone. Bone activity does not stop when a person reaches puberty. Throughout life, bone continues to form and reabsorb in a process called *remodeling*. In the young adult, approximately one-sixth of total skeletal calcium is turned over every year, but when a person reaches the fourth or fifth decade of life, reabsorption begins to outpace formation. Thus, after age 40, 0.5% to 1.0% of the total skeletal mass is lost yearly, with a great amount of individual variation.[11] Remodeling is influenced by many factors, including calcium and phosphorus metabolism, hormones, and the environment.

### Calcium, Phosphorus, and Parathyroid Hormone

The exact mechanism that causes calcium to deposit and new bone to form remains a mystery. Certain nutritional, endocrine, and environmental states must exist, however, for the process to occur in an orderly fashion.

For new bone to form, adequate amounts of calcium and phosphorus must be present in the plasma and interstitial fluid that bathes the osteoblasts. These critical the feces and, to a lesser extent, in urine.[13] Despite this large amount of calcium movement into and out of the body, the serum calcium level remains constant at about 10 mg/dL. The serum pH and albumin levels affect the amount of calcium in the blood.[13] Approximately one-half of circulating calcium is bound to serum albumin, but this calcium can be released when the serum pH drops.[24] The constancy of extracellular fluid calcium is also maintained by vitamin D, parathyroid hormone, and calcitonin (see p. 858).

Phosphorus is a major component of bone and also is involved in many metabolic processes. Serum levels of phosphorus vary according to intake, blood pH, and other factors. Serum samples are accurate only if drawn in the fasting state.[13] Phosphorus is efficiently absorbed by the intestines, and its excretion is regulated by the proximal tubules of the kidney nephrons.[13] If the renal capacity for excreting phosphorus is impaired, hyperphosphatemia results and there is an associated decrease in ionized serum calcium levels (see Chap. 38).[3]

In the diet, calcium and phosphate are supplied mainly by milk and meats. Phosphate is absorbed with calcium. When calcium is absorbed in abundance, so is phosphate. Excess phosphate is excreted along with excess calcium in the feces and urine.

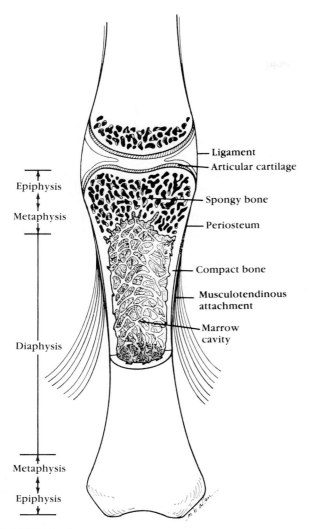

**FIGURE 45–4.**
A long bone and some of its relationships. (Source: M. Borysenko, et al., *Functional Histology* [2nd ed.]. Boston: Little, Brown, 1984.)

amounts are thought to be maintained in part by a partial membrane formed by osteoblasts. This membrane acts as a barrier between bone fluid and the extracellular fluid of the body (Figure 45-5).[9] The osteoblasts connect with other osteocytes deep in the bone where calcium can move into and out of the cell. Calcium salts precipitate on the surface of collagen fibers at periodic intervals. The initial calcium salts are a mixture of calcium and phosphate that become *hydroxyapatite crystals* through a process of resorption and reprecipitation, or substitution and addition of atoms.[10] Hydroxyapatite crystals ($Ca_{10}[PO_4]_6[OH]_2$) provide the crystalline structure of bone mineralization.

With a normal diet, a person takes in approximately 1000 mg of calcium, of which 300 mg is absorbed by the intestines into the bloodstream. From there it goes to the extracellular fluid, and some of it is returned to the intestinal tract through bile and pancreatic enzymes. A large amount of the daily calcium intake is excreted in

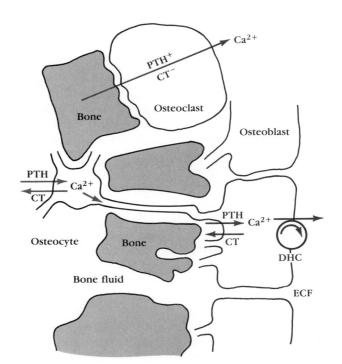

**FIGURE 45–5.**
Parathyroid hormone (PTH) increases and calcitonin (CT) decreases the permeability of bone cells to calcium, whereas 1,25-dihydroxycholecalciferol (DHC) facilitates the active transport of calcium from osteoblasts into extracellular fluid (ECF). (Source: W.F. Ganon, *Review of Medical Physiology* [12th ed.]. Los Altos, CA: Lange, 1985.)

When the serum calcium ion concentration is high, production of *parathyroid hormone (PTH)* is severely curtailed. This results in a lowered serum calcium level (see Chap. 38). Conversely, when serum calcium levels are lowered, parathyroid hormone secretion increases, which expands vitamin D activity and absorption of calcium in the intestinal tract. Parathyroid hormone promotes the formation of osteoclasts and retards the production of osteoblasts. The net result is increased reabsorption of bone, which causes the short-term effect of elevating serum calcium levels. Parathyroid hormone increases renal tubular reabsorption of calcium and decreases the reabsorption of phosphate ions.

## Vitamin D

Vitamin D is a steroid hormone that is taken in the diet and is formed in the skin by the action of the untraviolet rays of the sun. Vitamin D is designated as vitamins $D_2$ and $D_3$ according to their structural side chains, but they are metabolized identically and have equivalent biologic potencies.[13] For dietary vitamin D to be absorbed, bile must be present. Through a series of events in the liver and kidneys, vitamins $D_2$ and $D_3$ are converted to 1,25-dihydroxycholecalciferol $(1,25[OH]_2D_3)$, which is the active form of the vitamin. Other metabolites are formed in the complex conversions that take place, but only 1,25(OH)D is thought to have major physiologic action.[13] It affects serum calcium principally by controlling the absorption of calcium by the gut. The feedback mechanism involves increased PTH, increased production of $1,25(OH)_2D_3$, and increased calcium absorption from the ileum.[13] Vitamin D also increases calcium resorption in the kidney nephrons.[26] Renal failure depresses the reabsorption of calcium by the kidneys as well as curtailing the production of $1,25(OH)_2D_3$. In renal failure, vitamin D is virtually ineffective because of a decrease in the intestinal absorption of calcium.

Parathyroid hormone production increases when serum calcium levels drop, which increases 1,25-dihydroxycholecalciferol formation by the kidneys and leads to increased calcium absorption. These negative feedback mechanisms are important in ensuring an optimal amount of calcium and phosphate in the plasma. Lack of either calcium or active vitamin D over a period of time can alter bone formation and cause loss of bone mass.

## Calcitonin

Calcitonin is a hormone that is produced and secreted by parafollicular cells of the thyroid gland. The major stimulus for release of calcitonin is hypercalcemia, but its role in normal bone and kidney physiology is unclear.[13,21]Its immediate effect is to reduce bone reabsorption by decreasing osteoclast activity and increasing osteoblast activity. A more prolonged effect is to reduce the quantity of osteoclasts formed from the mesenchymal stem cells. Calcitonin does not significantly alter serum calcium levels in the adult; its effect is more significant in children, who have a more rapid rate of bone remodeling. Calcitonin has been administered in Paget's disease to reduce the rapid rate of bone turnover.[13] Increased calcitonin secretion is triggered by an increase in plasma calcium levels. The resulting decrease in serum calcium levels provides a second feedback mechanism for the control of blood calcium.

## Sex Hormones

*Estrogen* has an osteoblast-stimulating action. At puberty, a young girl has a rapid growth spurt before the epiphyseal plates close, which is attributed to estrogen. When growth plates close, girls stop growing, and this occurs a few years before their male counterparts on the average. Throughout the premenopausal period, estrogen promotes bone formation by increasing intestinal absorption of calcium and phosphorus and increasing calcitonin production. In the postmenopausal woman, osteoporosis can be caused by the lack of estrogen (see Chap. 56).

*Testosterone* in the boys and men increases bone length and thickness, and at the same time enhances epiphyseal closure. A decline in testosterone in the elderly man also can lead to osteoporosis.

## Growth Hormone

The anterior lobe of the pituitary gland secretes the growth hormone (somatotropin), which causes a linear increase in long bones by increasing cartilage formation, widening the epiphyseal plates, and increasing the amount of matrix laid down in the ends of the long bones (see Chap. 36). An excess of growth hormone in the growing person can cause gigantism. In the adult, whose epiphyseal plates are closed, the characteristic bone and soft tissue deformities of acromegaly result. Pituitary insufficiency can result in dwarfism in the child.

## Weight Bearing

It has long been observed that muscles atrophy and bones demineralize when a limb is immobilized. Weightlessness experienced by astronauts was noted to cause loss of bone calcium and bone weakness.[6] Physical compression stimulates osteoblastic deposition, probably by generating an electrical potential. This potential at the compression site stimulates osteoblastic activity and increases bone formation. Electrical signals can also stimulate epiphyseal growth. Studies in animals show that increased activity leads to an increase in bone mass, whereas inactivity, especially in growing animals, leads to a decrease in bone mass, decrease in the length and thickness of bones, and irregular articular surfaces and

## BOX 45-1.
### FACTORS THAT AFFECT BONE FORMATION

**FACILITATE BONE FORMATION**
Calcium
Phosphorus
Estrogen
Testosterone
Calcitonin
Vitamins D, A, and C
Growth hormone
Exercise
Insulin
**RETARD BONE FORMATION**
Estrogen/androgen deficiency
Vitamin deficiency
Starvation
Diabetes
Steroids
Inactivity/immobility
Heparin
Excess parathyroid level

epiphyseal lines.[28] Local skeletal mass increases in the bones most used in physical exertions such as playing tennis, weight lifting, and dancing.

### Other Factors

*Glucocorticoids* cause an increase in protein breakdown in all tissues of the body. Because bone matrix is a protein product, an increase in steroids, as in Cushing's disease, can decrease matrix formation and weaken the bones, causing osteoporosis. Steroids also have the specific effect of depressing osteoblastic activity.[10]

As was described earlier, two-thirds of the volume of bone is made up of osteoid organic material. Because all living tissues contain protein, anything that causes a decrease in protein in the body, such as starvation, retards bone formation and enhances bone loss. Lack of vitamins A and C also decreases the ground substance in bone and leads to decreased bone formation. Persons having long-term heparin therapy develop osteoporosis, because heparin apparently speeds up the breakdown of collagen.[16] Insulin increases the ability of the collagen matrix to produce osteoblasts. A summary of factors affecting bone growth is given in Box 45-1.

## NORMAL STRUCTURE AND FUNCTION OF JOINTS

### Types of Joints

Even though individual bones are hard and inflexible, the human body can make graceful, flowing movements. Any motion, whether writing a letter or playing football, is brought about by the simultaneous movement of several *articulations*, or joints. Almost all of the bones of the body are joined to each other in one way or another. Some permit a range of motion and some allow none at all. Joints are classified in several ways, but the most common grouping is according to the degree of movement they permit, as follows: *synarthroses*, immovable; *amphiarthroses*, somewhat movable; and *diarthroses*, freely movable. Joints may also be classified according to the material that connects them; for example, cartilaginous, fibrous, and synovial.

Using the degree of movement classification, the subgroups and their types are described in this section (Figure 45-6). Synarthroses provide little movement, have a rigid surface, and include the bones of the skull. The sutures of the cranial bones are joined together by fibrous tissue and interlocking projections and indentations. These joints are not completed at birth, and an infant has six gaps, or *fontanelles*, between bones. *Synchondrosis*, another type of immovable joint, is cartilage joining two bony surfaces. An example of synchrondrosis is the "joint" between the epiphysis and diaphysis of long bones that disappears after puberty. A third type of synarthrosis is a *gomphosis* (nail), which resembles a peg in a hole; an example is a tooth in the jaw.

Amphiarthroses are joints that permit very limited motion. A *symphysis* is a joint in which the bones are connected by disks of fibrocartilage. Examples are the symphysis pubis and the intervertebral disks between the vertebrae. One can see the benefits of such flexibility of the pelvis in childbirth and in the backbone with any movement. A *syndesmosis* is a slightly movable joint in which the bones are connected by ligaments permitting some bending and twisting; an example is the articulation between the tibia and fibula.

Diarthroses are often called *synovial* joints. They are freely movable and require lubrication to reduce the friction and abrasion that occur when one surface moves on another. The articulating surfaces of the bone are covered by a white, slick hyaline cartilage, and the entire joint is surrounded by an articular capsule that is filled with viscous synovial fluid. The inner layer of this capsule is a slippery, smooth membrane, whereas the outer layer is a tough, fibrous membrane. This inner, or *synovial*, membrane is rich in capillaries and cells, and is composed of secreting and phagocytic cells. The secretory cells produce synovial fluid, which contains water and protein. The glucose level of the fluid is similar to that of serum. The chief function of this fluid is to lubricate and supply nutrients to the cartilage. The excess protein it contains is returned to the blood by way of the lymphatic system that drains the area. Synovial joints are supplied with sensory nerves that cause pain when there is an accumulation of inflammatory cells in the synovial tissues.

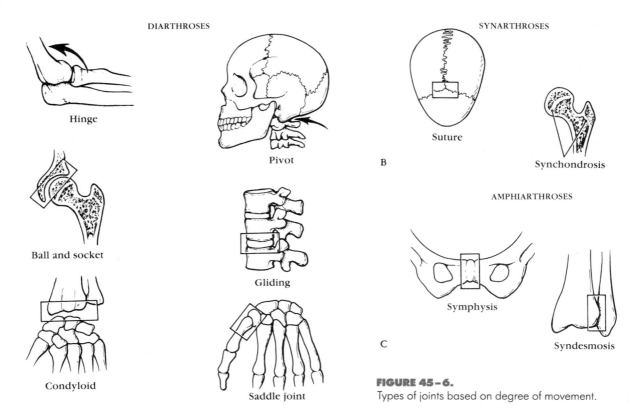

**FIGURE 45–6.**
Types of joints based on degree of movement.

## Classification of Synovial Joints

The synovial joints permit a variety of motion and are classified according to the shape of the articulation and the motion it facilitates. Figure 45-7 illustrates the various movements of major synovial joints. Table 45-2 summarizes joint movements and alteration affects. (See Figure 45-6 for illustration of the location and appearance of the joint types described below.)

## Ball-and-Socket Joints

These joints allow the greatest degree of motion and are formed by a bone fitting into a cup-shaped cavity of another bone. Examples are the hip and shoulder joints.

## Condyloid Joints

An oval-shaped articular surface fits into an elliptical cavity. These joints allow much movement, similar to the ball-and-socket, but abduction and adduction are limited. An example is the wrist between the radius and carpal bones.

## Hinge Joints

This type of joint permits movement in one plane only. The surface of one bone is convex, the other concave, and they fit together smoothly. Examples are the knee, elbow, and finger joints.

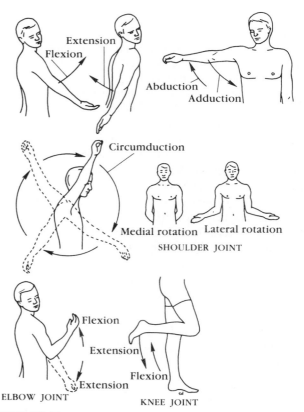

**FIGURE 45–7.**
Some anatomic terms used in relation to movement. (Source: R.S. Snell, *Clinical Anatomy for Medical Students* [2nd ed.]. Boston: Little, Brown, 1981.)

**TABLE 45-2.**
MOVEMENTS OF JOINTS

| JOINT | TYPE OF MOVEMENT | NORMAL MOVEMENTS | EFFECTS OF ALTERATIONS |
|---|---|---|---|
| Vertebral | Diarthrotic (may be classified as synarthrotic, cartilaginous, amphiarthrotic) | Bending, stretching, twisting of entire column; slight movement between vertebrae | Pain when moving or lifting; stiffness; low back pain |
| Clavicular | Diarthrotic | Elevating, protracting, retracting | Pain; inability to move shoulder forward or backward; inability to lift shoulder |
| Shoulder | Diarthrotic (ball-and-socket) | Flexion, extension, abduction; rotation; circumduction of upper arm | Pain; stiffness; immobility; heat; inability to lift objects; cannot bring arm in toward body; range of activity curtailed |
| Elbow | Diarthrotic (hinge-and-pivot) | Flexion, extension; supination of lower arm and hand; pronation of lower arm and hand | Immobility; pain; stiffness; heat; activities of daily living greatly diminished; swelling |
| Wrist | Diarthrotic | Flexion, extension; abduction of hand; adduction of hand | Pain; stiffness; swelling; common complaints of inability to do common activities of daily living such as cooking, opening lids, various grooming activities; may complain of dropping things |
| Hand | Diarthrotic | Flexion, extension, abduction, adduction, circumduction of thumb; thumb and finger apposition; flexion, extension, limited abduction and adduction of fingers; flexion, extension of fingers | Pain; swelling; stiffness; drops objects; deteriorating writing; ability to perform activities of daily living greatly diminished (buttoning clothes, tying knots or bows, combing hair) |
| Hip | Diarthrotic (ball-and-socket) | Flexion; extension; abduction; adduction; rotation; circumduction | Pain; stiffness; immobility; heat; limping; loss of range of motion; inability to put on garments that require lifting the legs; cannot climb stairs |
| Knee | Diarthrotic (hinge) | Flexion; extension; slight tibial rotation | Pain; stiffness; swelling; immobility; limping, falling; redness, swelling; heat |
| Ankle | Diarthrotic (hinge) | Dorsiflexion; plantar flexion | Pain; stiffness; immobility; limping; unusual discomfort with shoes; foot drop |
| Foot | Diarthrotic | Flexion; extension; gliding; inversion; slight abduction, adduction | Pain; stiffness; immobility; avoidance of standing and walking; shoes ill-fitting |

(Source: *Reprinted by permission of J. Moore.*)

## Pivot Joints

Pivot joints allow for rotation and supination and pronation. Examples are the atlas and axis joints of the head and the juncture between the head of the radius and the radial notch of the ulna.

## Saddle Joints

The articular surface of one bone is concave in one direction and convex in another; the other bone is just the opposite, so that the two sides fit together smoothly. An example is the carpometacarpal joint at the base of the thumb.

## Gliding Joints

The bone surfaces are flat or only slightly curved, thus permitting sliding movement in all directions. Examples of this type of joint are the carpal bones of wrist and the intervertebral joints.

Movements of joints may be classified as (1) gliding, producing some bone displacement; (2) angular, in which

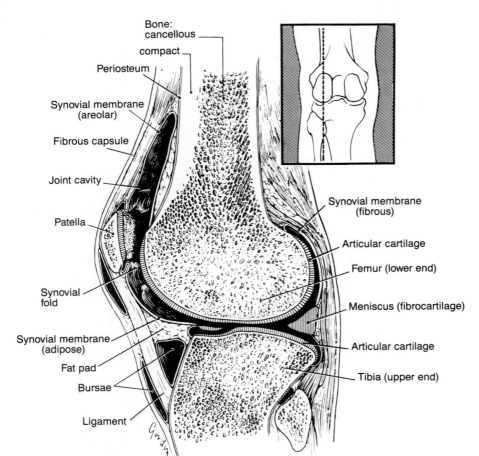

**FIGURE 45–8.**
Diagram of a knee joint cut in the sagittal plane indicated in the inset. (Source: D.H. Cormack, *Histology* [9th ed.]. Philadelphia: J.B. Lippincott, 1987.)

the angle between bones is changed; and (3) rotating, a twisting of a body part.

## Synovial Cavities

The joint capsule consists of an outer fibrous layer called the *fibrous capsule* and an inner layer called the *synovial membrane* (Figure 45-8). Ligaments may be incorporated into the capsule or separated from it by *bursae*, small, flat cavities filled with *synovial fluid*. Synovial fluid is like interstitial fluid except that it contains large quantities of mucopolysaccharides, which account for its viscosity and lubricative qualities.[5] The chief function of bursae is to reduce friction between moving parts.

## Ligaments and Tendons

Ligaments and tendons constitute the connective tissue that hold the body together. There are two types of ligaments, those that connect viscera to each other and those that connect one bone to another.[5] Tendons always connect voluntary muscle to another structure.

Ligaments are composed of distinct bands of connective tissue. Yellow ligaments are elastic (vertebral column) and allow for stretching. White ligaments, such as those in the knee, do not stretch, and they provide stability.

Tendons are actual extensions of muscles and attach muscle to bones or to other tissues. The thick, collagenous tissue has fibers that run in one direction so it can withstand a great deal of pull. These parallel bundles give tendons a glistening, shiny, white appearance. When part of broad and flat muscles, they have the same general appearance, and, similarly, when they are part of a long slender muscle, they are cordlike. The long, hard, cordlike tendons running into the hands and feet have been termed *leaders*. Tendons that cross bones or other tendons are lubricated by a slippery solution similar to synovial fluid that contains hyaluronic acid.[5] Tendons receive sensory fibers from muscle nerves, nearby deep nerves, and overlying superficial nerves. Blood supply to tendons is scarce, and it is for this reason that injured tendons heal slowly.

## FRACTURES AND ASSOCIATED SOFT TISSUE INJURIES

Fractures are most commonly defined as breaks in continuity of bone. They are ruptures of living tissue and

TYPES OF FRACTURE

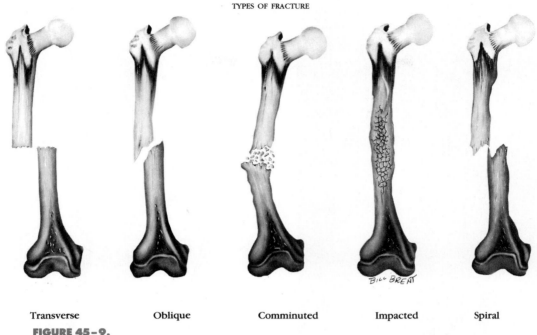

| Transverse | Oblique | Comminuted | Impacted | Spiral |

**FIGURE 45–9.**
Some terms used for different types of fractures. (Source: N. Caroline, *Emergency Care in the Streets* [2nd ed.]. Boston: Little, Brown, 1983.)

normally are the result of trauma, but they may be caused by repeated stress and fatigue (stress fracture) or an underlying disease (pathologic fracture). They may have associated extensive soft tissue damage with hemorrhage into muscles and joints, dislocation and rupture of tendons, nerve damage, and disruption of blood supply. Fractures occur when a force (energy) is imposed on a bone that is greater than it can absorb. Fractures are described in terms of types and directions of fracture lines (Figure 45-9).

## Classification of Fractures

*Simple fractures* do not disrupt the skin overlying the bone. *Compound fractures* break or tear the overlying skin.

Fractures are either *complete*, in which there is complete interruption in the continuity of bone, or *incomplete*, with some part of the bone intact (Figures 45-10 and 45-11). If a bone is broken in such a manner as to produce three or more fragments, it is called *comminuted* (Figure 45-12). An *impacted fracture* is one in which one fragment of bone is imbedded in the substance of the other. A fracture characterized by crushed bone is called a *compression* fracture and usually involves the spinal column (Figure 45-13). A *depressed fracture*, frequently seen in skull fractures, occurs when the bone is driven inward. Repeated mechanical stress and strain can result in a *stress fracture* (Figure 45-14).

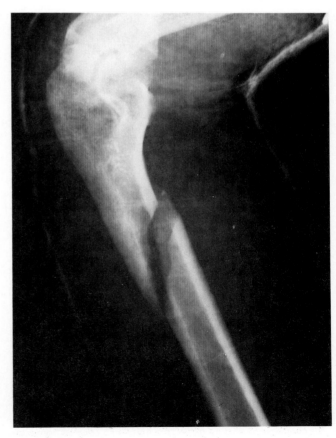

**FIGURE 45–10.**
Complete fracture of the humerus.

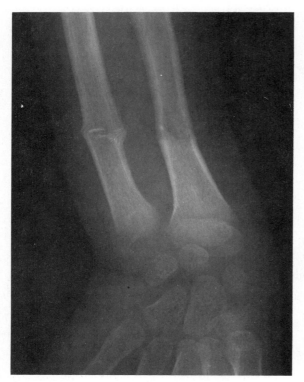

**FIGURE 45–11.**
The greenstick fracture of the radius and ulna usually occurs in children.

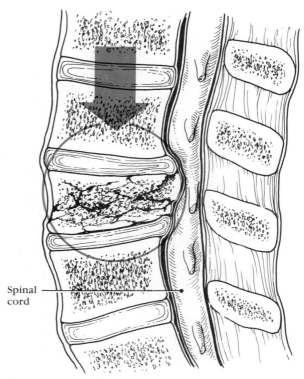

Spinal cord

**FIGURE 45–13.**
Compression fracture in the lumbar vertebrae.

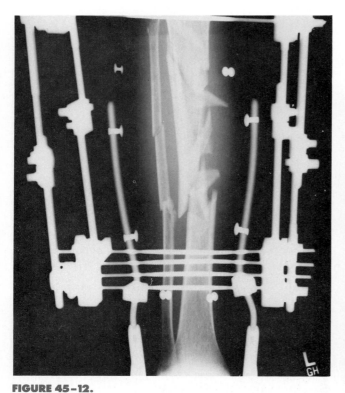

**FIGURE 45–12.**
This comminuted fracture of the tibia and fibula resulted from a direct blow from a car bumper. Radiograph shows the Hoffman apparatus used for treatment.

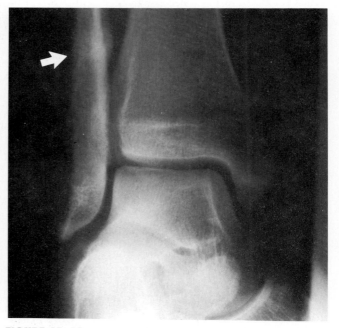

**FIGURE 45–14.**
Stress fracture of the fibula in a distance runner.

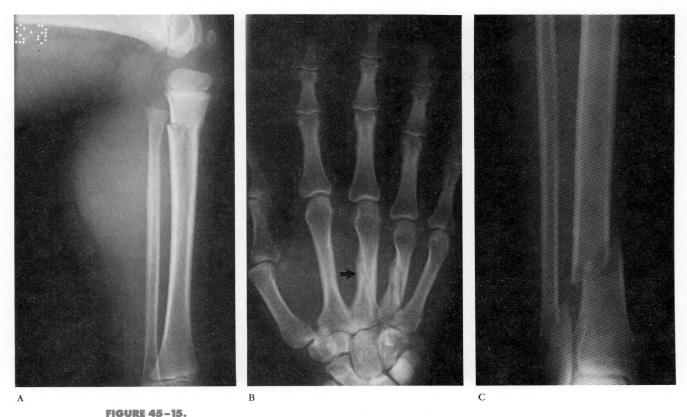

**FIGURE 45-15.**
**A.** Transverse fracture of the tibia. **B.** Oblique fracture of the third and fourth metacarpals. **C.** Spiral fracture of the tibia and fibula.

*Pathologic fractures* occur in diseased bone with little external force or with trivial trauma. Severe twisting or straining may cause a tendon or ligament to pull its bony attachment completely off the main part of the bone, producing an *avulsion* fracture. Fracture lines may be described as longitudinal, transverse, oblique, or spiral (Figure 45-15). Other descriptive terms include *overriding, angulation*, and *displacement* (Figure 45-16).

In general, soft tissue damage is greatest when a direct force is applied over the area, but is usually decreased when the force that breaks the bone is applied distal to the fracture. Table 45-3 lists mechanical forces and the types of fractures that may be associated with them. These relate primarily to the long bones.

## Signs and Symptoms of Fractures

Common signs associated with fractures include local swelling, loss of function or abnormal movement of the affected part, and deformities such as angulation, shortening, or rotation of the part. A *crepitation*, or grating sound, may be produced by bone fragments rubbing together. Pain or local tenderness is normally present. It is not uncommon, however, for local shock to cause complete anesthesia and flaccidity of the area for a period of a few minutes to a half-hour after a fracture. This is due to a temporary loss of nerve function at the site of the fracture. Associated vascular injury causes swelling, pallor, pain or numbness, and pulselessness. When the sharp burning pain becomes a deep throbbing sensation, tissue anoxia is suspected.[19]

## Fracture Healing

It normally takes a good deal of force to break a bone, and there is often associated soft tissue damage. Once a fracture has occurred, blood vessels and periosteum rupture, and blood seeps into the fracture site. This is called the *fracture hematoma*, which develops within 48 to 72 hours after injury. This hematoma surrounding the fracture site provides a loose fibrin mesh in which fibroblasts and capillary buds form a granulation tissue that replaces the blood clot. Osteoblasts and chondroblasts become active in forming new bone and cartilage, which within a week are dispersed throughout the soft tissue callus. This temporary bony union is called a provisional or primary union or *procallus*.[8,19] The procallus creates a balloon or collar over the fracture site and extends well past it. As healing continues, a *bridging external callus* is formed. New bone spicules proliferate as mineral salts

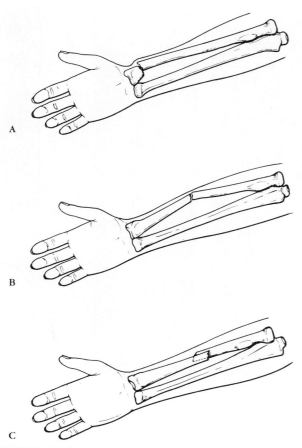

**FIGURE 45–16.**
Descriptive terms indicating types of fractures. **A.** Displacement.
**B.** Angulation. **C.** Overriding.

are laid down. The late medullary callus appears to be responsible for the slow growth of new bone across a fracture gap.[8] As the gap in fractured bone is bridged and fracture fragments become united, mature bone begins to replace the callus.[8] The excess callus already laid down is reabsorbed by the osteoclasts. The fracture site be-

**TABLE 45–3.**
MECHANICAL FORCES AND RELATED FRACTURES
OF LONG BONES

| FORCE | RESULTING FRACTURE |
| --- | --- |
| Twisting | Spiral |
| Angulation | Transverse |
| Angulation with axial compression | Transverse with separate triangular piece (butterfly) |
| Twisting, angulation, and compression | Short oblique |
| Direct blow | Transverse |
| Crushing blow | Comminuted |

comes firm in about 3 to 4 months, and radiographs show united bone (Figure 45-17).

The remodeling process is controlled by the weight-bearing and muscle stresses put on the bone. Through the processes of formation and resorption, bone returns to an architecturally sound state. *Wolff's law* describes a feedback system in which local instability stimulates bone formation and lack of stress stimulates bone reabsorption.[26] If aligned correctly, a simple bone fracture resumes an almost normal appearance within a period of 1 year (Figure 45-18).

## Conditions That Modify Healing

Because fracture healing is a continuous, sequential process, any interruption may modify the final result. This may be due to inadequate immobilization, poor blood supply, distraction of fragments, interposition of soft tissue, or infection.

When the bone is completely transected, *immobilization* is required to hold the fracture fragments rigidly in place. Any movement of the fragments could rupture the fracture hematoma. This reverses and thus prolongs the healing process because bleeding into the fracture site recurs. Immobilization is the first line of defense in ensuring a solid union.

A poor *blood supply* to the traumatized area can impair the healing process. All tissues of the body need nutrition provided through the bloodstream to maintain life. For the surrounding soft tissue and bones to heal, the blood supply must be adequate to provide the needed nutrition.

*Position* or *apposition* also can affect healing. *Distraction* describes a situation in which the fracture fragments are pulled apart from each other so that there is no bony contact. This may be caused by skeletal traction applied to align fragments or by muscle pull on individual fractures. If great enough, distraction may cause excessive tension on the capillaries and decrease the vital blood supply. An increased fracture gap must be bridged with granulation tissue, which increases healing time. When the healing time is increased, the chance of nonunion also increases. Distraction also is associated with the complication of separation of the fracture fragments by soft tissue that seals off the surface of one or both bones. This is known as *interposition of soft tissue*. If one or both of the fragments become covered with soft tissue, the hematoma is unable to form, and growth of granulation tissue is inhibited. This leads to a poor osseous union (Figure 45-19).

Compound fractures open internal structures to various microorganisms; therefore, *infection* becomes the major complication of bone healing. The open area is a rich culture medium for infection in the tissues and also for osteomyelitis (Figure 45-20). Osteomyelitis retards

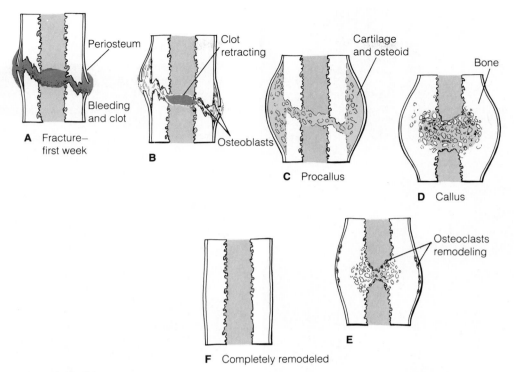

**FIGURE 45–17.**

Healing of a fracture. **A.** Immediately after fracture, blood seeps into the area and a hematoma forms. **B.** After 1 week, osteoblasts begin to form as clot retracts. **C.** After about 3 weeks, a procallus begins to form and stabilize the fracture. **D.** From 6 to 12 weeks, a callus forms with bone cells. **E.** In 3 to 4 months, osteoclasts begin to remodel the fracture site. **F.** With normal apposition, the bone will be completely remodeled in 12 months.

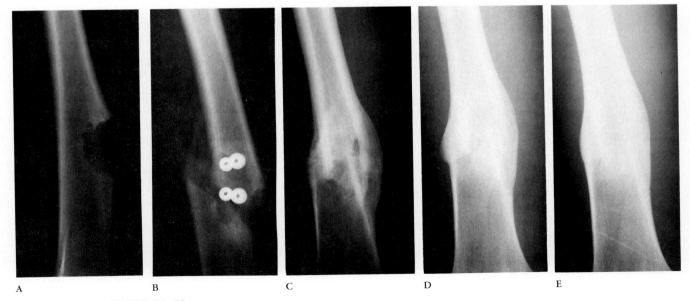

**FIGURE 45–18.**

The sequence of bone healing and remodeling is demonstrated in a 13-year-old bone with a chondromyxoid that was removed surgically. **A.** Initial appearance. **B.** Repaired pathologic fracture 1 month later. **C.** A procallus forms. **D.** Osteogenesis. **E.** Bone remodeling.

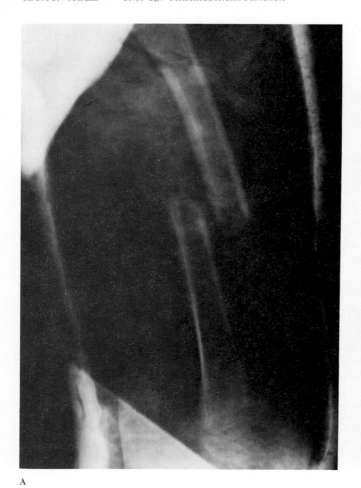

A

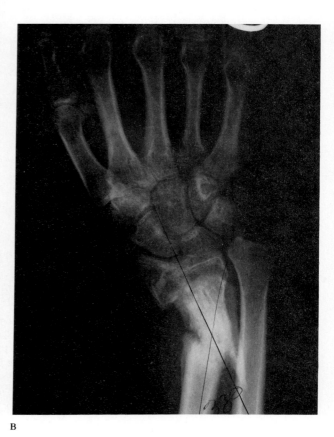

B

**FIGURE 45–19.**
**A.** Loss of apposition in this fractured femur increases the likelihood of soft tissue interposition and delayed union or nonunion. **B.** Malunion of the radius due to poor alignment during healing.

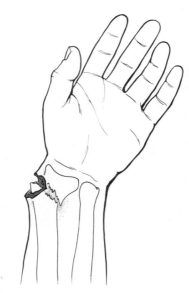

**FIGURE 45–20.**
Compound fracture of radius with surrounding soft tissue damage.

healing by destroying newly forming bone and interrupting its blood supply (see below).

*Delayed union* is a term used to denote an increased healing time. Although each person heals at a different pace, the average time needed to completely heal a fracture is generally consistent. A delayed union normally results from a breakdown in the early stages of healing; that is, inadequate immobilization, breakdown in hematoma formation, or poor alignment. Infection at the fracture site delays union, usually until the infectious process is stopped.

*Nonunion* occurs when the fragments fail to unite, usually because of infection and movement. Infection causes continuous bleeding and breakdown of osteoid matrix. Movement at the fracture site causes repeated bleeding episodes and decalcification at the fragment ends; it may cause the fracture gap to increase to such an extent that the ends no longer touch, leading to a permanent nonunion.

*Malunion* is union of the fragments in a position that

modifies function. The wrist fracture in Figure 45-19B was allowed to heal in poor alignment and resulted in shortening of the extremity and alteration of function.

Pulmonary fat emboli can be identified at autopsy in almost all persons dying soon after fractures of the long bones or pelvis. These may or may not have participated in the death of the individual.[6] The so-called *fat embolism syndrome* probably has multiple mechanisms of causation. These include chemical injury to the pulmonary vasculature and release of fat deposits from the stores in the fractured long bones. The clinical picture, although not clearly understood, involves the onset of the adult respiratory distress syndrome (ARDS) 24 to 72 hours after the traumatic event. Activation of cogaulation and the resultant disseminated intravascular coagulation (DIC) often complicates the picture, and it is not known if the DIC is directly related to the fat embolism (see Chap. 21 for a discussion of DIC). The cerebral edema and microembolic fat in the brain circulation are common, but, again, their source is not well understood.[6]

Because fat emboli also occur in persons with other conditions, other theories have emerged as to their cause. With any stress, catecholamines are released, mobilizing fatty acids and neutral fats into the bloodstream. These become coated with platelets to form larger emboli. Free fatty acids in the bloodstream have been noted to have a toxic effect on the capillaries, causing them to become blocked. The person experiences chest pain and sudden respiratory difficulty. A low-grade fever, mental confusion, petechiae, and fat globules in the urine support the diagnosis.[4,8]

### Alteration in Nerve Function Due to Bone Trauma

Soft tissue injuries such as laceration of a major artery, the insidious compartment syndrome, disabling tendon avulsion, and serious visceral injury are associated with fractures. These may be the primary focus of treatment in the emergency phase.

Sometimes a fracture causes an injury to adjacent structures. The fragments may rupture and compress nerves that may also be damaged by dislocation or direct trauma. Injuries of the axillary, radial, and peroneal nerves are described as *compartmental syndromes* (see below).

The axillary nerve may be damaged by fractures or dislocations around the shoulder or by penetrating wounds and direct blows. The axillary nerve is composed of C5 and C6 fibers and is a branch of the posterior cord of the brachial plexus. It emerges at the level of the humerus head and winds around the neck of the humerus. It supplies the deltoid and teres minor muscles. The deltoid muscle is used as an abductor for the shoulder; therefore, inability to abduct the shoulder indicates damage to the axillary nerve.

The radial nerve is commonly injured in spiral fractures of the humerus. It may be completely severed, impaled on a fractured fragment, or entrapped between the fragments. Lacerations of the arm and proximal forearm, and gunshot wounds are also common causes of radial nerve injury. Temporary nerve damage may also result from direct pressure from using crutches or hanging an arm on the back of a chair. The radial nerve is composed of the fibers from some of the cervical spinal nerves (C5, C6, C7, and C8) and, sometimes, the thoracic spinal nerve, T1. It is primarily a motor nerve that innervates the biceps, supinates the forearm, and extends the wrist, fingers, and thumb. Therefore, injury usually results in inability to extend the elbow or supinate the forearm. A typical wrist drop occurs that includes inability to extend the fingers. Complete return of function can be expected in most persons with temporary nerve damage. In others, function may not return for as long as 3 months to a year. When function does not return, surgery is usually indicated. However, the radial nerve has a greater ability to regenerate than all other large nerves. This is probably because the radial nerve is primarily a motor nerve that is involved mainly in gross muscle movements.

Peroneal nerves are classified as common, superficial, and deep. The common peroneal nerve emerges from the popliteal fossa and encircles the fibula neck. Damage may be the result of a direct blow; for example, a baseball bat hitting the fibula head with or without the presence of fractures. The result is a foot drop deformity in which the foot returns to normal in a few hours if the nerve is not ruptured.

### Compartmental Syndromes

Compartmental syndromes are uncommon complications of fractures and affect primarily the forearm and tibia. They are generally referred to as *Volkmann's ischemia* or *anterior tibial compartmental syndromes*. Volkmann's ischemia (volar compartmental syndrome) usually is related to the common supracondylar fracture of the humerus in children. Fracture of the tibia is common in anterior compartmental syndrome. Compartmental syndromes may result from a cast that is placed too tight, from intercompartmental bleeding, and from burns and snake or spider bites.

The compartments of the leg and forearm are composed of bones, muscles, nerves, and other associated structures encapsulated by the fascia and the skin, thus making a closed space (Figure 45-21). When injury occurs, the pressure builds within the compartment due to bleeding and soft tissue reaction. When the swelling reaches a point at which the fascia permits no further outward enlargement, the increasing pressure is directed inward and compresses blood vessels and other components of the compartment. When tissue pressure in-

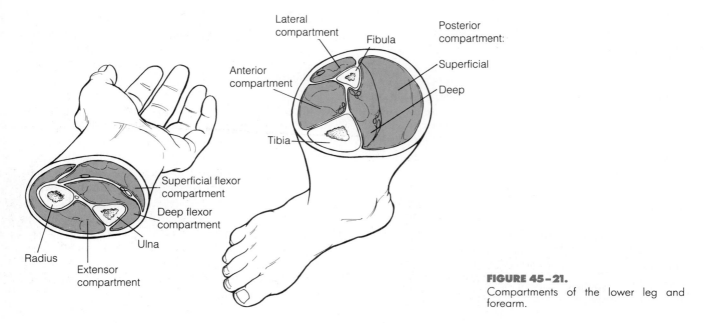

**FIGURE 45-21.**
Compartments of the lower leg and forearm.

creases to equal the diastolic pressure, the microcirculation ceases, although the peripheral pulse is unchanged. Within 30 minutes, damage to nerves begins, and if swelling is allowed to persist for 12 hours, irreversible functional loss occurs. Muscles require an abundant blood supply, and when the microcirculation is severely compromised they become ischemic, with onset of necrosis in 2 to 4 hours, becoming irreversible in 12 hours.

Anterior compartmental syndrome is heralded by pain in the anterior aspect of the tibia, paresthesia over the distribution of the deep peroneal nerve, and pain on passive dorsiflexion of the toes. The area appears swollen and blisters may develop on the skin. If the syndrome is allowed to proceed unchecked, paralysis, anesthesia, contractures, foot drop, and gangrene may develop, which in turn may lead to loss of the limb.

Volkmann's ischemia produces a disturbing contracture if untreated. Pain is the predominant symptom; it is referred to the palmar area and is exacerbated on passive extension of fingers. Some degree of sensory loss in the fingers occurs in the early stages. Contractures (clawlike deformities of the hand), wrist drop, and paralysis then result.

## Other Associated Soft Tissue Traumas

Tendons may also be damaged by fractures. When ligaments and tendons are involved in fractures, avulsion fractures may result. Damage to the extensor tendon of the distal phalanx can serve as an example. When a fracture occurs, it avulses (pulls apart) a small piece of bone to which the tendon is attached, leading to the inability to extend the distal phalanx. If left untreated, a mallet

deformity may result. A dysfunction of the bony attachment may occur in tendon damage that is left untreated.

*Visceral damage*, or damage to internal organs, may also occur from fractures. Examples include fracture of the pelvis in which the bladder is ruptured, and rib fractures causing perforation of the lung.

## ALTERATIONS IN CONNECTIVE TISSUE DEVELOPMENT

### Osteogenesis Imperfecta

Osteogenesis imperfecta is a group of hereditary disorders in which defective connective tissue formation leads to extremely fragile bones. The disorders have various severity of bone, eye, ear, dental, and cardiovascular involvement.[25] Different types are described, some of autosomal dominant inheritance and some of autosomal recessive.[25] The bones of the skull and face may be poorly ossified, with numerous fractures occurring in the long bones (Figure 45-22).[25] The skeletal aspect of this condition is a hereditary form of osteoporosis. Some types have few fractures but exhibit any combination of blue sclerae, deafness, short stature, joint dislocation, and opalescent teeth.[25] In severe cases, death of the infant during childbirth may occur due to trauma to the brain, which is relatively unprotected by the soft, membranous skull.

### Marfan's Syndrome

Marfan's syndrome is an autosomal dominant inheritance disorder characterized by abnormal body proportions

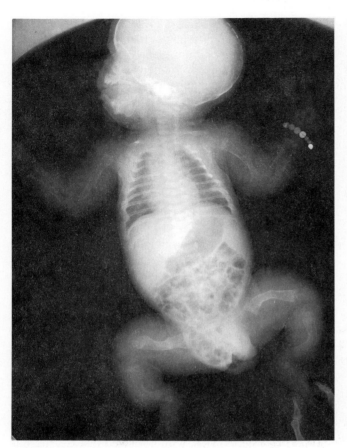

**FIGURE 45–22.**
Classic example of osteogenesis imperfecta in an infant. Diffuse osteoporosis with bone deformities of the extremities and pathologic fractures of the humeri, femora, and ribs.

with long arms, long digits, thoracic deformity such as pectus excavatum, curvature of the thoracic spine, and hyperextensibility of the joints.[25] Associated connective tissue defects result in dilatation and dissection of the aorta along with aortic insufficiency (see Chap. 25).

## Osteopetrosis (Marble Bones, or Albers-Schönberg Disease)

Osteopetrosis is a familial disease characterized by overgrowth and sclerosing of bone. Although the bones are heavy and thick, they tend to break rather than bend, and fractures often occur. When this disease is due to a recessive trait, it is called *malignant osteopetrosis* and can cause death *in utero* or in early life. The autosomal dominant trait causes less severe problems that may not be diagnosed until adulthood.[22]

Pathologic changes include an increase in cortical bone to nearly twice its normal density, with the growth almost exclusively endochondral. Crowding of the marrow cavity, often with complete marrow obliteration, re-

sults. The cause of the condition is a hereditary defect in osteoclast function with a resultant decrease in bone resorption.[4] Signs and symptoms of the disease relate to the skeletal malformations and the defects in hematopoiesis. Optic nerve impingement due to failure of modeling of the skull can result in blindness. Deafness can occur due to overgrowth of bone in the middle and inner ear. Cranial nerve palsies, nystagmus, and hydrocephalus may also be present. The teeth usually erupt late and develop cavities early; osteomyelitis of the jaw often develops. Anemia can be profound due to the small marrow spaces, and the enlarged liver and spleen are sources of extramedullary hematopoiesis. As in osteogenesis imperfecta, treatment is palliative, but children who reach adulthood can look forward to a relatively normal life span.

## IDIOPATHIC ALTERATIONS IN BONE

### Paget's Disease

As early as 1877, Sir James Paget described a disease of chronic bone inflammation that caused softening and bowing of the long bones. Paget's disease existed in ancient times, as shown by the study of bones in archaeologic collections. Evidence of the disease has been found in the skulls of American Indians and even Neanderthals.

The disease is rare in persons under 40 years of age, and men and women are equally affected. The frequency of the disease has ranged statistically from 3% to 4% of the population.[22] The figures include subclinical cases in which the disease was discovered microscopically on autopsy. The possible causes are many, but no exact etiology has been defined. Paget himself thought it was due to a chronic infection, and he called the disease *osteitis deformans*. Virus causation has been investigated, with antigens identical to the respiratory syncytial virus (RSV) and the measles virus identified.[6] Latent or slow virus causation is an appealing theory, but no virus has yet been isolated from affected tissue.[10] The disease occurs late in life, which allows time for a long period of latency. Other etiologic possibilities include hormonal dysfunction, autoimmune states, vascular disorders, and neoplastic disease.

Pathologically, Paget's disease is characterized by reabsorption of bone followed by rapid overgrowth, a phenomenon that can occur in different stages in the same person and even in the same bone. The histologic features are usually described in phases. The initial, osteolytic or destructive, phase is marked by extensive reabsorption of existing bone, with the presence of numerous multinucleated osteoclasts.[27] The mixed or active phase occurs when the osteoclasts destroy the ordered lamellar bone and osteoblasts respond to the destruction by rapid disposition of vascular connective tissue and remodeled lamellar bone. During this phase, the area appears to be highly vascular, with cement lines forming at sites where the lamellae are erratically joined, giving a mosaic appearance that may completely replace the preexisting bone.[6] The osteoblastic or sclerotic phase occurs when bone formation outstrips resorption, with lamellar bone as the predominant ingredient. Bone size and thickness are increased primarily in the head, femurs, humeri, and scapulae. This bone is soft, poorly mineralized, and subject to fractures. In individuals with widespread disease, almost every bone may be affected.[17]

The clinical features progress slowly and bone deformities can be considered part of the normal aging process. The condition is usually polyostotic (affecting more than one bone). The long bones of the legs become bowed and the pelvis misshapen. The thorax shortens, causing a loss of height. The bones of the skull are often affected, leading to symptoms of vertigo, headache, and progressive deafness due to compression of the eighth nerve. In the early stages of disease, pain in the affected bones may be experienced. Increased vascularity of the rebuilding bone, together with cutaneous vasodilatation, can produce warmth over affected bone, requiring an increase in cardiac output. Laboratory studies characteristically show elevation in levels of alkaline phosphatase that generally correlate with the extent of the process.[17] Roentgenographic appearance of the bone shows radiolucency with areas of density (Figure 45-23).

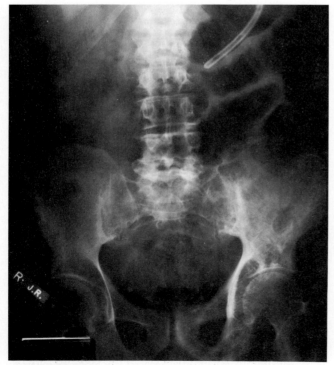

**FIGURE 45-23.**
Paget's disease of bone. Punched-out areas in the acetabular cavity, iliac wing, and ischial and pubic rami represent areas of resorption and remodeling that occur simultaneously.

No cure exists for Paget's disease, but newer therapies use calcitonin and diphosphates to inhibit osteoclastic activity.[20] Etidronate disodium, given orally, decreases bone reabsorption, and improvement may last for 6 months or more following discontinuation of therapy.[17] Mithramycin, a drug used in cancer therapy, may also be effective for patients with severe disease.[17] This suggests that the etiology is a virus-induced neoplastic process.

## von Recklinghausen's Disease

Osteitis fibrosa cystica, or von Recklinghausen's disease of the bone, is characterized by progressive resorption and destruction of bone brought about by long-standing hyperparathyroidism. Parathyroid hormone (PTH) excretion causes calcium and phosphorus to be removed from bone. Hyperplasia or neoplasia of the parathyroid glands may cause a hypersecretion of this hormone and thus demineralization of bone. Secondary hyperparathyroidism, as in chronic renal insufficiency, leads to decreased conversion of vitamin D to its active form in the kidneys and decreased absorption of calcium in the intestine. The low serum calcium level stimulates PTH secretion (see Chap. 38).

In the early stages of both primary and secondary hyperparathyroidism, changes in bone resemble osteomalacia or osteoporosis. With advanced disease, there is osteoclastic resorption of bone, which is replaced by fibrous tissue in the marrow spaces. The cancellous and cortical bones undergo thinning with resultant deformities. In focal areas of bone resorption, large fibrous scars develop, yielding minute to very large cysts, called *brown tumors*. These nonmalignant granulomas receive their brownish color from degeneration and hemorrhage into the site. Because of earlier diagnosis and treatment, only 10% to 15% of persons with primary hyperparathyroidism have significant skeletal changes.[6] Secondary hyperparathyroidism due to renal failure causes only a part of the syndrome of *renal osteodystrophy*, which also includes osteomalacia and osteosclerosis.

## Osteonecrosis

### Osteonecrosis in the Adult

*Osteonecrosis* is synonymous with avascular necrosis, aseptic necrosis, and ischemic necrosis of bone.[28] It has been identified as one of the most common causes of hip pain and incapacity. Table 45-4 lists some associated diseases.

Necrosis of femoral and humeral heads is secondary to various systemic diseases that affect blood supply to the bone. Pathologically the lesions occur primarily in subcortical areas of long bones that have a narrower

## TABLE 45-4.
DISEASES ASSOCIATED WITH OSTEONECROSIS

| ASSOCIATED DISEASE | NUMBER OF PATIENTS |
|---|---|
| Systemic lupus erythematosus | 82 |
| Rheumatoid arthritis | 26 |
| Renal transplant | 14 |
| Hemoglobinopathy | 12 |
| Trauma | 11 |
| Alcoholism | 10 |
| Solid tumors | 5 |
| Hodgkin's disease | 3 |
| Leukemia | 2 |
| Gout | 9 |
| Asthma | 8 |
| Polyarthritis—unknown etiology | 7 |
| Polymyositis/dermatomyositis | 4 |
| Undifferentiated connective tissue disease | 3 |
| Inflammatory bowel disease | 4 |
| Giant cell arteritis/polymyalgia rheumatica | 3 |
| Arteritis—unspecified | 2 |
| Sarcoidosis | 2 |
| Cushing's syndrome | 2 |
| Systemic sclerosis | 1 |
| Raynaud's disease | 1 |
| Idiopathic thrombocytopenia | 1 |
| Caisson's disease | 1 |
| Gaucher's disease | 1 |
| Juvenile rheumatoid arthritis | 1 |
| Ankylosing spondylitis | 1 |
| Sjögrne's syndrome | 1 |
| Other steroid | 4 |
| Nonassociated diseases | 61 |
| Ischemic necrosis of bone only | 91 |
| | 373 |

(Source: H.R. Schumacher, Primer on the Rheumatic Diseases. *Atlanta: Arthritis Foundation, 1988.*)

capillary circulation than other bones. The initial cause appears to be ischemia, which can be produced by obstruction or compression of the microcirculation.[6] A history of alcoholism has been reported in 10% to 39% of cases. *Traumatic osteonecrosis* usually occurs with impaired blood supply to femoral or humeral heads. *Nontraumatic osteonencrosis* occurs most frequently in persons treated with glucocorticoids, especially persons with systemic lupus erythematosus and renal transplants.[28] The most common symptom is pain on active motion. Pain at rest and at night is also very common. Limitation of motion also occurs as the disease progresses. Radiographic abnormalities may develop from several months to 5 years after pain is described.[28]

## Legg–Calvé–Perthes Disease

*Osteochondrosis* refers to a set of conditions affecting the epiphyseal region of bone in children during the growth period. The pathology is brought about by avascular necrosis in the area that causes the bone of the epiphysis to soften and die (Figure 45-24). Various names have been ascribed to avascular necrosis occurring in specific areas, but *Legg–Calvé–Perthes disease* is the most familiar.[8]

The onset of the condition appears to be growth-related. Until ages 3 and 4, the predominant blood supply to the femoral head comes across the growth plate from the metaphysis of the femur with other supply from the lateral epiphyseal vessels. At about 4 years of age, the growth plate begins to block the metaphyseal blood supply, and full development of the ligament artery supply to the femoral head is reached when a child is 7 or 8 years old. This leaves a period of time when the blood supply to the femoral head is dependent on the lateral epiphyseal vessels.

Precipitating causes of avascular necrosis may be trauma, infections, or inflammation. In the 2- to 4-year course of the disease, three stages occur:

1. Avascular necrosis causes the bone of the femoral head to soften and die, but the cartilage surrounding it, nourished by synovial fluid, remains viable.
2. Blood vessels from adjacent viable tissue grow in through the neck of the femur and begin the slow process of removing dead bone a little at a time, a process called *creeping substitution.*
3. Areas of reabsorbed bone are filled with new bone, and ossification occurs.

All three of these stages—necrosis, removal of dead bone, and reossification—may occur simultaneously within the same bone. Children may complain of aching pain and limited motion early in the disease, but later processes remain painless.

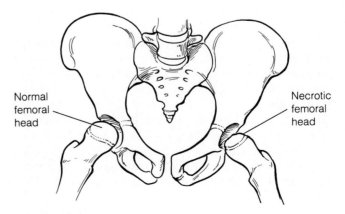

## FIGURE 45-24.
Legg–Calvé–Perthes disease. Flattened femoral head is the result of necrosis. Left femoral head is normal.

## Osgood-Schlatter Disease

Osgood-Schlatter disease usually occurs in boys from 10 to 15 years of age and is characterized by a painful, tender, and enlarged tibial tubercle. It is caused by a pull of the patellar tendon on the tibial tubercle epiphysis, caused by sudden or continuous strain during growth. The condition may not be a true osteochondrosis but may be due to injury.[8] Serial films show changes due to aseptic necrosis that results from avascular changes. As in Legg–Calvé–Perthes disease, pain disappears shortly after onset, but the tibial tubercle may remain enlarged.

## METABOLIC AND NUTRITIONAL BONE ALTERATIONS

### Osteoporosis

Osteoporosis is osteopenia due to reduction in both bone matrix and mineralization. *Osteopenia* is a reduction of bone mass greater than that expected for a given age, race, and sex.[11] It results in brittle bones that fracture quite easily. Because bone remodeling, with reabsorption balanced by formation, normally occurs throughout life, anything that either increases reabsorption or decreases formation causes loss of bone mass. The rate of reabsorption follows the surface-volume mass of bones. Therefore, because the trabeculae are composed of sheets of bone and have more surface volume than cortical bone, they are lost more rapidly. This loss leads to increased frequency of fractures in the weight-bearing bones where trabecular bone predominates. The vertebral bodies, radial head, and femoral neck are examples of this type of bone. Likewise, reabsorption is accelerated on the endosteal surfaces of trabecular bone while formation is occurring at the periosteal surfaces, thus leading to wider bones with a thinner, more porous cortex. The ratio of bone mineral to matrix formation is constant, but there is simply a reduction in both. This contrasts with osteomalacia, in which the matrix is normal but the mineralization is deficient.

Osteoporosis may be caused by genetic, nutritional, mobility, drug-related, hormonal, and age factors. Deficiencies in protein, vitamins C, D, and A, and calcium can lead to reduced matrix and mineralization.[11] Individuals with a family history of fractures due to osteoporosis have a greater risk of developing this condition. Estrogen and testosterone stimulate osteoblastic activity so that the frequency of osteoporosis increases with menopause. Theories suggest that estrogen may antagonize parathyroid hormone, which has a bone-resorption effect. Estrogen may also affect the absorption and excretion of calcium and phosphorus by direct action on the gastrointestinal tract, possibly through enhancing the metabolism of vitamin D.[6] Women with artificially induced menopause seem to develop the disease faster than those with normal, more slowly declining hormonal levels. Androgen deficiency in men also can lead to later onset osteoporosis. Endocrine changes such as diabetes mellitus and thyrotoxicosis, in which protein synthesis is decreased and catabolism is increased, respectively, also cause osteoporosis. Cushing's disease, with its protein catabolic loss, has the same bone results as prolonged steroid therapy. Prolonged therapy with heparin and certain cancer drugs may lead to osteoporosis. Smoking and excess alcohol ingestion increase the incidence of this condition. Irradiation, from radiographs or other exposure to radioactive materials, may affect bone by damage to the osteoblasts. Immobility of a limb and prolonged bed rest can also cause bone loss.

It has been estimated that osteoporosis affects 1 in 4 women over the age of 60. Bone loss begins in women at about age 45 and in men between 50 and 60 years of age.[11] Complications of the disorder, especially hip fractures, make it the 12th leading cause of death in the United States. Death usually results from respiratory complications secondary to immobility. The decline of estrogen after menopause combines with low bone mass to make certain groups of women more prone to the disease. White women tend to have less bone mass than black women, and thin women have less than obese women. Smokers seem to have less bone mass and tend to undergo menopause earlier than nonsmokers. In general, osteoporosis is most frequent in thin, small-built, fair-complexion, freckled, blond women with a sedentary lifestyle.[10]

Hip fractures account for more morbidity than all of the other osteoporotic fractures combined. More than 200,000 women suffer hip fractures in the United States each year.[7] In men, hip fractures are often related to long-term immobility such as after a stroke or head injury. Fractures of the distal forearm are common but rarely cause death. Vertebral fractures, either complete or compression, can occur with a minimal amount of trauma and may cause few symptoms. These vertebrae never regain their normal shape and account for the loss of height and the "dowager's hump" seen in older women and men.

Investigations of the appropriate prevention and treatment of osteoporosis have brought about much study and controversy. Studies suggest that various combinations of estrogen, calcium, vitamin D, and sodium fluoride seem to retard bone loss. These treatments are most effective when begun in the perimenopausal or early postmenopausal woman.[11] Estrogen appears to stop postmenopausal bone loss for as long as it is taken, although it is not without side effects. Calcium intake of 1.5 g/day is recommended either in the diet or as a supplement. In those with vertebral fractures, sodium fluoride induces the formation of new bone and decreases the frequency of other fractures. Vitamin D supplements may retard osteomalacia in the elderly who have deficient diets and minimal sunlight exposure. Studies suggest that regular exercise retards bone loss.[7]

## *Rickets/Osteomalacia*

Rickets is a disease in the infant or growing child that usually is caused by a lack of vitamin D. Osteomalacia, or adult rickets, results from a calcium or phosphorus deficiency, or both. In the United States, Vitamin D deficiency alone is rare in adults. The mineral deficiency can result either from a decrease in calcium absorption or an increase in phosphorus loss by the kidneys. In chronic renal failure, the kidneys are unable to activate vitamin D and excrete phosphate. The accompanying hyperparathyroidism increases bone reabsorption. In elderly individuals, low dietary intake of calcium and vitamin D combined with intestinal malabsorption can decrease bone mineralization.

The primary pathology consists of deficient mineralization of bone with a relative increase in uncalcified osteoid. The normal time required for osteoid calcification is 12 to 15 days, but in osteomalacia, the time interval lengthens to several months.[6] The lack of mineralization makes the bones soft, and they bow and break easily. Because bone formation in the growing child is most accelerated at the ends of the long bones, the epiphyseal tissue in rickets is soft, with the normally sharp, narrow line of ossification replaced by a wide, irregular zone of soft, gray tissue. Bowed legs and deformities of the costochondral junction (rachitic rosary) and thorax (pigeon breast), together with defective tooth enamel are evidence of rickets. In the adult, osteomalacia is displayed by mineral changes and pain in the lumbar vertebrae, pelvic girdle, and long bones of the lower limbs. Fractures occur with only minor trauma. Over time, the mineralization defect leads to decreased bone matrix and a hybrid state of osteomalacia-osteoporosis evolves.[6] Deformities can also occur in adults when the muscles and tendons change the shape of the softened bone.

## *Scurvy*

Vitamin C (ascorbic acid) is necessary for the production of the collagen of fibrous tissue and of bone matrix. A deficiency of vitamin C leads to scurvy, which is characterized by hemorrhages, anemia, and bone and teeth changes. Hemorrhages can occur in any organ and can vary from tiny petechiae to large hematomas. Bone disturbances are evidenced by a defective osteoid and a relative increase in reabsorption over formation. This leads to a decreased density of bone. Bleeding, spongy gums, and loose teeth are common. Scurvy in infants usually does not appear until after 6 months of age, and it takes from 3 months to 1 year of severe vitamin C deficiency to produce scurvy in an adult.

## INFECTIOUS DISEASES OF BONE

### *Osteomyelitis*

Osteomyelitis occurs when the bone and bone marrow are invaded by pyogenic organisms, almost always bacteria.[5] Infection of bone can come about in three ways: (1) through the bloodstream (hematogenous); (2) by extension of a contiguous infection; or (3) by direct surgical or traumatic introduction.[12]

In 60% to 70% of cases, the organism that causes osteomyelitis is hemolytic *Staphylococcus*, although streptococci, coliform bacteria, pneumococci, gonococci, or any bacterial or fungal agent may be involved. Immune suppressed or debilitated persons are at greater risk and may develop infections due to *Salmonella, Pseudomonas, Hemophilus influenzae*, and group B streptococci.[12] The infecting organism enters the bone through the nutrient or metaphyseal vessels and moves into the medullary canal. Vascularity increases, causing edema. Polymorphonuclear leukocytes accumulate in the area. In a few days, thrombosis of local vessels occurs, and ischemia results. Portions of bone tissue die. Pus in this confined space is under pressure and is pushed out through Volkmann's canals to the surface of the bone. It then spreads subperiosteally and can enter the bone at another level, or burst out into the surrounding tissue. In infants, before the epiphyseal cartilage seals off the metaphysis, spread can go directly to the joint and cause a suppurative arthritis. In older persons, if joint involvement does occur, it does so through subperiosteal spread. The dead bone is separated from viable tissue, and granulation tissue forms beneath the area of dead bone and infection. The necrotic bone, isolated from viable tissue, is termed *sequestrum*. New bone forms from the elevated periosteum. This bone, called the *involucrum*, envelopes the granulation tissue and sequestrum. Small sinuses permit the pus to escape.[12]

In chronic osteomyelitis, the granulation tissue becomes scar tissue and forms an impenetrable area around the infection. The localized area of suppuration is called *Brodie's abscess*.[12] A new area of bone develops to isolate the area further. The process is characterized by chronically draining sinuses with organisms that are resistant to antibiotic therapy.

Hematogenous osteomyelitis often follows urinary tract infection, bacterial endocarditis, respiratory infection, or a large soft tissue infection such as a decubitus ulcer. Immune suppressed individuals or those with a chronic disease are at high risk for bacteremias and osteomyelitis. Posttraumatic or spreading osteomyelitis are characterized by erythema, local pain, and draining sinuses. Infection of a joint prosthesis may be seen within a few days after surgery. Loosening of fixative appliances for fractures or prostheses in joint replacement is a typical finding, and radionuclide scans are nearly always positive.

The person with acute osteomyelitis appears acutely ill with fever, chills, and variable degrees of leukocytosis. If the osteomyelitis is in a limb, it becomes very painful. The pain is often described as a constant throbbing. Redness and swelling usually occur over the site, and sensitivity to the touch is characteristic. Radiologic evidence is noted after about 10 days and reflects bone destruction. Blood cultures may or may not be positive for the causative organism; massive antibiotic therapy usually arrests the disease. With vertebral osteomyelitis, blood cultures are usually negative and needle biopsy of infected bone is necessary.[12]

## Tuberculosis

Tuberculosis is a systemic disease caused by the tubercular bacillus, which spreads through the body through lymphatic or hematogenous routes (see Chap. 29). Skeletal involvement is rare now due to adequate therapy, but when it occurs it is often caused by seeding of the bacilli in the marrow cavity. The infection causes destruction of bone tissue and caseous necrosis that may enter the joint cavities or occur under the skin as an abscess with draining sinuses. Tubercular skeletal lesions usually do not wall themselves off, so invasion of joints and intervertebral disks may cause many deformities. Tuberculosis of the spine, called *Pott's disease*, most frequently occurs in children and can lead to kyphosis, scoliosis, or the hunchback deformity.

The onset of skeletal tuberculosis, in contrast to acute pyogenic osteomyelitis, is insidious, beginning with vague description of pain. Complications of tuberculosis of the spine include paraplegia and meningitis. Tuberculosis of the hip and knee joint is most frequent in children.

## Syphilis

Congenital or acquired syphilis of the bone is rare in the United States. In congenital syphilis, the spirochetes are delivered through the fetal bloodstream to the bones, where they inhibit osteogenesis. The epiphyseal plate is severely damaged and may actually be separated from the metaphysis. Bone syphilis is marked by endarteritis and periarteritis, and reactive bone forms from viable surrounding periosteum. Granulation tissue between the periosteum and cortical bone is laid down. In the tibia, a resulting "saber-shin" deformity gives a curved appearance to the anterior portion of the bone.

Acquired syphilis may also cause osteochondritis or periosteitis; there is a possibility that frank syphilitic lesions will appear within the medullary canal. The skull and vertebrae, as well as the long bones, can be affected in acquired syphilis.

# ALTERATIONS IN SKELETAL STRUCTURE

## Abnormal Spinal Curvatures

The normal spinal curvature is assessed in routine medical examinations (Figure 45-25). Changes in its contour give significant clues for underlying musculoskeletal disorders.

### Scoliosis

Scoliosis is a lateral curvature of the spine that can result from another disease such as polio or cerebral palsy. Most commonly it is an idiopathic disorder. It is estimated that over 1 million Americans have some degree of scoliosis, and girls are affected 8 times more often than boys. Scoliosis is most frequent in the early adolescent years.

The curvatures are classified according to location and consist of a primary, fixed curve with compensatory curves above and below (Figure 45-26). The deformity occurs slowly and is accelerated by the preadolescent growth spurt. The shoulder blade protrudes, the level of the iliac crests becomes unequal, and the curvature appears to be exaggerated when the individual bends over (Figure 45-27).[1] In general, the younger the age when the curvature is noticed and the higher up in the thorax it occurs, the poorer the prognosis.[7] Severe scoliosis can affect the heart and lungs by restrictive action. It may be markedly improved by surgical procedures.

### List

List is a lateral tilt of the spine from the T1 level (Figure 45-28). It may result from a herniated disk or a painful spasm of the muscles along the spine.[1]

### Gibbus

The angular deformity noted with a collapsed vertebra is a gibbus (Figure 45-29). Multiple causes include metastatic malignancy of the spine and tuberculosis.[1]

### Flattening of the Lumbar Curve

This contour change suggests a herniated lumbar disk or ankylosing spondylitis.[1] The normal curve in the lumbar area becomes straight (Figure 45-30).

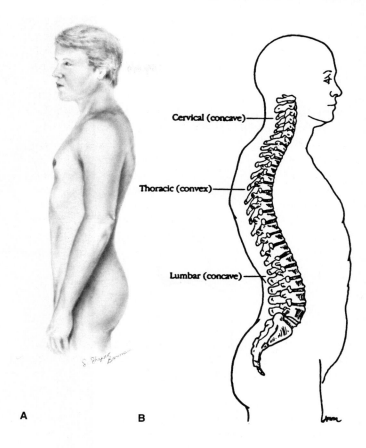

**FIGURE 45–25.**

Normal spine. (Source: B. Bates, *A Guide to Physical Examination and History Taking* [5th ed.]. Philadelphia: J.B. Lippincott, 1991.)

**A**                    **B**

## Lordosis

Lordosis is an accentuation of the normal lumbar curve (Figure 45-31). It often results from obesity or pregnancy as a compensation for the protuberant abdomen.[1]

## Kyphosis

Kyphosis may be the first indication of osteoporosis in the elderly person. It appears as a rounded thoracic convexity, especially in elderly women (Figure 45-32).[1] It may be accompanied by pain in the vertebral area and radiologic signs of osteoporosis.

## Clubfoot (Talipes)

Clubfoot deformities, the most frequent of the orthopedic congenital deformities of the lower extremities, occur with greatest frequency in boys. Two thirds of the cases are unilateral. Clubfoot may be caused by genetic and environmental factors. Generally, the talus points downward and the foot is adducted. The clinical varieties are *easy* and *resistant,* with the easy cases responding to strapping and stretching alone and the resistant cases requiring surgical intervention.

## Congenital Dislocation of the Hip

Congenital dislocation of the hip is probably caused by a combination of genetic and environmental factors. Genetic factors are linked to both joint laxity and acetabular dysplasia. Also, just prior to delivery of a full-term infant, the pregnant woman secretes a ligament-relaxing hormone that crosses the placental barrier and enhances joint laxity. This accounts for the relative rarity of hip dislocation in premature infants. Other environmental factors include intrauterine malposition, breech presentation during delivery, and, in some cultures, swaddling of neonates.

Pathologically, the acetabulum is defective and the femoral head is completely out of the joint, located posterior and superior to the acetabulum. Most frequently, this is a unilateral occurrence. Asymmetric groin skin creases are seen on examination, and the affected leg is shorter than the other. The leg cannot abduct completely. When it is extended and flexed at the hip, a click called *Ortolani's click* may be felt or heard. Because the femoral head must be in correct alignment with the acetabulum for the bones and joint to grow and develop normally, early detection is necessary. Reduction after age 6 years is almost impossible, and secondary bone changes occur that cause the child to walk with a typical lurching gait.

*(text continues on page 880)*

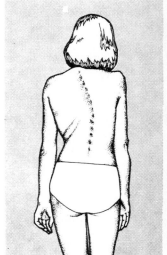

**A**

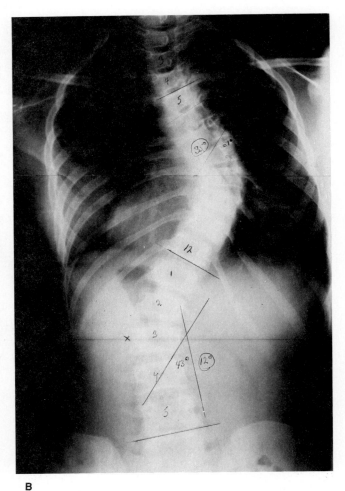

**B**

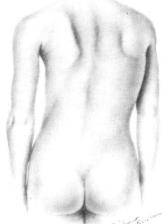

**C**

**FIGURE 45—26.**
**A.** Distortion of the rib cage resulting from scoliosis. **B.** Scoliosis of the spine with a thoracic primary curve and compensatory curve in the lumbar spine. Vertebral bodies are marked at the approximate beginning and end of each curve and are used to measure the degree of curvature. **C.** Scoliosis is shown here with a thoracic convexity to the right. Scoliosis may be structural (as illustrated) or functional, when it compensates for other abnormalities such as unequal leg lengths. Structural scoliosis is typically associated with rotation of the vertebrae upon each other, and the rib cage is accordingly deformed. (Source: **A:** C. Monk, *Orthopaedics for Undergraduates*, London: Oxford University Press, 1976, by permission of Oxford University Press. **C:** B. Bates, *A Guide to Physical Examination and History Taking* (3rd ed.), Philadelphia: J.B. Lippincott, 1983.)

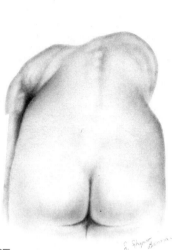

**FIGURE 45–27.**

The rotary deformity of scoliosis produces a hump or "razor back" deformity. This deviation is best demonstrated by asking the client to bend at the waist. (Source: B. Bates, *A Guide to Physical Examination* [5th ed.]. Philadelphia: J.B. Lippincott, 1991.)

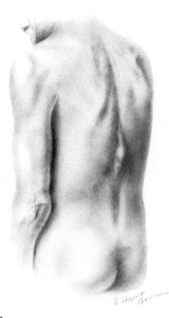

**FIGURE 45–29.**

Gibbus is an angular deformity of a collapsed vertebra. Causes include metastatic cancer and tuberculosis of the spine (Source: B. Bates, *A Guide to Physical Examination* [5th ed.]. Philadelphia: J.B. Lippincott, 1991.)

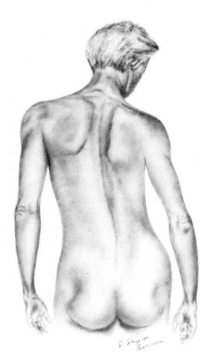

**FIGURE 45–28.**

List is a lateral tilt of the spine. When a plumb line dropped from the spinous process of T1 falls to one side of the gluteal cleft, a list is present. Causes include a herniated disc and painful spasms of the para vertebral muscles. Scoliosis (a lateral curve of the spine) is inherent in a list but has not been fully compensated for by a spinal deviation in the opposite direction. (Source: B. Bates, *A Guide to Physical Examination* [5th ed.]. Philadelphia: J.B. Lippincott, 1991.)

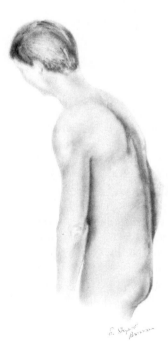

**FIGURE 45–30.**

Flattening of the lumbar curve, muscle spasm in the lumbar area, and decreased spinal mobility suggest the possibility of a herniated lumbar disk or, especially in men, ankylosing spondylitis. (Source: B. Bates, *A Guide to Physical Examination* [5th ed.]. Philadelphia: J.B. Lippincott, 1991.)

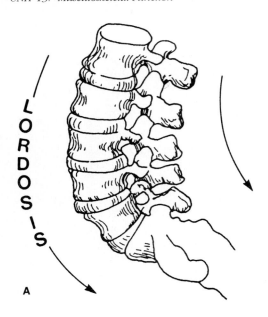

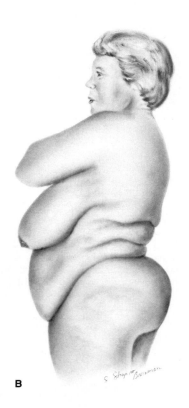

**FIGURE 45–31.**
**A.** The normal orientation of the lumbar spine is that of mild lordosis. Exaggerated lordosis may predispose the patient to mechanical back pain. **B.** Lordosis develops to compensate for the protuberant abdomen of pregnancy or marked obesity. It may also compensate for kyphosis and flexion deformities of the hips. A deep midline furrow may be seen between the lumbar paravertebral muscles. (Source: **A.** B. Reilly, *Practical Strategies in Outpatient Medicine* [2nd ed.]. Philadelphia: W.B. Saunders, 1991; **B.** B. Bates, *A Guide to Physical Examination and History Taking* [5th ed.]. Philadelphia: J.B. Lippincott, 1991.)

The earlier the child is treated, the more likely that complete hip function will be restored.

## ALTERATIONS IN JOINTS AND TENDONS

As discussed earlier, joints allow the body to be mobile. The synovial joints are most affected by alterations. Studies have shown that this type of articular cartilage, which is lubricated and nourished by synovial fluid, has many microscopic spaces filled with fluid, causing it to be elastic and to bounce back despite daily subjection to compression.

## Arthritis

The most frequent joint diseases are the arthritides, which effect 1 out of every 20 to 30 Americans and constitute a financial and health problem of considerable magnitude.

Arthritis simply means inflammation of a joint, and it occurs in many forms. Degenerative joint disease or trauma often are related to an increased incidence of osteoarthritis. Metabolic disturbances may cause gouty arthritis or it may be associated with conditions such as psoriasis or bursitis. Suppurative arthritis implies an infection of the joint with pyogenic organisms; tuberculous arthritis is inflammation secondary to tuberculosis. Autoimmune conditions produce many types of arthritis, the most crippling of which is rheumatoid arthritis, which has many forms.

### Rheumatoid Arthritis (RA)

Rheumatoid arthritis (RA) is an inflammatory disease that has been studied extensively in attempts to uncover an etiologic agent. In recent years, theories have supported an infectious cause or an autoimmune response. Many bacteria and viruses suspected of causing RA have been studied without success. The Epstein–Barr virus has been found to react with lymphocytes, transforming them into

the joint space. Pannus destroys the articular cartilage and underlying bone, resulting in loss of motion. The muscles that pull across the joint give rise to flexion and extension and subluxation deformities. Subcutaneous rheumatoid nodules, which are areas of necrosis surrounded by lymphocytes and plasma cells, are present in about one-fourth of persons affected. Figure 45-33 shows articular cortical reabsorption in the feet.

The fluid aspirated from the joint is thin and cloudy, and has an elevated white cell level. The lysosomal enzymes released from these neutrophils may be a factor in cartilage destruction. As the acute inflammatory process subsides, granulation tissue becomes scar tissue and eventually bone, causing a true ankylosis (a fixed, stiff joint). Local degenerative muscle is gradually replaced by fibrous tissue and the involved bones show osteoporosis.

Rheumatoid arthritis mostly affects the joints but can affect any system. Small and large arteries anywhere in the system can develop acute necrotizing vasculitis with thrombosis. The vasculitis can cause the vascular insufficiency of Raynaud's phenomenon or obliterative vasculitis from intimal proliferation. The manifestations of cardiac disease include conduction disturbances, pericardial adhesions, myocarditis, and valvular impingement.[2] In

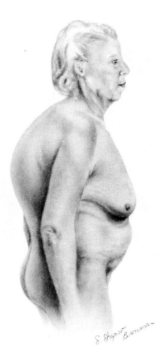

**FIGURE 45-32.**

Kyphosis, a rounded thoracic convexity, is common in aging, especially in women. (Source: B. Bates, *A Guide to Physical Examination* [5th ed.]. Philadelphia: J.B. Lippincott, 1991.)

immunogens.[5] A significant body of knowledge seems to support the immune response theory.

Antibodies known as *rheumatoid factor (RF)*, have been demonstrated in the sera of almost all individuals with RA. Synovial lymphocytes produce IgG, which is targeted as foreign, and production of IgG and IgM antiimmunoglobulins results. These antiimmunoglobulins are actually the rheumatoid factor. By binding with IgG, the antigenic target, the resulting complex activates the complement system in the joint. The RF titer is in direct relationship to the severity of the disease, although the actual stimulus for the formation of RF is unknown.

The numerous T lymphocytes in the joint may become sensitized to the joint collagens, causing an immunologic response that is enhanced by the release of lymphokines and the presence of prostaglandins.[6,29] Increased physical or emotional stress has always been recognized as a precipitator of acute exacerbations, but the mechanisms for the stress interaction are unknown.

Joint destruction is the primary pathology of RA and may affect any synovial membrane in the body. Joint inflammation with effusion is accompanied by capsular and periarticular soft tissue inflammation, causing swelling, redness, and painful motion of the joint. Proliferative synovitis persists, and the synovium becomes a thickened, hyperemic, densely cellular membrane called a *pannus*, which invades and erodes surrounding cartilage and bone.[29] Joint motion causes bleeding within the cavity. Clots of fibrin and newly formed granulation tissue fill

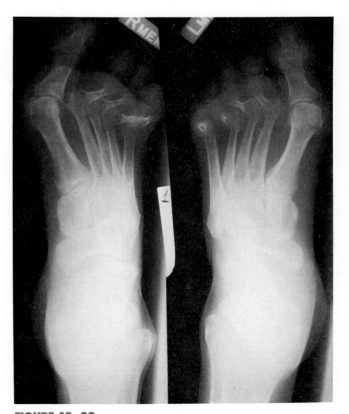

**FIGURE 45-33.**

Rheumatoid arthritis in the feet with ulnar deviation of the phalanges. Note the articular cortical resorption, which is common with RA.

the lungs, the person may exhibit pleuritis or interstitial pneumonitis. The eyes may show uveitis, keratoconjunctivitis, or chronic inflammation. Neuropathies, skeletal muscle inflammations, and spleen and liver enlargement may result.

The disease affects women in a ratio of 3:1 over men, and most often occurs between 20 and 50 years of age. The onset can be vague or acute. Fatigue, fever, and malaise may precede actual joint pain, or high fever and aching joints may herald the onset of the disease. Joint stiffness is more noticeable in the morning or after rest. The erythrocyte sedimentation rate is elevated. Clinical remission has been classified by the American Rheumatism Association in which five or more of the following requirements are fulfilled for at least 2 consecutive months:

▶ morning stiffness not exceeding 15 minutes;
▶ no fatigue
▶ no joint pain by history
▶ no joint pain on motion
▶ no soft tissue swelling in joints
▶ erythrocyte sedimentation rate less than 30 mm/hour for women or 20 mm/hour for men.[2]

Exacerbations are common and often cause increasing damage with greater stiffness and deformities. Any joint may be affected, and spinal cervical involvement may be seen. Hand and wrist deformities with swelling and a zig-zag appearance are common (Figure 45-34).[2]

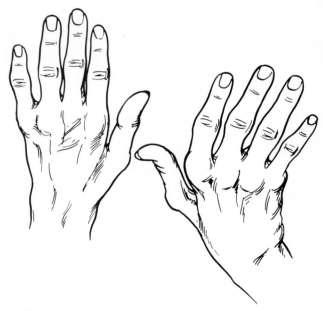

**FIGURE 45–34.**
Ulnar deviation and subluxation of the metacarpophalangeal joints have occurred in the patient's right hand. These joints also appear swollen. Muscle atrophy has developed in the dorsal musculature of both hands.

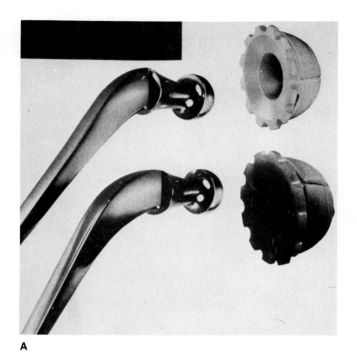

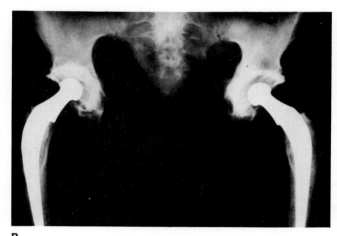

**FIGURE 45–35.**
**A.** Stainless steel femoral head and shaft fits into the artificial acetabulum, which is glued into correct placement. **B.** Total hip replacement with ball and socket.

Surgical procedures to replace dysfunctioning joints are often required (Figure 45-35).

A variant of rheumatoid arthritis is juvenile rheumatoid arthritis. The onset of juvenile RA in persons age 16 years or less is usually abrupt, with chills and high fever, or it may appear insidiously with typical stiffness of one or more joints. The joint pathology is similar to the adult form, and subcutaneous lesions may also be present. Fortunately, over one-half of these young persons have a complete remission. Permanent deformities are more common in those with acute febrile onset, multiple joint involvement, and a positive RF.[29]

**BOX 45-2.**
SERONEGATIVE SPONDYLARTHROPATHIES

Ankylosing spondylitis
Reiter's syndrome
Psoriatic arthropathy
Intestinal arthropathy
Juvenile ankylosing spondylitis
Reactive arthropathy

## Ankylosing Spondylitis

Ankylosing spondylitis is an arthritic condition that is classified as one of a group of seronegative spondylarthrides. Box 45-2 lists the conditions that are placed in this classification. Ankylosing spondylitis is characterized by sacroiliac joint involvement, peripheral inflammatory arthropathy, and the absence of the rheumatoid factor.[4] Destruction of cartilage and bone results in fibrous and bony ankylosing of the spine, giving the patient the typical stiff or "poker" spine (see Figure 45-30). Mobility of the spine is usually decreased symmetrically but does improve somewhat with exercise. Discomfort is insidious in onset and often described as morning stiffness.[4] If peripheral joints are affected early in the disease, joint replacement procedures may become necessary. The disease is only slightly more prevalent in men than in women, and the symptoms in men are more severe. The peak age range is from 20 to 40 years.[6] An elevated erythrocyte sedimentation rate (ESR) is characteristic, but evidence of immune complex formation is found less frequently than in rheumatoid disease.[4]

## Osteoarthritis

The term *osteoarthritis* is misleading because inflammation is not a usual component of this condition. The term *degenerative joint disease* more clearly describes the disease, which is the most common rheumatic disease.[23] The frequency usually is age-related, with most of those affected over 50 years old. Joints have a limited way in which to respond to the compressive forces in day-to-day living. In osteoarthritis, it has been found that the matrix in the articular cartilage is depleted, thus "unmasking" the basic collagen structure. Normally, the matrix spreads compression stress hydrostatically, but with its depletion the collagen fibers may rupture, causing flaking, fissuring, and eroding of the articular cartilage. These alterations are characteristic of the disorder. Laboratory studies rarely show increased ESR or synovial fluid inflammatory changes. Radiographs may appear normal or only show narrowing joint space or cyst formation. Osteoporosis is not a direct component of the disease, but because of age considerations it may also be seen.

The bone immediately under the affected area shows proliferation of fibroblasts and new bone formation. Periosteal bone growth also increases at the joint margins and at the site of ligament or tendon attachments, developing into bone spurs or ridges called *osteophytes*. The synovial capsule decreases in size, and movement is limited.

Degenerative joint disease generally affects joints that are under much pressure, especially the spine, fingers, knees, hips, and shoulders. Pain and stiffness early in the course occur after joint use and are relieved by rest. Later, pain occurs with motion or rest.[23] Spurs may be formed on the distal interphalangeal joints of the fingers and are termed *Heberden's nodes*. Flexor and lateral deviations of the fingers are common, especially in the elderly individual (see Chap. 7). Persons under occupational stress or who are obese or have faulty posture are at greatest risk for the disease. Trauma, such as sports injuries to a joint at an early age, can render the individual more susceptible to osteoarthritis with advancing years. Studies have shown a *wear-and-tear* process, with increased frequency in joints under stress.

## Gout

Gout is a general term for a group of diseases with one or more of the following manifestations: (1) increased serum urate concentration; (2) recurrent attacks of acute arthritis with urate crystals in synovial fluid; (3) aggregated deposits of urate in joints, leading to crippling and deformity; (4) renal disease; and (5) uric acid nephrolithiasis.[15] The prevalence of gout in the United States has been estimated at 275 per 100,000, with the risk increasing with age and serum urate concentrations.[27]

Gout is caused by monosodium urate crystals in the joints, which cause acute arthritis. These crystals precipitate in the joints when body fluids are supersaturated with uric acid. Gout is generally classified as primary or secondary. Primary gout is a genetic disorder in which the exact defect of uric acid metabolism is unknown in the vast majority of cases. Ninety percent of all gout is primary, with men most frequently affected. Secondary gout occurs whenever some superimposed condition either increases the production of uric acid or decreases its excretion.[14] Diseases characterized by rapid breakdown of cells (eg, leukemia), hemolytic anemia, cytolytic agents, and drugs that decrease excretion of urates (eg, thiazides and mercurial diuretics) have all been implicated in secondary gout.

In the body uric acid is made by the enzymatic breakdown of tissue and dietary purines. Gout, a hyperuricemic syndrome, can result from overproduction of uric acid, retention of uric acid due to renal malfunction, or both.[6] Normal purine metabolism is complicated, involving numerous enzymes and two pathways. Although the exact error of metabolism is unknown in most cases, the result is an abnormally large amount of uric acid in the blood. At an excessive point, uric acid crystals precipitate into the joint fluids, kidneys, heart, earlobes, and toes. The mass of urate crystals surrounded by inflammation with lymphocytes, plasma cells, and macrophages is called a *tophus*. Tophi may clump together and form large plaquelike encrustations that invade the articular surface and underlying bone causing deformities.

Gout is described in four clinical phases: asymptomatic hyperuricemia, acute gouty arthritis, intercritical gout, and chronic tophaceous gout.[27] In asymptomatic hyperuricemia, the serum urate level is elevated even though there are no symptoms. In acute gouty arthritis, there is a sudden onset of severe pain in the great toe or occasionally the heel, ankle, or instep. The affected joint becomes hot, red, and tender. The pain becomes intense and intolerable. It may be associated with chills and fever and resolve spontaneously or with treatment. The intervals between attacks are called *intercritical gout*. Crystal deposition persists during this phase. In the fourth phase, tophi occur in many locations, even in the aorta and heart valves. Deforming arthritis is common and can involve any joint.[27] The monosodium urate crystals (MSU) are deposited in the synovial fluids, and these can rapidly lyse neutrophils which release both lysosomal enzymes and crystals. This makes the inflammatory process continuous.[27]

The association of gout attacks with overeating and alcoholism is well-supported. About one-half of gouty individuals are more than 15% above their ideal weight and 75% exhibit hypertriglyceridemia.[27] Ethanol increases urate production through increasing blood lactate, which blocks the renal excretion of uric acid.[27] Therefore, the victim may describe an excessive consumption of rich foods or alcohol before an attack.

As stated before, acute gouty arthritis is heralded by the sudden onset of acute pain, usually in one joint in the lower extremity. Half of the attacks occur in the metatarsophalangeal joint of the great toe. Persons often relate unusual stress preceding an attack, which could include overeating, overindulgence in alcohol, emotional stress, or physical exertion.[6] A person may be asymptomatic for months or even years between attacks. Over many years, disabling, chronic, gouty arthritis may develop. Atherosclerosis becomes a problem in almost half of persons with gout, and death occurs most frequently from myocardial infarction or renal failure.[27] Treatment consists of a variety of drugs that inhibit uric acid production.

## Bursitis

Bursae are classically described as enclosed sacs containing a small amount of fluid that lubricates and cushions joints. Inflammation of a bursa is common and may be caused by unusual use of a part, by trauma, infection, or rheumatoid arthritis. The inflammation results in an excess production of fluid in the sac, which becomes distended and presses on sensory nerve endings causing pain. Commonly affected bursae are (1) the prepatellar bursa, caused by kneeling (housemaid's knee or nun's knee); (2) the olecranon bursa, subject to the repeated trauma of leaning on one's elbows (bartender's elbow); (3) the bursa located on the plantar aspect of the heel, which is subjected to repeated pressure (postman's heel); and (4) the bursa of the metatarsophalangeal joint of the great toe (bunion).

## Baker's Cyst

Baker's cyst is a firm, cystic mass along the medial border of the popliteal space. It occurs mostly in children, and is believed to be caused by fluid distention of the bursal sac associated with local muscles. Some cysts communicate directly with the joint cavity. Swelling is usually the only symptom, and surgical excision, although possible, is not often necessary.

## Tumors of Joints

### Synovial Sarcoma

Tumors of joints are uncommon, but they may occur on the tendon sheath, the bursae, and around the joints. Primitive mesenchymal cells, rather than synovial membrane cells, form the primary tumor. A gray-white mass invades along muscle and fascial planes, and although the tumor is slow-growing, it can metastasize to the lungs, bones, and brain.

### Tenosynovitis

Tenosynovitis is an inflammation of the tendon sheath and the enclosed tendon. It primarily affects the wrists, shoulders, and ankles. This condition is thought to be use-related, and occupational stresses, such as typing and heavy labor, may precipitate it. Synovial fluid and fibrin constituents within the tendon sheath may cause adhesions. These inflammations cause extreme pain on movement and may exhibit heat and redness or inflammation. Bacterial invasion of pyrogens and tuberculosis also have been implicated as causes of tenosynovitis.

### Fibromatosis

*Palmar fibromatosis* denotes chronic hyperplasia of the fascia in the palm of the hand, leading to fibrosis and a deformity called *Dupuytren's contracture*. The fingers, most often the ring and little fingers, contract into a fixed, flexed position. Usually bilateral, this condition is most frequent in middle-aged men. Heredity is believed to be a major factor in causation.

Plantar fibromatosis is similar to palmar fibromatosis, but it usually does not cause contractures. Nodular masses of fibrocytes arise from the plantar fascia, usually on the medial side of the foot. Trauma is thought to be the cause.

# BONE TUMORS

Tumors in the skeletal system can be either primary or secondary. Primary lesions can be benign or malignant. Of these, benign tumors are much more common and usually are self-limiting. Malignant tumors of the bone, although rare, are devastating and often fatal. Diagnosis is based on a careful history, tumor location, and radiographic appearance.

Benign bone tumors are usually slow-growing, noninvasive, and well-localized. Adolescents or young adults are usually affected most frequently, and the tumor growth stops when the skeletal system reaches maturity. Because of their noninvasive characteristics, benign tumors cause little or no pain and are often discovered secondarily to another complaint or a pathologic fracture.

Malignant neoplasms grow rapidly, spread and invade irregularly, and cause pain. Classic signs are constant or intermittant pain, usually worse at night; an unexplained swelling over a bone; a feeling of warmth of the skin over the bone, with prominent veins. Adolescents and young adults are most commonly affected. These tumors metastasize to other parts of the body and are usually fatal without early diagnosis and treatment.

Secondary tumors of the skeletal system are usually from primary sites in the breasts, lungs, kidneys, or other body systems. As the primary lesion grows and invades surrounding tissue, clumps of cancerous tissues are carried by the blood and lymphatic system to the bone, where they continue to grow and cause destruction.

The growth of tumors in the bone often causes increased radiodensities due to increased osteoblastic activity within the tumor. This can be seen on radiographs, which are helpful in diagnosis. Some tumors cause the bone to appear translucent, indicating increased osteoclast activity.

## Classification of Tumors

Primary bone neoplasm may be classified according to the skeletal tissue from which it arises: osseous, cartilage, or marrow. Tumors in each of these categories may be benign or malignant. Other bone tumors, such as giant-cell tumors, do not have these origins. This section discusses the more common benign and malignant tumors. These are grouped as osteoblastic (bone-forming), chondrogenic (tumors of marrow origin), and those of unknown origin.

## Fibrous Dysplasia

Fibrous dysplasia, which is characterized by replacement of cancellous bone by fibrous tissue, can affect one bone (monostotic), or many bones (polyostotic). Monostotic forms account for about 70% of cases, and these usually affect the ribs, femur, tibia, maxilla, mandible, or humerus.[6] The condition may be asymptomatic, or disfigurement from bony distortion may be seen. In the polyostotic form, the craniofacial bones are affected most frequently, but crippling deformities also may be associated.

The fibrous lesion begins in the medullary canal and spreads to the cortex, with cancellous bone and marrow replaced by yellow-gray, fibrous tissue. The cortex is thin, and bowing deformities and fractures are common. If this disease occurs in the monostotic form, the lesion grows slowly, but eventually deformity occurs unless the mass is surgically removed. If the polyostotic form of the disease is accompanied by extraskeletal signs and endocrine pathology, it is called *Albright's syndrome*.

Albright's syndrome is differentiated by precocious puberty in girls, café au lait pigmentation of the skin over the bone involvement, and predominant unilateral bone deformity, especially of the skull and long bones.[6] When the facial bones are affected, asymmetry of the face with distortions of the nose, jaw, and even severe displacement of an eye may occur. Although fibrous dysplasia has no proven genetic links, multisystem involvement of the polyostotic form does suggest some basic genetic defect. Many endocrine associations have been identified including hyperthyroidism, Cushing's syndrome, acromegaly, and hyperparathyroidism.[6]

## Bone-Forming Tumors

Benign osteoblastic tumors include *osteomas* and *osteoblastomas. Compact osteoma* is a benign tumor composed of dense bone with a well-circumscribed edge. It frequently arises in the cortical surface of bone of the skull and paranasal sinuses. Symptoms are caused from impingement of the tumor on the brain or sinuses. The tumors cause the face to become unfortunately distorted.[6]

*Osteoid osteoma* most commonly affects the femur and tibia, but can grow in any bone in the body except the skull. It is usually located in the diaphyses of long bones. It occurs predominantly in boys and young men between the ages of 5 and 25. The tumor consists of a well-rounded, central nidus that is sharply demarcated from a surrounding zone of bone. The nidus may range from a few millimeters to a centimeter and consists of osteoid tissue and trabeculae (Figure 45-36). The tissue is reddish-gray and is granular to the touch. It may be removed surgically because it causes localized pain, especially at night.

*Benign osteoblastoma* is a rare benign tumor that is sometimes confused with osteoid osteoma or even giant-

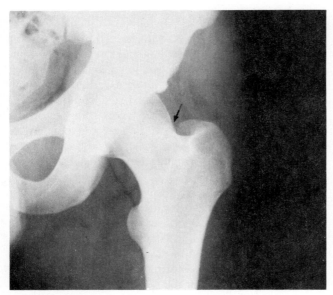

**FIGURE 45–36.**
Osteoid osteoma. Small transport area indicated by arrow represents the central nidus.

cell tumors. It occurs most frequently in boys and young men, usually in the first three decades of life. Its most common site is the spinal cord. Pain is a cardinal symptom, usually due to the pressure on adjacent structures, such as the spinal cord or nerve roots. It seems to be less severe than that caused by an osteoid osteoma and may be referred to a site distant from the tumor. Other symptoms depend on the location of the tumor and include weakness or even paraplegia. There is no characteristic radiographic appearance. In some cases, one may see bone destruction that is more or less demarcated from normal bone. Surgical removal usually relieves compression on the spinal column and nerve root. When the tumor is in a long bone, it may take on the appearance of an osteoid osteoma with a sclerotic border, except that the nidus may be many times longer.

The most prevalent malignant tumor of osteoid origin is the *osteogenic sarcoma* or *osteosarcoma*, in which tumor cells proliferate osteoid or immature bone. Osteosarcoma is the most common and most fatal primary bone tumor, often affecting people between the ages 10 and 20 years.[22] It occurs more often in young men than in young women, usually during periods of rapid skeletal growth. Irradiation and oncogenic viruses have been explored in its etiology.[22] When this lesion does occur in later years of life, it is usually related to Paget's disease. Radiation treatment for other tumors has also been indicated in the causation of osteogenic sarcoma in later life.

To be classified as a true osteogenic sarcoma, an osteoid substance must be produced. The tumor may show a predominance of elements, with osteoid, chondroid, or fibromatoid differentiation.[22] Bizarre pleomorphic cells with abundant mitoses or multinucleate giant cells are characteristic.[22]

Osteosarcomas usually occur in long tubular bones, but the skull, maxilla, spinal column, and clavicles, as well as other bones, are also affected. The femurs, tibia, and ulnae are the most frequent sites (Figure 45-37). After the age of 25, its frequency in flat and long bones is nearly equal.[6] The tumor usually is a localized swelling with tenderness associated with a large mass. Pain may or may not be present. Sometimes the tumor is found on incidental radiographic examination of an injury. It tends to recur within 1 to 2 years.

The survival rate of persons with osteosarcoma was dismal when resection or amputation alone was employed. Five-year survival of about 60% has been achieved using a combination of aggressive chemotherapy and surgery.[6]

## Tumors of Cartilaginous Origin

Benign chondrogenic tumors include osteochondroma and chondroblastoma. Many of these tumors are asymptomatic and are only discovered accidentally because of an injury to the area. *Osteochondromas* form a long mass produced by progressive endochondral ossification of a growing cartilaginous cap. The tumor is basically osseous and protrudes from the cortex of the bone with or without a stalk. The caps are usually cauliflower-shaped and occur mainly in persons between the first and second decades of life (Figure 45-38). The growth of the tumor parallels that of the adolescent, and once the epiphyses have closed, it normally stops. Multiple osteochondromas may occur when more than one bone is affected, with

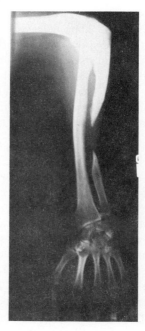

**FIGURE 45–37.**
Osteogenic sarcoma. Note the complete destruction of the ulna.

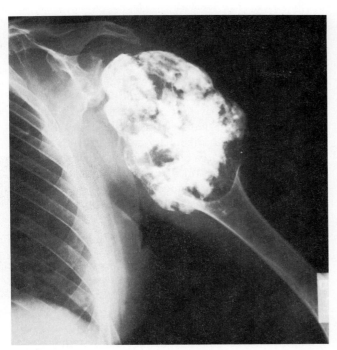

**FIGURE 45-38.**
Osteochondroma of the proximal right humerus is unusually large. Shows cartilaginous and osteoid matrix being laid down.

each growth having the same characteristics as the single osteochondroma.

Osteochondromas rarely undergo malignant change to osteosarcomas. This transformation may occur if there are multiple tumors or occasionally after surgical removal of an osteochondroma. The most common site for the tumorous mass is the metaphyseal region of long bones, specifically the femur and tibia, but it can affect any bone that develops by endochondral ossification.

*Endochondroma* is the term used to describe a tumor when it only involves the medulla and is encapsulated by an intact cortex. It commonly affects the small bones of the hands and feet, but may affect the ribs, sternum, spine, and long bones of persons between 20 and 30 years of age. The tumor usually affects the phalanges of the hand, producing a central area of rarefaction (decreasing density and weight) (Figure 45-39). Normally discovered during treatment of a fracture after a trivial injury, the tumor appears radiographically as a well-defined, translucent area with the cortex intact and areas of calcification.

Benign *chondroblastomas* closely resemble giant-cell tumors and affect mainly persons under age 20 years or before epiphyseal closure, whereas giant-cell tumors are rare under age 20 years. Histologically, chondroblastomas differ from giant-cell tumors in that they contain foci of calcification, trabeculae of osteoid tissue, and well-developed bone, as well as more or less well-defined areas of cartilaginous matrix, features that are not usually present in giant-cell tumors. Chondroblastomas are vir-

tually always benign, localized lesions that do not recur and do not invade.

Localized pain may be experienced and is often referred to the adjacent joint region. Wasting of muscle mass due to disuse caused by pain and limping may also be observed.

Radiographically, an area of central bone destruction is clearly demarcated by surrounding normal bone. There may be margins of increased bone density with mottled areas of calcification within the lesion. The tumor almost always involves the epiphyses and frequently the adjacent metaphyses, which are also seen on the films.[6]

*Chondrosarcoma* is a malignant bone tumor of cartilaginous origin. It can arise from benign chondrogenic origins, as described earlier, or may develop spontaneously. The tumor is rare; it occurs more frequently in men than in women.[10] It is primarily a condition of adulthood and old age, and rarely metastasizes until it has grown to a large size.[26]

Chondrosarcomas usually originate in the trunk and the upper ends of the femur and humerus, and points of attachments of muscle to bone at the knee, pelvis, shoulder, and hip are prevalent. Any bone of the body can be affected.

Physical symptoms may include pain, swelling, and a palpable mass due to the active invasive growth of the tumor. Tumors located in the trunk and long bones may be evidenced only by pain, which makes radiographic findings important. These usually include mottled areas of calcification and areas of osseous destruction (Figure 45-40). Even when treated with wide resection, recurrence has been encountered even after 10 years. Metastases may occur many years after initial diagnosis and treatment.

## Tumors of Undetermined Origin

*Ewing's sarcoma*, although rare, is one of the most lethal bone tumors. Approximately 90% of people affected are under age 30; the greatest number of tumors occur in the second decade of life. They affect men over women by a 2 to 1 margin.[4,22] The long tubular bones are most com-

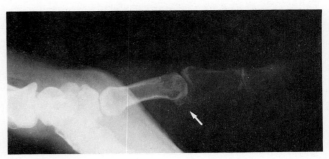

**FIGURE 45-39.**
Endochondroma of the thumb.

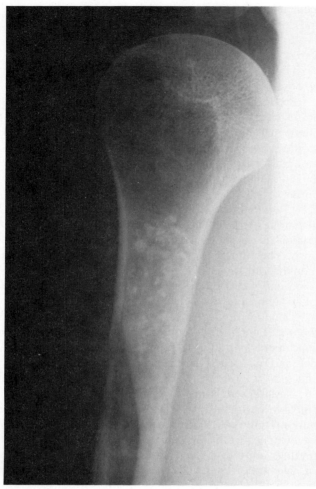

**FIGURE 45–40.**
Chondrosarcoma of the humerus. Mixed lytic and sclerotic areas give patchy appearance to bone.

monly involved, with the innominate bones–the pelvis, ischium, ribs, scapula, and sternum–following in that order, and then virtually any other bone in the body (Figure 45-41).

Ewing's sarcoma, like many other invasive tumors, results in pain, a tender mass, and venous distention. Some individuals may have anemia, temperature elevation, and sometimes leukocytosis.[22] This tumor generally has its origin in the medullary canal, growing outward and creating a lytic area on radiographs. Ewing's sarcoma is composed of nondistinctive, small, round cells that are not easily identified.[6] Some spicules of bone may be seen, but this is reactive bone and not part of the neoplasm. Elevation of the periosteum is typical, followed by periosteal bone formation, which creates what is known as an onion-skin appearance, seen radiologically.[6]

*Giant-cell tumors* are poorly understood, apparently malignant, distinct neoplasms. Cases of seemingly benign giant-cell tumors have been reported to undergo malignant transformation. For this reason, a histomorphic grading system has been developed, with grade I benign and grade II malignant.[10] Unfortunately, this system is not always accurate, as one part of the tumor may appear benign while another part may appear malignant.[26]

Giant-cell tumors generally affect individuals between ages 20 and 55 years. Peak occurrence is in the third decade of life. It affects women somewhat more frequently than men. Most giant-cell tumors arise in the epiphyses of long bones, with over one-half of the lesions close to the knee in the distal femur and proximal tibia; other sites include the sacrum, vertebrae, humerus, and radius.[22]

Giant-cell tumors usually begin forming within cancellous bone. As they grow and invade, the cortex may

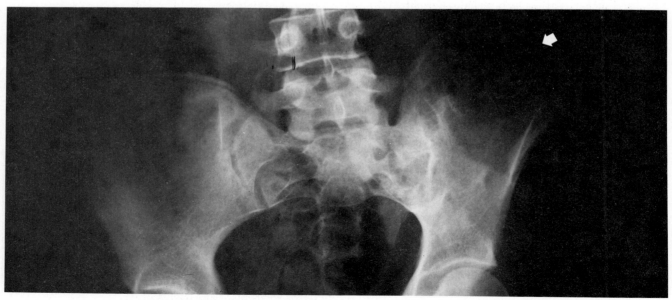

**FIGURE 45–41.**
Ewing's sarcoma. Note that the top of the ischium has been carved out by tumor.

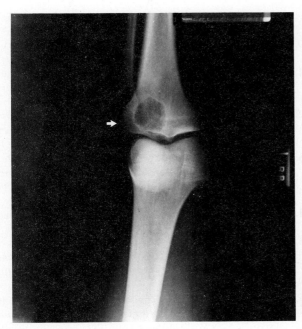

**FIGURE 45-42.**
Giant-cell tumor of the tibia (*arrow*).

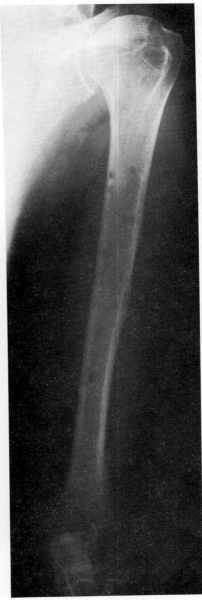

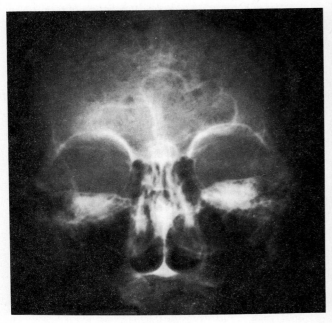

A

**FIGURE 45-43.**
Multiple myeloma of the skull **A.** and of the humerus **B.** Note the numerous lytic defects and diffuse osteoporosis characteristic of multiple myeloma.

B

be thinned or even broken, but new reactive bone generally preserves the cortex. The expansion of the tumor in the epiphyses classically forms a clublike deformity. Radiographs reveal a somewhat translucent area at the ends of the long bones, with a thin cortex (Figure 45-42).

## Hematogenic Tumors

*Multiple myeloma* is the most common neoplasm of the bone. It is composed of plasma cells showing variable degrees of differentiation (Figure 45-43). The skeletal effects of this condition are discussed in this section (see Chap. 20 for further discussion).

Multiple meyloma affects women and men equally, rarely occurs before the age of 50, and has its peak frequency in the fifth and sixth decades. It has a predilection for the vertebral column, but ribs, skull, pelvis, and virtually any bone in the body may be affected. Multiple myeloma appears radiographically as multifocal destructive bone lesions throughout the skeletal system, producing what appear to be rounded, punched-out areas.[6] These areas may measure up to 5 cm, with no surrounding zone of sclerosis. Pathologic fractures of the vertebrae are common.

The individual has a history of pain that is often referred to the spinal column. Neurologic symptoms occur because of compression of vertebral bodies or nerve roots due to extension of the neoplasm. Weakness, loss of weight, hemorrhagic disorders, and renal involvement are also associated with multiple myeloma. Hypercalcemia, hyperuricemia, and presence of Bence Jones proteins in the urine are frequently noted.

## REFERENCES

1. Bates, B. *A Guide to Physical Examination* (3rd ed.). Philadelphia: J.B. Lippincott, 1983.
2. Bennett, J.C. Clinical features of rheumatoid arthritis. In H.R. Schumacher, *Primer on the Rheumatic Diseases* (9th ed.). Atlanta: Arthritis Foundation, 1988.
3. Brautbar, N., and Kleeman, C.R. Hypophosphatemia and hyperphosphatemia: Clinical and pathophysiologic aspects. In M.H. Maxwell, C.R. Kleeman, and R.G. Narins, *Clinical Disorders of Fluid and Electrolyte Metabolism* (4th ed.). New York: McGraw-Hill, 1987.
4. Calin, A. Ankylosing spondylitis and the spondylarthropathies. In H.R. Schumacher, *Primer on the Rheumatic Diseases* (9th ed.). Atlanta: Arthritis Foundation, 1988.
5. Cormack, D.H. *Ham's Histology* (9th ed). Philadelphia: J.B. Lippincott, 1987.
6. Cotran, R.S., Kumar, V., and Robbins, S.L. *Pathologic Basis of Disease* (4th ed.). Philadelphia: W.B. Saunders, 1989.
7. Cummings, S.R., Nevitt, M.C., and Haber, R.J. Prevention of osteoporotic fractures. *West. J. Med.*, 134:5, 1985.
8. Duckworth, T. Lecture notes on orthopedics and fractures (2nd ed.). Boston: Blackwell, 1984.
9. Ganong, W. *Review of Medical Physiology* (12th ed.). Los Altos, Calif.: Lange, 1985.
10. Guyton, A.C. *Textbook of Medical Physiology* (8th ed.). Philadelphia: W.B. Saunders, 1990.
11. Hahn, B.H. Metabolic bone disease. In H.R. Schumacher, *Primer on the Rheumatic Diseases* (9th ed.). Atlanta: Arthritis Foundation, 1988.
12. Hirschmann, J.V. Osteomyelitis. In E. Braunwald et al., *Harrison's Principles of Internal Medicine* (11th ed.). New York: McGraw-Hill, 1987.
13. Holick, M.F., Krane, S.M., and Potts, J.T. Calcium, phosphorus and bone metabolism: Calcium-regulating hormones. In J. Wilson et al., *Harrison's Principles of Internal Medicine* (12th ed.). New York: McGraw-Hill, 1991.
14. Kelley, W.N. et al. *Textbook of Rheumatology*. Philadelphia: W.B. Saunders, 1985.
15. Kelley, W.N., and Palella, T.D. Gout and other disorders of purine metabolism. In J. Wilson et al., *Harrison's Principles of Internal Medicine* (12th ed.). New York: McGraw-Hill, 1991.
16. Krane, S.M., and Holick, M.F. Metabolic bone disease. In J. Wilson et al., *Harrison's Principles of Internal Medicine* (12th ed.). New York: McGraw-Hill, 1991.
17. Krane, S.M. Paget's disease of bone. In H.R. Schumacher, *Primer on the Rheumatic Diseases* (9th ed.). Atlanta: Arthritis Foundation, 1988.
18. Lane, J., and Vigorita, V. Osteoporosis. *Orthop. Clin. North Am.*, 15l:4, 1984.
19. Langer, R., and Bowen, B. Musculoskeletal trauma. In E. Howell, L. Widra, and M.G. Hill, *Comprehensive Trauma Nursing*. Glenview, Ill.: Scott, Foresman, 1988.
20. Markow, R., and Lane, J. Current concepts of Paget's disease of bone. *Orthop. Clin. North Am.*, 15:4, 1984.
21. Marx, S.J., and Bourdeau, J.E. Calcium metabolism. In M.H. Maxwell, C.R. Kleeman, and R.G. Narins, *Clinical Disorders of Fluid and Electrolyte Metabolism* (4th ed.). New York: McGraw-Hill, 1987.
22. Merino, M.J. Bones and joints. In V.A. LiVolsi et al., *Pathology* (2nd ed.). Media, Penn.: Harwal Publishing Co., 1989.
23. Moskowitz, R.W., and Goldberg, V.M. Osteoarthritis. In H.R. Schumacher, *Primer on the Rheumatic Diseases* (9th ed.). Atlanta: Arthritis Foundation, 1988.
24. Narins, R.G. et al. The metabolic acidoses. In M.H. Maxwell, C.R. Kleeman, and R.G. Narins, *Clinical Disorders of Fluid and Electrolyte Metabolism* (4th ed.). New York: McGraw-Hill, 1987.
25. Pyeritz, R.E. Heritable disorders of connective tissue. In H.R. Schumacher, *Primer on the Rheumatic Diseases* (9th ed.). Atlanta: Arthritis Foundation, 1988.
26. Rodrigo, J.J. *Orthopaedic Surgery: Basic Science and Clinical Science*. Boston: Little, Brown, 1986.
27. Tate, G., and Schumacher, H.R. Clinical features of gout. In H.R. Schumacher, *Primer on the Rheumatic Diseases* (9th ed.). Atlanta: Arthritis Foundation, 1988.
28. Zizic, T.M. Osteonecrosis. In H.R. Schumacher, *Primer on the Rheumatic Diseases* (9th ed.). Atlanta: Arthritis Foundation, 1988.
29. Zvaifler, N.J. Rheumatoid arthritis. In H.R. Schumacher, *Primer on the Rheumatic Diseases* (9th ed.). Atlanta: Arthritis Foundation, 1988.

# UNIT BIBLIOGRAPHY

Albright, J., and Miller, E. (eds.). Osteogenesis imperfecta. *Clin. Orthop.* 159:1, 1981.

Aloia, J.F. Estrogen and exercise in prevention and treatment of osteoporosis. *Geriatrics* 37(6):81, 1982.

Aroncheck, J.M., and Haddad, J.G. Paget's disease. *Orthop. Clin. North Am.* 14:1–3, 1983.

Beltran, J. *MRI: Musculoskeletal system*. Philadelphia: J.B. Lippincott, 1990.

Bowen, J.R., Foster, B.K., and Hartzell, C.R. Legg—Calvé—Perthes disease. *Clin. Orthop.* 185:97, 1984.

Clawson, D.K., and Frederick, A.M. Compartmental syndromes. *Clin. Orthop.* 113:2, 1975.

Cohen, A.S. *Progress in Clinical Rheumatology*, Vol. 1. Orlando, Fla.: Grune & Stratton, 1984.

Cotran, R., Kumar, V., and Robbins, S.L. *Robbins' Pathologic Basis of Disease* (4th ed.). Philadelphia: W.B. Saunders, 1989.

Duckworth, T. *Lecture Notes on Orthopaedics and Fractures* (2nd ed.). Boston: Blackwell, 1984.

Ferguson, A. Segmental vascular changes in the femoral head in children and adults. *Clin. Orthop.* 200:291, 1985.

Fox, J.H., and Kelly, W.N. Management of gout. *JAMA* 242:4, 1979.

Gould, J.A., and Davies, C.J. *Orthopaedic and Sports Physical Therapy*. St. Louis: Mosby, 1985.

Guyton, A. *Textbook of Medical Physiology* (8th ed.). Philadelphia: W.B. Saunders, 1990.

Harrison, M., and Burwell, R. Perthes' disease: A concept of pathogenesis. *Clin. Orthop.* 156:115, 1981.

Howell, E., Widra, L., and Hill, M.G. *Comprehensive Trauma Nursing*. Glenview, Ill.: Scott Foresman, 1988.

Kelley, W.N. *Textbook of Internal Medicine*. Philadelphia: J.B. Lippincott, 1989.

Kelley, W.N. *Textbook of Rheumatology*. Philadelphia: W.B. Saunders, 1985.

Kessler, R.M., and Hertling, D. *Management of Common Musculoskeletal Disorders*. Philadelphia: J.B. Lippincott, 1983.

Kuska, B. Acute onset compartment syndrome. *J. Emerg. Nurs.* 8:75, 1982.

LiVolsi, V.A. et al. *Pathology* (2nd ed.). Media, Penn.: Harwal Publ. Co., 1989.

Mankin, H.J., and Gebhardt, M. Advances in the management of bone tumors. *Clin. Orthop.* 200:73, 1985.

Marieb, E.N. *Essentials of Human Anatomy and Physiology*. Menlo Park, Calif.: Addison-Wesley, 1984.

Maxwell, M.H., Kleeman, C.R., and Narins, N.G. *Clinical Disorders of Fluid and Electrolyte Metabolism* (4th ed.). New York: McGraw-Hill, 1987.

Morizumi, H. Comparative study of alterations in skeletal muscle in Duchenne muscular dystrophy and polymyositis. *Acta Pathol. Jpn.* 34(6):1221, 1984.

Nachemson, A. Advances in low back pain. *Clin. Orthop.* 200:266, 1985.

Nordin, B. et al. New approaches to the problem of osteoporosis. *Clin. Orthop.* 200:181, 1985.

Pollock, M.I., Wilmore, J.H., and Fox, S.M. *Exercise in Health and Disease*. Philadelphia: W.B. Saunders, 1984.

Posner, A. The mineral of bone. *Clin. Orthop.* 200:87, 1985.

Rodman, G.P., and Schumacher, H.R. (eds.). *Primer on Rheumatic Disorders*. Atlanta: Arthritis Foundation, 1983.

Rodrigo, J.J. *Orthopaedic Surgery, Basic Science, and Clinical Science*. Boston: Little, Brown, 1986.

Salter, R.B. *Textbook of Disorders and Injuries to the Musculoskeletal System* (2nd ed.). Baltimore: Williams & Wilkins, 1983.

Schumacher, H.R. *Primer on the Rheumatic Diseases* (9th ed.). Atlanta: Arthritis Foundation, 1988.

Silverstein, A. *Human Anatomy and Physiology*. New York: Wiley, 1980.

Simmons, D. Fracture healing perspectives. *Clin. Orthop.* 200:100, 1985.

Turek, S.L. *Orthopaedics, Principles, and Their Application* (4th ed.). Philadelphia: J.B. Lippincott, 1984.

Turner, R.A., and Wise, C.M. *Textbook of Rheumatology*. Winston Salem, N.C.: Medical Examination, 1986.

Vander, A.J., Sherman, J.H., and Luciano, D.S. *Human Physiology: The Mechanisms of Body Function*. New York: McGraw-Hill, 1985.

Wilson, J.D. et al (eds.). *Harrison's Principles of Internal Medicine* (12th ed.). New York: McGraw-Hill, 1991.

# PROTECTIVE COVERINGS OF THE BODY

The skin is the largest and one of the most metabolically active organs of the body, but its function is often underestimated. It is a dynamic organ that regulates body temperature and fluid balance, and prevents microbial invasion. Hair and nails can also be considered as protective coverings to the body.

Chapter 46 discusses the protective and complex metabolic activities of skin. Chapter 47 describes common inflammatory processes, tumors, and traumatic alterations in skin integrity.

The reader is encouraged to use the learning objectives as guides to facilitate the study of this important organ. The bibliography at the end of the unit provides sources for further study of these topics.

# Normal Structure and Function of the Skin

Barbara L. Bullock

## Chapter Outline

## Learning Objectives

1. Describe the characteristics of the layers of the epidermis.
2. Describe the life cycle of the epidermal cell.
3. Discuss the chemical properties of the epidermis.
4. Describe the production of melanin.
5. Discuss the function of the dermis.
6. Describe the structure and function of the subcutaneous tissues.
7. Describe the process of sweat production and its function in regulating heat.
8. Compare the structure and function of sweat and sebaceous glands.
9. Discuss the growth and development of hair.
10. Describe the purposes for blood supply to the skin.
11. Explain the role of the different nerve receptors in the sensory function of skin.
12. Explain the role of the skin in vitamin D production.

The skin is the largest organ of the body, with a surface area of 1.8 m² and comprising 15% of total body weight in the average adult.[5] This surface area increases 7 times from birth to maturity. The skin's consistency ranges from the thick (0.25 in), tough, yet pliable covering of the body to the thin (0.007 in), delicate, mucous membranes of the mouth, nose, and eyelids. The skin is both pliable and durable, and allows for mobility and protection. At the same time it is one of the most sensitive organs of the body, capable of transmitting a variety of sensations, such as fine touch, pain, temperature, and pressure.[9] The skin functions as a barrier against pathogenic organisms and a protection against trauma from environmental forces.[3]

It is waterproof but can regulate body temperature through sweating. It protects the body from excessive ultraviolet light through production of the pigment melanin. The skin also gives an indication of the general health of a person through color, texture, and alterations in continuity.[3]

## ANATOMY AND PHYSIOLOGY

The skin is composed of three major layers that are, from the surface inward, the epidermis, dermis, and subcuta-

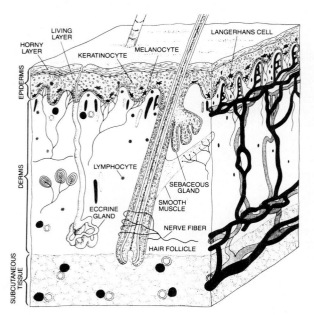

**FIGURE 46-1.**

Complex anatomy of the skin. The surface is covered by a horny layer of dead keratinocytes filled with the protein keratin. Living keratinocytes dominate the epidermis and proliferate as dead cells are lost from the surface. Melanocytes, which secrete pigment granules responsible for skin color, are at the base of the epidermis. Langerhans cells, dendritic cells that process antigens applied to the surface of the skin, lie above the basal layer of keratinocytes. The dermis is largely a network of connective tissue and is underlaid by fatty subcutaneous tissue. The specialized keratinocytes of the hair follicles form hair. The dermis is richly supplied with nerve fibers, some of which innervate sensory nerve endings, and with blood vessels. T lymphocytes are scattered through the skin, primarily in the epidermis and the upper dermis. (Source: R.I. Edelson and J.M. Fink. The immunologic function of the skin. *Sci. Am.* June, 1985; © Scientific American, Inc.)

neous tissues (Figure 46-1,). These layers have the following functions: (1) to protect against the external environment; (2) to maintain and regenerate layers; (3) to participate in defending the body against foreign substances; (4) to preserve the internal fluid environment; (5) to participate in excreting wastes; (6) to assist in regulating body temperature; (7) to produce vitamin D; and (8) to affect psychosocial aspects of daily living. The functions of the three layers of the skin are summarized in Table 46-1.

## Epidermis

The epidermis consists of stratified squamous epithelium that maintains its constant thickness through coordination of desquamation (loss or shedding) and growth.[5] The shedding property allows for cleansing of the surface while maintaining an intact layer for a protection and permeability barrier.[5]

## Layers of the Epidermis

The main layers, or *strata*, of the epidermis, from the dermis to the surface, are the stratum germinativum, stratum spinosum, stratum granulosum, stratum lucidum (present only on the palms and soles), and stratum corneum. These layers are more simply termed the basal, spinous, granular, and keratin layers (Figure 46-2).

The basal layer is one cell thick and lies in contact with the dermis. Within the basal layer are basal cells, which are cuboidal or columnar, have oval nuclei, and are united to each other by desmosomes, or bridges. These cells are attached to a basement membrane by tonofibrils, or half-desmosomes. The epidermis is also attached to the dermis by interlocking, irregularly shaped processes of basal cells with corresponding dermal processes that extend different depths into the dermis (dermoepidermal junction). Processes are present in varying numbers throughout the skin. For example, eyelids have few processes, while nipples have a complex system of ridges, and fingertips have parallel ridges that form cavernous valleys and tunnels.[7] The highly individualized patterns of fingerprints are the results of these valleys. In the normal epidermis, mitosis of new basal cells is limited to the basal layer. During regeneration, mitosis continues upward into the squamous layer.

Throughout the basal layer are dispersed melanocytes, which form melanin and are responsible for pigmentation of the skin. These cells are wedged between the basal cells. When stained, melanocytes have clear cytoplasm and small, dark nuclei.[2]

The spinous layer contains cells with a polygonal shape. Bridges hold the cells together. As these cells move toward the surface they begin to flatten. Within the cells, fibril or keratin precursors make a three-dimensional framework throughout the cytoplasm.[5]

The granular layer is from 2 to 4 cells thick and lies directly above the stratum spinosum. The cells become diamond-shaped and are filled with keratohyalin (hematoxylin) granules.[6] The stratum lucidum is not present in all skin sections but is in the thick epidermis, such as in the palms of the hands and soles of the feet. The cells in this layer are dead and are little more than cell membranes containing prekeratin filaments and protein.[3] This layer provides for toughness and friction.

The keratin layer varies in thickness from 0.02 mm on the forearm to 0.5 mm or more on the soles of the feet (see Figure 46-2). The cells of this layer are flat and without nuclei. Keratin is a tough, fibrous protein that resists chemical change. This layer shields the body from environmental damage and maintains the internal milieu. The skin has the lowest water permeability of any biologic membrane. This low permeability retards water loss and prevents most toxic agents from entering the body, although some substances are readily absorbed. The horny keratin cells are shed continuously, making way for new cells.

**TABLE 46-1.**
FUNCTIONS OF THE SKIN

| FUNCTION | EPIDERMIS | DERMIS | SUBCUTANEOUS TISSUE |
|---|---|---|---|
| Protection | Keratin provides protection from injury by corrosive materials. Inhibits proliferation of micro-organisms because of dry external surface. Mechanical strength through intracellular bonds. | Provides fibroblasts for wound healing. Provides mechanical strength through collagen fibers, elastic fibers, ground substance. Lymphatic and vascular tissues respond to inflammation, injury, and infection. | Absorbs mechanical shock. |
| Water balance | Low permeability to water and electrolytes prevents systemic dehydration and electrolyte loss. | | |
| Temperature regulation | Eccrine sweat glands allow dissipation of heat through evaporation of sweat secreted onto skin surface. | Cutaneous vasculature, through dilation or constriction, promotes or inhibits heat conduction from skin surface. | |
| Sensory organ | Transmits a variety of sensations through neuroreceptor system. | Encloses extensive network of free and encapsulated nerve endings for relaying sensations to the brain. | Contains large pressure receptors. |
| Vitamin synthesis | 7-Dehydrocholesterol present in large concentrations; photoconversion to vitamin D takes place. | | |
| Psychosocial | Body image alterations result with many epidermal diseases, such as generalized psoriasis. | Body image alterations occur with many dermal diseases, such as scleroderma. | |

(Source: T. Rosen, M. Lanning, and M. Hill, Nurse's Atlas of Dermatology. Boston: Little, Brown, 1983.)

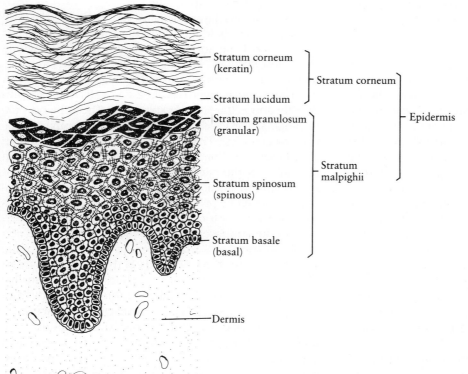

**FIGURE 46-2.**
Layers of the epidermis: Keratin, granular, spinous, and basal. These layers are also called the stratum corneum, stratum granulosum, stratum spinosum, and stratum basale. (Source: M. Borysenko et al. Functional Histology [2nd ed.]. Boston: Little, Brown, 1984.

## *Life Cycle of Epidermal Cells*

The life cycle of epidermal cells involves three phases: *mitosis, keratinization*, and *exfoliation*. The major epidermal cells are keratinocytes. Epidermal cells are continuously formed in the basal or germinative layer at a rate commensurate with the constant loss. New cells move from the basal layer to the stratum corneum in a random fashion that is influenced by the rate of keratinization and by the time that each cell left the basal layer. Transit time from basal layer to surface is anywhere from 12 to 25 days.

Mitosis is affected by two major factors: the diurnal cycle and hormones. Mitosis seems to occur at a greater rate during periods when the body is at rest or asleep. Hormonal influences include androgens, which cause the growth of hair in the typical masculine locations: over the pubis, on the face, on the chest, and on other locations of the body. Androgens aid in the formation of hair follicles and sebaceous glands. Estrogen hormones aid in the formation of the vaginal epithelium and provide for skin softness. Mitosis may be inhibited by adrenalin, levels of which are increased during times of wakefulness.

The second phase in the epidermal cell life cycle is keratinization. As the epidermal cell from the basal layer moves toward the surface, it loses its ability to undergo mitosis. Instead, it begins to synthesize fibrillar and amorphous proteins, keratin, and membrane-coating granules. The cell finally loses its nucleus and cellular organelles, becomes part of the keratin layer, and is shed. The fibrillar proteins make up the fibrils in the epidermal cell and give the layer strength and chemical inertness. As the cell moves toward the surface, more and more fibrils form, until they make up 50% of the protein in these cells. Amorphous proteins that make up the other 50% are embedded in a matrix and have no definite structure. Membrane-coating granules are formed and align near the apical part of the cell membrane. They fuse with the membrane, break it, and discharge their contents into the intercellular spaces in the granular layer. The function of membrane-coating granules is not clear, but they may bind cells together.

As the epidermal cell moves closer to the surface, keratohyalin granules form. These granules are present in cells immediately below the horny layer. When a cell reaches the horny layer, its membrane thickens. The nucleus and organelles disintegrate and are eliminated from the cell.

At the end of keratinization, cornified cells are cemented together in varying thicknesses. Those at the surface are shed, resulting in exfoliation, which is the last phase in the life of an epidermal cell.

Keratinocytes provide an environment for other cell types, including nonkeratinocytes such as melanocytes, Langerhans cells, Merkel cells, and possibly, lymphocytes.[6]

## *Nonkeratinocytes*

*Langerhans cells* are dendritic nonkeratinocytes that function as a part of the immune system. These cells promote the delayed hypersensitivity reactions seen in the skin.[3] They are present in the basal and suprabasal layers of the epidermis and occasionally in the dermis.[6] *Merkel cells* are present in the deep layers of the epidermis of the hands and feet. They are thought to be mechanoreceptors.[3] *Lymphocytes*, especially T lymphocytes, have been reported to be part of normal epidermis.[4] Other cells of the immune defense system are present in the dermis and subcutaneous tissues.

## *Skin Pigmentation*

The color of the skin is determined by *melanocytes*, which originate in the basal layer of the epidermis and in hair follicles. The main function of melanocytes is to synthesize pigment granules, or melanosomes. The main component of melanosomes is melanin, which provides the pigment for skin color. The melanocytes appear in the basal layer of the epidermis as clear cells before they begin to produce melanin.

Melanocytes produce and disperse melanin to keratinocytes (keratinizing basal cells) and hair cells.[1] Melanin is a biochrome of high molecular weight and is produced by oxidation of the amino acid tyrosine with tyrosinase. It forms with a protein matrix in the melanosome to make a melanoprotein. As more melanoprotein is formed, the melanosome grows to become a melanin granule and eventually loses the activity of the enzyme tyrosinase.

Formed melanin is transferred to keratinocytes by active phagocytosis of the distal end of the dendritic processes of the melanocyte.[3] The amount of melanin in these melanocyte dendrites determines skin color (Figure 46-3). In light-skinned individuals, melanin is present primarily in the basal layer of the epidermis. In dark- or black-skinned individuals, it is present throughout the epidermis, including the outermost horny layer. Melanogenesis increases after exposure to ultraviolet light or x-rays. After exposure, the melanocytes in the basal layer increase activity, become larger, develop longer dendrites, and produce more melanin. They may increase in number after exposure to ultraviolet light.[2,3] Melanin acts as a protective screen to protect the deep layers of the epidermis and the dermis from too much solar ultraviolet radiation.[2]

Skin pigmentation is controlled by genes and hormones. Genes regulate the number and shape of melanocytes in the epidermis and hair follicles. Hormonal influences have been demonstrated through the study of hyperpigmentation, as noted in hyperpituitarism and Addison's disease. Estrogen, progesterone, and melanocyte-stimulating hormone (MSH) contribute to increased pig-

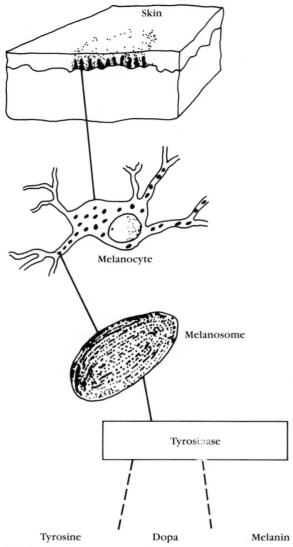

**Skin**

**Melanocyte**

**Melanosome**

**Tyrosinase**

**Tyrosine**          **Dopa**          **Melanin**

**FIGURE 46-3.**
Melanogenesis in human skin as seen in the light and electron microscopes and at the molecular level. (Source: E. Braunwald, *Harrison's Principles of Internal Medicine* [11th ed.]. New York: McGraw-Hill, 1987.)

mentation in various areas of the body during pregnancy. Apparently MSH does not play a major role in pigmentation in the human.[7] Excess amounts of MSH, however, produce a bronze discoloration of the skin. The exact hormonal mechanism for increasing pigmentation is not known.

### Chemical Properties of the Epidermis

The epidermis contains carbohydrates and various enzymes that influence skin cell activity. In normal skin, small amounts of glycogen are present, scattered in various areas of the body, such as the scrotum and scalp, and in cells surrounding pilosebaceous and sweat gland open-ings. After the skin has been traumatized, the amount of glycogen in the epidermis increases.

The epidermis also contains glucose, which diffuses easily into the cells, the amount depending on the serum glucose levels. Eighty percent to 90% of the energy in epidermal cells is derived from adenosine triphosphate (ATP), which is generated through respiration and glycolysis. Intense glycolytic activity in the presence of oxygen is a specific feature of the epidermis that is especially important during wound healing and skin regeneration.

Enzymes in the epidermis that influence all activity include alkaline phosphatase, acid phosphatase, and esterases. Alkaline phosphatase is not present in normal epidermal cells but is present in a damaged epidermis and disappears after healing. Acid phsophatase is a component of the normal epidermis.[7]

## Dermis

The dermis, or *corium*, lies between the epidermis and subcutaneous tissues (see Figure 46-1). It consists of a matrix of loose connective tissue, a fibrous protein embedded in an amorphous ground substance. The dermis is traversed by blood vessels, nerves, and lymphatics and is penetrated by epidermal appendages. The mass of the dermis accounts for 15% to 20% of total body weight.[6]

### Layers of the Dermis

The two main layers in the dermis are (1) the finely textured papillary dermis and (2) the deeper, thicker, coarsely textured reticular layer. The papillary layer lies directly beneath the epidermis. It is composed of thin fibers of collagen, reticular fibers, branching elastic fibers, fibroblasts, abundant ground substance, and capillaries. When the epidermis is removed, the upper surface of the papillary layer forms a negative image of the underside of the epidermis.

The reticular layer lies beneath the papillary layer and extends to the subcutaneous tissue. This layer is mainly composed of thick collagen bundles enmeshed in a network of coarse elastic fibers. It is responsible for the strength and toughness of the skin. There are fewer reticular fibers, blood vessels, fibroblasts, and ground substance in this layer than in the papillary layer.[2] Sensory nerve endings, hair follicles, sweat and sebaceous glands, and some smooth muscle are present in the reticular layer. The combined layers of the dermis vary in thickness. They are thinnest over the eyelids and thickest over the back.[6]

### Components of the Dermis

The two layers of the dermis are composed of varying amounts of collagen, elastic and reticular fibers, and ground substance. Collagen fibers lie at the lower portion of the dermis and make up most of this layer. The molecules form fibers that unite into bundles. These bundles are slightly extensible and wavy, allowing for a certain amount of stretching of the skin.

The elastic fibers are abundant in human skin, being entwined with collagen in the reticular layer of the dermis and extending into the papillary dermis. These fibers help secure the epidermis to the dermis and anchor blood vessels. They can be deformed by a small force and then easily recover their original dimensions.[7] Reticular fibers are young, finely formed fibers of collagen. They are present within and under the epidermal basement membrane and also help to secure the epidermis to the dermis.

Ground substance is present in small amounts in normal skin. It is the structureless portion of connective tissue lying outside of cells, fibers, vessels, and nerves that holds all these components together. Ground substance consists of water, electrolytes, glucose, plasma proteins, neutral and acid mucopolysaccharides, and mucoproteins.[7]

### Cellular Components of the Dermis

The three major cells that are present in the dermis are fibroblasts, macrophages, and mast cells. *Fibroblasts* are the most abundant of these cells; they secrete procollagen, proelastin, microfibrillar proteins, elastin, and components of ground substance.[1,6] *Macrophages* probably develop from the blood monocytes and can be fixed or ameboid cells that help rid the dermis of foreign substances and cell residue. Macrophages participate in the immune response and are vital to wound healing, inflammation, tissue resorption, and recycling of tissue components (see Chap. 13). *Mast cells* are present in perivascular connective tissue and their microscopic appearance shows the cytoplasm to be filled with large metachromatic granules. Under certain physical and chemical conditions, these cells degranulate. Such conditions include exposure to cold, heat, x-rays, ultraviolet light, toxins, certain peptides, and protamine sulfate. When degranulation occurs, the substances of heparin and histamine are released. Heparin prevents blood clotting and, in small amounts, accelerates lipid transportation. Histamine increases capillary permeability, contracts smooth muscle, increases chemotaxis, produces an itching sensation, and increases gastric secretion.[7]

### Functions of the Dermis

The dermis provides the main protection of the body from external injury. Its flexibility allows joint movement and localized stretching, but resists tearing, shearing, and local pressure. When skin is at rest, the protective collagen network is slack. When exposed to tension, the skin "gives" until the slack is taken up. Skin kept taut for long periods of time becomes fatigued, and stretching results. This is exhibited by the stretch marks or *striae gravidarum* (a pinkish-white or gray line seen where skin has been stretched by pregnancy, obesity, or tumor), which are irreversible. The skin also becomes thinner when compressed under force and wells up around the source of compression. Pressure damage may occur from long duration of pressure and distribution of force. Most damage is a result of long pressure, but severe point pressure can injure underlying and cutaneous tissues.

The dermis also provides the necessary base on which the epidermis receives nutrients and grows. It serves as a barrier to infection by way of hyaluronic acid in the ground substance, which prevents bacterial penetration.[6] Hyaluronic acid also binds water and helps maintain dermal turgor. The skin may also store water and electrolytes. Dermal concentrations of cations are slightly above those in blood, so that cations stored in the dermis may be tapped to maintain normal levels in blood.

### Subcutaneous Tissues

The third major layer of skin is the subcutaneous tissue. It is loose-textured, white, and fibrous. Fat and slender elastic fibers are intermingled. Subcutaneous papillae jut into the dermis. These papillae are larger and more dispersed than dermal papillae. It is through subcutaneous papillae that blood vessels and nerves enter the upper layers of skin.

The subcutaneous tissue layer contains blood and lymph vessels, roots of hair follicles, secretory portions of sweat glands, cutaneous and sensory nerve endings, and fat. Subcutaneous fat varies in amount throughout the body and is absent in the eyelids, penis, scrotum, nipples, and areolae. The unequal fat distribution between males and females is partially a result of hormonal influence. Strands or sheets of white, fibrous, connective tissue supports the fat tissue.

The subcutaneous tissue contains voluntary and involuntary muscles. Voluntary muscle is present on the scalp, face, and neck. Involuntary smooth muscle is present in the dartos muscle of the scrotum and in the muscle tissue of the areolae and nipples. Subcutaneous tissue is a heat insulator, shock absorber, and calorie-reserve depot.

### Epidermal Appendages

The sweat glands, sebaceous glands, hair, and nails compose the epidermal appendages. These extend through layers of the skin (Figure 46-4).

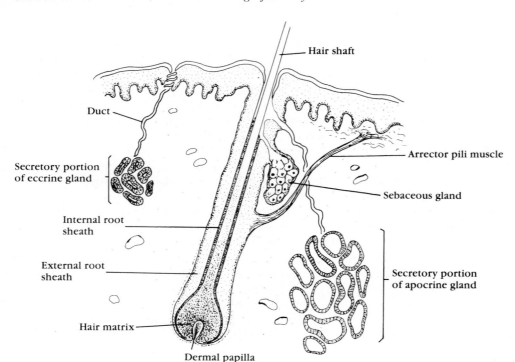

**FIGURE 46-4.**
Some cutaneous appendages. (Source: M. Borysenko, et al., *Functional Histology* [2nd ed.]. Boston: Little, Brown, 1984.)

## Sweat Glands

There are two types of sweat glands: eccrine and apocrine. The *eccrine* sweat glands are present all over the body and are most numerous in thick skin. They open to the surface epidermis and descend through the dermis to just above the subcutaneous layer of the skin. These glands are especially prominent on the soles of the feet, palms of the hand, and axillae.

Eccrine glands are simple, coiled, tubular glands that may be divided into four segments. The lowermost, or secretory, portion has two layers of cells. Of these, myoepithelial cells make up the outer layer and contract to facilitate sweat release. The inner layer is composed of clear large cells and dark small cells, which contain glycogen and polysaccharides, respectively. The secretory layer is one cell thick. In ascending order, the remaining portion of the eccrine unit includes the coiled dermal duct and a straight dermal duct, which opens on the surface of the epidermis through the spiraled intraepidermal duct (see Figure 46-4). The coiled and straight dermal ducts are two cells thick and are composed of cuboidal basophilic epithelium. The duct narrows as it ascends to the surface and widens again as it becomes the intraepidermal spiral duct. The cells lining the spiraling duct are keratinized but have no melanin.[6,7]

Eccrine glands produce sweat to aid in regulating of body temperature. Control of sweating is located in the hypothalamus, which responds to changes in body temperature.[7] Sweat is formed in the secretory coil of the eccrine unit. The solution here is isotonic or slightly hypertonic and contains lactate with small amounts of bicarbonate. In the dermal duct, sodium, chloride, and water are resorbed. As sweat exits onto the epidermis it is hypotonic. As the rate of sweating increases, sodium and chloride concentrations in the sweat also increase, whereas potassium, lactate, and urea concentrations decrease. Not all eccrine glands function all of the time, but they respond promptly to heat stress. The amount of sweat produced depends on the amount of heat to which the person is exposed. Two to three liters of sweat per hour may be produced in an adult exposed to extreme heat conditions. Eccrine sweat is a colorless and odorless hypotonic solution that is 99% water and 1% solutes, such as sodium chloride, potassium, urea, protein, lipids, amino acids, calcium, phosphorus, and iron. The specific gravity is 1.005, and the pH ranges from 4.5 to 7.0.

The skin plays passive and active roles in controlling body temperature. Passively, skin is a barrier to the external environment. Actively, the eccrine units, together with the cutaneous blood vessel network, participate in regulatory heat exchange. The sweat glands cool the surface of the skin with the liquid sweat, which evaporates, causing further cooling. The cutaneous vessels dilate or constrict to dissipate or conserve body heat. The control seat for this process is in the hypothalamus, the neural thermostat.

The hypothalamus is stimulated by changes in surface and blood temperatures. An increase in body temperature of 0.5°C causes the hypothalamus to send a message by way of cholinergic fibers of the sympathetic nervous system to the sweat glands, which pour sweat onto the body surface, causing cooling when it evaporates.[7]

Heat is the primary stimulus to eccrine sweat production, but other physiologic stimuli can stimulate sweating. Gustatory sweating occurs on the face and scalp after eating spicy foods. Emotional stress causes sweating on palms, soles, axillae, and forehead that may extend to the whole body. Pain, nausea, or vomiting also may cause localized or generalized sweating.

*Apocrine* sweat glands are present in the axillae, around the nipples, the anogenital region, external ear canals (ceruminous glands), eyelids (Moll's glands), and breasts (mammary glands). These glands make a secretion with an unknown function in humans. In animals, the secretion attracts animals of the opposite sex. The glands remain small until puberty, when they begin secreting.[3]

Apocrine gland ducts empty into the pilosebaceous follicle above the entrance of sebaceous gland ducts (see Figure 46-4). The coiled secretory gland is located in the lower dermis or subcutaneous tissues. The straight duct empties into the hair follicle. The apocrine coil has a larger diameter than the eccrine coil. The inner secretory layer of the coil is one cell thick. Surrounding the secretory cells are myoepithelial cells, basement membrane, and elastic and reticular fibers. The straight ductal portion of the gland has two cell layers with no myoepithelium and merges with the epithelium of the hair follicle.

Apocrine sweat has a milky color and contains protein and carbohydrates. In the duct, the sweat is sterile and odorless. Only after reaching the surface, where it contacts bacteria, does it take on an odor. Two steps are involved in the production of sweat from the apocrine glands, secretion and excretion. Sweat is secreted continuously and fills the duct before being excreted. When the duct is full, peristaltic waves produced by the myoepithelium propel the secretion outward. Excretion may be stimulated by emotional stress and hormones such as epinephrine.

## Sebaceous Glands

Sebaceous glands arise as epithelial buds from the outer root sheath of the hair follicle. The glands are present throughout the body, except in the palms of the hands and soles and dorsa of the feet. Because these glands develop as buds from the root sheath, they are almost always associated with hair follicles, but are found in some hairless skin, such as that of the nipples, prepuce, labia, and glans penis.[3] The size of sebaceous glands is inversely proportional with the diameter of hair in the follicles. They are largest where hair is sparse or absent, such as on the forehead, nose, chest, and back.

Several lobules compose the glands. The lobules are surrounded by a thin, vascular, fibrous, tissue capsule in the dermis. The cells next to the capsule provide the germinative layer and correspond to the germinative cells of the basal layer of epidermis (Figure 46-5). The germ cells

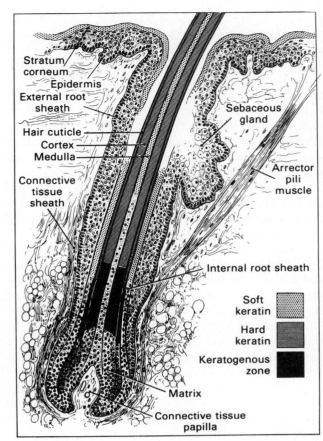

**FIGURE 46-5.**

Diagram of a hair follicle, showing the distribution of soft and hard keratin and the keratogenous zone in which the hard keratin of the hair is produced. (Source: Cormack, D.H., *Ham's Histology* [9th ed.]. Philadelphia: J.B. Lippincott, 1987. After C.P. Leblond. *Ann. NY Acad. Sci.* 53:464, 1951.)

change, taking up and filling with lipid, become bloated and disintegrate, and their contents of lipid and cell debris are discharged into the sebaceous duct as sebum. Other components of sebum include phospholipids, esterified cholesterol, triglycerides, and waxes. Sebum is then evacuated to the follicle and to the surface. It is sebum that produces oily skin; it lubricates the hair and skin and prevents drying. Sebaceous glands are holocrine glands, because they have no lumen and form secretions from decomposition of cells.[3]

## Hair

Human beings are covered with hair in all areas except the palms, soles, dorsum of digits, lips, glans penis, labia, and nipples. Hair is needed to screen the nasal passages and protect the scalp and eyes from sun and sweat.

There are several types of hair. Primary hair, or *lanugo*, is present on the human fetus and infant. These same fine hairs may be noted on the adult as *vellus* hairs. An example is the bald man who has fine vellus hair on his scalp. In the adult, coarse pigmented hair is most developed on the scalp, the beard and chest areas in men, and pubic and axillary areas.

Hair varies morphologically and biologically on different parts of the body. It also varies in structure, length, rate of growth, and response to stimuli. For instance, sex hormones govern hair growth in the pubic and axillary regions as part of the secondary sex characteristics. Sex hormones do not govern other hair growth. Morphologically, hair is divided into three types: straight, wavy, and woolly, depending on the angle of the hair follicles. Straight hair is found in American Indians, Chinese, and the Mongol races, and is coarse in nature.[3] Wavy hair is found in many ethnic groups, while woolly hair is found typically in black races.[2]

Hair originates in the hair follicle, and the two may be considered one structure. The hair bulb lies at the lower end of the follicle and encloses an ovoid, vascular papilla of connective tissue. The matrix cells of the bulb surround the papilla as it juts upward into the bulb (see Figure 46-5). At an outlet at the distal end of the bulb, the papilla emerges and is continuous with the connective tissue sheath that surrounds the follicle. The hair bulb is covered with concentric layers of tissue and enclosed by a thin outer root sheath. A basement membrane of reticular fibers and neutral mucopolysaccharides lies against the external root sheath. A fibrous sheath lies next to the basement membrane and is composed of collagen and fibroblasts. Melanocytes are present in the bulb and in the outer root sheath. The color of hair depends on the amount and distribution of melanin within it. The pigments of the melanin are black, brown, and yellow. The brown and black melanins are called *eumelanin*, while the yellow is called *pheomelanin*. The amounts produced are genetically controlled. It is thought that hair becomes gray when the melanocytes of the bulbs of the hair follicles fail to make tyrosinase.[3]

The mitotic activity of the matrix cells is very great, with hair matrix being replaced every 12 to 24 hours. The hair and inner root sheath are joined, so that they grow at the same rate. When the hair and inner sheath reach the external root sheath, the inner sheath disintegrates and the outer sheath begins to cornify. As the hair reaches the surface opening of the follicle, it is called a *hair shaft* and is a dead cornified structure extending out from the follicle.

The growth of hair occurs in cycles: *anagen*, growing; *catagen*, involuting; and *telogen*, resting. Anagen begins when a papilla joins with cells that enclose it. The papilla juts into the hair bulb, and new matrix cells in the bulb begin to form a hair and push toward the surface. As it pushes to the surface, the old hair in the follicle is loosened, pushed out, and lost. In catagen, the inferior portion disappears, the outer root sheath cornifies around the bulbous end of the hair shaft, melanin synthesis ceases, and the bulb turns white. A cord of epithelial cells replaces the inferior portion and connects the papilla to the bulb. In telogen, the epithelial cord shrinks away from the papilla and disconnects; the epithelial cells of the cord are undifferentiated and wait to join a new papilla and begin anagen. Each hair follicle operates independently; therefore, each hair may be in a different phase of the cycle from its neighbor. The life cycle of hair through the three stages varies in different parts of the body. Scalp hair–which is in anagen from 3 to 10 years, in catagen 3 weeks, and in telogen 3 months–has the longest growth period of any hair on the body. The longer the growing period, the longer the hair. Scalp hair grows about 0.4 to 0.5 mm daily and is influenced by factors such as nutrition, light, hormones, and temperature.[2] The phases of the hair cycle may be influenced by illness, which may place growing-phase hairs into resting-phase hairs that can be more easily lost or shed.[1]

Attached to the hair follicle is the arrectores pilorum, a smooth muscle attached to connective tissue hair sheath and inserted in the dermal papilla. Contraction of this muscle erects hair, squeezes out sebum, and creates goose flesh during the spasm.

## Nails

The nails are composed of specialized layers of epithelial cells and are protective coverings at the ends of fingers and toes (Figure 46-6). The rectangular nail plates on the dorsal surfaces of the ends of fingers and toes are composed of closely welded cells of cornified epithelium. They are semitransparent and allow the pink of the vascular nail bed to show. Each nail plate is surrounded by a fold of skin called the *nail bed*. The nail plate rests on top of the nail bed, where fibers attach the nail to the periosteum of the distal phalanx of each digit. The nail bed is abundant with blood vessels and sensory nerve endings. The distal edge of the nail is freely movable. The proximal edge is attached firmly at the base of the nail. The *lunula* is a white, half-moon-shaped area at the base of the nail and is the most actively growing portion of the nail. The epithelium in this area of the nail is thick, and

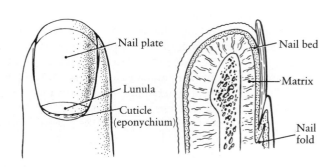

**FIGURE 46-6.**
Structure of the nail in cross-section of a finger.

the cells here become keratinized with harder keratin than that present in the hair or the epidermis. From the lunula the nail grows longitudinally over dermal ridges of the nail bed at a rate of about 0.5 mm per week.[3] The soft cuticle that forms over the proximal nail plate is called the *eponychium*.

## Blood Supply

Blood supply to the skin varies in different parts of the body, depending on factors such as the type of skin perfused, thickness of the skin's layers, and types and numbers of skin appendages. Common to skin throughout the body are deep subdermal arterial plexus and a superficial subpapillary plexus. Endothelial cells line all parts of the vasculature. In the small capillaries, one endothelial cell surrounds the lumen. Collagen or reticular fibers ensheath the capillaries. Arterioles have an intima, a smooth muscle layer, and an adventitia of collagen and elastic fibers. Venules consist of epithelium and collagen. In larger veins, smooth muscle and elastic fibers are present.

The number of blood vessels is greater than necessary to meet the biologic needs of the skin tissues. The vessels have two functions: (1) to provide oxygen and nutrients to skin cells, together with removing wastes, and (2) to aid in thermal regulation.

The vessels are arranged in a three-dimensional network consisting of the two plexuses (deep and superficial) and the vessels that connect them (Figure 46-7). The deep plexus is joined to larger vessels in the subcutaneous layer and lies in the lower portion of the dermis. The superficial plexus lies beneath the papillary dermis. A network of capillaries reaches up into the dermal papilla to nourish the upper layers of skin.

A second route of blood flow is through arteriovenous shunts located in the upper part of the reticular dermis. These shunts, known as *glomi*, are important in regulating heat. They are present throughout the skin but are particularly prevalent in the pads and nail beds of fingers and toes, soles and palms, ears, and center of the face. The shunts enable blood to bypass the capillaries and increase blood flow. The plexuses and arteriovenous shunts are controlled by the sympathetic nervous system and constrict and dilate in response to various chemical agents such as epinephrine and histamine. Under normal thermal conditions, the blood flow to the skin is about 250 mL/min/m$^2$ of body surface. This can decrease to 50 mL/min in severe cold, or increase to 2 to 3 L/min in extreme heat.[8] Vasodilation causes the skin to become hot and red, whereas vasoconstriction causes it to become cold, often with a pale or bluish hue.[8]

## Nervous Control

The skin is a major sensory organ. Dermal nerve endings receive stimuli from touch, pressure, temperature, pain, and itch. Nerve endings are most numerous on palms, soles, fingers, and mucocutaneous areas of lips, glans penis, and clitoris.

Temperature, pain, pressure, and itch are perceived

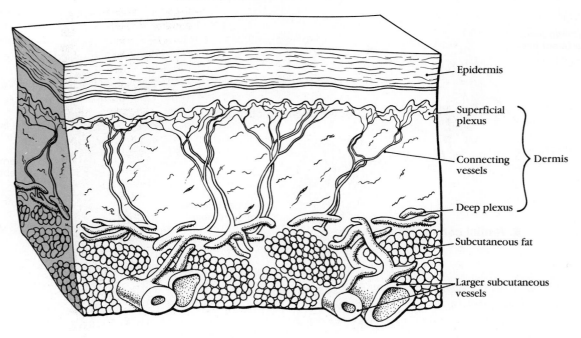

**FIGURE 46-7.**
Blood vessels of the subcutaneous tissue.

by nerves ending in the dermal papilla and surrounding hair follicles (Figure 46-8). Free nerve endings in the epidermis are both myelinated and unmyelinated, and respond to temperature, pain, and pressure.[2] *Merkel endings* are present in the deep layers of the epidermis. The cells have fingerlike cytoplasmic projections between the keratinocytes, and they attach to myelinated afferent fibers. They are thought to function as mechanoreceptors.[2]

*Meissner's corpuscles* receive touch stimuli. They lie in the papillary derma on the palms and soles, and consist of myelinated and unmyelinated nerve fibers. *Pacini's corpuscles* sense pressure and are located on the soles, palms, nipples, and genital and perianal regions. These encapsulated end organs of myelinated and unmyelinated fibers swiftly send messages to the central nervous system. Mucocutaneous end organs (*Krause end bulbs*)

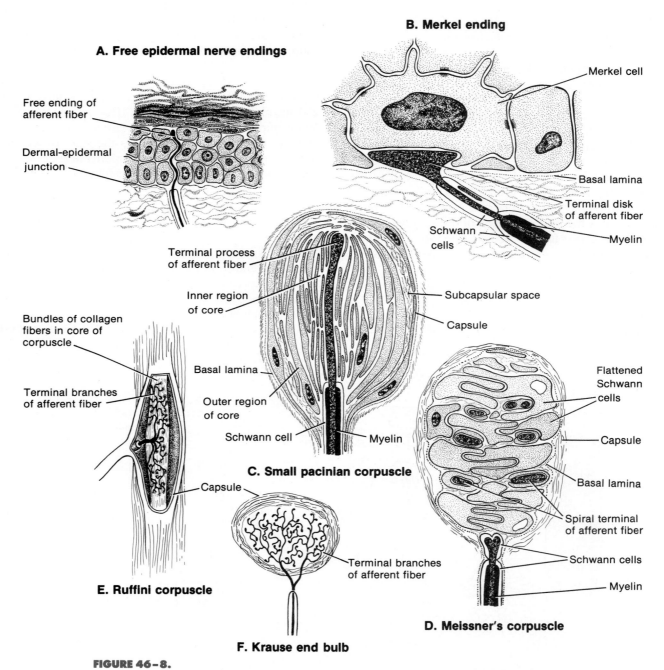

**FIGURE 46-8.**
Sensory receptors that are present in the skin. **A.** Free nerve ending in epidermis. **B.** Merkel ending in epidermis. **C.** Small pacinian corpuscle in dermis. **D.** Meissner's corpuscle in dermis. **E.** Ruffini corpuscle in dermis. **F.** Krause end bulb (mucocutaneous corpuscle) in dermis. (Source: D.H. Cormack, *Ham's Histology* [9th ed.]. Philadelphia: J.B. Lippincott, 1987.)

are present in regions such as lips, tongue, gums, eyelids, genitalia, and perianal area. These organs probably perceive general sensory stimuli and are present in the subpapillary dermis. Myelinated nerves enter the end organ, lose their myelin, and form numerous networks.

The mucocutaneous end organs, Meissner's and Pacini's corpuscles, are specialized sensory nerve end organs in areas of modified hairless skin. The remainder of skin over the body is supplied with sensory and autonomic nerve fibers located in the dermis. *Ruffini corpuscles* are found throughout the dermis, especially on the plantar surface of the feet. They are thought to be mechanoreceptors that respond to tension in the collagen fibers.[2] Sensory nerves are myelinated up to their terminal branches, are large in diameter, and extend toward the epidermis or hair follicle. These nerves arise from the spinal cord, return by way of the dorsal root ganglia, and receive sensations of temperature, pain, and itch on the unmyelinated nerve ends. Autonomic nerves to the skin are motor nerves, and they do not always have a myelin sheath. Branches of nerves from the sympathetic nervous system innervate blood vessels, arrectores pilorum muscles, and eccrine and apocrine glands.

## Vitamin D Synthesis in the Skin

Vitamin D is an essential fat-soluble vitamin that, when activated, aids in the absorption of calcium and phosphate in the intestine. The activated form of vitamin D (1,25-dihydroxycholecalciferol) is commonly referred to as vitamin D hormone. It improves mineralization of bone by increasing plasma calcium and phosphate concentrations to support forming bone.[8]

Vitamin D hormone is not a single compound but is a family of compounds, the two most important of which are vitamin $D_2$ and $D_3$. Vitamin $D_3$, or *cholecalciferol*, is produced in the skin when it is exposed to ultraviolet irradiation. The skin cells contain 7-dehydrocholesterol in the epidermis. Ultraviolet light penetrates the epidermis and causes 7-dehydrocholesterol to undergo photolysis to form previtamin D, which over a period of a few hours isomerizes to form vitamin $D_3$. Vitamin $D_3$ is then transported in the blood bound to serum protein. It is converted in two steps, first by the liver and then the kidneys, to vitamin D hormone and may then be stored in the liver and in body fat.[8] Vitamin $D_2$, or ergocalciferol, is the therapeutic form of vitamin D and, like vitamin $D_3$, is transported to the liver and kidneys, where it is converted to vitamin D hormone.[6]

## REFERENCES

1. Bauer, E., Tobas, M., and Goslen, J. Skin: Cells, matrix and function. In W. Kelley, *Textbook of Internal Medicine*. Philadelphia: J.B. Lippincott, 1989.
2. Bickers, D.R. Photosensitivity and other reactions to light. In J. Wilson et al. (eds.), *Harrison's Principles of Internal Medicine* (12th ed.). New York: McGraw-Hill, 1991.
3. Cormack, D. *Ham's Histology* (9th ed.). Philadelphia: J.B. Lippincott, 1987.
4. Edelson, R.L., and Fink, J.M. The immunologic function of the skin. *Sci. Am.*, 252(6):46, 1985.
5. Farmer, E.R. *Pathology of the Skin*. Norwalk, Conn.: Appleton-Lange, 1990.
6. Fitzpatrick, T.B. et al. *Dermatology in General Medicine* (3rd ed.). New York: McGraw-Hill, 1984.
7. Fitzpatrick, T.B., and Soter, N.A. Pathophysiology of skin. In N.A. Soter and H.R. Baden, *Pathophysiology of Dermatologic Diseases*. New York: McGraw-Hill, 1984.
8. Guyton, A. *Textbook of Medical Physiology*. Philadelphia: W.B. Saunders, 1990.
9. Rosen, K., Lanning, M., and Hill, M. *The Nurse's Atlas of Dermatology*. Boston: Little, Brown, 1983.

# chapter 47

Barbara L. Bullock

# Alterations in Skin Integrity

## Chapter Outline

## Learning Objectives

1. Identify the two types of skin sensitivity responses.
2. Explain the pathophysiologic process that results in acne.
3. Describe the three types of dermatitis/eczema disease.
4. List the complications of atopic dermatitis.
5. State the cause and precipitating factors of herpes simplex.
6. Describe the features and course of varicella virus disease.
7. Discuss the mechanism of activation of herpes zoster, its target population, and persons at greatest risk of infection.
8. Discuss the cause and treatment of warts (verrucae).
9. Describe the features of rubeola and rubella.
10. Review the common characteristics of impetigo.
11. Compare two examples of scaling disorders of the skin and their treatments.
12. State and discuss briefly the types of benign skin tumors.

13. Differentiate the three major types of malignant skin tumors.
14. Compare and contrast the differences between partial- and full-thickness burns.
15. Describe the changes that occur in the skin as a result of thermal therapy.
16. Discuss the systemic changes that occur as a result of burn injury.
17. Explain the causes, types of injuries, and effects of electrical and chemical burns.
18. Discuss the crucial factors in the formation of decubitus ulcers.
19. Describe the grading of decubitus ulcers.
20. Discuss the skin changes resulting from abrasions, incisions, puncture wounds, and lacerations.

To understand the pathophysiology of the skin and its diseases, one must be familiar with both the descriptive terms used to characterize skin lesions and the inflammatory processes that herald the diseases. A systematic approach to skin lesions prepares one to assess the extent of disease.

Important aspects for determining the pathophysiology of skin disease include the following: (1) characteristics of the lesion; (2) distribution of many lesions; (3) length of time present and recurrence; (4) medications taken, both systemic and topical; (5) family history of disease; and (6) environmental or personal exposure to hazardous material. Table 47-1 lists the basic nomenclature used to describe lesions. Figure 47-1 shows the

**TABLE 47–1.**
SKIN LESIONS

| LESION | DESCRIPTION |
| --- | --- |
| **Primary lesions** | |
| Macula | Flat (nonelevated) discoloration of the skin, less than 5 mm in diameter. |
| Patch | Similar to a macula, but more than 5 mm in diameter. |
| Papule | Solid, circumscribed, elevated lesion, less than 5 mm in diameter; often caused by accumulation of inflammatory cells, proliferation of neoplastic cells, or deposit of metabolic by-products. |
| Nodule | Similar to a papule, but 5 mm to 5 cm in diameter. |
| Tumor | Solid mass, more than 5 cm in diameter, usually extends deeper into the skin. |
| Plaque | A flattened, raised lesion with more lateral dimension (surface area) greater than height (elevation above the skin); sometimes the result of clustering of papules; has the feel of a thickened area of skin. |
| Vesicle | Small, circumscribed, elevated lesion containing fluid; diameter less than 5 mm. |
| Bulla | Larger version of a vesicle, more than 5 mm in diameter; alternatively called a *blister*. |
| Pustule | Yellow-white vesicle filled with pus. |
| Cyst | Semisolid or fluid-filled mass surrounded by a capsule; usually located in the deeper portions of the skin. |
| Wheal | Transient, round, irregularly shaped, faint pink elevation; caused by edema fluid in the dermis. |
| Comedo | Plugged, dilated pore, often called a *blackhead* or whitehead. |
| **Hemorrhagic flat lesions** | |
| Petechia | Hemorrhagic macula less than 5 mm. |
| Purpura | Hemorrhagic patch 5 mm to 5 cm. |
| Ecchymosis | Large hemorrhagic mark; black-and-blue spot. |
| **Secondary lesions** | |
| Scale | Excessive accumulation of loosely adherent keratin; usually seen in papules and plaques. |
| Erosion | Superficial loss of epidermis; not associated with scarring; often accompanies vesicles, bullae, or pustules. |
| Excoriation | Linear erosion caused by scratching. |
| Ulcer | Deep erosion resulting from loss of epidermis and part of dermis; often heals with a scar. |
| Crust | Accumulation of dried sebum, serum, cellular and bacterial debris over a damaged epidermis; often overlies erosion and is seen in vesicles, bullae, and pustules. |
| Lichenification | Thickened skin with accentuated markings; caused by chronic rubbing and scratching. |
| Fissure | Crack in the epidermis. |
| Atrophy | Thinning of the skin at site of disorder; appreciated best by palpation. |

(Source: T. Rosen, M. Lanning, and M. Hill, The Nurse's Atlas of Dermatology. Boston: Little, Brown, 1983.)

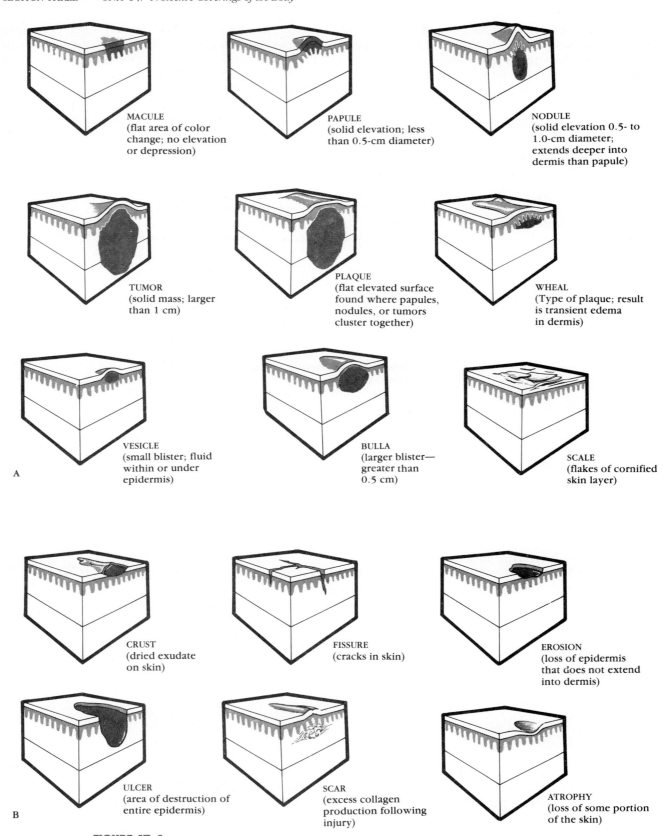

**FIGURE 47-1.**
**A.** Primary skin lesions and their characteristics. **B.** Secondary skin lesions and their characteristics. (Source: J. Sano and R. Judge, *Physical Assessment Skills for Nursing Practice* [2nd ed.]. Boston: Little, Brown, 1982.)

appearance of various lesions. Description of a lesion may require a combination of these terms.

# INFLAMMATION

The body's response to injury is to generate inflammation (see Chap. 13). Sources of injury to the skin include bacteria, viruses, temperature extremes, and chemical or mechanical irritants. Inflammation alters the surrounding blood vessels and adjacent tissues. Redness or erythema is the hallmark of inflammation. An irritant causes injury to the site, which results in a vascular reaction with fluid exudation and edema. Pressure from the edema or chemical irritation from the release of various mediator substances causes pain due to irritation of the nerve fibers in that area. The duration of the inflammatory response varies.

## Skin Sensitivity

Urticaria and angioedema can be classified as diseases or as reactions to injury or an allergen.

### Urticaria

This vascular reaction, commonly called *hives*, is manifested by transient erythema or whitish swellings (wheals) of the skin or mucous membranes.[1] Skin changes or lesions result from increased vascular permeability and local release of histamine and vasoactive mediators.[24] These changes may result in localized edema, which may begin to resolve within several hours. The lesions are usually erythematous, well-circumscribed wheals. A reddened halo of flare often surrounds the raised part of the lesion.[24] These lesions often cause pruritus and a stinging sensation. *Acute urticaria* can be defined as a cutaneous vascular reaction that evolves over a short period, from days to several weeks, and usually has a detectable cause. It resolves completely. Urticaria lasting longer than 6 weeks is classified as *chronic urticaria*. It may persist for years; it also may go away and then recur. The underlying cause is usually unknown.

The etiologies of urticaria are numerous and can include such components as foods, inhalants, drugs, injectants (eg, blood, vaccines), chemicals, mechanical and environmental irritants, and psychogenic factors. Cutaneous drug reactions occur in 1% to 3% of all hospitalized medical patients.[25] They usually occur within the first 4 to 6 days of drug treatment and have varying clinical features (Table 47-2).

Treatment involves removing the causative agent. Antihistamines are often used. Alleviating irritation factors, instituting elimination diets, and preventing and treating dry skin may be of benefit.

### Angioedema

Angioedema is a reaction that involves edema not only of the superficial skin but of the subcutaneous tissues. The differences between urticaria and angioedema are degree and location. Angioedema can be described as giant wheals, often involving the mucous membranes. It can cause many physical symptoms including severe respiratory distress, especially when it affects the larynx.

# COMMON INFLAMMATORY DISEASES OF THE SKIN

## Dry Skin

Dry skin in itself is a noninflammatory condition, but it can become reddened when it persists unrelieved. It is extremely common and consists of roughened, flaky skin with or without pruritus.[4]

The defect, which occurs commonly in the aging process, involves loss of water, electrolytes, and skin lipids. It is frequent in dry and cold climates, and environmental conditions aggravate the condition if it previously existed.

Dehydration after sweating dries out the surface keratin, and itching and inflammatory changes can be superimposed.[4] Treatment of dry skin involves rehydration with a moisturizer and water, together with barrier creams used consistently.

## Acne

Acne vulgaris is a common, chronic, inflammatory disease of the sebaceous glands and hair follicles of the skin, also known as the *pilosebaceous ducts* (Figure 47-2). It results from two factors: (1) accumulation of sebum, the fatty secretion liberated by the breakdown of sebaceous cells; and (2) irritation of the area around the hair follicle, leading to a perifolliculitis.

The exact etiology of acne is unknown, but it may be due to either increased activity of the sebaceous glands or inability of the material secreted to escape through a narrow opening. The resulting inflammation is precipitated by the combination of sebum, bacteria, and subsequent release of fatty acids. The last is caused by the hydrolytic action of the lipases, which are furnished by the bacteria on the sebum itself. The inflammatory reaction and resulting edema probably cause the sebaceous follicle to perforate its wall and develop perifolliculitis.

The development of acne depends on several factors, including heredity, use of oil-based cosmetics or skin treatments, ingestion of drugs (eg, steroids, androgens), and the presence of bacteria. Sebaceous glands are hormonally controlled, and the androgenic hormones may

**TABLE 47–2.**

CUTANEOUS DRUG REACTIONS

| TYPE OF ERUPTION | CLINICAL FEATURES | DRUGS POTENTIALLY CAUSING THE REACTION |
| --- | --- | --- |
| Morbilliform | Diffuse, confluent, macular, papular, erythematous<br>Often occur in first week | Penicillins<br>Sulfonamides<br>Phenytoin (with adenopathy, leukocytosis, liver function abnormalities in hypersensitivity syndrome)<br>Barbiturates<br>Ampicillin (up to 90% of patients with infectious mononucleosis) |
| Urticaria | Pruritic, erythematous, annular | Penicillins<br>Aspirin<br>Nonsteroidal antiinflammatory agents<br>Radiocontrast media |
| Erythema multiforme and toxic epidermal necrolysis | Erythematous target lesions with concentric rings that often become erosions that crust | Sulfonamides<br>Phenytoin<br>Penicillin derivatives<br>Phenyl butazone |
| Fixed drug reaction | Single (or at most a few) lesion, violaceous, annular with dusky center and hyperpigmentation; occasionally vesicular<br>Recur at same location with rechallenge | Phenolphthalein<br>Sulfonamides<br>Tetracyclines<br>Phenylbutazone<br>Barbiturates |
| Lichenoid | Papular with overlying fine silvery scale<br>Identical to true lichen planus | Gold<br>Antimalarials<br>Quinidine<br>Thiazides |
| Vasculitis | Palpable purpura<br>Extremities more than trunk | Penicillins<br>Thiazides<br>Allopurinol<br>Phenytoin |
| Erythema nodosum | Tender, erythematous nodules<br>Usually anterior tibial surface | Oral contraceptives |
| Vegetative | Nodular, crusted, purulent, often fungating lesions | Halogens (iodides, bromides) |
| Acneiform | Superficial papules, pustules | Corticosteroids<br>Phenytoin<br>Halogens |
| Pityriasis rosea | Oval, slightly scaly papules on trunk and proximal extremities | Gold |
| Pemphigus foliaceus | Erythematous, scaly, crusted, erosive lesions<br>Upper trunk, face | Penicillamine |

(Source: W.N. Kelley, Textbook of Internal Medicine. *Philadelphia: J.B. Lippincott, 1989.*)

increase the development and secretion of sebaceous glands. The lesions are located in the areas of predominant pilosebaceous glands—face, chest, back, neck, and upper arms.

The early, noninflammatory lesions are of two types, white (closed) and black comedones. The white comedo occurs in a closed excretory duct that has a very small, possibly microscopic, opening that prevents drainage. This lesion may lead to an inflammatory process and give rise to a papule or pustule. The black comedo (blackhead) is a widely dilated follicle filled with oxidized melanin that plugs an excretory duct of the skin.[15] Both

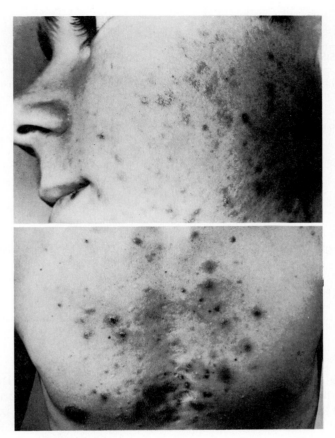

**FIGURE 47-2.**
Acne of the face and chest. (Source: G.C. Sauer, *Manual of Skin Diseases* [6th ed.]. Philadelphia: J.B. Lippincott, 1991.)

types of lesions obstruct the emptying of sebum to the surface, and may develop into small papules, pustules, nodules, or cysts. With time, most pustules and cysts open, drain, and heal. If severe, these lesions may result in scarring. The prevalence of acne is increased during adolescence and early adulthood, but it is usually self-limited. The central theme of medical treatment involves reducing the inflammation of the pilosebaceous glands by fostering their free drainage, avoiding rupture, and limiting bacterial growth.

## Acute Eczematous Dermatitis

Dermatitis and eczema are words that are used interchangeably. They constitute the superficial inflammatory diseases of the skin. There are five major classifications (Table 47-3). Morphologically, the changes of acute and chronic dermatitis are specific and recognizable.

### Contact Dermatitis

Contact dermatitis includes inflammations that are the result of contact with external agents, either chemical allergens or mechanical irritants. The lesion begins in the area of contact (Figure 47-3). The irritant removes some of the protective mechanisms of the skin, such as lipids and other hydrophilic material, and causes varying degrees of dryness. When contact is with strong compounds or is prolonged, lesions may evolve. If exposure is continued, acute dermatitis can progress to the chronic form. In most circumstances, complete tissue repair is possible if the irritant is removed and permanent changes in the skin have not taken place.[12]

Contact dermatitis is a delayed-hypersensitivity dermatitis. It results from exposure of a previously sensitized individual to contact allergens. Some of the causes include poison ivy antigens, many industrial chemicals, some drugs, and some metals. The clinical features include marked itching, burning with red blistering, or vesicles at the area of contact. Histologically there is papillary dermal edema and mast cell degranulation. The pattern is called spongiotic dermatitis.[15]

Removal of the sensitizer is necessary for treatment. The causative agent can be identified by a history, patch testing, or a use test. Unless the condition is severe, medical treatment includes soaks and corticosteroid creams. When dermatitis becomes severe and frequent, systemic steroids may be required.

**TABLE 47–3.**
CLASSIFICATION OF ECZEMATOUS DERMATITIS

| TYPE | CAUSE OR PATHOGENESIS | HISTOLOGY[a] | CLINICAL FEATURES |
|------|----------------------|-----------|-------------------|
| Contact dermatitis | Topically applied chemicals Pathogenesis: delayed hypersensitivity | Spongiotic dermatitis | Marked itching or burning or both; requires antecedent exposure |
| Atopic dermatitis | Unknown, may be heritable | Spongiotic dermatitis | Erythematous plaques in flexural areas; family history of eczema, hay fever, or asthma |
| Drug-related eczematous dermatitis | Systemically administered (eg, penicillin) | Spongiotic dermatitis; eosinophils often present in filfiltrate; deeper infiltrate | Eruption occurs with administration of drug; remits when drug is discontinued |
| Photoeczematous eruption | Ultraviolet light | Spongiotic dermatitis; deeper infiltrate | Occurs on sun-exposed skin; phototesting may help in diagnosis |
| Primary irritant dermatitis | Repeated trauma (rubbing) | Spongiotic dermatitis in early stages | Localized to site of trauma |

[a]All types, with time, may develop chronic changes.
(Source: R. Cotran, V. Kumar, and S. Robbins, Robbins' Pathologic Basis of Disease [4th ed.]. Philadelphia: W.B. Saunders, 1989.)

*Drug-related eczematous dermatitis* follows a specific hypersensitivity response to a particular drug (see Chap. 16). It causes a spongiotic dermatitis that usually goes away when the drug is discontinued.[15] In *photoeczematous* reactions, ultraviolet light causes a dermatitis reaction on sun-exposed areas.[15] Some individuals are very sensitive to the sun's rays and react with a significant dermatitis reaction.

*Primary irritant contact dermatitis* causes a nonallergic skin reaction. Repeated or extended contact by a mild irritant causes skin damage. Strong irritants cause immediate damage on initial contact. Mechanical irritation is due to inflammation from mechanical factors such as large-size particles of certain materials that cause pruritus. One example is wool, resulting in dermatitis that is due to the mechanical scratchiness of the irritant itself, not the mediation of a chemical substance.

The frequency of chemically caused contact dermatitis has increased. A basic substance such as water can indirectly be a chemical irritant through prolonged exposure and removal of the skin's protective barriers. Soaps and detergents increase the drying and facilitate the irritating action of water. Other chemicals and medications may cause an irritant dermatitis. Various biologic irritants, including human excrement, saliva, and tears, result in dermatitis after prolonged contact. Biologic irritants can also cause a predisposition to the development of yeast and bacterial infections, compounding the problem.

### Atopic Dermatitis

Atopic dermatitis is a highly specific disease that results from a genetically determined lowered threshold to pruritus and is characterized by intense itching. The affected areas include the flexural regions such as the antecubital fossa and wrists.[26] It may appear as a small papule, but there is evidence that scratching is the major factor producing the lesion. In acute atopic dermatitis, intense scratching leads to erythema, weeping, scaling, and lichenification. The histology is that of a nonspecific dermatitis. The list of exacerbating factors includes sudden changes in weather, psychologic stress, contact with wool or furs, and primary irritant chemicals.

Many complications can develop with atopic dermatitis, including an increase in the severity of viral infections. It is frequently associated with allergic rhinitis or asthma.[26] Affected persons should not be vaccinated against smallpox, as disseminated vaccinia can develop and cause a generalized infection of the skin. These persons are also prone to bacterial and fungal infections, ocular complications, and allergic contact dermatitis.

Treatment involves palliation by reducing or controlling precipitating events and providing symptomatic relief of pruritus. It does tend to decrease in severity as the person approaches adulthood.

## VIRAL INFECTIONS OF THE SKIN

### Herpes Simplex

Herpes simplex, also known as a fever blister or cold sore, is caused by type I herpes simplex virus. Initially, it is an acute condition with groups of vesicles on an erythematous base, which later become purulent and crust-

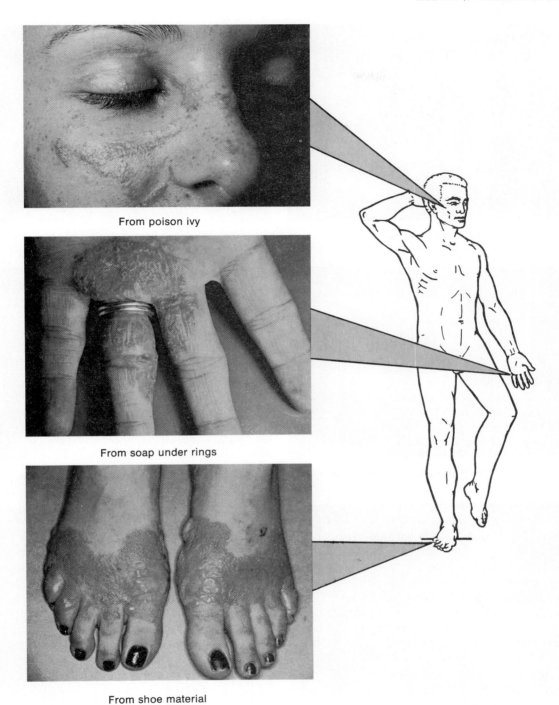

From poison ivy

From soap under rings

From shoe material

**FIGURE 47–3.**
Contact dermatitis. (Source: G.C. Sauer, *Manual of Skin Diseases* [6th ed.]. Philadelphia: J.B. Lippincott, 1991.)

ing. Distribution may occur to any area of the body, but the most frequently affected areas are the lips and perioral and genital areas; the lesions may be painful and pruritic (Figure 47-4). They resolve usually within 2 weeks.

It is believed that first exposure to infection occurs by the fifth year of life, but is not often observed. Nevertheless, the person has developed antibodies to the virus.

A small percentage of children have primary gingivostomatitis or vulvovaginitis as a result. Recurrence throughout life may result from either reactivation of the virus or reinoculation, and may be precipitated by stress-producing factors such as fever, excessive sun exposure, common cold, illness, and injury.

*Herpes progenitalis* has become a frequent infection

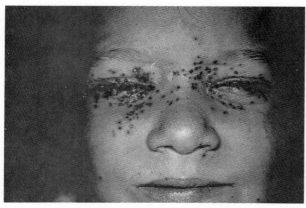

(A) Primary herpes simplex around the eyes
in a 5-year-old child

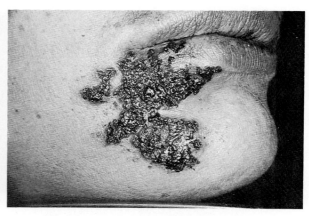

(B) Recurrent herpes simplex on chin with
secondary bacterial infection

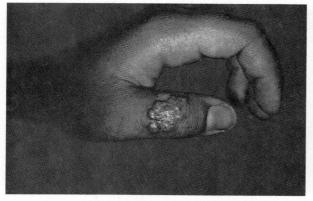

(C) Recurrent herpes simplex on a thumb

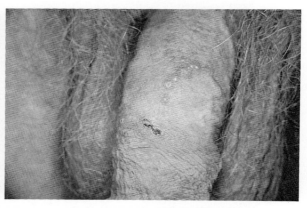

(D) Recurrent herpes simplex on the penis

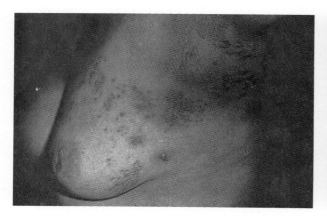

(E) Herpes zoster of left breast area

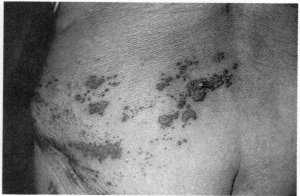

(F) Hemorrhagic zoster of left hip area

**FIGURE 47–4.**
Herpes simplex and zoster. (Source: G.C. Sauer, *Manual of Skin Diseases* [6th ed.]. Philadelphia: J.B. Lippincott, 1991.)

of the genital area and is caused by the type II herpes virus. It is usually sexually transmitted but can infect a baby during birth (see Chap. 57). Studies are currently investigating a relationship of this virus to cervical cancer.

Because no cure has been discovered, treatment of herpes simplex is basically symptomatic relief. Acyclovir (Zovirax), has been shown to be effective in shortening the duration of episodes; it may possibly decrease the number of recurrences. The long-term effects are being studied. Prevention can only be aimed at avoiding the identified precipitating factors.

## Varicella

Otherwise known as *chickenpox*, varicella is caused by the herpes zoster virus. An airborne, highly contagious virus in the prodromal and vesicular stages, it affects children more frequently than adults.

The varicella has an incubation period of 10 to 20 days. The prodromal stage often begins with moderate fever and malaise. Pink papules 2 to 4 mm in diameter are surrounded by a reddened halo (dew drop on a rose petal) that later dries and crusts. Lesions usually occur in groups; their distribution on the face, scalp, trunk, and arms is common. Generalized symptoms of headache, moderate fever, anorexia, and malaise may continue after the lesions erupt. Varicella in adults is much more severe than in children.

The usual treatment for varicella in children is aimed at keeping the skin lesions dry and relieving pruritus with lotion as necessary.

## Herpes Zoster

Herpes zoster is also produced by a varicella virus and it is often referred to as *shingles*. This acute inflammatory disease occurs when the dormant varicella virus is activated. It is most frequent in the elderly population, but it can occur in any age group. In the older person, pain usually precedes the lesion by 1 to 2 days.

The initial features are erythema and discomfort, followed in 1 to 7 days by grouped vesicles along a unilateral dermatome (Figure 47-5). These vesicles later crust and clear in 2 to 3 weeks.

Severe pain can result, and persistence is a feared complication. Although uncommon, generalized herpes zoster can result, a condition usually associated with a systemic malignancy of the lymphoma group.[21] A susceptible individual may develop chickenpox after exposure to this varicella virus.

## Warts (Verrucae)

Verrucae, or warts, are viral infections of the skin. There are three main types: verruca vulgaris (common wart), verruca plantaris (plantar wart), and condyloma acuminatum (venereal wart). It is believed that these are variations of the same virus.

The etiology of warts is not clearly understood, but they can be transmitted by contact from person to person. They are benign lesions and frequently occur at sites of injury or along a break in the skin.

*Verruca vulgaris* is a raised, well-circumscribed growth with an irregular gray surface, frequently present on the hands. Although treatment is often unsatisfactory,

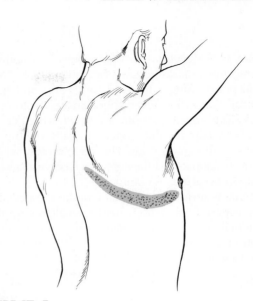

**FIGURE 47-5.**
Herpes zoster. The inflammatory lesions follow nerve distribution, especially in the thoracic region. Vesicles are apparent for 3 to 5 days and the crusted lesions remain for about 3 weeks.

surgical removal, electrosurgery, and cryosurgery have been used. Many warts resolve without treatment.

*Verruca plantaris* differs from the common wart by its location and the effect that pressure has on the lesion. The wart tends to grow on the soles of the feet, and pain is frequent due to the irritation of walking. As a result, the wart tends to grow inward.

*Condylomata acuminata* are lesions established primarily in warm, moist anogenital areas. Also known as venereal warts, they may or may not stem from sexual contact. They are large, pinkish or purplish projections with a rough surface.

## Rubeola (Measles)

Rubeola is a highly contagious infection caused by a myxovirus. The incubation period is approximately 10 to 14 days. Its course usually begins with fever and symptoms of upper respiratory infection that occur 6 to 7 days after inoculation and last 24 hours. The disease then enters what is known as the invasion phase, with development of high fever, chills, malaise, headache, photophobia, and dry cough. These symptoms last for 4 to 7 days. Lesions begin as inflammation or petechiae of the soft palate, followed by Koplik's spots, which are blue-white spots surrounded by a bright halo over the buccal mucosa. A macular eruption appears on the face, upper extremities, and trunk.

## Rubella

Also known as *German measles*, rubella is a common, acute, infectious disease caused by a myxovirus. The incubation period ranges from 12 to 25 days and begins with malaise and mild fever approximately 4 to 5 days before lesions appear. Lesions are small, irregular, pink macules and papules that appear initially on the face, spreading to the entire body. They fade rapidly within 2 to 3 days. Adenopathy of the superficial cervical and posterior auricular glands is common.

Rubella is serious in pregnant women, especially in the first trimester, when transmission to a fetus results in fetal anomalies. A titer is available to assess immunity. Vaccination is given to school-aged children and, with caution, to women of child-bearing age with low rubella titers.

## BACTERIAL INFECTIONS OF THE SKIN

### Impetigo

Impetigo is an acute bacterial infection that occurs superficially on the skin as serous and purulent vesicles that later rupture and form a golden crust. It frequently occurs in children, but persons in ill health are also predisposed to it. A common location for lesions is the face, but they may involve the extremities.

Causative organisms include $\beta$-hemolytic streptococci and coagulase-positive staphylococci. Impetigo is autoinoculable and can be transmitted among humans. Influencing factors include poor hygiene, tropical climates, and improper sanitation. A serious complication is glomerulonephritis, which may not be prevented by antibiotic treatment.

### Folliculitis

Folliculitis is a bacterial infection of the skin that originates within the hair follicle. Staphylococci are the usual causative organisms. Folliculitis appears as a pustule located at the opening of the hair follicle, predominantly on the scalp and extremities. The basic lesion is a reddened macule or papule surrounding the hair follicle. Predisposing factors include poor hygiene and maceration. Folliculitis can extend into the deeper skin layers if not treated promptly, and systemic antibiotics may be necessary.

### Furuncles and Carbuncles

Furuncles, also known as *boils*, frequently develop from a preceding staphylococcal folliculitis and are usually located in body areas containing hair follicles. Irritation, maceration, and lack of good hygiene are predisposing factors in their development. The lesions are nodules that are usually tender and red. They frequently remain tense for 2 to 4 days, become fluctuant, and later drain purulent material.[1]

Carbuncles are larger staphylococcal abscess that drain through various points. Some cases of furuncles and almost every case of carbuncles require systemic antibiotic therapy.

## FUNGAL DISEASES OF THE SKIN

Fungal diseases of the skin can be classified in three groups: superficial, intermediate, and deep. Some are *opportunistic* and affect a susceptible host, while some are truly *pathogenic* and can infect a healthy person.[15] The superficial diseases result in ringworm (tinea capitis), athlete's foot (tinea pedis), "jock itch" (tinea cruris), and tinea versicolor. These fungal diseases are primarily caused by dermatophytes that invade the superficial layers of the epidermis, hair, and nails. They are characterized by areas of scaling and erythema, and frequently exhibit vesicles and fissures.[21] Moisture, heat, and maceration are predisposing factors for growth; consequently, lesions appear in areas between toes, the axillae, nails, and groin. Treatment involves local therapy. With certain resistant fungi, griseofulvin, a fungostatic antibiotic, is used.

Intermediate fungal diseases invade both the superficial and deeper tissues. Moniliasis caused by *Candida albicans* is an example. This organism can also produce deep invasion when the host's resistance declines.[15]

Deep fungal infections invade deeper structures of living tissue and include diseases such as sporotrichosis, candidiasis, histoplasmosis, and aspergillosis (see Chap. 12). A much higher incidence of opportunistic deep fungal infections is being seen following the use of immunosuppressive drugs and invasive procedures.[15]

## SCALING DISORDERS OF THE SKIN

### Psoriasis

Psoriasis is a chronic, genetically determined disease of epidermal proliferation (Figure 47-6). The increased cell turnover rate and production of immature cells result in the classic features of sharply defined erythematous plaques covered by silvery white, loosely adherent scales.[2]

The precise etiology is not known, but genetic and environmental factors are of significance in its development. It is viewed as a chronic disease with much diversity in its location, severity, and frequency. Exacerbating

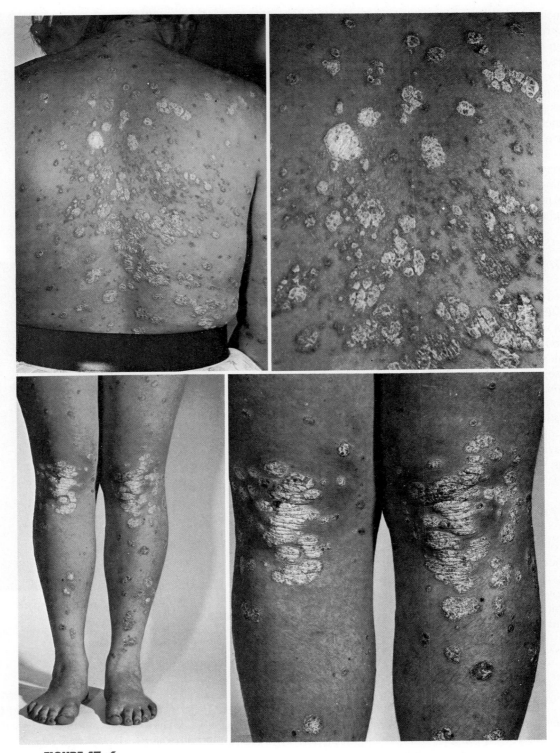

**FIGURE 47–6.**
Psoriasis of a 17-year-old girl. Moderately extensive psoriasis in classic distribution on back and knees. (Source: G.C. Sauer, *Manual of Skin Diseases* [6th ed.]. Philadelphia: J.B. Lippincott, 1991.)

factors include local trauma, overexposure to the sun, infection, stress, and physical illness.[18]

It can occur in all ages and is often distributed over the knees, elbows, scalp, and lumbosacral skin. When involved, the nails show pitting and dimpling. Psoriasis may be associated with arthritis. A serious but rare condition known as pustular psoriasis also can occur, causing sterile pustules, high fever, elevated white blood cell count, electrolyte imbalance, and malaise. This condition can be fatal.[2]

Psoriasis usually can be controlled, but remissions are common. Avoiding local skin injury, infection, and stress, maintaining good nutrition, and avoiding excessive weight gain improve the control of this disease.

## Pityriasis Rosea

Pityriasis rosea is a common, acute disease of the skin, usually affecting the adolescent and young adult. Its course is self-limited and thought to be infectious, possibly caused by a virus.

Clinical manifestations often arise after a prodrome of malaise, fatigue, and headache. The first lesion, known as the *herald patch*, is a single, oval, ringlike plaque that is later followed by lesions that are usually flat, erythematous patches covered by a fine scale; they resemble the primary plaque, but are smaller. Lesions are often pruritic. Distribution is most frequently on the neck, trunk, and arms.

## SKIN TUMORS

Tumors of the skin, like all tumors, are of two basic categories, benign and malignant. Benign tumors are slow-growing, and growth may stop entirely.[13] Malignant lesions show disorganization and abnormalities. They may grow rapidly and infiltrate surrounding tissues. Metastasis may occur depending on the origin of the tumor.

## Benign Tumors

### Seborrheic Keratosis

Seborrheic keratosis is the most common tumor in the elderly. A strong predisposing factor is prolonged exposure to the sun. The skin lesion is slightly raised, light brown, and sharply demarcated; pigmentation may deepen and the skin become thick (Figure 47-7). The lesion is covered with a greasy crust that is loosely attached. Locations include the trunk, shoulders, face, and scalp. Malignant transformation is quite uncommon, and most lesions do not require treatment unless they pose cosmetic difficulties or raise suspicions of malignancy.

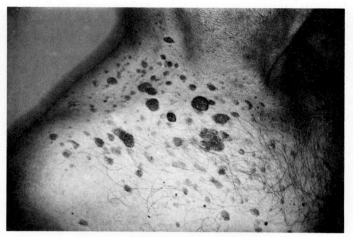

*(A)*  Seborrheic keratoses on the neck

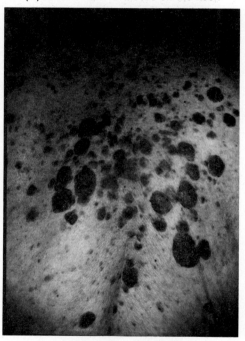

*(B)*  Seborrheic keratoses on back

**FIGURE 47-7.**
Epidermal tumors. (Source: G.C. Sauer, *Manual of Skin Diseases* [6th ed.]. Philadelphia: J.B. Lippincott, 1991.)

## Hemangioma

A hemangioma is a benign tumor of newly formed blood vessels. There are many different types. A strawberry hemangioma frequently appears as a dome-shaped, fully red, soft lesion with sharply demarcated edges. It has a tendency to grow slowly and usually regresses completely.

The *nevus flammeus* (ordinary birthmark) is a congenital vascular malformation that is usually unilateral and located on the face and neck. It appears as a light pink to dark purple patch that usually fades and regresses.[15] The *port wine stain* may grow with the child and become unsightly. It is often associated with mental retardation, seizures, hemiplegia, and other problems.[15]

*Cavernous hemangiomas* are large, cavernous, vascular channels that may occur in both the skin and subcutaneous tissues. The features of the lesions depend on their extent, varying from round to flat and from bright red to deep purple.

## Keratoacanthoma

Keratoacanthoma is a benign, cutaneous tumor with a central crater. Because it resembles squamous cell carcinoma, lesions are removed and examined histologically.

## Actinic Keratosis

Actinic keratosis is a premalignant lesion. Common names include "senile" or "solar" keratosis. Lesions are sharply demarcated, rough, red to brown or gray. At high risk to develop the condition are fair-skinned persons whose skin easily burns with sun exposure. Age of onset is related to the amount of sun exposure. Treatment is necessary, since a number of these lesions progress to squamous cell carcinoma. A variety of methods can be used to destroy them, including curettage, electrodesiccation, cryotherapy, topical chemotherapy, and excisional biopsy.

*Leukoplakia* is the most common premalignant lesion, occurring as a whitish patch on the mucosa of the oral cavity.[21] It occurs most frequently in elderly women.

# Malignant Disorders

## Basal Cell Carcinoma

Basal cell carcinoma is also known as *basal cell epithelioma* and is the most frequent type of skin cancer. Most basal cell carcinomas arise from the epidermis and hair follicles.[11] They tend to occur mainly in older persons, and the majority of lesions appear with cumulative, prolonged exposure to the sun. Persons who have had radiation therapy for breast, lung, or other types of internal malignancy have an increased risk. These common tumors are slow-growing, and although they rarely metastasize, treatment is necessary, for they may become locally destructive and can erode into vital areas.[15] Studies of T-lymphocyte depression in the cutaneous tissues of these individuals supports the theory that ultraviolet light impairs host defense mechanisms and allows the tumor to escape immune surveillance.[11,15]

Characteristically, the carcinoma has a smooth surface with a pearly border, often with ulceration of its center (Figure 47-8). Usually, numerous telangiectasias (localized groups of dilated, small blood vessels) are visible.[15] Treatments include cryotherapy, curettage, electrodesiccation, and topical chemotherapy.

## Squamous Cell Carcinoma

Squamous cell carcinoma is a malignant lesion that can affect both the skin and mucous membranes. It most frequently occurs in sun-damaged areas or areas exposed to irradiation or burns. The squamous cell carcinoma may also arise in scars, chronic ulcers, fistulas, and sinuses. The burn scar may serve as an initiator, or cocarcinogen, in the production of these malignancies.[11] Immune alterations have been described that include local imbalances of T-cell function that favor tumorigenesis in ultraviolet light-damaged skin.[15]

Characteristically, the carcinoma appears as a rough, hyperkeratotic nodule with an indurated base. It may ulcerate and can metastasize. Surgical excision is the treatment of choice. In some instances, curettage and electrodesiccation, irradiation, and chemotherapy can be used.

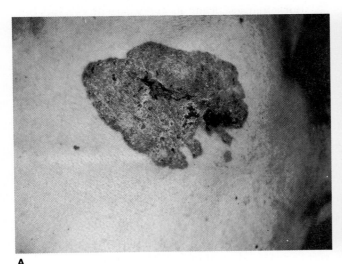

**A**

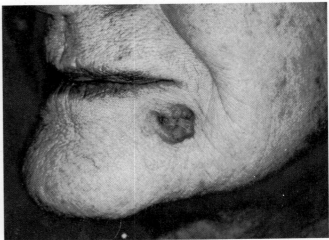

**B**

**FIGURE 47-8.**
**A.** A large superficial basal cell carcinoma on the back. **B.** Basal cell carcinoma on the chin. (Source: G.C. Sauer, *Manual of Skin Diseases* [6th ed.]. Philadelphia: J.B. Lippincott, 1991.)

## Malignant Melanoma

Malignant melanoma is a cancer arising from the melanin-producing cells. It is associated with a high risk for invasion and metastasis. Risk of developing some forms of the disease is increased with exposure to the sun. The worldwide frequency of this malignancy is rising more rapidly than any other cancer in white males and is the second most rapidly increasing cancer in white females.[10] Recognizing the lesion early is important, since prognosis is dependent on such factors as early removal, size, type, and extension. Five-year survival has improved, depending on the clinical type, to 90% to 100% when the tumor is less than 1 mm thick, and is about 50% when the tumor is larger than 3 mm in thickness.[10] All nevi should be inspected regularly, and self-examination should be taught.

Melanoma occurs most frequently in young and middle-aged adults. The most common location in men is the trunk and in women the legs.[7] The significant characterics are variable colors and irregular borders and surfaces. Nevi may have brown or black pigmentation with shades of red, white, or blue. Small satellite lesions 1 to 2 cm away from the primary lesion may be seen.

The precursor lesions to melanomas are the congenital nevi and the dysplastic nevi. The congenital nevus rarely becomes malignant if it is small (less than 1.5 cm in diameter). Large congenital nevi (larger than 20 cm in diameter) have a 5% to 20% risk of becoming malignant.[11] Dysplastic nevi are usually larger lesions of various colors with irregular borders and sometimes a central papule.[17] These often appear late in childhood or adolescence but may appear after age 35. When these develop in fair-skinned individuals, they will more likely develop into melanoma than the congenital nevi.[17]

Melanomas are of various types with the most common being the superficial spreading melanoma that usually arises within a nevus (Figure 47-9). Other types include *nodular*, which is darkly pigmented and may grow from normal skin; and *lentigo maligna melanoma*,

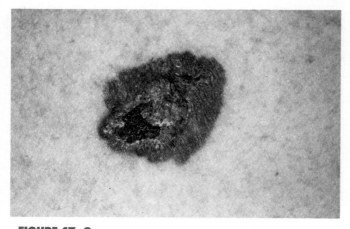

**FIGURE 47-9.**
Malignant melanoma in a nevus present since birth, on the scapular area. (Source: G.C. Sauer, *Manual of Skin Diseases* [6th ed.]. Philadelphia: J.B. Lippincott, 1991.)

which arises on a flat lesion, usually the sun-damaged face of an elderly person.[10,17] The classification of the tumor is crucial in determining the extent of the surgical dissection for removing it. The Clark classification is commonly used, as follows:[17]

Level I Confined to epidermis
Level II Partially penetrates papillary dermis
Level III Completely penetrates papillary dermis
Level IV Extends to reticular dermis
Level V Invades subcutaneous fat

Melanomas acquire new antigens, some of which are the oncofetal and histocompatibility antigens. The nevi often undergo several morphologic changes before exhibiting invasive, cancerous properties. Study of the relationship of melanomas to viral carcinogens is intriguing but not conclusive.[7,10] The malignant melanoma is highly invasive and spreads rapidly to the lymphatic system, and then may metastasize to any organ of the body.

## TRAUMATIC ALTERATIONS IN THE SKIN

### Burns

Burns are suffered by approximately 2 million persons annually, of which 130,000 persons require hospitalization and 10,000 die.[3] In a large 5-year study of adult burn patients, the average age was 44 years, 78% were black, and 62% were men. Major causes of burns included flames (44.8%), scalds (28.5%), and chemicals (9.7%). The injuries resulted from direct assault, cooking, smoking, explosion, house fire, contact with hot objects, bathtub accidents, house chores, and a variety of other factors, in that order. Individuals considered to be predisposed to burn injury were the elderly, those living alone, alcohol and drug abusers, and the physically and mentally ill.[3]

Burn injuries occur in every age group and both sexes. When they occur, they involve not only the skin tissue but all of the systems of the body. The depth of thermal injuries depends on the burning agent, temperature, and length of exposure to the heat.[14] The equilibrium point for skin is approximately 44°C (111.2°F). This temperature can be tolerated up to 6 hours without burning. The rate of skin destruction doubles with each degree rise, so that at 70°C (158°F), fleeting exposure will produce total epidermal necrosis.[14]

Burns are classified as first-, second-, and third-degree. A more precise classification may be made on the basis of partial-thickness, deep dermal, or full-thickness injury (Figure 47-10). It is often difficult to ascertain the depth of injury in the initial postburn period. To complicate matters further, a partial-thickness injury may convert to a deep dermal or full-thickness injury as a result of wound sepsis and microcirculatory insufficiency with delayed degeneration of deep epithelial appendages. As time progresses, the depth and extent of the burn become more apparent.

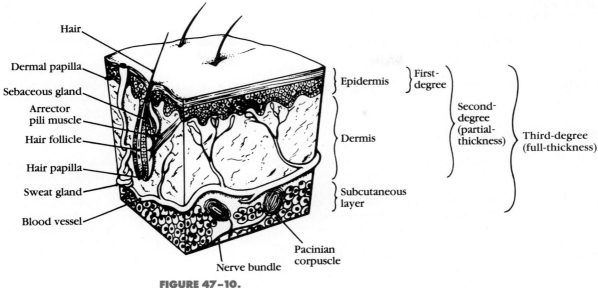

**FIGURE 47–10.**
Areas affected by first-, second-, and third-degree burns.

## Partial-Thickness Burns

Each degree of burn wound depth has various characteristics. Partial-thickness burns include first- and second-degree and deep dermal injuries (Table 47-4). The first-degree burn involves the epidermis. It may be caused by exposure to sunlight, brief exposures to a heat source, splashed hot liquid, high-intensity short-duration explosions, and chemical and electrical injury. A first-degree burn is pink to red, painful, and slightly edematous. The epidermis peels in 3 to 6 days, with itching and redness persisting a week or more. The wound leaves no scar when healed.[14]

The second-degree, partial-thickness burn may be superficial or deep dermal. It results from intense flash heat, hot liquid, contact with hot objects, chemicals, or electrical injury. The superficial burn involves the epidermis and dermis. It has a mottled pink to red color (Figure 47-11). It exhibits blistering and subcutaneous edema, is moist and very sensitive. This burn heals in 10 to 14 days without grafting. If it does not become infected or traumatized, usually no scar forms.

The deep dermal burn varies in color, being mottled with more white than red, a dull white, tan, or cherry red. The red areas blanch and refill. Dark streaks of coagulated capillaries may be seen. The burn extends down to the subcutaneous tissue. If epidermal appendages are intact, it has the potential to heal spontaneously without grafting, as viable skin cells are present in the appendages. It takes several months for a deep dermal burn to heal spontaneously. The wound may be blistered and moist, or it may be dry; it may or may not be sensitive; if a hair follicle remains, the hair will not pull out. The epithelium produced is extremely thin and may break down easily; the burn may convert to a full-thickness burn if it becomes infected. Many deep dermal burns are excised and grafted.[14]

## Full-Thickness Burns

These are full-thickness injuries that have no viable epithelial cells. The causes may be the same as for first- and second-degree burns. The wound appearance may vary, being white, tan, brown, black, or deep cherry red. The red areas do not blanch. The burn is usually dry and has a sunken, leathery appearance. The leathery covering is called *eschar*. A black network of coagulated capillaries may be seen (Figure 47-12). This wound itself is anesthetic and hair pulls out easily. Grafting is required to close the wound.[14]

The full-thickness burn may also involve the subcutaneous fat layer, fascia, muscle, and bone. Sometimes classified as a fourth-degree burn, it appears black and depressed. If bone shows through, it appears dry and dull. Grafting is necessary to close this wound. If a graft is required over bone, small perforations are made in the bone to the marrow. Granulation buds grow from these holes, coalesce, and form a bed to accept the graft.[14]

This degree of burn depends on the temperature of and duration of exposure to the heat source. The severity of the injury is dependent on the size of the burned area, its depth and location, the age of the victim, the presence of concomitant illness or injury, and the psychologic status of the victim. In assessing the burn situation further, it is helpful to know the circumstances surrounding the injury. Important information includes such aspects as place of injury, exposure to electricity, exposure to fumes, and other factors that may complicate the recovery.

**TABLE 47–4.**
CLASSIFICATION OF BURNS

|  | TISSUE | APPEARANCE | SYMPTOMS | RESOLUTION |
|---|---|---|---|---|
| **First-Degree** | | | | |
| Partial-thickness | Epidermis | Red, pink, slight edema | Pain | Epidermis peels in 3–6 days; itch, redness in a week or so; no scar |
| **Second-Degree** | | | | |
| Partial-thickness | | | | |
| Superficial | Epidermis and upper dermis | Mottled pink to red; blistering edema; moist | Sensitive | Heals in 10–14 days without grafting; no scar if no infection or trauma to wound |
| Deep dermal | Epidermis, dermis to subcutaneous tissue | Varies: white, tan, cherry red; red area blanches; dark, coagulated capillary streaks; blister and moist, or dry | May or may not be sensitive; if hair follicle present, hair does not pull out | Has potential to heal spontaneously over several months; may be excised or grafted |
| **Third-Degree** | | | | |
| Full-thickness | Epidermis; dermis; subcutaneous layer; no viable epithelial cells remain | White, tan, brown, black, deep cherry red; red areas do not blanch, wet or dry; sunken; eschar; coagulated capillaries | Anesthetic; hair pulls out | Grafting required after debridement |
| **Fourth-Degree** | | | | |
| Full-thickness | Epidermis; dermis; subcutaneous layer; fascia; muscle; bone | Blackened; depressed; bone is dull and dry | Anesthetic; hair pulls out | Grafting required |

Estimating the percentage of total body surface area that has been burned is crucial to determining fluid and nutritional requirements. The classic rule of nines has been a standard for estimating burn area (Figure 47-13).[16] This helpful method has some limitations, depending on the age of the burned patient (a child's head represents a greater percentage of body area than an adult's) and the extent of actual third-degree injury.[14]

## *Localized Changes Due to Burn Injury*

When skin is burned, many localized changes occur. Protein in cells is denatured and enzymes are inactivated. The tissue becomes coagulated, desiccated, or carbonized, depending on the temperature of the heat source and the length of exposure to it. Even with mild heat, the normal metabolic activity of a cell is altered. Burns caused by long exposure to low-intensity heat are characterized by major changes in deeper tissues.

The keratin layer is the water vapor barrier in the body. When it is destroyed, large amounts of fluid are lost. In a deep wound, the fluid loss is greater and often continues until the wound finally is closed, usually by grafting.

Burns extending down to and damaging the basal layer do not regenerate if all parts of this layer are destroyed. Heat extending to the "cement" that binds the epidermis to the dermis causes the epidermis to loosen; lost fluid fills in the space and a blister develops. When new epidermis is formed beneath the blister, the blister dries and peels off.

The dermis, composed of collagen fibers, elastin, and mast cells, is damaged when exposed to high de-

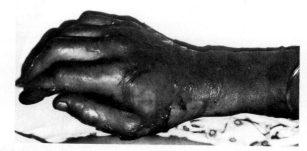

**FIGURE 47–11.**
Partial-thickness burn injury. (Source: C.V. Kenner, C.E. Guzzetta, and B.M. Dossey, *Critical Care Nursing* [2nd ed.]. Boston: Little, Brown, 1985.)

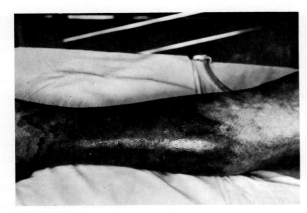

**FIGURE 47–12.**
Full-thickness burn injury of the right leg. (Source: C.V. Kenner, C.E. Guzzetta, and B.M. Dossey, *Critical Care Nursing* [2nd ed.]. Boston: Little, Brown, 1985.)

grees of heat. The epidermal appendages, if intact, contain epidermal cells in the external sheaths of the hair follicles. Glands can grow out and form new epithelium. When the burn extends to the subcutaneous tissues, the collagen fibers that normally anchor the dermis to the subcutaneous layer now hold the leathery burn eschar in place. Bacteria that form under the eschar release enzymes that lyse the collagen fibers, making it easier to remove eschar.

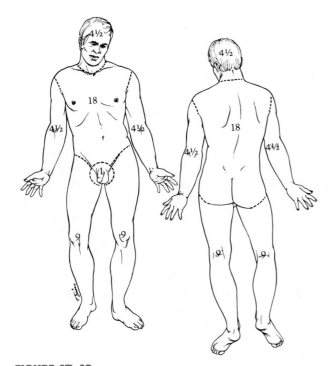

**FIGURE 47–13.**
The rule of nines. Each arm is 9%, the head 9%, the torso and abdomen 18%, the back 18%, and each leg 18%. (Source: C.V. Kenner, C.E. Guzzetta, and B.M. Dossey, *Critical Care Nursing* [2nd ed.]. Boston: Little, Brown, 1985.)

The melanocytes in the epidermis do not regenerate well, and in deep burns, the skin color usually does not return. As blood vessels are damaged from the thermal injury, color changes occur in the burn. In sunburn, the vessels in the subpapillary and papillary plexuses dilate, causing reddening. In a severe burn, coagulation of vessels causes the area to lose redness and become whiter, with the vessels themselves coagulating into blackened lines in the wound.

Plasma leaks from damaged blood vessels and provides the fluid for blisters. Lymph vessels, compressed by the edema from the wound, cannot drain the affected area. Escharotomy may become necessary if tissue swelling compromises the venous return and arterial blood supply, so that constricting burned skin and fluid cause ischemic changes in the involved area.[14] Escharotomy involves cutting or peeling away the constrictive eschar with a scalpel or dermatome to release the pressure on the underlying tissue.

## Systemic Changes Due to Burn Injury

Many changes occur throughout the body as a result of burn injury. Responses in the circulatory system account for color changes and the edema of burns. Contraction of the skin capillaries causes blanching. The wound appears white if the superficial dermis is coagulated. Later, when arterioles and capillaries dilate, it appears red. The capillaries lose protein-rich fluid through their abnormally permeable walls into the surrounding tissues, creating the most characteristic feature of the burn wound, *edema*.

Normally, plasma and interstitial fluid are chemically similar, except for blood cells and large plasma proteins, which elevate the colloid osmotic pressure in the blood. After burn injury, *colloids* (plasma proteins such as albumins and globulins) leak out of the damaged capillaries and into the interstitial spaces. The loss of protein-rich fluid decreases the intracapillary colloid osmotic pressure causing fluid to shift into the tissues (see Chap. 8). There is also an accompanying rise in intracapillary pressure as a result of capillary dilatation and increased blood flow of the inflammatory process. The loss of protein from capillaries is termed *capillary sieving*.[1] The amount of sieving is correlated with the severity of the burn. The more severe the burn, the more protein is lost. Capillary permeability also increases in tissues around the burn and other areas of the body.[14]

The permeability of tissue cells in and around the burn seems to allow abnormal interchange of fluids and electrolytes between cells and interstitial fluid. A limiting factor for extravasation of fluid is increased tissue pressure. Tissue pressure increases as fluid loss increases, and reaches a point at which the tissue can hold no more fluid.

The depth of the burn affects the volume and composition of edema fluid. In first-degree burns, protein loss is insignificant and edema slight, because vasodilatation is the only circulatory change. A second-degree burn has more severe capillary damage and more tissue damage. At first assessment, the surface area of a burn is easily seen, but the depth is not always immediately apparent. Large volumes of fluid can escape beneath the wound before swelling is noted. The third-degree burn has large injury to skin and area beneath and around it, which accounts for extensive fluid losses.

Edema can be displaced by pressure, move to dependent areas, and spread beyond the burn. The rate of edema formation depends on temperature of the injuring heat source, duration of exposure, area of the burn, and the time since injury. It is difficult to ascertain fluid loss by the amount of visible edema, because such loss occurs deep in the wound beneath it and in the vulnerable third spaces, such as the peritoneal cavity and even the lungs.[14] The leathery eschar does not expand with edema pressure, and large amounts of fluid collect beneath it, putting pressure on underlying tissues. The pressure may be relieved by escharotomy.

Studies show that fluid losses occur rapidly in the period immediately after the burn and decline in about 48 hours. The rate of loss slows when the capillary endothelium returns to its normal state, when the tissue pressure is in balance with capillary hydrostatic pressure, or when capillary stasis occurs. In minor uncomplicated burns, edema is chiefly resorbed by the lymphatic system and takes approximately as long as it took the edema to form. Lymphatics also drain larger burns, but this process may take weeks.

The amount of protein lost from plasma varies. Albumin and globulin are lost, with greater amounts of albumin lost than globulin owing to the smaller size of the albumin molecule. Immediately after the burn, the concentration of protein in plasma increases, because there is greater loss of water and electrolytes together with the protein loss. The following compensatory mechanisms exist to counteract fluid loss: interstitial fluid in unburned areas is absorbed by the blood; blood vessels in the spleen and unburned skin constrict, reducing the space the remaining blood volume must fill; and fluid is absorbed by the gut. Thirst may be intense. In minor burns, these mechanisms suffice. In major large burns, fluids and proteins must be replaced.[14]

Hemoconcentration is a sequel to capillary fluid loss. The fluid portion of the blood is lost to the tissues, allowing the cellular elements to concentrate. The hematocrit rises; blood flow becomes sluggish, compromising tissue nutrition and oxygenation. Thrombosis sometimes develops in these affected areas.

Water and electrolytes shift back and forth across normal capillary walls. Burn injury alters the shifts by increasing capillary permeability, causing protein loss and altered colloid osmotic pressure. Potassium is released from severely injured cells, causing elevated serum potassium levels and cardiac dysrhythmias (see Chap. 8). Sodium may increase in burn tissue, taking water with it. When the victim begins diuresis after 48 hours or so, potassium and sodium are excreted. Careful monitoring of electrolyte levels is important, so that replacement therapy may be initiated and electrolyte concentrations in replacement fluids, for example, may be reduced.

In some burns, there is a substantial loss of red blood cells, intensifying the effects of plasma loss. This usually occurs in deep burns and seems to be a gradual process. The loss of red blood cells is due in part to hemolysis in the burned area, which results in hemoglobinemia and hemoglobinuria soon after the burn occurs. Free hemoglobin in the plasma indicates a severe burn. For 24 to 48 hours, delayed hemolysis of partially damaged red blood cells occurs. Further decrease in red blood cells results from thrombosis and sludging. Anemia develops as a result of red cell loss as well as with bleeding during debridement and other causes.

Additional fluid is lost as insensible water loss from evaporation from the burn wound surface and through the respiratory system. Respiratory loss is greatest when a tracheostomy is required. Pulmonary dysfunction requiring tracheostomy is common in third-degree burns involving 25% to 70% of total body surface.[6]

Signs and symptoms of fluid deficiency include thirst, restlessness, and disorientation. Plain water given to relieve thirst may lead to water intoxication; to avoid this, solutions with balanced electrolytes must be administered. Fluids are usually given intravenously because of the frequency of vomiting after burn injury. Changes in the central nervous system are useful in following the progress of therapy. Restlessness is an early indication that fluid replacement therapy is ineffective. Disorientation in the first 24 hours usually means that more intensive treatment is needed.

The depletion of fluid to edema and insensible loss reduce circulatory blood volume and can result in reduced cardiac output and inadequate tissue perfusion. Tissue hypoxia may result, causing a shift to anaerobic cellular metabolism. Acidosis and irreversible burn shock can occur. The acid-base balance is disrupted because the buffering mechanism is upset by fluid shift in the body compartments, hyperventilation, and reduced renal function. Blood urea levels may rise if protein catabolism is excessive or large amounts of nitrogen are released from burned tissue in the presence of oliguria.

The respiratory system is often altered by burn injury, by inhalation injury, and by therapy. Heat exposure and irritants cause swelling and tissue breakdown. Respiratory tissues are irritated by gases from burning materials, such as carbon monoxide. Altered circulation may lead to inadequate pulmonary circulation. Hypoxia may result from the decreased amount of oxygen circulating. Aspiration pneumonia may develop from vomiting episodes. Tracheal or laryngeal obstruction may result from edema in the head and neck region, causing pressure against the trachea and larynx. Also, inflamed linings of trachea and larynx swell and block the airway. Edema under tight eschar in burns of the torso restricts chest movements, which also may lead to respiratory problems. The adult respiratory distress syndrome (ARDS) is an ominous complication of burn injury and may result after shock or severe hypoxia.[6] Finally, pulmonary emboli are always a danger as a result of changes in the vasculature, sepsis, and immobilization.

Physical findings in the respiratory system include singed nasal hairs and reddened or dark pharynx. Irritation and heat damage to respiratory tissue may lead to respiratory stridor, dyspnea, and copious secretions, often carbonaceous. Deep full-thickness burns of the face also cause burning of pharyngeal tissues. Laryngeal edema, focal erosion, focal laryngitis, and necrosis may be evident. Edema may be exhibited by hoarseness. Respiratory disorders that may occur during the course of therapy include pneumonia, atelectasis, obstruction from mucus plugs, ARDS, and septic emboli from infected venosections.

The gastrointestinal tract is also affected. Changes there include acute stress (Curling's) ulcers, gastric dilatation, paralytic ileus, and bleeding. Acute gastric and duodenal ulcers in burn victims are morphologically identical to acute stress ulcers in people without burns. Acute stress ulcers in individuals with and without burns are mostly gastric. They occur in 20% to 30% of persons with total body surface burns. Ulcers may occur in the stomach, duodenum, or both. The anatomic location of stress ulcers differs from that of peptic and duodenal ulcers not caused by stress. Stress gastric ulcers are present in the fundic mucosa as opposed to the pyloric mucosa of other gastric ulcers. Stress duodenal ulcers are located in the posterior, rather than the anterior duodenum. They have several foci when they occur in the stomach and a single focus when they occur in the duodenum.[2]

Gastric ulcers are generally smaller than duodenal ulcers. Those of 2 to 3 mm are difficult to see during gastroscopy, or even autopsy, but they are deep enough to cause significant bleeding. Many ulcers are hidden in the rugal folds. Stress ulcers exhibit a relative lack of inflammatory response, which may be due to the fact that many occur in the terminal stages of burn illness. Many of these stress ulcers are colonized with gram-negative bacilli. Vascular congestion and submucosal edema are often present. No single theory is held concerning pathogenesis of Curling's stress ulcers. They are similar morphologically to steroid-induced ulcers, but their pathogenesis is different from that of peptic ulcers. The most commonly held hypothesis for stress ulcers in postburn situations is ischemic hypoxia that may damage the mucosal barrier and allow back diffusion of hydrogen ions.[2] Bleeding and perforation are common complications.

Gastric dilatation and paralytic ileus may appear early

after burn injury. These conditions are neurologic in origin, may be secondary to fear or pain, or may occur as a result of hypovolemia or sepsis.

Liver dysfunction often occurs with burn injury. Factors that contribute to liver dysfunction include bacterial infection, lack of proper nutrition, drugs, anesthesia, blood transfusions leading to viral or serum hepatitis, and hepatic hypoxemia. Hepatic hypoxemia seems to be a result of a decrease in circulating fluid volume. The necrosis that results is usually minimal and focal, of a fatty nature, and reversible.

The kidney changes that occur may be permanent or temporary. Temporary kidney changes are manifested by oliguria, which results from a decreased glomerular filtration rate from the decreased circulatory volume. Blood urea nitrogen (BUN) and creatinine levels are elevated, and the level of antidiuretic hormone may be increased. Tubular damage may occur when the kidney is presented with an increased amount of protein breakdown products from the burn. If there is a history of kidney disorder, or if the person does not receive adequate treatment, permanent damage may occur. Hematuria may be present as a result of damaged red blood cells. Death may result from acute renal insufficiency despite adequate treatment.

Stress enhances the secretion of adrenocortical hormones. These hormones, especially cortisone, may help to stabilize the lysosome membranes, decrease inflammation, and prevent an overwhelming response. The down side of adrenocortical stimulation is that these hormones depress the immune response and make the person more vulnerable to infection. The adrenal medulla secretes large amounts of epinephrine and norepinephrine. These hormones also may be life-saving at a high energy cost to the body.

Problems in coagulation may occur after severe burn injury and may result from the burn, from complications secondary to the injury, or from therapy. Abnormalities include decreases in platelet count, clot retraction time, and partial thromboplastin and prothrombin times, along with elevated fibrinogen levels. A circulating heparinlike material that prolongs clotting times and depresses the prothrombin level is also present. These defects seem to occur in large burns involving large body surface areas, as well as in smaller burns. Consumption or use of clotting factors plays a role in coagulopathies. Coagulopathies, such as disseminated intravascular coagulation (DIC), frequently occur and are treated with transfusions of platelets, fresh-frozen plasma, whole blood, fibrinogen concentrations, and other clotting factors (see Chap. 21).

Wound infections are a major problem in burns and may lead to sepsis, which is the most common cause of death.[8,9] The frequency of infection is correlated with the extent and depth of the injury and with the success of treatment measures. Bacteria, both gram-positive and gram-negative, invade the wound surface and eventually reach the viable surrounding tissue. Products liberated by the bacteria can produce septic shock. In a large study of burn wound colonization and treatment, numerous strains of bacteria colonized the wounds within the first 24 hours. If treatment measures were not effective, penetration into the deeper tissues occurred and sepsis was a frequent result.[9] The study demonstrated the importance of decreasing the size of open, full-thickness wounds to prevent infection.

## Electrical Burn Injuries

Various lesions occur as a result of electrical burns. Six factors determine the extent of these injuries: type of current (direct or alternating); voltage of current; resistance of body tissues; value of current flowing through the tissues; pathway of the current through the body; and duration of the contact with the electrical source.

Direct current does not produce the same contraction of muscle and low-voltage direct current is not as dangerous as alternating current. High-voltage direct current, however, is often fatal.

Alternating current produces tetanic muscle contraction at low voltages which prevents the victim from releasing contact with the circuit. These low-voltage currents often result in ventricular fibrillation.[8] Low voltage means less than 500 volts, and high voltage is greater than 500 volts. Low-voltage injuries most often occur in the home and are likely to involve children and infants.[27] The usual source of current is a household plug; a curious child may stick a small object into the outlet. High-voltage injury commonly occurs in adults working with electric lines or equipment. These injuries have a high mortality, often due to cardiac asystole.

The body tissues offer varying degrees of resistance to electrical current. The resistance of tissues, in order of least to greatest, is as follows: nerves, blood, muscles, skin, tendons, fat, and bone. Skin resistance varies from person to person. The epidermis is nonvascular and offers high resistance when it is dry but, when wet, moisture decreases resistance and enhances the flow of current. The dermis offers low resistance because it is highly vascular.[27]

Thin skin is less resistant than thick skin, making the palms and soles most resistant. Usually, the greater the skin resistance, the greater the local burn, and the less the skin resistance, the more the internal injury. Current in contact with the skin eventually causes blistering. Blisters are moist and conduct current through the skin along the tissues of least resistance—blood vessels and nerves. Vessel walls are damaged and thrombi occur, often at a site far from the site of the electrical injury, making it difficult to evaluate the full extent of damage at the initial evaluation. Progressive tissue necrosis can occur for 12 to 14 days after the injury.[14]

Electric current may flow through the heart, producing ventricular fibrillation and often immediate death. High-voltage current often travels to the respiratory center of the brain, causing respiratory arrest and death.[14] Neurologic complications are the most common results of electrical injury and include varying levels of unconsciousness and spinal cord injuries.[8] In burned extremities, peripheral neuropathies are common.[8]

The value of the alternating current flowing through the body determines the resulting injury. Contact with a circuit produces muscle contraction, which may be severe enough to prevent the victim from releasing himself or herself from the source of current. If cardiac or respiratory arrest does not occur and the victim remains conscious, he or she may complain of ringing in the ears and deafness for a time, or visual disturbances such as flashes and brilliant luminous spots. The pathway through the body is also important in determining the extent of injury. The longer the contact, the greater amount of damage.

The injury in electrical burns may be one or more of three types: (1) entry and exit wounds, (2) electrothermal burns (flash or arc burns), and (3) flame burns. The *entry wound* occurs at the contact site. It may be small or large and usually appears as an ischemic, yellow-white, coagulated area, or it may be charred. It is dry and painless, and the edges are well-defined.[24] However, the extent of damage may be far greater than is evident on the surface. Necrosis of subcutaneous tissues and muscle from arterial thrombi may occur, or lack of thrombosis may cause hemorrhaging. Damage may be due to heat from the passage of current or due to the action of the current itself.[24] The *exit wound* appears as a blow-out type of injury caused by arcing current between victim and a nearby ground.[8] It is a dry area with depressed edges. This exit wound is usually more severe than the entry wound.[8]

*Electrothermal burns* are from the heat of the current passing near, but not through, the skin. The depth of the wound depends on the closeness to the electrical source. These are mainly associated with high-voltage current. The electricity arc leaping from the high current has a temperature of 2500°C. *Flame burns* occur when heat from an electrical current ignites clothing. They may cause more serious injury than the electric injury itself.

The tetanic contractions that lock the victim to the electric source may cause fractures and dislocations of joints. Cataracts often develop months to years after an electrical injury involving the head area. Abdominal injury may occur as a result of electrical trauma to the abdomen. The extent of injury is difficult to determine at first. Abdominal symptoms may not arise until days after the injury. Renal involvement seems to be more prevalent in electrical than in thermal injury. The damage may be caused by the initial electric shock, direct current damage to the kidneys or kidney vessels, abnormal protein breakdown in the damaged tissue, or a combination of all three.

## Chemical Burn Injuries

Chemical burns result from exposure to acids or alkaline chemicals (Table 47-5). Most lethal burns result from military conflict and industrial accidents. Domestic and laboratory accidents and criminal assaults usually result in smaller areas of damage.[14] The injury may result from chemical changes as well as from thermal injury to the tissues, depending on the nature of the chemical.

Tissue damage depends on five factors: (1) pH or concentration of the chemical; (2) amount of agent contacting the skin; (3) duration of contact; (4) amount of tissue penetration; and (5) mechanism of action of the chemical.[14] Chemical changes in tissues include denaturation, precipitation, alkalization, edema, separation of the epidermis from the dermis, disorganization of epidermal appendages, and widening and coalescence of collagen bundles.

Chemical agents are often classified by the way in which they affect protein. Oxidizing agents are corrosive and cause extensive protein denaturation. Some agents are desiccants and cause cellular dehydration. Others cause anoxic tissue damage.[14] The depth of chemical burns is often difficult to evaluate.

*Acid burns* most frequently occur in industrial plants as immersion injuries. They are often a result of splattering or spilling of an acid substance. The wound is painful and persists because of the chemical action. Its depth and appearance vary, depending on the amount of acid and length of exposure. Systemic changes are rare, but acid fumes may be inhaled. Treatment is best accomplished by initial dilution of the acid.

*Alkali burns* result from chemical irritation from a highly alkaline substance. One example is phosphorus burns, which are painful and often occur as a result of warfare. Phosphorus melts at body temperature and penetrates into tissue. When exposed to air, the wound smokes; in the dark, it glows bluish-green. Copper sulfate is used to treat these burns by inactivating the phosphorus. The chemical is then removed surgically. Caution must be used in working with copper, as its use may result in copper toxicity with massive hemolysis of red blood cells and acute renal tubular necrosis.

Complications of all types of burn wounds include infection, contractures from scarring, renal failure, ul-

## TABLE 47-5.
### CHEMICAL BURNS: PATHOPHYSIOLOGY AND TREATMENT

| | MECHANISM | APPEARANCE | TREATMENT | | |
| --- | --- | --- | --- | --- | --- |
| | | | Cleanse | Neutralize | Debride |
| **Acid burns** | | | | | |
| Sulfuric<br>Nitric<br>Hydrochloric<br>Trichloroacetic | Exothermic reaction; cell dehydration; protein precipitation | Gray, yellow; brown, black; soft to leathery eschar | Water | Sodium bicarbonate | Debride |
| Phenol<br>Hydrofluoric | | | Ethyl alcohol<br>Water | Sodium bicarbonate<br>Sodium bicarbonate; magnesium oxide; glycerin paste; calcium gluconate | Debride<br>Debride |
| **Alkali burns** | | | | | |
| Potassium hydroxide<br>Sodium hydroxide | Exothermic reaction; cellular dehydration; saponification of fat; protein precipitation | Erythema and blister; soapy, thick eschar; painful | Water | Acetic acid or ammonium chloride | Debride |
| Lime | | | Bursh off lime powder | Acetic acid or ammonium chloride | Debride |
| Ammonia | Same as above, plus laryngeal and pulmonary edema | Gray, yellow; brown, black; soft leathery texture | Water | Acetic acid or ammonium chloride | Debride |
| Phosphorous | Thermal effect; melts at body temperature; runs and ignites at 34°C | Gray blue green; flows in dark; depressed, leathery eschar | Water | Copper sulfate | Debride and remove phosphorous particles |

*(Source: K. Arndt, Manual of Dermatologic Therapeutics [4th ed.]. Boston: Little, Brown, 1989.)*

cers, liver failure, pneumonia, urinary tract infection, and acidosis. The frequency of complications increases with the severity of the burn.

## Decubitus Ulcers (Pressure Sores)

The word *decubitus* derives from the Latin *decumbo*, meaning "lying down."[22] During the late 19th and early 20th centuries, persons with decubitus ulcers generally had wasting diseases, such as tuberculosis, osteomyelitis, and chronic renal failure. Now, those persons at risk have conditions that alter mobility, including individuals with spinal cord injuries, the ill elderly who are incontinent, or persons who are bed- or wheelchair-bound. Decubitus ulcers are significant health problems because they increase the length of hospitalization, increase health care costs, and increase the chances of death. Four crucial factors play a role in decubitus formation: (1) pressure, (2) shearing forces, (3) friction, and (4) moisture. Pressure is the most crucial factor, and these ulcers are accurately called *pressure sores*.

*Pressure* is defined as the exertion of force on a surface by an object in contact with the surface.[22] The force is the weight of the individual applied onto the object upon which he or she is lying. Pressure is not evenly distributed over the body when lying or sitting. It is greatest over bony prominences, and it is over these areas that decubitus ulcers develop. A balance exists between interstitial pressure and solid tissue pressure to make a total tissue pressure of zero. With an increase in external pressure over an area, the interstitial fluid pressure increases, elevating total tissue pressure. As a result, capillary and arteriolar pressures rise, causing fluid to filter from capillaries. Edema and autolysis of cells follow. As the pressure continues, lymph vessels are occluded, resulting in accumulation of anaerobic metabolic wastes and tissue necrosis.[16] The duration and magnitude of pressure are key factors in the amount of tissue damage. With high pressure, it takes less time for tissue necrosis to occur. Constant pressure of 70 mm Hg for more than 1 to 6 hours produces irreversible tissue damage, depending on the condition of the skin and the person's nutritional status.[22] If pressure is intermittently relieved, tissue change is minimal.

As a pressure sore develops, the first sign is skin erythema from reactive hyperemia. Continuous pressure causes necrosis of tissue, and initially an eschar forms that covers and protects the wound. Loss of eschar allows bacterial invasion, and infection results.[22]

The sliding of adjacent tissue layers provides a progressive relative displacement of tissues. These *shearing forces* may be accentuated when the head of the bed is raised and the torso of the person slides down, exerting pressure to the sacrum and deep fascia while the posterior sacral skin is fixed. The shearing force in the deep superficial fascia stretches and angulates blood and lymph vessels, causes thrombosis, and undermines the dermis. The subcutaneous fat layer lacks tensile strength and is vulnerable to the mechanical shearing force. The two surfaces that are in contact move across each other, causing friction. This action removes the outer protective stratum corneum and hastens the onset of ulceration. The friction that occurs when a person is dragged across bed sheets is called *sheet burn*. The sacral ulcer commonly is formed in this way.[19]

Fecal matter, urine, and perspiration irritate and macerate the skin, softening it and making it more vulnerable to pressure sore formation.

### Classification and Treatment of Decubitus Ulcers

Decubitus ulcers are graded according to the depth of tissue loss. The usual scale is I to IV with III and IV putting the affected person at risk for infection and loss of function.[19,23] Table 47-6 describes these grades, and they are illustrated in Figure 47-14. In grade I, the sore is reversible. It resembles an abrasion of the epidermis, exposing the underlying dermis. An acute inflammatory response occurs; the wound is irregular in shape, is red, warm, and indurated, and is painful in a normally innervated person. Relief of pressure and local cleansing usually resolve the ulcer in 5 to 10 days.

A grade II decubitus ulcer is also reversible. As pressure continues, the entire dermis is affected. The wound appears as a shallow, full-thickness ulcer with distinct edges, early fibrosis, and skin color changes. The inflammatory response is present. Relief of pressure and local cleansing allow the wound to heal.

In grade III, the decubitus is extended downward, and the epidermis, dermis, and subcutaneous tissues are involved. This full-thickness skin defect spreads peripherally, because the fascia underlying the subcutaneous layer is resistant to pressure. A small broken area may appear on the surface, with a larger area beneath. The epidermis thickens and rolls over the wound edge toward the ulcer base. The ulcer has a dark-light pigmentation. The skin layers are completely distorted, and the wound begins to drain foul-smelling fluid (Figure 47-15). Systemic problems begin to occur in a grade III decubitus ulcer. As in a full-thickness burn injury, fluid and protein are lost. The person may experience fever, dehydration, anemia, and leukocytosis.

In a grade IV wound, the fascia underlying the subcutaneous tissue is penetrated and the wound is rapidly undermined. Complications include osteomyelitis of bone, sepsis, joint dislocations, and release of toxins. The condition may be fatal.[23]

A closed decubitus has no external opening but, inside, may act and appear as a grade III or IV lesion. These ulcers occur after long pressure insults with shear stress.

**TABLE 47–6.**
CLASSIFICATION OF DECUBITUS ULCERS

| GRADE | LAYERS OF SKIN | WOUND APPEARANCE | SYSTEMIC CHANGES | RESOLUTION |
|---|---|---|---|---|
| I | Partial-thickness | Irregular; warm; erythema; pain; edematous | None | Reversible with relief of pressure and local cleansing |
| II | Partial-thickness<br>Epidermis<br>Dermis | Shallow skin ulcer; edges distinct; fibrosis; skin color changes | None | Reversible with relief of pressure and local cleansing |
| III | Full-thickness<br>Epidermis<br>Dermis<br>Subcutaneous layer | Thick epidermal ulcer margin; light and dark pigmentation; skin layers distorted; drains foul-smelling fluid | Infection; fat necrosis; loss of fluid and protein; fever; dehydration; anemia; leukocytosis | Relief of pressure; systemic treatment with IV fluids; diet; medications; debridement and would graft |
| IV | Full-thickness<br>Epidermis<br>Dermis<br>Subcutaneous fat<br>Fascia<br>Muscle<br>Bone | Large open area; bone shows through | Osteomyelitis; sepsis; joint dislocation; toxic; fatal | Radical surgery to remove necrotic area; general support measures (IV; diet; medications) |
| | Closed subcutaneous tissue and deeper | No external sign until later, when skin ruptures; inside appears as a grade III or IV wound; bursalike cavity with necrotic debris | Infrequent infection | Wide excision; removal of bursal sac; flap graft with muscle |

A bursalike cavity forms and is filled with debris from the necrosis of subcutaneous and deeper areas. This type of decubitus ulcer often occurs over ischial tuberosities. Eventually, the overlying skin ruptures.

Another concept that forms the basis of wound care was developed by Marion Laboratories and uses a three-color concept for open wounds—red, yellow, and black. *Red* refers to the color of healthy granulation tissue and indicates that normal healing is occurring. *Yellow* is the color of suppurative exudate that results from microorganisms in the wound. The presence of this pus interferes with the normal healing process. *Black* is the color of necrotic tissue. The dead tissue also becomes a focus of infection and more tissue loss.[23] The black wound will require debridement, enzyme therapy, and moist dressings.

## Other Traumas

Other traumas to the skin include blunt wounds, abrasions (scrapes), incised wounds (as an incision), puncture wounds, and lacerations (cuts). An abrasion is a superficial open wound in which the outer surface layers of skin are scraped off. Nerve endings are exposed and bleeding is minimal. The wound often contains foreign matter that may initiate an inflammatory response. This type of wound normally heals spontaneously. An incision

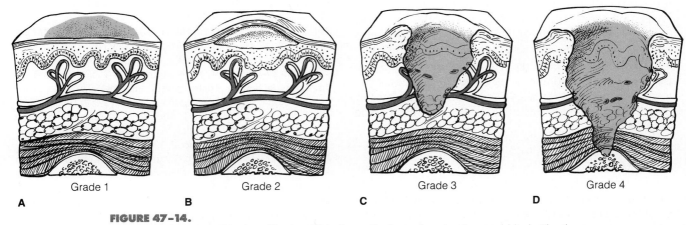

Grade 1   Grade 2   Grade 3   Grade 4

A         B         C         D

**FIGURE 47–14.**
How to grade a pressure ulcer. (Source: N.A. Stotts. Seeing red and yellow and black: The three color concept of wound care. *Nursing 90,* 20 (No. 2), 1990.)

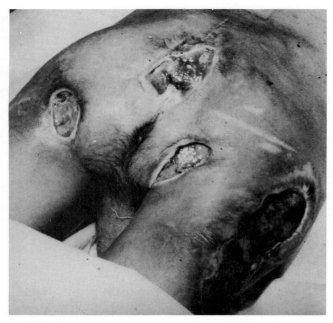

**FIGURE 47–15.**
Because of the widely undermined edges produced by shearing
forces, this sacral ulcer communicates with ischial and trochanteric
ulcers bilaterally. (Source: M.B. Constantian, *Pressure Ulcers.* Boston: Little, Brown, 1980.)

is a clean, straight-edged wound that goes through all
layers of skin; it bleeds freely and heals cleanly when
sutured.

Puncture or stab wounds are deeper than they are
wide and are caused by knives, pins, needles, spikes, and
so forth. Underlying structures may be damaged, with
concealed blood loss. A laceration is a cut or tear of tissues and is unlikely to heal without treatment.

In all traumatic skin wounds, tissue viability is crucial
and depends on circulation of blood to the area. All open
traumatic wounds are contaminated, and host resistance
must be supported.[20] The stages of wound healing, discussed in Chapter 13, involve a characteristic inflammatory response initiated by a vasoconstriction that decreases bleeding. This is followed by vasodilatation and
increased vascular permeability, leaking plasma proteins
into the wound. The final stage involves neutrophilic leukocytes that destroy bacteria.[5] This produces pus and suppuration of surrounding tissues. If the affected tissue can
totally regenerate, it replaces the necrotic tissue. Scar formation may become necessary to bridge an area of tissue
destruction.

## REFERENCES

1. Arndt, K. *Manual of Dermatologic Therapeutics* (4th ed.).
Boston: Little, Brown, 1989.
2. Bauer, E.F., Tabas, M., and Goslen, J.B. Psoriasis and other
proliferative disorders of epithelium. In W. Kelley, *Textbook of Internal Medicine.* Philadelphia: J.B. Lippincott,
1989.
3. Brodzka, W., Thornhill, H.L., and Howard, S. Burns: Causes
and risk factors. *Arch. Phys. Med. Rehab.* 66(11):746, 1985.
4. Bermuda Symposium on the Diagnosis and Management
of Dry Skin. New York: Chesebrough-Ponds, 1984.
5. Cuono, C.B. Physiology of wound healing. In F.J. Dagher
(ed.), *Cutaneous Wounds.* Mt. Kisco, N.Y.: Futura, 1985.
6. Demling, R.H. et al. Early lung dysfunction after major
burns: Role of edema and vasoactive mediators. *J. Trauma*
25(10):959, 1985.
7. Elder, D.E., and Clark, W.H. Malignant melanoma. In
B.H. Thiers and R.L. Dobson (eds.), *Pathogenesis of Skin
Disease.* New York: Churchill-Livingstone, 1986.
8. Heimbach, D.M. Electrical injury. In W.N. Kelley, *Textbook
of Internal Medicine.* Philadelphia: J.B. Lippincott, 1989.
9. Kagan, R.J. et al. Serious wound infections in burned patients. *Surgery* 98(4)10:640, 1985.
10. Katz, S. Approach to the management of skin cancers. In
W. Kelley, *Textbook of Internal Medicine.* Philadelphia: J.B.
Lippincott, 1989.
11. Lang, P.C. Nonmelanoma skin cancer. In B.H. Thiers and
R.L. Dobson (eds.), *Pathogenesis of Skin Disease.* New
York: Churchill-Livingstone, 1986.
12. Lawley, T.J., and Yancey, K.B. Examination of the skin. In
J. Wilson et al. (eds.), *Harrison's Principles of Internal
Medicine* (12th ed.). New York: McGraw-Hill, 1991.
13. Moschella, S.L., Pillsbury, D.M., and Hurley, H.J. *Dermatology* (2nd ed.). Philadelphia: W.B. Saunders, 1985.
14. Munster, A.M., and Ciccone, T.G. Burns. In F.J. Dagher (ed.),
*Cutaneous Wounds.* Mt. Kisco, N.Y.: Futura, 1985.
15. Murphy, G.F., and Mihm, M.C. The skin. In R. Cotran, V. Kumar, and S.L. Robbins (eds.), *Robbins' Pathologic Basis of
Disease* (4th ed.). Philadelphia: W.B. Saunders, 1989.
16. Nicher, L.S. et al. Improving the accuracy of burn-surface
estimation. *Plastic and Reconstr. Surg.* 76(3)9:425, 1985.
17. Prigel, C. How to spot melanoma. *Nursing 87* 17(6):60,
1987.
18. Sauer, G.C. *Manual of Skin Diseases* (6th ed.). Philadelphia: J.B. Lippincott, 1991.
19. Sebern, M. Home-team strategies for treating pressure
sores. *Nursing 87* 17(4):50, 1987.
20. Shack, R.B., and Manson, P.N. Traumatic wounds. In
F.J. Dagher (ed.), *Cutaneous Wounds.* Mt. Kisco, N.Y.: Futura, 1985.
21. Soter, N.A., and Baden, H.P. (eds.). *Pathophysiology of Dermatologic Diseases.* New York: McGraw-Hill, 1984.
22. Steuber, K., and Spence, R.J. Pressure sores. In F.J. Dagher
(ed.), *Cutaneous Wounds.* Mt. Kisco, N.Y.: Futura, 1985.
23. Stotts, N. Seeing red and yellow and black: The three color
concept of wound care. *Nursing 90* 20(2):59, 1990.
24. Udey, M., and Goslen, J. Allergic urticaria and erythema
multiforme. In W.N. Kelley, *Textbook of Internal Medicine.*
Philadelphia: J.B. Lippincott, 1989.
25. Udey, M., and Goslen, J. Cutaneous reactions to drugs. In
W.N. Kelley, *Textbook of Internal Medicine.* Philadelphia:
J.B. Lippincott, 1989.
26. Udey, M., Goslen, J., and Tabas, M. Immunologic and allergic cutaneous disorders. In W.N. Kelley, *Textbook of Internal Medicine.* Philadelphia: J.B. Lippincott, 1990.
27. Wallace, J. Electrical injuries. In J. Wilson et al (eds.), *Har-

rison's *Principles of Internal Medicine* (12th ed.). New York: McGraw-Hill, 1991.

## UNIT BIBLIOGRAPHY

Arndt, K. *Manual of Dermatologic Therapeutics* (4th ed.). Boston: Little, Brown, 1989.

Arnold, H.L., and Odom, R.B. *Andrew's Diseases of the Skin* (8th ed.). Philadelphia: W.B. Saunders, 1990.

Bauer, E., Tabas, M., and Goslen, J. Skin: Cells, matrix and function. In W.N. Kelley, *Textbook of Internal Medicine*. Philadelphia: J.B. Lippincott, 1989.

Binnick, S.A. *Skin Diseases: Diagnosis and Management in Clinical Practice*. Menlo Park, Calif.: Addison-Wesley, 1982.

Clark, R. Cutaneous tissue repair: Basic biologic considerations. *J. Am. Acad. Dermatol.* 13:701, 1985.

Cormack, D. *Ham's Histology* (9th ed.). Philadelphia: J.B. Lippincott, 1987.

Cotran, R.S., Kumar, V., and Robbins, S.L. *Robbins' Pathologic Basis of Disease* (4th ed.). Philadelphia: W.B. Saunders, 1989.

Daghar, F.J. (ed.). *Cutaneous Wounds*. Mt. Kisco, N.Y.: Futura, 1985.

Dobson, R.L., and Abele, D.C. *The Practice of Dermatology*. Philadelphia: Harper & Row, 1985.

Epstein, E. *Controversies in Dermatology*. Philadelphia: W.B. Saunders, 1984.

Farmer, E.R., and Hood, A.F. *Pathology of the Skin*. Norwalk, Conn.: Appleton-Lange, 1990.

Fry, L., Wojnaroska, F.T., and Shahrad, P. *Illustrated Encyclopedia of Dermatology*. Oradell, N.J.: Medical Economics, 1985.

Goldsmith, L.A. *Biochemistry and Physiology of the Skin*. New York: Oxford University Press, 1983.

Guyton, A.C. *Textbook of Medical Physiology* (8th ed.). Philadelphia: W.B. Saunders, 1990.

Habif, T.P. *Clinical Dermatology* (2nd ed.). St. Louis: Mosby, 1990.

Kaplan, E.N. *Emergency Management of Skin and Soft Tissue Wounds*. Boston: Little, Brown, 1984.

Lookingbill, D.P., and Marks, J.G. *Principles of Dermatology*. Philadelphia: W.B. Saunders, 1986.

Merino, M. Skin. In V.A. LiVolsi et al., *Pathology* (2nd ed.). Media, Penn.: Harwal, 1989.

Moschella, S., Pillsbury, D., and Hurley, H. *Dermatology* (2nd ed.). Philadelphia: W.B. Saunders, 1985.

Patterson, J.A. *Skin Disorders: Diagnosis and Treatment*. New York: Igaku-Shoin, 1989.

Patterson, J.W., and Blalock, W.K. *Dermatology: A Concise Textbook*. New York: Medical Exam, 1987.

Rosen, K., Lanning, M., and Hill, M. *The Nurse's Atlas of Dermatology*. Boston: Little, Brown, 1983.

Sams, W.M., and Lynch, P.J. *Principles and Practice of Dermatology*. Edinburgh: Churchill-Livingstone, 1990.

Sana, J., and Judge, R. *Physical Assessment Skills for Nursing Practice*. Boston: Little, Brown, 1982.

Sauer, G.C. *Manual of Skin Diseases* (6th ed.). Philadelphia: J.B. Lippincott, 1991.

Solomons, B.E. *Lecture Notes on Dermatology* (5th ed.). Oxford: Blackwell, 1983.

Soter, N.A., and Baden, H.P. (eds.). *Pathophysiology of Dermatologic Diseases*. New York: McGraw-Hill, 1984.

Stevens, A., Wheater, P., and Lowe, J.S. *Clinical Dermatopathology*. Edinburgh: Churchill-Livingstone, 1989.

Thiers, B.H., and Dobson, R.L. *Pathogenesis of Skin Disease*. Edinburgh: Churchill-Livingstone, 1986.

Wachtel, T.L., and Frank, D.H. *Burns of the Head and Neck*. Philadelphia: W.B. Saunders, 1984.

*unit*

**15**

# NEURAL CONTROL

The nervous system is incredibly complex and must be approached from an adequate basic knowledge of neural control. This approach considers the complicated system of connections and interconnections that allow for perception and movement. The advanced nervous system allows for the achievement of complicated thought and reasoning powers. Chapter 48 begins the discussion with the normal structure and function of the nervous system. Chapter 49 adds the normal and altered function of the special senses. Chapter 50 details some alterations that affect higher cortical functions, especially cerebrovascular accident, aphasia, agnosia, and epilepsy. Chapter 51 covers the physiologic phenomena of pain. Chapters 52, 53, and 54 detail traumatic alterations, tumors and infections, and degenerative alterations, respectively. Each chapter presents specific diagnostic tests that may be helpful in delineating these alterations. The most useful approach to the nervous system is to show how alterations in specific areas can disrupt function. Frequently, the location of the alterations rather than their size finally determines the degree of functional difficulty. The reader is again encouraged to use the learning objectives to organize study and to acquire a firm grasp of the material in Chapter 48 before considering the pathophysiology of the nervous sytem. The unit bibliography provides further resources for learning.

# Normal Structure and Function of the Central and Peripheral Nervous Systems

## Learning Objectives

1. Name the components of the neuron.
2. Describe variations in neuron morphology.
3. Classify neurons according to function.
4. Explain the events occurring with axon injury and regeneration.
5. Define *membrane potential*.
6. Discuss the events of the action potential.
7. List the major types of nerve fibers and their characteristics.
8. Identify factors that influence conduction velocity in nerve fibers.
9. Identify factors that increase neuron membrane excitability.
10. Identify factors that decrease neuron membrane excitability.
11. Define *sensory receptors*.
12. Explain types of sensory receptors.
13. Discuss the phenomenon of receptor adaptation.
14. Contrast receptor potential and generator potential.
15. Define *synapse*.
16. Discuss the events occurring at the chemical synapse.
17. Discuss characteristics of neurotransmitters.
18. List the major structures of the central nervous system in hierarchical order from spinal cord to cerebral cortex.
19. Identify the major functions of the central nervous system structures.
20. Trace the major ascending and descending spinal tracts.
21. Identify the major information transmitted by the ascending and descending spinal tracts.
22. List the components of the peripheral nervous system.
23. Differentiate between structure and function of the somatic efferent and the visceral efferent fibers.
24. Contrast the functions of the sympathetic and parasympathetic divisions of the autonomic nervous system.
25. Differentiate between adrenergic and cholinergic effector organs.
26. Describe the function, formation, and flow of cerebrospinal fluid.
27. Discuss the mechanism and function of the blood-brain barrier.
28. List the major arteries supplying blood to the brain.
29. Discuss the factors responsible for a constant cerebral blood supply in the healthy brain.
30. Describe the indications for and procedures performed in the following diagnostic studies in head and spine injuries: radiographs, angiography, computerized axial tomography scan, magnetic resonance imaging, echoencephalography, brain scan, pneumoencephalography, ventriculogram, myelography, and electroencephalography.

---

Humans interact with the environment through the nervous system, perceiving and responding to the stimuli that continually impinge on them. A complex system of connections and interconnections of nerve cells provides this perception, interim processing, and response. In addition, characteristics that endow humans with the ability to think, feel, reason, and remember evolve from these interacting neuronal networks of the brain.

## THE NEURON

The neuron is the structural and functional unit of nerve tissue, which has the capability to generate and conduct electrochemical impulses (Figure 48-1). Its cellular and cytoplasmic components and metabolic activities that maintain cell life are similar to those of other cells. The distinctive cellular shapes of neurons and their structural synapses that allow transmission of impulses from one to another are unique to the nerve cells. Unlike other cells, the mature neurons are unable to reproduce themselves. They lack centrosomes and, therefore, are incapable of mitosis. If the cell body dies, the entire neuron dies. Under certain circumstances, however, axons, peripheral nerves, regenerate if the cell body is preserved.

Incoming signals to the neuron may be transmitted to dendrites directly, to the cell body, or to the axon by the axon of another neuron (Figure 48-2). The area of contact between neurons is known as the *synapse*. Dendrites, together with the cell body, contain Nissl bodies, which synthesize cell protein and contain much of the ribonucleic acid (RNA) of the cytoplasm. Intracellular mitochondria produce adenosine triphosphate (ATP) for energy. Small vesicles and cisterns known as *Golgi apparatus* are present in the neuron and are thought to be involved in the condensing and storage of secretory substances, as well as in the formation of enzymatic substances which digest intracellular materials.

A fibrous axon (nerve fiber) originates from the axon hillock of the cell body (perikaryon) and transmits signals from the cell body to various parts of the nervous system. These long fibers differ from dendrites, which carry transmissions to the cell, in their branching and in composition of their outer membrane. Some axons are myelinated, while others have no myelin sheath. Myelin is a fatty layer that surrounds the nerve fiber and helps increase conduction of nerve impulses. The myelin sheath is interrupted by periodic gaps known as the *nodes of Ranvier*. Axon collaterals or fibers may emerge from these gaps. Exchange of metabolites takes place between

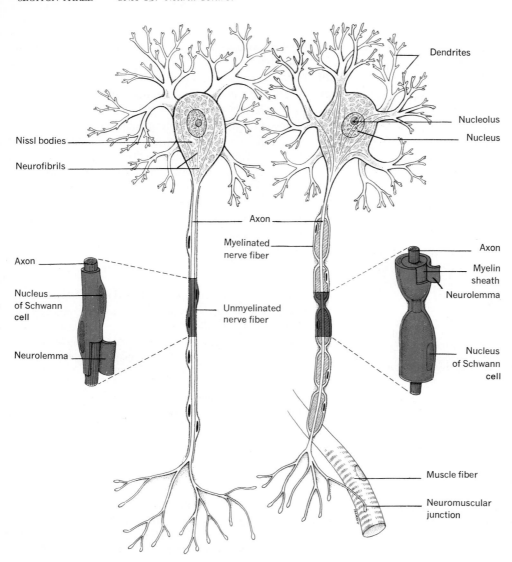

Nissl bodies

Neurofibrils

Axon

Nucleus
of Schwann
cell

Neurolemma

Dendrites

Nucleolus

Nucleus

Axon

Myelinated
nerve fiber

Unmyelinated
nerve fiber

Axon

Myelin
sheath

Neurolemma

Nucleus
of Schwann
cell

Muscle fiber

Neuromuscular
junction

**FIGURE 48-1.**

Typical efferent neurons: unmyelinated fiber (left), myelinated fiber (right). (Source: E.E. Chaffee, I.M. Lytle, *Basic Physiology and Anatomy.* Philadelphia: J.B. Lippincott, 1980.)

the axon and the extracellular environment at the nodes. The nodes of Ranvier are present in both central and peripheral nervous system neurons. However, they are much easier to identify in the peripheral nervous system. Schwann cells are located along the peripheral axons and produce the myelin sheath of lipoprotein that encases the fiber. Some of these cells produce numerous concentric wrappings around the central core axon and give the axon its characteristic white color (Figure 48-3). Unmyelinated fibers contain Schwann cells but lack the concentric wrappings. The outermost thin layer of myelin of the myelinated fibers is known as the *neurolemma* of the axon. This neurolemma is lacking in the myelinated fibers within the spinal cord and brain. Myelin provides protective, nutritive, and conductive functions for the axon.

In the central nervous system (CNS), glial cells, con-

stituent cells to the neurons, protect, nourish, and support the neurons. Collectively, they are referred to as *neuroglia.* Astrocytes, oligodendroglia, microglia, and ependymal are different types of glial cells (Figure 48-4).[10] Astrocytes, the most plentiful of the glial cells, provide structural support and nourishment for the neurons, and make up part of the blood-brain barrier. Oligodendroglia form myelin along axons, and the microglia have phagocytic properties. Ependymal cells line the ventricles of the brain and central canal of the spinal cord, and, in part, provide for the brain-cerebrospinal fluid barrier.

The billions of neurons in the nervous system may be identified according to their morphology and function. A variety of projections may arise from the body of the cell (Figure 48-5). Unipolar neurons possess a solitary axon, which divides near the cell body. Bipolar neurons project two axons and are unique to the olfactory

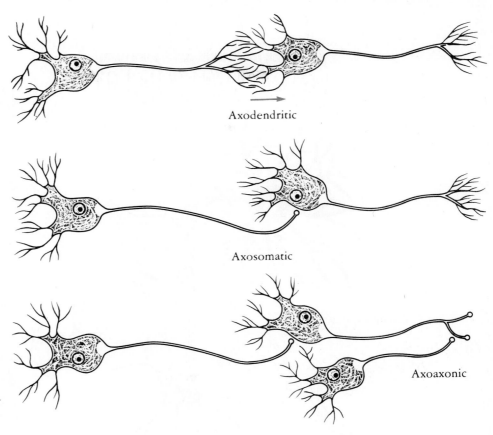

**FIGURE 48-2.**
Examples of various types of synaptic connections. (Source: R.S. Snell, *Clinical Neuroanatomy for Medical Students*. Boston: Little, Brown, 1980.)

Axodendritic

Axosomatic

Axoaxonic

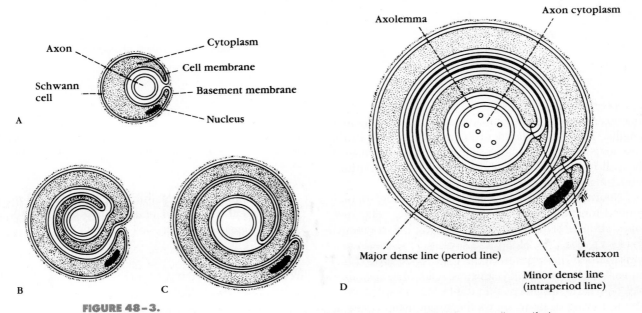

**FIGURE 48-3.**
Schematic representation of evolution of the myelin sheath of an axona: **A.** Schwann cell engulfs the axon, **B.** surrounds it, and **C.** wraps tight concentric layers around it (myelin sheath), **D.** appearance of a mature axon and myelinated sheath. (Source: R.S. Snell, *Clinical Neuroanatomy for Medical Students*. Boston: Little, Brown, 1980.)

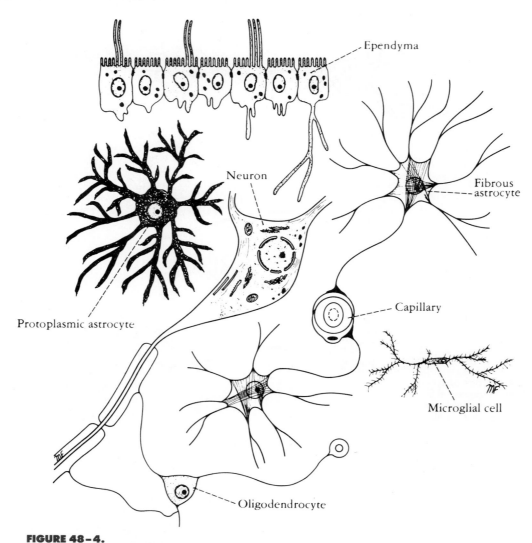

**FIGURE 48–4.**
Different types of neuroglial cells. (Source: R.S. Snell, *Clinical Neuroanatomy for Medical Students.* Boston: Little, Brown, 1980.)

mucous membrane, the retina, and spinal and vestibular ganglia. The multipolar neuron, most prevalent in the nervous system, consists of one major projection from the cell body, the axon, and generally multiple minor branchings (dendrites).

Neurons can also be classified according to their general function. Sensory (afferent) neurons relay messages about internal and external body environmental changes to the CNS. Motor and secretory (efferent) neurons transmit messages from the CNS. Association (internuncial or interneurons) neurons relay messages from one neuron to another within the brain and spinal cord. The following diagram shows the relationship of the afferent, association, and efferent neurons and their fibers as sensations are perceived from the somatic and visceral tissue and transmitted to glands and muscles.

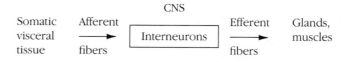

Clusters of neurons within the CNS are called *nuclei* (gray matter). Groups of neurons outside the CNS are known as *ganglia* (see pp. 967–968).

## Peripheral Axon Degeneration and Regeneration

As long as its cell body remains relatively unharmed, an injured neuron may regenerate. Serious damage to the cell body results in death of the entire neuron. A crushed

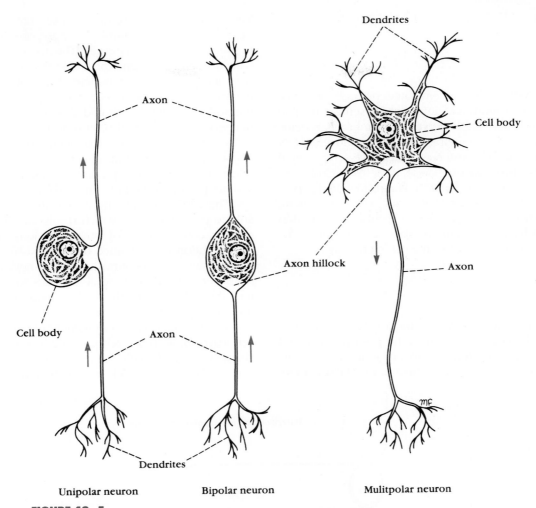

**FIGURE 48–5.**
Examples of morphologic variations in neurons related to the number of projections evolving from the cell. (Source: R.S. Snell, *Clinical Neuroanatomy for Medical Students.* Boston: Little, Brown, 1980.)

or severed axon of a peripheral nerve fiber triggers certain processes within a few hours of injury. Changes in the axon distal to the injury (wallerian degeneration) are particularly dramatic because that portion has been severed from the metabolic control of the cell body. Initially, the distal portion swells and the terminal neurofilaments hypertrophy. The myelin sheath shrinks and retracts at the nodes of Ranvier where the remaining nerve fiber becomes exposed. The axon gradually disappears and myelin disintegrates into fragments that are phagocytized.

Changes also occur proximal to the injury in both the axon and the cell body, itself (retrograde degeneration). Degenerative changes similar to those in the distal portion of the axon occur at the proximal portion for a few millimeters from the injury. The changes in the cell body (chromatolysis) are in response to repair of damages. The extent of cellular changes is related to the location

of the injury along the axon. An axon injury near the cell body produces greater changes in the cell than a more distant injury. The cellular cytoplasm swells and the nucleus is eccentrically placed toward the cell wall. Chromatolysis of Nissl bodies, suggestive of increased protein synthesis, takes place and the number of mitochondria increases. Injured neurofibrils (delicate threads projecting into the axon from the cell body) attempt to grow back into their original placements and begin sprouting from the proximal portion of the injured axon within 7 to 14 days after injury. If the fibrils are successful in finding their way into the neurolemma, they grow at a rate of 3 to 4 mm per day. The remaining Schwann cells form a sheet of myelin around the restored neurofibril, and the nodes of Ranvier are reformed as the nerve regenerates. Regeneration of injured nerves in the CNS is more difficult due to glial scarring, which frequently inhibits new fibrils from reaching their destinations.

# EXCITATION AND CONDUCTION IN NEURONS

## Membrane Potential

Membrane potentials are generated because of a disparity between cations and anions at the semipermeable and selectively permeable nerve cell membrane. Specific proteins at the cell membrane allow the movement of ions and facilitate the existence of the nerve cell potential and impulse propagation. These proteins include cell membrane pumps and channels. Pumps maintain appropriate ion concentrations in the cell side of the membrane by actively moving these ions against concentration gradients. Channel proteins provide selective paths for specific ions to diffuse across the cell membrane.

## Resting Potential

During the resting potential, the inner cell wall surface is negatively charged in relation to the positively charged outer surface as a result of disparity of sodium and potassium ions on either side of the membrane (Figure 48-6).

The extracellular fluid has a higher sodium concentration than the intracellular fluid, whereas potassium concentration is higher within the cell. The inside of the cell also contains anions (organic proteins) that are too large to pass across the cell membrane. These attract the positively charged sodium ions, some of which leak through the sodium channels. Should this movement continue unchecked, the influx of positively charged ions into the cell would soon result in electroneutrality in the cell. To counterbalance this diffusion of ions, a strong active transport system (sodium pump) continually pumps out sodium that has leaked into the cell (see Chap. 1).

The resting membrane is selectively more permeable to potassium ions, which results in a higher intracellular concentration of potassium ions. This higher concentration is maintained through passive movement of potassium and its attraction to the negative interior. A weaker potassium pump also moves some potassium into the cell. Due to the higher intracellular concentration, some diffusion of potassium out of the cell occurs continuously. This movement of potassium from the cell leaves more negatively charged ions than positively charged ions in the cell.[12] Also contributing to the imbalance of charges at the cell membrane is a strong sodium

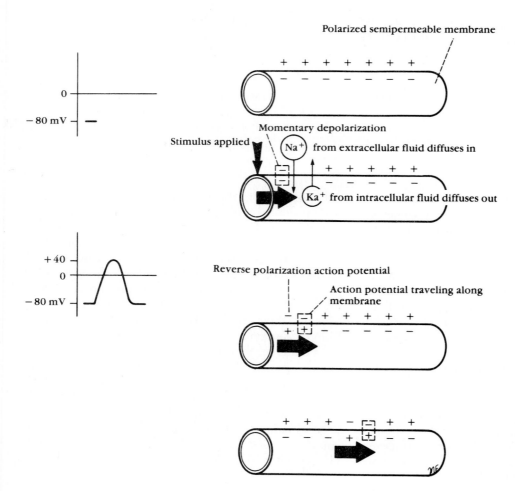

**FIGURE 48-6.**
Summary of electrical changes occurring in the axon during an action potential. (Source: R.S. Snell, *Clinical Neuroanatomy for Medical Students.* Boston: Little, Brown, 1980.)

pump that moves more sodium out of the cell than potassium is moved into the cell by the potassium pump. The inner surface remains electronegative and maintains a resting potential of approximately −70 to −90 mV. In this state, the cell is said to be polarized. Lacking a stimulus, the resting potential can remain unchanged for a long time.

## Action Potential

Unique to nerve, muscle, and gland cells is the change that can occur in a resting cell membrane potential when the cells are stimulated by electrical, chemical, or mechanical means. These stimuli can produce a sudden increase in cell membrane permeability to sodium, which results in a very brief, positive potential within the cell.

The sequence of physiochemical events that results in an alteration in the resting potential lasts a few milliseconds (msec) and is called the *action potential* (see Figure 48-6). In response to a stimulus, the cell membrane becomes much more permeable to sodium ions that rush into the cell through the opened sodium channels and cause the initial spike potential (Figure 48-7). Due to the positive charges carried into the cell by sodium, a change in voltage occurs inside the cell from approximately −70 mV at resting potential to about +40 mV at the height of the spike. This phase of the action potential is identified as *depolarization,* is self-propagating, and travels in both directions along the

entire fiber (Figure 48-8). As the current flows along the adjoining resting membrane, it increases the permeability of the membrane to sodium and thus depolarizes this area. The current flow is continuous until the action potential has propagated the entire length of the axon, very much as a flame travels the fuse of a firecracker.[11]

The influx of sodium is limited because permeability of the cell membrane to sodium is transient and the channels formerly open to it close. During a very brief time, called the *absolute refractory period,* the nerve cell responds to no further stimulus. After the absolute refractory period, the relative refractory period occurs, during which time the cell gradually resumes its excitability and is able to respond to stronger than normal stimuli. As sodium permeability decreases, potassium permeability increases, and there is an efflux of potassium from the cell, resulting in a transient increase in extracellular potassium. This is reflected by the negative afterpotential (after-depolarization) shown in Figure 48-7. The efflux of potassium after the spike potential allows the inside of the cell to become more negative once again (after-hyperpolarization).[12] The period of return to original potential is called the *repolarization phase.* The cell membrane becomes less permeable to potassium and the sodium pump transports sodium out of the cell. This pump is reflected by a positive afterpotential. Finally, potassium shifts into the cell through both membrane channels and pumps, returning the membrane to its resting potential.[5]

## Characteristics of the Action Potential

The point at which a stimulus can excite a fiber is known as the *threshold potential.* At this point, the sodium influx is equal to the potassium efflux. Threshold value differs with various types of nerve cells. For most neurons, the threshold potential is about 15 mV above the resting potential. For example, if the resting potential of a neuron is −80 mV, its threshold potential would be about −65 mV.

Once the threshold potential is reached, the stimulus travels until the axon is totally depolarized. The commencement of depolarization ensures propagation of the impulse along the entire axon, regardless of changes in the stimulus that originally initiated it. This phenomenon is known as the *all or none law,* which applies to excitable cells. Impulse propagation continues at the same speed and intensity and remains unchanged by increasing stimulus intensity. A stronger stimulus, however, increases the frequency of the impulses that are initiated during the relative refractory period. Once the impulse reaches the terminal bouton, one of a number of neurotransmitters is released into the synaptic cleft (see pp. 943–948). This neurotransmitter then diffuses to the postsynaptic membrane and brings about a voltage change.

Nerve trunks have many neurons that have varying

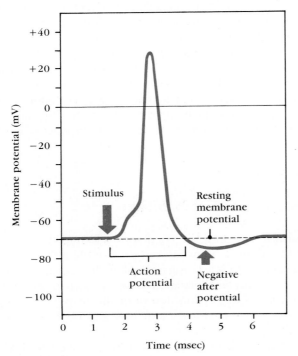

**FIGURE 48-7.**
Changes in membrane potential during an action potential.

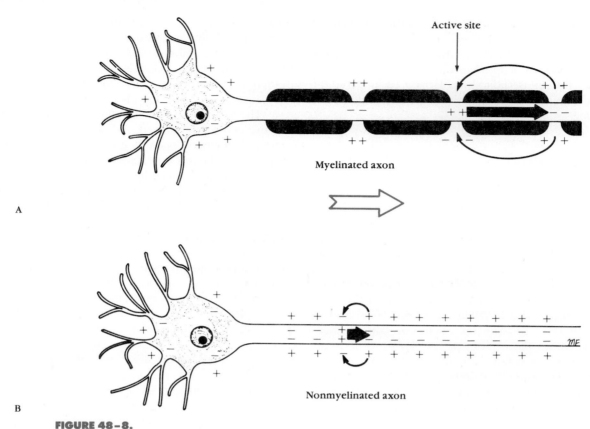

**FIGURE 48–8.**
Propagation of the action potential along **A.** myelinated and **B.** unmyelinated axons. (Source: R.S. Snell, *Clinical Neuroanatomy for Medical Students*. Boston: Little, Brown, 1980.)

independent threshold and velocity values, and the total action potential, known as the *compound action potential,* may depend on the number of neurons firing. A weak stimulus activates only a few neurons, while a strong stimulus excites more. The total action potential of the nerve trunk is the summation of the active neuron action potentials.

## Conduction Velocity in Nerve Fibers

The velocity of nerve conduction is influenced by the myelinization and diameter of the axon. Myelin acts as an effective insulator and inhibits electrochemical conduction. Therefore, the current passes over the myelin and through the extracellular fluid, and enters the nodes of Ranvier at 1-mm to 2-mm intervals, where the membrane is permeable to the ions. This type of current propagation is known as *saltatory conduction,* implying a leaping or hopping phenomenon (Figure 48-8A).

The myelin sheath enhances the velocity of current conduction as capacitance is reduced, which results in reduced numbers of charges propagating the length of the fiber. The heavily myelinated large motor fibers trans-

mit impulses at approximately 100 m per second. In contrast, small unmyelinated fibers may conduct impulses as slow as 0.5 m per second.

The diameter of the fiber is an additional important factor contributing to nerve conduction velocity. Velocity is increased in large-diameter nerve fibers due to lower internal resistance and a quicker depolarization time. Table 48-1 presents the relationship of sheathing and diameter to conduction velocities in various types of nerve fibers.

## Factors Increasing Membrane Excitability

Extrinsic and intrinsic conditions affecting the permeability of the sodium ion can profoundly influence cell excitability. Certain drugs can alter the sodium permeability so that facilitory and inhibitory mechanisms of the cell can no longer function normally. Diuretics, for example, can increase sodium loss and alter cell excitability.

Nerve cell membrane excitability is increased with low extracellular calcium levels. Normally, calcium binds

**TABLE 48-1.**

MAJOR NERVE FIBER CLASSIFICATION AND CONDUCTION SPEED

| FIBER TYPE | SHEATHING | DIAMETER | CONDUCTION SPEED (m/sec) | FUNCTION |
|---|---|---|---|---|
| A fibers | | | | |
| Alpha | Myelinated | 10–18 | 60–120 | Somatic motor, muscle proprioceptors |
| Beta | Myelinated | 5–10 | 38–70 | Rapid sensory touch, pressure, kinesthesia |
| Gamma | Myelinated | 1–5 | 15–45 | Motor to muscle spindle, rapid sensory (touch, pressure) |
| Delta | Myelinated | 2–5 | 5–30 | Pain, temperature, pressure |
| B fibers | Thinly myelinated | 3 | 3–15 | Autonomic preganglionic transmission |
| C fibers | Unmyelinated | 1–3 | 5–2 | Autonomic postganglionic transmission |

with some of the sodium channels and thereby reduces the movement of sodium across the membrane. With less calcium bound to the sodium channels, the movement of sodium becomes less restricted. This increased cell permeability to sodium results in progressively more excitable neuronal tissue. This is manifested clinically by a wide range of signs, including paresthesia, muscular twitching, carpopedal spasms, laryngeal stridor in children, bronchial spasms, tetanic spasms, and convulsions.

## *Factors Decreasing Membrane Excitability*

Increased calcium levels in the extracellular fluid decrease membrane excitability by reducing the membrane permeability that inhibits sodium passage through its channels. Calcium has high protein-binding power, as well as positive charges that facilitate repulsion of sodium at the cell membrane. This results in an inhibitory or stabilizing effect on the cell membrane. Clinically, elevated serum calcium levels are reflected by CNS depression.

Decreased levels of potassium in the extracellular fluids also decrease membrane excitability by increasing its resting potential. The resting potential is dependent on a constant concentration of potassium. A low extracellular potassium level is reflected clinically by depressed neuromuscular excitation, generalized weakness and fatigability of all muscles, diminished or absent reflexes, and paralytic ileus.

Local anesthetics, such as lidocaine and tetracaine, are other factors that can interfere with the initiation and transmission of the action potential. Depolarization is prevented by decreasing the membrane permeability to sodium, and the negative potential necessary for a propagated discharge does not develop or pass through the anesthetized area. The ease of achieving anesthesia is related to nerve fiber size. Small fibers associated with tem-

perature and superficial pain sensations are most easily anesthetized. Large fibers that transmit sensation of deep pain, touch, and pressure are anesthetized with more difficulty.

## *RECEPTORS*

### *Characteristics of Receptors*

Sensory receptors are specialized nerve cells that respond to specific information from the internal and external environments. The information is then transmitted by spinal or cranial nerves to specific areas of the CNS for interpretation. This is accomplished through conversion of various forms of natural energy from the environment into action potentials in neurons. Common to all receptors is this *transduction* of energy. Energy, converted by receptors, includes mechanical energy by *mechanoreceptors*, thermal energy by *thermoreceptors*, light energy by *photoreceptors*, and chemical energy by *chemoreceptors*. Receptors that respond to injury are known as *nociceptors*. *Exteroceptors* give information about the external environment and *interoceptors* and *proprioceptors* are sensitive to internal impulses and changes. *Teleceptors*, such as those found in the eyes and ears, provide information from more distant stimuli.

Receptor cells exhibit a wide range of morphologic and sensitivity differences (Figure 48-9).[5] Some have free nerve endings with coils, spirals, and branching networks; may be present throughout the body; and detect pain, cold, warmth, and crude touch. Some receptor cells are encased in variously shaped capsules and detect tissue deformation. Each receptor cell has adapted to respond to one specific type or modality of stimulus at a much lower threshold than do other receptors. This response in receptors is referred to as *adequate stimulus*. It remains the same no matter how the receptor is stimu-

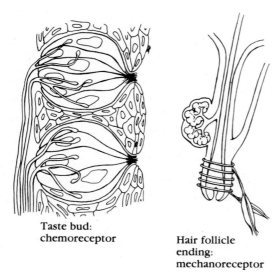

Taste bud:
chemoreceptor

Hair follicle
ending:
mechanoreceptor

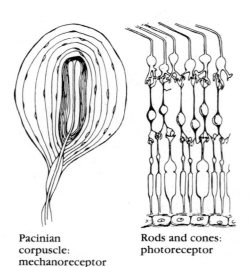

Pacinian
corpuscle:
mechanoreceptor

Rods and cones:
photoreceptor

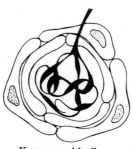

Krause end-bulb:
thermal receptor

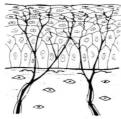

Free nerve ending:
thermal receptor

**FIGURE 48–9.**

Examples of variation in morphologic composition of somatic sensory receptors. (Source: D.M. McKeough, *The Neuroscience Coloring Book*. Boston: Little, Brown, 1982.)

lated. Each nerve tract terminates at a specific point in the CNS where the stimulus is interpreted.

When a constant stimulus is applied to a receptor, the frequency of action potentials initiated in the sensory nerve decreases. This phenomenon is known as *adaptation*. There is a wide variation in sensory organ adaptation. The pressure applied to a pacinian corpuscle results in a receptor potential that adapts rapidly. The fast-adapting receptors are called *phasic* receptors. In contrast, the muscle spindles and receptors for pain adapt very slowly. These receptors are known as *tonic* receptors.

## Receptor Potential

The modalities of sensation are converted by specific receptors into electrical energy by action potentials through graded potential changes. The receptor responses are not an all-or-nothing event like the action potentials of neurons. Rather, the magnitude is dependent on the intensity of the stimulus. As the magnitude of the stimulus is increased, the receptor potential increases. Receptor potentials are stationary, producing a local flow of current that spreads electrically to surrounding areas of the cell through a change of ionic conductance of the membrane of the nerve terminal. The ionic permeability change that initiates the receptor potential depends only on the stimulus, not on conductance changes through the function of the membrane potential as brought about in the action potentials. Because the receptor potential is not dependent on the membrane potential, it does not regenerate and remains stationary at the transducer area of the nerve terminal. If the receptor potential is great enough, the axon is depolarized and an action potential is triggered at the first node of Ranvier.

The mechanisms that generate receptor potentials vary with receptors.[5] For example, deformation generates receptor potential in the pacinian corpuscles, and chemicals initiate receptor potentials in the rods and cones of the eyes. Because most receptor terminals are minute in size and difficult to study, less information is available about their activity than about that of the action potentials.

## THE SYNAPSE

Information concerning the environment is relayed through a succession of neurons in contact with each other. These areas of contact are known as *synapses*. The terminal portion of the presynaptic axon, the *bouton* or *knob*, may synapse with the cell body, dendrites, axons of other nerve cells, or effector cells of muscles or glands. Impulses at the synapse can be transmitted through chemical or electrical means. Chemical synapses, by far the most common, involve the release of a chemical substance (neurotransmitter) in response to a stimulus. This substance may have an excitatory or inhibitory effect on the postsynaptic cell membrane. The electrical synapses present in invertebrate and lower vertebrates are fused synapses to propagate uninterrupted impulses. The discussion here is limited to chemical synapses.

Electron microscopy has considerably heightened our knowledge of the synaptic characteristics and properties. The anatomic structure of synapses varies widely in different parts of the human nervous system. Similarly, numerous functional differences exist.

The presynaptic fiber terminates in an enlarged knob called the *synaptic bouton, knob, end-foot,* or *button.* This presynaptic bouton is divided from the postsynaptic membrane by a narrow cleft of about 200 to 300 angstroms (A), known as the *synaptic cleft.* The presynaptic bouton contains stored particles of a transmitter substance that is released at the synapse in response to a stimulus. Vesicles open and empty the transmitter substance that then excites or inhibits the postsynaptic or effector neuron. Mitochondria in the presynaptic bouton provide the ATP for synthesizing the released substance that is continually regenerated. For example, the common transmitter substance acetylcholine is reduced to choline and acetic acid by the action of the enzyme cholinesterase. Choline and acetic acid are reabsorbed by the terminal bouton and, with the enzymatic assistance of choline acetylase, are resynthesized to acetylcholine, which is stored in the presynaptic vesicles until the next adequate stimulus.

Conduction of impulses through synapses is uni-directional. That is, impulses can be transmitted only through terminal boutons of presynaptic membranes to postsynaptic membranes.

## Events at the Chemical Synapse

As previously noted, the presynaptic terminal bouton contains vesicles with packets of appropriate transmitter substances. A very low level of spontaneous release of this transmitter substance occurs in the resting synapse. This causes spontaneous mini-depolarizations at the synapse. When an action potential spreads to the presynaptic bouton, as shown in Figure 48-10, depolarization of the membrane triggers release of this transmitter substance. It is thought that the trigger release at the terminal bouton requires calcium ions. This theory is supported by observations that low extracellular calcium levels result in diminished amounts of transmitter substance being released. The neurotransmitter substance then attaches to the postsynaptic receptor sites and the postsynaptic membrane potential is modified. The neurotransmitter substance not taken up by the postsynaptic receptors may be taken up by the presynaptic bouton and stored or inactivated by monoamine oxidase (MAO). Some of the unattached neurotransmitter is inactivated at the synaptic cleft or at the postsynaptic membrane by enzymes. In addition, some of the free neurotransmitter is lost through extracellular diffusion.[6]

The presynaptic release of an excitatory transmitter substance can initiate depolarizing response in the postsynaptic membrane that is referred to as the *excitatory postsynaptic potential* (EPSP).[4] The EPSP is graded, non-

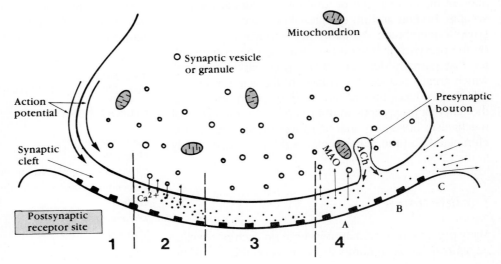

**FIGURE 48-10.**

Neurotransmitter action at the synapse. 1. Action potential depolarizes the presynaptic membrane. 2. Neurotransmitter, acetylcholine, is released into the synaptic cleft. Calcium ions are needed. 3. Neurotransmitter binds with receptors on the postsynaptic membrane. The potential of the postsynaptic membrane is modified. 4. The acetylcholine (ACh) is either taken up into presynaptic bouton or knob and stored, inactivated by acetylcholinesterase, or lost by extracellular diffusion. (Adapted from A. Lewis, *Mechanisms of Neurological Disease.* Boston: Little, Brown, 1980.)

propagative, and the result of an increase in the permeability of the postsynaptic membrane to sodium, potassium, chloride, and calcium ions. Sodium ions flow in across the membrane and decrease the negativity of the postsynaptic cell. The threshold voltage change produced in a motoneuron during depolarization in an EPSP is approximately 13 mV, from a resting potential of $-70$ to $-57$ mV.

The activity of one terminal bouton is not significant enough to initiate an action potential in the postsynaptic cell. It requires many active terminals discharging spontaneously to elicit an action potential. This phenomenon is known as *summation*.[11] Thus, the amplitude of the EPSP depends on the number of activated synapses, and if sufficient numbers are firing, an action potential results.

It has been shown that threshold is the lowest on the motoneuron at the axon hillock, and the thresholds of the cell body and dendrites are considerably higher. Therefore, action potentials initiated in most neurons originate in the axon hillock.

Some synapses release an inhibitory transmitter, thought to contain gamma-aminobutyric acid (GABA) at the postsynaptic membrane. This produces limited permeability to potassium and chloride. Potassium effluxes as chloride influxes, and no corresponding inflow of positive sodium ions occurs. This increases the negativity of the already negative postsysnaptic cell, and a state of hyperpolarization results. This is called an *inhibitory postsynaptic potential* (IPSP).[4] The permeability change is very brief because active transport of chloride out of the cell restores resting potential rapidly. Like the EPSP, the IPSP is graded and does not propagate. During the IPSP, the cell is less excitable as the membrane potential is more negative, and increased excitatory activity is needed to reach the threshold level.

In addition to the IPSP, another form of inhibition, called *presynaptic inhibition*, occurs throughout the nervous system. Although concentrated in the peripheral afferent fibers, this type of inhibition occurs at the presynaptic bouton and no change takes place in the postsynaptic membrane. An inhibitory terminal bouton acts on the presynaptic bouton by releasing a neurotransmitter that partially depolarizes the presynaptic terminal, which greatly reduces the voltage of the action potential and thus reduces the excitability in the membrane. It is thought that presynaptic inhibition provides for a control mechanism of sensory inflow, so less important input is eliminated and the major signal is relayed more clearly to the CNS.

## Facilitation

Many presynaptic terminals converge on each postsynaptic neuron. A certain number of action potentials must be transmitted simultaneously for a sufficient amount of neurotransmitter to be released to produce an action potential in the postsynaptic membrane. If an insufficient amount of a neurotransmitter is released, the postsynaptic membrane is excitatory, although not to threshold level, and it is said to be facilitated. It is above resting potential but below threshold value, and thus very receptive to a stimulus that can activate it with ease.

## Divergence and Convergence

Extremely complex networks of neurons exist in the nervous system. Extensive interactions among neurons are mediated through highly organized circuit connections. As axons emerge from the cell body, they divide and subdivide into many collateral branches that synapse with various numbers of other neurons. This presynaptic division is known as *divergence*. For example, the fibers of afferent neurons entering the spinal cord generally divide and subdivide into collateral branches that supply terminal boutons to many other postsynaptic spinal neurons. As a result, no one fiber contributes to an action potential but rather many fibers cooperatively produce the innervation. The repetitive subdivision strengthens the afferent information, which is made available to various parts of the CNS through the process of divergence.

Similarly, most postsynaptic neurons receive terminal boutons from presynaptic fibers. This postsynaptic anatomic phenomenon is known as *convergence*. Many axons may converge on a single neuron and the EPSP is dependent on sufficient amplitude of the active boutons converging upon it.

## Neurochemical Transmitter Substances

Presynaptic bouton vesicles store specific chemical substances that, when released into the synaptic cleft, either excite or inhibit other cells. Some transmitter substances are present only in the specific parts of the nervous system, while others are widely dispersed. Table 48-2 lists a

**TABLE 48–2.**
FUNCTIONS OF IDENTIFIED NEUROTRANSMITTERS

| NEUROTRANSMITTER | FUNCTION |
| --- | --- |
| Acetylcholine | Excitatory |
| Norepinephrine | Excitatory |
| 5-Hydroxytryptamine (serotonin) | Excitatory |
| Gamma-aminobutyric acid (GABA) | Inhibitory |
| Glycine | Inhibitory |
| Glutamic acid | Excitatory |
| Dopamine | Excitatory |

few neurochemical transmitters that have been identified with certainty. It is thought that many more will be identified in the future. It has been very difficult to pinpoint these substances because of the complex structure of the nervous system fibers.

Substances are considered to be neurochemical transmitters if they have the following general characteristics:[12] (1) are released by the presynaptic bouton on stimulation; (2) contain an enzyme in the presynaptic bouton for transmitter synthesis; (3) produce excitation or inhibition in the postsynaptic cell; and (4) have demonstrated a mechanism that diminishes the effects of the transmitter.

Acetylcholine is a well-established neurochemical transmitter and its activity at the neuromuscular junction is well understood. The terminal bouton of cholinergic nerve fibers contains vesicles, each of which holds about 10,000 molecules of acetylcholine. A vesicle fuses with the presynaptic membrane and results in the release of acetylcholine. This process is known as *exocytosis* (Figure 48-11). It is thought that the fusion of the vesicle to the presynaptic membrane is brought about by a sudden, transient increase in the concentration of calcium ions in the terminal bouton. The nerve impulse at the terminal bouton opens calcium channels to allow their flow into the bouton to facilitate exocytosis. The exact mechanism of the calcium activity in exocytosis is unknown. When the fused vesicle has discharged its acetylcholine at the presynaptic membrane, it is reclaimed by the bouton and restored with acetylcholine for its future use. The synthesis of acetylcholine occurs in the bouton in the following manner:[12]

Acetylcoenzyme A (acetate) + coline

$$\xrightarrow[\text{ATP}]{\text{choline acetyltransferase}} \text{acetylcholine}$$

The acetylcholine that diffuses across the synaptic cleft binds with an acetylcholine receptor on the postsynaptic membrane. This receptor is a channel protein that, in the presence of acetylcholine, lowers its energy state to an open conformation, allowing passage of sodium and potassium ions. Thus, a postsynaptic potential or voltage change is produced. The chemically gated postsynaptic potentials differ from action potentials of neurons in that their amplitude is smaller and their duration longer, and they are graded in accordance with the amount of transmitter released.

Within 2 or 3 msec of its release into the synaptic cleft, after it has depolarized the postsynaptic membrane, acetylcholine is hydrolyzed by the enzyme acetylcholinesterase:[12]

$$\text{Acetylcholine} \xrightarrow[\text{water}]{\text{acetylcholinesterase}} \text{choline + acetate}$$

Acetylcholinesterase is present abundantly in the membrane of the terminal bouton.

Insights into neurotransmitters and their inhibiting enzymes have been gained through the use of various pharmacologic agents that act on or compete with these substances. For example, the muscle relaxant curare competes with acetylcholine for receptor sites at the postsynaptic membrane. Thus, acetylcholine cannot bring about the membrane permeability for depolarization. Some drugs, such as nicotine, simulate acetylcholine action. Neostigmine and physostigmine inactivate the enzymatic action of acetylcholinesterase. Magnesium affects acetylcholine release. Elevated magnesium levels inhibit acetylcholine release by competing with the calcium ions that are necessary for the process.

Norepinephrine is the transmitter substance at all postganglionic sympathetic fibers, except those innervating sweat glands and skeletal muscle vasculature. This substance is formed through a series of steps catalyzed by enzymes with the initial active transport of tyrosine from the circulation into the nerve terminals as follows:[5]

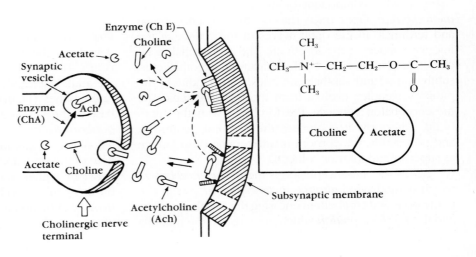

**FIGURE 48-11.**
Acetylcholine (ACh) exocytosis. Acetylcholine is formed in presynaptic bouton through enzyme action of choline acetyltransferase on acetate and choline. It is removed from the cleft by action of enzymes cholinesterase (ChE) which is present in subsynaptic membrane. (Source: E. Selkurt, *Basic Physiology for the Health Sciences* [2nd ed.]. Boston: Little, Brown, 1982.)

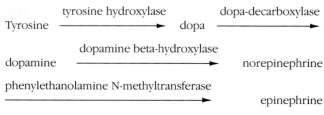

A nerve impulse initiates the release of norepinephrine into the cleft. Norepinephrine activity at the receptor is terminated primarily through its uptake into the terminal bouton and transport back into the vesicles for reuse. In addition, a small amount of norepinephrine is inactivated by the activity of MAO, and an additional small amount escapes the terminal bouton uptake and enters the systemic circulation, where it is primarily metabolized by the liver into vanillylmandelic acid (VMA) and excreted in the urine. Disease states exhibiting increased production of catecholamines characteristically show increased VMA urinary excretion. Minute amounts of released norepinephrine, which escape uptake and metabolic breakdown in the liver, appear unchanged in the urine.

## THE CENTRAL NERVOUS SYSTEM

### Phylogenetic Development

The human nervous system has a complex major processing system that lends control in a hierarchic manner. The highest level is the cerebral cortex, and the lowest, or most rudimentary, is the spinal reflex arc.

One can identify in the embryonic brain three distinct regions: the *rhombencephalon* or *hindbrain*, the *mesencephalon* or *midbrain*, and the *prosencephalon* or *forebrain* (Figure 48-12). The most sophisticated activities and complex subdividing occur in the prosencephalon, which includes the cerebral hemispheres, basal ganglia, and olfactory tract. This portion of the brain subdivided into the *telencephalon* or *endbrain* and the "deep inside" component of the prosencephalon, the *diencephalon*. Optic tracts traverse the prosencephalon and terminate in the optic nerves of the retinae at the inferior surface of the forebrain. The diencephalon includes structures such as the thalamus, hypothalamus, subthalamus, and subthalamic nucleus. In addition, the pituitary complex evolves from the hypothalamus. The mesencephalon connects the forebrain with the hindbrain. Anteriorly, it comprises the cerebral peduncles, and posteriorly, the corpora quadrigemina (also known as superior and inferior colliculi).

Below the mesencephalon is the *rhombencephalon*, which is subdivided into the *metencephalon*, giving rise to the pons and cerebellum encasing the fourth ventricle, and the *myelencephalon* which gives rise to the medulla

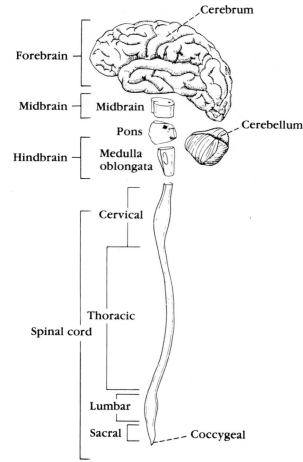

**FIGURE 48-12.**
The brain develops from three regions: hindbrain, midbrain, and forebrain. (Source: R.S. Snell, *Clinical Neuroanatomy for Medical Students*. Boston: Little, Brown, 1980.)

oblongata. Extending from the rhombencephalon inferiorly is the spinal cord.[7]

### Protective Coverings of the Brain and Spinal Cord

Protection is afforded the brain and spinal cord by bony coverings, the meninges, and the cerebrospinal fluid (CSF). The brain is encased within the skull, which in the adult is a nonflexible structure composed of several fused bones (Figure 48-13). Three depressions in the base of the skull are known as the *anterior, middle*, and *posterior fossae*.

A major opening, the *foramen magnum*, is at the base of the skull and allows information to be processed between higher and lower centers (Figure 48-14). At birth, openings within the skull, known as the *fontanelles*, can be noted. These generally close by 18 months of age.

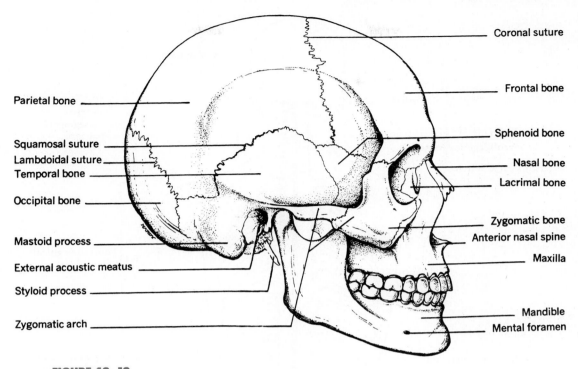

**FIGURE 48–13.**
Lateral view of the skull. (Source: J. Hickey, *The Clinical Practice of Neurological and Neurosurgical Nursing* [2nd ed.]. Philadelphia: J.B. Lippincott, 1986.)

The spinal cord is encased in the vertebral column that consists of 24 movable vertebrae: 7 cervical, 12 thoracic, and 5 lumbar, and the fused 5 sacral and 4 coccygeal vertebrae. Figure 48-15 shows the relationship of spinal nerves and vertebrae. Intravertebral disks separate each of the vertebrae. The central cartilaginous portion of the intervertebral disk is known as the *nucleus*

*pulposus* and the outer fibrous capsule as the *anulus fibrosus*.

In addition, the brain and spinal cord are protected by three connective tissue membranes called the *meninges*: the *dura mater*, the *arachnoid mater*, and the *pia mater*. The dura mater is a thick, tough, nonelastic fibrous membrane that lies directly below the skull. Its

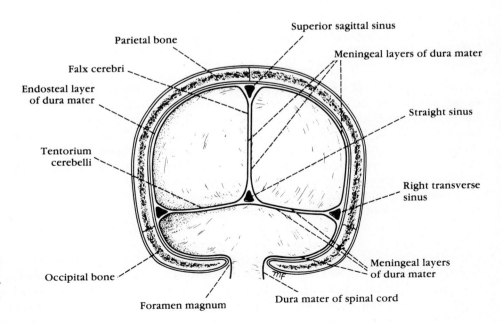

**FIGURE 48–14.**
Relationship of intracranial contents with the foramen magnum. (Source: R.S. Snell, *Clinical Neuroanatomy for Medical Students*. Boston: Little, Brown, 1980.)

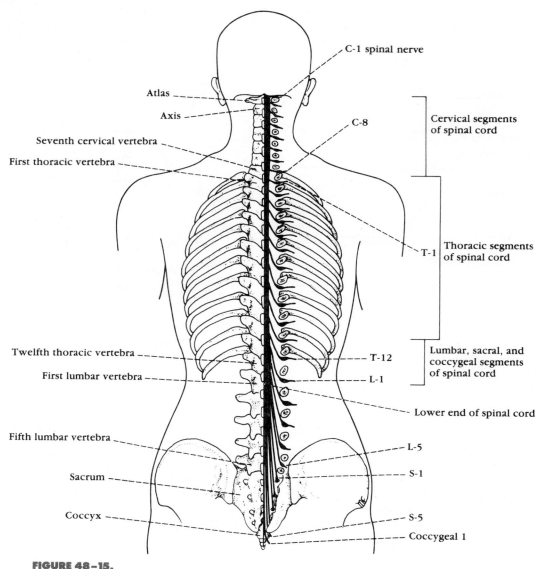

**FIGURE 48-15.**
Relationship of vertebral segments of cord with actual vertebrae. (Source: R.S. Snell, *Clinical Neuroanatomy for Medical Students.* Boston: Little, Brown, 1980.)

extension between the cerebral hemispheres is known as the *falx cerebri.* Between the cerebrum and cerebellum it is known as the *tentorium cerebelli*; between the lateral lobes of the cerebellum as the *falx cerebelli* and above the sella turcica as *diaphragma sellae*. A layer of the dura mater, together with the arachnoid and pia mater, extends through the foramen magnum and lines the vertebral column. The *epidural space* is between the inner surface of the skull and the dura mater. The space between the dura and arachnoid is known as the *subdural space.* A network of small blood vessels traverses this space. The delicate arachnoid, consisting of fibrous, weblike tissue, is the middle layer of the meninges wherein the CSF circulates and is reabsorbed. The area below the arachnoid membrane containing the CSF is known as the *subarachnoid* space. The innermost layer,

the pia mater, is a delicate, vascular, lacelike membrane directly adherent to the brain and spinal cord. The arachnoid layer projects small extensions called *arachnoid villi* into the dura mater that reabsorb CSF into the blood (Figure 48-16). Larger blood vessels lie in the subarachnoid space and branch into smaller vessels that pass through the pia mater as they enter the brain tissue.

## The Spinal Cord Processing System

The spinal cord, which is encased in the vertebral canal, transmits more complex signals from higher centers and responds spontaneously to local sensory information with automatic motor responses called *reflexes*. It is approximately 42 to 45 cm long in the adult and is segmented

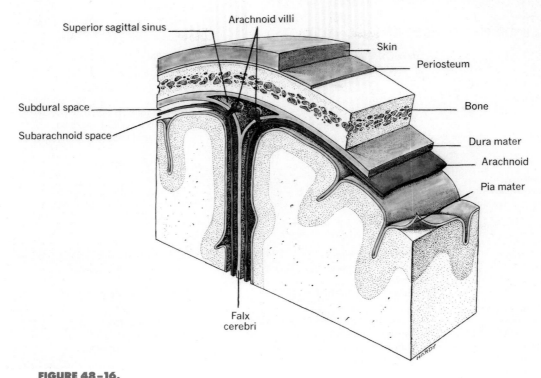

**FIGURE 48-16.**
The cranial meninges. Arachnoid villi shown within superior sagittal sinus are one site of passage of cerebrospinal fluid into the blood. (Source: E.E. Chaffee, I.M. Little, *Basic Physiology and Anatomy.* Philadelphia: J.B. Lippincott, 1980.)

into cervical, thoracic, lumbar, and sacral sections. Signals are received and transmitted through 31 pairs of spinal nerves, which are named for their corresponding vertebral level. Segments of the spinal cord do not correspond with vertebral levels (see Figure 48-15). The spinal cord is approximately 25 cm shorter than the vertebral canal and ends at the level of the first or second lumbar vertebra in the adult. It emerges from the base of the skull, the *foramen magnum*, and continues to the coccyx, where it ends in a tapered cone called *conus medullaris*. From the conus extends a thin filamentous connective tissue called the *filum terminale*. Together, the lumbosacral nerve roots project from the conus and are called the *cauda equina*.

The spinal cord enlarges at the lower cervical segments and again at the lower lumbar segments. These enlargements denote the origins of the *brachial* and *lumbar plexuses*, respectively. The brachial plexus, extending from C-5 to T-1, innervates the upper extremities; and the lumbar plexus, extending from L-3 to S-2, innervates lower extremities. The cell bodies are located in the inner, butterfly-shaped, gray portion of the spinal cord, and the ascending and descending projection nerve fibers form the outer white area. Major ascending and descending tracts and their transmissions are presented in Table 48-3. A small opening in the middle of the spinal cord, the *central canal*, is lined by ependymal cells and contains CSF. Afferent spinal nerves enter the cord at the posterior horn (somatic sensory and visceral) and efferent nerves emerge at the anterior horn (motor and autonomic) (Figure 48-17). The cell bodies of efferent motor fibers are located in the anterior horn and the cell bodies of the afferent sensory fibers are situated outside the spinal cord in the posterior root ganglion. Contact between the afferent and efferent fibers is made within the spinal cord through interneurons.

## Reflex Arc

A fundamental component of the nervous system is the reflex, which, in its simplest form, occurs in the spinal cord. A stimulus from the external environment may produce an immediate stereotypical reflex response from the CNS. For a reflex response to occur, the following mechanisms must be functional: an afferent neuron with its receptor, an area for the synapse transmission to occur (one or more central neurons), and an efferent neuron with its effector organ. The impulse passes from receptor to effector and commands a quick organ response. This simple chain of neuronal activity is known as a *reflex arc* and, at its most elemental level, is a *monosynaptic reflex* consisting of only one synapse and two neurons (see Figure 48-17). Most reflexes result from many more synaptic interconnections and are referred to as *polysynaptic reflexes*. The reflex activity encountered at higher levels in the CNS is considerably more complex.

**TABLE 48–3.**
MAJOR ASCENDING AND DESCENDING SPINAL TRACTS

| TRACTS | MAJOR TRANSMISSION INFORMATION | ORIGIN |
|---|---|---|
| **Anterior white column** | | |
| Descending (motor) | | |
| Ventral corticospinal | Voluntary movement | Pyramidal cells of motor cortex |
| Vestibulospinal | Posture and balance reflexes | Vestibular nuclei in medulla |
| Reticulospinal | Muscle tone controls activity of autonomic nervous system | Reticular of midbrain and medulla |
| Tectospinal | Audiovisual reflexes | Roof of the midbrain |
| Ascending (sensory) | | |
| Ventral spinothalamic | Light touch and pressure | Opposite posterior column |
| Spino-olivary | Reflex proprioception | Anterior marginal zone of spinal column |
| **Lateral white column** | | |
| Descending (motor) | | |
| Lateral corticospinal | Voluntary movement | Contralateral pyramidal cells of motor cortex |
| Rubrospinal | Muscle tone, head and upper trunk movement | Red nucleus of midbrain |
| Olivospinal | Facilitative and inhibitory reflexes | Inferior olivary nucleus |
| Ascending (sensory) | | |
| Dorsal spinocerebellar | Reflex proprioception to cerebellum | Ipsilateral dorsal nucleus |
| Ventral spinocerebellar | Reflex proprioception to cerebellum | Posterior white column |
| Lateral spinothalamic | Pain temperature tactile sensations | Contralateral dorsal column |
| **Posterior white column** | | |
| Descending (motor) | | |
| Fasciculus interfascicularis | Integration and association | Intraspinal and dorsal root |
| Ascending (sensory) | | |
| Fasciculus gracilis | Both transmit vibration, discriminative tactile senses, joint position, kinesthetic sensations | Posteromedian septum of low spinal cord |
| Fasciculus cuneatus | | Posterior nerve roots of thoraco-cervical cord |

Source: *D.G. Chusid, Correlative Neuroanatomy and Functional Neurology (19th ed.). Lange Medical Publishers,*
*1985. Reprinted by permission.*

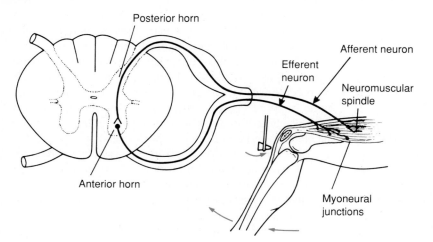

**FIGURE 48–17.**
A monosynaptic reflex arc. (Adapted from R.S. Snell, *Clinical Neuroanatomy for Medical Students.* Boston: Little, Brown, 1980.)

## Low-Brain Processing System (Rhombencephalon)

The next level of processing in the CNS takes place in the rhombencephalon. The major components of this region are the medulla oblongata, pons, cerebellum, and fourth ventricle (Figure 48-18). The processing encountered at this level occurs at the unconscious level and influences such vital activities as respiratory, cardiac, and vasomotor control.

## Medulla Oblongata

The medulla extends directly from the cervical spinal cord at the level of the foramen magnum and lies below the pons and fourth ventricle. The medulla is subdivided into three distinct sections: anterior, lateral, and posterior. Fissures and sulci provide landmarks that distinguish these divisions. The anterior portion contains two prominent ridges known as the *pyramids* that contain the *descending pyramidal tract*. These fibers project from the primary motor and somasthetic cortical areas and

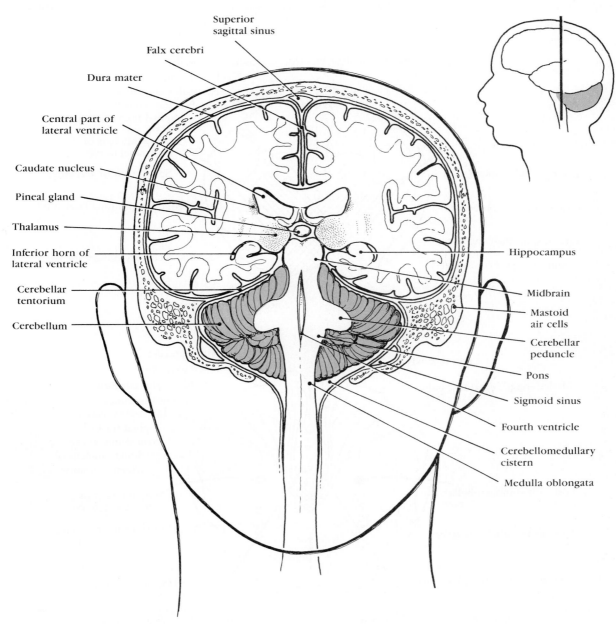

**FIGURE 48-18.**
The structures of the rhombencephalon, consisting of the medulla oblongata, the pons, and the cerebellum.

cross from one side to the other (pyramidal decussation) at the lower medulla before entering the spinal cord. By far, the majority of these fibers decussate and descend as the *lateral corticospinal* tract. The fibers from the motor cortex that remain uncrossed descend into the spinal cord as the *anterior corticospinal* tract. Injury anywhere along the corticospinal tract above the decussation results in motor deficits of the contralateral extremities.

The *olive*, a prominent mass, is located in the lateral section of the medulla. This structure gives rise to the *inferior olivary nuclear complex*, which is important in controlling movement, postural change, locomotion, and equilibrium through an interconnecting network

of fibers among the cerebral cortex, spinal cord, and cerebellum. This region contains nuclei for four cranial nerves: the 12th (hypoglossal), 11th (accessory), tenth (vagus), and ninth (glossopharyngeal). Cardiac and vasomotor control evolve from the reticular formation of this region. Respirations are controlled by the medullary center in coordination with the pneumotaxic center in the pons.

The posterior portion of the medulla forms a portion of the floor of the fourth ventricle. The ascending *medial lemniscus* tract arises here from the crossed over fasciculi cuneatus and gracilis fibers (Figure 48-19). The medial lemniscus is a major ascending brainstem tract that car-

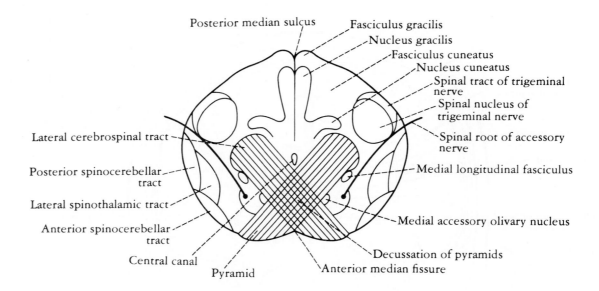

A

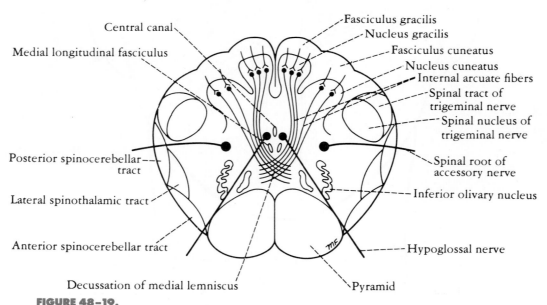

B

**FIGURE 48-19.**

Transverse sections of the medulla oblongata. A. Level of decussation of the pyramids. B. Level of decussation of the medial lemnisci. (Source: R.S. Snell, *Clinical Neuroanatomy for Medical Students.* Boston: Little, Brown, 1980.)

ries discriminative tactile information, proprioception, and vibration sensation to the sensory thalamic nucleus. Lesions in the medical lemniscus result in contralateral sensory deficits.

## Pons

The pons is continuous with the medulla and midbrain, separated by the pontine sulcus from the medulla and the superior pontine sulcus from the midbrain. The pons lies ventral to the cerebellum and is divided into two parts: a *dorsal* portion, the pontine tegmentum, and a *ventral* portion, the pons proper.[1] The dorsal portion is continuous with the medullary reticular formation and, together with the medulla, forms the floor and lateral wall of the fourth ventricle. This portion also contains important ascending and descending tracts and cranial nerve nuclei for the fifth (trigeminal), sixth (abducens), seventh (facial), and eighth (acoustic) cranial nerves (see p. 963). The pons regulates respiration through its pneumotaxic center.

The ventral portion of the pons consists of a large mass of orderly longitudinal and transverse fiber bundles that are interspersed with many pontine nuclei. The longitudinal fiber bundles traversing through this portion of the pons are the corticospinal, corticopontine, and corticobulbar. The ventral portion of the pons is an important relay center between the cerebral cortex and the opposite cerebellar hemisphere in providing smooth, coordinated movements. The transverse fibers arise from the pontine nuclei and cross to the opposite side to form the middle cerebellar peduncle.

## Cerebellar Processing

The cerebellum lies in the posterior cranial fossa and is separated from the cerebrum by the tentorium cerebelli (see Figure 48-18). The superior, middle, and inferior cerebellar peduncles connect the cerebellum to the midbrain, pons, and medulla, respectively. The cerebellum exerts ipsilateral control: the right side of the cerebellum controls the right side of the body and the left side of the cerebellum controls the left side of the body. As noted in Figure 48-20, the cerebellar structures are divided into two major lateral hemispheres and an intermediary section, the vermis. Fissures divide the hemispheres into three principal lobes: the *archicerebellum* (flocculonodular lobe), *paleocerebellum* (anterior lobe), and *neocerebellum* (posterior lobe). The archicerebellum is integrated with the vestibular system and is concerned with muscle tone, equilibrium, and position through its influence on the trunk musculature. The paleocerebellum consists of the cerebellum that lies anterior to the primary fissure, receiving most of the proprioceptive and interoceptive input from the head and body. It helps to maintain equilibrium and coordinate automatic movements, as well as to regulate muscle tone. The neocerebellum, phylogenetically the newest, consists of the cerebellum between the primary fissure and the posterior fissure. It coordinates voluntary movements and has extensive connections with the cerebral cortex.

The cerebellum processes and transmits information concerning current body movements, maintains posture, and regulates muscle tone. It does this through information it receives from the motor cortex of the cerebrum

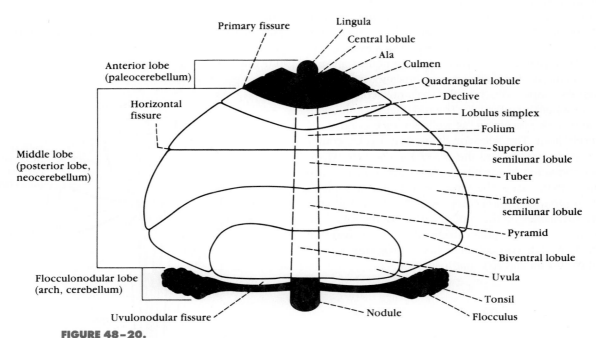

**FIGURE 48-20.**
Main cerebellar lobes, lobules, and fissures (Source: R.S. Snell, *Clinical Neuroanatomy for Medical Students.* Boston: Little, Brown, 1980.)

by way of the *corticocerebellar* pathway and from various sensory receptors by way of the *anterior* and *posterior spinocerebellar* tracts. Other significant tracts relaying this information to the cerebellum include the *spinoreticular* tract by the reticular area of the brainstem and the *spino-olivary* tract by the inferior olivary nucleus. Fiber-efferent tracts originate in various cerebellar nuclei and transmit information to the cerebral motor cortex, basal ganglia, red nucleus, reticular formation, and vestibular nuclei.[5]

Because the pathways from the cerebral cortex to the cerebellum are not direct, descending motor tracts, disruption of cerebellar function does not hinder voluntary movement, although movement no longer is smooth and coordinated. Disruption of cerebellar function can result in ataxia, intention tremor, adiadochokinesia (inability to perform rapid alternating movements), dysmetria (inability to judge distances when reaching out toward an object), hypotonia, tremor, and asthenia.

## Midbrain Processing System (Mesencephalon)

The midbrain extends from the pons and projects briefly between the two cerebral hemispheres, connecting the lower centers with the diencephalon. It, therefore, is a major motor and sensory fiber pathway between the higher and lower centers. The nuclei for third and fourth cranial nerves originate in this region. The *cerebral aqueduct (aqueduct of Sylvius)*, a small channel between the third and fourth ventricles, lies in the midbrain. The midbrain *tegmentum* is located ventral to the cerebral aqueduct and is continuous with the pontine tegmentum. The reticular formation in this region contains the *substantia nigra* and the *red* nucleus. The substantia nigra is a large pigmented mass containing neurotransmitters, particularly dopamine. It supports motor function through its connections with the thalamus, corpus striatum, and superior colliculus.[1] The red nucleus influences head and neck movement, as well as motor control, by the cerebellum. The *superior colliculus*, a relay center for the optic system, and the *inferior colliculus*, which relays information concerning auditory impulses, are also contained in this area. The superior and inferior colliculi (*corpora quadrigemina*) compose the tectum. The *crus cerebri* are masses on the ventral surface of the midbrain that comprise motor fibers originating in the cerebral cortex, as well as corticobulbar fibers projecting to cranial nerve nuclei and reticular formation.[1]

## Diencephalon Processing System

The diencephalon arises from the midbrain and is considered to be a part of the forebrain. It lies between the cerebral hemispheres and encases the third ventricle. Included in this area are the epithalamus, thalamus, hypothalamus, and subthalamus.

### Thalamic Processing

The thalamus, the largest portion of the diencephalon, is a major center for processing sensations and relaying these to the cerebral cortex. Input from all sensoria, except that for olfaction, is processed here. Numerous afferent nerve tracts from lower levels transmit information to the specific relay nuclei of the thalamus. The thalamus is divided into three sections: *lateral, medial*, and *anterior*, which are separated by the *internal medullary lamina*. Groups of nuclei within the internal medullary lamina are referred to as *intralaminar thalamic* nuclei. Sensory data are relayed through these nuclei.

The reticular activating system continues its upward projection to the thalamic nuclei. From the thalamic nuclei, fibers diffuse to all areas of the cerebral cortex. This system is known as the *diffuse thalamocortical system*. This system, which is also referred to as the nonspecific thalamocortical system, activates the first two layers of neurons of the cortex by partially depolarizing superficial cortical dendrites, resulting in increased facilitation of the cortex.[5] The *paleospinothalamic pathway*, which transmits burning and aching sensations, terminates in the diffuse thalamocortical system (Figure 48-21). Axons of the optic tract synapse in the lateral geniculate body, which projects from the thalamus. The fibers projecting from the lateral geniculate body pass posteriorly and terminate in the visual cortex.

### Hypothalamic Processing

The hypothalamus lies below the thalamus and forms part of the walls and floor of the third ventricle (Figure 48-22). It consists of a group of nuclei with specific functions and is divided into the anterior and posterior

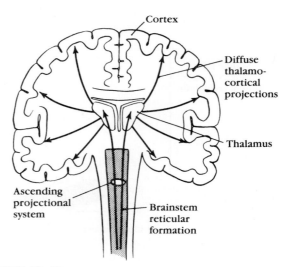

**FIGURE 48–21.**
The thalamocortical system.

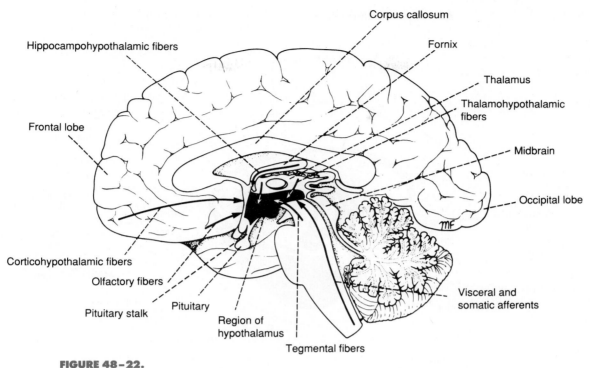

**FIGURE 48–22.**
Sagital section of brain showing main afferent pathways entering hypothalamus. (Adapted from R.S. Snell, *Clinical Neuroanatomy for Medical Students.* Boston: Little, Brown, 1980.)

portions. The pituitary stalk connects the hypothalamus to the pituitary gland, which provides the route for its neuroendocrine control.

Major processing of internal stimuli evoking the autonomic nervous system is concentrated in the hypothalamus. The functions that maintain the internal milieu processed by the hypothalamus include blood pressure, heart rate, respiratory rate, body temperature, water metabolism, and body fluid osmolality, feeding behavior, and neuroendocrine activity. The hypothalamus is a focal structure of the *limbic* system. Figure 48-23 illustrates the structures of the limbic system, which, in concert with the hypothalamus, perform an important role in overall behavior and emotions. Because vital autonomic functions are processed here, destruction of the hypothalamus results in death. The majority of the hypothalamic activity occurs at an unconscious level but excessive stimulation may evoke a conscious response. An example of this is a person who is chilled and consciously seeks warmth.

Responses to emotions of fear, anger, and excitement reflected by increased pulse rate, increased respiratory rate, increased gastric acidity, and sweating are communicated from the hypothalamus. Prolonged stimulation of the hypothalamus may result in hypertension or ulcers.

The *epithalamus* consists of the pineal body, habenular nuclei, stria medularis, and posterior commissure. It is located in the region above the thalamus and contains the roof of the third ventricle. Olfactory impulses are relayed through this region and visual reflexes are associated with certain fibers in the posterior commissure.

The function of the pineal body in the adult is uncertain. It becomes visible on skull films due to calcified material that accumulates with age, and it can provide useful information in the identification of space-occupying lesions.

## Basal Ganglia Processing

The basal ganglia (Figure 48-24), situated deep within the cerebral hemispheres, are responsible for motor control and information processing in the extrapyramidal system. The basal ganglia include the *caudate nucleus, putamen,* and *globus pallidus.* These nuclear masses have complex interconnections with the *subthalamic nucleus, red nucleus,* and *substantia nigra.* The claustrum and amygdaloid body, considered by some authors to be part of the basal ganglia, are not directly involved in motor control.

The basal ganglia are intimately related to the thalamus through circular neural pathways that control motor function. They inhibit muscle tone by transmitting inhibitory signals to the bulboreticular facilitory area and excitatory signals to the bulboreticular inhibitory area. Lesions in the basal ganglia result in an overactive facilitory area and underactive inhibitory area. Gross intentional movement that is performed without conscious thought is regulated by the caudate nucleus and putamen (collectively called the *striate body*).

Striate body transmissions are sent to the globus pallidus and relayed on to the ventrolateral nucleus of the thalamus and then on to the cerebral cortex. From the

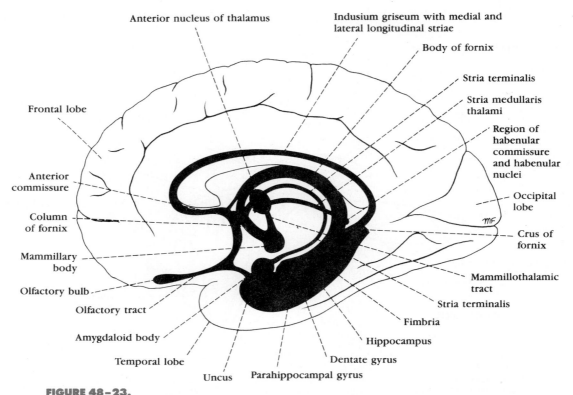

**FIGURE 48–23.**
Key structures of the limbic system (Source: R.S. Snell, *Clinical Neuroanatomy for Medical Students.* Boston: Little, Brown, 1980.)

cortex, the information travels through the pyramidal and extrapyramidal tracts to the spinal cord. Other impulses travel to the globus pallidus and then on to the substantia nigra and on to the reticular formation, where the final route transmits down through the reticulospinal tract.

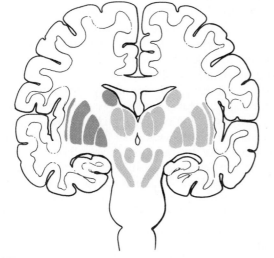

**FIGURE 48–24.**
Coronal section of brain showing basal ganglia.

The globus pallidus relays impulses through a similar feedback circuit to the ventrolateral nucleus of the thalamus and on to the cerebral cortex, and finally to the pyramidal and extrapyramidal tracts to the spinal cord. It also transmits by shorter circuits to the reticular formation and on to the reticulospinal tract of the spinal cord.[5]

The subthalamus nucleus, red nucleus, and substantia nigra are closely related to the globus pallidus and striate body. Their interactions, which control and coordinate motor function, are extremely complex and extensive, and little is known of the exact interconnections.

The neurons transmitting to the globus pallidus and striate body from the substantia nigra are inhibitory through *dopamine* secretion.[3]

Dysfunction or lesions in the region of the basal ganglia are manifested in involuntary tremor, athetosis, and torticollis (see Chap. 54).

## Forebrain (Prosencephalon)

Anatomically, the highest and largest portion of the brain, the cerebrum, is thought to be phylogenetically related to the thalamus because of its closely associated structure and function. All areas of the cerebral cortex have afferent and efferent fibers interconnecting with specific areas of the thalamus. As previously noted, this relationship is affirmed through the diffuse thalamocortical system.

The gray cerebral cortex is composed of five basic types of neurons: pyramidal cells, stellate cells, fusiform cells, horizontal cells, and the cells of Martinotti. The pyramidal and stellate cells are the most numerous. Pyramidal cells have pyramid-shaped bodies with axons that extend into the subcortical white matter. The stellate cells have a star-shaped body with short axons and dendrites. The horizontal cells lie entirely on the horizontal plane with axons and dendrites that are parallel in direction to the cortical surface. Polymorph or multiform cells may be modified types of pyramidal cells with a wide variety of shapes and contours. Dendrites often extend into the cortical layers, while axons project into the white matter. The cells of Martinotti are multipolar with short branch-

ing dendrites and myelinated axons. They may be modified stellate cells.[1]

The white matter of the cerebral hemispheres is composed of three types of myelinated nerve fibers: projection, transverse, and association. Projection fibers connect the cerebral cortex with lower centers of the brain and spinal cord, transverse fibers connect the two cerebral hemispheres, and association fibers provide interconnections within the same cerebral hemisphere.

The cerebrum appears as a series of convolutions (*gyri*) and grooves (*sulci*) that are instrumental in identifying the structural and functional geography of the cortex. Brodman is credited with mapping specific functional areas on the central cortex (Figure 48-25). Over

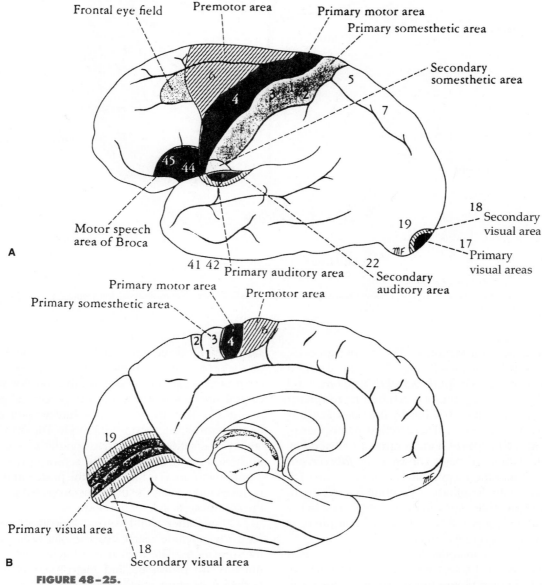

**FIGURE 48-25.**
Functional localization of the cerebral cortex based on Brodmann's cytoarchitectonic map. **A.** Lateral view of the left cerebral hemisphere; **B.** medial view of the left cerebral hemisphere. (Source: R.S. Snell, *Clinical Neuroanatomy for Medical Students.* Boston: Little, Brown, 1980.)

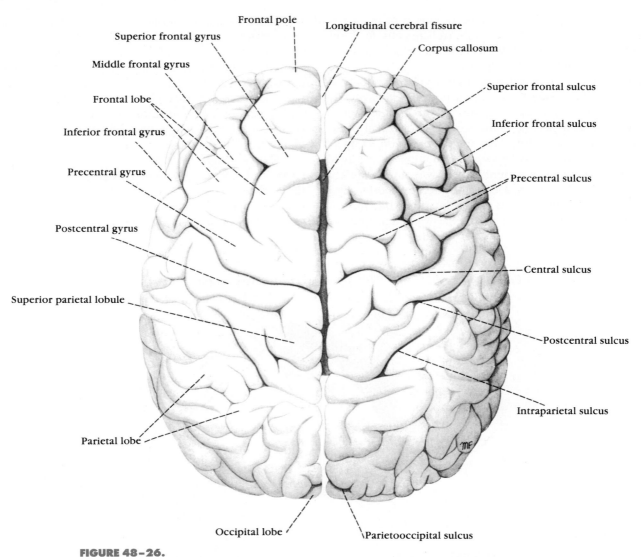

**FIGURE 48–26.**
Superior view of cerebral hemispheres (Source: R.S. Snell, *Clinical Neuroanatomy for Medical Students*. Boston: Little, Brown, 1980.)

100 of these have been identified. The deeper grooves, called *fissures*, assist in establishing the major cerebral regional divisions: the *frontal, parietal, temporal,* and *occipital* lobes. Similarly, the two cerebral hemispheres are distinguished from each other by the deep *longitudinal fissure* (Figure 48-26). The cerebral hemispheres, which exhibit *contralateral* body control, are divided by continuation of the dura mater known as the *falx cerebri*, which projects into the longitudinal cerebral fissure. Directly inferior to the longitudinal cerebral fissure, the fibers of the corpus collosum join the hemispheres. In the great majority of the population, the left hemisphere is dominant in the interpretive functions.

In addition to its anatomic superiority, the cerebral cortex maintains the highest level of information processing in the human. Some functional areas are localized; others are more general and widely dispersed. The

significant localized functional areas include the primary motor projection and sensory projection areas. The motor projection area is located on the anterior wall of the central sulcus and adjacent to the precentral gyrus (Figure 48-27). This area controls voluntary skeletal muscle movements of the contralateral body. The disproportionate representation of body parts on the sensory cortex is illustrated in Figure 48-28. The sensory projection area (somesthetic area) is located on the postcentral gyrus and receives input from the thalamus-projected sensations of the contralateral side of the body.

Other rather well-localized functions processed in the cortex include visual, hearing, olfaction, and somatic interpretations. The mental and intellectual activities in humans are processed and interpreted in widely dispersed association areas of the cortex.

A brief review of the function of the cerebral hemi-

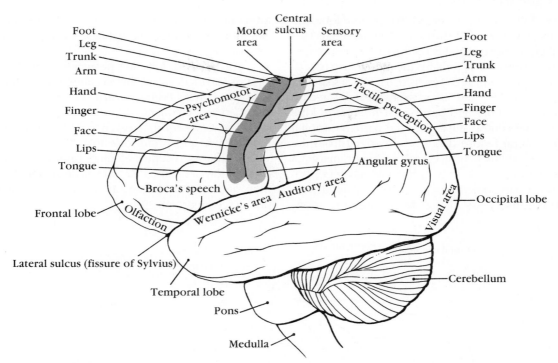

**FIGURE 48–27.**

Topographic organization of functions of control and interpretation on the precentral and postcentral gyri.

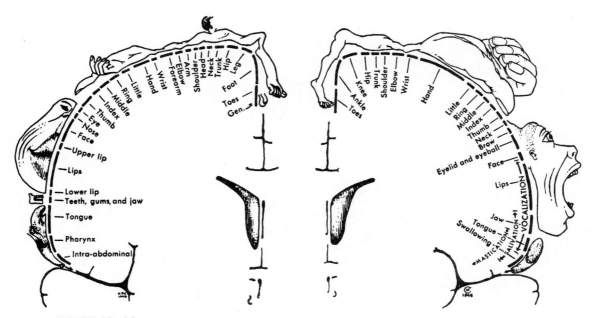

**FIGURE 48–28.**

Sensory (*left*) and motor (*right*) representations as determined by stimulation studies on the human cortex at surgery. Compart the sensory homunculus (*left*) to the motor homunculus (*right*). Note the relatively large areas devoted to the lips, thumb, and fingers. (Source: E. Penfield, T. Rasmussen, *The Cerebral Cortex of Man*. New York: Macmillan, 1955.)

sphere lobes follows (Figure 48-29). The *frontal* lobe, the largest of the lobes, extends from the central sulcus (fissure of Rolando) forward and from the lateral fissure (fissure of Sylvius) upward. It contains the motor strip (Brodman's area 4), premotor area (areas 6, 8), Broca's speech center (areas 44, 45), and association areas related to higher mental functions and behavior. The *parietal* lobe lies between the central sulcus and the parieto-occipital fissure. The lateral fissure divides the parietal from the temporal lobe. Angular, postcentral, and supramarginal gyri are significant landmarks in the parietal lobe. Primary and secondary somesthetic areas are contained here, as are many sensory association fibers. Interpretations of feeling and hearing are made here (areas 1, 2, 3). In addition, body image recognition evolves from the parietal lobe.

The *occipital* lobe lies posterior to the parietal lobe and is divided from the cerebellum by the parieto-occipital fissure. Primary visual centers and visual association areas are contained in the occipital lobe (areas 18, 19). The *temporal lobe* extends downward from the lateral fissure and posteriorly to the parieto-occipital fissure. Auditory receptive centers (areas 41, 42), auditory association area (area 22, Wernicke's), smell interpretation, and memory storage are contained in the temporal lobe (see Figure 48-29).

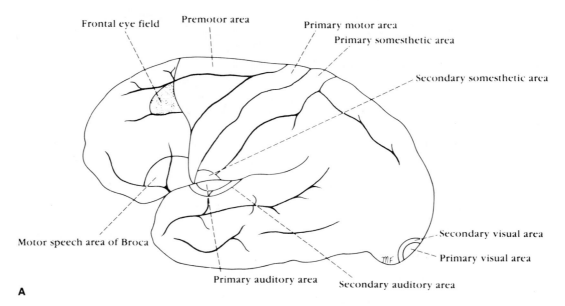

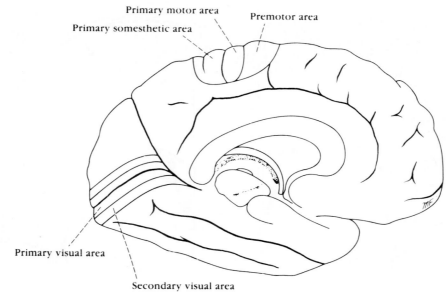

**FIGURE 48-29.**

Functional localization of the cerebral cortex: **A.** lateral view and **B.** medial view of the left cerebral hemisphere. (Source: R.S. Snell, *Clinical Neuroanatomy for Medical Students.* Boston: Little, Brown, 1980.)

# THE PERIPHERAL NERVOUS SYSTEM

The peripheral nervous system includes the nerve tissue outside the brain and spinal cord. It is composed of 31 paired spinal nerves and 12 cranial nerves, as well as numerous ganglia and plexuses. Every spinal nerve contains a dorsal (afferent) and ventral (efferent) root. The afferent nerve cells lie within the dorsal root ganglion and their fibers innervate through spinal nerves and through plexuses of the visceral nervous system. The efferent cell bodies lie within the ventral gray column of the spinal cord and innervate through ventral roots of all spinal nerves to the skeletal muscle and through ventral roots of spinal nerves of the thorax, upper lumbar, and middle sacral region to the viscera.

The cranial nerve nuclei are contained in the brainstem. The physiologic anatomy of the cranial nerves is not as clearly delineated as that of the spinal nerves. Some cranial nerves have only sensory components, some only motor components, and some contain both. Their names and general functions are presented in Table 48-4. Their functions and dysfunctions are further described in Chapter 52.

## Afferent (Sensory) Division

The afferent (sensory) division of the peripheral nervous system detects, transmits, and processes environmental information from internal and external sources through a variety of specific receptors. The *somatic afferent* fibers carry impulses from the skin, skeletal muscles, joints, and tendons to the CNS. The *visceral afferent* fibers carry impulses from the viscera to the CNS.

The receptors of afferent fibers transmit to the CNS by numerous converging fibers through peripheral nerves. As a result of this convergence of neurons, injury to a nerve fiber does not result in clearly defined sensory deficits. Rather, the area that responds in an altered manner is vaguely defined.

The areas in the skin innervated by specific spinal nerves are commonly called *dermatomes*. Traditionally, these have been arranged to correspond to the spinal cord segments. Thus, a rather loose topographic division of these segments includes the eight cervical, 12 thoracic, five lumbar, and five sacral cord regions. Considerable overlapping exists between the dermatomes and generally sensory deficits are identified when more than a single spinal nerve is interrupted. Dermatomes are mapped according to the segmentation of individual dorsal roots (Figure 48-30).

The afferent fibers carrying sensory data enter the spinal cord by way of the dorsal roots to the dorsal root ganglia and become dispersed according to function. Fibers that transmit pain and temperature are anatomically related and ascend through the *lateral spinothalamic tract* to the posterior ventral nucleus of the thalamus. The *ventral spinothalamic tracts* contain fibers from recep-

## TABLE 48-4.
### THE CRANIAL NERVES

| NUMBER | NAME OF NERVE | GENERAL FUNCTION |
|--------|---------------|------------------|
| I | Olfactory | Sense of smell |
| II | Optic | Vision |
| III | Oculomotor | Motor control and sensation for four eye muscles and upper eyelid elevator, pupillary constriction and accommodation |
| IV | Trochlear | Movement of major eyeball muscle |
| V | Trigeminal | Mastication and perception of facial sensations |
| VI | Abducens | Movement of eyeball |
| VII | Facial | Facial expression, salivation, cutaneous, and taste sensations |
| VIII | Acoustic | Equilibrium and hearing |
| IX | Glossopharyngeal | Salivation, movement of pharynx, sensations of skin, taste, and carotid baroreceptors |
| X | Vagus | Swallowing and laryngeal control, and parasympathetic innervation to thoracic and abdominal viscera |
| XI | Spinal accessory | Head and shoulder movement |
| XII | Hypoglossal | Movement of tongue |

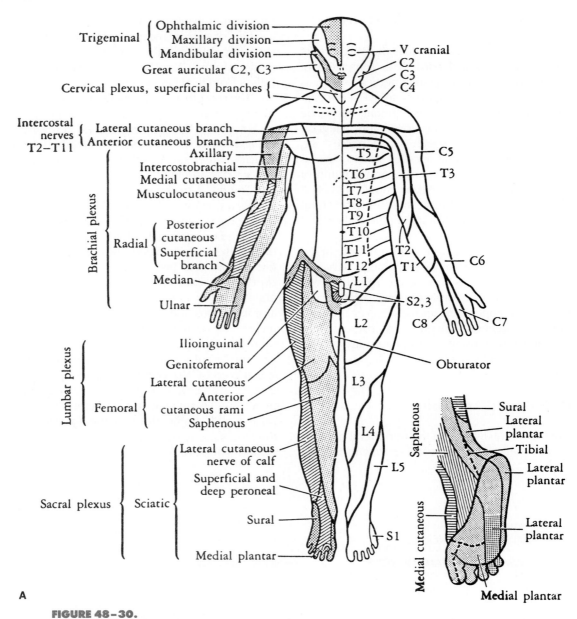

**FIGURE 48-30.**

Dermatomes. Cutaneous areas of distribution of spinal segments and the peripheral nerves: **A.** Anterior aspect of the body; **B.** posterior aspect of the body. (Source: J.N. Walton, *Brain's Diseases of the Nervous System* [8th ed.]. Oxford: Oxford University Press, 1977, Figures 7a and 7b.)

tors that are sensitive to touch and pressure (Figure 48-31). From here, they proceed to the somesthetic region of the cerebral postcentral gyrus. Impulses from muscles, tendons, ligaments, and joints (proprioceptive fibers) disperse in a variety of tracts. Some simply cross the cord to the anterior horn (stretch reflex). Others synapse with the posterior gray column and ascend the spinocerebellar tracts to the cerebellum, while yet others ascend by way of the posterior white columns, decussate at the medial lemniscus, and continue to the posterior ventral nucleus of the thalamus. The ascent from this region continues to the sensory cortex at the postcentral gyrus.

Figure 48-29 identifies the somesthetic projection areas on the postcentral gyrus. It is significant that the body areas that contain more sensory receptors are accorded a larger area on the surface of the sensory cortex. For example, the face and fingers, which are rife with receptors, occupy a larger neuronal area in the cortex than does the large body area of the trunk with its comparatively smaller receptor population.

As noted earlier, an important component of the afferent division is the thalamus, primarily because almost all sensory systems convey impulses to its specific nuclei through either the dorsal column or anterolateral tract.

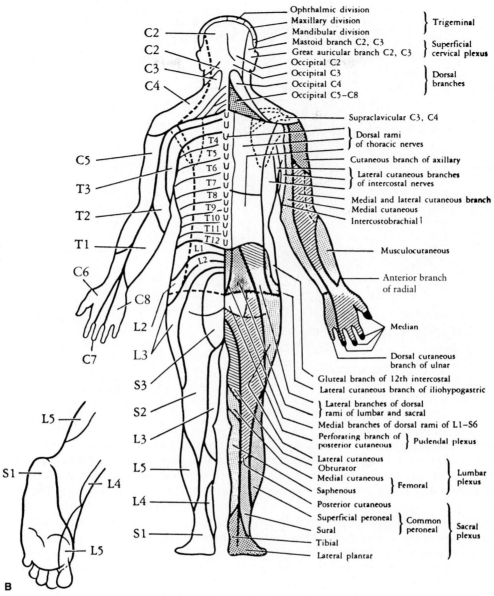

**FIGURE 48-30.** (Continued)

Together with the thalamus, the cortex is concerned with conscious perception of sensory stimuli that occur distantly from it. The thalamus provides perception of touch and pressure, whereas more complex discrimination sensations, such as texture, size, and weight of objects, are interpreted by the cortex.

## Efferent (Motor) Division

Voluntary and involuntary body activities initiated by the efferent division are transmitted as a response to the stimuli the CNS has received from the afferent division. These responses may be through the innervation of smooth muscles, cardiac muscle, and glands. This transmission arrives by way of the autonomic nervous system and is referred to as the *visceral efferent system*. The skeletal muscles, tendons, and joints receive innervation from the CNS by the *somatic efferent system*. The somatic responses at the lowest level occur in the spinal cord and are transmitted through the spinal reflex arc from each spinal segment. These responses are automatic and spontaneous.

The efferent fibers emerge from the ventral horn nu-

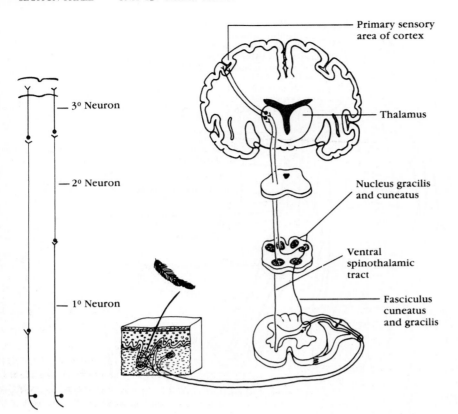

- 3° Neuron

- 2° Neuron

- 1° Neuron

Primary sensory
area of cortex

Thalamus

Nucleus gracilis
and cuneatus

Ventral
spinothalamic
tract

Fasciculus
cuneatus
and gracilis

**FIGURE 48–31.**

Touch-pressure pathways ascending to the thalamus by way of the ventral spinothalamic tract. Information is transmitted through a continuous neuron chain. (Source: I. Langley and F. Christensen, *Structure and Function of the Human Body*. Edina, MN: Burgess Publishing, 1978.)

clei (motor horn cells) and transmit impulses through the spinal nerves. Both efferent and afferent fibers transmit concurrently in most peripheral nerves. Thus, injury to one of these nerves may result in both sensory and motor deficits.

The efferent fibers receive their impulses from simple spinal reflex circuits or more complicated descending pathways from higher centers. The significant higher centers that are important in relaying efferent responses to the periphery include the precentral gyrus (motor cortex), basal ganglia, brainstem, and cerebellum. The fibers that transmit from these areas do so through two principal tracts: pyramidal and extrapyramidal.

### Pyramidal and Extrapyramidal Systems

The pyramidal tract (Figure 48-32), both lateral and ventral, originates in the motor cortex (precentral gyrus) of the cerebrum in large pyramid-shaped cells called *Betz cells*. It transmits, uninterrupted, in a descending manner through the basal ganglia and brainstem. The area where it joins other projection fibers, between the basal ganglia and the thalamus, is known as the *internal capsule*. In the brainstem, most of the fibers decussate and project through a structure known as the *pyramid*. The crossed fibers then continue to descend as the *lateral corticospinal tract* and terminate in the ventral horn of the gray

matter at a specific spinal cord level. A few fibers continue to descend without decussation by way of the *ventral corticospinal tract* and cross near the level of their termination in the ventral horn. The fibers of the pyramidal tract compose the *upper motor neuron*. The pyramidal fibers synapse with segmental anterior horn cells (motor neurons), which, in turn, synapse with peripheral efferent fibers innervating specific muscles, tendons, and joints. The neurons innervating skeletal muscle are known as the *lower motor neurons*.[3]

The remaining efferent fibers that do not traverse the pyramid in the brainstem are part of the extrapyramidal systems. Unlike the pyramidal tract, the extrapyramidal tracts do not continue to the cord uninterrupted. The system is more complex, less directed, and highly interconnected, and is considered by some authors to be a functional, rather than an anatomic, entity.[1,2] Many of the fibers descend from the cortex directly to specific areas in the basal ganglia and brainstem, while others make intermediate synapses. Several extrapyramidal tracts originate in the brainstem and are named for their site of origin. These include the *vestibulospinal tract* from the lateral vestibular nucleus in the medulla, the *rubrospinal tract* from the red nucleus in the midbrain, the *tectospinal tract* from the roof (superior colliculus) of the midbrain, and the *reticulospinal tract* from the reticular formation in the pons and medulla. The majority of the extrapy-

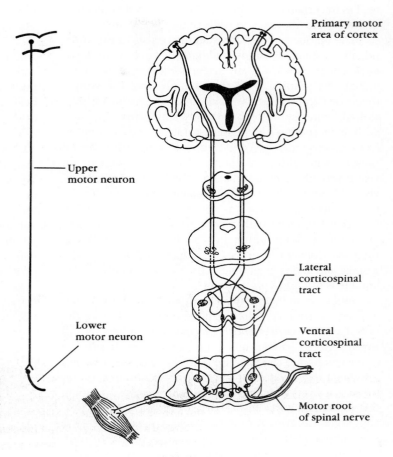

**FIGURE 48–32.**
Pyramidal motor pathways originating at the primary motor area. The lateral corticospinal tract crosses at the level of the medulla and the ventral corticospinal tract descends uncrossed. The pyramidal tract is composed of the upper and lower motor neurons. (Source: I. Langley and F. Christensen, *Structure and Function of the Human Body.* Edina, MN: Burgess Publishing, 1978.)

ramidal fibers decussate with the reticulospinal tract. In addition to the named tracts, important fibers of the extrapyramidal system originate in the cerebellum and the vestibular apparatus.

The pyramidal tract processes information regarding voluntary movement dealing with precise and specific activities of muscles, whereas the extrapyramidal tracts provide the "supporting" type of movement that accompanies the more precise movements afforded by the pyramidal tract. For example, the gross movements necessary to engage in the activity of writing are influenced by the extrapyramidal tracts. Included here are such movements as might be necessary for proper body positioning, particularly of the upper arm and shoulder. The more precise movement of holding the pencil effectively is controlled by the corticospinal tract.

## THE AUTONOMIC NERVOUS SYSTEM

The autonomic nervous system, also referred to as the general visceral efferent system, maintains the internal environment in a relatively steady state. Though it is outside the CNS, it is influenced by the CNS and is distinct from the peripheral nervous system. Autonomic fibers project innervations, which are activated from the CNS to smooth muscles, cardiac muscle, and glands in an involuntary manner to regulate activities related to respiration, cardiovascular function, digestion, excretion, body temperature, and sexual function. Centers in the hypothalamus, brainstem, and spinal cord transmit reflex responses to visceral organs to regulate the internal environment. Autonomic fibers differ from somatic efferent fibers in that they consist of a double neuron chain from the CNS to the visceral effectors, whereas the somatic efferents transmit through one neuron. Visceral efferent fibers transmit in spinal nerves and in several cranial nerves. Visceral efferent innervation frequently accompanies somatic efferent activity. For example, a jogger receives innervation from the somatic efferent fibers to provide the skeletal muscle responses required in the jogging activity. Simultaneously, the somatic efferent system innervates the cardiac and smooth muscle. The somatic efferent responses can be observed readily, whereas the visceral efferent responses are less obvious.

In addition to the autonomic efferent fibers, certain afferent fibers are sometimes assigned to the autonomic nervous system. These are present in spinal nerves, as well as in certain cranial nerves. They innervate receptors in the viscera, thorax, and walls of the blood vessels.

The autonomic nervous system consists of two functionally distinct divisions: *sympathetic* and *parasympathetic* (Figure 48-33). Many visceral effector organs have a dual nerve supply, one from each division. The sympathetic division assists the body into action during physiologic and psychologic stress by supportive activities, such as increasing heart and respiratory rates and mobilizing glucose from glycogen stores to supply the skeletal muscles with additional energy. The parasympathetic division provides a counterbalance for the sympathetic division. Nerve cells of both divisions group outside the CNS in structures known as *autonomic ganglia*. Cell fibers that terminate with a synapse at these ganglia and retain the cell body within the CNS are the *preganglionic neurons*. Conversely, nerve cells having cell bodies in the ganglia and axons extending to the organs and glands are known as the *postganglionic neurons*.

As shown in Figure 48-34, the sympathetic system has a chain or trunk of paired ganglia on either side of the spinal cord (*paravertebral ganglia*), extending its full length. These ganglia are connected on each side by nerve trunks and together are referred to as the right and left *sympathetic chains* or *sympathetic trunks*. In addition to these paired ganglia, single ganglia exist surrounding the abdominal aorta and its larger branches, where preganglionic neurons terminate without synapsing in the sympathetic chain. These are known as *collateral (prevertebral) ganglia* and include the celiac and superior and inferior mesenteric ganglia. The terminal ganglia are parasympathetic and are located in proximity to the effector organs.

## Sympathetic Division (Thoracolumbar)

The cell bodies of the short preganglionic sympathetic neurons arise from the sympathetic motoneurons of the intermediolateral horns of the spinal cord between the first thoracic and second lumbar vertebrae (see Figure 48-33). The fibers of these neurons pass through the intervertebral foramina in conjunction with respective spinal nerves. Shortly, the sympathetic fibers (preganglionic) depart from the spinal nerve and enter a sympathetic chain through the white rami communicans (see Figure 48-34). They may synapse here immediately with a postganglion neuron or pass directly through the sympathetic chain to synapse with a single sympathetic ganglion, or pass up or down the sympathetic chain and synapse at a different level.

Some postganglionic sympathetic fibers, after having synapsed in the sympathetic chain, pass back into the spinal nerve through the gray rami communicans and accompany the spinal nerve to innervate blood vessels, sweat glands, and piloerector muscles in the skin.

## Parasympathetic Division (Craniosacral)

The autonomic fibers that arise from the cranial and sacral portions of the CNS compose the parasympathetic nervous system (see Figure 48-33). Somatic efferent fibers in the cranial region arise in conjunction with the oculomotor (third), facial (seventh), glossopharyngeal (ninth), and vagus (tenth) nerves. The vagus transmits the majority of the parasympathetic impulses through its wide distribution in the thoracic and abdominal viscera. The remaining cranial nerves innervate organs of the head. The sacral fibers arise from the anterior roots of the second, third, and fourth sacral spinal nerves and innervate pelvic organs and the colon. Most of the preganglionic fibers transmit without interruption to the organs they innervate, where they synapse with the parasympathetic ganglia that are located in the area of the effector organ. In contrast to the sympathetic fibers, the parasympathetic preganglionic fibers are long and the postganglionic fibers are short.

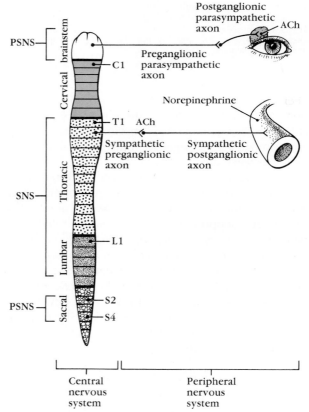

**FIGURE 48-33.**

Schematic overview of the origins of sympathetic (SNS) and parasympathetic (PSNS) nervous systems with corresponding major transmitter substances at the synapses: acetylcholine (ACh) and norepinephrine (noradrenalin).

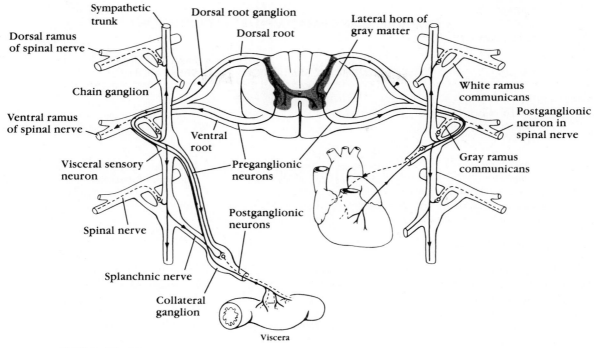

**FIGURE 48-34.**

Sympathetic fibers emerge from the spinal cord in conjunction with respective spinal nerves and transmit to autonomic ganglia by way of white rami. (Source: A. Spence and E. Mason, *Human Anatomy and Physiology*. Menlo Park, CA: Benjamin/Cummings, 1979.)

## Transmitter Substances of the Autonomic Nervous System

Chemical mediation is necessary for neuronal transmission between neurons and between neurons and their effector organs. Excitation results from chemical release of transmitter substances between preganglionic and postganglionic neurons and their effectors in the autonomic nervous system. The transmitter substance in the autonomic nervous system from the preganglionic neurons to the postganglionic neurons in both the sympathetic and parasympathetic nervous systems is *acetylcholine (ACh)*. Acetylcholine continues to be the transmitter substance from the parasympathetic postganglionic neurons. Because of the secretion of ACh, these fibers are known as *cholinergic* and their receptors are *cholinoceptive*.

The primary transmitter substance secreted by the postganglionic fibers of the sympathetic nervous system to its effector organs is *norepinephrine (NE)*. The fibers are referred to as *adrenergic* and terminate on *adrenoceptive* receptors (alpha and beta). A few of the fibers of the postganglionic sympathetic nervous system secrete ACh at their terminal fibers, including fibers to sweat glands and postganglionic sympathetic vasodilator fibers to skeletal muscle vasculature.[2] A single postganglionic sympathetic nerve may innervate thousands of receptor sites. This is demonstrated by the diffuse response to the sympathetic nervous system excitation, in contrast to the more localized responses characteristic of parasympathetic activity.

## Receptor Substances of the Effector Organs

The effector organs secrete substances that react with terminal bouton secretions. The exact nature of these substances is uncertain. It has been theorized that the combination of the autonomic nervous system transmitter substance and receptor substances alters the permeability of the cell membrane to certain ions. This alteration may result in changes in membrane potential, eliciting either action potentials or tonic effects. In addition to changes in the cell membrane, receptor substances may initiate chemical reactions within the cell.

## Stimulation and Inhibition of the Autonomic Nervous System

The actions of the sympathetic and parasympathetic nervous systems on various receptor organs are summarized in Table 48-5.

**TABLE 48–5.**

THE EFFECTS OF SYMPATHETIC AND PARASYMPATHETIC STIMULATION ON EFFECTOR ORGANS

| ORGAN | SYMPATHETIC STIMULATION | PARASYMPATHETIC STIMULATION |
|---|---|---|
| Eye | | |
| Radial muscle of iris | Dilates | |
| Sphincter muscle of iris | | Constricts |
| Heart | | |
| SA node | Increases rate | Decreases rate |
| Atria | Increases contractility | Decreases contractility |
| Ventricles | Increases contractility, conduction, automaticity | Decreases contractility |
| Coronary blood vessels | Dilates | Constricts |
| Systemic blood vessels | | |
| Abdominal | | Constricts |
| Skeletal muscle | Dilates | |
| Lungs | | |
| Bronchial muscle | Dilates (relaxes) | Constricts |
| Bronchial secretions | Decreases | Increases |
| Bronchial vessels | Constricts mildly | None |
| Skin | | |
| Sweat glands | Copious generalized secretion | Slight localized secretion |
| Blood vessels | Constricts (adrenergic) Dilates (cholinergic) | Dilates |
| Intestine | | |
| Motility | Decreases | Increases |
| Sphincters | Contracts | Relaxes |
| Liver | Glycogenolysis | None |
| Gallbladder and ducts | Relaxes | Constricts |
| Pancreas | | |
| Acini cells | None | Secrete |
| Islet cells | Inhibits alpha-receptors, stimulates beta-receptors to secrete | Secrete |
| Salivary glands | Thick secretions | Thin secretions |
| Fat cells | Lipolysis | None |
| Bladder | | |
| Detrusor muscle | Relaxes | Contracts |
| Trigone | Contracts | Relaxes |
| Penis | Ejaculation | Erection |
| Basal metabolism | Increased | None |
| Adrenal medulla | Increased secretion | None |
| Mentation | Increased | None |

The dual actions are a cooperative effort to maintain a constant internal environment in response to the ever-changing external world. General responses of the sympathetic nervous system are activated under emergency situations to make internal adjustments that facilitate an appropriate response by the body. For example, in response to stressful exercise, the cardiovascular system is stimulated by the sympathetic system to increase cardiac output by increasing heart rate and force, thus providing additional perfusion to skeletal muscle, brain, and liver, while simultaneously reducing the blood supply to the viscera. The parasympathetic system, in contrast, promotes activities that maintain body function from day to day, including digestion and elimination.

The visceral effectors that receive stimulation from both the sympathetic and parasympathetic systems generally receive antagonistic stimulation. An example of this includes the effect on bronchial secretions. Sympathetic stimulation decreases bronchial secretions and parasympathetic stimulation increases them. In another example, the sympathetic system dilates the pupils, while the parasympathetic system constricts them. The dual system does not function consistently in a cooperative balance since some organs receive innervation primarily from only one system. Examples include the smooth muscles of the skin, hair, sweat glands, and cutaneous blood vessels, which are primarily innervated from the sympathetic system. The detrusor muscle of the bladder receives parasympathetic innervation only.

The inhibitory actions of the autonomic nervous system occur both directly and indirectly on the effector organs. For example, vagal stimulation (parasympathetic) slows the heart through a direct inhibitory action of the cholinergic postganglionic neurons on the sinoatrial node. On the other hand, vasodilation of the peripheral arterioles occurs indirectly through a decrease in impulse transmission in the sympathetic effector fibers.

While most organs and viscera receive innervation from both sympathetic and parasympathetic systems, one of these generally has an inhibitory effect and the other an excitatory effect. There is no consistent rule of thumb for guidance as to which system stimulates and which inhibits.

## Effects of Sympathetic and Parasympathetic Stimulation on Various Structures

### Lacrimal Glands

The parasympathetic system vasodilates and stimulates secretion of the lacrimal glands through the postganglionic axons from the sphenopalatine ganglion by the maxillary division of the fifth cranial nerve. The preganglionic axons originate in the superior salivatory nucleus and follow the route of the seventh cranial nerve. The sympathetic system has a vasoconstrictive effect on the lacrimal glands and transmits its impulses through preganglionic neurons, which originate from the intermediolateral cells in the thoracic spinal column, and through postganglionic neurons of the superior cervical ganglion. The impulses reach the glands through the maxillary division of the fifth cranial nerve.[9]

### Eyes

Pupillary constriction and near-vision accommodation are accomplished through parasympathetic stimulation. The oculomotor nucleus sends preganglionic axons by the oculomotor nerve to the ciliary ganglion. From here the postganglionic axons reach the ciliary muscle and constrictor muscle of the iris by the ciliary nerve. When pupils are reflexively stimulated with light, the pupillary openings decrease and reduce the amount of light reaching the retinae.

The sympathetic stimulation dilates the pupils, constricts vessels, elevates the eyelids, and provides far-vision accommodation. The preganglionic axons of fibers accomplishing these activities originate in the thoracic spinal segments and ascend by the sympathetic chain to the superior cervical ganglion where they synapse with the postganglionic neurons. The postganglionic axons travel through divisions of the fifth nerve to the dilator muscles of the irises (levator palpebrae superioris), and radial fibers of the ciliary muscles. Innervation of blood vessels of the retinae, orbits, and conjunctivae is accomplished in the same manner.[8]

### Salivary Glands

The superior salivary nucleus projects the preganglionic axons for the submaxillary and sublingual glands, and the inferior salivary nucleus projects preganglionic axons for the parotid gland. The axons from the superior salivary nucleus travel through a branch of the seventh cranial nerve to the submaxillary and sublingual ganglia, and those from the inferior salivary nucleus travel through a branch of the ninth cranial nerve to the otic ganglia. From the submaxillary and sublingual ganglia, axons project to their glands and from the otic ganglia to the parotid gland through the fifth cranial nerve. The parasympathetic system activates these glands to vasodilate and secrete.

The sympathetic system vasoconstricts and promotes secretion of salivary glands. Its preganglionic axons ascend from the upper thoracic spinal cord to the superior cervical ganglia to synapse with the postganglionic neurons. These axons reach the glands along the external carotid and external maxillary arteries.[9]

### Heart

The overall effects of the parasympathetic system on the heart are deceleration and coronary artery vasoconstriction. Its stimulation of the heart decreases its effectiveness. However, in the process, it does slow the metabolism and oxygen requirements, and thus provides some rest for the cardiac muscle. The parasympathetic preganglionic fibers pass from the dorsal motor nucleus of the vagus and synapse with the postganglionic neurons through the vagal trunk at cardiac plexus ganglia in the atrial walls.

In contrast, the sympathetic system increases the overall activity of the heart, produces both positive chronotropic and inotropic effects, and dilates the coronary arteries. In essence, the sympathetic system makes the heart more effective, although it simultaneously increases workload and metabolic requirements. The upper thoracic spinal cord provides the origin of the preganglionic neurons, which project their axons from the ventral roots and white rami to the sympathetic chain. The postganglionic neurons emerge from higher thoracic and lower cervical ganglia and travel to the cardiac plexus.[12]

## Bronchi

The bronchi are constricted by the parasympathetic system. The origin of the parasympathetic neurons and the course of their preganglionic and postganglionic fibers are similar to those of the parasympathetic fibers innervating the heart. The preganglionic fibers synapse with the postganglionic fibers in the pulmonary plexus. The axons of the postganglionic cells terminate in the bronchi and blood vessels.

The sympathetic system dilates the bronchi. The neurons originate in thoracic segments 2 through 6 and their axons enter the pulmonary plexus in a manner similar to that of the parasympathetic system.[5]

## Esophagus

The parasympathetic system exerts the main autonomic influence over the function of the esophagus. Stimulation causes smooth muscle of the esophagus to constrict, increasing its overall activity in propelling ingested materials along its course. This stimulation comes from various branches of the vagus nerve.[12]

## Abdominal Viscera, Glands, and Vessels

Stimulation of the parasympathetic system promotes peristalsis and increases in secretion by the various gastrointestinal glands. The preganglionic fibers originate from the vagus and synapse with the postganglionic fibers of the various visceral organs in their intrinsic plexus.

In contrast, the sympathetic system inhibits peristalsis and enhances vasoconstriction. The lower thoracic and upper lumbar cord segments provide the origin of the preganglionic neurons. Their axons traverse the splanchnic nerves to synapse with the postganglionic neurons in the prevertebral ganglion plexus. Innervation is provided to the visceral smooth muscle and blood vessels.[9]

## Pelvic Viscera

Stimulation of the parasympathetic system assists in urination and defecation by contracting the bladder and lower colon. Penile erection is also facilitated by the parasympathetic system. The neurons that accomplish these functions originate in the sacral cord segments and their axons transmit to the various organs.

Stimulation of the sympathetic system promotes contraction of the vesicle sphincter, vasoconstriction, and ejaculation. The preganglionic neurons originate in the lower thoracic and upper lumbar segments and travel along the splanchnic nerves similarly to those of the abdominal viscera. The postganglionic fibers travel along the hypogastric nerves of the organs innervated.[9]

## Peripheral Vessels and Sweat Glands

The major effect of the autonomic nervous system on the peripheral and deep vessels is stimulation of the sympathetic system. This results in vasoconstriction of cutaneous vessels, as well as deep visceral vessels. Sweat glands secrete in response to sympathetic stimulation. The postganglionic fibers to the sweat glands are cholinergic in contrast with other sympathetic fibers, which are adrenergic. For this reason, many sources classify sweat secretion as a sympathetic function.[5]

## Adrenal Medulla

In response to sympathetic stimulation, the adrenal medulla secretes epinephrine and norepinephrine into the circulating blood, which reaches all cells and produces an excitatory effect. This mechanism is part of the diffuse sympathoadrenal system, which is activated in response to stress. In addition to the stimulatory effect on the nervous system, epinephrine and norepinephrine affect metabolism through glycogenolysis in the liver and skeletal muscle and mobilization of fatty acids.

Distinct effects of circulating epinephrine and norepinephrine on heart function include increased force and rate of contraction, as well as increased excitability of the myocardium. Norepinephrine produces vasoconstriction in most organs, whereas epinephrine has a dilating effect on the vessels of the liver and skeletal muscle. Other effects observed in response to circulating epinephrine and norepinephrine include increased mental acuity, inhibition of the gastrointestinal tract, and pupillary dilation. Thus, the circulating catecholamines released by the adrenal medulla have functions similar to those of the adrenergic nerve discharges and, indeed, enhance their action. The effects of the circulating catecholamines linger because their metabolism or removal from blood takes longer than it does in those released at the adrenergic nerve terminals.[5]

Minimal secretion of epinephrine and norepinephrine occurs at basal conditions as in sleep. During increased activity and stress, or when adrenergic stimulation is increased in such conditions as pain, cold, hypoglycemia, and emotional excitement, secretion is considerably increased. This stimulation is transmitted to the adrenal medulla by the hypothalamic nervous centers, as well as by direct sympathetic innervation of the medulla.

The effects of epinephrine and norepinephrine vary on different types of adrenergic receptor cells. *Alpha-adrenergic receptors* mediate vasoconstriction when acted on by both norepinephrine and epinephrine; *beta-adrenergic receptors* mediate vasodilation and increase rate and strength of the cardiac function. The latter is in response to the action of epinephrine on these receptors. Alpha-adrenergic receptors are dispersed widely in various organs but predominate in the precapillary sphincters of smooth muscles of blood vessels.

Beta-adrenergic receptors predominate in the heart, coronary arteries, lungs, bronchi, liver, and brain.

## Autonomic Reflexes

In response to certain environmental conditions, autonomic reflexes maintain the internal environment appropriate to the demand, that of either action or repair. For the most part, the actions occur at an unconscious level and involve functions such as control of pupillary size,

cardiovascular status, and variations in respiratory, gastrointestinal, and genitourinary systems.

# THE VENTRICULAR AND CEREBROSPINAL FLUID SYSTEMS

## Function of Cerebrospinal Fluid

The CSF that circulates in the subarachnoid space around the brain and spinal cord (Figure 48-35) provides an important supportive and protective mechanism for the

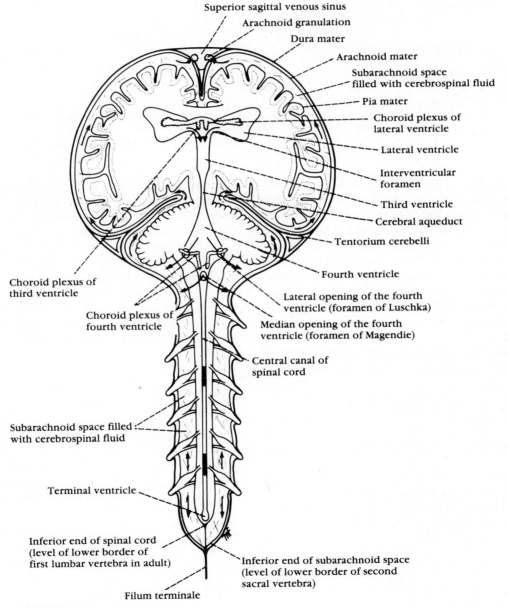

**FIGURE 48–35.**

Formation of CSF in choroid plexuses; circulation and absorption into the arachnoid villi. (Source: R.S. Snell, *Clinical Neuroanatomy for Medical Students*. Boston: Little, Brown, 1980.)

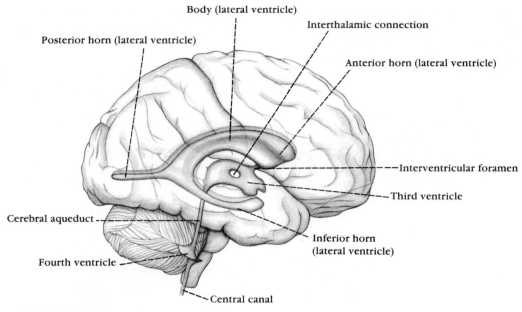

**FIGURE 48-36.**
The lateral third and fourth ventricles. (Source: R.S. Snell, *Clinical Neuroanatomy for Medical Students.*
Boston: Little, Brown, 1980.)

CNS. Together with support from blood vessels, nerve roots, and fine fibrous arachnoid trabeculae, the brain is directly encased within the subarachnoid CSF and receives buoyancy from it that prevents the vessels and nerve roots from stretching in response to movements of the head. The average weight of the adult brain is approximately 1450 gm in the air, although in the buoyant CSF bath, its weight is reduced to approximately 50 gm. This buoyancy allows for relatively effective suspension of the brain and assists in preventing lethal damage under daily traumas.

*Pneumoencephalography* demonstrated the effects of CSF deficiency on the brain. This diagnostic procedure, rarely performed today, visualizes structural elements of the brain when CSF is removed and replaced by air. Thus, the weight of the brain rests on the vascular, nervous, and meningeal structures and results in a severe headache that is greatly intensified by the slightest jarring of the head.

In addition to its mechanical function, CSF provides a medium for passage of substances between blood and the extracellular fluid of the brain. It probably also nourishes brain tissues and removes the metabolites of nerve cell function.

## *Formation and Absorption of Cerebrospinal Fluid*

The CSF is produced, circulated, and reabsorbed continuously. Its principal formation site is in the *choroid plexus*

of the lateral ventricle, with most of the remainder being formed in the third and fourth ventricles (Figure 48-36). Box 48-1 lists the normal composition and pressure of CSF. The choroid plexus is a network of capillary tufts surrounded by cuboidal epithelium (Figure 48-37). The fluid is produced through filtration, diffusion, and active transport from the blood. A second lesser source of CSF is from the ependymal cells lining the ventricles and meningeal blood vessels. In the adult human, approximately 500 ml of fluid is produced per 24 hours and approximately 125 ml is circulating at any given time. Wide

**BOX 48-1.**
NORMAL VALUES OF CEREBROSPINAL FLUID

| | |
|---|---|
| Appearance | Clear, colorless, odorless |
| Specific gravity | 1.007 |
| pH | 7.35 |
| Protein | 14–45 mg/dl |
| Glucose | 40–80 mg/dl (60% of serum glucose level) |
| Lymphocytes | 0–5 |
| Erythrocytes | 0 |
| Chlorides | 120–130 mEq/L |
| Sodium | 140 mEq/L |
| Potassium | 3.0 mEq/L |
| Bicarbonate | 23.6 mEq/L |
| Pressure | 80–180 mm $H_2O$ (in side recumbent position) |

fluctuations may occur in the amount produced during any given 24-hour period. Sodium ions are actively transported across the epithelial cells into CSF from blood. This results in a greater osmotic force in the CSF; therefore, to maintain osmotic equilibrium, water passively follows the ions. Thus, water is extracted from the capillaries and is responsible for the secretory function of the choroid plexus. Facilitated diffusion allows transportation of glucose in both directions.

The CSF is absorbed into the venous circulation through *arachnoid villi* (see Figure 48-16), granulations that project from the cerebral subarachnoid space into the venous sinuses. The CSF is passively absorbed because its hydrostatic pressure is greater than that of venous blood in the venous sinuses. Certain particles, such as red blood cells and creatinine, pass unimpeded through the arachnoid villi.

## Flow and Obstruction of Flow of Cerebrospinal Fluid

The origin of CSF in the choroid plexus of the ventricles and its normal flow to the arachnoid villi are illustrated in Figure 48-35. The fluid arrives in the third ventricle from the lateral ventricles through the interventricular foramen, flows on to the fourth ventricle through the cerebral aqueduct, and then goes on to the subarachnoid cisterns through the foramina of Magendie and Luschka. As the fluid flows over the cerebral hemispheres, it passes into the sagittal sinus for rapid reabsorption through the arachnoid villi.

Interference along the pathway of the flow of CSF results in ventricular enlargement and a condition known as *hydrocephalus*. The two types of hydrocephalus are *communicating* and *noncommunicating*. If CSF flows freely between the ventricles and lumbar subarachnoid space, it is communicating hydrocephalus. A problem exists with reabsorption of CSF in this condition. Blockage within the ventricular system that prevents free flow of CSF from one or more ventricles results in noncommunicating hydrocephalus. Ventricular dilation results in both types and leads to increased intracranial pressure (see Chap. 54).

## Brain Barriers

Brain cell function is dependent on a closely controlled environment. Not all circulating substances in the blood pass freely to the brain or CSF. This occurs either because their molecules are too large or the molecules they bind with are too large to cross the CNS membranes. This has been demonstrated with the injection of certain acidic dyes, such as trypan blue, which stain other body tissues but not most brain tissue. The molecules these dyes bind with are too large to enter the brain or CSF. Substances pass into the brain from the blood through capillaries to

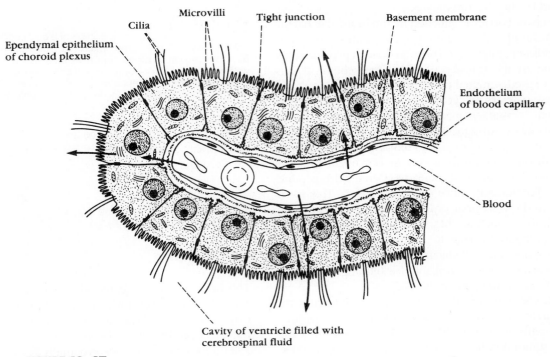

**FIGURE 48–37.**
Microscopic structure of the choroid plexus (Source: R.S. Snell, *Clinical Neuroanatomy for Medical Students.* Boston: Little, Brown, 1980.)

the extracellular space of the brain, or through the choroid plexus into the CSF from which small amounts are passed into the brain. Barriers exist between the blood and brain, blood and CSF, and the brain and CSF.

The materials separating the various cerebral compartments, in essence, are responsible for the entrance and exit of materials to and from the CSF and brain. The choroid plexus and the brain parenchyma (except the hypothalamus) provide the barriers to free movement of substances into the brain. Molecular size, charge, and lipid solubility affect the rate of diffusion across the cerebral membranes and cells. Small molecules and lipid-soluble substances penetrate more rapidly than large molecules and water-soluble polar compounds. Plasma proteins are excluded from the CNS because of their large molecular size. Nonionized substances pass more readily into the brain and CSF than ionized substances. Substances that penetrate rapidly into the CSF and brain include water, carbon dioxide, and oxygen.

The endothelia of capillary cells of the brain overlap and are fused together by tight junctions, creating a common, thickened, basement membrane with adjacent glia and neurons. This dense basement membrane, in conjunction with an additional layer of neuroglial cells surrounding the capillaries, restricts diffusion of large-molecular substances between the blood and brain (Figure 48-38). This capillary structure is equated with the blood-brain barrier. The blood-CSF barrier exists as a result of the secretory function of the choroid plexus. This is evidenced by different concentrations of certain substances in the CSF and in plasma, indicating a selective transport by the choroid plexus.

A weaker barrier is afforded by the brain-CSF barrier through the ependymal lining of the ventricular system and its adjacent glial cells. These structures provide some limitation in the transfer of fluids and chemical substances to the interstitial fluids from the CSF.

These barriers protect the brain by inhibiting potentially toxic substances from entering and facilitating entrance to those substances essential for its metabolism. Substances, such as glucose and oxygen, pass to the brain rapidly through the capillary system to maintain constant environment for the CNS neurons. Certain drugs penetrate the barrier with more ease than others. This is important in the treatment of CNS infections because certain antibiotics, such as chlortetracyclines and penicillin, have very limited access to the brain. Others, such as erythromycin and sulfadiazine, enter readily. Because proteins are not readily available for binding, drugs generally do not accumulate in the CSF.

Radiotherapy, infections, and tumors interrupt the brain-barrier systems and allow transport of materials that normally are not readily accorded entrance. For this reason, tumor localization with brain scanning is effective. Intravenous radioactive substances are injected into the individual and monitored with a scanner. The gamma

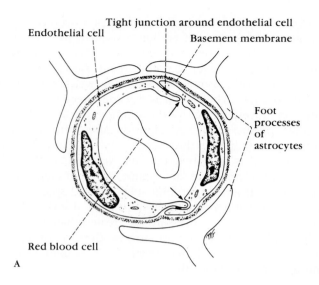

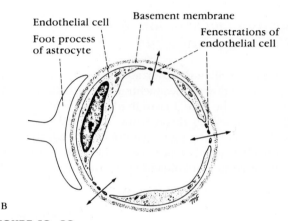

**FIGURE 48–38.**
Blood-brain barrier. **A.** Cross section of blood capillary of the central nervous system in area where the blood-brain barrier exists. **B.** Cross section of blood capillary of the central nervous system where the blood-brain barrier appears to be absent. Note the presence of fenestrations in endothelial cells. (Source: R.S. Snell, *Clinical Neuroanatomy for Medical Students.* Boston: Little, Brown, 1980.)

rays emitted by the substance are recorded on x-ray film and appear as dark areas in the regions of the barrier breakdown.

## BRAIN BLOOD SUPPLY AND REGULATION

### Arterial and Venous Circulation

The brain receives the blood supply from the internal carotid arteries anteriorly and vertebral arteries posteriorly. As the internal carotid arteries, which originate from the aorta on the left and common carotid on the right, ascend into the brain, they eventually branch into the anterior and middle cerebral arteries. The vertebral arteries, originating from the subclavian arteries, ascend and become the basilar artery at the pons level. The basilar artery terminates in the right and left posterior cerebral arteries, which supply the posterior regions of the cerebrum. The anterior and posterior cerebral arteries are joined by smaller communicating arteries and form a ring known as the *circle of Willis* (Figure 48-39). The blood supply to both cerebral hemispheres is identical. Although anomalies are common, for the most part, they are clinically insignificant. The venous system drains the blood from the cerebrum and cerebellum through deep veins and dural sinuses that ultimately empty into the internal jugular veins.

## Autoregulation and Cerebral Blood Flow

The healthy brain has the ability to maintain a fairly constant blood flow (approximately 50 ml/100 gm/minute),

even within widely fluctuating physiological conditions. Normal cerebral blood flow is provided when the cerebral perfusion pressure (CPP) is maintained between 40 to 130 mm Hg. The CPP commonly ranges around 80 to 90 mm Hg. Cerebral perfusion pressure is obtained by subtracting the mean intracranial pressure (MICP) from the mean systemic arterial pressure (MSAP): CPP = MSAP − MICP.

Autoregulatory mechanisms in the healthy brain maintain the relatively constant blood flow through metabolic and pressure autoregulatory mechanisms. The metabolic autoregulatory mechanism operates in response to increases in carbon dioxide tension and decreases in oxygen tension. Carbon dioxide is the most potent cerebral vessel vasodilator and its presence in increased amounts results in increased CBF. This allows for removal of excess carbon dioxide and restoration of oxygen levels toward normal. Hypercapnea and hypoxia have significant effects on the vessel caliber and, thus, on

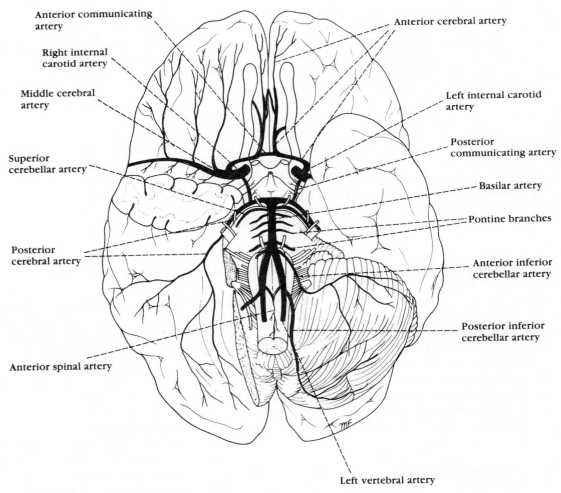

**FIGURE 48–39.**
The arteries on the inferior surface of the brain. Note the formation of the circulus arteriosus (circle of Willis). (Source: R.S. Snell, *Clinical Neuroanatomy for Medical Students.* Boston: Little, Brown, 1980.)

the intrinsic control of the cerebral blood flow. Likewise, the pH level affects cerebral arteries. Increased hydrogen ion concentrations have a powerful dilating effect on the cerebral vessels.

Pressure autoregulation responds to vessel resistance as a result of changes in intracranial pressure of systemic blood pressure. As a result of this mechanism, a relatively constant blood flow is maintained in the presence of wide fluctuations in arterial blood pressure. Cerebral vessels constrict in response to increased systemic arterial pressure and dilate when the systemic pressure lowers. A mean systemic arterial blood pressure below 60 mm Hg results in decreased cerebral perfusion. Pressure autoregulation is maintained in the healthy brain when ICP is below 30 mm Hg, MAP is between 60 to 160 mm Hg, and cerebral perfusion pressure ranges 50 to 150 mm Hg. Autoregulation ceases when the CPP is less than 40 mm Hg. When the ICP increases significantly and equals the MAP, CPP and CBF become zero. Marked reduction of CBF occurs when intracranial pressure rises rapidly to about 35 mm Hg.

Other factors that affect cerebral blood flow include cerebral outflow, blood viscosity, and cardiac output. Impedance in cerebral outflow may result in increased intracranial pressure and compromise autoregulation. Increases in blood viscosity decreases CBF, and decreased blood viscosity increases CBF. Cerebral blood flow is reduced when cardiac output is decreased by one third.

## DIAGNOSTIC STUDIES OF NERVOUS SYSTEM ALTERATIONS

A variety of studies may be undertaken to support and expand the impression given by the clinical signs. The diagnostic studies commonly used are described in this section.

### Lateral and Posteroanterior Radiographs of Skull and Cervical Spine

Radiographs are generally done initially because they give certain vital information and can be completed with relative ease. The films can reveal skull fractures and shifting of the calcified pineal gland, thereby indicating the presence of mass lesions, such as subdural hematomas. Fractures, fracture compressions, and subluxations of the cervical spine can be revealed by plain films.

### Cerebral Angiography

Angiography is particularly useful in diagnosing vascular lesions such as aneurysms, arteriovenous malformations, vasospasm, and occlusions of cerebral vessels. Angiogra-

phy also identifies vessels that have been displaced by hematomas and other mass lesions. This invasive procedure involves injecting a radiopaque dye into an arterial blood vessel to allow visualization of the cerebral circulation. The material that passes through the intracranial and extracranial circulations outlines the arterial, capillary, and venous structures. Usual injection sites of the contrast media are the common carotid, femoral, and brachial arteries. The area of the suspected lesion largely influences the selection of the injection site.

### Computerized Axial Tomography

Computerized tomography (CT) scanning is a very useful, effective, and rapid radiographic modality used for the diagnosis of nervous system lesions. The scans distinguish white matter from gray matter, identify the ventricles and sulci, and with administration of intravenous contrast media, reveal major vessels of the brain. A narrow moving beam of X ray is passed through successive layers of the head around a 360-degree axis. A small computer processes the accumulated data by calculating the differences in tissue density in contiguous tissue slices. Pathologic changes can be constructed from the density data in terms of shape, size, and position of structures of the brain. A wide variety of intracranial disorders may be demonstrated by the CT scan, including traumatic intracranial hematomas, neoplasms, cerebral infarctions, hydrocephalus, intracerebral hemorrhage, intracranial shifts, and brain abscesses. Certain spinal disorders, such as fractures, cord tumors, and disk abnormalities, can be effectively diagnosed by scanning.

As a neurodiagnostic tool, tomography has proved to be more efficient in many situations than conventional radiologic and air studies by virtue of its rapidity, noninvasiveness, and relative reliability in diagnosis.

### Magnetic Resonance Imaging

Magnetic resonance imaging (MRI) is the most recently developed diagnostic tool. It provides views of the successive layers of the brain in any plane within a powerful magnetic field. Protons of brain tissue and CSF align themselves in the orientation of the magnetic field. A specific radio frequency is introduced into the field that causes protons to resonate and change their alignment. A computer analyzes the absorbed radio frequency energy and projects it as an image on a screen.

The MRI has some distinct advantages over the CT scan. It projects images more clearly in that the gray and white matter are more precisely distinguished, posterior fossa and brainstem tissues are viewed more accurately, and certain lesions involving white matter are more readily identified. Like the CT scan, MRI is noninvasive and poses less hazard to the individual because it does not use radiation. Due to its powerful magnetic field, however, the equipment requires special housing.

## Echoencephalography

Echoencephalography is a safe, noninvasive neurologic diagnostic tool that involves the use of an ultrasound generator and receiver that display echo pulsations on an oscilloscope. Permanent recording is done through an attached camera. Echoes from deep within the skull visualize shifts in midline structures that may reflect intracranial trauma, cerebrovascular alterations, or space-occupying lesions. Lateral shifts of the pineal gland are also determined by echoencephalography, as well as by plain radiographs. The echoencephalogram has been useful as an adjunct to more conventional and accurate neurodiagnostic studies, such as the CT scan and angiography. The limitations in echoencephalography lie in the many chances for error in administering and interpreting the test.

## Brain Scan

The brain scan is a safe neurodiagnostic technique used primarily to detect intracranial tumors, abscesses, and some subdural hematomas. A radioactive substance is injected intravenously and accumulates in abnormal areas of the brain as a result of breakdown of the blood-brain barrier. It is not particularly useful in diagnosis of an acute head injury because the radioactive substance must be injected 1 to 2 hours before scanning. This time span is excessive in persons who require rapid diagnosis and treatment. Positive brain scans result when scalp contusions are present. Because many acute head injuries are accompanied by scalp contusions, the scan findings may not present an accurate picture of the underlying brain pathology.

## Pneumoencephalography

This procedure is used to diagnose space-occupying lesions and morphologic changes within the ventricular system. It is not feasible for diagnosis in acute head injuries because of its complex invasive nature. It is contraindicated in persons with papilledema and increased intracranial pressure.

This test involves replacing CSF with air or oxygen by means of lumbar puncture or, rarely, cisternal puncture. The air enters the ventricular system primarily through the foramen of Magendie, and serial films are taken to visualize the cerebral structures. This procedure is used infrequently because it has been replaced by other diagnostic tests that are less invasive and allow adequate visualization of the cerebral structures.

## Ventriculography

Ventriculography is a variation of the pneumoencephalogram in which CSF is replaced with air or oxygen directly in the lateral ventricles. This procedure is performed in the operating room through skull burr holes and under local anesthesia. The ventriculogram is done for the diagnosis of expanding intracranial lesions and cerebral anomalies because it determines the patency of the ventricles.

## Myelography

In myelography, radiopaque substance is introduced into the spinal subarachnoid space for the purpose of visualizing the vertebral canal. Prior to the injection of the contrast media into the subarachnoid space through lumbar puncture, Queckenstedt's test may be done to determine patency of the spinal canal. This is performed by compressing the jugular veins when a lumbar puncture has been made. When the compression is maintained, the CSF pressure is elevated. Unilateral compression results in moderate elevation of CSF pressure, whereas bilateral compression shows an even higher rise. When the compression is terminated, the CSF pressure returns to normal. Failure of the pressure to rise and fall indicates some obstruction within the spinal canal above the lumbar puncture site.

Myelography is carried out in the radiology department on a tilt-table so that the person can be manipulated to allow the spinal canal to fill in several positions. With the person in position and lumbar puncture accomplished, approximately 10 ml of CSF is withdrawn and the radiopaque material is injected slowly. Serial films are then taken in various parts of the vertebral canal. On completion of the films, the contrast media is removed.

Myelography is most commonly used for the diagnosis of intravertebral disk protrusions of herniations. Abnormal results indicate incomplete canal filling with contrast media or total obstruction of its flow. In addition to disk abnormalities, tumors and adhesions encroaching on the spinal canal can be demonstrated.

## Electroencephalography

The electroencephalogram (EEG) is recorded from the surface of the scalp and is a significant tool in assessing the continuing, spontaneous electrical activity of the cerebral cortex. Electrodes are placed on the skull and variations in potential are recorded between two cortical electrodes (bipolar record) or between a cortical electrode and an indifferent electrode usually placed on the ear (unipolar record). Simultaneous recordings from numerous portions of the cranium are accomplished by systematic electrode placement. The EEG activity reflects the graded potential changes in the cortical neurons. This cortical activity, in turn, is dependent on stimuli reaching it from deeper brain structures, as has been demonstrated by studies that indicate that the cerebral cortex separated from these structures lacks the normal EEG patterns. Additional support for deep structure effect on the EEG recording is the fact that both cerebral hemispheres generally demonstrate synchronous activity, suggesting a pacemaker mechanism in the deeper structures of the brain.

The changes observed in the EEG patterns in response to afferent stimulation are referred to as desynchronization of the EEG. This occurs whenever eyes are opened and alpha rhythm is replaced by a high-frequency, low-amplitude activity that exhibits no dominant pattern. Synchronized alpha activity indicates that many dendrite units are firing simultaneously, resulting in a rhythmic discharge. The frequency and amplitude of the EEG are affected by electrode placement, the activity or behavior and emotional status of the subject, and biochemical and structural status of the cortex. Oscillations vary from 1 to 50 Hz, and scalp voltage amplitude ranges widely according to internal and external environmental conditions.

## Types of Brain Waves

The normal EEG depends on the integrity and normal functioning of the cerebral cortex, as well as certain structures deep in the brain. Four principal wavebands are commonly recorded in the normal individual's brain function: alpha, beta, theta, and delta.

The alpha waves make up alpha rhythm, which ranges at frequencies of 8 to 13 per second but most commonly occurs at frequencies of 9 to 10 per second (Figure 48-40). Alpha waves are recorded symmetrically in most healthy adults from both the occipital and parietal regions. These are not fully developed until about age 13

years and may exhibit greater amplitude on the right side in younger individuals. Alpha waves are present only in the resting person whose eyes are closed. When eyes are open, the alpha waves disappear and are replaced by an asynchronous rhythm of low voltage. Metabolic aberrations, such as anoxia and hypoglycemia, slow alpha frequency.

Beta waves are recorded from the frontal lobe of the brain and represent activity of the motor cortex (see Figure 48-40). Their frequency is above 13 cycles per second (cps) and the amplitude is generally low. Beta activity may predominate in some people and is seen to replace alpha waves in those who are tense and anxious. Voluntary movement can block beta wave activity. Closely related to beta waves and recorded from central regions of the brain are mu waves. These have a relatively high amplitude and a frequency of about one half that of beta waves. Like beta waves, their activity is blocked by voluntary movement.

Theta waves project a frequency between 4 and 7 cps and an amplitude comparable to that of beta waves (see Figure 48-40). These are recorded primarily in children and in some adults in emotional distress from the parietal and frontotemporal regions of the brain. Visual attention may block theta wave activity.

Delta waves encompass all the electrical rhythms of less than 4 cps (see Figure 48-40). This pattern is observed normally in individuals in deeper stages of sleep and in young children, and is the dominant rhythm in infants. Presence of delta waves in the awake adult may signify organic brain pathology.

A significant correlation exists between an individual's level of arousal and the dominant frequency of the EEG. Waves appear at 3 or fewer per second in deep sleep states. As sleep lightens, bursts of 10 to 12 waves per second begin to appear at shorter and shorter intervals until the waking state when a continuous, more rapid frequency and lower-amplitude rhythm dominate. Thus, a direct correlation can be observed in the person's state of arousal and the cortical electrical activity recorded on the EEG.

The EEG evaluations contribute to the diagnostic process of patients with cranial neurologic problems. Characteristic rhythms are observed with the various epileptic seizures, as well as during the intervals between the attacks (see Figure 48-40 and Chap. 50). Focal damage to the cortex, either of internal or external origin, is usually reflected by an irregular and abnormal rhythm, which generally is slow and asymmetric with its corresponding hemispheric position. The EEG is also useful in the diagnosis of cerebral death.

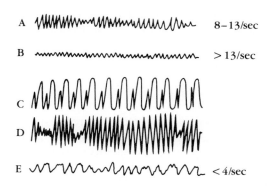

**FIGURE 48-40.**
EEG waves. **A.** Alpha waves. **B.** Beta waves. **C.** Spike and dome waves during petit mal seizures. **D.** High-frequency spike waves during grand mal seizure. **E.** Delta waves. **F.** Theta waves.

## Evoked Potentials

Evoked potentials are recorded on the EEG when an external stimulus has been applied to a specific sense organ. These have been useful in demonstrating abnormal sensory organ function. Commonly used evoked potentials are to test the integrity of the visual pathways (pattern-shift visual evoked response; PSVER), the brainstem (far field brainstem auditory evoked response; BAER), and the somatosensory system (short-latency somatosensory evoked potentials; SLSEP). A computer is used to average and maximize the responses.

The PSVER is particularly useful in diagnosing lesions of the optic nerve and its pathways. It is an effective test to detect optic neuritis, optic nerve compression, and demylinization of the optic pathways, such as is associated with multiple sclerosis. Each eye is tested separately as the individual views a pattern of light while recordings are made on the electroencephalograph.

The BAER tests auditory stimuli on the cerebral cortex and is useful for diagnosing peripheral hearing loss and lesions in the auditory tracts and brainstem. A series of clicks is administered to one ear through earphones while an EEG is recorded. This is repeated on the other ear. The ear that is not being tested at the time receives white noise.

The SLSEP diagnoses nerve conduction defects of the somatic sensory system. Peripheral nerves are stimulated by electrodes on overlying skin and EEG electrodes are placed peripherally and on the scalp. Common stimulation sites are the wrist and ankle. The SLSEP is most useful in diagnoses of lesions in spinal roots, posterior columns, and brainstem involvement, such as may occur with Guillain-Barré syndrome and multiple sclerosis.

## REFERENCES

1. Carpenter, M., and Sutin, J. *Human Neuroanatomy* (8th ed.). Baltimore: Williams & Wilkins, 1983.
2. Chusid, J. *Correlative Neuroanatomy and Functional Neurology* (19th ed.). Los Altos, Calif.: Lange, 1985.
3. Clark, R. *Essentials of Clinical Neuroanatomy and Neurophysiology* (5th ed.). Philadelphia: F.A. Davis, 1975.
4. Eccles, J. *The Understanding of the Brain.* New York: McGraw-Hill, 1973.
5. Guyton, A.C. *Textbook of Medical Physiology* (7th ed.). Philadelphia: W.B. Saunders, 1986.
6. Iverson, L. The chemistry of the brain. *Sci. Am.* 241:134, 1979.
7. Nauta, W., and Feirtag, M. The organization of the brain. *Sci. Am.* 241:88, 1979.
8. Peele, T. *The Neuroanatomic Basis for Clinical Neurology* (3rd ed.). New York: McGraw-Hill, 1977.
9. Ruch, T., and Patton, H. *Physiology and Biophysics* (20th ed.). Philadelphia: W.B. Saunders, 1973.
10. Snell, R.S. *Clinical Neuroanatomy for Medical Students.* Boston: Little, Brown, 1980.
11. Stevens, C. The neuron. *Sci. Am.* 241:54, 1979.
12. Willis, W., and Grossman, R. *Medical Neurobiology* (3rd ed.). St. Louis: Mosby, 1981.

# chapter 49

Reet Henze

# Adaptations and Alterations in the Special Senses

## Chapter Outline

▶ **Vision**
  **Structure and Function**
  **Visual Pathways**
  **Image Formation**
  **Accommodation**
  **Pupillary Aperture**
  **Physiology of Vision**
  **Color Vision**
  **Color Blindness**
  **Dark Adaptation**
  **Refraction Defects**
  **Measurement of Visual Acuity**
  **Visual Field Defects**
  **Other Disturbances of Vision**
    Glaucoma
    Cataracts
    Retinal Detachment
    Retinitis Pigmentosa

▶ **Hearing**
  **Structure and Function**
  **Sound Conduction Through the Ear**
  **Hearing Pathways**
  **Hearing Loss**
  **The Vestibular System**
    Vertigo
    Meniere's Disease
    Nystagmus
    Labyrinthine Ataxia
  **Assessment of Hearing and Balance**
  **Sound Amplification**

▶ **Taste**
  **Structure and Function**
  **Taste Pathways**
  **Taste Disturbances**
  **Taste Assessment**
▶ **Smell**
  **Structure and Function**
  **Smell Disturbances**
  **Smell Assessment**

## Learning Objectives

1. Name the structures of the eye.
2. State the normal intraocular pressure.
3. Trace the visual pathways from the optic disk to the occipital lobe.
4. Discuss the mechanism of image formation in the eye.
5. Define *refraction index*.
6. Explain the process of accommodation.
7. Discuss factors that influence the pupillary aperture.
8. Identify the functions of rods and cones.
9. Discuss the initiation of receptor potential of the retina.
10. Explain the trichromic theory of color vision.
11. Contrast myopia and hypermetropia.
12. Define *astigmatism*.
13. Discuss the pathologic basis of the hemianopsias.
14. Discuss the mechanisms maintaining normal intraocular pressure.
15. Identify conditions that lead to increased intraocular pressure.
16. Differentiate between chronic simple and acute glaucoma.
17. Identify the structures of the ear.
18. Trace sound conduction through the ear and the fiber pathways to the auditory cortex.
19. Differentiate between conduction deafness and sensorineural deafness.
20. Discuss the role of the vestibular system with respect to changes of position and movement.
21. Discuss common clinical findings associated with Meniere's disease.
22. Identify three tests that might be performed to detect hearing loss.
23. Locate the primary sensations of taste on the tongue.
24. Trace taste pathways from innervation of taste buds to cerebral cortex.
25. Discuss pathogenesis of taste disturbance.
26. Identify the receptor cell for the sense of smell.
27. Discuss adaptation of smell receptors.
28. Identify potential causes of anosmia.

The senses of vision, hearing, taste, and smell provide humans with the means to perceive the environment and respond in a way that supports adaptation and, at times, even survival. The receptors of the eyes, ears, tongue, and nose are stimulated and messages are transmitted to specific regions of the cerebral cortex for processing. Alterations in the function of these senses, particularly vision and hearing, can result in physiologic, psychologic, sociologic, and economic difficulties. Common alterations are described in this chapter; others can be found in specialized texts.

# VISION

## Structure and Function

The eye is a complex peripheral structure that transmits vision to the visual area of the occipital lobe of the cerebral cortex. It nestles in the orbit, a cone-shaped cavity with fragile walls composed of the frontal, maxillary, zygomatic, sphenoid, ethmoid, lacrimal, and palatine bones. The thinness of the orbital wall makes this area particularly susceptible to fractures. The eyeball occupies the anterior portion of the orbital cavity; its principle

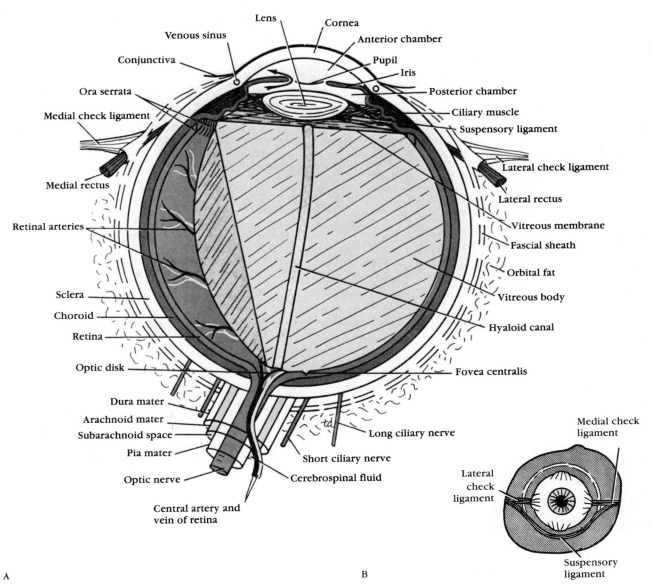

A                                                                                          B

**FIGURE 49–1.**
**A.** Horizontal section through eyeball and optic nerve. Note that central artery and vein of the retina cross the subarachnoid space to reach the optic nerve. **B.** The check ligaments and suspensory ligaments of the eyeball. (From R.S. Snell, *Clinical Anatomy for Medical Students* [2nd ed.]. Boston: Little, Brown, 1981.)

structures are identified in Figure 49-1. The area of the orbit not occupied by the eyeball is filled with fascia, fat, nerves, blood vessels, muscle, and the lacrimal gland. Six extrinsic muscles, most of which arise from the apex of the orbit and insert into the scleral lining, allow for the movement and rotation of the eyeball. These include the superior rectus, inferior rectus, medial rectus, lateral rectus, superior oblique, and inferior oblique muscles. Innervation for these muscles arrives from the third, fourth, and sixth cranial nerves.

The three layers of the eyeball are the sclera, choroid, and retina. The outermost supportive and protective layer, the sclera, is composed of dense fibrous tissue and forms a white, opaque membrane around the eyeball except at the cornea, where it becomes transparent. It is through this transparent area that light rays enter the eye to stimulate the rods and cones. The second (middle) layer of the eyeball is the vascular choroid. Nutrients are exchanged in this heavily pigmented layer. The ciliary muscle, which is important in facilitating light and accommodation reflexes, lies between the sclera and choroid layers. The choroid also contains the iris, the center of which is the pupil. The sphincter and dilator muscles of the iris, together with the ciliary muscle, are known as the intrinsic muscles of the eye. They control the amount of light admitted into the eye. Innervation to these muscles comes from the third cranial nerve and the superior cervical ganglion. The crystalline lens, which is suspended by the suspensory ligament from the inner surface of the ciliary body, bends the rays of light so that they are projected properly on the retina. The anterior chamber is a fluid-filled space anterior to the iris and lens. The posterior chamber, behind the iris and fluid-filled as well, together with the anterior chamber, assists in maintaining constant pressure in the eyeball. Normal intraocular pressure is between 10 and 22 mm Hg, with the most common pressures being 15 or 16 mm Hg. Glaucoma results if drainage of this aqueous humor is insufficient and intraocular pressure rises (Figure 49-2). Vitreous humor, which is soft and gelatinous, fills the space behind the lens and helps maintain the shape of the eyeball.

The third layer of the eyeball, the retina, consists of two parts. The outer pigmented layer is attached to the choroid. The inner layer consists of a synaptic series of nervous tissue. The macula lutea, a yellowish spot near the center of the retina, encompasses a small depression in its center called the fovea centralis. This is an area consisting only of cones and projecting the most acute vision. Medial to the fovea centralis is the optic disk. It is at this whitish spot that the optic nerve exits from the eyeball. Because this area contains no sensory receptors, it is known as the physiologic blind spot of the retina. Increased intraocular pressure is reflected in the optic disk by its cupped shape, that is, the disk appears pushed backward. In contrast, increased intracranial pressure

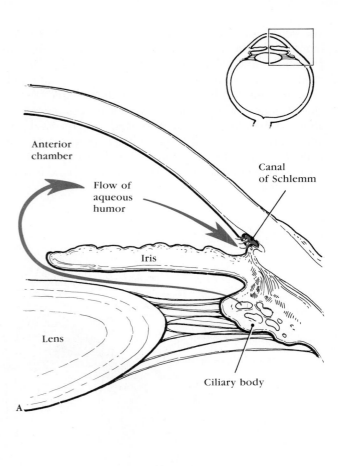

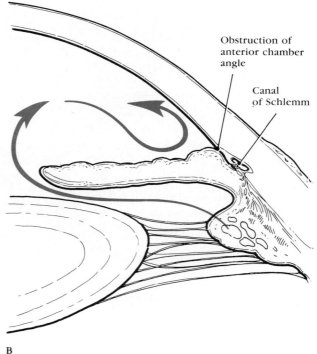

**FIGURE 49–2.**

**A.** Normal flow of aqueous humor. **B.** Obstructed flow in acute (closed- or narrow-angle) glaucoma. (Adapted from M. Lechiger and F. Moya, *Introduction to the Practice of Anesthesia* [2nd ed.]. New York: Harper & Row, 1978.)

produces the opposite effect, that is, an optic disk that is pushed inward, called a *choked disk,* or *papilledema* (see Chap. 52).

The blood supply to the retina enters through the central artery, a branch of the ophthalmic artery, which enters the eyeball with the optic nerve and runs with it to the retina where it divides in the middle of the disk into superior and inferior branches. The veins in the eyeball are anatomically related to the arteries and empty into the ophthalmic veins.

## Visual Pathways

The ganglionic cell axons of the retina emerge from the optic disk as the optic nerve. Axons from the nasal half of each eye cross in the optic chiasm and terminate in the opposite occipital lobe. Axons from the temporal half of each eye do not cross but terminate on their respective sides in the superior colliculus and lateral geniculate body (Figure 49-3).[3] Those fibers terminating in the lateral geniculate body seem to be associated with visual perception and those terminating in the superior colliculus excite reflex activity.[10] The fibers from the lateral geniculate body emerge as the optic radiation and continue to the striate cortex in the occipital lobe.

## Image Formation

The refractive surfaces of the cornea and lens initiate the mechanism for image formation. These surfaces and the aqueous and vitreous humors provide varying densities for the light to pass through. This accounts for the refractive phenomenon. If a light ray passes into denser medium, it is bent toward the perpendicular and the speed of transmission is slowed. A less dense medium bends the light ray away from the perpendicular and speeds its transmission. The degree of light impediment, or the power of a substance to bend light, is its *refractive index.* The refractive index of air is 1.0; of water, 1.33; of the cornea, 1.38; and of the crystalline lens, 1.40.[8]

Light strikes the cornea at different angles and is bent in different amounts depending on the curvature and refractive indexes of the interposed structures. Refraction of light occurs at the corneal interface, aqueous humor, and crystalline lens, and is projected on the retina in an inverted and reverted manner that is perceived by the brain as upright.

## Accommodation

Adjustments for distant vision are made by the lens. Normally, parallel light rays from distant objects are focused on the retina. The ciliary muscle contracts to increase the curvature of the lens to view objects closer to the eye. The increased curvature of the lens increases its power, shortens focal length, and focuses near objects on the retina. This is the process of accommodation. The closest point at which a person can clearly focus an object is called the *near point*. This point recedes with advancing age. For example, the near point for a normal eye of an 8-year-old is approximately 8.6 cm; for a 20-year-old, it is 10.4 cm; and for a 60-year-old, it is approximately 83 cm from the eye. Ocular convergence and pupillary constriction (miosis) are associated with the accommodation reflex. Convergence ensures that images recorded are focused on the macular area at the fovea centralis.[10]

The accommodation reflex is mediated by the third cranial nerve through parasympathetic postganglionic fibers. The stimulus that triggers the accommodation response is perception of an image out of focus. The parasympathetic impulses on the ciliary muscle must, therefore, increase progressively to maintain the image in focus continually.

Progressive age reduces the efficiency of accommodation due to the loss of elasticity of the lens. The eye may remain focused almost permanently on a constant distance. This deterioration is known as *presbyopia*. It is readily corrected with proper bifocal lenses for far and near vision.

## Pupillary Aperture

The iris controls the amount of light that enters the eye through the action of its two sets of smooth muscles: the sphincter and dilator muscles. Miosis is accomplished through the contraction of the sphincter muscle, and mydriasis is facilitated through the contraction of the dilator muscle. Innervation for the sphincter muscles comes from the postganglionic parasympathetic neurons in the ciliary ganglion. The preganglionic neurons transmit to the ganglion by the third cranial nerve. Innervation for the dilator muscle arrives from the sympathetic postganglionic neurons of the superior cervical ganglion, and reaches the eye through a series of progressively smaller arteries.

The pupillary aperture in the human eye can vary from 1.5 to 8.0 mm in diameter. In normal eyes, the aperture is a reflex response to change in light intensity. Pupils constrict in response to increased light intensities and dilate to decreased light intensities (pupillary light reflex). If illumination enters only one eye, both pupils constrict. This simultaneous constriction of the contralateral eye is referred to as the *consensual light reflex*. Photoreceptors of the retina, including rods and cones, are receptors for the light reflex.

Emotional states of alarm produce pupillary dilation. This reaction is initiated by stimulation of the sympathetic fibers and inhibition of the parasympathetic fibers. Darkness inhibits the parasympathetic supply and results in pupil dilation.

## VISUAL PATHWAYS

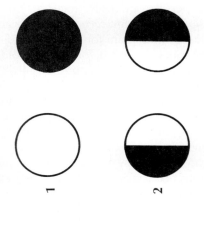

Left Visual Field | Right Visual Field

Temporal | Nasal | Temporal

Right eye

Left eye

Optic nerve

Optic tract

Optic radiation

## VISUAL FIELDS

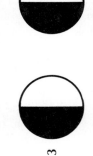

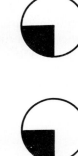

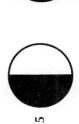

**BLACKENED FIELD INDICATES AREA OF NO VISION**

**1**

**BLIND RIGHT EYE** (*right optic nerve*)
A lesion of the optic nerve, and of course of the eye itself, produces unilateral blindness.

**2**

**BITEMPORAL HEMIANOPSIA** (*optic chiasm*)
A lesion at the optic chiasm may involve only those fibers that are crossing over to the opposite side. Since these fibers originate in the nasal half of each retina, visual loss involves the temporal half of each field.

**3**

**LEFT HOMONYMOUS HEMIANOPSIA** (*right optic tract*)
A lesion of the optic tract interrupts fibers originating on the same side of both eyes. Visual loss in the eyes is therefore similar (homonymous) and involves half of each field (hemianopsia).

**4**

**HOMONYMOUS LEFT UPPER QUADRANTIC DEFECT** (*optic radiation, partial*)
A partial lesion of the optic radiation may involve only a portion of the nerve fibers, producing, for example, a homonymous quadrantic defect.

**5**

**LEFT HOMONYMOUS HEMIANOPSIA** (*right optic radiation*)
A complete interruption of fibers in the optic radiation produces a visual defect similar to that produced by a lesion of the optic tract.

LEFT | RIGHT

## FIGURE 49–3.

Visual pathways. (Source: B. Bates, *A Guide to Physical Examination and History Taking* [4th ed.]. Philadelphia: J.B. Lippincott, 1987.)

986

Light reflex of the pupil and miosis of accommodation are not identical mechanisms and can occur independently of each other. An example of this occurs with the Argyll Robertson pupil, which may occur as a complication of syphilis. In this phenomenon, the pupil remains constricted and unresponsive to light but does respond to the accommodation mechanism.[2]

## Physiology of Vision

Rods and cones are receptors of the retina and have distinctly different morphologic compositions and functions (Figure 49-4). The cones mediate daylight vision, allowing perception of detail and color of objects. The rods mediate night vision, allowing visualization of outlines of objects without revealing color or detail. The rods, however, are very sensitive to movement of objects in the visual field.

The retina is formed by numerous layers of cells, fibers, and ganglia (Figure 49-5). The nerve cells in the retina include bipolar cells, ganglion cells, horizontal cells, and amacrine cells. The rods and cones, which are adjacent to the pigment epithelium of the choroid, synapse with the bipolar cells, which, in turn, synapse with dendrites of the ganglion cells. Horizontal cells connect receptor cells (rods and cones) and amacrine cells connect ganglion cells to each other and to bipolar cells. The dendrites of the ganglion cells synapse with bipolar cell axons in the inner plexiform layer (see Figure 49-5), and their axons converge to enter the optic nerve. The fovea centralis is composed of tightly packed cones that connect individually to the optic nerve, whereas in other parts of the retina they share fibers with many other rods and cones. The pigmented layer of the retina is the outermost layer, which decreases light reflexion. This pigment layer is directly adjacent to the choroid and receives much of its nutritive needs from the choroid vascular supply. Melanin is the black pigment that gives this layer its characteristic dark color.

As light passes through the layers of the retina to reach the light-sensitive portion of the rods and cones deep in the retina, light energy is absorbed by the pigment rhodopsin, or visual purple. Rhodopsin is a light-sensitive protein and aldehyde of vitamin A compound contained in rods that breaks down when light reaches it. This is the initial activity in producing the generator potential. The breakdown of rhodopsin can be visualized by the change in the dark-adapted retina from a dark purple to lack of color on exposure to light. The breakdown of rhodopsin results in the formation of a protein, scotopsin, and a carotene pigment, retinene.[4] In darkness, scotopsin and retinene recombine through a series of intermediary steps and form rhodopsin again, which is stored in the outer segments of the rods and is again photoexcitable.

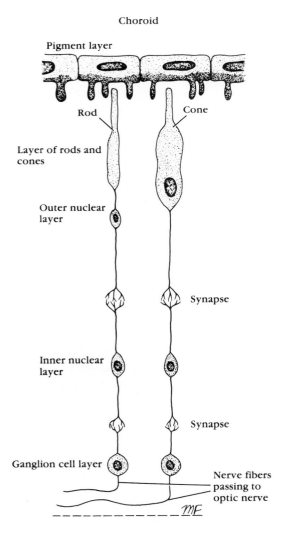

**FIGURE 49-4.**
Rods and cones.

$$\text{Rhodopsin} \xrightarrow[\text{dark}]{\text{light}} \text{retinene} + \text{scotopsin}$$

$$\longrightarrow \text{generator potential}$$

Knowledge about the pigments in the cones is somewhat speculative. Reflexion densitometry has demonstrated the presence of pigments in the foveal region of the retina that peak in the blue, green, and red parts of the spectrum. This is accomplished by shining light in the eye and measuring the intensity of energy at different wave lengths in the light reflected from the retina. In this manner, the amount of light absorbed by the visual receptor cells can be determined. Erythrolobe is a pigment identified in the fovea that absorbs light in the red part of the spectrum; chlorolobe is a pigment that absorbs light in the green part of the spectrum in the fovea.

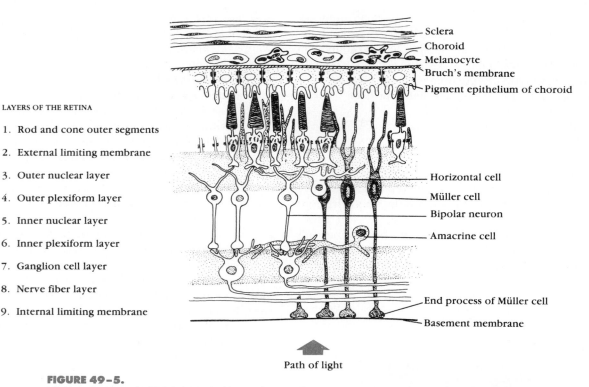

LAYERS OF THE RETINA

1.  Rod and cone outer segments

2.  External limiting membrane

3.  Outer nuclear layer

4.  Outer plexiform layer

5.  Inner nuclear layer

6.  Inner plexiform layer

7.  Ganglion cell layer

8.  Nerve fiber layer

9.  Internal limiting membrane

Sclera
Choroid
Melanocyte
Bruch's membrane
Pigment epithelium of choroid

Horizontal cell
Müller cell
Bipolar neuron
Amacrine cell

End process of Müller cell
Basement membrane

Path of light

**FIGURE 49–5.**
Highly schematic diagram showing the nine layers of the retina and their connections, using a few cells of each type as examples. Note that light must pass through the entire thickness of the retina before it finally triggers a photochemical reaction in the rod and cone outer segments. This "backward" retina is typical of all vertebrates. (From M. Borysenko et al., *Functional Histology* [2nd ed.]. Boston: Little, Brown, 1984.)

A third cone pigment, iodopsin, a violet-sensitive substance, has been isolated from the retinae of chickens and is also thought to exist in the human eye cones. A pigment receptor for blue substances has also been identified. The composition of the cone pigments is similar to rhodopsin, although in varying degrees. Thus, cone pigments absorb a variety of colors to different extents, and color-dependent nerve impulses result. These impulses are interpreted by the visual cortex as color sensations.

The photochemical decomposition that occurs in response to light striking either the cones or rods produces a receptor potential that remains for the duration of the stimulus. The receptor potentials of the retina differ from other receptor potentials in that hyperpolarization is produced rather than depolarization. Each optic nerve fiber connects with many receptors by ganglionic cells. The number of receptor cells on the retina is much greater than the number in the optic nerve. This convergence on ganglionic cells allows summation to occur; therefore, light falling on different parts of the retina together may cause excitation. Thus, the more rods and cones that are excited, the more intense the signal. The ganglion cells receive the excitation impulses from the rods and cones through the bipolar cells.

The ganglionic cells produce synaptic depolarization and stimulate threshold spikes that are all or nothing and are propagated along their axons to the lateral geniculate body. Three types of responses are observed in ganglionic cells. One fires only in response to light stimulus on the retina and is known as the on fiber; another discharges only in response to light off and is known as the off fiber. The third, most numerous type, responds to both light on and off and is called the on-off fiber.

The horizontal cells transmit inhibitory impulses laterally from rods and cones to bipolar cells and become most important in detecting visual contrasts and color differentiations. Amacrine cells have a very transient inhibitory effect on the ganglionic cells in response to stimulation from bipolar cells and possibly rods and cones. Amacrine cell inhibition seems to enhance the contrast experienced in visual images. The neural pathways from the retina to the visual cortex are identified in Figure 49-3.

## Color Vision

The differentiation of wave lengths of the visible spectrum allows the human eye to detect color in the environment. The precise mechanism that is responsible for color detection has been theorized by numerous researchers throughout the past century. Most of the investigation seems to be based on the *trichromatic theory*, which assumes that there are three variations in cones, each containing a different photochemical substance. One type of cone is responsible for red color, another for blue, and the third for green.[4] This theory, also known as the *Young-Helmholtz theory*, named after its originators over a century ago, is widely accepted today. Each of these cones gives rise to a distinct impulse that travels to the visual cortex of the occipital lobe. Red, blue, and green are colors that may produce any color in the spectrum by correct proportionate mixture. When all of the cones are stimulated equally, the sensation of white results. In contrast, when no stimulation of the three types of cones occurs, black is experienced. Other colors are perceived as a result of the combined stimulation of the three types of cones to varying degrees.

In summary, color vision evolves from the spectral sensitivity of cones and is most highly developed in the fovea where cones are concentrated. Each cone is maximally stimulated by a specific color. Color information is transmitted to the brain by common cone pathways of the optic fibers, and the transmission of specific colors is monitored by the stimulation of horizontal cells.

## Color Blindness

Many forms of color blindness exist but the most common variety is the inability to distinguish red from green. These may be hereditary, congenital, or acquired. The most common of these is hereditary through the male sex-linked recessive gene. Congenital color vision defects also tend to be red-green defects with intact yellow-blue vision. Acquired defects involve a variety of color defects.[1] Acquired visual defects may be lost partially, such as in a quadrant or half of the visual field, or they may involve the entire visual field. When a certain group of color receptors is not present in the retinae, all colors appear the same in the range of missing cones.

Individuals can be assessed for color blindness by numerous tests. Those most commonly used are the polychromatic charts and the yarn-matching tests. The former presents a chart, known as the *Ishihara* chart, with numerous look-alike, colored spots in a figuration that a person with normal vision can identify easily. The yarn-matching test involves asking the person to match a skein of yarn with strands from a pile of variously colored yarn.

## Dark Adaptation

The eyes are said to be *dark adapted* after a period of time in darkness. This decline in visual threshold is at its maximum after approximately 20 minutes in the dark environment. When one returns to the light environment, the uncomfortable brightness requires the eyes to adapt to light again. This adaptation takes about 5 minutes and is called *light adaptation*. Dark adaptation occurs, in part, as rhodopsin stores are rebuilt in the rods and some

similar, yet unknown, process occurs in the cones.[4] Dark adaptation is most effectively maintained by avoiding exposure to light. When visual acuity is necessary in a dark environment, such as for viewing a fluoroscopy screen and radiographs, red goggles may be worn on returning to bright light to avoid having to wait 20 minutes for adaptation. The light wavelengths in the red part of the spectrum allow cone vision to continue while stimulating rods only to a slight degree.

Only the periphery of the retina of the human eye is sensitive to light in the dark-adapted eye and, therefore, the sensitivity to darkness is much greater in the rods than the cones. Rods are not exclusively responsible for dark adaptation, however. Because of the presence of both rods and cones, dark adaptation takes place in two stages. First, a small increase in sensitivity, which is accomplished in about 7 minutes, is attributed in dark adaptation of cones. After this, a less rapid, but quantitatively greater rod adaptation occurs in rods.[5]

## Refraction Defects

*Emmetropia* (normal refraction) occurs when the relaxed eye is capable of clearly focusing distant parallel light rays on the retina (Figure 49-6). Nearby vision requires contraction of the ciliary muscle to bring the ob-

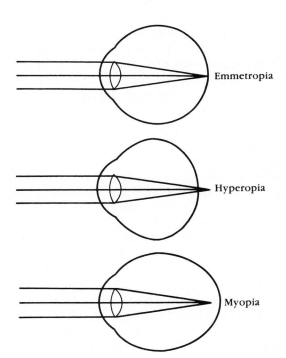

**FIGURE 49-6.**
Common defects in the optical system of the eye. Emmetropia is normal refraction. A shortened eyeball gives rise to hyperopia (farsightedness). An abnormally long eyeball may characterize myopia (nearsightedness). Adjustments should be made in the lens selection on the ophthalmoscope for these anatomic differences. (From R. Judge, G. Zuidema, and F. Fitzgerald, *Clinical Diagnosis: A Physiologic Approach*. Boston: Little, Brown, 1982.)

ject to focus. Defects of vision are present if the light rays converge either in front of or behind the retina, or if the eyeball is abnormally shaped.[4]

*Myopia* (nearsightedness) is a result of an object focusing in front of the retina due to increased anteroposterior diameter (see Figure 49-6). Myopic individuals cannot focus a distant object sharply; however, as they move closer to the object, it becomes more focused and eventually falls on the retina. The excessive refraction of myopia is readily corrected by a *concave* diverging lens, which produces a longer than normal focal point.

*Hyperopia* (farsightedness) occurs with an abnormally short eyeball; the parallel light rays are focused beyond the retina in the relaxed eye (see Figure 49-6). Through the mechanism of accommodation, the hyperopic person can focus on distant objects. As objects move closer to the eye, images become blurred and accommodation can no longer compensate. The near point in this individual is abnormally distant. Hyperopia is corrected by using the refraction of light rays through a *convex* lens and shortening the normal focal point.

*Astigmatism* is a defect of the curvature of the cornea and lens that produces refractive errors where parallel light rays are imperfectly focused on the retina. Clear focusing requires a spherical cornea and lens on all meridians. In the presence of irregular curvature of these structures, light striking peripheral areas is bent at different angles and is not focused on a single point on the retina. Astigmatism can be corrected with lenses that are cut from a piece of cylindric instead of spheric glass. The axis of the cylinder is placed approximately in relation to the meridian of the eye lens.

## Measurement of Visual Acuity

Individual visual acuity, the degrees to which a person can recognize contours and details of objects, can be readily measured by such instruments as the *Snellen letter chart*. The subject is asked to read the chart from the distance of 20 feet and identify the smallest line that can be seen. This is tested with each eye, one at a time. The results are recorded as a fraction, with 20 as its numerator for the distance from which the person views the chart. The denominator is the distance from which the smallest line is seen. Normal visual acuity is considered to be 20/20.

Visual acuity is dependent on a number of factors, including brightness of the stimulus, density of the receptor cells, state of the cones, contrasting illumination between background and the stimulus, and length of exposure to the stimulus.

## Visual Field Defects

Normally an individual's visual field extends approximately 90 degrees to the temporal side, 60 degrees to the nasal side, and 130 degrees vertically. The *confrontation test* can be used as a crude assessment of visual field acuity. In this test, the examiner positions himself or herself about 2 feet away from the individual and the person is asked to cover one eye and fix his or her gaze with the other eye on the examiner's eye directly opposite. The examiner closes his or her eye so that it roughly superimposes on the person's and then introduces a small object, such as a pencil, from beyond the visual field and asks the patient to indicate when he or she first sees the object. If abnormalities are detected, a standard perimetric test is performed.

Visual field defects occur as a result of lesions in the visual pathway. The specific defect reflects the region of the lesion on the visual pathway (see Figure 49-3). Blindness in one half of the visual field is known as *hemianopsia* (henianopsia). Lesions of the decussating fibers of the optic chiasm are commonly a result of pituitary tumors and reflect a *bitemporal hemianopsia*, a mirror image defect on one side of both visual fields. *Heteronymous* defects are asymmetrical defects in the eyes and usually indicate involvement of the optic chiasm region. Loss of vision in corresponding halves of the visual fields are known as *homonymous hemianopsia* and suggest lesions posterior to the optic chiasm in the optic tracts originating on the same side of both eyes. When homonymous hemianopsias can be superimposed on each other accurately, they are said to be *congruous* and the lesion is likely in the calcarine cortex and subcortical white matter of the occipital lobe.[1] Those homonymous hemianopsias whose boundaries differ are *incongruous* and more likely involve lesions in the parietal or temporal lobe.[1]

Defects that affect one quadrant of the visual field are described as *quadrantic hemianopsia* and involve only a partial area of the optic radiation.

## Other Disturbances of Vision

Decreased visual acuity may be associated with various lesions, syndromes, drug therapies, and nutritional deficiencies. Specific types of impairments result from lesions in different locations along the visual pathways.

*Scotomas* are abnormal blind spots in the visual field which are surrounded by normal vision. They are referred to by their shape and position. These may exist with a person's knowledge (positive scotomas) or without his or her knowledge (negative scotomas). Scotomas may result from vascular disease, toxic effect of certain drugs, nutritional deficiencies, demyelinating diseases, certain hereditary conditions, and glaucoma. *Diplopia*, double vision, results from an eye muscle imbalance between the eyes, resulting in image reception at different spots on each retina.

*Papilledema* (choked disk) is most common with increased intracranial pressure due to brain tumors, trauma, hemorrhage, infections, and other causes. In its early stages, minor visual changes, such as fuzziness in vision and slight elevation of the optic disk, may be visualized. As the condition progresses, the entire disk and surrounding tissue become severely elevated and edematous, obscuring its peripheral blood vessels.

*Optic atrophy* results in slow, progressive failure in visual acuity. It may be associated with multiple sclerosis, tabes dorsalis, neuritis, glaucoma, increased intracranial pressure, trauma, vascular occlusion, or congenital and hereditary conditions. The optic disk affected usually appears chalky white with clearly delineated margins. *Degeneration of the retina* may result from drug therapy (particularly the phenothiazine group), infections, and various metabolic or endocrine disorders.

Cerebral tumors, aneurysms, vascular diseases, infections, and degenerative processes may lead to visual defects, producing a variety of symptoms associated with a specific region. Defects may result in ocular movement, visual acuity, or interpretation of what is seen.

## Glaucoma

Increased intraocular pressure and loss in the visual field are hallmarks of glaucoma. Several underlying conditions can result in increased intraocular pressure. The most common of these is blockage or stenosis of aqueous outflow channels.[7] Normally, the aqueous humor, which is produced by the ciliary epithelium, flows from the posterior chamber of the eye through the pupil into the anterior chamber. Aqueous humor then leaves the anterior chamber and returns to the venous system by passing through the trabecular mesh of the anterior chamber into Schlemm's canal. A balance between production and absorption of aqueous humor provides for normal intraocular pressure.

Other potential causes of increased intraocular pressure in glaucoma include increases in systemic vascular pressure, which is reflected in venous engorgement, and decreased drainage through aqueous drainage channels. Increased production of aqueous humor is thought to contribute to a small proportion of those suffering from glaucoma.[7] The increased intraocular pressure associated with glaucoma may result in atrophy and degeneration of the optic nerve.

Glaucoma is described as *chronic simple* (open-angle) or *acute* (closed-angle or narrow-angle). The angle refers to the area where the iris meets the cornea in the anterior chamber (see Figure 49-2). Chronic simple glaucoma is thought to have a hereditary basis and is a common cause of blindness. It may be asymptomatic for years and finally reveal itself when the individual experiences peripheral vision loss, difficulty with dark adaptation, blurring of vision, seeing halos around lights, and difficulty focusing on near objects. Although the anterior chamber angle is open in chronic simple glaucoma, an obstruction exists for the flow of aqueous

humor through the trabecular mesh. Once this type of glaucoma has been diagnosed, the existing visual defects cannot be corrected. Further deterioration can be controlled with miotic drugs.

Acute glaucoma is manifested when an obstruction, either complete or partial, in the flow of aqueous humor is produced by closure of the anterior chamber angle (see Figure 49-2). This may result from an anteroposterior thickening of the lens or a forward movement of the lens that causes the iris to press against the lens capsule and prevent outflow of aqueous humor. Complete closure of the angle presents a dramatic clinical picture of severe eye pain, blurred or cloudy vision, halos around lights, a hard red eye with cloudy cornea, and nausea and vomiting. Intraocular pressure is elevated.

Glaucoma may be primary or secondary to eye conditions associated with infection, tumors, hemorrhage, and trauma. Diagnosis is based on clinical features and tonometry, tonography, and peripheral vision testing.

## Cataracts

As noted earlier, the normal lens is clear and transparent, and acts as a major refractive structure. Certain conditions may cause clouding of the lens and result in loss of vision associated with cataracts. These may result from trauma to the eye, elevated glucose levels in the aqueous humor (diabetes mellitus), irradiation to the lens, viruses, chemicals, and amino acid or vitamin deficiencies. Occasionally, cataracts may be congenital, but more commonly they are associated with advancing age (*senile cataracts*). Also, they have been associated with certain disease processes of the skin, skeleton, and nervous system, and chromosomal abnormalities.

Senile cataracts result from the aging process as the lens undergoes changes. New fibers develop continually in the lens and these slowly increase the lens size. Older lens fibers become dehydrated, compressed, and sclerosed, forming a yellowish brown pigment that becomes so dense as to result in nuclear sclerosis and decreased transparency. Cataracts may produce visual abnormalities as a result of decreased light transmission, abnormal morphology, or biochemistry and optical aberrations.[7] Diagnosis of cataracts is confirmed by the clinical features, usual eye tests, and ophthalmoscopic examination.

## Retinal Detachment

The separation of the retina from the choroid is generally spontaneous, although it may occur secondary to trauma. Retinal detachment is common in older individuals because aging may cause the vitreous body to shrink, resulting in retinal tearing. As the tear occurs in the retina, choroid vessels transudate and vitreous humor seeps under the retina, stripping it from the choroid.

The individual with a detached retina experiences "floaters" and lines in the visual field. In addition, flashes of light and blurred black spots appear suddenly in conjunction with defects in vision. If the macula is involved, severe vision loss results. The person often complains of a sensation of a curtain coming over the eye. Generally, there is no pain or redness of the eye.

Diagnosis of retinal detachment is made by clinical symptoms and ophthalmoscopy. A biocular indirect ophthalmoscope and scleral depressor are used to produce a three-dimensional view of the retina and its damage.

### Retinitis Pigmentosa

Retinitis pigmentosa is a degenerative inherited disease of the eyes that manifests itself initially by night blindness. Persons may inherit the disease through an autosomal dominant, autosomal recessive, or X-linked gene.[9] Progression of symptoms may be so slow that it may be difficult to detail an accurate course of the disease. Visual field constriction (tunnel vision) is commonly associated with the night blindness. Other symptoms include photophobia and disturbance in color vision. The disease may progress to total blindness, although some persons retain reading vision in a small central part of the visual field. Changes in the fundus may be identified early in the course of the disease by a disturbance in the pigment epithelium of the retina. Areas of hyperpigmentation and atrophy may be identified by angiography, although the hallmark of retinitis pigmentosa is degeneration of the rods and cones associated with loss of pigmentation.[9] The waxy-appearing optic disk, thinning of retinal arteries, and choriocapillary atrophy are other associated changes.

Diagnosis of retinitis pigmentosa is based on signs and symptoms of the disease, characteristic changes of the fundus, and a family history of the disease.

## HEARING

### Structure and Function

The ear is a mechanoreceptor; it is sensitive to rapid changes in pressure that are transmitted to its fluid medium. In essence, the ear is a mechanical transducer as sound at various frequencies is converted into nerve impulses through the cochlear component of the acoustic (eighth cranial nerve) nerve, that are transmitted into the central nervous system for interpretation. Sound is conducted through air, ossicles, and fluid, and is measured in number in vibrations per second, which are recorded as *cycles per second (cps)* or *Hertz (Hz)*. The human ear is able to perceive frequencies to 20,000 Hz. Aging reduces the number of frequencies perceived. The greatest sensitivity of the human ear is in the range of 1000 to 4000 Hz.

In addition to the hearing function of the ears, their receptors mediate a sense of position and equilibrium through the vestibular component of the eighth cranial nerve.

## Sound Conduction Through the Ear

The ear is anatomically segmented into the *outer, middle*, and *inner* areas (Figure 49-7). The outer ear funnels sound waves to the *tympanic membrane* (eardrum). Its canal is an S-shaped, 3-cm tube that is supplied with ceruminous and sebaceous glands, as well as hair follicles. The canal has resonance properties as sound waves are reflected from the tympanic membrane. It may enhance or dampen incoming waves. The external canal is lined with squamous epithelium, cartilage, and bone that provide support and maintain its patency.

At the terminal end of the external ear, the tympanic membrane separates it from the middle ear. This fibrous tissue vibrates freely with all audible sound frequencies and transmits these to the three auditory ossicles of the middle ear: the *malleus, incus*, and *stapes*. The middle ear with its three ossicles is situated in an air cavity of the temporal bone. It communicates with the nasopharynx by means of the auditory or Eustachian tube; the mucous membrane that lines the middle ear continues to line the pharynx, as well as the air cells of the mastoid. The auditory tube also equalizes pressure in the middle ear with that of atmospheric pressure. Swallowing and yawning open the tube; high atmospheric pressures tend to close the tube. Microorganisms from the oropharynx often travel through the auditory tube to the middle ear, causing infections in this area.

The manubrium of the malleus is attached to the tympanic membrane, and its short process articulates with the incus to produce vibratory movements in the stapes, which is attached to the walls of the oval window (Figure 49-8). The *tensor tympani* and *stapedius muscles* of the middle ear prevent the bones from transmitting excessive vibrations by pulling on the bones to decrease contact with the tympanic membrane and oval window. The former is innervated by the fifth cranial nerve and the latter by the seventh.

The inner ear is encased in the petrous part of the temporal bone and mediates sound-induced nerve impulses, position orientation, and balance. It is composed of two labyrinths, one within the other. The outer labyrinth is bony and separated from the inner membranous one by perilymph fluid; it contains the cochlea, vestibule, and the three semicircular canals. The membranous labyrinth contains fluid called *endolymph*. The anterior portion of the membranous labyrinth contains the cochlea, which receives the sound waves from the oval window. The cochlea, a small, shell-shaped structure, is divided into three chambers by the *basilar* and *Reissner's membranes*. These chambers are the *scala vestibuli, scala*

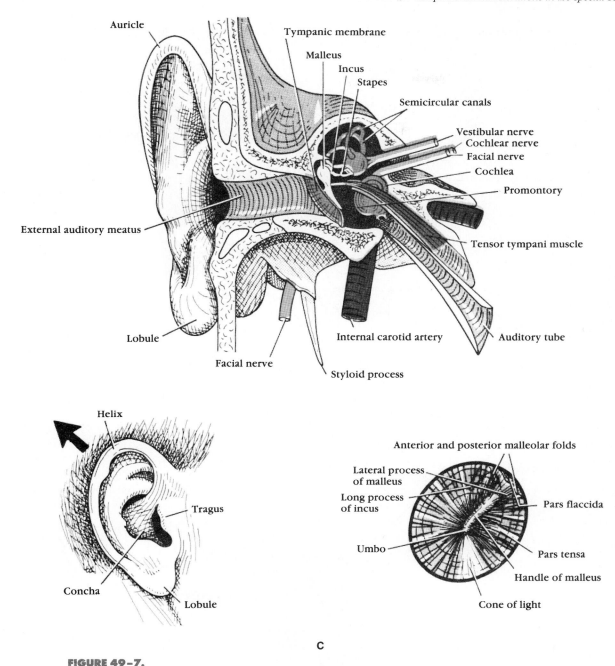

**FIGURE 49-7.**
Parts of the ear. **A.** Outer or external ear. **B.** Middle ear components. **C.** Inner ear components.
(From R.S. Snell, *Clinical Anatomy for Medical Students* [2nd ed.]. Boston: Little, Brown, 1981.)

*tympani,* and *cochlear duct.* Posteriorly, the cochlea opens into the osseous vestibule, which, in turn, extends to the three semicircular canals.

The *organ of Corti,* located on the basilar membrane, contains the receptor cells of audition. These are hair cells that generate nerve impulses in response to sound vibrations from the oscillations of the oval window. Impulses that stimulate the dendrites of the cochlear division of the acoustic nerve are transmitted to

the hearing center in the temporal lobe of the cortex. The various frequencies of sound generate different patterns of vibrations and allow sounds to be discriminated from each other. Subjective interpretation of the frequency of sound waves results in the recognition of *pitch.* The higher frequencies are identified as higher pitch. In addition to frequency, the location of the stimulation of cells on the basilar membrane affects pitch. Low-frequency sounds generate greater activity of the basilar

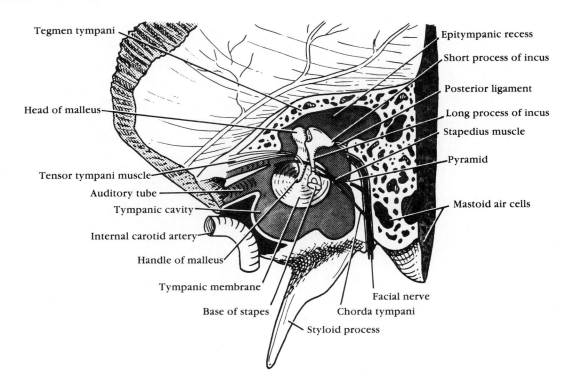

Tegmen tympani

Head of malleus

Tensor tympani muscle

Auditory tube

Tympanic cavity

Internal carotid artery

Handle of malleus

Tympanic membrane

Base of stapes

Styloid process

Epitympanic recess

Short process of incus

Posterior ligament

Long process of incus

Stapedius muscle

Pyramid

Mastoid air cells

Facial nerve

Chorda tympani

A

Geniculate ganglion

Aditus to mastoid antrum

Lateral semicircular canal

Tensor tympani muscle

Processus cochleariformis

Zygomatic arch

Facial nerve in canal

Pyramid

Mastoid antrum

Fenestra vestibuli

Promontory

Fenestra cochleae

Mastoid air cells

Facial nerve

Styloid process

B

**FIGURE 49–8.**
**A.** Lateral wall of right middle ear viewed from medial side. Note the position of ossicles and mastoid antrum. **B.** Medial wall of right middle ear viewed from lateral side. Note the position of the facial nerve in its bony canal. (From R.S. Snell, *Clinical Anatomy for Medical Students* [2nd ed.]. Boston: Little, Brown, 1981.)

membrane near the apex of the cochlea, and high-frequency sounds activate the basilar membrane near the base of the cochlea. Other frequencies fall between these extremes. This explanation of pitch discrimination is known as the *place theory.*

The amplitude of vibrations affects the perception of loudness at a constant frequency in that greater amplitude produces greater loudness. This does not hold true when two sounds of different frequency are contrasted simultaneously, however, because auditory sensitivity is a function of frequency. Thus, frequency and amplitude are both significant in determining the perception of loudness in two or more simultaneous sounds.

## Hearing Pathways

The axons of bipolar neurons from the cochlea enter the pons and divide into the dorsal and ventral cochlear nuclei. Second-order neurons cross here and ascend by the lateral lemniscus to the inferior colliculus. From there, they transmit to the medial geniculate body and on to the auditory cortex in the temporal lobe by the auditory radiations (Figure 49-9).

The auditory cortex allows a person to recognize tone patterns, analyze characteristics of sound, and localize sound. Low-frequency tones are recognized anteriorly and high-frequency tones, posteriorly, in the audi-

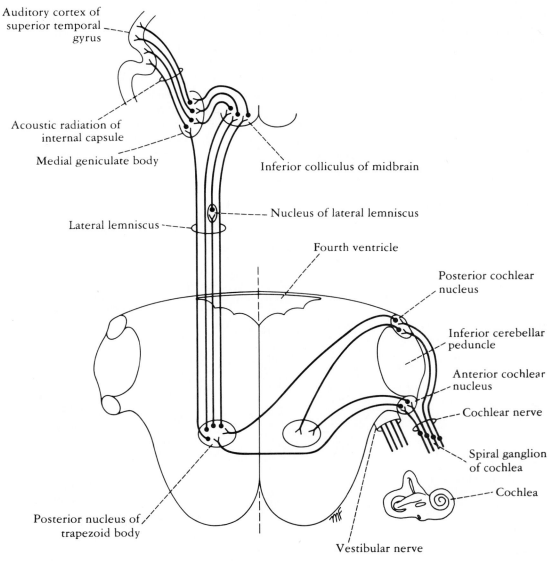

**FIGURE 49-9.**
Cochlear nerve nuclei and their central connections. (From R.S. Snell, *Clinical Neuroanatomy for Medical Students.* Boston: Little, Brown, 1980.)

tory cortex. Neurons throughout the auditory cortex respond to onset, duration, and direction of stimulus.

The auditory association area lies inferior to the primary auditory center and is thought to associate auditory information with other sensations, as well as different sound frequencies with each other. Lesions in this area prevent a person from comprehending the meaning of sounds heard; words can be heard but not understood. The origin (location) of sound is determined by the sound's arrival to the two ears. One ear receives information before the other, and the ear that is closer to the sound source receives a louder sound.

## Hearing Loss

Hearing loss can result from disorders of the central hearing mechanisms or the peripheral pathways. Peripheral hearing loss involves impairment of sound transmission in the external and middle ear and is referred to as *conduction deafness*. Lesions in the neural pathway produce *sensorineural deafness*. Lesions in the cochlear nuclei and their connections result in *central deafness*.[1]

Conduction deafness can result from obstruction of the external canal by cerumen or foreign objects, damage to the tympanic membrane, cholesteatoma, or immobility of the tympanic membrane or ossicles sec-

ondary to chronic otitis media. *Otosclerosis* results in conduction deafness by immobilizing of the stapes in the oval window.

Sensorineural deafness can be caused by long-term therapy with certain antibiotics in the mycin group, pathology of the hair cells of the cochlea, or disease processes in the auditory nerve pathway.

## The Vestibular System

Disorders of coordination may result from the vestibular system through the labyrinthine and righting reflexes. Lesions may occur in the labyrinths, vestibular nerve, vestibular pathways within the brainstem, cerebrum, or cerebellum. Figure 49-10 shows the pathways of the vestibular nerve and its interconnections with the cerebellum, parts of the labyrinths, and the cerebrum. The vestibular system maintains equilibrium, preserves head position, and directs the gaze of the eyes.

The vestibular portion of the eighth nerve has its peripheral endings on the hair cells of the maculae of the *utricle* and *saccule* and on the cristae in the ampullae of the three *semicircular canals* (Figure 49-11). The utricle and saccule record linear acceleration and static phenomena; the semicircular canals record angular acceleration.[6] Recent evidence implies that the utricle may be

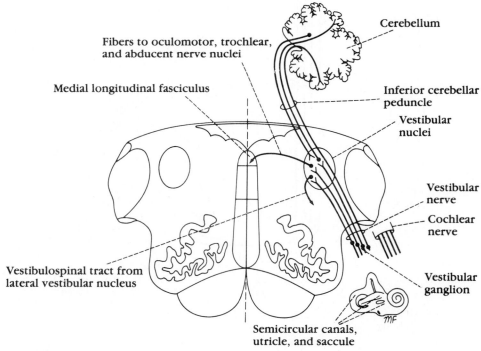

**FIGURE 49–10.**
Vestibular nerve nuclei and their central connections (Source: R.S. Snell, *Clinical Neuroanatomy for Medical Students*. Boston: Little, Brown, 1980.)

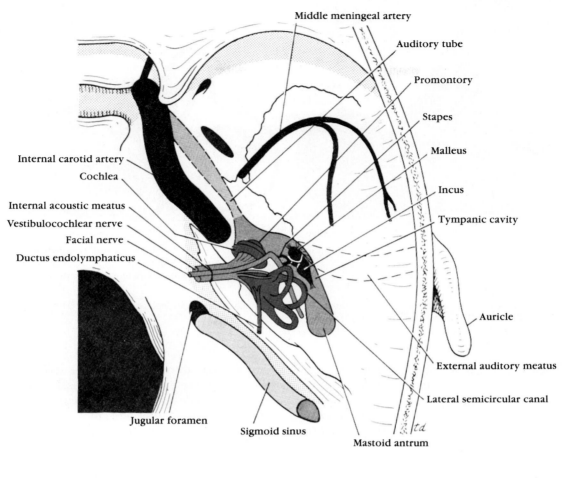

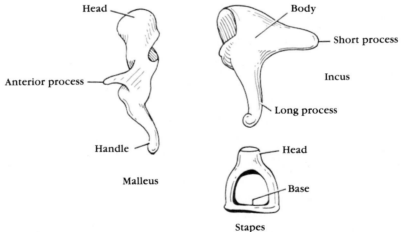

**FIGURE 49–11.**
**A.** Parts of the right ear in relation to temporal bone as viewed from above. **B.** The auditory ossicles (Source: R.S. Snell, *Clinical Anatomy for Medical Students* [2nd ed.]. Boston: Little, Brown, 1981.)

more related to the semicircular canals' vestibular functions while the saccule has a closer association with hearing.

The *utricle, saccule,* and *semicircular canals* function together to maintain equilibrium. These structures are housed in a bony labyrinth that contains a membranous labyrinth composed of the semicircular canals and the two chambers: the utricle and the saccule (Figure 49-12). Within the utricle and saccule are maculae that provide sensory areas that detect the relationship of the head

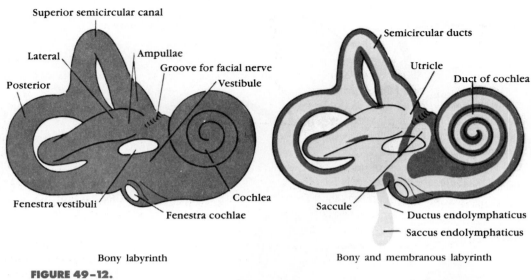

**FIGURE 49–12.**

Bony and membranous labyrinths (Source: R.S. Snell, *Clinical Anatomy for Medical Students* [2nd ed.]. Boston: Little, Brown, 1981.)

to gravitational pull and other forces. The maculae operate in conditions of acceleration and in static equilibrium. Internal and external hair cells synapse with a network of cochlear nerve endings, which terminate in the *cochlear nerve*. Within the semicircular canals, endolymph flows and stimulates the sensory nerve fibers that join up with the vestibular nerve. Fluid flow in the opposite direction inhibits these sensory nerve fibers.

The ganglion cells of the vestibular division of the eighth nerve are in the internal auditory meatus, and the dendrites end in the specialized epithelium of the hair cells. The axons pass back to the upper medulla, accompanied by the cochlear nerve. On entering the medulla, the fibers pass directly to the cerebellum and to four vestibular nuclei that communicate with the medial longitudinal fasciculus and with the nuclei of the third, fourth, and sixth cranial nerves and the upper cervical and accessory nerves. This connection results in vestibular influence on movement of the neck, eyes, and head.

A close interrelationship exists between the vestibular nerves and the cerebellum. This relationship accounts for the equilibrium changes that occur with rapid changes in direction. The maculae of the utricle and saccule provide vestibular input to the cerebellum. The influence of the two-way input and output results in coordination of the muscles of the neck and in the coordination required for posture. Interconnection of vestibular nerves to the reticular system may account for the nausea, vomiting, and sweating that results when the vestibular system is stimulated.

Two vestibulospinal tracts arise from the vestibular nuclei. The lateral tract comes from the lateral vestibular nucleus and extends to the sacral level of the cord. The medial tract comes from the medial vestibular nucleus

and extends through the cervical level. Impulses descending in these tracts assist in local myotactic (muscle stretching) reflexes and reinforce the tonus of the extensor muscles of the trunk and limbs, producing extra force to support the body against gravity and to maintain an upright posture.

Communication between the vestibular nuclei and the cerebral nuclei is not established but may exist because vertigo and dizziness have resulted from cortical stimulation of posterior aspects of the temporal lobe. Disturbances of function of the vestibular system may result in vertigo, nystagmus, and ataxia.

## Vertigo

Vertigo is a disturbance of equilibrium resulting in a variety of sensations of whirling, rotation, weakness, lightheadedness, or faintness. Posture is maintained by the normal interaction of several structures: labyrinths, eyes, muscles, joints, and higher neural centers. Causes of vertigo are multitudinous and include disorders of the labyrinth, vestibular nerve, vestibular nuclei, cerebellum, brainstem, eyes, and cerebral cortex.

There are several types of vertigo: acute paroxysmal, chronic, and benign positional. Acute paroxysmal vertigo is exemplified by sudden onset of acute movement and is sensed as rotatory, either objective or subjective. If rotatory and objective, external objects seem to be rotating while the person is stationary. If subjective, the person seems to be rotating in relation to the external environment. In addition to rotation, sensations of spinning, falling through space, or being pushed are experienced. Movement of objects or of oneself may appear in any plane—horizontal, oblique, or vertical.

Single attacks of vertigo may occur in acute labyrinthitis. Chronic vertigo is experienced as transient sensations of rotation with sudden head turning. Another type of attack, which may persist for months, is a constant sense of imbalance. Benign positional vertigo occurs only when the head is in certain postures and ceases when the head is moved out of these positions. An attack may occur with the head in a forward or backward position, or turned to one side. Affected persons learn to avoid the particular posture that causes the attack.

Attacks of vertigo can be disabling because the person may be thrown to the ground in reaction to false clues of movement. Nausea, vomiting, pallor, nystagmus, sweating, hypotension, excessive salivation, and difficulty with walking may accompany acute attacks of vertigo.

Rapid destruction of one labyrinth causes vertigo, nystagmus, and occasionally, some temporary nausea and vomiting. The vestibular nuclei seem to work by comparing signals from both labyrinths. Whenever a labyrinth is destroyed, the other side overcompensates for the input. Bilateral destruction of the labyrinths does not cause nystagmus or vertigo but the equilibrium may be disturbed for many months.

## Meniere's Disease

Meniere's disease is a classic example of vertigo as a result of labyrinthine disease. It is characterized by recurrent attacks of vertigo associated with disordered autonomic activity and gradual loss of hearing, which frequently begins before the appearance of the first bout of vertigo. Vertigo, which is of the whirling and rotation type, appears abruptly and lasts from minutes to more than an hour. It is usually severe enough to cause the person to lie down. Nausea, vomiting, tinnitus, feeling of fullness in ears, hypotension, sweating, and nystagmus may accompany the attacks. Considerable variation exists in the frequency and severity of the attacks. These may occur for a while and then go into remission for a considerable time.

The mechanism of vertigo is unknown at this time, although it is theorized that the autonomic nervous system control of the labyrinthine circulation is impaired. Caloric testing (irrigation of the ear canal) reveals loss of thermally induced nystagmus on the involved side, and audiometry shows decreased air and bone conduction. Meniere's disease affects both sexes equally and generally appears in the fifth decade.

## Nystagmus

Nystagmus is characterized by rhythmic oscillation of the eyes, and occurs both in physiologic and pathologic circumstances. Nystagmus can be induced in healthy persons by irrigating the external auditory canal with hot or cold water or by rotation in a revolving chair. One form

of physiologic nystagmus is *opticokinetic nystagmus*, which is induced by having the person look at a repeating pattern passed in a horizontal or vertical direction in front of the eyes.

Pathologically, *vestibular nystagmus* occurs as a response to some disturbance of the synergistic action of the two vestibular organs or their central connections. The nystagmus is always phasic. There is a slow phase in one direction of the eyes and then an opposing quick phase. The direction of nystagmus is based on the direction of the fast component. If the slow phase is to the right and the quick one is to the left, the person is said to exhibit nystagmus to the left. The movement of the eye may be horizontal, vertical, or rotary. The rotary tendency is most prominent whenever a lesion involves the labyrinth.

Vestibular nystagmus is associated with vertigo and is increased on turning the head or eyes in the direction of the quick phase. This occurs in dysfunction of the semicircular canals or their peripheral neurons. It is limited in duration because central compensation occurs. If it should persist longer than a few weeks, it is usually because of change in the vestibular pathway.[3] Other causes of pathologic nystagmus are abnormal retinal or labyrinthine impulses, lesions of the cervical spinal cord, lesions involving the central paths concerned in ocular posture, particularly those in the midbrain and midbrain tegmentum, weakness of the ocular muscles, drug treatment, and congenital abnormalities of unknown etiology.

## Labyrinthine Ataxia

Ataxia is often striking in vestibular disease. It is characterized by disturbances of equilibrium in standing and walking, and does not affect isolated limb movements. It has many features of cerebellar ataxia, such as the broad-based, staggering gait, leaning over backward or to one side, and deviation from direction of gait. It can usually be differentiated from cerebellar ataxia through association with nystagmus and vertigo. Causes of ataxia differ. Some are caused by degenerative, demyelinating, or inflammatory lesions and others by lesions in the thalamus and subthalamic region near the main cerebellar and sensory pathways. The most common mixed ataxias are the cerebellar and vestibular, and the posterior column and cerebellar forms. In multiple sclerosis, for example, symptoms of ataxia are mainly of the cerebellar and vestibular forms.

## Assessment of Hearing and Balance

A single effective means of assessing hearing ability is to have the person cover one ear with the hand and whisper a few words softly near the opposite ear; this is repeated for the other ear. If the person is able to perceive these words, the hearing is probably normal. In addition, auditory loss can be determined through the use of equipment, such as the tuning fork and audiometer. These tools can assist in distinguishing sensorineural hearing loss from conductive loss.

A simple test for conductive loss can be demonstrated through the use of a tuning fork. A vibrating tuning fork of 256 Hz is placed on the mastoid process until the individual no longer hears it and is then held in the air next to the external auditory meatus. This is known as the *Rinne test*. In persons with normal hearing, air conduction is acute and vibrations are heard after bone conduction has ceased. If vibrations are not heard in the air after bone conduction has ceased, the person has conductive deafness. If the vibrating tuning fork is heard at the ear canal after no longer being heard on the mastoid process, the conducting mechanisms through the middle ear are intact and the problem is in the inner ear or its transmissions; the person then has sensorineural loss.

*Weber's test* is also effective in identifying hearing loss. A vibrating tuning fork is placed at the vertex of the head; normal perception of the sound is equal in both ears. If conductive loss is present, the sound is louder in the affected ear due to the masking effect of the environmental noise. In the presence of sensorineural damage, sound is heard better in the normal ear.

*Audiometry* tests the sensitivity of the ear to pure tones at different frequencies through earphones. The audiometer, which is an electronic oscillator, measures hearing objectively and plots it on a graph that represents the percentage of normal hearing based on the average threshold of normal hearing of a population. Conductive and sensorineural hearing impairments can be distinguished by this means.

The vestibular component of the eighth cranial nerve may be assessed if the person's history reveals vertigo with nausea and vomiting. Vestibular function is evaluated by the *caloric test*. The subject is supine at a 30-degree elevation. After ascertaining no observable defects of the external auditory canal, first cold and then warm water is introduced alternately into the canal. The ear is irrigated with water at 30°C and 44°C with a minimal pause of 5 minutes between each irrigations. Tonic deviation of the eyes is normally induced to the side being irrigated with cold water. After a short latent period, nystagmus occurs toward the opposite side. Warm-water irrigation produces nystagmus toward the irrigated side. An absent or decreased response indicates impairment of the vestibular system.

## Sound Amplification

Sound may be amplified for some individuals through the use of a hearing aid. Some persons with hearing impairments may benefit more from a hearing aid than others. Those with middle ear disturbances generally receive the greatest improvement, while those with inner ear or nerve damage receive less. Hearing aids improve hearing through the mechanical amplification of sound. The person's ability to hear per se is not improved.

## TASTE

### Structure and Function

The sense of taste is a specialized function that is concerned with identification of food. The four primary taste sensations are *sweet, sour, bitter*, and *salt*. The other, more complex sensations that humans perceive are combinations of the primary sensations together with the olfactory sensation. Even though the tip of the tongue perceives all four sensations, specific areas of the tongue are more sensitive to particular sensations (Figure 49-13).

*Taste buds* are the organs of taste (Figure 49-14). These oval structures are located most numerously in the fungiform papillae of the tongue and are also present in the palate, pharynx, and epiglottis. Microvilli project from the buds to the surface and come into contact with the substances dissolved in the fluids of the mouth. This contact is thought to be the basis for the generator potentials. Innervation for the taste buds arrives from their base through small myelinated fibers. Each taste bud is innervated by several nerve fibers and each receives innervation from several taste buds. The life span of a taste bud is approximately 5 to 10 days. As buds degenerate, new buds are being formed and innervated. The total number

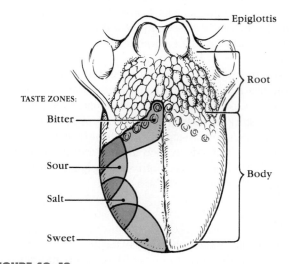

**FIGURE 49–13.**
The dorsal surface of the tongue showing the areas for perception of sweet, sour, bitter, and salt tastes.

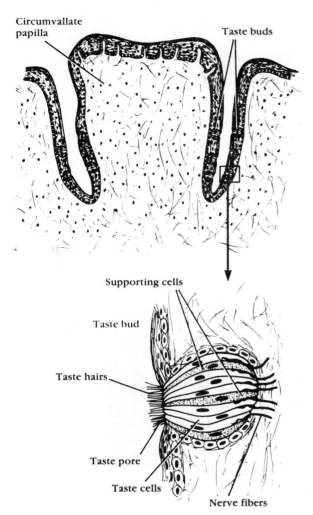

Circumvallate papilla

Taste buds

Supporting cells

Taste bud

Taste hairs

Taste pore

Taste cells

Nerve fibers

**FIGURE 49-14.**
Microscopic appearance of a taste bud.

of taste buds diminish as individuals age, accounting for the diminished sense of taste in the elderly.

In addition to taste buds, the sense of smell contributes significantly to taste perception. Odors of substances taken into the mouth pass to the nasopharynx and stimulate olfactory receptors. Consistency and temperature of ingested substances also contribute to the overall taste perception.

Because taste affects what is consumed, it contributes significantly to the nutritional status and internal environment of the body. Nutritional needs are not solely dependent on taste, however. Researchers have shown that people tend to select foods and liquids containing substances in which they may be deficient. This is supported by studies on adrenalectomized animals, which tend to develop a preference for salty substances. Animals that have had the parathyroid gland removed usually show an increased appetite for calcium-containing substances.[4]

## Taste Pathways

Innervation from the taste buds to the central nervous system is through the seventh, ninth, and tenth cranial nerves. The taste buds of the anterior two thirds of the tongue transmit by way of the lingual nerve and then diverge into the chorda tympani, a branch of the seventh cranial nerve. The posterior one third of the tongue, the soft palate, transmits through the ninth cranial nerve, and the remainder of the areas (extreme dorsal portion of tongue, pharynx, and larynx) are transmitted by the 10th cranial nerve. All three of these nerves terminate in the medulla oblongata and form the *tractus solitarius*. From this region, second-order neurons transmit to the thalamus and then on to the postcentral gyrus of the cerebral cortex, where taste sensation shares projection sites with other somatic sensations.

## Taste Disturbances

The sense of taste may be diminished (hypogeusia) secondary to other underlying problems, such as dryness of the tongue, irradiation of the head, respiratory infections, and aging. It occurs with heavy smoking, as well as unilaterally in accompaniment with Bell's palsy. Lesions of the thalamus and parietal lobe may result in impairment or loss of taste on the opposite side of the tongue, and parietal lobe seizures may be heralded by an aura of a specific taste. Certain medications may alter the interpretation of taste.

*Idiopathic hypogeusia* is a syndrome associated with hyposmia, dysomia, and dysgeusia, in conjunction with diminished taste acuity. The smell and taste of food are most unpleasant for these people. They often experience weight loss, depression, and anxiety. One identified cause of this syndrome is depression of zinc content in the parotid saliva.[1]

## Taste Assessment

To assess taste, one examines the function of the eighth, ninth, and tenth cranial nerves. The discrimination of taste in humans is relatively crude, and approximately a 30% concentration of a substance is necessary before discrimination is detected. Thresholds of response to substances vary and sensitivity to bitter tastes, in particular, is much higher than to other tastes. This protective mechanism is significant in that many poisonous alkaloids are characteristically bitter.

In assessing taste, substances that are sweet, sour, salty, and bitter are assembled. They are individually swabbed on the appropriate area of the tongue and the person is asked to identify the taste sensation. To prevent mixing of the substances applied to the tongue, the individual is asked to rinse the mouth after each sensation has been identified.

## SMELL

### Structure and Function

In humans, the sense of smell is closely associated physiologically with the sense of taste. Many foods are perceived partially by both senses, which are chemoreceptors that are stimulated by substances in the nose and mouth. Anatomically, they differ in that the apparatus perceiving smell is not relayed to the thalamus or a cortical projection area.

The receptor cells of olfaction are the *bipolar olfactory cells*, which are located in the olfactory mucous membrane. Unlike other nerve cells, the olfactory cells are continuously dying and generating new ones. Peripherally, these cells have dendrites that terminate on the surface of the mucus of the nasal cavity and project a group of cilia. The axons of the olfactory neurons pass through the *cribriform plate* of the ethmoid bone and enter the olfactory bulb. Here they synapse with second-order neurons, the *mitral cells*, and form a plexus of fibers called the *olfactory glomeruli* or *synaptic glomeruli* (Figure 49-15). Olfactory signals are transmitted from here through the olfactory tract of the axons of the mitral cells and terminate in two principle areas: the prepyriform area and parts of the amygdaloid complex.

Olfactory receptors are stimulated by volatile lipids and water-soluble substances that are inhaled into the mucosa of the nasal cavity. Little is known about the excitatory process of the individual receptor cells, although researchers have elicited several potentials in response to different odors.

Although the physiologic basis for odor discrimination and differentiation is still unknown, several theories have been proposed. Some physiologists have proposed the existence of primary odors that excite specific cells. An attempt to explain how this excitation takes place is proposed by the proponents of the *stereochemical* theory. They believe that the odor molecules fit into specifically shaped receptor sites on the surface of the olfactory microvilli membrane. Other theorists have attempted to explain odor discrimination by the physical properties of the stimulant, such as its molecular vibrations. Electrophysiologic studies have ascertained that different odors stimulate different parts of the olfactory mucosa to varying degrees. On the basis of this, it would appear that olfactory receptors are not specific for a single odor but for a variety of odors to a different degree.[1]

Adaptation is quite rapid in the sense of smell because receptors are readily fatigued by persistent odors. Newly appearing odors may be detected rapidly, however. It requires only a small amount of volatile substance

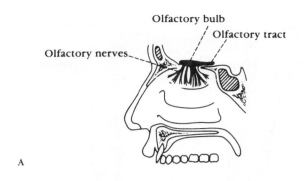

A

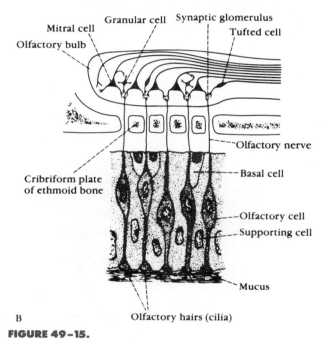

B

**FIGURE 49-15.**
**A.** Distribution of olfactory nerves on lateral wall of the nose.
**B.** Connections between olfactory cells and neurons of the olfactory bulb (Source: R.S. Snell, *Clinical Neuroanatomy for Medical Students.* Boston: Little, Brown, 1980.)

to stimulate the olfactory receptors. Inhalation of irritating substances, such as ammonium salts, produces pain through stimulation of the trigeminal nerve. In addition, certain respiratory reflexes are initiated by its odors.

### Smell Disturbances

*Anosmia*, the loss of smell, is the most frequent disturbance associated with the sense of smell and may accompany such disorders as hypertrophy of nasal mucosa, sinusitis, upper respiratory infections, and allergies. *Hyposmia* is a reduced sense of smell and is most frequently associated with heavy smoking. Facial injuries involving the cribriform plate and certain tumors involving the olfactory groove may result in the loss of smell. Hysteria may be accompanied by anosmia or *hyperosmia* (increased acuity of smell). Olfactory hallucinations and delusions may occur with certain mental illnesses, as well as temporal lobe disorders. Specific smells may precede seizures arising from the uncal region. *Dysosmia* or *parosmia* is a distortion of a smell and may occur as a result of local nasopharyngeal conditions, such as empyema or partial injuries.

## Smell Assessment

The sense of smell can be assessed simply by requesting the individual to identify common aromatic substances, such as coffee, vanilla, and cologne. When doing this, the person is asked to close his or her eyes and occlude the opposite nostril. Although the individual is requested to identify the odor if possible, this ability is less significant than the perception of the odor. Therefore, the individual is asked to identify when he or she initially perceives the odor. The procedure is then repeated for the other nostril and perception is compared.

## REFERENCES

1. Adams, R., and Mauria, V. *Principles of Neurology* (4th ed.). New York: McGraw-Hill, 1989.
2. Carpenter, M., and Sutin, J. *Human Neuroanatomy* (8th ed.). Baltimore: Williams and Wilkins, 1983.
3. Clark, R.G. *Essentials of Clinical Neuroanatomy and Neurophysiology* (5th ed.). Philadelphia: Davis, 1975.
4. Guyton, A.C. *Textbook of Medical Physiology* (8th ed.). Philadelphia: W.B. Saunders, 1990.
5. Hubel, D.H., and Wiesel, T.N. Brain mechanisms of vision. *Sci. Am.* 241:150, 1979.
6. Hudspeth, A.J. The hair cells of the inner ear. *Sci. Am.* 248:59, 1983.
7. Moses, R. *Adler's Physiology of the Eye* (7th ed.). St. Louis: Mosby, 1981.
8. Nauta, W.J., and Feirtag, M. The organization of the brain. *Sci. Am.* 241:99, 1979.
9. Rose, F.C. *The Eye in General Practice.* Baltimore: University Park Press, 1983.
10. Walton, J. *Brain Diseases of the Nervous System* (9th ed.). Oxford: Oxford University Press, 1985.

# chapter 50

Reet Henze

# Common Adaptations and Alterations in Higher Neurologic Function

## Chapter Outline

## Learning Objectives

1. Discuss the major classifications of cerebrovascular disease.

2. Describe the pathologic changes that occur with intracerebral hemorrhages, cerebral thrombosis, and embolism.

3. Locate and discuss cerebral aneurysms and arteriovenous malformations.

4. Relate the clinical manifestations of stroke to the underlying pathologic bases.

5. List clinical findings associated with occlusion of each of the major cerebral arteries.

6. Define *thrombotic stroke in evolution*.

7. List the etiologic factors of stroke.

8. Explain why bleeding is a common complication after initial rupture of an intracerebral aneurysm.

9. Describe the neurologic findings in each of the gradations of ruptured cerebral aneurysms.

10. Discuss the implications of vasospasm with ruptured cerebral aneurysms.

11. Draw or describe the appearance of arteriovenous malformation.

12. Explain why arteriovenous malformations rupture and the significance of the location of the bleeding.

13. Define *aphasia*.

14. Differentiate Wernicke's aphasia, Broca's aphasia, and global aphasia.

15. Define the disorders of speech: *anarthria, agraphia, alexia,* and *word-deafness*.

16. Define *apraxia*.

17. Define *agnosia*.

18. Discuss the various types of agnosia.

19. Define *Gerstmann's syndrome*.

20. Discuss the pathophysiology of epilepsy.

(continued)

## Learning Objectives (Continued)

**21.** Differentiate between primary or idiopathic and secondary or symptomatic seizures.

**22.** Discuss partial versus generalized seizures.

**23.** List some precipitating factors that may initiate seizures.

**24.** Describe changes on the electroencephalogram that correlate with three different types of seizures.

---

Cerebrovascular disease leads to hospitalization for more persons than any other neurologic disorder. Cerebrovascular accidents (CVAs) are the third leading cause of death (after heart disease and cancer) in the United States. Major disabilities frequently remain in those who survive the initial assault. Paresis, aphasia, agnosia, and apraxia are among common associated impairments. Epilepsy is another major neurologic disorder. It ranks second only to CVAs in numbers of persons with neurologic disease in the United States.

## CEREBROVASCULAR DISEASE: PATHOLOGY AND RELATED CLINICAL SIGNS

Cerebrovascular disease results either directly or indirectly, suddenly or over time, from a disruption of cerebral blood flow that causes a variety of brain dysfunctions. The brain does not tolerate anoxia because there exists no oxygen reserve. Therefore, permanent cell damage can occur rather rapidly with a disruption of cerebral blood flow. Short periods of hypoxia (15 minutes or less) generally result in reversible neurologic deficits, whereas those lasting longer can lead to permanent neurologic deficits and cerebral infarction. Those neurologic impairments that result from a sudden disruption of the blood supply to a specific area of the brain are referred to as CVAs or strokes.

Cerebrovascular disease is commonly associated with hypertensive and atherosclerotic disease. Both of these conditions are closely linked with other conditions and risk factors: hypercholesterolemia, arteriovenous malformations (AVMs), arteritis, vasospasm, cigarette smoking, obesity, diabetes mellitus, physical inactivity, emotional stress, and family history of premature atherosclerosis.

As is the case with most neuropathology, the site of a cerebral vascular lesion is more critical in the production of pathologic signs and symptoms than is its pathology. The area of the brain involved is dependent on the specific cerebral vessel affected. Table 50-1 lists major cerebral arteries and the effects associated with their involvement.

**TABLE 50-1.**
CLINICAL FINDINGS WITH OCCLUSION OF MAJOR CEREBRAL ARTERIES

| OCCLUDED ARTERIES | ASSOCIATED FINDINGS |
|---|---|
| Internal carotid system | Contralateral hemiplegia<br>Aphasia with dominant side involvement<br>Blindness, visual blurring<br>Agnosia<br>Hemianopia<br>Cranial nerve deficits<br>Contralateral anosognosia<br>Bruit over occluded artery |
| Middle cerebral artery | Contralateral arm and leg weakness or paralysis<br>Homonymous hemianopia<br>Eye deviation to opposite side<br>Dysphagia or aphasia with dominant side involvement<br>Anosognosia with nondominant hemisphere involvement<br>Contralateral sensory impairment<br>Apraxia with nondominant side involvement |
| Anterior cerebral artery | Contralateral paralysis of leg, foot, and arm (lesser degree)<br>Bladder incontinence<br>Sensory deficit in leg, foot, toes<br>Akinetic mutism<br>Gait impairment<br>Mood disturbance, personality change |
| Vertebral-basilar system | Variations in level of consciousness<br>Hemianopia<br>Possible quadriplegia<br>Eye muscle paralysis<br>Headache<br>Limb weakness<br>Nystagmus<br>Diplopia<br>Mutism<br>Dysarthria<br>Ataxia<br>Dysphagia<br>Varying sensory deficits (numbness)<br>Vertigo<br>Varying cranial nerve deficits |

Cerebrovascular disease is also associated with its etiologic basis: occlusion of cerebral arteries or hemorrhage. Occlusive disease results from thrombosis and embolism. Hemorrhagic disease results from intracerebral, subarachnoid, or AVM bleeding into the brain parenchyma or spaces. Whatever the cause, necrosis of the brain parenchyma may result. Cerebrovascular accidents also can be described according to onset and duration: completed, progressing or evolving, and transient ischemic attack (TIA). A stroke is said to be completed when the blood supply has been cut off to a portion of the brain and permanent neurologic alterations follow. Progressing or evolving stroke progresses over hours or days and finally results in permanent deficits. Transient ischemic attacks are strokes that generally last a few minutes to a few hours and the neurologic deficits resolve.

## Transient Ischemic Attacks

Transient ischemic attacks result in a temporary episode of neurologic dysfunction as a result of a diminished blood supply to a specific area of the brain, generally from thrombotic origins secondary to atherosclerosis (atheroma). Transient ischemic attacks usually last no longer than 15 minutes, although some may exhibit signs up to 24 hours.

Virtually any cerebral artery may be involved and symptoms vary according to the area of involvement. They may be minor focal deficits or major deficits resulting in complete loss of consciousness. Common findings with TIAs include transient episodes of contralateral weakness of the face, arms, and legs (hemiparesis), as well as sensory deficits (hemiparesthesias) and visual impairments. Involvement of the ophthalmic artery results in unilateral visual symptoms, known as amaurosis fugax. In this condition, the individual loses sight in one eye for 2 to 3 minutes as a result of a transient ischemia of the retina.

Transient ischemic attacks may be associated with the development of collateral communicating vessels in the intracerebral arterial system that compensate in a short time for the deficits from the occlusion of one arterial source. Nevertheless, in one study, the findings indicated that 75% of those individuals experiencing a TIA proceeded to have a stroke at a later time.[1]

Diagnosis of TIAs usually requires angiographic evaluation of the location, size, and pathologic process in the cerebral arteries. Radiopaque substances are injected to outline the cerebral vasculature to locate areas of narrowing or disease.

## Occlusive Cerebrovascular Disease

Occlusive cerebrovascular disease results from thrombosis and emboli formation in the cerebral vessels. The effects of occlusion vary with its extent of involvement, time, and location. In addition, the collateral vessels available to divert the remaining circulation affect the blood flow to a specific area of the brain. Obstruction of the flow to any region rapidly results in cell ischemia, and potentially irreversible necrosis and cerebral infarction.

### Cerebral Thrombosis

Ischemic infarction in the brain is often due to cerebral thrombosis that occurs on an atherosclerotic plaque. Atherosclerotic thrombosis is the leading cause of CVAs. The most common areas of thrombosis formation are those where atheromatous plaques have already resulted in narrowing of the vessels. The sites most frequently affected are the internal carotid artery in the region of the carotid sinus, the junction of the vertebral and basilar arteries, the bifurcation of the middle cerebral artery, the posterior cerebral artery in the area of the cerebral peduncle, and the anterior cerebral artery in the area of the corpus collosum.[4]

Wide variations may be observed in clinical signs resulting from disruption of blood flow to specific regions of the brain.

Occlusions of major arteries manifest the clinical findings given in Table 50-1. The resulting obstruction to blood flow may cause infarction to the area supplied by the artery. This type of lesion may be referred to as an atherothrombotic brain infarction (ABI).

Infarcts are often described as red (hemorrhagic) or white (anemia). In the first few days, the pale or white infarcts assume a muddy, mottled appearance that is associated with surrounding tissue edema. After about 10 days, liquefaction of the area becomes evident from the release of neuronal lysosomes and other lytic substances into the brain parenchyma.[2] Scar tissue begins to form at the margins of the necrotic area. The necrotic tissue is removed and replaced by cystic scar tissue. Gliosis (proliferation of glial cells) around the area is characteristic and this is followed by polymorphonuclear leukocyte (PMN) exudation, leading to removal of the necrotic debris. Therefore, characteristic scar tissue is laid down after the acute inflammation subsides.

Red infarcts also cause tissue destruction. Red blood cells are broken down and removed. The necrotic parenchyma undergoes liquefaction, and characteristic scar tissue is formed at the margins of the affected area. Cerebral edema accompanies cerebral infarction and is maximal 3 to 5 days after an acute stroke.[6] It is a major cause of death after acute stroke.

The onset of cerebral thrombosis is usually gradual with periods of progression and periods of improvement. This is apparently due to spread of the thrombus and is called a *thrombotic stroke in evolution*. This thrombosis causes the cerebral infarction, and it may be associated with a hemorrhage into the brain parenchyma.

Symptoms often begin or are noted in the early morning. These may consist of headache, vertigo, mental confusion, aphasia, and focal neurologic signs, which may occur weeks to months before the stroke is completed.

Recovery is variable and depends on the location and the amount of intracerebral damage. Function in an affected leg usually is recovered prior to arm and hand function, which may not return at all.

## Cerebral Embolism

Cerebral embolism is second only to thrombosis as a cause of stroke. The main source of an embolus is the heart. Heart conditions that predispose an individual to cerebral embolization include atrial fibrillation, bacterial endocarditis, rheumatic endocarditis and the valvular diseases that may follow it, and congenital heart disease.[4] Less common sources of emboli are fat or tumor cell emboli. The embolus frequently lodges in the middle cerebral artery, which is a direct continuation of the carotid artery. Massive brain infarction occurs where a large embolus lodges in a major cerebral vessel. Frequently, however, large thrombi break into smaller clots that travel to occlude more distal branches.

The onset of embolic infarction is always very sudden and the effect is immediate. It usually has no warning signs. The clinical features depend on the artery affected and the amount and location of brain infarction (see Table 50-1). Aggressive treatment of the underlying cause must ensue to prevent subsequent episodes.

## Hemorrhagic Cerebrovascular Disease

Cerebrovascular disease as a result of intracranial bleeds is the third leading cause of CVAs. Bleeds may occur in vessels deep within the parenchyma or on the surface of the brain.

### Intracerebral Hemorrhage

Hypertension is the major cause of spontaneous bleeding into the brain parenchyma. Continued grossly elevated blood pressure weakens the vessel and eventually causes its rupture. It is thought that microaneurysms called *Charcot-Buchard aneurysms* form at bifurcations of small intracerebral arteries, probably as a result of the sustained hypertension.[2] The severity of the hemorrhage is related to the amount of blood extravasated and the region of the brain affected. Intracerebral bleeds generally tend to occur deep within the brain substance (Figure 50-1A). The most common areas of bleed in the brain secondary to hypertension are the putamen and the adjacent internal capsule. These areas account for about 50% of cases.[1,2] Other potential areas include the central white matter of the temporal, parietal, and frontal lobes, the thalamus, cerebellum, and pons.

In large bleeds, the extravasation of blood forms a circular type mass that disrupts and compresses surrounding brain tissue, resulting in infarction and tissue necrosis. These hemorrhages may displace midline structures that can compress vital centers, lead to coma, and eventually, death. Commonly, blood seeps into the ventricular

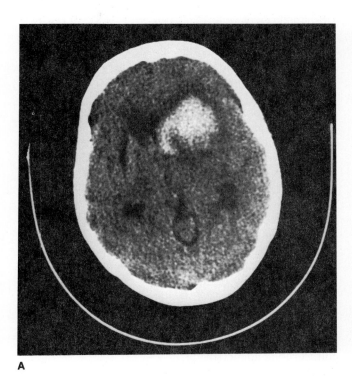

**A**

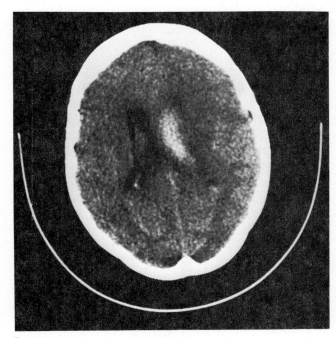

**B**

**FIGURE 50-1.**
**A.** CT scan showing large, right hemispheric intracerebral bleed.
**B.** Same bleed showing intraventricular involvement.

system (Figure 50-1B). Analysis of cerebrospinal fluid (CSF) reflects presence of blood in the great majority of those who have suffered large hemorrhages. Intracerebral hemorrhages may also be small, single bleeds or have several foci. Some may reflect no obvious neurologic deficits, whereas a large number of small hemorrhages in the parenchyma may result in severe neurologic impairment.

Intracerebral bleeds occur abruptly and the symptoms evolve rather rapidly. Prodromal symptoms are generally absent. Severe headache occurs fairly consistently. Other symptoms relate to the region of the brain involved.

Intracerebral hemorrhages commonly occur deep within the brain substance, in the region of the basal ganglia. The bleeding may be massive or have numerous foci. The blood in the parenchyma causes extensive neuronal destruction, and the central area of hemorrhage is often surrounded by small hemorrhages. The blood is treated like foreign material and eventually is broken down, phagocytized by macrophages, and removed from the area. Many mechanisms appear to cause intracerebral hemorrhage, for example, a sudden elevation of blood pressure in the presence of diseased intracranial vessels may cause rupture of the vessels.

Ischemia secondary to arterial spasm may be followed by rupture of the diseased vessels. The most common cause of subarachnoid hemorrhage (bleeding into the ventricles and subarachnoid space) is rupture of an intracerebral aneurysm.

## Aneurysms

The etiology of cerebral aneurysms is mainly related to developmental defects and the resulting aneurysms account for 95% of aneurysms that rupture.[2] Developmental defects involve a weakness in the middle coat (tunica media) of the vessel that results in a saccular outpouching at the weakened area. These so-called *berry aneurysms* can vary from one to several centimeters in size and generally have a well-defined neck that originates most often near bifurcations in the anterior vessels of the circle of Willis (Figures 50-2 and 50-3).[5] Berry aneurysms have the highest frequency of rupture in persons between 30 and 60 years of age, and both sexes are affected equally. Of individuals with developmental cerebral aneurysms, about one fifth demonstrate numerous aneurysms.

Less common than developmental aneurysms are those associated with atherosclerotic degenerative changes of the cerebral vasculature. They are known as fusiform aneurysms and result from weakening of the tunica media secondary to degenerative atherosclerotic processes. The arteries become thin and fibrous, often apparently as a result of long-term hypertension. Al-

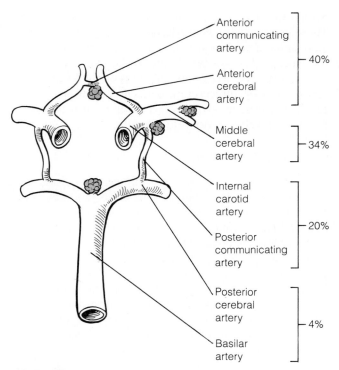

**FIGURE 50-2.**
Common sites for berry aneurysms in the circle of Willis.

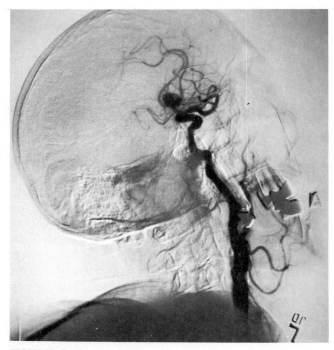

**FIGURE 50-3.**
Anteriogram showing cerebral aneurysm involving the anterior communicating artery.

though fusiform aneurysms of cerebral arteries may occur in some younger individuals, they generally affect those over age 50 years.

Cerebral aneurysms can remain silent for many years, often going undetected throughout life and being discovered only on routine postmortem examination. They become evident during life when they rupture or compress adjacent nerve tissue, causing focal cerebral disturbances.

The signs and symptoms of subarachnoid bleeding from a ruptured aneurysm may be localized from the pressure exerted on surrounding tissue. Focal localizing signs are related to the region of the brain involved and may include visual defects, cranial nerve paralysis, hemiparesis, and focal seizures. Generalized signs of subarachnoid bleeding reflect meningeal irritation and include photophobia, fever, malaise, vomiting, abnormal mentation with disorientation, and nuchal rigidity. If conscious, the person complains of a severe headache of a different nature from any experienced previously. Transitory unconsciousness or extended coma may accompany bleeding from ruptured aneurysms. Initial and prolonged coma generally indicates an unfavorable outcome. It is common to assess neurologic findings after a ruptured cerebral aneurysm according to grade (Table 50-2).

The aneurysm decreases in size after rupture and a fibrin clot forms over the site of the rupture. The individual is at risk of a recurrence of bleeding during the first few weeks after the initial bleed, during the period of clot lysis or breakdown. Recurrent bleeding in cerebral aneurysms considerably increases mortality risk.

Diagnosis of ruptured cerebral aneurysms is based on history, clinical examination, lumbar puncture, cerebral angiography, computed axial tomographic (CT) scans, and magnetic resonance imaging (MRI). Treatment is conservative initially in an effort to stabilize the pathologic processes. When stabilization has been accomplished, surgical intervention is generally necessary to resolve the aneurysm.

Vasospasm frequently accompanies ruptured cerebral aneurysms. It accounts for 50% of the morbidity and mortality of individuals who survive the initial bleed.[3] Because spasm develops within a week or two after the rupture, it results in narrowing of the vessel lumen. This may lead to cerebral ischemia and clinically evident neurologic deficits. The precise cause of vasospasm is unknown but is thought to be related to certain intrinsic chemicals associated with lysis of the clot. These include substances such as serotonin, prostaglandins, catecholamines, histamine, angiotensin, and oxyhemoglobin.[3] In most cases, surgery is delayed until the spasm subsides.

## Arteriovenous Malformations

Vascular malformations usually result from developmental defects of the cerebral veins, capillaries, or arteries in certain localized regions of the brain. These defects have very few distinguishing characteristics with respect to their location. The AVMs may also be secondary to trauma or injury.

The veins appear to connect to the arteries without an intermediate capillary bed (Figure 50-4). The vessel walls are very thin and lack the normal structure of arter-

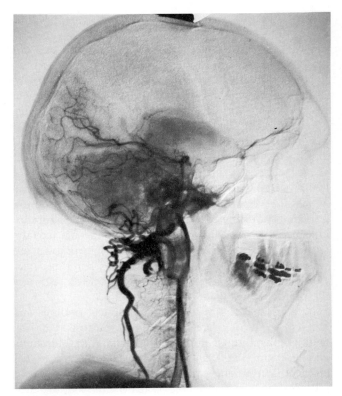

**FIGURE 50-4.**
Arteriogram showing an arteriovenous malformation that is fed by the vertebral artery and drains into superficial veins and internal jugular vein.

**TABLE 50-2.**
GRADES OF RUPTURED CEREBRAL ANEURYSMS

| GRADE | NEUROLOGIC FINDINGS |
|---|---|
| I | Alert and oriented, mild headache, no neurologic deficits |
| II | Alert and oriented, moderate to severe headache, signs of meningeal irritation, minimal neurologic deficits |
| III | Drowsy and confused, pronounced focal neurologic deficits, signs of meningeal irritation |
| IV | Stuperous or unresponsive, major neurologic deficits may be present, mild decerebrate rigidity |
| V | Coma and decerebrate rigidity |

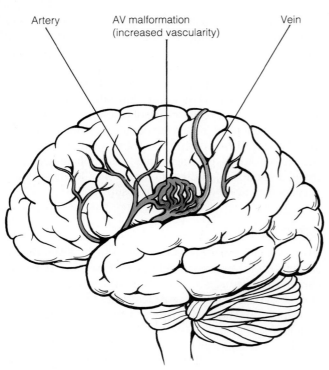

**FIGURE 50-5.**
Appearance of superficial arteriovenous malformation. Vessels are dilated and tortuous.

ies and veins. The malformations are referred to as AVMs or, less appropriately, aneurysms or angiomas (Figure 50-5). They are present most commonly on the surface of the cerebral hemispheres, although they may appear deeper within the cerebral lobes, brainstem, or spinal cord. Although many AVMs are present from birth, they may not become evident until young adulthood or later. Their presence is manifested by symptoms of hemorrhage, seizures, headaches, or focal neurologic deficits. A bruit may be audible over the area of the malformation.

As the very thin walls of these vessels become engorged, the vessels are particularly vulnerable to rupture and bleeding. Bleeding most commonly occurs into the subarachnoid space and, therefore, the symptoms are similar to those observed with ruptured cerebral aneurysms. In addition, specific findings reflect the region of the brain that is involved.

Diagnosis of AVM is based on clinical findings and results of one or more of the following tests: cerebral angiography, lumbar puncture, CT scan, MRI, electroencephalogram (EEG), and radioactive scan. Treatment is surgical ligation and excision of the feeder vessels into the area, whenever possible. If the location of the AVM does not permit surgical excision, embolization may be performed to occlude the feeder vessels in an attempt to reduce the blood flow to the AVM.

## SPEECH DISORDERS

*Language* is defined as audible, articulate human speech produced by the action of the tongue and adjacent vocal cords. *Speech* may be the act of speaking, the result of speaking, the utterance of vocal sounds that convey ideas, or the ability to express thoughts by words. Mechanisms of speech are accomplished through internal symbolization and thought. Language is dependent on retention, recall, visualization, and the integration of symbols. Speech depends on the interpretation of auditory and visual images, which reach the higher human processes during differing states of consciousness and, to some degree, the lower states of consciousness.

Language is a function primarily of the left cerebral hemisphere. Figure 50-6 shows the approximate location of the speech centers in the brain. The ability to produce language is dependent on the normal function and integrity of the primary receptive areas in the temporal and occipital lobes and the expressive areas in the inferior part of the frontal lobe of the dominant hemisphere. To speak, one must initially formulate the thought to be expressed, choose appropriate words, and then control the motor activity of the muscles of phonation and articulation. Simultaneously, accurate recording of visual and auditory stimuli is necessary before the significance of the words used can be appreciated. Language and speech may become impaired in many ways. Regardless of the cause, the results are generally similar when the brain is damaged.

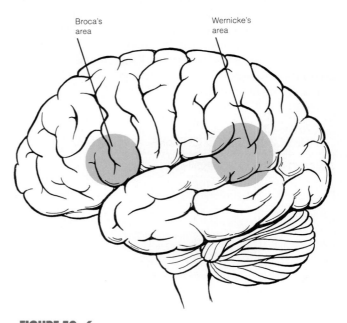

**FIGURE 50-6.**
Location of speech centers in the brain.

# Aphasia

Aphasia is a neurologic defect in speech. The ability either to comprehend and integrate *receptive language* or to formulate and use *expressive language*, or both is impaired. The receptive language modalities are *reading*, which requires visual integration and comprehension of the printed word, and *listening*, which necessitates auditory integration and comprehension of the verbal word. The expressive language modalities are *writing*, which requires visual-motor formulation and use of the printed word, and *speaking*, which requires oral-motor formulation and the use of verbal words. The aphasic individual usually has some impairment of all language modalities.

Aphasia is usually caused by organic disease of the brain that results from a lesion in the left cerebral hemisphere. This hemisphere is considered to be dominant in the reception and expression of language. Infrequently, aphasia has occurred in right-sided lesions associated with right-handed individuals. However, their right-handedness has sometimes been forced or induced. In left-handed persons, lesions of the left or of the right hemispheres may cause aphasia, but most frequently the left.

When certain portions of the cortex and subcortical associated pathways of the dominant hemisphere are altered by lack of blood supply (loss of oxygen or hemorrhage to the brain tissue), speech patterns become altered, limited, or destroyed, depending on the magnitude of the pathology. Vascular disturbances are the most common cause of aphasia. Infarction, caused by thrombotic embolic occlusion of the middle cerebral artery or the left internal carotid artery, is the etiology in the majority of cases, and impairs both spoken and written language. Transient ischemic attacks and migraine headache may trigger transitory speech disorders.

Space-occupying lesions, such as intracerebral hemorrhage, intracranial tumors, and infections, also may cause aphasia. Left hemisphere aphasia results from damage to a specific region of the brain, the first and second temporal gyri, the insula, and the posterior part of the third convolution. Visual and auditory impulses reach the cerebral cortex posteriorly through the occipital lobe and anteroinferiorly through the temporal lobe. There is extraction of the semantic value of the auditory and visual message and of the symbolic formation of the expressed message in the posterior portion of the temporal convolutions. The anterior part of the region is necessary for the motor realization of the expressed message. Many cortical areas and association pathways are concerned in the integration of the function of speech.

Many combinations of vascular, neoplastic, and traumatic causes and locations of lesions lead to different language patterns. Classifications have been developed to define prominent characteristics, to localize position and size of cerebral lesions, and to assess the language deficit pattern in each category of aphasia. The primary types of speech disorders are: (1) Wernicke's aphasia, which causes disturbances of all language activities except articulation; (2) Broca's aphasia, involving disturbances in spoken and written language with dysarthria (disorder of articulation); and (3) selective disorders of receptive and expressive activities of spoken or written language.

## Wernicke's Aphasia

The posterior one third of the superior temporal convolution of the dominant hemisphere is called Wernicke's area (see Figure 50-6). Wernicke's area influences the understanding and interpretation of word symbols. Lesions in other areas, particularly in the posterior half of the dominant hemisphere, angular gyrus, and supramarginal gyrus, influence speech function through the involvement of association fibers.

Wernicke's aphasia is an impairment in comprehension of speech and includes central, receptive, cortical, sensory, auditory, semantic, and conduction aphasia. Affected persons have fluent, spontaneous speech with normal rhythm and articulation but comprehension, repetition, and naming are impaired. Speech appears devoid of meaning despite the fluency and spontaneity. Expression is hindered by difficulty in the choice of words to speak and to write. Repetition, reading aloud, and writing from dictation are deranged. Understanding of spoken language is disturbed. The speech of others is heard but the words are not comprehended. Speech lacks content and contains much meaningless expression.

Lesions in the Wernicke's area inhibit comprehension in spoken and written language because of their interconnections with the angular gyrus. Lesions of the angular gyrus and posteroinferior part of the parietal lobe may cause acalculia, autotopanosia, and disorientation for right and left sides (Table 50-3).

## Broca's Aphasia

The lesion in Broca's aphasia is located in the caudal part of the inferior frontal gyrus rostral to the motor area of the tongue, pharynx, or larynx, or involves the pathways carrying impulses from the temporal lobe to this area (see Figure 50-6). Broca's aphasia includes disorders described as cortical motor, expressive, and verbal aphasias, and disorders in expression of spoken language. The person may not be able to utter a word or may have extremely limited speech. The speech is generally nonfluent, slow, and poorly articulated. Small words are frequently omitted from sentences. Simultaneously, the person fully comprehends the spoken word and obeys commands. Efforts to speak are frustrated by inability to find appropriate words. Agraphia, reduction of written language, coexists

**TABLE 50–3.**
TERMS USED TO DESCRIBE SOME DISORDERS OF HIGHER CORTICAL FUNCTION

| TERM | DEFINITION |
|---|---|
| Acalculia | Inability to solve mathematical problems |
| Agnosia | Loss of comprehension of auditory, tactile, visual, or other sensations although the sensations and the sensory system are intact |
| Auditory agnosia | Inability to recognize auditory objects |
| Tactile agnosia | Inability to identify objects by touch |
| Visual agnosia | Inability to recognize objects seen |
| Verbal agnosia | Inability to recognize spoken language |
| Agrammatism | Inability to arrange words in grammatic sequence or to form a grammatic or intelligent sentence |
| Anosognosia | Lack of awareness of presence of disease, eg, paralysis |
| Apraxia | Inability to carry out a voluntary movement, although the conductive systems are intact |
| Constructional apraxia | Inability to construct models with matchsticks, cubes, etc., to assemble puzzles, or to draw |
| Dressing apraxia | Inability to dress or undress |
| Autotopagnosia | Inability to orient various parts of the body correctly |
| Dysarthria | Disorder of articulation |
| Prosopagnosia | Inability to recognize faces and one's own face |

with aphasia and can be more severe in some individuals. Agrammatism, when present in spoken language, is present in written language (see Table 50-3). The individual is aware of the problem; this frequently leads to feelings of frustration and depression.

### Global Aphasia

Global aphasia is caused by large lesions involving both Broca's and Wernicke's areas of the dominant cerebral hemisphere. Commonly, the lesion is an occlusion of the left internal carotid artery or middle cerebral artery. Blood supply to the language areas of the brain is supplied almost exclusively through the middle cerebral artery.

As the term implies, *global aphasia* affects all aspects of speech. Individuals with global aphasia generally have hemiplegia and are unable to comprehend or speak. At best, they may be able to utter an occasional isolated word or well-known cliche. They are unable to repeat what is said to them and are unable to read and write.

### Selective Disorders of Receptive or Expressive Activities of Spoken and Written Language

The pure disorders of receptive and expressive speech include anarthria, agraphia, alexia, and word-deafness.

In *anarthria*, reading aloud and voluntary speech repetition are disturbed, whereas understanding of spo-

ken and written language and writing remain normal. It usually appears as a sequela of Broca's aphasia.

In *agraphia*, all forms of writing are defective. The lesion may be located in the posterior part of the second frontal gyrus.

*Alexia* severely impairs reading of words, and reading of letters is less obstructed. Language activities may be normal except for the recognition of written symbols. The lesion is located in the lingual and fusiform gyri.

*Word-deafness* is impairment in the understanding of spoken language, repetition, and writing from dictation but all other speech activities are normal. The lesion is in the superior aspect of the temporal lobe.

## APRAXIA

Apraxia is the inability to carry out a voluntary movement, although the conductive systems are intact, indicating cerebral cortical integrative impairment. The person is able to make the individual movements that comprise executing a certain act but cannot execute the total act. There is no paralysis, ataxia, abnormal movement, or sensory loss.

To execute a skilled movement, one must use a logical routine. First, the command is received at the primary auditory cortex and relayed to the auditory association areas for comprehension. The information is relayed by the association fiber systems to the motor association areas in the premotor cortex of the dominant hemisphere. From the dominant premotor cortex, information is conveyed to the premotor and motor cortexes of the nondominant hemisphere to enable the nondominant hand to perform the learned skilled movement.

Apraxia is caused by damage to the association areas or fibers concerned with voluntary motor activity. Lesions in these areas cause impairment in accordance with their locations. Those between the supramarginal gyrus and premotor regions of the dominant parietal lobe may produce bilateral apraxia (see Figure 50-6). They usually also result in an aphasia. Lesions of the dominant premotor association areas may produce bilateral impairment in certain tongue and hand movements. Those of the anterior half of the corpus callosum result in an apraxia of the nondominant hand.

Apraxia of the lips and tongue is fairly common and may occur with lesions of the left supramarginal gyrus or the left motor association cortex, and frequently accompanies apraxia of the limbs. Apraxia of the limbs may be revealed as dressing apraxia (inability to dress or undress), and constructional apraxia (inability to construct models with matchsticks or cubes, assemble puzzles, or draw).

The location of lesions producing the various apraxias is somewhat controversial. All forms of apraxia may occur in cases of diffuse brain damage leading to dementia, which suggests that symptoms may be caused by the mass effect of a lesion rather than its location.

## AGNOSIA

Perception occurs when sensory data originating at sensory receptors are forwarded by peripheral and spinal pathways to the primary sensory cortex for analysis and sorting. These data are dispatched to the association areas that contain the memory banks for higher-order interpretation, and there they are translated into codes and symbols of language. This process of recognizing the significance of sensory stimuli is known as *gnosia*. *Agnosia*, impairment of this faculty of recognition, is caused by lesions of the visual association areas of the cerebral cortex, although the primary sensory pathway is intact.

### Types of Agnosia

The three types of agnosia are: (1) visual agnosia, an inability to recognize objects seen; (2) tactile agnosia, an inability to identify objects by touch; and (3) auditory agnosia (inability to recognize sounds although auditory sensation is intact). A person with visual agnosia may not recognize a safety pin just by looking at it but can name it instantaneously if it is placed in the hand. Conversely, one with tactile agnosia visually identifies the safety pin that one was unable to recognize when it was placed in the hand.

### Visual Agnosia

Visual agnosia is caused by a lesion of the visual association areas. Lesions limited to these areas do not cause blindness. Objects are clearly seen but are not recognized or identified. Visual agnosia is characterized by inability to recognize any object or shape by sight, although it can be recognized through other senses, such as touch or smell. Categories include agnosia for objects, colors, and physiognomies.

Persons suffering from the rare object agnosia are not able to recognize objects visually. Those with color agnosia are unable to recognize colors, a defect that may be confined to one half of the visual fields (called *hemiagnosia* for colors). Agnosia for physiognomies, or prosopagnosia renders the person unable to recognize faces, sometimes even his or her own face in the mirror. The individual is unable to recognize a familiar face but can identify a person once that person starts to speak.

### Tactile Agnosia

Normal tactile recognition is the ability to identify an object by feeling without the help of other sensory information. Feeling movements provide impressions until the object is identified. Lesions of the parietal lobe posterior to the somesthetic area produce tactile agnosia, or the inability to identify objects by touch and feeling. It is often called *astereognosis*. Some previously acquired factual information is lost from the brain's memory stores. Therefore, one cannot compare present sensory phenomena with past experience.

### Auditory Agnosia

Auditory agnosia is the inability to recognize sounds. The auditory sensation is intact but the difficulty is in separating them from the sensory aphasias. The first temporal convolution and part of the second temporal convolution of the dominant hemisphere are considered important for auditory recognition.

From the descriptive point of view, auditory agnosia is the inability to recognize familiar concrete sounds, such as animal noises, a sounding bell, or the ticking of a clock (agnosia for nonlinguistic sounds). Other auditory perceptual disorders include verbal agnosia (the inability to recognize spoken language), sensory amusia (the inability to recognize music), and congenital auditory agnosia (primary retardation of speech development, usually associated with mental retardation).

## BODY IMAGE

Humans build images of their bodies from sensory impulses from the special senses (skin, muscles, bones, and joints) that provide information of relationships with the body and the external environment. This concept of body image is stored in the association areas of the parietal lobes.

Lesions of the nondominant parietal lobe, particularly the inferior parietal lobe, may create abnormalities in concepts of body image. Lack of awareness of the left side of the body despite intact cortical and primary sensation is exhibited. Lack of awareness of hemiparesis may be noted. The person may perceive sensory stimuli applied independently to the two sides of the body but if sensory stimuli are applied bilaterally simultaneously, one is generally ignored.

### Gerstmann's Syndrome

Lesions of the left (dominant) parietal lobe, particularly the supramarginal and angular gyrus areas, may produce one or more of a complex of symptoms known as Gerstmann's syndrome (bilateral asomatognosia). It includes right-left disorientation, that is, inability to distinguish right from left. Finger agnosia is exhibited by failure to recognize one's fingers in the presence of intact sensation and is associated with constructional apraxia. Acalculia (inability to solve mathematical problems) and dyslexia (inability to read) are common when the lesion involves the angular gyrus.

## SEIZURE DISORDERS

*Epilepsy*, a general term used synonymously in this chapter with seizure disorders, is characterized by sudden, excessive discharges of electrical energy in neurons. These may occur within a structurally normal or diseased central nervous system. The discharge may trigger a convulsive movement, interrupt sensation, alter consciousness, or lead to some combination of these disturbances. Seizures may originate from diverse factors that are metabolic, toxic, degenerative, genetic, infectious, neoplastic, and traumatic, as well as from unknown factors.

Seizures may be linked with increased local excitability (epileptogenic focus), reduced inhibition, or a combination of both. Some neurons in focal lesions have been identified as hypersensitive and remain in a state of partial depolarization. Increased permeability of their cytoplasmic membranes makes these neurons susceptible to activation by hyperthermia, hypoglycemia, hyponatremia, hypoxia, repeated sensory stimulation, and even certain phases of sleep. Reduced inhibition may be caused by a lesion of the cortex.

Once the intensity of a seizure discharge has progressed sufficiently, it may spread to adjacent cortical, thalamic, brainstem nuclei, as well as other regions of the brain. Excitement feeds back from the thalamus to the primary focus and to other parts of the brain. This process is evidenced by the high-frequency discharge shown on

evidenced by the high-frequency discharge shown on EEG. Within the process, a diencephalocortical inhibition intermittently interrupts the discharge and converts the tonic phase (neuron depolarization) to the clonic phase and polarized cell membranes. The discharges become less and less frequent until they cease.

Severe seizures may cause systemic hypoxia with accompanying acidosis from increased lactic acid, which may result from respiratory spasms, airway blockage, and excessive muscular activity that accompanies seizures. An extremely severe prolonged seizure can cause respiratory arrest or cardiac standstill. Metabolic needs increase markedly during a seizure, causing increased cerebral blood flow, glycolysis, and tissue respiration.

### Electroencephalography in Seizures

The EEG is a sensitive tool for diagnosis and clinical evaluation of epilepsy. Despite its value, the diagnosis of epilepsy should not be based solely on the EEG findings because some individuals have abnormal EEGs without clinical signs of seizure activity and a significant number of those exhibiting clinical signs of epilepsy present normal EEGs.

The electrical discharges produced by the brain's electrical activity are called *brain waves* and are recorded by electrodes placed on the surface of the scalp. Because the EEG is a surface recording, it reflects the most superficial activity, especially that of the cerebral cortex. The waves are recorded while the person is awake and resting in a darkened room or with the eyes closed. Movements and external distractions are minimized. During a recording of the brain's waves, the subject may be asked to hyperventilate to stimulate characteristic seizure activity secondary to alkalosis and vasoconstriction. Certain provocative techniques, photic stimulation, and sleep deprivation may be useful in initiating abnormal electrical activity in some persons. Electroencephalographic recording during sleep may also be useful in detecting abnormalities.

In normal adults, the dominant activity in the parietal occipital areas occurs at 8 to 13 cycles per second (cps),

**Number of complete cycles of a rhythm in one second (cps)**

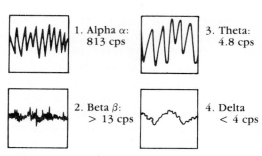

1. Alpha α: 813 cps
2. Beta β: > 13 cps
3. Theta: 4.8 cps
4. Delta < 4 cps

**FIGURE 50-7.**
Frequency of brain waves.

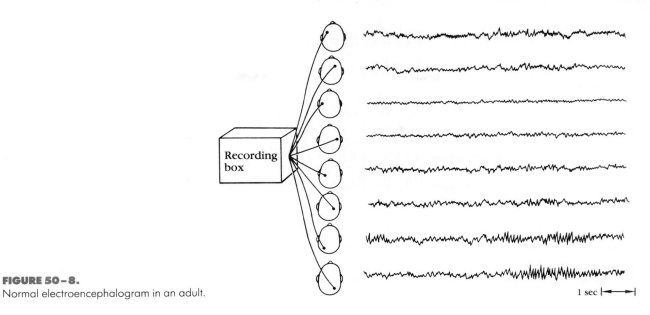

**FIGURE 50–8.**

Normal electroencephalogram in an adult.

1 sec |◄————►|

identified as *alpha rhythm*. In the frontal areas, the dominant activity is of lower amplitude and faster frequency (greater than 13 cps), and is known as *beta rhythm*. Slower frequencies than alpha rhythm are recognized as slow waves. Those 4 to 7 cps are *theta rhythms*, and 1 to 3 cps are *delta rhythms* (Figure 50-7). Theta waves are considered abnormal sometimes, whereas delta waves are always abnormal EEG waves, indicating injury to brain tissue. Other abnormalities are spike, high voltage waves, and asymmetrical frequency and amplitude between the hemispheres. Normal EEG variations occur in individuals. Age differences are noted on the EEG (Figures 50-8 and 50-9). An infant at 13 months has dominant awakened activity of 4 to 5 cps; at age 5 years, 6 to 7 cps; and at age 12 years, 8 to 9 cps (alpha rhythm).

Abnormalities in EEGs are useful in diagnosing epilepsy, particularly if recorded during the seizure activity. During petit mal epilepsy, one can observe repetitive slow regular rhythmic outbursts consisting of spike and delta waves at a frequency of 3 Hz (Figure 50-10). Grand mal epilepsy reflects high frequency spikes (Figure 50-11), and temporal lobe seizures may demonstrate spikes or rhythmical outbursts of the slower delta or theta waves. Electroencephalograms may be normal between seizures. Brain masses such as tumors, hematomas, and abscesses may demonstrate localized slow-wave (delta)

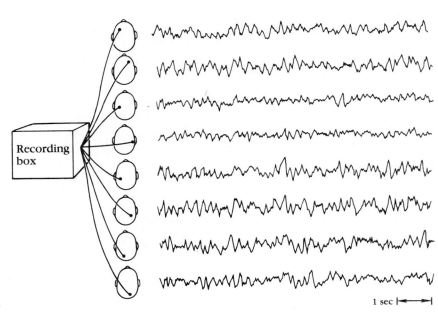

**FIGURE 50–9.**

Normal electroencephalogram in a child.

1 sec |◄————►|

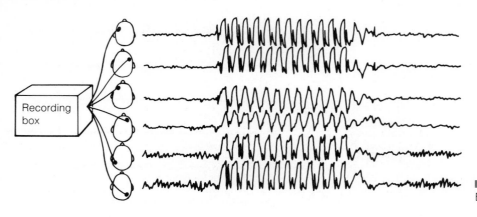

**FIGURE 50–10.**
EEG appearance during petit mal seizure.

activity. Stupor and coma produce widespread, diffuse slow-wave activity.

Encephalopathy may produce theta waves. Asymmetrical, localized spike and wave patterns are recorded over areas of involvement in partial seizures. In some neurologic degenerative conditions, such as Parkinson's and muscular dystrophy, the EEG may remain normal.

The EEG is useful in determining brain death. Electrocerebral silence (isoelectric EEG) is indicative of irreversible coma associated with global cerebral ischemia.

## Classification of Seizures

Seizures have been classified according to location of the focus, etiologic basis, and clinical features. The International Classification System listed in Box 50-1 has been adopted worldwide and is used in this chapter. It is based on clinical features and associated EEG findings in seizures that are generalized or partial. *Generalized seizures* have bilaterally symmetric epileptigenic foci originating within deep subcortical diencephalic structures,

whereas partial seizures usually begin in a cortical focus but may arise from subcortical structures. Seizures may be *primary* or *idiopathic* if their origin is unknown, or *secondary* or *symptomatic* if a definitive diagnosis is determined.

## Generalized Seizures

Generalized seizures involve both cerebral hemispheres and commonly result in loss of consciousness, which may vary from a very brief episode to a more prolonged time. Anterograde and retrograde amnesia frequently accompany the loss of consciousness. The most common forms of generalized seizures are petit mal (absence) and grand mal (tonic-clonic). Generalized seizures also include myoclonic and akinetic types.

### Absence Seizures (Petit Mal)

These seizures exhibit a characteristic spike-and-wave pattern with 3 cps on the EEG. The term *absence seizure*

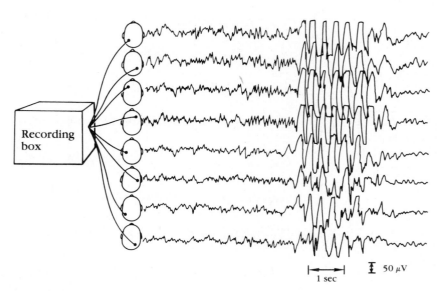

1 sec    ⬍ 50 µV

**FIGURE 50–11.**
EEG appearance during grand mal seizure.

**BOX 50–1.**
INTERNATIONAL CLASSIFICATION OF SEIZURES

I. Partial seizures (focal origin)
   A. Simple
      1. Motor (Jacksonian)
      2. Sensory (visual, auditory, olfactory, gustatory, vertiginous)
      3. Autonomic
      4. Psychic
   B. Complex (impaired consciousness)
      1. Temporal lobe (psychomotor)
   C. Secondary generalization
      1. Simple or complex
II. Generalized seizures (symmetrical bilaterally, no focal onset)
   A. Tonic-clonic (grand mal)
   B. Absence (petit mal)
      1. Simple—loss of consciousness
      2. Complex—brief tonic, clonic, or automatic movement
   C. Myoclonic
   D. Infantile spasms
   E. Atonic (astatic, akinetic)
   F. Lennox–Gestaut syndrome
III. Unilateral tonic, clonic seizures.
   A. With impaired consciousness
   B. Without impaired consciousness
IV. Unclassified epileptic seizures

is used because the person, although present physically, is absent with respect to higher cortical functions during the episode. The majority of such persons have normal intelligence and have no significant abnormal physical findings on neurologic examination. Onset is usually about age 5 years and attacks are most prevalent in childhood. Absence seizures decrease after puberty.

Petit mal seizures are characterized by a loss of awareness that may be accompanied by automatisms, such as flicking of the eyelids, twitching of facial muscles, or staring into space while general postural tone is preserved. They may be precipitated by seeing bright or flashing lights or hearing loud noises, and may be preceded by hyperventilation. Attacks may recur numerous times during the day. They may last from 5 to 10 seconds, after which consciousness is abruptly restored and the interrupted activity is promptly resumed. Memory may be defective only through the seizure. As the person reaches adolescence, frequency decreases and the individual may develop other types of seizures, usually grand mal.

### Tonic-Clonic Seizures (Grand Mal)

Electrical disruption with grand mal seizures originates anywhere in the forebrain and usually engulfs the whole forebrain. The epileptic discharge shows nonfocal changes of high amplitude and rapid synchronous bursts on the EEG. For several hours preceding the seizure, vague prodomal sensations, such as epigastric distress, muscular twitching, or other unnatural sensations, may occur. Commonly, a brief aura consisting of a specific movement or unnatural sensation is the last thing the individual remembers before losing consciousness.

After the aura, if present, the individual abruptly loses consciousness, falls to the ground, and suffers generalized tonic contractions, followed by clonic contractions of all muscles. Muscle contraction in the tonic phase lasts for a few seconds. The entire body becomes rigid with the arms and legs extended. The jaws become clenched, the head may be retracted, and the eyeballs are rolled backward. As air is forced through the closed vocal cords, a loud cry may emit. Breathing usually ceases during this time. Movements become jerky in the clonic phase as muscle groups contract and relax. The arms and legs contract and relax forcibly. Breathing becomes noisy and stertorous, and profuse perspiration is noted. Excessive salivation and loss of bladder or bowel sphincter control may also occur.

Contractions become slower, sometimes irregular, and then stop. The entire seizure may last up to 10 minutes. Spasms of the tongue and jaw may cause biting injuries to the tongue or cheeks. Unconsciousness for the entire seizure is characteristic and may continue up to one-half hour after the episode. As consciousness is regained, the individual is often briefly confused, fatigued, and drowsy, and complains of muscle soreness. The individual has no memory of the seizure attack but usually remembers the aura. In the early part of the postseizure period, there may be reflex signs characteristic of upper motor neuron disorder (see Chap. 52). Paralysis may follow the attack for a short time and is described as post-convulsive (*postictal*) or *Todd's paralysis*.

Febrile grand mal convulsions frequently occur in children under age 5 years, predominantly between 6 months and 3 years of age. They are generalized and of short duration. These children have a high familial frequency of this type of seizure and may suffer from nonfebrile convulsions in later life.

Grand mal seizures that follow one another without restoration of consciousness are called *status epilepticus*, or seizures without interruption. This disorder is serious, producing exhaustion, hypoxia, acidosis, and other metabolic derangements. Hospitalization and prompt pharmacotherapy are urgent to prevent irreversible brain damage or death.

### Myoclonic Seizures

Individuals with myoclonic seizures have sudden rapid flexion of the limbs and trunk singularly or repeatedly, generally with a momentary loss of consciousness.

Loud sounds or bright lights may precipitate the episodes. Intentional movement worsens them. These disorders occur with greatest frequency in childhood but may continue after puberty. Bilateral, synchronous 3 cps discharges are noted on EEG during each episode.

Myoclonic spasms occurring in infancy, called *massive spasms,* are first noted at 6 to 9 months of age, and continue to age 2 or 3 years. There is usually associated retardation of psychomotor development, and the spasms may be related to other conditions, such as phenylketonuria, perinatal brain damage, pyridoxine deficiency, or tuberous sclerosis. Myoclonic spasms may be generalized or multifocal and tend to disappear with growth but other seizure patterns may emerge. In adults, myoclonic seizures may accompany dementia in conditions such as Creutzfeldt-Jacob disease and certain acute conditions, such as acute viral encephalitis (see Chap. 53). A benign form of myoclonus has been described that is associated with sudden myoclonic jerks when falling asleep or awakening.

### Akinetic Seizures

In these seizures, persons experience sudden loss of consciousness and fall to the ground without contraction or motion. Muscle tone is lost briefly but stance is resumed almost immediately. A history of infantile spasms and mental retardation is often present.

### Infantile Spasms

Characteristically, infantile spasms affect children in the 3-month to 2-year-old group. These seizures may be associated with an unknown metabolic disturbance (primary infantile spasms) or caused by a variety of known degenerative, structural birth injuries or developmental conditions: amino acid abnormalities, phenylketonuria, and tuberous sclerosis (secondary infantile spasms). The seizures are characterized by flexor spasms of the extremities and frequently are associated with mental retardation.

### Lennox-Gestaut Syndrome

The Lennox-Gestaut seizures occurring in childhood are associated with prolonged seizures in a febrile episode of acute encephalitis or encephalopathy. These seizures may recur spontaneously or with subsequent infections and febrile illnesses. These febrile-associated seizures may be compounded with atonic and ataxic spells, tonic seizures, as well as atypical petit mal and psychomotor seizures. Mental retardation is a common finding with this syndrome.

## Partial Seizures

Partial seizures arise from a focal area and progress in a manner consistent to the area of irritation. They are char-acterized by specific, repeated patterns of activity and are of two general types: *simple* or *elementary*, in which consciousness remains unimpaired, and *complex*, in which there is accompanying alteration in consciousness. Partial seizures may have a motor, sensory, or varied complex focus.

### Focal Motor Seizures (Jacksonian Seizures)

Focal motor seizures usually originate in the premotor cortex and cause involuntary movements of the contra-lateral limbs. A common manifestation is the turning of the individual's head and eyes away from the irritable focus (contraversive movement). This may be the extent of the seizure or it may start in one portion of the pre-motor cortex and spread gradually in clonic movements to the adjacent region. The clinical manifestations change accordingly.

Typically, the convulsive movement in Jacksonian seizures begins in the distal portion of an extremity and progresses medially. For example, a seizure starting in the foot may move up the leg, down the arm, and to the face; or it may begin in the hand, spread to the face, and then to the leg. This is called *jacksonian march*. The seizure begins with a tonic contraction and rapidly progresses to a clonic movement. The episode may last 20 to 30 seconds without loss of consciousness. Conversely, it may spread to the opposite hemisphere with resultant loss of consciousness, thus becoming a generalized seizure. Despite the greater frequency of focal seizures in young children, the jacksonian march appears most often in adults and adolescents; focal motor seizures may also occur in certain metabolic derangements.

### Focal Sensory Seizures

A lesion in the postcentral or precentral convolution of the sensory cortex in the parietal lobe provokes focal sensory seizures. A simple, uniform, tactile, auditory, or visual experience with complaints of numbness, tingling, pins-and-needles sensation, coldness, or a sensation of water running over a portion of the body may be described. This type of seizure usually begins in the lips, fingers, and toes, and remains localized or progresses to adjacent body parts. If the lesion is in the sensory association area, the experience is more complex and may be visual or auditory. If visual, sensations of light, darkness, or color may be experienced. If auditory, the person may complain of buzzing, roaring in the ears, or hearing voices or words. Consciousness and memory are preserved.

### Complex Partial Seizures (Psychomotor)

Temporal lobe structures, the medial surface of the hemispheres, and the limbic system are involved with this disorder. However, certain psychomotor seizures may arise from the frontal lobe. Children, as well as adults, are affected with this form of seizure. The person may exhibit bizarre behavior and exaggerated emotionality. These seizures may be characterized by slow, paroxysmal waves in either the anterior or posterior leads of the EEG. Episodic fluctuations in attitude, attention, behavior, or memory occur. The individual seems to interact in a purposeful, although inappropriate, manner. Seizures may begin with an olfactory aura or an unpleasant smell or taste. On other occasions, the person may experience hallucinations or perceptual illusions, or perceive strange objects or people as familiar (*deja vu*) and familiar objects and people as strange (*jamais vu*). The person appears to be in a dreamy state and may be unresponsive to vocal stimulation but mechanically performs a task while the seizure is progressing (automatisms). These abnormal movements and inappropriate speech may also be associated characteristics. Strong epigastric and abdominal sensations commonly occur.

Later, episodic recall is lost and the individual is amnesic to the aberrant behavior. Automatisms, when present, include chewing, smacking, licking of the lips, or clapping of the hands. Less frequently, the head and eyes may turn to one side, or tonic spasms of the limbs may occur. Some psychomotor seizures last about a minute, some may continue for hours, and others may progress to tonic, tonic-clonic, or other forms of generalized seizures.

## Secondary or Symptomatic Generalized Seizures

Secondary seizures are caused by some metabolic or structural underlying disorder. Metabolic disturbances can result from conditions such as renal failure, hypoglycemia, hypoxia, hyponatremia, hypernatremia, hypercalcemia, hepatic failure, or withdrawal of drugs.

Meningitis and encephalitis in children lead to strong convulsive tendencies. After recovery, there may be residual recurrent generalized, focal, or psychomotor seizures.

Many structural lesions are caused by disorders in cerebral blood supply, intracranial tumors, or scarring of the brain. These can produce various types of seizure activity.

## REFERENCES

1. Adams, R., and Maurice, V. *Principles of Neurology* (4th ed.). New York: McGraw-Hill, 1989.
2. Cotran, R.S., Kumar, V., and Robbins, S.J. *Pathologic Basis of Disease* (4th ed.). Philadelphia: W.B. Saunders, 1989.
3. Jackson, L. Cerebral vasospasm after intracranial aneurysmal subarachnoid hemorrhage: A nursing perspective. *Heart Lung* 15:14, 1986.
4. Pallett, P., and O'Brien, M. *Textbook of Neurological Nursing.* Boston: Little, Brown, 1985.
5. Stein, J.H. (ed.). *Internal Medicine.* Boston: Little, Brown, 1983.
6. Wall, M. Cerebral thrombosis: Assessment and nursing management of acute phase. *J. Neurosci. Nurs.* 18:36, 1986.

# chapter 51

Barbara L. Bullock

# Pain

## Chapter Outline

▶ **Neurophysiology of Pain**
　　**Pain Receptors and Pathways**
　　**Endogenous Pain Control**
　　　**System**
▶ **Pain Theory**
　　**Gate-Control Theory**

▶ **Acute Versus Chronic Pain**
　　**Acute Pain**
　　**Chronic Pain**
　　　Possible Physiologic Changes
　　　Classifying Chronic Pain
　　　　*Pain Sensation*
　　　　*Pain Behavior*
　　　　*Functional Status at Work*
　　　　　*or Home*
　　　　*Emotional State*
　　　　*Somatic Preoccupation*

▶ **Specific Types of Pain**
　　**Cutaneous Pain**
　　**Visceral Pain**
　　**Referred Pain**
　　**Headache**
　　**Phantom Limb Pain**
　　**Hyperalgesia**

## Learning Objectives

1. Define *pain* in terms of cause and individual effect.
2. Describe the pain receptors through which pain perception is achieved.
3. Differentiate between fast or acute pain and slow or dull pain.
4. Define the purposes of the neospinothalamic and paleospinothalamic tracts.
5. Describe the spinoreticular system.
6. Describe the important chemical transmitters involved in pain modulation.
7. Discriminate between cutaneous pain and deep somatic pain.

8. Explain the gate-control theory.
9. Discriminate between the causes of and reactions to acute and chronic pain.
10. Discuss the effects of chronic pain on human physiology and psychosocial interactions.
11. Locate the sites of referred pain according to the affected deep organ.
12. Compare intracranial and extracranial headache regarding cause and clinical picture.
13. Define *hyperalgesia, neuralgia,* and *causalgia.*

Pain is a sensation caused by some type of noxious stimulation. It is described with many terms such as mild, severe, chronic, acute, burning, dull, sharp, referred, localized, throbbing, or crushing. Because pain makes a person aware of something that may cause tissue damage, it is considered to be a protective mechanism. Pain is usually perceived as a warning that something is amiss, and it prompts the individual to take some action, such as seeking medical help. Pain is always subjective in nature. The response to the painful sensation is also subjective and individual, highly influenced by the person's culture, so-

ciety, race, and sex. Study of the pain response has led to some understanding of the mechanisms by which pain is perceived, mediated, and transported. There is less understanding concerning the highly individual responses to the painful experience. Table 51-1 gives some definitions that are helpful in sorting out the various components of pain perception and response. These help to keep the concept in perspective while indicating the psychological and physiological natures of the phenomenon.

　　Pain signals the person that an injured (damaged) part of the body needs attention or rest, and the person

**TABLE 51–1.**
DEFINITIONS OF PAIN

| TERM | DEFINITION |
| --- | --- |
| Pain | An unpleasant sensory and emotional experience associated with actual or potential tissue damage, or described in terms of such damage |
| Pain receptor | A primitive, unorganized, weedlike nerve ending with many overlapping branches from receptors above and below it |
| Afferent pain fibers | Pain-conducting fibers for both fast and slow pain signals; A fibers are rapid conducting; C delta fibers are slow conducting |
| Epicritic pain | Specific, localized, cutaneous conducting from a specific skin area, usually referred to as a dermatome |
| Protopathic pain | Deep somatic and visceral pain conducted through larger, more diffuse pathways causing a generalized, poorly localized pain |
| Spinothalamic tracts | Principal pain conducting pathways in the spinal cord |
| Reticulospinal tract | Pain conducting pathway of more diffuse nature still passing through segments of sympathetic ganglia to the thalamus and cerebral cortex |
| Pain stimuli | May be detectable injury or may not be known; the stimuli cause a reported pain sensation; the effect depends on the presence of other peripheral stimuli and on CNS activity; stimuli differ in their effectiveness according to changes in the CNS response |
| Impairment | Loss or abnormality of psychologic, physiologic, or anatomic structure or function |
| Functional limitation | Restriction or inability to perform an activity in the manner considered normal for a human being; includes loss of capabilities due to inability to integrate physical and psychologic function due to pain or other impairment |
| Disability | A disadvantage for an individual that limits or prevents fulfillment of a normal role |
| Operational definitions | Considering the presenting complaints in terms of pain sensation and behavior, functional status at work and home, emotional state, and somatic preoccupation |

Sources: *P. Wall and R. Melzack, Textbook of Pain (2nd ed.). Edinburgh: Churchill-Livingstone, 1989; M. Fuerstein, Definitions of pain, in C.D. Tollison, Handbook of Chronic Pain Management, Baltimore: Williams & Wilkins, 1989; H. Mersky, Classifications of chronic pain: Descriptions of chronic pain syndromes and definitions of pain terms, Pain Suppl. 3, S217, 1986: and M. Osterweis, A. Kleinman, and D. Mechanic, Pain and Disability: Clinical, Behavioral and Public Policy Perspectives, Washington, D.C.: National Academy Press, 1987.*

takes action to decrease the perception of pain.[17] The pain signal also may be present to facilitate stillness to allow an injured part to heal.[14] These concepts are valid for acute, short-term pain but do not help to explain the suffering of long-term or chronic pain. As is discussed later in this chapter, there is a significant difference in pain types and, thus, in the pain response.

## NEUROPHYSIOLOGY OF PAIN

### Pain Receptors and Pathways

Pain receptors, also called *nociceptors,* are naked nerve endings found in nearly every tissue of the body.[3] These respond to thermal, chemical, and mechanical stimulation. The degree or amplitude of the stimulation determines whether the perception is pleasurable or painful. The two major types of receptors are small myelinated A delta fibers and larger unmyelinated C fibers. The A delta fibers conduct impulses at a very rapid rate and are responsible for transmitting acute sharp pain signals from the peripheral nerves to the spinal cord.[4] The A delta fibers are activated by thermal and mechanical stimuli.[10] The type C fibers transmit sensory input at a much slower rate and probably produce slow chronic type of pain. The C fibers respond to thermal, mechanical, and chemical stimulation.[10] The usual initiating process for the acute pain response involves a traumatic event (such as cutting the finger), which produces a bright, sudden, sharp pain

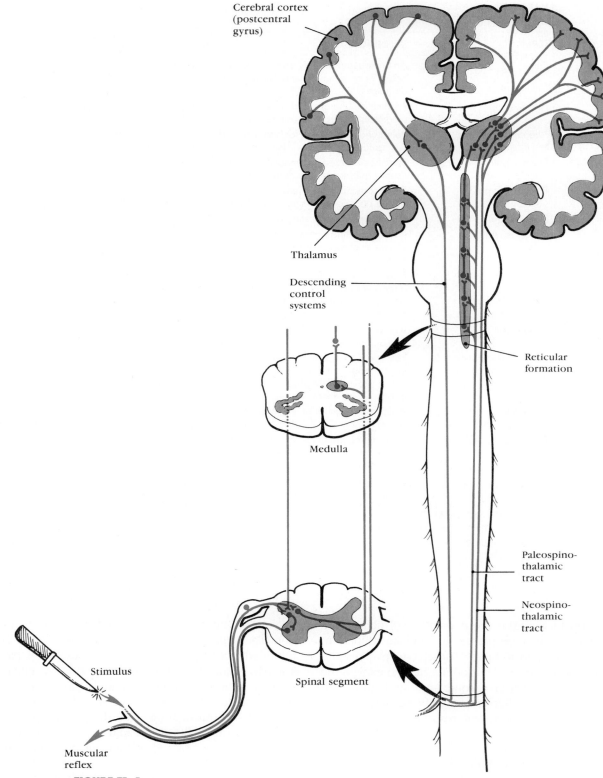

**Cerebral cortex (postcentral gyrus)**

**Thalamus**

**Descending control systems**

**Reticular formation**

**Medulla**

**Paleospino-thalamic tract**

**Neospino-thalamic tract**

**Stimulus**

**Spinal segment**

**Muscular reflex**

**FIGURE 51–1.**
The CNS pathways. Sensory nerves transmit stimuli from pain receptors into the dorsal root ganglia. The impulses travel to the spinal cord, synapse, cross the cord, and ascend to either the neospino-thalamic or paleospinothalamic branch of the spinothalamic tract. The tract rises to the medulla, where the paleospinothalamic projects a branch into the brainstem reticular formation. Branches also enter the pons and midbrain. The neospinothalamic branch proceeds directly into the cortex, synapsing in the midbrain and transmitting impulses into the postcentral gyrus, where pain is perceived. (Adapted from C. Chapman and J. Bonica, *Acute Pain,* Kalamazoo, MI: Scope, 1983.)

that is followed in a second or so by a slow, burning, throbbing pain. As the slow pain continues, the pain is usually perceived to be more severe, and after a variable period of time it may be perceived as intolerable.

Pain is perceived when the tolerance at the site is reached and the impulses are sent along the sensory pathway to the dorsal root ganglia, then to the spinal cord, after which they cross over into the spinothalamic tract. *Pain tolerance* refers to that variable period of time of pain endurance before a pain response is initiated. As described above, when the pain stimulus is repetitive or continuous, the tolerance for it usually decreases. Pain tolerance is a very individual characteristic for persons and is influenced by family, race, culture, personality, and by life situations. *Pain threshold*, on the other hand, is the point at which the noxious stimulus is perceived as pain. Acute painful stimuli will take precedence over long-term or chronic pain. Thus, the description of the pain is often localized to the acute pain, with later description of other painful sites when the acute pain subsides.

The spinothalamic tract is divided into two parts: the neospinothalamic and paleospinothalamic tracts (Figure 51-1). The neospinothalamic tract begins at the synapse in the dorsal horn, and crosses and ascends to the lateral side of the spinal cord with fibers synapsing in the thalamus, and then to the cortex. It transmits sharp, localized pain, which can be specifically recognized by the person experiencing it. The paleospinothalamic tract carries less localized pain. It arises in the lamina regions of the spinal cord and sends branches to the reticular formation of the brain-stem structures, then finally to the structures of the forebrain. It is thought to transmit burning and dull pain. When pain becomes chronic, there may be associated peripheral factors or it may be due to central nervous system damage or psychological abnormalities in a histologically normal brain.[6]

The dorsal root ganglia, described in detail in Chapter 48, are found on the dorsal or posterior root of all spinal nerves and conduct impulses into the spinal cord. The spinal or segmental nerve conducts the epicritic (discriminated, usually acute) pain from a specific area on the skin called a *dermatome*.[5] The dermatomes are described and illustrated in Chapter 48. The dermatomes usually have distinct boundaries but a ganglion may carry some information from the dermatome immediately above or below it.[5] Deep somatic and visceral pain is usually poorly localized and discriminated. It is also called *protopathic pain* and is not as rigidly related to the nerve roots. It may travel with the autonomic nerve fibers that supply the affected area.[5]

The processing in the cortex allows for discriminative, exact, and meaningful interpretation of pain but this processing is not necessary to the perception of pain.[3] In other words, pain can be experienced without precise processing in the cerebral cortex as has been noted in

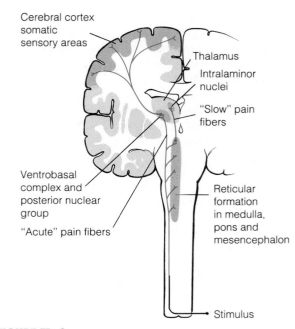

**FIGURE 51–2.**
Perception of pain may occur in the mesencephalon and/or higher cortical levels.

cases of severe head injury. About three fourths to nine tenths of pain fibers terminate in the medulla, pons, and mesencephalon; from these areas, higher order neurons are transmitted to the thalamus, hypothalamus, and cerebrum (Figure 51-2).[4] A small number of acute pain fibers pass directly to the thalamus and are then transmitted to the cerebral cortex to precisely localize the pain source. A great number of slow-chronic pain fibers terminate in the reticular formation of the brain stem and excite the reticular activating system (see Chap. 48). These then serve the function of arousing and promoting actions to rid the body of the painful stimulus.[4] These pathways are localized only to gross areas of the body.

Pain response is never simple. Despite extensive research, the mechanism and perception is still not totally understood. The acute response previously described is relatively predictable in that there is a tissue damaging stimulus that usually provokes a physical, as well as a subjective, response. The physical response to a pin-prick, for example, is reflex withdrawal from the pin, while pain from deep tissue damage usually causes tonic muscle contractions and immobility to splint the area.[17] In the pin-prick example, the information is projected to the postcentral gyrus, which then allows for cognitive discrimination of the source of tissue injury.

The known stimuli that produce the response from nociceptors are released in damaged tissue. These tissues release substances such as *prostaglandins, bradykinins, histamines,* and other chemotactic substances. These substances cause the stimulation of the nociceptors, and the pain persists as long as the stimuli are in the tissues. *Substance P*, present in synaptic vesicles of the unmyelinated fibers, activates the pain response when it is released after injury. An attempt has been made to link the magnitude of the pain response to the amount of substance P released into the tissues. This view is very poorly substantiated in actual clinical practice and underscores the fact that the pain response is unique to the individual perceiving it.

## Endogenous Pain Control System

The brain has the capability to control the intensity of pain signals by activation of an endogenous pain control system. This system, illustrated in Figure 51-3, consists of three major parts: the *periaqueductal gray area* of the mesencephalon and upper pons, the *raphe magnus nucleus*, and a *pain inhibitory complex* located in the dorsal horns of the spinal cord.[4] Many of the nerve fibers secrete *enkephalin*, and the fibers originating in the raphe magnus nucleus that terminate in the dorsal horns of the spinal cord secrete *serotonin*. Serotonin acts on another set of local cord neurons that secrete enkephalin.[4] Enkephalins bind to specific receptors and inhibit the release of substance P, thus providing analgesia for nociceptive stimulation. The analgesia system can block both fast and slow types of pain signals at the initial entry point to the spinal cord. The central pain control system also includes multiple areas within the brain that have opiate receptors. These areas secrete opiatelike substances that include *Beta endorphin, met-enkephalin, leu-enkephalin*, and *dynorphin*. These substances can block pain signals entering through the peripheral nerves (Figure 51-4).

Therapeutic devices are being used to suppress pain by stimulating large sensory nerve fibers. *Transcutaneous electric nerve stimulation (TENS)* has been used in cases of acute postoperative and severe, persistent pain. It employs a battery-operated portable unit with electrodes that may be attached to the skin near the source of pain.[8] Theoretically, the TENS unit works using the closing of the gates as described by the gate-control theory (see below). This is achieved by overstimulation of large diameter sensory neurons to flood the central gates in the spinal cord and block the perception of pain sensation carried by unmyelinated fibers (Figure 51-5). Counter irritation (sensory stimulation) has been used for many years to relieve pain. The methods employed include rubbing, massaging, mildly painful stimuli, electroanalgesia, and even acupuncture.[12,13]

## PAIN THEORY

To explain the universal phenomenon of pain, numerous theories concerning its origin, transmission, perception, and manifestation have been offered. The *specificity theory* was an early attempt to explain all pain physiologically. It simply related the amount of pain to the amount of noxious stimulation and tissue damage. It failed to address chronic pain and individual variations in the pain response. The *pattern theory* related pain intensity to the strength of the stimulus and the summative effect of continued stimulation. The *gate-control theory* was published by Melzack and Wall in 1965. Because its concepts have been usable in treating pain, it is still considered to be reliable, especially in the understanding of the acute pain response.

## Gate-Control Theory

The gate-control theory proposed the presence of neural gating mechanisms at different levels of the central nervous system to account for interactions between pain and other sensory modalities. It used aspects of the specificity and pattern theories with an explanation for the pain perception and response differences among individuals. The theory recognizes three factors concerned with pain transmission and modulation: (1) the arrival of nociceptive stimuli; (2) the effect of other converging peripheral stimuli that may exaggerate or diminish the effect of the nociceptive stimuli; and (3) the presence of central nervous system control systems that influence the input.[16,17]

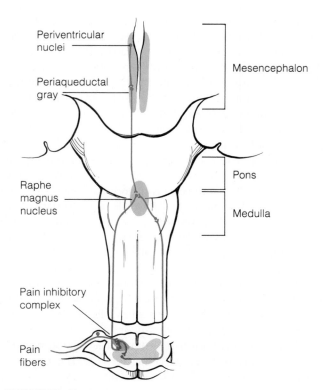

Periventricular nuclei

Periaqueductal gray

Mesencephalon

Raphe magnus nucleus

Pons

Medulla

Pain inhibitory complex

Pain fibers

**FIGURE 51-3.**
Endogenous pain control system of the brain.

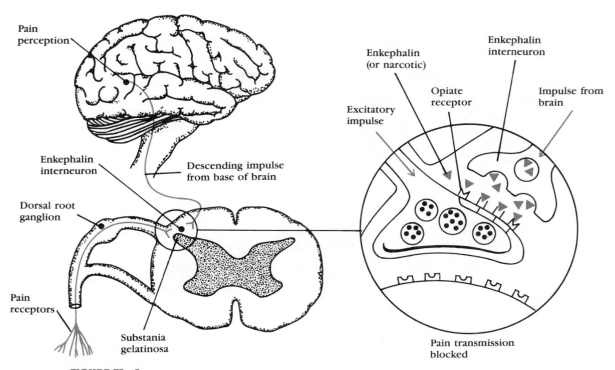

**FIGURE 51–4.**
The biologic receptors of the endorphin system. (Source: K. Foley, *The Management of Cancer Pain: A Symposium.* New York: HP Publishing, 1984.)

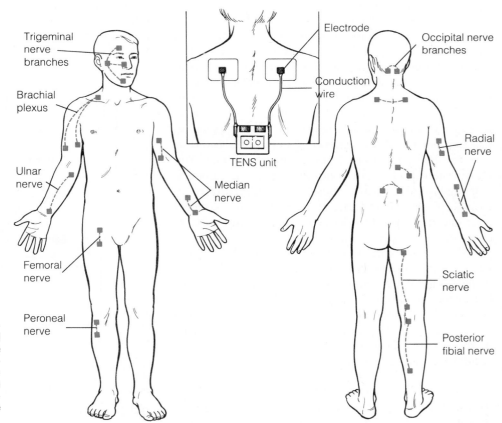

**FIGURE 51–5.**
Transcutaneous electric nerve stimulation (TENS) unit may be placed close to source of pain to activate various sensory nerves. The purpose is to flood the gates in the spinal cord and block the perception of pain. Various sites are used depending on the location of the painful stimulus.

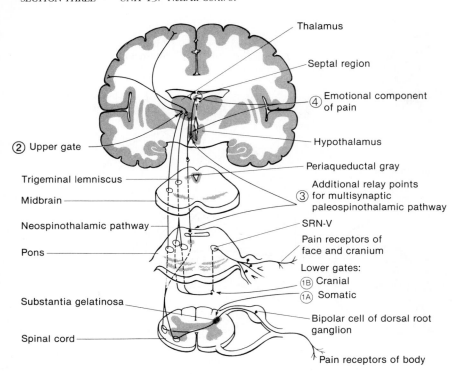

**FIGURE 51–6.**

The pain pathways illustrating the lower (1A and 1B) and upper (2) gates where pain impulses are subject to modulation; additional relay points (3) of paleospinothalamic pathway and brain centers that contribute the affective quality to pain (4) (Source: A.K. Swonger and L.L. Constantine, *Drugs and Therapy* [2nd ed.]. Boston: Little, Brown, 1988.)

The theory proposes that peripheral stimulation produces nerve impulses that are projected to three spinal cord systems: (1) the cells of the *substantia gelatinosa (SG)* in the dorsal horn; (2) the *dorsal column fibers*; and (3) the *central transmission cells (T cells)* in the dorsal horn (Figure 51-6). The SG acts as a gate-control system to modulate (inhibit) the flow of nerve impulses from peripheral fibers to the central nervous system.[15] The dorsal column fibers act as a central nervous system control trigger to stimulate selective brain processes that influence the gate-control system. The T cells activate neural mechanisms in the brain that are responsible for pain perception and response (Figure 51-7). When pain signals are persistent, the fraction of impulses allowed to pass through the various gates gradually declines. The lower gate (SG) is partly controlled by the transmitters, enkephalin and serotonin. These transmitters partly regulate the release of substance P, the peptide that conveys pain information. Activation of the A delta and C fibers decreases the inhibitory effect of the SG.

The *central control system (CCS)* rapidly activates two cognitive subsystems in the brain. This activation selectively modulates or inhibits peripheral nerve impulses before they are projected to the brain. Specifically, the CCS activates the descending efferent fibers in the brainstem reticular formation and cortex. The CCS regulates activity in the *sensory-discriminative, motivation-affective,* and *cognitive-evaluative* systems. These systems determine pain response. The sensory-discriminative system is mediated through the brainstem and cerebral processing centers. It processes pain intensity and strength along with the character of the event producing the experience. The

motivational-affective component appears to be mediated through the brainstem and reticular system. It is manifested by emotional features that lead to typical defense or escape behaviors. The cognitive-evaluative system processes pain meaning in the cerebral cortex. It is the learned response to the perception of pain and is thought to be the area where pain modulation may be enhanced. It is this system that relates to central control activities,

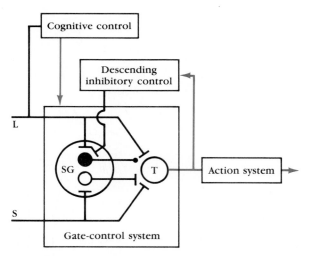

**FIGURE 51–7.**

The gate-control theory. The SG contains both excitatory (white circle) and inhibitory (black circle) links. The action of the inhibitory link could be presynaptic, postsynaptic, or both (round knob). The brainstem inhibitory system is influenced by the sensory input after transmission through the gate and projects back to the dorsal horn. The system is a separate input to the gate. (Source: R. Melzack and P.D. Wall, *The Challenge of Pain,* London: Basic Books, Inc. 1973.)

**TABLE 51–2.**
ACUTE VERSUS CHRONIC PAIN

| ACUTE | CHRONIC |
|---|---|
| **Characteristics** | |
| Limited duration | Prolonged, generally lasting more than 6 mo |
| Purposeful, serves as a sign of impending tissue damage | Serves no useful purpose |
| Gradually subsides | Often progresses in severity as pathology increases |
| Can generally localize pain | Localization imprecise; often pain is described as ache or soreness |
| Behavior usually restless, thrashing, pacing, rubbing body part, grimacing, and other facial expression of pain | Apt to be tired-looking, may or may not have facial expression of pain, often depressed. Suffering causes exhaustion of physical and mental capabilities<br>Pain becomes a central life focus<br>Accommodates behavior to pain |
| Usually signaled by a rise in pulse rate, decrease in blood pressure, and onset of sweating (diaphoresis) | Often have complex history of surgical procedures and therapies and a history of dependence on medications |
| **Responsiveness to analgesics** | |
| Usually readily responsive | Less responsive |
| Tolerance usually does not develop | Tolerance usually develops |
| Sedative effect of analgesic is an advantage | Sedative effect of analgesic is a disadvantage |
| Oral or parenteral routes | Usually oral route is employed |
| Standard doses can be used | Doses must be titrated to needs and level of tolerance of individual |
| Additional drugs are seldom required to manage pain | Additional drugs are often required to manage pain (tricyclic antidepressants or amphetamine) |

Source: A. Swonger and M. Matejski, Nursing Pharmacology, *Glenview, Ill.: Scott, Foresman, 1988.*

such as distraction, fear, and anxiety, may intervene between stimulus and response.[9,15] Thus, once activated, the CCS can inhibit or facilitate pain perception.[17] The mechanism used has to do with unique individuality relating to emotional, cognitive, and attentional factors that influence the perception of the nociceptive stimulus.[17]

## *ACUTE VERSUS CHRONIC PAIN*

The main clinical distinction between acute and chronic pain is primarily based on the duration of the pain problem. Table 51-2 indicates the differences between the two processes. Actually, the acute pain problem is more similar to the acute illness model, while the chronic pain problem tends to be the disease state itself.[6] In acute illness, the following four features apply:

1. The illness is symptomatic and can be labeled.
2. The illness is caused by external disease agents.
3. The illness is short term.
4. Treatment can cure the problem and eliminate symptoms.[6]

Chronic pain does not seem to be a continuation of acute pain but is thought to involve changes in either the peripheral or central nervous systems, or both.[15,17]

In chronic pain, the assumption that the pain is temporary becomes unbelievable for the individual as each day passes. Secondly, the assumption that treatment will result in a cure is challenged because the pain may continue without an "organic" cause.[6] Many factors enter into the adjustment of persons suffering chronic pain, many of which decrease pain tolerance and interfere with the normal activities of life.

## *Acute Pain*

Acute pain is viewed as a reaction to a stimulus that produces a generalized response. Sympathetic (adrenergic) reactions increase the energy necessary to mobilize an emergency response.[14] The characteristic pain response includes:

1. Marked elevation of systolic and diastolic blood pressure
2. Tachycardia

3. Peripheral vasoconstriction
4. Pupillary dilatation
5. Sweating
6. Hyperventilation
7. Inhibition of gastrointestinal motility
8. Muscle tension increase and hypermotility of muscles
9. Extreme anxiety
10. Hostility
11. Glycogen outpouring from the liver to increase blood sugar

Acute pain sensations and complaints are usually appropriate to the tissue damaging response. It may be related to an observable injury which, when natural healing or medical treatment has been employed, abates. The amount of pain expected is often inferred by the diagnosis of the causative agent.[6] The person may be asked to rate the pain on a numerical or word-associated basis. The visual analog scale (VAS) is used to progress from an anchor of no pain to pain of maximal intensity. The McGill Pain Questionnaire consists of words arranged into classes that describe the pain experience as to its sensory quality, affective quality, and overall evaluative quality. This scale has been used to distinguish among pain syndromes.[13] The tool provides information on pain quality and intensity as well as affective components. Figure 51-8 provides a sample of the McGill Pain Questionnaire. Judgments concerning the amount of pain to be expected are made, and the response of the affected person to treatment measures and analgesia are evaluated.

## Chronic Pain

Chronic pain is defined as pain that persists more or less continually over 6 months. It causes a change in the pattern of physiologic and psychologic responses. While sympathetic nervous system responses predominate in acute pain, these become habitual in the chronic state with an emergence of vegetative signs.[15] These signs include sleep disturbances (delayed onset and frequent awakening), lack of energy, depression, and irritability.[15] Pain tolerance for other, even minor injuries, is lessened. A change in eating habits is often described; weight loss or gain is reported. Interestingly, the vegetative signs may relate to a depletion of central serotonin, which has been shown to cause sleep disturbances, lowered pain tolerance, and depression.[15]

### Possible Physiologic Changes

While none of the physiologic changes of chronic pain are precisely identified, it is proposed that changes after an injury can occur in the nerve terminals, afferent fibers, and central system. Some of these changes can contribute to chronic pain.[18] Impulse conduction patterns may be changed by injury through sensitization of nerve endings.[17] These nerve endings may suffer changes in structure due to tissue breakdown products. Also, if there has been severance of a nerve axon, as it regenerates, false signals may be sent to the central system and be interpreted as pain. Peripheral nerve damage may cause central change in the dorsal root ganglia, which then are sensitive to circulating adrenalin and mechanical distortion.[18] The neurotransmitters in the SG may become depleted, causing less resistance to painful input.[11] The C fibers that are intimately involved with slow pain transmission have terminal arbors that innervate some cell regions not normally excited. With damage, these regions may be enlarged.[17,18] When a nociceptive stimulus is received with a warning event (eg, knowing that a certain movement causes pain), the central system may learn to respond to the expected stimulus, as well as the actual pain stimulus.[17,18]

### Classifying Chronic Pain

To classify chronic pain precisely, the following characteristics are considered: (1) region affected, (2) system affected, (3) pattern or temporal characteristics, (4) time since onset, and (5) suspected etiology. These give a pattern and provide the clinician with a basis for prognosis and treatment.[2] Often, however, there is no clear-cut diagnosis or treatment. An operational definition of chronic pain must then be developed in order to deal constructively with the individual problem.

The following are components of an operational definition of chronic pain: pain sensation, pain behavior, functional status at work and home, emotional state, and somatic preoccupation.[2] These are briefly considered below.

*PAIN SENSATION.*    This is the actual experience of pain that includes location, pain quality, and activities that aggravate or cause the pain. This mainly requires subjective reporting by the person.

*PAIN BEHAVIOR.*    This refers to a complex set of expressions that indicate that the person is experiencing pain. These include direct observation and reports by the person.[2] Individuals experiencing chronic pain tend to be less active and have less interpersonal interactions than their normal counterparts.[15] The tendency is to solicit more medical interventions and to overuse analgesics and other drugs.[15] The chronic invalid behaviors include adopting the sick role that includes a preoccupation with the symptom of pain. These persons often are dissatisfied with medical care and are looking for a cure. Conversely, when the medical practitioner cannot discover a pathologic reason for the pain, he or she may categorize the pain as psychogenic. This attitude is frustrating for the sufferer and counterproductive in pain management.

# McGill Pain Questionnaire

Patient's Name _____ Date _____ Time_____am/pm

PRI: S_____ A _____ E _____ M_____ PRI(T)_____ PPI_____
(1-10)      (11-15)      (16)      (17-20)      (1-20)

**1 FLICKERING**
QUIVERING
PULSING
THROBBING
BEATING
POUNDING

**2 JUMPING**
FLASHING
SHOOTING

**3 PRICKING**
BORING
DRILLING
STABBING
LANCINATING

**4 SHARP**
CUTTING
LACERATING

**5 PINCHING**
PRESSING
GNAWING
CRAMPING
CRUSHING

**6 TUGGING**
PULLING
WRENCHING

**7 HOT**
BURNING
SCALDING
SEARING

**8 TINGLING**
ITCHY
SMARTING
STINGING

**9 DULL**
SORE
HURTING
ACHING
HEAVY

**10 TENDER**
TAUT
RASPING
SPLITTING

**11 TIRING**
EXHAUSTING

**12 SICKENING**
SUFFOCATING

**13 FEARFUL**
FRIGHTFUL
TERRIFYING

**14 PUNISHING**
GRUELLING
CRUEL
VICIOUS
KILLING

**15 WRETCHED**
BLINDING

**16 ANNOYING**
TROUBLESOME
MISERABLE
INTENSE
UNBEARABLE

**17 SPREADING**
RADIATING
PENETRATING
PIERCING

**18 TIGHT**
NUMB
DRAWING
SQUEEZING
TEARING

**19 COOL**
COLD
FREEZING

**20 NAGGING**
NAUSEATING
AGONIZING
DREADFUL
TORTURING

**PPI**
0 NO PAIN
1 MILD
2 DISCOMFORTING
3 DISTRESSING
4 HORRIBLE
5 EXCRUCIATING

BRIEF __   RHYTHMIC __   CONTINUOUS __
MOMENTARY __   PERIODIC __   STEADY __
TRANSIENT __   INTERMITTENT __   CONSTANT __

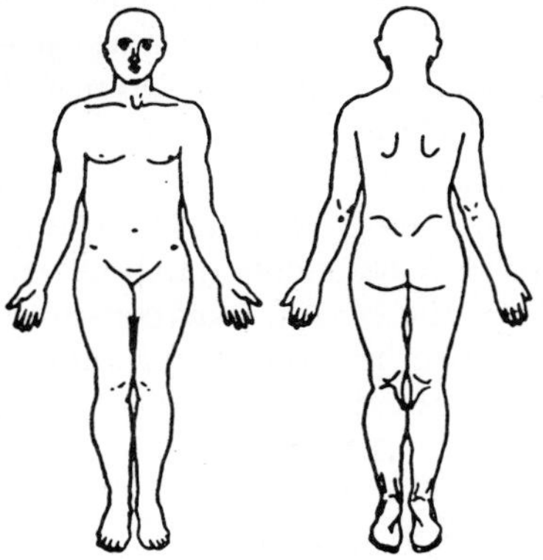

E = EXTERNAL
I = INTERNAL

COMMENTS:

**FIGURE 51-8.**
The McGill Pain Questionnaire. The numbers of descriptors in each category are noted. S = subjective 1–10; A = affective 11–15; E = evaluative 16; M = miscellaneous 17–20; PRI = pain rating index computed by the chosen words; PPI = present pain index, which is the rate of the pain intensity. A descriptor of the nature of the pain is checked and the pain is located on the figure with E or I for external or internal pain. Comments include response to pain medications. (Source: R. Melzack, The McGill Pain Questionnaire. In R. Melzack, [ed.]. *Pain Measurement and Assessment.* New York: Raven Press, 1983.)

*FUNCTIONAL STATUS AT WORK OR HOME.* Job performance usually declines because there is increasing preoccupation with the pain sensation. Functional abilities (rather than disabilities) must be assessed to prevent the loss of employment or the placement on medical disability.

In home or interpersonal relationships, loss of control is exhibited by increasing reliance on the sick role to manipulate or tyrannize others.[15] Roles are shifted and guilt arises in family members who cannot help the sufferer.

*EMOTIONAL STATE.* Depression is the most common result of chronic pain. Anxiety, fatigue, and irritability also can play a role in enhancing the pain experience. If the pain has a definite source, such as cancer pain, the focus is on the source and the person may not be incapacitated by it.

*SOMATIC PREOCCUPATION.* This term refers to heightened sensitivity or selective attention to bodily discomfort.[1] This means that the person may consciously dwell on the pain experience. This preoccupation often results in heightened pain response.

## SPECIFIC TYPES OF PAIN

The material in the previous pages discusses pain that is carried through "acute" pain fibers and "slow" pain fibers, as well as the knotty problem of how chronic pain is transmitted. The following section presents specific types of pain, some of which are mainly acute and some which are chronic. A complete listing of pain-producing conditions is not presented and the reader is referred to other areas of this text and the bibliography at the end of the unit for further detail.

### Cutaneous Pain

*Cutaneous pain* is usually direct, acute pain that is precisely localized from the skin. The area of nerve segment affected is along a distinct dermatome (see Chap. 48). The nerve fibers between the dermatome actually overlap to some extent. For example, T6 stimulus reception results in pain being experienced in the T5, T6, and T7 dermatome areas.[1] The three distinct skin layers produce pain sensation that differs. The epidermis produces itching and burning pain. The dermis produces localized, superficial pain. Damage in the subcutaneous tissues produces an aching, throbbing type pain.[8]

### Visceral Pain

The *visceral type* of pain tends to be diffuse or poorly localized. Sufferers rarely can precisely localize the pain

or identify any potential causative factors. Some visceral pain is *referred* in nature.

### Referred Pain

Referred pain refers to a felt pain sensation that is in a part of the body considerably removed from the area initiating the pain.[4] Normally, the pain arises in a deep organ and is felt on an area of body surface.

Reflex muscular spasm is a common cause of referred pain. The muscle spasm will initiate severe back pain, headaches, and other painful reactions.[4]

Visceral or deep organ pain may be produced by ischemia, chemical stimuli, spasm, or overdistention of a hollow viscus (gut, gallbladder, etc.). The pain may be referred through particular parietal transmission pathways to other areas on the skin and perceived as sharp, burning, and often excruciating.[4] The visceral nerve transmission is usually through slow C pain fibers, while the interconnecting parietal pathways are transmitted through A delta fibers, which accounts for how they are perceived. Figure 51-9 shows surface areas of referred pain and

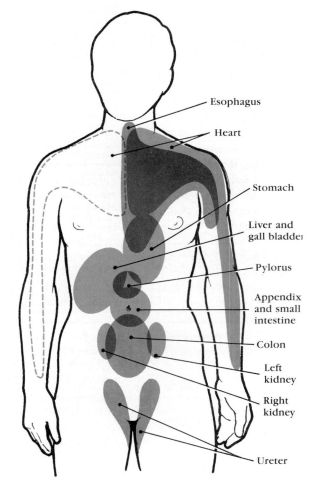

**FIGURE 51-9.**
Typical areas of referred pain from visceral organs.

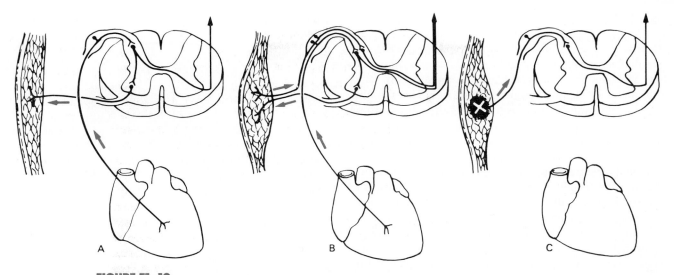

**FIGURE 51–10.**
Sequence of development of somatic components of cardiac pain. **A.** Nociceptive afferent input into dorsal horn causes efferent stimulation of muscles in the chest wall, which leads to muscle spasm. **B.** Muscle spasm acts as a new source of noxious input that produces trigger areas, and thus a vicious cycle develops. **C.** Nociceptive input from muscle continues after healing of the heart lesion. Injection of trigger areas with a local anesthetic eliminates the pain. (Source: J. Bonica, *The Management of Pain* [2nd ed.]. Lea and Febiger, 1990.)

their usual source of origin. *Chest pain* that arises from cardiac ischemia is discussed in detail in Chapter 25. The pain impulses are conducted through sympathetic nerves to the first four or five thoracic ganglia and to the spinal cord through second, third, fourth, and fifth spinal nerves.[4] The oppression and substernal pain felt may be due to blood vessel spasm or muscle reaction.[1] Figure 51-10 illustrates a vicious cycle that can be set up and even persist after cardiac healing. Esophageal, gastric, and gallbladder pain may all be confused with cardiac pain due to the overlapping areas of referral. Kidney, colon, and small intestine pain may have abdominal areas of referral, whereas uterus and ureter pain often are referred into the groin. Table 51-3 indicates some common referral sites from visceral structure damage.

**TABLE 51–3.**
LOCALIZATION OF REFERRED PAIN FROM VISCERAL STRUCTURE DAMAGE

| VISCERAL STRUCTURE DAMAGE | AREA OF SKIN EXPERIENCING PAIN |
| --- | --- |
| Diaphragm | Skin of ipsilateral shoulder and outer surface of upper arm |
| Heart | Dermatomes C3–T8, with resulting pain in left arm and hand, especially in distribution of ulnar nerve; shoulder, back, substernal region, neck, axilla, and jaw; occasionally stomach, with "indigestion" symptoms noted |
| Stomach | Dermatomes T6–T9; chest and substernal region |
| Ovaries | Dermatome T10; periumbilical |
| Uterus | Dermatomes S1–S2, sometimes manifesting as pain in lower back |
| Prostate | Dermatomes T10–T12, manifesting as pain in periumbilical and inguinal areas, tip of penis, and occasionally scrotum |
| Kidneys | Dermatomes T10–L1; lower back and umbilical area |
| Rectum | Dermatomes S2–S4; low sacral back pain and sciatic pain in upper thigh or calf on dorsum of leg |

Source: N. Hendler, Diagnosis and Nonsurgical Management of Chronic Pain. New York: Raven Press, 1981. Reprinted by permission of Raven Press.

## *Headache*

Headaches are extremely common phenomena that may result from stimuli inside and outside of the cranium. Figure 51-11 shows areas of headache that result from different causes. Intracranial origins include vascular stretching, meningeal trauma, low cerebrospinal fluid pressure, alcohol, and constipation.[7] Stimulation of pain receptors above the tentorium causes referred headaches to the front half of the head. Those beneath the tentorium cause occipital headaches, which are usually intense in nature.[4] Alcohol is thought to be a direct chemical irritator of the meninges, while constipation probably causes toxic products or circulatory system changes.[4]

*Migraine* headaches are thought to be due to vasospasm of certain cerebral arteries that produce intracerebral ischemia, followed by vasodilation and stretching of arterial walls. The precise mechanism of production is unknown but disturbance in the trigeminal pathways may be a major factor.[7] Table 51-4 describes the characteristics of vascular or migraine headaches.

Extracranial origins for headache include nasal sinus disorders, eye changes, and the so-called *tension headache*. Nasal congestion and pressure are caused from infection and congestion of the frontal and maxillary sinuses with pain in the eyes, forehead, and scalp. Eye changes may cause headache through excessive irradiation, eye muscle fatigue, conjunctival irritation, and glau-

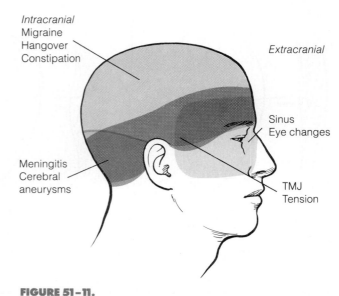

**FIGURE 51-11.**
Areas of headache from different causes. Areas of overlap often make the source of the headache difficult to identify.

coma.[4,7] The tension headache is probably the most common cause of headache and usually is described as a headache resulting from emotional stress or fatigue.[7] The associated muscle spasms are thought to be of the neck muscles because they are attached to the base of the

**TABLE 51-4.**
CHARACTERISTICS OF VASCULAR OR MIGRAINE HEADACHES

| CHARACTERISTICS | DESCRIPTION |
| --- | --- |
| Onset | Childhood through puberty, plus family history |
| Location | 70–80% temple or forehead<br>Unilateral, spread to occiput, neck, shoulder<br>Whole head; one side more painful |
| Intensity | Mild to severe |
| Quality | Throbbing, pulsing |
| Pattern | Stage I—prodromal (aura); stage II—headache<br>Scintillating scotoma; visual disturbances; paresthesia; dizziness; head noises |
| Duration | Stage I, 20–30 min; stage II, 12–24 h |
| Frequency | Several times per day, week, or year |
| Associated symptoms | Increased urination, nervousness, colitis, abdominal pain, nasal symptoms, dyspepsia, diarrhea, constipation, sweating, exhaustion, pallor, fever, red dull eyes, awaken 3–4 AM |
| Chronology | 3–9% of population; onset as early as age 8 mo; in children females and males are equal; 23% onset before age 40 y; more common in females |
| Aggravating/easing factors | Menstruation aggravates, contraceptives aggravate<br>Pregnancy eases, tryptophan eases |
| Precipitating factors | Glare, dust, odors, temperature changes, barometric pressure and humidity changes, stress—physical and psychologic, lack of oxygen, hunger, smoking, decrease in blood serotonin |

Source: J. Mannheimer and B. Lampe, Clinical Transcutaneous Electrical Nerve Stimulation. *Philadelphia: F.A. Davis, 1989. Reprinted by permission.*

skull.[4] Another common cause of headache is the *temporomandibular joint (TMJ) syndrome*. The pain results from a joint problem in the mandible usually caused by poor bite or joint problems. This difficult problem often causes intermittent or chronic pain.

## Phantom Limb Pain

Phantom limb pain is felt after the amputation of a limb and is not universal to all affected persons. It is characterized by tingling, burning, or intolerable pain in the amputated extremity. It may be due to a self-perpetuating, closed-loop type nervous stimulation similar to that described with chronic chest pain. The pain may remit in weeks or months, or may continue for years. Nerve blocks or TENS units may be used to stop the pain.

## Hyperalgesia

*Hyperalgesia* is the term used for an excessively excitable pain pathway. The basic causes include excessive sensitivity of pain receptors (primary hyperalgesia) or facilitation of sensory transmission (secondary hyperalgesia). Primary hyperalgesia results from stimulation of numerous cutaneous receptors, such as with sunburned skin. Secondary hyperalgesia frequently results from spinal cord or thalamic lesions.[4] Other terms used for this syndrome are *neuralgia* and *causalgia*.

In neuralgia, a severe, shooting, or throbbing pain results from light or normal stimulation of superficial areas. The pain follows the areas supplied by specific spinal or cranial nerve roots. A common type of neuralgia, trigeminal neuralgia (tic douloureux), causes lightning-like stabs of pain involving the second or third divisions of the trigeminal nerve.[10] Other types of neuralgias include postherpetic neuralgia, which causes shocklike pains along a dermatome after an attack of herpes zoster, and glossopharyngeal neuralgia, which is felt in the tonsil and posterior pharynx.[10]

Causalgia results from actual damage to any of the peripheral nerves. The pain is continuous and often exacerbated by emotional stress.[10] It is probably generated by excess sympathetic nervous system activity on the already damaged nerves. These syndromes may respond well to sympathetic blockage and early mobilization.[10]

## REFERENCES

1. Bonica, J. *The Management of Pain* (2nd ed.). Philadelphia: Lea & Febiger, 1990.
2. Feuerstein, M. Definitions of pain. In C.D. Tollison, *Handbook of Chronic Pain Management*. Baltimore: Williams & Wilkins, 1989.
3. Ganong, W.F. *Review of Medical Physiology* (12th ed.). Los Altos, Calif.: Lange, 1985.
4. Guyton, A. *Textbook of Physiology* (8th ed.). Philadelphia: W.B. Saunders, 1990.
5. Hall, J.L. Anatomy of pain. In C.D. Tollison, *Handbook of Chronic Pain Management*. Baltimore: Williams & Wilkins, 1989.
6. Hanson, R.S., and Gerber, R.F. *Coping with Chronic Pain*. New York: Guilford Press, 1990.
7. Lance, J. Approach to the patient with headaches. In W.N. Kelley, *Textbook of Internal Medicine*. Philadelphia: J.B. Lippincott, 1989.
8. Mannheimer, J., and Lampe, G. *Clinical Transcutaneous Electrical Nerve Stimulation*. Philadelphia: F.A. Davis, 1989.
9. McCaffrey, M., and Beebe, A. *Pain: A Clinical Manual for Nursing Practice*. St. Louis: Mosby, 1989.
10. Moulin, D. Approach to the patient with chronic pain syndromes. In W.N. Kelley, *Textbook of Internal Medicine*. Philadelphia: J.B. Lippincott, 1989.
11. North, R.B. Neural stimulation. In C.D. Tollison, *Handbook of Chronic Pain Management*. Baltimore: Williams & Wilkins, 1989.
12. Pinals, R.S. Management of neck, back, and extraarticular pain syndromes. In W.N. Kelley, *Textbook of Internal Medicine*. Philadelphia: J.B. Lippincott, 1989.
13. Rosenzweig, M.R., and Leiman, A.L. *Physiological Psychology* (2nd ed.). New York: Random House, 1989.
14. Sjolund, B., Eriksson, M., and Loese, J. Transcutaneous and implanted electric stimulation of peripheral nerves. In J. Bonica, *The Management of Pain* (2nd ed.). Philadelphia: Lea & Febiger, 1990.
15. Sternbach, R.A. Acute versus chronic pain. In P. Wall and R. Melzack, *Textbook of Pain* (2nd ed.). Edinburgh: Churchill-Livingstone, 1989.
16. Wall, P.D. Introduction. In P. Wall and R. Melzack, *Textbook of Pain* (2nd ed.). Edinburgh: Churchill-Livingstone, 1989.
17. Wall, P.D. The dorsal horn. In P. Wall and R. Melzack, *Textbook of Pain* (2nd ed.). Edinburgh: Churchill-Livingstone, 1989.
18. Whitehead, W., and Kuhn, W. Chronic pain: An overview. In T.W. Miller, *Chronic Pain*. Madison, Conn.: International University Press, 1990.

# chapter 52

Reet Henze

# Traumatic Alterations in the Nervous System

## Chapter Outline

## Learning Objectives

1. Distinguish the two aspects of consciousness.
2. Describe the role of the reticular activating system in modulating consciousness.
3. Explain the basis for alterations in the level of consciousness.
4. Explain the etiologic basis of coma.
5. Contrast coma of metabolic origin with coma of structural injury.
6. Discuss the basis of coma from supratentorial and infratentorial lesions.
7. Describe associated functional disturbances common in comatose persons, including altered motor and pupillary responses, respiratory patterns, and eye movements.
8. Differentiate between upper and lower motor neuron lesions.
9. Explain the various types of skull fractures.
10. Differentiate between cerebral concussion and contusion.

11. Discuss type of injury, early and progressive clinical signs and symptoms, and treatment of epidural hematomas, subdural hematomas, subdural hygromas, subarachnoid hemorrhage, and intracerebral hematoma.
12. Describe the effect produced by cerebral vasospasm associated with subarachnoid hemorrhage.
13. Differentiate between cytotoxic and vasogenic cerebral edema.
14. Discuss how traumatic injury may occur to each of the cranial nerves and the clinical findings associated with these injuries.
15. State the normal intracranial pressure.
16. Discuss the etiology of increased intracranial pressure.
17. Describe how intracranial pressure can be measured.
18. Discuss the major types of brain shifts that can occur with increased intracranial pressure.

*(continued)*

Trauma to the nervous system can result in major changes in physiologic and psychologic functioning. Damage secondary to a primary injury of the nervous system, such as cerebral edema and increased intracranial pressure (ICP), may be potentially more devastating than the original injury. Many structural and metabolic processes impinging on the brain lead to alterations in consciousness and varying degrees of brain dysfunction. This chapter begins with a focus on consciousness and its varying levels reflective of clinical findings.

## CONSCIOUSNESS

The conscious state of human existence involves complex neural phenomena that provide for wakefulness and an awareness of self and environment. Two aspects of consciousness are content of consciousness and arousal. The former relates to mental activities such as perception of self and memory, and the latter relates to a state of wakefulness. The levels of function of the nervous system can be roughly related clinically to varying levels of consciousness. In essence, when higher levels no longer function due to various disease or traumatic processes, lower levels can be observed functioning. Content of consciousness activities (mental activities) is carried out at the highest level: the cerebral cortex. The arousal phenomenon arises from a much lower level in the brainstem structures. Within the two components of consciousness, there exists in each varying degrees of function. The structures necessary for consciousness include the intact central structures of the diencephalon and projections from it, the thalamocortical system, and the reticular activating system (RAS) of the brainstem. The cerebral cortex provides perception to the neural basis of consciousness that evolves from the lower levels of the brain.[1]

The RAS is important in modulating wakefulness, arousal, and conscious perception of the environment. It evolves from the deep structures of the brain and brainstem to project onto the cortex. This portion of the RAS is known as the *ascending reticular activating system*. A portion of the RAS bypasses the thalamus on its projectory route, whereas another part terminates in the specific nuclei of the thalamus and from these, projects diffusely to the entire cortex. The former is referred to as the nonspecific or diffuse thalamocortical system and the latter as the specific thalamocortical system.[2]

Peripheral stimulation is transmitted by the afferent pathways to projection areas on the cerebral cortex by the specific and nonspecific thalamic nuclei for the perception of consciousness. Chapter 48 details the important functions of the thalamus in receiving sensory information from various parts of the body and relaying these onto specific areas of the cortex. This relay involves a three-synapse transmission to its projection site on the cortex and is part of the specific thalamocortical system. Stimulation of the specific thalamic nuclei gives rise to localized primary responses that may not, in themselves, be sufficient to produce conscious perception.

The nonspecific thalamocortical system, on the other hand, does not project to specific nuclei of the thalamus but bypasses the thalamus region in groups of nuclei, including the midline nuclei, intralaminar nuclei, and reticular thalamic nucleus. Nonspecific system conduction involves a multisynaptic path with indistinct boundaries and numerous interconnections with the specific thalamic nuclei before finally projecting to widely distributed cortical receiving areas.

During sleep and anesthesia, transmission of the specific thalamic nuclei remains unchanged, whereas the nonspecific system becomes suppressed. In normal, wakeful brain functioning, a continuous activating flow from the nonspecific system controls the state of consciousness or wakefulness at any given time. This flow is known as the RAS. As the activating afferent flow diminishes, sleep states ensue. Major damage to the RAS anywhere rostral to the pons results in greatly diminished cortical activation, which affects the conscious state.

Investigators have applied electrical stimulation to different areas of the RAS in an attempt to understand its function better. Electrical stimulation of the upper brainstem portion of the RAS demonstrates immediate waking in the sleeping animal and general activation of the entire central nervous system. In contrast, electrical stimulation of the RAS as it evolves from the thalamic nuclei results in more specific activation of the cortex, which allows for mental activities requiring a more direct focus. During sleep, the RAS may be activated by various external and internal stimuli. Some of these are more potent activators than others, for example, pain is a strong activator.

In addition to stimulation of the RAS from the afferent ascending system, stimulation may also descend from all areas of the cerebral cortex. Particularly strong stimulation arrives from the cortical motor projection areas. It is well-known that activity such as walking wards off sleep, which might otherwise overtake the individual during sitting or reclining.

## ALTERATIONS IN CONSCIOUSNESS

The most sensitive indicator of brain function is level of consciousness. A wide range of consciousness may be observed from an alert state to deep coma. Subtle changes that affect diagnosis and management can occur within short time spans.

A person with a normal level of consciousness is awake, aware, and interacting appropriately with the environment when not engaged in normal sleep. Alertness; orientation to time, place, and person; and general responses to the surroundings are evaluated frequently in individuals with cerebral neurologic disturbances. A person whose level of consciousness deteriorates from a normal interaction with the environment may lapse slowly or very rapidly to a totally unresponsive state, depending on the underlying neurologic pathology.

Slow deterioration of the level of consciousness reveals different levels of response that can be observed clinically. Subjective observations may be described: the lethargic person is somnolent and drowsy, and responds sluggishly to verbal and painful stimuli. Heightened stimuli may be necessary to evoke a response and the person may drift back into sleep soon after the stimulation. The individual may be oriented or exhibit occasional disorientation. As brain function deteriorates, lethargy becomes stupor. Vigorous and persistent noxious stimuli are applied to evoke a response because verbal stimuli generally produce little response. The attention span is very short and excessive motor responses may be exhibited.

Further deterioration of brain function is reflected in ensuing coma. The first sign is a light coma or semicoma in which no responses are made to ordinary verbal and tactile stimuli. However, motor responses do occur in a reflexive manner to noxious stimuli. Deepening coma is observed when reflexive motor responses are no longer elicited in response to vigorous noxious stimulation, and flaccidity of the extremities predominates. Pupillary, pha-ryngeal, and corneal responses may be minimal or absent. Thermoregulatory mechanisms become erratic and respiratory patterns become irregular.

## Coma

The importance of an intact and functioning ascending RAS extending from the midbrain to the hypothalamus, thalamus, and finally to the cerebral cortex was discussed in Chapter 48. Disruption of the conscious state is commonly viewed from an etiologic basis of structural or metabolic/toxic origin. Uncommonly, coma has a psychogenic basis.

Persons whose coma is as a result of structural processes have incurred physical damage to the brain, such as a contusion, infection, intracerebral bleeding, tumor, or edema. Coma results from structural causes when damage occurs to both cerebral cortices or the brainstem. Brain expansion, such as that which occurs in the herniation syndromes, may cause secondary damage to the structures necessary for consciousness and result in coma. The distinguishing characteristics of structurally induced coma are focal signs that reflect the area of the brain involved.[10] These focal signs are usually initially unilateral processes, such as hemiparesis and unilateral pupillary dilation. Without intervention, the focal signs may become bilateral.

Toxic and metabolically induced coma results from ingestion of exogenous nervous system poisons (toxic) or from disease processes producing endogenous materials that interfere with normal brain metabolism.[10]

In addition, coma may have psychogenic origins. These can be distinguished from organic basis by attempting to open an eyelid. Active resistance to eyelid opening occurs with psychogenic coma. With true coma, the eyelid is readily opened, falls back into prior position slowly, and remains slightly open. The cold caloric test is another effective means to distinguish psychogenic coma from organic coma (see Chap. 48). If nystagmus occurs during the test, the unresponsiveness is psychogenic.[2] The common causes of coma are summarized in Table 52-1.

### Clinical Findings

Coma has been likened to sleep. Similarities do exist, for example, both lack conscious behavior, and electroencephalogram (EEG) recordings tend to show slow rhythms. Nevertheless, the differences are striking. Humans may be aroused from sleep but those in profound coma cannot be aroused. Eye movements may be lacking in coma resulting from acute neurologic processes, and rapid eye movement (REM) sleep patterns are not present. As coma becomes chronic, some individuals display periods of restlessness that may be equated with sleep-wakefulness cycles.

## TABLE 52–1.
### COMMON ETIOLOGIC BASES FOR COMA

**Structural Processes**

Supratentorial lesions
  Epidural hematomas
  Tumors
  Infections
  Hemorrhage
  Subdural hematomas
  Contusions
  Edema
Infratentorial lesions
  Hemorrhage
  Infarction
  Aneurysms
  Tumors
  Contusions

**Endogenous Metabolic Processes**

Renal failure (uremia)
Diabetic ketoacidosis
Electrolyte imbalances
Hyperosmolarity

**Acidosis**

Hepatic encephalopathy
Hypoxia
Hypercarbia
Hypoglycemia

**Exogenous Toxic Poisons**

Sedative drugs
Alcohol

**Psychogenic Disorders**

Fainting
Hysteria
Catatonia

### Supratentorially Induced Coma

Isolated, small lesions of the cerebral hemispheres are not sufficient to cause coma as long as the ascending RAS and its connections to the cortex are intact. With progressively larger hemispheric lesions in regions above the tentorium, behavior becomes dulled until maximum obliteration of the cortex occurs and no content of consciousness is preserved. Supratentorial hemispheric lesions produce coma by enlarging sufficiently to cross midline structures and compress the opposite hemisphere (Figure 52-1) or by caudal compression of the diencephalon and midbrain. Dangerous manifestations of hemispheric compressions include herniations of the diencephalon or uncus through the tentorial notch, which results in aggravating vascular obstruction and accentuation of already present ischemia. Similarly, circulation of cerebrospinal fluid (CSF) is blocked with transtentorial herniations and the pressure in the cranium rises. Transtentorial herniation is also accompanied by brainstem hemorrhages and ischemia that is thought to be caused by the midbrain and pons stretching the medial branches of the basilar artery.

### Infratentorially Induced Coma

Coma as a result of dysfunction or destruction of areas below the tentorium may evolve from within the brainstem structures and produce destructive effects directly on the paramedian midbrain-pontine reticular formation. Lesions external to the brainstem may compress the re-

ticular formation and may involve direct invasive destruction or compression of its blood supply, resulting in brainstem ischemia and eventual necrosis. The brainstem may be destroyed by cerebrovascular accident, neoplasm, aneurysms, hematomas, infectious processes, and head trauma.

Lesions external to the brainstem may compress the tegmentum, resulting in damage to the neural tissue. This may compromise the vascular supply and result in ischemia. In addition, the mesencephalic tegmentum may be compressed through an upward herniation of the cerebellum and midbrain through the tentorial notch. This compression results in tissue distortion and vascular obstruction with eventual coma. Expanding lesions of the posterior fossa (cerebellum) are a common cause of upward herniation of structures through the tentorial notch. Downward compression of the brainstem may result from the herniation of the cerebellar tonsils through the foramen magnum. This results in compression and ischemia of the medulla with resultant circulatory and respiratory aberrations.

### Functional Disturbances Associated with Coma

Certain clinical alterations in function may reflect the level and extent of underlying brain pathology. These include alterations in consciousness, motor responses, respiratory patterns, pupillary responses, and eye movements.

In evaluating level of consciousness, the individual's motor responses may be significant in relation to the extent of pathology and depth of coma. Limb movement

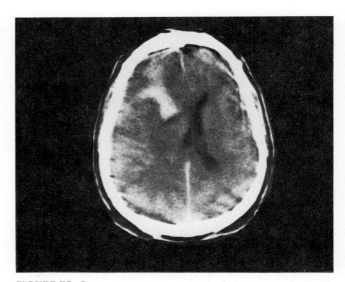

### FIGURE 52–1.
Intracerebral bleeding in left frontal lobe (light area). Compression of left lateral ventricle with slight compression of midline structures.

is a means of assessing asymmetry of function in the nervous system. A consistently justifiable correlation between the level of consciousness and motor responses should not be made because each of these functions is controlled by separate pathways and stands apart. Nevertheless, lesions at certain levels within the central nervous system result in specific types of motor responses that are readily observable clinically and support the region of the pathology.

If no response is elicited to verbal stimuli, other stimuli are used to arouse a response. The responses are significant in that they may indicate the extent of damage by their purposefulness. Purposeful motor responses to noxious stimuli in the comatose person indicate that the sensory pathways and corticospinal pathways are functioning. An example is an attempt to push the noxious stimulus away. Inappropriate motor responses are stereotyped patterns commonly indicating the level or region of damage. Decorticate and decerebrate motor responses are examples of inappropriate involuntary responses (Figure 52-2).

The decorticate response denotes supratentorial dysfunction commonly observed with the interruption of the corticospinal pathways by lesions of the internal capsule or cerebral hemispheric. It is clinically manifested by a flexion response of the upper extremities and an extension response of the lower extremities. The arms are adducted and in rigid flexion, with the hands rotated internally and fingers flexed. The decerebrate response is elicited in persons with extensive brainstem damage to the midpontine level, as well as large cerebral lesions that compress the lower thalamus and midbrain. Severe metabolic disorders, such as hypoglycemia, hepatic coma,

and certain drug intoxications, may diminish brainstem function and induce a decerebrate response. Characteristic musculoskeletal patterns include extension responses of both upper and lower extremities.

Fully expressed, the decerebrate individual exhibits opisthotonos (head extended, body arched) posturing with clenched teeth and arms rigidly extended, adducted, and hyperpronated. The legs are stiffly extended and feet plantar flexed. The extent of the decerebrate response correlates with severity of the pathology and is occasionally seen as wavering back and forth between decorticate and decerebrate, reflecting physiologic changes.

Decerebrate responses of the upper extremities, together with flaccidity of the lower extremities, indicates more extensive brainstem damage extending even beyond the pons level. In certain persons, asymmetry of abnormal responses and normal responses may reflect underlying cerebral pathology. For example, a person may exhibit unilateral decorticate response, or decorticate response on one side and decerebrate on the other side.

Unilaterally absent motor responses to noxious stimuli indicates interruption in the corticospinal pathways, damage to the RAS at the pontomedullary level, or psychogenic disruption. Hyperreflexia and the presence of the Babinski's response support structural lesions of the central nervous system as the origin of the coma. Certain metabolic abnormalities, such as hypoglycemia and uremia, may exhibit the same signs but can be quickly confirmed by laboratory studies.

## Paralysis

Paralysis, the loss of voluntary movement, is relatively common with trauma to the nervous system. Lesions involving the corticobulbar and corticospinal tracts are known as *upper motor neuron lesions* and result in *spastic paralysis* (Figure 52-3). Lesions involving motor cranial nerves, whose cell bodies are in the brainstem nuclei, and spinal nerves, whose cell bodies are in the anterior horn of the spinal cord, are referred to as *lower motor neuron lesions* and result in *flaccid paralysis* (see Figure 52-3). Motor and sensory losses may coexist and indicate mixed motor and sensory nerve involvement or involvement of both the anterior and posterior roots.

The activity of the reflex arc provides the muscle with tone. Interruption of the arc associated with lower motor neuron lesions results in atony and soft, unresponsive muscle. Voluntary activity and reflex action cannot be elicited when the final common pathway of the lower motor neuron is severed. Deep tendon reflexes are absent also.

In lesions of the upper motor neuron, the activity of the reflex arc remains intact, although voluntary control of movement is lost. The pyramidal tract and its collaterals, as well as other descending tracts that influence lower motor neurons, may be involved in the paralysis.

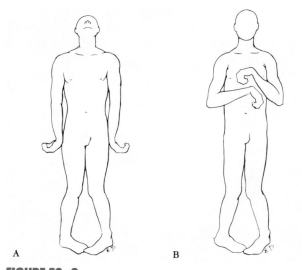

**FIGURE 52-2.**
Abnormal posturing. **A.** Decerebrate position **B.** Decorticate position. (Source: C.V. Kenner, C.E. Guzzetta, and B.M. Dossey, *Critical Care Nursing* [2nd ed.]. Boston: Little, Brown, 1985.)

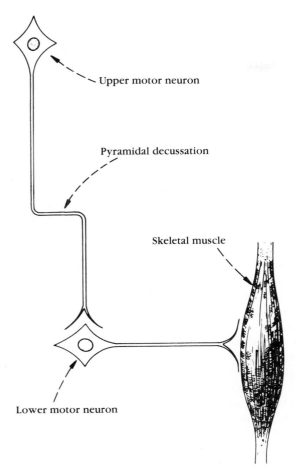

**FIGURE 52–3.**

Traditional concept of motor control. Upper motor neuron lesions produce paralysis, hypertonia, and hyperreflexia. Lower motor neuron lesions produce paralysis, hypotonia, areflexia, and muscle wasting (Source: M.A. Samuels, *Manual of Neurologic Therapeutics* [2nd ed.]. Boston: Little, Brown, 1982.)

The muscle feels hard, is very sensitive to stretch, and is said to be *hypertonic.* Deep tendon reflexes are increased after a period of areflexia immediately after this type of lesion. The characteristics of upper and lower motor neuron lesions are summarized in Table 52-2.

**TABLE 52–2.**
CHARACTERISTICS OF UPPER MOTOR NEURON AND LOWER MOTOR NEURON LESIONS

| UPPER MOTOR NEURON | LOWER MOTOR NEURON |
|---|---|
| Spastic paralysis | Flaccid paralysis |
| Hyperreflexia (increased deep tendon reflexes) | Hyporeflexia (decreased deep tendon reflexes) |
| Unilaterally upgoing great toe (Babinski's sign) | Absent or normal plantar response |
| Minimal or no muscle atrophy | Significant muscle atrophy |
| Fasciculations absent | Fasciculations present |

## Pupillary Responses in Altered States of Consciousness

The close anatomic relationship of fibers that control pupillary reactions and consciousness provides a valuable guide to the location of the pathologic processes causing coma. Other origins of coma also may be assessed by the pupillary responses because metabolic aberrations leave little effect on the pupils whereas certain structural pathology produces distinct changes.

Pupillary responses are regulated by sympathetic and parasympathetic nervous systems. A balance is normally maintained by the two systems to produce a pupillary aperture appropriate to the prevailing environment. *Mydriasis* (dilation) is produced by the sympathetic nervous system and *miosis* (constriction) by the parasympathetic nervous system. The parasympathetic impulses arrive through the third nerve from the *Edinger-Westphal nuclei* in the midbrain. The sympathetic innervation arrives by a more complex route that originates in the hypothalamus, traverses the brainstem, and travels along with the internal carotid artery into the skull where it reaches the eye through the filaments of the ophthalmic artery and a division of the fifth nerve. Damage to specific areas of the brain produces characteristic pupillary responses that are valuable for diagnostic purposes.

Pupils' size, position, and response to bright light are observed in assessing the neurologic status of the comatose individual. Normal response to bright light in a partially darkened room is a brisk constriction of the pupil. Other responses may indicate abnormal neurologic processes. In addition, simultaneous constriction occurs in the opposite pupil (*consensual reflex*). Pupils normally are at midposition and *conjugate* (equally coupled) at rest. Conjugated pupils can be noted by shining a bright light into both eyes simultaneously and observing the light reflection on the same area in each eye. In coma, eyes may exhibit slow, random, roving movements that may be conjugate or dysconjugate. These movements cannot be mimicked voluntarily; hence, they are valuable in differential diagnosis.

Damage to the midbrain results in fixed pupils that are not reactive to light but do fluctuate in size. Pupils that react imply a functioning midbrain because midbrain lesions generally impinge on both the sympathetic and parasympathetic eye pathways. Lesions affecting the midbrain most commonly result from transtentorial herniation. Other causes include neoplasms and vascular abnormalities affecting the midbrain. Involvement of the sympathetic fibers, either centrally between the hypothalamus and spinal cord or peripherally at the superior cervical ganglion, cervical sympathetic chain, or along the carotid artery, results in ipsilateral pupillary constriction, ptosis (drooping eyelids), and anhidrosis (absence of sweat) of the ipsilateral side of the face (*Horner's syndrome*). Pupillary light reflex remains intact with hypothalamic damage. The combinations of symptoms indicating Horner's syndrome with central involvement are significant in that they may lead to progressive neurologic deterioration resulting in transtentorial herniation (see p. 1053).

Pontine lesions interfere with descending sympathetic pathways and thus produce bilateral small pupils. Generally, pupils with pontine involvement react to light but this may be difficult to discern without a magnifying glass.

Involvement of the third nerve may be observed in comatose persons when lesions compress the temporal uncus sufficiently to cause herniation and the resultant third nerve compression against the tentorium. Initially, a unilateral, dilated, nonreactive pupil is observed, which may progress to bilateral involvement with expanding cranial pathology.

In assessing pupillary size and reactivity to determine the origin of coma, awareness of certain pharmacologic effects may be useful. Heroin, morphine, and other opiates produce pupils characteristic of pontine lesions; that is, pupils become pinpoint and difficult to assess for light reactivity. Cocaine dilates pupils through interference with norepinephrine absorption by nerve endings. Ingestion of large amounts of atropine and scopolamine results in dilated, nonreactive pupils, which may give a false impression of a structural lesion. Glutethimide-produced (nonbarbiturate sedative; Doriden) coma results in moderately dilated, nonreactive pupils.

Profound anoxia, usually secondary to severely diminished cardiac output, results in dilated, nonreactive pupils. Metabolically produced coma generally results in pupils that are reactive until the terminal stage and thus provide significant data in differential diagnosis of coma.

### Eye Movements in Altered States of Consciousness

Vestibuloreflex pathways proximate areas controlling consciousness and, therefore, provide for a useful assessment guide. The *oculocephalic reflex (doll's head response)* is assessed by rotating the head from side to side with eyelids kept open. In the positive response, eyes deviate conjugatively opposite the head deviation. As the neck is extended, the eyes deviate to a downward gaze; as it is flexed, the eyes deviate to an upward gaze. The precise physiologic mechanism responsible for this response remains obscure, although it is hypothesized that it involves either the vestibular system or the proprioceptive afferents from the neck, or both. The presence of the doll's head response indicates an intact brainstem and intact cranial nerves controlling eye movement. The oculocephalic reflex is tested in individuals whose voluntary eye responses cannot be tested due to coma. Absence of the doll's head response indicates severe brainstem dysfunction.

*Oculovestibular reflex (cold caloric stimulation)* is

obtained by introducing cold water slowly into the intact, patent ear canal. Normal response implies that some intact brainstem function is present and is reflected by an intermittent tonic deviation of the eyes to the side of the irrigated ear.

### Respiratory Patterns in Altered States of Consciousness

Because of the neurologic influences on respiration in various regions of the brain, respiratory patterns observed during coma are useful in diagnosis (Figure 52-4). *Central neurogenic hyperventilation* is deep, rapid breathing that generally indicates dysfunction in the brainstem tegmentum between the midbrain and pons. Respiratory alkalosis is revealed by laboratory findings of low carbon dioxide tension and high pH. *Apneustic* breathing consists of a prolonged inspiratory phase followed by an expiratory pause. This pattern reflects pontine-level damage, most generally pontine infarctions secondary to basilar artery occlusions.

*Ataxic* breathing results from lesions in the RAS of the dorsomedial portion of the medulla and is characteristically a very irregular breathing pattern with irregularly interspersed pauses. The respiratory center tends to be rather hyposensitive, and minimal depression, either with mild sedation or sleep, may lead to apnea. Generally, individuals with ataxic respirations who are apneic secondary to depressant drugs or sleep respond to verbal commands to resume breathing. In severe medullary compression or lesions, ataxic breathing is viewed as a preterminal event.

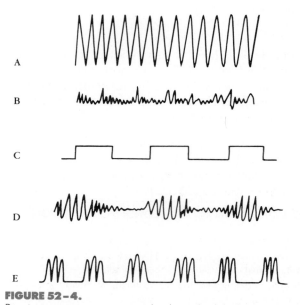

**FIGURE 52–4.**

Respiratory patterns associated with cerebral dysfunction at various levels. **A.** Central neurogenic hyperventilation (diencephalon); **B.** Ataxic (medullary); **C.** Apneustic (pontine); **D.** Cheyne-Stokes (diencephalon); **E.** Cluster (high medulla, low pons).

**TABLE 52–3.**
GLASCOW COMA SCALE

| COMA SCALE CRITERIA | | | TIME (O'CLOCK) | | | | | | | | | | | | | | | | | | | | | | | |
|---|---|---|---|---|---|---|---|---|---|---|---|---|---|---|---|---|---|---|---|---|---|---|---|---|---|---|---|
| | | | 7 | 8 | 9 | 10 | 11 | N | 1 | 2 | 3 | 4 | 5 | 6 | 7 | 8 | 9 | 10 | 11 | M | 1 | 2 | 3 | 4 | 5 | 6 |
| Eyes open | Spontaneously | 4 | | | | | | | | | | | | | | | | | | | | | | | | |
| | To speech | 3 | × | × | | | | | | | | | | | | | | | | | | | | | | |
| | To pain | 2 | | | × | | | | | | | | | | | | | | | | | | | | | |
| | None | 1 | | | | × | | | | | | | | | | | | | | | | | | | | |
| Best verbal response | Oriented | 5 | | | | | | | | | | | | | | | | | | | | | | | | |
| | Confused | 4 | × | × | | | | | | | | | | | | | | | | | | | | | | |
| | Inappropriate words | 3 | | | | | | | | | | | | | | | | | | | | | | | | | |
| | Incomprehensible sounds | 2 | | | × | | | | | | | | | | | | | | | | | | | | | | |
| | None | 1 | | | | × | | | | | | | | | | | | | | | | | | | | | |
| Best motor response | Obey commands | 5 | × | × | | | | | | | | | | | | | | | | | | | | | | | |
| | Localize pain | 4 | | | × | | | | | | | | | | | | | | | | | | | | | | |
| | Flexion to pain | 3 | | | | | | | | | | | | | | | | | | | | | | | | | |
| | Extension to pain | 2 | | | | × | | | | | | | | | | | | | | | | | | | | | |
| | None | 1 | | | | | | | | | | | | | | | | | | | | | | | | | |
| Glascow coma score (Example findings) | | | 12 | 12 | 8 | 4 | | | | | | | | | | | | | | | | | | | | |

*Cheyne-Stokes* respiration consists of a regular crescendo-decrescendo pattern altering with periods of apnea. It reflects bilateral hemispheric dysfunction with a brainstem that is essentially intact. The hemispheric disturbances resulting in Cheyne-Stokes respiration are generally deep within the brain, involving the basal ganglia and internal capsule. This respiratory pattern also accompanies disturbances of metabolic pathogenesis affecting similar cerebral regions, such as occurs with congestive heart failure. Cheyne-Stokes respiration results from an increased sensitivity to carbon dioxide levels, which leads to hyperpnea (increased respiratory rate). As a result, the blood carbon dioxide level falls to below the stimulatory level and results in a period of apnea. During the apneic period, the carbon dioxide again accumulates to the respiratory threshold level, and the cyclic hyperpnea and apnea continue.

Cluster breathing, such as *Biot's* breathing, which is not associated with a regular pattern, may result from damage in the high medulla or low pons region. Lesions in the low brainstem also may lead to frequent yawning and hiccups. The underlying mechanism for this is not clearly understood.

### Recording Assessments

Accurate neurologic assessment of the person in a coma is crucial to the correct treatment and best possible outcome. Initial assessment provides a comparative basis for subsequent observations. Changes in neurologic status are particularly important and may reveal serious pathologic processes within the nervous system.

The *Glasgow coma scale* is an assessment tool that has received wide acceptance in both the United States and Europe (Table 52-3). It provides an objective means for making and recording standardized observations with respect to eye opening, verbal responses, and motor responses. The best response in each of these categories is checked at regular time intervals and given a numeric value that, when totaled in all categories, can range from a low of three to 14 for healthy persons. It also provides a prognostic guide in that individuals with a Glasgow coma scale score of seven or below generally have a guarded prognosis, and those having a score above seven have a more favorable prognosis.

## TRAUMATIC HEAD INJURY

Our highly mechanized society has created an appalling number of traumatic injuries, a great majority resulting from use of the automobile. Many of these injuries involve the head. The resulting mortality is associated with injury and compression of the brainstem, cerebral contusions and lacerations, large expanding hemispheric lesions, and cerebral edema.

The cranial vault affords protection to the brain with the hair, skin, bone, meninges, and CSF. When force is applied, these protective encasements absorb energy that would normally be transmitted to the skull. When the force exceeds absorption capacity, it is transmitted to the cranial contents, and tissue damage results. The resultant injury frequently correlates with the amount of force applied to the cranial contents. The effect of head trauma

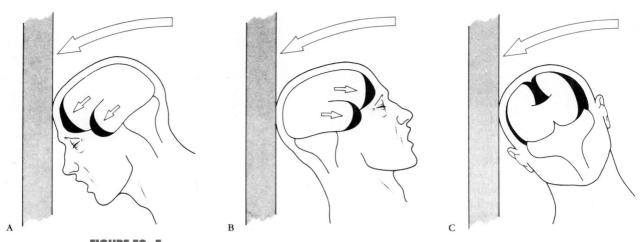

**FIGURE 52–5.**
Cortical contusion with respect to direction of head movement. **A.** Head moving forward and striking stationary surface: major injury at tips of frontal and temporal poles. **B.** Head moving backward and striking stationary surface: major injury in frontal and temporal lobes (contrecoup). **C.** Head moving laterally and striking stationary surface: major injury on side opposite that which strikes surface (contrecoup). Medial surfaces of hemispheres are also injured by impingement on relatively rigid falx (Source: S. Budassi and J. Barber, *Emergency Nursing Principles and Practice.* St. Louis: Mosby, 1981.)

may be a direct result of the injury or a secondary tissue response.

Head injuries with no obvious external damage but with an intact skull are referred to as *closed.* In contrast, *open head injuries* may reveal penetration of the scalp, skull, meninges, or brain tissue. Closed head injuries frequently result from sudden acceleration-deceleration accidents (Figure 52-5). The cranial contents shift to the opposite side of the impact within the rigid skull. This is known as the *contrecoup* injury and may lead to contusions and lacerations as the semisolid brain moves over rough projections within the cranial cavity. In addition, the cerebrum may rotate with trauma, and result in damage to the upper midbrain, as well as areas of the frontal, temporal, and occipital lobes.

## Skull Fractures

A blow to the head may result in one of several or combination of these types of skull fractures. Skull fractures may lack significance in themselves unless communication results and the cranial contents or bone fragments are driven into the neural tissue of the brain. These injuries show that a severe blow has occurred to the head and potentially severe injury has been incurred by the brain. Skull fractures may be *linear, comminuted, compound,* and *depressed.* The most common linear fractures are simply line fractures without displacement or communication with cranial contents. Comminuted fractures are multiple linear fractures and have the same characteristics. Compound fractures provide communication of the cranial contents with the lacerated scalp and are more

serious than linear and comminuted fractures. These require debridement and wound closure within 48 hours. Depressed skull fractures result in deformation of the cranial tissue by bone fragments. They decrease the volume of the cranial cavity and may produce uncal herniation. Venous return may be impeded, and secondary hemorrhages in the midbrain and pons may result. Cranial nerves may also be injured by skull fractures.

Basilar skull fractures involve the base of the skull at either the anterior, middle, or posterior fossa or combinations of the three regions. Although basilar skull fractures may be difficult to detect on radiographs, they do present some characteristic clinical signs. Fractures of the anterior and middle fossae in association with severe head trauma are more common than those of the posterior fossa. Persons with anterior fossa basilar skull fractures may exhibit periorbital ecchymosis, cranial nerve injury reflecting anosmia (first cranial nerve), and visual and pupil abnormalities (second and third cranial nerves). The presence of CSF rhinorrhea strongly suggests an anterior fossa basilar skull fracture. The signs of middle fossa basilar skull fractures include CSF otorrhea, hemotympanium, ecchymosis over the mastoid bone (Battle's sign), and facial paralysis (seventh cranial nerve injury). Involvement of the posterior fossa basilar skull may be indicated by signs of medullary failure.

## Concussions

Concussions result in a diffuse, transient and reversible injury to the brain caused by sudden movement of the brain. Damage may occur in many areas, and the extent of involvement is very variable, ranging from very mild dysfunction to severe involvement characterized by neurologic dysfunction, unconsciousness, and traumatic amnesia. Involvement of the brainstem RAS and certain subcortical areas may result in prolonged unconsciousness. This relatively minor concussion as a result of mild blows to the head may lead to brief loss of consciousness due to the temporary physiologic disruption of the RAS. If present, the period of unconsciousness ranges from seconds to as long as a few hours or more in more severe cases. No anatomic injury is sustained, and the process is reversible when neuronal function returns.

Persons suffering concussions are amnesic to the accident and may appear confused for a short period after the accident. The memory loss associated with events prior to the time of injury are referred to as *retrograde amnesia* and those associated to events after the time of injury are noted as *antegrade amnesia*. Those individuals suffering from both retrograde and antegrade amnesia are said to have *traumatic amnesia*. The length of unconsciousness and amnesia is generally proportional to the severity of the concussion. The longer the period of unconsciousness and amnesia, the more severe the injury.

Generally, neurologic signs return to normal rapidly and further deterioration does not result from the concussion after the initial impact. Invariably, headaches and dizziness accompany concussions and may persist for a long time after the injury. Some individuals also continue to experience problems with attention, memory, judgment, and concentration.

## Contusions

Contusions occur as a result of blunt trauma in closed head injuries and brain tissue destruction occurs at the area of the blow (*coup area*) or at the opposite side of the blow (*contrecoup area*). Contrecoup injuries may occur as a result of deceleration (impact stopping a moving head) or acceleration (object strikes relatively stationary head) injuries. The cerebral hemispheres, particularly the basal anterior portions of frontal and temporal lobes, as well as posterior portions of the occipital lobe, are frequently involved because these areas slide over bony irregularities of the base of the skull. Blows to the back of the head may result in contrecoup injuries to frontal and temporal lobes. A variety of neurologic abnormalities may result from *hemispheric contusions*, even though consciousness may be retained. In contrast, *brainstem contusions* result in loss of consciousness from tissue injury to the brainstem RAS. The period of unconsciousness may range from hours to a lifetime.

Cerebral lacerations involve traumatic disruption in continuity of brain tissue. Cerebral lacerations are inevitably associated with severe head injuries and occur as a result of closed blunt trauma, depressed skull fractures, or penetrating trauma. Frequently, they may be accompanied by cerebral contusions and concussions. Clinical findings and recovery are dependent on the region involved and the extent of tissue injured.

Visible bruising occurs with cerebral contusions due to the petechial hemorrhage that results from the blow to the head. The injured area swells and becomes visibly red and progressively purple due to venous obstruction and local edema. With large hemorrhages or clusters of small hemorrhages, ICP increases. The EEG recordings directly over an area of contusion reveal progressive abnormalities with the appearance of high-amplitude theta and delta waves (see Chap. 50). Regional hypoxia and acidosis may result in the contused area and produce hyperemia. Cerebral oxygen consumption is reduced by contusions, and cerebral lactate production is greatly increased, probably due to increased regional hypoxia and the resultant anaerobic metabolism.

Contusions may be partially reversible, depending on the severity of the blow and the amount of tissue injury. Lighter blows usually result in faster recovery.

## Vascular Injuries of the Brain

Potentially catastrophic intracranial processes may result from hemorrhage into the cranial vault from epidural, subdural, subarachnoid, and intracerebral vascular sources. Individuals who are lucid for a period of time after trauma and then begin to deteriorate neurologically are, in all probability, suffering from cerebrovascular injury and bleeding into the cranial contents. Bleeding into the rigid cranium results in increased ICP, which is manifested by its localized or generalized effects on the brain (see p. 1051).

### Epidural Hematoma

A serious sequela of head injuries is the epidural hematoma, venous or arterial bleeding into the extradural space resulting in compression of the brain toward the opposite side (Figure 52-6). These bleeds can arise in various regions of the brain. Those occurring in the lateral brain tend to be most severe, running a course more rapid than other, more slowly developing epidural hematomas in the frontal and occipital areas. A common epidural bleed occurs as the result of middle meningeal artery or vein injury in the parietotemporal area. This bleed is frequently accompanied by linear fractures of the skull at the temporal region over the middle meningeal artery and vein. As the blood volume increases within the cranium from the lacerated vessel, the brain is subjected to increasing pressure and distortion, which generally results in a fatal outcome within 24 hours without surgical intervention.

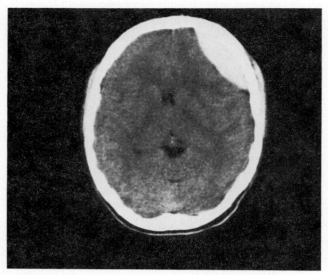

**FIGURE 52-6.**
Epidural hematoma (light area in well-contained round configuration) in right frontal lobe.

The individual with a parietotemporal epidural hematoma follows a rather predictable course. After the initial blow to the head, a lucid interval of varying length follows, although a brief period of unconsciousness frequently precedes the lucid interval, reflecting the concussive effects of head injury. The lucid interval may vary from 10 to 15 minutes to hours and, rarely, days. During this period, a severe headache often occurs. Progressive loss of consciousness and deterioration in neurologic signs follow as a result of the expanding lesion and extrusion of the temporal lobe through the tentorial opening. *Temporal lobe (uncal) herniation* compresses the brainstem and presents a rather distinct clinical picture. Deterioration of the level of consciousness results from the compression of the brainstem RAS as the temporal lobe herniates on its upper portion. Respirations become deep and labored initially and later, shallow and irregular. Contralateral motor deficiencies result due to compression of the corticospinal tracts that pass through the brainstem. Distinct ipsilateral pupillary changes can be observed as the nucleus of the third nerve originates in the brainstem and traverses upward through the tentorial opening. Seizures may present at any time during this progressive course. Without intervention, continual bleeding leads to progressive neurologic degeneration as evidenced by bilateral pupillary dilation, bilateral decerebrate response, and profound coma with irregular respiratory patterns.

Epidural hematomas are identified by the initial clinical picture, computed axial tomographic (CT) scan, roentgenograms, and EEG changes. The CT scans provide the most useful information. If a scanner is unavailable, carotid arteriography is used to outline the hematoma. Radiographs frequently reveal the linear fracture in the

parietotemporal area and displacement of the pineal gland by the hematoma. The scan identifies any abnormal masses and structural shifts within the cranium. Electroencephalographic readings may reveal diffuse slowing in the waves over the hematoma, reflecting compression of the underlying structures.

## Subdural Hematoma

Subdural hematomas are the most frequently encountered meningeal hemorrhages and occur in the *acute, subacute,* and *chronic* forms (Figures 52-7A-C). They may be unilateral or bilateral. Bleeding into the subdural space (between dura mater and arachnoid mater) as a result of injury to vessels may be from either venous or arterial sources, although the venous source is more common.

Acute subdural hematomas result from severe head injuries and may accompany other manifestations of cerebral trauma, such as contusions and lacerations. They may resemble epidural hematomas in their neurologic deficits with rapid deterioration without prompt intervention. The appearance of the symptoms is usually within 48 hours of injury. The person may be unconscious and rapidly deteriorate, or may be in a lucid state that deteriorates to drowsiness, agitation, stupor, and coma. Signs of brainstem compression may be evidenced by a unilaterally dilated pupil and contralateral hemiparesis. Acute subdural hematomas are identified in the same manner as epidural hematomas. Once diagnosed, they constitute a surgical emergency and must be treated promptly. The hematomas can be evacuated through burr holes or by craniotomy. Unfortunately, acute hematomas carry a high mortality, even with surgical intervention.

Subacute subdural hematomas have an improved prognosis because the venous bleeding tends to be slower than in the acute form. Symptoms generally appear within 2 days to 2 weeks after injury. The individual is usually lucid after the head injury; this state degenerates to drowsiness, stupor, and coma. The person may stabilize into a coma for a few days and not exhibit the steady deterioration that accompanies the epidural hematomas. The period of stability is followed by a period of fluctuating neurologic signs that progress to increasing ICP and eventual fatal outcome without surgical interventions. The presence of subacute subdural hematomas is established by the clinical signs, MRIs, CT scans, or roentgenograms.

Chronic subdural hematomas result from very slow bleeding as a result of an insignificant injury. This type of injury is most common in infants, the elderly, and apparently demented or alcoholic individuals. Symptoms appear over a wide time span from 2 weeks to several months. Because the bleeding slowly accumulates as a clot within the subdural space, a period of hemolysis follows. Cerebrospinal fluid is attracted to the lysed blood through osmosis through the arachnoid membrane. The

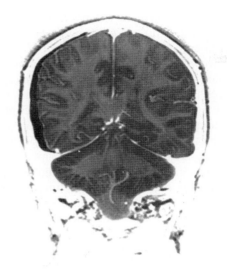

**A**

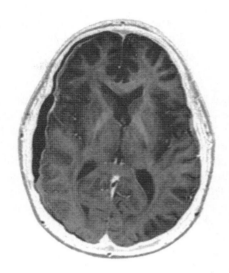

**B**

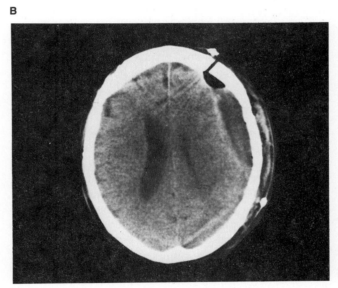

**C**

**FIGURE 52–7.**
**A.** Subdural hematoma coronal view. **B.** Subdural hematoma transverse view. **C.** Subdural hematoma recurring after craniotomy (darker area in right frontoparietal region) showing compression of right ventricle.

increasing size of the subdural hematoma impinges further on surrounding capillaries, tearing some of these and initiating more bleeding. This increases the osmotic force even further and contributes to the increase in the overall size of the hematoma. The hematoma may eventually form an encasing membrane around it that may calcify, or it may continue its slow bleed and, lacking proper intervention, result in transtentorial herniation and a fatal outcome.

An individual with chronic subdural hematoma may or may not recall injury to the head. A period of weeks may follow during which the person experiences headache, slowness of thinking, apathy, drowsiness, and confusion. He or she is usually conscious on admission to the hospital and may complain of a generalized dull headache. In the early stages, the individual may exhibit

some hemiparesis on the contralateral side. With progressive changes, focal seizures, papilledema, homonymous hemianopsia, aphasia, and waxing and waning of the level of consciousness may develop.

Chronic subdural hematomas may be identified by the xanthochromic (yellow appearance) and relatively low protein content of the CSF. The EEG may show increased slow activity in the theta and delta waves with diminished voltage in the region of the hematoma. Tomographic scans, radiographs, and arteriography may be helpful in confirming the presence of the hematoma. Chronic subdural hematomas are generally drained through burr holes. This may be followed by turning a bone flap to remove any thickened membranes to diminish the possibility of recurrence. Small chronic subdural hematomas may be managed without surgery. The prognosis is considerably better when proper intervention has been instituted than for the more acute forms of this hematoma or the epidural hematoma.

## Subdural Hygroma

Subdural hygroma is an excessive collection of fluid under the dura mater, which most commonly results from trauma. Subsequent tearing of the arachnoid allows CSF to escape into the subdural space. Due to the vascularity of the arachnoid, some vessels are generally damaged, also allowing CSF to mix with blood in the subdural space. This CSF-blood mixing produces a highly osmotic fluid that continues to pull in fluid; it slowly expands in size.

The diagnosis is confirmed with certainty by burr hole skull opening, although these hygromas may be revealed by CT scan and other radiologic procedures. Developing signs and symptoms of subdural hygromas after trauma are very similar to those of the chronic subdural hematomas. Symptoms are relieved by draining the fluid if a large collection of fluid-produced neurologic deficits and other pathologic processes are not present.

## Subarachnoid Hemorrhage

Subarachnoid hemorrhage refers to bleeding into the subarachnoid space (Figure 52-8). It may occur spontaneously with a disruption in the vascular integrity, or most commonly, as a result of congenital malformations of cerebrovascular beds, such as arteriovenous malformations or cerebral aneurysms. These may also be associated with developmental defects in the media and elastica of vessels. It may also result from trauma. Bleeding into the subarachnoid space originates from arterial sources

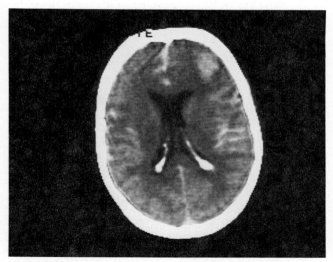

**FIGURE 52–8.**
Subarachnoid bleeding (light diffuse areas throughout brain).

and mixes freely with the circulating CSF, irritating the contacting central nervous system structures.

The clinical signs in subarachnoid hemorrhage are generalized and in most situations do not focus in the area of involvement; therefore, they are not significant in localizing the site of hemorrhage. They include headache, which is frequently described as severe, violent, or excruciating. Some individuals retain consciousness initially, although about one half experience a delayed-onset coma. Conscious individuals complain of visual disturbances, such as photophobia or diplopia and deterioration of vision. Fever, malaise, vomiting, and nuchal rigidity may be additional clinical findings. Abnormal mentation with disorientation is not uncommon. The spinal fluid is grossly bloody and exhibits increased pressure. Xanthochromia is noted within a few hours of the bleed and persists for about 20 to 30 days. The spinal fluid also shows increased monocytes and protein. Other helpful diagnostic procedures are cerebral angiography and CT scan.

Cerebral vasospasm is a frequent and potentially serious complication associated with subarachnoid hemorrhage. It may accompany the hemorrhage from ruptured cerebral aneurysm, trauma, tumors, or arteriovenous malformations to a lesser degree. Cerebral vasospasm is the angiographically demonstrated narrowing of portions of the involved arteries.[6] Symptomatic vasospasm becomes evident about 4 to 12 days after the hemorrhage and generally resolves within 3 weeks. The symptoms include worsening headache, low grade fever, change in level of consciousness, aphasia, and hemiparesis.[13] The focal deficits are related to the area involved. The exact cause of cerebral vasospasm remains unknown but it is hypothesized that certain substances, such as serotonin, prostaglandins, and catecholamines released from platelets and erythrocytes, as well as histamine, oxyhemoglobin, and angiotensin have spasmogenic properties.[6]

Subarachnoid hemorrhage may be treated surgically or conservatively, depending on the general overall condition of the individual. Those who are obtunded and experiencing significant vasospasm are generally not good surgical risks and are treated conservatively with strict bedrest until the condition improves or vasospasm decreases. Recurrence of bleeding is always a possibility, and much of the focus of care is directed at preventing this.

## Intracerebral Hematoma

Traumatic disruption of cerebral vessels within the cerebral substance may result in neurologic deficits, depending on the location and amount of bleeding. The shearing forces resulting from brain movement within the skull frequently lead to laceration of the vessels and hemorrhage into the parenchyma. Common sites of intracerebral bleeding are the frontal and temporal lobes.

Those intracerebral hematomas associated with trauma comprise a very small percentage of all intracerebral hematomas.

Individuals with intracerebral bleeding may be comatose or may have a lucid period before lapsing into a coma. Motor deficits may be present, and decorticate or decerebrate responses may occur. The bleeding site may be identified by CT scan, as shown in Figure 52-1, or by cerebral arteriography. The CSF pressure may be elevated and the fluid may appear bloody and xanthochromic.

Intracerebral hematomas may be treated by surgical decompression through burr holes or by removing a bone flap. Surgical evacuation frequently is impossible due to location of the hematomas. Even with successful surgical evacuation, neurologic deficits frequently remain due to residual effects of the hematoma and trauma. Conservative treatment focuses on minimizing cerebral edema and increased ICP through medications, posturing, and supportive therapy.

## Cerebral Edema

A common and serious sequela of head injury is cerebral edema, wherein the total water content in the brain parenchyma becomes excessive. In addition to head injury, cerebral edema may also occur with intracranial surgery, brain tumors, hypoxemia, infarctions, and infections. Two distinct types have been identified: *cytotoxic* and *vasogenic*. Cytotoxic cerebral edema reflects cellular dysfunction or injury and occurs secondarily to conditions that result in the accumulation of metabolic waste products associated with cerebral hypoxia. Cytotoxic edema affects primarily the gray matter of the brain. The fluid collection is intracellular within most of the cell components of the brain. The sodium pump is not able to remove accumulating intracellular sodium due to adenosine triphosphate (ATP) deficiency that results from hypoxia. The accumulated intracellular sodium pulls water into the cell, and waste products of anaerobic metabolism accumulate, rendering the cell dysfunctional. Cytotoxic edema occurs with certain intoxications, hypoxia, some metabolic disorders, and water overload.

Vasogenic edema is a result of damage to or dysfunction in the cerebral blood vessels. The fluid forms intercellularly and its composition is very similar to plasma. This type of cerebral edema results from increased permeability of the capillary membranes and widening of the junctions between the cells (breakdown of blood-brain barrier). The widening of these normally tight junctions allows plasma proteins from the blood to pass into the extracellular spaces. Vasogenic edema occurs commonly with trauma, including surgical trauma, contusions, inflammatory processes, neoplasms, and subdural and epidural hematomas.

It is thought that alteration in the blood-brain barrier occurs in both types of cerebral edema. The mechanism of the alteration is not known but it has been proposed to be associated with loss of cerebral autoregulation. As a result of malfunction of the blood-brain barrier, the brain becomes more permeable to molecules that normally do not cross this barrier.

As cerebral edema increases within the nonflexible skull, clinical signs indicate increased ICP. If edema progresses, neurologic function continues to deteriorate due to intracranial shifts or herniations. The signs indicating increased ICP, brain shifts, and herniations are discussed on pp. 1051–1054.

The morphologic changes in the edematous brain as seen at surgery or autopsy are characteristic and striking. The brain appears heavy and boggy. The gyri have lost their normal triangular appearance and the sulci have been obliterated. Brain sections reveal flattened ventricles and an indiscernible subarachnoid space.[6]

## Initial Assessment and Management of Head Injuries

After the initial assurance of an adequate airway, effective respiratory exchange, and absence of acute shock, a careful history is obtained. If possible, the nature of the accident is determined and the lapse of time since the accident is noted. This information may assist in localizing the site of injury and give some indication of its degree. Neurologic evaluation of the level of consciousness, pupillary responses, motor activity, respiratory patterns, and vital signs is obtained for a baseline assessment. In addition, the head is examined carefully to determine the presence of lacerations, foreign objects, or depressed skull fractures. The ear canals are evaluated for the presence of blood, and otoscopic examination of the tympanic membrane is carried out to assess for a bluish coloration indicating bleeding into the middle ear. The presence of ecchymosis over the mastoid area (*Battle's sign*) is evaluated and may indicate the possibility of a basilar skull fracture. Blood from the ear, if mixed with CSF (*otorrhea*), will not clot and leaves a halo effect at the periphery of the drainage on dressings or pillow. Drainage of mixed blood and CSF from the nose (*rhinorrhea*) has characteristics similar to those of otorrhea.[12]

Individuals with acute head injuries should be treated as if they also sustained a cervical spine injury until it is proven otherwise. Pain, if present, may be associated with the area of neck injury. However, this is not a totally reliable indicator of the presence of spinal cord injury (SCI) because pain may not be exhibited and cannot be verified in the unconscious person. Careful palpation of the neck and alignment of the spinous process at the midline of the posterior neck should be done to evaluate for possible cervical cord injury. The neck is immobilized with sandbags, cervical collars, or head straps until cervical radiographs indicate no abnormalities.

Vital signs reflect the status of the head-injured person and may support the late findings of increased ICP or the presence of shock. Elevated temperature may indicate small brainstem hemorrhages or trauma directly to the thermoregulatory mechanisms of the hypothalamus. Focal seizures may accompany acute head injuries and help to localize the site of the lesion. Observations of the nature and origin of the onset of the seizures are invaluable to the overall assessment of the head-injured individual.

## ASSESSMENT OF TRAUMATIC DISRUPTION TO CRANIAL NERVES

A person with a head injury may suffer partial or total loss of function of cranial nerves in the area of the lesion. If the individual is conscious, the function of each of the nerves can be assessed briefly. In addition, the integrity of several of the cranial nerves can be assessed grossly in the unconscious individual.

### Olfactory Nerve

The first cranial nerve extends from the inferior surface of the frontal lobe and mediates the sense of smell. Disruption of the olfactory nerve may accompany acute head injury, particularly in the presence of basilar skull fractures involving the anterior fossa and fractures of the cribriform plate. Nerve filaments may be damaged in contrecoup injuries after trauma to the occipital or parietotemporal region. Other disorders responsible for disruption of the sense of smell (*anosmia*) include upper respiratory infections, rhinitis, tumors, meningitis, and subarachnoid hemorrhages.

The first cranial nerve can be assessed simply by requesting the individual to close his or her eyes and identify some common odors such as soap, coffee, and alcohol. Each nostril is tested individually and the person is asked to occlude one nostril while the other is being tested. First cranial nerve function cannot be evaluated in the unconscious individual.

### Optic Nerve

The second cranial nerve is necessary for vision. Visual impulses originate in the photoreceptors of the retinas and are transmitted by the optic nerve to the optic chiasm and to the various parts of the occipital cortex for recognition and interpretation. Lesions from trauma or intrinsic origins anywhere along these pathways cause specific patterns of visual loss (see Figure 49-3). Damage to the optic nerve generally results from force to the frontal area of the skull. Vision defects may also result from injury to the vessels supplying the optic nerve. Vision loss is maximal directly after injury. If vision is to be recovered, it may be anticipated within the first month after injury because optic nerve atrophy begins within this time. Injury to the occipital lobe may also result in impaired vision. However, commonly pupillary light reflexes in this situation remain intact and prognosis generally is favorable.

Careful clinical evaluation of the visual fields can be very significant in determining the site of a lesion. The quadrants of each eye of the cooperative person can be examined individually by superimposing the examiner's eye directly in the visual field of the individual. The examiner closes the eye directly across from the individual's closed eye. The person is instructed to look directly into the examiner's eye and is asked to signal on first seeing the examiner's finger move into the visual field. This is repeated from each of the four quadrants of each eye: superior, inferior, temporal, and nasal. Assuming the examiner's vision to be normal, the injured person should see the finger at the same time the examiner does. A more rudimentary assessment is simply to ask the person to count the number of fingers the examiner is holding out. The unresponsive or uncooperative individual may respond with a blink to a threatened motion toward the head if visual fields are at least partially intact. An unconscious person's ability to perceive light can be assessed during examination of the direct light reflex, because the second cranial nerve forms the afferent nerve for this reflex arc.

A frequently encountered vision disturbance is *homonymous hemianopsia* in which corresponding halves of bilateral vision are lost. In addition to trauma, cerebral infarctions, tumors, and abscesses may cause homonymous hemianopsia. This defect can be recognized by having the individual count all 10 fingers held out by the examiner. Wide turning of the individual's head to visualize all fingers may indicate a homonymous hemianopsia.

### Oculomotor, Trochlear, and Abducens Nerves

The third, fourth, and sixth nerves are generally examined together because of their cooperative function in controlling the movements of the eyes. In addition, the oculomotor nerve innervates the levator palpebrae superioris muscle, which mediates elevation of the eyelids, and the constrictor muscle of the iris, which alters pupillary aperture in accordance with the degree of illumination. Similarly, convergence and accommodation are mediated by the third nerve. Pupillary responses are more fully discussed in Chapter 49.

The nuclei of the oculomotor nerve are in the midbrain. The axons traverse ventrally to emerge from the midbrain at the level of the tentorial notch and pass through a portion of the cerebral peduncle. At this level, the nerve is particularly vulnerable to compression from other cerebral structures, and its encroachment is reflected by unilateral pupil change on the ipsilateral side.

The third cranial nerve innervates the levator of the eyelid, superior and inferior recti, inferior oblique, and medial rectus. It moves the eyes up, down, obliquely, and medially. The nuclei of the trochlear nerve also are in the midbrain caudal to the oculomotor nucleus, and transmit impulses to the superior oblique muscle to move the eye down and out. The abducens nuclei are in the lower pons below the fourth ventricle floor and control lateral eye movements by innervating superior, inferior, and medial rectus muscles and the inferior oblique muscle.

Trauma of the frontal region of the skull may cause injury to the third, fourth, and sixth nerves. Brainstem trauma may result in difficulties with conjugate movement, and paralysis of individual nerves may ensue in some persons. Upward gaze and convergence and lateral eye movements may be interrupted with brainstem lesions. Numerous combinations of third, fourth, and sixth nerve palsies may accompany injuries to the nerves of the superior orbital fissure. Frequently, these injuries are accompanied by diplopia.

In assessing extraocular eye movements, the eyes are observed for conjugate gaze. They are examined with respect to each other and should be aligned parallel in the visual axis when the individual is gazing straight ahead. Extraocular function is evaluated by asking the person to follow the examiner's finger in six cardinal positions. In the comatose individual, spontaneous eye movement may be noted. Eye movement also may be noted by assessing the oculocephalic reflex (doll's head maneuver).

## Trigeminal Nerve

The fifth cranial nerve is a mixed sensory motor nerve and mediates sensations from over the entire face and scalp to the vertex, the paranasal sinuses, the nasal and oral cavities, and the corneae. The motor component of the fifth nerve innervates the muscles of mastication. The sensory nuclei of the trigeminal nerve are in the gasserian ganglion anterior to the pons, and the motor nuclei arise in the midpons region.

The extracranial portions of the fifth nerve are most frequently involved in traumatic injuries. Scalp wounds or compression fractures of the supraorbital area may sever its supraorbital portion of the fifth nerve. This may be identified by the paresthesias, hyperesthesias, and neuralgic pain that lingers in the affected scalp and forehead. The infraorbital portion may also be severed and result in anesthesia of the affected cheek and upper lip.

Causes of disruption of parts of the fifth nerve include tumors arising in the posterior fossa, as well as generalized trauma to the cerebellopontile region or local trauma to the face. *Tic douloureux*, or *trigeminal neuralgia*, occurs primarily in women in the fifth and sixth decades of life and is manifested by excruciating, unpredictable, paroxysmal pain along part or all of the divisions of the fifth nerve. The cause of this condition remains obscure but it has been known to be exacerbated by infections, emotional upset, facial movements, and drafts.

Three major divisions of the fifth nerve are the *ophthalmic, maxillary*, and *mandibular*. Each of these divisions is examined for touch perception and discrimination on both sides of the face. With the individual's eyes closed, the examiner tests areas with a wisp of cotton and a pin, asking the person to identify which area is touched. The afferent limb of the corneal reflex is mediated by the fifth cranial nerve. The *corneal reflex* is assessed by stroking the cornea with a wisp of cotton from the side while the person's eyes are turned to the opposite side to avoid an involuntary blink.

The motor component of the fifth nerve is examined by having the person clench the teeth and open the mouth while the examiner palpates the jaw. Deviation occurs to the affected side in presence of weakness.

Most of the assessment of the fifth cranial nerve requires cooperation by the person; however, a few aspects may be assessed in the comatose individual. The chin can be pushed down and resistance noted. The corneal reflex also can be assessed.

## Facial Nerve

The seventh cranial nerve is a mixed motor and sensory nerve, although its primary innervation is motor control of the muscles of facial expression. Its sensory component mediates taste perception in the anterior two thirds of the tongue and innervates the lacrimal and certain salivary glands. The nucleus for the seventh nerve is in the lower pons. Certain cortical innervation of the voluntary movement of the face is transmitted to portions of the seventh nerve nucleus by way of the corticobulbar tract. Some of these axons cross to the contralateral nuclei and others terminate in the ipsilateral nuclei. High face muscles are innervated by fibers from both contralateral and ipsilateral fibers, and the lower muscles are innervated by fibers from the contralateral cortex only. Weakness generated from the effects on the corticobulbar tract are of central origin (upper motor neuron) and cause only contralateral lower face weakness. Ipsilateral weakness of an entire side of the face is of peripheral origin (lower motor neuron) from a lesion at the nucleus or the peripheral axon of the seventh nerve.

Dysfunction of the seventh nerve may occur with basilar skull fractures because its location traversing the temporal bone makes it particularly susceptible to injury. Fractures of the petrous portions of the temporal bone may result in injury to the seventh nerve and resultant facial paralysis. In such situations, the prognosis is generally favorable, and function returns with slow recovery that may last for months.

Proximity of the seventh nerve to the middle ear increases the injurious effects of middle ear infections and tumors of the region on the nerve. Central facial paralysis can result from infarctions, lesions, and abscesses of the contralateral cerebral cortex. *Bell's palsy* is an inflammatory response to infections and allergies affecting the seventh nerve within the temporal bone, which results in ipsilateral facial paralysis.

Assessment of the facial nerve includes examining facial tone and symmetry by requesting the person to wrinkle the forehead, smile, whistle, close the eyes, and show the teeth. The sensory component can be assessed by applying sweet, sour, salty, and bitter substances to the appropriate areas of the anterior tongue and having the person identify the tastes. The mouth is rinsed between applications of the substances.

In the comatose person, the corneal reflex may be assessed as the efferent limb of the reflex is mediated by the facial nerve. In addition, facial grimacing can be noted in response to noxious stimulation.

## Vestibulocochlear Nerve

The eighth cranial nerve is composed of the vestibular and cochlear divisions, the former mediating balance and equilibrium and the latter, hearing. Nuclei of the acoustic nerve are in the lower pons (see Chap. 50).

Traumatic head injury may result in loss of hearing due to fractures extending through the middle ear. Severing of the nerve results in permanent deafness. Hemorrhage into the middle ear also compromises hearing; however, it does carry a prognosis of some recovery of hearing as the blood clot is absorbed. Edema and contusions of the eighth nerve result in hearing impairments that recover with the healing process. Vertigo results from edema or hemorrhage into the labyrinth, which is aggravated by head movement and associated with nausea and vomiting. Although vertigo may be resolved within 2 or 3 weeks, the person may continue to feel lightheaded and reveal signs of ataxia for months after the injury. True vertigo results from labyrinthine disease. The classic type is Meniere's disease (see Chap. 50).

Hearing can be assessed simply by covering one of the person's ears and whispering softly near the other. This is repeated in the other ear. Ability to hear whispering is fairly indicative of normal hearing. Should whispering not be audible, further testing is indicated. The vestibular component is investigated primarily through a described history of vertigo, unsteadiness of gait, and nausea. Testing is undertaken on the basis of the presence of the above symptoms.

Hearing can be assessed grossly in the comatose individual by noting the response to noise or verbal stimuli. Lack of response may also indicate deep coma. The vestibular component may be assessed by the oculocephalic or oculovestibular reflexes.

## Glossopharyngeal and Vagus Nerves

The ninth and tenth nerves are anatomically and structurally similar and, therefore, are examined together. The glossopharyngeal nerve innervates the muscles of the pharynx, posterior one third of the taste sensation of the tongue, sensations of the tonsils, pharynx, and carotid sinuses, and carotid body. The vagus nerve has widespread innervation of the thoracic and abdominal visceral organs, as well as the larynx and pharynx. The nuclei of these nerves are in the medulla.

Traumatic injury to the lower brainstem, fractures of the posterior fossa, and vascular injuries at the base of the skull may injure the ninth and tenth nerves. This is reflected in dysphagia and a diminished or absent gag reflex.

Assessment of the ninth and tenth cranial nerves involves an initial inspection of the soft palate for symmetry. A gag reflex is elicited with a tongue blade in contact with the posterior oropharynx. Normally, the palate elevates and the pharyngeal muscles contract. The person is asked to swallow water, and the ability to do this without regurgitating is assessed. Speech is noted for signs of abnormal phonation and hoarseness. The gag and swallowing reflexes are routinely assessed in the comatose individual by noting the ability to handle secretions. This indicates gross function of the ninth and tenth cranial nerves.

## Accessory Nerve

The 11th cranial nerve nuclei are in the anterior gray column of the first few segments of the cervical spinal cord and transmit to innervate the sternocleidomastoid and trapezius muscles to allow lifting or shrugging of shoulders, head rotation, and neck extension. Low brainstem injuries and fractures of the posterior fossa and basilar skull may result in injury and paralysis of the 11th nerve. In addition, trauma to the neck region may result in impairment of the spinal accessory nerve. Weakness on one side may be suggestive of a stroke, whereas bilateral weakness may support motor neuron diseases or neuromuscular problems.

The functioning of this motor nerve in innervating the sternocleidomastoid is evaluated by having the individual turn the head toward the shoulder while the examiner puts resistance on the movement and assesses the strength of the muscle. This test is repeated on the other side. The functioning of the trapezius is evaluated by having the person raise the shoulders against the resistance applied by the examiner. Assessment of this cranial nerve requires cooperation and, therefore, its integrity cannot be determined in a comatose individual.

## Hypoglossal Nerve

The 12th cranial nerve is a motor nerve innervating the musculature of the tongue to allow normal articulation and food management in the mouth. Its nucleus is in the floor of the fourth ventricle. The function of the hypoglossal nerve may be jeopardized by trauma to the neck, as well as to the regions described in the 11th nerve injuries. Traumatic lesion here may result in unilateral tongue weakness, which is evidenced by deviation of the protruding tongue to the weak side. Bilateral tongue weakness is most commonly associated with disease processes, such as amyotrophic lateral sclerosis and poliomyelitis.

The function of the hypoglossal nerve is evaluated by having the individual protrude the tongue and observing for any deviation. The strength of the muscles of the tongue is assessed by the examiner by pushing against the cheek that the person is pressing outward with the tongue. Notation is made of any difficulty with articulation during conversation. In the comatose individual, one can note the position and movement of the tongue when the mouth is opened. The tongue normally lies in the midline and deviation to either side is abnormal.

## INCREASED INTRACRANIAL PRESSURE (INTRACRANIAL HYPERTENSION)

Head injuries may lead to increased ICP due to expanding brain volume, increased blood volume, or increased accumulation of CSF. Without treatment, this may compromise neurologic function, as well as life, itself. Therefore, early diagnosis and treatment are essential. In addition to trauma, increased ICP accompanies many neurologic problems and conditions.

In the adult, the cranial vault affords a nonflexible encasement around the brain tissue and extracellular fluid, which is primarily blood and CSF. Although total intracranial volume varies slightly, ICP remains relatively constant. Small increases in volume of one of the cranial components are compensated normally by a decrease in the volume of another (Monro-Kellie hypothesis). Intracranial CSF may be shifted to the subarachnoid space of the spine, and the vascular bed of the brain may be reduced by shifting the blood to areas of less resistance.[4] A measure of stiffness of the brain is known as *elastance* and indicates the brain's tolerance for increases in volume. Elastance is described by the formula: $E = P/V$ where $E$ = elastance; $P$ = pressure; and $V$ = volume.

Intracranial *compliance*, the ability of the cranial contents to adapt to changes in volume, is determined by the volume and rate of displacement of intracranial tissue, blood, and CSF. Compliance is the reciprocal of elastance and can be described by the following formula: $C = V/P$.

During the period of compensation when the volume/pressure curve is increasing slowly, large intracranial volume increases can be tolerated without significant ICP changes (adequate compliance, low elastance).[4] When the small margin of compensation within the cranium is exhausted, however, the ICP rises, and small increases in volume at this point result in large rises in ICP (decreased compliance, high elastance) (Figure 52-9). Without intervention, decompensation and death ensue.

When present, clinical indicators of increased ICP include headache, recurrent vomiting, decreased level of consciousness, papilledema, pupillary dilation, peripheral motor changes, and respiratory irregularities. Decreasing pulse, elevated systolic pressure, and widening pulse pressure (Cushing's response) are compensatory signs supportive of maintaining cerebral blood flow. The varying presence of these signs indicates the level of brain dysfunction that has occurred as a result of the

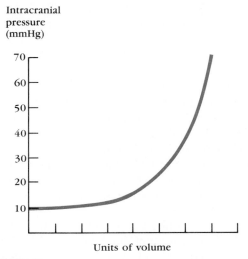

**FIGURE 52-9.**
Compliance curve: intracranial volume/pressure relationship. Compensation rapidly falls as volume rises. (Source: B. Jennett, *An Introduction to Neurosurgery* [3rd ed.]. London: Heinemann, 1977.)

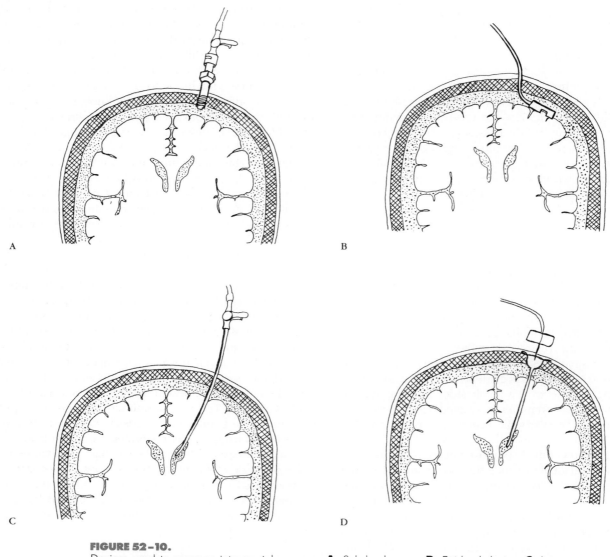

**FIGURE 52-10.**
Devices used to measure intracranial pressure. **A.** Subdural screw. **B.** Epidural device. **C.** Intraventricular catheter. **D.** Intraventricular cannula (Source: *Massachusetts General Hospital Department of Nursing Manual of Nursing Procedures* [2nd ed.]. Boston: Little, Brown, 1980.)

pathologic process that led to the increased ICP. Generally, when the clinical signs indicating brain stem involvement (hypertension, bradycardia, irregular respirations) are present, the individual has reached a state of decompensation and has a poor prognosis for recovery. Treatment is most effective while the brain is in a compensatory state because once compensatory mechanisms have been used up, the pressure within the cranium rises rapidly.

Intracranial monitoring provides a reliable means to detect changes in ICP before clinical signs are evident. This is most conveniently done by measuring CSF as pressure is equally transmitted in all directions in fluid.[3] Changes in ICP can be monitored by the use of a sub-

dural screw, an epidural device, through the lateral ventricles with an intraventricular cannula, or directly in the brain parenchyma through a transducer tipped pressure monitor catheter (Figure 52-10). Normal ICP is less than 13 mm Hg or 200 mm of water. Some fluctuations over the narrow normal range are common. The pressures measured by these methods are transmitted to a pressure transducer and recording instrument. The mechanical impulses transmitted to the transducer are converted into electrical impulses that appear on an oscilloscope as varying wave patterns (Figure 52-11). The most significant of these are the plateau waves (A waves) that are recorded with advanced stages of increased ICP.

The pressure in the cranium may rise rather abruptly

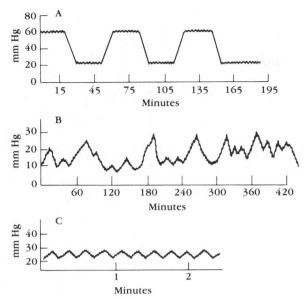

**FIGURE 52–11.**

Generalized shapes of the three types of ICP waves; A, or plateau waves (top), B waves (middle) and C waves (bottom). Source: A. Hamilton, *Critical Care Nursing Skills.* New York: Appleton-Century-Crofts, 1981.)

or insidiously. Severely head-injured individuals with rapidly increasing ICP and intracranial bleeding frequently have escape of blood into the CSF, which results in an increased osmotic force, thus increasing CSF volume. Increased ICP also occurs with infections, tumors, and hypercapnia. Tissue expands with inflammatory and neoplastic processes, and the cerebral vasculature increases in size in response to elevated carbon dioxide levels. Expansion of the volume of tissue and CSF results in compression of cerebral vessels and, in turn, a reflexively higher systemic blood pressure, resulting in a compensatory lower pulse rate. Without adequate intervention, the cerebral structures shift and decompensation is noted by a decrease in the systemic blood pressure and rapid, irregular, weak pulse.

## *Intracranial Shifts (Herniation Syndromes)*

Major brain shifts that can occur in response to expanding cerebral pathology are *cingulate herniation, transcalvarial herniation, central transtentorial herniation, uncal herniation*, and *cerebellar foramen magnum herniation* (Figure 52-12). These develop in response to intracranial hypertension in a cranium that is subdivided into compartments by a rather rigid membrane, the dura mater. The falx cerebri divides the cerebral hemispheres, and the tentorium cerebelli divides the cerebrum from the cerebellum. The tentorial notch is the oval-shaped opening in the tentorium cerebelli that allows the passage of nerve tracts and blood vessels. Expanding cerebral pathology in any one of the compartments will shift pressure to a compartment of lesser pressure. The signs and symptoms associated with intracranial shifts are dependent on the amount of compensation; the compartment involved, eg, supratentorial or infratentorial; and the location of the lesion in that compartment.

In cingulate herniation, lateral displacement of expanding cerebral mass compresses the cingulate gyrus under the falx cerebri, which displaces the internal cerebral vein. This displacement results in the vessel compression and leads to ischemia and edema, thus potentially further increasing the ICP. Transcalvarial herniation occurs with open head injuries where the brain tissue extrudes through an unstable fractured skull.

Central transtentorial herniation (a rostral-caudal displacement) may result from supratentorial lesions; however, they are more commonly a result of diffuse increased ICP, such as in Reye's syndrome. Pressure is exerted centrally and downward displacement occurs, encroaching on the diencephalon and midbrain. Cingulate herniation may precede the central transtentorial herniation.

Clinical signs of central transtentorial herniation reflect increasing ICP and include changes in alertness and visual acuity. Papilledema results from optic nerve compression because interference occurs with venous return from the optic disk. As central expansion progresses caudally, brainstem compression is reflected clinically by a further deteriorating level of consciousness. With compression of the corticospinal tract, the Babinski's

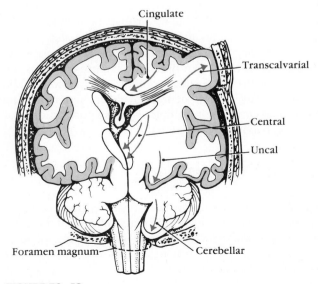

**FIGURE 52–12.**

Major types of intracranial herniations.

response is elicited and the extremities become rigid and deteriorate to a decortication or decerebration (see pp. 1036–1039). Early central herniation exhibits pupillary constriction, which leads to moderate dilation without light reflex response as increasing pressure is exerted on the midbrain region. Wide, fixed dilation is a terminal sign. Respiratory patterns initially may be periodic with yawning and sighing interruptions. This changes to a persistent hyperventilation as central compression continues caudally and, in terminal stages, becomes an ataxic pattern prior to respiratory arrest.

Lesions in the lateral middle fossa or medial part of one temporal lobe result in *uncal herniation*. Crowding in the uncus and hippocampal gyrus at the tentorial notch compresses the ipsilateral third nerve, which results in a unilaterally dilated pupil. In cases where the uncus compresses and displaces the diencephalon and midbrain to the opposite side, pupillary dilation and motor changes occur opposite the side of the lesion. Neurologic deterioration may progress rapidly without successful intervention after the initial pupillary dilation, to stupor, absence of extraocular movement, hemiplegia, and decerebrate posturing. Terminal stages of uncal herniation resemble central herniation.

Cerebellar foramen magnum herniation results from the expanding lesions of the cerebellum and may be unilateral or bilateral displacement. The expanding lesions may be caused by centrally placed frontal tumors or generalized brain swelling, such as in Reye's syndrome, or arise in association with uncal herniation. The effects of cerebellar foramen magnum herniation and traumatic, rapidly expanding lesions below the tentorium result in brainstem dysfunction with a rapid loss of consciousness and other neurologic deficits indicating severe dysfunction. The dysfunction is caused by the direct effects on the vital centers in the brainstem and the inability of the subtentorial contents to compensate adequately. Motor responses vary from flaccidity to flexor to extension responses. Low brainstem breathing patterns, such as apneustic and ataxic breathing, predominate. Lesions of the medulla result in rapid neurologic deterioration, leading to death as centers controlling respiratory and vasomotor function become dysfunctional.

## SPINAL CORD INJURY

Injuries of the spinal cord as a result of trauma are increasing every year due to the extensive use of the automobile and increased amount of time persons spend in recreation and sports activities. Figures 52-13 and 52-14 show the relationship of SCI to traumatic events and its incidence in the younger population. Additionally, SCI affects the male population much more frequently than females by an 82% to 18% margin.[11] The extent and level

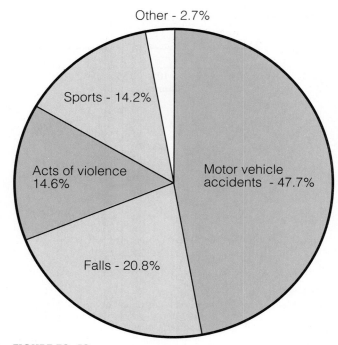

**FIGURE 52–13.**

Distribution of SCI by etiology (Source: S.L. Stover and P.R. Fine, *Spinal Cord Injury: The Facts and Figures.* Birmingham: University of Alabama at Birmingham, 1985.)

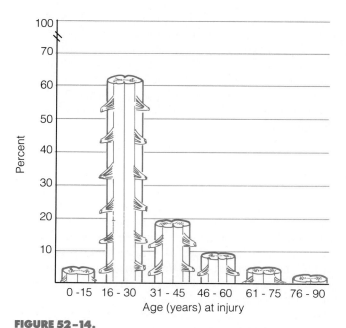

**FIGURE 52–14.**

Age at injury. (Source: S.L. Stover and P.R. Fine, *Spinal Cord Injury: The Facts and Figures.* Birmingham: University of Alabama at Birmingham, 1985.)

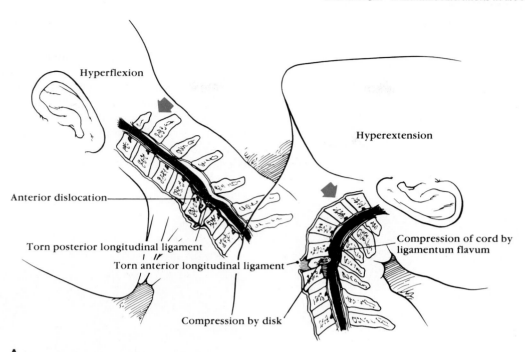

Hyperflexion

Hyperextension

Anterior dislocation

Compression of cord by
ligamentum flavum

Torn posterior longitudinal ligament

Torn anterior longitudinal ligament

Compression by disk

**A**

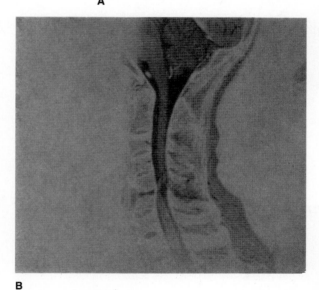

**B**

**FIGURE 52-15.**
**A.** Mechanism of spinal injury (Source: C.V. Kenner, C.E. Guzzetta, and B.M. Dossey, *Critical Care Nursing* [2nd ed.]. Boston: Little, Brown, 1985.) **B.** CT scan of cervical injury.

of SCI vary widely. Whiplash occurs in acceleration injuries and may result in very minor discomfort from the mild hyperextension type of cord injuries, whereas total quadriplegia may result from severe fracture dislocations of the cervical vertebral column and serious cord damage. Trauma to the spinal cord can occur at any level, although the areas most frequently damaged are the lower cervical spine, particularly the C-5, C-6 region (Figure 52-15), and the upper thoracic spine.

Common mechanisms of SCI from traumatic impact include the hyperextension or hyperflexion injuries (Figure 52-16), frequently accompanied by rotational movement, vertical compression, lateral flexion, and penetrating injuries. The resultant spinal cord damage may be transient or permanent depending on the extent of parenchymal damage. Injuries similar to those that occur to the brain can also occur to the spinal cord, including concussion, contusion, hemorrhage, lacerations, and compression. Associated vertebral injuries may lead to spinal cord damage in subluxation, compression fractures, and

to result in irreversible total paraplegia causes severe edema and hemorrhage within a few hours, which then leads to massive necrosis and finally, parenchymal and vessel destruction.

Immediately after cord injury, focal hemorrhages begin in the gray matter and rapidly increase in size until the entire gray matter is hemorrhagic and necrotic. The hemorrhages in the white matter proximal to the gray matter do not coalesce but are associated with massive edema that envelops all of the white matter. It has been

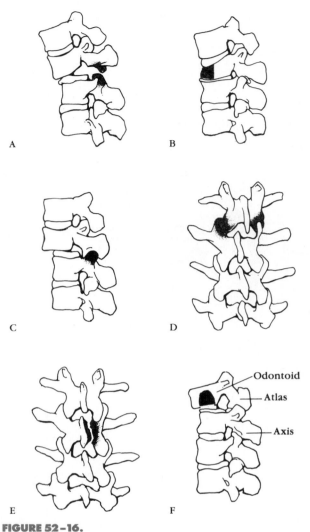

**FIGURE 52–16.**
Common types of vertebral injury: **A.** Subluxation, **B.** Compression fracture, **C.** Bilateral fracture, joint dislocation, **D.** Unilateral facet joint dislocation, **E.** Posterior arch fracture, **F.** Odontoid fracture. (Source: R. Judge, G.F. Zuidema, and F. Fitzgerald, *Clinical Diagnosis, A Physiologic Approach.* Boston: Little, Brown, 1982.)

fracture dislocations, as well as the other vertebral injuries noted in Figure 52-17. The extent of cord damage in vertebral injuries is related to the degree of bony encroachment or compression on the cord. Severe injuries result in partial or complete functional transection of the spinal cord.

## *Morphologic Changes Associated with Irreversible Cord Damage*

Experimentally induced SCI in laboratory animals has provided insight into the structural changes occurring at varying times after injury. A force strong enough

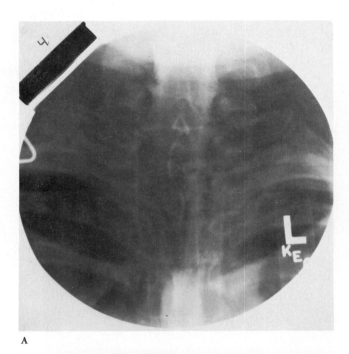

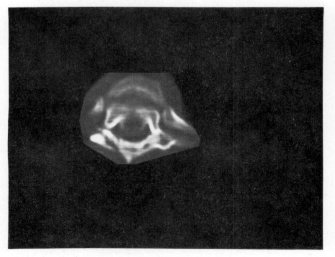

**FIGURE 52–17.**
**A.** Myelogram showing cord injury at level T-2 and T-3. Area of decreased contrast shows cord contusion and edema. **B.** CT scan of same person showing numerous vertebral fractures and cord edema.

speculated that norepinephrine, which is released in large amounts by the traumatized cord, contributes to the hemorrhagic necrosis caused by direct physical damage.[3] The lesion is progressive for several hours. After the injury, the hemorrhage into the gray matter is present in 15 minutes, and disintegration of the myelin sheath and axonal shrinkage occurs within 1 to 4 hours.[9]

## Functional Alterations Related to Level of Injury

Cervical spine injuries occurring above the fourth cervical segment (C-4) may be fatal because innervation of the diaphragm and intercostal muscles may be obliterated by the injury and the individual dies from respiratory failure.[5] With increasing sophistication of the public in knowledge and technique of cardiopulmonary resuscitation, increasing numbers of these victims arrive at emergency medical facilities. However, with improved medical technology, life expectancy has improved significantly.[11] High cervical cord transection results in quadriplegia.

Persons with transection injuries below the fifth cervical segment (C-5) have full innervation of the sternocleidomastoid, trapezius, and other muscles, and, therefore, retain neck, shoulder, and scapula movement. Individuals with lesions at the sixth cervical segment (C-6) have the function of the shoulder and elbow, and partial function of the wrist. Complete innervation of the rotator muscles of the shoulder is retained and partial innervation is transmitted to the serratus, pectoralis major, and latissimus dorsi muscles. Wrist muscles and the biceps retain innervation allowing for elbow and wrist flexion.

Persons with injuries at the seventh (C-7) and eighth (C-8) cord segments exhibit additional elbow, wrist, and hand function. Innervation is intact to the triceps and common and long finger extensors, enabling elbow extension and flexion, and functional, although weak, finger extension and flexion.

Transection injuries to the region of the *thoracic* and *lumbar* cord render the victim paraplegic (Figure 52-18A). Those with high thoracic injury, of first thoracic segment (T-1), retain full innervation of upper extremity musculature. Injuries experienced at the sixth thoracic segment (T-6) allow the person to have an increased respiratory reserve as intercostal innervation is intact. Those experiencing 12th thoracic segment (T-12) lesions have partial innervation to the lower extremities and may, in fact, regain ambulation when supported by long-leg braces and assisted by crutches.

Persons who sustain *low lumbar* and *sacral* cord lesions have full innervation to upper extremities and trunk, hip flexors and extensors, knee extensors, and ankle movement. Therefore, they are able to ambulate with minimal supportive devices.

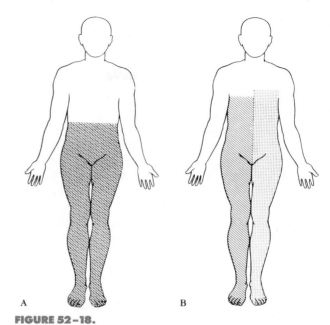

**FIGURE 52–18.**
**A.** Complete transverse lesion of the spinal cord. **B.** Brown-Sequard syndrome: lesion of the left side of the spinal cord (Source: J. Simpson and K. Magee, *Clinical Evaluation of the Nervous System.* Boston: Little, Brown, 1973.)

## Functional Alterations Related to Incomplete Cord Injuries (Cord Syndrome)

Central cord syndrome occurs commonly as a result of hyperextension injuries secondary to trauma of the cervical cord. To a lesser extent, it is also associated with disruption in cervical cord blood supply and degenerative processes of the spine. Central cord syndrome symptoms vary with the extent of trauma and edema, as well as the specific location. Motor weakness occurs in this syndrome in both upper and lower extremities, although it is generally greater in the upper extremities due to the fact that more damage occurs to the centrally located cervical tracts which supply the upper extremities. Loss of pain and temperature sensation varies, although greater losses occur in the upper extremities.

Brown-Sequard syndrome results from injury to one side of the spinal cord (Figure 52-18B). This may occur as a result of a transverse hemisection secondary to stab or missile injury, trauma resulting in fracture-dislocation of a spinous process, or acute herniated intervertebral disk. The clinical findings reveal ipsilateral paralysis, loss of proprioception touch, and vibratory sense, in conjunction with contralateral loss of pain and temperature sensation below the level of the lesion. Horner's syndrome may accompany Brown-Sequard cord injuries at or above the T-1 level. This is supported by findings of ptosis, pupillary constriction, and anhidrosis on the affected side.

In this syndrome, the preganglionic sympathetic neurons are involved at the level of injury.[11,14]

Anterior cord syndrome occurs as a result of injury to the anterior portion of the cord. The fact that the spinothalamic and corticospinal tracts project through this area of the cord produce clinical findings that are associated with disruption of these tracts. There occurs complete motor loss (corticospinal tract), as well as loss of pain, touch, and temperature sensations (spinothalamic tract) below the level of the lesion. Proprioception, light touch, and vibratory sensations remain intact.[11] Anterior cord syndrome injuries occur as a result of forward dislocation or subluxation of vertebrae, acute intravertebral herniations, flexion injuries, and conditions that compress arteries supplying the anterior spinal cord.

## Spinal Cord Transection

Total spinal cord transection results in immediate loss of all voluntary movement from the segments below the transection. The skin and other tissues become permanently anesthetized. Initially, reflex activity is abolished; however, it does recover and eventually may become hyperactive.

### Spinal Shock

The rapid depression of cord reflex activity after cord injury is referred to as spinal shock or posttransectional areflexia. It results from the interruption of neural pathways with the remainder of the central nervous system. The exact mechanisms causing spinal shock and recovery of reflexes are still elusive. It has been speculated that the excitatory effects of alpha and gamma motoneurons on other spinal motoneurons have been lost due to transection of the descending pathways, and that inhibitory spinal internuncial neurons become disinhibited, thus resulting in diminished reflexes. Considerable variability of the duration of spinal shock exists in humans. Some reflexes may reappear as early as 2 or 3 days after transection whereas others may not return for 6 weeks or longer. The earliest indicator of resolution of spinal shock is the return of perianal reflexes. Spinal shock is more pronounced in the cord segments surrounding the lesion, and recovery of reflexes generally occurs last there.

In addition to areflexia in spinal shock, clinical signs include autonomic deficits, which are reflected in a hypotension, bradycardia as well as loss of sweating, piloerection, and body temperature control below the area of transection. The body tends to assume the temperature of the environment (poikilothermia). Because of the depressed vasoconstrictive action below the level of the lesion by the sympathetic nervous system, individuals are susceptible to severe postural hypotension. Bowel and bladder reflexes from the sacrum are inhibited, and control over their functions is temporarily lost during spinal shock. Loss of sensation and flaccid paralysis occur below the transection site. Considerable variation exists with individual functional capacity after cord injury and, therefore, variation is observed in the extent of spinal shock.

### Reflex Return in Cord Injuries: Flexion-Extension Reflexes

Recovery from spinal shock generally is a long and slow process. The return of stretch and flexion reflexes after severe cord injury is first noted in response to noxious stimulation. An example of this response is the dorsiflexion of the great toe (Babinski's sign) in response to stimulation of the sole of the foot. Complications, such as infection and malnutrition, may delay the return of the flexor responses. As the flexor reflex recovers, it gradually becomes excited more readily from wider areas of the skin.

As recovery progresses after cord injury, flexor reflexes are interspersed with extensor spasms with ultimate progression to predominantly extensor activity. Individuals with partial cord transection generally exhibit strong extensor spasticity, whereas this seldom occurs with complete transection.

### Autonomic Reflexes

The autonomic spinal reflexes include those that control reflexive action of vasomotor activity, diaphoresis, and emptying of the bladder and rectum. Vasomotor reflexes are abolished below the level of transection during spinal shock, but with time, tonic autonomic activity returns and wide fluctuations in arterial pressure diminish. Temperature control by the skin is essentially abolished for a time after spinal transection as autonomic innervation for sweating is suppressed.

Reflex emptying of the bladder and rectum does occur in individuals with spinal transections after a period of initial atony and increased sphincter tone. Dilation of the bladder with urine eventually overcomes sphincter resistance and overflow incontinence occurs. With progression of time, spontaneous, brief contractions of the bladder evolve into larger contractions that are accompanied by bladder sphincter opening and brief micturition. Thus, small amounts of urine are voided with varying amounts of residual urine retained. Sensory stimuli may be used to precipitate micturition, such as tapping on the abdomen, anal stimulation, or stroking the inner aspect of the upper thigh. Downward manual pressure on the lower abdomen over the bladder (Crede's maneuver) is also used to initiate micturition.

*Autonomic dysreflexia* or *autonomic hyperreflexia* constitutes a cluster of symptoms in which many spinal cord autonomic responses are discharging simultaneously and excessively. This syndrome occurs in persons with high spinal cord injuries above the level of the sixth or seventh thoracic segment.[7] Its occurrence is highly unpredictable and it can arise unexpectedly for years after the injury. The symptoms occur in response to a specific noxious stimuli, appear quickly, and may lead to life-threatening conditions, such as severe hypertension, seizures, cerebral hemorrhages, and myocardial infarction.[11] Therefore, measures must be taken rapidly to identify the precipitating cause and remove it.

The symptoms of autonomic dysreflexia occur as a result of blockage of the afferent sensory transmissions at the level of the lesion. The transmission in autonomic dysreflexia is as a result of mass discharge due to a large portion of the sympathetic nervous system being stimulated by sensory receptors. Noxious agents stimulate sensory receptors, which transmit to the spinal cord and ascend the posterior columns and spinothalamic tracts. As the impulses ascend the cord, they reflexively stimulate the neurons of the sympathetic nervous system in the lateral horn of the cord. Since the modulating effects from higher centers are blocked, the sympathetic reflex activity continues unabated, causing arteriolar spasm of the skin, pelvic viscera, and arterioles, and resulting in vasoconstriction.[8] As a result, the individual may experience a pounding headache, blurred vision, and severe hypertension that may rise as high as 300 mm Hg systolic. The increased blood pressure distends the carotid sinus and aortic arch baroreceptors, which, in turn, stimulate the vagus nerve to decrease the heart rate and dilate the skin vessels above the level of the lesion in an attempt to lower the blood pressure. The dilated vessels produce flushing and profuse diaphoresis above the level. Because these impulses from higher centers are blocked to the lower body, the vessels remain vasoconstricted and the individual exhibits *cutes anserina* (goose flesh) and pale skin below the lesion. Other symptoms include restlessness, nasal congestion, and nausea.[8,14]

Precipitating factors leading to autonomic dysreflexia most commonly include bladder and bowel distention or manipulation. Other triggering stimuli may include decubitus ulcers, spasticity, stimulation of pain receptors, pressure on the penis, and strong uterine contractions.[11]

When the symptoms occur, rapid intervention is necessary to lower the blood pressure. The head of the bed is elevated since persons with high cord injuries usually have lower blood pressure in the sitting position. The source of stimulation must be found rapidly and removed. If these measures are not successful in reducing hypertension, ganglionic-blocking agents or other antihypertensive drugs are given intravenously.

## Intervertebral Disc Herniation

Herniation or rupture of the nucleus pulposus of the intervertebral disk is caused by minor or major trauma in about half of the cases of herniation (Figure 52-19). In other cases, however, onset is acute with no history of

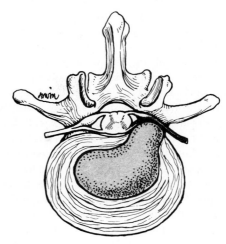

**FIGURE 52–19.**
Herniated disk showing compression of the spinal root by the herniated nucleus pulposus. (Source: R. Judge, G.F. Zuidema, and F. Fitzgerald, *Clinical Diagnosis, A Physiologic Approach.* Boston: Little, Brown, 1982.)

serious trauma. Sudden straining of the back in an unusual position and lifting while bending forward are frequently reported to be associated with disk herniation. Herniation of the nucleus pulposus produces pain, sensory loss, and paralysis by pressure on the spinal nerve roots or on the spinal cord. The most common injury occurs in the lumbosacral intervertebral disks (L4-L5 and L5-S1), which reflects a clinical picture of sciatica. Herniations of the cervical disks occur occasionally, and those in the thoracic region are rare.

Clinical findings associated with ruptured or herniated disks are related to the size and location of the extruded material. Single nerve roots may be involved in small lesions; however, several roots may be compressed. The spinal cord may be compressed by large, centrally situated cervical disks, and symptoms are reflective of spinal cord tumors or degenerative diseases.

The vast majority of the *lumbosacral herniations* occur between the fourth or fifth lumbar and first sacral interspaces. Sciatic symptoms associated with the lumbosacral herniation include pain in the lower back radiating down the posterior surface of one or both legs. The pain occurs as a result of posterior displacement of the disk and compression on the pain sensory pathways of the cord or sensory part of the compressed nerve. In unilateral involvement, scoliosis occurs toward the opposite side of sciatic pain, and movement of the lumbar spine is limited. Paresthesias in the leg or foot are common. Tenderness is experienced on palpation along the course of the sciatic nerve. Motor weakness occurs in a small percentage of cases. Hypoesthesia to touch or pinprick is present in about one-half of cases. A decreased or absent ankle reflex is common with herniation of the lumbosacral disk. Coughing, sneezing, or straining may produce radiation of pain along the course of the sciatic nerve.

Generally, symptoms are unilateral; however, with large central protrusions, they may be bilateral.

Herniation of the cervical disks occurs most commonly at the level of the fifth through seventh cervical roots. Displacement of the disk in this region causes stiffness of the neck and shoulder pain that radiates down the arm into the hand. Paresthesias may accompany the pain. Weakness and atrophy of the biceps and diminution of the biceps reflex may be present with sixth cervical root damage. Paresthesias and sensory loss in the index finger, weakness of the triceps muscle, and loss of triceps reflex are indicative of involvement of the seventh cervical root. Eighth cervical root compression reflects forearm pain along the medial side, as well as sensory loss along the medial cutaneous nerve of the forearm and ulnar nerve distribution in the hand.

## Diagnosis and Management

Differential diagnosis must be undertaken with a person presenting with symptoms of herniated disk because other conditions have similar symptoms including spinal cord tumors, syringomyelia, spine arthritis, and other disk degenerative conditions. Radiologic findings supportive of a herniated disk show loss of normal curvature of the spine, scoliosis, and narrowing of intervertebral spaces. Diagnosis is most conclusively demonstrated by contrast myelography, which reveals defects in outline of the subarachnoid space or interruption of the flow of the dye in the presence of herniated disks. In addition, CT scanning or MRI is effective in visualizing defective disks. Other diagnostic tools used for a definitive diagnosis include electromyography, discograms, and nerve root infiltration. Elevated protein content of CSF is another supportive finding; CSF may be completely or partially blocked with extrusions in the thoracic or cervical regions.

Conservative treatment in the acute stage is focused on bedrest, local heat application, and analgesics. Traction to lower extremities may be applied initially with lumbosacral disk herniations. Cervical halter traction is indicated for cervical disk involvement. Surgical intervention is indicated if conservative modes of treatment fail and signs of cord compression develop. Simple removal of the disk is commonly performed to relieve the symptoms.

## REFERENCES

1. Adams, R., and Victor, M. *Principles of Neurology* (4th ed.). New York: McGraw-Hill, 1989.
2. Finkelstein, S., and Ropper, A. The diagnoses of coma: Its pitfalls and limitations. *Heart Lung* 8:1059, 1979.
3. Gilliam, E.E. Intracranial hypertension: Advances in intracranial pressure monitoring. *Crit. Care Nurs. Clin. N. Am.* 2(1):21, March 1990.
4. Guyton, A. *Textbook of Medical Physiology* (7th ed.). Philadelphia: W.B. Saunders, 1986.
5. Hughes, M.C. Critical care nursing for the patient with a spinal cord injury. *Crit. Care Nurs. Clin. N. Am.* 2(1):33, March 1990.
6. Jackson, L. Cerebral vasospasm after an intracranial aneurysmal subarachnoid hemorrhage: A nursing perspective. *Heart Lung* 1:14, 1986.
7. Kidd, P.S. Emergency management of spinal cord injuries. *Crit. Care Nurs. Clin. N. Am.* 2(3):349, Sept. 1990.
8. Lazure, L. Defusing the dangers of autonomic dysreflexia. *Nurs. 80* 8:52, 1980.
9. Lewis, A. *Mechanisms of Neurologic Disease.* Boston: Little, Brown, 1976.
10. Plum, F., and Posner, J. *The Diagnosis of Stupor and Coma* (3rd ed.). Philadelphia: Davis, 1980.
11. Stelling, J. Spinal Cord Injury. In E. Howell, L. Widra, and M.G. Hill (eds.), *Comprehensive Trauma Nursing.* Glenview, Ill.: Scott Foresman, 1988.
12. Stewart-Amidei, C., and Hill, M.G. Head Trauma. In E. Howell, L. Widra, and M.G. Hill (eds.), *Comprehensive Trauma Nursing.* Glenview, Ill.: Scott Foresman, 1988.
13. Susi, E.A., and Walls, S.K. Traumatic cerebral vasospasms and secondary head injury. *Crit. Care Nurs. Clin. N. Am.* 2(1):15—20, March 1990.
14. Walleck, C.A. Neurologic considerations in the critical care phase. *Crit. Care Nurs. Clin. N. Am.* 2(3):357, Sept. 1990.

# Tumors and Infections of the Central Nervous System

### Learning Objectives

1. Identify the tissues from which central nervous system tumors may originate.

2. Describe the classification systems for cranial and spinal tumors.

3. Compare the frequency and malignancy of brain and spinal tumors.

4. Describe central nervous system alterations that lead to focal disturbances and increased intracranial pressure.

5. State what is thought to be the basis for the localized cerebral edema that surrounds brain tumors.

6. Describe central nervous system alterations that lead to the development of papilledema.

7. State the body's compensatory mechanisms for dealing with increased intracranial pressure.

8. Describe the clinical manifestations associated with brain tumors.

9. Discuss the clinical manifestations associated with tumors of the frontal, temporal, parietal, and occipital lobes, cerebellum, and brainstem.

10. Discuss clinical manifestations associated with the various types of spinal tumors, as well as with different levels of compression by spinal tumors.

11. Describe techniques used to diagnose brain and spinal tumors.

12. Compare and contrast characteristics of the central nervous system tumors: tissue type, appearance, rate of growth, invasive qualities, central nervous system alterations, and pertinent clinical manifestations.

13. State the two most common primary sites from which metastasis occurs to the brain.

14. State the various routes by which microorganisms reach the central nervous system.

15. List the ways in which viruses gain access to the body.

16. State the ways in which viruses invade the central nervous system.

17. Compare and contrast characteristics of the central nervous system infections: routes of infection, central nervous system alterations, pertinent clinical manifestations, and prognosis.

---

Tumors of the central nervous system (CNS) and the invasion of this system by infectious organisms are discussed in this chapter. Frequency, alterations within the CNS, resultant clinical manifestations, and relevant diagnostic studies are reviewed. The topic is vast, and the reader is referred to special texts for additional information and study of the subject.

## TUMORS

### General Considerations

Tumors of the CNS include both benign and malignant neoplasms within the brain and the spinal cord. The location, size, invasiveness, and rate of growth of these tumors are frequently more crucial to the ultimate course of the disease than the degree of malignancy. Virtually all brain tumors are potentially life-threatening. They can arise from the glial cells, blood vessels and connective tissue, meninges, pituitary gland, and pineal gland (Figure 53-1). Metastatic tumors from primary sites throughout the body are also encountered within the CNS.

With their variety and complexity, classification of intracranial tumors becomes a problem. An adaptation of the Kernahan and Sayre classification is found in Table 53-1. It is based on naming the tumor with respect to cells present in the adult nervous system, vascular tissue, and developmental defects.

A single tumor may contain more than one cell type.

A malignancy grading of I to IV is also included, with I being the least malignant.

Intraspinal tumors are classified in accordance with their location in relation to the dura and spinal cord, as well as histologic type. Thus, two groups are generally considered: extradural, those arising from the extradural space or vertebral bodies, and intradural, those arising from the blood vessels, meninges, or nerve roots (extramedullary), and those arising from within the substance of the spinal cord, itself (intramedullary). Intramedullary tumors are intradural, while extramedullary tumors can be either extradural or intradural.

Generally speaking, the location, size, and invasive quality of intracranial and intraspinal neoplasms are responsible for certain neurologic symptoms. The destruction and displacement of tissue, in addition to increased intracranial pressure, cause specific symptoms (Figure 53-2). Morbidity and mortality associated with intracranial tumors are high but advancements in diagnostic techniques, medical therapeutics, and neurosurgical techniques have improved the prognosis. Spinal cord tumors are more easily removed surgically than brain tumors. Thus, if recognized early and removed, prognosis for persons with intraspinal tumors is quite favorable.

### Frequency

Primary CNS tumors are not rare. As an intracranial disease, they are second in frequency only to stroke. They

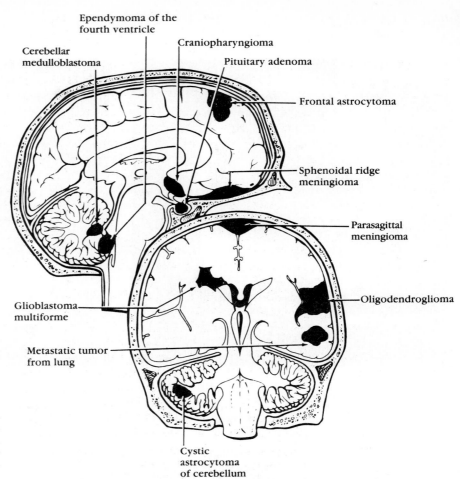

**FIGURE 53-1.**

Common intracranial tumors and the positions in which they frequently occur. Metastatic tumors may localize anywhere. (Source: M. Snyder and M. Jackle, *Neurologic Nursing: A Critical Care Nursing Focus.* Bowie, MD: Brady, 1981.)

**TABLE 53-1.**
CLASSIFICATION AND OCCURRENCES OF BRAIN TUMORS

|  | PERCENT |
|---|---|
| Gliomas | 40-50 |
| Astrocytoma, grade I | 5-10 |
| Astrocytoma, grade II | 2-5 |
| Astrocytoma, grades III and IV (glioblastoma multiforme) | 20-30 |
| Medulloblastoma | 3-5 |
| Oligodendroglioma | 1-4 |
| Ependymoma, grades I-V | 1-3 |
| Meningioma | 12-20 |
| Pituitary tumors | 5-15 |
| Neurolemmomas (mainly eighth nerve) | 3-10 |
| Metastatic tumors | 5-10 |
| Blood vessel tumors | |
| Arteriovenous malformations | |
| Hemangioblastomas | |
| Endotheliomas | 0.5-1 |
| Tumors of developmental defects | 2-3 |
| Dermoids, epidermoids, teratomas | |
| Chordomas, paraphyseal cysts | |
| Craniopharyngiomas | 3-8 |
| Pinealomas | 0.5-0.8 |
| Miscellaneous | |
| Sarcomas, papillomas of the choroid plexus, lipomas, unclassified, etc. | 1-3 |

Source: *S.I. Schwartz (ed.).* Principles of Surgery (5th ed.). New York: McGraw-Hill, 1989.

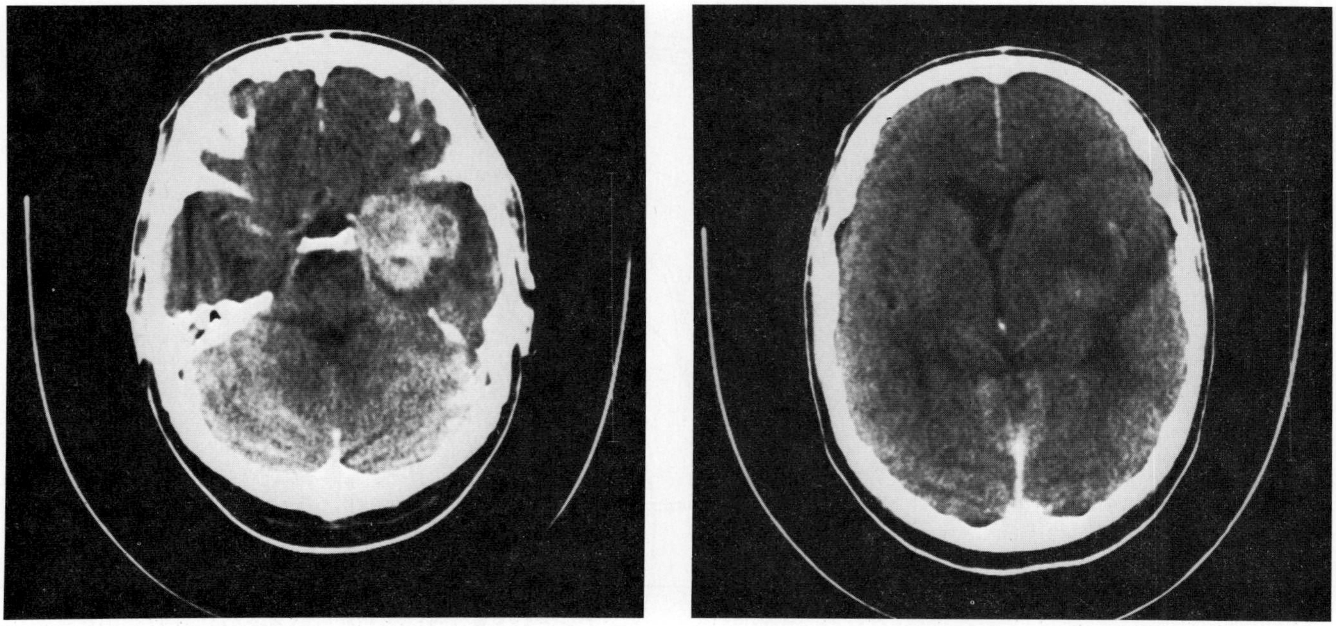

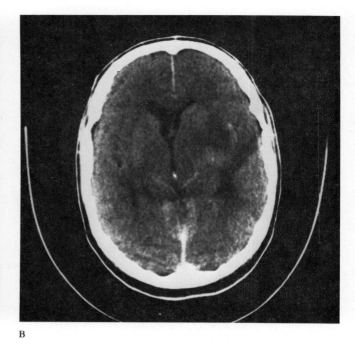

A                                    B

**FIGURE 53-2.**
**A.** Contrast-enhanced CT scan showing right cerebral metastatic tumor. **B.** View of compression and shift of midline structures by same tumor.

occur in all age groups and in both sexes. The usual range and peak incidence of cerebral tumors, according to age of clinical presentation, are shown in Figure 53-3.

Although it is difficult to establish accurate incidence of primary tumors in the general population, Table 53-1 presents widely accepted percentages of occurrence for

the various types of intracranial neoplasms. The brain and its coverings are also involved by neoplasm in 20% of all persons who have cancer at some time in the course of the illness.[1] Approximately 1% of all autopsied deaths indicate the presence of CNS tumors.[6]

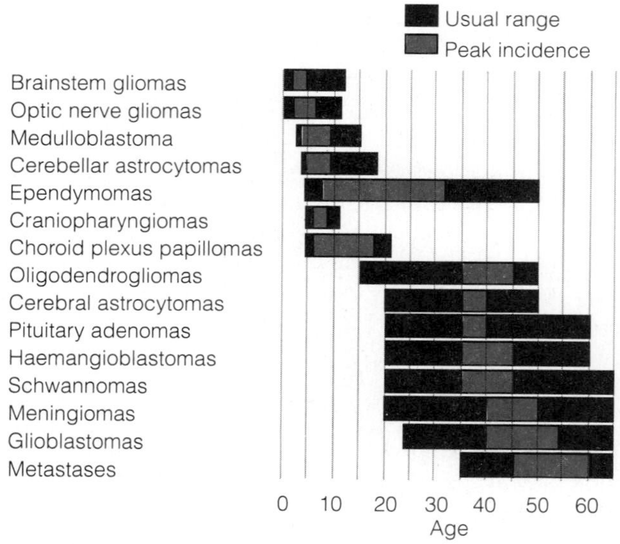

Although intracranial tumors can occur at any age, their frequency seems to be increased in young children and again in the fifth and sixth decades of life. In children, brain tumors are the most common solid tumors and the second most common malignancy after leukemia.[6,10] The most common brain tumors of childhood include craniopharyngiomas, ependymomas, medulloblastomas, cerebellar astrocytomas, brainstem gliomas, optic path gliomas, and pinealomas. In adults, gliomas account for approximately one half of all brain tumors.[13] Pituitary adenomas, acoustic neuromas, and meningiomas are prevalent during adulthood and almost completely absent during childhood (see Figure 53-3).

Intraspinal tumors occur less frequently than those that involve the brain and are rare in children. Intraspinal tumors account for approximately 15% of all primary tumors in hospitalized neurosurgical patients.[12] Twenty-five percent of intraspinal tumors are extradural and are generally metastatic. Seventy-five percent are intradural. Of these, extramedullary lesions are more frequent than intramedullary lesions. Extramedullary tumors are usually meningiomas or neurofibromas and are easily removed surgically. Intramedullary tumors have the same cellular origins as intracranial tumors and generally infiltrate surrounding tissue. These intramedullary tumors are fre-

■ Usual range
■ Peak incidence

Brainstem gliomas
Optic nerve gliomas
Medulloblastoma
Cerebellar astrocytomas
Ependymomas
Craniopharyngiomas
Choroid plexus papillomas
Oligodendrogliomas
Cerebral astrocytomas
Pituitary adenomas
Haemangioblastomas
Schwannomas
Meningiomas
Glioblastomas
Metastases

0   10   20   30   40   50   60
Age

**FIGURE 53-3.**
Usual range and peak incidence of cerebral tumor according to age of clinical presentation (Source: J.R. Youmans, *Neurological Surgery* [2nd ed.]. Philadelphia: W.B. Saunders, 1982.)

quently gliomas (particularly ependymomas), which commonly arise from the cauda equina and lumbar areas. Astrocytomas, oligodendrogliomas, glioblastomas, hemangioblastomas, and medulloblastomas occur less frequently and can arise in any of the spinal segments.

## Alterations in the Central Nervous System Due to Tumors

Brain tumors may be benign or malignant with regard to histology and morphology of their cellular components. It must be remembered, however, that all tumors of the brain are potentially harmful due to their relationship to vital structures. Thus, malignant or harmful effects may be produced by histologically benign lesions.

Brain tumors rarely metastasize to extraneural tissue; however, they infiltrate into surrounding nervous tissue, into the meninges, or through the ependymal layer into the ventricles. Once the tumor gains access to the subarachnoid space or ventricular system, and thus the cerebrospinal fluid (CSF) pathways, it may spread throughout the entire CNS. This may include the spinal cord and peripheral nerve roots.[6]

Within the confined space of the skull, a growing tumor alters the normally stable volume of the brain, blood, and CSF. Thus, as the mass grows, compression of brain tissue, as well as alterations in blood and CSF circulation, lead to focal disturbances and increased intracranial pressure. More specifically, tumor growth can produce any of several alterations. Compression of brain tissue and invasion of brain parenchyma cause destruction of neural tissue. Blood circulation may be decreased to such an extent that necrosis of brain tissue occurs. Compression, infiltration of neural tissue, and decreased blood supply may also lead to altered neural excitability with resultant seizure activity. Elevation of capillary pressure, due to compression of venules in the area adjacent to the tumor, is thought to be the basis for localized cerebral edema that frequently surrounds the tumor.

As the volume of the intracranial contents is increased, CSF is displaced from the subarachnoid space and ventricles through the foramen magnum to the spinal subarachnoid space. The CSF is also displaced through the optic foramen to the perioptic subarachnoid space. With elevations in CSF pressure, particularly in the perioptic subarachnoid space, venous drainage from the optic nerve head and retina is impaired. This is manifested by papilledema or choked disk. Growth of the mass may also obstruct CSF circulation from the lateral ventricles to the subarachnoid space with resultant hydrocephalus.

Rapid development of any of the previously discussed situations causes a life-threatening increase in intracranial pressure. Compensatory mechanisms exist and include decreased parenchymal cell numbers, decreased intracellular fluid contents, decreased CSF volume, and decreased intracranial blood volume. These compensatory mechanisms may take days or months to be effective and are thus not useful with rapidly developing intracranial pressure.[13] Untreated increased intracranial pressure may cause brain herniation.

Alterations as a result of intraspinal tumors are largely due to compression of the spinal cord, interference with circulation, and pressure on veins or arteries. Ischemia of cord segments occurs, as well as edema below the level of compression. Extradural spinal tumors usually result from extraneural metastases, particularly from the breast or lung, and cause rapid compression of the spinal cord. Hemorrhage due to the metastases, as well as vertebral column collapse, add to the compressive effects of extradural tumors.

Extramedullary tumors are basically of two types, neurofibromas and meningiomas, and are generally benign. Neurofibromas grow in the nerve root and often form an hourglass-like expansion that extends into the extradural space.

Meningiomas grow from the arachnoid membrane. These tumors are commonly present in the posterolateral aspect of the cord. They often result in the Brown-Sequard syndrome, due to the compressive damage to one half of the spinal cord (see Chap. 52).

As mentioned previously, intramedullary tumors are histologically the same as intracranial tumors. These lesions damage sensory fibers that cross each other in the center of the cord. They also destroy neurons. There is a frequent association between intramedullary tumors and syringomyelia.[1]

## Clinical Manifestations

The symptoms produced by intracranial tumors are extremely variable and depend on characteristics of the neoplasm, invasive qualities, location, and rate of growth. Because these tumors eventually give rise to an increase in intracranial pressure, three symptoms may occur: headache, vomiting, and papilledema. Additionally, changes in mental function and seizures often occur as a result of CNS tumors.

Headache is a common symptom of intracranial tumors. Early in the course of tumor growth, headache is thought to result from local displacement and traction of pain-sensitive structures within the skull–cranial nerves, arteries, veins, and venous sinuses. As the tumor grows, the pain is reflective of generalized increased intracranial pressure. The headache may be dull and is usually temporary, although it may be severe, dull or sharp, and intermittent. It is generally most severe on awakening and tends to improve throughout the day. Typically, it is aggravated by stooping, coughing, or straining to have a bowel movement. In general, the headache has little localizing value with regard to tumor site.

Vomiting is also experienced by many persons with intracranial tumors, particularly those who suffer from tumors of the posterior fossa. It is a result of stimulation of the emetic center in the medulla. Vomiting associated with tumors is not necessarily preceded by nausea and is not related to ingestion of food. It often occurs before breakfast and is frequently projectile.

Papilledema may not be present in the early stages of tumor growth but occurs as intracranial pressure increases. In some persons, papilledema does not develop even when the intracranial pressure becomes greatly elevated. Hemorrhages may be noted around the optic disk in association with papilledema. Complaints of blurred vision and halos around lights with enlargement of a blind spot and fleeting moments of dimmed vision (amaurosis fugax) may be elicited.

Local effects of intracranial tumors occur due to irritation, destruction, or compression of neural tissue in the location of the tumor. Generally speaking, supratentorial lesions give rise to paralysis, seizures, memory loss, visual field defects, and impairment in consciousness; infratentorial lesions give rise to cranial nerve dysfunction and ataxia.

Frontal lobe tumors cause disturbed mental status, speech disturbances, generalized or focal seizures, hemiparesis, and ataxia. Mental symptoms are manifested by progressive apathy, mild dementia with impairment of memory and intellect, decreased judgment, altered social adaptation, labile emotions, and depression. Aphasia or apraxia may occur when the left or dominant frontal lobe is affected. Pressure on motor areas produces hemiparesis and may result in jacksonian seizures, which may progress to generalized seizures. The unsteady gait associated with frontal lobe tumors may resemble cerebellar ataxia.

Involvement of the dominant temporal lobe may cause sensory aphasia, which begins with difficulty in naming objects. The individual has difficulty comprehending the spoken word and speaks in jargon. Tinnitus occurs as a result of irritation to the adjacent cortex or temporal auditory receptor. Anterior temporal lobe tumors cause visual field changes that may progress to complete hemianopsia. Psychomotor seizures may occur.

Parietal lobe involvement may include motor-sensory focal seizures, agnosia, hypoesthesia (decreased sensitivity to touch), paresthesia, and dyslexia. Visual defects may also occur. Tumors of the parietal lobe in the dominant hemisphere may result in difficulty comprehending language. Those in the nondominant hemisphere parietal lobe may interfere with awareness of contralateral body parts.

Involvement of the occipital lobe may produce visual field disturbances in the form of homonymous hemianopsia and quadratic defects. This may be associated with visual agnosia (loss of comprehension of visual sensation) on the dominant side, hallucinations, and convulsive seizures that are preceded by an aura.

Cerebellar tumors produce disturbances in equilibrium and coordination. The specific disorder depends on the location and size of the tumor. Disorders of movement may include nystagmus, adiadochokinesis (inability to make rapid alternative movements), asynergia (incoordination of muscle groups), dysmetria (abnormal force of muscular movements), intention tremor, and deviation from a line of movement.[9] Hypotonia may be present. Speech disturbances may be noted with tendency toward staccato or scanning speech. Papilledema often occurs with a cerebellar tumor. Cerebellar tumors may exert pressure on the brainstem and result in cranial nerve deficits.

Brainstem involvement produces varied effects. There is increasing paralysis of the cranial nerves with paralysis of eye movements, loss of facial sensation, and difficulty swallowing. Motor deficits reflect involvement of the descending and ascending motor tracts. Lesions of the hypothalamus may produce diabetes insipidus, obesity, disturbances of temperature regulation, and somnolence.

Clinical manifestations associated with spinal cord tumors depend on the type of lesion and the level at which the lesion occurs (Table 53-2). Generally speaking, a soft, slow-growing mass causes gradual compression of the spinal cord with gradually increasing neurologic signs. Malignant and metastatic tumors cause rapid compression of the spinal cord and destruction of the neural tissue.

Extradural tumors usually result from metastasis from primary tumor sites. Local, dull pain is often the first symptom; it is intensified with movements of the spine. Later, due to rapid growth, the spinal cord becomes compressed and severe pain occurs. Early signs of cord compression include loss of joint position sense, loss of vibration, and spastic weakness below the level at which the lesion occurs. Without surgical removal of the tumor, irreversible damage that may include irreversible paraplegia occurs.

Extramedullary lesions, primarily neurofibromas and meningiomas, are usually benign and early in their growth involve the periphery of the cord. There is pain in the back and along the spinal roots. The pain is worse at night and is aggravated by movement or straining. Posteriorly situated tumors produce sensory losses including paresthesia and loss of proprioceptive sense. Sensory loss first occurs below the level of the lesion. Anterior compression of the cord causes severe motor dysfunctions. Lateral cord compression may produce the Brown-Sequard syndrome, in which there is ipsilateral motor weakness and deep sensory loss, as well as contralateral loss of pain and temperature perception below the level of the lesion. Early diagnosis and surgical removal produce good prognoses.

**TABLE 53-2.**
COMMON SYMPTOMS OF SPINAL CORD TUMORS

| SYMPTOM | DESCRIPTION |
|---|---|
| Pain in spine, neck, back | Usually gradual onset; may occur suddenly with sudden movement or injury; aggravated by Valsalva maneuver; nocturnal pain predominates due to recumbency (patient may prefer to sleep upright) |
| Radicular pain | Occurs in the distribution of segmental innervation; aggravated by movement that alters anatomic relationships; causes diagnostic confusion (T-8 root involvement may be misinterpreted as ulcer disease) |
| Medullary referred pain | Shooting or burning over peripheral areas; often bilateral; not influenced by Valsalva maneuver; appears at different sites |
| Motor disturbances | Motor deficits are caused by lesions of the pyramidal or corticospinal tracts, causing spasticity and increased reflexes and spastic gait; weakness may present as a limp in the guise of muscle stiffness or rigidity |
| Nonspecific sensory disturbances | Numbness; tingling; coldness |

Source: F. McQuat, The insidious spinal cord tumor. Reprinted with permission from Journal of Neurosurgical Nursing 13:18, 1981. By permission of the American Association of Neuroscience Nurses.

Intramedullary tumors tend to be more histologically benign, are slow growing, and have a more benign course than similar intracranial tumors. There is usually a dull, aching pain in the area of the lesion. A dissociated sensory loss occurs in which there is a bilateral sensory loss of pain and temperature that extends through all involved segments. However, the senses of touch, motion, position, and vibration are usually preserved. Intramedullary tumors may extend through several spinal cord segments, making surgical removal difficult.

The various levels of compression by spinal cord tu-

mors are as follows: foramen magnum, cervical region, thoracic region, lumbar-sacral region, and cauda equina. A summary of signs and symptoms of common root lesions appears in Table 53-3.

A tumor in the area of the foramen magnum compresses intracranial contents, nerve roots, and the spinal cord. This causes suboccipital pain. Dermatomes C-2 and C-3 are compressed, which produces weakness of the head and neck. As the tumor extends into the intracranial cavity, increased pressure is produced, as well as pressure on the cerebellum and cranial nerve nuclei.

**TABLE 53-3.**
SYMPTOMS AND SIGNS OF COMMON ROOT LESIONS

| ROOT | LOCATION OF PAIN | SENSORY LOSS | REFLEX LOSS | WEAKNESS AND ATROPHY |
|---|---|---|---|---|
| C-5 | Lower neck, tip of shoulder, arm | Deltoid area (inconsistent) | Biceps | Shoulder abductors, biceps |
| C-6 | Lower neck, medial scapula, arm, radial side of forearm | Radial side of hand, thumb, index finger | Biceps | Biceps |
| C-7 | Lower neck, medial scapula, precordium, arm, forearm | Index finger, middle finger | Triceps | Triceps |
| C-8 | Lower neck, medial arm and forearm, ulnar side of hand, fourth and fifth fingers | Ulnar side of hand, fourth and fifth fingers | | Intrinsic hand muscles |
| L-4 | Low back, anterior and medial thigh | Anterior thigh | Quadriceps | Quadriceps |
| L-5 | Low back, lateral thigh, lateral leg, dorsum of foot, great toe | Great toe, medial side of dorsum of foot, lateral leg, and thigh | | Toe extensors, ankle dorsiflexors, and evertors |
| S-1 | Low back, posterior thigh, posterior leg, lateral side of foot, heel | Lateral foot, heel, posterior leg | Achilles | Ankle dorsiflexion and plantar flexion |

Source: J. Simpson and K. Magee, Clinical Evaluation of the Nervous System. Boston: Little, Brown, 1970.

Tumors in the cervical region produce motor and sensory losses in the shoulders, arms, and hands. Bicep, tricep, and brachioradial tendon reflexes may be lost, and varying motor and sensory deficits of the upper extremities arise if the lesion occurs in the lower cervical region. High cervical tumors compress the diaphragmatic nerves and result in paralysis of the diaphragm.

Thoracic lesions may produce pain and tightness across the chest and abdomen. Lower-extremity paresthesia may develop with the loss of abdominal reflexes when the lesion is in the lower thoracic area. Paralysis of the intercostal muscles results at the involved region.

Upper lumbar lesions cause hip flexion weakness, lower leg spasticity, loss of knee jerk reflexes, brisk ankle reflexes, and bilateral Babinski's signs. With extensive involvement of the high lumbar cord, movement and sensation are lost in the lower limbs. Sensory deficits result in the area of the perineum.

Lower lumbar and upper sacral lesions cause weakness of perineal, calf, and foot muscles. There is often loss of the Achilles reflex. Lower sacral lesions cause sensation losses in the buttocks and perianal area. Bladder and bowel control may be impaired. Lesions in the cauda equina region cause impotence and loss of sphincter control; pain in the sacral and perineal areas often radiates to the legs.

## Diagnosis

Two basic steps are used to diagnose CNS tumors. First, a detailed history is elicited and careful neurologic examination is performed. Second, radiologic investigations are performed depending on the findings of the neurologic examination. Films of the skull do not visualize the brain, itself, but reflect changes caused by chronically increased intracranial pressure. These changes include erosion of the sella turcica, calcification of the pineal body or of a lesion, increased density of surrounding bone, and destruction of vertebrae associated with spinal tumors.

Air encephalography (AEG) performed through a lumbar puncture is useful in outlining tumors that impinge on CSF pathways or displace and distort the ventricles. Ventriculography is used to outline the ventricular system through the use of contrast material or air introduced directly into the lateral ventricle. This procedure is useful especially for persons with increased intracranial pressure in whom a lumbar puncture for the AEG could cause a cerebellar foramen magnum herniation. Angiography detects displacement of vessels from their normal position due to tumor growth. It also provides information concerning the intrinsic vasculature of the tumor.

Isotopes injected intravenously break down the blood-brain barrier, which allows an abnormal amount of radioactive material to accumulate in the area of the tumor. With isotope scanning, blood supply to the tumor is important and avascular or small tumors may not be detected. The computerized axial tomography (CT) scan is the screening procedure of choice because it is noninvasive and nonpainful. It involves the use of a computer, which because of various absorptive characteristics of brain tissue, blood, CSF, cyst fluid, and tumors, can process numerous high-speed films to produce a pictorial print of transverse sections of the body.

Magnetic resonance imaging (MRI) is an instrument that views the brain in successive layers within a powerful magnetic field. Images are clear and more precisely identified than with CT scanning (see Chap. 52). An electroencephalogram (EEG) gives valuable information concerning altered neuron excitability in the region of the tumor and shows abnormalities in 75% of tumors.[9] An echoencephalogram shows shifts in intracranial contents. A myelogram is useful in localizing tumors of the spinal cord.

Lumbar puncture may be performed to examine the CSF. In the presence of tumors, this test usually reveals a normal CSF glucose, an elevated protein level, and sometimes tumor cells. During lumbar puncture, Queckenstedt's jugular compression test can demonstrate a spinal subarachnoid block. Due to the danger of brain herniation, lumbar puncture is not performed when there is obvious evidence of increased intracranial pressure.

Somatosensory evoked potentials (SSEPs) is a neurodiagnostic test which may be done to localize sensory deficits. This test evaluates the functions of sensory pathways from a peripheral nerve to the sensory cortex by electrically stimulating the relevant nerve and recording afferent activity at various levels. Brain tumors may cause delays in sensory pathway conduction as a result of brain tissue compression and abnormal vascularization.[4]

Finally, to make a diagnosis, tumor histology must be determined. This usually requires surgery and tumor tissue examination.

## Tumors of the Neuroglia Cells (Gliomas)

The glial cells provide support and protection for nerve cells and include astrocytes, oligodendroglia, and ependymal cells. Gliomas, as a group, are the most common primary intracranial tumors found in adults. Approximately 8000 people are diagnosed with gliomas each year in the United States.[7] The tumors are named and classified according to cell type: astrocytomas, oligodendrogliomas, and ependymomas. Gliomas may invade any area of the CNS and are infiltrating by nature. They may also spread from one area of the brain or spinal cord to another.

## Astrocytomas

Astrocytomas develop from astrocytes. These spider-shaped or star-shaped cells infiltrate brain tissue and are frequently associated with cysts of various sizes. Their invasive nature usually makes surgical removal difficult. An exception is the pilocytic astrocytoma that grows in the cerebellum and optic nerve and has a good prognosis after removal.[5]

Astrocytomas have varying degrees of malignancy. Some are well-differentiated and grow slowly for many years but may become more anaplastic over time and are classified as anaplastic astrocytomas and glioblastomas. Gross inspection usually reveals poorly defined, gray-white, infiltrative masses that enlarge and distort underlying CNS tissue. The initial symptom frequently is a focal or generalized seizure. Headaches, mental disturbances, and signs of increased intracranial pressure may develop several years later.

Other astrocytomas are very poorly differentiated, anaplastic tumors that have a rapid rate of growth. On gross inspection, they are large, infiltrative lesions. Their prognosis is dismal; death occurs within months to a few years after diagnosis.

Due to variations in anaplasia, a malignancy grading system of I to IV is used. Differentiated astrocytomas are referred to as grade I or II, anaplastic astrocytomas as grade III, and glioblastoma multiforme as grade IV. Rating systems are highly subjective and their clinical usefulness is limited.

## Glioblastoma Multiforme

Glioblastoma multiforme is an extremely malignant, highly vascular glioma that frequently arises from undifferentiated astrocytomas (Figure 53-4). The appearance on gross inspection varies according to the region of the brain in which it arises, the degree of necrosis, and the presence of hemorrhage. Glioblastomas grow very rapidly, are invasive, and are resistant to various combinations of surgery, radiotherapy, and chemotherapy. Tissue necrosis and brain edema are characteristic, thus prognosis is poor. Ninety percent of these patients die within 2 years after diagnosis.[5]

## Oligodendrogliomas

Oligodendrogliomas arise from oligodendroglia, a neuroglia with vinelike processes present sporadically throughout the CNS. The frontal lobe is the most common site for this tumor in 40% to 70% of the cases.[1] Gross examination usually reveals well-defined, gray, globular masses. These may contain cystic foci, calcifications, and hemorrhagic areas.[12] These tumors are similar in behavior to astrocytomas in that they generally grow slowly. On occasion, however, rapid growth occurs and

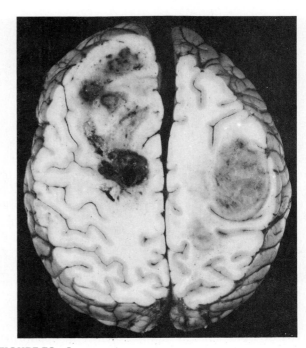

**FIGURE 53–4.**
Glioblastoma multiforme. This extremely anaplastic tumor of the astrocytic series is represented by a necrotic, hemorrhagic lesion that has crossed the corpus callosum and has spread throughout both hemispheres. (From E. Rubin and J. Farber, *Pathology*. Philadelphia: J.B. Lippincott, 1988.)

these tumors may imitate the glioblastomas. Distinction may be made only on histologic examination. Oligodendrogliomas also have a tendency to form focal calcification.

## Ependymomas

Ependymal cells line the ventricular walls and form the central canal in the spinal cord. Generally, cranial ependymomas appear as fairly well-defined masses that grow by expansion.[5] Ependymomas tend to form small canals (rosettes) within the tumor. The tumor cells also align themselves around blood vessels (pseudorosettes). Those that arise from ependymal cells lining the walls of the ventricular system fill and obstruct the ventricles and invade adjacent tissue. This can obstruct CSF passage and lead to the development of hydrocephalus. The most common site of ependymomas is the fourth ventricle.

Ependymomas that arise within the spinal cord represent a large percentage of intraspinal gliomas. Symptoms are related to the spinal level at which they occur. The location of these tumors often makes them inaccessible to removal by surgery. Thus, even though they grow slowly, the prognosis is poor and death occurs in a few years.

Variants of ependymomas include subependymomas and myxopapillary ependymomas. Subependymo-

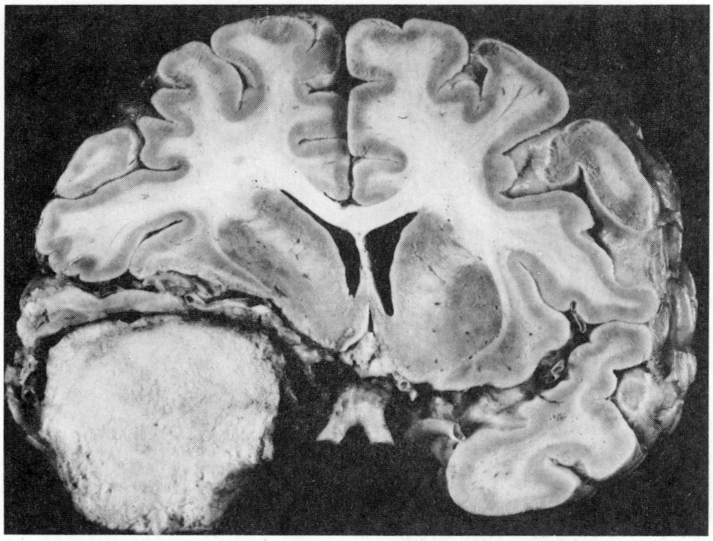

**FIGURE 53–5.**

Meningioma. This globoid tumor, which underlies the temporal lobe, compresses but does not infiltrate this portion of the brain. The presence of the meningioma "irritated" the cortex, initiating a seizure disorder. (From E. Rubin and J. Farber, *Pathology*. Philadelphia: J.B. Lippincott, 1988.)

mas arise from neuroglial tissue beneath the ependymal lining and are composed of astrocytic and ependymal elements. These small, hard, lobular tumors rarely grow large enough to cause symptoms. Myxopapillary ependymomas are composed mostly of ependymal cells arising almost exclusively in the filum terminale.

## Tumors of Neuronal Origin

*Cerebral neuroblastomas* arise in precursor cells of neurons. Gross examination reveals well-defined, gray, granular masses that may contain areas of necrosis, hemorrhage, and cysts.[5] Neuroblastomas are rare and usually occur during the first decade of life. Their rate of growth is rapid and they commonly recur after surgery.

*Gangliogliomas* are very rare tumors composed of neuroglial tissue. Gross inspection reveals well-defined masses with granular surfaces. Calcifications and small cysts may be present within the mass. These tumors are most common in children and young adults. If the location permits surgical excision, the prognosis is good.

## Tumors of Embryonic Origin

Medulloblastomas arise predominantly from primitive cells in the cerebellum. Thus, they have the potential to develop along neuronal or neuroglial lines. Gross inspection generally reveals fairly well-demarcated, gray-white masses with indistinct edges.[5] Medulloblastomas occur almost exclusively in children and account for approximately 20% of pediatric brain tumors.[10] This tumor type has been found in adults in rare situations up to the sixth decade of life. They most frequently affect

males. They are highly malignant, grow rapidly, and infiltrate throughout the subarachnoid space with resultant widespread meningeal foci. The CSF pathways become blocked and signs of increased intracranial pressure develop. These tumors are associated with increasing ataxia, headaches, and forceful vomiting. The prognosis is dismal but combinations of surgery, radiotherapy, and chemotherapy can prolong survival.

## Tumors of the Meninges

### Meningiomas

Meningiomas are primary tumors arising from the meninges (Figure 53-5). They are most common in females and occur generally in the seventh decade of life.[12] These tumors comprise approximately 15% of all primary intracranial tumors.[1] Meningeal constituents that may be involved include arachnoid cells, fibroblasts, and blood vessels. Gross inspection tends to reveal tough, gray-white, irregular to round, lobular masses.[5] Meningiomas are quite vascular and are seen readily on radioisotope scans. They are usually well-circumscribed, encapsulated, and press into surrounding tissue. The tumors may penetrate adjacent bone but widespread infiltration of surrounding nervous tissue is not common. Most of these tumors are benign and grow slowly so that initial symptoms may be overlooked. As they continue to grow, symptoms include seizures, headache, visual impairment, hemiparesis, and aphasia. If they are diagnosed early and are in an area accessible to surgery, complete excision is possible and a good prognosis results. If these tumors are not completely resected, they may recur. Prognosis of meningiomas is largely dependent on the location of the tumor.[6]

# Tumors of the Pituitary Gland

Pituitary adenomas are a special group of nervous system tumors that produce neurologic signs and symptoms when they put pressure on the hypothalamus, optic chiasm, third ventricle, and medial temporal lobe. The initial symptoms are hormonal disturbances or visual field defects. These tumors arise from the three cell types in the anterior pituitary: basophil cells, which stain blue; eosinophil cells, which stain red; and chromophobe cells, which do not stain. Although pituitary tumors have usually been classified according to cell type, it is more accurate to identify them as functioning (secreting a hormone) or nonfunctioning (nonsecreting). They usually contain a predominant cell type, however, and the chromophobe cells give rise to these tumors most frequently (see Chap. 36). Prognosis depends on the success of treatment, which may include irradiation, hypophysectomy, or hormone replacement. Treatment is considerably more successful when the tumor is still confined to the sella.

*Adrenocorticotropic hormone (ACTH)-producing pituitary adenomas* are primarily composed of basophil cells and are usually so small that adjacent tissue is not compressed. They have powerful effects, however, due to hypersecretion of ACTH, which is one of several mechanisms that produce Cushing's syndrome. Symptoms of Cushing's syndrome include weakness, emotional lability, moon face, obesity of the torso, hypertension, salt and water retention, diabetes mellitus, glycosuria, osteoporosis, skin striae over the abdomen, hirsutism, and amenorrhea (see Chap. 37).

*Pituitary adenomas inducing gigantism and acromegaly* are primarily composed of acidophilic cells, and are small and rather slow-growing. They cause an increase in the output of growth hormone. If they develop before bone growth is complete, gigantism results. Tumor development after bone growth has stopped produces the clinical picture called *acromegaly.* These adenomas may grow to such size that they press on the optic chiasm, causing complete or parial bitemporal hemianopsia or other visual disturbances.

*Nonsecreting pituitary adenomas* are the most common pituitary tumors and are composed primarily of chromophobe cells. Although these cells have no known special function, tumors arising from them are rather large and produce symptoms by compressing the pituitary gland, optic chiasm, hypothalamus, and adjacent brain tissue. These tumors usually produce hypopituitarism. Signs and symptoms include a sallow appearance, loss of body hair, weakness, amenorrhea, loss of sexual desire, low basal metabolism, hypoglycemia, hypotension, and electrolyte disturbances. As thetumor presses on the optic chiasm, bitemporal hemianopsia is produced and blindness may result (see Chap. 36).

# Tumors of the Cranial and Peripheral Nerves and Nerve Roots

Neurilemmomas (schwannomas) and neurofibromas arise from cells that ensheath cranial nerves, peripheral nerves, cauda equina, and nerve roots. The three types of cells within the nerve sheaths include *Schwann cells, perineural cells,* and *fibroblasts* in the epineurium and endoneurium. Although the three cells are similar morphologically, Schwann cells are generally the primary source of tumors.

Neurilemmomas are tumors that arise from the Schwann cells and occur on any of the nerves or nerve roots. The tumors are firm, circumscribed, well-encapsulated, and white to gray.[5] Many lesions may be present on the same nerve or throughout the body. They often involve the vestibulocochlear division of the acoustic (eighth) nerve (acoustic neuroma), most frequently at the cerebellopontile angle, or where the acoustic nerve enters the internal auditory meatus. Bilateral involvement of the acoustic nerve occurs in von Recklinghausen's neurofibromatosis, type 2.

Acoustic neuromas produce the following symptoms due to position or disruption in function: impaired hearing; tinnitus; vertigo; balance and coordination difficulties; ataxia; loss of caloric vestibular reactivity with horizontal nystagmus; palsies of the third, fifth, and seventh cranial nerves; and signs of increased intracranial pressure as the normal flow of CSF is obstructed. Complete surgical removal is usually attempted to prevent recurrence of the tumor but this often produces cranial nerve dysfunctions, such as deafness or facial paralysis.

Neurofibromas arise primarily from Schwann cells and fibroblasts and generally tend to be multiple and encapsulated. Gross examination reveals enlargement of the affected nerve or nerve root. Numerous tumors are often present, especially when associated with the hereditary disease, von Recklinghausen's neurofibromatosis.

# Tumors of the Blood Vessels

Blood vessel tumors include arteriovenous malformations (AVMs), hemangioblastomas, and endotheliomas. They account for only a very small percentage of brain tumors.

## Arteriovenous Malformations

These malformations consist of an abnormal collection of blood vessels in which arteries join veins directly rather than through capillaries. The majority of angiomas are in the posterior half of the cerebral hemispheres. The abnormal vessels are present at birth and enlarge with the passage of time. Thus, symptoms may not occur for years although manifestations are often noted between the ages 10 and 30 years. As the vessels grow, they may compress the normal brain, and weak walls may bleed into the cerebral or subarachnoid spaces. Mortality associated with the first hemorrhage is about 10%.[12] Recurrence of hemorrhage is a constant danger and various modes of treatment have been used. Symptoms vary according to the region of involvement and size of the AVM. In some cases, there are no clinical symptoms and the AVM is found only on autopsy.

### Hemangioblastomas

Hemangioblastomas are neoplasms made up of an aggregation of blood vessels that may also be cystic. These arise most commonly in the cerebellum but may occur in the cerebrum. Symptoms include ataxia, dizziness, and signs of increased intracranial pressure. Because erythropoietin is often secreted from these tumors, polycythemia may be exhibited. If the cerebellar cyst can be opened and the hemangioblastomatous nodule excised, the prognosis is good. A combination of cerebellar hemangioblastoma in association with cysts of the kidneys and pancreas, together with angiomatosis of the retinae, is known as *von Hippel-Lindau syndrome*. This disease is inherited as a dominant trait.[6]

## Tumors of Developmental Defects

Developmental tumors arise from cells that have developed abnormally and persist throughout prenatal growth. These include dermoids, teratomas, cholesteatomas, chordomas, and craniopharyngiomas.

### Dermoids and Teratomas

Dermoids and teratomas may occur anywhere in the CNS but frequently arise in the ventricular system. They may obstruct the third ventricle, the aqueduct of Sylvius, or the fourth ventricle. As a result of embryonic displacement of tissue, these tumors may contain bits of hair, primitive teeth, or other material.

### Cholesteatomas

These relatively rare growths are also known as *epidermoid tumors* or *cysts* and occur most commonly in the young adult. They consist of encapsulated epithelial debris and are most frequently located in the cerebellopontine angle. They simulate acoustic neuromas when located there. Other areas that may give rise to cholesteatomas include the fourth ventricle, supraseller region, and the pineal recession.

Although they are benign tumors, they may enlarge and cause erosion of adjacent bones.

### Chordomas

These are rare, congenital, malignant tumors that are derived from remnants of the primitive notochord. They are jellylike, gray-pink growths and grow near the sella turcica, at the base of the brain, or at the cervical or the sacrococcygeal areas. These tumors erode the bone and invade the dura. Total surgical removal is impossible due to their highly invasive nature. Symptoms of congenital tumors usually develop within the first 10 years of life and depend on the size and location of the lesion.

### Craniopharyngiomas (Rathke's Pouch Tumors)

These are tumors derived from Rathke's pouch, a pouch in the embryonic membrane that develops into the anterior lobe of the pituitary. They are most often located above the sella turcica. This tumor is encapsulated and grows as a solid mass or more frequently as a cyst. The cyst often contains thick, brown, oily fluid and often has some degree of calcification. Rupture of the cystic fluid into the subarachnoid space may cause recurrent bouts of "sterile" meningitis or, in some cases, bacterial meningitis. As the craniopharyngioma grows, pressure is applied to the pituitary gland, the optic chiasm, and sometimes the base of the brain. Erosion of the sella wall may occur. Symptoms most commonly occur in children and young adults, and reflect signs and symptoms of pituitary hypofunction, hydrocephalus, visual disturbances, and diabetes insipidus. Surgical removal is possible if the site is accessible.

## Tumors of Adenexal Structures

Pinealomas are rare tumors composed of large epithelial cells present in the adult pineal gland. Cell differentiation divides pinealomas into pinecytomas and pineablastomas. Pinealomas cause symptoms by compressing the aqueduct of Sylvius, causing hydrocephalus and increased intracranial pressure. Treatment may include a combination of surgery, atrioventricular shunt, and radiotherapy.

Choroid plexus papillomas are rare tumors that occur primarily in children. Gross inspection reveals well-defined, cauliflower-like, papillary masses that often protrude into the fourth ventricle.[6,12] Although histologically benign, they may cause intraventricular bleeding, papilledema, hydrocephalus, and increased intracranial pressure. Treatment includes surgery followed by radiotherapy.

## Metastatic Tumors

Metastases most commonly occur from primary sites in the lungs (45%) and breast (20%) but neoplasms of the gastrointestinal tract, genitourinary tract, bone, thyroid gland, and nasal sinuses can also metastasize to the brain and spinal cord.[6] Metastatic tumors are generally solid, circumscribed masses that are surrounded by vasogenic edema. They may be solitary tumors or multiple small masses scattered throughout the CNS. Signs and symptoms vary with the location, size, and number of lesions. Intracranial metastases most often appear in individuals who already have symptoms of far-advanced cancers but occasionally produce the initial symptoms. Even with combinations of surgery, radiotherapy, and chemotherapy, prognosis is poor.

## INFECTIONS

### General Considerations

Central nervous system tissue is not immune to viral, bacterial, or other infections. The infections usually arise initially in another region of the body. Organisms can gain access to the CNS in several ways: (1) by spread from adjacent structures—nasal sinuses, skull, middle ear; (2) by entrance through penetrating wounds; and (3) through the bloodstream. Once infectious organisms enter the CNS, they can spread rapidly by way of the CSF, leading to widespread, devastating results.

Diagnosis of any CNS infections depends on evidence of the infective organism, together with changes in pressure, glucose, and protein levels of the CSF. Magnetic resonance imaging may provide evidence of focal inflammatory disease. The CNS alterations and clinical manifestations vary according to the type of infection.

### Viral Infections

Viruses may gain access to the body orally, through the respiratory system, by animal or mosquito bites, or across the placenta to the fetus. Once inside the body, they make their way to the CNS through the hematogenous route by the cerebral capillaries and the choroid plexus. Other entry routes include the peripheral nerves and possibly, penetrating the olfactory mucosa.[1]

Within the CNS, viruses apparently affect specific, susceptible cells. Thus, the pathologic effects are considerably different. Damage to the CNS may be due to direct viral invasion of cells with subsequent lysis (acute encephalitis); to selective lysis with resulting demyelination (progressive multifocal leukoencephalopathy); to immune responses to viral antigens (acute disseminated encephalomyelitis); and, in some cases, to cellular destruction without apparent inflammatory or immune response. Viruses may also remain latent in cells for months or years until circumstances trigger acute infections (see Chap. 12).

Innumerable viruses are known to invade the nervous system, and only a representative sample of the most frequently encountered viruses is presented in the following section.

### Acute Encephalitis

*Encephalitis* is a general term that encompasses infections of the brain parenchyma in which a wide range of symptoms is manifested. Although encephalitis may be caused by bacteria, rickettsia, parasites, and fungi, viral infections are most common. Presented in Box 53-1 are a variety of causes of viral encephalitis and virus-related acute encephalopathies. Symptoms include headache, high fever, confusion, convulsions, and restlessness that progresses to stupor and coma. There may also be focal

---

**BOX 53-1.**
CAUSES OF VIRAL ENCEPHALITIS AND VIRUS-RELATED ACUTE ENCEPHALOPATHIES

Viral encephalitis
  Sporadic
    Mumps
    Herpes simplex viruses
    Lymphocytic choriomeningitis virus
    Cytomegalovirus
    Epstein–Barr virus
    Adenovirus
    Rabies
  Epidemic
    Arboviruses (St. Louis, Eastern, Western, California, Venezuelan Equine, Colorado tick fever)
    Enteroviruses (coxsackievirus and echoviruses)
Postinfectious encephalomyelitis
  Measles
  Varicella
  Mumps
  Rubella
  Influenza
Viral infections in immunocompromised patients
  Cytomegalovirus
  Herpes simplex viruses
  Enteroviruses
  Adenoviruses
  Measles
  JC virus (Progressive multifocal leukoencephalopathy)
  Human immunodeficiency viruses (HIV)
Virus-associated encephalopathy
  Reye's syndrome

Source: *L.P. Weiner. Viral encephalitis.* In: R.T. Johnson (ed.), Current Therapy in Neurologic Disease-3. *Philadelphia: B.C. Decker, 1990.*

CNS impairment, such as hemiparesis, asymmetry of tendon reflexes, Babinski's sign, involuntary movements, ataxia, and difficulty in speaking or understanding. Brainstem involvement may be manifested by facial weakness or ocular palsies. Analysis of CSF usually reveals increased numbers of lymphocytes, normal to slightly increased pressure, slightly increased protein, normal glucose, and normal chloride levels. A comatose state may persist for days, weeks, or months after the acute infection. Residual effects may include behavior and personality changes, mental deterioration, parkinsonism, paralysis, and persistent seizures. The specific signs and symptoms that predominate depend on the causative organism. A wide variety of viruses cause encephalitis and a discussion of the more common ones follows.

*ARTHROPOD-BORNE (ARBO) VIRUS ENCEPHALITIS.*    This large group of viruses commonly causes encephalitis. The organisms seem to occur in certain geographic locations and during certain seasons, especially summer and early fall when mosquitoes are biting. Except for tick-borne arboviruses, all of these viruses have vertebrate hosts with mosquito vectors. The principal site of infection is the brain. Clinical manifestations among the different arboviruses are similar; however, they may vary with age of the afflicted individual. For example, onset of fever and convulsions is most abrupt in children.

*Eastern equine encephalitis*, occurring primarily in the eastern states, is an infrequent cause of encephalitis. It is the most serious of the arboviruses because it causes extensive destruction of the cerebral cortex and white matter. When there is clinical evidence (one in 19 cases) of encephalitis due to this virus, mortality is close to 80%.[5] Those who survive often have residual effects that include blindness, deafness, mental retardation, emotional disorders, and hemiplegia. The greatest change in CSF is large numbers of polymorphonuclear leukocytes.

*Western equine encephalitis* may involve the upper spinal cord, as well as large portions of the brain. It is most common in the western region of the country. Fever, stupor, dizziness, confusion, and headache are common factors. Mortality is lower than with eastern equine encephalitis. Postencephalitic parkinsonism is a frequent sequela of this type of encephalitis.

*St. Louis encephalitis* is a milder form of the disease and may involve both the brain and spinal cord. It occurs primarily in the central and western states. Prominent meningeal involvement accompanies St. Louis encephalitis. Other findings include fever, athetosis, drowsiness or stupor, tremors, and, more commonly, seizures. Any age group may develop this infection and recovery is generally good.

*California encephalitis* affects children more frequently than adults. Its onset is insidious and its signs include headache, fever, vomiting, mental confusion, seizures, and stupor that may deteriorate to coma. Although

recovery from the acute episode is common, residual learning difficulties, emotional lability, and seizures may remain as long-term problems.

*HERPES SIMPLEX.*    Herpes simplex virus (HSV) is a very serious and common form of encephalitis that may produce illness in any age group. This type of encephalitis has been reported in all parts of the world. Most frequently, the disease is associated with type I HSV, which is also the common cause of oral mucosal lesions. The virus may be introduced from a primary lip infection to the brainstem by the trigeminal nerve. Type II HSV causes genital infection and, when present in the mother, produces acute encephalitis in the neonate, acquired during passage through an infected birth canal.[1]

Alterations in the CNS are more common in the medial and inferior portions of the temporal lobes and orbital gyri of the frontal lobes. The lesions include hemorrhagic necrosis, inflammation, and perivascular infiltrates. The CSF reveals an increased pressure, increased protein level, increased number of lymphocytes, and the presence of red cells due to the hemorrhagic nature of the lesions. Serologic tests and brain biopsy confirm a diagnosis of herpes simplex encephalitis. Clinical manifestations include acute onset with headache, fever, convulsions, confusion, stupor, and coma, in addition to focal disturbances related to lesions in specific portions of the temporal and frontal lobes. Once a diagnosis of HSV is made, treatment with acyclovir is instituted.[14]

*RABIES.*    Clinical cases of rabies in humans are rare, but once the disease is established, it is almost always fatal. This dreaded viral disease can affect anyone who has sustained a bite through the skin by a rabid animal (usually dogs, cats, bats, foxes, raccoons, or skunks). Its incubation period varies from 14 days to 3 months. Survival of inoculated victims depends on specific postexposure prophylaxis.

The virus makes its way from the wound to the CNS through the peripheral nerves, producing degenerative changes in these neurons. Alterations in the CNS include brain edema, neuron degeneration, and vascular congestion. Inflammatory reactions seem to be greatest in the basal nuclei, midbrain, and medulla. The spinal cord, sympathetic ganglia, and dorsal root ganglia may also be involved. Negri bodies, which are oval-shaped, eosinophilic, cytoplasmic inclusions, are a characteristic histologic feature of rabies.

Clinical manifestations occur in stages, beginning with generalized malaise, apathy, fever, and headache. These general symptoms, together with pain and numbness in the area of the wound, are diagnostic of the illness in its early stage. Within 24 to 72 hours after the general symptoms, there is an excitement phase marked by extreme fear, violent spasms of the larynx when swallowing that lead to hydrophobia, and dysphagia that leads to salivating with frothing from the mouth. Heightened sensitivity to external stimuli can produce localized twitching and generalized seizures. Facial numbness, dysarthria, hallucinations, and a confusional psychosis accompany this phase. Finally, there are alternating periods of stupor and mania, high fever, flaccid paralysis, coma, and respiratory failure. Death usually occurs from respiratory center failure within 2 to 7 days after the onset of neurologic symptoms.

## Slow Virus Disease

Unlike the acute encephalitides, the slow virus diseases go through a long latent period lasting from months to years before they manifest symptoms. Once symptoms have appeared, these diseases tend to progress at a slower pace. Two general types of slow infections are: (1) true slow virus infections, which include subacute sclerosing panencephalitis (SSPE), progressive multifocal leukoencephalopathy (PML), and progressive rubella panencephalitis; and (2) unconventional agent infections (spongiform), which include Creutzfeldt-Jakob disease and kuru.[1] The former are caused by known, conventional viruses; the latter are caused by yet unidentified agents that have some resemblance to viruses but do not produce an immune reaction in the host.

*SUBACUTE SCLEROSING PANENCEPHALITIS.* This illness usually occurs in children and is related to a prior infection by the measles virus. Granular regions, areas of focal destruction, and proliferation of neuroglial cells are present in the CNS. The CSF reveals increased protein, increased gamma globulin fraction, and high levels of measles antibody. There is also evidence of measles antigen in neurons and glial cells. Bursts of high-voltage and sharp waves are noted on EEG examination. The illness occurs in stages over several years: (1) initially, personality changes occur; (2) intellectual deterioration, seizures, ataxia, and visual disturbances follow; and (3) rigidity, progressive unresponsiveness, and signs of autonomic dysfunction cause death within a few months or 1 to 3 years.

*PROGRESSIVE MULTIFOCAL LEUKOENCEPHALOPATHY.* This condition most often occurs in middle-aged persons who have a chronic debilitating disease such as rheumatoid arthritis, acquired immune deficiency syndrome (AIDS), or neoplastic disease, or in those who are receiving immunosuppressive therapy. Opportunistic viruses, such as C-J cirus or simian virus 40 (SV-40), cause CNS alterations, including widespread demyelinization of white matter, particularly of the cerebral hemispheres, brainstem, cerebellum, and rarely, the spinal cord. The CSF usually remains normal. Diagnosis of lesions may be facilitated by computerized axial tomography.[1] Symptoms of PML include hemiparesis, visual field defects, aphasia,

ataxia, dysarthria, confusion, and eventually coma. Death occurs within 3 to 20 months after onset of symptoms.

*PROGRESSIVE RUBELLA PANENCEPHALITIS.* This type of encephalitis, associated with rubella either of congenital or childhood origin, appears after a long latent period and continues on a progressive course. Initial symptoms are subtle changes in behavior and intellectual performance. Seizures arise in association with progressive mental deterioration, motor incoordination and spasicity; mutism, quadriplegia, and ophthalmoplegia mark the terminal stages of the disease. Progressive rubella panencephalitis seems to affect the white matter primarily, destroying nerve cells and attracting lymphocytes and mononuclear cells.

*SUBACUTE SPONGIFORM ENCEPHALOPATHY (CREUTZFELDT-JAKOB DISEASE, TRANSMISSIBLE VIRAL DEMENTIA).* This rare, rapidly progressive disease, which usually occurs in late middle age, produces CNS alterations mainly in the cerebral and cerebellar cortices and occasionally the basal ganglia. Alterations include neural degeneration, gliosis, and a spongelike condition in affected areas. Although serologic studies and CSF are normal, there is usually an associated, distinctive EEG pattern of diffuse nonspecific slowing, which changes to sharp waves or spikes on an increasingly flat background.[1]

The early clinical manifestations include personality changes, memory loss, visual abnormalities (distortions of shape, decreased visual acuity), and delirium. These symptoms are followed rapidly by dementia, myoclonic contractions, dysarthria, and ataxia, which eventually give way to stupor and coma, although myoclonic contractions continue. To date there is no effective treatment. Death usually occurs within 1 to 2 years after onset of symptoms.

*KURU.* *Kuru,* the first slow viral infection documented in humans, occurs in the Fore natives of Papua, New Guinea. The disease is associated with cannibalism in this tribe. Although the CNS alterations are similar to those associated with subacute spongiform encephalopathy, in kuru the spongelike conditions are more prominent in the corpus striatum and cerebellum.[12] Clinical manifestations include progressive cerebellar ataxia, shivering tremors, abnormal extraocular movement, incontinence, progression to complete immobility, and dementia in the terminal stage. After the onset of symptoms, death usually occurs within 3 to 6 months.

## Human Immunodeficiency Virus-Type 1

All parts of the CNS may be involved in the course of human immunodeficiency virus-type 1 (HIV-1). One or more neurologic syndromes have been reported in ap-

**TABLE 53–4.**
MAJOR NEUROLOGIC COMPLICATIONS OF HIV-1 INFECTION

| HIV-1 RELATED | OPPORTUNISTIC PROCESSES |
|---|---|
| Acute aseptic meningitis | Cryptococcal meningitis* |
| Chronic pleocytosis | Toxoplasmosis* |
| HIV-1 encephalopathy* | CMV retinitis/encephalitis* |
| Vacuolar myelopathy | Other CNS opportunistic infections* |
| Predominantly sensory neuropathy | Herpes group radiculitis |
| Inflammatory demyelinating polyneuropathy | Progressive multifocal leukoencephalopathy* |
| Mononeuritis multiplex | Primary CNS lymphoma* |
| Myopathy | Systemic lymphoma* |
| | Neurosyphilis |

*AIDS-defining condition.
Source: J. McArthur, Neurologic diseases associated with HIV-1 infection. In R.T. Johnson (ed.). Current Therapy in Neurologic Disease-3. Philadelphia: B.C. Decker, 1990.

proximately 40% of persons who have AIDS or AIDS-related complex (ARC) (see Chap. 15).[3] Neurologic complaints are the initial symptoms in 10% of all AIDS patients.[8] Nervous system involvement may result from primary HIV infection, secondary to immunosuppression, or both. The major neurologic complications associated with HIV-1 infection are presented in Table 53-4.

*DIRECT NEUROLOGIC EFFECTS OF HIV-1.* Persons initially infected with the HIV-1 virus may develop *acute aseptic meningitis* as a result of CNS response to viral invasion. A mild lymphocytic pleocytosis and modest CSF protein elevation may occur.[1] Clinical manifestations include headache, cranial neuropathies, and symptoms associated with meningeal irritation and transient encephalopathies.

*HIV-1 encephalopathy* and *encephalitis* have been described as the most common neurologic pathologies associated with AIDS. One third of AIDS patients develop these conditions early in the course of the disease, while two thirds develop them late in the illness.[1] Also known as *AIDS dementia complex*, HIV encephalopathy occurs as a result of direct HIV invasion of the CNS through infected macrophages or through the blood-brain barrier by endothelial cells.[3] Computerized tomography scans or MRI reveal mild to moderate brain atrophy and white matter changes. Examination of CSF reveals pleocytosis and elevated protein. In adults, clinical manifestations include progressive dementia with memory loss, disorientation, intellectual impairment, and psychotic behavior. Headache, ataxia, and aphasia are also frequent symptoms. In infants and children, manifestations of HIV encephalopathy include developmental delays, cognitive deterioration, corticospinal tract signs, or microencephaly.

Temporary improvement in dementia may occur with administration of zidovadine. However, there is rarely improvement in patients with far-advanced dementia.[8]

*Myelopathy* associated with HIV-1 is a spinal cord disorder taking the form of vacuolar degeneration. This problem occurs in approximately 20% of AIDS patients and is manifested by progressive spastic paraparesis and sensory ataxia.[8] The myelopathy is progressive and shows little response to zidovadine therapy. Spasticity may be relieved with antispasticity agents.

*Sensory neuropathies* occur in 30% of AIDS patients, usually late in the course of the illness and associated with systemic opportunistic infections.[8] Painful sensory symptoms in the feet include contact hypersensitivity, reduced or absent ankle reflexes, and elevated sensory thresholds. Pain-modifying agents may be used to provide symptomatic relief.

In contrast to sensory neuropathies, *inflammatory demyelinating polyneuropathies (IDP)* occur early in the course of HIV infection, prior to developing immunodeficiency. Inflammatory demyelinating polyneuropathy may be evident as acute (Guillain-Barré) or chronic types. In the acute type, profound motor weakness develops rapidly and there is associated CSF pleocytosis. Inflammatory demyelinating polyneuropathy is often more of a chronic, relapsing process.[8]

*Myopathy* taking the form of *inflammatory polymyositis* has been described as an uncommon complication of HIV-1. There is an elevation in serum creatine phosphokinase (CPK), and muscle biopsy reveals inflammatory infiltrates and fiber necrosis. The major clinical manifestation is moderate to severe weakness. Myopathy may be improved with corticosteroid therapy.[1]

*HIV-1 ASSOCIATED OPPORTUNISTIC PROCESSES OF THE CNS.* A number of opportunistic processes involving the CNS affect AIDS patients (see Table 53-4). These processes reflect the underlying immune deficiency produced by HIV and lysis of CD4 lymphocytes by this virus.[8] During the course of the AIDS illness, opportunistic processes may be multiple and occur concurrently with each other, and thus complicate diagnosis and treatment.

The most common and treatable intracranial focal complication is *cerebral toxoplasmosis*. The obligate intracellular protozoan, *Toxoplasma gondii*, produces multiple inflammatory and necrotic abscesses throughout the cerebral hemispheres, especially in the basal ganglia. These abnormalities are present in CT and MRI studies. Cerebrospinal fluid reveals elevated protein, decreased glucose levels, and pleocytosis. Long-term, suppressive therapy is required with clindamycin and pyrimethamine.

*Cryptococcus neoformans*, a yeast, is the most frequent fungal infection affecting the CNS in 6% to 11% of AIDS patients.[3] Clinical manifestations are typical of meningitis symptoms and include headache, neck stiffness, fever, altered mentation, and nausea. Actual culture isolation of the cryptococci may be found in CSF. Treatment with flucrylate and itraconazole has shown promise as primary therapy and as maintenance agents.[8]

Encephalitis in AIDS patients may also be produced by *cytomegalovirus (CMV)* and *human papovavirus*, producing PML. Cytomegalovirus may cause infection in the retina and visual loss in 20% of AIDS patients.[8] Progressive multifocal leukoencephalopathy is evident initially as a progressive accumulation of focal neurologic deficits. Approximately 2% of people with AIDS develop PML.

Additional opportunistic infections include *herpes zoster* and *neurosyphilis*. *Herpes zoster radiculitis* occurs in 5% to 10% of AIDS patients.[8] Treatment may not be required unless cervical or lumbar dermatomes are involved and produce severe myeloradiculitis with permanent motor deficits. While neurosyphilis is not strictly an opportunistic infection, it has been suggested that the course of syphilis is accelerated in AIDS patients.[8] Also, there appears to be an increase in frequency of syphilitic meningitis and meningovascular syphilis in AIDS patients.

In addition to opportunistic infections, it has been suggested that primary CNS lymphomas develop in 5% of AIDS patients.[3] Unifocal or multifocal lesions are present on CT scans. Clinical manifestations include focal neurologic dysfunction with dementia, confusion, or lethargy. Radiotherapy is used to reduce tumor size and manage symptoms.

## Aseptic Meningitis Complex (Benign Viral Meningitis)

These are general names for disorders in which there is evidence of meningeal irritation, although pyogenic organisms, parasites, or fungi are not present in CSF. Lymphocytes are commonly present in the CSF in individuals with aseptic meningitis. A virus is expected to be the causative agent, and the following viruses have been found in over one third of the individuals with aseptic

meningitis complex: mumps, herpes simplex, Coxsackievirus, lymphocytic choriomeningitis virus, and ECHO virus. More recently, it has been recognized that human immunodeficiency virus (HIV) may produce an acute aseptic meningitis with an infectious mononucleosis-like clinical picture.[1] The symptoms are mild, and most individuals recover from these illnesses without significant residual effects.

## Viruses Acquired Congenitally

Viruses are capable of crossing the placenta to reach the fetus, especially during the first trimester of pregnancy. They often produce devastating effects on the fetus. Although it is possible for many types of viruses to infect the fetus, the most common ones are *rubella* and *CMV*.

Congenital rubella often occurs during the first 10 weeks of gestation. The virus invades the brain of the fetus and contributes to the establishment of severe mental retardation, seizures, and motor defects. Other manifestations may include low birth weight, abnormally small eyeballs, pigmentary retinal degeneration, glaucoma, cloudy cornea, cataracts, neurocochlear deafness, enlarged liver and spleen, jaundice, and patent ductus arteriosus or intraventricular septal defects.[1] These severe effects are preventable by ensuring that women receive the rubella vaccine prior to becoming pregnant. Congenital rubella syndrome has been reduced by 96% in the United States as a result of immmunization programs.[2]

Cytomegaloviruses usually infect the fetus early during the first trimester of pregnancy and may produce cerebral malformation. Later, although the brain is normally formed, CMV may produce inflammatory necrosis in various parts of the brain. Nervous system effects of this infection may include mental defects, convulsions, microcephaly, and often hydrocephalus. Other manifestations include enlarged liver and spleen, jaundice, melena, hematemesis, and petechiae.[1] Cytomegalovirus affects approximately 3000 children annually in the United States.[14] Whether a fetus has been infected by CMV cannot be determined until birth (and in some cases, several years later) because the infection is not apparent in pregnant women.

## Myelitis

Poliomyelitis and herpes zoster are the two principal types of myelitis (inflammation of the spinal cord).

*POLIOMYELITIS.* Since the advent of the Salk vaccine in 1955 and the oral Sabin vaccine in 1958, cases of paralytic poliomyelitis are uncommon. The synonym for poliomyelitis is *infantile paralysis;* however, the disease occurs in all age groups. The disease is known to occur throughout the world and peak frequency is during the summer months. Approximately 15 cases are reported each year in the United States.[1]

The human intestinal tract is the main viral reservoir for the ribonucleic acid (RNA) virus, which infects through the fecal-oral route. Incubation lasts from 1 to 3 weeks. The virus then penetrates intestinal walls, invades the bloodstream, and is carried throughout the body.

Alterations in the CNS include destruction of nerve cells, as well as cellular infiltration, edema, and severe inflammatory processes that produce tissue necrosis and hemorrhages. Although the entire CNS may be involved, the predominant site of alterations is the anterior horn of the spinal cord. Examination of CSF usually shows no evidence of the virus during the clinical disease; however, protein levels are elevated, glucose level is normal, and the number of lymphocytes is increased.

The majority of persons infected with the virus experience no symptoms, or only a vague illness because of the failure of the virus to invade the CNS. Even after CNS invasion, however, clinical effects range from a mild, nonparalytic form of the disease to a severe, paralytic form. This variation in symptoms is related to the severity of the inflammatory response and to the degree to which nerve cells are injured.

Nonparalytic poliomyelitis produces general symptoms of fever, headache, listlessness, anorexia, nausea, vomiting, sore throat, and aching muscles. At this point, the disease may be resolved. With increasing irritability, restlessness, muscle tenderness and spasms, neck and back pain, and neck stiffness, in addition to Kernig's and Brudzinski's signs, the paralytic form of the disease is often imminent.

Paralytic poliomyelitis is often divided into three types: *spinal, bulbar,* and *encephalitic.* This division is primarily useful as a descriptive mechanism since these types are often combined during the course of the disease. Spinal involvement may include muscle weakness with fasciculations, diminished reflexes in association with progressive abdominal and limb muscle weakness, eventual paralysis (the level varying among different age groups), and muscle atrophy. Bulbar involvement impairs the ability to swallow, disturbs respiration and vasomotor control, and progressively slows respirations. Cyanosis and hypertension may occur, followed by hypotension and circulatory collapse. Mortality is as high as 75% when there is accompanying paralysis of phrenic and intercostal muscles.[1] Involvement of the high brainstem and hypothalamus produces encephalitic symptoms that include restlessness, confusion, and anxiety initially, progressing to stupor and coma.[1]

HERPES ZOSTER (SHINGLES).    Herpes zoster infection, caused by the varicella zoster virus, occurs most commonly in adulthood, particularly with advancing age, and in persons with underlying systemic diseases, such as the leukemias or lymphomas. The development of this illness is not completely understood. It is thought that herpes zoster infection represents a reactivation of varicella virus infection that persists in the nerve ganglia after a primary infection with chickenpox. Herpes zoster is not communicable, except possibly to people who have not had chickenpox.[1] Individuals who have herpes zoster infection usually have a past history of chickenpox. Nervous system alterations include congested, edematous, and hemorrhagic dorsal root ganglion. There is also disintegration of ganglion cells. Painful, vesicular skin eruptions, which harbor varicella zoster virus, are associated with involvement of the corresponding dorsal root ganglion or gasserian ganglion. The most frequently involved dermatomes are T-5 to T-10; however, any dermatome may be involved. In some cases, accompanying sensory loss and motor palsies occur. Although most individuals recover, the process is often slow and painful. The pain may persist for months or even years, causing much despair for the person.

## Postinfectious/Postvaccinal Diseases

Acute disseminated (postinfectious) encephalomyelitis, acute inflammatory polyradiculoneuropathy (Guillain-Barré syndrome), and Reye's syndrome often occur during or shortly after viral infection, or rarely after vaccinations for smallpox, rabies, or typhoid. These conditions often require individual susceptibility to the virus or viral effects.

ACUTE DISSEMINATED (POSTINFECTIOUS) ENCEPHALOMYELITIS.    Postinfectious encephalomyelitis develops 2 to 4 days after a rash and is thought to be an autoimmune response to myelin, which is triggered by a virus.[5] Demyelination occurs in the region of the brainstem and spinal cord. In addition, the meninges are infiltrated by inflammatory cells. Clinical manifestations include headaches, stiffness of the neck, lethargy, and eventually coma. Ten to 20% of affected persons die in the acute phase of the illness.[1] Neurologic residual effects are severe in those who survive.

GUILLAIN-BARRÉ SYNDROME (ACUTE IDIOPATHIC NEUROPATHY).    This syndrome is thought to be the result of an autoimmune reaction triggered by a virus in the peripheral nerves. Nervous system alterations include inflammatory infiltrate around vessels throughout the cranial and spinal nerves, demyelination, and axon destruction. The CSF reveals an elevated protein level and pleocytosis. Clinical manifestations include proximal and distal weakness or paralysis of extremities, hypotonia, areflexia, pain, and paresthesias. Weakness that progresses to total motor paralysis of respiratory muscles can result in death. Autonomic dysfunction may occur with resultant sudden fluctuations in blood pressure and heart rate, orthostatic hypotension, and cessation of sweating. Individuals who survive the acute phase of the disease usually recover completely; however, some have residual motor or reflex deficits (see Chap. 29).

*REYE'S SYNDROME.* Reye's syndrome seems to occur after viral infections, such as influenza B and varicella infections, although the relationship between the virus and pathologic changes is not understood. Whether the condition results from the viral infection or from treatment with aspirin is under investigation. The probability is high that the syndrome is produced in concert with aspirin ingestion.[5] Many factors, including genetic and environmental, apparently function together in the production of this catastrophic disorder. It occurs predominantly in children between ages 6 months and 15 years.[5] It is characterized by the onset of acute encephalopathy 10 days to 2 weeks after a viral infection. Cerebral edema is produced, as well as fatty changes in the liver and renal tubules. The disease is also characterized by hypoglycemia, increased serum aminotransferases, and serum ammonia levels. Clinical manifestations include persistent vomiting, delirium, seizures, stupor, and eventual coma. Respiratory distress, tachypnea, and apnea are prominent features in infants. Full-blown disease with encephalopathy and liver involvement carries 40% to 60% mortality but this appears to be improving due to earlier diagnosis and supportive treatment. The initiation of treatment before the occurrence of coma has reduced associated fatality to 5% to 10%.[1]

## Bacterial Infections

### Pyogenic Infections

The brain or its coverings can be infected by pyogenic (pus-forming) microorganisms. The most common organisms that are responsible for bacterial infections are normally harbored in the nasopharynx in the general population. Bacteria enter the CNS by spread from adjacent cranial structures, through the bloodstream. In a few unfortunate cases, the infection is iatrogenic, for example, from a lumbar puncture or contaminated scapel. It is frequently difficult to determine the exact entry route of the organism. Once within the CNS, the effects of pyogenic microorganisms may be disastrous.

*BACTERIAL MENINGITIS (LEPTOMENINGITIS).* The leptomeninges and subarachnoid space are primary targets for invasion by pyogenic microorganisms. Once an infection enters any part of the subarachnoid space, it spreads quickly throughout CSF pathways in the brain and spinal cord. Thus, an inflammatory reaction is set up in the pia and arachnoid, and in the ventricles. Any microorganisms entering the body may cause meningitis. However, some bacteria are more prominent and seem to be more prevalent in certain age groups. Pneumococcus organisms are commonly cultured in very young patients and in adults over 40 years of age, *Escherichia coli* in the neonatal period, *Hemophilus influenzae* in infants and young children, and *Neisseria meningitidis* in adolescents and young adults. Fifty percent of the cases in infants and young children are attributed to *H. influenzae.*[11] Spinal fluid cultures usually reveal the causative agent.

Meningococcal infections develop more rapidly and distinctly than other forms of meningitis. They may occur singularly or in epidemics where overcrowding exists. The organism is spread by droplet infection from those who harbor the meningococcus in their nasal passages. Disease onset is heralded by a distinctive petechial or purpuric rash. A particularly disastrous event (Waterhouse-Friderichsen syndrome) may occur after any bacterial meningitis, although it is most commonly associated with fulminant meningococcemia. This condition is manifested by overwhelming bacteremia, adrenocortical necrosis, and vasomotor collapse. Hemophilus influenzae meningitis commonly follows ear and upper respiratory infections in the young. Pneumococcal meningitis can be related to prior infections in the lungs, nasal sinuses, and heart valves.

Alterations occurring with the various bacterial infections include swelling and congestion of the brain and spinal cord, as well as exudate within the subarachnoid space. In severe cases, inflammatory cells can occlude vessels that penetrate the brain, resulting in areas of necrosis. The CSF reveals elevated protein, decreased glucose, and decreased chloride levels, elevated pressure (above 180 mm of water), and the presence of large numbers of leukocytes.

Clinical manifestations of acute pyogenic meningitis are fever, headache, pain with eye movement, photophobia, neck and back stiffness, positive Kernig's and Brudzinski's signs, generalized convulsions, drowsiness, and confusion. Focal signs may be observed with some bacterial infections as a result of occlusion of vessels and regional brain necrosis. Stupor, followed by coma and death, may occur without prompt and adequate treatment.

Residual effects are also a danger due to destruction or fibrotic thickening of the meningeal framework. Potential residual effects include optic arachnoiditis, meningomyelitis, and chronic meningoencephalitis with hydrocephalus. Again, with prompt diagnosis and antibiotic therapy, these residual effects are less common than they once were.

*BRAIN ABSCESS.* Approximately one half of all brain abscesses are secondary to infection in the nasal cavity, middle ear, and mastoid cells. The remaining cases are due to primary focus of infection elsewhere in the body, particularly the lungs or pleura, heart, and distal bones (Figure 53-6). Streptococci, staphylococci, and

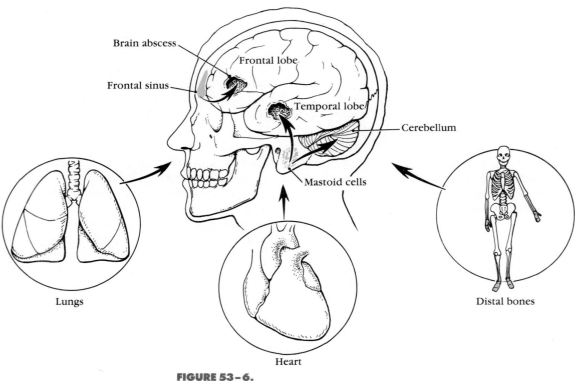

**FIGURE 53–6.**
Origins and locations of cerebral abscesses.

pneumococci are often the causative organisms. A small proportion (about 10%) of cases result from infection being introduced through compound skull fractures or intracranial operations.[1]

An abscess is formed when an inflammation, caused by an invading organism, liquefies and begins to accumulate white blood cells. A fibrous capsule is formed in an effort to contain the pus. As the abscess expands, nerve tissue is compressed and destroyed. Chronic inflammation and pronounced edema surround the abscess. The CSF reveals a normal glucose level, increased protein level, and increased white cell count. The CSF pressure is often moderately elevated early in the abscess formation and markedly elevated in the later stages. If the abscess ruptures into the subarachnoid space or ventricles, organisms can be cultured from CSF. Other diagnostic techniques that may be used are skull films, CT scans, EEG, and ventriculography.

The most frequent initial clinical manifestation is headache, with other symptoms being similar to those produced by growing masses within the brain. Notably, the increased intracranial pressure and focal complaints related to the location of the abscess are important. In addition, a brain abscess can rupture and lead to other complications, such as sinus thrombosis, ventriculitis, or meningitis. Mortality from brain abscesses has been greatly reduced due to successful combinations of antibiotic therapy and surgery.

*SUBDURAL EMPYEMA.* *Empyema* refers to pus in a body cavity; thus, subdural empyema is a suppurative process in the subdural space. It usually occurs between the dura's inner surface and the outer surface of the arachnoid. The most common causative organisms are streptococci or bacteroides, and less often *Staphylococcus aureus, E. coli*, and pseudomonas.[1] Infective organisms usually travel to the subdural space by spread from thrombophlebitis or by erosion through bone or dura from the frontal sinuses, ethmoid sinuses, middle ear, or mastoid cells. Exudate is present on the undersurface of the dura. As the empyema grows, pressure is applied to the underlying cerebral hemisphere. Thrombophlebitis of cerebral veins that are near the subdural empyema can contribute to ischemic necrosis of the cortex. The CSF reveals elevated pressure, increased protein and normal glucose levels, and an increased number of lymphocytes.

Many affected persons have a history of chronic mastoiditis or sinusitis. Clinical manifestations indicating that the infection has spread to the subdural space include fever, general malaise, a localized headache that becomes generalized, associated vomiting, and neck stiffness. As the empyema enlarges, focal neurologic signs, lethargy, and coma develop. Prognosis depends on the success of surgery and antibiotic therapy, as well as the extent to which neurologic deficits have occurred.

## Tuberculous Infections

Tuberculous meningitis and tuberculomas of the brain and spinal cord are usually secondary to a tuberculous focus in another part of the body. Thus, as better public health measures and modern therapy help control the frequency of tuberculosis, the frequency of tuberculous meningitis and tuberculomas of the brain and cord are decreased.

*TUBERCULOUS MENINGITIS.* Tuberculous meningitis occurs in areas of high tuberculosis prevalence, primarily in young children. In low-frequency areas, it occurs mostly in the elderly population as a result of reactivation of dormant organisms. Tuberculous meningitis is caused by *Mycobacterium tuberculosis*. This condition has a slower onset and more chronic course than pyogenic meningitis.

The base of the brain and the spinal cord become compressed by shaggy, necrotic, fibrinous, yellow exudate. There may also be large areas of caseation and tiny tubercles around the blood vessels.[1] The CSF reveals increased pressure, elevated protein, and decreased glucose levels (but not as low as values observed in pyogenic meningitis), and the presence of polymorphonuclear leukocytes and lymphocytes. With careful technique in obtaining a specimen, tubercle bacilli may be recovered from CSF.

Clinical manifestations depend on the chronicity of the disease and the extent of pathologic processes. In general, adults have headache, fever, lethargy, confusion, neck stiffness, positive Kernig's and Brudzinski's signs, weight loss, and night sweats. Young children frequently experience vomiting, irritability, and seizures.

Due to the slow onset of this illness, neurologic damage may be present before treatment is sought. Then, even though the person survives, there may be lasting effects, such as recurrent seizures, retarded intellectual development, mental disturbances, visual disturbances, deafness, and hemiparesis.

*TUBERCULOMAS OF BRAIN AND SPINAL CORD.* Tuberculomas (tuberculous granulation masses), although rare in the United States, constitute from 5% to 30% of all intracranial space-occupying lesions in underdeveloped countries.[1] Tuberculomas may be single or multiple and contain a core of caseation necrosis surrounded by a fibrous capsule. Within the brain and spinal cord, they produce neurologic effects similar to those of other expanding intracranial and intraspinal lesions. The CSF reveals increased protein levels and a small number of lymphocytes. Tuberculomas of the brain and spinal cord have been known to calcify while still small before any neurologic changes have occurred. These are often found at autopsy.

Tuberculous infection may affect the spinal cord in a number of ways, causing spinal block. Evidence of spinal root disease may be the result of inflammatory meningeal exudate invasion of the underlying parenchyma. Compression by an epidural mass of granulation tissue produces spinal symptoms and Pott's paraplegia.[1]

## Neurosyphilis

The frequency of neurosyphilis (tertiary stage of syphilis) has decreased in the last several decades due to prompt diagnosis and treatment of early syphilis. The overall frequency of syphilis is increasing, however, particularly in young persons.

*Treponema pallidum* is a spiral, motile organism that causes syphilis. Once this organism is introduced into the body, it usually invades the CNS within 3 to 18 months. Neurosyphilis is progressive in the large majority of individuals and includes several forms: asymptomatic neurosyphilis, meningovascular syphilis, general paresis, and tabes dorsalis (see Chap. 57).

Meningitis is the initial event in all forms of neurosyphilis but the severity of symptoms varies among the different forms and it may remain asymptomatic for several years. The CSF is the most accurate, sensitive indicator that an active neurosyphilitic infection is present. Changes in CSF include positive serologic tests: the Veneral Disease Research Laboratory slide test, Kolmer test, fluorescent treponemal antibody absorption test, and treponema immobilization test; increased protein level; presence of increased lymphocytes, plasma cells, and mononuclear cells; and an abnormal colloidal gold curve.

*ASYMPTOMATIC NEUROSYPHILIS.* As the name *asymptomatic neurosyphilis* implies, there are usually no physical signs or symptoms of the meningitis. This form of the disease is recognized by the changes in CSF listed above. Treatment prevents further development of the disease.

*MENINGOVASCULAR NEUROSYPHILIS.* This form of neurosyphilis commonly develops 6 to 7 years after the original infection. The CNS alterations include infiltration of meninges and blood vessels with plasma cells and lymphocytes, inflammation of arteries, and fibrosis that leads to occlusion of vessels. The vascular lesions are referred to as Heubner's arteritis. Miliary gummas may also be seen in the meninges.

Clinical manifestations are similar to those of low-grade meningitis, as well as cerebrovascular accident and mental derangement. Unless treated, neurologic deficits continue to progress.

*GENERAL PARESIS.*    This form of neurosyphilis usually develops 15 to 20 years after the original infection. Early treatment of syphilis has decreased the frequency of general paresis. In this form of neurosyphilis, the parenchyma of the brain is involved due to the presence of spirochetes. There is a diffuse destruction of cortical neurons and proliferation of astrocytes. Plasma cells and lymphocytes accumulate around blood vessels.

Clinical manifestations are those of progressive mental and physical deterioration. Initially, slight memory loss, changes in behavior, and decreased ability to reason occur. Later, the individual develops a severe dementia with elaborate delusional systems and disregard for moral and social standards. Physically, the individual experiences dysarthria, tremor of the tongue and hands, myoclonic jerks, muscular hypotonia, hyperactive tendon reflexes, Babinski's signs, seizures, and Argyll Robertson pupils. Without treatment, the prognosis is poor and death occurs in a few years.

*TABES DORSALIS.*    Tabes dorsalis, like general paresis, occurs many years after the onset of infection. This form of neurosyphilis is also uncommon now due to improved, early treatment with penicillin.

The CNS alterations include degeneration of the posterior columns, fibrosis around the posterior roots, and destruction of proprioceptive fibers in the radicular nerves. These changes produce various symptoms, the most common being ataxia. Other features of this type of neurosyphilis are lightening pains (sudden sharp pains lasting only a portion of a second), ataxia due to sensory defects, and urinary incontinence. Visceral symptoms include vomiting and bouts of sharp epigastric pain that extend around the body. Other clinical manifestations may include Argyll Robertson pupils, Charcot's joints due to repeated injury to insensitive joints, absence of a vibration sense, and deep tendon reflexes, as well as Romberg's sign. Romberg's sign is the inability to maintain balance with the eyes closed and the feet together. Although treatment with penicillin can arrest the disease process, residual effects, such as urinary incontinence, lightening pains, visceral crises, and Charcot's joints, may persist indefinitely.

## Disorders Due to Bacterial Exotoxins

Bacterial exotoxins can have powerful effects on the CNS and can result in life-threatening motor problems. The major diseases produced by these toxins are tetanus, diphtheria, and botulism.

*TETANUS.*    *Clostridium tetani* produces tetanus after contaminating penetrating wounds or the umbilical cord of the newborn with spores. These anaerobic, spore-forming bacilli produce two exotoxins: a tetanolysin and a tetanospasmin. Neurotoxic effects are produced by tetanospasmin. Most of the toxin enters the peripheral endings of motor neurons from the bloodstream, travels up the fibers to the spinal cord and brainstem, and crosses the synaptic cleft to the inhibitory neurons, where it prevents the release of glycine. Glycine is a neuromuscular transmitter secreted mainly in the synapses of the spinal cord; it acts as an inhibitor. The action of tetanospasmin is through an affinity for the sympathetic nervous system, the medullary centers, the anterior horn cells of the spinal cord, and the motor end plates in skeletal muscle. It produces uninhibited motor responses leading to the typical muscle spasm.

The incubation period varies from several days to several months. Usually, symptoms occur within 2 weeks after wound contamination. The initial manifestation is usually difficulty opening the jaw (trismus); thus, the synonym *lockjaw*. There is generalized muscle stiffness with eventual muscle spasms (tetanic seizures or convulsions). These convulsions are very painful and can occur spontaneously or in response to the slightest stimuli. Facial spasms produce a characteristic sardonic smile (risus sardonicus). Contractions of back muscles produce a forward arching of the back (opisthotonos). Spasms of glottal, laryngeal, and respiratory muscles cause difficulty in breathing and frequently lead to death due to asphyxia. In established clinical cases of tetanus, overall mortality is 50%.[1] The toxin is not able to cross the blood-brain barrier, which accounts for the normal mentation in these individuals.[5] The disease is prevented with active immunization with tetanus toxoid. Also, prompt administration of antitoxin may prevent progression of symptoms.

*DIPHTHERIA.*    *Corynebacterium diphtheriae* produces an acute infection: diphtheria. Although open wounds in any part of the body can provide entry for this organism, the usual portal of entry is the oral cavity. The incubation period is 1 to 7 days. During this time, the organism becomes established and proliferates at the site of implantation, usually the throat and trachea. The bacteria produce exotoxin that is absorbed by the blood and carried to the CNS and heart. Early general manifestations of the disease are fever, sore throat, chills, and malaise. Local neurologic manifestations occur within 5 to 12 days and include vomiting, dysphagia, possible cranial nerve involvement, and nasal voice due to palatal paralysis. Blurred vision and loss of accommodation occur in the second or third week due to ciliary paralysis. Between the fifth and sixth weeks, weakness and paralysis of the extremities may occur. Most neurologic disturbances disappear slowly, and individuals usually improve completely if respiratory obstruction or cardiac failure does not supervene. The disease is prevented by immunization; prompt administration of antitoxin may prevent clinical manifestations.

*BOTULISM.* *Clostridium botulinum* can contaminate and produce exotoxins in food, such as fruits, vegetables, and meats that are kept for long periods of time without refrigeration. When ingested, the toxin resists gastric digestion, is absorbed by the blood, and then travels to the nervous system. The botulinus toxin acts only on the presynaptic endings of neuromuscular junctions and autonomic ganglia. It prevents the release of acetylcholine and causes symptoms resembling those of myasthenia gravis. The result is a descending form of paralysis from the cranial nerves downward. Symptoms occur within 12 to 36 hours after ingestion of the contaminated food.[1] Neural symptoms may or may not be preceded by nausea and vomiting. The individual may develop cranial nerve palsies, blurred vision, diplopia, ptosis, strabismus, hoarseness, dysarthria, dysphagia, vertigo, deafness, constipation, and progressive muscle weakness. Tendon reflexes may be absent. Sensation remains intact and the person is conscious throughout the illness. Even with prompt administration of *C. botulinum* antitoxins, death occurs in about 15% of cases due to paralysis of respiratory muscles and respiratory infections. Those who survive generally recover completely with effective supportive care over a long, slow course.[5]

## Fungal Infections

Fungi infect the CNS less commonly than bacteria and viruses. Their effects can be similar to bacterial infection but more difficult to treat. Fungal infections may produce brain abscesses, meningitis, meningoencephalitis, and thrombophlebitis of vessels within the CNS. As with other infections, fungal infections of the CNS are usually secondary to a primary source of infection elsewhere in the body. In addition, they may be a complication of another disease process, such as cancer, or related to immunosuppressant drugs.

Fungi usually spread to the CNS by the bloodstream. Once in the CNS, they cause an inflammatory reaction, and a purulent exudate involves the meninges. In some cases, invasion of vessel walls results in vasculitis and thrombosis with subsequent nervous tissue infarction. The process develops slowly over days or weeks. Clinical manifestations are similar to those of tuberculous meningitis. In addition, hydrocephalus is a frequent related complication. The CSF reveals elevated pressure, increased protein and decreased glucose levels, moderate pleocytosis (increased number of lymphocytes), and often the isolation of the infective organism.

Many types of fungi may invade the CNS. The most common infections are candidiasis, cryptococcosis, coccidioidomycosis, and mucormycosis.

## Cryptococcosis (Torulosis)

Common in soil and bird droppings, cryptococci are the most frequent cause of fungal infection of the CNS. The fungus is transmitted to humans through the respiratory tract. Cryptococcosis, which usually arises secondary to a pulmonary infection, produces cysts and granulomas in the cortex and occasionally in the deep white matter and basal ganglia. These cysts contain large numbers of organisms. *Cryptococcus neoformans* is recovered from spinal fluid. Mortality, even in the absence of preexisting diseases (lymphomas and Hodgkin's disease), is nearly 40%.[1] Clinical features are similar to those of subacute meningitis or encephalitis.

## Coccidioidomycosis

*Coccidioides immitis* produces a relatively mild, flulike illness involving the respiratory organs. Common in the southwestern United States, coccidioidomycosis may become a chronic, diffuse, granulomatous disease that spreads throughout the body. The meninges and CSF become involved with resultant pathologic and clinical manifestations similar to those of tuberculous meningitis. When the meninges become involved, treatment is difficult. Amphotericin B is the only effective drug; even with this treatment, the disease is often fatal.

## Mucormycosis (Zygomycosis, Phycomycosis)

Mucormycosis, caused by one of the mucorales, is a rare opportunistic infection occurring in very debilitated persons. One of the primary sites of invasion is the nasal sinuses. From the nasal sinuses, the organism may spread along invaded vessels to periorbital tissue and the cranial vault. Nervous tissue infarctions occur as a result of vascular occlusion. Once the mucorales organism has invaded the brain, prognosis is very poor.

## Protozoal Infections

### Malaria

*Plasmodium vivax* produces the most common form of malaria. This organism does not actually invade brain tissue but the parasitized red blood cells block microcirculation, thus leading to tissue hypoxia and ischemic necrosis. The vessel blockage within the brain leads to glial necrosis, which causes drowsiness, confusion, and seizures. Quinine is used for treatment and is helpful unless the cerebral symptoms are far advanced.

*Plasmodium falciparum* produces a form of malaria that has more severe symptoms. The parasite fills capillaries, and Durck's nodes (small foci of necrosis surrounded by glia) are present in brain tissue. The CSF reveals elevated pressure and contains white blood cells. Clinical manifestations include focal neurologic signs, headache, seizures, aphasia, cerebellar ataxia, hemiplegia, hemianopsia and, eventually, coma. Cerebral malaria due to *P. falciparum* is usually rapidly fatal.

### Toxoplasmosis

*Toxoplasma gondii* produces an infection that is either acquired or congenital. The organism is acquired congenitally, by eating raw beef, or by contact with cat feces.

Acquired toxoplasmosis that produces clinical effects is rare. In clinical cases, the white and gray matter contain necrotic lesions that harbor *T. gondii*. Symptoms are similar to meningoencephalitis. Acquired toxoplasmosis is observed rather frequently in persons with AIDS.

Congenital toxoplasmosis causes much destruction of the neonatal brain. Signs of infection are fever, rash, seizures, and enlarged liver and spleen that may be present at birth. Slow psychomotor development becomes evident early in life. In some cases, clinical manifestations of the illness are not present for days, weeks, or months. These clinical effects include hydrocephalus, retardation, cerebral calcification, and chorioretinitis.

### Amebiasis

Infection with amoebae may occur after swimming in lakes or ponds. The causative organisms are usually of the *Naegleria* genus, and there is a prevalence of cases in the southeastern United States.

The CNS alterations include abscesses in the cortex and purulent exudate involving the meninges. The CSF findings are similar to those of bacterial meningitis. The disease is rapidly progressive with the symptoms of nausea, vomiting, fever, neck stiffness, focal neurologic signs, seizures, and eventually coma. This illness is usually fatal within a week of onset due to the resistance of *Naegleria* to treatment.

### Trypanosomiasis

Several strains of *Trypanosoma brucei* produce African sleeping sickness, which is transmitted by the tsetse fly. Two epidemiologic patterns are described: Gambian (Middle and West African) and Rhodesian (East African). The Rhodesian type is more severe, with intercurrent infections and myocarditis dominating the clinical picture. Within 2 years after infection with the Gambian form, trypanosomes produce meningoencephalitis, with thickening of the meninges and cerebral edema. Symptoms range from somnolence to convulsions and coma. Mortality depends on the effectiveness of treatment and the degree of CNS involvement.

*Trypanosoma cruzi* produces Chagas' disease in Central and South America, rarely in North America. The organism is transmitted by biting bugs commonly called assassin bugs. Chagas' disease is either acute or chronic. The acute form is prevalent in children and produces fever, enlarged liver and spleen, myocardial involvement with congestive failure, and eventually involvement of the lungs, meninges, and brain. Months or years after an acute attack, the chronic form may develop with subsequent meningoencephalitis. Pentavalent arsenicals have shown some success in the treatment of both types of trypanosomiasis.

### Trichinosis

*Trichinella spiralis* enters the body when raw or insufficiently cooked pork is eaten. Within 2 to 3 days, early symptoms of the disease are apparent and are mainly due to the invasion of muscle by larvae, producing mild gastroenteritis, muscle weakness, and tenderness. Three to 6 weeks after ingestion, larvae invade the nervous system. Lymphocytic and mononuclear infiltration of the meninges, as well as focal gliosis, occur. Symptoms of CNS involvement include headache, confusion, neck stiffness, seizures, and occasionally coma. Although trichinosis is usually not fatal, seizures and neurologic deficits may continue indefinitely.

## Metazoal Infections

### Cysticercosis

Ingestion of encysted eggs of pork tapeworm, *Taenia solium*, produce cysticercosis. This disease is most common in South American countries. The larvae spread throughout the body and develop cysts in any body tissue. Cystic nodules within the brain produce symptoms similar to those of brain tumors. Jacksonian seizures are common manifestations. Prognosis depends on the extent of neurologic damage and effective therapy with praziquantel, an antihelminthic agent.

### Echinococcosis (Hydatid Disease)

This disease is caused by the ingestion of larvae of the canine tapeworm, *Echinococcus granulosus*. The larvae invade the liver, lungs, bones, and less frequently, the brain. The larvae become encysted and are at first microscopic. However, within 5 or more years, the cysts may grow to massive sizes of 10 cm or more.[5] Thus, within the brain, symptoms are similar to those associated with brain tumors. The amount of local destruction throughout the body determines the prognosis.

## Rickettsial Infections

Rickettsial infections are relatively rare in the United States. They are caused by microorganisms that are obligate intracellular parasites with multiplication occurring only within living cells of susceptible hosts. Their cycle involves an animal reservoir and an insect vector (ticks, fleas, lice, mites, and humans). Epidemic typhus involves only a cycle with lice and humans.

Major rickettsial diseases include epidemic (primary) typhus, louse-borne; murine (endemic) typhus, flea-borne; scrub typhus or tsutsugamushi fever, mite-borne; Rocky Mountain spotted fever, tick-borne; and Q fever, tick-borne and airborne. Within the CNS, rickettsial diseases can produce lesions in the gray and white matter. Focal gliosis, together with mononuclear leukocytes, produce characteristic typhus nodules.

All the rickettsial diseases except Q fever have similar pathologic and clinical effects. A 3-day to 18-day incubation period is followed by the abrupt onset of high fever, chills, headache, and weakness followed by a generalized macular rash. During the second week after the onset of fever, the CNS becomes involved, producing apathy, dullness, intermittent episodes of delirium, and eventually stupor and coma. Occasionally, in untreated cases, there are focal neurologic manifestations and optic neuritis. The CSF may be completely normal. Q fever is not accompanied by a rash and produces symptoms similar to those of a low-grade meningitis.

Mortality due to typhus is greatest during epidemics. Early antibiotic therapy has reduced fatality rates to less than 10% for typhus and 5% for Rocky Mountain spotted fever.[1] Fatalities are rarely associated with scrub typhus and Q fever.

## REFERENCES

1. Adams, R., and Victor, M. *Principles of Neurology* (4th ed.). New York: McGraw-Hill, 1989.
2. Bale, J.F. Viral infection. In R.T. Johnson (ed.), *Current Therapy in Neurologic Disease-3*. Philadelphia: B.C. Decker, 1990.
3. Beckham, M.M. Neurologic manifestations of AIDS. *Crit. Care Nurs. Clin. N. Am.* 2:29, 1990.
4. Berkshire, J., and Watson-Evans, H. Meningioma: A nursing perspective. *J Neurosci. Nurs.* 21(2):233, 1989.
5. Cotran, R.S., Kumar, V., and Robbins, S.L. *Robbins' Pathologic Basis of Disease* (4th ed.). Philadelphia: W.B. Saunders, 1989.
6. Davidson, G. Nervous system. In J. Walker (ed.), *Pathology of Human Disease*. Philadelphia: Lea & Febiger, 1989.
7. Dropcho, E.J. Glioma. In R.T. Johnson (ed.), *Current Therapy in Neurologic Disease-3*. Philadelphia: B.C. Decker, 1990.
8. McArthur, J. Neurologic diseases associated with HIV-1 infection. In R.T. Johnson (ed.), *Current Therapy in Neurologic Disease-3*. Philadelphia: B.C. Decker, 1990.
9. McDonald J., et al. *Central Nervous System Tumors in Clinical Oncology for Medical Students and Physicians: A Multidisciplinary Approach* (6th ed.). New York: American Cancer Society, 1983.
10. Phillips, P.C. Brain tumors in children. In R.T. Johnson (ed.), *Current Therapy in Neurologic Disease-3*. Philadelphia: B.C. Decker, 1990.
11. Prendergast, V. Bacterial meningitis update. *J. Neurosci. Nurs.* 19:2, 1987.
12. Russel, D., and Rubinstein, L. *Pathology of Tumors of the Nervous System* (5th ed.). Baltimore: Williams & Wilkins, 1989.
13. Schwartz, S.I. (ed.). *Principles of Surgery* (5th ed.). New York: McGraw-Hill, 1989.
14. Weiner, L.P. Viral encephalitis. In R.T. Johnson (ed.), *Current Therapy in Neurologic Disease-3*. Philadelphia: B.C. Decker, 1990.

# chapter 54

Reet Henze
Barbara L. Bullock

# Degenerative and Chronic Alterations in the Nervous System

## Chapter Outline

▶ **Progressive Neurologic Disabilities**
  **Primary Disabilities**
  **Secondary Disabilities**
▶ **Paralyzing Developmental or Congenital Disorders**
  **Spina Bifida**
  **Syringomyelia**
  **Hydrocephalus**
    Pseudotumor Cerebri
  **Cranial Malformations**
  **Cerebral Palsy**

▶ **Disorders Characterized by Progressive Weakness or Paralysis**
  **Myasthenia Gravis**
  **Subacute Combined Degeneration of the Cord**
  **Guillain-Barré Syndrome**
  **Multiple Sclerosis**
  **Amyotrophic Lateral Sclerosis**

▶ **Disorders Characterized by Abnormal Movements**
  **Parkinson's Disease**
  **Drug-Induced Dyskinesias and Dystonias**
  **Torticollis**
  **Huntington's Chorea**
▶ **Disorders Characterized by Memory and Judgment Deficits**
  **Atherosclerotic Dementia**
  **Alzheimer's Disease**
  **Pick's Disease**
  **Neurosyphilis**

## Learning Objectives

1. Differentiate between primary and secondary disabilities.
2. Identify examples of developmental, congenital, and degenerative alterations in the nervous system.
3. Explain why the site of a neurologic alteration has a greater impact on the production of clinical signs than does the nature of the lesion.
4. Identify examples of congenital and developmental alterations in the motor areas of the brain and cord.
5. Identify examples of developmental and degenerative alterations in the upper voluntary motor areas of the nervous system leading to progressive weakness, tremor, or spastic paralysis.
6. Contrast upper and lower motor neuron paralysis.
7. Describe alterations in the lower voluntary motor areas of the nervous system leading to transient or permanent sensory or motor changes, or flaccid paralysis.

8. Describe the structural basis for signs and symptoms of bulbar palsy.
9. Explain the physiologic basis for medical treatment of muscle weakness and fatigue related to inadequate transmission of impulses across the myoneural junction.
10. Describe pathologic changes in the extrapyramidal motor system resulting in the loss of normal automatic or spontaneous body movements.
11. Describe pathologic changes in the extrapyramidal system resulting in the generation or facilitation of abnormal movements.
12. Identify examples of structural alterations that affect higher cerebral functions, such as memory and judgment.
13. Define prognostic terms such as *recovery, stabilization, progression, recurrence, remission,* and *exacerbation.*

## PROGRESSIVE NEUROLOGIC DISABILITIES

### Primary Disabilities

A primary disability is a structural and functional alteration that results directly from a pathologic process. Primary disabilities may be due to congenital disorders, genetic disorders, injuries, or disease, and unlike cardiovascular or skeletal disorders, they usually are referred to in terms of the functional, rather than structural, alteration. For example, terms such as *spastic quadriplegia* and *right homonymous hemianopsia* are more frequently used than such phrases as *demyelination of the . . . tracts* or *anoxia of the . . . branch of the . . . nerve.*

A reason for referring to primary neurologic alterations in functional terms is that often the nature of the lesion is hard to identify early in the course of the disease. Also, the description of the dysfunction helps to pinpoint the site of the lesion, even if it does not give much evidence as to its nature. The location of changes in the nervous system reflects the clinical signs and symptoms no matter whether the lesion that interrupts the generation of transmission of nerve impulses is developmental, infectious, degenerative, vascular, neoplastic, or traumatic. Therefore, a lesion that interrupts the pyramidal tracts in the brain or cord may produce spastic paralysis whether it is due to neuronal anoxia or to an inborn metabolic defect in the nerve cells. Similarly, an imbalance between the neurotransmitters in the basal ganglia results in abnormalities of movement whether it is due to degeneration of dopamine-releasing neurons after carbon monoxide poisoning or to the dopamine-blocking or -binding effects of phenothiazine drugs.

The degenerative and other neurologic disorders selected as examples in this chapter share common signs and symptoms because they cause structural or chemical alterations in common locations in the brain. Because their etiologies vary greatly, their treatment and prognosis are quite different, even when initial symptoms seem similar.

## Secondary Disabilities

Secondary disabilities are caused by restrictions or conditions imposed because of the presence or treatment of primary neurologic disability. These secondary conditions may arise from forced inactivity, such as a muscle contracture that occurs in a paralyzed limb. They also may arise from injury; for example, when a paralyzed extremity is not properly supported, its weight may cause subluxation of the associated joint. Most of the secondary disabilities associated with primary neurologic disease are progressive, and may be threatening to function and indeed to life, even if the primary disorder is resolved. Secondary disabilities often are as preventable as they are crippling.

Organic disease of the nervous system usually is long-term and does not always end with recovery. If a person does recover from a neurologic disease, such as neurosyphilis, full function may not be regained, even though the causative agent has been eliminated. Residual primary damage or secondary disabilities may linger or become permanent. Even if recovery is possible or when a disorder such as Guillain-Barré syndrome is self-limiting, it usually takes considerable time for full function to return.

# PARALYZING DEVELOPMENTAL OR CONGENITAL DISORDERS

Developmental disorders occur when neurologic structures fail to develop to full size or mature function, or when they develop abnormally. Their causes usually are not known. Congenital diseases are those present at birth; the classification includes clinically apparent genetic disease and that which occurs during fetal life as a result of infection, anoxia, malnutrition, or some other traumatic or toxic factor.

## Spina Bifida

Spina bifida is a developmental disorder of the vertebral arches. During embryogenesis, the bony arch of the canal fails to close completely. If this is the only defect, it is called *spina bifida occulta* because there are no signs of neurologic deficit to signify its presence. The bony defect is identifiable only by radiography or palpation. The site of the lesion may be marked by dimpling and wisps of hair on the skin surface. The cause of this defect is unknown, although various theories link it with prenatal infection, prenatal drug usage, or heredity.[19]

Unfortunately, spina bifida often is associated with a defect in the closure of the neural tube (Figure 54-1). This can range from a closed but dilated central cord canal *(syringomyelocele)* to a sac protruding through the bony defect that contains meninges *(meningocele)* or, more commonly, elements of the spinal cord *(meningomyelocele)*. These sacs may leak cerebrospinal fluid (CSF) if the skin covering is incomplete. Other defects, such as abnormal neural tissue or a fistula, may be associated with this type of spina bifida. In the occipital area, brain elements may protrude through a defect in the skull; this impairment is referred to as an *encephalocele*.

Spina bifida occulta may occur with no clinical signs or symptoms. It is possible for late signs such as persistent or intermittent eneuresis (the most common symptom), late walking, or even chronic cold feet to be traced to a previously undetected lesion.

Several forms of spina bifida can be diagnosed in utero by amniocentesis and ultrasonography or at birth by the presence of the sac protruding through the defect in the vertebral arch. If the sac is a meningocele, it is possible for the infant to show no signs of neurologic deficit, although hydrocephalus may occur after surgical repair. The meningomyelocele is accompanied by signs of neurologic damage, the extent of which is dependent on the size and level of the lesion and the presence of dysplastic neural tissue. If the defect occurs in the lumbosacral area, flaccid paralysis of the lower limbs and absence of sensation below the level of the lesion usually are present. Sphincter control also is affected in both

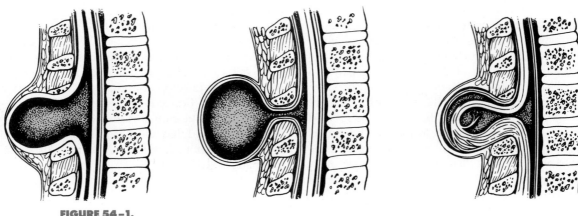

**FIGURE 54–1.**
Types of spina bifida: syringomyelocele, meningocele, and meningomyelocele.

bowel and bladder. These neurologic deficits occur because the defect and abnormal tissue often involve all or most of the lumbosacral spinal cord together with the nerve roots entering and exiting in the lumbosacral area. Alteration in blood supply because of pressure, trauma, or infection also may contribute to the interruption of the reflex arcs in the area. If the tip end of the conus terminalis is intact, some external bowel sphincter control may be present because of an intact reflex arc.[19] The frequency of accompanying mental retardation with severe developmental spinal defects is high.

Prognosis for life and function are excellent with spina bifida occulta and after surgical repair of a meningocele, especially in the absence of hydrocephalus. Surgical repair commonly is undertaken with serious developmental spinal defects to avoid the dangerous complication of ascending meningitis. About 50% of children who survive surgical treatment for meningomyelocele reach adulthood, and some may learn to walk with braces and crutches. The primary disabilities of meningomyelocele may be resolved, but complications result from secondary disabilities, especially immobility.

## Syringomyelia

Syringomyelia refers to the development of a *syrinx*, which is an abnormal cleft or cavity in cord tissue.[14] The cause of primary syringomyelia remains unknown, although considerable attention has been given to its origin as a congenital neural tube defect. Unlike spina bifida, syringomyelia is characterized by the onset of progressive motor symptoms in the adult. Weakness and spastic paralysis as well as alterations in sensory function all may progress steadily or intermittently throughout the remainder of life. These symptoms are similar to those of some spinal cord tumors.

Syringomyelia is considered to be a developmental disorder that involves enlargement of affected segments

of the spinal cord and development of tubular fluid cavities. It may be a developmental defect that involves disruption of CSF flow through the outlets of the fourth ventricle. It is present throughout embryogenesis but does not become symptomatic until the normally microscopic central canal of the spinal cord balloons and forms fluid-filled cavities in the nervous tissue of the cord itself (Figure 54-2). A pathologic cavity caused by retained CSF, called a syrinx, results, thus the name syringomyelia.

Syringomyelia may occur in association with other developmental defects such as spina bifida, Chiari malformation, and hydrocephalus. Secondary syringomyelia may accompany tumors, infections, trauma, bleeding, and infarction in the central nervous system. Signs and symptoms of syrinx formation normally occur sometime after age 30 years, although they may begin at any age. The nature of the clinical signs depends on the level and size of the cavities and which structures are affected. The syrinx typically develops from the center of the cord outward, in the direction of the dorsal gray horns (Figure 54-3). Because pain and temperature fibers cross immediately in the cord and are relayed by the cells in the

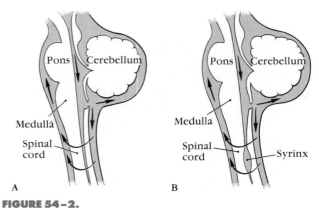

**FIGURE 54–2.**
Syringomyelia. **A.** Normal circulation. **B.** Presence of syrinx in the spinal column.

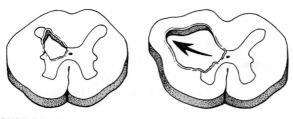

**FIGURE 54–3.**
Development of a syrinx from the center outward into the dorsal gray horns.

dorsal gray horns of the cord, the loss of these sensations with analgesia, thermoanesthesia, and preservation of the touch sensation are early signs of the onset of syringomyelia. Accompanying these early signs are weakness and wasting of hands and arms. If the syrinx spreads anteriorly toward the anterior horn cells, signs of lower motor neuron damage with small-muscle atrophy occur. Signs and symptoms develop asymmetrically at first, but cord compression may become so severe that complete paraplegia results.

The lower cervical and upper thoracic areas of the cord most frequently develop syrinx-related alterations. If the brain stem is affected initially or by extension, it is termed *syringobulbia*. Characteristic symptoms of medullary involvement result from cranial nerve damage, and include weakness of facial and palatal muscles, laryngeal palsy, wasting and weakness of the tongue, loss of pain and temperature sensation, and onset of trigeminal pain. Dizziness may occur. Severe involvement of the medulla oblongata may be lethal.

In primary syringomyelia, the CSF remains normal unless its circulation becomes obstructed. The protein content is high in CSF of syringomyelia associated with tumor growth. The cord enlarges in the areas of syrinx

formation, and signs and symptoms may be suggestive of spinal cord tumor, multiple sclerosis, or amyotrophic lateral sclerosis. Later, manifestations of poorly healed, painless injuries with trophic skin lesions confirm the diagnosis of syringomyelia.

Clinical manifestations may be stationary for years, or slow progression may lead to death from brain stem involvement or from secondary problems such as extensive decubitus ulcers, renal infection, and pneumonia. Symptomatic treatment is aimed at preventing lethal and crippling secondary disabilities. If attempted early in primary syringomyelia, surgical decompression of the medulla and fourth ventricle by removal of the posterior rim of the foramen magnum has yielded promising results in arresting and, occasionally, reversing the sensory losses. Some patients with associated hydrocephalus benefit from ventriculoperitoneal shunting. If the outlets in the fourth ventricle are occluded, they are opened, and the central canal may be aspirated at the time of surgery.[7]

## Hydrocephalus

The word *hydrocephalus* refers to an increased quantity of CSF within the ventricles of the cerebrum. If CSF pressure is normal or only sporadically increased with gradual cortical atrophy, the symptoms begin slowly, and relate to memory and judgment deficits, speech disorders, alterations in gait, some spasticity, incontinence, and the signs of progressive dementia. If the pressure is elevated because of excess formation, faulty circulation, or inadequate reabsorption of CSF, the symptoms are more abrupt in onset and more severe.

The most common cause of hydrocephalus is obstruction to the flow of CSF (Figure 54-4). In the fetus or neonate, the obstruction may result from cerebellar dys-

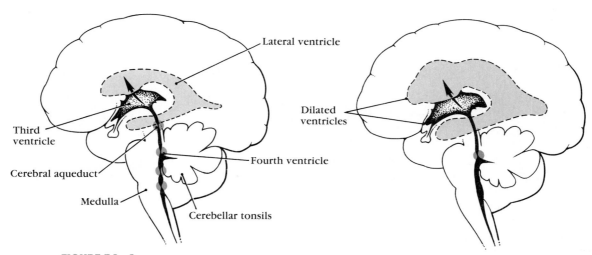

**FIGURE 54–4.**
Schematic representation of areas of possible obstruction to spinal fluid and resulting ventricular enlargement.

plasia, tumor, subarachnoid hemorrhage, or infectious or developmental abnormalities of the cerebellar tonsils, medulla, cerebral aqueduct, or fourth ventricle. In the older person, the obstruction may be due to trauma, infection, or tumor. If the obstruction is within the CSF pathways, the disorder is classified as *noncommunicating* or *obstructive hydrocephalus*. If CSF can gain access to the subarachnoid space and is then not absorbed by the arachnoid villi, it is classified as a *communicating hydrocephalus*. This type of hydrocephalus may be associated with postmeningitic or posthemorrhagic states. Excess formation of CSF is rare, and may be caused by choroid plexus tumors. Noncommunicating hydrocephalus caused by faulty circulation or obstruction results in enlargement of the ventricular system. This eventually leads to signs of increased intracranial pressure in adults and to bulging fontanelles and an enlarged head in infants. The treatment of choice is the removal of the obstruction. Prognosis depends on the cause and severity of the obstruction and on the timing and effectiveness of the treatment.

Clinical manifestations of hydrocephalus depend on the age and rapidity of onset, as well as on the nature and success of the treatment. A newborn infant who exhibits a grossly enlarged head, widely separated cranial sutures, and protruding eyes usually has irreversible signs of prolonged pressure, such as blindness from optic atrophy, paralysis, and mental retardation. In other infants, rapidly increasing head circumference, feeding problems, irritability, delayed motor skills, high-pitched cry, and turned down (setting-sun) eyes are signs of progressive hydrocephalus (Figure 54-5B). Because cerebral expansion is permitted by the open sutures and fontanelles in infancy, classic signs of increasing intracranial pressure, such as headache, vomiting, and altered vital signs, usually are minimal or absent. In older children or adults whose cranial sutures have closed, headache and vomiting often are early signs, and develop with much less trapping of CSF and greater increases in CSF.

Diagnosis is based on clinical observation of head circumference increase in infants and on demonstration of dilated ventricles. Magnetic resonance imaging (MRI) or computed tomography (CT) scan often demonstrates the ventricular dilatation and the cause. In the absence of available MRI or CT scanning, a combination of skull films, angiography, and air studies can identify hydrocephalus.

### Pseudotumor Cerebri

A condition that most frequently occurs in young, obese women, pseudotumor cerebri is related to hydrocephalus and is associated with CSF increases. Intracranial pressure is greatly elevated, usually to 250 to 400 mm $H_2O$, and may be as high as 600 mm $H_2O$. Persons with this benign intracranial hypertension have headache and papilledema. Focal signs and other neurologic deficits usually are absent. Treatment focuses on serial lumbar punctures to drain CSF, to maintain intracranial pressure near normal. In many instances, these persons recover after repeated lumbar punctures have restored the balance of CSF formation and absorption.

### Cranial Malformations

Arrested brain growth is the cause of the cranial malformation called *microcephaly vera*, or small head. Premature suture closure frequently associated with microcephaly results from arrested brain growth and is not a cause of it. This is an inherited defect of the autosomal recessive or sex-linked gene. There is no treatment for the severe mental retardation of microcephaly, which often is accompanied by cerebral palsy or seizure activity.

*Craniostenosis* is early closure and ossification of one or more of the sutures in the skull that occurs before brain growth is arrested. Early recognition and immediate surgery to create artificial sutures are necessary

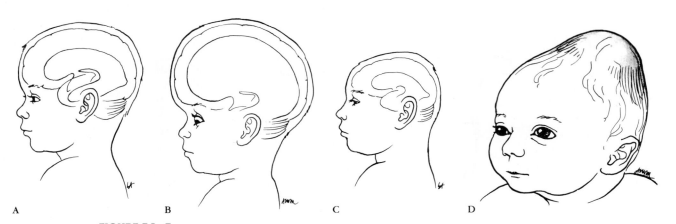

**FIGURE 54–5.**
Some cephalic shapes. **A.** Normal. **B.** Hydrocephalus. **C.** Microcephalus. **D.** Molding. (Source: R. Judge, G. Zuidema, and F. Fitzgerald, *Clinical Diagnosis: A Physiologic Approach.* Boston: Little, Brown, 1982.)

**TABLE 54–1.**
TYPES AND CLINICAL MANIFESTATIONS OF CEREBRAL PALSIES (CP)

| TYPE | PERCENTAGE | CLINICAL MANIFESTATIONS |
|---|---|---|
| Spastic, Paralytic | | |
| Diplegia | 50 | Spasticity predominates, especially in the legs. Mental retardation occurs only in a small percent. Walking is delayed and the gait is stiff and awkward, often with crossing of the legs, called scissors gait. Lower legs often are splayed outward and feet flexed. Speech may be markedly impaired or unaffected. Sphincter control is usually attained, though delayed. |
| Quadriplegia | 30 | Spasticity of all four extremities is common. Often associated with marked retardation. Children are nonambulatory and attain little or no speech or sphincter control. |
| Hemiplegia | 10 | Spasticity and control affects one side of the body. The clinical picture varies according to associated mental retardation. Two-thirds to three-fourths have normal intelligence. Seizures are common with one-third. |
| Dyskinetic CP Ataxic CP | 10 | Dyskinetic CP exhibits elements of extrapyramidal system dysfunction. Abnormal movements (choreoathetotic) may predominate, increase or decrease as the child grows older. Mental retardation is frequent. Ataxic CP indicates cerebellar damage and ataxic gait, and incoordination is characteristic. Either dyskinetic or ataxic CP may be associated with other forms and is difficult to clearly distinguish. When it is clearly identified, it is classified as mixed CP. Mixed CP may refer to any combination of the clinical manifestations. |

to decompress the brain and to limit the extent of neurologic damage caused by increasing intracranial pressure. If treatment is absent or delayed, this pressure can cause exophthalmos, optic atrophy, seizures, and mental retardation.

## Cerebral Palsy

The term *cerebral palsy* (CP) includes a wide variety of nonprogressive brain disorders that occur during intrauterine life, during delivery, or during early infancy. CP, by definition, is a syndrome of motor disabilities, although it may be accompanied by mental retardation or seizure disorders, or both. Causes are many, and include cerebral developmental disorders such as microcephaly, intracranial hemorrhage, and cerebral anoxia, and poisoning by toxins such as excessive bilirubin in the blood (kernicterus). Prenatal factors include infection with rubella, nutritional deficiency, and blood factor incompatibility. Asphyxia may produce CP prenatally or during labor or delivery. Intrapartum production of CP also may be related to anesthesia or various metabolic disturbances. Postpartum development of CP is relatively uncommon but may develop after central nervous system infections, asphyxia, or head trauma.[5]

Clinical manifestations of CP depend on the areas of the brain that sustain damage. Three main groups of CP

have been described according to the dominant signs (Table 54-1). The *paralytic cerebral palsies* are the result of damage to the cortical motor cells and the pyramidal tracts in the brain. These typically are manifested as spastic diplegias, quadriplegias, or hemiplegias. The *dyskinetic cerebral palsies* are caused by damage to the extrapyramidal system, and are characterized by abnormal movements of athetoid, choreiform, or dystonic nature (see p. 1096). The *ataxic cerebral palsies* indicate cerebellar damage, and typically involve incoordination and gait disturbances. Mixed CP may combine any of the these.

Symptoms are present and nonprogressive from birth or early infancy, and diagnosis usually is made early in the preschool years. Treatment is aimed at preventing crippling secondary disabilities and providing special education to ensure the greatest possible function.

## DISORDERS CHARACTERIZED BY PROGRESSIVE WEAKNESS OR PARALYSIS

Progressively paralyzing neurologic disorders affect the pyramidal system of the brain or cord, or the final common pathway between the cord and the muscle. They may result from dietary deficiencies, autoimmune disorders, genetic defects, and infectious diseases, or they may be idiopathic. If the reflex arc remains intact, the usual sign is a spastic paresis or paralysis with normal or hyperactive reflexes. If the lower motor neuron or final common pathway is interrupted, the result is flaccid paralysis with diminished or absent reflexes. If the damage is spread throughout the motor system, as in amyotrophic lateral sclerosis, spasticity is present until the final common pathway is interrupted, when characteristic flaccidity and atrophic wasting of muscles predominate. Prognosis and treatment depend on the nature of the disease and the availability and use of treatment.

## Myasthenia Gravis

Myasthenia gravis (MG) is a chronic disease that destroys the acetylcholine (ACh) receptors of the neuromuscular junction. The result of this destruction is impairment of nerve impulse passage (Figure 54-6).[6] MG most commonly occurs in young adults, and progresses with remissions and exacerbations. It is characterized by activity-induced abnormal muscle fatigability. The fatigue results in typical drooping of eyelids (ptosis) and jaw, nasal voice, slurred speech, and weakness of the proximal extremities; all symptoms worsen during the day but improve with rest or with the use of anticholinesterase drugs, such as neostigmine. Muscle fibers eventually may degenerate, and weakness, especially of the muscles of the head, neck, trunk, and limbs, may become irreversible. Hyperplasia of the thymus frequently is associated, and about 12% of persons with MG have a thymoma (benign thymic tumor). Reflexes may remain normal or reflect fatigue, decreasing with each repeated test. There appears to be no sensory alteration.

Several primary muscle disorders cause clinically similar fatigue in the muscles, but only MG responds to anticholinesterase drugs. MG involves progressive failure of impulse conduction at the neuromuscular junction. It is an autoimmune disease, with cellular and humoral factors that contribute to the disease. The triggering mechanism for the autoimmune response remains elusive. Circulating ACh-receptor antibodies have been identified that link themselves to receptor sites in the voluntary muscles, damaging and blocking the receptors. In some cases, aggregates of lymphocytes are present in the muscles and other organs. Postsynaptic membrane abnormalities result in muscles becoming less responsive to nerve impulses. ACh is less effective in producing

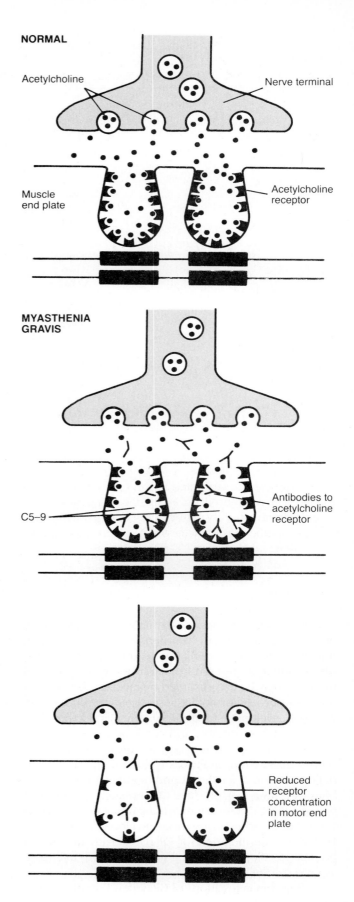

**FIGURE 54-6.**

A schematic representation of the neuromuscular junction in myasthenia gravis showing degradation of acetylcholine receptors by specific antibodies and complement. (Source: R. Cotran, V. Kumar, S. Robbins, *Robbins' Pathologic Basis of Disease* [4th ed.]. Philadelphia: W.B. Saunders, 1989.)

the desired depolarization in the affected muscles, and muscle contractions become le..s effective with each rapidly succeeding nerve impulse.

The observed relation between MG and disorders of the thyroid, such as thyroiditis and thyrotoxicosis, is believed to be due to a common disturbance of the immune system, expressed in different ways. The nature of these disturbances is not fully understood, nor is their relation clear. Many experts postulate that genetic characteristics may constitute risk factors for autoimmune disorders such as MG, thyroiditis, and even diabetes mellitus.[2]

During the early active stage of MG, although the characteristic remissions and exacerbations are occurring and before muscle atrophy sets in, some patients may respond well to surgical removal of the thymus. Many believe that early thymectomy may decrease the level of autoimmune activity before much permanent damage is sustained by the ACh-receptor sites in the voluntary muscles. Plasmapheresis is another method of treatment aimed at removing anti—ACh-receptor antibodies from the blood to decrease the autoimmune activity.[2] Steroids usually are given to suppress the production of antibodies. Other immunosuppressive drugs, such as azathioprine, have been beneficial in some cases. Anticholinesterase drugs are administered to prevent the breakdown of the ACh at the myoneural junction. Too much anticholinesterase drug activity may produce skeletal muscle weakness that resembles the myasthenic defect. Additional clinical signs include nausea, vomiting, gastrointestinal irritability, bradycardia, diarrhea, pallor, miosis, and excessive salivation. This phenomenon is called *cholinergic crisis* or *depolarization block.*[1] It is hard to differentiate clinically between a cholinergic crisis and a myasthenic crisis, or disease exacerbation. Most persons who are in a crisis state are treated for cholinergic crisis, withdrawn from the anticholinesterase drugs, and maintained on assisted respiration until the type of crisis can be identified.

The course of MG is variable. Some people do not develop any symptoms other than the initial ocular muscle fatigue and weakness. Others who exhibit more generalized symptoms respond well to standard treatment for years. A small percentage suffer the acute, fulminating disease accompanied by muscle atrophy with poor response to all treatment. Death from MG usually occurs within the first 5 to 10 years of onset, when the disease is most acute. Lethal crises do not usually occur late in the disease, and the damage sustained tends to remain constant or to be compensated for by other muscles. Death that occurs after many years usually is due to the secondary problem of immobility, which leads to pneumonia.

Myasthenic mothers may pass the antibodies to their infants through the placenta. These infants may experience spontaneous recovery from the myasthenia symptoms within 1 to 3 months, or they may persist with the disease for their lifetime.

## Subacute Combined Degeneration of the Cord

Vitamin $B_{12}$ deficiency, which usually occurs as part of pernicious anemia (see Chap. 19), can lead to degeneration of the white matter in the lateral and posterior spinal cord, as well as peripheral polyneuropathy and slight cerebral atrophy. Neurologic manifestations begin gradually and usually are accompanied by the classic megaloblastic anemia. Unusual sensations such as tingling, numbness, and pain often are the first symptoms of neurologic degeneration. These paresthesias are followed by motor signs of weakness and incoordination. The paresthesias and motor signs both tend to begin in the lower limbs and move to the upper limbs and trunk as the disease spreads up the posterior and lateral cord. With progressive and untreated degeneration of the cord, sensory ataxia and either spastic paralysis with hyperactive reflexes or flaccid paralysis with absent reflexes may occur in all four limbs, with the most pronounced symptoms in the lower limbs. If degeneration is confined to the posterior columns, incoordination is predominant. If it is more lateral, weakness and paralysis are most characteristic. The nature of the paralysis is influenced by the presence or absence of peripheral neuropathy and the status of the reflex arc. In addition to these motor signs, persons may suffer optic atrophy or nystagmus if the second or third cranial nerve is affected. The other cranial nerves seldom are affected. Cerebral atrophy may result in impaired memory, confusion, paranoid behavior, irritability, and depression.

The damaged peripheral nerves eventually regenerate, with improvement in sensory symptoms, coordination, and reflexes, but spasticity and signs of cerebral atrophy are not likely to disappear, since central nervous system damage is not reversible. Early diagnosis is important because the condition is treatable and reversible if symptoms have been present for only a short duration.

Clinically similar disorders, such as neurosyphilis and multiple sclerosis, must be ruled out by gastric acid evaluation, blood tests for megaloblastic anemia, and bone marrow evaluation for abnormalities of red cells. Serum $B_{12}$ may be evaluated or tests may be made of vitamin $B_{12}$ absorption using radioactive vitamin $B_{12}$.

## Guillain-Barré Syndrome

An acute, frequently postinfectious polyneuritis, Guillain-Barré syndrome may be due to an allergic response or to some type of hypersensitivity reaction. The specific triggering mechanism for this disturbance in the immune response remains unknown, but the lymphocytes become sensitized and destroy myelin.[14] The onset usually occurs a few days or weeks after a febrile illness, vaccination, injury, or surgery. Guillain-Barré syndrome has no predilection for age-group, sex, or race, and when an infectious cause—most often respiratory or gastrointestinal—can be demonstrated, it usually is viral. It also has occurred after immunizations.

Demyelination and degeneration of the myelin sheath and axon occur in the segmental peripheral nerves and the anterior and posterior spinal nerve roots. Cranial nerve involvement often is observed. Lymphocytes and macrophages infiltrate the myelin sheath initially, and later, if disease progression continues, the axon is involved.[6] Inflammation, edema, and damaged nerves result in both sensory and motor dysfunction.

Initial clinical symptoms are general bilateral weakness, first manifested by difficulty in walking. These symptoms become progressive and accompanied by paresthesias and, possibly, pain in the back. The symptoms progress in an ascending manner to involve the muscles of the trunk, upper extremities, and cranial nerves. Complete flaccid paralysis may or may not occur. Maximum manifestations of the disease occur in about 3 weeks, although the rate of spread varies. In severe cases, total paralysis develops rapidly, and serious respiratory involvement requires artificial ventilation. The sensory involvement usually is less profound than the motor involvement. Proprioception and vibratory sense are the most commonly observed sensory deficits, but deficits in light touch, pinprick, muscle sensitivity, and temperature sensations may occur.

Variant autonomic dysfunctions may occur: postural hypotension, tachycardia, arrhythmias, diaphoresis, and other manifestations. Reflexes normally are diminished or lost, but occasionally remain normal, even with severe muscle weakness. When the onset of flaccid paralysis is sudden and symmetric, and when it is accompanied by sensory changes, diagnosis of Guillain-Barré syndrome can be made by clinical observation and history alone. Muscle atrophy is not common but may result when axon loss is severe. Electrodiagnostic studies show slowing of nerve conduction in most affected persons. CSF protein level becomes markedly elevated after the first few days of illness, whereas the cell count remains negative (albuminocytologic dissociation).[6]

When death occurs, it usually is due to respiratory arrest or pneumonia. For survivors of respiratory problems, the prognosis for life and for eventual recovery of function is good. Eighty-five percent make a complete recovery in 4 to 6 months, but others may have severe residual disabilities. The rate of recovery depends on the extent of neural and axonal regeneration required. Treatment with steroids, adrenocorticotropic hormone, or other immunosuppressant drugs may or may not be beneficial in altering the course of the disease.

## Multiple Sclerosis

Multiple sclerosis (MS) is a relatively common chronic and progressive inflammatory, demyelinating disease of the central nervous system. It results in diverse manifestations of neurologic alteration. Its basic cause or causes are unknown, but it probably is an autoimmune disorder influenced by a genetic susceptibility. Although no single virus has been incriminated in its causation, MS has been associated with human leukocyte antigens (HLA), particularly HLA-B7 and HLA DW2.[3] This suggests the possibility that a latent viral infection precipitates the disease. Dietary deficiencies and acute viral infections also have been studied as causative agents.[13] Stress and trauma seem to play a role in precipitating the onset of MS or in exacerbating the symptoms. MS is most common in colder climates, and its onset usually is between ages 20 and 40 years. Women have a higher incidence than men.[6] The incidence of MS is much higher in people of European origin, with a much lower incidence among Orientals, Africans, and native Americans.[3,6]

The disease normally begins rather suddenly with the occurrence of a set of focal symptoms of visual disturbance or of motor dysfunction in one or two limbs. The causative lesion or plaque is present predominantly in the white matter of the central nervous system, and the myelin sheaths that normally act as insulation around nerve fibers are lost. Loss of myelin slows, blocks, or distorts transmission of nerve impulses. During the course of the disease, some of the myelinated fibers may regenerate and associated symptoms disappear. Gliosis eventually occurs in the lesions, and scar tissue replaces myelin and may replace the axis cylinders themselves. From this gliosis comes the term *sclerosis,* meaning induration or scarring. Oligodendrocytes disappear and astrocytes proliferate.

Initial symptoms may be transient, and frequently are followed by complete, or nearly complete, recovery as the myelin is replaced. Periods of remission are common. Later alterations become permanent, with remissions and exacerbations limited to new symptoms superimposed on a baseline of disability. This permanence in symptoms is due to eventual disruption and destruction of the nerve cells themselves, even though this is initially a disease of the myelin sheath rather than of the cells.[3] If the lesions are predominantly in the pyramidal tracts of the cerebrum or spinal cord, the symptoms are motor. If they affect the lateral spinothalamic or posterior tracts of the cord, sensory changes are noted. Weakness or spastic paralysis of the limbs and sphincters with hyperactive reflexes is common. Sexual dysfunction, with impotence in men and alteration in vaginal sensations in women, is a common and disturbing aspect of sensorimotor changes. Paresthesias such as pain, numbness, and tingling may be noted in the limbs or the face. Emotional changes may range from emotional lability to sustained euphoria or severe depression.[3]

Brain stem lesions often contribute to emotional lability and also produce symptoms of cranial nerve injury. The optic, oculomotor, trochlear, and abducens nerves and the vestibular branch of the auditory nerve are especially common sites of damage. Visual signs and symptoms range from nystagmus to diplopia to visual dimness to patchy or complete blindness. Pupillary abnormalities may be noted. Dizziness may be mild, or it may be severe and associated with nausea and vomiting. Speech may be difficult because of spastic weakness of facial and speech muscles. Dysphagia makes eating difficult, with increased danger of aspiration. Cerebellar lesions also affect speech, producing slurred, uncoordinated articulation. Other signs such as intention tremor of the hands, head tremor, and staggering gait are indicative of cerebellar lesions.

Although early clinical manifestations may be limited to effects of alteration in the cerebellar area, the brain stem, or the cerebrum, late MS usually affects all parts of the central nervous system. The classic triad of Charcot described in 1868, which occurs late in the disease, includes nystagmus, intention tremor, and speech disorders.[4] Spastic paraplegia, incontinence, and extreme emotional lability also are typical of the late stages of MS.

The diagnosis is based on clinical features, observing the pattern of remission and exacerbation of symptoms, and ruling out other diseases such as subacute combined degeneration of the cord (see p. 1093). Studies of antibodies in the blood or CSF often show gamma globulin abnormalities in those with established MS. The most consistent CSF finding is the presence of oligoclonal bands of IgG.[13] These bands are immunoglobulins directed against the various antigens of the measles virus, but no specific antigen has been isolated in MS.[6] Other changes in the CSF are inconsistent and nonspecific.

The prognosis varies from progression to death in less than 6 months (acute MS) to a benign course for more than 20 years without shortening or altering productive life. Fulminant cases that are fatal within weeks to months show intense inflammatory response in the lesions.[3] Even when the person survives to old age, the last years often are spent as a spastic paraplegic, with visual disorders, incontinence, dysarthria, and lack of emotional control. Death often is due to secondary disorders, such as pneumonia or septic decubitus ulcers.

Treatment of MS usually is symptomatic and focused on preventing complications. Special high-vitamin, low-fat diets, steroids, and core-cooling of the body have failed to consistently influence the course of the disease. Immunosuppression using plasma exchange, steroids, azathioprine, and cyclophosphamide has provided encouraging results.[10]

## Amyotrophic Lateral Sclerosis

Amyotrophic lateral sclerosis (ALS, or progressive muscle atrophy) is another primary neurologic disease that affects motor function and results in alterations of gait and paralysis. It is a noninflammatory disease of the upper and lower motor neurons, with demyelination secondary to axon degeneration. Unlike MS, which classically is characterized by remissions and exacerbations, ALS usually steadily progresses to death within 2 to 6 years of diagnosis.[6] Premature aging of nerve cells caused by some environmental or genetic factor, nutritional deficiencies, heavy-metal poisoning, an autoimmune response, metabolic defects, and even a dormant virus have all been identified as possible causes or contributors to ALS.[18]

Loss of the motor cells in the cerebral cortex can result in signs of upper motor neuron damage, with weakness or spastic paralysis and hyperactive reflexes. This is especially likely to occur in the lower limbs. Damage to cranial nerves in the medulla produces signs of *bulbar palsy*, either of the spastic or flaccid type. Bulbar palsy refers to weakness or paralysis of the muscles supplied by the motor cranial nerves. Commonly, upper and lower motor neuron damage are mixed in ALS. Lower motor signs predominate in the upper extremities and upper motor signs predominate in the lower extremities. When reflexes are interrupted, muscles atrophy secondary to denervation and loss of muscle tone. In these areas, diminished reflexes or flaccid paralysis occurs. Muscle atrophy often is present in the upper limbs and tongue.

Degeneration may occur anywhere within the pyramidal system, in the anterior motor cells of the spinal cord, or in the ventral nerve roots. It is most severe in the cervical cord.[14] It characteristically does not affect peripheral nerves. The muscle fasciculations or twitching frequently seen in the upper limbs or tongue are thought to be caused by accumulating excessive neurotransmitter at the myoneural junction rather than by abnormal spontaneous discharges of degenerating nerve cells.[9]

The onset of ALS usually occurs after age 50, with 2:1 occurrence in men over women. One common early sign may be muscle fasciculations of the tongue when the brain stem is involved. Fasciculations also may be seen in the hands or upper limbs, and are small local muscle contractions that occur when a muscle is tapped or moved passively. Whenever the brain stem is affected, slurred speech and weakness of the palate and facial muscles may occur. Reflexes may be normal, hyperactive, or diminished, depending on whether there is lower motor neuron damage. If lower motor neuron damage is present, muscle wasting occurs in the tongue or other muscles. Swallowing eventually is affected, and speech may become unintelligible.

Weakness and clumsiness are first noted in the distal portions of the upper limbs, and wasting of the muscles of the hand is characteristic. Sexual dysfunction, such as impotence, is an early sign; bowel and bladder sphincters usually are not affected until late in the disease. Lower-extremity function is retained longer than upper-extremity function, but as the disease progresses, the latter also is lost. Characteristically, there is no sensory alteration in ALS. Paralysis of the trunk and respiratory muscles occurs late in the course of the disease if bulbar palsy does not cause death first. Death often is due to pneumonia or respiratory failure.[14]

Diagnosis is based on characteristic clinical signs, such as upper limb weakness, wasting of hand muscles, and muscle fasciculations. Disorders such as syringomyelia, cord tumors, and neurosyphilis may cause similar clinical signs, but they usually have pain and sensory changes associated with them. The absence of muscle atrophy and lack of muscle response to edrophonium hydrochloride rule out a diagnosis of MG. Biopsy of muscle and electromyography show denervation atrophy in ALS.

Prognosis is worst when the brain stem is affected first. Life expectancy is best when the degeneration remains confined to the lower motor neurons of the middle and lower spinal cord. Affected persons seldom survive longer than 10 years after onset, but death can occur within a year. Treatment is symptomatic, with no beneficial effects from antiinflammatory and immunosuppressive drugs.

## DISORDERS CHARACTERIZED BY ABNORMAL MOVEMENTS

Abnormal movements often indicate alterations in the extrapyramidal motor system. This system is not clearly understood, so that the relation of the pathology and structural alterations with the clinical manifestations is not clear. Abnormal movements often result from alterations, and reflect a disturbance in the balance between the excitatory and inhibitory neurotransmitters in the basal ganglia. The neurotransmitters involved apparently are dopamine, ACh, and gamma-aminobutyric acid (GABA). The basal ganglia most often affected are the four that make up the corpus striatum: caudate, putamen, globus pallidus, and claustrum. In some disorders, such as early parkinsonism, conscious effort can temporarily suppress these movements, but typically they return when the person relaxes or is distracted.

The abnormal movements that result are of different types but may be painful or incapacitating. Abnormal movements range from the fine, rhythmic quivering of tremor to the violent, irregular jerking or twisting movements of *ballismus*. *Dyskinesias*, or alterations in voluntary muscle movement, and *dystonias*, or alterations in muscle tone (such as rigidity), are both classified as abnormalities of movement. *Fixed* or *intermittent muscle spasms*, such as are characteristic of torticollis, may be included unless they are due to muscle rather than nerve damage. *Choreas* are irregular muscle twitchings that may become so severe that they contribute to death from exhaustion. *Athetosis*, or athetoid movements, is slow, repeated, purposeless muscle movements that may affect the digits only or the entire body.

There are many causes of extrapyramidal dysfunction. Cerebral anoxia or trauma in utero or during delivery may produce an athetoid cerebral palsy, spastic cerebral palsy, or both. The characteristic tremors of parkinsonism may be produced by therapy with the major tranquilizers of the phenothiazine family or by carbon monoxide poisoning. The exhausting muscle twitchings of chorea may be due to a genetic defect or an infectious disease. As with all neurologic disorders, abnormal movements give more clues about which structures are damaged than about what has damaged them. Therefore, a complete physical examination and a thorough family history may be more important than laboratory test results in identifying the source of the problem.

## Parkinson's Disease

Parkinson's disease, also known as paralysis agitans, is a common, chronic degenerative disease of the elderly population. This disease occurs between ages 50 and 80, with onset of symptoms most often observed around age 60. It is a disorder of the basal ganglia, specifically, loss of pigmented cells in the substantia nigra.[4]

Dopamine is one of the chemical transmitters in the brain that is stored in the cells of the basal ganglia. It is depleted in Parkinson's disease, particularly in the substantia nigra and corpus striatum. It has been suggested that 80% depletion of dopamine has occurred before clinical signs of parkinsonism become evident.[15] Dopamine-containing neurons project to the corpus striatum through fibers called the nigrostriatal pathway. In the corpus striatum, dopamine, together with ACh, is important in controlling complex movements. Dopamine acts as an inhibitory transmitter and ACh acts as an excitatory transmitter. Coordinated voluntary motor activity occurs as a result of a balance between the excitatory cholinergic and inhibitory dopaminergic secretions. With dopamine depletion in Parkinson's disease, the classic triad of Parkinson's appears: tremors, rigidity, and bradykinesia (slow movement).

The clinical signs of Parkinson's disease apparently arise from progressive degeneration of the pigmented cells of the substantia nigra (Figure 54-7).[6] The underlying cause of this cellular destruction is unknown. The dopaminergic cells synthesize and secrete the neurotransmitter dopamine, and their degeneration results in a subsequent decrease of dopamine transmitted to the corpus striatum. As a result, the striatal cells, under the predominance of ACh, initiate action potentials more rapidly because the counterbalance of dopamine is decreased or absent. If the dopamine fibers projecting to the corpus striatum degenerate, permanent or progressive muscle rigidity or the tremors of parkinsonism result. If the dopamine in the corpus striatum is blocked or bound temporarily by a drug such as chlorpromazine, the typically reversible rigidity or tremors of the parkinsonian syndrome occur.

In addition to tremors, rigidity, and bradykinesia, Parkinson's disease is characterized by a masklike facial ex-

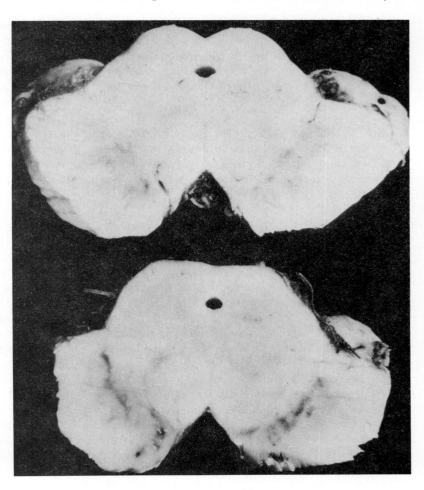

**FIGURE 54-7.**
Brainstem in parkinsonism. Pigmentation is decreased in the substantia nigra as compared with normal (below). (F. Miller, *Peery and Miller's Pathology* [3rd ed.]. Boston: Little, Brown, 1978.)

pression and infrequent blinking caused by diminished automatic movements. Speech is quiet and monotonous. Cognitive and perceptual abilities reflect deterioration in memory and problem-solving in many persons. Spontaneous, automatic movements, such as swinging the arms when walking, also diminish and cease. The body posture becomes stooped, with apparent flexion of the limbs. The characteristic gait progresses with small, shuffling steps that pick up speed as the person travels. Increasing muscle rigidity in both extensor and flexor muscles may cause jerky or spastic movements. Rather than losing voluntary function, the person finds it increasingly difficult to initiate voluntary acts (akinesia), and the actions tend to be slow and clumsy.

The tremors of parkinsonism commonly occur in the hands initially and then progress to involve the ankles, head, or mouth. The tremors are most prominent during rest. They can be suppressed with conscious effort for brief periods and usually disappear with sleep. If the index finger and thumb are both involved, the tremors may be described as "pill-rolling." Intention tremors, which refer to tremors that occur during the performance of a precise movement, also can occur. Both resting and intention tremors worsen under emotional stress, although extreme provocation may result in the quick,

efficient performance of complex motor functions. Other symptoms, such as heat intolerance, excessive salivation, diaphoresis, and urinary incontinence, are due to autonomic nervous system dysfunction. Intellectual deterioration and dementia are common when Parkinson's disease becomes advanced.[4]

If the symptoms of parkinsonism are due to dopamine binding or blocking by drugs such as chlorpromazine, they usually disappear when the drug is withdrawn or decreased. If the symptoms are due to a discrete episode of cerebral anoxia or trauma, such as carbon monoxide poisoning or head injury, they may stabilize. Most cases are characterized by progressive disability until death occurs from secondary problems such as pneumonia in 10 or more years after onset of the disease. Diagnosis is based on signs and symptoms and on ruling out other diseases associated with muscle rigidity or tremors, such as multiple sclerosis and neurosyphilis.[12]

## Drug-Induced Dyskinesias and Dystonias

The major tranquilizers have many effects on the extrapyramidal nervous system. Besides the drug-induced parkinsonian syndrome, which usually occurs early in therapy, there may be a number of other effects, some of which are reversible and some permanent. Dyskinesias are rhythmic, involuntary movements such as chewing or smacking. Dystonias are painful, distorted movements of the face, head, or limbs. Variation exists in severity of dystonias.

Both dyskinesias and dystonias can occur alone or in association with more typically parkinsonian symptoms soon after major tranquilizer therapy is begun. They usually respond well to anticholinergic therapy, and are probably caused by a relative increase in cholinergic activity in the presence of a sudden reduction in the level of dopamine in the basal ganglia. The anticholinergic therapy seems temporarily to restore the balance.[16] *Akathisia*, or restlessness in the muscles, is more difficult to treat, and may require dosage reduction or a change in drugs.[8]

Dyskinesias and dystonias also may occur during levodopa therapy. They usually disappear as the drug is decreased. Unfortunately these symptoms may appear before the tremors of parkinsonism are under control, which means that if the dosage of levodopa is increased enough to control the tremors, the dyskinesias or dystonias may become intolerable. If the dosage is decreased to eliminate the dystonias, the tremors may become much worse.

When dyskinesias occur late in a tranquilizer therapy or after the drug has been discontinued (tardive dyskinesias), they may be evidence of permanent, irreversible change in the extrapyramidal nervous system. This change may be in the dopamine receptors themselves. Tardive dyskinesias do not respond well to anticholinergic therapy, as do early dyskinesias, although they also seem to be due to a disturbed balance in the brain between ACh and dopamine.[16]

## Torticollis

Torticollis, or wryneck, is an intermittent or sustained dystonic contraction of the cervical muscles on one side of the neck caused by hysteria, drug therapy, or organic neurologic disease. It may occur as one of the painful dystonias in early phenothiazine therapy or, rarely, it may accompany primary parkinsonism. When it occurs in association with primary or secondary parkinsonism, it may be due to a relative increase in cholinergic activity in the brain associated with a striatal dopamine deficiency.[11]

The angle of head rotation depends on which muscles are affected; the affected muscles often hypertrophy in response to the constant or frequent powerful muscle contractions. The muscles most commonly involved are the scalene, sternocleidomastoid, and trapezius. The spasm may occur suddenly and painfully, which is characteristic of the drug-induced dystonias and hysteria. The contraction also can occur slowly. Primary muscle fibrosis after trauma and abnormalities of the cervical spine must be ruled out as the cause of this disorder. If major tranquilizers are being used, reduction in dose or anticholinergic therapy may prove useful. Psychotherapy or relaxation therapy may be helpful for hysterical torticollis. Unfortunately if the cause is a lesion in the corpus striatum, the prognosis for cure is poor.[20]

In severe cases, the only successful treatment is to transect the upper anterior cervical roots and spinal accessory nerves.

## Huntington's Chorea

Huntington's chorea is an inherited autosomal dominant disorder characterized by a progressive degeneration of the cerebral cortex as well as of the basal ganglia, particularly the caudate nucleus and putamen. In addition to the dramatic choreiform movements for which it is named, there is progressive deterioration of higher intellectual functions, such as memory and judgment, to the point of severe dementia and death.

In Huntington's chorea, the neurotransmitter GABA is markedly reduced in the degenerating areas of the brain. ACh also seems to be reduced, resulting in an imbalance among the three transmitters—GABA, ACh, and dopamine. When dopamine predominates, chorea results, indicating heightened dopamine sensitivity of the striated receptors.[17] When chorea is the major motor symptom, degenerative lesions are especially common in the caudate. In those occasional persons in whom rigidity and tremors predominate, lesions seem to be more likely in the putamen. In many cases of Huntington's chorea, lesions are common throughout the corpus striatum and in the thalamus as well.[20] As is usual with extrapyramidal disorders, the full significance of these lesions is not totally understood.

It is believed that GABA is an inhibitory transmitter and that the neurons that degenerate in the corpus striatum are inhibitory neurons.[11] As a result, increasingly violent choreiform movements begin to occur in the face, neck, and arms during middle age, and may be the first signs of neurologic disease. In addition to the chorea or, less commonly, widespread muscle rigidity and tremors, dementia develops that is characterized by impulsiveness, paranoia, neurosis, emotional outbursts, loss of judgment and memory, irritability or apathy, delusions or hallucinations, and suicidal tendencies. The dementia seems to result from atrophy of the cerebral cortex, especially over the frontal and parietal lobes.[20]

When a family history of Huntington's chorea exists, diagnosis is made by this history and confirming physical examination. With a negative family history, diseases such as neurosyphilis must be ruled out. Huntington's chorea normally progresses to death from pneumonia or heart failure in 10 to 20 years. No treatment is known to have an effect on the progression of the disease. Drugs that stimulate GABA and ACh synthesis have proved ineffective in treatment of this disease.

## DISORDERS CHARACTERIZED BY MEMORY AND JUDGMENT DEFICITS

Dementia refers to an organically caused syndrome of impaired intellectual functions. There is widespread deterioration in the cerebral cortex, especially in the frontal lobes. Characteristically, decreasing quality of judgment, loss of abstract thinking and reasoning, and diminished memory are accompanied by emotional changes ranging from apathy to lability.

There are many causes of dementia, but there is no theory for the etiology or pathophysiology for most of these diseases.[4] The examples presented here have been selected because dementia is the prime symptom and demonstrates similarity between vascular, infectious, and other types of lesions. No cure exists, but the pathologic process may be arrested with subsequent therapy for residual problems.

### Atherosclerotic Dementia

Cerebral atherosclerosis may contribute to the development of transient ischemic attacks or cerebrovascular accidents of a focal nature (see Chap. 50). Cerebral atherosclerosis also can produce the symptoms of dementia secondary to diffuse, small cerebral infarctions and widespread cerebral anoxia. About 15% to 20% of dementias are attributed to cerebral atherosclerosis.[16] The term *senile dementia* may be used for the results of diffuse cerebral atherosclerosis; it usually refers to a condition of decreasing intellectual capability with increasing disorientation and emotional lability beginning in the aged person. The disorder most frequently seems to be due to a decreasing blood supply and cerebral anoxia resulting in cortical degeneration. Sensory deprivation and overmedication in the institutionalized elderly may be contributing factors to the progression of senile dementia.

### Alzheimer's Disease

A common, progressive cerebral degeneration, Alzheimer's disease begins to be symptomatic between ages 50 and 65.[6] The causative basis for Alzheimer's disease remains unknown. Much research has been conducted in an attempt to better understand this devastating disease. Several models have been proposed as basis for the disease, including decreased ACh, abnormal glutamate system, genetics, abnormal proteins, infectious agents, toxins, and inadequate blood flow.[21] Future research may elucidate a cause of and appropriate therapy for this condition.

Pathologic changes include cortical degeneration that is most marked in frontal, temporal, and parietal lobes. Extensive convolutional atrophy of the brain with enlargement of the ventricular system is seen.[4] Characteristic degeneration includes a decrease in neurons most pronounced in regions of the brain that are responsible for cognition, memory, and other thought processes. Neurons accumulate as characteristic fiberlike strands, known as *neurofibrillary tangles*. The blood vessels contain and are surrounded by amorphous aggregates of protein. In addition, deposits of cellular debris and amyloid (neuritic plaques) are present throughout the brain. Finally, there is marked reduction in the production of neurotransmitters, particularly ACh.[20]

Early symptoms are insidious, and include loss of memory, carelessness about personal appearance, emotional disturbances that progress to complete disorientation, severe deterioration in speech, incontinence, and stereotyped, repetitive movements. Depression is common as the person recognizes the cognitive decline that is occurring. Progression to severe dementia is relentless and occurs over a period of 5 to 10 years, although the rate of progression varies. Terminally, the person loses all cognitive ability and cannot perceive, think, speak, or move.[15] Death results from secondary causes, such as septic decubitus ulcers, dehydration, and pneumonia. Diagnosis of Alzheimer's disease usually is made after other conditions that can cause dementia have been ruled out. No treatment seems to have a significant effect on the course of the disease.

### Pick's Disease

Pick's disease, a degenerative neurologic disease of the fourth and fifth decades, is thought to be passed on by an autosomal dominant gene. It affects women more than men and may occur in families.[4] The clinical picture is similar to that of Alzheimer's disease. Degeneration occurs, with atrophy of the frontal and temporal lobes. The first three cortical layers are most severely involved, and the gyri are dramatically atrophied so as to give this area of the brain the appearance of a dried walnut. The unaffected cells frequently swell, and contain cytoplasmic filamentous inclusions known as *Pick bodies*.[4]

The initial signs and symptoms reflect personality changes that, unlike Alzheimer's disease and Huntington's chorea, elude the person's awareness. The behavioral deterioration is evidenced by disinterest in surroundings, forgetfulness, confusion, cognitive sluggishness, and apathy and dementia. As the disease progresses, language deteriorates to echolalia (parrotlike repetition of words) and stereotyped words and phrases to incomprehensible jargon and, finally, to mutism. Motor deterioration begins with gait disturbances, weakness, and rigidity and progresses to flexion contractions and paraplegia.

There is no known effective treatment of Pick's disease. Supportive and symptomatic treatment is the mainstay of care. Death occurs after a 2- to 10-year course with the disease.[4]

## Neurosyphilis

Neurosyphilis seldom is seen, except in primitive cultures.[6] It is thought that the causative spirochete, *Treponema pallidum*, reaches the nervous system during the second stage of a syphilitic infection, although neurologic symptoms may not occur for months or years. If neurologic symptoms appear within a few years of the initial infection, they tend to be focal, and respond well to antibiotic therapy. When the onset of neurologic symptoms is delayed for a longer period, the earliest signs reveal widespread pathology and do not respond as well to therapy.

In the second stage of syphilis, the symptoms of neurosyphilis are transient and vague, including headache and intermittent pains in the trunk and limbs. Rarely, acute meningitis or encephalitis occurs and may result in seizures or coma.[20] A few years after this early stage, inflammation of arterial walls and meningitis often occur, occasionally manifesting a communicating hydrocephalus. Symptoms of the vascular pathology and meningitis include seizures, headache, anxiety, and signs of cranial nerve damage, such as palsies, neuralgia, dizziness, and deafness.[20]

Blood tests for syphilis usually are positive in secondary and early tertiary neurosyphilis. The CSF is positive for *T. pallidum* and the serum protein level and mononuclear cell count are elevated. These tests, used to confirm the diagnosis of neurosyphilis and to monitor the response to antibiotic therapy, indicate success when the cell count falls, the protein content decreases, and changes eventually occur in the VDRL test.

General paresis develops about 20 years after the initial infection, and the spirochetes seem to invade the brain parenchyma and cord tissue rather than stay in the meninges and blood vessels. As a result, lesions are spread diffusely over the cerebral cortex, basal ganglia, and sometimes the cerebellar cortex. Early symptoms include impaired memory and concentration. Later, characteristic personal carelessness, impulsiveness, incontinence, and signs of both receptive and expressive aphasia develop. Seizures are common, as are irregular and miotic pupils. Pupils' reaction to light is diminished or absent even though they may accommodate to distance changes; this condition is called *Argyll Robertson pupils*, which signifies midbrain damage. It is especially suggestive of neurosyphilis, although similar pupil changes may be seen in other disorders, such as alcoholic polyneuropathy. Because of damage to the cortical motor cells and pyramidal tracts, voluntary motor function decreases, and reflexes become hyperactive unless the cord is invaded, in which case reflexes may diminish or disappear. The untreated end result of general paresis usually is a bedridden, incontinent, confused, hallucinating person who is susceptible to all the secondary problems of immobility. Penicillin and erythromycin are curative for syphilis, and no tolerance to the drugs appears to be developed by the organism.

## REFERENCES

1.  Albanese, J.A. *Nurses' Drug Reference*. New York: McGraw-Hill, 1982.
2.  Anchi, T. Plasmapheresis as a treatment of myasthenia gravis. *J. Neurosurg. Nurs.* 13:23, 1981.
3.  Antel, J.P., and Arnasan, B.G. Demyelinating Diseases. In J. Wilson et al. (eds.), *Harrison's Principles of Internal Medicine* (12th ed.). New York: McGraw-Hill, 1991.
4.  Beal, M.F., Richardson, E.P., and Martin, J.B. Degenerative diseases of the nervous system. In J. Wilson et al. (eds.), *Harrison's Principles of Internal Medicine* (12th ed.). New York: McGraw-Hill, 1991.
5.  Caviness, V.S. Neurocutaneous syndromes and other developmental disorders of the central nervous system. In J. Wilson et al. (eds.), *Harrison's Principles of Internal Medicine* (12th ed.). New York: McGraw-Hill, 1991.
6.  Cotran, R.S., Kumar, V., and Robbins, S. *Robbins' Pathologic Basis of Disease* (4th ed.). Philadelphia: W.B. Saunders, 1989.
7.  Haerer, A., and Currier, R.D. *Neurology Notes* (5th ed.). Jackson, Miss.: University of Mississippi Medical School, 1974.
8.  Harris, E. Extrapyramidal side effects of antipsychotic medication. *Am. J. Nurs.* 81:1324, 1981.
9.  Hartley, F.D. A nurse's view: Amyotrophic lateral sclerosis. *J. Neurosurg. Nurs.* 13:89, 1981.
10. Hartshorn, I. Immunosuppressive treatment of multiple sclerosis. *J. Neurosurg. Nurs.* 16:275, 1984.
11. Iverson, L. The chemistry of the brain. *Sci. Am.* 9:141, 1979.
12. Lannon, M., et al. Comprehensive care of the patient with Parkinson's disease. *J. Neurosurg. Nurs.* 18:121, 1986.
13. Lewis, S. Viral and immunopathology in multiple sclerosis. *J. Neurosurg. Nurs.* 15:346, 1983.
14. LiVolsi, V.A. Nervous system. In V.A. LiVolsi et al. (eds.), *Pathology* (2nd ed.). New York: John Wiley & Sons, 1989.
15. Perkin, G. *Basic Neurology*. Chichester, Engl.: Ellis Horwood Ltd., 1986.
16. Rosal-Greif, V. Drug-induced dyskinesias. *Am. J. Nurs.* 82:66, 1982.
17. Stripe, J., et al. Huntington's disease. *Am. J. Nurs.* 79:1428, 1979.
18. Tandon, R., and Bradley, W.G. Amyotrophic lateral sclerosis: Pt. 2 Etiopathogenesis. *Ann. Neurol.* 18:419, 1985.

**19.** Vigliarolo, D. Managing bowel incontinence in children with meningomyelocele. *Am. J. Nurs.* 80:105, 1980.

**20.** Walton, J.N. *Brain's Diseases of the Nervous System* (8th ed.). New York: Oxford University Press, 1977.

**21.** Wurtman, R. Alzheimer's disease. *Sci. Am.* 252:62, 1985.

# UNIT BIBLIOGRAPHY

Adams, R., and Maurice, V. *Principles of Neurology* (4th ed.). New York: McGraw-Hill, 1989.

Appel, S.H., et al. Amyotrophic lateral sclerosis. *Arch. Neurol.* 3:234, 1986.

Barnett, H., Mohr, J., Bennett, M., and Frank, M. *Stroke: Pathophysiology, Diagnosis, and Management* (Vol. 1). New York: Churchill Livingstone, 1986.

Beekham, M.M. Neurologic manifestations of AIDS. *Crit. Care Nurs. Clin. North Am.* 2:29, 1990.

Bonica, J. *The Management of Pain* (2nd ed.). Philadelphia: Lea & Febiger, 1990.

Byers, V., and Guthrie, M. The limbic system and behavior. *J. Neurosurg. Nurs.* 16:80, 1984.

Carpenter, M., and Sutin, J. *Human Neuroanatomy* (8th ed.). Baltimore: Williams & Wilkins, 1983.

Cormack, D.H. *Ham's Histology* (9th ed.). Philadelphia: J.B. Lippincott, 1987.

Cotran, R.S., Kumar, V., and Robbins, S.L. *Robbins' Pathologic Basis of Disease* (4th ed.). Philadelphia: W.B. Saunders, 1989.

Dodson, J. The slow death: Alzheimer's disease. *J. Neurosurg. Nurs.* 16:270, 1984.

Dudas, S., and Stevens, K. Central cord injury: Implications for nursing. *J. Neurosurg. Nurs.* 16:84, 1984.

Dunant, Y., and Maurice, I. The release of acetylcholine. *Sci. Am.* 252:58, 1985.

Ganong, W.F. *Review of Medical Physiology* (12th ed.). Los Altos, Calif.: Lange, 1985.

Germon, K. Interpretation of ICP pulse waves to determine intracerebral compliance. *J. Neurosci. Nurs.* 20:6, 1988.

Guyton, A.C. *Textbook of Medical Physiology* (8th ed.). Philadelphia: W.B. Saunders, 1990.

Hachinski, V., and Norris, J. *The Acute Stroke*. Philadelphia: F.A. Davis, 1985.

Hanneman, E. Brain resuscitation. *Heart Lung* 15:3, 1986.

Hanson, R.S., and Gerber, R.F. *Coping with Chronic Pain*. New York: Guilford Press, 1990.

Harthorn, J. Immunosuppressive treatment of multiple sclerosis. *J. Neurosurg. Nurs.* 16:275, 1984.

Hickey, J. *The Clinical Practice of Neurological and Neurosurgical Nursing* (2nd ed.). Philadelphia: J.B. Lippincott, 1986.

Hudspeth, A. The hair cells of the inner ear. *Sci. Am.* 248:54, 1983.

Jackson, L. Cerebral vasospasm after intracranial aneurysmal subarachnoid hemorrhage: A nursing perspective. *Heart Lung* 15:14, 1986.

Jankovic, J., and Tolosa, E. *Parkinson's Disease and Movement Disorders*. Baltimore: Munich, Urban & Schwarzenberg, 1988.

Johnson, R.T. *Current Therapy in Neurologic Disease 3*. Philadelphia: B.C. Decker, 1990.

Kelley, W.N. (ed.). *Textbook of Internal Medicine*. Philadelphia: J.B. Lippincott, 1989.

King, L.R., et al. Pituitary hormone response to head injury. *Neurosurgery* 9:229, 1981.

Lannon, M., et al. Comprehensive care of the patient with Parkinson's disease. *J. Neurosci. Nurs.* 18:121, 1986.

Leina's, R. Calcium in synaptic transmission. *Sci. Am.* 247:56, 1983.

Leverenz, J., and Sumi, S. Parkinson's disease in patients with Alzheimer's. *Arch. Neurol.* 7:662, 1986.

Lewis, S. Viral and immunopathology in multiple sclerosis. *J. Neurosurg. Nurs.* 15:346, 1983.

Mannheimer, J., and Lampe, G. *Clinical Transcutaneous Electrical Nerve Stimulation*. Philadelphia: F.A. Davis, 1989.

McCaffrey, M., and Beebe, A. *Pain: A Clinical Manual for Nursing Practice*. St. Louis: C.V. Mosby, 1989.

Miller, T.W. *Chronic Pain*. Madison, Conn.: International University Press, 1990.

Mitchell, S., and Yates, R. Extracranial-intracranial bypass surgery. *J. Neurosurg. Nurs.* 17:288, 1985.

Moses, R. (ed.). *Adler's Physiology of the Eye* (7th ed.). St. Louis: C.V. Mosby, 1981.

Perkin, G. *Basic Neurology*. Chichester, Engl.: Elles Hardwood Ltd., 1986.

Richmond, T. A critical care challenge: The patient with a cervical spinal cord injury. *Focus* 12:23, 1985.

Schwartz, S.I. *Principles of Surgery* (5th ed.). New York: McGraw-Hill, 1989.

Shoemaker, W.C. (ed.). *Textbook of Critical Care* (2nd ed.). Philadelphia: W.B. Saunders, 1989.

Taylor, J. Increased intracranial pressure. *Nurs.83* 13:44, 1983.

Tollison, C.D. *Handbook of Chronic Pain Management*. Baltimore: Williams & Wilkins, 1989.

Wald, M. Cerebral thrombosis: Assessment and nursing management of the acute phase. *J. Neurosci. Nurs.* 18:36, 1986.

Wall, P., and Melzack, R. *Textbook of Pain* (2nd ed.). Edinburgh: Churchill Livingstone, 1989.

Walter, J. *Pathology of Human Disease*. Philadelphia: Lea & Febiger, 1989.

Walton, J. *Brains Diseases of the Nervous System* (9th ed.). Oxford: Oxford University Press, 1985.

Wang, C., et al. Brain injury due to head trauma. *Arch. Neurol.* 6:570, 1986.

Weisberg, L. Subdural empyema. *Arch. Neurol.* 5:49, 1986.

Wilson, J. et al. (eds.), Harrison's Principles of Internal Medicine (12th ed.). New York: McGraw-Hill, 1991.

Wurtman, R. Alzheimer's disease. *Sci. Am.* 252:62, 1985.

Wurtz, R., Goldberg, M., and Robinson, D. Brain mechanisms in visual attention. *Sci. Am.* 246:124, 1982.

Yanoff, M., and Fine, B. *Ocular Pathology* (2nd ed.). Philadelphia: Harper & Row, 1982.

Zuidema, G., Rutherford, R., and Ballenger, W. *The Management of Trauma* (4th ed.). Philadelphia: W.B. Saunders, 1985.

# unit

# 16

# REPRODUCTION

Unit 16 discusses reproductive physiology and the common pathologic problems associated with both the male and the female reproductive systems. Chapter 55 provides an overview of normal male as well as altered male reproductive function. A discussion of normal and altered female reproductive function is presented in Chapter 56. Included in both chapters are an overview of the anatomy and physiology of each system and laboratory and diagnostic aids in the examination of these systems. Chapter 57 presents a discussion of those sexually transmitted diseases that affect reproductive function.

The reader is encouraged to use the learning objectives as a study guide outline. The unit bibliography gives direction for further research.

# chapter 55

Sharron P. Schlosser

# Normal and Altered Male Reproductive Function

## Learning Objectives

1. Describe the development and function of the male sex organs.
2. List three functions of the male reproductive system.
3. Discuss spermatogenesis.
4. List and discuss the factors involved in determining male fertility.
5. List and discuss the stages of male response in the sex act.
6. Differentiate erection, emission, and ejaculation in the sex act.
7. Identify the functions of testosterone.
8. Describe the production and degradation of testosterone.
9. Discuss the influence of the hypothalamus and anterior pituitary on the production of testosterone and spermatogenesis.
10. Briefly describe three diagnostic tests used to determine alterations in male reproductive function.
11. Differentiate prostatitis, benign prostatic hyperplasia, and carcinoma of the prostate.
12. Discuss the staging of prostatic carcinoma.
13. Define *phimosis, paraphimosis, hypospadias, epispadias, balanitis, priapism, hydrocele, varicocele, torsion of testis, cryptorchidism, orchitis,* and *epididymitis.*
14. Describe the four types of testicular germ cell tumors.
15. List and describe the three major stages of testicular tumors.
16. Discuss the possible influence on male offspring of in utero exposure to diethylstilbestrol (DES).

Reproductive function is an integral facet of the human being. Survival of the species depends on proper functioning of the reproductive system. Alterations in male function may be disturbing, since they often represent a threat to this reproductive function and a man's self-image. Alterations can occur in any reproductive organ at virtually any age. This chapter provides an overview of both normal and altered male reproductive function, including congenital anomalies, infections, and cancers.

## ANATOMY

The male reproductive system includes both essential and accessory organs (Figure 55-1). The essential organs are the testes, which produce sperm; accessory organs include the epididymis, vas deferens, seminal vesicles, ejaculatory ducts, prostate gland, and urethra. The sup-

porting structures of the scrotum, penis, and spermatic cords also are considered accessory organs.

## Scrotum

The scrotum is a saclike structure suspended between the penis and anus in the perineal area. It is composed of fascial connective tissue, which contains smooth muscle known as dartos fascia, and two lateral compartments. The testes are located within these compartments, and the left testis usually is lower than the right one. In the mature male, the scrotum is covered with sparse hair and is darker than adjacent skin. It is sensitive to touch, temperature, pain, and pressure.

The scrotum functions to protect and support the testes and sperm. The cremaster, a thin skeletal muscle, and the dartos contract when cold to draw the testes closer to

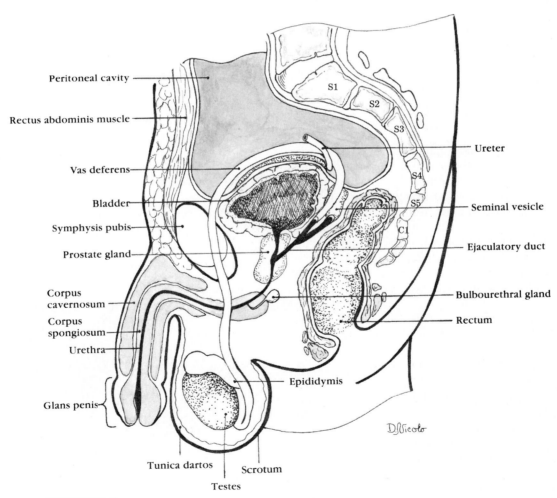

**FIGURE 55-1.**
Side view of male genitourinary anatomy. (M.A. Miller, D.A. Brooten, *The Childbearing Family: A Nursing Perspective* [2nd ed.]. Boston: Little, Brown, 1983.)

the body. When warm, the muscles relax, allowing the testes to drop away from the body. This process permits the testes to maintain a more constant environmental temperature, which is about 3°F lower than normal body temperature. When the environmental temperature is too high, spermatogenesis is impaired.

## Testes

The testes are two ovoid glands suspended in the scrotum by attachment to both scrotal tissue and spermatic cords. The testes measure 4 to 5 cm in length and 2 to 3 cm in diameter, and weigh 10 to 15 g. The testes consist of two layers of tissue–the tunica vaginalis and the tunica albuginea. The tunica vaginalis is a thin, serous covering acquired from the peritoneum during descent. The tunica albuginea is a tough, fibrous membrane that encapsulates the testes. Extensions of the tunica albuginea divide the testes into lobules. Each lobule contains *seminiferous tubules* and *interstitial cells of Leydig.* The seminiferous tubules function as the site for spermatogenesis. Sertoli cells, located in the walls of the tubules, serve to produce and secrete nutrients for spermatogonia in the tubules. Testosterone, the male hormone, is secreted by the interstitial cells (see p. 1112).

## Epididymis

The epididymis is a tortuous genital duct, about 6 m in length, that connects the testis and vas deferens and serves as a passageway for spermatozoa. It is located on top of the testis, and is divided into three parts: (1) the head, which is connected to the testis; (2) the body; and (3) the tail, which is continuous with the vas deferens (Figure 55-2). Sperm are stored in the epididymis up to 2 weeks. During this time, they mature, develop the power of motility, and become capable of fertilizing an ovum.

## Vas Deferens

The vas deferens is an uncoiled, fibromuscular tube or duct that is about 45 cm long and 2.5 mm thick. This duct ascends from the tail of the epididymis in the scrotum into the abdomen, where it passes over the bladder. On the posterior of the bladder, the duct enlarges into the ampulla of the vas deferens and joins with the duct from the seminal vesicle to form the ejaculatory duct (Figure 55-3).

The vas deferens stores the majority of the sperm. During the storage period, sperm metabolism continues, and large amounts of carbon dioxide are produced and

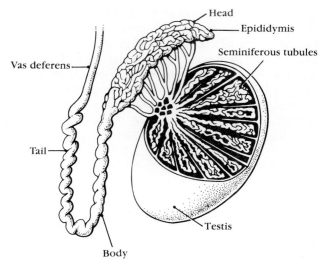

**FIGURE 55–2.**
The vas deferens in relation to the tubules of the testis and epididymis.

secreted into the surrounding fluid. The resulting acidic pH inhibits activity of the sperm during storage. When stimulated, the sympathetic nerves from the pelvic plexus cause peristaltic contractions of the muscular layer and result in emission of stored sperm into the ejaculatory ducts. On release to the exterior, the sperm again exhibit the power of motility.[4]

## Seminal Vesicles

The seminal vesicles are two saclike structures about 5 cm long, lined with secretory epithelium, and located

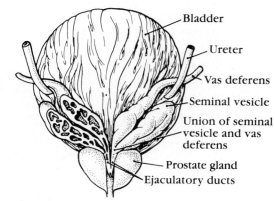

**FIGURE 55–3.**
Union of the seminal vesicles with the vas deferens and entrance into the prostate gland.

directly behind the urinary bladder (see Figure 55-3). They produce a viscous, alkaline, yellowish fluid that makes up a large part of the seminal fluid volume. This fluid is rich in fructose, an energy source for sperm metabolism. Fluid from the seminal vesicles also contains citric acid, five amino acids, and prostaglandins. Sympathetic stimulation produces contractions of the seminal vesicles and emission of the contents.

## Ejaculatory Ducts

The ejaculatory ducts, two short tubes about 2 cm in length, are formed by union of the ampulla of the vas deferens and the ducts of the seminal vesicles. The ejaculatory ducts descend through the prostate gland and terminate in the prostatic urethra, where sperm and secretions from the seminal vesicles and prostate are emitted.

## Prostate Gland

The prostate gland is a walnut-sized gland about 4 cm in diameter and 3 cm thick, and weighs about 20 g. It is located just below the bladder, and surrounds the ejaculatory duct and about an inch of the urethra. The gland is divided into five lobules by the urethra and the ejaculatory duct. Its primary function is to secrete a thin, milky, alkaline fluid that constitutes a large part of the seminal fluid volume. This fluid is discharged into the urethra during emission, and helps to neutralize the acidic fluid of the male urethra and female vagina. Additionally, the prostate gland secretes acid phosphatase, which can be used in assessment of prostatic function.

## Urethra

The urethra is the terminal portion of the seminal fluid passageway. It is about 18 to 20 cm long and divided into three areas: (1) the prostatic urethra, (2) the membranous urethra, and (3) the penile urethra. The prostatic urethra is the proximal portion, and is about 2.5 cm in length. The membranous urethra is the shortest and central section; it measures 0.5 cm and contains the external sphincter. The distal portion is the longest at about 15 cm and constitutes the penile urethra.

## Bulbourethral Glands

The bulbourethral (Cowper's) glands are two pea-sized, brownish glands located just below the prostate. These glands are about 1 cm in diameter and drain into the urethra. On sexual stimulation, these glands secrete a clear, viscous, alkaline fluid that lines the urethra, neutralizes the pH, and lubricates the tip of the penis in preparation for intercourse.

## Penis

The penis is a long, cylinderlike structure covered by a loose layer of skin. It consists of the body and the glans. The body contains three compartments of erectile tissue: two corpora cavernosa and the corpus spongiosum (see Figure 55-1). The corpora cavernosa are large and parallel to each other. The corpus spongiosum is smaller, lower than the corpora cavernosa, and contains the urethra. Distally, the corpus spongiosum expands to form the glans penis. In the uncircumcised male, a fold of loose skin, the prepuce, covers the glans. The erectile tissue is spongelike, and contains large venous sinuses interspersed with arteries and veins. Sexual stimulation results in dilation of the arteries and arterioles and distention of the cavernous spaces with blood. Filling of the erectile tissue results in erection of the penis. The penis serves two functions: (1) it contains the urethra, which is the passageway for urine, and (2) it is the male organ of copulation.

# MALE REPRODUCTIVE FUNCTIONS

The male reproductive system serves the following primary functions: (1) spermatogenesis, (2) performance of the sex act, and (3) hormonal regulation of male sexual function.

## Spermatogenesis

The seminiferous tubules of the newborn male's testes contain primitive sex cells called *spermatogonia*. They are located in two to three layers in the outer border of the tubular epithelium (Figure 55-4). At puberty (about age 13), spermatogenesis begins in all the seminiferous tubules as a result of stimulation by the adenohypophyseal (anterior pituitary) gonadotropic hormones (see Chap. 36).

During spermatogenesis, a series of meiotic divisions occurs. The primary spermatocyte divides into two secondary spermatocytes, which subsequently divide and produce four spermatids (Figure 55-5). During this process, each cell retains one of each pair of 23 chromosomes. Of the 23 chromosomes, one is the sex chromosome.

In the process of spermatid production, each cell loses most of its cytoplasm and elongates into a sperm,

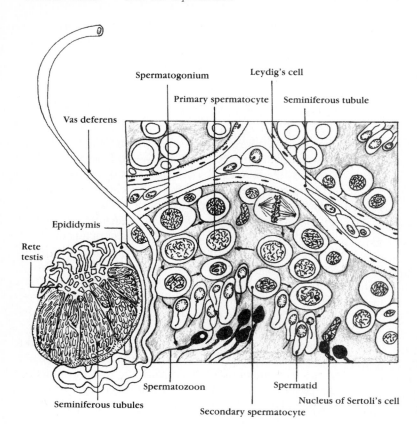

**FIGURE 55–4.**
Male ductal system and developing reproductive cells. The detail on the right shows spermatogenesis and the seminiferous tubule. (M.A. Miller, D.A. Brooten, *The Childbearing Family: A Nursing Perspective* [2nd ed.]. Boston: Little, Brown, 1983.)

which consists of a head, a neck, a body, and a tail (Figure 55-6). The head is formed when nuclear material rearranges and the cell membrane contracts around it. This part of the sperm fertilizes the ovum and the tail portion provides rapid motility.

## Fertility

Actual male fertility depends on (1) the quantity of semen ejaculated, (2) the number of sperm per milliliter, and (3) the motility and morphology of the sperm. The seminal fluid ejaculated with each coitus averages 400 million sperm in a fluid volume of about 3 mL. When the number of sperm in each milliliter drops below 20 to 50 million, *infertility* (defined as the inability to conceive after 12 months of adequate exposure in unprotected intercourse) or *sterility* (absolute inability to conceive) frequently results.

The acrosome on the head of the sperm produces the enzymes *hyaluronidase* and several proteinases. It is believed that these enzymes are necessary to remove the outer cell layers of the ovum. Only one sperm is responsible for the actual fertilization (Figure 55-7).

## Male Function in the Sex Act

With respect to sexual behavior, humans differ from all other living creatures. In animals, for example, sex drive and behavior are instinctual and depend on hormones. With humans, the initiation of the sex act may begin through physical or mental stimulation (Figure 55-8). Erotic thoughts and dreams may produce erection and ejaculation in the male.

The most important area of sexual stimulation in the male is the glans penis. Sexual sensations produced by the massage of intercourse pass through the pudendal nerve, into the sacral portion of the spinal cord, and on to the cerebrum. Physical stimulation also may occur with touching the anal epithelium, perineum, or scrotum. These sexual sensations enter the pudendal nerve from the perineal and scrotal nerves and then enter the sacral portion of the spinal cord to be transmitted to the cerebrum.

The first effect of sexual stimulation is *erection* of the penis. The penis normally is flaccid because of constriction of the arterioles that supply its vascular spaces (Figure 55-9). Sexual stimulation results in a stimulation of parasympathetic nerves and inhibition of sympathetic

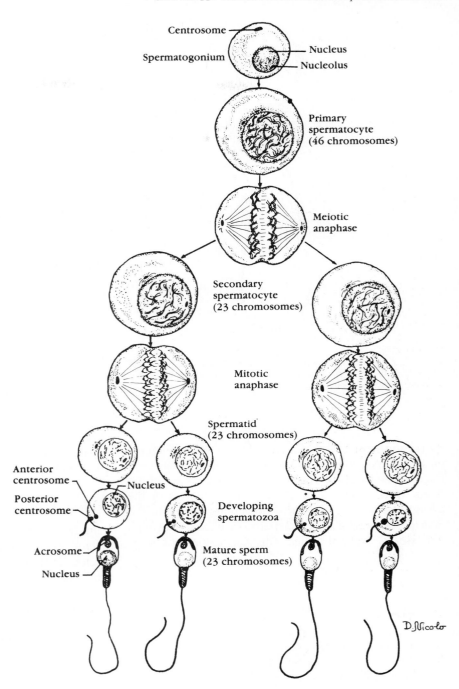

**FIGURE 55–5.**
Maturation of male reproductive cells. (M.A. Miller, and D.A. Brooten, *The Child-bearing Family: A Nursing Perspective* [2nd ed.]. Boston: Little, Brown, 1983.)

nerves to the arterioles. As a result, the penile arterioles dilate and the veins constrict. Blood is forced into the vascular spaces and erectile tissue. The blood flow, under pressure, produces a ballooning effect of the erectile tissue and results in a hard, elongated penis.

During this first stage of the male sexual response, lubricating fluid is discharged mainly from the bulbo-urethral glands, which results from parasympathetic stimulation.

The second stage involves two processes: *emission* and *ejaculation* (Figure 55-10). Emission is initiated when sympathetic impulses are emitted by reflex centers in the spinal cord, which pass to the smooth muscle of the genital ducts, producing contractions and forcing the

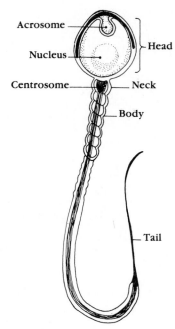

**FIGURE 55–6.**
The mature sperm, consisting of head, neck, body, and tail. (M.A. Miller, D.A. Brooten, *The Childbearing Family: A Nursing Perspective* [2nd ed.]. Boston: Little, Brown, 1983.)

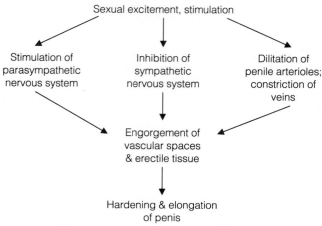

**FIGURE 55–8.**
Mechanism of erection of the penis.

a parasympathetic response and culminates the sex act for the male.

## Hormonal Regulation of Male Sexual Function

Male sexual function is regulated by a complex feedback mechanism that involves hormones secreted by the hypothalamus, anterior pituitary, and testes.

### Hypothalamus and Pituitary

The hypothalamus secretes two gonadotropin releasing factors (GnRFs)—follicle-stimulating hormone releasing factor (FSH-RF) and luteinizing hormone releasing factor (LH-RF) (Figure 55-11). When secreted by the hypothalamus, these releasing factors are conducted through the blood flow channels, called the hypothalamicohypophyseal portal system, to the pituitary. Elevated levels of FSH-RF and LH-RF stimulate the anterior pituitary

sperm and seminal fluid into the internal urethra. Filling of the internal urethra then initiates impulses that result in contractions of the skeletal muscle at the base of the penis. During these contractions, the sphincter at the base of the bladder constricts, preventing the expulsion of urine, as seminal fluid and sperm are expelled through the external urethral orifice. This ejaculation represents

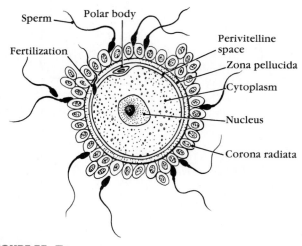

**FIGURE 55–7.**
Fertilization of an ovum.

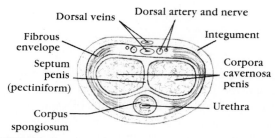

**FIGURE 55–9.**
Vascular supply to penis. (W.H. Masters and V.E. Johnson, *Human Sexual Response*. Boston: Little, Brown, 1966.)

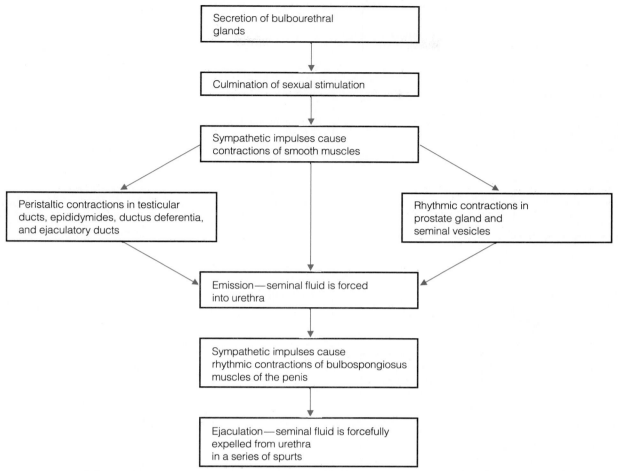

**FIGURE 55–10.**

The mechanism of emission and ejaculation. (K.M. Van De Graaff and S.I. Fox, *Concepts of Human Anatomy and Physiology.* Dubuque, IA: Wm. C. Brown, 1989.)

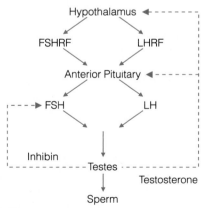

**FIGURE 55–11.**

Feedback relation of FSH secretion. The two gonadotropic hormone releasing factors are follicle-stimulating hormone releasing factor (FSHRF) and luteinizing hormone releasing factor (LHRF). They are secreted by the hypothalamus and cause the release of follicle-stimulating hormone (FSH) and luteinizing hormone (LH), which stimulate the Leydig cells of the testes to produce testosterone.

to secrete two sex hormones: follicle-stimulating hormone (FSH) and luteinizing hormone (LH), also referred to as interstitial cell-stimulating hormone (ICSH).

ICSH then stimulates Leydig cells to produce testosterone. A rise in the blood level of testosterone provides negative feedback to the hypothalamus and anterior pituitary, thus reducing the levels of FSH-RF and LH- RF from the hypothalamus and inhibiting the pituitary's response to these GnRFs. A drop in FSH-RF and LH-RF stimulates a reduction in the secretion of FSH and ICSH. A drop in the ICSH then inhibits secretion of testosterone. As testosterone levels drop, the hypothalamus and anterior pituitary are again triggered to secrete ICSH (Figure 55-12). It also is believed that the testes are responsible for the secretion of inhibin, a polypeptide hormone. This hormone seems to inhibit production of FSH without affecting the production of LH.

FSH is responsible for conversion of spermatogonia into sperm, and ICSH stimulates the production of testosterone. Without FSH, spermatogenesis does not occur,

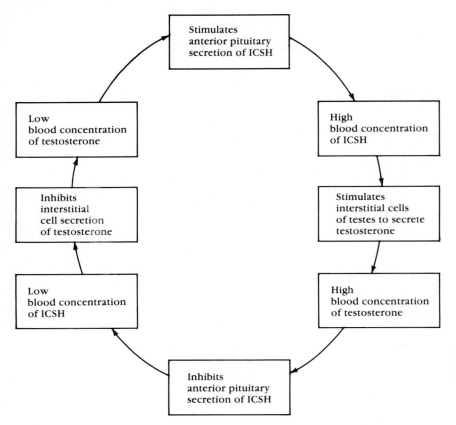

**FIGURE 55-12.**

Negative feedback mechanism for the secretion of interstitial cell-stimulating hormone (ICSH) and interstitial cell secretion of testosterone. (C. Anthony, *Textbook of Anatomy and Physiology.* St. Louis: C.V. Mosby, 1979.)

and without testosterone, the sperm do not mature. Thus the secretion of FSH and ICSH is controlled not only by testosterone, but also by FSH-RF and LH-RF. Stress and emotions affect secretory function of the hypothalamus and usually decrease secretion of the releasing factors.

During fetal life, the production of human chorionic gonadotropin (HCG) also is important in the development of male sex organs. HCG possesses properties that are similar to those of ICSH. Thus it stimulates the interstitial cells in the fetal testes to produce testosterone, which is then responsible for the development of the male organs.

## Male Sex Hormones

The male sex hormones, also known as androgens, are secreted primarily by the *interstitial cells of Leydig* in the testes and in smaller amounts by the adrenals. The testosterone released by these cells circulates in the bloodstream for only 15 to 30 minutes before it is fixed in tissues to perform intracellular functions or is degraded by the liver. Once testosterone enters the cells, it is converted to *dihydrotestosterone.* Dihydrotestosterone combines with nuclear protein, and promotes messenger ribonucleic acid synthesis, which then enhances cellular protein production. Testosterone not fixed in tissues is converted in the liver into androsterone and dehydroepiandrosterone. These forms are conjugated into glucuronides or sulfates and are excreted in bile or urine as 17-ketosteroids (Figure 55-13). The inactivation process for testosterone accounts for the ineffectiveness of oral administration of this hormone. Testosterone functions to (1) control development of male secondary sex characteristics, (2) regulate metabolism, (3) affect fluid and electrolyte balance, and (4) inhibit anterior pituitary secretion of gonadotropins.

The influence of testosterone on male secondary sex characteristics begins as early as the second month of embryonic life, when HCG from the placenta stimulates production of small amounts of testosterone. This testosterone is thought to affect the development of the penis, scrotum, prostate gland, seminal vesicles, and genital ducts in the fetus. During childhood, virtually no testosterone is produced until puberty, at which time secretion rapidly increases. After puberty and continuing until maturity at about age 20, testosterone stimulates enlargement of the penis, scrotum, and testes.

Testosterone also stimulates protein anabolism, which is directly responsible for virilization of the male. The secondary sex characteristics—muscular development

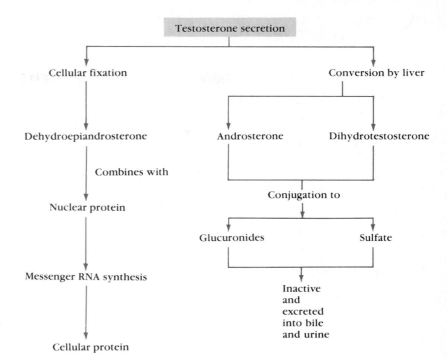

**FIGURE 55-13.**

Paths of testosterone after secretion by testes. Part of the hormone becomes fixed in tissues to perform intracellular functions and part is degraded by the liver.

and strength; hair growth on the face, axillae, and chest; bone growth; and deepening of the voice—are manifestations of this process. In affecting bone growth, testosterone also functions in early uniting of the epiphyses and shafts of long bones, which stops the growth process. The basal metabolic rate increases under the influence of this hormone.

Testosterone secondarily increases retention of sodium, potassium, calcium, and water. The hormone levels can affect the fluid balance through influencing iron retention by the kidneys. It is a method to retain substances necessary to effect the anabolic process. High levels of testosterone inhibit secretion of gonadotropins by the anterior pituitary.

# PHYSICAL, LABORATORY, AND DIAGNOSTIC TESTS

Physical examination, computed tomographic (CT) scanning, ultrasonography, and laboratory evaluation are all important in assessing male reproductive function. These assessments aid in diagnosing infectious disorders, infertility, and neoplastic disease. Physical examination detects redness, swelling, discharge, and abnormal masses; laboratory evaluation centers on testicular function, cultures, and serology testing. Primary laboratory studies include measurement of testosterone secretion, examination of seminal fluid, serology, and cultures for infectious disorders.

## Physical Examination

The physical examination includes inspection and palpation of the external genitalia and a rectal examination. After visual examination of the external genitalia, the examiner palpates the scrotal contents for abnormal masses. A rectal examination is performed to detect the size and texture of the prostate or the presence and location of masses. Prostatic massage also may be performed to obtain a sample of prostatic secretions.

## Testosterone Measurement

Testosterone, a 19-carbon hormone that affects the development of male sex characteristics, degrades into androsterone and dehydroepiandrosterone, which can be measured as *17-ketosteroids*. About one third of 17-ketosteroid excretion in the male can be attributed to testosterone and its products.

Testosterone levels, measured directly, are particularly helpful in assessing hypogonadism, impotence, cryptorchidism, and pituitary gonadotropin functions in the male. Male hypogonadism and Klinefelter's syndrome can be associated with a decreased testosterone level.

In women, testosterone measurement may assist in the diagnosis of ovarian and adrenal tumors. Adrenal neoplasms, benign and malignant ovarian tumors, adrenogenital syndrome, and Stein-Leventhal syndrome with virilization frequently are associated with an increased

**TABLE 55–1.**

NORMAL HORMONE LEVELS

| HORMONE | AGE | BLOOD | URINE |
| --- | --- | --- | --- |
| Testosterone | | | |
| Male | Adult | 0.3–1.0 g/dL (average = 0.7) | 47–156 g/24 h (average = 70) |
| | Adolescent | 0.10 g/dL | |
| Female | All ages | 0–0.1 g/dL (average = 0.04) | 0–15 g/24 h (average = 6) |
| 17-Ketosteroids | | | |
| Male and female | All ages | 25–125 g/dL | |
| Male | 10 y | | 1–4 mg/24 h |
| | 20–30 y | | 6–26 mg/24 h |
| | 50 y | | 5–18 mg/24 h |
| | 70 y | | 2–10 mg/24 h |
| Female | 10 y | | 1–4 mg/24 h |
| | 20–30 y | | 4–14 mg/24 h |
| | 50 y | | 3–9 mg/24 h |
| | 70 y | | 1–7 mg/24 h |
| Chorionic gonadotropin | | | |
| Male | | | 0 |

testosterone level. Table 55-1 depicts normal laboratory values for testosterone production; these values may vary slightly from institution to institution.

Levels of 17-ketosteroids may be high in testicular tumors and adrenal cortical hyperplasia. Before puberty, spermatogenesis seldom occurs as a result of testosterone production.

## Semen Examination

Semen examination is of particular importance in evaluating infertility. Seminal fluid for examination is best collected through masturbation, which provides a complete specimen of ejaculate. This method also protects sperm morphology and motility, which may be affected by rubber condoms.

Both the sperm and the quantity of fluid are examined. Semen viscosity and morphology and motility of the sperm are assessed. The normal sperm count varies widely. Most authorities consider greater than 50 million sperm per milliliter to be normal; however, pregnancies have been documented with lower levels. The normal volume of ejaculate is 3 to 5 mL. Infertility has been associated with both lower and higher volumes.

The morphology and motility of sperm may be factors in infertility even when the count is normal. High percentages of inactive or abnormally formed sperm are associated with infertility. Viscosity of seminal fluid may vary. Initially thick, the fluid must liquefy to allow normal motility of the sperm. This liquefaction usually is complete in 15 to 20 minutes. Normal semen test results are summarized in Table 55-2.

## Tissue Biopsy

Testicular biopsy may be indicated if the semen examination reveals no sperm or to aid in the diagnosis of testicular atrophy. If a testicular tumor is suspected, biopsy usually is performed only after orchiectomy, to prevent dissemination of the tumor cells. Tissue biopsy is helpful in diagnosing cancer of the penis and prostate.

## Prostate Ultrasonography

Prostate ultrasonography is a relatively new procedure used in the diagnosis and early detection of prostate cancer. It involves the use of ultrasonic waves from a rectal probe to produce an image of the prostate. This procedure may prove most beneficial in detecting cancers that are too small to be noted on physical examination.

**TABLE 55–2.**

SEMEN EXAMINATION

| TEST | NORMAL RESULTS |
| --- | --- |
| Sperm count | 50–60 million/mL or more |
| Volume | 3–6 mL |
| Morphology | 60% of sperm motile; 50% of normal morphology |
| Liquefaction | Complete in 15–20 min |
| pH | 7.2–7.8 |
| Leukocyte count | 0–2000/mL |

# ALTERATIONS IN MALE FUNCTION

## Penis

Alterations in the penis and penile function can be divided into those alterations related to congenital anomalies and those that affect the adult. Congenital and childhood alterations include phimosis and paraphimosis, hypospadias, and epispadias. Adult alterations include Peyronie's disease, priapism, balanitis, and carcinoma.

### Phimosis and Paraphimosis

Phimosis is a condition in which the prepuce is too narrow or stenosed to retract over the glans penis. In more severe cases, urinary flow may be obstructed. It frequently is congenital, but it may occur after infection or injury. If manual retraction is unsuccessful in treating the condition, surgical intervention is indicated. When untreated, this condition predisposes the man to secondary infection, scarring, and perhaps cancer because secretions and smegma accumulate under the prepuce and cannot be cleaned away. Forcible retraction of the foreskin may lead to constriction, swelling, and pain of the glans penis. Circumcision may be performed to correct the problem.

Paraphimosis occurs when the foreskin is retracted behind the corona of the glans. Impaired blood flow results in edema of the glans. Surgical intervention is indicated when manual correction fails.

### Hypospadias

At about 7 to 8 weeks' gestation, the embryo develops a genital tubercle and two genital swellings. In the male fetus, the genital tubercle develops into the penis. The two swellings develop into two folds (urethral and scrotal), which descend and fuse. This fusion closes the urethra in the penis and forms the scrotum. Failure of these folds to fuse on the ventral side results in the congenital anomaly of hypospadias. The urethral orifice is located on the under side of the penis from close to the normal opening all the way to the perineum (Figure 55-14). The foreskin on the ventral side usually is absent.

The condition also is associated with undescended testes and chordee. Chordee occurs when a fibrous band of tissue replaces the normal skin and produces a ventral curvature of the penis (Figure 55-14B). If the anomaly is so severe that the infant's sex is questionable, chromosomal studies are initiated. Surgical repair is aimed at straightening the penis and forming a urethra that terminates as centrally as possible.

### Epispadias

Epispadias, a rare congenital anomaly, results from failure of the dorsal side of the penis to fuse. The urethral opening is located on this surface rather than in the center. The urethral opening may be found just behind the glans, or it may extend the length of the penis when associated with exstrophy of the bladder. Surgical repair is

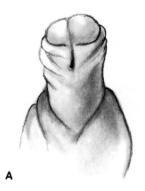

**A**

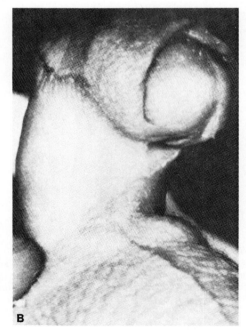

**B**

**FIGURE 55–14.**
**A.** Hypospadias is a congenital displacement of the urethral meatus to the inferior surface of the penis. A groove extends from the actual urethral meatus to its normal location on the tip of the glans. **B.** Hypospadias with significant chordee. (B. Bates, *A Guide to Physical Examination and History Taking* [5th ed.]. Philadelphia: J.B. Lippincott, 1991.)

aimed at establishing a normally functioning urethra and penis.

## Balanitis

Balanitis is an inflammation of the glans penis. It most frequently occurs in uncircumcised males who exercise poor hygiene. It also may result from venereal disease. Clinical manifestations include redness, swelling, pain, and purulent drainage. Infection may cause adhesions and scarring. Cultures and sensitivity are performed to diagnose the organism so as to initiate antibiotic therapy. Circumcision may be indicated in uncircumcised males.

## Peyronie's Disease

Peyronie's disease is a condition characterized by the formation of fibrous plaques on the dorsal side of the penis (Figure 55-15). It also is accompanied by penile curvature and pain during erection. It frequently is associated with Dupuytren's contracture of hand tendons. The condition is found primarily in middle-aged and older men.

## Priapism

Priapism refers to prolonged, persistent penile erection in the absence of sexual stimulation. The condition is extremely painful and may last from hours to several days. The cause is unknown; however, it has been associated with leukemia and sickle cell anemia. Surgical interven-

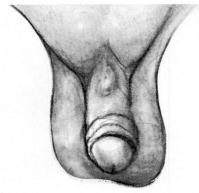

**FIGURE 55–15.**
Peyronie's disease. In Peyronie's disease, there are palpable nontender hard plaques just beneath the skin, usually along the dorsum of the penis. The patient complains of crooked, painful erections. (B. Bates, *A Guide to Physical Examination and History Taking* [5th ed.]. Philadelphia: J.B. Lippincott, 1991.)

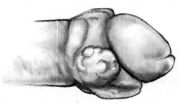

**FIGURE 55–16.**
Carcinoma of the penis. Carcinoma may present as an indurated nodule or ulcer that usually is nontender. Limited almost completely to men who are not circumcised in childhood, it may be masked by the prepuce. Any persistent penile sore must be considered suspicious. (B. Bates, *A Guide to Physical Examination and History Taking* [5th ed.]. Philadelphia: J.B. Lippincott, 1991.)

tion within the first few hours provides drainage from the corpora cavernosa and helps to prevent impotence.

## Penile Carcinoma

Penile carcinoma (Figure 55-16), a rare condition that tends to progress slowly, includes two neoplastic lesions: (1) carcinoma in situ, or Bowen's disease, and (2) invasive carcinoma. Carcinoma in situ appears as a smooth, red lesion with a well-demarcated border. There also is the potential for conversion to invasive squamous cell carcinoma. Surgical excision is the treatment of choice. Prophylactic treatment may include radiation and administration of 5-fluorouracil.

Invasive squamous cell carcinoma primarily affects the prepuce and glans. The lesion appears as a small, gray, crusted papule that gradually enlarges and produces necrotic ulceration in the center. Larger lesions that involve the shaft of the penis or the inguinal nodes may require penile resection or amputation. A summary of the staging and tissue involvement is provided in Table 55-3.

Radiation therapy and chemotherapy are used increasingly as palliative and curative treatments. Early

**TABLE 55–3.**
STAGING OF PENILE CARCINOMA

| STAGE | INVOLVEMENT |
| --- | --- |
| I | Glans or prepuce |
| II | Shaft of penis |
| III | Inguinal lymph nodes (operable) |
| IV | Inguinal lymph nodes (inoperable) Metastasis |

**FIGURE 55-17.**
**A.** Hydrocele. A hydrocele is a nontender, fluid-filled mass that occupies the space within the tunica vaginalis. The examining fingers can get above the mass within the scrotum. The mass transilluminates. **B.** Varicocele refers to varicose veins of the spermatic cord, usually found on the left. It feels like a soft "bag of worms" separate from the testis, and slowly collapses when the scrotum is elevated in the supine patient. Infertility may be associated. (B. Bates, *A Guide to Physical Examination and History Taking* [5th ed.]. Philadelphia: J.B. Lippincott, 1991.)

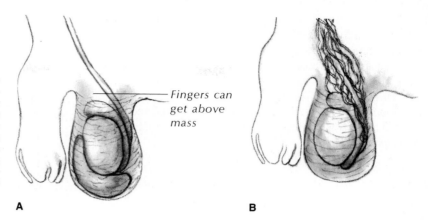

*Fingers can get above mass*

A                                                    B

circumcision seems to prevent development of the squamous cell carcinoma, whereas chronic infection and infection from the human papillomavirus increase the risk of developing penile carcinoma.

## Scrotum, Testes, and Epididymis

### Hydrocele

A hydrocele is an accumulation of clear or straw-colored fluid within the tunica vaginalis sac that encloses the testis (Figure 55-17A). It is the most common cause of scrotal enlargement.[3] It frequently develops without a known cause, but it may occur after epididymitis, orchitis, injury, or neoplasm. In the newborn, it results from late closure of the tunica vaginalis. The condition may be asymptomatic or cause pain or tension in the scrotal sac. Treatment may include aspiration or incision if the hydrocele is large or uncomfortable, or if the testis cannot be palpated. Transillumination provides a differential diagnosis between hydrocele and solid testicular masses.

### Varicocele

Varicocele most often occurs in young men between the ages of 15 and 25. It refers to the abnormal dilation of the venous plexus of the testis, and most often is found on the left side. Occurrence on the right side is strongly suggestive of a tumor obstructing a vein above the scrotum. Palpation reveals dilated and tortuous veins often described as a "bag of worms" (Figure 55-17B). Clinically, the primary concern relates to potential infertility. Both motility and number of sperm are decreased because of the increased warmth created by vascular engorgement. The condition usually is asymptomatic, but the person may complain of a dragging sensation or dull pain in the

scrotum. Scrotal support is the treatment of choice. Surgical ligation of the internal spermatic vein is reserved for severe conditions or when an increased sperm count is desired.

### Torsion of the Testis

Torsion of the testis (Figure 55-18), an infrequent cause of testicular enlargement, primarily occurs during adolescence. It may occur spontaneously or after physical exercise. This condition results from rotation of the testis within the tunica vaginalis, which cuts off the blood supply to the testis. With twisting of the spermatic cord and testis, venous obstruction results in vascular engorgement and sometimes extravasation of blood into the scrotal sac.

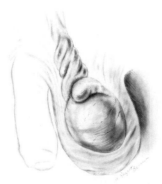

**FIGURE 55-18.**
Torsion or twisting of the testis on its spermatic cord produces an acutely painful, tender, and swollen organ that is retracted upward in the scrotum. The scrotum becomes red and edematous. There is no associated urinary infection. Torsion, most common in adolescents, is a surgical emergency because of obstructed circulation. (B. Bates, *A Guide to Physical Examination and History Taking* [5th ed.]. Philadelphia: J.B. Lippincott, 1991.)

The first symptom normally is sudden onset of severe pain in the testicular area. It is unrelieved by rest or scrotal support and may radiate into the groin. Other manifestations include scrotal edema, testicular tenderness, and perhaps nausea and vomiting. If the torsion cannot be reduced, surgical intervention to untwist the spermatic cord and immobilize the testis is indicated. Untreated torsion of the testis may result in atrophy, abscess, or infertility.

## Cryptorchidism

During fetal development, the testes form in the abdomen and normally descend into the scrotum during the last trimester of pregnancy. Incomplete or maldescent of the testis results in cryptorchidism (Figure 55-19). The testis may remain in the abdomen, or be arrested in the inguinal canal, low pelvis, or high in the scrotum (see Figure 55-19). It may be unilateral or bilateral, and when unilateral, it is somewhat more common on the right.[3] Retractile testis refers to a testis that normally descends into the scrotum but occasionally is pulled back into the inguinal canal. Ectopic testis is one that descends to the wrong area, such as the perineum.

The cause of cryptorchidism is unknown; however, it has been associated with a shortened spermatic cord, testosterone deficiencies, narrowed inguinal canal, and adhesions of the pathway. It is necessary to correct the condition if sterility is to be avoided because after puberty, the testes atrophy progressively. Spermatogenesis decreases, and the cells may be replaced by collagenous fibrous tissue. Because there is a direct relation between cryptorchidism and testicular cancer, surgical placement in the scrotum is recommended.

## Orchitis

Orchitis, inflammation of the testes, may be acquired (1) as an ascending infection of the genital tract, (2) through lymphatic spread, or (3) as a complication of mumps, since the mumps virus is excreted through the urine. Infection may be bilateral or unilateral, and most often is caused by ascending bacteria, including *Staphylococcus, Streptococcus, Escherichia coli, Klebsiella pneumoniae*, and *Pseudomonas aeruginosa*. Orchitis, as a complication of mumps, occurs in about 18% of men with mumps and primarily affects adults.[3]

Clinical manifestations include severe testicular pain, swelling, chills, and fever (Figure 55-20). On examination, the testis appears swollen and tender with a swollen and red scrotum. Complications, including hydrocele and abscess, may result in sterility or impotence. Treatment includes bed rest, scrotal support, warm compresses, and antibiotics, if indicated. Analgesics may be indicated for relief of pain. Surgical intervention may be

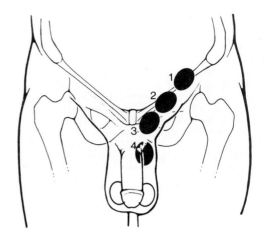

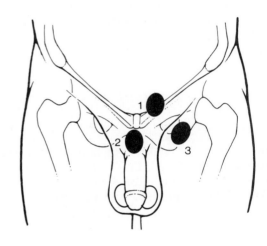

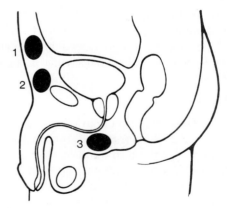

**FIGURE 55–19.**

Cryptorchidism. (a) Incomplete descent of a testis may involve four separate regions: (1) in the pelvic cavity, (2) in the inguinal canal, (3) at the superficial inguinal ring, and (4) in the upper scrotum. (b) An ectopic testis may be (1) in the superficial fascia of the anterior pelvic wall, (2) at the root of the penis, or (3) in the perineum, in the thigh alongside the femoral vessels. (K.M. Van De Graaff and S.I. Fox, *Concepts of Human Anatomy and Physiology.* Dubuque, IA: Wm. C. Brown, 1989.)

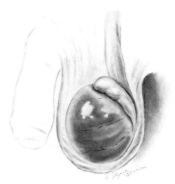

**FIGURE 55–20.**
Acute orchitis. An acutely inflamed testis is painful, tender, and swollen. The testis may be difficult to distinguish from the epididymis. The scrotum may be reddened. Look for evidence of postpubertal mumps or other, less common infectious causes. (B. Bates, *A Guide to Physical Examination and History Taking* [4th ed.]. Philadelphia: J.B. Lippincott, 1987.)

indicated for drainage of the hydrocele. Abscess formation usually results in surgical removal of the testis.

## Testicular Tumors

Testicular tumors, the most common cancer in men between ages 15 and 25, also are the most common cause of testicular enlargement (Figure 55-21).[5] These tumors are predominantly malignant, often metastasize before diagnosis, and arise from germ cells in 95% of cases.[3] The benign tumors usually arise from the interstitial cells of Leydig or Sertoli cells.

Although several classifications have been used with testicular cancer, the most frequently used one was proposed by the Armed Forces Institute of Pathology and modified by the World Health Organization. This classification proposes two groups based on histologic pattern type: (1) those tumors with one histologic pattern type present and (2) those tumors with more than one histologic pattern type present. Tumors of a single histologic pattern type can be further classified as to seminoma and nonseminomatous tumors. Table 55-4 provides a summary of this classification with the associated appearance, incidence, and site of metastasis.

Seminomas are the most common tumor and appear as gray-white, fleshy masses. Most seminomas remain localized until late in the course of the disease when metastases occur to regional and aortic lymph nodes. Because of their sensitivity to irradiation, pure seminomas confined to the testis with no apparent metastases or elevated biochemical markers are best treated with this modality postoperatively. Even when retroperitoneal metastasis of less than 5 cm is confirmed by lymphangiography or CT scanning, radiation therapy is the treatment of choice. When HCG levels remain elevated or alphafetoprotein (AFP) levels are elevated, chemotherapy, retroperitoneal lymphadenectomy, or both are considered in determining appropriate treatment.

Embryonal carcinomas are highly malignant tumors that exhibit a wide variety of cell types. They may occur in both adults and children. Small, gray-white nodules are formed, which usually do not invade the entire testis. Metastasis to the lymph nodes, liver, lungs, and bones is frequent. Elevated serum levels of AFP or HCG help to differentiate these tumors from other testicular tumors.[3]

Choriocarcinomas are small, gray tumors that frequently are not palpable. Characteristically, they produce both cytotrophoblastic and syncytiotrophoblastic cells identical to those formed in the placenta. These cells secrete HCG, which, when found, aids in the diagnosis of choriocarcinoma. Early, distant metastasis usually causes death within a year of diagnosis.

Teratoma and teratocarcinoma are tumors with various cellular types. Teratomas are composed of tissues

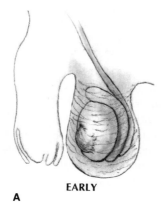

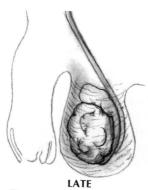

**FIGURE 55–21.**
Tumor of the testis. **A.** Early. A tumor of the testis usually appears as a painless nodule. It does not transilluminate. Any nodule within the testis must raise the suspicion of cancer. **B.** Late. As a testicular neoplasm grows and spreads, it may seem to replace the entire organ. The testis characteristically feels heavier than normal. (B. Bates, *A Guide to Physical Examination and History Taking* [5th ed.]. Philadelphia: J.B. Lippincott, 1991.)

**A**      EARLY

**B**      LATE

**TABLE 55–4.**
CLASSIFICATION OF TESTICULAR GERM CELL TUMORS

| CLASSIFICATION | APPEARANCE | INCIDENCE % | METASTASES |
|---|---|---|---|
| **Single Histologic Pattern** | | 60 | |
| Seminoma | Large, gray, white fleshy mass | 40 | Regional aortic lymph nodes |
| Nonseminomas | Small, gray, white nodule | 10–20 | Lymph nodes, liver, lungs, bones |
|   Embryonal carcinoma | | | |
|   Choriocarcinoma | Small, gray; frequently not palpable; contains both cytotrophoblast & syncytiotrophoblastic cells | 1 | Organ by way of bloodstream |
| Teratoma | Variable | 10 | Lymphatic |
| **Multiple Histologic Pattern** | | 40 | |
| Teratocarcinoma (teratoma & embryonal carcinoma) | | | |
| Seminoma plus others | | | |
| Choriocarcinoma plus others | | | |
| Any combination | | | |

normally derived from the primary germ layers (ectoderm, mesoderm, endoderm) of the embryo. Teratocarcinoma contains both embryonal carcinoma and teratoma cells. Metastases normally follow the lymphatic system but may involve many other structures.

The exact cause of testicular cancer has not been determined. Predisposing factors that seem to contribute to its development include cryptorchidism, genetic influence, age, and race. The genetic influence is evidenced in a higher incidence in brothers and in contralateral tumors in unilateral cryptorchidism. Testicular cancer more frequently occurs in Caucasian men than in Afro-American men. The incidence of testicular cancer decreases with age.

The most frequent symptom of a testicular tumor is painless enlargement of the testis. On examination, the mass does not transilluminate, and lymphadenopathy may be noted. The male may complain of a feeling of heaviness or a dull ache. Gynecomastia is associated with tumors that produce HCG and estrogen. Low back pain may be associated with retroperitoneal lymph node involvement. Other symptoms may be present, and vary with the site of metastasis.

Diagnosis and staging are based on physical examination, protein biochemical markers in serum, CT scanning, and biopsy only after removal of the entire testis (Table 55-5). In addition to manual palpation of the tumor, two protein biochemical markers in serum are especially beneficial in diagnosing and staging testicular tumors. These markers are the beta subunit of HCG and AFP. Tumors with trophoblastic elements are responsible for the beta subunit HCG, although this marker may be present even when these elements are apparently absent. AFP levels are elevated in about 60% of men with nonseminomatous germ cell tumors.

Treatment varies with the type and stage of disease, and includes surgery, radiation, and chemotherapy, either alone or in various combinations. Pure seminomas without evidence of metastasis usually are treated with radiation. In the United States, nonseminomatous tumors most often are treated with orchiectomy, retroperitoneal resection, or chemotherapy. The most commonly used chemotherapeutic agents include vinblastine, bleomycin, cisplatin, dactinomycin, doxorubicin, and cyclophosphamide. Various combinations of these drugs are being used in cancer treatment centers across the nation.

Prognosis depends on the histologic type of the tumor, stage of disease, and utilization of appropriate therapy. Pure seminoma in the earlier stages is associated with a cure rate as high as 100%. Metastatic disease of a

**TABLE 55–5.**
STAGING OF TESTICULAR CANCER

| STAGE | INVOLVEMENT |
|---|---|
| I | Testis |
| II | Primary regional retroperitoneal lymph nodes |
| IIa | Metastases usually <5 cm |
| IIb | Metastases >5 cm |
| III | Visceral metastases below diaphragm; metastases above diaphragm |

differing histologic type, not sensitive to radiation, usually accounts for failure. The cure rate associated with stages I and IIa nonseminomatous tumors is 95%. Because of the progress made in recent years in treatment, patients with stages IIb and III disease now see a cure rate of 80% to 90%.[1]

## Epididymitis

Epididymitis occurs when disease-producing organisms in the urine, urethra, prostate gland, or seminal vesicles spread to the epididymis (Figure 55-22). Acute epididymitis may result from sexually transmitted organisms, *Pseudomonas aeruginosa*, or enteric bacteria. The most common sexually transmitted organisms are *Neisseria gonorrhoeae* and *Chlamydia trachomatis*. It also may occur as a complication of prostatectomy.

Symptoms include pain, chills, fever, and malaise, with scrotal swelling so great that it interferes with ambulation and produces congestion of the testes. Necrosis and fibrosis may occlude the genital ducts and result in sterility. Treatment includes bed rest, scrotal elevation, sitz baths, hot or cold applications, and antibiotics appropriate for the organism.

## Prostate Gland

The prostate gland maintains its normal size until about age 50. At this point, in some men, it begins to decrease in size. This atrophy is associated with a decrease in testosterone level and usually produces no symptoms. Other alterations in prostate function normally occur in adult life and involve an enlargement of the prostate gland. These conditions include prostatitis, benign prostatic hyperplasia (BPH), and carcinoma.

## Prostatitis

Prostatitis, inflammation of the prostate gland, usually results from ascending infection of the urethra; it also may result from (1) descending infection from the bladder or kidneys; (2) hematogenous spread from teeth, skin, or gastrointestinal or respiratory system; or (3) lymphogenous spread from rectal bacteria. This condition occurs in three forms: (1) acute bacterial, (2) chronic bacterial, and (3) chronic abacterial.

*Acute bacterial prostatitis* is caused by the same organisms that produce urinary tract infections. The most frequent causative organism is *E. coli*, which ascends from the urethra.

Manifestations of acute bacterial prostatitis include chills and fever, dysuria, urinary frequency and urgency, and hematuria. It also may be associated with suprapubic, perineal, or scrotal pain and purulent urethral discharge. On rectal examination, the prostate is enlarged, tender,

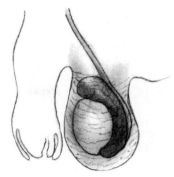

**FIGURE 55-22.**
Acute epididymitis. An acute inflamed epididymis is tender and swollen, and may be difficult to distinguish from the testis. The scrotum may be reddened, and the vas deferens also may be inflamed. Epididymitis chiefly occurs in adults. Coexisting urinary tract infection or prostatitis supports the diagnosis. (B. Bates, *A Guide to Physical Examination and History Taking* [5th ed.]. Philadelphia: J.B. Lippincott, 1991.)

and warm. The seminal vesicles also may be palpated, since infection of these organs frequently accompanies prostatitis. Urinalysis may be positive for blood and pus cells. Urine cultures aid in diagnosis of the specific organism. Although prostate massage can aid in identification of the organism, it should be used judiciously, since it can precipitate bacteremia. Catheterization, if performed on a man with acute prostatitis, may be responsible for spreading the inflammation into the bladder. Appropriate antibiotics, analgesics, and sitz baths, if instituted early, usually resolve the condition. The infection may become chronic if it is not adequately treated.

*Chronic bacterial prostatitis* may represent a continuation of acute prostatitis that did not completely respond to antibiotics. Some men are asymptomatic, with diagnosis occurring on routine urinalysis. Clinical manifestations in other men include low-grade fever, dull perineal pain, nocturia, and dysuria. Inflammatory cells and bacteria usually are found in prostatic secretions. The infection may be resistant to antibiotics because the antibiotics do not adequately penetrate the prostate.

*Abacterial prostatitis* is the most common form of prostatitis.[3] Symptoms are mild, and include low back pain and urinary frequency and urgency with rectal, urethral, or perineal discomfort. Physical examination usually reveals a nontender prostate with normal urine and prostate fluid. Evidence of inflammation (ie, lymphocytes) may be present. Chronic abacterial prostatitis may be related to excessive alcohol or caffeine intake.

## Benign Prostatic Hyperplasia

BPH, enlargement of the prostate, is a common condition that affects most men over age 50. As many as 95% of men over age 70 are affected.[3] Hyperplasia occurs, and produces large, fairly discrete nodules located in the median and lateral lobes. Enlarging nodules compress the prostatic portion of the urethra, producing symptoms of urinary obstruction. Because of the obstructive nature of BPH, the pathogenesis and clinical manifestations are discussed in Chapter 34, with obstructions of the genitourinary tract.

## Cancer of the Prostate

The American Cancer Society estimated an incidence of 106,000 new cases of prostate cancer in 1990. When skin cancer is excluded, prostate cancer is the most common cancer in men.[2] It also is the second leading cause of cancer deaths in men.[2] Prostate cancer primarily occurs in men over age 50, with a peak incidence at about age 75.

Adenocarcinoma, with varying degrees of differentiation, from well differentiated to poorly differentiated, is the usual form of prostate cancer. Tumors that are poorly differentiated are more invasive. The disease most frequently occurs in the posterior lobe; hard, fixed nodules can be palpated on rectal examination. In the early stages, it produces no symptoms. For this reason, metastasis is common, with the most frequent sites being bones, lungs, lymph nodes, and liver. Early symptoms are those of urethral obstruction, and by this time, it usually is associated with metastasis.

Based on inconclusive data, risk factors associated with increased incidence of prostate cancer include age, race, genetic predisposition, hormonal influences, venereal disease, and environmental factors (dietary fat and chemical carcinogens). As noted earlier, the incidence of prostate cancer increases with age. It occurs more often in Afro-Americans than in Caucasians.

Research studies indicate that among environmental factors, dietary fat may be important. The incidence of prostate cancer among Japanese and Polish men is very low. When these men immigrate to parts of the world that have a higher incidence, their chance of developing prostate cancer increases.[1]

As in other forms of cancer, disease staging becomes important in determining appropriate therapy. Although a number of staging classifications have been proposed, the tumor-node-metastasis (TNM) staging classification for cancer of the prostate is summarized in Table 55-6.[1]

Stage I represents a small, localized lesion. It is clinically unsuspected and not detectable on rectal examina-

**TABLE 55–6.**
STAGING OF PROSTATE CANCER

| STAGE | OCCURRENCE (%) | INVOLVEMENT |
|---|---|---|
| **Primary Cancer** | | |
| T1 | 5–10 | Rectal examination reveals no palpable tumor |
| a | | Microscopic examination—≤3 high-power fields of carcinoma |
| b | | Microscopic examination—>3 high-power fields of carcinoma |
| T2 | 20 | Tumor palpable on examination |
| a | | Diameter <1.5 cm; surrounded by normal tissue; confined to single lateral lobe |
| b | | Diameter >1.5 cm; involves both lobes |
| T3 | 40–45 | Tumor progression into or beyond capsule |
| a | | Periprostatic tissues; seminal vesicle |
| b | | Tumor >6 cm; extension into periprostatic tissues; one or both seminal vesicles |
| T4 | | Fixed or adjacent structures |
| **Regional Lymph Nodes**[a] | | |
| N0 | | Pelvic lymph nodes not involved |
| N1 | | Single pelvic node on same side |
| N2 | | Bilateral, multiple or lymph node oposite tumor site |
| N3 | | Mass fixed on pelvic wall |
| **Distant Metastasis** | | |
| M0 | | None |
| M1 | | Present |

[a]*Staging based on histologic examination.*

tion. This stage frequently is found at autopsy or during surgery for BPH. Stage II represents a localized lesion that is palpable rectally. Stage III indicates extracapsular extension of the lesion. It is palpable on rectal examination and may involve the seminal vesicles. The acid phosphatase level may be elevated. In stage IV, metastases to various organs, pelvic nodes, and distant lymph nodes have occurred. Bone metastasis frequently results in elevation of alkaline phosphatase levels.

Probably the most beneficial of all diagnostic tools is the rectal examination. It should be performed during annual examinations in all men over age 40. Because most tumors arise in the posterior lobe, palpation usually is easy. A relatively new procedure aimed at diagnosing prostate cancer in the early stages is prostate ultrasonography. Additional diagnostic studies include measuring levels of acid phosphatase and alkaline phosphatase, biopsy of detectable lesions of the posterior lobe, and CT scanning or radiography of the spine and pelvis if scans are unavailable. Cystoscopy and lymphangiography also aid in diagnosing the extent of the disease.

Treatment depends on the stage of the disease and the person's age and symptoms. Options include surgery or radiation therapy or both, hormones, and chemotherapy. Hormonal therapy is aimed at decreasing testosterone levels and consists of estrogens. Gonadotropin releasing hormone analogues may be used to decrease production of pituitary gonadotropin and testicular androgens. These analogues have an associated decrease in the risk of cardiovascular disease and thromboembolism. The 5-year survival rate is 84% when diagnosis of a localized lesion is made. The overall 5-year survival rate for all stages has increased to 70%.[2]

## Diethylstilbestrol Exposure

The use of DES in the treatment of threatened spontaneous abortion rapidly increased from the late 1940s through the 1960s. The effects of in utero exposure of the female fetus to this drug has been known and publicized for years. It was not until the late 1970s that evidence associating in utero exposure of the male fetus to DES with certain reproductive anomalies began to emerge.

Reported anomalies involve the urethra, epididymis, testes, and semen. Urethral anomalies include meatal stenosis and hypospadias. More specifically, DES exposure has been associated with low sperm counts, abnormally shaped sperm, and decreased ejaculate volume. Congenital anomalies in males include undescended as well as underdeveloped testes, testicular cysts, and abnormal meatal openings.

## REFERENCES

1. American Cancer Society, Massachusetts Division. *Cancer Manual* (7th ed.). Boston: American Cancer Society, 1986.
2. American Cancer Society. *Cancer Facts & Figures—1990.* Atlanta: American Cancer Society, 1990.
3. Cotran, R.S., Kumar, V., and Robbins, S.L. *Robbin's Pathologic Basis of Disease* (4th ed.). Philadelphia: W.B. Saunders, 1989.
4. Guyton, A.C. *Textbook of Medical Physiology* (8th ed.). Philadelphia: W.B. Saunders, 1990.
5. Higgs, D.J. The patient with testicular cancer: Nursing management of chemotherapy. *Oncol. Nurs. Forum* 17(2):243-249, 1990.

# chapter 56

Sharron P. Schlosser

# Normal and Altered Female Reproductive Function

## Chapter Outline

## Learning Objectives

1. Describe the development and function of the female sex organs.
2. List the functions of estrogen, progesterone, prolactin, and prostaglandins.
3. Describe hypothalamic and pituitary influence on the menstrual cycle.
4. List and discuss the three phases of the menstrual cycle.
5. Describe the phases involved in the female response in the sex act.
6. Discuss oogenesis.
7. Describe fertilization and implantation.
8. Define *menopause* and discuss the physiologic basis for the associated symptoms.
9. Define the various diagnostic tests used in diagnosis of female reproductive alterations.
10. Give the normal values for laboratory tests used in the diagnosis of alterations in female reproduction.
11. Define *endometriosis*.

(continued)

## Learning Objectives (Continued)

**12.** List the clinical manifestations of endometriosis and its pathologic basis.

**13.** Distinguish between primary and secondary dysmenorrhea.

**14.** Discuss the role of prostaglandins in dysmenorrhea.

**15.** Define *dysfunctional uterine bleeding.*

**16.** Distinguish between primary and secondary amenorrhea.

**17.** Compare and contrast the forms of vaginitis with respect to causative organisms, clinical manifestations, and diagnostic studies.

**18.** Distinguish between cervical erosion and eversion.

**19.** Define *toxic shock syndrome* and give its clinical manifestations.

**20.** Compare and contrast uterine fibroids and endometrial cancer.

**21.** Distinguish between functional ovarian cysts, benign neoplastic tumors of the ovary, and ovarian cancer.

**22.** Compare and contrast the three types of trophoblastic disease.

**23.** Discuss the sequential process of cellular proliferation of cervical cancer.

**24.** Describe the effects of diethylstilbestrol (DES) administration on mothers and offspring.

**25.** Describe the staging systems of cancer of the ovary, breast, cervix, and endometrium.

**26.** List the three influences on breast cancer currently under study.

For many women, the ability to conceive and bear children is an essential part of being a woman. Alterations in this function represent a threat to body image and self-concept. Alterations may occur in all reproductive organs and with no consideration of age. This chapter provides an overview of the anatomy and physiology fundamental to understanding alterations in female reproduction as well as a discussion of these alterations.

## ANATOMY

The female reproductive organs include both essential and accessory organs (Figures 56-1 and 56-2). The essential organs are the ovaries, which produce ova. The accessory organs include the fallopian tubes, uterus, and vagina, which serve as ducts; Bartholin's, Skene's, and mammary glands; and external genitalia.

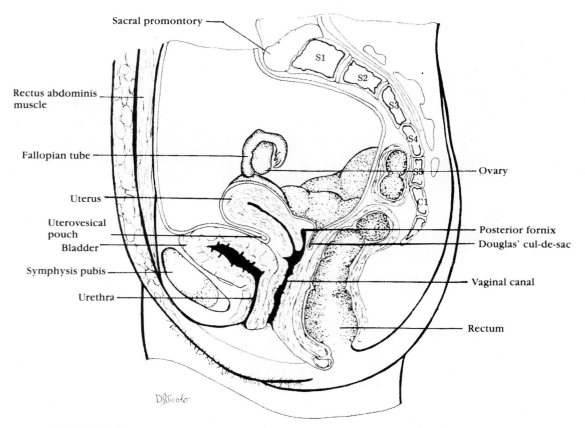

**FIGURE 56–1.**
Side view of female genitourinary anatomy. (M.A. Miller and D.A. Brooten, *The Childbearing Family: A Nursing Perspective* [2nd ed.]. Boston: Little, Brown, 1983.)

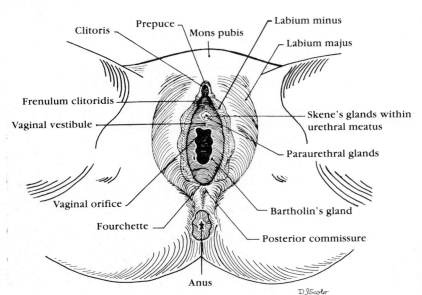

**FIGURE 56–2.**
External female genitalia. (M.A. Miller and D.A. Brooten, *The Childbearing Family: A Nursing Perspective* [2nd ed.]. Boston: Little, Brown, 1983.)

## Ovaries

The ovaries are two nodular, ovoid glands located on either side of the uterus. Each ovary is 3.5 cm long, 2 cm wide, and 1 cm thick and is attached by three ligaments: mesovarium, ovarian, and suspensory (Figure 56-3). The mesovarium ligament, an extension of the broad liga-

ment, attaches the ovary to the back of the broad ligament, and the ovarian ligament attaches the ovary to the uterus. The suspensory ligament is an extension of the broad ligament beyond the fallopian tubes, and attaches the ovary to the pelvic wall. The broad ligament is an extension of the parietal peritoneum, and supports the fallopian tubes and uterus. The ovaries perform the vital

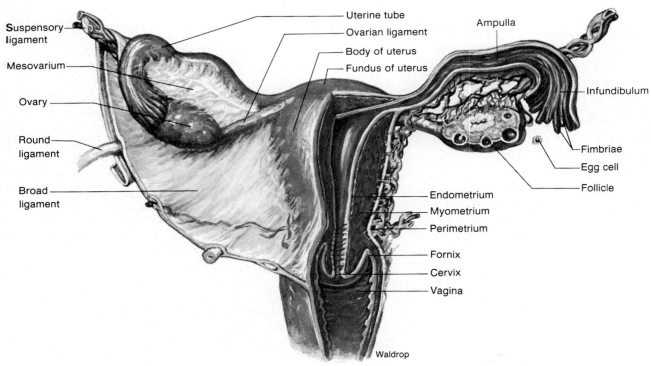

**FIGURE 56–3.**
Anterior view of female reproductive organs showing the relation of the ovaries, uterine tubes, uterus, cervix, and vagina. (K.M. Van DeGraaff and S.I. Fox, *Concepts of Human Anatomy and Physiology* [2nd ed.]. Dubuque, IA: Wm. C. Brown, 1989.)

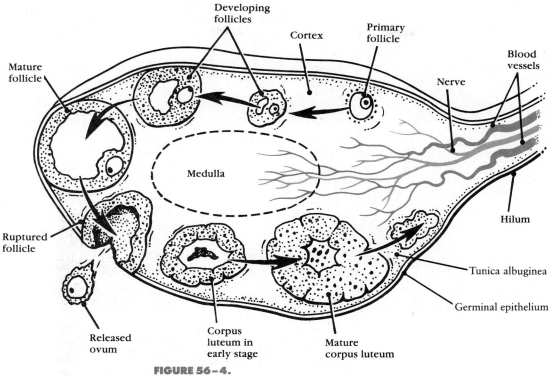

**FIGURE 56-4.**
Three layers of the ovary: cortex, medulla, and hilum.

functions of ovulation and hormone secretion. The regulation of these functions are discussed in more depth in Chapter 36.

The ovary consists of four layers: (1) the germinal epithelium, (2) the tunica albuginea, (3) the cortex, and (4) the medulla (Figure 56-4). The germinal epithelium is the covering on the outer portion of the ovary. The tunica albuginea is a layer of collagenous connective tissue just below the germinal epithelium. The cortex is composed of fine areolar stroma, blood vessels, and follicles containing ova at various stages of development. The medial portion of the ovary is the hilum, where nerves and blood vessels enter the ovary. It is composed of connective tissue and hilar cells, which secrete steroid hormones. The inner portion is the medulla, which is composed of stroma or connective tissue, smooth muscle, blood and lymph vessels, and nerves.

## Uterus

The uterus is a hollow, pear-shaped, highly muscular organ that, in the nonpregnant state, is 7 cm long, 5 cm wide, and 2.5 cm in diameter. It consists of three parts: (1) the dome-shaped fundus, located above the entrance of the tubes; (2) the corpus, or body, located below the entrance of the tubes; and (3) the cervix, which is the lowest and narrowest portion (Figure 56-5). The uterus

is located posterior to the bladder and anterior to the rectum. It is essential in menstruation, pregnancy, and labor.

The uterine walls are composed of three layers: (1) endometrium, (2) myometrium, and (3) peritoneum, also known as the perimetrium (see Figure 56-5). The endometrium is the mucous membrane lining of the body of the uterus. It consists of three layers of tissue: (1) stratum compactum, (2) stratum spongiosum, and (3) stratum basale. The *stratum compactum* is the surface layer, and consists of partially ciliated simple columnar epithelium. The *stratum spongiosum* is the spongy middle layer of loose connective tissue. Both the stratum compactum and the stratum spongiosum slough during menstruation and after delivery. The *stratum basale* is the dense inner layer that attaches to the myometrium.

The myometrium is the thick middle layer that consists of three layers of smooth-muscle fibers supported by connective tissue. This layer blends into the endometrium and provides great strength for the uterus. The myometrial layer is thickest in the fundus, which allows for more force during the contractions of labor, aiding in delivery.

The third layer of the uterine wall, the peritoneum, consists of a thin, serous membrane covering almost all of the uterus. On the anterior surface, the peritoneum is reflected onto the bladder below the internal os of the cervix.

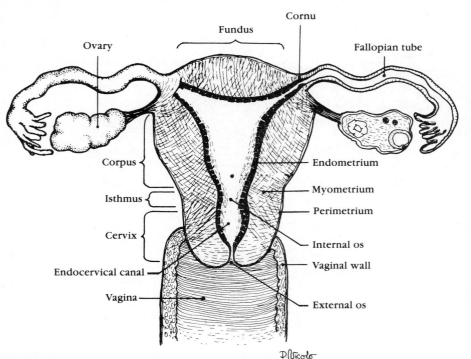

**FIGURE 56–5.**
Internal female reproductive organs. (M.A. Miller and D.A. Brooten, *The Childbearing Family: A Nursing Perspective* [2nd ed.]. Boston: Little, Brown, 1983.)

The uterus is mainly supported by the levator ani muscles and eight ligaments, which include two broad ligaments, two uterosacral ligaments, and a posterior, an anterior, and two round ligaments. The broad ligaments are extensions of the parietal peritoneum that extend from the walls and floor of the pelvis to the lateral walls of the uterus. The uterosacral ligaments also are extensions of the peritoneum. They connect the uterus and sacrum by extending from the pelvic floor around the rectum to the sacrum. The round ligaments are fibromuscular cords that extend from the upper outer portion of the uterus through the inguinal canals and terminate in the labia majora. The outer ligaments are extensions of the peritoneum (Figure 56-6).

Two of these ligaments are of particular importance because of the pouches they form. The posterior ligament forms the rectouterine pouch (or cul-de-sac of Douglas) as it extends from the posterior surface of the uterus to the rectum (see Figure 56-1). This is the lowest point of the pelvic cavity.

The anterior ligament forms the uterovesical pouch as it extends from the anterior uterus to the posterior bladder. This pouch is not as deep as the rectouterine pouch.

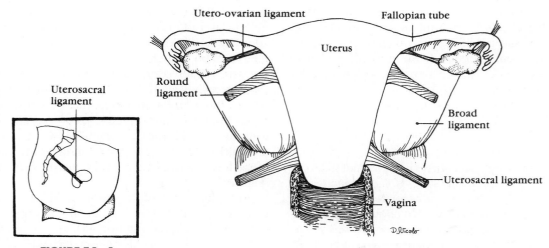

**FIGURE 56–6.**
Ligaments supporting the uterus in the pelvic cavity. (M.A. Miller and D.A. Brooten, *The Childbearing Family: A Nursing Perspective* [2nd ed.]. Boston: Little, Brown, 1983.)

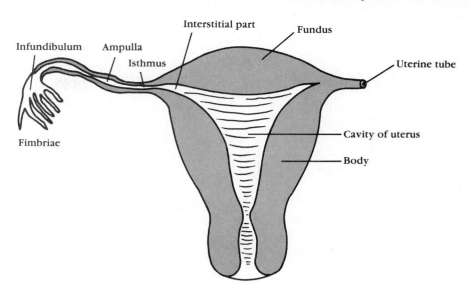

**FIGURE 56-7.**
Fallopian tube and uterus. (R.S. Snell, *Clinical Anatomy for Medical Students* [2nd ed.]. Boston: Little, Brown, 1981.)

## Fallopian Tubes

The fallopian tubes are slender, muscular tubes about 10 cm in length and 0.7 cm in diameter. They are located in the folds of the broad ligaments and attached at the upper outer angles of the uterus. These structures are the passageway through which the ova travel to the uterus and are the normal site for conception.

The fallopian tubes consist of four sections: (1) interstitial section, (2) isthmus, (3) ampulla, and (4) infundibulum (Figure 56-7). The interstitial section is short and narrow, and lies within the muscular wall of the uterus. The isthmus is the straight part with a thick, muscular wall and narrow lumen. It is adjacent to the uterus and is the usual site for tubal ligation. The ampulla, the longest, widest section, is thin-walled with a highly folded lining. The wide distal opening near the ovary is the infundibulum, or fimbriated end. Through muscular action, the fimbriae wave back and forth to create a current that moves ova toward the infundibulum.

Three histologic layers compose the wall of the fallopian tube: (1) serous, (2) muscularis, and (3) mucosa. The serous layer is the outer lubricative layer formed by part of the visceral peritoneum. The muscularis layer consists of two layers of smooth muscle whose peristaltic contractions aid in movement of the ovum through the tube. The mucosa layer is the inner lining and consists of ciliated columnar cells.

## Vagina

The vagina is a musculomembranous canal located anterior to the rectum and posterior to the urethra. It is about 9 cm long and extends upward from the vulva to the mid-point of the cervix. It is the passageway both for menstrual flow and for the fetus during delivery, and is the recipient for the penis during sexual intercourse.

The wall of the vagina is composed of three layers: (1) mucosal, (2) muscularis, and (3) fibrous. The mucosal layer consists of stratified squamous epithelial cells arranged in small transverse folds called rugae. The muscularis is composed of smooth muscle and connective tissue with the ability to distend. The fibrous layer is the outer layer that attaches to the pelvic organs. It is composed of dense fibrous connective tissue and elastic fibers. The vagina contains no glands, but the epithelial cells of the mucosa undergo changes in response to estrogen. Without the influence of estrogen, the epithelium is thin and consists almost entirely of basal cells. The mucosal cells also contain a considerable amount of glycogen.

## Bartholin's Glands

The Bartholin's (or greater vestibular) glands are two bean-shaped, mucus-secreting glands located on each side of the vaginal orifice (Figure 56-8). Secretion is increased during sexual excitement and moistens the inner surface of the labia in preparation for intercourse. The duct may become obstructed or infected, particularly by gonococci, and Bartholin's cyst or abscess may be formed (Figure 56-9).

## Skene's Glands

Skene's glands are tiny, mucus-secreting glands located just posterior to the external urethral meatus (see Fig-

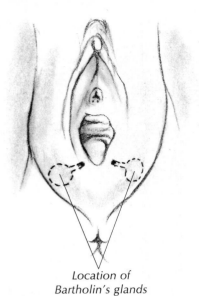

Location of
Bartholin's glands

**FIGURE 56-8.**
Location of Bartholin's glands. (B. Bates, *A Guide to Physical Examination and History Taking* [4th ed.]. Philadelphia: J.B. Lippincott, 1987.)

ure 56-2). The mucus from the Skene's glands, together with mucus from glands in the urethra, keeps the urethral opening moist and lubricated. The Skene's glands also are susceptible to infection by gonococci, which are difficult to eradicate from this location.

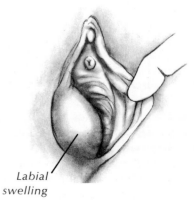

Labial
swelling

**FIGURE 56-9.**
Inflammation of Bartholin's gland. Inflammation of Bartholin's glands may be acute or chronic. Causes include gonococci, *Chlamydia trachomatis*, and other organisms. Acutely, it appears as a tense, hot, tender abscess. Look for pus coming out of the duct or erythema around the duct opening. Chronically, a nontender cyst occupies the posterior labium. It may be large or small. (B. Bates, *A Guide to Physical Examination and History Taking* [5th ed.]. Philadelphia: J.B. Lippincott, 1991.)

## Breasts

The breasts, which contain the mammary glands, are two skin glands located over the pectoral muscles between the second and sixth ribs. The breasts extend from the lateral sternum to the anterior border of the axilla. The portion of the breast that extends upward and laterally to the axilla is called the breast tail, and lies in proximity to blood and lymph vessels. The breasts are attached by a layer of connective tissue. Each breast consists of a nipple and surrounding areola, lobes, ducts, and fibrous and fatty tissue (Figure 56-10). The function of the breast is to secrete milk to nourish the newborn infant.

The nipple, a cylindric projection near the center of the breast, is located approximately in the fourth intercostal space. It is surrounded by a pigmented, circular area, the areola, and is perforated by ductal openings. Sexual stimulation results in engorgement and muscle contraction, which causes the nipple to become erect.

The mature female breast is made up of 15 to 20 lobes arranged around the nipple. Each lobe is further composed of a number of lobules. Inside each lobule are the alveoli, which contain both myoepithelial and acinar cells. The acinar cells are secretory cells in lactation, and the myoepithelial cells contract to force milk into the ducts.

Each lobule is drained by intralobular ducts that empty into the lactiferous duct. These ducts dilate into a reservoir, called the lactiferous sinus or ampulla, just before they open in the nipple. Lobes and ducts are separated by fibrous tissue. Fatty tissue contributes to breast size.

Lymph drainage of the breast is important, especially in breast cancer. Lymph vessels normally follow the lactiferous ducts and eventually drain into the central axillary nodes (Figure 56-11). This creates drainage of the superficial and areolar as well as glandular parts of the breast. Blood is supplied by branches of the thoracic artery.

During puberty, breast development is controlled by estrogen and progesterone. Estrogen stimulates deposits of adipose tissue and growth of the glands and ducts, and progesterone stimulates development of the secreting cells. Pregnancy and lactation are associated with hypertrophy of the breasts; menopause may produce an atrophy of the breasts.

## External Genitalia

The external genitalia, commonly called the vulva, consists of the mons pubis, labia majora, labia minora, clitoris, urinary meatus, vaginal orifice, and vestibule (see Figure 56-2). Sometimes Bartholin's glands are considered part of the vulva. The *mons pubis* is a subcutaneous pad of adipose connective tissue that covers the symphysis. It

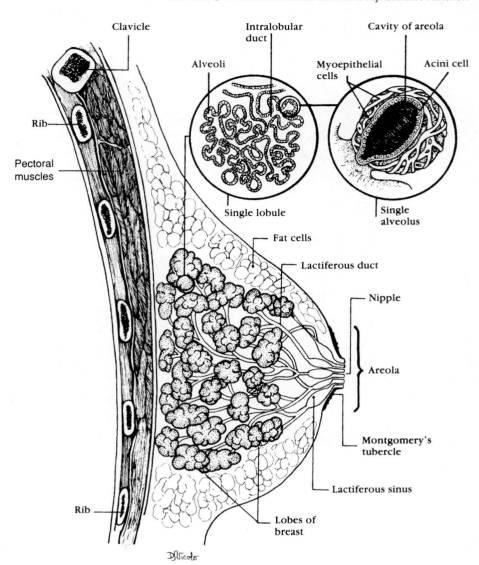

**FIGURE 56–10.**
Breast and ductal system. (Adapted from
M.A. Miller and D.A. Brooten, *The Childbearing Family: A Nursing Perspective*
[2nd ed.]. Boston: Little, Brown, 1983.)

is covered with coarse pubic hair at puberty. The *labia
majora* consists of two prominent longitudinal folds of
pigmented skin that extend down and back from the
mons pubis. They are 7 to 8 cm in length and 2 to 3 cm
wide. The labia majora are composed of areolar and
adipose tissue as well as extensive lymph vessels, and
are covered on the outside with hair. Both sebaceous
and sweat glands are contained within the labia majora.
On the inside, the labia majora are smooth and moist.
The labia majora are synonymous with the scrotum in
the male.

The *labia minora* are two smaller thin folds that lie
within the labia majora. They extend down and back from
the clitoris. The labia minora contain no hair but are rich
in sebaceous glands. The *clitoris* is a small, rounded projection, highly sensitive to touch. It is 5 to 6 mm long and
6 to 8 mm wide. The clitoris is composed of erectile tissue and is synonymous in origin with the penis. The *ves-

tibule* is an almond-shaped flat area that extends from the
clitoris to the fourchette. It is bordered by the labia minora, and contains openings to the urethral orifice, vaginal orifice, Bartholin's glands, and Skene's glands.

## FEMALE REPRODUCTIVE FUNCTIONS

Female reproductive functions, which begin with puberty
and end with menopause, fall into two phases: (1) preparation of the body for conception and gestation, and
(2) gestation. The specific functions include the reproductive cycle, production of female hormones, the sex
act, and gestation.

The female reproductive cycle involves many periodic changes throughout the life span or from menarche
to menopause. Successful reproductive function depends
on changes that occur in the ovaries, endometrium, myo-

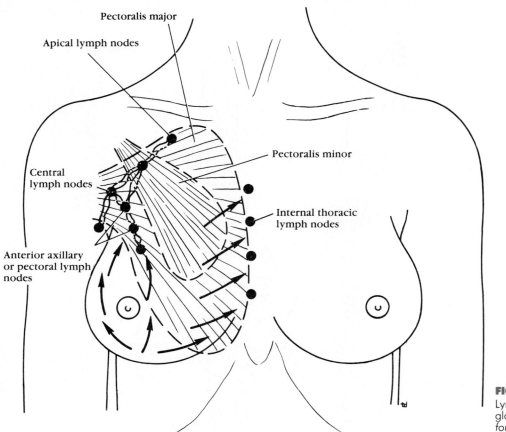

**FIGURE 56–11.**
Lymphatic drainage of mammary glands. (R.S. Snell, *Clinical Anatomy for Medical Students* [2nd ed.]. Boston: Little, Brown, 1981.)

metrium, breasts, vagina, and endocrine glands, and on changes in body temperature. Even the woman's emotions are affected by these changes. Various organs respond differently to the changes, but all can be related to the menstrual cycle.

## Hypothalamic Influence

Cyclic changes in the reproductive cycle begin with hormonal changes initiated by the hypothalamus, which is considered to be part of both the nervous and the endocrine systems. Both physical and emotional stressors can affect menstrual regularity through the nervous control of the hypothalamus. Depending on the messages it receives, the hypothalamus then secretes hormones called *releasing* or *inhibiting factors*, which act directly on the pituitary gland (Figure 56-12). Neurosecretory substances that are secreted by the hypothalamus and transported through the hypothalamic-hypophyseal portal system to the anterior pituitary include (1) follicle-stimulating hormone releasing factor, (2) luteinizing hormone releasing factor, and (3) luteotropic hormone inhibiting

factor. These factors act on the anterior pituitary to control the gland's secretion. *Oxytocin*, secreted by the posterior pituitary, increases uterine contractions during labor and moves milk from breast glands to nipples during sucking.

## Pituitary Influence

The anterior pituitary secretes two hormones that directly influence reproductive function: follicle-stimulating hormone (FSH) and luteinizing hormone (LH). Together with estrogen and progesterone, FSH and LH act directly on the ovaries to control ovulation. The release of FSH and LH is regulated by feedback effects of estrogen and progesterone on the hypothalamus (see Figure 56-12).

Additionally, the anterior pituitary secretes *prolactin*, also called luteotropic hormone. Prolactin acts on the breasts to control lactation after delivery. The release of prolactin is prevented by the prolactin inhibiting factor, which is controlled by high levels of estrogen or progesterone. Suckling and low estrogen levels stimulate prolactin production.

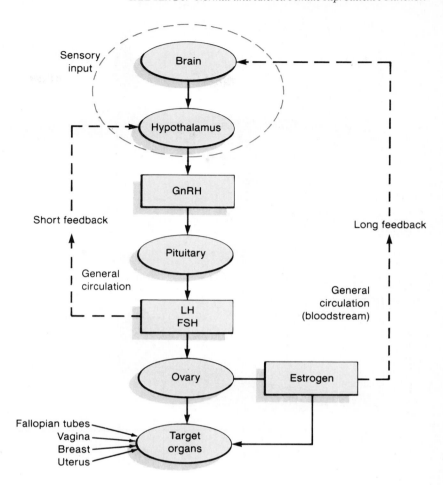

**FIGURE 56–12.**
Diagrammatic representation of the neuroendo-
crine feedback mechanisms. (K.A. May and L.R.
Mahlmeister, *Comprehensive Maternity Nursing*.
Philadelphia: J.B. Lippincott, 1990.)

## Menstrual Cycle

The menstrual cycle involves regular changes that are
repeated about every 28 days. This process may vary in
individual women but has three phases: (1) menstrual,
(2) proliferative, and (3) secretory. The proliferative
and secretory phases are separated by ovulation (Figure 56-13).

### Menstrual Phase

The menstrual phase begins with the onset of the menses
and lasts about 5 days. Average blood loss is 30 to 150 mL,
the amount varying widely among individual women.
During the menstrual phase, the blood levels of both estrogen and progesterone are low. This phase also involves degeneration and sloughing of the stratum compactum and most of the stratum spongiosum.

### Proliferative Phase

The proliferative phase follows the menstrual phase and
is accompanied by changes in the endometrium, myome-

trium, and ovaries. The cyclic changes in these organs
result from fluctuation in gonadotropin and estrogen levels. Changes in the endometrium and myometrium are
primarily controlled by blood levels of estrogen. With increasing levels of estrogen, the endometrium thickens as
the endometrial cells and arterioles grow longer and
more coiled. The water content of the endometrium and
contractions of the myometrium also increase. These
changes in the endometrium and myometrium prepare
the uterus for implantation of the fertilized ovum.

Changes in the ovaries occur in what is referred to
as the follicular phase. This ovarian phase encompasses
both the menstrual and the proliferative phases of the
menstrual cycle. Low levels of estrogen in the menstrual
phase signal the production of FSH by the anterior pituitary. In the ovaries, FSH production then stimulates the
primary follicles. At that time, a number of follicles begin
to mature. Soon only one, the *graafian follicle*, begins to
dominate while the others recede. This follicle gradually
moves to the surface of the ovary (Figure 56-14). The follicle contains the ovum, and is surrounded by a layer of
granulosa cells, which are further surrounded by specialized cells called the *theca interna* and *theca externa*. Es-

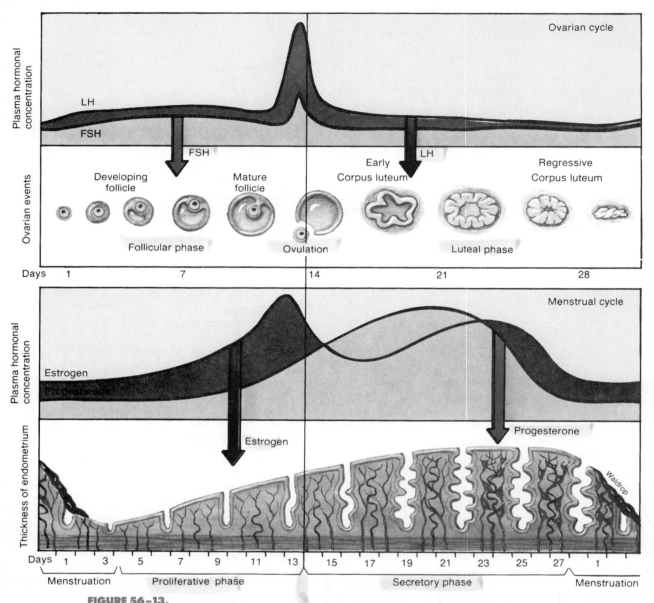

**FIGURE 56–13.**
Phases of the menstrual cycle in relation to ovarian changes and hormone secretion, and the relation between changes in the ovaries and the endometrium of the uterus during different phases of the menstrual cycle. (K.M. VanDeGraaff and S.I. Fox, *Concepts of Human Anatomy and Physiology* [2nd ed.]. Dubuque, IA: Wm. C. Brown, 1988.)

trogen is secreted by the theca interna, and the granulosa cells supply nutrition for the ova.

As the follicle enlarges, fluid begins to collect inside, pushing the ovum to one side. It is surrounded on the outside by granulosa cells called the cumulus oophorus. A clear membrane also develops and surrounds the ovum. This inner surrounding is termed the zona pellucida. Outside the zona pellucida and inside the cumulus oophorus is a single layer of cells called the corona radiata. While these changes are occurring within the follicle, the anterior pituitary begins gradual secretion of LH, which stimulates the follicles to increase estrogen production.

High levels of estrogen then signal the hypothalamus to stop producing FSH releasing factor. Production of LH continues, resulting in a surge of LH about 12 hours before ovulation. This increase triggers ovulation within 1 to 24 hours. The mature ovum is then extruded from the ovary with both the zona pellucida and corona radiata surrounding it.

## Ovulation

Ovulation divides the proliferative and secretory phases of the menstrual cycle, and usually occurs 14 days before

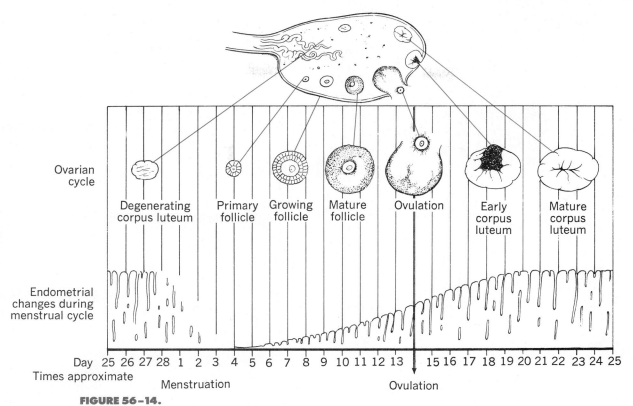

**FIGURE 56–14.**

Schematic representation of one ovarian cycle and the corresponding changes in thickness of the endometrium. It is thickest just before the onset of menstruation and thinnest just as it ceases. (S.J. Reeder and L.L. Martin, *Maternity Nursing: Family Newborn, and Women's Health Care* [16th ed.]. Philadelphia, J.B. Lippincott, 1987.)

the onset of the next menstrual cycle. In a number of women it is accompanied by low abdominal pain, termed *mittelschmerz*. The escape of fluid or blood from the follicle is believed to produce peritoneal irritation that causes the pain.

Ovulation also is accompanied by changes in cervical mucus. Cervical mucus increases in amount as it becomes clear and thin. Under the influence of high estrogen levels, it forms a ferning pattern when allowed to dry on a slide (Figure 56-15).

## Oogenesis

Unlike spermatogenesis, which continuously produces many sperm, oogenesis is the cyclic production of a single ovum. Immediately before ovulation, the primary oocyte undergoes its first meiotic division, resulting in a secondary oocyte that contains 23 chromosomes and most of the cytoplasm. A second body is formed, and is referred to as a first polar body. This first polar body receives 23 chromosomes but little cytoplasm. The secondary oocyte then undergoes a second meiotic division. Both cells again contain 23 chromosomes but only one receives the majority of cytoplasm. This cell is the *mature ovum*. The second cell is known as a second polar body. Meiosis is arrested at this phase if fertilization does not

occur. Figure 56-16 shows the maturation of one mature ovum.

## Secretory Phase

The secretory phase begins with ovulation, and is characterized by (1) formation of the corpus luteum in

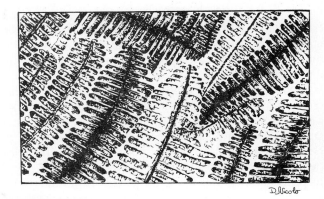

**FIGURE 56–15.**

Fern pattern seen on microscopic examination of cervical mucus at midcycle in normal menstruating women. (M.A. Miller and D.A. Brooten, *The Childbearing Family: A Nursing Perspective* [2nd ed.]. Boston: Little, Brown, 1983.)

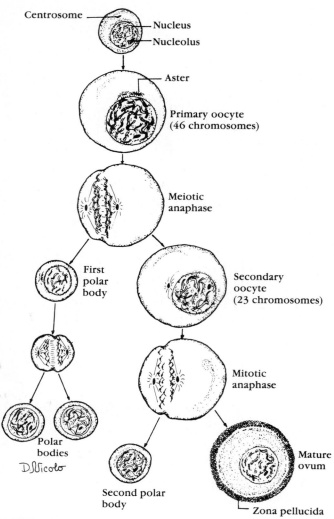

**FIGURE 56-16.**
Maturation of female reproductive cells resulting in formation of one mature ovum. (M.A. Miller and D.A. Brooten, *The Childbearing Family: A Nursing Perspective* [2nd ed.]. Boston: Little, Brown, 1983.)

the ovary, (2) production of progesterone and estrogen, (3) secretory changes in the endometrium, and (4) decreased contractions in the myometrium. This phase of the menstrual cycle corresponds with the luteal phase in the ovary.

During the luteal phase in the ovary, follicle walls collapse with some hemorrhage into the cavity, forming a corpus hemorrhagia. Under the influence of LH, the granulosa cells hypertrophy, take on a yellow color, and become known as luteal cells. This golden body, the corpus luteum, continues to function for about 7 to 8 days. Its primary function is to secrete progesterone and some estrogen. These hormones initiate the negative feedback loop to the hypothalamus and pituitary gland that prevents further ovulation within the cycle.

In the absence of fertilization, luteal cells begin to degenerate, causing a decrease in estrogen and proges-

terone levels. The corpus luteum eventually is converted into the corpus albicans, which moves to the center of the ovary and finally disappears.

The production of progesterone by the corpus luteum leads to secretory changes in the endometrium that create a favorable environment for pregnancy. Increase in the endometrium at this time is believed to be due to swelling from increased water content rather than cellular proliferation. The endometrium becomes more vascular, with coiled spiral arteries located close to the surface. The changes produce a thick, succulent environment, rich in glycogen and ideal for implantation of the fertilized ovum.

Progesterone also is associated with a decrease in myometrial contractions. In addition, women may notice fluid retention, breast tenderness and fullness, as well as moodiness and premenstrual tension from the high levels of progesterone. Increased levels of progesterone also cause an increase in basal body temperature during the secretory phase of the menstrual cycle. This characteristic of progesterone provides the basis for basal temperature studies for women with fertility problems.

In the absence of fertilization and implantation, progesterone secretion falls, which is a signal for the beginning of a new cycle. Degenerated endometrium sloughs, the hypothalamus begins to secrete releasing factors, and the cycle begins again.

## Production of Female Hormones

Estrogen and progesterone are the two primary female hormones. Others are androgen, prolactin, and the prostaglandins.

### Estrogen

Estrogen is a general term for a class of hormones predominantly present in the female. It is a steroid hormone primarily secreted by the ovaries and by the placenta during pregnancy, with a small amount being secreted by the adrenal cortices. There are a number of natural estrogens, but only three are potent enough to produce physiologic effects: estradiol, estrone, and estriol. The major estrogen, estradiol, is the most potent (12 times more than estrone), but the ovaries secrete about 4 times more estrone. Both estradiol and estrone can be identified in venous blood from the ovary, and estriol is oxidized mainly in the liver from estradiol and estrone.

After being secreted by the ovaries, estradiol and estrone either enter cells to perform their functions or are oxidized principally in the liver to estriol. Estrogens are inactivated in the liver through conjugation with sulfuric acid and glucuronic acid. The glucuronides and sulfates are then excreted in the bile. Estrogens in extracellular fluids are primarily in the form of estroprotein, another process accomplished in the liver. This inactivation process accounts for the ineffectiveness of the natural estrogens when administered orally. Conditions that depress liver function also may be associated with increased estrogen levels because of the absence of the inactivation process.

In the clinical setting, two other forms of estrogen may be used: synthetic and conjugated. The synthetic estrogens are of particular importance because of their potency when administered orally. Estrogen affects cell proliferation and development of the female secondary sex characteristics as well as the previously described effect on the menstrual cycle.

Throughout childhood, small quantities of estrogen are produced, but at puberty, the levels greatly increase. As a result of estrogen influence, the sex organs, including external genitalia, breasts, ovaries, fallopian tubes, uterus, and vagina, increase in size. Vaginal epithelium thickens and differentiates into layers that increase the resistance of the vagina to injury and infection. The epithelium also increases its glycogen levels. Estrogens also affect the fat deposits in the vulva and mons pubis, growth of the pelvis, and distribution of axillary and pubic hair.

The onset of puberty is associated with a rapid growth rate in the female. Estrogens cause early uniting of the epiphyses and shafts of the long bones, causing female growth to cease earlier than male growth. They also affect calcium and phosphate retention, which is important in menopause when estrogen levels are greatly reduced.

Estrogens influence the skin and capillary walls. With increased levels of estrogen, the skin becomes soft, smooth, and thicker than that of a child. It also is more vascular. For this reason, women may bleed more when cut or note increased skin warmth. In addition, the capillary walls become stronger. When estrogen levels are low, there is a greater tendency toward bruising.

### Progesterone

Progesterone often is considered the hormone of pregnancy because of its effect on the endometrium and myometrium (see Chap. 36). It is produced almost exclusively by the corpus luteum in the nonpregnant female and by the placenta during pregnancy. Chemically, natural progesterone is similar to estrogen. It is less potent than estrogen, and is secreted in larger amounts. Shortly after secretion, it is degraded to pregnanediol and excreted in this form in the urine.

In addition to its uterine effects, progesterone affects the breasts. Whereas estrogen is responsible for breast growth, progesterone is responsible for maturation of lobules and alveoli, so that they may become secretory when stimulated by prolactin.

### Androgens

Female androgens are secreted in small amounts by the adrenal glands and ovaries. In disruptions of female function, the amount of secretions can become significant and result in masculine hair distribution, acne, and deepening of the voice.

### Prolactin

Prolactin is a protein hormone secreted by the anterior pituitary. Suckling during breastfeeding and low estrogen levels stimulate its release. High estrogen and progesterone levels trigger the release of prolactin inhibiting factor from the hypothalamus, thus preventing its secretion. Prolactin stimulates production of milk by the acinar cells in the alveoli. Pituitary gland tumors can cause milk production, even in the absence of pregnancy.

### Prostaglandins

Prostaglandins are a group of potent lipids that function as local hormones. They are considered important in reproductive physiology.

Prostaglandins have been separated into three groups: prostaglandin A, E, and F (PGA, PGE, and PGF). Each group exerts different actions on systems of the body. Prostaglandins are synthesized from phospholipids in various body tissues.[6] Phospholipase A, an enzyme, is responsible for liberation of essential fatty acids from the phospholipids. The essential fatty acids are then converted to PGE or PGF by prostaglandin synthetase. Prostaglandin A is the result of additional metabolism of PGE (Figure 56-17).

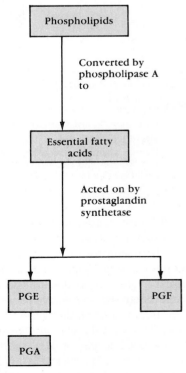

**FIGURE 56-17.**
Synthesis of prostaglandins.

**Excitement Stage**                    **Plateau Stage**

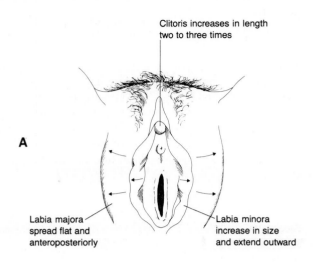

Clitoris increases in length
two to three times

Clitoris retracts under hood
(it is difficult to locate and
so tender that efforts to touch it
directly may cause discomfort)

**A**

Labia majora
spread flat and
anteroposteriorly

Labia minora
increase in size
and extend outward

Labia majora
(no further response)

Bartholin glands
secrete 1 to 3
drops

Labia minora turn bright red and increase
in size (if stimulation continues, orgasm
occurs 1 minute or 1½ minutes after
the bright red color appears)

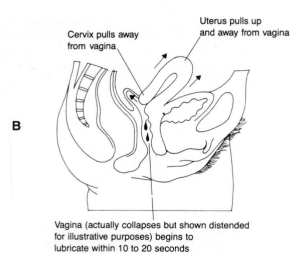

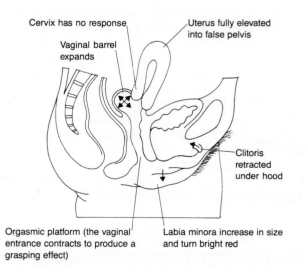

Uterus pulls up
and away from vagina

Cervix pulls away
from vagina

Cervix has no response

Uterus fully elevated
into false pelvis

Vaginal barrel
expands

**B**

Clitoris
retracted
under hood

Vagina (actually collapses but shown distended
for illustrative purposes) begins to
lubricate within 10 to 20 seconds

Inner ⅔ of vagina lengthens and distends

Orgasmic platform (the vaginal
entrance contracts to produce a
grasping effect)

Labia minora increase in size
and turn bright red

**FIGURE 56–18.**
Female sexual response cycle. **A.** Changes in external genitalia. **B.** Changes in internal genitalia.
(S.J. Reeder and L.L. Martin, *Maternity Nursing: Family, Newborn, and Women's Health Care* [16th
ed.]. Philadelphia, J.B. Lippincott, 1987.)

Prostaglandins are degraded primarily in the lungs soon after they enter the circulation. For this reason, their actions seem to be mainly local.

Although there are many prostaglandins, only $PGE_2$ and $PGF_2$ primarily affect reproduction. Both have been identified in endometrial tissue, where they exert a stimulating effect on the uterus.[9] Studies have confirmed that levels of prostaglandins vary with the menstrual cycle (Table 56-1). Elevated levels of $PGE_2$ and $PGF_2$ have been identified as a possible factor in primary dysmenorrhea. $PGE_2$ is used to induce uterine contractions for

intrauterine fetal death, missed abortion, and hydatidiform mole.

## Female Response in the Sex Act

The female response in the sex act is a normal physiologic process. Although every woman has different levels of response, the physiologic events of response occur in an orderly sequence: (1) excitation, (2) plateau, (3) orgasm, and (4) resolution (Figure 56-18).

**Orgasm Stage**

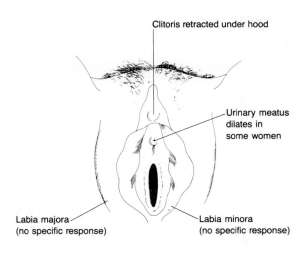

**Resolution Stage**

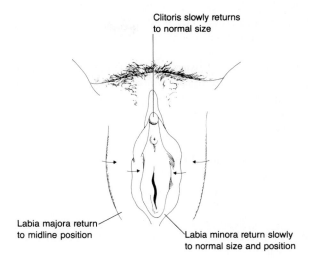

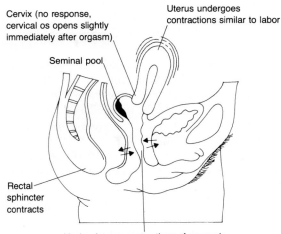

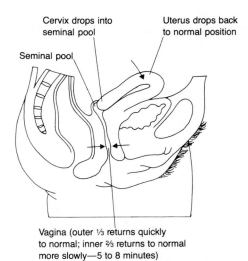

**FIGURE 56–18.** (Continued)

**TABLE 56–1.**

LEVELS OF PROSTAGLANDINS IN DIFFERENT PHASES OF THE MENSTRUAL CYCLE (ng/100 ng TISSUE)

| PROSTAGLANDIN | PROLIFERATIVE PHASE | MIDLUTEAL PHASE | MENSES |
|---|---|---|---|
| $PGE_2$ | 13–26 | 13–26 | 52 |
| $PGF_{2\alpha}$ | 10–25 | 67 | 67, maintained |

*Clithroe, H.J., and Pickles, V.R. The separation of the smooth muscle stimulants in menstrual fluid. J. Physiol. (Lond.) 156:225, 1961; and Downie, J., Poyser, N.L., and Wunderlick, M. Levels of prostaglandins in the human endometrium during the normal menstrual cycle. J. Physiol. (Lond.) 236:456, 1974.*

Excitation begins with either physical or emotional stimulation. The first response to sexual stimulation is vaginal lubrication. This is a result of vasodilatation and congestion, and can occur within 10 to 30 seconds of stimulation. Transudation of fluid, not secretion, accounts for lubrication because the vagina contains no secretory glands. Other characteristics of the excitement phase include (1) engorgement and enlargement of the labia, clitoris, and uterus; (2) enlargement and ballooning of the vagina; (3) elevation of the uterus and cervix; and (4) nipple erection. Blood pressure and pulse increase, and the "sex flush" may appear as a measleslike rash on epigastrium, chest, and throat.

The plateau phase is reached as sexual arousal is increased. Characteristics of this phase include retraction of the clitoris against the symphysis, narrowing of the vaginal opening, increased length and diameter of the vagina, deep red coloring of the labia minora, and complete elevation of the uterus. Breast size may increase in the plateau phase, and the sex flush may spread over the shoulders, inner surface of arms, and perhaps abdomen, back, and thighs. Respiratory rate also increases late in the plateau phase.

During orgasm, vasocongestion reaches its maximum and stimulates the reflex stretch mechanism. As a result, rhythmic contractions occur in the clitoris, uterus, outer one-third of the vagina, and perhaps the rectal sphincter. Rhythmic contractions also may be noted in the arms, legs, abdomen, and buttocks.

During resolution, the final phase of sexual response, the body returns to its preexcitement phase. Within 10 to 15 seconds, the clitoris returns to normal and normal color returns to the labia minora. Ten to 15 minutes are required for the vagina to return to normal, and the cervical os remains open for about 30 minutes. Unlike the male, who experiences a refractory period during resolution when he is incapable of sexual stimulation, some women are capable of several orgasms without dropping below the plateau phase. Resolution then follows the last orgasm.

## Gestation

Gestation begins with fertilization of the ovum and continues throughout the development of the fetus. A concise discussion of the biophysical development of reproduction as a basis for discussion of the alterations in normal pregnancy is provided in Chapter 4.

## Menopause

Menopause, the cessation of menstruation, marks the final phase of female reproductive function. The transition or gradual change in ovarian function is termed *climac-*

*teric*. The average age of menopause for women in the United States is 50 years. Menopause is complete when the woman has experienced no menstrual periods for 1 year.

In some women, menopause occurs abruptly with complete cessation of menstruation after normal periods. In others, gradual cessation is characterized by decreased amounts of bleeding with monthly cycles, periods of amenorrhea, and finally complete cessation of normal periods. Menopause is accompanied by decreased estrogen levels and reversal in estrogen forms. The production of all estrogens by the ovaries decreases. The primary estrogen in menopause is estrone, which is derived from androstenedione and fat conversion.

Menopause frequently is associated with other physiologic changes and symptoms. These include hot flashes, changes in reproductive organs, cardiovascular disease, osteoporosis, and nervousness and psychologic problems.[6] The most common symptom is hot flashes. These begin as a feeling of warmth in the chest and progress upward over the neck and face. They may be accompanied by flushing of the skin in these areas and profuse diaphoresis. The exact cause has not been determined, but they appear to be related to estrogen withdrawal.

Changes in reproductive organs include atrophy of the labia; dryness and thinning of vaginal walls; decreased support of bladder, rectum, and uterus; and decreased size of the uterus and cervix. These changes are all associated with lower estrogen levels, and account for such complaints as dyspareunia, stress incontinence, and vaginal itching and burning.

Evidence supports increased frequency of hypertension, stroke, and heart disease after menopause.[11] Decreased estrogen levels also are linked to osteoporosis and increased bone fragility. Estrogen administration has been shown to halt the process in young women who undergo surgical removal of the ovaries.

Psychologic symptoms associated with menopause include nervousness, depression, headache, insomnia, decreased sex drive, memory loss, vertigo, and a feeling of worthlessness and hopelessness. No connection has been identified between these symptoms and estrogen levels. Therefore, basic personality and cultural influences are of more importance in determining treatment.

## LABORATORY AND DIAGNOSTIC AIDS

### Gynecologic Examination

The most important of all diagnostic tools available is the physical examination. Gynecologic examination of the female reproductive system involves three steps: (1) external examination, (2) speculum examination, and (3) bimanual examination. External examination includes inspection and palpation of the breasts, palpation of the

**TABLE 56-2.**
NORMAL HORMONE LEVELS

| HORMONE | BLOOD | URINE |
|---|---|---|
| Pregnanediol | | |
|   Male | | <1.5 mg/24 h |
|   Female | | |
|     Proliferative phase | | 0.5–1.5 mg/24 h |
|     Luteal phase | | 2–7 mg/24 h |
|     Postmenopausal | | 0.2–1.0 mg/24 h |
| Estrogens (total) | | |
|   Male | | 4–25 μg/24 h |
|   Female | | 4–60 μg/24 h with increase in pregnancy |
| Prolactin | <20 ng/mL | |
| Progesterone | | |
|   Proliferative phase | <1.0 ng/mL | |
|   Luteal phase | <2.0 ng/mL | |
| FSH | | 6–50 mouse uterine units/24 h |
| Luteinizing hormone | | |
|   Proliferative phase | <70 mIU/mL | |
|   Luteal phase | >70 mIU/mL | |
| Estriol | | 10–20 mg/24 h |

abdomen, and inspection of the external genitalia. With these procedures, one can detect masses, redness, and swelling or lesions of the breasts and external genitalia.

The speculum examination allows for visualization of the cervix and vaginal wall and detection of redness, lesions, swelling, or unusual discharge. Specimens for laboratory tests, including Papanicolaou smear, wet smear, gonorrhea cultures, and biopsies, also may be collected at this time.

The final step is the bimanual examination, in which the uterus, ovaries, and fallopian tubes are palpated. It also usually involves either a rectal or a rectovaginal examination by which the examiner is able to palpate such pelvic structures as the posterior surface of the uterus, the uterosacral ligaments, and the cul-de-sac of Douglas.

## Hormone Levels

Both bioassay and chemical methods are available for determining ovarian hormone levels. These tests are time-consuming, difficult to perform or to standardize, and expensive. Therefore, most of the studies to detect hormone levels are indirect.

### Progesterone

Progesterone is a steroid that is degraded shortly after secretion. Most of this degradation occurs in the liver, with the major end product being pregnanediol. Because pregnanediol is excreted in the urine, its rate of excretion can be used to estimate progesterone formation. This estimation must be done by chemical means be-

cause pregnanediol exerts no progesteronic effects. Results are difficult to standardize, but the generally accepted normal values are summarized in Table 56-2.

Increased levels of progesterone may be associated with luteal cysts of the ovary, arrhenoblastoma of the ovary, and hyperadrenocorticism. Decreased levels may occur in amenorrhea, threatened abortion, fetal death, and toxemia of pregnancy.

Indirect methods of determining progesterone levels include endometrial biopsy and basal body temperature. An endometrial biopsy is useful in determining the stage of the menstrual cycle and, therefore, infers the level of hormone production. In studying basal body temperature charts, a sustained rise of 1°F implies that ovulation has taken place and that progesterone secretion is adequate.

### Estrogen

One useful laboratory test in the study of estrogen levels is measurement of 24-hour urinary estriol excretion. Because estriol is produced by the placenta, it represents both fetal and placental activity. A significant drop (40% less than the mean of three previous values) may indicate that the fetus is in jeopardy because urinary estriol excretion increases as pregnancy progresses. Incomplete 24-hour urine specimens as well as pyelonephritis have been known to affect the results. Normal findings are 10 to 20 mg/24 h.

Changes in cervical mucus and epithelial cells of the vagina are good indicators of estrogen production. Cervical mucus undergoes definite changes in response to estrogen and progesterone production. Spinnbarkeit and ferning are two characteristics of cervical mucus that can easily be studied. Spinnbarkeit refers to the elasticity of cervical mucus at the time of ovulation that allows the examiner to draw it out into a long, thin thread of 15 to 20 cm. During minimal estrogen production, threads reach only 1 to 2 cm.

Ferning refers to the pattern created when cervical mucus, under the influence of estrogen, dries (see Figure 56-15). Ferning results when sodium chloride in the mucus crystallizes. Estrogen secretion increases the sodium chloride content of cervical mucus, whereas progesterone decreases it. Therefore, the level of estrogen without progesterone determines the presence of a ferning pattern. This pattern is fullest and most complete at the time of ovulation.

Vaginal smears also are useful in determining estrogen levels because the vaginal cells undergo cyclic changes. Estrogen thickens the vaginal epithelium. Glucose excretion also corresponds to estrogen secretion. Both are highest at the time of ovulation.

## Smears

### Papanicolaou Smear

A specimen for Papanicolaou (Pap) smear is best collected from the cervical canal and the squamocolumnar junction near the external os during the speculum examination. Dry cotton swabs are used to collect cervical canal secretions, and a small wooden spatula is used for the squamocolumnar specimen (Figure 56-19). The specimen is then transferred to a glass slide where it is fixed for staining and microscopic examination. The primary purpose of a Pap smear is to screen for abnormal cervical

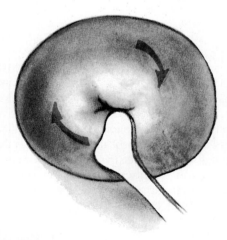

**FIGURE 56-19.**
Cervical and vaginal diagnostic tests. (B. Bates, *A Guide to Physical Examination and History Taking* [5th ed.]. Philadelphia: J.B. Lippincott, 1991.)

cells and indicate the need for more extensive testing. It also may help to detect cancer of the endometrium and vagina.

Classification of Pap smear results varies widely from institution to institution. The original system identified five classes of smears ranging from I, which was normal, to V, definitely malignant. A more recent method uses three major classifications: (1) benign, (2) precancerous, and (3) malignant. The precancerous classification includes cervical intraepithelial neoplasia, also referred to as dysplasia. Other clinicians use a verbal description to indicate their findings. A summary of the various classifications is shown in Table 56-3.

### Wet Smear

Wet smears are especially beneficial in diagnosing the cause of vaginitis. In this procedure, a specimen of vaginal discharge is placed on a slide, mixed with a drop of saline solution or potassium hydroxide, and examined under the microscope for *Candida, Trichomonas*, or other organisms. It is not conclusive for gonorrhea.

## Biopsy

### Endometrial Biopsy

To take an endometrial biopsy, a curet is inserted through the cervix, placed against the uterine wall, and slowly withdrawn. It is best to repeat the procedure on different walls of the uterus to obtain enough tissue to represent a major portion of the uterus.

Endometrial biopsy is especially useful in evaluating dysfunctional bleeding. It may be helpful in diagnosis of endometrial cancer; there is a chance, however, that scattered growths may be missed. Another use for endometrial biopsy is in infertility studies. It is best performed just before the onset of menses or day 22 of the menstrual cycle. It can interfere with pregnancy if conception has occurred.

### Cervical Biopsy

A punch biopsy instrument is used in the physician's office to obtain samples of cervical tissue. This can aid in more precise diagnosis of questionable lesions. It also is helpful in removing small polyps.

### Cone Biopsy

Cone biopsy, also referred to as conization, involves removing a cone-shaped specimen of cervical tissue, any visible lesions, and tissue specimens of the squamocolumnar junction and cervical canal. It may be used as follow-up to Pap smear or punch biopsy.

**TABLE 56–3.**
CLASSIFICATIONS OF PAP SMEAR FINDINGS

| CLASS | ORIGINAL | CIN SYSTEM | CATEGORY | OTHER DESCRIPTIVE TERMS |
|---|---|---|---|---|
| I | Absence of atypical or abnormal cells | Normal | Benign | Negative |
| II | Atypical cytologic picture, but no evidence of cancer | Inflammatory | Benign | Atypical |
| III | Cytologic picture suggestive of but not conclusive for cancer | Mild CIN | Mild CIN | Mild dysplasia |
| IV | Cytologic picture strongly suggestive for cancer | Severe CIN | Severe CIN | Carcinoma in situ |
| V | Ctyologic picture conclusive for cancer | Cancer | Malignant | Invasive cancer |

CIN, Cervical intraepithelial neoplasia.

## Open Breast Biopsy

Breast biopsy is surgical intervention to remove a lump. A frozen section can be examined for immediate classification; more extensive pathologic studies require additional time.

## Needle Biopsy

The physician inserts a needle into a breast lesion and aspirates its contents. This procedure may be performed in the office and is followed-up as necessary.

## Vulvar Biopsy

Punch biopsy forceps can be used to obtain vulvar tissue. The gross appearance frequently is normal, and staining procedures must be used to identify pathology.

# Radiography

## Hysterosalpingography

Hysterosalpingography is a radiographic examination of the uterus and fallopian tubes. A small cannula is inserted through the cervix, and radiopaque dye is injected into the uterus and fallopian tubes. Filling of the uterus and tubes can be observed on the fluoroscopy screen. Spot films also may be made. Hysterosalpingography is especially useful in noting the size and shape of the uterus and tubes as well as tubal obstruction.

## Mammography

Mammography is a radiologic examination of the breasts. It is useful to detect early lesions that cannot be palpated and the exact location of deep tumors. It may be useful in predicting cancer. With the refinement of this procedure, radiation exposure is minimal and is now considered safe for routine screening. The American Cancer Society recommends a baseline mammogram on all women between ages 35 and 40, routine mammograms every 2 years between ages 40 and 49, and annual examinations for women age 50 or older. For women at increased risk for breast cancer, mammography may be initiated on an annual basis at age 40.

# Other Procedures

## Colposcopy

The colposcope is a binocular diagnostic instrument that provides a magnified (19 to 20×) view of the cervix and vaginal walls. It is mounted on a tripod, and maintains no contact with the patient. Colposcopy is useful in follow-up of abnormal results of Pap smears, to identify abnormal areas for biopsy, and to examine lesions on the vulva. Colposcopy also is recommended in follow-up of women whose mothers took DES during pregnancy; it also may be used for women with dyspareunia and bleeding with intercourse. Each procedure involves the following five observations: (1) vascular pattern, (2) color tone, (3) intercapillary distance, (4) borderline versus normal tissue, and (5) surface pattern.[9]

## Laparoscopy and Culdoscopy

Both laparoscopy and culdoscopy are surgical procedures that allow the physician to visualize the pelvic area through a lighted tube. The procedures are performed to note the condition and position of the various organs, as well as scarring, presence of endometrial tissue, and in-fection. A tubal ligation also may be performed through the laparoscope.

## Hysteroscopy

Hysteroscopy is an office procedure that can be used in follow-up to hysterosalpingography findings of abnormal uterine contour or in treatment of certain uterine fi-broids and polyps.[12] This procedure allows the physician to visualize the inner portion of the uterus and to collect a biopsy specimen from any abnormal area.

## Ultrasonography

Ultrasonography, also referred to as sonography, is a non-invasive technique that is particularly useful in providing pictures of soft tissues of the body. Little preparation is necessary for pelvic ultrasonography except that the per-son must have a full bladder. The bladder distended with 200 to 400 mL of urine is used as a reference point and to displace the pelvic organs for better visualization. Over-distention can distort the findings.

An ultrasound transducer serves as both a transmitter and a receiver. It converts an electrical signal into ultra-sound energy, which is transmitted into the body and then reflected from tissues of different densities. These reflections of ultrasound energy are then received by the transducer and converted again to electrical energy for recording. The procedure is painless and takes about 5 to 30 minutes to complete.

Ultrasonography has become a valuable diagnostic tool in both obstetrics and gynecology. In obstetrics, it is especially useful to confirm pregnancy, to establish or confirm dates or placental location, to rule out large or small size for gestational age, to determine fetal position, and to detect hydrops. Gynecologists use ultrasonogra-phy to assist in the diagnosis of uterine malformation, hydatidiform mole, tumors, ovarian masses, pelvic in-flammatory disease, tubal malformations, and pelvic ab-scess or hematoma.

## Schiller's Test

The Schiller's test is a simple procedure that involves painting the cervix with Schiller's solution or similar io-dine solution. A normal cervix, which contains glycogen, appears mahogany brown from absorption of the iodine. Abnormal areas that contain no glycogen remain a light brown. The primary usefulness of the test is to locate ex-act areas for biopsy (Figure 56-20).

## Cultures

Cultures are most helpful in the diagnosis of the specific organism responsible for an infection. A specimen is col-lected from the infection site with a sterile cotton swab

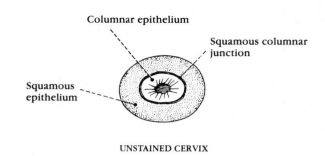

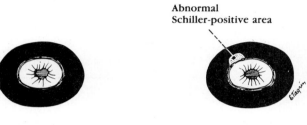

**FIGURE 56-20.**
Schiller's test. (T.H. Green, Jr., and R.C. Knapp, Gynecology, in G.I. Nardi and G.D. Zuidema, (eds.), *Surgery: A Concise Guide to Clini-cal Practice* [4th ed.]. Boston: Little, Brown, 1982.)

and immediately placed in an appropriate medium. The specimen is then incubated and checked for growth and sensitivity. If gonorrhea is suspected, special precautions should be undertaken to ensure an anaerobic environ-ment. Special media also may be used to reduce growth of other bacteria.

## Thermography

Thermography is the photographic display of infrared rays from skin temperature over the breast. Skin tem-perature is elevated in breast cancer because of increased blood flow in the tumor area. This procedure does not always detect early cancers, and false-positive results are common.

## Rubin's Test

In the Rubin's test, carbon dioxide is injected through a cannula into the uterus. If one or both fallopian tubes are open, the woman feels referred shoulder pain. The value of this test is to determine the patency of at least one tube.

## Huhner Test

The Huhner test, also called the postcoital test, is an ex-amination of cervical mucus. Ideally, it is performed dur-ing ovulation and within several hours of intercourse. Cervical mucus is collected with an eyedropper or cotton

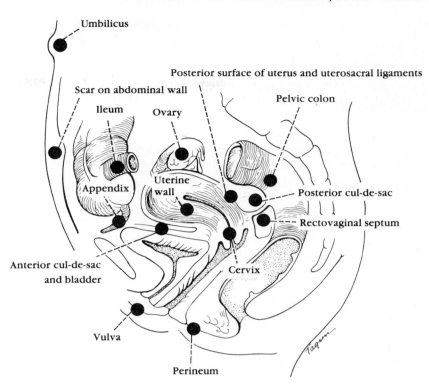

**FIGURE 56–21.**
Sites of occurrence of endometriosis. (T.H. Green, Jr., *Gynecology Essentials of Clinical Practice* [3rd ed.]. Boston: Little, Brown, 1977.)

swab and examined under a microscope. It is a simple procedure used in screening for infertility because the examiner can note the characteristics of the cervical mucus as well as the number and activity of sperm present.

## ALTERATIONS IN FEMALE FUNCTION

### Menstrual Problems

#### Endometriosis

Endometriosis refers to the abnormal location of endometrial tissue. Two types of endometriosis, internal and external, are described. *Internal endometriosis*, or adenomyosis, refers to the location of aberrant endometrial tissue within the myometrium. *External endometriosis* refers to the location of endometrial tissue outside the uterus. Sites for external endometriosis include the outer surface or perimetrium of the uterus, fallopian tubes, ovaries (most common site), bladder and rectal surfaces, uterine ligaments, cul-de-sac, rectovaginal septum, appendix, and bowel. Aberrant tissue also may be found in laparotomy scars, vulva, vagina, and umbilicus (Figure 56-21). In this chapter, the term *adenomyosis* is used to refer to the internal condition and *endometriosis* is used to refer to the external condition.

Endometriosis is characterized by functional aberrant endometrium that responds to hormonal stimulation as normal uterine endometrium does. This tissue grows and thickens under cyclic hormonal influence; as estrogen

and progesterone are withdrawn, it reacts with bleeding. Early lesions appear as tiny red-blue spots surrounded by puckered scar tissue. Larger masses may form when the smaller lesions coalesce. These usually are located on the serosal layer of the involved organs. In the ovaries, lesions may take the form of *endometriomas*, cystic lesions lined with functioning endometrium. Bleeding within the cysts results in thick, chocolate-colored fluid, thus the term *chocolate cysts* (Figure 56-22). Adhesions result when bleeding occurs into the peritoneal cavity, and

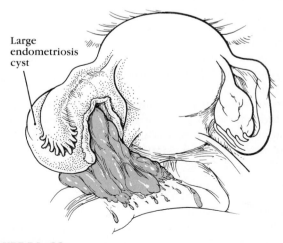

**FIGURE 56–22.**
Endometriomas with cyst formation.

lead to fixation of involved pelvic structures. Infertility has been reported in 40% of women diagnosed with endometriosis.[19]

The exact cause of endometriosis is unknown, but two primary theories are accepted: retrograde menstruation and metaplasia.[9] The *retrograde menstruation* theory, known as Samson's theory, states that during menstruation, endometrial tissue is regurgitated through the fallopian tubes into the pelvic cavity where it implants. The *metaplasia* theory suggests that the undifferentiated coelomic epithelia of the embryo remain dormant until menarche. This tissue then begins to respond to estrogen and progesterone in a way that is similar to that of other endometrial tissue.

Clinical manifestations depend on the locations of lesions. The most common symptom is low abdominal or pelvic pain associated with the menstrual period, such as backache and cramps beginning just before or with the onset of menses. The pain increases throughout menstruation and subsides afterward. It is commonly described as a dull, bearing-down type of pain. Its cause is irritation from hemorrhage of the aberrant tissue, or distention. A chocolate cyst may rupture with signs of acute abdomen. Sterility or infertility may result from extensive scarring of the ovaries and tubes. Dyspareunia reflects uterine involvement, dysuria reflects bladder involvement, and pain on defecation occurs with rectal involvement.

No specific laboratory test is available for diagnosis of endometriosis. Physical examination may reveal small nodular masses on pelvic organs that enlarge during menstruation and seldom are movable (Figure 56-23). Laparoscopy and exploratory surgery are the most beneficial because they allow direct visualization of the lesion.

Treatment depends on the woman's symptoms, age, and childbearing desires. In early endometriosis, treatment consists of analgesia and regular follow-up care. With severe symptoms, surgery is indicated. Surgery in women who desire children usually is aimed at removing as much endometrial tissue as possible while preserving the uterus and ovaries. Hormonal therapy that prevents ovulation or produces pseudopregnancy also may help in the younger woman.

In adenomyosis, endometrial tissue has invaded the myometrium. The invasion may be diffuse or localized, and results in an enlarged uterus (Figure 56-24). This buried endometrium usually is nonfunctional. Symptoms include menorrhagia, dyspareunia, dysmenorrhea, and generalized pelvic discomfort. The usual treatment is hysterectomy, which is indicated by symptoms.

## Premenstrual Syndrome

Premenstrual syndrome is a term used to cover collectively the discomforts noted before the onset of menses. The symptoms vary with individuals but most frequently include headache, breast tenderness, abdominal heavi-

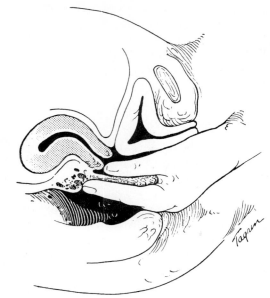

**FIGURE 56–23.**

Rectal examination in the patient with typical pelvic endometriosis. The tender nodularity of the uterosacral ligaments and cul-de-sac and the fixed retroversion of the uterus are almost diagnostic of the disease. (T.H. Green, Jr., *Gynecology: Essentials of Clinical Practice* [3rd ed.]. Boston: Little, Brown, 1977.)

ness and bloating, edema, weight gain, backache, nervous irritability, mood changes, crying spells, depression, insomnia, and anxiety. These symptoms worsen 7 to 10 days before menses and subside when the menstrual flow is well established. The exact cause of premenstrual

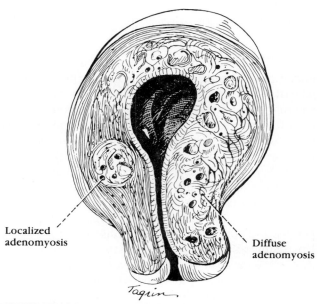

Localized adenomyosis

Diffuse adenomyosis

**FIGURE 56–24.**

Adenomyosis of the uterus. Diffuse involvement of the uterine wall (right) and the localized form, the so-called adenomyoma (left). (T.H. Green, Jr., *Gynecology: Essentials of Clinical Practice* [3rd ed.]. Boston: Little, Brown, 1977.)

discomfort is unknown, but it is believed to be associated with estrogen and progesterone levels.

Treatment is symptomatic and varies with individuals. The most frequently used treatments include vitamins, diuretics, dietary restriction of sodium and carbohydrates, exercise, tranquilizers, and sedatives.

## Dysmenorrhea

Dysmenorrhea may occur as a single entity or as part of the premenstrual syndrome. Dysmenorrhea means painful menstruation and is commonly referred to as cramps. There are two types of dysmenorrhea: primary and secondary. *Secondary dysmenorrhea* is caused by organic pelvic disease such as cancer of the uterus, bladder, or intestinal tract. Primary dysmenorrhea refers to painful menses unrelated to an obvious physical cause. It usually begins with the establishment of the ovulatory cycle. Spasmodic primary dysmenorrhea usually is characterized by sharp cramping sensations the first day or two of menses. It may improve as cycles are reestablished after pregnancy. Congestive primary dysmenorrhea frequently occurs in association with premenstrual syndrome. It is characterized by a dull, aching pain before the onset of menses.

The cause of primary dysmenorrhea remains unknown. One theory attributes it to the secretion of prostaglandins, especially $PGE_2$, which have a stimulating effect on uterine muscle. Nausea, vomiting, and diarrhea associated with dysmenorrhea also have been attributed to prostaglandins. Other possible factors include acute anteflexion of the uterus, estrogen—progesterone imbalance, and hypersensitivity of the person to pain.

The most common treatments include hormones, analgesics, prostaglandin synthetase, optimum health maintenance, and psychotherapy. Hormonal therapy is aimed at preventing ovulation because anovulatory cycles seldom are painful. Antiprostaglandins, such as aspirin, indomethacin, naproxen, and ibuprofen, may be administered before the onset of menses to inhibit prostaglandin synthesis. The drugs may not only inhibit prostaglandin synthesis, but also block its action. Mild analgesics also may be administered.

## Abnormal Uterine Bleeding

Abnormal uterine bleeding is the most common reason women visit the gynecologist and the leading indication for dilatation and curettage.[14] This condition usually is a symptom of some underlying disease process rather than a disease entity itself. Terms used to describe abnormal uterine bleeding are defined in Table 56-4.

The many causes of abnormal uterine bleeding can be grouped into four major categories: (1) complications of pregnancy, (2) organic lesions, (3) constitutional diseases, and (4) true dysfunctional uterine bleeding. Complications of pregnancy include abortion, trophoblastic disease, and ectopic pregnancy. Organic lesions include conditions associated with pelvic diseases, such as infections, tumors, and polyps. Constitutional diseases are conditions such as hypertension, blood dyscrasias, and hormonal dysfunction. No pelvic disease is present, but symptoms are reflected through abnormal uterine bleeding. The last category represents abnormal bleeding associated with endocrine dysfunction.

*DYSFUNCTIONAL UTERINE BLEEDING.* The term *dysfunctional uterine bleeding* refers to abnormal bleeding that is the result of endocrine dysfunction. Fifty percent of dysfunctional uterine bleeding occurs in women over age 40, and 20% occurs in adolescents under age 20.[14] It often is associated with absence of ovulation, but it also is seen in ovulatory cycles. In anovulatory cycles, no corpus luteum is formed, no progesterone produced, and no secretory changes occur in the endometrium. The endometrium becomes hyperplastic. As estrogen levels decrease from degenerating follicles, withdrawal bleeding occurs. Dysfunctional uterine bleeding occasionally results from inadequate production of progesterone after ovulation.

Psychogenic uterine bleeding may be included in dysfunctional uterine bleeding when both organic and

**TABLE 56-4.**
TERMINOLOGY ASSOCIATED WITH ABNORMAL UTERINE BLEEDING

| TERM | DEFINITION |
| --- | --- |
| Metrorrhagia or intermenstrual bleeding | Bleeding between periods |
| Menorrhagia or hypermenorrhea | Excessive menstrual flow |
| Polymenorrhea | Abnormally frequent menstrual bleeding |
| Oligomenorrhea | Abnormally infrequent menses |
| Hypomenorrhea | Deficient menstrual flow |
| Amenorrhea | Absence of menstrual flow |
| Perimenopausal bleeding | Irregular bleeding before menopause |
| Postmenopausal bleeding | Bleeding that occurs 1 or more years after menopause |

constitutional causes have been ruled out. The influence of emotional stimulation on the hypothalamus and the resultant influence on the gonadotropic hormones are discussed in Chapter 36. Emotions also may directly affect the uterine blood vessels and produce bleeding.

Diagnosis is made after a complete and thorough menstrual history. Physical examination reveals pelvic lesions and aids in the diagnosis of constitutional diseases. Laboratory studies include thyroid function, complete blood count (CBC), and platelet count to rule out blood dyscrasias. Studies to determine the presence of ovulation include measurements of estrogen and progesterone levels, endometrial biopsy, and spinnbarkeit and ferning studies of cervical mucus. During the climacteric, both cytologic studies and biopsy are important to rule out cancer.

AMENORRHEA.    Amenorrhea is not a disease entity. It may indicate a serious condition or be completely normal, as in pregnancy. It may be either primary or secondary. *Primary amenorrhea* refers to a failure to begin menstrual cycles. *Secondary amenorrhea* occurs after a variable period of normal function. Causes of amenorrhea may be physiologic, anatomic, genetic, endocrinologic, constitutional, or psychogenic. Physiologic causes include pregnancy, lactation, menopause, and adolescence. Anatomic factors include congenital anomalies, hysterectomy, and endometrial destruction. Genetic factors include Turner's syndrome and hermaphroditism. Dysfunction of the hypothalamus, pituitary, ovary, thyroid, or adrenal glands also may produce amenorrhea. Malnutrition, obesity, drug addiction, diabetes, and anemia are all constitutional problems that can prevent menstrual periods. Psychogenic factors include psychosis and anorexia nervosa. Menstrual dysfunction also is seen in athletes as a result of physical and emotional stress, changes in body composition and weight, and alteration in hormonal secretions.

Specific diagnostic tools, in addition to history and physical examination, include thyroid function studies, serum prolactin level, buccal smear, skull radiography, progesterone challenge test, and hormone values.

## Reproductive Tract Infections

### Atrophic Vaginitis

Atrophic vaginitis refers to inflammation of the atrophied epithelium in postmenopausal women. It produces an irritating vaginal discharge with pruritus and swelling, and secondary dyspareunia and dysuria. Red strawberry spots may be noted on the vaginal wall. Bleeding may occur from trauma to the thin epithelium, but cancer must be ruled out as its cause. Estrogen therapy is used to convert the epithelium to the more normal, thick, stratified, squamous layer.

### Cervicitis

Cervicitis refers to inflammation of the cervix, which may be acute or chronic. Acute cervicitis usually occurs with other acute reproductive tract infections. Causative organisms include *Gonococcus, Staphylococcus,* and *Streptococcus* species and *Escherichia coli.* Speculum examination reveals an edematous, congested cervix with purulent discharge. Symptoms may include dyspareunia, backache, dull pain in the lower abdomen, and urinary frequency and urgency. Pain may be noted on palpation. Cultures and smears identify the causative organism, and appropriate antibiotic therapy is then instituted.

Many women exhibit some form of chronic cervicitis. It may occur after acute infections, childbirth trauma, or abortion. The cervical canal is primarily affected, but there are no characteristic findings of the cervix. The only symptom may be a mucopurulent vaginal discharge or, occasionally, paracervical or low back pain. Abnormal bleeding is rare and often indicates cervical cancer. Physical examination may reveal cervical erosions, cervical eversions, or nabothian cysts.

*Cervical erosion* refers to an area of the surface of the cervix in which the surface epithelia are partially or totally absent (Figure 56-25A). It appears red and raw. Columnar cells are more likely to exhibit this characteristic than squamous cells, and they are not as curable. *Cervical eversion* refers to a portion of the cervix in which columnar epithelium of the cervical canal extends outward (Figure 56-25B). The characteristic squamocolumnar junction is then located along the outer edge of the lesion. Eversion most frequently occurs in women who are taking oral contraceptives, young women who have never been pregnant, and the daughters of women who took DES during pregnancy. There is an increase in mucoid secretions. In an attempt to repair the eversion,

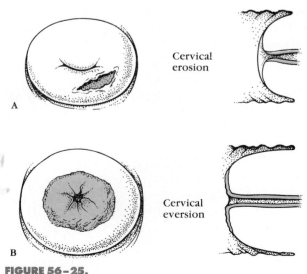

**FIGURE 56–25.**
**A.** Cervical erosion. **B.** Cervical eversion.

the squamous cells begin to grow inward. As this invasion progresses, the mucus-secreting glands are obliterated. Their secretions are then trapped beneath the epithelium, producing *nabothian cysts*. These cysts are filled with normal mucus, are not infected, and produce no symptoms.

The primary concern in diagnosing cervicitis is screening for cervical cancer because the lesions are not easily differentiated by the naked eye. In addition to cultures, Pap smear, colposcopy, and biopsy are the most important screening aids.

Silver nitrate, douches, and antibiotics are relatively ineffective methods of treatment because of the depth of the lesions. Small areas may be treated with thermal cautery or cryosurgery. Entire areas are treated in depth; healing and reepithelialization then take place. The sloughing cervical tissue produces an annoying discharge that may be treated with antibiotic creams for 7 to 10 days. Complete healing may take 6 to 8 weeks.

## Toxic Shock Syndrome

Toxic shock syndrome (TSS) is an entity first recognized and reported in 1978. At that time, it was thought to be related to *Staphylococcus aureus*. Since then it has gained notoriety as a condition that most often occurs in menstruating women who use tampons. Nonmenstrual TSS has been associated with vaginal and cesarean delivery, therapeutic abortion, and infected wounds and skin lesions. The causative agent is believed to be a toxin produced by *S. aureus*.

The link with tampons is most interesting because the unused tampons of women who develop TSS contained no *S. aureus*.[4] Two theories support the tampon link. One states that bacteria are nourished by carboxymethyl cellulose, which is present in many tampons.[4] The other theory indicates that conditions for bacterial growth are improved through the use of superabsorbent tampons.

Clinical manifestations of TSS include (1) elevated temperature, sudden in onset; (2) vomiting and diarrhea; and (3) an erythematous macular rash that is present especially on the palms and soles. The sunburn-like rash progresses to peeling of palms and soles about 10 days later. Renal dysfunction may develop, with decreased urine output. Hypotension and shock may develop. Laboratory studies usually reveal elevated blood urea nitrogen, serum creatinine, bilirubin, and creatine phosphokinase levels. Additional complications associated with TSS include disseminated intravascular coagulation, adult respiratory distress syndrome, and acidosis. Box 56-1 summarizes criteria for diagnosis.

Treatment varies, depending on the extent of symptoms. It may include antibiotics (penicillinase-resistant penicillin) or cephalosporins, intravenous colloid to prevent fluid loss from blood vessels, ventilation therapy, heparin, blood transfusion, and correction of acid-base imbalance.

## Pelvic Inflammatory Disease

Pelvic inflammatory disease (PID) is a general term used to refer to any infection of the upper reproductive tract (above the cervix). More precise terms such as endometritis, endoparametritis, salpingitis, oophoritis, and pelvic

---

**BOX 56–1.**
TOXIC SHOCK SYNDROME CASE DEFINITION

Fever (temperature ≥38.9°C [102°F])
Rash (diffuse macular erythroderma)
Desquamation, 1–2 wk after onset of illness, particularly of palms and soles
Hypotension (systolic blood pressure ≤90 mm Hg for adults or <fifth percentile by age for children <16 years old, or orthostatic syncope)
Involvement of three or more of the following organ systems:
    GI (vomiting or diarrhea at onset of illness)
    Muscular (severe myalgia or creatine phosphokinase level ≥2 × ULN)
    Mucous membrane (vaginal, oropharyngeal, or conjunctival) hyperemia
    Renal (BUN or Cr ≥2 × ULN or ≥5 white blood cells/high-power field—in the absence of a
        urinary tract infection)
    Hepatic (total bilirubin, SGOT, or SGPT ≥2 × ULN)
    Hematologic (platelets ≤100,000/μL)
    Central nervous system (disorientation or alterations in consciousness without focal neurologic
        signs when fever and hypotension are absent)
Negative results on the following tests, if obtained:
    Blood, throat, or cerebrospinal fluid cultures
    Serologic tests for Rocky Mountain spotted fever, leptospirosis, or measles

*UNL, upper limits of normal.*
*Centers for Disease Control, M.M.W.R. 29:442, 1980.*

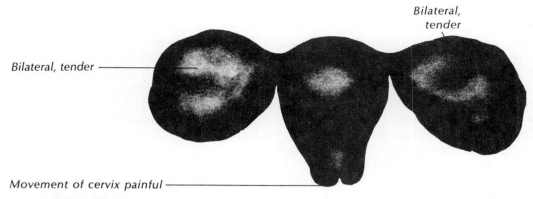

**FIGURE 56–26.**

Pelvic inflammatory disease. Acute pelvic inflammatory disease is associated with tender, bilateral adnexal masses, although pain and muscle spasm usually make it impossible to delineate them. Movement of the cervix produces pain. Chronic pelvic inflammatory disease is manifested by bilateral, tender, usually irregular and fairly fixed adnexal masses. (B. Bates, *A Guide to Physical Examination and History Taking* [4th ed.]. Philadelphia: J.B. Lippincott, 1987.)

peritonitis indicate specific areas of involvement (Figure 56-26). Common causes of PID include *Gonococcus, Staphylococcus*, and *Streptococcus* species, and *Chlamydia trachomatis* (see Chap. 57). It often occurs after delivery or abortion and in women who use intrauterine devices (IUDs) as a means of contraception.

Symptoms include the sudden onset of severe pelvic pain, chills and fever, nausea, vomiting, and a heavy, purulent vaginal discharge with foul odor. Vaginal bleeding also may be present.

One of the most important diagnostic tools in PID is a complete and thorough history. Specific information of most importance relates to previous reproductive tract infection, delivery, abortion, pelvic surgery, onset of pain, date of last menses, sexual history, and type of contraceptive used. Specific diagnostic tests include cultures of any discharge, CBC, and possible ultrasound studies if pelvic abscess is suspected.

Medical regimen depends on the cause, acuteness, and extent of the infection. Hospitalization with bed rest and appropriate intravenous antibiotics may be indicated. Analgesics may be ordered for pain. Removal of an IUD is indicated when one is present. Surgical drainage usually is recommended for an abscess. The importance of follow-up care cannot be overemphasized. Untreated or inadequately treated PID may result in infertility or sterility.

## Benign Conditions of the Female Reproductive Tract

### Uterine Fibroids

Uterine fibroids, also referred to as *leiomyomas, myomas*, or *fibromyomas*, are second only to pregnancy as the most common cause of uterine enlargement. Twenty percent to 50% of women between ages 30 and 50 have some evidence of these growths. Fibroids are masses of muscle and connective tissue that are stimulated by estrogen, thereby increasing in size with pregnancy and decreasing in size with menopause. Diagnosis most often is made on the basis of physical examination. Ultrasonography, radiography, hysteroscopy, and dilatation and curettage may aid in the diagnosis.

The tumors occur singly or in groups, and vary from the size of peas to that of an apple or a cantaloupe. They are firm, smooth, and spheric. Sectioning of a fibroid tumor reveals a pinkish white, whorled, and lined muscle bundle.

Position in the uterine wall determines the type of classification of fibroids (Figure 56-27). Intramural or interstitial tumors are present in central portions of the uterine wall; these are the most common. Submucosal tumors are located between the endometrium and the uterine lining. Projection into the uterine cavity with subsequent distortion and enlargement of the endometrium may cause excessive menstrual bleeding and habitual abortion. Subserous fibroids lie beneath the serous lining of the uterus and project outward into the abdominal cavity. If a subserous tumor extends outward on a stalk, it is called *pedunculated*.

Many fibroids are asymptomatic. As they enlarge, the woman may experience excessive or prolonged bleeding during regular monthly cycles, urinary frequency, constipation, abdominal fullness, low abdominal pain, dysmenorrhea, and infertility. Abnormal bleeding usually occurs with submucous tumors because of the increased amount of endometrium to build and slough. Enlargement of fibroids can produce pressure on the bladder, urethra, rectum, or nerves. Infertility and habitual abortion most frequently occur with submucous

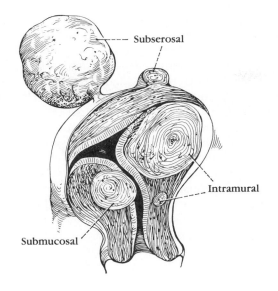

A

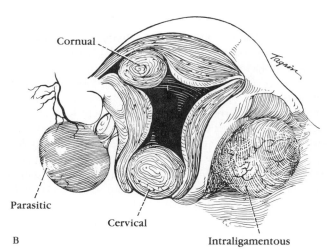

B

**FIGURE 56–27.**
Uterine fibroids. **A.** Types. **B.** Various locations. (T.H. Green, Jr., *Gynecology: Essentials of Clinical Practice* [3rd ed.]. Boston: Little, Brown, 1977.)

tumors because of distortion of the endometrium and uterine cavity. Enlarging fibroids have been known to interfere with delivery of a full-term fetus.

The course of treatment is determined by age, parity, symptoms, and condition of the woman and by size and location of tumors. No treatment is necessary for asymptomatic patients. Women who are approaching menopause usually are observed at regular intervals because withdrawal of estrogen results in a stationary or decreasing size of the fibroids. Hysteroscopic surgery may be most beneficial for women with submucosal myomas,[12] whereas hysterectomy may be indicated for the woman who does not want additional children. It is advisable to delay surgery in the woman who is anemic. The administration of gonadotropin releasing hormone agonist usually produces amenorrhea, which allows spontaneous recovery from the anemia. Intramural tumors also may shrink during this time.[12]

## *Functional Ovarian Cysts*

Functional ovarian cysts are the result of normal ovarian function, and account for more than 50% of ovarian enlargements (Figure 56-28). A functional follicular cyst results when a maturing follicle fails to rupture an ovum. Instead, it continues to enlarge and produce estrogen. A corpus luteum cyst occurs when the corpus luteum fails to degenerate normally. It continues to grow and produce progesterone.

Functional ovarian cysts ordinarily produce no symptoms. They may be noted on periodic examination, and usually disappear after the next menstrual cycle. When a functional cyst ruptures, it may tear an ovarian vessel. Intraperitoneal bleeding occurs, and the extent of symptoms is related to the amount of hemorrhage. With excessive bleeding, abdominal pain may be severe in onset, requiring hospitalization and surgery.

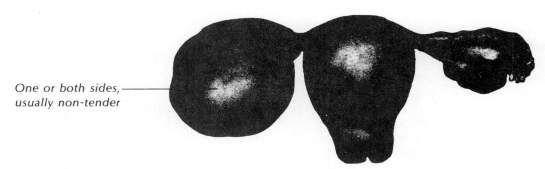

*One or both sides, usually non-tender*

**FIGURE 56–28.**
Ovarian cysts and tumors may be detected as adnexal masses on one or both sides. Later they may grow up out of the pelvis. Cysts tend to be smooth and compressible; tumors are more solid and often nodular. Uncomplicated cysts and tumors usually are not tender. (B. Bates, *A Guide to Physical Examination and History Taking* [4th ed.]. Philadelphia: J.B. Lippincott, 1987.)

## Benign Neoplastic Tumors of the Ovaries

Benign neoplasms are more important than functional cysts, although they occur less frequently. They may grow to be quite large and secrete hormones. Classification is by cellular origin: (1) germ cell, (2) germinal epithelium, (3) gonadal stroma, and (4) nonspecialized stroma. Three of the most common benign neoplasms are cystic teratomas or dermoid cysts, serous cystadenomas, and mucinous cystadenomas.

Dermoid cysts represent about 15% to 20% of all ovarian neoplasms and arise from germ cells. They are most frequent in women aged 18 to 35. The tumor is gray and smooth, and contains tissue from all three germ layers—commonly skin, hair, and sebaceous glands.

Benign serous cystadenomas arise from germinal epithelium and, with mucinous cystadenomas, account for about 50% of benign ovarian neoplasms. They most frequently affect women between ages 40 and 50. The tumors may be unilateral or bilateral. They are pearly gray, lobulated, and filled with a clear, yellow fluid that becomes brown if there is bleeding in the cyst. *Psammoma bodies*, which are small, calcified granules, may be present in the cell wall. Papillary serous cystadenomas may develop into cancers.

Mucinous cystadenomas also arise from germinal epithelium and usually are unilateral. Most are larger than serous cystadenomas, contain no psammoma bodies, and contain thick, straw-colored fluid

Most ovarian tumors are asymptomatic and noted on routine pelvic examination. Once they are enlarged enough to produce pressure, the woman may complain of pain on defecation, dyspareunia, heaviness, and sterility. Increased enlargement may result in abdominal distention, dyspnea, and anorexia. Menstrual irregularities, masculinization, and feminization may occur if hormones are produced. Complications include rupture, hemorrhage, possible infection, and torsion of pedicle cyst. The treatment of choice is surgical removal, since the tumors increase in size and may undergo malignant changes.

## Benign Breast Alterations

The two most common benign breast alterations are fibrocystic disease and fibroadenoma. Fibrocystic disease is the most common of all female breast lesions, affecting 50% of women of childbearing age. The peak incidence is noted at about age 40.[16] It is a benign neoplasm that consists of proliferative ductal epithelium and fibrous stroma. Characteristically, the lesion becomes nodular from fibrous thickening. It may be tender, especially before menstruation, and exhibit cystic formation. Complaints of dull, heavy pain and a sense of fullness that increases before menstruation are characteristic. The nodule most often is located in the upper outer quadrant.

Fibrocystic disease tends to follow a progressive

course of three stages.[16] The first stage occurs in young women from the late teen years to the early 30s. At this time, there is tenderness and fullness but minimal lumpiness the week premenstrually. The second stage appears in women in their mid-30s and 40s. Nodules may be noted, causing the woman to see a physician. Discomfort is greater and occurs for a longer period. During the third stage, lesions appear suddenly and are painful. Biopsy often is implemented to differentiate this lesion from breast cancer.

The exact cause is unknown, but it is thought to result from abnormal or exaggerated response of breast tissue to cyclic hormonal stimulation. Methylxanthines, which include caffeine, also have been implicated as a possible cause. These substances are responsible for inhibiting an enzyme that breaks down cyclic adenosine monophosphate (cAMP).[16] As a result, cAMP levels rise. Levels of cAMP also have been found to be higher in women with fibrocystic disease.

Medical management of fibrocystic disease includes administration of oral contraceptives and progestins. Danazol and bromocriptine therapy have been used to obtain subjective relief of symptoms.[16]

The second most common benign breast tumor is fibroadenoma. Physical examination reveals a well-outlined, solid, firm lump that moves freely. It most often occurs in the upper outer quadrant in women aged 15 to 40, being the most common breast lesion in the adolescent female. The cause of this condition is unknown, but estrogen stimulation is suspected because it primarily occurs in younger women and seldom after menopause. Treatment is surgical removal of the lump. Recurrence is common.

## Premalignant and Malignant Conditions

### Trophoblastic Disease

The term *trophoblastic disease* refers to three complications of uterine pregnancy: (1) hydatidiform mole, (2) chorioadenoma destruens, and (3) choriocarcinoma. Hydatidiform mole usually is benign with malignant potential, whereas choriocarcinoma is a highly aggressive cancer.

*HYDATIDIFORM MOLE.*  Hydatidiform mole represents a malformation of the placenta. It is characterized by absence of embryo development; conversion of the chorionic villi into marked vesicles with clear, thick, sticky fluid; and production of human chorionic gonadotropin (HCG). Molar pregnancies are classified as partial or complete, based on morphology, chromosomal pattern, and histopathology.[3]

Clinical manifestations of complete moles include intermittent bleeding, excessive increase in uterine size, no evidence of fetal development, markedly elevated HCG levels, and spontaneous abortion. The woman may experience intermittent bleeding after amenorrhea. A dark brown vaginal discharge may be accompanied by passage of watery fluid that contains characteristic vesicles. Even by the 16th to 20th week, no fetal heart tones are noted and no fetal movement is felt; ultrasonography reveals no fetal skeleton. Levels of HCG are higher than those associated with normal pregnancy. Hyperemesis gravidarum, bilateral ovarian cysts, and toxemia of pregnancy before the 24th week also have been noted with hydatidiform mole.

In contrast, the partial mole is characterized by embryonic or fetal tissue as well as chorionic villi swelling. Most women present with signs and symptoms of incomplete or missed abortion. No fetal heart tones are noted, and the size of the uterus usually is appropriate for gestational age.[3]

Diagnostic tools include dilatation and curettage, histologic studies, measurement of HCG levels, and ultrasonography. Histologic studies can be performed on tissue that is passed spontaneously or obtained from dilatation and curettage. Curettage scrapings usually include both superficial and deep tissue to determine invasiveness. Ultrasonography reveals a characteristic pattern of hydatidiform mole, which helps in differentiation (Figure 56-29).

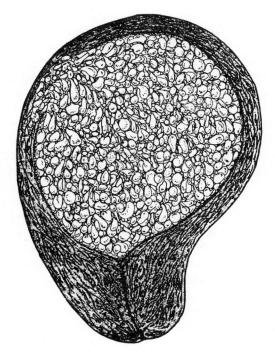

**FIGURE 56-29.**
Hydatidiform mole. (M.A. Miller and D.A. Brooten, *The Childbearing Family: A Nursing Perspective* [2nd ed.]. Boston: Little, Brown, 1983.)

Treatment of choice is evacuation of the uterus as soon as possible after diagnosis. Possible means for evacuation of uterine contents include dilatation and curettage, suction curettage, and hysterectomy. About 80% are benign and cured by these procedures. Overall, 15% become invasive, with 2% to 3% progressing to choriocarcinoma.[5]

After evacuation, HCG levels (especially the beta subunit) are initially checked every week, gradually moving to every other week, and finally monthly for 1 year. HCG levels ordinarily return to normal within a week or so. If they are still elevated at 4 weeks, about 50% of affected women develop choriocarcinoma unless chemotherapy is instituted. Chemotherapy may be instituted as a prophylactic measure. Chemotherapeutic agents include the folic acid antagonists methotrexate and dactinomycin.

*CHORIOADENOMA DESTRUENS.* Chorioadenoma destruens is an invasive hydatidiform mole. It is characterized by the presence of chorionic villi deep within the myometrium. Penetration of the uterine wall with rupture and hemorrhage is possible.

Curettage may not be successful in removing the lesion because of the depth of invasion. Chemotherapy with methotrexate or dactinomycin usually is initiated. Levels of HCG are measured regularly until they return to normal. Thereafter, they are measured at monthly intervals for 1 year.

*CHORIOCARCINOMA.* Choriocarcinoma is a rare, malignant tumor of the trophoblast that most frequently occurs in the uterus. It affects 1 in 40,000 to 70,000 pregnancies in the United States.[5] Additionally, it primarily affects women under age 20 and over age 40. It is characterized by sheets of immature cells (cytotrophoblasts and syncytiotrophoblasts) that invade the uterine wall and produce necrosis and hemorrhage. Chorionic villi are not present. Choriocarcinoma may occur in the ovaries.

The only symptom noticed may be a bloody, brownish discharge associated with irregular bleeding or continual bleeding after a delivery or abortion. The first symptoms frequently are related to metastasis. Because the most common site of metastasis is the lung, hemoptysis may be the first complaint. Other metastatic sites include the vagina, brain, liver, and kidneys. Levels of HCG remain markedly elevated.

Before the use of chemotherapeutic agents, the prognosis for a woman with choriocarcinoma was extremely grim, with death occurring within 1 to 2 years. The *1990 Cancer Facts and Figures* lists choriocarcinoma as one cancer that today often is cured.[1] Among the agents used are methotrexate, dactinomycin, chlorambucil, and vincristine. The response of lung metastasis also is very good, but lesions in the brain and liver respond poorly. Prognosis continues to be directly related to the degree of metastasis, duration of disease, and HCG titer. A cure rate approaching 100% may be obtained when metastasis is limited to the pelvis, vagina, and lungs.[5]

### Diethylstilbestrol Exposure

The first synthetic estrogen was released in the 1940s. It was used to prevent miscarriage and lactation after delivery, and as hormonal therapy for dysfunctional uterine bleeding after menopause. In the late 1960s, it became linked with adenocarcinoma of the vagina, vaginal adenosis, squamous cell carcinoma of the cervix and vagina, and cervical dysplasia, as well as congenital abnormalities of both male and female offspring and impaired sperm production.

Cancer of the vagina is a rare condition, most frequently occurring in women over age 50. It usually is the squamous cell type, but adenocarcinoma has been identified in a number of adolescent girls whose mothers received DES during pregnancy.

Vaginal adenosis is a benign condition in which the transformation zone of the squamocolumnar junction extends over the vaginal portion of the cervix and may involve the vaginal walls. This condition is extremely common in daughters of mothers who took DES and may predispose them to adenocarcinoma. A question also arises as to whether adenosis may progress to squamous cell cancer of the cervix or vagina.

Additionally, DES has been associated with congenital anomalies, including cervical anomalies such as collars, hoods, and ridges and altered fallopian tube structure. Based on hysterosalpingography findings, the most common uterine anomaly is a T-shaped uterus.[10]

Lowered fertility rates have been identified in both male and female offspring of mothers who took DES. Irregular or infrequent menstrual periods as well as increased incidence of incompetent cervix have been associated with in utero exposure of females to DES. There also is an increased rate of spontaneous abortion and premature delivery in women exposed to DES.

The most important factors in treatment of DES problems are identification of those exposed and follow-up care every 6 to 12 months. Children of women known or suspected of DES exposure should have regular examinations beginning at puberty. Routine procedures should include Pap smears and colposcopy. Precancerous cell changes can be found early and appropriate therapy initiated. Reproductive tract surgery should be used cautiously in women exposed to DES because of the increased risk of cervical stenosis. Controversy continues over the use of cerclage procedures in an attempt to decrease spontaneous abortion caused by incompetent cervix.[10]

### Endometrial Carcinoma

During the past 40 years, the death rate from uterine cancer has decreased more than 70%. It currently accounts for about 7% of all cancer in females, with a frequency in women that is surpassed by cancer of breast, colon and rectum, and lung. It primarily affects postmenopausal women, with peak occurrence in the 50s and 60s.[1,2]

Experimental evidence has linked endometrial cancer with ingestion of exogenous estrogens. Endogenous estrogen production unbalanced by progesterone may contribute to its frequency in early menopause. Recent evidence, however, indicates a decreased risk of endometrial cancer when estrogen therapy is supplemented with progesterone for 2 weeks. Additional factors that seem to increase the risk of endometrial cancer include history of infertility, anovulation, nulliparity, obesity, diabetes, and hypertension. Demographics indicate a higher incidence in urban, white, and Jewish women.[1,2]

In many cases, malignant changes are preceded by abnormal cell maturation. Adenomatous hyperplasia has been known to occur both spontaneously and as a result of estrogen drugs. If untreated, the process progresses to an in situ lesion in which the cells are larger and more disoriented. Nuclei may be present in different locations with varying size and staining characteristics. About 85% of endometrial cancer is adenocarcinoma. Cells may be well differentiated or so undifferentiated that no glandular pattern is evident. The lesion usually represents a slow-growing tumor with late metastasis. Metastasis occurs first to the cervix and myometrium, and later involves the vagina, pelvis, and lungs. Increased risk of vaginal recurrence, myometrial invasion, and nodal spread is associated with poorly differentiated tumor patterns.

Staging or extension of the lesion from the site of origin and grading of cellular differentiation of endometrial cancer are possible only after removal of the uterus and subsequent pathologic studies. Therefore, grading is of little value in determining initial therapy. The grades of endometrial cancer are I through III, with grade I representing well-differentiated cells and grade II, undifferentiated.

The staging process varies within institutions and parts of the nation. The Federation Internationale de Gynecologic et Obstetrique (FIGO) has adopted a system of five major stages (Table 56-5). Other staging procedures divide the disease into fewer stages: stages I and II with confinement to the uterus, and stage III limited to pelvic spread. The staging and grading procedures are most important in determining appropriate therapy, which includes surgery, radiation, or a combination. Progesterone therapy, when instituted, should be continued indefinitely, since recurrences after discontinued therapy may not respond to medication. Chemotherapy is used less frequently but, when instituted, includes doxorubicin, cyclophosphamide, and cisplatin.

The first sign of endometrial cancer is abnormal uterine bleeding. It may range from light, irregular bleeding with intermenstrual spotting to heavy, prolonged periods when it occurs before menopause. After menopause, any bleeding should be suspicious. Another early

**TABLE 56-5.**
STAGES OF ENDOMETRIAL CARCINOMA AS DEVISED BY FIGO

| STAGE | DESCRIPTION |
|---|---|
| 0 | Carcinoma in situ |
| I | Tumor confined to the corpus uteri |
| II | Tumor involves both the corpus and the cervix |
| III | Tumor extends outside the uterus, but not outside the true pelvis |
| IV | Tumor involves bladder or rectum, or extends outside the true pelvis |

*FIGO, Federation Internationale de Gynecologic et Obstetrique.*

sign may be marked leukorrhea. Both signs reflect erosion and ulceration of the endometrium. Later signs include cramping, pelvic discomfort, lower abdominal or bladder pressure, bleeding after intercourse, and swollen lymph nodes.

The most important diagnostic tool is probably dilatation and curettage because it allows the most comprehensive study. Routine Pap smears have limited usefulness unless metastasis has occurred. Both endometrial biopsy and washing may reveal abnormal endometrial tissue.

The American Cancer Society reports an overall survival rate of 85% with endometrial cancer.[1] This survival rate rises to 92% if diagnosed in the early stages and to about 100% when discovered in the precancerous stage.

## Cervical Cancer

The American Cancer Society reports that in recent years, the incidence of invasive cervical cancer has decreased, whereas that of carcinoma in situ has slightly increased. Cervical cancer usually occurs between ages 30 and 50 in women (1) who began intercourse before age 20, (2) who are of low socioeconomic status, (3) who are black, (4) who received DES during pregnancy, (5) who have had many sexual partners, and (6) who are multiparous.[1] There also seems to be an emerging link between cigarette smoking[18] and certain sexually transmitted diseases, especially genital herpes and human papillomavirus (see Chap. 57).[1] Chronic cervicitis and unrepaired cervical lacerations also seem to predispose to cancer.

Cancer of the cervix normally is of the squamous cell type, and represents a sequential process of cellular proliferation. It usually begins in the transformation zone of the squamocolumnar junction as a basal cell hyperplasia (Figure 56-30). As the hyperplasia extends toward the surface, it becomes known as dysplasia, which refers to the disorderly cellular arrangement in the upper layers of the epithelium. The nuclei of these cells are enlarged and stain darkly. Some cells may be multinucleated. The

number of atypical cells determines the classification: mild, moderate, or severe.

The next stage in the sequential process is carcinoma in situ. This stage represents an involvement of the entire epithelial cell layer, and is referred to as intraepithelial neoplasm. The term *cervical intraepithelial neoplasia (CIN)* refers to all dysplasia and carcinoma in situ, since the potential for progression and metastasis exists.

There are three forms of invasive cervical cancer: fungating, ulcerative, and infiltrative. The fungating tumor is a nodular thickening of the epithelium that may project above the mucosa. The ulcerative lesion represents a sloughing necrosis of the central portion of the tumor. Infiltrative invasion represents downward growth into the stroma. As metastasis continues, there is spread to the bladder, rectum, and lymph nodes; the lungs, bones, and liver eventually may be involved. The slow process of metastasis is believed to occur as long as 10 to 30 years after the precursor of carcinoma in situ.[2] In more rapidly growing lesions, invasion can occur in 3 to 4 years.

Because early cervical cancer is asymptomatic, early diagnosis and staging of the lesion are essential (Table 56-6). Routine Pap smears have probably done more than any other diagnostic tool to detect early cervical cancer. Early CIN also can be detected by Pap smears. Histologic confirmation is obtained through colposcopy, cervical biopsy, and conization.

Laser surgery, electrocautery, and cryosurgery are procedures aimed at treating the neoplasia or removing the lesion in early-stage cancer. Total hysterectomy, radical hysterectomy, radiation therapy, or pelvic exenteration may be indicated as the extent of cancer increases.

The survival rate with cervical cancer continues to be less than that with endometrial cancer. The American Cancer Society reports an overall survival rate of 67% for cervical cancer patients.[1] The survival rate increases sig-

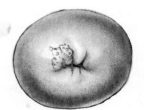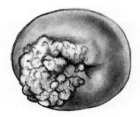

**FIGURE 56-30.**
Carcinoma of the cervix usually begins at or near the cervical os. It often has a hard, granular surface that bleeds easily. In later stages, an extensive irregular cauliflower-type growth may develop. Early carcinomas are clinically indistinguishable from ectropions, and may even be present in a cervix that appears normal. (B. Bates, *A Guide to Physical Examination and History Taking* [5th ed.]. Philadelphia: J.B. Lippincott, 1991.)

**TABLE 56-6.**
FIGO RECOMMENDATIONS FOR STAGING
CERVICAL CANCER

| STAGE | DESCRIPTION |
|---|---|
| 0 | Carcinoma in situ |
| I | Carcinoma limited to the cervix |
| II | Carcinoma extends beyond the cervix and involves the upper two thirds of the vagina |
| III | Carcinoma involves the lower one third of the vagina and has become fixed to the pelvic wall |
| IV | Carcinoma involves the rectum or bladder, or extends beyond the true pelvis |

FIGO, Federation Internationale de Gynecologic et Obstetrique.

nificantly with early diagnosis (88%) and with carcinoma in situ (100%).

## Ovarian Cancer

Ovarian cancer is the most lethal of all cancers that affect the female reproductive system; however, it accounts for only 4% of all cancers among women.[1] The reason for its lethality is the advanced stage when diagnosis is made. It most frequently occurs in women over age 60.

There is no diagnostic tool for early detection of ovarian cancer. If detected early, it is by chance and on routine periodic examinations. Any ovarian enlargement in the postmenopausal woman and any ovarian mass larger than 5 cm in diameter, regardless of age, should be suspected. Palpation of the ovaries after menopause is abnormal and another indication for further study. In middle-aged women, vague complaints of bowel or bladder dysfunction without definitive diagnosis may be additional indication for further study.

Ovarian tumors may be epithelial, germ cell, or stromal in origin. The most common is epithelial, with both germ cell and stromal tumors being uncommon. Epithelial tumors may be further classified as serous, mucinous, endometroid, clear cell, and undifferentiated.[2]

Ovarian cancer is difficult to diagnose from gross inspection until it invades the ovarian wall or seeds tumor cells in the peritoneal cavity. The epithelial form usually is cystic, whereas the appearance is a solid form when it involves the stroma and connective tissue.[20]

The risk associated with ovarian cancer increases with age. There also is increased risk associated with nulliparity and breast, endometrial, or colorectal cancer. Age at first pregnancy and first live birth, as well as the number of children, may affect the risk of ovarian cancer.

Several serum markers are helpful when dealing with ovarian cancer. These include CA-125, carcinoembryonic antigen (CEA), HCG, and alpha-fetoprotein (AFP). CA-125 uses a monoclonal antibody to detect antigens in the blood. CA-125 is found in 85% of women with advanced ovarian cancer. HCG and AFP levels aid in diagnosis of germ cell tumors. Other diagnostic aids include chest radiography, computed tomographic scanning of the abdomen and pelvis, and ultrasonography.

Initial treatment in any woman with ovarian cancer is surgical. Total hysterectomy with bilateral salpingo-oophorectomy and omentectomy is recommended. Supplementary therapy, when indicated, includes irradiation and chemotherapy. Chemotherapy treatment for epithelial tumors includes cisplatin in combination with cyclophosphamide, doxorubicin, or both.

Treatment of germ cell tumors, which occur unilaterally and in girls and young women, is aimed at preserving fertility. Unilateral oophorectomy is the primary treatment for stage I disease. Adjuvant chemotherapy includes the use of vincristine—dactinomycin—cyclophosphamide and vinblastine—bleomycin—cisplatin. Dysgerminomas are highly sensitive to radiation and are thus treated with radiation therapy.

Grading and staging systems also are used in ovarian cancer. The tumors are graded I through IV, from well differentiated to undifferentiated (Table 56-7).

The American Cancer Society reports an overall survival rate with ovarian cancer of only 38%.[1] With early diagnosis and treatment, the survival rate may approach 85%. Survival rate associated with regional metastasis is 45% compared with only 18% with distant metastasis.

## Breast Cancer

The most frequent site of cancer in the woman continues to be in the breast. This disease is second only to lung cancer as a cause of death from cancer in women. The condition occurs only rarely in men but will strike about 1 in 10 women.[1]

The cause is still unknown, but three theories have been put forth: (1) viral influence, (2) hormonal influence, and (3) genetic influence. It has been discovered that mouse mammary tumor virus can be transmitted through mother's milk and can produce cancer in suck-

**TABLE 56-7.**
ACCEPTED STAGING CLASSIFICATION FOR
OVARIAN CARCINOMA

| STAGE | DESCRIPTION |
|---|---|
| I | Tumor limited to one or both ovaries |
| II | Tumor involves one or both ovaries with pelvic extension |
| III | Tumor growth with widespread intraperitoneal metastasis |
| IV | Tumor growth involves metastasis outside the peritoneal cavity |

ling mice. The enzyme, reverse transcriptase, present in oncogenic virus particles, also has been identified in human milk samples with viruslike particles. Support for the other two theories can be found in risk factors associated with breast cancer.

The frequency of breast cancer increases with age, with the greatest incidence occurring in women over age 50. Personal or family history of breast cancer, especially a mother or sister, greatly increases one's chances of developing breast cancer. Nulliparas, women who deliver their first term pregnancy after age 30, and women with late menopause (after age 45) are at increased risk for breast cancer. Although findings are inconclusive and need additional study, obesity, high-fat diet, oral contraceptives, and estrogen replacement may influence the risk of developing breast cancer.

Breast cancer usually is discovered by the woman. She notes a single lump that is painless, nontender, and movable. It most frequently is found in the upper outer quadrant. The tumor may arise in either the ducts or lobules, and may be either infiltrating or noninfiltrating. As the condition progresses, the tumor becomes adherent to the pectoral muscles and fixed. Dimpling and retraction of the skin and nipple may develop. Peau d'orange skin may be noted, with dimpling that resembles the skin of an orange in the area of tumor involvement. Breast distortion or change in breast contour as well as axillary adenopathy may be noted. Nipple discharge that is unilateral and serous may indicate intraductal papilloma or chronic cystic mastopathy. Definitive diagnosis should be made, since nipple discharge may occur in breast cancer. Histologic types include ductal, lobular, and medullary. Infiltrating ductal is the most common, accounting for about 70% of breast cancers. Primary metastatic sites include lymph nodes, lungs, bones, liver, and pleura, although it may occur anywhere.

Breast self-examination is widely taught to detect lumps in the breast, and should be done on a monthly basis by all women over age 18. In addition to monthly self-examination, all women between ages 18 and 35 should have breast examinations performed by the professional at least every 3 years. Professional examination should be done annually in women over age 40. Ultrasonography is especially helpful in differentiating cystic lesions and solid masses. Thermography continues to be used in some screening procedures; however, the only effective technique for locating nonpalpable lesions is mammography. The American Cancer Society recommends that a baseline mammogram be obtained on all women between ages 35 and 39. Women between 40 and 49 should have a mammogram at least every 2 years and annually if at high risk. All women age 50 or older should have a mammogram on an annual basis.[1]

Definitive diagnosis is necessary whenever a breast mass is identified. Needle aspiration usually is sufficient when benign cysts are suspected. Nonpalpable areas of

**TABLE 56-8.**
ESTROGEN AND PROGESTERONE RECEPTOR PROTEIN VALUES

| VALUES | INTERPRETATION |
|---|---|
| <3 femtomoles/mg | Negative |
| 3–10 femtomoles/mg | Suggestive, borderline |
| >10 femtomoles/mg | Positive |

density or microcalcifications identified on mammogram can be localized by use of fine wire placement for biopsy. Definitive diagnosis can be made when the mass is excised and biopsy performed.

When a cancer has been diagnosed, all women should be screened for metastasis before implementation of a specific treatment regimen. This screening may include bone scans, liver function studies, and determination of alkaline phosphatase, serum calcium, and phosphorus levels.

Additional screening measures used to determine the appropriate therapy for the individual woman include tumor study for estrogen and progesterone receptor protein levels, serum marker levels, and flow cytometry. Estrogen and progesterone receptor protein levels are helpful in determining the prognosis as well as predicting response to hormonal therapy. Levels vary in premenopausal and postmenopausal women. Table 56-8 reflects values and their meaning in premenopausal women. Because these values increase with age, postmenopausal women may demonstrate levels as high as 200 femtomoles per milligram. Studies indicate that the prognosis is better in those patients with receptor-positive tumors. Researchers believe that receptor-positive tumors also are more susceptible to hormonal therapy with tamoxifen.

The two serum markers used in determining therapy in breast cancer are CEA and cystic disease protein. CEA levels greater than 10 mg/mL and cystic disease protein values greater than 150 mg/mL provide presumptive evidence of recurrent disease or metastasis to distant organs.

Flow cytometry is perhaps the newest technique being used with breast cancer patients. Flow cytometry can be completed on frozen tissue or paraffin-embedded specimens. Using paraffin-embedded samples avoids some problems encountered with frozen specimens.[7] Flow cytometry analysis provides information on tumor DNA index (ploidy) and the percentage of cells in S-phase. This procedure is being used in clinical areas across the nation in an attempt to identify women at high-risk for breast cancer.

Staging of breast cancer is based on the tumor-node-metastasis classification. In this process, the tumor is evaluated for size and extent of involvement in surrounding tissue and lymph nodes as well as distant metastasis.

**TABLE 56–9.**
STAGING OF BREAST CANCER

| STAGE | CLASS | DESCRIPTION |
|---|---|---|
| I | T1 | Tumor 2 cm or less |
| | N0 | No palpable axillary nodes |
| | M0 | No evident metastasis |
| II | T0 | No palpable tumor |
| | T1 | Tumor 2 cm or less |
| | T2 | Tumor less than 5 cm |
| | N1 | Palpable axillary nodes with histologic evidence of breast cancer |
| | M0 | No evidence of metastasis |
| III | T3 | Tumor more than 5 cm; may be fixed to muscle or fascia |
| | N1 or N2 | Fixed nodes |
| | M0 | No evidence of metastasis |
| IV | T4 | Tumor any size with fixation to chest wall or skin; presence of edema, including peau d'orange; ulceration; skin nodules; inflammatory carcinoma |
| | N3 | Supraclavicular or intraclavicular nodes or arm edema |
| | M1 | Distant metastasis present or suspected |

*Modified from American Cancer Society Staging, 1986.*

The summary of this process presented in Table 56-9 is modified from the American Cancer Society staging.[2] No standard has been established regarding the number of nodes involved for positive versus negative grading.

The treatment for breast cancer is highly individualized. Most women with early disease are given the option of lumpectomy with radiation, or total mastectomy. Axillary node resection should accompany both procedures. Results of follow-up screening then can be used in determining the need for adjuvant chemotherapy or hormonal therapy. Lumpectomy without radiation is associated with a failure rate greater than 30% and should not be considered a viable alternative.[2] Chemotherapy and tamoxifen can decrease the risk of relapse or recurrent disease even when nodes are negative. Therefore, the decision regarding adjuvant therapy should be made only after thorough discussion with the patient regarding the chance of relapse without treatment, expected decrease in risk associated with the therapy, and the expected side effects of therapy.[15] Tamoxifen is less toxic than the chemotherapy but should be taken for 5 years. The most frequently used chemotherapeutic drugs include doxorubicin, cyclophosphamide, methotrexate, 5-fluorouracil, prednisone, and vincristine. Combination chemotherapy includes cyclophosphamide—doxorubicin—5-fluorouracil, cyclophosphamide—methotrexate—5-fluorouracil, and cyclophosphamide—methotrexate—5-fluorouracil—vincristine—prednisone.

The American Cancer Society reports a 90% 5-year survival rate for breast cancer that is still localized. The survival rate drops to 68% with regional spread and to only 18% with distant metastases.[1]

## Vulvar Cancer

The incidence of vulvar cancer is increasing, with about 1.5 per 100,000 women being affected.[13] This increased incidence is believed to be the result of improved attention to and diagnosis of obvious lesions and chronic pruritus of the vulva. Obvious lesions and chronic pruritus that do not respond promptly to local therapy should be biopsied to aid in early diagnosis. Historically, vulvar cancer has been considered to be a disease that primarily affects older women between ages 50 and 60. One clinic, however, reported that almost 80% of cases in their clinic were women under age 50.[17] Another factor that contributes to the increased rate of vulvar cancer is the high rate of infection with the human papillomavirus among women.

Vulvar intraepithelial neoplasia (VIN) may appear as white, red, blue, or brown pigmented lesions. The lesions may occur singly or as multiple papules or macules (Figure 56-31). Lesions also may be found on perianal skin. Most often the patient is asymptomatic. When symptoms are present, they include complaints of pruritus and vulvar burning.

Diagnosis is based on biopsy findings. To aid in identification of areas in need of biopsy, the skin is washed with 1% acetic acid, dried, and covered with an application of toluidine blue dye. After several minutes, the skin is again washed with 1% acetic acid. Areas where biopsy should be performed retain the purple color. The rate of false-positives as well as false-negatives with this proce-

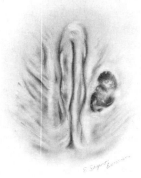

**FIGURE 56–31.**
An ulcerated or raised, red vulvar lesion in an elderly woman may indicate vulvar carcinoma. (B. Bates, *A Guide to Physical Examination and History Taking* [5th ed.]. Philadelphia: J.B. Lippincott, 1991.)

dure is high.[17] A hand magnifying lens as well as the lens of the colposcope may be helpful in identifying biopsy sites.

Treatment choices of VIN include local excision, laser vaporization, cryotherapy, and electrocautery. In cases of local invasion, local excision is the treatment of choice

There is no consensus regarding the management of vulvar cancer. With more and more younger women being affected, there is growing concern for conservative treatment that limits anatomic deformity, preserves psychosexual function, promotes a positive self-image, and at the same time provides adequate treatment of the cancer.

The Gynecologic Oncology Group has concluded that treatment for vulvar cancer must be determined on an individual basis.[8] Factors to consider in determining individual treatment include depth of invasion, midline location, histologic grade, and vascular space involvement. Treatment regimens include surgery with and without node resection, radiation therapy, and chemotherapy. Chemotherapeutic agents used include 5-fluorouracil, cisplatin, and carboplatin. Radiation therapy may include intracavitary radium as well as external radiation.[8]

# REFERENCES

1. American Cancer Society. *Cancer Facts & Figures—1990.* Atlanta: American Cancer Society, 1990.
2. American Cancer Society, Massachusetts Division. *Cancer Manual* (7th ed.). Boston: American Cancer Society, 1986.
3. Berkowitz, R.S., Goldstein, D.P., and Bernstein, M.R. Partial molar pregnancy: A separate entity. *Contemp. OB/GYN* 31(6):99, 1988.
4. Centers for Disease Control. Follow-up on toxic-shock syndrome. *MMWR* 29:441, 1980.
5. Cotran, R.S., Kumar, V., and Robbins, S.L. *Robbins' Pathologic Basis of Disease* (4th ed.). Philadelphia: W.B. Saunders, 1989.
6. Guyton, A.C. *Textbook of Medical Physiology* (8th ed.). Philadelphia: W.B. Saunders, 1990.
7. Hedley, D.W. Measurement of DNA content of archival material as a guide to prognosis. In J. Ragaz and I.M. Ariel (eds.), *High Risk Breast Cancer Diagnosis.* New York: Springer-Verlag, 1989.
8. Karlan, B.Y., and Lagasse, L.D. Conservative management of vulvar cancer. *Contemp. OB/GYN* 35(6):27, 1990.
9. Kistner, R.W. *Gynecology: Principles and Practice* (4th ed.). Chicago: Yearbook, 1986.
10. Levy, M.J., and Stillman, R.J. Reproductive surgery and the DES uterus. *Contemp. OB/GYN* 35:97, 1990.
11. London, R.S., and Hammond, C.B. The climacteric. In D.N. Danforth and J.R. Scott (eds.), *Obstetrics and Gynecology* (5th ed.). Philadelphia: J.B. Lippincott, 1986.
12. March, C.M. Hysteroscopic resection of submucous myomas. *Contemp. OB/GYN* 35:59, 1990.
13. Morgan, L.S., and Wilkinson, E.J. Meeting the challenge of superficially invasive vulvar carcinoma. *Contemp. OB/GYN* 31(5):181, 1988.
14. Murata, J.M. Abnormal genital bleeding and secondary amenorrhea: Common gynecological problems. *J. Obstet. Gynecol. Neonatal Nurs.* 19:26, 1990.
15. National Institute of Health. Consensus development conference statement on the treatment of early stage breast cancer, June 18-21, 1990. Sponsored by National Cancer Institute and the Office of Medical Applications of Research of the National Institutes of Health, 1990.
16. Norwood, S.L. Fibrocystic breast disease: An update and review. *J. Obstet. Gynecol. Neonatal Nurs.* 19:116, 1990.
17. Roy, M. VIN—Latest management approaches. *Contemp. OB/GYN* 31(5):170, 1988.
18. Slattery, M.L., Robison, L.M., Schuman, K.L., et al. Cigarette smoking and exposure to passive smoke are risk factors for cervical cancer. *J.A.M.A.* 261:1593, 1989.
19. Wedell, M.A., Billings, P., and Fayez, J.A. Endometriosis and the infertile patient. *J. Obstet. Gynecol. Neonatal Nurs.* 14:280, 1985.
20. Zaloudek, C., Tavassoli, F.A., and Kurman, R.J. Malignant lesions of the ovary. In D.N. Danforth and J.R. Scott (eds.), *Obstetrics and Gynecology* (5th ed.). Philadelphia: J.B. Lippincott, 1986.

# Sexually Transmitted Diseases

## Chapter Outline

▶ **Bacterial Sexually Transmitted Diseases**
    **Gonorrhea**
    **Syphilis**
    **Chancroid**
    **Granuloma Inguinale**
    **Lymphogranuloma Venereum**
    ***Haemophilus vaginalis* Vaginitis**
    ***Chlamydia trachomatis***

▶ **Viral Sexually Transmitted Diseases**
    **Genital Herpes**
    **Condylomata Acuminata**
    **Acquired Immune Deficiency Syndrome**
▶ **Fungal Sexually Transmitted Disease**
    **Candidiasis**
▶ **Protozoal Sexually Transmitted Disease**
    **Trichomonal Vaginitis**

## Learning Objectives

1. Identify the causative organism for each of the sexually transmitted diseases (STDs).
2. Discuss the clinical manifestations of each STD.
3. Identify the three most prevalent STDs.
4. Discuss the impact of each STD on the fetus or neonate.
5. Discuss the appropriate diagnostic aids and treatment for each STD.

---

Sexually transmitted disease (STD) refers to those conditions that can be transmitted through sexual intercourse or intimate contact. For many years, these conditions were referred to as venereal disease, and primarily included gonorrhea and syphilis. The term STD is more inclusive, and refers to many more conditions (Table 57-1) so classified by the Centers for Disease Control (CDC).

In addition to the classic venereal diseases of gonorrhea and syphilis, other prime STDs include genital herpes, chancroid, granuloma inguinale, and lymphogranuloma venereum. The term STD also has been used to refer to several infections that affect reproductive function. Among these infections are trichomonal and candidal infections, those caused by *Haemophilus vaginalis* and *Chlamydia trachomatis*, and condylomata acuminata.

Another group of conditions considered to be STDs are those infections caused by enteric pathogens. These organisms are believed to be transmitted by oral-anal sex, and include *Shigella, Entamoeba histolytica*, and *Giardia lamblia*.

The most recent alteration in reproductive function to be recognized as sexually transmitted is infection with the human immunodeficiency virus (HIV). Viral infections currently recognized as STDs include hepatitis B and cytomegalovirus. Additionally, the CDC also recognizes scabies, pediculosis pubis, *Campylobacter,* and shigellosis as being sexually transmitted. A review of Table 57-1 indicates that STDs can be classified by the causative organism as to bacterial, viral, protozoal, parasitic, or fungal.

The STDs discussed in this chapter include those diseases that occur most frequently as well as those with the greatest impact on reproductive function. Conditions not discussed in this chapter include *Campylobacter* enteritis, cytomegalovirus, shigellosis, scabies, and pediculosis pubis. More information on these infections can

**TABLE 57-1.**
SEXUALLY TRANSMITTED DISEASES

| DISEASE | ORGANISM | MORPHOLOGY |
|---|---|---|
| **Bacterial** | | |
| Gonorrhea | *Neisseria gonorrhoeae* | Gram-negative diplococcus |
| Syphilis | *Treponema pallidum* | Spirochete |
| Chancroid | *Haemophilus ducreyi* | Gram-negative bacillus |
| Granuloma inguinale | *Donovania granulomatis* | Gram-negative bacillus |
| Lymphogranuloma venereum | *Chlamydia* | |
| Chlamydia | *Chlamydia trachomatis* | |
| Vaginitis | *Haemophilus vaginalis* | Gram-negative bacillus |
| Shigellosis | *Shigella* | Gram-negative aerobic, bacillus |
| **Viral** | | |
| Genital herpes | Herpesvirus hominis type 2 | DNA present |
| Condylomata acuminata | Human papillomavirus | DNA present |
| Acquired immune deficiency syndrome | Human immunodeficiency virus | RNA retrovirus |
| Cytomegalovirus | Cytomegalovirus | DNA present |
| Hepatitis B | Hepatitis B | DNA type |
| **Fungal** | | |
| Trichomoniasis | *Trichomonas vaginalis* | Flagellate |
| Amebiasis | *Entamoeba histolytica* | Anaerobic motile trophozoite (active); cysts transmission |
| Giardiasis | *Giardia lamblia* | Flagellate |
| **Parasites** | | |
| Scabies | *Sarcoptes scabiei* | |
| Pediculosis pubis | *Phthirius pubis* | |

be found in Chapter 12; hepatitis B is discussed in Chapter 43.

## BACTERIAL SEXUALLY TRANSMITTED DISEASES

### Gonorrhea

Gonorrhea is the second most common STD. Although it continues to occur in epidemic proportions in the United States, it is estimated that the 1990 reduction goal of 280 cases per 100,000 population will be met.[5] Even with this goal, two concerns remain: (1) the stable rate in the black population and the slow decline of adolescent infection when compared with the older adult population, and (2) the increasing number of penicillin-resistant strains of the gonococcus.[5]

The causative organism in gonorrhea is *Neisseria gonorrhoeae,* which is a gram-negative diplococcus. This organism thrives in the warm, moist environment of mucous membranes. It may spread rapidly during menstruation because of the favorable environment produced by the blood. It does not survive well outside the body, and exhibits increasing resistance to penicillin. It is almost exclusively an STD, but it can be contracted by the fetus during delivery or by people who have skin breaks that come in contact with contaminated discharge. It may occur in the throat, eyes, or rectum as the result of oral-anal sex, anal sex, or contamination during the birth process. The clinical spectrum of gonococcal infection is shown in Figure 57-1.

Women who contract gonorrhea frequently are asymptomatic. When symptoms are present, they may include green or yellow vaginal discharge, dysuria, urinary frequency, pruritus, and red swollen vulva. Rectal discharge may be noted with rectal infection. Additionally, Skene's glands and Bartholin's glands may be involved (Figure 57-2A).

In the male, urethritis occurs 2 to 10 days after exposure. At this time, a purulent discharge from the urethral meatus is noted (Figure 57-2B). The discharge is clear at first but soon becomes white or even green. It may be accompanied by itching, burning, and pain around the meatal opening, especially during voiding. Ten percent to 20% of males with gonorrhea may have

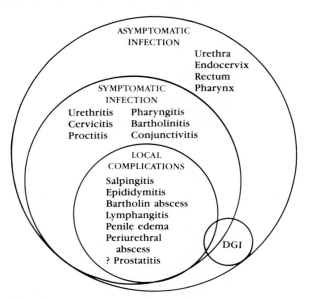

**FIGURE 57-1.**
Spectrum of gonococcal manifestations. DGI, disseminated gono-coccal infection. (K.K. Holmes et al., *Sexually Transmitted Diseases.* New York: McGraw-Hill, 1984.)

Conclusive diagnosis must be made on the basis of cultures because there are no serology tests for diagnosis. Culture media usually contain antibiotics to inhibit other bacterial growth, and these are placed in an atmosphere of increased carbon dioxide. Bacterial growth should be apparent within 24 to 48 hours if gonorrheal organisms are present.

Treatment with ceftriaxone plus doxycycline is instituted immediately and usually is curative.[4] A follow-up culture should be done to document eradication of the organism. In people who are sensitive to penicillin or with gonococcal strains that are resistant to penicillin, other antibiotics such as tetracycline may be used. Sexual partners should be treated concurrently, and intercourse should be avoided until repeat cultures indicate a cure. Single infection with the gonococcus organism does not confer immunity.

no symptoms. In the absence of prompt treatment, infection is likely to spread to involve the prostate, seminal vesicles, and epididymis. With chronic or prolonged infection, abscesses, tissue destruction, and scarring may result. Urethral strictures may lead to hydronephrosis, and epididymitis may cause sterility. Other complications that may occur from gonococcal bacteremia include suppurative arthritis, acute bacterial endocarditis, and suppurative meningitis.

## Syphilis

Syphilis is less common than gonorrhea but more serious. Serologic screening has been successful in detecting syphilis, resulting in a dramatic decline of the disease in the 1950s. The incidence of syphilis is now on the increase, with more than 105,000 cases reported in 1989.[10] This number represents the most reported cases in 40 years. The increased incidence also has been associated with the rising incidence of HIV infection. The rate of infectious syphilis reflects a decrease among homosexual men and an increase among black men as well as heterosexual men and women.

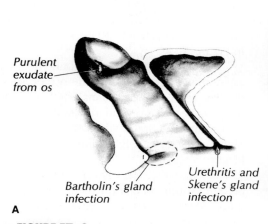

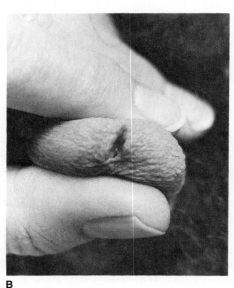

**FIGURE 57-2.**
**A.** Early gonorrhea. (B. Bates, *A Guide to Physical Examination and History Taking* [4th ed.]. Philadelphia: J.B. Lippincott, 1987.) **B.** The discharge of gonococcal urethritis tends to be profuse and yellow, whereas that of nongonococcal urethritis tends to be scanty and white or clear. Definitive diagnosis requires a Gram stain and culture. (B. Bates, *A Guide to Physical Examination and History Taking* [5th ed.]. Philadelphia: J.B. Lippincott, 1991.)

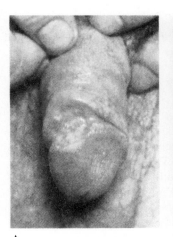
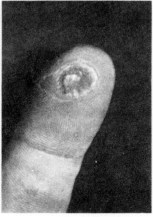

**FIGURE 57–3.**
**A.** Primary-stage syphilis chancre on the penis. **B.** Primary chancre on a finger. (*Sexually Transmitted Diseases* by D. Barlow, photographed by Tom Treasure. Published by Oxford University Press. © 1979 by David Barlow.)

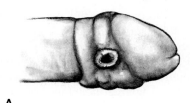

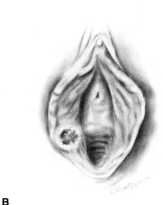

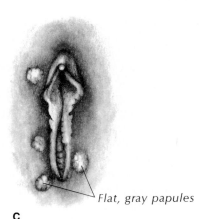

*Flat, gray papules*

**FIGURE 57–4.**
**A.** Syphilitic chancre. **B.** Syphilitic chancre on vulva. **C.** Secondary syphilis. (B. Bates, *A Guide to Physical Examination and History Taking* [5th ed.]. Philadelphia, J.B. Lippincott, 1991.)

The causative organism in syphilis is the spirochete *Treponema pallidum*. Because of its size, the spirochete is visible only with darkfield microscopy. It is sensitive to both drying and temperature, and normally enters the skin through moist mucous membranes. It also has been known to enter through breaks in the skin. Transmission may be through sexual contact, by personal contact, or by an infected mother to her unborn fetus.

The course of untreated syphilis progresses in three stages: primary, secondary, and tertiary. Within 24 hours after the spirochete has entered the body, it spreads throughout. Primary syphilis develops after an incubation period of 10 days to 3 months. The first symptom, a chancre, appears at the site of entry (Figure 57-3). The chancre usually is a painless, red, hardened lesion that may resemble a pimple and often is accompanied by regional lymphadenopathy (Figure 57-4A and B). Because the person feels well, the infection may go undetected at this stage, and results of serology tests are normal. The infection, as well as blood, is highly contagious at this time. The chancre usually disappears within 2 to 6 weeks with or without treatment. Diagnosis is based on identification of the spirochete from the ulceration.

The second stage appears at variable times up to 6 months later. It begins with the development of a generalized, usually maculopapular rash, especially on the palms and soles. Other lesions may be follicular, pustular, or scaling. Large elevated plaques, termed condylomata lata (wartlike, flattened areas), develop on the genitalia (Figure 57-4C). Secondary syphilis also may be characterized by fever, headaches, loss of appetite, sore mouth, and alopecia. Generalized lymphadenopathy, hepatitis, and nephrosis may occur. Spirochetes are present in all lesions, especially condylomata lata. Syphilis in this stage remains highly contagious, and spiro-

chetes may even cross the placenta to an unborn baby. About 4 to 12 weeks after the beginning of the second stage, all symptoms disappear and the disease enters a latent period. Results of serology tests at this time usually are positive. The course of the disease is variable at this stage. After the latent period, syphilis may be cured spontaneously, remain latent permanently, relapse, or enter the third stage.

After a period of years, the condition progresses to tertiary syphilis and eventually is no longer contagious. Fifty percent of those with tertiary syphilis remain symptom-free; however, results of serology tests may remain positive and the spirochetes can affect an unborn fetus if an infected woman becomes pregnant. For the other infected people, the disease progresses and develops into late clinical syphilis. It can affect any body part, especially the heart (80% to 85%) and central nervous system (5% to 10%).[8]

Chronic inflammation of bones and joints may occur. Gummas, large necrotic areas, may develop in the liver, bones, and testes, producing a nodular pattern of cirrhosis, joint destruction, and enlargement resembling a tumor. Gummatous lesions in the central nervous system are rare, but meningovascular syphilis commonly causes infiltration of the meninges and blood vessels by lymphocytes and plasma cells.[8] Neurosyphilis involves the loss of cortical neurons because of the large number of spirochetes throughout the brain parenchyma. The effect of neurosyphilis is dementia, and behavioral changes that progress to psychotic behavior and ataxic paresthesia. Finally, loss of position, deep pain, and temperature sensation occur. The average interval from infection to symptomatic neurosyphilis is 20 to 30 years.

Infection with *T. pallidum* confers immunity on the infected person. Both syphilitic reagin and treponemal immobilizing serum antibodies are produced after 1 to 4 months. Treponemal immobilizing antibodies are specific, and probably account for the active immunity. Syphilitic reagin is the basis for both the complement fixation and flocculation diagnostic tests.

In the early stage, diagnosis is made only by darkfield microscopy. After the antigen—antibody reaction has occurred, serology tests such as the VDRL (Venereal Disease Research Laboratory), FTA-ABS (fluorescent treponemal antibody-absorption), TPI (*Treponema pallidum* immobilization), TPHA (*Treponema pallidum* hemoagglutinin assay), and RPR (rapid plasma reagin) are commonly used to confirm the diagnosis. The VDRL is the most widely used because of cost and simplicity; however, both false-positive and false-negative results are likely to occur with this test. The next most favorable test is the PTA-ABS. The TPHA and RPR are used for screening large populations.

Penicillin continues to be the drug of choice for treating people with syphilis. It must be given in doses appropriate to the stage of disease. In people with known sensitivity to penicillin, the choice is tetracycline. Because of its teratogenic effect, tetracycline should not be administered to pregnant women. In these cases, the treatment of choice becomes erythromycin. Treatment should be initiated at any point of diagnosis during pregnancy to prevent additional damage to the fetus. Transplacental transmission of the disease leads to death or extensive infection in the infant. Eyes, liver, teeth, and lungs can be affected, leading to dysfunction of the organs in the infant.

## Chancroid

Chancroid is an acute disease process that produces a soft chancre or shallow, ragged ulcer after an incubation period of up to 10 days. This condition is prevalent worldwide, especially in Southeast Asia, Africa, and South America. It is caused by the gram-negative bacillus *Haemophilus ducreyi*.

Within 3 to 5 days of exposure, a maculopapular lesion appears on the penis or vulva. This lesion progresses to pustular lesions and eventually sloughing of the skin. This process results in a painful ulcer 1 to 3 cm in diameter. Self-inoculation with the causative organism results in the appearance of numerous lesions. Inguinal lymph nodes become swollen and tender. Suppuration from lymph nodes and the necrotic chancre occur. Gram's stain of exudate, culture, and biopsy aid in diagnosis. Erythromycin, ceftriaxone, or sulfisoxazole (Gantrisin) and good hygiene allow healing in 2 to 4 weeks.

## Granuloma Inguinale

Granuloma inguinale (Donovanosis) is a chronic disease process caused by the gram-negative bacillus *Calymmatobacterium granulomatis*. It begins as a papule and progresses to a spreading necrotic ulcer with extensive scarring. It has a low degree of infectivity and progressively involves the skin and lymphatics of the groin and inguinal areas. Smears and biopsy aid in identification of Donovan bodies and differentiation from other STDs. Antibiotic treatment with tetracycline usually results in complete healing. Gentamicin and chloramphenicol also have been used in treatment of granuloma inguinale.

## Lymphogranuloma Venereum

This condition is caused by a strain of *Chlamydia* organisms. It is characterized by a small, painless papule or vesicle that appears after an incubation of less than 3 weeks. Spontaneous healing usually occurs after several days. Within 2 to 8 weeks, painful lymphatic involvement occurs with possible obstruction. Malaise, fever, and headache may be noted. In addition to history and physical examination, aspiration of lymph for complement fixation and skin test with Frei antigen may be performed to confirm the diagnosis. Treatment of lymphogranuloma venereum includes erythromycin and tetracycline.

# Haemophilus vaginalis *Vaginitis*

*Haemophilus vaginalis,* also referred to as *Gardnerella,* has now been identified as one causative organism in vaginitis previously referred to as nonspecific vaginitis. It is a gram-negative bacillus similar to *Corynebacterium vaginalis.* It is spread through sexual contact, and elimination of the infection requires treatment of both sexual partners.

The most outstanding symptom is a thin, heavy, gray discharge with the presence of only mild irritation (Figure 57-5). Diagnosis is made by identifying cells dotted with small, short bacilli. Cultures may be done for additional confirmation. Ampicillin or tetracycline may be administered orally for systemic effect. Milder cases may be treated with sulfonamide creams or suppositories such as sulfathiazole, sulfisoxazole, or nitrofurazone. Metronidazole also may be used.

## NONSPECIFIC VAGINITIS
(*Associated with Gardnerella Vaginalis*)

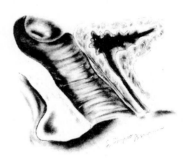

**Discharge**
Gray, thin, homogeneous, malodorous, occasionally somewhat frothy; not so profuse as in Trichomonas or Monilia infections, may be minimal

**Vulva**
Usually normal

**Urethritis**
Absent

**Bartholin Gland Infection**
Absent

**Vaginal Mucosa**
Usually normal; occasionally may be red or swollen

**Cervix**
Normal

**FIGURE 57–5.**
Nonspecific vaginitis (associated with *Gardnerella vaginalis*). (B. Bates, *A Guide to Physical Examination and History Taking* [4th ed.]. Philadelphia: J.B. Lippincott, 1987.)

# Chlamydia trachomatis

Chlamydia are the most common sexually transmitted organisms in the United States today, having surpassed even gonorrhea. An estimated 3 to 4 million cases occur per year.[11] It has been noted most often in the younger population, especially in sexually active adolescents. People considered to be at increased risk for chlamydial infection include those (1) with more than one current sex partner, (2) with a history of multiple partners, (3) aged 15 to 24, (4) using a nonbarrier contraceptive, and (5) from lower socioeconomic status.

The causative organism in chlamydial infections is *Chlamydia trachomatis,* an intracellular bacterial parasite. Physical examination with cultures and Papanicolaou smears aid in ruling out herpes and gonorrhea as well as other conditions. Clinical diagnosis often is based on documentation of urethritis with discharge or symptoms of cervicitis when gonorrhea has been ruled out. Gram's stains may indicate the presence of polymorphonuclear leukocytes. Many women who are infected with the organism remain asymptomatic for years.

Definitive diagnosis of chlamydial infection is based on tissue culture taken from endocervical secretions. This technique is time-consuming and expensive, and requires meticulous care in transporting the specimen to a laboratory equipped to perform the examination. To avoid the problems associated with chlamydial cultures, two new tests have been developed and approved by the Food and Drug Administration.[2] These tests are Chlamydiazyme and Microtract. The Chlamydiazyme test is an enzyme-linked immunoassay that depends on an antigen—antibody reaction. The results are read on a spectrophotometer. Results greater than 0.1 are considered positive. The Microtract test uses a fluorescein-labeled monoclonal antibody. Specimens are collected from the endocervix or anterior urethra in males, placed on a slide, and fixed before transporting to the laboratory. A fluorescent microscope is used to read the stained and incubated slide.

The most outstanding symptoms involve the genitourinary system. As much as 50% of nongonococcal urethritis in men and cervicitis in women may be caused by *C. trachomatis.*[2] Although women frequently are asymptomatic, symptoms, when present, include lower abdominal pain, vaginal discharge, dysuria, urinary frequency, and vaginal bleeding. Discharge, when present, may be heavy with a fishy odor. The discharge is gray-white and creamy, and usually is not accompanied by itching or irritation. Examination of the cervix, the most common site of female infection, may reveal congestion, mucopurulent discharge, or ectopy. Acute salpingitis, conjunctivitis, and repeated sore throats may be noted in women. If left untreated, the infection can result in pelvic inflammatory disease with salpingitis and even sterility. Chlamydial infection also has been associated with increased incidence of ectopic pregnancy.[6]

Chlamydial infections usually are controlled with antibiotics, which include doxycycline, erythromycin, and tetracycline. During pregnancy, untreated infection is associated with increased frequencies of premature rupture of the membranes, premature contractions, and small-for-gestational-age infants.[7] A newborn may acquire the disease through contact with an infected birth canal. The disease in the newborn may result in conjunctivitis or pneumonia. Prophylactic treatment of the newborn with erythromycin ophthalmic ointment helps to prevent neonatal conjunctivitis. Treatment of chlamydial infection also requires treatment of the sexual partner. Lack of treatment in the partner may result in reinfection of the patient.

## VIRAL SEXUALLY TRANSMITTED DISEASES

### Genital Herpes

Genital herpes, one of the most common of the primary STDs, is a highly contagious condition caused by the herpesvirus hominis (HVH) type 2, one of the herpes simplex viruses. Type 1 refers to the common cold sore or fever blister that primarily occurs above the waist. The condition occurs in two forms: primary and recurrent. After incubation of 3 to 7 days, HVH type 2 produces single or multiple vesicles greater than 1 mm in diameter that rupture spontaneously after 24 to 72 hours. These vesicles are accompanied by redness and swelling. After rupture of the vesicles, painful, reddened ulcers develop that eventually scab, heal, and disappear (Figure 57-6). The primary attack usually lasts for 3 to 4 weeks before

the virus and then becomes dormant in the nerve cells. Sores reappear whenever triggered to multiply. Factors known to trigger outbreak of symptoms include colds, fever, severe sunburn, menstruation, gastrointestinal upset, and stress. Recurrent attacks produce less edema and inflammation, and lesions usually disappear in 7 to 10 days. An estimated 80% or more of infected people experience annual recurrences.

The first attack of genital herpes usually is the worst, and is characterized by small, extremely painful blisters. Before the appearance of blisters, the person may notice a tingling or burning sensation possibly followed by intense itching. In the male, lesions of 0.5 to 1.5 cm are present on the glans penis, prepuce, buttocks, and inner thighs (Figure 57-7). In the female, 90% of the lesions appear on the cervix. Contamination of other body parts may lead to lesions on the thighs, buttocks, and fingers. Secondary infection may occur when the blisters rupture. In both sexes, the initial infection may be accompanied by fever, swelling, enlarged painful lymph nodes, and, in the male, dysuria. Fever and enlarged lymph nodes are less likely to occur with subsequent attacks. Infected people should be cautioned that shedding of the virus may occur even in the absence of symptoms.[3]

There is no known cure for herpes. Several agents have been used with varying success in the treatment of lesions. These include iodine solutions, chloroform, immunotherapy, bacillus Calmette-Guérin vaccine, nitrous oxide, ether, and photoinactivation with a light-sensitive dye and fluorescent light. The only effective antiviral drug in the United States is acyclovir (Zovirax). Alone it is inactive, but when in contact with the virus, it is converted to an active form by an enzyme, thymidine kinase, produced by the virus. It hastens healing and decreases transmissibility but has no effect on recurrence.

Herpes infection can be painful and annoying to the man or woman, but it can represent a life-threatening situation to an unborn fetus. This disease can produce abortion or premature delivery. Genital herpes is highly contagious when the vesicles rupture, and delivery through an infected vagina increases the chance that the infection will be passed to the infant.[1] Herpes infection in a newborn can produce brain damage or death. Therefore, a cesarean birth is advisable in any woman with active genital herpes. Another primary concern for women with herpesvirus is the increased risk of cervical cancer. It is now suspected that herpes may be a factor in the development of cervical and vulvar cancer.

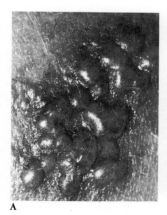 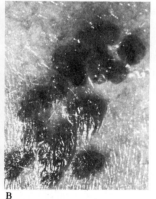

A                                              B

**FIGURE 57-6.**
**A.** Genital herpes blisters before treatment. **B.** Blisters after 4 days of treatment with intravaginal and topical 2-deoxy-D-glucose. (H. Blough and R. Giuntoli, Successful treatment of human genital herpes with 2-deoxy-D-glucose. *J.A.M.A.* 241:2798, 1979.)

### Condylomata Acuminata

Condylomata acuminata, referred to as venereal warts, are caused by the *human papillomavirus*. Infection often coexists with other STDs such as *Trichomonas, Monilia,* and gonorrhea. The incubation period between infection

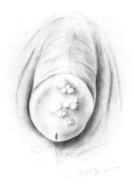

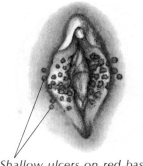

Shallow ulcers on red bases

A                                                                    B

**FIGURE 57–7.**
**A.** Genital herpes on penis. **B.** Genital herpes on vulva. (B. Bates, *A Guide to Physical Examination and History Taking* [5th ed.]. Philadelphia: J.B. Lippincott, 1991.)

and development of the lesions is 1 to 3 months. The characteristic cauliflower-like lesions (Figure 57-8) are estrogen-dependent and located on the introitus, vulva, or rectum. These lesions may be associated with heavy vaginal discharge, foul odor, and bleeding. Anyone with external growths should be examined for lesions within the vagina, cervix, or rectum. Women with a history of infection caused by human papillomavirus are at increased risk for cancer of the cervix, vulva, and vagina. A relation also has been established between both penile and anal cancer and papillomavirus infection.[9]

Diagnosis is based on clinical appearance or history of sexual contact with an infected person. Biopsy may be performed to rule out vulvar tumors, and a VDRL test may be performed to rule out the condylomata lata found in secondary syphilis.

Condylomata acuminata lesions are treated with podophyllin (20% to 25%) in tincture of benzoin. This solution should be applied to all lesions at weekly intervals until the lesions are resolved. Podophyllin is a corrosive solution, and should be washed off within 2 to 4 hours of the initial application. Length of application may be increased with subsequent treatments, provided there is no adverse effect. Petroleum jelly may be used to protect the surrounding normal tissue. Cautery, cryotherapy, carbon dioxide laser surgery, or 5-fluorouracil cream may be used, depending on the size of the lesions. Radiation therapy may be indicated. If lesions measure more than 1.5 to 2 cm, surgical excision, cryotherapy, or cautery usually are used. Concurrent treatment of sexual partners may help to prevent recurrence.

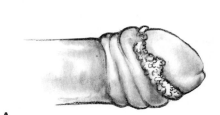

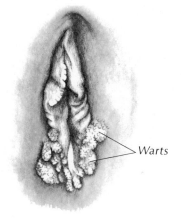

Warts

A                                                                    B

**FIGURE 57–8.**
**A.** Venereal wart (condyloma acuminatum) on penis. **B.** Venereal wart on vulva. (B. Bates, *A Guide to Physical Examination and History Taking* [5th ed.]. Philadelphia: J.B. Lippincott, 1991.)

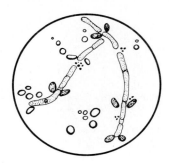

**FIGURE 57–9.**

Fresh vaginal smear preparation. Microscopic picture in candidal vaginitis. (T.H. Green, Jr., *Gynecology: Essentials of Clinical Practice* [3rd ed.]. Boston: Little, Brown, 1977.)

## *Acquired Immune Deficiency Syndrome*

The multiplicity of transmission routes has contributed to the controversy over the status of acquired immune deficiency syndrome (AIDS) as an STD. This syndrome, first identified in 1979, has received much medical attention during recent years. Although more extensive discussion of the pathophysiology of HIV infection, including AIDS, is found in Chapter 15, a brief discussion of the sexual nature and the impact of AIDS on pregnancy and the neonate is provided here.

The causative organism of AIDS is an infectious agent, HIV (formerly called human T cell lymphotrophic virus, or HTLV III). Routes of transmission appear to be intimate sexual contact and inoculation with contaminated blood or blood products. Homosexual or bisexual men, hemophiliacs, and intravenous drug users seem to be especially at risk. The CDC have now reported the presence of opportunistic infections typical of AIDS, including *Pneumocystis carinii* pneumonia, in heterosexual women. Most of these women had been associated with sexual partners in the high-risk group.

When AIDS occurs in children, mortality is extremely high. Many of these children are hemophiliacs who contracted the disease through transfusions with contami-

nated blood before the time of proper blood screening. The incidence of AIDS now being confirmed in newborns indicates the transmission of the virus during pregnancy, labor and delivery, and shortly after birth from infected women to their fetuses or offspring. Transmission of the virus through breast milk continues to be the subject of research.

## *FUNGAL SEXUALLY TRANSMITTED DISEASE*

### *Candidiasis*

Candidiasis is a vaginal infection produced by the fungus *Candida albicans* (Figure 57-9). It also is referred to as moniliasis, thrush, and yeast infection. The organism normally is present on the skin and in the digestive tract, and may colonize the vagina of some asymptomatic women. Symptoms arise when there is an overgrowth of the organism, which most frequently occurs during pregnancy, after antibiotic therapy, in diabetics, and in women taking oral contraceptives. Infants may become infected at delivery and develop thrush. In pregnant women and those taking oral contraceptives, estrogen levels are high, resulting in high glycogen levels that produce a favorable environment for fungal growth. It is believed that systemic antibiotics also suppress the normal bacterial flora in the vagina, and in diabetics, the vaginal environment is "sweeter," both of which encourage fungal growth. The yeast infection produces a heavy, white, cottage cheese—like discharge that is odorless. Complaints of severe itching, dysuria, dyspareunia, and perineal burning are common. The vulva appears erythematous and inflamed (Figure 57-10). Speculum examination may reveal white plaques on the vaginal wall. Diagnosis is confirmed by wet smear examination with potassium hydroxide.

Antifungal preparations such as nystatin, miconazole, and clotrimazole are the treatments of choice. These

*Monilia (Candida) vaginitis*

Discharge—may be thin but characteristically thick, white and curdy

Vaginal mucosa—in severe cases, red and inflamed

Cervix—may show patches of discharge

Vulva—often reddened, itchy and swollen

Urethra—no infection

Bartholin gland—no infection

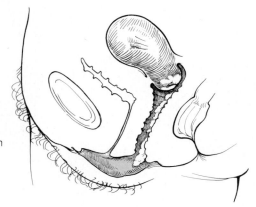

**FIGURE 57–10.**

Candidal vaginitis.

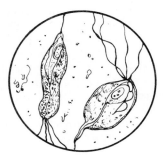

**FIGURE 57-11.**

Microscopic appearance of *Trichomonas vaginalis* organisms. (T.H. Green, Jr., *Gynecology: Essentials of Clinical Practice* [3rd ed.]. Boston: Little, Brown, 1977.)

medications are used as topical drugs and are inserted into the vagina, where they exert a local action on the organism. Absorption is poor from the skin and mucous membrane in the vagina. In the past, gentian violet swabs and suppositories have been used, but they produce staining and sometimes allergic reactions. Taking lactobacillus tablets and eating yogurt may be helpful in restoring the normal bacterial flora after antibiotic therapy. Correction of any abnormally high blood glucose levels in the diabetic is essential in control of the disease. Treatment of the male partner may be necessary to break the reinfection cycle.

## PROTOZOAL SEXUALLY TRANSMITTED DISEASE

### Trichomonal Vaginitis

Trichomoniasis is a vaginal infection caused by the single-celled protozoan, *Trichomonas vaginalis* (Figure 57-11). The organism may remain dormant for extended periods and prefers a basic vaginal pH. It has been identified in the male urethra and prostate, so sexual contact serves as a frequent source of reinfection for the female. The frequency of *Trichomonas* infection is highest in women with many sexual partners.

The organism produces an intense itching and burning of the vulva and vagina. It is accompanied by a moderate to profuse discharge that is thin, frothy, and greenish yellow to greenish white with a foul odor. Examination of the cervix may reveal small, deep, red spots referred to as strawberry spots. Microscopic examination of a wet smear reveals a one-cell protozoan with four flagellae. Cultures seldom are done to confirm the diagnosis.

The treatment of choice is a trichomonacidal drug, metronidazole. It is effective in eradicating the organism in 90% of cases. It may be accompanied by severe side effects and should be used only after confirmed diagnosis of *Trichomonas*. Side effects of metronidazole include

leukopenia, nausea, diarrhea, headache, and alcohol intolerance. The drug has been found to produce cancer in mice and birth defects in guinea pigs and mice. Therefore, its use is avoided in pregnant women or in those suspected of being pregnant. Alternative treatment includes AVC cream or suppositories, Aci-Jel, and iodoquinol. Again, treatment of the male partner may be necessary to prevent the reinfection cycle.

## REFERENCES

1. Bates, B. *A Guide to Physical Examination and History Taking* (5th ed.). Philadelphia: J.B. Lippincott, 1991.
2. Bourcier, K.M., and Seidler, A.J. Chlamydia and condylomata acuminata: An update for the nurse practitioner. *J. Obstet. Gynecol. Neonatal Nurs.* 16:17, 1987.
3. Brock, B.V., Selke, S., Benedetti, J., et al. Frequency of asymptomatic shedding of herpes simplex virus in women with genital herpes. *J.A.M.A.* 263:418, 1990.
4. Centers for Disease Control. Sexually transmitted diseases: Treatment guidelines. *M.M.W.R.* 38(5-8):1, 1989.
5. Centers for Disease Control. Progress toward achieving the 1990 objectives for the nation for sexually transmitted diseases. *M.M.W.R.* 39(4):53, 1990.
6. Chow, J.M., Yonekura, M.L., Richwald, G.A., et al. The association between *Chlamydia trachomatis* and ectopic pregnancy: A matched-pair, case-control study. *J.A.M.A.* 263:3164, 1990.
7. Cohen, I., Veille, J., and Calkins, B.M. Improved pregnancy outcome following successful treatment of chlamydial infection. *J.A.M.A.* 263:3160, 1990.
8. Cotran, R.S., Kumar, V., and Robbins, S.L. *Robbins' Pathologic Basis of Disease* (4th ed.). Philadelphia: W.B. Saunders, 1989.
9. Palefsky, J.M., Gonzales, J., Greenblatt, R.M., et al. Anal intraepithelial neoplasia and anal papillomavirus infection among homosexual males with group IV HIV disease. *J.A.M.A.* 263:2911, 1990.
10. Wendel, G.D., Jr., and Gilstrap, L.C. III. Syphilis rise calls for accurate diagnosis. *Contemp. OB/GYN* 35(6):37, 1990.
11. Woolard, D.G., Larson, J., and Hudson, L. Screening for *Chlamydia trachomatis* at a university health service. *J. Obstet. Gynecol. Neonatal Nurs.* 18:145, 1989.

## UNIT BIBLIOGRAPHY

Adami, H., Bergstrom, R., Holmberg, L., et al. The effect of female sex hormones on cancer survival: A register-based study in patients younger than 20 years at diagnosis. *J.A.M.A.* 263:2189, 1990.

Almadrones, L., and Yerys, C. Problems associated with the administration of intraperitoneal therapy using the port-a-cath system. *Oncol. Nurs. Forum* 17:75, 1990.

American Cancer Society. *Cancer Facts & Figures—1990.* Atlanta: American Cancer Society, 1990.

American Cancer Society, Massachusetts Division. *Cancer Manual* (7th ed.). Boston: American Cancer Society, 1986.

Averette, H.E., Lewis, J.L., Jr., Coppleson, M., and Richart, R.M. Redefining microinvasive cervical carcinoma. *Contemp. OB/GYN* 31(5):187, 1988.

Azziz, R. Determining the cause of hirsutism and anovulation. *Contemp. OB/GYN* 31(5):126, 1988.

Bates, B. *A Guide to Physical Examination and History Taking* (4th ed.). Philadelphia: J.B. Lippincott, 1987.

Berek, J.S., Bagshawe, K.D., and Bast, R.C. Monoclonal antibodies' role in combating gyn malignancies. *Contemp. OB/GYN* 35(2):109, 1990.

Bergkvist, L., Adami, H., Persson, I., et al. The risk of breast cancer after estrogen and estrogen-progestin replacement. *N. Engl. J. Med.* 321:293, 1989.

Berkowitz, R.S., Goldstein, D.P., and Bernstein, M.R. Partial molar pregnancy: A separate entity. *Contemp. OB/GYN* 31(6): 99, 1988.

Bourcier, K.M., and Seidler, A.J. Chlamydia and condylomata acuminata: An update for the nurse practitioner. *J. Obstet. Gynecol. Neonatal Nurs.* 16:17, 1987.

Brock, B.V., Selke, S., Benedetti, J., et al. Frequency of asymptomatic shedding of herpes simplex virus in women with genital herpes. *J.A.M.A.* 263:418, 1990.

Burnhill, M.S. Treating persistent and recurrent vulvovaginitis. *Contemp. OB/GYN* 31(3):71, 1988.

Burnhill, M.S. Clinician's guide to counseling patients with chronic vaginitis. *Contemp. OB/GYN* 35(1):37, 1990.

Carney-Gersten, P., Moore, M.D., and Giuffre, M. *Oncol. Nurs. Forum* 17:403, 1990.

Centers for Disease Control. Follow-up on toxic-shock syndrome. *M.M.W.R.* 29:441, 1980.

Centers for Disease Control. Sexually transmitted diseases: Treatment guidelines. *M.M.W.R.* 38(5-8):1, 1989.

Centers for Disease Control. Progress toward achieving the 1990 objectives for the nation for sexually transmitted diseases. *M.M.W.R.* 39(4):53, 1990.

Chow, J.M., Yonekura, M.L., Richwald, G.A., et al. The association between *Chlamydia trachomatis* and ectopic pregnancy: A matched-pair, case-control study. *J.A.M.A.* 263:3164, 1990.

Cohen, I., Veille, J., and Calkins, B.M. Improved pregnancy outcome following successful treatment of chlamydial infection. *J.A.M.A.* 263:3160, 1990.

Cotran, R.S., Kumar, V., and Robbins, S.L. *Robbins' Pathologic Basis of Disease* (4th ed.). Philadelphia: W.B. Saunders, 1989.

DeGeorge, D., Gray, J.J., Fetting, J.H., and Rolls, B.J. Weight gain in patients with breast cancer receiving adjuvant treatment as a function of restraint, disinhibition, and hunger. *Oncol. Nurs. Forum* 17(3) Supplement: 23, 1990.

Deitch, D.V., and Smith, J.E. Symptoms of chronic vaginal infection and microscopic condyloma in women. *J. Obstet. Gynecol. Neonatal Nurs.* 19:133, 1990.

Guyton, A.C. *Textbook of Medical Physiology* (7th ed.). Philadelphia: W.B. Saunders, 1986.

Harger, J.H. Genital herpes infections. *Contemp. OB/GYN* 35(5): 83, 1990.

Hedley, D.W. Measurement of DNA content of archival material as a guide to prognosis. In J. Ragaz and I.M. Ariel (eds.), *High Risk Breast Cancer Diagnosis.* New York: Springer-Verlag, 1989.

Higgs, D.J. The patient with testicular cancer: Nursing management of chemotherapy. *Oncol. Nurs. Forum* 17(2):243, 1990.

Hillard, P.A., and Rebar, R.W. Abnormal uterine bleeding needs a special approach. *Contemp. OB/GYN* 35(5):51, 1990.

Indman, P.D. An individual approach to office laser surgery for vulvovaginal disease. *Contemp. OB/GYN* 31(5):160, 1988.

Karlan, B.Y., and Lagasse, L.D. Conservative management of vulvar cancer. *Contemp. OB/GYN* 35(6):27, 1990.

Kistner, R.W. *Gynecology: Principles and Practice* (4th ed.). Chicago: Yearbook, 1986.

Levy, M.J., and Stillman, R.J. Reproductive surgery and the DES uterus. Update on Surgery 1990. *Contemp. OB/GYN* 35:97, 1990.

London, S.N., and Hammond, C.B. The climacteric. In D.N. Danforth and J.R. Scott (eds.), *Obstetrics and Gynecology* (5th ed.). Philadelphia: J.B. Lippincott, 1986.

Maloney, M.E. Exploring the common vulvar dermatoses. *Contemp. OB/GYN* 31(4):91, 1988.

March, C.M. Hysteroscopic resection of submucous myomas. Update on Surgery 1990. *Contemp. OB/GYN* 35:59, 1990.

Martin, J.P. Male cancer awareness: Impact of an employee education program. *Oncol. Nurs. Forum* 17(1):59, 1990.

Mason, D.R. Erectile dysfunctions: Assessment and care. *Nurse Pract.* 14(12):23, 1989.

Minkoff, H.L. Preventing damage from nonviral STDs. *Contemp. OB/GYN* 31(2):139, 1988.

Morgan, L.S., and Wilkinson, E.J. Meeting the challenge of superficially invasive vulvar carcinoma. *Contemp. OB/GYN* 31(5):181, 1988.

Murata, J.M. Abnormal genital bleeding and secondary amenorrhea: Common gynecological problems. *J. Obstet. Gynecol. Neonatal Nurs.* 19:26, 1990.

National Institute of Health. Consensus development conference statement on the treatment of early stage breast cancer, June 18–21, 1990. Sponsored by National Cancer Institute and the Office of Medical Applications of Research of the National Institutes of Health, 1990.

Nettles-Carlson, B. Early detection of breast cancer. *J. Obstet. Gynecol. Neonatal Nurs.* 18:373, 1989.

Northouse, L. A longitudinal study of the adjustment of patients and husbands to breast cancer. *Oncol. Nurs. Forum* 17(3) Supplement:39, 1990.

Norwood, S.L. Fibrocystic breast disease: An update and review. *J. Obstet. Gynecol. Neonatal Nurs.* 19:116, 1990.

Nuovo, G.J., and Pedemonte, B.M. Human papillomavirus types and recurrent cervical warts. *J.A.M.A.* 263:1223, 1990.

Palefsky, J.M., Gonzales, J., Greenblatt, R.M., et al. Anal intraepithelial neoplasia and anal papillomavirus infection among homosexual males with group IV HIV disease. *J.A.M.A.* 263:2911, 1990.

Reid, R. How HPV testing helps the clinician. Issues in OB/GYN. *Contemp. OB/GYN* 31(3): 34, 1988.

Richart, R.M., Aalders, J.G., Boronow, R.C., and Morrow, C.P. Endometrial cancer: State of the art. *Contemp. OB/GYN* 31(6): 107, 1988.

Richart, R.M., Gomez-Carrion, Y., and Kaufman, R.H. Treatment priorities for vulvar neoplasia. *Contemp. OB/GYN* 31(2):79, 1988.

Roy, M. VIN–Latest management approaches. *Contemp. OB/GYN* 31(5):170, 1988.

Schiffman, M. Arguments against routine clinical use of HPV assays. Issues in OB/GYN. *Contemp. OB/GYN* 34(2): 46, 1990.

Schlaff, W.D. Treating myomas and endometriosis with GnRH analogs. *Contemp. OB/GYN* 35(2):26, 1990.

Shangold, M., Rebar, R.W., Wentz, A.C., and Schiff, I. Evaluation and management of menstrual dysfunction in athletes. *J.A.M.A.* 263:1665, 1990.

Slattery, M.L., Robison, L.M., Schuman, K.L., et al. Cigarette smoking and exposure to passive smoke are risk factors for cervical cancer. *J.A.M.A.* 261:1593, 1989.

Speroff, L. Breast cancer and postmenopausal hormone therapy. *Contemp. OB/GYN* 35(1):71, 1990.

Styrt, B., and Gorbach, S.L. Recent developments in the understanding of the pathogenesis and treatment of anaerobic infections. *N. Engl. J. Med.* 321:298, 1989.

Timor-Tritsch, I.E., and Rottem, S. High-frequency transvaginal sonography: New diagnostic boon. *Contemp. OB/GYN* 31(4): 111, 1988.

Toole, K.A., and Vigilante, P. Cervical dysplasia and condyloma as risks for carcinoma: Two case studies. *M.C.N.* 15:170, 1990.

Vieiralves-Wiltgen, C., and Engle, V.F. Identification and management of DES-exposed women. *Nurse Pract.* 13(11):15, 1988.

Ward, S., Heidrich, S., and Wolberg, W. Factors women take into account when deciding upon type of surgery for breast cancer. *Cancer Nurs.* 12:344, 1989.

Wedell, M.A., Billings, P., and Fayez, J.A. Endometriosis and the infertile patient. *J. Obstet. Gynecol. Neonatal Nurs.* 14:280, 1985.

Wendel, G.D., Jr., and Gilstrap, L.C. III. Syphilis rise calls for accurate diagnosis. *Contemp. OB/GYN* 35(6):37, 1990.

Wolner-Hanssen, P., Eschenbach, D.A., Paavonen, J., et al. Decreased risk of symptomatic chlamydial pelvic inflammatory disease associated with oral contraceptive use. *J.A.M.A.* 263:54, 1990.

Woolard, D.G., Larson, J., and Hudson, L. Screening for *Chlamydia trachomatis* at a university health service. *J. Obstet. Gynecol. Neonatal Nurs.* 18:145, 1989.

Yoder, L.H. The epidemiology of ovarian cancer: A review. *Oncol. Nurs. Forum* 17:411, 1990.

Zaloudek, C., Tavassoli, F.A., and Kurman, R.J. Malignant lesions of the ovary. In D.H. Danforth and J.R. Scott (eds.), *Obstetric and Gynecology* (5th ed.). Philadelphia: J.B. Lippincott, 1986.

# Index

NOTE: A *t* following a page number indicates tabular material and an *f* following a page number indicates an illustration. Drugs are listed under their generic names. When a drug trade name is listed, the reader is referred to the generic name.